Help your students learn to **Think Like a Nurse** with **new digital learning resources** in Maternal and Pediatric Nursing!

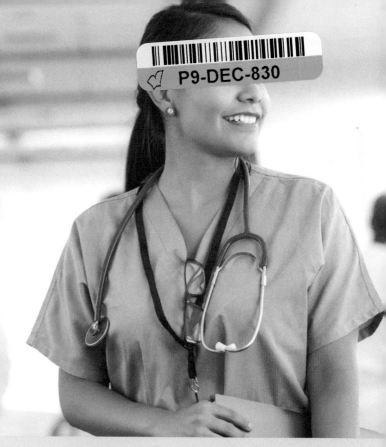

MyNursingLab®

MyNursingLab's personalized learning path helps students master and retain course information more quickly so they can focus on higher-level decision-making skills.

NEW! Clinical Decision-Making Cases in MyNursingLab provide opportunities for students to practice analyzing information and making important decisions at key moments in patient care scenarios.

Learn more at mynursinglab.com

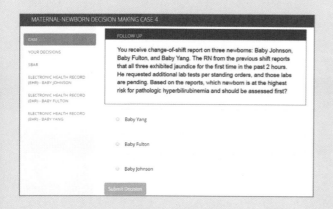

NEW! Maternity & Pediatric Nursing Reference App

The Maternity & Pediatric Nursing Reference App provides a collection of handy tools and additional content, previously only available in text format, for quick reference in the clinical setting. Students can now easily access this vital content in a useful mobile format wherever and whenever they need it! Now available for free on both the Apple App Store and Google Play.

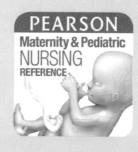

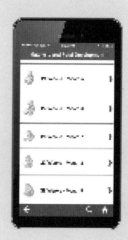

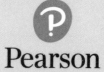
Pearson

Principles of Pediatric Nursing
Caring for Children

Seventh Edition

Jane W. Ball, RN, CPNP, DrPH
Consultant, Trauma System Development, Gaithersburg, Maryland

Ruth C. Bindler, RNC, PhD
Professor Emeritus, Washington State University College of Nursing, Spokane, Washington

Kay J. Cowen, RN-BC, MSN, CNE
Clinical Professor, University of North Carolina at Greensboro School of Nursing, Greensboro, North Carolina

Michele R. Shaw, RN, PhD
Associate Professor, Washington State University College of Nursing, Spokane, Washington

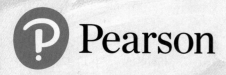

330 Hudson Street, NY NY 10013

Publisher: Julie Levin Alexander
Editorial Coordinator: Sarah Henrich
Portfolio Manager: Katrin Beacom
Content Producer: Erin Rafferty
Editorial Assistant: Erin Sullivan
Vice President of Sales & Marketing: David Gesell
Vice President, Director of Marketing: Margaret Waples
Senior Product Marketing Manager: Christopher Barry
Field Marketing Manager: Brittany Hammond
Director, Publishing Operations: Paul DeLuca
Team Lead, Project Management: Cynthia Zonneveld
Team Lead, Program Management: Melissa Bashe
Development Editor: Mary Cook

Full-Service Vendor: SPi Global
Full-Service Senior Production Editor: Patty Donovan, SPi Global
Manufacturing Manager: Maura Zaldivar-Garcia
Senior Producer: Amy Peltier
Media Producer and Project Manager: Lisa Rinaldi
Art Director: Mary Siener
Cover Credit: *A Day In May*, painting used with permission from Katie m. Berggren, www.KmBerggren.com
Printer/Binder: LSC Communications
Cover Printer: Phoenix

Notice: Care has been taken to confirm the accuracy of information presented in this book. The authors, editors, and the publisher, however, cannot accept any responsibility for errors or omissions or for consequences from application of the information in this book and make no warranty, express or implied, with respect to its contents.

The authors and publisher have exerted every effort to ensure that drug selections and dosages set forth in this text are in accord with current recommendations and practice at time of publication. However, in view of ongoing research, changes in government regulations, and the constant flow of information relating to drug therapy and reactions, the reader is urged to check the package inserts, pharmacy information, or current online information of all drugs for any change in indications or dosage and for added warning and precautions. This is particularly important when the recommended agent is a new and/or infrequently administered drug.

A note about nursing diagnoses: Nursing diagnoses in this text are taken from *Nursing Diagnoses—Definitions and Classification 2015–2017*. Copyright © 2014, 1994–2012 by NANDA International. Used by arrangement with John Wiley & Sons Limited. In order to make safe and effective judgments using NANDA-I nursing diagnoses it is essential that nurses refer to the definitions and defining characteristics of the diagnoses listed in this work.

Library of Congress Cataloging-in-Publication Data
Names: Ball, Jane (Jane W.), author. | Bindler, Ruth McGillis, author. |
    Cowen, Kay J., author. | Shaw, Michele R., author.
Title: Principles of pediatric nursing: caring for children / Jane W. Ball,
    Ruth C. Bindler, Kay J. Cowen, Michele R. Shaw.
Description: Seventh edition. | Hoboken, NJ : Pearson Education, [2017] |
    Includes bibliographical references and index.
Identifiers: LCCN 2016035091| ISBN 9780134257013 | ISBN 0134257014
Subjects: | MESH: Pediatric Nursing | Nursing Assessment--methods | Child |
    Infant
Classification: LCC RJ245 | NLM WY 159 | DDC 618.92/00231—dc23 LC
record available at https://lccn.loc.gov/2016035091

2014017177

2 16

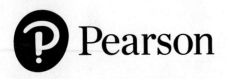

ISBN-13: 978-0-13-425701-3
ISBN-10:   0-13-425701-4

Dedication

We dedicate this book to:

- Our families who are ever supportive and understanding about our passion for children and writing,

- Our mentors, colleagues, and students who inspire us to apply our knowledge and challenge our thinking,

- The children, adolescents, and families with whom we work and who foster our philosophy of pediatric nursing.

About the Authors

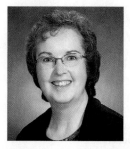

JANE W. BALL graduated from the Johns Hopkins Hospital School of Nursing and subsequently received a BS from the Johns Hopkins University. She began her nursing career working in the pediatric surgical inpatient, emergency department, and outpatient clinic of the Johns Hopkins Medical Center, first as a staff nurse and then as a pediatric nurse practitioner. After recognizing a need to focus on the health of children, she returned to school and obtained both a master's degree of public health and a doctorate of public health degree from the Johns Hopkins University Bloomberg School of Public Health with a focus on maternal and child health. After graduation, Dr. Ball became the chief of child health services for the Commonwealth of Pennsylvania Department of Health. In this capacity she oversaw the state-funded well-child clinics and explored ways to improve education for the state's community health nurses. After relocating to Texas, she joined the faculty at the University of Texas at Arlington School of Nursing to teach community pediatrics to registered nurses returning to school for a BSN. During this time Dr. Ball became involved in writing her first textbook, *Mosby's Guide to Physical Examination*, which is currently in its eighth edition. After relocating to the Washington, DC, area, she worked at Children's National Medical Center on a number of federally funded projects. The first project in 1986, teaching instructors of emergency medical technicians from all states about the special care children need during an emergency, revealed the shortcomings of the emergency medical services system for children. This exposure was a career-changing event. A textbook titled *Pediatric Emergencies: A Manual for Prehospital Providers* was subsequently developed. A second project led to the development of a pediatric emergency education program for nurses in emergency departments to promote improved care for children. Both of these programs served as a foundation for other pediatric emergency education developed and sponsored by national organizations. For 15 years Dr. Ball managed the federally funded Emergency Medical Services for Children's National Resource Center. As executive director, she provided and directed the provision of consultation and resource development for state health agencies, health professionals, families, and advocates about successful methods to improve the healthcare system so that children get optimal emergency care in all healthcare settings. After leaving that position, she continues to be engaged in many projects with a focus on the emergency care system. She is a consultant to the American College of Surgeons Committee on Trauma, supporting state trauma system development. She recently completed a federally funded project to study whether the implementation of a statewide pediatric emergency department recognition program improved pediatric emergency care. In 2010, Dr. Ball received the Distinguished Alumna Award from the Johns Hopkins University.

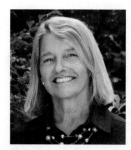

RUTH C. MCGILLIS BINDLER received her BSN from Cornell University—New York Hospital School of Nursing. She worked in oncology nursing at Memorial-Sloan Kettering Cancer Center in New York, and then as a public health nurse in Dane County, Wisconsin. Thus began her commitment to work with children as she visited children and their families at home and served as a school nurse. Due to this interest in child healthcare needs, she earned her MS in child development from the University of Wisconsin. A move to Washington State was accompanied by a new job as a faculty member at the Intercollegiate Center for Nursing Education in Spokane. Dr. Bindler was fortunate to be involved for over 38 years in the growth of this nursing education consortium, which is a combination of public and private universities and colleges and is now the Washington State University (WSU) College of Nursing. She obtained a PhD in human nutrition at WSU, where she taught theory and clinical courses in child health nursing, cultural diversity and health, graduate research, pharmacology, and assessment, and served as lead faculty for child health nursing. Dr. Bindler was the first director of the PhD in Nursing program at WSU and most recently served as Associate Dean for Graduate Programs, which include Master of Nursing, Post-Masters certificates, PhD, and Doctor of Nursing Practice (DNP) programs. She recently retired and serves the college and profession as a professor emeritus, continuing work with graduate students and research. Her first professional book, *Pediatric Medications*, was published in 1981, and she has continued to publish articles and books in the areas of pediatric medications and pediatric health. Research foci have been childhood obesity, type 2 diabetes, metabolic syndrome, and cardiometabolic risk factors in children. Ethnic diversity and interprofessional collaboration have been additional themes in her work. Dr. Bindler believes that her role as a faculty member and administrator enabled her to learn continually, foster the development of students in nursing, lead and mentor junior faculty into the teaching role, and participate fully in the profession of nursing. In addition to teaching, research, publication, and leadership, she enhances her life by professional and community service and by activities with her family.

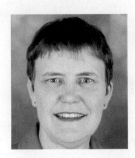

KAY J. COWEN received her BSN from East Carolina University in Greenville, North Carolina, and began her career as a staff nurse on the pediatric unit of North Carolina Baptist Hospital in Winston-Salem. She developed a special interest in the psychosocial needs of hospitalized children and preparing them for hospitalization. This led to the focus of her master's thesis at the University of North Carolina at Greensboro (UNCG), where she received a master of science in nursing education degree with a focus in maternal child nursing.

Mrs. Cowen began her teaching career in 1984 at UNCG, where she continues today as clinical professor in the Parent Child Department. Her primary responsibilities include coordinating the pediatric nursing course, teaching classroom content, and supervising a clinical group of students. Mrs. Cowen shared her passion for the psychosocial care of children and the needs of their families through her first experience as an author in the chapter "Hospital Care for Children" in Jackson and Saunders' *Child Health Nursing: A Comprehensive Approach to the Care of Children and Their Families* published in 1993.

In the classroom, Mrs. Cowen realized that students learn through a variety of teaching strategies and became especially interested in the strategy of gaming. She led a research study to evaluate the effectiveness of gaming in the classroom and subsequently continues to incorporate gaming in her teaching. In the clinical setting, Mrs. Cowen teaches her students the skills needed to care for patients and the importance of family-centered care, focusing not only on the physical needs of the child but also on the psychosocial needs of the child and family. During her teaching career, Mrs. Cowen has continued to work part time as a staff nurse, first on the pediatric unit of Moses Cone Hospital in Greensboro and then at Brenner Children's Hospital in Winston-Salem. In 2006, she became the part-time pediatric nurse educator in Brenner's Family Resource Center. Through Mrs. Cowen's expertise, she is able to extend her love of teaching to children and families, and through her role as an author, she is able to extend her dedication to pediatric nursing and nursing education.

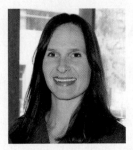

MICHELE R. SHAW received her BSN from Pacific Lutheran University in Tacoma, Washington. She began her career as a nurse at a long-term care facility and then as a home healthcare nurse in Spokane, Washington. While making home visits, she became interested in the nursing care needs of children and families. She realized the importance of educating the family about their child's condition and to include family members while planning and carrying out the nursing care plan. This interest in family nursing led her into the area of maternal-child nursing, where she served as a postpartum nurse for nearly 18 years. Her experience with providing nursing care to families in various settings has highlighted her belief in the need of a family-centered approach in order to provide optimal nursing care. Dr. Shaw began her teaching career as a teaching assistant in 2001 at the Washington State University (WSU) College of Nursing, where she continues today as an associate professor. It was during those early years as a teaching assistant that she began to realize her passion for educating nursing students. This interest led to her completing a master's degree in nursing with an emphasis on education at WSU. Knowing that she wanted to continue working in nursing academia, Dr. Shaw went on to receive her PhD in nursing from the University of Arizona in Tucson. She has taught theory, seminar, and clinical courses in maternal-child nursing, family health, evidence-based practice, ethical decision making, physical assessment, and professional practice. Dr. Shaw recently assisted in the development of the Bachelor of Science-to-PhD in Nursing program at WSU. This fast-track program will enable students with an earned bachelor's degree to complete a PhD in nursing in four years.

Dr. Shaw enjoys working with undergraduate and graduate students and encourages active participation in research. Her research interests include children with asthma and their families, childbearing women and their families, and substance use among youth and childbearing women. She is particularly interested in children's and families' unique perspectives, and thus much of her research uses qualitative approaches. She continues to publish articles in the areas of pediatric asthma and substance use among childbearing women. Dr. Shaw believes her active role in nursing academia and research allows her to stay current in various pedagogical approaches to enhance nursing students' learning experiences, as well as continuous learning about evidence-based interventions to provide nursing care to children and families.

Thank You!

We are forever grateful to nurse geneticist Linda D. Ward, PhD, APRN, the author of this book's genetics chapter, Chapter 3, "Genetic and Genomic Influences." We appreciate her expertise in genetic and genomic science, her superb writing skills, and her willingness to contribute such an essential chapter to our text. We are also thankful to Brenda Senger, RN, PhD, for contributing the content on mitochondrial diseases in Chapter 30.

We are grateful to all the nurses, both clinicians and educators, who reviewed the manuscript of this text. Their insights, suggestions, and eye for detail helped us prepare a more relevant, useful, and current book, reflective of the present time and of the essential components of learning in the field of child health nursing.

Mary Armstrong, MSN, RN, CCRN, CPN
Carson Newman University
Jefferson City, Tennessee

Elizabeth Bettini, APRN, MSN, PCNS-BC, CHPPN
Division of Anesthesiology & Pain Medicine
Children's National Medical Center
Washington, D.C.

Melissa Black, PhDc, MSN, FNP, RN
NCLEX Review Nurse
Kaplan
Greenville, South Carolina

Ann M. Bowling, PhD, RN, CPNP-PC, CNE
Assistant Professor
Wright State University
Dayton, Ohio

Michele I. Bracken, PhD, WHNP-BC
Associate Professor
Clinical Coordinator Maternal/Newborn/Women's Health
Salisbury University
Salisbury, Maryland

Robin Caldwell, RNC-OB
Instructor
Catawba Valley Community College
Hickory, North Carolina

Karan Dublin, MEd, RN
Professor
Tyler Junior College
Tyler, Texas

Barbara S. Edwards, RN, CPN
Staff Nurse
Brenner Children's Hospital
Winston-Salem, North Carolina

Linda B. Esposito, MSN, RN, CCRN
Nurse Practice Specialist
Brenner Children's Hospital
Wake Forest Baptist Medical Center
Winston-Salem, North Carolina

Julie Fitzgerald, PhD, RN, CNE
Assistant Professor
Ramapo College of New Jersey
Mahwah, New Jersey

Niki Fogg, MS, RN, CPN
Assistant Clinical Professor
Texas Woman's University
Dallas, Texas

Vivienne Friday, EdD, RN
Nurse Educator
Bridgeport Hospital School of Nursing
Bridgeport, Connecticut

Deborah Henry, MSN, RN
Nursing Faculty
Blue Ridge Community College
Flat Rock, North Carolina

Indra Hershorin, PhD, RN, CNE
Assistant Professor
Barry University
Miami Shores, Florida

Karen L. Hessler, PhD, FNP-C
Assistant Professor
University of Northern Colorado
Greeley, Colorado

Catherine Hrycyk, MScN, RN
Faculty, Pediatric Nursing and Pharmacology
De Anza College
Cupertino, California

Gina Idol, RN, BSN, CPN
Wake Forest Baptist Health
Brenner Children's Hospital
Winston-Salem, North Carolina

Laura Kubin, PhD, RN, CPN, CHES
Assistant Professor
Texas Woman's University
Dallas, Texas

Meredith Lahl, MSN, PCNS-BC, PPCNP-BC, CPON
Senior Director of Advanced Practice Nursing
Cleveland Clinic
Cleveland, Ohio

Robyn Leo, MS, RN
Associate Professor and Chairperson for Nursing
Worcester State University
Worcester, Massachusetts

Angela P. Lukomski, RN, DNP, CPNP
Associate Professor
Eastern Michigan University
Ypsilanti, Michigan

Patricia Novak, RN, BSN, MSN
Faculty
Gateway Community College
Phoenix, Arizona

Gloanna J. Peek, PhD, RN, CPNP
Clinical Associate Professor
PNP Specialty Option Coordinator
The University of Arizona
Tucson, Arizona

Susan Perkins, MSN, RN
Senior Instructor
Washington State University
Spokane, Washington

Linda Sue Pippin, MSN, RN-BC
Adjunct Faculty
Newberry College
Newberry, South Carolina

Theresa Puckett, RN, CNE
Instructor
Stark State College
North Canton, Ohio

Colleen Quinn, RN, MSN, EdD
Professor
Broward College
Davie, Florida

JoAnne Silbert-Flagg, DNP, PNP, IBCLC
Assistant Professor
Johns Hopkins University
Baltimore, Maryland

Jennifer S. Simmons, MSN, RN, CPNP-AC/PC, CPON
Pediatric Oncology Nurse Practitioner
Brenner Children's Hospital
Wake Forest Baptist Medical Center
Winston-Salem, North Carolina

Anita Smith, CPNP
Nurse Practitioner
Department of Pediatric
Hematology
Wake Forest Health Sciences
Winston-Salem, North
Carolina

**Charla Smith, MSN, RN,
CPN, CNE**
Associate Professor
Jackson State Community
College
Jackson, Tennessee

**Nancy M. Smith, DNP,
CRNP, FNP-BC**
Assistant Professor
Salisbury University
Salisbury, Maryland

**Maureen P. Tippen, RN, C,
MS**
Clinical Assistant Professor
University of Michigan
Flint, Michigan

Teresa Tyson, RN, PhD
Assistant Professor
Winston-Salem State
University
Winston-Salem, North
Carolina

Diane K. Van Os, MS, RN
Professor
Westminster College
Salt Lake City, Utah

Amber Welborn, RN, MSN
Lecturer
University of North Carolina
Greensboro, North Carolina

**Cecilia Wilson, PhD, RN,
CPN**
Associate Clinical Professor
Texas Woman's University
Dallas, Texas

Preface

Health care and healthcare delivery systems are changing dramatically. The Affordable Care Act, a focus on interprofessional collaboration, an emphasis on patient safety, and evidence-based practice will contribute to ongoing challenges and evolution in health care in the coming years. Pediatric nurses must respond to and integrate these changes into their practice. In addition, pediatric nursing presents its own unique challenges for practitioners of health care. Student nurses must learn what helps them to provide safe, effective, and excellent care today, while integrating new knowledge and skills needed as nursing practice continues to develop and respond to healthcare needs. Students must learn how to think and apply information as new knowledge becomes available. "As the student uses knowledge in situations of practice, new understanding is gained as well as knowing how, when, and why it is relevant in particular situations. . . . We call this teaching for a sense of salience."*

Faculty are responsible for selecting patient care assignments that assist the student in applying knowledge in the clinical setting, as well as utilizing various pedagogies to assist the student in focusing on the patient experience. We have integrated concepts from the Carnegie Report that foster clinical expertise by offering a variety of critical thinking and clinical reasoning questions, patient care scenarios, and research and evidence-based practice features. Information technology plays a major role in both health care and teaching, and therefore features in this text encourage the student to use and analyze content available through information technology.

Preparation for Nursing Excellence

The goal of this seventh edition of *Principles of Pediatric Nursing* is to provide core pediatric nursing knowledge that prepares students for excellence in nursing and to offer the tools of scholarship and critical thinking needed to apply this learning in the future. Students must learn to question, evaluate the research evidence available, apply pertinent information in clinical settings, and constantly adapt to growing knowledge and an evolving healthcare system.

This text reflects a multitude of approaches to learning that can be helpful to all students. We acknowledge that many students learn pediatric nursing in a very short time period. Therefore, the approaches in this text are designed to assist students to assess the child's needs, take into account population-based practice, and make care decisions based on the standards of pediatric nursing practice.

Realities of Pediatric Nursing

Pediatric nursing occurs in many acute care and community healthcare settings, such as hospitals, homes, schools, and health centers. Procedures may be performed in short-stay units, and long-term care is often provided at home for children with complex health conditions. Families are often the providers of care as well as the case managers for these children. Technologic advances are resulting in earlier diagnoses and new therapies; these technologic approaches are integrated whenever pertinent throughout the text.

Pediatric nursing care is provided within the context of a rapidly changing society. An examination of the major morbidities and mortalities of childhood guided the revision of material and topics throughout the text. Specific chapters focus on the family, health promotion across the life span, pediatric nutrition, and care for children with chronic conditions. Chapter 2 addresses cultural influences on health care and provides guidance for students caring for children in our growing intercultural society. Chapter 3, on genetics and genomics, is intended to help students recognize the impact of such knowledge on pediatric nursing and apply these concepts when working with families. Current social and environmental challenges for children have guided the further development of Chapter 17, which covers societal and environmental influences on child health.

Many graduating nurses practice in acute care facilities; this text continues to emphasize the information necessary to prepare students for working in hospitals. In addition, the information provided here will enable graduates to assume positions in ambulatory care facilities, home health nursing, schools, and a variety of other settings. Effective communication methods, principles of working with families, and knowledge of pathophysiologic, psychologic, developmental, and environmental factors found in these chapters can all be applied in a wide variety of settings. The importance of interprofessional care is recognized; therefore, collaboration and communication with various health professionals is emphasized.

Another major evolution involves access to information and reliance on the Internet. Nurses must learn to obtain information and then analyze and judge the quality of information they find. Increasingly, nurses need experience with information technology and management. Nurses must also advise children and family members to use the Internet wisely to help them in making healthcare choices. This text will assist the student in making practice decisions based on scholarship and evidence-based research.

Organization and Integrated Themes

We have organized *Principles of Pediatric Nursing: Caring for Children*, Seventh Edition, to present important information on growth and development, family-centered care, culture, genetics, physical assessment, health promotion, nutrition, health issues in today's world, and children's responses to illness and injury. This information is needed to care for children in the many healthcare settings where pediatric nursing care is provided. Following the foundational chapters, this book is

*Benner, P., Sutphen, M., Leonard, V., & Day, L. (2010). *Educating nurses: A call for radical transformation* (p. 94). San Francisco, CA: Jossey-Bass.

organized by body systems to facilitate the student's ability to locate information, focus studying, and prepare for clinical experiences with children and families. The organizational framework also eliminates redundancy, so that the student uses time efficiently. **Learning Outcomes** begin the chapter, and **Chapter Highlights** end the chapter.

The **Bindler-Ball Child Healthcare Model** is used to illustrate the important core value that all children need health promotion and health maintenance interventions, no matter where they seek health care or what health conditions they may be experiencing.

The nursing process is used as the framework for nursing care. **Nursing Management** is the major heading, with subheadings of **Nursing Assessment and Diagnosis, Planning and Implementation,** and **Evaluation**. When it is appropriate to focus on care in a specific setting, Hospital-Based Care, Discharge Planning, and Community Care are separated into sections. We feature nursing care plans throughout the text to help students approach care from the nursing process perspective. Some have an acute care hospitalization focus, whereas others have a community-based focus. **Nursing Care Plans** include nursing diagnoses, goals, interventions, and rationales.

Several major concepts are integrated throughout the text to encourage the student to think creatively and critically about nursing care. These major themes are interwoven throughout the text through the many features and supplements, including:

- *Nursing care* is the critical and central core of this text. Nursing assessment and management are emphasized in all sections of the book, with examples of nurses providing care in a number of different settings. Nurses apply a variety of guidelines related to the profession and to health conditions. The new feature, **Professionalism in Practice**, relates guidelines important to nursing care.

- *Collaborative care* descriptions of the diagnostic and therapeutic care for various health conditions reflect the interprofessional team role of nurses with other healthcare professionals (e.g., physicians, physical therapists, mental health counselors, pharmacists, and others) as described in *The Essentials of Baccalaureate Education for Professional Nursing Practice* (American Association of Colleges of Nursing, 2008).

- *Clinical reasoning and problem-solving principles* are integrated in the organization, pedagogy, and writing style. Examples include the evidence-based practice features, clinical reasoning boxes, the end-of-chapter **Clinical Reasoning in Action** feature, and art captions. Students practice clinical reasoning and critical thinking in their everyday lives, but they need help to apply these concepts to the practice of nursing. This text and the accompanying learning materials help students understand how their normal curiosity and problem-solving ability can be applied to pediatric nursing.

- *Communication* is one of the most important skills that students need to learn. Effective communication with children is challenging because they communicate differently, according to their developmental levels. Family members have communication needs in addition to those of their children. Effective communication with a variety of healthcare providers is essential for effective care. This book integrates communication skills by applied examples that help the student communicate effectively with children, their families, and other health professionals.

- *Patient safety* is emphasized in nursing management sections and in the **Safety Alert!** boxes.

- *Family and patient education* about health care is an integral part of the pediatric nurse's responsibilities. Because hospitalizations are often brief, leaving families increasingly responsible for caring for recuperating children at home, information about healthcare needs and procedures has become even more important. The **Families Want to Know** feature describes teaching strategies and content for various patient conditions.

- *Developing cultural competence* is critical for all nurses in the increasingly diverse community of today's world. Students have met people from different ethnic and cultural groups, but they need help to understand, respect, and integrate differing beliefs, practices, and healthcare needs when providing care.

- *Growth and development considerations and physical assessment* are central to the effective practice of pediatric nursing. A separate chapter is devoted to each area (Chapters 4 and 5, respectively). In addition, both topics are integrated where appropriate in narrative, growth and development boxes, figures, and captions.

- *Health promotion* is an important focus of nursing care for children with acute and chronic health conditions. Four chapters focus on health promotion. One provides an overview of concepts related to health promotion; the other three address health promotion principles for children of different ages. In addition, a **Health Promotion** feature helps illustrate opportunities for maintaining and improving the health of children with certain health conditions.

- *Community care* is an increasing part of nursing responsibilities. To assist students in transferring knowledge to caring for children in community settings, information is provided in the nursing management sections of chapters. In addition, an entire chapter is devoted to nursing care in the community and directly addresses the nurse's roles in several community settings.

These themes and others are interwoven in the narrative of most chapters and are reflected in the art as well as in the supplements that students can use to augment their learning.

Resources for Student Success

- **Online Resources** are available at www.pearsonhighered.com/nursingresources and aim to further enhance the student's learning experience, build on knowledge gained from this textbook, prepare students for the NCLEX-RN® examination, and foster clinical reasoning.

- The *Clinical Skills Manual for Maternity and Pediatric Nursing,* ISBN 0134257006, is a useful resource to assist students in successful planning and performance of essential nursing skills. This manual helps translate theoretic concepts into performance while caring for health clients in a variety of settings.

- **NEW! Pearson's** *Maternity and Pediatric Nursing Reference App,* now available for both iPhone and Android devices, provides a collection of handy tools and additional content for students and professionals looking for a quick reference in maternity or pediatrics nursing. The pediatric content provided in the **Guidance for Children and Families** section includes insight into the issues related to health maintenance, development, and family that may present from birth to adolescence.

- **MyNursingLab for Pediatric Nursing** is designed to engage students with pediatric content while offering data-driven guidance that helps them better absorb course material and understand difficult concepts. The Pearson eText version of *Principles of Pediatric Nursing*, Seventh Edition, is available with MyNursingLab for Pediatric Nursing.

Resources for Faculty Success

Pearson is pleased to offer a complete suite of resources to support teaching and learning, including:

- **TestGen Test Bank**
- **Lecture Note PowerPoints**
- **Classroom Response System PowerPoints**
- **Instructor's Resource Manual**

Acknowledgments

It is both exciting and challenging to have the opportunity to write a textbook and to keep it updated with each revision. It is inspiring to observe the evolution of pediatric nursing practice and to encourage nursing students to share the excitement and enthusiasm we feel for working with children and their families. Although each edition carries its own unique set of challenges and circumstances, it continues to be a privilege to contribute to the education of the new generation of student nurses.

This seventh edition integrates new features and digital approaches developed in collaboration with Pearson Nursing. Erin Rafferty, content producer at Pearson, has been responsive and receptive, as well as an effective collaborator with us in this new edition. We are grateful for the support of our portfolio manager at Pearson, Katrin Beacom. The vice president and publisher, Julie Alexander, enthusiastically supported this venture and has supported us in decisions regarding changes, updates, and features for the text.

For this edition, we have been blessed to have Mary Cook as a development editor. Mary challenged us creatively, ensured consistency, and kept us on track. She has been supportive, innovative, and composed during the long months of hard work.

We are grateful to the families and many healthcare facilities that have permitted us to capture the images used in photographs throughout the book. George Dodson provided us with much of the photography to help illustrate current nursing concepts.

We also gratefully acknowledge the contributions of Linda Ward, a nurse leader who authored Chapter 3, "Genetic and Genomic Influences," and Brenda Senger, who contributed the mitochondrial disease content in Chapter 30.

Our thanks also go to Mary Siener, art director, for guiding all aspects of the design for this edition. At SPi Global, it has been a pleasure to work with Patty Donovan, who coordinated production.

A special thank you goes to Katie m. Berggren, who gave permission to use her painting *A Day In May* for the cover of this edition. This work and others can be viewed at www.Km-Berggren.com.

Finally, our families once again have supported us tirelessly through the revision process. They sacrificed by allowing us to work on the book when we could have been with them. Yet, they show others the book with pride. We could not have accomplished this without their love and patience.

Jane W. Ball

Ruth C. Bindler

Kay J. Cowen

Michele R. Shaw

Features to Help You Use This Textbook Successfully

Instructors and students alike value the in-text learning aids that we include in our textbooks. The following guide will help you use the features and resources from *Principles of Pediatric Nursing*, Seventh Edition, to be successful in the classroom, in the clinical setting, on the NCLEX-RN® examination, and in nursing practice.

Each chapter begins with **Learning Outcomes** and a chapter-opening **Quote**. These personal stories illustrate the diversity of cultures, parental concerns, and family situations that nurses will encounter throughout the course of their careers. A **Focus On** section appears at the beginning of each systems chapter as a reference to use while reading the chapter. Each Focus On section includes the following:

- **Anatomy and Physiology** provides a quick review of the body system.

- **Pediatric Differences** will help you recognize physiologic and mental differences in children at various ages.

- **Diagnostic Tests and Laboratory Procedures** offer information related to the specific body system to assist in clinical application.

- **Assessment Guides** assist with diagnoses by incorporating physical assessment and normal findings, alterations and possible causes, and guidelines for nursing interventions.

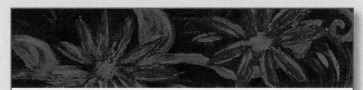

Chapter 11
Nursing Considerations for the Hospitalized Child

We live 50 miles from the hospital and have three other children. We were worried about how we were going to be able to stay with Sabrina. She's only 4, and it's her first time in the hospital. Fortunately, they have beds for parents, so one of us can always be by her side throughout her procedure and recuperation.

—Mother of Sabrina, 4 years old

Mel Curtis/Getty Images

⌄ Learning Outcomes

11.1 Compare and contrast the child's understanding of health and illness according to the child's developmental level.

11.2 Explain the effect of hospitalization on the child and family.

11.3 Describe the child's and family's adaption to hospitalization.

11.4 Apply family-centered care principles to the hospital setting.

11.5 Identify nursing strategies to minimize the stressors related to hospitalization.

11.6 Integrate the concept of family presence during procedures and nursing strategies used to prepare the family.

11.7 Summarize strategies for preparing children and families for discharge from the hospital setting.

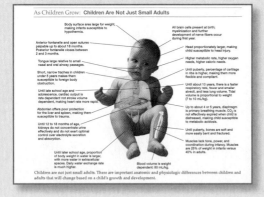

As Children Grow: Children Are Not Just Small Adults

As Children Grow boxes illustrate the anatomic and physiologic differences between children and adults. These features illustrate how the child progresses through developmental stages and the important ways in which a child's development influences healthcare needs.

Clinical Reasoning boxes provide brief case scenarios that ask students to determine the appropriate response.

Clinical Reasoning Health Promotion
The pediatric nurse should apply concepts of health promotion and maintenance in all healthcare settings. If the child is seen in an emergency room for treatment of a fracture, what questions should the nurse ask about immunization status and safety issues? If the nurse sees a child with a chronic disorder of cerebral palsy in the outpatient clinic at an orthopedic hospital, what health promotion and health maintenance services should be integrated?

Clinical Tip

Explain to the child and parents, in easy-to-understand terms, the purpose of equipment that is being used. Answer alarms quickly regardless of the reason for the alarm. Follow with an explanation of why alarms sound, including the fact that many times monitor alarms will sound when the child moves, if the monitor becomes disconnected, or if the monitor patches are loose.

Clinical Tip features offer hands-on suggestions and clinical advice. These are placed at locations in the text that will help students apply them. They include topics such as legal and ethical considerations, nursing alerts, and home and community care considerations.

Developing Cultural Competence boxes highlight specific cultural issues and their application to nursing care.

Developing Cultural Competence Smoking Rates Among Youth

Among youth in the United States, White youth are significantly more likely to smoke than either Hispanic or African American peers. About 19% of White students reported smoking in the previous month, while 14% of Hispanic and 8% of African American students reported this behavior (CDC, 2014a). American Indian and Alaska Natives also have high smoking rates, while Asian Americans have low rates. Youth smoking rates also vary by state, ranging from 4% to 20% among various states (CDC, 2014a; USDHHS, 2011).

EVIDENCE-BASED PRACTICE | Infant Sleep

Clinical Question

Many babies have limited sleeping periods during the night, and their night awakenings disturb parents' sleep. Parents may have busy days and be unable to nap and, hence, possibly not be able to perform at a safe and productive level during the day. Parental stress and depression are associated with frequent child awakenings. What strategies are needed to assist them in supporting the infant's sleep?

The Evidence

Sleep of the infant is an important concern for many parents, but there is little research-based evidence about what strategies really improve infant sleep. A study of 314 twin pairs found that most sleep disturbances in early childhood are linked to environmental factors, and thus behavioral interventions with parents are suggested for altering infant sleep patterns (Brescianini, Volzone, Fagnani, et al., 2011). Consistent with these findings, a study evaluating 170 parents for knowledge of child sleep found that most parents could not answer the majority of questions correctly. The researchers suggested that evaluating parental knowledge and teaching about developmental progression of sleep patterns should occur during health visits

(Schreck & Richdale, 2011). A cross-cultural study found that parents from predominantly Asian countries were more likely to identify sleep disturbance in their children than those from countries with a majority of White parents. These findings suggest that information is needed about cultural differences in sleep expectations of parents (Sadeh, Mindell, & Rivera, 2011).

Best Practice

This evidence-based practice provides implications for nursing care. Ask parents of young newborns to record the infant sleep patterns. As the infant nears 3 to 4 months of age, patterns should demonstrate few night wakenings and feedings. Teach parents about how to minimize stimulation and interaction at night. Provide opportunities to review results at future health supervision visits, or offer telephone or other support to parents.

Clinical Reasoning

What reasons might working parents have for responding eagerly and interacting with an infant who awakens at night? Do you think there are other reasons why infants awake at night? What clues help you to decide if an infant sleep problem exists?

Evidence-Based Practice boxes present recent nursing research, discuss implications, and challenge students to incorporate this information into nursing practice through nursing actions.

Families Want to Know

Ways to Decrease the Incidence of Cancer in Children

Many parents ask what they can do to decrease the incidence of cancer in children as they grow into adulthood. Three major teaching areas should be addressed:

1. Have children increase intake of fruits and vegetables. Most children do not eat enough of these foods, and increased intake is associated with lower rates of many cancers. Aim for a minimum of five servings daily.

2. Protect skin with sunscreen. Early excessive exposure to sun, and having had one or repeated severe sunburns during childhood, increases chances of skin cancers developing in adulthood. Tanning bed exposure is a prime risk factor for skin cancer; all children and adolescents, and particularly those with cancer, should strictly avoid tanning beds (Greinert & Boniol, 2011).

3. Discourage smoking among children and be sure children are not exposed to environmental tobacco smoke. This will decrease the future chance of developing lung cancer.

When there is a history of cancer in the family, particularly of a type associated with familial incidence such as some breast or ovarian cancers, encourage the family to learn more about the cancer and teach their children to receive regular surveillance as they enter young adulthood.

Inform youth in all families about screening, such as the Papanicolaou test, breast self-examination, and testicular examination that can lead to early detection. Encourage youth to receive the human papillomavirus quadrivalent vaccine recombinant (Gardasil) to prevent cervical cancers and other health problems caused by human papillomavirus (HPV). (See Chapter 16 for further information.)

Families Want to Know features present special healthcare issues or problems and the related key teaching points to address with the family.

Growth and Development

Children with chronic illnesses such as JIA may develop increased dependence on their parents. It is essential that school-age children maintain as much independence as possible to promote their development of industry. These children should also have some responsibility for their treatment plan. Children with JIA may also need to miss school for periods of time. A plan should be developed so that the child is able to keep up with school assignments. In addition, ongoing contact with peers should be maintained to promote the child's social development.

Growth and Development boxes provide information about the different responses of children at various ages to health conditions.

Healthy People 2020

(MICH-30.1) Increase the proportion of children who have access to a medical home

- While 57.5% of children under age 18 years had an established medical home in 2007, the objective of 63.3% of children with such access is the present goal (U.S. Department of Health and Human Services, 2011).

Healthy People 2020 goals are cited throughout the text to acquaint students with national public health efforts and to assist them in making connections between care of individual families and broad-based community health care and public policy. The coding in front of each objective identifies the specific chapter—for example, "Maternal, Infant, and Child Health" (MICH); "Adolescent Health" (AH); and "Injury and Violence Prevention" (IVP)—and number for the initiative. See the *Healthy People 2020* website to find the chapter abbreviations for all objectives listed in our text.

A feature titled **Health Promotion** summarizes the needs of children with specific chronic conditions, such as asthma or diabetes. These overviews teach students that children with chronic conditions, like all children, have health maintenance and promotion needs that require prevention and education to maximize potential.

Health Promotion   **The Child With Bronchopulmonary Dysplasia**

Health Supervision
- Assess blood pressure to detect abnormal findings associated with pulmonary hypertension.
- Coordinate vision screening by an ophthalmologist every 2 to 3 months during the first year of life. Myopia and strabismus are common in children who were born prematurely.
- Coordinate pulmonary function tests annually or as needed for clinical condition.
- Perform hearing and other screening tests as recommended for age.

Growth and Developmental Surveillance
- Assess growth and plot measurements on a growth chart corrected for gestational age. Even if length and weight are lower than normal, monitor for continued growth following the growth curves.
- Perform a developmental assessment, correcting for gestational age.

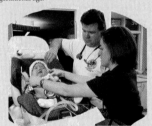

Nutrition
- Review caloric intake. Ensure that increased calories are provided to support growth. Assess feeding difficulties related to oral motor function associated with long-term enteral feeding. Refer to a nutritionist as necessary.

Physical Activity
- Organize care to provide rest periods during the day.
- Give parents ideas for promoting the infant's motor development, such as reaching for and moving toward toys and objects of interest.

Family Interactions
- Identify ways to coordinate nighttime care to reduce child and family sleep disturbances.
- Provide discipline appropriate for developmental age.

Disease Prevention Strategies
- Reduce exposure to infections. Encourage selection of a childcare provider who cares for a small number of children, if one is used. If possible, avoid the use of childcare centers during respiratory syncytial virus (RSV) season.
- Immunize the child with the routine vaccine schedule based on chronologic age.
- Administer the 23-valent pneumococcal vaccine at 2 years of age.
- Provide monthly injections of palivizumab throughout the RSV season.

Condition-Specific Guidance
- Develop an emergency care plan for times when the infant's condition rapidly worsens.

Medications Used for Infective Endocarditis: Prophylaxis for Dental and Invasive Respiratory Procedures

ANTIBIOTIC RECOMMENDATIONS	NURSING MANAGEMENT

Amoxicillin for oral use
Ampicillin for IM or IV use
If allergic to penicillin:
    Cephalexin
    Clindamycin
    Azithromycin
    Clarithromycin
	• Give 1 large dose 30–60 min before procedures, or up to 2 hr after the procedure if preprocedure dose is missed.
	• Teach parents and the child to keep at least 1 dose in the home for dental visits or emergencies.
	• Have parents inform each healthcare provider of the child's need for prophylaxis.

Source: Data from American Academy of Pediatrics (AAP). (2015). *Red book: 2015 report of the Committee on Infectious Diseases* (30th ed., p. 971). Elk Grove Village, IL: Author; Sabe, M. A., Shrestha, N. K., & Menon, V. (2013). Contemporary drug treatment of infective endocarditis. *American Journal of Cardiovascular Drugs, 13*, 251–258; Park, M. K. (2014). *Pediatric cardiology for practitioners* (6th ed., p. 349). Philadelphia: Elsevier Saunders.

A **Medications Used to Treat** feature in tabular format provides an overview of the types of medications that can be used for a specific condition and nursing considerations associated with their use.

Nursing Care Plan: The Child With a Visual Impairment Secondary to Retinopathy of Prematurity

1. Nursing Diagnosis: *Communication, Readiness for Enhanced,* related to altered reception, transmission, and integration resulting of visual images (NANDA-I © 2014)

GOAL: The child will receive adequate sensory input.

INTERVENTION	RATIONALE
• Provide kinesthetic, tactile, and auditory stimulation during play and in daily care (e.g., talking and playing). Provide music while bathing an infant, using bells and other noises on each side of infant. Verbally describe to a child all actions being carried out by adult.	• Because visual sensory input is not present, the child needs input from all other senses to compensate and provide adequate sensory stimulation.

EXPECTED OUTCOME: Child will demonstrate minimal signs of sensory deprivation.

2. Nursing Diagnosis: *Injury, Risk for,* related to impaired vision (NANDA-I © 2014)

GOAL: The child will be protected from safety hazards that can lead to injury.

INTERVENTION	RATIONALE
• Evaluate environment for potential safety hazards based on age of child and degree of impairment. Be particularly alert to objects that give visual cues to their dangers (e.g., stairs, stoves, fireplaces, candles). Eliminate safety hazards and protect the child from exposure. Take the child on a tour of new rooms, explaining safety hazards (e.g., schools, hotel room, hospital room).	• The child may be at risk for injury related both to developmental stage and to inability to visualize hazards.

EXPECTED OUTCOME: Child will experience no injuries.

3. Nursing Diagnosis: *Development: Delayed, Risk for,* related to impaired vision (NANDA-I © 2014)

GOAL: The child has experiences necessary to foster normal growth and development.

INTERVENTION	RATIONALE
• Help parents plan early, regular social activities with other children.	• The child with a visual impairment benefits developmentally from contact with other children.
• Provide opportunities and encourage self-feeding activities.	• To obtain adequate nutrients, the child needs to feel comfortable feeding self.
• Provide an environment rich in sensory input.	• Sensory input is needed for normal development to occur.
• Assess growth and development during regular examinations to identify the child's strengths and needs.	• Regular examinations aid in early identification of growth problems or developmental delays, so that appropriate interventions can be planned.

EXPECTED OUTCOME: Child will demonstrate normal growth and development milestones.

4. Nursing Diagnosis: *Family Processes, Interrupted,* related to child's prolonged disability from sensory impairment (NANDA-I © 2014)

GOAL: The family will identify methods for coping with their child with a visual impairment.

INTERVENTION	RATIONALE
• Provide explanation of visual impairment as appropriate.	• The parents may feel guilt about the child's visual impairment, which can be allayed by knowledge of the cause.
• Refer parents to organizations, early intervention programs, and other parents of children with visual impairments.	• The parents will receive needed information and support from others.
• Assist parents to plan for meeting the developmental, educational, and safety needs of their child with a visual impairment. Offer resources for changing home environment to assist child.	• The child may require an enhanced environment in order to foster developmental progress.

EXPECTED OUTCOME: Family will successfully cope with the experience of having a child with a visual impairment.

Nursing Care Plans are also provided. They address health conditions and illustrate the conceptual approach that nurses need in caring for children, including assessment, NANDA nursing diagnoses, goals, plans, and interventions.

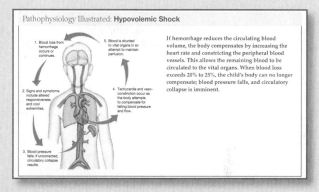

Pathophysiology Illustrated: **Hypovolemic Shock**

Pathophysiology Illustrated boxes feature unique drawings that illustrate conditions on a cellular or organ level, and may also portray the step-by-step process of a disease. These images visually explain the pathophysiology of certain conditions to increase students' understanding of the condition and its treatment.

Professionalism in Practice **Accommodations for Children With JIA**

Section 504 of the Rehabilitation Act of 1973 and the Individuals with Disabilities Education Act (IDEA) protect children with disabilities from discrimination. A formal plan such as an individualized education plan (IEP) should be developed for the child with arthritis that outlines accommodations and modifications that are needed at school (Solomon, 2014). The school nurse can work with the family and school administration to determine the plan. Accommodations at school may include providing a set of books for the home so that the child is not required to carry the books home daily. Additional time may be required for the child to move from class to class. The school nurse can refer parents and children to the Arthritis Foundation and the American Juvenile Arthritis Organization for further information and support. The adolescent should also be referred for vocational counseling and offered support for transition to adult services.

Professionalism in Practice boxes focus on important topics related to contemporary nursing practice issues, including legal and ethical considerations. This feature reflects a commitment to quality improvement in all aspects of care.

SAFETY ALERT!
If you feel a mass during palpation of a child's abdomen, stop palpating immediately and report the finding to the child's primary healthcare provider. Never palpate the liver or abdomen of a child with Wilms tumor as this could cause a piece of the tumor to dislodge. Place a sign on the child's bed and in the chart alerting healthcare providers not to palpate the abdomen.

The **SAFETY ALERT!** features present essential information that calls attention to issues that could place a patient or a nurse at risk and provide guidance on maintaining a safe environment for all patients and healthcare providers.

Each chapter ends with **Chapter Highlights** that outline the main points of the chapter and a list of **References** from which students can locate additional resources. In addition, the **Clinical Reasoning in Action** features at the end of each chapter propose a real-life scenario and a series of clinical reasoning questions so that you can apply to the clinical setting what you learned in class.

Where relevant, SKILLS found in the companion book, *Clinical Skills Manual for Maternity and Pediatric Nursing*, Fifth Edition, are cited.

Chapter Highlights

- The hypothalamic-pituitary axis produces several releasing and inhibiting hormones that regulate the function of many endocrine glands.

- Puberty is the process of sexual maturation that occurs when the gonads secrete increased amounts of the sex hormones estrogen and testosterone, resulting in the development of primary and secondary sexual characteristics.

- Children with hypopituitarism have short stature as a result of growth hormone deficiency. Treatment with growth hormone early in life enables these children to potentially attain genetically appropriate heights.

- An excessive secretion of growth hormone or hyperpituitarism may cause children to have tall stature, growing up to 7 or 8 feet in height if no intervention is provided before the epiphyseal plates close.

- Diabetes insipidus is a disorder of the posterior pituitary gland and is defined as an inability of the kidneys to concentrate urine.

- Syndrome of inappropriate antidiuretic hormone (SIADH) results from an excessive amount of serum antidiuretic hormone (ADH), leading to water intoxication and hyponatremia.

- Precocious puberty is defined as the appearance of any secondary sexual characteristics before 8 years in girls and 9 years in boys. If no treatment is provided, the hormones will stimulate closure of the epiphyseal plates and the child will have short stature as an adult.

- Untreated or ineffectively treated congenital hypothyroidism results in impaired growth and intellectual disability.

- Signs of hyperthyroidism include an enlarged, nontender thyroid gland (goiter), prominent or bulging eyes, eyelid lag, tachycardia, nervousness, increased appetite with weight loss, emotional lability, moodiness, heat intolerance, hypertension, hyperactivity, irregular menses, insomnia, tremor, and muscle weakness.

- During infancy, most cases of endogenous Cushing disease are due to a functioning adrenocortical tumor. The most common cause of endogenous Cushing syndrome in children older than 7 years of age is Cushing disease, in which a pituitary tumor (adenoma) secretes excess ACTH.

- Congenital adrenal hyperplasia has two forms, salt-losing or non–salt-losing with virilization. The salt-losing form accounts for 75% of cases and is caused by aldosterone deficiency and overproduction of androgen. The non–salt-losing form accounts for the other 25% of cases.

- Congenital adrenal hyperplasia is the most common cause of pseudohermaphroditism (ambiguous genitalia) in newborn girls.

- Adrenal insufficiency, also known as *Addison disease*, is a rare disorder in childhood characterized by a deficiency of glucocorticoids (cortisone) and mineralocorticoids (aldosterone). Symptoms include weakness, fatigue, weight loss, and gastrointestinal symptoms such as nausea, vomiting, diarrhea, constipation, and abdominal pain. Other symptoms include hyperpigmentation, hypotension, dizziness, joint pain, salt cravings, and hypoglycemia.

- Pheochromocytoma is a tumor that arises from the adrenal gland and causes an excessive release of catecholamines. Clinical manifestations include hypertension, palpitations sweating, anxiety, tremors, and headache.

- Diabetes mellitus type 1 is the most common metabolic disease in children and one of the most common chronic diseases in school-age children. It is a disorder of carbohydrate, protein, and fat metabolism.

- Treatment of the child with diabetic ketoacidosis includes intravenous fluids and electrolytes for dehydration and acidosis. Insulin is given by continuous infusion pump to decrease the serum glucose level at a slow but steady rate to prevent the development of cerebral edema.

- Common causes of hypoglycemia in children with type 1 diabetes include an error in insulin dosage, inadequate calories because of missed meals, or exercise without a corresponding increase in caloric intake.

- Type 2 diabetes mellitus is a condition that results from insulin resistance. Children most commonly affected are obese, and many have family members with the same type of diabetes.

- Secondary amenorrhea is the cessation of spontaneous menstrual periods for at least 120 days and occurs 6 months or 3 cycles after menarche.

Contents

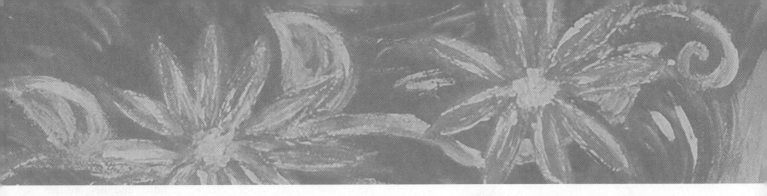

Chapter 1
Nurse's Role in Care of the Child: Hospital, Community, and Home

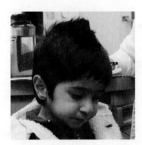

Manny takes medication for seizures, and he is in the health clinic because he had a seizure last week. I will help the parents learn more about seizures, how they are treated, and what they should do when Manny has a seizure.

—Nurse caring for Manny, 3 years old

Learning Outcomes

1.1 Describe the continuum of pediatric health care.

1.2 Compare the roles of nurses in child health care.

1.3 Analyze the current societal influences on pediatric health care and nursing practice.

1.4 Report the most common causes of child mortality by age group and reasons for hospitalization.

1.5 Contrast the policies for obtaining informed consent of minors to policies for adults.

1.6 Examine three unique pediatric legal and ethical issues in pediatric nursing practice.

Pediatric Healthcare Overview

Nurses provide care to healthy children as well as to those with illnesses, injuries, and chronic conditions such as seizures, in a wide variety of settings. They contribute to the health and welfare of children as they monitor their growth and development, and help them adapt to and manage their health conditions. Fortunately, most children are healthy, experiencing only occasional short-term health problems, and nurses have the opportunity to help children and families prevent disease and promote a healthy lifestyle. However, children with special healthcare needs require frequent contact with the healthcare system to achieve and maintain their optimal level of health.

Pediatric health care occurs along a continuum that reflects not only the various settings of care but also the complexity and range of care needed by individual children and their families. For example, all children need health promotion and health maintenance services, but some children will need care for chronic conditions, acute illnesses and injuries, and even end-of-life care. See Figure 1–1 for the model of pediatric health care on which this text is based.

The range of healthcare settings in which pediatric nurses work includes the following:

- The hospital, including pediatric wards, intensive care units, newborn nursery, emergency department, radiology, and specialty clinics
- Physician offices, clinics, and healthcare centers
- The child's home
- Rehabilitation centers and residential treatment centers
- Schools, childcare centers, and camps
- The community

Without a doubt, nurses play a significant role in the provision of health care for children. Their responsibilities vary in the

1

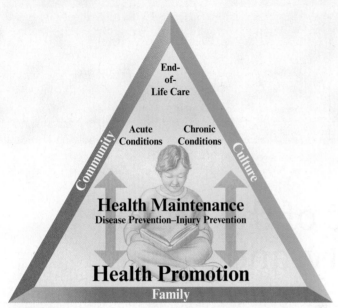

Figure 1–1 The Bindler-Ball Continuum of Pediatric Health Care for Children and Their Families. The outer bars represent the family, cultural, and community influence on the care that the child receives, either through the services sought by the family or the services provided in the community. Cultural influences include the family's values and beliefs, and the cultural competence of the nurse in caring for a child and family.

The inner categories represent the range of health care needed by children. All children need health promotion and health maintenance services, represented by the base of the triangle. Notice the arrows representing the upward and downward movement between the levels of care as the child's condition changes.

Children may be healthy with episodic acute illnesses and injuries. Some children develop a chronic condition for which specialized health care is needed. A child's chronic condition may be well controlled, but acute episodes (such as with asthma) or other illnesses and injuries may occur, thus prompting additional health promotion and health maintenance services. Some children develop a life-threatening illness and ultimately need end-of-life care. A healthy child may also experience a catastrophic injury leading to death, thereby requiring supportive end-of-life care for the family.

SOURCE: Bindler, R. C., & Ball, J. W. (2007). The Binder-Ball healthcare model: A new paradigm for health promotion. *Pediatric Nursing, 22*(2).

different clinical settings as they collaborate with other healthcare providers, such as physicians, social workers, pharmacists, optometrists, psychologists, dentists, nutritionists, speech therapists, and physical and occupational therapists.

Assessment, nursing care interventions, and client education are universal roles for nurses regardless of the setting in which they work. This chapter defines the various roles for the nursing care of children and reviews concepts important to pediatric nursing.

Role of the Nurse in Pediatrics

Pediatric nursing, using a family-centered care approach, focuses on promoting the health of children of newborn age through young adulthood; protecting them from illness and injury; recognizing the differences in presentation of diseases between children and adults; adapting nursing care to the age, development, social factors, and health status of the child; assisting and educating the family to care for their child's health condition needs; and advocating for the care of children and their families in all healthcare settings and the community. The nursing roles in caring for children and their families include direct care, client education, advocacy, and case management. Pediatric nurses collaborate with other healthcare professionals as a team member while performing each of these nursing roles.

Nurses who specialize in pediatrics apply foundational knowledge learned during their nursing education, such as the nursing process, anatomy and physiology, physical assessment, healthcare condition recognition and management, and the full range of nursing skills. Pediatric nurses then add additional competencies related to the care of children and their families, such as the following:

- Interacting effectively with children of different ages and their families
- Modifying physical assessment techniques for the age and development of the child
- Identifying strategies to reduce the child's pain and stress
- Accurately calculating medication dosages and volume for administration
- Considering the child's developmental status for client safety and injury prevention activities
- Adapting nursing procedures to the developmental age of the child

Several nursing organizations have collaborated to develop standards of practice for pediatric nurses.

Professionalism in Practice **Standards for Pediatric Nursing Practice**

The American Nurses Association, the National Association of Pediatric Nurse Practitioners, and the Society of Pediatric Nurses jointly developed *Pediatric Nursing: Scope and Standards of Practice* (2015). These standards describe the expectations for professional performance during care to children and their families. Practicing nurses have an obligation to maintain competence, update their knowledge of new research and practice changes, and practice in an ethical manner when assessing, planning, and evaluating the care provided to children and their families. Collaboration with the family and other healthcare professionals as well as advocating for the child and family are additional expectations when providing nursing care.

Direct Nursing Care

The nursing process provides the framework for delivery of direct pediatric nursing care. The nurse assesses the child, identifies the health concerns, and lists the nursing diagnoses describing the responses of the child and family to those health concerns in the nursing care plan. The nurse then implements and evaluates nursing care. This care is designed to meet the physical and emotional needs of the child and family. It is tailored to the child's developmental stage, giving the child additional responsibility for self-care with increasing age. Planned care is offered in a sensitive manner, compatible with the cultural beliefs of the child and family in collaboration with the family, using family-centered care principles (see Chapter 2).

Nurses play an important role in minimizing the psychologic and physical distress experienced by children and their families. Providing support to children as well as their families is one component of direct nursing care. This often involves listening to their concerns, being present during stressful or emotional experiences, and implementing strategies to help children and family members cope (see Chapter 2). Nurses can also help families by suggesting ways to support their children in all healthcare settings, including the home.

Patient Education

The education of children and their families improves treatment results. In pediatric nursing, patient education may be challenging, because nurses work with children at various levels of understanding. Rather than giving simple facts, the goal of client education is to help the child and parents or guardians make informed choices about health and healthy behaviors.

As patient educators, nurses help children adapt to the hospital setting and prepare them for procedures (Figure 1–2). Most hospitals encourage a parent to stay with the child and to provide much of the direct and supportive care. Nurses teach parents to watch for important signs and responses to therapies, to increase the child's comfort, and even to provide advanced care. Taking an active role prepares the parent to assume total responsibility for care after the child leaves the hospital.

Planning and preparation, as well as an understanding of the child's developmental level, are needed to effectively educate children and parents. An assessment of the knowledge the child and family have about health conditions or health practices, their past experiences, and their attitudes and beliefs is a starting point for education. The nurse needs to think about strategies

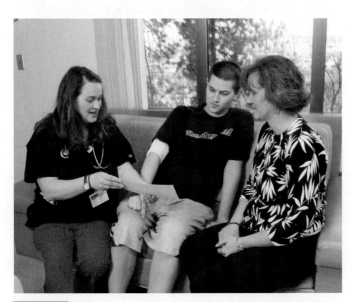

Figure 1–2 Explaining procedures can reduce this adolescent's and family's fears and anxieties about what to expect as well as teach procedures and proper home care.

and resources available to help the child and family learn about the current health condition. See *Developing Cultural Competence: Adapting the Reading Level of Patient Education Materials*. Education can be evaluated during future visits of children receiving ongoing health promotion and health maintenance care and of those with a chronic condition that requires home management.

Developing Cultural Competence Adapting the Reading Level of Patient Education Materials

Understanding written information in patient care instructions, education materials, and even prescription labels is important to promote **adherence** (the extent to which a client or parent follows recommended care for the health problem). Among U.S. adults, 20% read at a fifth-grade level or below; however, this rate varies by cultural group with higher rates of poor literacy among Latinos, Blacks, and Asians (Pontius, 2013). This means that many parents have difficulty using and understanding health information. Healthcare materials must be provided in the appropriate language and at the appropriate reading level (e.g., sixth-grade reading level for low literacy individuals) (Pontius, 2014). Printed materials to educate children and families about a health condition might be readily available, but they may be written at a reading level that is too high. Even though printed material may be available in the primary language of the client and family, do not assume that the family has reading skills in that language.

When developing patient education materials with a lower reading level:

- Use short familiar words with one or two syllables in short sentences.
- Substitute simple language that defines a medical term rather than using the term.
- Use pictures or graphics to give instructions when possible.
- Use active voice rather than passive voice.
- Use the term *must* to express a requirement.
- Divide the content into small sections and use headers.
- Use lists and tables to simplify content.
- Use a computer program to evaluate the reading level of the materials you develop.

Patient Advocacy

Advocacy—acting to safeguard and advance the interests of another—is directed at enabling the child and family to adjust to the changes in the child's health in their own way. To be an effective advocate, the nurse must be aware of the needs of the child and family, the family's resources, and the healthcare services available in the community. The nurse can then assist the family and the child to make informed choices about these services and to act in the child's best interests.

As advocates, nurses often serve on committees to ensure that the policies and resources of healthcare agencies meet the psychosocial needs of children and their families. The nurse must also protect the child and family by taking appropriate actions related to any incidents of incompetent, unethical, or illegal practices by any member of the healthcare team.

Case Management

What happens when a child has significant health problems? Can one nurse handle it all? When a child has a significant chronic health condition, healthcare professionals (physicians, nurses, social workers, physical and occupational therapists, and other specialists) often create an interdisciplinary plan to meet the child's medical, nursing, developmental, educational, and psychosocial needs. Because nurses spend time with the child and family while providing nursing care, they often know about the family's wishes and resources. As a member of the interprofessional team, the nurse can serve as the family's advocate to ensure that the care plan considers the family's wishes and contains appropriate services. A nurse may become the child's case manager, coordinating the implementation of the interdisciplinary care plan. Sometimes the parent or a social worker becomes the case manager.

Case management is a process that involves the assessment, planning, facilitation, and delivery of healthcare services, including healthcare options by the interprofessional team to promote quality and cost effectiveness of care (Woodward & Rice, 2015). This practice promotes **continuity of care**, the process of facilitating a client's care between and among healthcare providers and settings based on health needs and available resources. The nurse case manager has control over the use of healthcare resources that are considered appropriate for the child's condition and links the child and family to these services. Case management may be used for care of the patient when hospitalized and for long-term care of chronic conditions.

Discharge planning is a form of case management. Good discharge planning promotes a smooth, rapid, and safe transition into the community and improves the results of treatment begun in the hospital. To be a discharge planner, the nurse needs to know about community medical resources, home care agencies qualified to care for children, educational interventions, and services reimbursed by the child's health plan or other financial resources.

Research

Clinical research helps develop, refine, and expand knowledge that advances the science of pediatric nursing care and improves the nursing care provided to children (Christian, 2012). Research can focus on evaluating innovations in care to determine if practice is improved. Pediatric nurses read and analyze new research findings and apply those findings to practice. Such findings may potentially advance healthcare outcomes, improve comfort, or even reduce the cost of care. This research may also be used in developing specific healthcare facility evidence-based clinical practice guidelines. For example, pediatric nurses may identify issues in client care processes that involve clinical practice, education, ethical issues, and specific needs of particular populations of children.

Nursing Process in Pediatric Care

Clinical Reasoning

Clinical reasoning is the analytical process used when assessing client cues and information, synthesizing that information and applying it to understand a child's or family's problem or concern, and then using the nursing process to plan and evaluate the child's care. **Critical thinking** is an individualized, creative thinking or reasoning process that nurses use to solve problems. Both of these reasoning skills are essential for nurses. For example, the child's condition can change during a hospitalization, requiring nurses to recognize subtle cues that need attention to prevent the child's deterioration.

The nursing process involves clinical reasoning and critical thinking when planning nursing care for infants, children, and adolescents. Consider how the five steps of the nursing process relate to children:

- *Assessment* involves collecting client and family data and performing physical examinations in all healthcare settings. The nurse analyzes and synthesizes data to make a judgment about the child's problems.

- *Nursing diagnoses* describe the health promotion and health patterns that nurses can identify and manage by developing a plan for specific nursing actions. The North American Nursing Diagnosis Association (NANDA) has established the standard language for these nursing diagnoses. Each nursing diagnosis has defining characteristics, related factors or risk factors, nursing intervention classifications (NIC), and nursing outcome classifications (NOC).

- *Nursing care plans* are based on the identification of desired outcomes or goals that will improve the child's or family's healthy or dysfunctional health patterns. The nurse creates a nursing care plan in collaboration with the child and family or customizes standard care plans for specific diagnoses that may be used in all healthcare settings. Standard care plans are customized based on data collected from the child's assessment and an evaluation of the child's response to care. The family (and the child, when old enough) and the nurse should agree with the care plan goals.

- *Implementation* is performing the interventions or specific action steps outlined in the nursing care plan.

- *Evaluation* is the use of specific objective and subjective measures (often called *outcome measures* or *outcome criteria*) to measure the progress of the child and family in reaching the goals defined in the nursing care plan. As the child's condition improves and goals are attained, the nursing care plan is modified with new goals and nursing actions based on data from ongoing assessments.

Evidence-Based Practice

Evidence-based practice (EBP) is a problem-solving approach that integrates the best research evidence with a healthcare professional's clinical expertise and the client's values or preferences (Ritt, 2013). It provides a bridge between research and practice by using a systematic search for the most relevant evidence related to a clinical question or problem, followed by a critical review of that evidence to help answer it. Evidence-based practice is one strategy to keep nursing practice current and to promote positive outcomes for children and their families. It has become an important strategy used by healthcare institutions to improve client safety and quality of care. Use of EBP requires the nurse to be a lifelong learner.

Several steps are involved in the EBP (Lockwood, Aromataris, & Munn, 2014):

1. Ask and clearly describe the specific clinical question.

2. Collect the most relevant and best evidence from well-designed studies.

3. Critically review, synthesize, and analyze the evidence for quality and application to the clinical question and population served.

4. Integrate the evidence with your clinical experience and the client's preferences and values, often providing the development of a practice guideline for nursing practice.

5. Evaluate the nursing practice change resulting from the EBP process for its impact on quality of care.

Nurses often collaborate with an interprofessional team to investigate EBP clinical questions to develop a **clinical practice guideline**, a consensus of evidence-based and expert opinion statements about the care for a specific diagnosis used to assist the interprofessional team of healthcare providers to make decisions about the appropriate care of a child who has that condition (Keiffer, 2015). Some practice guidelines are developed by government agencies and national professional organizations. These guidelines encourage practice changes that improve quality and encourage more cost-effective care. Practice guidelines are tools that promote uniformity in care so that client outcomes and healthcare professional performance can be measured. One example is the pediatric asthma guidelines developed by the National Asthma Education Program.

Practice guidelines help promote **collaborative practice**, a comprehensive model of health care that uses an interprofessional team of health professionals to provide high-quality, cost-effective care. Other examples of practice guidelines include the care of a child with type 1 diabetes and traumatic brain injury.

Settings for Pediatric Nursing Care

Pediatric nurses function in a variety of settings within the hospital. Acute care may be provided in the emergency department, observation or short-stay unit, postanesthesia unit, intensive care unit, general pediatric inpatient unit, and various outpatient clinics. In rehabilitation centers, nurses provide inpatient and ambulatory care to help restore children to an optimal state and plan for discharge management of chronic conditions. Pediatric nurses working with children and families on a general pediatric hospital unit promote health improvement in the following ways:

- Gathering data and assessing the health of children and their families
- Providing ordered medical therapies
- Delivering nursing care in a manner that preserves as many of the child's and family's normal routines as possible while maintaining the family unit
- Working with the family and healthcare team to develop an individualized healthcare plan and a discharge plan, or to implement a clinical practice guideline

The hospital stay is part of a care continuum that allows children to complete therapy at home, at school, or in other community settings. Pediatric nurses assist families in transitioning from the acute hospital setting to the home or other facility, such as a rehabilitation center or long-term care facility. Managing the child's transition from acute care to another setting involves discharge planning that integrates interdisciplinary care plans and collaboration with a broad range of healthcare professionals. The nurse may assist the family of a child with significant health problems to prepare for the child's return home and to develop an emergency care plan in case the child has an unexpected healthcare crisis. See Chapter 11 for more information on caring for children in the hospital setting.

Pediatric nurses also work in several community healthcare settings such as physician offices, health centers, specialty care clinics, home health agencies, and schools. See Chapter 10 for more information about nursing care in community settings.

Contemporary Climate for Pediatric Nursing Care

In 2014, more than 73.6 million children under the age of 18 years lived in the United States. They accounted for 23.1% of the population (U.S. Census Bureau, Population Division, 2015). (See Figure 1–3 for a distribution of the population by age group.) The racial and ethnic diversity of children under 18 years of age in the United States continues to increase and is currently estimated as follows (Federal Interagency Forum on Child and Family Statistics, 2014):

- White, non-Hispanic: 52.4%
- Black, non-Hispanic: 13.8%
- Hispanic: 24.1%
- Asian: 4.6%
- All other races: 5.1%

Culturally Sensitive Care

The U.S. population has a varied mix of cultural groups, with ever-increasing diversity. In 2012, approximately 47.6% of all children under age 18 years were from families of minority populations. By the year 2050, it is expected that the proportion of children who are of Hispanic origin will increase to 36%, equaling the proportion of non-Hispanic White children (Federal Interagency Forum on Child and Family Statistics, 2013). Diversity also exists among the non-Hispanic White population, representing many cultural groups who have immigrated from European and former Soviet bloc countries. See Chapter 2 for more information on cultures.

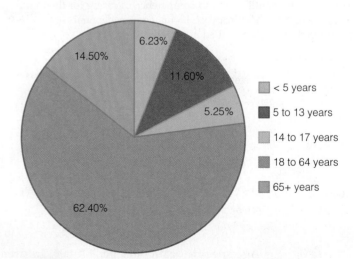

Figure 1–3 **The population of children under age 18 years was estimated in 2014 to account for 23.1% of the population in the United States. Note the comparison of the pediatric population size with other population age groups.**

SOURCE: Data from U.S. Census Bureau, Population Division. (2015). *Annual estimates of the resident population for selected age groups by sex for the United States, states, counties, and Puerto Rico Commonwealth and municipios: April 1, 2010, to July 1, 2014.* Retrieved from http://factfinder.census.gov

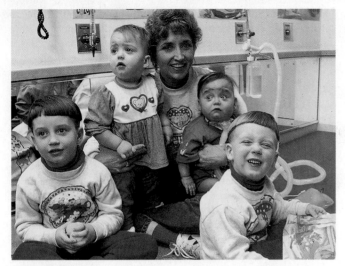

TABLE 1–1 Five Leading Causes of Infant Mortality, 2013

CAUSE OF INFANT MORTALITY	RATE PER 1000 LIVE BIRTHS
Congenital malformations	121.0
Low birth weight	106.9
Maternal complications	40.6
Sudden infant death syndrome	39.7
Unintentional injuries	29.6

Source: Adapted from Kochanek, K. D., Murphy, S. L., Xu, J., & Arias, E. (2014). Mortality in the United States, 2013. *NCHS Data Brief, No. 178*. Retrieved from http://www.cdc.gov/nchs/data/databriefs/db178.pdf

Figure 1–4 Many facilities now encourage family visitation for children with health problems that require long-term hospitalization. Extended family visits enable parents to learn about the child's care, and provide siblings with opportunities to interact with the hospitalized child.

Family-Centered Care

Recognizing the family as the constant influence and support in a child's life is the foundation for developing a trusting relationship with families. The family is the principal caregiver and support for the child, and the family is important in helping the child recover from an illness or injury (Figure 1–4). The effort to address and meet the emotional, social, and developmental needs of children and families seeking health care in all settings is a concept known as **family-centered care**. Families are often considered partners in care, learning about children's conditions and participating in decisions regarding their care. Thus, families gain greater confidence and competence in caring for their children who have healthcare problems. The key elements of family-centered care are described in Chapter 2.

Pediatric Health Statistics

Mortality

Children have different healthcare problems than adults, and the problems may be related to stage of development or other factors. The **infant mortality** (death in infants under 12 months of age) rate was 5.96 deaths per 1000 live births in the United States in 2013 (Kochanek, Murphy, Xu, et al., 2014). See Table 1–1 for the leading causes of infant mortality in 2013. The mortality rate for non-Hispanic Black infants is more than twice the rate of non-Hispanic Whites (U.S. Department of Health and Human Services, 2013). The leading causes of infant mortality vary according to the age of the infant. For example, the leading causes of death in the neonatal period (birth to 28 days of age) are short gestation, low birth weight, and congenital malformations. The leading causes of mortality in the postneonatal period (between 1 and 12 months of age) are sudden infant death syndrome, congenital malformations, and unintentional injuries (U.S. Department of Health and Human Services, 2013).

The most common cause of death for children between 1 and 19 years of age is unintentional injury. Congenital malformations, cancer, and diseases of the heart are among the most common medical causes of death in children and adolescents. Figure 1–5

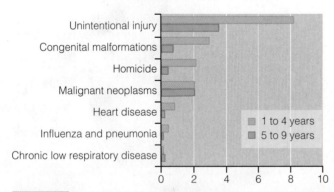

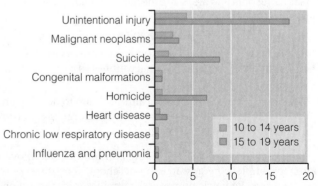

Figure 1–5 Age-specific death rates per 100,000 children for the leading causes of mortality in the United States in 2013. *A,* Leading causes of death and death rates for children between 1 and 9 years of age. *B,* Leading causes of death and death rates for children between 10 and 19 years of age. The leading cause of death in children in all age groups was unintentional injury. Why do you think that is? Which type of unintentional injury has the highest rate of death? Drowning? Fires and burns? Motor vehicle crashes? What about intentional injury? See Table 1–2 for the answers.

SOURCE: Data from Centers for Disease Control and Prevention, National Center for Health Statistics. (2015a). *Health data interactive*. Retrieved from www.cdc.gov/nchs/hdi.htm

shows the age-specific mortality rates for the leading causes of death by age group.

Healthy People 2020

(MICH-3) Reduce the rate of child deaths

Injury accounted for an alarming percentage of deaths to children and youth in 2013: children 1 to 4 years—40.7%, children 5 to 9 years—35.9%, youth 10 to 14 years—45.1%, and adolescents 15 to 19 years—71.7% (Centers for Disease Control and Prevention, National Center for Health Statistics, 2015b). Although unintentional injury is the leading cause of death for children and youth, intentional injury (homicide and suicide) is among the top five major causes of death for our nation's children. The major causes of unintentional injury mortality in childhood include motor vehicle (passengers and pedestrians), drowning, fires and burns, suffocation, and poisoning. Table 1–2 illustrates the leading causes of injury deaths by age group. Many injury prevention programs have been implemented by state health departments, healthcare facilities, and national organizations to reduce the number of children who die unnecessarily.

The U.S. government set objectives to improve the health of children and young adults in the 21st century in the report titled *Healthy People 2020*. These national health objectives focus on reducing the incidence of death and disability from the major causes of death shown in Figure 1–5 and Tables 1–1 and 1–2. *Healthy People 2020*'s overarching goals are listed in Box 1–1. Often federal funding in grants is linked to the development of programs aimed at reducing the number of deaths from these factors in specific high-risk groups. Throughout this text, *Healthy People 2020* objectives related to health promotion and specific conditions are identified in specially designed "speed bumps." The coding in front of each objective identifies the specific topic area and objective number for the *Healthy People 2020* initiative. Pediatric nurses focus directly on many of these topic areas, including the following:

- Maternal, infant, and child health (MICH)
- Adolescent health (AH)
- Injury and violence prevention (IVP)
- Nutrition and weight status (NWS)
- Educational and community-based programs (ECBP)

> **Box 1–1** *Healthy People 2020* **Overarching Goals**
> Goal 1: Attain high-quality, longer lives free of disease, disability, injury, and premature death.
> Goal 2: Achieve health equity, eliminate disparities, and improve the health of all groups.
> Goal 3: Create social and physical environments that promote good health for all.
> Goal 4: Promote quality of life, healthy development, and healthy behaviors across all life stages.
>
> **SOURCE:** U.S. Department of Health and Human Services. (2015). *Healthy People 2020*. Retrieved from http://www.healthypeople.gov/2020/about/default.aspx

- Vision (V)
- Substance abuse (SA)
- Tobacco use (TU)
- Environmental health (EH)
- Physical activity (PA)
- Immunization and infectious diseases (IID)
- Respiratory diseases (RD)
- Disability and health (DH)

Morbidity

Morbidity is an illness or injury that limits activity, requires medical attention or hospitalization, or results in a chronic condition. Morbidity varies according to the age of the child. In 2011, children under 18 years of age accounted for more than 5.6 million hospitalizations, and the number of hospitalizations in this age group had decreased 26% since 1997. Infants less than 1 year of age accounted for 4.2 million of these hospitalizations. Most of these hospitalizations were related to live birth, but other leading causes of hospitalization included acute bronchitis, hemolytic jaundice, pneumonia, and short gestation/low birth weight (Pfuntner, Wier, & Stocks, 2013). Figure 1–6 illustrates the five leading causes of hospitalization of children 1 through 17 years of age in 2011. Diseases of the respiratory system account for the greatest number of hospitalizations when pneumonia and asthma hospitalizations are combined. Hospitalizations for mood disorders have increased 68% since 1997. What do you think could account for the increase in hospitalizations for mood disorders? See Chapter 17.

TABLE 1–2 Five Leading Causes of Injury Death by Age Group, 2013[*]

AGE GROUP	RANKING				
	FIRST	**SECOND**	**THIRD**	**FOURTH**	**FIFTH**
Under 1 year	Suffocation	Homicide, unspecified cause	Homicide, specified cause	Motor vehicle	Undetermined suffocation
1 to 4 years	Drowning	Motor vehicle	Suffocation	Homicide	Fire, burns
5 to 9 years	Motor vehicle	Drowning	Fire, burns	Homicide, firearms	Suffocation
10 to 14 years	Motor vehicle	Suicide, suffocation	Suicide, firearms	Homicide, firearms	Drowning
15 to 19 years	Motor vehicle	Homicide, firearms	Suicide, suffocation	Suicide, firearms	Poisoning

*Darker shading indicates unintentional injuries.

Source: Data from National Center for Health Statistics. (2015). 10 leading causes of injury deaths, United States 2013. Retrieved from http://www.cdc.gov/injury/wisqars/fatal.html

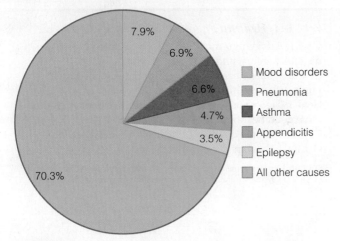

Figure 1–6 The five leading causes of hospitalization for children 1 to 17 years of age in the United States in 2011 are presented as a percentage of all causes of hospitalization in this age group.

SOURCE: Data from Pfuntner, A., Wier, L. M., & Stocks, C. (2013). Most frequent conditions in U.S. hospitals, 2011. *H-CUP Statistical Brief, No. 162.* Retrieved from http://www.hcup-us.ahrq.gov/reports/statbriefs/sb162.pdf

Healthcare Issues

Healthcare Financing

Cost and access to health care are important policy issues. Congress created the Children's Health Insurance Program (CHIP) in 1997 to serve uninsured children up to age 19 years. This program was reauthorized in 2009 to provide health insurance for children when their family's income is too high to qualify for Medicaid but inadequate to pay for private insurance coverage. Medicaid and the State Children's Health Insurance Program (SCHIP) provide health coverage to more than 31 million children, including half of all low-income children in the United States (Centers for Medicare and Medicaid Services, 2014a). See Figure 1–7 for the distribution of children's health insurance status.

Clinical Tip

The federal poverty rate is used to determine eligibility for many health and welfare services. The rate is a sliding scale based on the number of persons in the family, and it is updated annually. For example, in 2013, the Affordable Care Act specified that 133% of the federal poverty level ($31,321.50 for a family of four) be used as the eligibility criteria for Medicaid. Eligibility for CHIP begins at 200% of the federal poverty level, but some states set a higher level for eligibility (Centers for Medicare and Medicaid Services, 2014b).

The Patient Protection and Affordable Care Act (ACA) bridges a portion of the gap for children whose family income is too low for private health insurance but too high to qualify for Medicaid and SCHIP. It ends preexisting condition exclusions for children, eliminates annual limits on insurance coverage, and keeps young adults covered for a longer period on their parents' health insurance policy (U.S. Department of Health and Human Services, 2015). Pediatric healthcare professionals continue to have concerns regarding the need to have pediatric service

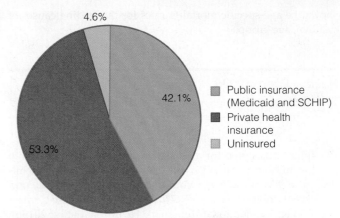

Figure 1–7 In the United States, how is health care of children through age 18 years paid for? These data from 2014 show that U.S. taxes support 42.1% of the costs. What can you do to help? Something as simple as counseling parents about injury prevention and providing immunizations while a child is under care for other problems can prevent potential health problems. Part of good nursing care is supporting the well-being of the child in addition to caring for the presenting problem.

SOURCE: Data from Martinez, M., & Cohen, R. A. (2015). *Health insurance coverage: Early release of estimates from the National Health Interview Survey, January–September 2014.* National Center for Health Statistics. Retrieved from http://www.cdc.gov/nchs/data/nhis/earlyrelease/insur201503.pdf

requirements similar to the essential services required by Medicaid and SCHIP, especially if the SCHIP program is not reauthorized. Services for children with special healthcare needs and rehabilitation included in large-group private health plans may potentially be threatened if these health payers modify benefits to fit the ACA requirements (Fry-Bowers, 2015).

Despite the availability of SCHIP, many eligible children are not enrolled. The expectation is that when parents contact their state Affordable Care Act Health Insurance Marketplace, qualifications for Medicaid or SCHIP will be identified and parents will be directed to enroll their children in those programs. Nurses can play an important role in encouraging families to investigate their eligibility for the program. Obtain current guidelines in your state about eligibility requirements and coverage benefits.

Healthcare Technology

Research and technology have enabled many children with congenital anomalies and low birth weights to survive, with and without chronic conditions. Technologic advances have led to the development of portable medical equipment for home care that children use to support physiologic functions. For example, approximately 9 million U.S. children have special healthcare needs requiring complex care or specialized equipment (e.g., ventilators, feeding tubes, intravenous or central lines and their associated pumps, cardiorespiratory monitors, peritoneal dialysis, and pacemakers) (Baker & Cormier, 2013). The number of children assisted by technology continues to increase as scientific and technologic advances grow. However, this technology also adds burdens to the family, such as stresses on family functioning, preparation for power outages, and higher costs for health care. Some families have regained control over their lives by creating intensive care units in their homes (Figure 1–8). See Chapter 12 for more information on children with special healthcare needs.

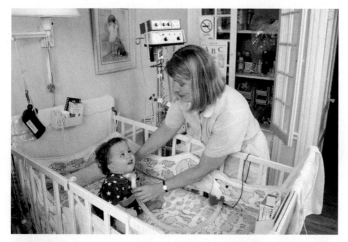

Figure 1–8 It is often desirable from a family and cost perspective to provide health care in the home, and technologic advances have made this possible. But is it less costly to provide care in the home for a child with technology assistance? Are the parents' out-of-pocket expenses for medical supplies considered? What about a parent's need to discontinue employment to care for the child? What is the emotional strain on families who care for their child 24 hours a day, 7 days a week? What support is needed by these families to continue providing this level of care at home? See Chapters 10 and 12 for answers.

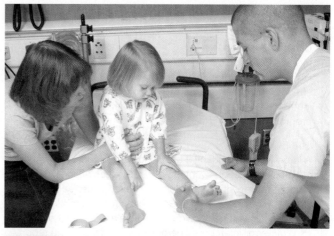

Figure 1–9 An important client safety action is to verify the identity of the child prior to performing any procedure or administering medication. The nurse needs two forms of identification. In this case the child's identification bracelet is compared to the name and birth date on the laboratory test form, and the parent also confirms the child's identity.

Legal Concepts and Responsibilities

Regulation of Nursing Practice

Nurses are accountable for their professional actions, and each state regulates nursing practice with a nurse practice act. A state's nurse practice act defines the legal roles and responsibilities of nurses. As professionals, nurses set standards for education and practice that conform to state regulations. Standards for nursing education are modified as the science of nursing progresses.

Accountability and Risk Management

ACCOUNTABILITY
The family entrusts the child's care to the healthcare team. Family members expect this team to provide good medical and nursing care and to avoid mistakes that cause harm. The Quality and Safety Education for Nurses (QSEN) project, established in 2005, is designed "to meet the challenge of preparing future nurses who will have the knowledge, skills and attitudes (KSAs) necessary to continuously improve the quality and safety of the healthcare systems within which they work" (QSEN, 2014). The project focuses on competencies in six areas: patient-centered care, teamwork and collaboration, evidence-based practice, quality improvement, safety, and informatics.

PATIENT SAFETY
Patient safety is defined as the freedom from unintentional injury caused by medical care; it includes freedom from harm by death-related or adverse drug events, misidentification of the

patient, and healthcare-associated infections (AAP, 2011b). Correct client identification is essential prior to all procedures and medication administration. See Figure 1–9. Some aspects of pediatric care increase the risk for medical error, such as medication dosages that must be calculated for the child's weight and liquid medications that require an additional calculation for volume per dose. The young child's immature physiology may also affect the ability to metabolize and excrete certain medications.

Clinical Tip
Parents play an important role in their child's safety as a partner with the child's healthcare team. Recognize their role and encourage parents to collaborate with healthcare professionals to keep their child safe in the clinical setting. Encourage them to ask questions and to persist until they understand and agree with the proposed outcome of care. Parents also help prevent injuries to their child in the clinical setting, and they may identify potential deficiencies or errors in care, such as failure to perform hand hygiene.

Many medical errors within hospitals are "systems errors," such as medication prescription and dispensing errors, rather than being the error of a single individual. (See *Evidence-Based Practice: Medication Errors.*) The Joint Commission has National Patient Safety Goals (NPSG) that focus on correct identification of patients, improved staff communication, safe medication administration, infection control, safe use of alarms, identifying patients at risk for suicide, and preventing mistakes in surgery (The Joint Commission, 2014).

Reasons for the higher rate of medication error in children may include the following:

• Medication dosage is based on weight or body surface area, often making dosage calculations more complex. This means the optimal dose is based on mg/kg and divided by number of doses to be given a day. When suspensions or liquid preparations are used, dosage calculation increases

EVIDENCE-BASED PRACTICE | Medication Errors

Clinical Question

Medication error is a significant problem in pediatric nursing because children are at higher risk for serious adverse effects. What characteristics of medication errors involving nurses need more attention by hospital patient safety programs?

The Evidence

A large children's hospital used anonymous reporting of adverse medication events to evaluate medication errors and to identify prevention strategies; however, underreporting by RNs was suspected. When RNs were surveyed to identify situations in which they would not file a safety event or near miss (an error intercepted before it reached the client) report, responses included not enough time and not being aware of a need to report near miss events. The RNs were then educated to recognize events that should be reported and tips to decrease the time needed to report events. Next, they were given data about trends in reported medication errors and near-miss events (e.g., incorrect intravenous fluid use, the need for better storage supply bin labeling, and separation of similarly named fluids). Efforts resulted in an increased event reporting, but nurses still reported inadequate time to submit reports (Hession-Laband & Mantell, 2011).

A prospective study was conducted in three tertiary pediatric hospitals in Canada to review anonymously reported pediatric medication administration errors by nurses working on 18 medical/surgical and critical care units. A total of 372 occurrences of potential errors (34.1%) and actual errors (65.9%) were reported over a 3-month period. The majority occurred on medical/surgical units (74%) compared to critical care units (26%). Three primary factors contributed to medication errors: workload, distraction, and ineffective communication (Sears, O'Brien-Pallas, Stevens, et al., 2013).

A meta-analysis of 63 research studies was conducted and aimed at reducing medication errors in children under age 19 years cared for in the hospital and ambulatory settings. Studies focused on preventable events that could lead to inappropriate medication use or potential harm as well as events that caused harm. The events were associated with prescribing, administering, and dispensing medications. Studies that included voluntary reporting of medication errors or near-miss events were excluded, as it was believed underreporting would exist. Problems identified in studies that affect their usefulness included lack of uniformity in definitions of medication error causes, as well as variations in data collection methods and how outcomes were reported. Although medication error reductions were reported, these problems prevented the identification of good evidence regarding medication error interventions that healthcare facilities should implement (Rinke, Bundy, Velasquez, et al., 2014).

Best Practice

Nurses need to learn about the system problems that contribute to medication error, so they can help identify strategies to reduce the risk for error, such as ways to reduce distraction during medication preparation and administration. New hospital systems are being implemented to reduce medication error, and strategies to successfully encourage reporting of actual and potential medication errors continue to be needed. Increased reporting by nurses, physicians, and pharmacists would help identify additional factors contributing to medication errors in different units and the effectiveness of new strategies to reduce errors.

Clinical Reasoning

Identify the medication error reduction policies and strategies for the inpatient pediatric unit. What medication safety practices have resulted from a review of error reports? Identify two potential strategies to improve medication safety in this setting.

---

in complexity. Then both the correct dose and the amount of liquid preparation (mg/mL) for that dose must be calculated. Some medications are in concentrations that require dilution, further complicating the accurate medication dosage calculation.

- A misplaced decimal when calculating a medication dosage may result in a harmful overdose or ineffective dose. Children with a critical illness or injury do not have the reserves to deal with a medication overdose.

- Off-label medications (not approved for use in children by the U.S. Food and Drug Administration) are sometimes prescribed, so the appropriate pediatric dose and adverse effects are unknown.

- Young children cannot communicate well regarding the adverse effects of medication.

RISK MANAGEMENT

Healthcare facilities are challenged to promote optimal patient care and to reduce liability by implementing strategies to reduce medical errors in all child patients. **Risk management** is a process established by a healthcare institution to identify, evaluate, and reduce the risk of injury to patients, staff, and visitors,

and thus reduce the institution's liability. This involves the study of causes of medical errors and near-miss errors within a healthcare facility and implementing system changes to prevent future errors similar to those studied. Box 1–2 explains several strategies that have been developed to reduce medication errors in children.

Quality improvement is the continuous study of systems, services, and processes of care, and using that information to improve healthcare processes, services, and patient outcomes. Nurses participate in the development of institutional policies and standards of nursing practice. Hospitals and home health agencies encourage the development of diagnosis-specific nursing care plans and interdisciplinary clinical practice guidelines that serve as minimal standards of care for the facility.

During the development of standards of care for the facility, indicators of effective care by pediatric nurses and other providers are identified. These indicators may measure either the process of care, the facility's systems, or the expected outcome of care for a specific patient condition. Client records are regularly reviewed to identify deviations from the facility standards or clinical practice guidelines. When deviations from expected processes and outcomes are identified, opportunities to improve the system or processes of care provision are explored with all

Box 1–2 System Strategies to Reduce Pediatric Medication Errors

- Use the child's weight in kilograms in all healthcare settings as the standard weight for prescriptions.
- Look for the child's weight and age, the calculated dose, and mg/kg dose on every prescription. Unit dose dispensing systems should be used. The administration rate for all IV medications should be specified.
- Do not use a zero after a whole number (e.g., 5.0 could be misread as 50) because an error with a 10-fold dosage increase could occur. Use a leading zero before a decimal point when the dose is less than a whole unit to ensure that the decimal is seen (e.g., 0.5 rather than .5).
- Do not store medications with similar sounding names close together. Look at labels for capital letters that a pharmacy may use to help distinguish between medications with similar sounding names (e.g., DOBUTamine and DOPamine).
- Expect prescriptions to be typed or written legibly with printed letters. Milliliter rather than teaspoon volume measurement should be used. Electronic prescription systems supported by the American Academy of Pediatrics may improve legibility, require all needed prescribing information, and actually calculate the correct dosage for the prescriber (American Academy of Pediatrics, 2013).
- Follow all guidelines for patient identification before administering the medication, even if bar coding is used.

care providers. Recommendations for the revision of institutional standards to further improve care by nurses and other health providers in the institution often result.

Policy and procedure manuals should be current and have evidence incorporated to provide guidance on nursing procedures, use of technology, patient education, and evaluation of interventions to promote client safety. Nurses often participate as committee members in the development and revision of these policy and procedure manuals.

Documentation of nursing care is an essential part of risk management and quality improvement. If a patient record is subpoenaed, documented care is considered the only care provided, regardless of the quality of undocumented care. The patient assessment, the nursing care plan, and the child's responses to medical therapies and nursing care, including the regularly scheduled evaluation of the client's progress toward nursing goals, must all be documented accurately and sequentially. Nurses must also report any untoward incidents that could inhibit the client's recovery.

Clinical Tip

The patient's record is a legal document that is admissible evidence in court. Information in the patient's record must be written in objective terms or appropriately recorded in the electronic medical record. When recording a client's response to therapy, the nurse must include physiologic responses and exact quotes. The date, time, and nurse's signature and title are required.

Legal and Ethical Issues in Pediatric Care

Marvin, a 15-year-old boy with acute nonlymphocytic leukemia, has relapsed after a second remission with an acute onset of fever, joint pain, and petechiae (Figure 1–10). A hematopoietic stem cell (bone marrow) transplant is one of his therapeutic options. Although Marvin has agreed to a transplant if a suitable donor is found, he does not want to be resuscitated and placed on life support equipment if he has a cardiac arrest. Marvin has experienced all the burdens of therapy up to this point. He has talked extensively with the hospital chaplain and social worker and feels comfortable with his decision. His parents want an all-out effort to sustain his life until a donor is located.

Marvin's case illustrates the legal and ethical dilemmas in caring for older children and adolescents, especially since he has the ability to understand and make reasonable decisions. At what age can children make an informed decision about whether to accept or refuse treatment? What happens when the parents and child have conflicting opinions about treatment? How are ethical decisions resolved?

Informed Consent

Informed consent is a formal authorization by the child's parent or guardian allowing an invasive procedure to be performed or for participation in research. Information that must be provided to obtain informed consent includes the following:

- An explanation of the child's diagnosis
- A description of the proposed treatment or research; possible outcome, benefits, and significant risks associated with the proposed treatment or research
- Alternative treatments and their potential outcome, benefits, and significant risks
- Answers to questions
- Informing a parent or guardian about the right to refuse treatment or research participation on behalf of the child

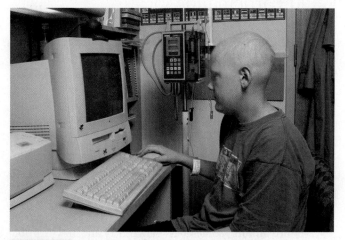

Figure 1–10 Marvin, a 15-year-old boy with acute nonlymphocytic leukemia, has definite opinions about his treatment. His parents have a difficult time accepting his opinions when they differ from their own. At what age can children make an informed decision about whether to accept or refuse treatment?

The physician is legally responsible for obtaining informed consent. In the case of research, the investigative researcher may formally designate a person to obtain informed consent. The nurse should verify that informed consent has been obtained prior to any procedure or research participation, alert physicians to the need for informed consent, serve as a witness for informed consent, and respond to questions asked by parents and children.

Consent must be given voluntarily and prior to the procedure or research. Parents, as the legal custodians of minor children, are customarily requested to give informed consent on behalf of a child. Both children and parents must understand that they have the right to refuse treatment at any time.

When parents are divorced and have joint custody, in most cases either may give informed consent. When parents are divorced and one parent has custody, some states limit the parental rights to give informed consent to the parent with custody. Obtain information about your state law regarding custody and who can provide informed consent for healthcare procedures and treatments.

Clinical Tip

Obtain legal advice for complex family issues related to guardianship, divorced parents disagreeing over care, or a caregiver who is not the legal guardian. Each agency should have designated legal experts or consultants for provision of such legal advice.

Many children live in homes with a parent and other adult (stepparent, cohabiting unmarried adult, or grandparent) who does not have legal authority to sign consent. Proxy consent can be granted in writing by the parent to another adult so that children can obtain health care when needed. In an emergency, treatment to preserve life or limb does not require consent, if it cannot be immediately obtained. After examining the child and determining that an emergency condition does not exist, nonurgent treatment should not be provided until the parent or guardian with legal authority can be reached (even if by telephone) (AAP, 2011a).

Child Participation in Healthcare Decisions

Older children and adolescents often have the cognitive capacity to participate in or make medical decisions, but their rights to make most medical decisions are controlled by state law. Adolescents under the age of majority, as defined by state law, are considered minor children, and parental consent is required for medical treatment in the majority of states. Adolescents can legally give informed consent in the following special circumstances:

- **Emancipated minors** (economically self-supporting adolescents under 18 years of age [e.g., married, pregnant, enlisted, or incarcerated] not subject to parental control) and minor parents of a child patient can legally give informed consent.
- **Mature minors** (adolescents between 14 and 18 years able to understand treatment risks) may give independent consent to receive or refuse treatment for limited conditions by federal law, such as testing and treating sexually transmitted infections, contraception services, substance abuse, and mental health care. However, mature minors do not have authority to consent for general medical treatment in most states (Coleman & Rosoff, 2013).

Despite these limitations in informed consent, children and adolescents should have an opportunity to participate in treatment decisions with their parents as reasoning skills develop. **Assent** is the voluntary agreement to accept treatment or to participate in a research project. To give assent, the child needs a basic understanding of what will be done and what is required for participation. The child must also know that he or she can say no (dissent). Parents may wish to actively involve the child in listening to the informed consent information and permit them to express agreement or disagreement with treatment. Nurses can help parents recognize when the child is ready to participate in care decisions and help answer questions the child has about the condition and treatment. The parents, however, make final decisions regarding the treatment or research participation. The child's dissent to participate in research should be respected.

Growth and Development Consent Considerations

By 7 to 8 years of age, a child is usually able to understand concrete explanations about assent for research participation. Generally, by age 11 years, a child's abstract reasoning and logic are advanced. By age 14 years, an adolescent can usually weigh options and make decisions regarding consent as capably as an adult.

Child's Rights Versus Parents' Rights

Parents or guardians have the authority to make choices about their child's health care except in the following cases:

- The parents' choice of treatment does not permit lifesaving treatment for the child. See *Developing Cultural Competence* for information about religious beliefs and emergency treatment.
- There is a potential conflict of interest between the child and parents, such as with suspected child abuse or neglect.
- The child and parents do not agree on major treatment options.

Developing Cultural Competence Religious Beliefs

Jehovah's Witnesses oppose transfusions of blood products for themselves and their children because they believe transfusions are equivalent to the oral intake of blood, which is morally and spiritually wrong according to their interpretation of the Bible (Leviticus 17:13–14). A Jehovah's Witness who receives a transfusion believes he or she has committed a sin and may have forfeited everlasting life. Most healthcare facilities have policies to address the care of these children. Every effort is made to avoid the use of blood products with alternative therapies, except when a blood product will be lifesaving. Then a judicial order is sought.

Healthcare providers involve adolescents in decision making about major treatment interventions in an effort to promote agreement about the treatment plan. In some cases, adolescents and parents or guardians disagree about a major treatment intervention (e.g., bone marrow transplant, heart transplant). Healthcare providers may try negotiation and compromise as a first step to help adolescents and parents reach agreement about interventions so that the adolescent's voice and opinion are considered. Medical consultation may be sought to identify other treatment options that might be acceptable to both the adolescent and parents. The facility's ethics committee (often composed of healthcare professionals, clergy, consumer representatives, and an ethics expert) usually becomes involved to help resolve the issue. If agreement cannot be reached, the adolescent may need to seek designation as an emancipated minor or ultimately follow the parents' decision regarding treatment.

CONFIDENTIALITY

The Health Insurance Portability and Accountability Act (HIPAA), P.L. 104-191, was enacted by Congress in 1996. One goal of the law is to protect the privacy of citizens by establishing standards for the management of confidential electronic medical information. Healthcare organizations have developed policies to prevent the inappropriate disclosure of protected health information. Patients have the right to determine who can have access to their health information. Sharing protected patient information in the hospital within the hearing of others as well as on social media is a violation of confidentiality. Be aware of policies that hospitals and other health facilities have regarding guidelines for confidentiality with electronic medical records and for the use of social media.

Confidentiality is an agreement between a client and a provider that information discussed during the healthcare encounter will not be shared without the client's permission. Adolescents often do not want their parents informed about sensitive healthcare information. Their concerns about confidentiality may influence whether or not they seek health care. The electronic medical record systems are an additional challenge to adolescent confidentiality, even if seeking care for contraception or a condition such as a sexually transmitted infection. Healthcare systems are developing electronic health record (EHR) systems that can be accessed by parents of adolescents. Guidelines for controlled access to sensitive information are not uniformly built in to those EHR systems so that individual healthcare providers can code some information as private (Daniel, Malvin, Jasik, et al., 2014). The issue of confidentiality for adolescents is further complicated because the parents are responsible for the financial costs of the healthcare services. In some cases parents may get indirect information from health insurance bills. See *Families Want to Know: Adolescents and Confidentiality* for ways to promote confidentiality.

Patient Self-Determination Act

The federal Patient Self-Determination Act directs healthcare institutions to inform hospitalized patients about their rights, which include making **advance directives** (writing a living will or authorizing a durable power of attorney for healthcare decisions on the client's behalf). An adolescent with a serious or life-limiting condition, such as Marvin presented earlier, has a strong and legitimate interest in expressing an opinion about aggressive therapy. The adolescent and parents should be encouraged to talk and reach a joint therapy decision. If the parents and adolescent are unable to agree, the legal issues become complex, as previously described.

Do-not-attempt-resuscitation (or allow natural death) orders have become more common for children with terminal illnesses in which no further aggressive treatments are available or desired. In some cases these children are cared for at home. State health policies and guidelines must be in place for an emergency care provider in the community to honor a written do-not-resuscitate order for a child who has a life-threatening event (Abbott & Stone, 2014). See Chapter 13 for issues related to palliative and end-of-life care.

Ethical Issues

Major advances in medical technology—such as the ability to save the lives of severely impaired newborns, to extend the lives of chronically ill and seriously injured children, to perform genetic testing, and to provide gene therapy—have led to challenges for healthcare professionals and parents to make the best decision for the child's condition. For example, limiting or withdrawing life-sustaining treatment may be appropriate for the child who is severely ill or injured at the end of life to promote comfort, or making a decision not to attempt cardiopulmonary resuscitation (Kodish & Weise, 2016). Healthcare professionals have a moral obligation to deliver care with compassion and respect for the worth and uniqueness of each individual; they must understand and respect religious and cultural differences that impact parental decisions about requesting or refusing a treatment.

Ethics is the philosophic study of morality, and the analysis of moral problems and moral judgments. It is an inquiry into the justification of particular actions. Ethical issues may arise from a **moral dilemma**—a conflict involving individual beliefs, social values, and ethical principles. Each side of the conflict may support different courses of action (e.g., performing or refraining

Families Want to Know
Adolescents and Confidentiality

Adolescents need a safe and confidential environment to discuss healthcare issues so they will seek health care when needed. Ways to promote confidentiality include the following actions:

- Discuss the importance to the adolescent and parents about giving adolescents, and the parents, an opportunity to talk in private with the healthcare provider about their concerns.
  - Adolescents learn how to speak for themselves about their health concerns.
  - This becomes the basis for a trusting relationship with the healthcare professional.

- Explain the limits of confidentiality.
  - Privacy will be maintained unless something dangerous or life threatening regarding the adolescent is revealed.
  - The electronic health record and health insurance billing information may reveal some private information to the parents.
  - Some conditions require mandatory reporting to the health department, such as tuberculosis and the human immunodeficiency virus (HIV).

- Obtain the phone number or other contact information so the adolescent may be contacted to share laboratory test results or to check on response to treatment.

- Make sure clinic literature is small enough to fit discreetly into a purse or wallet.

from performing a therapy). Emotions play a significant role in the development of ethical dilemmas. Parents want to protect the child, and they have their vision of what is good for the child. Healthcare professionals have different values than families because of their culture and life experiences. Differences in values may also exist between members of the healthcare team caring for the child. Regardless, all healthcare professionals want the child to benefit from the care they give.

Nurses may face ethical dilemmas when providing pediatric care. They witness parents struggling to decide among treatment options. Pediatric nurses have a responsibility to become knowledgeable about the moral and legal rights of their patients and families and to protect and support those rights. They must work with parents to form a therapeutic alliance, and attempt to prevent conflicts when the values of the family and healthcare professionals do not match. Pediatric nurses work to find out what is important to the parents in the care of their child. The parents may be able to describe what they wish to avoid having happen to their child, and this could become a starting point for discussion about the child's care with healthcare professionals.

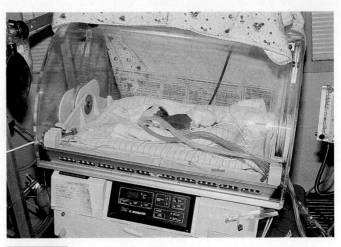

Figure 1–11 Due to technological advances that sustain life, parents must sometimes face difficult decisions. If a newborn is certain to have severe disabilities, at what point should parents decide to withhold or withdraw treatment?

SOURCE: Courtesy of Carol Harrigan, RNC, MSN, NNP.

Clinical Tip

No matter what decision parents make about their child's care, they need to be reassured that they are trying to do what they think is best for their child.

Healthcare facilities have an ethics committee to resolve conflicts about treatment decisions between healthcare professionals and the child and family, or to resolve a dispute between healthcare professionals about the care to provide a child. The ethics committee resolves the conflict or dispute by performing an individual case consultation. A healthcare provider or the family can request a consultation.

WITHHOLDING OR WITHDRAWING MEDICAL TREATMENT

Newborn John, at 5 days of age, has a birth weight of 1200 grams, acute respiratory distress, and a severe intraventricular hemorrhage. See Figure 1–11. Consent is being sought by the physician for surgical placement of a ventriculoperitoneal shunt. Regardless of intensive medical care and planned surgical intervention, the newborn is expected to have a severe disability if he survives. The newborn's condition is critical, and it is not certain how well he will respond to surgery.

The Child Abuse and Treatment Act of 1984, also known as the Baby Doe Regulations, defines withholding of medically indicated treatment for a child with a life-threatening condition as medical neglect, except when care is futile (Douglas & Dahnke, 2013). This act was enacted to protect the rights of newborns with severe defects. **Futility** is a situation in which treatments do not provide a clear clinical benefit. Physicians are not obligated to offer interventions that cause extreme pain and suffering when there is no or limited potential benefit.

Parents are participants in the decisions made about care for infants with severe disabilities and children with life-limiting conditions. They are entitled to full information about the risks and benefits of a procedure and the child's long-term prognosis. Parents should have clear information on the seriousness of the child's condition and prognosis, the child's potential quality of life, the degree of pain and suffering, and physician recommendations. Efforts should be made to understand the perspective and values of the parents, especially when their decision does not match the healthcare provider's recommendations. Conflict may arise when parents choose to withdraw therapy or request aggressive therapy when the healthcare providers' recommendations differ. An ethical consultation may be needed to resolve conflicts.

GENETIC TESTING OF CHILDREN

With advances in genetics research, it is now possible to test infants and children for the presence of a genetic condition carrier status. It is also possible to conduct presymptomatic testing for a specific condition, such as Huntington disease or Duchenne muscular dystrophy. Genetic screening of newborns, such as for inborn errors of metabolism, cystic fibrosis, sickle cell anemia, and other conditions, routinely occurs. In this case, the early identification of the genetic condition benefits the infant. A system is in place to confirm the diagnosis, and treatment and follow-up care are available to affected newborns. See Chapter 3 for additional information about ethical issues associated with genetic testing.

ORGAN TRANSPLANTATION ISSUES

The death of a child can benefit several other children through organ transplantation, which has become an accepted therapeutic option for some life-threatening conditions. The limited supply of organs has created numerous ethical issues. Which patients on the waiting list should receive the organs available? Should a patient with multiple congenital anomalies, disabilities, or abnormal chromosomes be eligible for a transplant? Should families be permitted to pay donor families for organs? Should the family's ability to pay for an organ transplant give a child higher priority for an organ? Should a patient receive a second organ transplant, replacing an organ deteriorating because of rejection? Should parents conceive another child, hoping that the new baby is a potential stem-cell donor for a child with an illness? If so, what pressures does this place on both children as they grow older? Each institution performing organ transplants develops guidelines for ethical decision making regarding these and other questions.

The Children's Health Act, P.L.106-310 passed in 2000, directed the development of specific criteria, policies, and procedures to address the specific needs of children regarding priorities for organ allocation. Guidelines for the allocation of hearts, lungs, livers, and kidneys for children have been developed that give preference to children based on factors in addition to time on the waiting list (Workman, Myrick, Meyers, et al., 2013).

Partnering With Families

The topics discussed in this chapter reflect the current challenges children and their families face in the healthcare system—access to health care, specific disease and injury risks, and ethical and legal concerns. A nurse in collaboration with parents and children is essential every step of the way regarding:

- Obtaining informed consent and assent
- Respecting that the parent is an expert with regard to the child's care
- Acknowledging and supporting cultural values in the provision of care
- Preparing parents to assume ongoing complex healthcare responsibilities for their child

Developing relationships with children and families is challenging, exciting, and ultimately gratifying for nurses who choose to specialize in pediatrics.

Chapter Highlights

- Roles of nurses in caring for children include direct patient care, patient education, patient advocacy, case management, and research.
- Nurses care for children in many different settings: the emergency department, radiology, inpatient units, critical care units, postanesthesia units, outpatient clinics, schools, childcare centers, physician offices, community health centers, rehabilitation centers, and the home.
- Family-centered care is a method designed to meet the emotional, social, and developmental needs of children and families needing health care.
- Nurses must identify culturally relevant facts about their clients to provide appropriate and competent care to an increasingly diverse population.
- Unintentional injury is the leading cause of death for children between 1 and 19 years of age.
- The State Children's Health Insurance Program (SCHIP) and the Patient Protection and Affordable Care Act are programs that make health insurance more affordable for families with limited incomes.
- Documentation of nursing care is essential for risk management and quality improvement. Be sure to include the patient assessment, the nursing care plan, the child's responses to medical therapies and nursing care, and a regular evaluation of the child's progress in meeting nursing goals.
- Informed consent is the formal preauthorization for an invasive procedure or participation in research. Parents typically give informed consent for children under 18 years of age unless the child is an emancipated minor (a self-supporting adolescent not subject to parental control).
- Children should be actively involved in decisions about their care as their decision-making abilities develop. Although they cannot provide informed consent to participate in research, children should receive information about a research project and be asked their opinion about participation.
- Because adolescents fear disclosure of confidential information, they may avoid seeking health care. It is important to tell adolescents when confidentiality cannot be maintained, such as when a reportable disease must be reported to a public health agency or when an electronic health record may be reviewed by parents.
- Adolescents with a potentially life-limiting health condition should be encouraged to talk with their parents and to make joint decisions about future care.
- A formalized ethical decision-making process may assist healthcare providers and families in making important decisions about withholding, withdrawing, or limiting a child's therapy.

Clinical Reasoning in Action

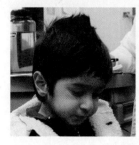

Recall 3-year-old Manny, at the beginning of the chapter, who has a seizure disorder. He receives his care in a mobile van sent to his community by the local children's hospital. Manny has a regular source of care because his family income qualifies him for the state's Child Health Insurance Program (CHIP).

1. List at least five competencies nurses need to care for children.
2. Identify at least four different settings in which a child with a seizure disorder could receive health care.
3. List three specific injury prevention messages for a child of Manny's age that should be provided to Manny's parents to reduce his risk for morbidity and mortality.
4. List specific steps the nurse should use in the healthcare setting to ensure that an error is avoided for Manny's prescribed seizure medication and administration by his parents.

References

Abbott, J. T., & Stone, S. (2014). End of life. In J. A. Marx, R. S. Hockberger, & R. M. Walls (Eds.), *Rosen's emergency medicine—Concepts and clinical practice* (8th ed., pp. e47–e58). Philadelphia, PA: Elsevier Saunders.

American Academy of Pediatrics (AAP) Committee on Pediatric Emergency Medicine and Committee on Bioethics. (2011a). Policy statement—Consent for emergency medical services for children and adolescents. *Pediatrics, 128*(2), 427–433.

American Academy of Pediatrics (AAP), Steering Committee on Quality Improvement and Management, & Committee on Hospital Care. (2011b). Policy statement—Principles of pediatric patient safety: Reducing harm due to medical care. *Pediatrics, 127*(6), 1199–1210.

American Academy of Pediatrics (AAP). (2013). Electronic prescribing in pediatrics: Toward safer and more effective medication management. *Pediatrics, 131*(4), e1350–e1356.

American Nurses Association, National Association of Pediatric Nurse Practitioners, & Society of Pediatric Nurses. (2015). *Pediatric nursing: Scope and standards of practice* (2nd ed.). Silver Spring, MD: NursesBooks.org.

Baker, L. R., & Cormier, L. A. (2013). Disaster preparedness and families of children with special healthcare needs: A geographic comparison. *Journal of Community Health, 38*, 106–112.

Bindler, R. C., & Ball, J. W. (2007). The Bindler-Ball healthcare model: A new paradigm for health promotion. *Pediatric Nursing, 22*(2), 121–126.

Centers for Disease Control and Prevention, National Center for Health Statistics. (2015a). *Health data interactive.* Retrieved from www.cdc.gov/nchs/hdi.htm

Centers for Disease Control and Prevention, National Center for Health Statistics. (2015b). *Ten leading causes of injury deaths, United States, 2013.* Retrieved from http://www.cdc.gov/injury/wisqars/leading_causes_death.html

Centers for Medicare and Medicaid Services. (2014a). *Medicaid: Children.* Retrieved from http://www.medicaid.gov/Medicaid-CHIP-Program-Information/By-Population/Children/Children.html

Centers for Medicare and Medicaid Services. (2014b). *2013 poverty level guidelines.* Retrieved from http://www.medicaid.gov/Medicaid-CHIP-Program-Information/By-Topics/Eligibility/Downloads/2013-Federal-Poverty-level-charts.pdf

Christian, B. J. (2012). Translational research—Improving everyday pediatric nursing practice through research and evidence-based practice. *Journal of Pediatric Nursing, 27*, 280–282.

Coleman, D. L., & Rosoff, P. M. (2013). The legal authority of mature minors to consent to general medical treatment. *Pediatrics, 131*(4), 786–793.

Daniel, S., Malvin J., Jasik, C. B., & Brindis, C. D. (2014). *Sensitive health care services in the era of electronic health records: Challenges and opportunities in protecting confidentiality for adolescents and young adults.* Retrieved from http://bit.ly/ElectronicHealthRecord-Brief

Douglas, S. M., & Dahnke, M. D. (2013). Creating an ethical environment for parents and health providers dealing with the treatment dilemmas of neonates at the edge of viability. *Journal of Neonatal Nursing, 19*, 33–37.

Federal Interagency Forum on Child and Family Statistics. (2013). *America's children: Key national indicators of well-being, 2013.* Retrieved from http://childstats.gov/americaschildren/index.asp

Federal Interagency Forum on Child and Family Statistics. (2014). *At a glance for 2014: America's children: Key national indicators of well-being.* Retrieved from http://childstats.gov/americaschildren/index.asp

Fry-Bowers, E. K. (2015). The ACA and insurance implications for children with special health care needs. *Journal of Pediatric Health Care, 29*(2), 212–215.

Hession-Laband, E., & Mantell, P. (2011). Lessons learned: Use of event reporting by nurses to improve patient safety and quality. *Journal of Pediatric Nursing, 26*(2), 149–155.

The Joint Commission. (2014). *2014 Hospital National Patient Safety Goals.* Retrieved from http://www.jointcommission.org/assets/1/6/2014_HAP_NPSG_E.pdf

Keiffer, M. R. (2015). Utilization of clinical practice guidelines: Barriers and facilitators. *Nursing Clinics of North America, 50*, 327–347.

Kochanek, K. D., Murphy, S. L., Xu, J., & Arias, E. (2014). Mortality in the United States, 2013. *NCHS Data Brief, No. 178.* Retrieved from http://www.cdc.gov/nchs/data/databriefs/db178.pdf

Kodish, E., & Weise, K. (2016). Ethics in pediatric care. In R. M. Kliegman, B. F. Stanton, J. W. St. Geme, & N. F. Schor (Eds.), *Nelson textbook of pediatrics* (20th ed., pp. 27–33). Philadelphia, PA: Elsevier.

Lockwood, C., Aromataris, E., & Munn, Z. (2014). Translating evidence into policy and practice. *Nursing Clinics of North America, 48*, 555–566.

Martinez, M., & Cohen, R. A. (2015). *Health insurance coverage: Early release of estimates from the National Health Interview Survey, January–September 2014.* National Center for Health Statistics. Retrieved from http://www.cdc.gov/nchs/data/nhis/earlyrelease/insur201503.pdf

Pfuntner, A., Wier, L. M., & Stocks, C. (2013). Most frequent conditions in U.S. hospitals, 2011. *H-CUP Statistical Brief, No. 162.* Retrieved from http://www.hcup-us.ahrq.gov/reports/statbriefs/sb162.pdf

Pontius, D. J. (2013). Health literacy part 1: Practical techniques for getting your message home. *NASN School Nurse, 28*(5), 246–252.

Pontius, D. J. (2014). Health literacy part 2: Practical techniques for getting your message home. *NASN School Nurse, 29*(1), 30–42.

Quality and Safety Education for Nurses (QSEN). (2014). *About QSEN.* Retrieved from www.qsen.org/about_qsen.php

Rinke, M. L., Bundy, D. G., Velasquez, C. A., Rao, S., Zerhouni, Y., Lobner, K., . . . Miller, M. R. (2014). Interventions to reduce pediatric medication errors: A systematic review. *Pediatrics, 134*(2), 338–360.

Ritt, E. (2013). Embedding a culture of analytics in nursing practice. *Nurse Leader, 11*(3), 48–50.

Sears, K., O'Brien-Pallas, L., Stevens, B., & Murphy, G. T. (2013). The relationship between the nursing work environment and the occurrence of reported paediatric medication administration errors: A pan Canadian study. *Journal of Pediatric Nursing, 28*, 351–356.

U.S. Census Bureau, Population Division. (2015). *Annual estimates of the resident population for selected age groups by sex for the United States, states, counties, and Puerto Rico Commonwealth and municipios: April 1, 2010, to July 1, 2014.* Retrieved from http://factfindercensus.gov

U.S. Department of Health and Human Services. (2013). *Child Health USA 2013.* Retrieved from http://www.mchb.hrsa.gov/publications/pdfs/childhealth2013.pdf

U.S. Department of Health and Human Services. (2015). *Healthy People 2020.* Retrieved from http://www.healthypeople.gov/2020/about/default.aspx

U.S. Department of Health and Human Services. (2015). *Key features of the Affordable Care Act by year.* Retrieved from http://www.hhs.gov/healthcare/facts/timeline/timeline-text.html.

Woodward, J., & Rice, E. (2015). Case management. *Nursing Clinics of North America, 50*, 109–121.

Workman, J. K., Myrick, C. W., Meyers, R. L., Bratton, S. L., & Nakagawa, T. A., (2013). Pediatric organ donation and transplantation. *Pediatrics, 131*(6), e1723–e1730.

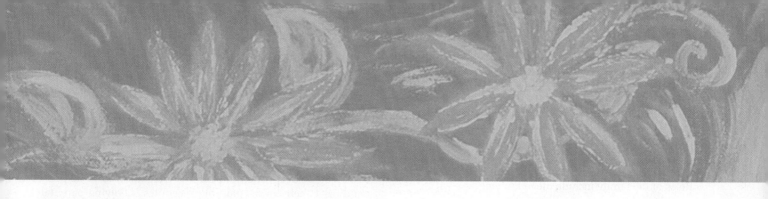

Chapter 2
Family-Centered Care and Cultural Considerations

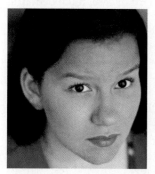

Casey has made a lot of progress since the car accident, but the doctors have told us that the recovery process will take a very long time. I know he will depend on us to take care of him when he is discharged from the hospital.

—Mother of Casey, 16 years old

Ryan McVay/Stockbyte/Getty Images

⌄ Learning Outcomes

2.1 Describe key concepts of family-centered care.

2.2 Compare the characteristics of different types of families.

2.3 Contrast four different parenting styles and analyze their impact on child personality development.

2.4 Explain the effects of major family changes on children.

2.5 List the categories of family strengths that help families develop and cope with stressors.

2.6 Summarize the advantages of using a family or cultural assessment tool.

2.7 Develop a family-centered nursing care plan for the child and family.

2.8 Describe cultural influences on the family's beliefs about health, illness, and treatments.

2.9 Discuss nursing interventions for providing culturally sensitive and competent care to the child and family.

Family and Family Roles

The U.S. Census Bureau defines a **family** as two or more individuals who are joined together by marriage, birth, or adoption and live together in the same household (U.S. Census Bureau, 2013). More broadly, however, a family may be a self-identified group of two or more persons joined together by shared resources and emotional closeness, whether or not they are related by blood, marriage, or adoption, or even living in the same household. The family, as defined by its members, is likely to be dynamic,

because membership often changes over time. For example, second marriages often integrate children into a newly formed family, and spouses of married children are integrated into an existing family while the newly married couple begins a new family. Family members may live in different cities, states, or even countries. So, there is no *typical* family.

Generally, family members depend on each other for emotional, physical, and economic support. Families are guided by a common set of values or beliefs about the worth and importance of certain ideas and traditions. These values often bind family members together. These beliefs are greatly influenced by external factors, including cultural background, social norms, education, environmental influences, socioeconomic status, and beliefs held by peers, coworkers, political and community leaders, and other individuals outside the family unit. Because of the influence of these external factors, a family's values may change considerably over the years, or members within a family may hold values that conflict with those of other family members.

Roles of the family include the following:

- Caring, nurturing, and educating children
- Maintaining the continuity of society by transmitting the family's knowledge, customs, values, and beliefs to children
- Receiving and giving love
- Preparing children to become productive members of society
- Meeting the needs of its members
- Serving as a buffer between its members and environmental and societal demands while advocating or addressing the interests and needs of the individual family members

Individual family members take on certain social and gender roles and hold a designated status within the family based on the values and beliefs that bind extended families together. These values and beliefs may evolve from the family's cultural values and practices, social norms, education, and other influences to which parents were exposed during childhood, adolescence, and early adult years. Parental roles, including childrearing practices and beliefs, are usually learned through a socialization process during childhood and adolescence.

Parents have important roles that involve childrearing and the long-term care of children until they reach adulthood. Depending on their other roles in society, parents work to successfully nurture and rear children and to help them meet role expectations. Parents must also meet the needs of the family unit and provide economic support for the family. Children also learn specific roles through a socialization process. Parents set expectations of behavior with discipline and modeling of appropriate behavior.

Ideally the family is a child's source of strength and support, the major constant in the child's life. Families are intimately involved in their children's physical and psychologic well-being, and they play a vital role in the health promotion and health maintenance of their children. By respecting the family's role, strengths, and experiences with the healthcare system, nurses have an opportunity to develop an effective partnership with the child and family as they make healthcare decisions that promote the child's health. This partnership between nurses and families is known as family-centered care.

Family-Centered Care

Family-centered care is a philosophy of health care in which a mutually beneficial partnership develops between families and the nurse, and also other health professionals. In this way the priorities and needs of the family are addressed when the family seeks health care for the child. Each party respects the knowledge, skills, experience, and cultural beliefs that the other brings to the healthcare encounter. This is in contrast to family-focused care, in which the role of the health professional is that of an expert who directs care, tells the family what to do, and intervenes on behalf of the family.

History of Family-Centered Care

Family-centered care became integral to the nursing care of children when it was recognized that families had a significant role in promoting the psychosocial and developmental needs of children in the hospital. When parents were initially allowed to stay with hospitalized children, nurses and other health professionals noticed that children were quieter, happier, and recovering sooner. Research confirmed that children as well as parents had decreased anxiety when the parents were allowed to be present during their child's painful procedures. Allowing parental involvement in the plan of care is beneficial to both the hospitalized child and the family (Committee on Hospital Care & Institute for Patient and Family-Centered Care, 2012).

Nurses have long embraced the family-centered care philosophy. This philosophy is also becoming more widely accepted by other health professionals. Parents are now recognized as partners in their child's care (see Figure 2–1), not as visitors in the healthcare setting, as patient- and family-centered care has become the standard of care in the pediatric setting (Dokken & Buell, 2011). The Society of Pediatric Nurses and the American Nurses Association have developed nursing practice guidelines for family-centered care, as shown in Box 2–1. For additional information related to the hospitalized child, see Chapter 11.

Promoting Family-Centered Care

Collaborating with families in the provision of health care is essential to promote the best outcome when caring for children. Families have important knowledge to share about their child, their child's health condition, and how their child responds to various actions and events. They also need access to information that will make it possible for them to fully participate in planning and decision making. Parents have a role in developing an effective collaborative relationship with nurses and other health professionals. Parents often become experts in their child's health condition and learn to advocate for their child. They also must learn to communicate effectively with the health professionals caring for their child, and in the process develop a trusting relationship.

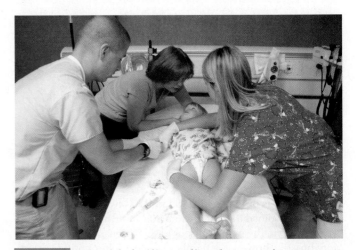

Figure 2–1 **A health facility policy that permits a parent to be present during a procedure performed on a child is an example of a family-centered care policy. The parent plays an important role in providing security and comfort to this child who is having blood drawn.**

Box 2–1 Concepts of Family-Centered Care

- The family is acknowledged as the constant in the child's life and a partner in the child's health care.
- The family, child, and health professionals work together in the best interest of the child and the family. Over time, the child assumes a partnership role in his or her health care.
- Health professionals listen to and respect the skills and expertise that the family brings to the relationship.
- Trust is a fundamental element of the relationship between the family, child, and health professionals.
- Communication occurs in an open, unbiased manner and is ongoing.
- Families, children, and health professionals make decisions regarding the child's care in a collaborative manner in all healthcare settings and for all types of health care needed (e.g., health promotion, health maintenance, acute care, chronic condition care, and end-of-life care). Negotiation may be involved in collaborative decision making.
- The child is supported to learn about and participate in his or her health care and decision making. The adolescent is supported to assume a partnership role in his or her health care and in the transition to adult health care.
- The racial, ethnic, cultural, and socioeconomic background of the family and child, as well as family traditions, are honored. Health professionals work to integrate these values and the preferences of the family and child when planning and providing health care.
- Family-to-family and peer support are encouraged.
- Healthcare settings develop policies, procedures, practices, and systems that are family friendly and family centered; they support the choices the family and child make regarding care.
- Health information for children and families is available and provided to match the range of cultural and linguistic diversity in the community as well as the health literacy levels.

SOURCE: Data from Lewandowski, L. A., & Tesler, M. D. (Eds.). (2008). *Family-centered care: Putting it into action. The SPN/ANA Guide to Family-Centered Care.* Washington, DC: American Nurses Publishing; Committee on Hospital Care & Institute for Patient and Family-Centered Care. (2012). Patient and family-centered care and the pediatrician's role. *Pediatrics, 129*(2), 394–404; Hughs, D. (2014). *A review of the literature pertaining to family-centered care for children with special health care needs.* Retrieved from http://lpfch-cshcn.org/publications/research-reports/a-review-of-the-literature-pertaining-to-family-centered-care-for-children-with-special-health-care-needs/

Clinical Tip

Some healthcare facilities are developing family resource centers to provide consumer information and support (Figure 2–2). In most cases, the resource center is a consumer-oriented health library with staffing, but peer support services may also be coordinated through the center. Families can be supported to access useful information that helps them become informed participants in decision making about their child's care. In addition, the family resource center may serve as a place for family members to read, rest, and reflect (Institute for Patient- and Family-Centered Care, 2013).

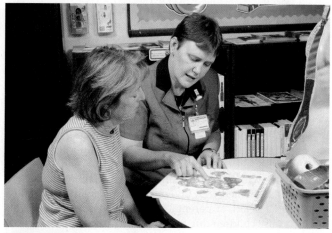

Figure 2–2 The family resource center provides an opportunity for family members to obtain more information about their child's illness from the pediatric nurse educator. This nurse uses pictures from a chart to explain a child's illness to the parent.

Beyond the provision of nursing care itself, children and parents can participate in the development of policies and guidelines for family-centered care in all types of healthcare settings. Their experiences while receiving care in the healthcare setting may reveal valuable insights. Taking parents' perspectives into consideration can be critical for staff and hospital administrators in providing quality patient care and achieving successful patient satisfaction. Parents who exhibit leadership qualities can be empowered to serve on advisory boards or councils, representing the family and community perspective.

Parents can also serve a valuable role in family-to-family support networks as mentors to new families entering the healthcare system for a new chronic condition. Some parents may help raise awareness about specific healthcare issues, serve as advocates for public policy issues, and assist with fundraising activities. Guidelines for working with families as advisors and tools for assessing the family-centered policies in various healthcare settings are available from the Institute for Patient- and Family-Centered Care.

It is important to consider how a healthcare setting's written policies, procedures, and literature for families refer to families and what attitudes these materials convey. Words such as *policies, allowed,* and *not permitted* imply that hospital personnel have authority over families in matters concerning their children. Words such as *guidelines, working together,* and *welcome* communicate an openness and appreciation for families in the care of their children.

Family Composition

Families are diverse in structure, roles, and relationships. Various types of families—both those considered traditional and nontraditional—exist in contemporary U.S. society. This section identifies common types of family structures:

- In the *nuclear family,* children live in a household with both biologic parents and no other relatives or persons. One parent may stay home to rear the children while one parent works, but more commonly, both parents are employed by choice or necessity. Two-income families must address important issues such as childcare arrangements, household chores, and how to ensure quality family time. *Dual-career/dual-earner families* are now considered the norm in modern society.

- The *child-free family* is a growing trend. In some cases, a family is child free by choice; in other cases, a family is child free because of issues related to infertility.

- In an *extended family*, a couple shares household and child-rearing responsibilities with parents, siblings, or other relatives. Families may reside together to share housing expenses and child care. However, in many cases, the child may be residing with the grandparent and one parent because of issues associated with unemployment, parental separation, parental death, or parental substance abuse. Grandparents may raise children due to the inability of parents to care for their own children (see Figure 2–3).

- An *extended kin network family* is a specific form of an extended family in which two nuclear families of primary or unmarried kin live in proximity to each other. The family shares a social support network, chores, goods, and services.

- The *single-parent family* is becoming increasingly common. In some cases, the head of the household is widowed, divorced, abandoned, or separated. In other cases, the head of the household, most often the mother, remains unmarried. Single-parent families often face difficulties because the sole parent may lack social and emotional support, need assistance with childrearing issues, and face financial strain (see Figure 2–4).

- The *single-mother-by-choice family* represents a family composed of an unmarried woman who chooses to conceive or adopt without a life partner (Maggio, 2013). Although these families are included in the single-parent family statistics, they differ significantly in that these women typically are older, college educated, and financially stable and have contemplated pregnancy significantly prior to conceiving (Single Mothers by Choice, 2013).

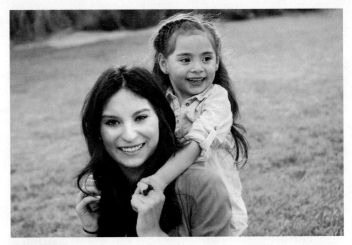

Figure 2–4 **Single-parent families account for nearly one third of all U.S. families. What types of challenges do single-parent families face?**

SOURCE: © Phase4Photography/Fotolia.

- The *blended or reconstituted nuclear family* includes two parents with biologic children from a previous marriage or relationship who marry or cohabit. This family structure has become increasingly common due to high rates of divorce and remarriage. Potential advantages to the children may include better financial support and a new supportive role model. Stresses can include lack of a clear role for the stepparent, lack of acceptance of the stepparent, financial stresses when two families must be supported by stepparents, and communication problems.

- A *binuclear family* is a postdivorce family in which the biologic children are members of two nuclear households, with coparenting by the father and the mother. The children alternate between the two homes, spending varying amounts of time with each parent in a situation called *coparenting*, usually involving joint custody. **Joint custody** is a legal situation in which both parents have equal responsibility and legal rights, regardless of where the children live. The binuclear family is a model for effective communication. It enables both biologic parents to be involved in a child's upbringing and provides additional support and role models in the form of extended family members.

- A *heterosexual cohabiting family* describes a heterosexual couple who may or may not have children and who live together outside of marriage. This may include never-married individuals as well as divorced or widowed persons. Some individuals choose this model for personal reasons; others do so for financial reasons or to seek companionship.

- *Gay and lesbian families* include those in which two adults of the same gender live together as domestic partners with or without children, and those in which a gay or lesbian single parent rears a child. Children in these families may be from a previous heterosexual union, or be born to or adopted by one or both member(s) of the same-sex couple. A biologic child may be born to one of the partners through artificial insemination or through a surrogate mother. Children who are adopted or born into lesbian and gay families are highly valued, as with heterosexual families (see Figure 2–5). Evidence suggests that children reared by same-sex couples are as well adjusted as those born into heterosexual families and have positive peer relationships (Haney-Caron & Heilbrun, 2014).

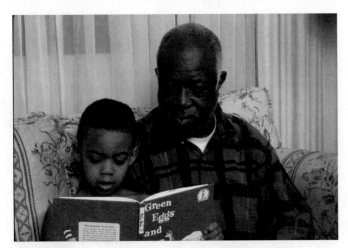

Figure 2–3 **This child lives with his mother and grandparents following the divorce of his parents. The special attention provided by his grandfather is helping him adapt to the change in his family, and it enables the mother to go to work feeling confident that her son is safely cared for before and after school.**

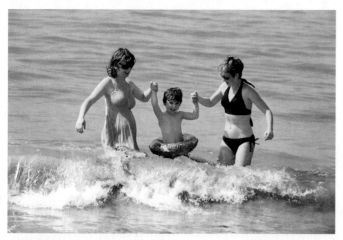

Figure 2–5 Children raised in a homosexual family have been found to do as well emotionally, behaviorally, and socially as those born into heterosexual families (Haney-Caron & Heilbrun, 2014). These parents are as dedicated as heterosexual parents to promoting the growth and development of their children.

SOURCE: Galina Barskaya/Fotolia.

Clinical Tip

It is important to establish which parent has legal custody, current visitation policies, and other variables (e.g., restraining orders and supervised visitation) when communicating information to parents about their children. Certain legal issues may prohibit the nurse from sharing some information with the noncustodial parent.

Family Functioning

Transition to Parenthood

Choosing to become a parent is a major life change for adults. Many couples experience significant family and cultural pressure to have a baby. Mothers may be eager to have a child but be concerned about fulfilling all the expectations of others (father, the baby, other children, her parents, close friends, and employer). Fathers anticipate increased responsibility and many are concerned about their ability to provide adequate support for the family.

At the time of birth, the parents experience stresses and challenges along with feelings of pride and excitement. Both mothers and fathers make adjustments to their lifestyles to give priority to parenting. The baby is dependent for total care 24 hours a day, and this often results in sleep deprivation, irritability, less personal time, and less time for the couple's relationship. In addition, the family often experiences a change in financial status.

Several factors influence how well the parents adjust to their new role. Social support provided to the mother, especially by the father, is important for the mother's adjustment. Marital happiness during pregnancy is an important adjustment factor for both parents. Infants with significant health conditions or those with difficult temperaments can cause extra stress for the parents and affect their adjustment to the parenting role.

With the birth of the first child, both mothers and fathers have challenges related to renegotiating their employment to accommodate family and childcare time. Fathers are sometimes additionally challenged to develop closeness with the infant and to learn how to care for the infant, especially when they may not have had role models or any childcare experience. Most parents find that caring for infants and children takes more time than anticipated.

Nurses can help new parents through this important transition by listening to the challenges they describe during the infant's first health visits. Encourage fathers and mothers to attend and participate in health promotion visits with the healthcare provider so that positive parenting can be supported. Answer questions and offer ideas to address described problems that the parents may be too tired to solve on their own. Help them recognize that frustrations and feelings they have regarding the challenges of infant care are normal and expected. Encourage both parents to become active in caring for the infant and to gain comfort in that care. Help each parent find activities that she or he enjoys with regard to infant care to encourage interaction and bonding with the infant.

Clinical Tip

Eligible parents of newborns and adopted children are entitled to 12 work-weeks of unpaid leave during a 12-month period initially authorized under the federal Family and Medical Leave Act of 1993. Vacation or sick leave may often be used to pay for time away from work. This act also applies if a child, spouse, or parent of the employee develops a serious health condition. The employee is entitled to return to the previous position or an equivalent position with the same pay, benefits, and other conditions (U.S. Department of Labor, 2012).

Parental Influences on the Child

The qualities of family relationships and of family behaviors are important aspects of family strengths and family functioning. Positive family relationships are characterized by parent–child warmth and supportiveness. Warm parent–child relationships can buffer children from stress and promote positive cognitive and social outcomes. Parents who are warm and place high demands on their children for appropriate behavior have children who tend to be content, self-reliant, self-controlled, and open to learning in school.

Mothers and fathers each contribute to the psychologic, emotional, and social health and development of their children. Both parents provide affection, nurturing, and comfort. They teach children life skills and healthy lifestyles. Although focus is frequently on the role of the mother, research has demonstrated that fathers too are important in the child's development (Bright Futures, 2012).

Family Size

The size of the family influences the amount of attention given to children. In small families, parents often have more time to give attention to the children, to encourage achievement, to meet family expectations, and to support involvement in community activities. Children in larger families are encouraged to be cooperative so that the family group functions well. The child usually receives less personal attention from the parents and must often turn to others in the family for support. Family finances may be more limited in large families. Children may adopt a specialized family role to gain recognition, such as the "responsible one," "the clown," or "the black sheep."

Sibling Relationships

Siblings are the first peers of a child and often have a lifelong relationship lasting up to 70 or more years. Siblings, especially those of the same gender, who are closer in age tend to have a closer relationship because they often share many common experiences through childhood and adolescence. In general, for children who are more widely spaced in age, the parents have greater influence than do the siblings. However, the older sibling may be a strong role model for younger brothers and sisters.

Sibling rivalry exists between children at times in all families, but most children learn to share, compete, and compromise with their siblings. Some sisters and brothers take on roles such as protector, problem solver, friend, and supporter for dealing with issues in the family and in the environment. Some siblings learn to work well together to maintain privacy or to form a coalition for negotiating with the parents. Usually, an older sister or brother helps reinforce rules and roles in the family by prompting and inhibiting certain patterns of behavior in the younger siblings. However, one sibling may test the waters by breaking a previously implicit rule to determine how much flexibility is allowed in certain family rules.

Children develop different personalities because of the need to establish a distinct identity for themselves and to be seen as unique in the family. Siblings may share some experiences, but they are often exposed to different environmental experiences that also help shape their personalities. Few if any personality differences tend to result solely from the birth order of the child. Firstborn children, on average, have slightly higher IQs and greater achievement in school and in their careers, which may be related to the fact that they have all the attention of the parents until the next baby comes along (Craig & Dunn, 2013).

Parenting

The family is an important component in the lives of all children, and it plays an essential role in fostering the development of infants, children, and youth. A significant concept in families is that of parenting. **Parenting** is a leadership role in the family in which children are guided to learn acceptable behaviors, beliefs, morals, and rituals of the family and to become socially responsible contributing members of society. The manner in which children are parented, in combination with their individual personality traits and characteristics, influences their developmental outcomes.

Parents have responsibility for providing stability to children with a nurturing, safe, and structured environment. Every child needs to have physical and emotional space in which to grow and develop. This space enables the child to personally find the relationship balance between closeness and distance, as well as safety and risk. Parents also provide their children with the values, beliefs, rituals, and behaviors learned and transmitted across family generations. See *Developing Cultural Competence: Family Structure and Roles*. To be successful in parenting, parents must have a certain flexibility that enables the family to adapt and adjust to family changes with time and other significant stressors and challenges.

Developing Cultural Competence Family Structure and Roles

A family's structure and roles are largely dependent on cultural influence. For example, culture may determine who has authority (head of household) and is the primary decision maker for other members of the family. Sometimes the decision maker role varies by the type of decisions to be made. For example, in some cultures, such as Hispanic, decisions regarding the health care of children are primarily the responsibility of the female, whereas other decisions are male dominated. Family dominance patterns may be *patriarchal*, as may be seen in Appalachian cultures; *matriarchal*, as may be seen in African American cultures; or more *egalitarian*, as may be seen in European American cultures.

To be successful parents, implement reasonable **limit setting** (established rules or guidelines for behavior) on children's autonomy while they learn values and self-control. At the same time, parents need to foster the child's curiosity, initiative, and sense of competence. Parents use different styles to parent their children. Parental warmth and control are two major factors that are important in the development of children. *Parental warmth* refers to the amount of affection and approval displayed. *Parental control* refers to how restrictive the parents are regarding rules. See Table 2–1 for the characteristics associated with parental warmth and control.

Diana Baumrind identified three parenting styles (*authoritarian, authoritative,* and *permissive*) and described the influences each style has on children. This proposed classification is still useful in identifying parenting behavior (Baumrind, 2012, 2013), as is another parenting style, called *indifferent*, that exists in some families (Craig & Dunn, 2013). Although families generally exhibit one style, they may vary their style for certain situations. Table 2–2 shows characteristics or parenting styles by levels of warmth and control.

TABLE 2–1 Characteristics of Significant Parenting Attributes

PARENTING ATTRIBUTE	PARENTAL WARMTH	PARENTAL CONTROL
High level	Warm, nurturing Express affection and smile at children frequently Limit criticism, punishment Express approval of child	Restrictive control of behavior Survey and enforce compliance with rules Encourage children to fulfill their responsibilities May limit freedom of expression
Low level	Cool, hostile Quick to criticize or punish Ignore children Rarely express affection or approval Rejection may be seen	Permissive, minimally controlling Make fewer demands Fewer restrictions on behavior or expression of emotion Permit freedom in exploring environment

TABLE 2–2 Parenting Styles by Level of Warmth and Control

PARENTING STYLE	WARMTH/CONTROL	BEHAVIOR OF PARENT	CHILD OUTCOMES
Authoritarian	High control Low warmth	Highly controlling, issues commands and expects them to be obeyed Little communication with the child Inflexible rules Permits little independence	May become fearful, withdrawn, and unassertive Girls often passive and dependent during adolescence Boys often rebellious and aggressive
Authoritative	Moderately high control High warmth	Accepts and encourages growing autonomy of the child Open communication with the child Flexible rules	Tends to be best adjusted, self-reliant, self-controlled, and socially competent Higher self-esteem Better school performance
Permissive	Low control High warmth	Few or no restraints Unconditional love Communication flows from child to parent Much freedom and little guidance	May become rebellious, aggressive, socially inept, self-indulgent, or impulsive May be creative, active, and outgoing
Indifferent	Low control Low warmth	No limit setting Lacks affection for the child Focused on stress in own life	May show a high expression of destructive impulses and delinquent behavior

Source: Adapted from Craig, G. J., & Dunn, W. L. (2013). *Understanding human development* (3rd ed., p. 206). Upper Saddle River, NJ: Pearson.

Authoritarian Parents

Authoritarian parents tend to be punitive and adhere to rigid rules, or be more dictatorial. Parents who use this style might say, "Because I'm your parent, that's why," "A rule is a rule," or "Just do what I say." While this style sets firm limits, those limits or rules are not negotiable or open to any discussion. Parents expect family beliefs and principles to be accepted without question. Children have no opportunity to participate in the family decision-making process. Children with authoritarian parents do not develop the skills to examine why a certain behavior is desirable or how their actions might influence others.

Authoritative Parents

Authoritative parents use firm control to set limits, but they establish an atmosphere with open discussion, or are more democratic. Although the limits for behavior are clear and reasonable, the child is encouraged to talk about why certain behaviors occurred and how the situations might be handled differently another time. Parents provide explanations about inappropriate behaviors at the child's level of understanding. Children are allowed to express their opinions and objections, and some flexibility is permitted when appropriate. However, parents make it clear that they are the ultimate authority for decisions. Children with authoritative parents develop a sense of social responsibility because they converse about their responsibilities and approaches.

Permissive Parents

Permissive parents show a great deal of warmth but set few controls or restraints on the child's behavior. Parents are so intent on showing unconditional love that they fail in performing some important parenting functions. Children are allowed to regulate their own behavior. Discipline is inconsistent, and parents may threaten punishment but not follow through. Both extremes result in excessive permissiveness, and the child does not learn socially acceptable limits of behavior. When the parents do not impose any controls on the child, the child ends up controlling the parents.

Indifferent Parents

Indifferent parents display little interest in their children or in their roles as parents. They do not demonstrate affection or approval of the children, nor do they set limits or controls on the children. This may occur because of disinterest, or because their lives are busy and stress filled, leaving little time or energy for their children. Children who experience this style of parenting often have the worst outcomes, such as destructive impulses and delinquent behavior. If the parents are also hostile, the child often develops delinquent behavior (Craig & Dunn, 2013).

Parent Adaptability

Parents who are able to adapt their behavior to meet the needs of children at different developmental stages are also more effective. Parenting styles may change as the child grows older. For example, parents may use negotiation to help the child develop problem-solving skills and learn how to compromise and get along with others. This enables the child to have more self-control and self-responsibility over time. Parents and some children can develop shared goals and jointly participate in decision making, whereas other children require constant negotiation for decision making. See *Families Want to Know: Guidelines for Promoting Acceptable Behavior in Children.*

Assessing Parenting Styles

Nurses can assess parenting styles by asking families how they handle situations that require setting limits. The nurse in all settings is often in a position to discuss parenting styles and to offer suggestions for managing certain types of child behaviors that are frustrating to the family. Keep in mind that no two children are alike, and parents often must vary their parenting styles for different children in the family. For example, children's temperaments are often tied to their behavioral style. (See Chapter 4 for more information on child temperament.) One child may need very clear limits set with discussion and reinforcement, whereas a sibling may immediately respond to the parents' limit setting without a need for discussion. See *Developing Cultural Competence: Cultural Influences on Parenting.*

Families Want to Know
Guidelines for Promoting Acceptable Behavior in Children

- Set realistic expectations and directions for behavior based on the child's age and understanding; consistently enforce the expected directions and behaviors.
- Focus on promoting appropriate and desirable behaviors in the child:
  - Model or suggest appropriate behavior;
  - Review expected behavior for special situations, such as a family party, going to the movies, or other social events;
  - Help the child distinguish between inside and outside voice and behaviors; and
  - Praise or reward the child for using appropriate behaviors.
- As soon as any inappropriate behavior begins, tell the child and offer guidelines for behavior change or provide a distraction.
- When reprimanding the child, focus on the behavior rather than stating that the child is bad. Explain how the behavior is inappropriate; how it makes you, as the parent, and any other person involved feel. Avoid ridicule or accusation that can take the form of shame or criticism. These actions can have an impact on the child's self-esteem if repeated often enough.
- Be alert for situations when the child could potentially misbehave, such as when the child is tired or overexcited. Use a distraction to control or calm the child.
- Help the child gain self-control with friendly reminders (e.g., count to three, as soon as the clothes are on the doll, as soon as you finish the game) regarding the timing for transition to the next event of the day, such as bedtime, putting the toys away, or washing hands before dinner.
- Discuss reasons and social rules for expected behaviors when the child is old enough to understand.

Developing Cultural Competence Cultural Influences on Parenting

Some cultural influences on parenting are associated with chosen lifestyle. For example, living in a predominantly ethnic neighborhood makes it possible to participate in special events that support children in learning about their culture. Parents use the community for social contacts that help reinforce patterns of parenting and establish behavioral expectations of their children. Frequent contact or living with the extended family also helps the children learn family and ethnic traditions, behaviors, and values. Additionally, children may be sent to faith-based schools that foster values important to the family.

Discipline and Limit Setting

Discipline is a method for teaching the rules that govern behavior or conduct. **Punishment** is the action taken to enforce the rules when the child misbehaves. Parenting styles play an important role in the type of discipline and punishment used with children. When clear limits are set and consistently maintained, as with authoritative parenting, punishment may be needed less often. Limit setting and firm control of those limits are important discipline methods used so children learn to what extent they can safely and independently operate within the environment. Firm limits also help children feel secure because they are reassured by consistency and the sense of protection perceived by the limits. Punishment helps children learn that there are consequences for misbehavior, and that other individuals may be affected by that behavior. This helps children develop a sense of responsibility for their behavior.

Clinical Tip

Nurses have an important educational role in helping parents identify an appropriate discipline method and how to take an authoritative role with their children. Encourage and educate parents about the need to be in charge, to set the rules, and to stand by those rules so that children learn how to behave.

Parents use various strategies for the discipline and punishment of children. Factors that affect what type of discipline is used are related to gender of the child, education level and age of the parents, family income, and culture. In addition, the type of misbehavior and the location in which it occurs affects the type of discipline used. Various discipline strategies that are used with children include the following:

- *Reasoning:* Explaining why a behavior or action is inappropriate or describing how limit setting is important. By reasoning, parents can help the child understand why certain behaviors are wrong. Similarly, parents can share personal stories and fables to help children understand social and moral values or to better understand acceptable behavior.
- *Behavior modification:* Giving positive rewards (such as treats or privileges) or reinforcement for good behavior or consistently ignoring inappropriate behavior to minimize the behavior. This encourages children to behave in specified ways.
- *Experiencing consequences:* Allowing the child to learn important lessons associated with misbehavior, such as taking away a toy, using a time-out, withholding privileges, or providing no dessert if the child misses dinner or does not eat nutritious foods (see Figure 2–6).
- *Corporal punishment:* Spanking, slapping, or inflicting pain with a paddle, whip, or other object. This type of punishment is not recommended by the American Academy of Pediatrics and is considered an aversive strategy (AAP, 2015; Theunissen, Vogels, & Reijneveld, 2015).
- *Scolding or yelling:* Using harsh language to verbally reprimand the child. This is not a recommended strategy as this may decrease the child's self-esteem. See Chapters 7 through 9 for age-specific discipline strategies.

Clinical Tip

Time-out is a punishment method of placing the child in a location away from toys and attention as a consequence of misbehavior. The general rule for the length of time-out is 1 minute per year of age (AAP, 2015).

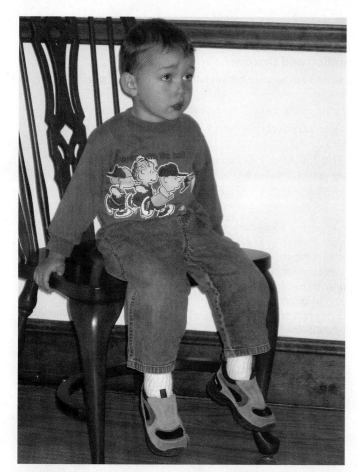

Figure 2–6 One effective discipline method is to remove the child to an isolated area where no interaction with children and adults can occur and no toys are present. This is used to demonstrate that there is a consequence to misbehavior. For older children, consider the loss of phone, computer, or other privileges.

Special Family Considerations

Divorce and Its Effects on Children

It is estimated that approximately half of all children in the United States will experience divorce of their parents at some point (Anthony, DiPerna, & Amato, 2014). Children are affected in many ways when the family breaks apart, even if the divorce was preceded by periods of stress and tension in the home. Many children believe they are at fault for the separation and divorce, having said or done something to make the parent leave. When one parent leaves, the children may feel abandoned and divorced by that parent. They may also fear being abandoned by the remaining parent. Children might become engaged in the disputes of parents, and they experience conflicts of loyalty when parents fight for their affection.

In divorces involving a lot of conflict and hostility, the children might experience increased problems with adjustment. When they must make a lot of changes in their lives in addition to the parents' separation (new home, different school), their adjustment is made more difficult because their sense of order is upset. Predictable routines have changed, and children may test limits to see if they still apply. The more changes they must make in the period immediately after the divorce, the more challenging is their adjustment. The disruption associated with divorce is also linked to academic and behavior problems among children (Arkes, 2015). See Table 2–3 for potential effects of divorce on children of different ages.

Sometimes parents are so stressed that their customary parenting styles become inconsistent. They may be unable to provide the warmth, affection, and support that the children need during this time. Battles over custody, child support, property division, and visitation rights all cause more distress for the children.

Nurses can assist families who are experiencing divorce by inquiring about the circumstances and changes that the child is undergoing. Talk with parents about the child's fears of abandonment and concerns, reminding parents that even

TABLE 2–3 Potential Effects of Divorce on Children of Different Ages

AGE	BEHAVIOR*
Preschool	Fear, anxiety, worry Self-blame Sorrow and grief Anger Regression Searching and questioning Temper tantrums Increased crankiness and aggression Loneliness Unhappiness Depression
School age	Worry, anxiety, depression Sadness Insecurity Fantasy Grief Guilt Self-blame Inability to concentrate on schoolwork Lower academic achievement Regression Aggression Confusion Anger Resentment Behavioral problems at school and home Manipulation of parents Withdrawal from friends and activities Fear Loneliness
Adolescence	Panic Fear Depression Guilt Risk taking Fear of loneliness and abandonment Denial Anger Sadness Aggressiveness Skipping or dropping out of school Use of drugs and alcohol Sexual acting out

*This table lists some of the behaviors that could potentially be seen with different age groups and is not all-inclusive. Many other behaviors may be present as well, depending on the individual child.

Source: Data from Anthony, C. J., DiPerna, J. C., & Amato, P. R. (2014). Divorce, approaches to learning, and children's academic achievement: A longitudinal analysis of mediated and moderated effects. *Journal of School Psychology, 52,* 249–261; Craig, G. J., & Dunn, W. L. (2013). *Understanding human development* (3rd ed.). Upper Saddle River, NJ: Pearson; Gross, G. (2015). *The impact of divorce on children of different ages.* Retrieved from http://www.huffingtonpost.com/dr-gail-gross/the-impact-of-divorce-on-children-of-different-ages_b_6820636.html; Mazjub, R. M., & Mansor, S. (2012). Perception and adjustment of adolescents towards divorce. *Procedia—Social and Behavioral Sciences, 46,* 3530–3534.

infants and toddlers can sense tensions in the home. Remind parents about the need to keep children out of the middle of confrontations and to maintain limits of acceptable behavior. Encourage parents to avoid saying negative statements about the other parent and encourage them to make every effort to maintain the relationship with the children. Help parents recognize their child(ren)'s needs for love and security during this difficult period.

The quality of the relationship between the divorced parents has an important impact on the future relationships their children have with them as adults. Children do better when both parents remain involved with their children and cooperate with each other after divorce (American Academy of Child and Adolescent Psychiatry, 2011).

Fathers who do not live with their children but live nearby are more likely to have involvement with their children if they have a good relationship with the child's mother, financial resources, and work experience. The relationship between father and child may be improved when the father can interact with the child in a conflict-free environment. See *Families Want to Know: Promoting Relationships With Parents Following Separation and Divorce.*

Stepparenting

When divorced or widowed parents remarry, the child may respond with ambivalence, divided loyalty, anger, or uncertainty. Parents should anticipate how the child and the entire family will respond to changes in lifestyles, routines, and interaction patterns and address them early in the formation of the new family relationship. When a stepparent joins a ready-made family, opportunities for improved emotional and financial support of the child can result, but the development of a new cohesive family requires many adjustments by all family members.

Blending two families often results in the need to identify or negotiate new customs, traditions, rituals, and routines for the family. Children may fear or experience losses such as a close relationship with the noncustodial parent, neighborhood friends (if a move was required), contact with grandparents, and family traditions. Discussions with children about their feelings may help the new family develop plans that ease the transition.

Stepparents must adjust to the habits and personality of the child and then work to gain trust and acceptance. If the child has not accepted the divorce or loss of a biologic parent, the stepparent faces more challenges in developing a trusting, affectionate, and respectful relationship. Sharing in childrearing decisions and responsibilities is an important task for stepparents, but their roles and the role of the joint or noncustodial parent need to be discussed and negotiated.

Stepparents are additional parents, not replacement parents. The stepparent and the child need to adjust to each other. The stepparent should try to establish a position in the child's life that is different from that of the missing biologic parent, rather than competing with the biologic parent. Stepmothers often have more challenges than stepfathers adjusting to their new role. This may be because they spend more time with the children.

In most stepparent families, discipline is a challenge. Family members must agree on standards of behavior, as well as the type of discipline and who carries it out; these guidelines need to be consistently maintained. Discipline by a stepparent is difficult until a bond develops between the stepparent and stepchild. The development of this bond cannot be forced. Time and honest communication are needed to gain the child's trust.

Clinical Tip

Identify the parent who can legally provide consent for medical treatment when there has been a divorce and potentially a remarriage. In some states the noncustodial parent cannot give consent. The stepparent cannot give consent unless the custodial parent grants written permission. Stepparents or other family members may also not know the child's medical history. Identify the legal framework for informed consent with regard to these children so that care is provided in an appropriate and responsible manner.

Contact with the biologic parent often continues through custody arrangements, financial support, and visitation. Children may actually move between two households, adding to the complexity and stressors in their lives. Power conflicts may emerge if the biologic parents do not make efforts to cooperate in parenting decisions. When parents agree to work together for the child's benefit, a parenting coalition between all parents in the two families can reduce the conflicts and tensions that can emerge.

Foster Care

Foster care is the provision of protection and shelter for a child in an approved living situation away from the family of origin. It is legally coordinated by the state's child welfare system. The goal of foster care is to ensure the safety and well-being of vulnerable children. During 2014, 265,000 children entered foster care, and 238,000 exited. As of September 30, 2014, 415,000 children were in foster care (U.S. Department of Health and Human Services, 2015).

Children enter the foster care system for many reasons. The primary reason is child abuse and neglect. Other reasons include parental problems such as abandonment, illness, alcohol/substance abuse, incarceration, and death. Severe behavioral problems in the child can also lead to placement in foster care

(American Academy of Child and Adolescent Psychiatry, 2013). Each state has guidelines regarding qualifications and standards for foster care parents and the process for becoming a foster parent. In an effort to ensure that the child is placed in a safe and nurturing environment, state guidelines that are used when investigating the home often include an interview with the interested adults to check for readiness to be a foster parent, health of all family members, legal background checks, and safety of the residence. Foster parents are also required to have initial training and annual continuing education.

Foster parents may be relatives (kinship care) or unrelated families with whom the child has a strong emotional bond. However, many children needing foster care are placed in extended families because there are fewer suitable nonkinship family foster homes. Kinship placement is frequently viewed as a better alternative, providing a more stable environment for the child. When children are placed with relatives, some sense of continuity and connectedness is maintained for these children (Fusco & Cahalane, 2015). Kinship care is generally perceived as more normative with fewer stigmas attached to it than nonkinship placement. Additionally, children in kinship care have been shown to have better outcomes in relation to safety, stability, and well-being (Font, 2014). Kinship providers are frequently older, in poorer health, have less income, and more likely to be single than nonkinship foster parents (Nesmith, 2015). Also, kinship foster parents receive fewer support services (Soine, 2013).

Foster Parenting

Foster parenting is very demanding, as they must provide for daily needs of children as well as support them emotionally. Foster parents provide transportation to medical and mental health counseling appointments, coordinate visits with birth parents and caseworkers, and advocate for the child in school settings. When the child has complex problems or needs, the challenge of caring for the foster child is even greater. Foster parents do receive some funding to care for the foster child, but it is often inadequate for the child's needs; therefore, the foster parents subsidize the child's care from their own funds. Some foster parents leave the system due to lack of adequate support. When the child must be moved to a different foster family, this may further exacerbate the ongoing stress that the individual child experiences in the foster care system.

Much of the child's adjustment rests with the stability of the family and available resources. Even though foster care is intended to be a temporary short placement—until the child can be returned home or an adoptive home is found—placed children may actually reside with the foster family for a lengthy time, sometimes for years. For children who have come from an environment that has been unstable, abusive, or neglectful, the foster care home can be supportive to the child's health status, development, and academic achievement.

Foster parents caring for children need to provide continuity, consistency, and predictability. It is essential that foster parents provide a nurturing environment for these children and show love and affection toward them. Developmentally appropriate activities are also essential to foster the child's long-term physical and emotional development.

Health Status of Foster Children

Physical health problems, as well as developmental, behavioral, and emotional problems, are common in children in foster care (American Academy of Child and Adolescent Psychiatry, 2013). Efforts to ensure that children receive appropriate health care

while in foster care are challenged by various barriers, such as lack of coordination between healthcare providers and social workers.

Every child entering foster care should receive an initial health screening, followed by a more comprehensive health assessment within a month. Findings and recommendations from the health assessment and additional health evaluations should be incorporated into the child's social service case plan. Nurses can play an important role in partnering with foster parents to arrange for and obtain the services needed by the child. Foster parents need to be supported in their efforts to care for these children, helping them to develop self-esteem and resilience.

Transition to Permanent Placement

Although many children are reunited with birth parents, other children cannot be. The Adoption and Safe Families Act of 1997 (P.L. 105-89) led to significant changes in child welfare and was enacted to increase well-being, safety, and permanence. Timelines were shortened for decision making about permanent placement of children, and incentives were established for states to encourage adoption. States were given guidelines regarding when reasonable efforts to reunite children with birth parents are no longer necessary, and when action is required in certain circumstances to terminate parental rights (Phillips & Mann, 2013). Kinship foster care was formally recognized. **Legal guardianship** (a permanent placement option for the child, often with relatives, in which parental rights are not terminated) was established as an alternative to **adoption** (a legal relationship between the child and parents not related by birth in which the adoptive parents assume all legal and financial responsibility for the child). Long-term foster care was eliminated as a permanent placement option in nonkinship care, but it could continue for kinship foster care to promote stability for the involved children (Adoption.com, 2013).

Clinical Tip

The Foster Care Independence Act of 1999 (P.L. 106-169) requires states to provide youth 18 to 21 years of age with services to help them make the transition to self-sufficiency. These services include training and education, financial support, and employment services (U.S. Department of Health and Human Services, 2012).

For those children with kinship foster care, adoption is often not perceived as the best option. Legal guardianship enables the child to retain legal connections with the birth family and relationships with the extended family. The guardian assumes limited financial liability for the child's care. Legal guardianship can be reversed at a future time if the birth parents petition the court.

Adoption

Motivations for adoption of a child vary with the families seeking adoption. In some cases, couples have infertility problems and are unable to have a biologic child. In a family that already has biologic children, the reasons could include the following:

- A desire to provide a home to a child who needs one or to have a larger family without additional biologic children
- Fertility issues requiring invasive medical procedures that are too extensive, expensive, or psychologically overwhelming for a subsequent pregnancy

- Adoption of a foster child with whom the family has established strong bonds
- Adoption by a family relative or stepparent

The supply of healthy infants available for adoption is much smaller than the number of families who want to adopt. Most children in the United States available for adoption are older children, often of minority populations or of mixed races, and those with special healthcare needs. In 2012, the number of children waiting to be adopted was 102,000. This number increased to 108,000 in 2014 (U.S. Department of Health and Human Services, 2015). Because most families choosing to adopt prefer to have an infant, many children have been adopted from foreign nations. Today, adopted children account for approximately 2% of all children in the United States (Jones, Schulte, & Committee on Early Childhood and Council on Foster Care, Adoption, and Kinship Care, 2012).

Legal Aspects of Adoption

Adoption is controlled by individual state law. Most adoptions are arranged through an authorized agency, such as a licensed social service agency. Others are provided by independent agencies in collaboration with physicians, lawyers, nurses, and members of the clergy. State laws require any family who wants to adopt a child to undergo a home study, a process in which parents are interviewed about a large number of topics and issues and are provided education and guidelines to prepare for the adoption. The National Adoption Information Clearinghouse provides information about state adoption laws.

Birth mothers and birth fathers are each required to relinquish legal rights to a child before an adoption can occur. The legal period between the child's birth and when the birth mother relinquishes legal rights varies by state. Efforts are made to ensure that the birth mother is not coerced into relinquishing legal rights to the child immediately after birth. In an open adoption, the birth mother and adoptive parents often have contact with each other prior to the birth and have jointly planned potential future contacts between the child and biologic mother. In some adoptions, birth mothers write a letter to the child that is given to the child at an appropriate age.

Preparation for Adoption

Adopting parents often benefit from preadoption counseling, which may help provide the support and reassurance needed about parenting and the adoptive process, as well as make connections with support groups or other families with adopted children. Preadoptive parents may wonder about their ability to love and parent the child and may have concerns about the responses of relatives, other children, and friends, especially if the child is from a different ethnic or racial group. Children already present in the family need to be reassured that they will not be displaced by the new child. Families need information about the child's understanding of what adoption means and guidance to help inform the child about being adopted.

Responses by Adopted Children

Children vary in their understanding and response to adoption by age (Jones et al., 2012):

- Children under 3 years of age do not recognize a difference between being adopted into a family versus being a biologic child in the family.
- Starting at about 3 years of age, children like to hear about their adoption story and they begin to ask what adoption means. Children adopted at this age may experience the separation from their other family and relatives. They are aware of physical differences between themselves and the adoptive family when they are of a different race or ethnic group. They may be fearful of abandonment by the adoptive family.
- By 5 years of age, adopted children begin to recognize they are different from most of their peers who were not adopted. Some children develop a feeling of responsibility for their biologic parents' decision not to keep them.
- School-age children may fantasize about their biologic family and what their life might have been like if they were not adopted. Their self-esteem may be affected if they think there was a flaw in them that caused their biologic parents to give them up for adoption.
- Adolescents may continue to fantasize about the "ideal" biologic family and try out identities similar to what they know or imagine about their biologic parents. They may also become angry that their own life experience is different from societal norms. Adolescents and young adults may seek information about their biologic family through a reunion registry. See *Families Want to Know: Informing the Child About Adoption.*

Families Want to Know
Informing the Child About Adoption

Most parents have anxiety about when and how to tell the child that he or she was adopted. There is no perfect age to approach this topic, so consider the child's age and developmental stage when sharing information.

- Some authorities believe the child should be told at such a young age that the child will always know that he or she is adopted. This may be especially important when the child is of a different ethnic or racial group or has very different physical characteristics than the parents.
- The terms *adoption, adopted, birth family,* or *biologic family* should be part of the family's natural conversation (Jones et al., 2012).
- Decide when you and the child are most ready to introduce the topic of adoption—such as when a discussion of babies and where they come from occurs. However, avoid waiting for "just the right moment" because children may wonder what other information has not yet been shared.
- Make sure the child is told *before* a third party is likely to say something. The chances of this happening increase as the child enters school.

- Tell the child in a matter-of-fact manner about the adoption. Let the child know how much he or she was wanted and that some personal qualities of the child made the selection special. Avoid phrases such as "given up" for adoption. A more positive phrase to use is that the biologic family made an adoption plan in the best interest of the child's future.

- Make sure the child understands that his or her place in the family is permanent. The adoptive family's commitment to the child should be repeated frequently.

- Be willing to honestly discuss the child's biologic family and the adoption process so the child feels comfortable asking questions. More discussion about adoption will be needed as the child grows older, especially when the child begins to ask at about 5 to 6 years of age why she or he was not wanted by the biologic parents. Anticipate that the child will grieve about the loss of the birth parents.

- As the child grows older and asks for more information about the birth parents, provide what information is known and try to help the child deal with information that is difficult to hear. Help the child decide what information to share with strangers, friends, and extended family members.

- Recognize that the adolescent may fantasize about the birth parents and want to find them. Listening to the adolescent's concerns and providing support during this challenging time of development is important.

Children who are older when adopted must also make the commitment to the family relationship. They often have a memory of parents and other caregivers, so developing a close relationship with the adoptive parents takes more time. It may also be more challenging for the adoptive parents to develop as strong an emotional bond to the older child as occurs when an infant is adopted. Even when a serious commitment has been made to adopt an older child, adjustment of the family and child may be difficult for everyone. Counseling may be helpful to some families during the transition process.

International Adoptions

International adoption is relatively common in the United States. Often, internationally adopted children need special healthcare services. Nurses work with families that have adopted children from other countries to provide a comprehensive evaluation of the child to detect potential developmental problems and health conditions as soon as the child is brought into the country.

Emotional and psychologic problems may be the result of long-term institutionalization in an orphanage, such as inconsistency in interpersonal development and delayed developmental milestones. The child and family may need counseling and support to help the child adjust to being part of a family. For the child who has been in an orphanage, his or her initial response to the new parents may be crying or turning away. Children need a transition period of several months to adjust to a different daily routine and to bond with the parents. Exposing the child to large numbers of family members or to busy environments may be stressful to the child. The nurse may become involved in providing counseling to the family when it is trying to integrate the adopted child into the family's life and routine (see Figure 2–7). As the child grows, efforts to help the child understand the cultural birth heritage are also important. See Chapter 4 for additional information about international adoption.

Family Theories

Families must be understood in their own context. It is important, for example, to understand each family's strengths and uniqueness and how the family and its members respond to the complex and often conflicting demands for time and attention.

Family theories are helpful in comprehending family functioning, environment–family interchange, family changes over time, and family response to health and illness. A brief review

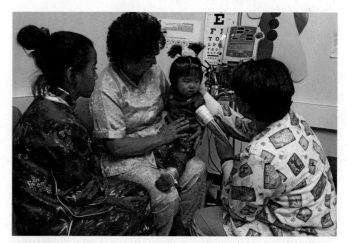

Figure 2–7   Adopted children who are of mixed race or a different ethnic group than the parents may cause a few additional challenges for the adoptive parents. Family members may be less supportive of the adoption initially. Because the children may have different physical characteristics, the family may capture more attention than it wishes. The family needs to learn to appreciate the different cultures represented in the newly formed family.

of family theories provides a context about family functioning that can assist with planning nursing care and developing future partnerships with families and their children.

Each family has structure and functions to help it maintain stability while responding continuously to various stresses and strains within the family and in the family's interactions and functioning within the community. Families develop and modify their responses and functioning over time to adapt or be tolerant of family, community, and environmental changes. Family processes include the behaviors and strategies that help regulate space, time, energy, and other aspects of family functioning to promote family stability, growth, and control.

Family Development Theory

Family development theories use a framework to categorize a family's progression over time according to specific, typical stages in family life. These are predictable stages in the life cycle

TABLE 2-4 Eight-Stage Family Life Cycle

STAGES	CHARACTERISTICS
Stage I	Beginning family, newly married couples*
Stage II	Childbearing family (oldest child is an infant through 30 months of age)
Stage III	Families with preschool children (oldest child is between 2.5 and 6 years of age)
Stage IV	Families with school-age children (oldest child is between 6 and 13 years of age)
Stage V	Families with teenagers (oldest child is between 13 and 20 years of age)
Stage VI	Families launching young adults (all children leave home)
Stage VII	Middle-aged parents (empty nest through retirement)
Stage VIII	Family in retirement and old age (retirement to death of both spouses)

*Keep in mind that this was the norm at the time the model was developed, but today families form through many different types of relationships.

Source: Adapted from Duvall, E. M. (1977). Marriage and family development (5th ed.). Philadelphia, PA: Lippincott; Duvall, E. M., & Miller, B. C. (1985). Marriage and family development (6th ed.). New York, NY: Harper Row; Coehlo, D. P. (2015). Family child health nursing. In J. R. Kaakinen, D. P. Coehlo, R. Steele, A. Tabacco, & S. M. H. Hanson, Family health care nursing: Theory, practice, and research (5th ed., pp. 387–432). Philadelphia, PA: F. A. Davis

of every family, but they follow no rigid pattern. Duvall's (1977) eight stages in the family life cycle of a traditional nuclear family have been used as the foundation for contemporary models of the family life cycle that describe the developmental processes and role expectations for different family types. Table 2–4 lists the eight stages of Duvall's family life cycle to illustrate important developmental transitions that occur at some point in most families.

Other family development models have been developed to address the stages and developmental tasks facing the unattached young adult, the gay and lesbian family, those who divorce, and those who remarry. Textbooks on families and developmental psychology provide further information on this topic.

Nurses can assess families by their developmental stage, how well they are fulfilling the tasks of that stage, and the availability of resources to accomplish developmental tasks. The stages provide a method for anticipating transitions and potential stressors with family role changes that occur at different points along the developmental continuum for different family types. By understanding the family's developmental stage, the nurse can analyze the family growth and health promotion needs and identify developmental transitions and potential stressors. This enables the nurse to identify the types of teaching and anticipatory guidance that might be needed.

Family Systems Theory

Family systems theory focuses on the family as an "organized whole and/or as individuals within family units who form an interactive and interdependent system" (Kaakinen & Hanson, 2015, p. 76). A family is a living social system, consisting of a small group of individuals who are closely interrelated and interdependent while collaborating to attain family functions and goals. In short, the family is more than the sum of its members (Clark, 2015; Kaakinen & Hanson, 2015). In family systems theory, due to the amount of interrelationship and interdependence

in the family, any change or stressor experienced by one or more family members affects the entire family and causes disruption. Families are adaptable and can change interactions and behaviors associated with the disruption in response to positive feedback.

From a systems perspective, the family may or may not exchange materials, energy, and information with its physical, social, and cultural environments. An *open family* seeks information and resources and actively interacts with the community to solve problems. A *closed family* views change and offered support as a threat, and resistance to outside influences is a strategy the family uses to maintain control. These attributes have an effect on the capacity of the family to adapt—to modify behavior and change as the situation demands (Clark, 2015; Kaakinen & Hanson, 2015).

Family systems theory encourages nurses to see the child and parents as participating members of a whole family (Kaakinen & Hanson, 2015). It encourages looking at the processes within the family and the relationships between subsystems (spouse, parent–child, and siblings) and suprasystems (the community within which it is embedded). Stress and crises motivate the family to mobilize its resources and to begin problem solving.

Using this perspective, the nurse can assess the effects of illness or injury on the entire family system and the reciprocal effects of the family on the illness or injury. Assessing how open or closed the family is to information and resources is important in planning nursing care. Open families will be more receptive to referrals and interventions from health professionals. The nurse will need to work with the closed family to establish trust and acceptance before the family is receptive to ideas and interventions proposed.

Family Stress Theory

Family stress theory focuses on the family's ability to cope and adjust to stressful events, such as having a child with a significant health condition (Ramisch, 2012). Most families know their resources and have developed coping strategies to deal with daily routine stressors (e.g., completion of household chores, homework). Family stressors may pile up from many sources, such as work demands, school issues, extended family demands, the desire to achieve quality family time, and community roles. Additional stressors may include inadequate finances, healthcare concerns, and relationship challenges.

Nonroutine stressors (such as surgery or the birth of a child) and unexpected events (a child's sudden illness or injury) are often more stressful because the family has not had time to review resources and prepare a response. A child's illness or injury affects every member of the family. Family members respond to this stress, sometimes in a way that changes interactions among family members and with the environment. By identifying how families respond to the stress of a child's illness or injury, nurses can provide support that may reduce the impact on the entire family.

No one theory is sufficient for viewing the needs and behaviors of all families. The theories previously described herein continue to evolve as researchers identify new or broadened explanations for behaviors, so it is difficult to attach one specific theorist to each family theory. When assessing families, you may find it useful to consider more than one of these theories to help you understand the full set of behaviors associated with individual families and to plan effective nursing interventions.

Family Assessment

To identify strategies for **coping** (the use of learned behavioral and cognitive strategies to manage or relieve perceived stress), nurses must be able to assess family strengths and support mechanisms and to determine when families have overextended their resources and need additional support. In some cases, nurses can provide the additional support needed. At other times, referral to other health professionals is appropriate to address the family's needs.

Children and families live within a variety of settings and interact with those settings in ways that directly or indirectly influence behaviors and learning. Because of these environmental influences on the family, it is important to consider the relationship of the family with the social networks within the community.

Family Stressors

A child's illness or injury affects every member of the family. Such a stressor demands a response from the family members that can change the way they interact with each other and with other people. Nurses need to identify and assess how families respond to the stress of illness or injury of a child or other family members because of the potential hardships it causes the entire family.

Family Strengths

Family strengths are the relationships, processes, and resources that families can use during times of adversity and change to manage stressors. Nurses can support families by helping them identify and use these strengths to manage the stressors associated with family challenges or crises. Strengths that enable families to develop and adapt to stressors include (Lester et al., 2013):

- Resources such as education, prior experiences, and finances
- Effective communication and collaborative problem solving
- Being emotionally aware and working to maintain emotional stability
- Developing shared meaning about the experience

Identify a family's **resilience**—the family's capacity to develop strengths and abilities to "bounce back" from stress and challenges. Resilience is often a dynamic interaction between protective processes (strengths and capacities) and vulnerabilities, such as life-event stressors, health status, or environmental risks (Herrman, Stewart, Diaz-Granados, et al., 2011). When a family can control and deal with events satisfactorily, its members gain a sense of competence, making them more resilient, in contrast to families who are overwhelmed by traumatic experiences. Resilience of children is discussed in Chapter 17.

Most families have the capacity to develop resilience. Nursing support may be needed to help family members learn new skills, make adaptations, and gain confidence in their abilities to manage the challenges of the child's health condition. Potential resources to foster resilience include the faith community, finances, social support, physical health, family flexibility, and family coping mechanisms. Families with fewer resources will be more susceptible to disruption when a healthcare crisis or event occurs.

Family strengths helpful in managing stressors include the following:

- *Communication skills:* The ability of family members to listen, gather information, and discuss their concerns in an honest and open manner
- *Shared family values and beliefs:* The family's common perceptions of reality and willingness to have hope and to appreciate that change is possible; family celebrations; family traditions
- *Intrafamily support:* The provision of support and reinforcement by extended family members to promote family cohesion and an atmosphere of belonging; family time and routines
- *Self-care abilities:* The family's ability to take responsibility for health problems and the demonstrated willingness of individual members to take good care of themselves
- *Problem-solving skills:* The family's use of negotiation in problem solving, using daily and prior life experiences as resources, and focusing on the present rather than past events or disappointments; effective utilization of healthcare resources
- *Community linkages:* Maintenance of active linkages with the community; reaching out to others in the social network including extended family and friends

Functional families use their strengths and a variety of coping strategies to successfully reduce stress. Coping strategies of dysfunctional families are generally defensive (e.g., denial of family problems, exploiting a family member, use of threats or withdrawal of affection and support, dominance and submissive patterns, and family substance abuse).

After developing a rapport and relationship with the family, the nurse can help families identify their strengths and areas for improvement that can lead to increased resilience. Focus on family competence and acknowledge and validate family members' emotions. Help families recognize that strengths and strategies used in prior life experiences may transfer to the current healthcare experience. When family members recognize the strengths they bring to the management of their child's healthcare problem, the family is more likely to become an effective partner in the process.

Collecting Data for Family Assessment

Establish a trusting relationship with the child and family to obtain an accurate and concise family assessment. Identify the primary concerns of the parent(s) and child, noting that they may be different. Acknowledge these multiple concerns and demonstrate respect for the diversity of the family. The goal is to obtain family information to plan nursing interventions that help the family care for the child and improve the child's outcomes while valuing each family member.

Information about the family is collected continuously during the healthcare process, through interviews, observations of family interactions, reports from other healthcare providers or agencies working with the family, and with a family assessment tool.

Additional data for the family assessment include the psychosocial history and daily living patterns (see Chapter 5). Observation of the home and family members is recommended in some cases to obtain valuable information about family functioning.

Family Assessment Tools

Family assessment tools help in gathering information about the family's functioning. Some tools specifically focus on family strengths, coping strategies, and family stresses. Learning about how the family nurtures its members, solves problems, and communicates may help identify strategies that can be effective for managing the child's health care. The nurse may learn how to work more effectively with the family, such as by collaborating with the family in planning for health maintenance and health promotion strategies.

GENOGRAM

Information about family structure can be illustrated on a **genogram** (a pedigree that displays information about a family's health history over at least three generations). (See Chapter 3 for examples of pedigrees.) Additional identifying features such as social class, occupation, place of residence, faith, and ethnicity may be added for the family assessment process.

FAMILY ECOMAP

An **ecomap** is an illustration of a family's relationships and social networks that may be prepared by nurses in partnership with family members. The nurse may learn information about how the family perceives or receives social support and the strength of family relationships with significant other persons and organizations. Community resources being used by the family and other potential community resources that may help promote the family's health may be identified. Figure 2–8 shows a sample ecomap.

Clinical Tip

Family assessment data that may be helpful include:

- Name, age, gender, and family relationship of all people residing in the household
- Family type, structure, roles, and values
- Cultural associations, including cultural norms and customs related to childrearing and infant feeding
- Faith-based group participation
- Support systems network, including extended family, friends, faith-based affiliations, and community associations
- Communication patterns, including language barriers
- Environmental data—place of residence, housing condition, number of persons living in the residence, sleeping arrangements, play areas, neighborhood characteristics

CALGARY FAMILY ASSESSMENT MODEL

Developed by Lorraine Wright and Maureen Leahey (2013), the Calgary Family Assessment Model uses three categories of information (structural, developmental, and functional family data) to assess a family's strengths and problems. The complete model is available in their textbook, *Nurses and Families: A Guide to Family Assessment and Intervention*. The model enables collection of extensive family information, and it can facilitate

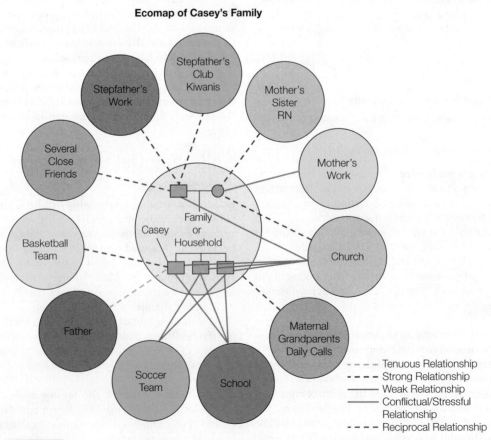

Ecomap of Casey's Family

Figure 2–8 An ecomap illustrates the family's relationships and interactions with groups and individuals in the immediate external environment.

assessment of family challenges, such as problems integrating a treatment plan in family routines. A family genogram or eco-map may also be helpful in completing the assessment (Wright & Leahey, 2013).

HOME OBSERVATION FOR MEASUREMENT OF THE ENVIRONMENT (HOME)

The HOME Inventory is an assessment tool developed to measure the quality and quantity of stimulation and support available to a child in the home environment (Caldwell & Bradley, 1984). The tool is used to identify relationships between the home environment, child care, and a child's development (Hackman et al., 2013; Sarsour et al., 2011). Four age-specific scales are available (birth to 3 years, 3 to 6 years, 6 to 10 years, and 10 to 15 years). Examples of subscales contained in each age-specific HOME Inventory include parental responsivity, acceptance of child, the physical environment, learning materials, variety in experience, and parental involvement. Data are collected during an informal, low-stress interview and observation over 45 to 90 minutes in the home setting. The child's primary caregiver and the child must be present and awake so their interaction can be observed. Family members are encouraged to act normally. Assessment of the home environment may help identify nursing interventions that promote the child's growth and development, such as items in the home that can be used for toys and strategies for parent interaction with the child to promote learning.

Cultural Considerations

When caring for families, it is critical to consider the influence of culture, which may affect how a family responds to health-related issues. **Culture** has many definitions and is currently described as

> the combination of a body of knowledge, a body of belief, and a body of behavior. It involves a number of elements, including personal identification, language, thoughts, communications, actions, customs, beliefs, values, and institutions that are often specific to ethnic, racial, religious, geographic, or social groups. (U.S. Department of Health and Human Services, National Institutes of Health, 2013)

Culture is characterized by certain key elements, including the following:

- Culture is based on shared values and beliefs. Expected behaviors and roles emerge that are consistent with those values and beliefs. A belief system suggests what preventive health measures and treatment for diseases are sought and accepted. It may also state the importance of children, the family, other individuals, and the collective group, all of which can influence the choices people in the culture make regarding health.

- Culture is learned and dynamic. A child is born into a culture and starts learning the beliefs and practices of the group from birth. Children who are members of two cultural groups, such as African and immigrant, learn about both groups as they grow and develop. Immigrants have moved from one country to another to live and may face challenges when integrating the rules of the dominant culture. Children who have family members from two or more cultural groups integrate parts of the worldview from each group. Therefore, although culture is connected with

groups, each individual's manifestation of his or her own cultural background will be unique. Culture evolves and adapts as new members are born into or join the group and as the surrounding social and physical environments change. For example, as first-generation immigrants enter a new country, they generally closely follow the cultural patterns of their native lands. As their children grow, the youth maintain some of the family cultural patterns but begin to incorporate some of the new culture (Figure 2–9).

- Culture is integrated into life and uses symbols. It is integrated through social institutions such as schools, houses of worship, friendships, families, and occupations. This provides a variety of opportunities for learning about one's culture. The sense of integration may be disrupted or harder to maintain if individuals move frequently and as cultures intertwine with each other. Symbols are an important way that many cultures communicate with each other and with the outside world. Language, dress, music, tools, and non-verbal gestures are symbols a culture uses to display and transmit the culture.

Race refers to a group of people who share biologic similarities such as skin color, bone structure, and genetic traits. Examples of races include White (sometimes called Caucasian or European American), Black (sometimes called African American in the United States), Hispanic, Natives (such as Native Americans, Alaskan Native, Hawaiian Native, and First Nation people of Canada), and Asian.

Ethnicity describes a "cultural group's sense of identification associated with the group's common social and cultural heritage" (Spector, 2013, p. 357). Examples of ethnic groups include Hmong, Jews, and Irish Americans. Even the mainstream or majority of groups usually identify with an ethnic group. Some beliefs and practices are common among certain ethnic groups, but it is important to avoid **stereotyping** individuals—that is, assuming that all members of a group have the same characteristics. The nurse should assess the woman or child and family to see which characteristics common to a group are possessed by

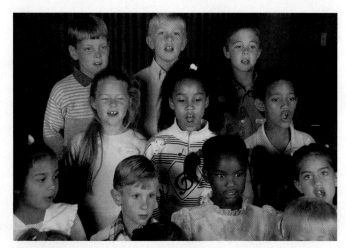

Figure 2–9 Today very few communities are limited to one culture. The children in this multicultural choir are representative of the changes in demographics of many Western countries. Even though they may differ in cultural background, a common thread is found in their religious preference.

SOURCE: Myrleen Pearson/PhotoEdit.

the patient rather than assume that because individuals identify themselves as a specific ethnicity they must practice certain customs.

Acculturation refers to the process of modifying one's culture to fit within the new or dominant culture. **Assimilation** is related to acculturation and is described as adopting and incorporating traits of the new culture within one's practice (Spector, 2013). Acculturation frequently occurs when people leave their country of origin and immigrate to a new country. Often, acculturation is associated with improved health status and health behaviors, especially if the immigration is associated with improved socioeconomic status, which leads to better nutrition and access to health care. This is frequently true for people who immigrate to the United States from a developing country. On the other hand, health sometimes declines with acculturation. For example, obesity is a problem that is growing rapidly within the United States and particularly among immigrant populations.

Cultural Assessment

In addition to the family assessment tools referred to earlier in this chapter, there are several tools (see Table 2–5) that can be used for cultural assessment of the family. Nurses must also consider contexts, such as the person's family, culture, work, community, history, and environment. The person must be in a state of balance within all personal and contextual parts. Illness occurs as a result of imbalance of one or all parts of the person (mind, body, spirit).

TABLE 2–5 Cultural Assessment Models

THEORIST	MODEL	DESCRIPTION	COMPONENTS/CONCEPTS
Dr. Madeleine Leininger	Sunrise Enabler	This guide can be used to examine a variety of influences on care and culture.	• Cultural values and lifeways • Political and legal factors • Economic factors • Educational factors • Kinship and social factors • Religious and philosophical factors • Technological factors (McFarland & Wehbe-Alamah, 2015, p. 25)
Dr. Larry Purnell	Model for Cultural Competence	Twelve major concepts are common to all cultures and can be assessed to provide important information about an individual family or group (Purnell, 2013).	• Overview, inhabited localities, and topography • Communication • Family roles and organization • Workforce issues • Biocultural ecology • High-risk behaviors • Nutrition • Pregnancy and childbearing practices • Death rituals • Spirituality • Healthcare practices • Healthcare providers (Purnell, 2013, p. 18)
Dr. Joyce Newman Giger and Dr. Ruth Davidhizar	Transcultural Assessment Model	The client is the center of care and culturally unique. Knowledge of the cultural heritage, beliefs, attitudes, and behaviors of the client is required to provide culturally competent care. This model is based on six phenomena that nurses must assess.	• Communication • Space • Social organization • Time • Environmental control • Biologic variations (Giger & Davidhizar, 2013, p. 5)
Dr. Rachel Spector	HEALTH Traditions Model	This model is predicated on the concept of holistic health and describes practices that can be used to maintain, protect, and restore health. Health is a complex, interrelated, and balanced state of the physical, mental, and spiritual.	• Physical—all physical aspects, such as anatomic organs, gender, age, nutrition, genetic inheritance, body chemistry, and physical condition • Mental—cognitive processes, such as memories, thoughts, and knowledge of such emotional processes as feelings, self-esteem, and defenses • Spiritual—both positive and negative learned spiritual practices and teachings, dreams, stories, and symbols; protecting forces; and metaphysical or innate forces (Spector, 2013, p. 91)

Sources: Data from Giger, J. N., & Davidhizar, R. E. (2013). *Transcultural nursing: Assessment & intervention* (6th ed.). St. Louis, MO: Mosby Elsevier; McFarland, M. R., & Wehbe-Alamah, H. B. (2015). The theory of culture care diversity and universality. In M. R. McFarland & H. B. Weheb-Alamah (Eds.), *Leininger's culture care diversity and universality: A worldwide nursing theory* (3rd ed., pp. 1–34). Burlington, MA: Jones and Bartlett; Purnell, L. D. (2013). *Transcultural health care: A culturally competent approach* (4th ed.). Philadelphia, PA: F. A. Davis; Spector, R. E. (2013). *Cultural diversity in health and illness* (8th ed.). Upper Saddle River, NJ: Pearson.

Cultural Practices That Influence Health Care

FAMILY ROLES AND ORGANIZATION

A family's organization and the roles played by individual family members are largely dependent on cultural influence. For example, culture may determine who has authority (head of household) and is the primary decision maker for other members of the family. Nurses should be alert for roles and functions in families. Teaching may need to be directed to those responsible for decision making in order to effectively promote the child's health.

Culture also defines gender roles and the roles of the elderly and of extended family. In some cultures, major decisions for the family, including a child's health care, involve input from grandparents and other extended family members (Figure 2–10). Grandparents may even assume responsibility for care of the children in the family. In these cases, nurses must direct teaching for health promotion and demonstration for treatment procedures to the grandparent.

Family goals are also determined by cultural values and practices, as are family member roles and childrearing practices and beliefs. In some families, children are expected to take on responsibilities early and may be expected to perform tasks such as management of their own chronic disease and nutritional intake. In other families, children are given long periods to grow up and are not expected to manage healthcare needs. Examples

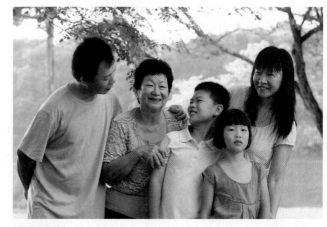

Figure 2–10 **Many cultures value the input of grandparents and other elders in the family or group. For example, in this multigenerational family, the grandmother's guidance is highly valued and significantly influences the family's childrearing practices.**

SOURCE: Wong yu liang/Fotolia

of childrearing practices common to particular cultures are listed in Table 2–6. Realize that the practices listed are common in these cultures but not necessarily practiced by all members of that culture.

TABLE 2–6 Childrearing Practices of Selected Cultures

CULTURE	CHILDREARING PRACTICES
African American	Grandmothers play an important role in the care of children. Children are expected to demonstrate respectfulness, conformity to rules, obedience, and good behavior. Extended family is very important.
Amish	The family contains, on average, seven children. Childrearing is regarded as the highest priority for parents. Grandparents often provide care to children. Children are expected to continue with the Amish tradition. Children are expected to follow the rules as prescribed by the church district.
Appalachian	Large families are common. Strict parenting practices and physical punishment are common. Grandparents frequently provide care to children.
Arab American	The father is typically the disciplinarian. The child's character is considered a reflection of the family's influence. Children are expected to respect their elders and to have good behavior. Adolescents are expected to do well in their studies. Discipline may include physical punishment and shaming.
Chinese American	The family may lavish resources on the child. Children typically depend on family for all needs and may not be expected to earn their own money as adolescents. Male children are often more valued than female children. Children may be taught to avoid displaying their emotions/feelings. Children are expected to assist parents in the home (chores). High educational achievement is expected.
Mexican American	Children are closely protected and are not encouraged to leave the home. Extended family members frequently live close by. Children are expected to demonstrate respect for parents and elderly family members. Discipline may include physical punishment. Education is a priority.
Navajo Indian	Large families are important. Grandmothers are important decision makers in the family. Children are encouraged to make decisions and live and learn from those decisions. Children are taught to respect their elders and be respectful of traditions.

Sources: Data from Purnell, L. D. (2013). Transcultural health care: A culturally competent approach (4th ed.). Philadelphia, PA: F. A. Davis; Purnell, L. D. (2014). Guide to culturally competent health care (3rd ed.). Philadelphia, PA: F. A. Davis

COMMUNICATION

Communication is the method by which members of cultural groups share information and preserve their beliefs, values, norms, and practices. Information is transmitted through both verbal and nonverbal methods. Verbal communication consists of spoken or written words, including tone and level of voice, language, verbal style and dialect, and written material.

Obviously, verbal communication is improved when a healthcare provider speaks the same language as the patient and family. Children are most likely to speak both the language of the parents and the healthcare providers and may appear to be likely interpreters. However, it is recommended that children never be used to interpret in healthcare situations due to the confidentiality needs of both parent and child. Additionally, if children are used as interpreters, it can create an imbalance in power that could adversely affect parental authority. Signs, posted literature, and brochures should be available in the languages of the children and families served. Even when children speak the language of the healthcare providers, written material must be provided at a level that the family can read and understand.

Language can also affect health literacy skills, as a large number of instructions are given in writing, including prescriptions and directions on medication bottles, signs hanging in health facilities, consent forms for procedures and surgery, insurance forms, directions for techniques or procedures, future appointment dates, and health promotion materials. Verify what the child and family can read and whether alternative methods should be used. Nurses can verbally give the information and provide paper and pencil so the family can take notes in their own language. Translation services should be available in all healthcare settings, including the pharmacy, the appointment desk, and for phone calls, to ensure access to services for all children and families served.

Clinical Tip

Speaking and reading may not occur in the same language. For example, an immigrant may read and speak fluently in a primary language and speak but not read the language of the new country. The immigrant's child may read and speak the language of the present country and speak but not read the native language of the family. Always ask about both reading and speaking preferences.

Nonverbal communication refers to body language such as posture, gestures, facial expressions, eye contact, and touch, as well as the use of silence. The nurse's use of nonverbal communication may hinder or help communication. Gestures and body language may be misunderstood or misinterpreted. For example, eye contact has different meanings among cultures. Silence is considered a sign of respect in some cultures. Watch for patterns in various cultures and alter your approach to be more congruent.

Touch is another form of nonverbal communication. The appropriateness of touch varies by culture. Adults commonly feel that it is acceptable to touch children of all ages, but this may not be accurate. Watch for responses from the child and family. Nurses must touch children to weigh them, take blood pressures, and give immunizations, but this does not mean that close touch is appropriate at all times.

TIME ORIENTATION

Cultures have specific values and meanings regarding time orientation. Cultural groups may place emphasis on the events of the past, those events that occur in the present, or those events that will occur in the future. Children reflect the time orientation of their families and the cultures in which they live. Time is also influenced by development so that young children sometimes do not understand the use of clocks, the importance ascribed to being "on time," or other time orientations.

Cultures that are oriented predominantly to the past may want to begin healthcare encounters with lengthy descriptions of past healthcare treatments, family history of diseases, or individual past experiences with health. There may be little interest in learning methods of adapting to or maintaining a new plan of care.

For cultures that are oriented predominantly to the present, little consideration may be given to either the past or the future. For example, adolescents commonly focus on the present and may not engage in preventive health practices for long-term health. Therefore, short-term goals often provide more incentive to adolescents.

Cultures that are oriented predominantly to the future, such as European American, may not focus on what is important at the present time. For example, the family focusing on the future may focus on the dreams they had for a child's education or sports performance and have trouble setting present goals for treatment of a disease such as juvenile arthritis. One commonly hears that it was a big adjustment to learn to "take one day at a time." Not living up to the family's expectation for his or her future success may be difficult for a child who has developed an illness that has a chronic course.

Time also refers to punctuality about schedules and appointments. In the United States, the predominant culture respects being on time and considers time valuable and not to be wasted. Other cultures may not emphasize a concern for time. This may be manifested by a family's inability to follow timed medication schedules or treatments or to show up as scheduled for an appointment. In these cases it is not intended as a sign of disrespect.

NUTRITION

Nutritional practices begin even before birth, as many cultural groups have beliefs that determine foods that are healthy to eat or should be avoided during pregnancy. Nutritional habits and patterns vary among cultures and are related to both religious practices and health beliefs. Certain cultures and religions have restrictions on or prescriptions about specific foods and preparation methods. Ritualistic behaviors involving eating and drinking—for example, on special occasions and holidays—are observed by most cultures. Many religions recommend fasts during specific holy seasons, such as Lent for Roman Catholics, Yom Kippur for Jews, and Ramadan for Muslims; however, in most cases, small children, pregnant women, the elderly, and sick individuals are not required to fast.

Additionally, some cultures value large size or may associate a healthy child with being "large." Other cultures value slimness and look down on individuals who are obese. Both of these views influence family eating patterns and expectations for the child; the child's self-esteem can therefore be influenced. The U.S. culture honors being slim in the media but reinforces eating and large size by the availability of fast food and positive image of large sports stars such as some football players, which can result in confusion about health and body image.

Nutrition may also be essential to the culture's practices for health promotion and care during illness. Health problems associated with specific cultures that may require dietary changes are also identified. Nutrition can be closely related to environmental situations, and families with few resources may not be able to obtain or eat cultural foods due to access or financial issues. Nutrition plays a powerful role in maintaining health, so resources for nutritious and desired foods may be needed.

HEALTH BELIEFS, APPROACHES, AND PRACTICES

The family members' health beliefs influence their approaches and practices regarding health and illness. The young child has a view of health and illness connected with developmental understanding and gradually takes on the family's cultural view while growing older. Additionally, some families, when faced with a life-threatening illness of their child, may seek alternative health practices that are not considered part of their cultural heritage. This is especially true if the family becomes frustrated with traditional biomedical treatments that are unable to cure their child. See Table 2–7 for examples of health practices common to specific cultures. Nurses and other healthcare professionals should learn about the family's belief system and integrate all types of care that the family wishes as long as there is no danger to the child.

Clinical Tip

Some families believe in the hot and cold theory of disease, which subscribes to the thought that illnesses and diseases are a result of disruption in the hot and cold balance of the body. Therefore, consuming foods of the opposite variety can cure or prevent specific hot and cold illnesses. Hot and cold therapies related to healing are practiced in some African American, Asian, Latino, Arab, Muslim, and Caribbean cultures (Andrews & Boyle, 2012); see Table 2–8.

Faith-based belief and practice is an integral part of culture for some families. Views of religion and spirituality can shape their approaches and responses to a child's illness and guide practices to maintain health. Religious beliefs may influence the family's explanation of the cause of a child's illness, their perception of the severity of the illness, and choices of treatments for the illness, and can offer solace to the family and child. For these reasons, it is important to determine the influence of religion and spirituality within the family.

Faith and spirituality can be a source of great comfort and support for children who are ill and their families. Conversely, conflicts may arise between the family's religion or spirituality and biomedical care for the child. For example, the family's pursuit of specific religious therapies can serve as a barrier to biomedical care, because some parents may believe that their spiritual practices can substitute for medical treatment of the child. **Religion**, commonly referred to as **faith-based belief**, is an organized system of shared beliefs regarding the significance of the nature, cause, and purpose of life and of the universe. Religion is usually centered on the belief in or the worshipping of a supernatural or Supreme Being (such as God or Allah).

Spirituality refers to an individual's experience and own interpretation of a relationship with a Supreme Being. Children are spiritual beings and generally express their spirituality through behavior such as imaginative play, art, dance, and song (Lascar, 2013). Prayer, one of the most common expressions of religious faith, is a frequently used therapy in which many children and families engage (Lambert, Fincham, & Graham, 2011; Wachholtz & Sambamoorthi, 2011).

Specific differences in beliefs between families and healthcare providers are common in the following areas: help-seeking behaviors, causes of diseases or illnesses, death and dying, caretaking and caregiving, and childrearing practices.

TABLE 2–7 Health Practices of Selected Cultures

CULTURE	HEALTH PRACTICES

African American	Religious healing (laying on hands)
	Talismans (amulets or lucky charms)
	Herbal remedies/oils
	Use of healers:
	  "Old woman" healers
	  Voodoo healers
	  Shamans
	  Spiritualists
	  Root doctors

Asian American	Acupuncture/acupressure
	Coin rubbing
	Cupping
	Herbs
	Hot and cold foods
	Massage
	Meditation
	Moxibustion (heat therapy)
	Qigong (combines meditation, movement, and regulation of breathing)
	Restoring energy between yin and yang
	Tai chi
	Tiger balm
	Use of healers:
	  Physicians
	  Herbalists
	  Acupuncturists

European American	Amulets Healing rituals Dietary modifications Exercise Traditional medicine Use of healers: Traditional healthcare providers: physicians, nurses, and nurse practitioners

Hispanic or Latin American	Hot and cold foods
	Herbs
	Massage
	Prayers
	Religious medals
	Use of healers:
	  Curanderos/curanderas
	  Yerberos or jerberos (herbalists)
	  Brujos/brujas (witches)
	  Espiritistas (spiritualists)
	  Sobadores

Native American	Ceremony
	Counseling
	Herbs and plants
	Healing touch/acupressure
	Medicine bundle
	Singing
	Pipe ceremony
	Drumming and chanting (prayer)
	Smudging
	Sun dance
	Sweat lodge (purification ceremony)
	Vision quest (a powerful ceremony)
	Use of healers:
	  Medicine men or women
	  Shamans

Source: Data from Andrews, M. M., & Boyle, J. S. (2012). *Transcultural concepts in nursing care* (6th ed.). Philadelphia, PA: Lippincott Williams & Wilkins; Fontaine, K. L. (2015). *Complementary and alternative therapies for nursing practice* (4th ed.). Upper Saddle River, NJ: Pearson; Giger, J. N., & Davidhizar, R. E. (2013). *Transcultural nursing: Assessment & intervention* (6th ed.). St. Louis, MO: Mosby Elsevier; Spector, R. E. (2013). *Cultural diversity in health and illness* (8th ed.). Upper Saddle River, NJ: Pearson.

TABLE 2–8 Hot and Cold Conditions and Foods

HOT CONDITIONS	COLD FOODS USED TO TREAT HOT CONDITIONS	COLD CONDITIONS	HOT FOODS USED TO TREAT COLD CONDITIONS
Diarrhea	Barley water	Cancer	Beef
Fever	Chicken	Earaches	Cheese
Constipation	Dairy products	Headaches	Eggs
Infection	Raisins	Musculoskeletal conditions	Grains (other than barley)
Kidney problems	Fish	Pneumonia	Liquor
Liver conditions	Cucumber	Menstrual cramps	Pork
Sore throats	Fresh fruits	Malaria	Onions
Stomach ulcers	Fresh vegetables	Arthritis	Spicy foods
	Goat meat	Rhinitis	Chocolate
		Colic	Warm water with honey

Source: Data from Purnell, L. D. (2014). *Guide to culturally competent health care* (3rd ed.). Philadelphia, PA: F. A. Davis; Purnell, L. D. (2013). *Transcultural health care: A culturally competent approach* (4th ed.). Philadelphia, PA: F. A. Davis; Spector, R. E. (2013). *Cultural diversity in health and illness* (8th ed.). Upper Saddle River, NJ: Pearson.

In differing degrees these elements influence the cultural beliefs and values of an ethnic group, making the group unique. Misunderstandings may occur when the healthcare professional and the family come from different cultural groups. In addition, past experiences with health care may have made the family angry or suspicious of providers. Nurses must be able to recognize, respect, and respond to ethnic diversity in a way that leads to a mutually desirable outcome. The nurse must identify culturally relevant facts about the patient to provide culturally appropriate and competent care. For example, some cultural groups practice complementary and alternative therapies that are unknown to the nurse (see the section titled "Complementary and Alternative Modalities"). Although some of these therapies are beneficial or cause no harm, others may interact with prescribed medications and be harmful.

Clinical Tip

Avoid imposing your personal cultural values on the children and families in your care. By learning about the values of the different ethnic groups in the community—religious beliefs that have an impact on healthcare practices, beliefs about common illnesses, and specific healing practices—you can develop an individualized nursing care plan for each child and family.

Cultural competence refers to the ability of the nurse to understand and effectively respond to the needs of patients and families from different cultural backgrounds (Spector, 2013). Recognizing the influence of culture on one's beliefs, values, and healthcare practices is essential for the nurse in order to deliver culturally competent care. The nurse should also consider the potential that an extended family member may need to be consulted regarding the treatment plan for the child,

Professionalism in Practice Standards of Practice for Culturally Competent Nursing

Standards of Practice for Culturally Competent Nursing were developed to guide nursing practice. These standards focus on clinical practice, education, administration, and research. Emphasis is placed on the importance of provided culturally competent care to all patients and families (Douglas, Pierce, Rosenkoetter, et al., 2011). Identify and learn more about the cultures in the community where you provide nursing care so that you provide culturally competent care to your patients.

especially if the child spends a lot of time with extended family members.

Nurses demonstrate appropriate strategies for delivering culturally sensitive care when they develop techniques in assessing the influence of culture on the child and family and incorporate that information into an individualized plan of care. When the family's cultural values are incorporated into the care plan, the family is more likely to accept and adhere to the recommended care, especially in the home care setting.

Culturally competent nurses find effective ways to work with the family to determine how they can incorporate prescribed therapies with their healthcare practices. Ensure that the child and family understand the problem or illness, treatment, and health promotion activities. Apply culturally sensitive techniques when dispelling any cultural myths. See *Developing Cultural Competence: Traditional Healthcare Providers.*

Developing Cultural Competence Traditional Healthcare Providers

When appropriate, collaborate with the family to determine the role traditional healthcare providers and other practitioners (e.g., folk healers, spiritualists) will have in the care of the child. Encourage collaboration and communication between practitioners to ensure continuity of care.

Nurses can also collaborate with a multidisciplinary team including social workers and language specialists to assist the family in receiving assistance with barriers to care such as transportation, financial issues, remote access, and others.

Complementary and Alternative Modalities

Complementary and alternative modalities (CAM) are generally described as healthcare approaches that are not considered to be part of conventional Western medicine (National Center for Complementary and Alternative Medicine [NCCAM], 2013a). Although the terms *complementary* and *alternative* are often used interchangeably, they have different meanings and applications. A **complementary therapy** may be defined as any procedure or product that is used as an adjunct to conventional medical treatment (Mitchell, 2013; NCCAM, 2013a). An example of a complementary therapy is the use of massage therapy in conjunction with biomedical therapy, such as narcotic analgesics, for a child with cancer pain.

In contrast, an **alternative therapy** is usually considered a substance or procedure that is used in place of conventional medicine (NCCAM, 2013a). An example of an alternative therapy is the use of herbal medicines instead of traditional Western medical care for a child's health condition, such as surgery, radiation, prescribed medications, or other medical interventions.

The dramatic increase in complementary and alternative therapies that began in the final decade of the 20th century was probably the result of a combination of several factors:

- Increased consumer awareness of the limitations of conventional Western medicine
- Increased international travel
- Increased media attention
- Advent of the Internet

The NCCAM (2013a) classifies complementary health approaches into two main subgroups: natural products and mind and body practices. *Natural products* include herbs, vitamins, minerals, and probiotics (also referred to as dietary supplements). Examples of *mind and body practices* include acupuncture, massage therapy, meditation, relaxation, yoga, healing (therapeutic) touch, and hypnotherapy. Some examples of complementary and alternative modalities are provided in Table 2–9.

Safety Issues Concerning CAM Therapies

The misleading claims of usefulness, dosing safety of some products, and lack of manufacturing standards of natural products are just a few of the issues raised with the use of herbs and natural products. Parents often believe that herbs and natural products are less likely to be harmful than prescribed medications, failing to

TABLE 2–9 Selected Types of Complementary and Alternative Modalities

THERAPY	DESCRIPTION	POTENTIAL USE IN CHILDREN	NURSING IMPLICATIONS
Aromatherapy	Essential oils (extracts or essences) from flowers, herbs, and trees provide strong, pleasant odors to promote relaxation, health, and well-being.	The family may use candles or oils to promote a child's pain relief or to encourage the child's relaxation. Use of aromatherapy in the hospital may reduce nausea due to hospital odors.	Few side effects when used as directed; however, allergies to oils may worsen symptoms in a child with asthma and other pulmonary disorders. Caution families to avoid aromatherapy.
Dietary supplements	A product (other than tobacco) is taken by mouth that contains an ingredient intended to supplement the diet, such as vitamins, minerals, herbs or other botanicals, amino acids, and substances such as enzymes, organ tissues, and metabolites. Dietary supplements come in many forms, such as extracts, tablets, capsules, liquids, and powders. They have special labeling requirements.	Many parents administer daily multiple vitamins to their children. For example, echinacea is an herb that is used to treat colds and the flu and stimulate the immune system.	Assess the family's use of dietary supplements for the child. Determine potential interactions between supplements and prescribed medications. Teach parents about safe dosages and safe storage of vitamins and other dietary supplements for children. Herbs must be used with caution in children.
Massage	Therapists press, rub, and manipulate muscle and soft tissues to enhance function of those tissues and promote relaxation, well-being, and relief from pain.	Massage is beneficial in children who have discomfort related to teething; it reduces colic, promotes sleep, reduces pain related to procedures such as immunizations, and promotes growth of preterm infants (Fontaine, 2015). See Figure 2–11.	Assess the child for benefits of massage. Potential contraindications to massage therapy may include bleeding disorders, fractures, and an open or healing wound.
Therapeutic touch	In therapeutic touch, the healing force of the therapist affects the patient's recovery. Healing is promoted when the body's energies are in balance. By passing their hands over the patient, without touching the patient, healers can identify energy imbalances.	The family may enlist a spiritualist or other practitioner to perform therapeutic touch on the child to promote pain relief or a quicker recovery.	Assess the benefits of therapeutic touch on the child (e.g., pain relief). Partner with the family to establish other methods of pain relief if therapeutic touch is not effective.
Faith-based therapies	Prayer is a commonly used form of complementary therapy. Other faith-based therapies include faith healing, lying on hands, meditation, and anointing.	Families may include a variety of faith-based therapies, depending on the child's condition. Spiritual health may help improve quality of care, decrease anxiety, and increase positive feelings, such as hope, optimism, and freedom from regret.	Provide the child and family a private environment for faith-based practices. Assess for benefits of the therapies. Partner with the family to determine alternative methods of therapy if needed.

Sources: Data from Fontaine, K. L. (2015). *Complementary and alternative therapies for nursing practice* (4th ed.). Upper Saddle River, NJ: Pearson; National Center for Complementary and Alternative Medicine (NCCAM). (2013a). *Complementary, alternative, or integrative health: What's in a name?* Retrieved from http://nccam.nih.gov/health/whatiscam/D347.pdf; National Cancer Institute. (2012). *Spirituality in cancer care.* Retrieved from http://www.cancer.gov/cancertopics/pdq/supportivecare/spirituality/Patient/

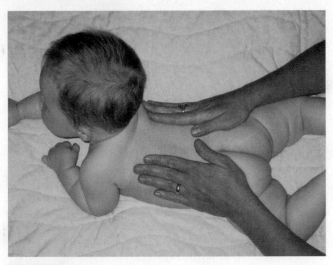

Figure 2–11 Infant massage.

recognize that safety concerns exist. However, "natural" is not the same as safe, and many CAM products have not been evaluated for use in children. Examples of problems that may occur with the use of complementary and alternative modalities include:

- Interaction with prescribed medications (interferes with metabolism of medication or increases the effect of the prescribed medication, like an overdose)

- Side effect or allergic reaction directly associated with the product

- Substitution of the product for a prescribed medication that is potentially lifesaving

- Toxic effects because of contaminants or other additives in the product, or if the plant used for the herb was incorrectly identified

The use of CAM in the care of children must be addressed because of the limited research with this age group and developmental variations that may influence efficacy and safety. Although many CAM therapies may have been proven effective in adults, they may have little effect on children, or even be harmful. The National Institutes of Health and the Agency for Healthcare Research and Quality have set research agendas to investigate the effectiveness of CAM therapies for treatment.

Complementary and alternative modalities must be assessed for safety, including positive and negative benefits, cost, efficacy, and clinical usefulness. The use of herbs and natural products raises many issues, such as standards of products, misleading claims, safety related to megadoses of some products, and standardization of natural products. Determine the family's use of complementary and/or alternative medicine such as the type of remedies and healthcare practices used. Also determine the side effects, risks, and other implications to the child receiving this type of therapy. Partner with the family to ensure safe practices with the use of CAM products.

SAFETY ALERT!
Complementary and alternative therapies must be assessed for safety, including positive and negative benefits, cost, efficacy, and clinical usefulness. The use of herbs and natural products raises many issues, of which these are just a few: standards of products, misleading claims, and safety related to megadoses of some products. When the family does not disclose CAM use to the healthcare provider, the risk of interaction with conventional medicines and harm to the patient increases (Adams et al., 2013). See *Families Want to Know: CAM Therapies*.

Nursing Management

The goal of culturally competent family-centered nursing management is to assess and help families recognize their strengths and resilience. This information can then be used in collaboratively planning the nursing care with the child and family. See *Evidence-Based Practice: Investigating Culture and Healthcare Barriers*.

Nursing Assessment and Diagnosis

The presence of a newly acquired disability adds a dimension of developmental risk. The child and family members may respond with either psychologic or behavioral problems, or they may respond in a more positive manner.

Collect the psychosocial history and daily living patterns data from the family and child. Assessment of the culturally diverse child and family includes determining the family's healthcare practices such as health traditions, health beliefs, health-seeking behaviors, healthcare practitioner, and religion or spirituality.

Select the appropriate family assessment tool to collect information that can help evaluate the family's strengths and resources. Analyze the information collected and focus on key information that will help develop a plan of care for the child and family. Follow these steps:

- Determine how this condition influences family functioning.

- Identify how all the family members have responded to the child's acute condition and disability.

Families Want to Know

CAM Therapies

Once the nurse has been informed about CAM therapies used, potential side effects and risks can be considered, such as interactions between an herb and a prescribed medication. Partner with the family to promote the following safe practices for CAM use (NCCAM, 2013b):

- Ensure that your child has received an accurate diagnosis from a licensed healthcare provider and that CAM use does not replace or delay conventional medical care.

- If you decide to use CAM for your child, do not increase the dose or length of treatment beyond what is recommended. More is not necessarily better.

- If your child experiences an effect from a CAM therapy that concerns you, contact your child's healthcare provider.

- Store herbal and other dietary supplements out of the sight and reach of children.

- Obtain information about how the family is considering management of the child's care at home.

- Determine if other family issues or stressors must be integrated into the plan of care.

- Identify the family's expectations of different health professionals and facilities to help manage the child's care.

- Prepare an ecomap and genogram.

Examples of nursing diagnoses that may result from the family and home assessment include the following (NANDA-I © 2014):

- *Coping: Family, Compromised,* related to multiple simultaneous stressors

- *Family Processes, Interrupted,* related to child with a significant disability requiring alteration in family functioning

- *Caregiver Role Strain, Risk for,* related to child with a newly acquired disability and the associated financial burden

- *Social Interaction, Impaired (Parents and Child),* related to lack of family or respite support

Planning and Implementation

Families need support to increase resources and coping behaviors so they can successfully manage the multiple stressors of daily living along with a child's chronic condition.

Establishing a therapeutic relationship with the family is an important intervention. This relationship should be characterized by empathy and trust, as well as the development of mutually identified goals for the child's care. To help families develop resilience, focus on family competence and strengths. Acknowledge and validate their emotions. Provide information in a clear, timely, and sensitive manner. Ask questions that help direct the family's thinking rather than providing them with all the answers. Teach families to identify solutions until they are able to independently problem solve. Linkage with other families who have faced similar situations may be helpful.

EVIDENCE-BASED PRACTICE | Investigating Culture and Healthcare Barriers

Clinical Question
What barriers to providing accessible health care exist among ethnically diverse families with children?

The Evidence
Ferayorni, Sinha, and McDonald (2011) examined demographic characteristics, socioeconomic status, access to care, perceived barriers to care, compliance with follow-up care, and unmet health needs in foreign-born children who visited a pediatric emergency department. Parents of 385 children were interviewed during a visit to the emergency department and over the telephone 1 week after the visit. Twenty-three percent of these children did not have health insurance. Compared to children with health insurance, those who did not have coverage were less likely to have a regular healthcare provider and a regular place for health and dental care. Parents of 31% of uninsured children cited a perceived barrier to care. Barriers reported most often were language, lack of insurance and inability to pay, and transportation. Parents of 26 children reported unmet healthcare needs, with a slightly higher prevalence among uninsured children as opposed to insured children. Dental care was the most commonly reported unmet healthcare need. Uninsured children who were foreign born were primarily Spanish speaking, poorer, and had poor access to health care. This population was also more likely to use the emergency department for its healthcare needs.

Adorador, McNulty, Hart, and Fitzpatrick (2011) examined perceived barriers to immunizations in 108 Latino mothers of children in a low-income clinic. Results of the immunization survey revealed that 92% of mothers thought their children were up to date on their immunizations when health records indicated that only 42% were up to date. Barriers to immunizations identified by these mothers included the child being sick, transportation issues, no health insurance, affordability, language concerns, and childcare issues.

Taylor, Nicolle, and Maguire (2013) conducted interviews with 38 healthcare professionals to determine their perceptions of the barriers that ethnic minorities who spoke poor or no English encountered when seeking health care. Five key themes emerged from the interviews: language; low literacy; retention of information; lack of understanding; and attitudes, gender attitudes, and health beliefs.

Best Practice
Socioeconomic status is a theme in two of these studies. These families may not have health insurance, a regular healthcare provider, or adequate transportation. Nurses need to refer families to sources for healthcare services and then follow up to be sure the families were able to access care. Referrals to community health centers and instructions for transportation to the health setting are important for many families. A need for understandable information is another theme among most groups. Explaining why an immunization is needed as well as providing information about the child's condition are important nursing roles. Interpreters may be needed to provide this information. Referring the family to others from the same ethnic or racial group and assisting them in navigating complex systems such as school and social services may also be necessary. Cultural differences and practices were also cited as a barrier to health care. It is essential that healthcare providers become familiar with other cultures and be accepting of practices that are safe for the child. By being open to practices of other cultures, healthcare providers will find families more willing to share openly about how they treat their children. This may lead to an opportunity for education related to unsafe practices.

Clinical Reasoning
What is the process that immigrant families in your state or province must follow to secure health care for their children? How would you help to guide someone through this process? What cultural groups are common in your community? Do you speak their language? If not, what measures should you take to ensure that they understand the teaching offered in clinical settings? What type of support groups will be helpful for families when they have a child with special healthcare needs?

Assist the family to begin planning for ongoing care using family-centered principles:

- Identify the primary decision maker for the child's health care.

- Discuss the family's goals for managing the child's care in the home setting.

- Consider how the family's strengths and previous problem-solving experiences can be integrated into the intervention.

- Consider the family's ethnic and religious background in developing intervention recommendations. Assist the child and family to determine how they can incorporate prescribed therapies with their healthcare practices. Ensure that the child and family understand the child's illness, treatment, or health promotion. Apply culturally sensitive techniques when dispelling any cultural myths.

- Ask questions in a respectful and nonjudgmental manner to help identify a family's use of CAM, encouraging the parent to share the information.

- Offer the family one or more potential interventions rather than trying to force one intervention. Be open to modifying the intervention or devising an alternative intervention to better match the family's lifestyle or cultural preferences.

- Identify the type of support or assistance the family would like to have.

- Identify potential resources in the community that match the child's and family's needs for support. Collaborate with the family to discuss those resources and to select those that are acceptable to the family.

- Make sure the family has a care coordinator, especially when a family member seems to be unable to assume the case management role initially. Assist families in obtaining resources through such actions as role rehearsal, providing instructions and support when making an initial call, or connecting with another family support person who can help with resource linkage.

- Refer families with moderate or severe dysfunction to community resources for social support and counseling, as appropriate.

Evaluation

Expected outcomes of nursing care include:

- Collaboration of the child and family with an assigned case manager so that interventions are implemented as recommended by the nurse and healthcare team

- Appropriate care provided by the family to the child with an acquired disability

Chapter Highlights

- The family is defined as two or more individuals who are joined together by marriage, birth, or adoption and live together in the same household.

- Family-centered care is a philosophy of health care in which a mutually beneficial partnership develops between families and the nurse and also other health professionals. In this way, the priorities and needs of the family are addressed when the family seeks health care for the child.

- Various types of families exist and include the nuclear family, dual-career/dual-earner family, child-free family, extended family, extended kin network family, single-parent family, single-mother-by-choice family, blended or reconstituted nuclear family, binuclear family, heterosexual cohabitating family, and the gay and lesbian family.

- Parenting is a leadership role in the family in which children are guided to learn acceptable behaviors, beliefs, morals, and rituals of the family, and to become socially responsible contributing members of society.

- Discipline is a method for teaching rules that govern behavior or conduct. Punishment is the action taken to enforce the rules when a child misbehaves.

- The quality of the relationship between divorced parents has an important impact on their future relationships with their children. Better maintenance of family and kinship ties results

when divorced parents are able to minimize the conflict and continue sharing parenting.

- The goal of foster care is to ensure the safety and well-being of vulnerable children by placing them in an approved living situation, away from the family of origin, that is legally coordinated by the state's child welfare system.

- Adoption is a legal relationship between a child and parents not related by birth in which the parents assume legal and financial responsibility for the child. Many children are adopted from foreign nations.

- Family theories help in understanding family functioning, environment–family interchange, family changes over time, and the family response to health and illness.

- Family development theories use a framework to categorize a family's progression over time according to specific, typical stages in family life.

- Family assessment tools are used to gather information about the family's functioning with regard to characteristics such as nurturing its members, problem solving, and communication. Information gathered helps the nurse work more effectively with the family in meeting the child's healthcare needs.

- Resilience is the family's capacity to develop strengths and abilities to bounce back from the stresses and challenges faced, and to eliminate or minimize negative concerns.

- Family strengths are the relationships and processes that support and protect families and family members during times of adversity and change. These strengths enable families to develop, adapt to change, and cope with challenges.

- Culture is a significant determinant of an individual's beliefs, behavior, and response to health and illness. Parental beliefs and behaviors can either promote the child's health care or impede preventive care, delay or complicate medical care, or result in the use of ineffective or harmful remedies.

- Cultural competence refers to the ability of the nurse to understand and respond effectively to the cultural needs of the child and family.

- A cultural assessment can assist the nurse in identifying cultural norms and in providing culturally appropriate nursing care. Providing spiritually sensitive care involves determining the current spiritual and religious beliefs and practices that will affect the child and family, accommodating these practices where possible, and examining one's own spiritual or religious beliefs to be more aware and able to provide nonjudgmental care.

- Complementary and alternative therapies are defined as diverse medical and healthcare systems, practices, and products that are not presently considered to be part of conventional medicine.

Clinical Reasoning in Action

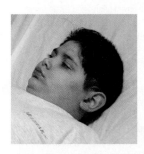

Sixteen-year-old Casey is recuperating from injuries sustained in a motor vehicle crash in which he was the passenger. He was not wearing a seat belt and experienced a brain injury after striking the windshield. His cognitive and motor functions are impaired. Following a 7-day acute care hospital stay, he was moved to an inpatient rehabilitation hospital where he has been for the past 5 days. He is much more responsive to stimuli and to family members 12 days after his injury. Physical therapy is provided twice a day to promote range of motion and muscle tone and to prevent contractures. Plans are being made to discharge him to his home and provide him with outpatient rehabilitation care within the next 5 days. A case manager will be assigned to coordinate his healthcare services.

Casey lives with his mother, two half-brothers (10 and 6 years old), and stepfather. Both his mother and stepfather are employed full time and are trying to determine how to manage care for the teen when he returns home. Casey's grandparents live nearby and may provide some support to the family. Because Spanish is the language spoken primarily by the family, teaching materials are provided in both Spanish and English.

Casey is totally dependent for care, including bathing, toileting, feeding, and mobilizing. Although he is expected to regain self-care abilities, the impact of the injury on his cognitive ability and future functioning is unknown.

During the past 12 days, Casey's extended family has provided support to the family, but the level of support in the future weeks will decrease because of other family obligations. Casey's mother has already initiated a leave of absence from work so she can care for him when he returns home; however, this will mean the family has reduced income during that time period. Casey's younger brothers have been able to visit him, and they are very anxious because Casey cannot talk with them. They have been trying to avoid bothering their mother and father during this time, but they are wondering when life will be more normal and they can again participate in their usual after-school activities.

1. What information about the family strengths, needs, and resilience can be identified from the information just given?

2. What additional information would be helpful to know about family strengths and needs prior to developing a nursing care plan?

3. Based on your assessment of the family and the challenges facing the family members, list at least one nursing diagnosis that addresses issues important for planning nursing care for Casey and his family.

4. Describe the use of family-centered care principles in planning Casey's nursing care in collaboration with the family.

References

Adams, D., Dagenais, S., Clifford, T., Baydala, L., King, W. J., Hervas-Malo, M., . . . Vohra, S. (2013). Complementary and alternative medicine use by pediatric specialty outpatients. *Pediatrics, 131*(2), 225–232.

Adoption.com. (2013). *Summary of the Adoption and Safe Families Act of 1997.* Retrieved from http://library.adoption.com/articles/summary-of-the-adoption-and-safe-families-act-of-1997.html

Adorador, A., McNulty, R., Hart, D., & Fitzpatrick, J. J. (2011). Perceived barriers to immunizations as identified by Latino mothers. *Journal of the Academy of Nurse Practitioners, 23,* 501–508.

American Academy of Child and Adolescent Psychiatry. (2011). *Children and divorce.* Retrieved from https://www.aacap.org/App_Themes/AACAP/docs/facts_for_families/01_children_and_divorce.pdf

American Academy of Child and Adolescent Psychiatry. (2013). *Facts for families guide: Foster care.* Retrieved from http://www.aacap.org/AACAP/Families_and_Youth/Facts_for_Families/Facts_for_families_Pages/Foster_Care_64.aspx

American Academy of Pediatrics (AAP). (2015). *Disciplining your child.* Retrieved from https://www.healthychildren.org/English/family-life/family-dynamics/communication-discipline/Pages/Disciplining-Your-Child.aspx

Andrews, M. M., & Boyle, J. S. (2012). *Transcultural concepts in nursing care* (6th ed.). Philadelphia, PA: Lippincott Williams & Wilkins.

Anthony, C. J., DiPerna, J. C., & Amato, P. R. (2014). Divorce, approaches to learning, and children's academic achievement: A longitudinal analysis of mediated and moderated effects. *Journal of School Psychology, 52,* 249–261.

Arkes, J. (2015). The temporal effects of divorces and separations on children's academic achievement and problem behavior. *Journal of Divorce and Remarriage, 56,* 25–42.

Baumrind, D. (2012). Differentiating between confrontive and coercive kinds of parental power-assertive disciplinary practices. *Human Development, 55,* 35–51.

Baumrind, D. (2013). Authoritative parenting revisited: History and current status. In R. E Larzelere, A. S. Morris, & A.W. Harrist (Eds.), *Authoritative parenting: Synthesizing nurturance and discipline for optimal child development* (pp. 11–34). Washington, DC: American Psychological Association.

Bright Futures. (2012). *The role of fathers: Family support.* Retrieved from http://www.healthyfuturesva.com/detail.aspx?id=218

Caldwell, B. M., & Bradley, R. H. (1984). *The Home Observation for Measurement of the Environment.* Little Rock: University of Arkansas.

Coehlo, D. P. (2015). Family child health nursing. In J. R. Kaakinen, D. P. Coehlo, R. Steele, A. Tabacco, & S. M. H. Hanson (Eds.), *Family health care nursing: Theory, practice, and research* (5th ed., pp. 387–432). Philadelphia, PA: F. A. Davis.

Committee on Hospital Care & Institute for Patient and Family-Centered Care. (2012). Patient and family-centered care and the pediatrician's role. *Pediatrics, 129*(2), 394–404.

Clark, M. J. (2015). Care of families. In M. J. Clark (Ed.), *Population and community health nursing* (6th ed., pp. 326–351). Hoboken, NJ: Pearson.

Craig, G. J., & Dunn, W. L. (2013). *Understanding human development* (3rd ed., p. 206). Upper Saddle River, NJ: Pearson.

Dokken, D. L., & Buell, L. D. (2011). Families as educators: Guidance for implementation. *Pediatric Nursing, 37*(1), 41–43.

Douglas, M. K., Pierce, J. U., Rosenkoetter, M., Pacquiao, D., Callister, L. C., Hattar-Pollara, M., . . . Purnell, L. (2011). Standards of Practice for Culturally Competent Nursing Care: 2011 update. *Journal of Transcultural Nursing, 22*(4), 317–333.

Duvall, E. M. (1977). *Marriage and family development* (5th ed.). Philadelphia, PA: Lippincott.

Duvall, E. M., & Miller, B. C. (1985). *Marriage and family development* (6th ed.). New York, NY: HarperCollins.

Ferayorni, A., Sinha, M., & McDonald, F. W. (2011). Health issues among foreign born uninsured children visiting an inner city pediatric emergency department. *Journal of Immigrant and Minority Health, 13*(3), 434–444.

Font, S. A. (2014). Kinship and nonrelative foster care: The effect of placement type on child well-being. *Child Development, 85*(5), 2074–2090.

Fontaine, K. L. (2015). *Complementary and alternative therapies for nursing practice* (4th ed.). Upper Saddle River, NJ: Pearson.

Fusco, R. A., & Cahalane, H. (2015). Socioemotional problems among young children in out-of-home care: A comparison of kinship and foster care placement. *Journal of Family Social Work, 18*(3), 183–201.

Giger, J. N., & Davidhizar, R. E. (2013). *Transcultural nursing: Assessment & intervention* (6th ed.). St. Louis, MO: Mosby Elsevier.

Gross, G. (2015). *The impact of divorce on children of different ages.* Retrieved from http://www.huffingtonpost.com/dr-gail-gross/the-impact-of-divorce-on-children-of-different-ages_b_6820636.html

Hackman, D. A., Betancourt, L. M., Brodsky, N. L., Kobrin, L., Hurt, H., & Farah, M. J. (2013). Selective impact of early parental responsivity on adolescent stress reactivity. *PLOS One, 8*(3), e58250

Haney-Caron, E., & Heilbrun, K. (2014). Lesbian and gay parents and determination of child custody: The changing legal landscape and implications for policy and practice. *Psychology of Sexual Orientation and Gender Diversity, 1*(1), 19–29.

Herrman, H., Stewart, D. E., Diaz-Granados, N., Berger, E. L., Jackson, B., & Yuen, T. (2011). What is resilience? *Canadian Journal of Psychiatry, 56*(5), 258–265.

Hughs, D. (2014). *A review of the literature pertaining to family-centered care for children with special health care needs.* Retrieved from http://lpfch-cshcn.org/publications/research-reports/a-review-of-the-literature-pertaining-to-family-centered-care-for-children-with-special-health-care-needs/

Institute for Patient- and Family-Centered Care. (2013). *Patient and family resource centers.* Retrieved from http://www.ipfcc.org/advance/topics/pafam-resource.html

Jones, V. F., Schulte, E. E., & Committee on Early Childhood and Council on Foster Care, Adoption, and Kinship Care. (2012). The pediatrician's role in supporting adoptive families. *Pediatrics, 130*(4), e1040–e1049.

Kaakinen, J. R., & Hanson, S. M. H. (2015). Theoretical foundations for the nursing of families. In J. R. Kaakinen, D. P. Coehlo, R. Steele, A. Tabacco, & S. M. H. Hanson (Eds.), *Family health care nursing: Theory, practice, and research* (5th ed., pp. 67–104). Philadelphia, PA: F. A. Davis.

Lambert, N. M., Fincham, F. D., & Graham, S. M. (2011). Understanding the layperson's perception of prayer: A prototype analysis of prayer. *Psychology of Religion and Spirituality, 3*(1), 55–65.

Lascar, E. (2013). *The role of spiritual care in CPC programs.* Retrieved from http://www.ehospice.com/internationalchildrens/ArticleView/tabid/10670/ArticleId/3929/language/en-GB/Default.aspx

Lester, P., Stein, J. A., Saltzman, W., Woodward, K., McDermid, S. W., Milburn, N., . . . Beardslee, W. (2013). Psychological health of military children: Longitudinal evaluation of a family-centered prevention program to enhance family resilience. *Military Medicine, 178*(8), 838–845.

Lewandowski, L. A., & Tesler, M. D. (Eds.). (2008). Family-centered care: Putting it into action. *The SPN/ANA Guide to Family-Centered Care.* Washington, DC: American Nurses Publishing.

Maggio, J. (2013). *Peace and the single mom.* New York, NY: Choose NOW Publishing.

Mazjub, R. M., & Mansor, S. (2012). Perception and adjustment of adolescents towards divorce. *Procedia—Social and Behavioral Sciences, 46*, 3530–3534.

McFarland, M. R., & Wehbe-Alamah, H. B. (2015). The theory of culture care diversity and universality. In M. R. McFarland & H. B. Weheb-Alamah (Eds.), *Leininger's culture care diversity and universality: A worldwide nursing theory* (3rd ed., pp. 1–34). Burlington, MA: Jones and Bartlett.

Mitchell, M. (2013). Women's use of complementary and alternative medicine in pregnancy: A journey to normal birth. *British Journal of Midwifery, 21*(2), 100–106.

National Cancer Institute (2012). *Spirituality in cancer care.* Retrieved from http://www.cancer.gov/cancertopics/pdq/supportivecare/spirituality/Patient/

National Center for Complementary and Alternative Medicine (NCCAM). (2013a). *Complementary, alternative, or integrative health: What's in a name?* Retrieved from http://www.nccam.nih.gov/health/whatiscam/

National Center for Complementary and Alternative Medicine (NCCAM). (2013b). *Children and complementary health approaches.* Retrieved from http://www.nccam.nih.gov/health/children

Nesmith, A. (2015). Factors influencing the regularity of parental visits with children in foster care. *Child and Adolescent Social Work Journal, 32,* 219–228.

Phillips, C. M., & Mann, A. (2013). Historical analysis of the Adoption and Safe Families Act of 1997. *Journal of Human Behavior in the Social Environment. 23,* 862–868.

Purnell, L. D. (2013). *Transcultural health care: A culturally competent approach* (4th ed.). Philadelphia, PA: F. A. Davis.

Purnell, L. D. (2014). *Guide to culturally competent health care* (3rd ed.). Philadelphia, PA: F. A. Davis.

Ramisch, J. (2012). Marriage and family therapists working with couples who have children with autism. *Journal of Marital and Family Therapy, 38*(2), 305–316.

Sarsour, K., Sheridan, M., Jutte, D., Nuru-Jeter, A., Hinshaw, S., & Boyce, W. T. (2011). Family socioeconomic status and child executive functions: The roles of language, home environment, and single parenthood. *Journal of the International Neuropsychological Society, 17,* 120–132.

Single Mothers by Choice. (2013). *About single mothers by choice.* Retrieved from http://www.singlemothersbychoice.org/

Soine, L. (2013). Kinship foster caregivers—Partners for permanency. *Social Work Today, 13*(5), 12.

Spector, R. E. (2013). *Cultural diversity in health and illness* (8th ed.). Upper Saddle River, NJ: Pearson.

Taylor, S. P., Nicolle, C., & Maguire, M. (2013). Cross-cultural communication barriers in health care. *Nursing Standard, 27*(31), 35–43.

Theunissen, M. H. C., Vogels, A. G. C., & Reijneveld, S. A. (2015). Punishment and reward in parental discipline for children aged 5 to 6 years: Prevalence and groups at risk. *Academic Pediatrics, 15*(1), 96–102.

U.S. Census Bureau. (2013). *Current population survey (CPS)—Definitions.* Retrieved from http://www.census.gov/cps/about/cpsdef.html

U.S. Department of Health and Human Services. (2012). *Foster Care Independence Act of 1999 P.L. 106–169.* Retrieved from https://www.childwelfare.gov/pubPDFs/majorfedlegis.pdf

U.S. Department of Health and Human Services, National Institutes of Health. (2013). *Cultural competency.* Retrieved from http://www.nih.gov/clearcommunication/culturalcompetency.htm

U.S. Department of Health and Human Services. (2015). *Trends in foster care and adoption: FY 2005–FY 2014.* Retrieved from http://www.acf.hhs.gov/sites/default/files/cb/trends_fostercare_adoption2014.pdf

U.S. Department of Labor. (2012). *Fact Sheet No. 28: The Family and Medical Leave Act of 1993.* Retrieved from http://www.dol.gov/whd/regs/compliance/whdfs28.pdf

Wachholtz, A., & Sambamoorthi, U. (2011). National trends in prayer use as a coping mechanism for health concerns: Changes from 2002 to 2007. *Psychology of Religion and Spirituality, 3*(2), 67–77.

Wright, L. M., & Leahey, M. (2013). *Nurses and families: A guide to family assessment and intervention* (6th ed.). Philadelphia, PA: F. A. Davis.

Zoucha, R., & Zamarripa, C. A. (2013). People of Mexican heritage. In L. D. Purnell (Ed.), *Transcultural health care: A culturally competent approach* (4th ed., pp. 374–390). Philadelphia, PA: F. A. Davis.

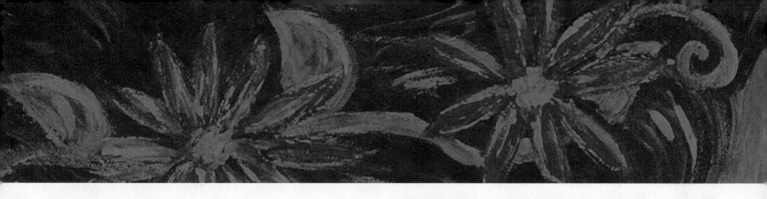

Chapter 3
Genetic and Genomic Influences

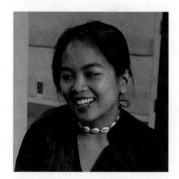

I came in for a sports physical, but I really want to be tested for Huntington disease. My mom's father died from Huntington when I was 8. My mom won't really talk about it, but I know she doesn't want to be tested. I have been doing some reading about Huntington disease, and I want to be tested. I mean, how can I plan my life if I don't know how long I'm going to be able to enjoy it?

—Sarah, 16 years old

Learning Outcomes

3.1 Explain the role of genetic and genomic concepts in health promotion, disease prevention, screening, diagnostics, selection of treatment, and monitoring of treatment effectiveness.

3.2 Elicit a family health history and construct a genetic pedigree.

3.3 Incorporate knowledge of genetic and genomic influences and risk factors into assessment, planning, and implementation of nursing care.

3.4 Integrate basic genetic and genomic concepts into child and family education.

3.5 Understand implications of genome science on the nursing role with particular attention to ethical, legal, and social issues.

3.6 Discuss the significance of recent advances in human genetics and genomics and their impact on healthcare delivery.

Partnering With Families: Meeting the Standard of Genetic Nursing Care Delivery

Completion of the Human Genome Project in 2003 heralded the dawn of the genomic era of health care. It has long been known that some diseases occur due to specific gene defects. **Genetic diseases** have traditionally been thought of as inherited diseases caused by a defect in a single gene. Although "typical" genetic diseases have enormous health consequences for affected individuals and families, they have relatively little impact on the health of most people. The Human Genome Project decoded human deoxyribonucleic acid (DNA), revealing the sequence of its 3 billion "letters" (also called bases or nucleotides). Research associated with the Human Genome Project has revealed virtually all diseases to have a genetic component. The human **genome** is the entire DNA sequence of an individual, and the study of **genomics** takes a holistic view of gene function. Human genomics is the study of all DNA in the human genome, including how genes interact with each other and with environmental, psychosocial, and cultural factors. Essentially all diseases and health conditions have both genetic and environmental components, but the genetic contribution to various diseases varies widely (Figure 3–1).

45

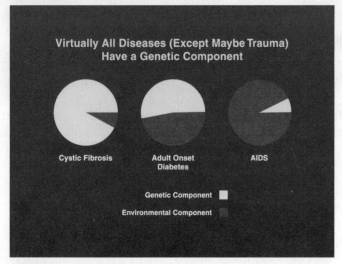

Virtually All Diseases (Except Maybe Trauma) Have a Genetic Component

Cystic Fibrosis Adult Onset Diabetes AIDS

Genetic Component
Environmental Component

Figure 3–1 Although the causes for nearly all diseases and health conditions have both genetic and environmental components, the relative contribution of genetic and environmental influences varies widely. At one end of the spectrum lie "traditional" genetic diseases, such as cystic fibrosis (CF). Although CF is caused by a gene alteration, its morbidity and mortality vary according to environmental effects such as medical management. On the other hand, AIDS is an infectious disease that will not occur without environmental exposure to HIV. Still, there are genetic alterations that cause some people to be resistant to HIV infection. In type 2 diabetes, the genetic and environmental contributions are fairly equivalent.

SOURCE: Copyright © by Francis Collins. Used by permission of Francis Collins.

DNA is central to our state of health because of its role in determining the set of proteins an individual has available to carry out specific physiologic functions. There are about 21,000 genes in the human genome, and each gene directs the formation of one or more proteins (Lander, 2011). Proteins include enzymes, cell receptors, ion channels, structural molecules, antibodies, and other molecules necessary for biologic function. Good health is dependent on normal gene structure (or sequence) and normal gene function (or expression). Gene sequence, which is the order of the gene's nucleotides or bases, determines whether a protein encoded by the gene has the correct amino acid sequence so that it can function normally. Normal gene function means that genes are expressed (i.e., translated and transcribed to make proteins) at the appropriate time and in appropriate amounts to support normal physiologic function.

Gene expression, which is affected by all manners of environmental and **epigenetic** effects, is therefore just as important as gene sequence. Genetic abnormalities may cause too much or too little of a specific protein, or perhaps a dysfunctional protein, to be formed. Sometimes the altered protein is sufficient to cause disease; this is the case with traditional genetic diseases such as cystic fibrosis and sickle cell disease. More often, multiple genetic variations, together with environmental factors, increase risk for disease. Both traditional genetic disorders and common complex diseases such as heart disease,

stroke, diabetes, and cancer are now known to be related to variation in gene sequence and gene expression. Research has uncovered many of the genetic and environmental factors that increase risk for disease, leading to development of new treatments that range in scope from promoting healthy lifestyles to specific genetic therapies. Knowledge gained from human genome research is anticipated to transform health care across the entire continuum of care, allowing care to be tailored to each person's individual risk for disease. Genomic information is already being used to personalize health promotion and disease prevention, screening, treatment, and monitoring of treatment effectiveness (Green, Guyer, & National Human Genome Research Institute, 2011).

Nurses must be prepared to deliver genetically competent care in many healthcare settings to individuals, families, communities, and populations. Nurses in newborn nurseries and mother–baby units may be the first to suspect a newborn has a genetic condition. Pediatric nurses often care for children with genetic conditions who may require frequent hospitalization. Nurses in general and specialty clinics must be prepared to help asymptomatic individuals and families who are increasingly seeking information about their risk for an inherited disease or condition. Parents who order direct-to-consumer genetic tests may bring questions about their results to nurses. For these and other reasons, nurses must achieve genetic and genomic literacy in order to deliver competent care in the genomic era.

The translation of genetic and genomic knowledge to clinical care requires nurses to integrate new genetic knowledge into their nursing practice. This expectation was formally established in 2007 by the American Nurses Association (ANA) and the International Society of Nurses in Genetics (ISONG) in a joint statement, *Genetics/Genomics Nursing: Scope and Standards of Practice*. This document, now in its second edition (2016), outlines the levels of genetic knowledge required of all registered nurses, including basic and advanced practice nurses in general practice as well as those who specialize in providing genetics services. In addition, a set of essential competencies in genetics and genomics has been defined and endorsed by nearly 50 nursing organizations. These competencies represent the minimal level of genetic and genomic competency expected of every registered nurse across all practice settings (Consensus Panel on Genetic/Genomic Nursing Competencies, 2009). Examples of nursing activities that reflect genetic and genomic competence include:

- Identifying risk for disease by collecting a family history and drawing a three-generation pedigree
- Helping individuals and families to understand the implications and limitations of genetic testing
- Administering gene-based therapies
- Providing nondirective counseling to assist families who have questions or concerns about their reproductive risks
- Recognizing signs and symptoms, such as dysmorphic features or hypotonia, that may indicate a genetic condition in a newborn
- Anticipating variable responses among individuals to "standard" medication doses, due to pharmacogenetic effects
- Ensuring the delivery of genetically competent care for the child and family—for example, ensuring that a child about to start thiopurine treatment has completed pharmacogenetic testing

- Helping individuals and families identify credible sources of genetic information
- Applying concepts of health promotion and health maintenance to assist children and families who are at increased risk to develop common chronic conditions, such as heart disease, to make informed lifestyle choices
- Partnering with families affected by genetic conditions, including providing advocacy, supporting the child's and family's decisions, teaching, facilitating appropriate referrals, clarifying information, and providing further information about available resources and services
- Partnering with the community to educate the public about genetics
- Supporting legislation to protect genetic information and to protect those with genetic conditions from discrimination
- Applying knowledge of the ethical, legal, and social implications of genetic information

Through informed application of fundamental genetic and genomic concepts, nurses can significantly improve the nursing care provided to children and their families. In fact, understanding and applying these concepts is an essential part of child and family nursing.

Impact of Genetic Advances on Health Promotion and Health Maintenance

Health promotion and health maintenance for children and their families are foundational for all nursing care (see Chapters 6 through 9). The genomic era offers a promise of precision health care based on an individual's or a population's risk for disease, which varies according to the set of genes they inherited, cultural influences, and a multitude of environmental factors to which they are exposed. Although some people may be aware that they carry an altered gene associated with a specific disease, most individuals do not know details of their genetic makeup or how their genetic inheritance influences their future health. This is particularly true for common conditions such as heart disease and diabetes, for which risk varies with inheritance of a number of altered genes and is modified by lifestyle factors such as diet and physical activity. Having specific knowledge about one's genetic makeup and associated increased risk for disease provides a basis for health screening and may provide motivation for people to maintain a healthy lifestyle. Imagine, then, if people knew their statistical risks for inheriting or developing disease, based on their specific genotype. Health promotion and health maintenance teaching and nursing interventions would be targeted to individuals according to their disease risk. Children and families may experience increased motivation to adhere to lifestyle choices and health screenings that are personalized according to their disease risk. Precision health care is a major goal in the genomic era (Collins & Varmus, 2015).

With knowledge of how genetic variations influence health, the pediatric nurse can ensure health teaching and early detection of complications from genetic conditions with emphasis on primary and secondary health promotion and disease prevention. For example:

- Nurses should ensure informed consent for newborn screening and provide teaching and support to families whose infants have positive screens.

- Nurses should recognize hypotonia (reduced muscle tone, limited voluntary movement, reduced strength, and joints with increased range of motion) in newborns and advocate for a referral for the infant to be evaluated by a genetic specialist (Prows, Hopkin, Barnoy, et al., 2013).
- A child who screens positive for scoliosis (see Chapter 29) should be assessed for axillary freckling and café au lait spots, due to the relationship between scoliosis and neurofibromatosis.
- Screening for Marfan syndrome (see Chapter 21) should be a part of all sports physicals, due to the lethal cardiovascular complication of aortic dilation. This can be accomplished by assessing for common characteristics such as myopia, scoliosis, tall stature, long fingers and thumbs, a hollow chest, and an arm span greater than the height.
- Nurses should both teach and support families regarding any specific interventions necessary to avoid complications in children with genetic conditions. Examples are the importance for children with phenylketonuria (PKU) to maintain a phenylalanine-free diet for life, and the need to maintain children with sickle cell disease (see Chapter 23) on penicillin.

> **Professionalism in Practice** **Using the People-First Approach**
>
> The nurse must incorporate a person-first philosophy and use genetic terminology that promotes an individual's positive self-image. When communicating genetic concerns to children, families, other healthcare providers, or the public, take care to use words that do not reflect value.
>
> Use the term **wild type gene** or *expected gene* or *unaltered gene* (rather than "normal" gene) and *altered gene* or *disease-producing gene* (rather than "mutated" or "abnormal" gene).
>
> Name the diagnosis rather than apply the label. For example, newborn Sammy, who exhibits Down syndrome, should not be identified as the "Down baby" but as Sammy who has Down syndrome. And describe Sally as having (a diagnosis of) autism, not as being autistic.
>
> Also, the term *cognitive disability* or *intellectual disability* is preferred (rather than "mental retardation").
>
> Source: Adapted from Snow, K. (n.d.). *People first language.* Retrieved from http://www.disabilityisnatural.com/images/PDF/pfl09.pdf

- When caring for the child with Down syndrome (see Chapter 28), the pediatric nurse can help the parents shift from the more expected and traditional focus of disease management to health promotion and protection by teaching parents about the established guidelines for exams and screenings specific to children with Down syndrome.

Early diagnosis allows early intervention with health-promoting care specific to a genetic diagnosis, promoting achievement of maximal function, better health, and improved quality of life for children affected with genetic alterations. The pediatric nurse must be able to identify available community-based and genetic-based resources to assist the child or adolescent and the family with strategies to support both health promotion and health maintenance activities.

Genetic Basics

A basic knowledge of the cell, DNA, cell division, chromosomes, and genes is essential to deliver the genetic standard of care to children, adolescents, and their families.

The **cell** is the basic unit of life and the working unit of all living systems. Life starts as a single cell, but the developed human body is made up of trillions of cells. These cells share common features such as a nucleus that contains 46 chromosomes and **organelles** such as mitochondria. Cells are specialized in appearance and function, according to their location. For example, pancreatic cells function much differently than nerve cells.

All human cells, except red blood cells, contain a complete set of DNA molecules, which are long sequences of nucleotides. A nucleotide is a base with an attached sugar and phosphate group. Four different bases, designated A, C, T, and G, make up DNA. The order, or sequence, of these bases provides exact instructions for protein building. The entire DNA in a human cell is referred to as the **human genome**. Most of the DNA is organized into chromosomes, which are contained in the cell nucleus. A small amount of DNA is found in the mitochondria, which is discussed later in this section. Each person's genome is unique, with the exception of monozygotic twins, who are derived from the same fertilized ovum and therefore share identical DNA.

Each cell nucleus contains about 6 feet of DNA that is tightly wound and packaged into 23 pairs of chromosomes, making a complete set of 46 chromosomes. The set includes 22 pairs of **autosomes**, which are by tradition numbered according to size, with chromosome 1 being the largest. There are two copies of each autosome, one inherited from the mother and the other from the father. Copies of a chromosome pair are called **homologous chromosomes**. The 23rd chromosome pair, the **sex chromosomes**, determines an individual's sex. A female has two copies of the X chromosome (one copy inherited from each parent), and a male has one X chromosome (inherited from his mother) and one Y chromosome (inherited from his father). The structure and number of chromosomes can be shown by preparing a **karyotype**, or picture of an individual's chromosomes (Figure 3–2). Sperm and ova represent exceptions to the 23–pair rule because each contains only a single chromosome from each homologous pair.

Cell Division

Mitosis and meiosis are the two types of cell division in humans. **Mitosis** takes place in somatic or tissue cells of the body, allowing the formation of new cells. Cell division by mitosis results in two cells called daughter cells that are genetically identical to the original cell and to each other. Mitosis is responsible for rapid human growth in early life and also replaces cells lost daily from skin surfaces and the lining of gastrointestinal and respiratory tracts.

Meiosis is also known as reduction cell division. Meiosis occurs only in the reproductive cells of the testes and ovaries and results in the formation of sperm and oocytes (**gametes**). Meiosis is similar to mitosis in that it is a form of cell division; however, through a series of complex mechanisms, the amount of genetic material is reduced to half. Each gamete contains a single copy of each of the 22 autosomes, plus a single sex chromosome. This is critical to ensure that when two gametes combine during fertilization, the correct total number of chromosomes (46) is present in the offspring's cells. The other purpose of meiosis is to make new combinations of genetic material through processes of crossing over and independent assortment. New combinations are necessary to promote diversity in the human population. **Crossing over** results from an exchange or shuffling of material between homologous chromosomes inherited from the father and mother. This exchange results in new intact chromosomes that represent a patchwork of maternal and paternal genetic material. Only the Y chromosome does not have the ability to cross over, since it lacks a homologous mate. **Independent assortment** means that chromosome pairs segregate randomly into one or another gamete, further enhancing the genetic diversity that is possible at fertilization.

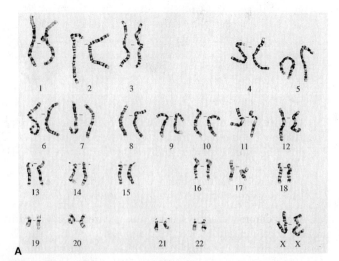
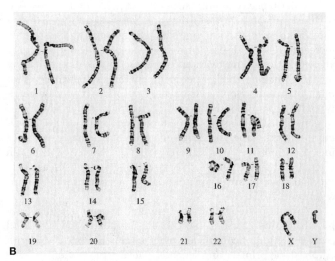

Figure 3–2 A karyotype is a picture of an individual's chromosomes. It depicts the number and structure of the 22 pairs of autosomes and the sex chromosomes. *A*, Female. *B*, Male.

SOURCE: Greenwood Genetic Center.

Chromosomal Alterations

Alterations in chromosomes sometimes occur during cell division (meiosis or mitosis) and are classified as alterations in either chromosome number or chromosome structure. The clinical consequences of both types of alterations vary according to the amount of DNA involved.

ALTERATIONS IN CHROMOSOME NUMBER

An increase or decrease in chromosome number is called **aneuploidy**. Aneuploidy is the result of an error during cell division, most often when **nondisjunction** occurs during meiosis. With nondisjunction, paired homologous chromosomes do not separate before migrating into egg or sperm cells. This creates a gamete with either two copies or no copies of a particular chromosome. When such a gamete is fertilized by a normal gamete with all 23 chromosomes, a **zygote** that is **monosomic** (missing one member of a chromosome pair) or **trisomic** (having three homologous chromosomes instead of the usual two) results.

In general, humans do not tolerate either extra or missing DNA very well. Most monosomic or trisomic conceptions result in early pregnancy loss. For example, Turner syndrome is the only monosomic condition that is compatible with life. Trisomies involving chromosomes with small numbers of genes may result in live births. Examples are trisomy 13 (Patau syndrome), trisomy 18 (Edwards syndrome), and trisomy 21 (Down syndrome). Each of these aneuploidies produces clinical features that vary according to the chromosome that is duplicated. It is not a coincidence that the three trisomic conditions that are not universally lethal involve duplication of chromosomes containing the smallest number of genes (Pierce, 2014).

Mosaicism. Monosomy and/or trisomy can also occur during mitosis, resulting in an individual with two, or occasionally more, separate cell lines with different chromosomal makeup. This is known as **mosaicism**. The earlier in development the error occurs, the more cells that will be abnormal. The converse is also true. The degree to which a person is affected by this chromosomal error varies. For example, individuals with mosaic Turner syndrome may show varying degrees of infertility or short stature, and an individual with mosaic Down syndrome may have a higher intelligence level than children whose every cell has three copies of chromosome 21.

STRUCTURAL CHROMOSOMAL ALTERATIONS

Inversion. A chromosomal **inversion** occurs when a chromosome breaks in two places and the piece between the breaks turns end for end and reattaches within the same chromosome. An inversion changes the DNA sequence for that portion of the chromosome. Inversion often results in *balanced* rearrangements, because the amount of DNA in the chromosome remains normal. The clinical consequences of an inversion depend on how much chromosomal material is involved and where the inversion occurs. For example, an inversion that occurs between genes may have no effect on health, whereas an inversion within the gene that codes for factor VIII, a clotting factor, is an important cause of hemophilia A.

Deletion and Duplication. Chromosomal alterations sometimes occur when unequal crossing over or abnormal segregation causes a chromosome to have a missing segment (deletion) or an additional segment (duplication) of genetic material. These are called *unbalanced* rearrangements. Conditions associated with unbalanced rearrangements may be incompatible with life or cause altered physical and/or mental development. An example is cri du chat syndrome, caused by a large deletion on chromosome 5. Children with cri du chat have microcephaly (a small head), significant intellectual disability, and a peculiar cry during infancy that sounds like a cat mewing (Schaaf, Zschocke, & Potocki, 2012).

Translocation. **Translocation** occurs when two, usually nonhomologous, chromosomes exchange segments of DNA. A translocation that results in a correct amount of chromosomal material but a new arrangement is a *balanced translocation*. The individual who has a balanced rearrangement has all the chromosomal material present and therefore does not usually have any physical or mental disabilities. However, individuals with a balanced translocation are at high risk to produce gametes with unbalanced rearrangements. This leads to increased risk of pregnancy loss or having children with mental and/or physical disabilities due to missing or extra genetic material. In about 4% of cases of Down syndrome, the extra chromosome 21 is due to a translocation (Schaaf, Zschocke, & Potocki, 2012). When a child with Down syndrome is born, it is important to conduct a chromosome study to determine if the cause is nondisjunction or translocation. Translocation is unrelated to maternal age, but it carries a significantly greater recurrence risk with subsequent pregnancies.

Genes

In addition to understanding chromosomal alterations, the nurse must have knowledge of genes—what they are, their function, and the consequences of gene alterations. The nurse must understand the inheritance of gene alterations in order to design appropriate nursing interventions and teach the child, adolescent, and family at risk for or with a known genetic condition. Also, as genetic influences on common chronic disease are better understood, knowledge of gene function and inheritance has become increasingly relevant in health promotion and health maintenance.

A **gene** is a small segment of a chromosome that can be identified with a particular function, most commonly protein production. Each chromosome contains many genes arranged in a linear order. Genes that reside on autosomes (i.e., chromosomes 1 through 22) come in pairs, with one copy on each homologous chromosome. Each gene copy, or **allele**, is inherited from a different parent; therefore, pairs of alleles likely have differences in their nucleotide sequence. These differences may be so minor that they don't affect gene function at all, or they may disrupt or totally disable the gene. An individual who has two functionally identical alleles of a gene is said to be **homozygous** (*homo* = same) for that gene. An individual whose alleles for a particular gene function differently is said to be **heterozygous** (*hetero* = different) for that gene. As previously discussed, genes on the sex chromosomes of males are unpaired, because the X and Y chromosomes contain different genes.

Genes have a specific location on a designated chromosome; this is called the *genetic locus*. Gene mapping has documented the locus for most human genes. For example, it is known that the Huntington gene is located at the tip of chromosome 4, whereas the gene associated with cystic fibrosis is on chromosome 7. It is important to remember that all people share the same set of genes. For example, not only people with Huntington disease have the Huntington gene. All people (with probable rare exceptions) have two copies of the Huntington gene, and people who carry a particular mutation in one of their Huntington genes will develop disease. In everyday language, people tend to use a kind of shorthand that infers that particular genes are "disease genes." Someone might say, for example, "I have the *BRCA* gene" when they mean their *BRCA* gene has a mutation that increases their risk for cancer. The *BRCA* gene itself is a tumor suppressor gene found in all people that, when functioning normally, protects against cancer. Nurses should try to be precise in their language to avoid reinforcing common misconceptions.

Genes are described as *altered* or *mutated* when a change has taken place in their nucleotide sequence. Such a change may or may not result in an altered protein product; a gene alteration that does not change the protein product is called a *polymorphism* or *silent mutation*. Other changes in nucleotide sequence, perhaps at a locus some distance from the gene itself, may affect gene expression—a gene's activity in making protein. Smaller, non-DNA molecules are also involved in gene expression; these epigenetic effects can cause genes to be overexpressed (making more than expected protein product), underexpressed (making less than expected), or expressed at a time in development when the gene is normally inactive. The observable, outward expression of an individual's entire physical, biochemical, and physiologic makeup, as determined by the person's genotype and environmental factors, is referred to as **phenotype**. Phenotype may be expressed as physical appearance such as curly or straight hair or physiologic function such as signs or symptoms of a disease.

FUNCTION AND DISTRIBUTION OF GENES

It is believed that only about 1% of the human genome is actually represented by genes (McCarthy, McLeod, & Ginsburg, 2013). The vast majority of human DNA does not encode proteins. In humans, protein-coding DNA is organized into about 21,000 genes (Lander, 2011); each individual's particular set of genes represents his or her **genotype**. These 21,000 genes are responsible for encoding hundreds of thousands of proteins that carry out all physiologic functions. An error, or mutation, in a gene can disrupt the order of amino acids that make up that gene's protein product. A protein with an incorrect amino acid may assume the wrong three-dimensional shape and, because protein function is dependent on protein shape (or configuration), the protein may not function as expected. Proteins are highly specialized and perform virtually all cellular functions. They form structures, transmit messages between cells, fight infection, direct genes to turn on or off, metabolize nutrients and drugs, and sense light, taste, and smell. Drug receptors, antibodies, and ion channels are proteins. When proteins do not function normally, health may be impaired.

Gene activity in making proteins (gene expression) can change moment to moment in response to thousands of intra- and extracellular signals. An example is the mechanism that stimulates cells to produce insulin after eating a candy bar. After eating, a gene on chromosome 11 of pancreatic cells is activated and produces insulin. Although the insulin gene is present in all nucleated cells of the body, it is functional only in insulin-secreting pancreatic cells.

MITOCHONDRIAL GENES

Chromosomes in the cell nucleus are not the only site where genes reside. Mitochondria (organelles involved in energy metabolism, known as the "powerhouse" of the cell) also contain a small amount of DNA. Mitochondrial DNA (mtDNA) contains 37 genes with roles in generating energy (in the form of adenosine triphosphate [ATP]) from glucose (Turnpenny & Ellard, 2012). Cells requiring large amounts of energy contain more mitochondria than other cells. Mitochondrial DNA is inherited from the mother in a unique *matrilineal* pattern. This occurs because mitochondria are located in the tail of the sperm, which detaches at fertilization. A female with a mitochondrial gene mutation will consequently pass that mutation to all her children, whereas an affected male will not pass a mtDNA mutation to any of his children (Turnpenny & Ellard, 2012). Clinical manifestations occurring as a result of mitochondrial gene alterations primarily affect high-energy tissues such as brain and cardiac and skeletal muscle.

HUMAN GENETIC VARIATION

The Human Genome Project and other genetic studies have shown that humans are remarkably similar to each other at the DNA level. On average, any two humans vary in less than 1% of their nucleotide sequence. Much of human variation can be attributed to single-nucleotide (or "single-letter") changes in DNA sequence. DNA sequencing of hundreds of individuals around the globe has shown that single nucleotide changes occur at about 38 million sites (or loci) across the genome (The 1000 Genomes Project Consortium, 2012); the rest of the genome is identical in ≥99% of individuals. These single-letter variations are called **single nucleotide polymorphisms** or SNPs (pronounced "snips"). Most SNPs are benign, although collectively they account for much phenotypic variation in appearance and risk for disease. They have been mapped to the human genome, and the resulting SNP maps are of enormous value to researchers. For example, scientists studying the genetics of type 2 diabetes mellitus have compared SNP patterns in large numbers of individuals with and without the disease to identify genetic variations associated with this common multifactorial disease. Such **genome-wide association studies** (GWAS) are uncovering the genetic contribution to common chronic conditions that cause most of the disease burden in developed countries.

In recent years, DNA research has identified **copy number variation** as an additional source of human genetic variation. In some individuals, stretches of DNA of variable size (up to 3 million bases and sometimes containing entire genes) are missing or replicated one or more times. Copy number variants (CNVs) appear to be fairly common; on average, each person is believed to have about 100 CNVs of various sizes (Lander, 2011). A CNV that contains an entire gene may result in more than expected gene product. In some cases, copy number variation has been associated with disease, birth defects, or the rate of metabolism of some drugs (Pierce, 2014).

GENE ALTERATIONS AND DISEASE

An alteration in the DNA sequence of a gene may cause a defective protein to be formed, which may have clinical significance. Gene alterations can be inherited, or they can be acquired. Mutations inherited from one or both parents (hereditary mutations) are also known as *germline mutations* because the mutation exists in the reproductive cells or gametes. Consequently, the DNA in every cell of that offspring will have the gene alteration, which can then be transmitted to following generations.

The second kind of gene alteration is an acquired, or somatic, mutation. These are mutations that occur in the DNA of cells of an individual at any time throughout a lifetime. They result from errors during cell division (mitosis) or from environmental influences such as radiation, toxins, or viral infections. Acquired mutations are also called sporadic or *de novo* mutations. Most cases of cancer, for example, are due to somatic mutations. Somatic mutations are not passed from one generation to another.

Single-gene alterations are responsible for more than 5000 hereditary diseases such as cystic fibrosis, Duchenne muscular dystrophy, and phenylketonuria (Online Mendelian Inheritance in Man [OMIM], 2014). Each of these disorders is relatively rare, although collectively they affect 1 of every 200 newborns (Schaaf, Zschocke, & Potocki, 2012). Although they are of enormous consequence to affected families, they constitute a relatively small portion of the total public health burden.

Genes vary enormously in size, but all are very long, containing tens of thousands or even hundreds of thousands of base pairs. Consequently, mutations can occur at various different loci within a gene and result in a wide variety of signs and symptoms. For example, the cystic fibrosis transmembrane conductance regulator (CFTR) gene on chromosome 7 contains about 250,000 base pairs and encodes a protein that forms a chloride channel. More than 1000 different CFTR mutations that disrupt the chloride channel have been identified (Turnpenny & Ellard, 2012). Some of these mutations cause cystic fibrosis; others are associated with milder disorders such as absence of the vas deferens, pancreatitis, and rhinosinusitis. Most genetic tests for cystic fibrosis will detect only the most common CFTR mutations.

Alterations as small as a single nucleotide are known to cause disease. Sickle cell disease is such a disorder: A single A-for-T substitution in the HBB gene causes an incorrect amino acid (valine) to be inserted at a site in the protein product (β-globin) normally occupied by a different amino acid (glutamic acid). The altered β-globin protein is then incorporated into hemoglobin molecules. Under conditions of low oxygen tension, the altered β-globin causes red blood cells to assume an abnormal, sickle-like shape. This leads to vascular occlusion and hemolytic anemia (Turnpenny & Ellard, 2012).

In other situations, multiple gene alterations along with environmental factors contribute to disease or health conditions. These conditions are said to be **multifactorial**. Most common chronic disorders—including hypertension, heart disease, type 2 diabetes, and most cancers—are multifactorial, as are several birth defects. Alterations in regulatory genes may also occur. Regulatory elements are stretches of DNA sequence, usually located between genes, which control gene expression or activity in making proteins. They include gene promoters, enhancers, silencers, and other control mechanisms and are important in maintaining homeostasis. Mutation of a regulatory gene might lead to the loss of expression of a gene, unexpected expression in a tissue in which it is usually silent, or a change in the time when a gene is expressed. Small, non-DNA molecules are also known to affect gene function; these epigenetic factors are of great interest in genetics research.

GENE ALTERATIONS THAT DECREASE RISK OF DISEASE

Although gene mutations are commonly associated with disease, they can also be helpful and decrease the risk of disease. For example, having a single copy of some genes known to cause autosomal recessive disorders can provide protection against disease. Individuals with a single altered sickle cell disease (SCD) gene are less likely to develop malaria. Another protective gene alteration involves a deletion in the CCR5 gene, which encodes a cell receptor to which the human immunodeficiency virus (HIV) binds. Persons who have two copies of the altered CCR5 gene are almost completely resistant to infection with HIV type 1, and those who are heterozygous for the deletion (have one copy of

the altered gene) experience markedly delayed progression from the point of HIV infection to the development of AIDS (Lewis, 2015). As genome research continues, more beneficial gene alterations are being identified.

Principles of Inheritance

Knowledge of inheritance prepares nurses to offer and reinforce genetic information to children, adolescents, and their families. Genetic knowledge may be important in assisting patients with care management and reproductive decision making. Nurses should apply basic principles of inheritance to risk assessment and teaching; these include (a) nearly all genes are paired, (b) only one gene of each pair is transmitted (passed on) from each parent to an offspring, and (c) one copy of each gene in the offspring comes from the mother and the other copy comes from the father. Understanding of Mendelian patterns of inheritance is based on these principles.

Classic Mendelian Patterns of Inheritance

Conditions that are caused by a mutation or alteration of a single gene are known as *monogenic* or *single-gene disorders.* More than 5000 known single-gene disorders have been catalogued, with detailed information posted to a searchable public database, the Online Mendelian Inheritance in Man (OMIM, 2014). Single-gene disorders are known as *Mendelian disorders* because they are predictably passed on from generation to generation following Mendel's laws of inheritance. Monogenic disorders that occur due to a mutation on an autosome (chromosome numbers 1 through 22) are most commonly inherited in an autosomal dominant or autosomal recessive pattern. Disorders due to a mutation on one of the sex chromosomes are inherited in an X-linked, or occasionally Y-linked, pattern. See Table 3–1.

DOMINANT VERSUS RECESSIVE DISORDERS

For some disorders, the presence of a single altered gene allele is enough to cause disease; these disorders are said to be **dominant**. An individual who is heterozygous for a dominant disorder will therefore have (or express) the disorder, despite the presence of one normally functioning allele. Other disorders occur only when both alleles of a gene pair are altered. In these **recessive** disorders, the gene product produced from a single unaltered gene is sufficient to perform the expected function and maintain homeostasis. Because most human genes reside on autosomes, the most common inheritance patterns are therefore called *autosomal dominant* or *autosomal recessive.*

AUTOSOMAL DOMINANT

More than half of the known Mendelian conditions are autosomal dominant (AD). Examples include neurofibromatosis, achondroplasia (dwarfism), Marfan syndrome, Huntington disease, and familial hypercholesterolemia. By definition, AD disorders involve altered genes on autosomes rather than the sex chromosomes X and Y. Disease occurs in AD disorders despite the presence of one unaltered gene, and most individuals with AD disorders are heterozygous for the disease-producing gene. Homozygous dominant conditions can occur, but they are generally much more severe or lethal and frequently result in early pregnancy loss. For example, the child who is born homozygous for achondroplasia (dwarfism with short stature and short limbs) is much more severely affected than a heterozygous child and usually will not survive early infancy.

TABLE 3–1 Selected Genetic Conditions Inherited in a Mendelian Pattern

GENETIC CONDITION	DESCRIPTION	INHERITANCE PATTERN
Achondroplasia	Abnormal bone growth resulting in short stature	Autosomal dominant More than 80% of cases represent a new mutation
Beta-thalassemia	Reduced synthesis of hemoglobin A resulting in anemia	Autosomal recessive
Cystic fibrosis	Complex multisystem disease leading to end-stage lung disease	Autosomal recessive
Duchenne muscular dystrophy	Progressive disease leading to atrophy of skeletal and/or cardiac muscle	X-linked recessive
Fragile X syndrome	Minimal-to-moderate intellectual disability due to trinucleotide repeat expansion	X-linked recessive Anticipation is demonstrated
Gaucher disease	Several subtypes, but all are lipid storage diseases due to enzyme deficiency	Autosomal recessive
Hemophilia A	Bleeding disorder due to deficient factor VIII clotting activity	X-linked recessive About 30% of cases represent a new mutation
Marfan syndrome	Connective tissue disorder with cardiovascular, ocular, and skeletal involvement	Autosomal dominant 25% of cases represent a new mutation
Neurofibromatosis (NF-1)	Variable expression with café au lait spots and benign cutaneous and subcutaneous neurofibromas	Autosomal dominant 50% of cases represent a new mutation
Phenylketonuria (PKU)	Enzyme deficiency results in accumulation of phenylalanine, inhibiting brain and cognitive development	Autosomal recessive
Sickle cell disease	Abnormal hemoglobin causes vaso-occlusive events and chronic anemia	Autosomal recessive
Tay-Sachs disease	Fatal neurodegenerative disorder of lipid accumulation due to enzyme deficiency	Autosomal recessive

Source: Information adapted from Online Mendelian Inheritance in Man (OMIM). Retrieved March 14, 2014, from http://omim.org/

Inheritance Risk in Autosomal Dominant Conditions.   Because the gene alteration in AD conditions occurs on an autosome rather than a sex chromosome, both males and females have an equal chance of being affected. There is a 50% chance that an affected parent will pass the altered disease-producing gene on to a child. Nurses must remember and teach families that each pregnancy is an independent event with a 50% chance of an affected child, no matter how many of a couple's previous children inherited the altered gene. Family histories will often reflect this 50% inheritance rate as well as both males and females being affected. An affected child always has an affected parent, who in turn also has an affected parent (Figure 3–3). Exceptions to this inheritance pattern occur when the condition is due to a spontaneous new mutation, as discussed later in this chapter.

AUTOSOMAL RECESSIVE

Autosomal recessive (AR) conditions occur when both copies of the same gene in an individual are altered. Generally, AR conditions are more severe and have an earlier onset than conditions with other patterns of inheritance. Examples of AR conditions include cystic fibrosis, sickle cell disease, Tay-Sachs disease, and most inborn errors of metabolism. Like autosomal dominant disorders, AR conditions involve genes on one of the 22 autosomes. A condition is called "recessive" when two altered copies of a gene are needed to express the condition. A child born with a recessive condition has therefore inherited one altered gene from each parent. Both parents are **carriers** of the condition. Usually carriers do not exhibit signs or symptoms; however, exceptions to this general rule are increasingly being discovered. Sickle cell

disease (SCD) provides an example: Although individuals with a single copy of the altered gene are usually asymptomatic, they can develop symptoms in situations of extreme physical exertion, dehydration, or high altitude (Bender & Seibel, 2014). The heterozygous or carrier state for SCD (known as sickle cell trait) actually affords some evolutionary benefit, because a single copy of the altered gene provides some resistance to malaria. Individuals

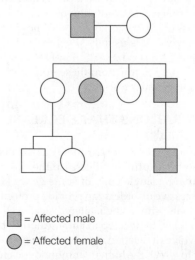

= Affected male

= Affected female

Figure 3–3   **Autosomal dominant pedigree: One parent is affected. Statistically, 50% of offspring will be affected, regardless of gender.**

whose ancestors are from malaria-endemic areas are therefore more likely to carry an altered sickle cell gene. See *Developing Cultural Competence: Ancestral or Ethnic Groups and Autosomal Recessive Inheritance.* Because carrier status usually confers no symptoms, parents are often unaware of their carrier status until they have an affected child.

Developing Cultural Competence Ancestral or Ethnic Groups and Autosomal Recessive Inheritance

Because the prevalence of autosomal recessive conditions varies around the globe, certain recessive genetic conditions are more common in particular populations. This is why nurses should ask about the country of origin of an individual's ancestors when collecting a family history. In populations in which individuals tend to marry within their own community or even their own extended family, autosomal recessive conditions are especially common. This is known as the "founder effect." For example, Ellis-van Creveld syndrome, an inherited condition in which polydactyly (extra fingers) and other structural defects occur, is commonly found among the Old Order Amish population of Pennsylvania (OMIM, 2014).

Examples of disorders that occur more frequently in specific populations are as follows.

Ashkenazi Jewish—Tay-Sachs Disease, Gaucher Disease, Cystic Fibrosis

Carrier rates for several autosomal recessive diseases are particularly high in the Ashkenazi (Eastern European) Jewish population. For example, carrier frequency for Tay-Sachs disease and cystic fibrosis are approximately 100 times higher in this group compared to non-Jewish populations. Specific carrier screening is often targeted to individuals of Ashkenazi Jewish descent.

Turkish, Irish, East Asian Populations, Pennsylvania Amish—Phenylketonuria (PKU)

Carrier rates as high as 1 in 26 have been found in Turkish populations. The PKU gene is rare in Japanese, Finnish, Ashkenazi Jewish, and African populations (Mitchell, 2013).

Mediterranean (Italians, Greeks), Middle Eastern, Central and Southeast Asian, Indian, Far East, African—β-Thalassemia

High gene frequency of β-Thalassemia in these populations is most likely related to selective pressure from malaria. The highest incidences are reported in Cyprus and Sardinia (with 12% to 14% carrier rates) and southeast Asia (Origa, 2015).

Northern European—Cystic Fibrosis (CF)

Cystic fibrosis is the most common life-limiting autosomal recessive condition in individuals with Northern European ancestors. Carrier rates among Caucasians in North America are about 1:25, compared to 1:65 for African Americans (Strom et al., 2011).

Sub-Saharan African, Mediterranean, Middle Eastern, Indian, Caribbean, and Populations from Parts of Central and South America—Sickle Cell Disease

The prevalence of sickle cell trait is about 10% among African Americans. Approximately one in every 300 to 500 African American infants born in the United States has sickle cell disease (Bender & Seibel, 2014).

Inheritance Risk in Autosomal Recessive Conditions.   Because AR conditions do not involve genetic material on the sex chromosomes, males and females have an equal chance of inheriting the altered genes and exhibiting the condition. When both parents are carriers of an autosomal recessive gene alteration, each pregnancy presents the same inheritance risks. Each child born to carrier parents has a 25% chance of inheriting two copies of the altered gene and having the condition, a 50% chance of inheriting only one altered gene copy and being a carrier, and a 25% chance of inheriting two unaltered genes and thus neither being affected nor being a carrier (Figure 3–4). Remembering that each pregnancy is an independent event, these probability percentages remain constant with each pregnancy, no matter how many affected or unaffected children a family already has. This is often a difficult concept for parents to grasp, and the nurse should carefully evaluate the parent's level of understanding of this important detail about inheritance.

The transmission percentages stated previously apply when both parents are carriers of an autosomal recessive condition. Percentages will change if only one parent is a carrier or if a parent is homozygous for the condition. The nurse must be able to teach a parent about these simple inheritance percentages.

X-LINKED

X-linked conditions are the result of an altered gene on the X chromosome. Examples include hemophilia A and Duchenne muscular dystrophy. Recall that the sex chromosomes are unevenly represented in males and females. Males, with their single X chromosome, have just one copy of each gene that resides on the X chromosome. Any altered X gene will consequently be expressed in males, because an unaltered allele is not present for "backup." Females have two copies of each X gene, and the unaltered gene generally compensates for an altered allele, making the female a carrier.

Inheritance Risk in X-Linked Conditions.   In families with X-linked disorders, a pattern of maternal transmission is seen. Females who are carriers of X-linked conditions have a 50% chance of passing the altered gene to their offspring. Any daughter who receives the altered gene is likely to receive an unaltered X chromosome from her father and therefore be a carrier like

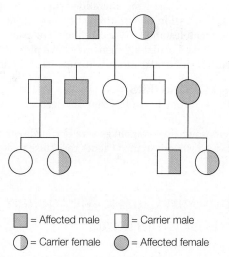

■ = Affected male   ▯ = Carrier male

◯ = Carrier female   ⬤ = Affected female

Figure 3–4 **Autosomal recessive pedigree: Both parents are carriers. Statistically, 25% of offspring will be affected, regardless of gender.**

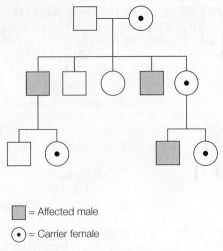

= Affected male

⊙ = Carrier female

Figure 3–5 X-linked recessive pedigree: The mother is the carrier. Statistically, 50% of male offspring will be affected, and 50% of female offspring will be carriers.

her mother. Sons of carrier mothers, however, have no backup X chromosome. Therefore, a son who inherits the altered X will display the condition and go on to pass that altered X to each of his daughters, who will then be carriers of the altered gene. A male can never transmit an altered gene on the X chromosome to his sons, because only Y chromosomes are transmitted from fathers to sons (Figure 3–5).

X Inactivation. Early in embryonic life, within a week of fertilization, one of the X chromosomes inherited by females is inactivated. This process results in equalizing the expression of X-linked genes in the two genders. Each female receives an X chromosome from her mother (maternal X) and one from her father (paternal X). The inactivation of either the maternal or paternal X chromosome is random. However, once that X has been inactivated in any given cell, all the cell's descendants (through mitosis) contain the same inactive X chromosome. Therefore, females are mosaic for X-linked genes; some cells will express genes from the maternal X chromosome, whereas other cells will express genes from the paternal X. Females who inherit altered genes on an X chromosome therefore show variable expression, because the gene alteration will be present in only some cells. Expression of symptoms can vary from extremely mild to a full manifestation of the condition. For example, female carriers of X-linked ocular albinism may have pigment deficiencies of their iris and ocular fundus (Turnpenny & Ellard, 2012).

Y-LINKED DISORDERS

Because the Y chromosome has very few genes, alterations on the Y chromosome are not often associated with health problems. The Y chromosome does contain genes associated with spermatogenesis, and alterations in those genes can cause male infertility (Turnpenny & Ellard, 2012).

Variability in Classic Mendelian Patterns of Inheritance

In addition to classic Mendelian inheritance patterns, nurses must be prepared to help families understand several other concepts that affect risk for inheriting a genetic disorder. These concepts include the following common variations in traditional Mendelian patterns of inheritance.

PENETRANCE

Penetrance is the probability that a gene will be expressed phenotypically. It is an "all or none" concept in that a gene is considered to be penetrant if it is expressed to any degree (Lewis, 2015). Penetrance can be measured in the following way. In a certain group of individuals with the same genotype, what percentage of them will exhibit any signs or symptoms of the condition? If the number is less than 100%, then that condition is said to show *reduced* or *incomplete penetrance*. For example, both achondroplasia and Huntington disease exhibit 100% penetrance, because every individual with one copy of the altered gene will exhibit signs and symptoms of the disease.

VARIABLE EXPRESSIVITY

The term *expressivity* is used to describe the degree to which a phenotype is expressed. When people with the same genetic makeup (genotype) exhibit signs or symptoms with varying degrees of severity, the phenotype is described as showing *variable expression*. Variable expression is common in the autosomal dominant condition neurofibromatosis (NF-1). Although neurofibromatosis has 100% penetrance, members of the same affected family often exhibit variation in degree of signs or symptoms (Friedman, 2014).

NEW MUTATION

When there is no previous family history of a condition, the disease may be caused by a spontaneous new mutation. A new mutation is said to be sporadic, or *de novo*. Mutation rates have been estimated for a number of inherited disorders and vary widely due to a number of factors, only some of which are understood. Diseases with high new mutation rates include neurofibromatosis type 1, achondroplasia, Duchenne muscular dystrophy, and hemophilia A and B. Determining whether a genetic condition is due to an inherited or a *de novo* mutation has important implications in calculating a family's recurrence risk.

ANTICIPATION

Anticipation is said to occur when successive generations in a family exhibit earlier onset of symptoms and more severe signs and symptoms of certain diseases. Anticipation occurs in disorders characterized by unstable repeat expansions, which are DNA sequences that consist of repeating units of three or more nucleotides, for example CAGCAG . . . CAG. Repeat units have a tendency to expand, or accumulate repeats, during meiosis, especially during spermatogenesis. As a result, the number of repeats tends to increase in successive generations. More than a dozen diseases, most neurologic in nature, result from unstable repeat expansions. These include Huntington disease, fragile X syndrome, and myotonic dystrophy (Schaaf, Zschocke, & Potocki, 2012).

IMPRINTING

The expression of a few genetic conditions varies depending on whether the altered gene is inherited from the mother or the father. This differential gene expression is due to genomic imprinting. Imprinting takes place before gametes are formed, when certain genes are chemically marked as having maternal or paternal origin. After conception, the imprint controls gene expression so that only one allele, either maternal or paternal, is expressed. If the unsilenced (active) allele carries a mutation, disease may result. A well-studied example of imprinting involves a deletion in a gene on chromosome 15 that causes two very different disorders depending on whether the altered gene comes from the mother or the father. Prader-Willi syndrome, characterized by hypotonia in infancy, excessive eating habits

TABLE 3–2 Common Birth Defects and Conditions With a Multifactorial Cause

Neural tube defects	A neural tube defect (NTD) is a condition that occurs early during fetal development with incomplete closure of the neural tube. Severity of the disorder varies, depending on which part of the tube does not close. Anencephaly, meningomyelocele, and spina bifida are examples of NTD. Recurrence risk is increased in families with an affected child, but that risk can be modified by maternal dietary folic acid supplementation (Turnpenny & Ellard, 2012).
Congenital heart defects	Most congenital heart defects are thought to be of multifactorial cause. A number of genes have been associated with patent ductus arteriosus, atrial or ventricular septal defects, and other heart defects. In some states, newborn screening for critical congenital heart disease is performed routinely using pulse oximetry (Bradshaw & Martin, 2012).
Cleft lip and palate	Cleft lip and/or palate (CL/P) occur due to failure of bony fusion early in gestation. While rare gene mutations can cause CL/P, most cases are thought to be multifactorial. The more severe the malformation, the higher the family's recurrence risk is for future pregnancies (Tobias, Connor, & Ferguson-Smith, 2011).
Autism spectrum disorder	Although the etiology of autism spectrum disorder remains poorly understood, most experts believe it to be multifactorial. Twin studies suggest a strong genetic component, with 60% to 90% concordance between identical twins. A number of environmental influences have been suspected to influence the development of autism as well, including environmental exposures, viral infections, and maternal stress (Johnson, Giarelli, Lewis, et al., 2013).

leading to obesity, and mild-to-moderate intellectual disability, is due to a deletion on chromosome 15 that is inherited from the father. Angelman syndrome is due to a similar deletion in the same gene on chromosome 15, but it is inherited from the mother. The clinical presentation is very different. Individuals with Angelman syndrome have severe intellectual disability, absent speech, an uncoordinated gait, seizures, and a happy, sociable disposition (Schaaf, Zschocke, & Potocki, 2012).

UNIPARENTAL DISOMY
In cases of uniparental disomy, the child inherits both copies of a chromosome pair (or homologous parts of a chromosome pair) from the same parent instead of one copy from each parent. If there are no altered genes on these chromosomes, the child may not be affected by this event. However, if the chromosomes contain an altered gene for an autosomal recessive disease, the child will receive both altered genes and express the disease. For instance, if a child inherits two altered copies of chromosome 7 from a mother who is a carrier for cystic fibrosis, the child will then exhibit signs and symptoms of cystic fibrosis.

Multifactorial Inheritance
Most inherited traits, such as eye and skin color, are polygenic. That is, they occur as a result of variations on several genes. Most diseases and health conditions are polygenic as well, and the expression of those altered genes is often modified by environmental influences. These are called *multifactorial conditions* and include many birth defects such as cleft lip and palate, pediatric conditions such as autism and asthma, and adult-onset conditions such as cancer and heart disease. Because the term *polygenic* does not imply the influence of the environment, the term *multifactorial* is preferred terminology. The relative contribution of genetic and environmental influences varies across disorders.

Multifactorial conditions aggregate in families but do not follow the characteristic Mendelian patterns of inheritance seen with single-gene conditions. Recurrence risk varies among multifactorial conditions, but is usually less than that of Mendelian conditions. Recurrence risk is calculated from population studies and expressed as a percentage; for some disorders, recurrence risk is not easily predicted. Recurrence risk varies according to the number of affected family members, the degree of relationship, and sometimes the severity of the defect. As examples, the recurrence risk for cleft lip or cleft palate in a family with one

affected child is 4%, whereas recurrence risk for pyloric stenosis is as high as 10% (Turnpenny & Ellard, 2012). See Table 3–2.

Collaborative Care
Many health professionals work together in the screening, diagnosis, identification, and treatment of genetic disorders. The goals of collaborative care are early diagnosis through assessment and testing, development of an effective treatment plan combined with psychosocial support to enhance coping, and referral to a genetic specialist when needed.

Diagnostic Procedures
Genetic testing is available for both chromosomal and gene-based alterations, and the entire landscape of genetic testing is changing rapidly. New methodologies have not only expanded the number of conditions for which genetic testing is available, but, to an even greater degree, reduced the cost. Increasingly, genetic testing is offered directly to consumers, who receive limited counseling about test results. Patients and families are likely to have limited or incorrect understanding about the types of genetic tests available and what information those tests are able and not able to provide, and they may access unreliable sources for information. Further, interpreting results of genetic testing can be complex. As described later in this chapter, a test for cystic fibrosis may be reported as negative, but the significance of that finding depends on how many of the multiple CF-causing mutations were included in the test. The pediatric nurse needs knowledge of available genetic tests and their implications to assist patients and their families as they weigh choices regarding genetic testing. See Box 3–1.

Box 3–1 What Is a Genetic Test?
A genetic test involves the analysis of chromosomes, DNA, RNA, genes, or gene products (e.g., enzymes and other proteins) to detect variations related to disease or health. Whether a laboratory method is considered a genetic test also depends on the intended use, claim, or purpose of a test. For example, amino acid analysis to detect metabolic disorders such as PKU is considered a genetic test, but the use of this same analysis to monitor general nutritional status is not (U.S. Department of Health and Human Services, 2008).

RECOMMENDATIONS FOR GENETIC TESTING

Genetic tests are useful to diagnose disease, predict risk of future disease, inform reproductive decision making, and manage patient care. Guidelines regarding who should be tested and when to test are available for some genetic conditions. However, new knowledge accumulates rapidly, and recommendations for practice often lag behind research findings by several years.

CATEGORIES OF GENETIC TESTS

Genetic tests have been used for some time to detect heritable conditions that are passed from generation to generation. In general, genetic tests are categorized based on their intended use or purpose and the approach or methodology they utilize. Categories of genetic tests according to their purpose are displayed in Table 3–3. Genetic tests may analyze DNA, products of DNA, or other substances that indicate a genetic defect. DNA itself can be analyzed on a number of levels, from karyotyping an entire set of chromosomes to examining a specific gene for a mutation. Tests of DNA products (RNA or proteins) are sometimes done to measure gene function or expression. Some genetic tests measure metabolites that accumulate when individuals lack a specific enzyme due to a gene mutation.

It is especially important for the pediatric nurse to understand the difference between screening tests, which are used in populations to find individuals at risk for a disorder, and diagnostic tests, which are required to make a diagnosis. Newborn screening is carried out on most newborns in developed countries to identify children who may have a genetic disease such as a metabolic or endocrine disease or hemoglobinopathy. Many of these disorders are exceedingly rare. In recent years, a laboratory technique called *tandem mass spectrometry* has allowed greatly expanded newborn screening with little increase in laboratory cost. Issues around expanded newborn screening are of considerable interest, in part due to issues of follow-up. Even the most specific of screening tests will result in false-positive results, which must be followed up with a diagnostic test. The cost of follow-up testing is significant both in terms of parental anxiety and financial burden (DeLuca, Zanni, Bonhomme, et al., 2013). See Chapter 7 for further description of newborn screening.

Diagnostic tests are performed to confirm a diagnosis in a symptomatic child or adult. Diagnostic tests may be ordered when a child is suspected of having a specific disorder based on clinical presentation or screening test results. Sometimes diagnostic testing is carried out prenatally to identify genetic disease such as a trisomy in a fetus.

DIAGNOSING CHROMOSOMAL ALTERATIONS

Cytogenetics describes the microscopic examination of chromosomes to reveal large alterations such as additions, deletions, breaks, and rearrangements or rejoinings (translocations). Prenatally, amniocentesis and chorionic villi sampling (CVS) can be undertaken to provide specimens for cytogenetic examination. After a child is born, chromosomal diagnostic examination can be accomplished with a blood, skin, or buccal cell sample. Cytogenetic testing includes karyotyping, as described earlier in this chapter, and molecular cytogenetic techniques, which are capable of detecting submicroscopic DNA variations too small to be seen on a karyotype.

DIAGNOSING GENE ALTERATIONS

Recent advances in molecular genetic technology along with the mapping of the human genome have resulted in tremendous expansion of available genetic testing. Genetic testing is currently available for more than 4000 disorders, with new tests constantly being added (GeneTests, 2015). DNA-based tests involve sophisticated new technology that permits the detection of DNA sequence changes as small as a single nucleotide. These tests can be performed on blood, bone marrow, amniotic fluid, fibroblast cells of the skin, or buccal cells from the mouth. Genetic testing can examine DNA (to determine specific nucleotide sequence), RNA (to measure gene expression), or proteins (to analyze gene products). Some tests can be performed quickly; others require several days to weeks, or occasionally several months, before results are reported. Test results may be delayed because of the complexities of interpreting test data, rather than delays in the laboratory testing itself.

Genes are very long DNA sequences made up of hundreds of thousands of nucleotides (or base pairs). Alterations at various sites along a gene may alter its function and cause disease. As an example, the *CFTR* gene (which in an altered form causes cystic fibrosis) is 230,000 base pairs long, and nearly 2000 different *CFTR* mutations have been identified (U.S. CF Foundation, 2011). Most of these mutations are exceedingly rare; the most common (named delta F508) is found in about two thirds of affected individuals (Schaaf, Zschocke, & Potocki, 2012). Although DNA testing is capable of detecting any of these alterations in DNA sequence, it is not feasible to test for all of them. Currently available *CFTR* tests detect up to 98 different mutations; most panels test for 23 to 25 mutations. Thus, the chance of missing an uncommon mutation varies, depending on which test is selected. Also, mutation detection rates are higher in patients of European ancestry than other populations. Therefore, a "negative" CF

TABLE 3–3 Categories of Genetic Tests

TYPE OF TEST	DESCRIPTION
Diagnostic testing	Used to establish a diagnosis of a genetic disorder in an individual who is symptomatic or has had a positive screening test.
Prenatal testing	Testing to identify a fetus with a genetic disease or condition. Some prenatal testing is offered routinely; other testing may be initiated due to family history or maternal factors.
Newborn screening	Testing of a newborn to identify babies at risk for a condition that may require immediate initiation of treatment to prevent death or disability.
Preimplantation testing	Following in vitro fertilization (IVF), testing to identify embryos with a particular genetic condition.
Carrier testing	Testing in an asymptomatic individual to identify carrier status for a genetic condition.
Presymptomatic and predictive testing	Offered usually to asymptomatic individuals to detect genetic conditions that occur later in life. • *Presymptomatic testing* detects mutations that, if present, are likely or certain to eventually cause symptoms (an example is Huntington disease). • *Predictive or predispositional testing* detects mutations that increase the likelihood that symptoms will develop (such as *BRCA1* and *BRCA2* testing).

test must be interpreted with caution and an eye on how many mutations were included in the test. This is just one of the limitations of genetic testing that nurses must understand in order to provide genetically competent care. See *The Role of the Nurse in Genetic Testing* later in this chapter.

Tests of gene expression are available as well. For example, **microarray analysis** can detect levels of messenger RNA in cells, which indicates which genes are "turned on" or actively being expressed. Microarray analysis is especially useful to examine tumor cells—for example, to see if an oncogene is being overexpressed and thereby stimulating proliferation of cancer cells.

Other genetic tests examine gene products or metabolites of gene products, rather than the makeup of the gene itself. One example is a biochemical test for PKU. PKU is caused by an alteration in the gene encoding the enzyme phenylalanine hydroxylase (PAH), which breaks down dietary phenylalanine. The PKU test actually measures phenylalanine levels, which are markedly elevated in individuals with PAH deficiency. Many of these biochemical tests have been in use for years.

Quality and Accuracy of Genetic Tests

Genetic nurses express concern that genetic tests are becoming available very quickly with little regulation of the companies offering them. The quality, accuracy, and reliability of genetic test results are not measured against any common standard. Of perhaps greater concern is the interpretation of genetic test results. Even if a test per se is accurate and reliable, companies are free to apply their own criteria to interpret the results. Growth in direct-to-consumer marketing of genetic tests has resulted in increasingly accessible and affordable testing without the benefit of oversight by a healthcare provider. In most cases, little or no education is provided for the individual undergoing testing, nor is counseling or follow-up uniformly provided. Individuals may make hard and irrevocable life-altering decisions after receiving test results, so accuracy and reliability, along with professional counseling, are essential (Beery & Workman, 2012).

Professionalism in Practice ELSI

Since its inception, the National Human Genome Research Institute has designated a percentage of its budget to examining the ethical, legal, and social implications (ELSI) of genetic and genomic information. Genetic testing raises many questions that have been addressed by ELSI. Genetic exceptionalism, the idea that genetic information should be treated differently than other health information, continues to be a subject of great interest and little consensus. Proponents of genetic exceptionalism point out that genetic information is unique and deserving of special consideration and protection because it is predictive, is potentially stigmatizing, and may reveal information about family members other than the patient undergoing testing. The contrasting view points out that other information is also predictive (consider blood cholesterol and risk for cardiovascular disease) and stigmatizing (for example, information about sexually transmitted infections).

Federal health privacy protection, as mandated under the federal Health Insurance Portability and Accountability Act (HIPAA) privacy rule, does not afford special protection to genetic information, treating it as being no more sensitive than other health-related information. However, by 2008 the majority of states had enacted legislation taking the exceptionalist view, providing protection against discrimination based on genetic information and penalties for violating genetic privacy (U.S. Department of Health and Human Services, 2008). These laws were implemented in response to public concerns that individuals might be reluctant to seek potentially beneficial genetic testing without some guarantee about the confidentiality, privacy, and security of that information. For example, an individual may have health coverage for a genetic test but be unwilling to submit the claim due to concerns about the insurance company "owning" the information in the test result. Federal legislation to prohibit discrimination based on genetic information in health insurance and employment (the Genetic Information Nondiscrimination Act, or GINA) was implemented in November 2009. As a federal law, GINA offers protection to Americans in all states.

Nursing Management

By simply integrating genetic and genomic concepts into assessment, observation, and history gathering, the pediatric nurse can improve the standard of care delivered and have a positive impact on the child and family. The pediatric nurse does not need to be a genetic expert, but baseline knowledge and heightened awareness of genetic and genomic issues will support appropriate assessment and referral to genetic specialists as needed.

Family Risk Assessment

GENETIC FAMILY HISTORY

While gathering a family history, the nurse must look for genetic information that might indicate the need for referral to a genetic specialist. Examples that would indicate a family may benefit from a genetic referral include a family history of conditions known or suspected to be genetic, several family members with the same condition, intellectual disability or learning difficulties, dysmorphic features or congenital anomalies, neonatal or pediatric death of unknown cause, recurrent miscarriage, or established genetic carrier status.

PEDIGREES

Pediatric nurses and all other health professionals should know how to collect a three-generation family history, record the history in a pedigree, and "think genetic." Information to document in a family history includes:

- First name of all family members with age or year of birth
- Any medical conditions or diseases, including age at diagnosis
- Age and cause of death
- Infertility or no children by choice
- Pregnancy complications with gestational age indicated
- Adoption status
- Ancestry
- Consanguinity

A **pedigree** is a graphic representation or diagram of a family's medical history and genetic relationships (Figure 3–6). Standard format, nomenclature, and symbols for pedigrees were adopted in 2008 (Bennett, French, Resta, et al., 2008). A pedigree is constructed around a designated "index" patient, called the **proband** (if the patient is affected with the genetic disorder of interest) or **consultand** (if the patient seeks genetic counseling without being known to have the disorder). A finished pedigree provides a clear, visual representation of a family's medical data and biologic relationships at a glance. A pedigree identifies affected individuals in the immediate and extended family and can identify family members who might benefit from a genetic consultation. A pedigree can also illustrate patterns of inheritance and clusters of multifactorial conditions. On the basis of the pedigree, risk assessment, genetic referral and/or reproductive risk teaching for the individual and family can occur. The visual nature of a pedigree enhances a family's learning and can be used to clarify misunderstandings or misconceptions about inheritance. If completed correctly and comprehensively, a pedigree allows all healthcare professionals working with the child or family to quickly see what history and background information has been collected.

All registered nurses, regardless of academic preparation, practice setting, role, or specialty, are expected to be able to elicit a three-generation family history and document that information in the form of a pedigree, using standardized symbols and terminology (Consensus Panel on Genetic/Genomic Nursing Competencies, 2009). It is important to gather a three-generation family pedigree even if the nurse believes this is a first occasion of the condition within a family. A condition without any identifiable inheritance pattern on the pedigree may be due to a new mutation or variable expressivity. Throughout the process of gathering family history assessment data, the nurse must protect family confidentiality at all times. A pedigree is different from a personal health history in that it reflects information about multiple individuals, which greatly increases the risk for harm if confidentiality is broken. A pedigree may reveal sensitive details that include infertility problems, reproductive decisions, or incorrectly assigned paternity that may not be known by a current partner or other family members. Other sensitive issues include pregnancies conceived by technology, a history of suicides, drug or alcohol abuse, and same-sex relationships.

Challenges inherent in recalling the family history include the parents' inability to remember conditions that have been surgically repaired and then forgotten. Parents may fail to report conditions thought not to be genetic or that have been attributed incorrectly to other causes. Also, parents may be reluctant to reveal sensitive information, particularly information unknown to other family members.

Instructions for creating a pedigree from family history information are beyond the scope of this text but are readily available online. See the National Human Genome Research Institute's website. Nurses should be able to identify and access resources for pedigree construction for their own use or for families to use. In fact, families are encouraged to collect and record their own family history in a form that can be shared within the family as well as with healthcare providers. The U.S. Surgeon General's Family History Initiative is a national campaign to promote the collection of family histories. The Initiative provides a web-based program that allows individuals to easily record and save their information, as well as print their family pedigree (http://www.hhs.gov/familyhistory/).

GENETIC PHYSICAL ASSESSMENT

The pediatric nurse in any healthcare setting should also "think genetic" when performing physical assessment (see Chapter 5). An early finding by the nurse will provide the child and family with an opportunity for a genetic referral and more specialized health care.

Major and Minor Anomalies

Dysmorphology refers to the study of human congenital defects or abnormalities of body structure that begin before birth. Traditionally, congenital anomalies have been included under the umbrella of genetic disorders whether they occur due to a gene alteration or another cause of abnormal embryonic or fetal development. Dysmorphic anomalies can occur anywhere in the body, but are perhaps most often associated with facial features. As a routine part of patient assessment, the nurse should screen for both minor and major anomalies. A **minor anomaly** or malformation is an unusual morphologic feature that in itself is of no serious medical or cosmetic concern to the individual or family. The presence of a single minor anomaly is relatively common, occurring in approximately 10% of newborns, and is usually of no consequence (Turnpenny & Ellard, 2012). Some minor anomalies

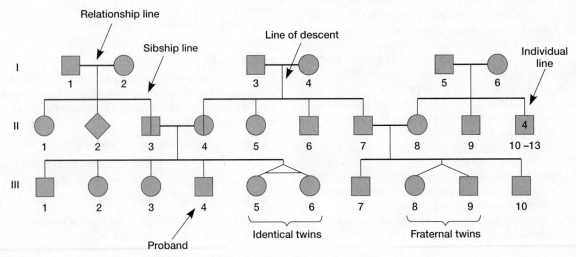

Figure 3–6 **Sample three-generation pedigree.**

are merely family traits or are present in certain ethnic groups. Minor anomalies include such traits as wide-set eyes, single palmar creases, café au lait patches, low anterior hairline, preauricular (in front of the ears) pits and tags, broad face, or mild proportionate short stature. Examples of variations associated with ethnic origin include upward-slanting eyes or prominent epicanthal folds among individuals of Asian descent.

The appearance of multiple minor anomalies in an infant is of greater concern. Fewer than 1% of newborns have two minor anomalies, and fewer still have three or more. But of those infants who do have multiple minor anomalies, many will also have a major anomaly or an underlying genetic condition. Therefore, the nurse who notes multiple minor anomalies in a newborn or child should consider the possibility of a major anomaly or an underlying genetic condition and advocate for a genetic referral. For example, a newborn who is hypotonic and has a single palmar crease with up-slanting eyes that do not resemble his parent's eyes should be evaluated for Down syndrome.

About 2% to 3% of all children have a **major anomaly**, defined as a serious structural defect present at birth that may have severe medical or cosmetic consequences, interfere with normal functioning of body systems, lead to a lifelong disability, or even cause an early death. Congenital heart defects, cleft lip and/or palate, myelomeningocele, duodenal atresia, and craniosynostosis are considered major anomalies, as is developmental disability. Some major anomalies are present at birth but are not apparent, such as deafness, various skeletal dysplasias, and some types of congenital heart defects (Turnpenny & Ellard, 2012).

A **syndrome** is a collection of multiple anomalies, major or minor, that occur in a consistent pattern and have a common cause. For example, Down syndrome is the cause of a variety of anomalies that can appear in multiple body systems, including the eyes, ears, hair, mouth and tongue, heart, and brain. A **sequence** is a collection of anomalies that occur as a chain of events initiated by a single problem. As an example, Potter sequence begins with prenatal failure of renal development, which leads to small amounts of amniotic fluid, which in turn causes growth restriction. An **association** is a group of abnormalities of unknown cause that occur together more often than is expected by chance (Schaaf, Zschocke, & Potocki, 2012).

The nurse can identify clues to genetic problems by examining the child and considering the physical characteristics of the parents and other family members (see *Assessment Guide: The Child With Selected Dysmorphic Physical Features*). Nurses may even ask to look at family photographs and examine them for common dysmorphic features and family traits. Several standardized craniofacial measurements have been defined, and tables are available displaying normal values according to age, so that dysmorphic facial features are more easily identified (Figure 3–7). By advocating for a genetic referral, the pediatric nurse can make a difference in the child's state of health.

THE ROLE OF THE NURSE IN GENETIC TESTING

Many people have misconceptions about genetic testing. Nurses play an important role in teaching parents and children about the implications and limitations of genetic tests to ensure that they make informed decisions. The nurse should promote communication, autonomy, and privacy when helping families. Recognizing that genetic testing affects families, and not just individuals, the nurse should use a family perspective when assisting parents and children who are making decisions about genetic testing. Not all family members will want to know their genetic risks. All voices should be heard, and each family member's decision

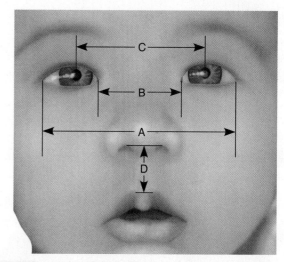

Figure 3–7 **Classic facial measurements for genetic assessment with a focus on facial features.** *A*, **Outer intercanthal distance.** *B*, **Intercanthal distance.** *C*, **Interpupillary distance.** *D*, **Philtrum length.**

should be respected, whether it is to participate in genetic testing or to decline. To ensure autonomy, a nondirective approach is critical. Nurses must take care to avoid imposing their own values or personal opinions onto patients and families. Finally, as with all aspects of delivering genetic nursing care, privacy and confidentiality are paramount.

Genetic Testing Issues of Minors

In order to support, advocate for, and educate children, adolescents, and their families, the pediatric nurse must have knowledge of issues related to genetic testing of minor children. Parents may request genetic testing for their minor children without foreseeing the consequences associated with a positive finding. Nurses have a critical role in providing information and anticipatory guidance for families considering genetic testing.

The primary focus of genetic testing in children is to promote the child's well-being, and guidelines generally recommend that genetic testing in children only be conducted if the results would affect medical management soon after testing. With this in mind, nurses should help families to clearly understand why a genetic test is being done.

In general, four reasons have been suggested to consider genetic testing of minors. The first is if the testing offers an immediate medical benefit for the child in terms of disease prevention or early treatment. Newborn screening is an example of testing designed to promote the health of children, and consensus statements by several professional groups support mandatory offering of newborn screening for all children (Ross, Saal, David, et al., 2013). Diagnostic genetic testing for children with symptoms of a genetic condition is also broadly supported, because establishing a diagnosis informs health management for the child as well as reproductive decision making by the family. Predictive testing in asymptomatic children for conditions that cause morbidity at a young age or for specific health promotion, screening, or treatment is also recommended. An example is familial adenomatous polyposis (FAP). Children with a family history of FAP should be tested for the altered gene, because screening by colonoscopy is recommended for affected individuals during adolescence (Munck, Gargouri, Alberti, et al., 2011). Genetic counseling and informed consent are essential prior to predictive genetic testing in minors (Ross et al., 2013).

ASSESSMENT GUIDE | The Child With Selected Dysmorphic Physical Features*

Skull	Asymmetric head/face	Fontanels too large or small
	Brachycephaly (short, broad head shape) (see Figure 27–11)	Frontal bossing (prominent central forehead)
		Microcephaly or macrocephaly
	Craniosynostosis (premature closing of skull sutures)	Micrognathia (small jaw)
	Flattened or prominent occiput	Prognathism (projection of jaw beyond that of the forehead)
Extremities	Abnormally positioned feet	Hypoplastic (very small) or absent nails
	Arachnodactyly (long fingers or toes)	Hypotonia (diminished muscle tone)
	Brachydactyly (short fingers or toes)	Loose joints
	Camptodactyly (permanent flexion of fingers or toes)	Polydactyly (extra fingers and/or toes)
	Clinodactyly (curved fingers or toes, most often the fifth finger)	Rocker bottom feet
		Single transverse palmar crease (see Figure 5–33)
	Edema of the hands or feet	Syndactyly (webbing between fingers and toes)
	Extremely long/thin or short extremities	
Ears	Ear tags or pits	Hearing loss
	Ears that are posteriorly rotated	Low-set or malformed ears
Hair	Excessive body hair	Large section of white hair in otherwise pigmented hair
	Unusual hairline or hair distribution	Sparse or brittle hair
Eyes	Blue sclera	Extreme myopia (nearsightedness)
	Different colored eyes	Hypertelorism (widely spaced eyes)
	Down-slanting eyes	Hypotelorism (closely spaced eyes)
	Epicanthal folds inconsistent with ethnicity (see Figure 5–7)	Short palpebral fissures (distance between inner and outer canthus of eyes)
	Extreme hyperopia (farsightedness)	Up-slanting eyes (see Figure 5–8)
Skin	Axillary freckling (see Figure 27–12)	Hirsutism (excessive hair)
	Café au lait spots (see Figure 27–12)	Hyperelastic skin
	Excessive skin	Leaf-shaped white markings
	Extremely loose or thin skin	Syndactyly (webbing between fingers and toes)
Mouth	Cleft lip with or without cleft palate (see Figure 25–1)	Early loss of teeth
	Large or small tongue	Late eruption of teeth
	Misshapen, missing, or extra teeth	Smooth or abnormal philtrum
		Thin upper lip
Other	Abdominal wall defect	Seizures
	Ambiguous genitalia	Short, webbed neck
	Cryptorchidism (undescended testicle)	Single umbilical artery
	Hernia (inguinal or umbilical)	Small or widely spaced nipples
	Hypospadias	Multiple fractures
	Hypogonadism	Unusual cry (catlike/mewing, hoarse, weak)
	Obesity	Unusually tall or short stature
	Scoliosis	Webbed neck

*This list is not all-inclusive but is meant to increase the nurse's awareness of assessment findings that may be significant and require a referral to a genetic specialist.

A second kind of situation occurs when an adolescent is facing a reproductive decision of his or her own. If the adolescent has a family history of a genetic condition, the individual might be interested in genetic testing such as carrier screening that offers no specific medical benefit to the adolescent other than family planning. Recall Sarah, the young woman in the opening scenario who wanted to be tested for Huntington disease. Might genetic testing affect her reproductive decisions?

A third situation occurs when a parent or child requests predictive genetic testing for future planning in the absence of any immediate benefit. This situation may arise with inherited adult-onset disorders such as Huntington disease, certain cancers, or familial (early-onset) Alzheimer disease. An older child who has a relative with such a disorder may wish to know whether he or she carries the altered gene to plan for a life career or to make relationship decisions such as marriage. Parents sometimes request predictive or carrier testing for their children who are well below reproductive age. In the genetics community, there is widespread consensus that predictive genetic testing for minors in the absence of targeted preventive, surveillance, or treatment interventions should be deferred until a child reaches the age of majority (Ross et al., 2013). In most states that age is 18 years.

Finally, a family member may request genetic testing for a child when the test results are entirely for the benefit of another family member, with no direct benefit to the child. This may occur during DNA linkage studies, in which multiple blood samples from both affected and unaffected individuals within a family are analyzed and compared to identify a specific DNA alteration for diagnosing a genetic condition in that particular family. Another example is genetic testing for the purpose of human leukocyte antigen (HLA) matching prior to stem cell donation. Because HLA-matched siblings are often preferred as stem cell donors, parents may request this testing, which offers no clinical benefit for the child but may benefit immediate family members. Such testing is supported by consensus in pediatric and genetic communities (Ross et al., 2013).

In recent years, advances in genomic knowledge and increasing availability of genomic testing have blurred the issues around testing in minors. Consider, for example, carrier screening. It is generally agreed that when carrier status is identified on newborn screening, those results should be communicated to the family (Ross et al., 2013). While routine carrier testing when carrier status has no medical relevance during minority is not recommended, carrier screening may be appropriate for adolescents under certain circumstances. Examples are sickle cell trait screening for some athletes and carrier screening for adolescents who are pregnant or considering reproduction. Predispositional testing, which can be ordered direct-to-consumer (i.e., without benefit of professional guidance), is also complex. Consider a child who is tested and found to have a genetic predisposition to type 2 diabetes. Typically, the disease risk is moderately elevated—perhaps two to three times the population risk. Does knowledge of that genetic test have immediate medical benefit for the child? Does the potential benefit outweigh any harm that may accompany the knowledge? Issues such as these are of great interest in genomic medicine, but clear guidelines have yet to be established.

The pediatric nurse must be aware of these potential situations and know that decisions to perform genetic tests on children and adolescents are not made easily. Unless the potential benefits of testing outweigh the potential harms to the child, a genetic test is not justified and should be postponed until the child is capable of making an informed decision. Amidst a rapidly changing landscape of genomic testing, and recognizing the difficult issues and lack of consensus around genetic testing in children and minors, the genetics community is working to develop standardized practice recommendations to guide clinical decision making (Ross et al., 2013).

Communication with the child and family about genetic testing should include an assessment of the positive and negative outcomes of the test. Are there existing treatments for the condition being tested? What are the potential psychologic issues associated with a positive or negative test? Who will be affected by the test results? Will the test results be shared with extended family members? The nurse has an important role in educating adolescents and parents about issues around genetic testing to ensure that they are making informed decisions. The nurse should also consider the decision-making ability of the child. There is little consensus regarding the age at which children may be able to take part in a decision-making process involving genetic testing, and it is imperative for the nurse to be an advocate for the child.

Ensuring Informed Consent for Genetic Testing

The pediatric nurse is responsible for alerting children and their families of their right to make an informed decision prior to *any* genetic testing, with consideration of the special circumstances arising from the family's social, cultural, and community life. All genetic testing should be voluntary, and it is the nurse's responsibility to ensure that the consent process includes discussion of the risks and benefits of the test, including potential physical or psychological harm or societal injury due to stigmatization or discrimination. Ross and colleagues (2013) suggest using a consent process similar to that conducted before an elective medical procedure. Providing informed consent involves more than just presenting a form and asking patients to sign; rather, nurses must ensure patients fully understand both the process of the testing and potential implications (Badzek, Henaghan, Turner, et al., 2012). For example, tests may reveal unexpected genetic alterations unrelated to the indication for which the test was ordered, and the management of such **incidental findings** should be explained during the consent process. The nurse should be aware that health insurance policies may not cover genetic testing, which is often very expensive. Even if the insurance benefit will cover the test, and despite protections afforded by law, many individuals are fearful of discrimination based on genetic test results that are included in their medical record. The pediatric nurse should inform the child and the family of their right to know who will have access to the genetic test results.

Ensuring Confidentiality and Privacy for Genetic Testing

Issues of confidentiality and privacy are of particular concern when genetic information is involved. Results of genetic tests can be far reaching beyond usual concerns about health information. Tests may reveal information about other family members who did not consent to testing and who may not want to know (or have other family members know) that information. Current legal protection of genetic information is limited to health insurance and employment, but other concerns remain. Can genetic information be released to the courts, military, schools, or adoption agencies? Would a child with a known gene alteration for Huntington disease be offered a college scholarship for the best law school? The technology that has made genetic testing possible has far outpaced the ability of health policy makers and legislators to put in place systems to protect genetic information. Not only should nurses be diligent about protecting patients' genetic information but they should also discuss with patients and families the potential implications when sensitive test results are shared, either intentionally or inadvertently. Such anticipatory guidance is a key nursing role in patient advocacy (Consensus Panel on Genetic/Genomic Nursing Competencies, 2009).

Psychosocial Issues

Pediatric nurses must be prepared to assist children and families to manage anxiety related to genetic testing. Uncertainty and stress associated with making a decision to undertake genetic testing may extend into weeks or even months before results are available. That stress may be increased or relieved once test results are known. Although receiving favorable test results may decrease anxiety for the family or the individual, problems may occur and the pediatric nurse must be prepared to address them. For example, concerns about carrier status may interfere with development of intimacy and interpersonal relationships. A positive test result may lead to feelings of unworthiness or disturbed self-image. Survivor guilt may affect children with negative results if their siblings test positive. Younger children may blame themselves, thinking they did or said something to cause the gene alteration. The adolescent carrying a gene alteration for a late-onset disease may have an increased tendency for risky behaviors. The adolescent who has inherited an altered disease-producing gene may foster resentment toward the parent who carries the altered gene. Parental guilt may exist for passing the altered gene to the child. Finally, parent–child bonds may be altered if parents become either overprotective or overly permissive. The parent and other family members may unconsciously form lowered expectations for the child or adolescent. Nurses must use counseling interventions to assist patients to process, adjust to, and use genetic information.

Planning and Implementation

The pediatric nurse is responsible for comprehensively delivering the standard of care to children and families, while being aware of limitations of his or her own knowledge and expertise (Consensus Panel on Genetic/Genomic Nursing Competencies, 2009). Although nurses without specialized training and credentialing in genetics are not expected to assume the role of genetic professionals, they do have critical roles in providing genomic health care. Often, nurses have more direct patient interaction than other health professionals and maintain a particularly high level of trust with patients. Nurses therefore are well positioned to recognize a patient or family who may be at increased risk for a genetic condition. In general, nurses are expected to (1) integrate genetic and genomic concepts into a comprehensive nursing assessment including documenting that history in the form of a pedigree, (2) recognize significant genomic information in the family history, (3) apply knowledge of local or regional services to explain available genetic services to patients, and (4) facilitate a genetic referral when appropriate (Consensus Panel on Genetic/Genomic Nursing Competencies, 2009; Jacobs & Patch, 2013).

GENETIC REFERRALS AND COUNSELING

After gathering assessment data that incorporate genetic concepts, the pediatric nurse is able to partner with children and their families by initiating a referral to genetic specialists if there are indicators for a genetic referral (see Clinical Tip). The nurse should provide the family with information about the advantages of a referral to a genetic specialist and the disadvantages of not following through with the referral. The nurse should inform the child and family that a genetic referral can provide information and answer questions they may have concerning genetic health. Families should be encouraged to address all their concerns with the genetic specialist, who will be able to answer questions regarding genetic conditions, inheritance, availability of treatment, and economic, insurance, and future implications of genetic conditions. Initiating or facilitating the referral of a child with a suspected genetic problem to a geneticist, genetic clinical nurse specialist, or genetic clinic is an expected nursing responsibility in the same way as referrals to a dietitian or a social worker. When in doubt, the pediatric nurse should contact the advanced practice genetic clinical nurse, genetic counselor, or geneticist to discuss concerns.

Clinical Tip

The following are indications for pediatric referral to a genetic specialist:

- If the child or family reports a known or "believed" genetic condition in the family
- Single major or multiple minor congenital anomalies
- Dysmorphic features that are not familial
- Developmental delay or regression
- A known or suspected metabolic disorder
- Speech problems
- Learning disability
- Failure to thrive
- Delays in physical growth, unusual body proportions, or low muscle tone
- Abnormal or delayed development of secondary sex characteristics or sex organs
- Extremely short or tall stature
- Blindness or cataracts in infants or children
- Deafness
- Hypotonia in an infant or child
- Seizures in newborns or infants
- Skin lesions such as café au lait spots

FAMILY PREPARATION FOR GENETIC REFERRALS AND GENETIC COUNSELING

Not knowing what to expect from a genetic referral is common, and fear of the unknown may cause anxiety for both the child and family. To facilitate a genetic referral to genetic specialists, the pediatric nurse should educate the child and family so they know what to expect during and after a genetic evaluation.

Usually before the first genetic evaluation visit, the parents will be contacted to provide a detailed medical and family history and to make an appointment for genetic consultation. The parent should be prepared to give as exact a family history as possible so that a detailed three-generation pedigree can be constructed. The parents should be informed that a genetic consultation can last several hours. During the appointment, a genetic clinical nurse, genetic counselor, and/or physician will perform an initial interview with the parents and their child. A geneticist will examine the child and possibly the parent(s) in order to establish an accurate diagnosis. Tests may be ordered. These may include chromosome analysis, DNA-based testing, radiographs, biopsy, biochemical tests, developmental testing, or linkage studies.

After the exam and the completion of any applicable testing, the geneticist or genetic counselor will discuss the findings with the parents and/or child and make recommendations. The discussion will include the natural history of the condition, its pattern of inheritance, current preventive or treatment options, and risks to the child or family. The visit will include opportunities for questions and answers and assessment and evaluation of the family's understanding. It is typical for information retention to be very low for a family facing a new genetic diagnosis. This makes it imperative for the nurse to reinforce genetic concepts at a later time when the individual or family is ready.

As the visit concludes, the child and parents can expect that appropriate referrals will be made, available services will be discussed, and a follow-up visit may be scheduled. A summary of the information is usually sent to the family. The child's healthcare provider will receive a report if requested by the individual or parents.

Genetic healthcare providers present the individual and the family with information to promote informed decisions. They are also sensitive to the importance of protecting the individual's autonomy. A challenge during any visit to a genetic specialist is in providing nondirective counseling. Families should be permitted to make decisions that are not influenced by any biases or values from the nurse, counselor, or geneticist. Many families are accustomed to practitioners and nurses providing direction and guidance in their decision making, and families may be uncomfortable with a nondirectional approach. They might believe that the nurse or healthcare provider is withholding very bad news. Health professionals should present all indicated options and discuss the positive and negative aspects of each option, employing therapeutic listening and communication skills.

FAMILY TEACHING

The pediatric nurse must be aware of available genetic resources and participate in education about genetic disorders and health promotion and prevention. Informing children and their families of what to expect from a genetic referral and clarifying and reinforcing information obtained during a genetic referral or genetic test results are also important.

Cultural and religious beliefs and values of the individual and family must be assessed by the nurse prior to teaching. Gene alterations may be viewed as uncontrollable, as occurring secondary to cultural beliefs such as a stranger looking at the infant, or as a "punishment." A family's readiness to learn can be influenced by cultural or religious beliefs and values. Obtaining educational materials in the primary language of the child or family will help facilitate the teaching–learning experience.

The nurse must be aware of common inheritance misconceptions such as a parent's belief that with a 25% recurrence risk, after one child is affected the next three children will be unaffected, or with a 50% recurrence risk every other child will be affected. The recurrence risk *for each pregnancy* should be continually stressed by the nurse. Families often believe that certain family members have inherited a genetic condition because they look like or "take after" a relative with a genetic condition. When new gene alterations or mutations are found or even discussed, families will often express surprise. Because no one else in the family has the condition, they perceive the trait or condition cannot be inherited. Helping families understand basic, relevant genetic concepts is fundamental to delivering competent genetic nursing care.

Psychosocial Care

In order to provide holistic care, the nurse should identify the psychosocial needs and expectations of the child and family, as well as their cultural, spiritual, value, and belief systems. Denial of a genetic diagnosis is common, and nurses must be aware of the family's state of acceptance. Nurses must often help alleviate anxiety or guilt in the child or family. Anxiety related to uncertainty is common when awaiting diagnosis or test results, but individuals also experience anxiety from not understanding the future implications of a confirmed genetic disease. Guilt may be associated with knowledge of a genetic condition being "in the family." It is important for the nurse to reassure parents that the genetic condition is not the result of something they did or did not do during pregnancy. The nurse should encourage open discussion and free expression of fears and concerns. Guilt and shame are common as a family deals with the loss of the expectation and dream of a healthy child, grandchild, niece, or nephew. Reinforce to parents that genetic alterations are caused by changes within a gene and not by superstitions related to sin or other cultural beliefs. As mothers, fathers, and extended family members provide continuous care for the individual with a genetic condition, depression can result. Depression can also occur in the individual with the condition. The nurse must maintain awareness of the possibility of depression and be proactive in obtaining support for the individual or family. See Chapter 28.

The nurse also is responsible for assessing the family's coping mechanisms and available family, spiritual, cultural, and community support systems. The nurse can refer the individual or family to a support group; however, it is important to have permission from the child or family before providing a support group with their names and contact information. Electronic sources of genetic information abound and are unregulated; many of them are proprietary, offering expensive genetic testing that may have little scientific basis. Nurses should help families select and evaluate credible websites and online discussion groups.

Another key role for the nurse is to help families with the often difficult task of communicating genetic information such as inheritance patterns to extended family members. Cultural values of autonomy and privacy come into play when a person considers whether to communicate genetic information to extended family members who may also carry the altered gene. Family members often have difficulty understanding that some genetic conditions have variable expressivity. Members of the extended family often feel shock and profound guilt upon learning that they carry the gene alteration that has caused their loved one to have a genetic condition.

Managing Care Through Advocacy

The pediatric nurse must continually advocate for the child and family and support their decisions even if the decisions contradict the nurse's own ideals and morals. Therefore, careful self-assessment of feelings is essential for nurses to recognize when their own attitudes and values may affect care (Consensus Panel on Genetic/Genomic Nursing Competencies, 2009). Coping with genetic revelations and making genetic-related treatment decisions are difficult activities for everyone. The nurse must remember that families will need resources and support and also help in gathering information about reproductive options.

Evaluation

Expected outcomes of delivering nursing care with a genetic focus include:

- The child and family will make informed and voluntary decisions related to genetic health issues.

- The child and family will accurately identify:

  - Basic genetic concepts and simple inheritance risk probabilities

  - What to expect from a genetic referral

  - The influence of genetic factors in health promotion and health maintenance

  - Social, legal, and ethical issues related to genetic testing

Visions for the Future

Nurses are often the primary caregivers to whom children and their families turn for information, guidance, and clarification of ideas. Genetic and genomic competency among nurses is essential, not only to provide direct care but also to function as informed members of the community and greater society. As advances in genome science are increasingly translated to health care, the role of nurses not only remains vital but also increases in breadth. For example, the Precision Medicine Initiative, launched in the United States in 2015, aims to tailor health care to people's unique characteristics, including their personal genome (Collins & Varmus, 2015). Precision medicine will target care, including health promotion and disease prevention plans, pharmacotherapeutics, and cancer treatment, based on each person's unique genome. Genome-based care is anticipated to expand genetic testing and include new interventions such as gene therapy. As genomic health care becomes the standard of care, the nurse's role expands not only to delivering that care, but also to explaining the care and the implications of care to clients and families. Nurses must acquire foundational understanding of genetic and genomic concepts, maintain currency as genomic discovery is translated to practice, and be ready to discuss trends and changes with children, adolescents, and their families.

Chapter Highlights

- All diseases and health conditions have both genetic and environmental influences.

- Recent advances in genome science are expected to transform health care to "precision" care, which applies genomic knowledge about an individual to individualize health care.

- Nurses are expected to achieve competency in delivering genome-based care.

- Human DNA is organized into 46 chromosomes—44 autosomes and 2 sex chromosomes, which contain about 21,000 genes.

- Errors in chromosome number (aneuploidy) or chromosome structure (e.g., deletions) can impair health.

- Having the correct amount of DNA is critical to health; in most cases, having an extra or a missing chromosome is lethal.

- Large chromosomal alterations can be seen in a karyotype; very small alterations can be detected using molecular methods.

- The primary function of the human genome, which contains about 21,000 genes, is to encode proteins that carry out all physiologic functions.

- Different forms of a gene that occupy the same place on a pair of chromosomes are alleles. Humans normally have two alleles for each gene—one inherited from each parent.

- More than 99% of DNA sequence (i.e., the order of the A-T-C-G bases) is identical between individuals.

- Errors or mutations in DNA can disrupt health by encoding faulty proteins that do not function as expected, by causing too much or too little of a protein to be formed, or by causing a protein to be formed at the wrong time during development.

- When both alleles for particular gene function the same, the individual is said to be homozygous for that gene; if the alleles function differently, the individual is heterozygous for the gene.

- Single-gene (Mendelian) diseases are typically rare and occur when specific genes are altered; environmental influences usually contribute minimally to the disease process.

- Complex (multifactorial) diseases and health conditions are common and usually occur when multiple gene alterations collectively increase or disease risk; environmental influences usually have significant impact, which can increase risk or be protective.

- Most DNA is located in the cell nucleus, but mitochondria also have a small amount of DNA that encodes proteins critical to energy production. Mitochondrial DNA is inherited from the mother.

- Single-gene conditions follow Mendelian patterns of inheritance; multifactorial conditions do not.

- Several types of genetic tests are available and vary in intended use, implications, and limitations.

- The nurse must be aware of the ethical, social, legal, cultural, and spiritual issues related to the delivery of genetic care.

- A federal law (GINA) offers special protections regarding genetic information in the areas of health care and employment.

- A genetic pedigree is a graphic representation of a family's medical history that is used increasingly as a screening tool to identify people who may be at increased risk for disease.

- All registered nurses should be able to elicit and depict a three-generation family health history in the form of a genetic pedigree, using standard format, symbols, and terminology.

- Congenital anomalies may indicate a genetic condition is present, and nurses should carefully assess newborns and children for dysmorphic features.

- Nurses have an important role in educating clients about genetic testing, promoting informed decision making, and obtaining informed consent.

- Genetic testing of minors has particular implications that require careful consideration.

- Basic genetic nursing involves initiating a referral to genetic specialists.

- Providing psychosocial support is a critical part of genome-based nursing care.

Clinical Reasoning in Action

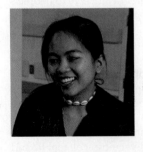

Recall 16-year-old Sarah from the chapter-opening scenario. While at the sports clinic for a routine physical, she questions the nurse about being tested for Huntington disease. Huntington disease (HD) is a progressive disorder of motor, cognitive, and psychiatric disturbances. Symptoms typically present between ages 35 and 44 years, with a median survival time of 15 to 18 years after onset. HD is inherited in an autosomal dominant pattern. Sarah's maternal grandfather died from HD. Sarah has been reading about HD and is

interested in being tested. Her mother strongly objects; she does not want to know her own Huntington status.

Sarah's mother, Diane, is of western European Caucasian descent. Sarah's knowledge about her father is limited. She knows that he is a third-generation Filipino American but has no medical information on him or his extended family.

Sarah's grandmother on her mother's side has three sisters and two brothers. The two brothers died of myocardial infarctions at the ages of 37 and 55 years, respectively. Sarah's maternal grandfather had no brothers but had two sisters. Her maternal grandfather died at age 62 years of Huntington disease. The sisters are alive and well and have no medical problems.

Diane has two brothers and two sisters. She is the youngest of the siblings. Her oldest brother, Ken, was diagnosed 10 years ago with Huntington disease at age 41 years. Ken has two daughters ages 21 and 25 years. Sarah is very close to these cousins, and she knows that they have no medical problems beyond seasonal allergies and migraine headaches. Diane's other brother, Brian (age 38 years), has recently had bouts of depression and has noticed slight difficulties in coordination and involuntary movements. Brian and his wife, Sally, adopted a son, Dave, with Down syndrome, and he is 19 years old. Sarah's brother is age 12 years and does not have any medical problems.

1. What further data would you gather from Sarah before referring her to a genetic specialist?

2. What are the signs and symptoms of Huntington disease? The prognosis? Is it linked to any ethnic group?

3. Create a family pedigree for Sarah based on the family information she has provided. What does the pedigree reveal, and what nursing actions would you plan for Sarah?

4. What are the implications for Sarah's family if her test is positive for HD? What if her result is negative?

5. Should Sarah be tested at this time? Give a rationale for your answer.

References

American Nurses Association (ANA), & International Society of Nurses in Genetics (ISONG). (2016). *Genetics/genomics nursing: Scope and standards of practice* (2nd ed.). Silver Spring, MD: NursesBooks.org.

Badzek, L., Henaghan, M., Turner, M., & Monsen, R. (2012). Ethical, legal, and social issues in the translation of genomics into health care. *Journal of Nursing Scholarship, 4*(1), 15–24.

Beery, T. A., & Workman, M. L. (2012). *Genetics and genomics in nursing and health care.* Philadelphia, PA: F. A. Davis.

Bender, M. A., & Seibel, G. D. (2014). *Sickle cell disease.* Retrieved July 25, 2015, from http://www.ncbi.nlm.nih.gov/books/NBK1377/

Bennett, R. L., French, K. S., Resta, R. G., & Doyle, D. L. (2008). Standardized human pedigree nomenclature: Update and assessment of the recommendations of the National Society of Genetic Counselors. *Journal of Genetic Counseling, 17*(5), 424–433.

Bradshaw, E. A., & Martin, G. R. (2012). Screening for critical congenital heart disease: Advancing detection in the newborn. *Current Opinion in Pediatrics, 24*(5), 603–608.

Collins, F. S., & Varmus, H. (2015). A new initiative on precision medicine. *The New England Journal of Medicine, 372*(9), 793–795. doi:10.1056. NEJMp1500523

Consensus Panel on Genetic/Genomic Nursing Competencies. (2009). *Essentials of genetic and genomic nursing: Competencies, curricula guidelines, and outcome indicators* (2nd ed.). Silver Spring, MD: American Nurses Association.

DeLuca, J., Zanni, K. L., Bonhomme, N., & Kemper, A. R. (2013). Implications of newborn screening for nurses. *Journal of Nursing Scholarship, 45*(1), 25–33.

Friedman, J. M. (2014). *Neurofibromatosis 1.* Retrieved from http://www.ncbi.nlm.nih.gov/books/NBK1109/

GeneTests. (2015). Retrieved July 26, 2015, from https://www.genetests.org/

Green, E. D., Guyer, M. S., & National Human Genome Research Institute. (2011). Charting a course for genomic medicine from base pairs to bedside. *Nature, 470*(7333), 204–213. doi:10.1038/nature09764

Jacobs, C., & Patch, C. (2013). Identifying individuals who might benefit from genetic services and information. *Nursing Standard, 28*(9), 37–42.

Johnson, N. L., Giarelli, E., Lewis, C., & Rice, C. E. (2013). Genomics and autism spectrum disorder. *Journal of Nursing Scholarship, 45*(1), 1–10.

Lander, E. S. (2011). Initial impact of the sequencing of the human genome. *Nature, 470,* 187–197. doi:10.1038/nature09792

Lewis, R. (2015). *Human genetics* (11th ed.). New York, NY: McGraw Hill Education.

McCarthy, J. J., McLeod, H. L., & Ginsburg, G. S. (2013). Genomic medicine: A decade of successes, challenges, and opportunities. *Science Translational Medicine, 5*(189), 1–17. doi:10.1126/scitranslmed.3005785

Mitchell, J. J. (2013). *Phenylalanine hydroxylase deficiency.* Retrieved July 25, 2015, from http://www.ncbi.nlm.nih.gov/books/NBK1504/

Munck, A., Gargouri, L., Alberti, C., Viala, J., Peuchmaur, M., & Lenaerts, C. (2011). Evaluation of guidelines for management of familial adenomatous polyposis in a multicenter pediatric cohort. *Journal of Pediatric Gastroenterology and Nutrition, 53*(3), 296–302.

Online Mendelian Inheritance in Man (OMIM®). (2014). Baltimore, MD: Johns Hopkins University. Retrieved from http://omim.org/

Origa, R. (2015). *Beta-thalassemia.* Retrieved from http://www.ncbi.nlm.nih.gov/books/NBK1426/

Pierce, B. A. (2014). *Genetics: A conceptual approach* (5th ed.). New York: W. H. Freeman and Company.

Prows, C. A., Hopkin, R. J., Barnoy, S., & Van Riper, M. (2013). An update of childhood genetic disorders. *Journal of Nursing Scholarship, 45*(1), 34–42.

Ross, L. F., Saal, H. M., David, K. L., Anderson, R. R., American Academy of Pediatrics, & American College of Medical Genetics and Genomics. (2013). Technical report: Ethical and policy issues in genetic testing and screening of children. *Genetics in Medicine, 15*(3), 234–245.

Schaaf, C. P., Zschocke, J., & Potocki, L. (2012). *Human genetics: From molecules to medicine.* Baltimore, MD: Lippincott Williams & Wilkins.

Snow, K. (n.d.). *People first language.* Retrieved from http://www.disabilityisnatural.com/images/PDF/pfl09.pdf

Strom, C. M., Crossley, B., Buller-Buerkle, A., Jarvis, M., Quan, F., Peng, M., . . . Sun, W. (2011). Cystic fibrosis testing 8 years on: Lessons learned from carrier screening and sequencing analysis. *Genetics in Medicine, 13*(2), 166–172. doi:strom10.1097/GIM.0b013e3181fa24c4

The 1000 Genomes Project Consortium. (2012). An integrated map of genetic variation from 1,092 human genomes. *Nature, 491,* 56–65. doi:10.1038/nature11632

Tobias, E. S., Connor, M., & Ferguson-Smith, M. (2011). *Essential medical genetics* (6th ed.). West Sussex, England: Wiley-Blackwell.

Turnpenny, P., & Ellard, S. (2012). *Emery's elements of medical genetics.* Philadelphia, PA: Elsevier Churchill Livingstone.

U.S. CF Foundation. (2011). *The clinical and functional translation of CFTR (CFTR2).* Retrieved July 26, 2015, from http://www.cftr2.org

U.S. Department of Health and Human Services. (2008). *United States system of oversight of genetic testing: A response to the charge of the Secretary of Health and Human Services. Report of the Secretary's Advisory Committee on Genetics, Health, and Society (SACGHS).* Retrieved March 15, 2014, from http://osp.od.nih.gov/sites/default/files/SACGHS_oversight_report.pdf

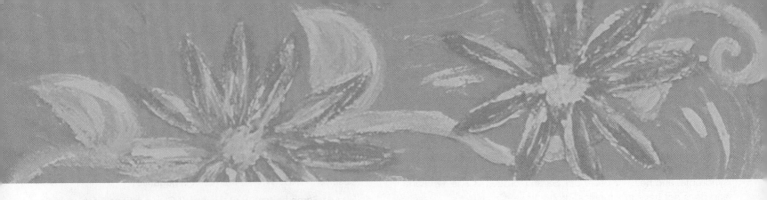

Chapter 4
Growth and Development

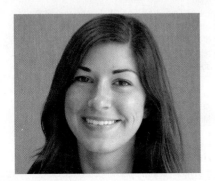

We want to help our adopted daughter Irena grow into a healthy and special child. She had challenges in her short life in Romania that we can only imagine. We worry about how we can help her grow and develop.

—Mother of Irena, age 2

∨ Learning Outcomes

4.1 Describe the major theories of development as formulated by Freud, Erikson, Piaget, Kohlberg, social learning theorists, and behaviorists.

4.2 Recognize risks to developmental progression and factors that protect against those risks.

4.3 Plan nursing interventions for children that are appropriate for each child's developmental state based on theoretical frameworks.

4.4 Explain contemporary developmental approaches such as temperament theory, ecologic theory, and the resilience framework.

4.5 Identify major developmental milestones for infants, toddlers, preschoolers, school-age children, and adolescents.

4.6 Synthesize information from several theoretical approaches to plan assessments of the child's physical growth and developmental milestones.

4.7 Describe the role of play in the growth and development of children.

4.8 Use data collected during developmental assessments to implement activities that promote development of children and adolescents.

Children develop as they interact with their surroundings. They learn skills at different ages, but the order in which they learn them is universal. Development is affected by factors such as nutrition and cultural practices, as well as the social situation in the country or neighborhood. While each child will develop in a unique manner influenced by genetic makeup, life experiences, and the interactions among these factors, certain principles of development assist parents and the nurse in fostering positive adaptations for the child.

This chapter covers general principles of growth and development and explores several theories related to childhood development, as well as their nursing applications. Each age group, from infancy through adolescence, is described in detail. Developmental milestones, physical and cognitive characteristics,

play patterns, and communication strategies are presented, as are conditions that interfere with usual developmental progression. The information provided helps guide developmentally appropriate care for children in each age group and in a variety of situations. These concepts can be applied when caring for all children, including those in special situations.

Principles of Growth and Development

It is essential to understand the concepts of growth and development when learning to care for children. A skilled pediatric nurse integrates knowledge of physical growth and psychosocial development into each child healthcare encounter. **Growth** refers to an increase in physical size. It represents quantitative changes such as height, weight, blood pressure, and number of words in the child's vocabulary. **Development** refers to a qualitative increase in capability or function. Developmental skills, such as the ability to sit without support or to throw a ball overhand, unfold in a complex manner influenced by the relationship between the child's innate capabilities and the stimuli and support provided in the environment. The quantitative and qualitative changes in body organ functioning, ability to communicate, and performance of motor skills develop over time and are key components in the process of planning pediatric health care.

Each child displays a unique maturational pattern during the process of development. Although the exact age at which skills emerge differs, the sequence or order of skill performance is uniform among children. Skill development proceeds according to two processes: from the head downward, and from the center of the body outward.

- **Cephalocaudal development** (Figure 4–1) proceeds from the head downward through the body and toward the feet. For example, at birth an infant's head is much larger proportionately than the trunk or extremities. Similarly, infants learn to hold up their heads before sitting and to sit before standing. Skills such as walking that involve the legs and feet develop last in infancy.

- **Proximodistal development** (see Figure 4–1) proceeds from the center of the body outward toward the extremities. For example, infants are first able to control the trunk, then the arms; only later are fine motor movements of the fingers possible. As the child grows, both physical and cognitive skills differentiate from general to more specific skills. Pediatric nurses use these concepts of predictable and sequential developmental direction to analyze the infant's and child's present

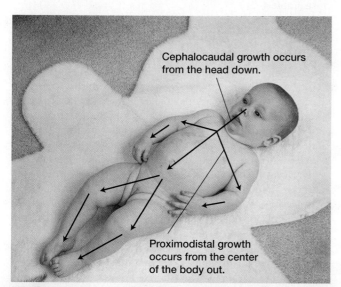

Figure 4–1 **Cephalocaudal and proximodistal development. In normal cephalocaudal growth, the child gains control of the head and neck before the trunk and limbs. In normal proximodistal growth, the child controls arm movements before hand movements. For example, the child reaches for objects before being able to grasp them. Children gain control of their hands before their fingers; that is, they can hold things with the entire hand before they can pick something up with just their fingers.**

state and to partner with parents to plan ways to encourage and support the next emerging developmental abilities.

During the childhood years, extraordinary changes occur in all aspects of development. Physical size, motor skills, cognitive ability, language, sensory ability, and psychosocial patterns all undergo major transformations. Nurses study normal patterns of development to identify children who demonstrate unexpected developmental findings. These assessments can guide the nurse in planning interventions for the child and family, such as referring the child for a diagnostic evaluation or rehabilitation, or teaching the parents how to provide adequate stimulation for the child. Nurses use **anticipatory guidance** to predict upcoming developmental tasks or needs of a child and to perform appropriate teaching related to them. When development is proceeding normally, nurses use their knowledge of these normal patterns to provide approaches based on the child's cognitive and language ability, to offer appropriate toys and activities during illness, and to respond therapeutically during interactions with the child. See Chapters 7 to 9 for specific application of developmental surveillance into health promotion visits. For situations with special challenges, such as in adoptions, additional interventions may be needed (see *Growth and Development*).

Growth and Development

About 15% of annual adoptions in the United States, or over 7000, are international adoptions. China, South Korea, Russia, Ethiopia, Uganda, Ukraine, and Haiti are among the most common countries of origin for orphans being adopted in the United States (U.S. Department of State, 2015). All adoptions can be stressful for the new parents and child, but international adoptions pose a unique set of circumstances that influence the child's development.

Parents need to protect themselves and others from infectious diseases when traveling to bring home a child from another country. They should consult their local health district and healthcare providers for a list of recommended immunizations for the country they are visiting. They should also obtain a list of medications and supplies to carry for themselves and the child, such as antidiarrheal medicine, decongestants, analgesics, bandages, and hand sanitizer (Children's Hospital of Philadelphia, 2012).

Parents require counseling to learn about cultural practices, language, and other differences they may encounter. Once they bring the child home, they will need support as the child grows to integrate the child's history and culture into their family. The moment when the child meets an adoptive parent may be seen as joyous by the parent but it can be traumatic for the young child, who is being separated from familiar adults. Parents need preparation for establishing trust with the child (Children's Hospital of Philadelphia, 2012).

The adopted child should be examined once home for length, weight, and head circumference. If growth is delayed, continued monitoring and dietary interventions will be needed. The psychosocially based problem of *avoidant/restrictive food intake disorder* (formerly called *eating disorder of infancy and childhood* or *failure to thrive*) should also be considered. (See Chapter 14 for a thorough discussion of this condition.) Parasitic infection and chronic diseases are possible causes of continuing growth abnormalities. Perform developmental screening to provide a baseline for future developmental observations. Frequent physical and psychosocial assessments will be needed, and teaching is provided for parents to enhance development.

SAFETY ALERT!

Although a primary purpose of understanding and monitoring development is to be able to apply anticipatory guidance so that parents and nurses can provide the child with appropriate toys and experiences, there is also a very important link between safety and development. Developmental knowledge provides information about the major illness and accident risks for each age group as well as preventive techniques. For example, a 6-month-old child should never be left alone on a high surface, preschoolers must be carefully monitored while playing, and teenagers must demonstrate responsibility before being allowed to drive. As you read this chapter, try to identify the physical, cognitive, and social reasons that guide the safety precautions to be taken with children of various ages.

Major Theories of Development

Child development is a complex process. Many theorists have attempted to organize their observations of behavior into a description of principles or a set of stages. Each theory focuses on a particular facet of development. Most developmental theorists separate children into age groups by common characteristics (Table 4–1).

Freud's Theory of Psychosexual Development

THEORETICAL FRAMEWORK

Sigmund Freud (1856–1939) was a physician in Vienna, Austria. His work with adults experiencing a variety of neurologic disorders led him to develop an approach called *psychoanalysis*, which explored the driving forces of the unconscious mind. These psychoanalytic techniques led Freud to believe that early childhood experiences form the unconscious motivation for actions in later life. He believed that sexual energy is centered in specific parts

TABLE 4–1 Developmental Age Groups

DEVELOPMENTAL STAGE	AGE GROUP	CHARACTERISTICS
Infancy	Birth to 12 months	Includes infants or babies up to 1 year of age, all of whom require a high level of care in daily activities.
Toddlerhood	1–3 years	Characterized by increased motor ability and independent behavior.
Preschool	3–6 years	The preschooler refines gross and fine motor ability and language skills and often participates in a preschool learning program.
School age	6–12 years	Begins with entry into a school system and is characterized by growing intellectual skills, physical ability, and independence.
Adolescence	12–18 years	Begins with entry into the teen years. Mature cognitive thought, formation of identity, and influence of peers are important characteristics of adolescence.

TABLE 4–2 Common Defense Mechanisms Used by Children

DEFENSE MECHANISM	DEFINITION	EXAMPLE
Regression	Return to an earlier behavior	A child who has been previously toilet trained becomes incontinent when a new infant is born into the family.
Repression	Involuntary forgetting of uncomfortable situations	An abused child cannot consciously recall episodes of abuse.
Rationalization	An attempt to make unacceptable feelings acceptable	A child explains hitting another because "he took my toy."
Fantasy	A creation of the mind to help deal with unacceptable fear	A hospitalized child who is weak pretends to be Superman.

of the body at certain ages. Unresolved conflict and unmet needs at a certain stage lead to a fixation of development at that stage (Dunn & Craig, 2013).

Freud viewed the personality as a structure with three parts: The *id* is the basic sexual energy that is present at birth and drives the individual to seek pleasure; the *ego* is the realistic part of the person, which develops during infancy and searches for acceptable methods of meeting impulses; and the *superego* is the moral/ethical system, which develops in childhood and contains a set of values and a conscience (Dunn & Craig, 2013). The ego diverts impulses and protects itself from excess anxiety by use of **defense mechanisms**, including regression to earlier stages and repression or forgetting of painful experiences such as child abuse (Table 4–2).

Clinical Reasoning International Adoption Counseling

Michael and Alyssa had tried for several years to have a biologic child. After an unsuccessful in vitro fertilization, they decided to try to adopt a child. They explored opportunities with adoption agencies and learned that international adoption would be possible for them. They adopted 2-year-old Irena from Romania several months ago. Irena appears small for her age, but she seems to be thriving in her new environment. She is learning to say a few English words and is responding appropriately to care and interactions.

Despite thorough investigation of Michael and Alyssa by the adoption agency, they received only scant information about Irena's history. They were told that she was left at an orphanage by her birth mother when she was about 7 months old; the birth mother stated that the pregnancy and birth were normal. According to reports, the birth mother had decided to relinquish the child because she had two older children to care for and her husband had left home nearly a year before and had not been heard from since.

How can you work with Michael and Alyssa to ensure special attention to Irena's growth and healthcare needs, such as physical growth, language, and social skills? Consider both assessment and planned interventions.

What will Irena's cultural needs be as she grows older? How can Michael and Alyssa prepare to tell her about her adoption and background someday?

STAGES

Oral (Birth to 1 Year). The infant derives pleasure largely from the mouth, with sucking and eating as primary desires.

Anal (1 to 3 Years). The young child's pleasure is centered in the anal area, with control over body secretions as a prime force in behavior.

Phallic (3 to 6 Years). Sexual energy becomes centered in the genitalia as the child works out relationships with parents of the same and opposite sexes.

Latency (6 to 12 Years). Sexual energy is at rest in the passage between earlier stages and adolescence.

Genital (12 Years to Adulthood). Mature sexuality is achieved as physical growth is completed and relationships with others occur.

NURSING APPLICATION

Freud emphasized the importance of meeting the needs of each stage in order to move successfully into future developmental stages. The crisis of illness can interfere with normal developmental processes and add challenges for the nurse striving to meet an ill child's needs. For example, the importance of sucking in infancy guides the nurse to provide a pacifier for the infant who cannot have oral fluids. The preschool child's concern about sexuality guides the nurse to provide privacy and clear explanations during any procedures involving the genital area. It may be necessary to teach parents that masturbation by the young child is normal and to help parents deal with it through distraction or refocusing. The adolescent's focus on relationships suggests that the nurse should include questions about significant friends during history taking. Table 4–3 summarizes techniques the nurse can use to apply these theoretical concepts to the care of children.

Erikson's Theory of Psychosocial Development

THEORETICAL FRAMEWORK

Erik Erikson (1902–1994) studied Freud's theory of psychoanalysis under Freud's daughter, Anna. He later established his own developmental theory, which describes psychosocial stages during eight periods of human life. Five of Erikson's eight stages apply to children and are described below. For each stage, Erikson identified a crisis—that is, a particular challenge that exists for healthy personality development to occur (Erikson, 1963, 1968). The word *crisis* in this context refers to normal maturational social needs rather than to a single critical event. Each developmental crisis has two possible outcomes. When needs are met, the consequence is healthy and the individual moves on to future stages with particular strengths. When needs are not met, an unhealthy outcome occurs that will influence future social relationships.

STAGES

Trust Versus Mistrust (Birth to 1 Year). The task of the first year of life is to establish trust in the people providing care. Trust is fostered by provision of food, clean clothing, touch, and comfort. If basic needs are not met, the infant will eventually learn to mistrust others.

Autonomy Versus Shame and Doubt (1 to 3 Years). The toddler's sense of autonomy or independence is shown by controlling body excretions, saying no when asked to do something,

and directing motor activity and play. Children who are consistently criticized for expressions of autonomy or for lack of control—for example, during toilet training—will develop a sense of shame about themselves and doubt in their abilities.

Initiative Versus Guilt (3 to 6 Years). The young child initiates new activities and considers new ideas. This interest in exploring the world creates a child who is involved and busy. Constant criticism, on the other hand, leads to feelings of guilt and a lack of purpose.

Industry Versus Inferiority (6 to 12 Years). The middle years of childhood are characterized by development of new interests and by involvement in activities. The child takes pride in accomplishments in sports, school, home, and community. If the child cannot accomplish what is expected, however, the result will be a sense of inferiority.

Identity Versus Role Confusion (12 to 18 Years). In adolescence, as the body matures and thought processes become more complex, a new sense of identity, or self, is established. The self, family, peer group, and community are all examined and redefined. The adolescent who is unable to establish a meaningful definition of self will experience confusion in one or more roles of life.

NURSING APPLICATION

Erikson's theory is directly applicable to the nursing care of children. Health promotion and health maintenance visits in the community provide opportunities for helping caregivers meet children's needs. Parents benefit from learning what the child's developmental tasks are at each stage and from discussing ideas about how to encourage healthy psychosocial development. Such discussions also may highlight parental concerns and provide a forum for reassurance about normal developmental characteristics, such as a child who does not follow through on each activity as a preschooler or tries different hairstyles each month as an adolescent.

The child's usual support from family, peers, and others is interrupted by hospitalization. The challenge of hospitalization also adds a situational crisis to the normal developmental crisis a child is experiencing. Although the nurse may meet many of the hospitalized child's needs, continued parental involvement is necessary both during and after hospitalization to ensure progression through expected developmental stages (see Table 4–3).

Piaget's Theory of Cognitive Development

THEORETICAL FRAMEWORK

Jean Piaget (1896–1980) was a Swiss scientist who wrote detailed observations of the behavior of his own and other children. Based on these observations, Piaget formulated a theory of cognitive (or intellectual) development. He believed that the child's view of the world is influenced largely by age and maturational ability. Given nurturing experiences, the child's ability to think matures naturally (Ginsberg & Opper, 1988; Piaget, 1972). The child incorporates new experiences via **assimilation** and changes to deal with these experiences by the process of **accommodation**. An example of assimilation occurs when the infant uses reflexes to suck on objects that touch the lips. With more experience the infant accommodates to learn that not all objects are pleasant to suck and cognitive structures change to integrate and learn from the experiences.

TABLE 4–3 Nursing Applications of Theories of Freud, Erikson, and Piaget

AGE GROUP	THEORIST/DEVELOPMENTAL STAGE	CHARACTERISTICS OF STAGE	NURSING APPLICATIONS
Infant (birth to 1 year)	Freud: Oral stage	The baby obtains pleasure and comfort through the mouth.	When a baby is not able to take foods or fluids, offer a pacifier if not contraindicated. After painful procedures, offer a baby a bottle or pacifier or have the mother breastfeed.
	Erikson: Trust versus mistrust stage	The baby establishes a sense of trust when basic needs are met.	Hold the hospitalized baby often. Offer comfort after painful procedures. Meet the baby's needs for food and hygiene. Encourage parents to room in. Manage pain effectively with use of pain medications and other measures.
	Piaget: Sensorimotor stage	The baby learns from movement and sensory input.	Use crib mobiles, manipulative toys, wall murals, and bright colors to provide interesting stimuli and comfort. Use toys to distract the baby during procedures and assessments.
Toddler (1–3 years)	Freud: Anal stage	The child derives gratification from control over body excretions.	Ask about toilet training and the child's rituals and words for elimination during admission history. Continue child's normal patterns of elimination in the hospital. Do not begin toilet training during illness or hospitalization. Accept regression in toileting during illness or hospitalization. Have potty chairs available in hospital and childcare centers.
	Erikson: Autonomy versus shame and doubt stage	The child is increasingly independent in many spheres of life.	Allow self-feeding opportunities. Encourage child to remove and put on own clothes, brush teeth, or assist with hygiene. (A) If immobilization for a procedure is necessary, proceed quickly, providing explanations and comfort.
	Piaget: Sensorimotor stage (end); preoperational stage (beginning)	The child shows increasing curiosity and explorative behavior. Language skills improve.	Ensure safe surroundings to allow opportunities to manipulate objects. Name objects and give simple explanations.
Preschooler (3–6 years)	Freud: Phallic stage	The child initially identifies with the parent of the opposite sex but by the end of this stage identifies with the same-sex parent.	Be alert for children who appear more comfortable with male or female nurses, and attempt to accommodate them. Encourage parental involvement in care. Plan for playtime and offer a variety of materials from which to choose.
	Erikson: Initiative versus guilt stage	The child likes to initiate play activities.	Offer medical equipment for play to lessen anxiety about strange objects. (B) Assess children's concerns as expressed through their drawings. Accept the child's choices and expressions of feelings.

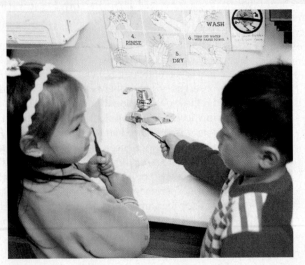

A

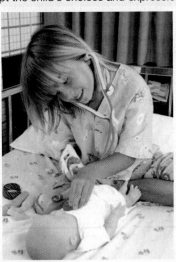

B

AGE GROUP	THEORIST/DEVELOPMENTAL STAGE	CHARACTERISTICS OF STAGE	NURSING APPLICATIONS
	Piaget: Preoperational stage	The child is increasingly verbal but has some limitations in thought processes. Causality is often confused, so the child may feel responsible for causing an illness.	Offer explanations about all procedures and treatments. Clearly explain that the child is not responsible for causing an illness in self or family member.
School age (6–12 years)	Freud: Latency stage	The child places importance on privacy and understanding the body.	Provide gowns, covers, and underwear. Knock on door before entering. Explain treatments and procedures.
	Erikson: Industry versus inferiority stage	The child gains a sense of self-worth from involvement in activities.	Encourage the child to continue schoolwork while hospitalized. Encourage the child to bring favorite pastimes to the hospital. (C) Help the child adjust to limitations on favorite activities.
	Piaget: Concrete operational stage	The child is capable of mature thought when allowed to manipulate and see objects.	Give clear instructions about details of treatment. Show the child equipment that will be used in treatment.
Adolescent (12–18 years)	Freud: Genital stage	The adolescent's focus is on genital function and relationships.	Ensure access to gynecologic care for adolescent females and testicular examinations for adolescent males. Provide information on sexuality. Ensure privacy during health care. Have brochures and videos available for teaching about sexuality.
	Erikson: Identity versus role confusion stage	The adolescent's search for self-identity leads to independence from parents and reliance on peers.	Provide a separate recreation room for teens who are hospitalized. (D) Take health history and perform examinations without parents present. Introduce adolescent to other teens with same health problem.
	Piaget: Formal operational stage	The adolescent is capable of mature, abstract thought.	Give clear and complete information about health care and treatments. Offer both written and verbal instructions. Continue to provide education about the disease to the adolescent with a chronic illness, as mature thought now leads to greater understanding.

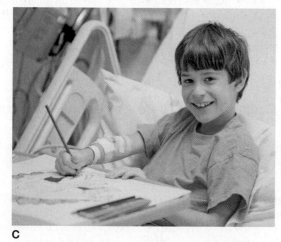

C

SOURCE: iStock/Getty Images

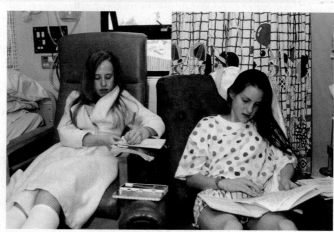

D

SOURCE: Photofusion Picture Library/Alamy

STAGES

Sensorimotor (Birth to 2 Years).   Infants learn about the world by input obtained through the senses and by their motor activity. Six substages are characteristic of this stage.

Use of Reflexes (Birth to 1 Month).   The infant begins life with a set of reflexes such as sucking, rooting, and grasping. By using these reflexes, the infant receives stimulation via touch, sound, smell, and vision. The reflexes thus pave the way for the first learning to occur.

Primary Circular Reactions (1 to 4 Months).   Once the infant responds reflexively, the pleasure gained from that response causes repetition of the behavior. For example, if a toy grasped reflexively makes noise and is interesting to look at, the infant will grasp it again.

Secondary Circular Reactions (4 to 8 Months).   Awareness of the environment grows as the infant begins to connect cause and effect. The sounds of bottle preparation will lead to excited behavior. If an object is partially hidden, the infant will attempt to uncover and retrieve it.

Coordination of Secondary Schemes (8 to 12 Months).   Intentional behavior is observed as the infant uses learned behavior to obtain objects, create sounds, or engage in other pleasurable activities. **Object permanence** (the knowledge that something continues to exist even when out of sight) begins when the infant remembers where a hidden object is likely to be found; it is no longer "out of sight, out of mind." However, the concept of object permanence is not fully developed. The infant knows the parent well, objects to new people, and seems very worried when the parent leaves. Other caretakers may be rejected because the infant does not understand that the parent will return. This phase of "stranger anxiety" is quite common and heralds the infant's growing recognition of and desire to be cared for by the parent.

Tertiary Circular Reactions (12 to 18 Months).   Curiosity, experimentation, and exploration dominate as the toddler tries out actions to learn results. At this age, children turn objects in every direction, place them in their mouths, use them for banging, and insert them in containers as they explore their qualities and uses.

Mental Combinations (18 to 24 Months).   Language provides a new tool for the toddler to use in understanding the world. Language enables the child to think about events and objects before or after they occur. Object permanence is now fully developed as the child actively searches for objects in various locations and out of view. The child who has had successful separations from the parents followed by their return, such as hours spent in another's home or childcare center, begins to understand that the missing parent will return.

Preoperational (2 to 7 Years).   The young child thinks by using words as symbols, but logic is not well developed. Two substages characterize this stage.

Preconceptual Substage.   During the preconceptual substage (2 to 4 years), vocabulary and comprehension increase greatly but the child is egocentric (i.e., unable to see things from the perspective of another).

Intuitive Substage.   In the intuitive substage (4 to 7 years), the child relies on transductive reasoning (drawing conclusions from one general fact to another). For example, when a child disobeys a parent and then falls and breaks an arm that same day, the child may ascribe the broken arm to bad behavior.

Cause-and-effect relationships are often unrealistic or a result of magical thinking (the belief that events occur because of thoughts or wishes).

Additional characteristics noted in the thought of preschoolers include *centration*, or the ability to consider only one aspect of a situation at a time, and *animism*, or giving life to inanimate objects because they move, make noise, or have certain other qualities.

Concrete Operational (7 to 11 Years).   Transductive reasoning has given way to a more accurate understanding of cause and effect. The child can reason quite well if concrete objects are used in teaching or experimentation. The concept of conservation (that matter does not change when its form is altered) is learned at this age.

Formal Operational (11 Years to Adulthood).   Fully mature intellectual thought has now been attained. The adolescent can think abstractly about objects or concepts and consider different alternatives or outcomes.

NURSING APPLICATION

Piaget's theory is essential to pediatric nursing. The nurse must understand a child's thought processes in order to design stimulating activities and meaningful, appropriate teaching plans. What activities could be planned for a hospitalized child based on his or her expected cognitive level? How can cognitive development be encouraged in a school-age child receiving home health services? Understanding a child's concept of time suggests how far in advance to prepare that child for procedures. Similarly, decisions about offering manipulative toys, reading stories, drawing pictures, or giving the child reading material to explain healthcare measures depend on the child's cognitive stage of development (see Table 4–3).

Kohlberg's Theory of Moral Development

THEORETICAL FRAMEWORK

Lawrence Kohlberg (1927–1987) was a German theorist who used Piaget's cognitive theory as a basis for his theory of moral development. He presented stories involving moral dilemmas to children and adults and asked them to solve the dilemmas. Kohlberg then analyzed the motives they expressed when making decisions about the best course to take. Based on the explanations given, Kohlberg established three levels of moral reasoning. Although he provided age guidelines, he stated that they are approximate and that many people never reach the highest (postconventional) stage of development (Santrock, 2012).

STAGES

Preconventional (4 to 7 Years).   Decisions are based on the desire to please others and to avoid punishment.

Conventional (7 to 12 Years).   Conscience, or an internal set of standards, becomes important. Rules are important and must be followed to please other people and "be good."

Postconventional (12 Years and Older).   The individual has internalized ethical standards on which to base decisions. Social responsibility is recognized. The value in each of two differing moral approaches can be considered and a decision made.

NURSING APPLICATION

Decision making is required in many areas of health care. Children can be assisted to make decisions about health care and to consider alternatives when available. Keep in mind that young children may agree to participate in research simply because they want to comply with adults and appear cooperative. Guidelines for child participation in research are available (see Chapter 1).

Parents can be provided with information so that they can assist their children in moral judgments. Encourage talking with a child or adolescent about how a particular decision was made. Parents can then add information and help the child learn to integrate more factors into decision making. Talking about the process is important in helping children progress to higher moral development stages. Focusing on the feelings of others, using positive discipline techniques, and clearly identifying positive and negative behaviors are important.

Social Learning Theory

THEORETICAL FRAMEWORK

Originally from Canada, psychologist Albert Bandura (1925–) has conducted research at Stanford University for many years. He believes that children learn attitudes, beliefs, customs, and values through their social contacts with adults and other children. Children imitate (or model) the behavior they see; if the behavior is positively reinforced, they tend to repeat it. The external environment and the child's internal processes are key elements in social learning theory (Bandura, 1986, 1997a).

Bandura believes that an important determinant of behavior is self-efficacy, or the expectation that someone can produce a desired outcome. For example, if adolescents believe they can avoid use of drugs or alcohol, they are more likely to do so. A child who has confidence in his or her ability to exercise regularly or lose weight has a greater chance of success with these behavior changes. Parents who have confidence in their ability to care adequately for their infants are more likely to do so (Bandura, 1997b). See *Evidence-Based Practice: Concept of Self-Efficacy* for further examples of application of the concept of self-efficacy.

NURSING APPLICATION

The importance of modeling behavior can readily be applied in health care. Children are more likely to cooperate if they see adults or other children performing a task willingly. A frightened child may watch another child perform vision screening or have blood drawn and then decide to allow the procedure to take place. Contact with positive role models is useful when teaching children and adolescents self-care for chronic diseases such as diabetes. Give positive reinforcement for desired performance.

Nurses can use the concept of self-efficacy to increase the chance of success with lifestyle behavior changes. For example, encouraging youth who are trying to quit smoking, providing them with role models, and pointing out parental successes with their children all demonstrate methods of fostering self-efficacy.

Behaviorism

THEORETICAL FRAMEWORK

John Watson (1878–1958) was an American scientist who applied the research of animal behaviorists, such as Pavlov and Skinner, to children. Pavlov and, later, Skinner worked with animals, presenting a stimulus such as food and pairing it with another stimulus such as a ringing bell. Eventually the animal being fed began to salivate when the bell rang. As Skinner and, then, Watson began to apply these concepts to children, they showed that behaviors can be elicited by positive reinforcement, such as a food treat, or extinguished by negative reinforcement, such as

---

EVIDENCE-BASED PRACTICE | Concept of Self-Efficacy

Clinical Question
How can nurses use the concept of self-efficacy when planning interventions for children and families?

The Evidence
Parental self-efficacy is the belief that parents can manage a range of tasks and situations in caring for their children. Higher self-efficacy scores in parents were predictive of greater success in treatment of young children who were overweight (Davies, Terhorts, Nakonechny, et al., 2014). The authors of this literature review also established an Internet site to provide information and enhance self-efficacy in parents regarding healthy lifestyles for children (Davies et al., 2014).

Mothers who have a greater degree of self-efficacy about ability to breastfeed are significantly more likely to begin and to continue breastfeeding. A Breastfeeding Self-Efficacy Scale has been developed to identify risk and protective factors that influence the self-efficacy of new mothers. Evaluating breastfeeding self-efficacy in Hispanic women was able to inform the topics for teaching that would best promote breastfeeding (Joshi, Trout, Aguirre, et al., 2014).

An intervention with over 1000 students in grades 5 and 6 was effective in increasing youth self-efficacy regarding television viewing time and decreasing television viewing time (Salmon et al., 2011).

Best Practice
In addition to providing information about health behaviors, nurses need to integrate methods to increase self-efficacy in teaching projects with families. Assessments should be designed to identify self-efficacy of parents and children around health topics of interest. When planning interventions to encourage health behaviors in children and adolescents, assess the youth's beliefs that the new behaviors are important and that they can be adopted. Include interventions that demonstrate that others have adopted the health behaviors and plan approaches to enhance the child's belief in ability to change.

Clinical Reasoning
Plan a teaching project about the importance of physical activity and healthy eating for presentation to a group of 12-year-olds. What approaches will enhance the self-efficacy of the children? How would interventions to enhance self-efficacy differ for young elementary school children from those in middle or high school? What theoretical approaches discussed earlier in this chapter help you understand the cognitive abilities of children at various ages and suggest ways to influence their self-efficacy?

scolding or withdrawal of attention. Watson believed that he could make a child into anyone he desired—from a professional to a thief or beggar—simply by reinforcing behavior in certain ways (Santrock, 2012).

NURSING APPLICATION

Behaviorism has been criticized for being simplistic and for its denial of people's inherent capacity to respond willfully to events in the environment. However, this theory does have some use in health care. When particular behaviors are desired, healthcare providers can establish positive reinforcement to encourage these behaviors. Using behavioral techniques, nurses may influence the behavior of children by giving a sticker to a child after a physical examination or a blood draw. Parents often use reinforcement in toilet training and other skills learned in childhood.

Ecologic Theory

THEORETICAL FRAMEWORK

There is controversy among theorists concerning the relative importance of heredity versus environment—or nature versus nurture—in human development. **Nature** refers to the genetic or hereditary capability of an individual. **Nurture** refers to the effects of the environment on a person's performance (Figure 4–2). Piaget believed in the importance of internal cognitive structures that unfold at their appointed times, given any environment that provides basic opportunities. He emphasized the strength of nature. The behaviorist John Watson, on the other hand, believed that behaviors are primarily shaped by environmental responses; he thus stressed the predominance of nurture. Contemporary developmental theories increasingly recognize the interaction of nature and nurture in determining the child's development.

Urie Bronfenbrenner (1917–2005), a professor at Cornell University, formulated the ecologic theory of development to explain the unique relationship of the child with all of life's experiences or systems (Bronfenbrenner, 1986, 2005; Bronfenbrenner, McClelland, Ceci, et al., 1996). **Ecologic theory**

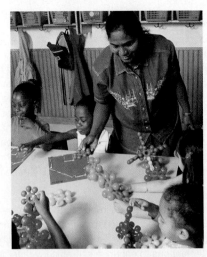

Figure 4–2 An example of nurturing. Children exposed to pleasant stimulation and who are supported by an adult will develop and refine their skills faster. Group activities such as these provide an opportunity for both motor skill and psychosocial development. Can you identify which skills are being developed?

emphasizes the presence of mutual interactions between the child and these various settings or systems. Neither nature nor nurture is considered of more importance. Bronfenbrenner believed each child brings a unique set of genes—as well as specific attributes such as age, gender, health, and other characteristics—to his or her interactions with the environment. The child then interacts in many settings at different levels or systems (Figure 4–3).

LEVELS/SYSTEMS

Microsystem. This level is defined as the daily, consistent, close relationships such as home, child care, school, friends, and neighbors. For the child with a chronic illness requiring regular care, the healthcare providers may even be part of the microsystem. In the ecologic model, the child influences each of the settings in the microsystem, in addition to being influenced by them, with reciprocal interactions.

Mesosystem. This level includes relationships of microsystems with one another. For example, two microsystems for most children are the home and the school. The relationships between these microsystems are shown by parents' involvement in their children's school. This involvement, in turn, influences the effects of the home and school settings on the children.

Exosystem. This level is composed of those settings that influence the child even though the child is not in close daily contact with the system. Examples include the parents' jobs and the governing board of the local school district. Although the child may not go to the parents' workplaces, the child can be influenced by policies related to health care, sick leave, inflexible work hours, overtime, or travel, or even by the mood of the boss (through its impact on the parent). Likewise, when a local school board votes to ban certain books or to finance a field trip, the child is influenced by these decisions; the child, in turn, can help establish an atmosphere that will guide future school board decisions.

Macrosystem. This level includes the beliefs, values, and behaviors expressed in the child's environment. Culture is a powerful influence in the macrosystem, as is the political system. For instance, a democratic system creates different beliefs, values, and even eating practices than an anarchic system.

Chronosystem. This final level brings the perspective of time to the previous settings. The time period during which the child grows up influences views of health and illness. For example, the experiences of children with influenza in the 19th versus the 20th century were quite different. The age of the parent, child, and other family members also influences views of health.

NURSING APPLICATION

Nurses use ecologic theory when they assess the child's settings to identify influences on development. Table 4–4 provides an assessment tool based on this theory. Interventions are planned to enhance the strengths of the child's settings and to improve on areas that are not supportive.

Temperament Theory

THEORETICAL FRAMEWORK

In contrast to behaviorists such as Watson or maturational theorists such as Piaget, Stella Chess and Alexander Thomas recognize the innate qualities of personality that each individual brings to the events of daily life. They, like Bronfenbrenner, believe the

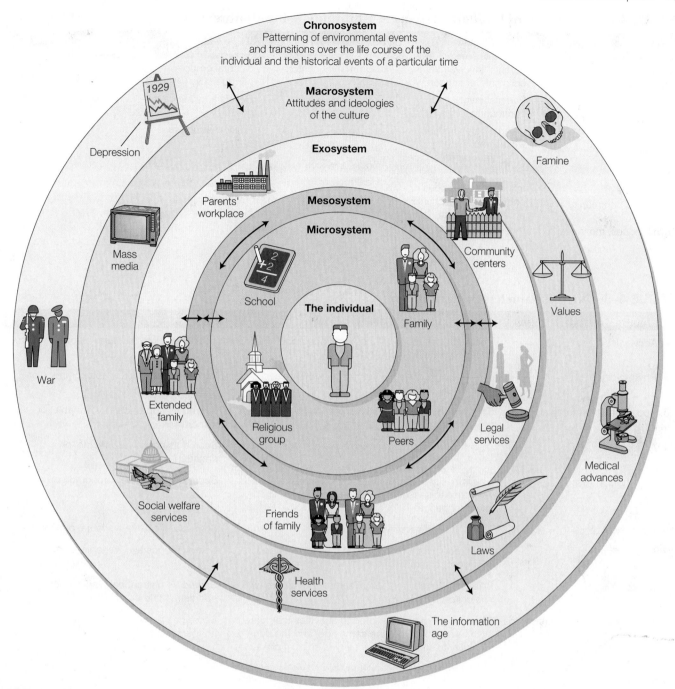

Figure 4–3 Bronfenbrenner's ecologic theory of development views the individual as interacting within five levels or systems.

SOURCE: Data from Santrock, J. W. (2007). *Life-span development.* Madison, WI: Brown & Benchmark. Based on Bronfenbrenner's (1979, 1986) works in Contexts of child rearing: Problems and prospects. *American Psychologist, 34,* 844–850; Ecology of the family as a context for human development: Research perspectives. *Developmental Psychology, 22,* 723–742.

child is an individual who both influences and is influenced by the environment. However, Chess and Thomas focus on one specific aspect of development—the wide spectrum of behaviors possible in children—identifying nine parameters of response to daily events (Table 4–5). Their theory is based on a research study titled the New York Longitudinal Study, which began with infants in 1956 and has continued into the adulthood of these participating individuals. By careful observations of responses to life events, Chess and Thomas identified characteristics of personality that provide the basis for the study on temperament.

Infants generally display clusters of responses, which are classified into three major personality types (Table 4–6). Although most children do not demonstrate all behaviors described for a particular type, they usually show a grouping indicative of one personality type (Chess & Thomas, 1995, 1996, 1999).

Recent research demonstrates that personality characteristics displayed during infancy are often consistent with those seen later in life. Predicting future characteristics is not possible, however, because of the complex and dynamic interaction of personality traits and environmental reactions.

TABLE 4–4 Assessment of Ecologic Systems in Childhood—Bronfenbrenner

MICROSYSTEMS	MESOSYSTEMS	EXOSYSTEMS	MACROSYSTEMS	CHRONOSYSTEMS
Parents	Parents' involvement in child care or school	Community centers	Cultural group membership	Child's and parents' ages
Significant others in close contact	Parents' involvement in community	Local political influences	Beliefs and values of group	Period in historic time
Childcare arrangements	Parents' relationships with significant others (e.g., grandparents, care providers)	Parents' work	Political structure	
School		Parents' friends and activities		
Neighborhood contacts		Social services		
Clubs	Influences of religious community (e.g., church, synagogue, mosque) or parents and school	Health care		
Friends, peers		Libraries		
Religious community (e.g., churches, synagogues, mosques)				

TABLE 4–5 Nine Parameters of Personality

PARAMETER	DESCRIPTION	SCORING
1. Activity level	The degree of motion during eating, playing, sleeping, bathing	Scored as high, medium, or low
2. Rhythmicity	The regularity of schedule maintained for sleep, hunger, elimination	Scored as regular, variable, or irregular
3. Approach or withdrawal	The response to a new stimulus such as a food, activity, or person	Scored as approachable, variable, or withdrawn
4. Adaptability	The degree of adaptation to new situations	Scored as adaptive, variable, or nonadaptive
5. Threshold of responsiveness	The intensity of stimulation needed to elicit a response to sensory input, objects in the environment, or people	Scored as high, medium, or low
6. Intensity of reaction	The degree of response to situations	Scored as positive, variable, or negative
7. Quality of mood	The predominant mood during daily activity and in response to stimuli	Scored as positive, variable, or negative
8. Distractibility	The ability of environmental stimuli to interfere with the child's activity	Scored as distractible, variable, or nondistractible
9. Attention span and persistence	The amount of time devoted to activities (compared with other children of the same age) and the degree of ability to stick with an activity in spite of obstacles	Scored as persistent, variable, or nonpersistent

Source: Data from Chess, S., & Thomas, A. (1996). *Temperament: Theory and practice.* Philadelphia, PA: Brunner/Mazel, Publishers.

Many other researchers have expanded the work of Chess and Thomas, developing assessment tools for temperament types. The concept of "goodness of fit" is an outgrowth of this theory. *Goodness of fit* refers to whether parents' expectations of their child's behavior are consistent with the child's temperament type. There is a "good fit" when the properties of the environment are in accord with the child's capabilities, characteristics, and style of behavior, and when the people in the environment know how to best support the child (The Center for Parenting Education, 2014). For example, an infant who is very active and reacts strongly to verbal stimuli may be unable to sleep well when placed in a room with older siblings. A child who is slow to warm up may not perform well in the first few months at a new school, much to the parents' disappointment. When parents understand a child's temperament characteristics, they are better able to shape the environment to meet the child's needs.

NURSING APPLICATION

The concept of personality type or temperament is a useful one for nurses. Nurses can assess the temperament of young children and alter the environment to meet their needs. This may involve moving a hospitalized child to a single room to ensure adequate rest if the child is easily stimulated, or allowing a shy child time to become accustomed to new surroundings and equipment before beginning procedures or treatments.

Parents are often relieved to learn about temperament characteristics. They learn to appreciate their children's qualities and to adapt the environment to meet the children's needs. A burden of guilt can also be lifted from parents who feel that they are responsible for their child's actions. Parents may be taught ways to enhance goodness of fit between the child's personality and the environment (Chess & Thomas, 1999) (Table 4–7).

TABLE 4–6 Patterns of Temperament

PATTERN	DESCRIPTION	% OF N.Y. LONGITUDINAL STUDY PARTICIPANTS
The "easy" child	Generally moderate in activity Shows regularity in patterns of eating, sleeping, and elimination Usually positive in mood Adapts to new situations when subjected to new stimuli Able to accept rules Works well with others	Approximately 40%
The "difficult" child	Displays irregular schedules for eating, sleeping, and elimination Adapts slowly to new situations and persons Displays a predominantly negative mood Intense reactions to the environment common	Approximately 10%
The "slow-to-warm-up" child	Initial withdrawal, followed by gradual, quiet, slow interaction with the environment Adapts slowly to new situations Mild reactions to environment	Approximately 15%
Mixed	Some of each personality type's characteristics apparent	Approximately 35%

Source: Chess, S., & Thomas, A. (1995). *Temperament in clinical practice*. New York, NY: Guilford Press.

TABLE 4–7 Ways to Improve Goodness of Fit Between Parents and Child

CHILD'S BEHAVIOR	PARENTS' ADAPTATIONS
Extremely active	Plan periods of active play several times a day. Have restful periods before bedtime to foster sleep.
Shy	Allow time to adapt at own pace to new people and situations.
Easily stimulated	Have quiet room for sleeping for an infant. Have quiet room for homework for a school-age child.
Short attention span	Provide projects that can be completed in a short period. Gradually encourage longer periods at activities.

Resiliency Theory

THEORETICAL FRAMEWORK

Why do some children coming from similar backgrounds have such different behavioral outcomes? The resiliency theory examines the individual's characteristics as well as the interaction of these characteristics with the environment. **Resilience** is the ability to function with healthy responses even when faced with significant stress and adversity (Benard, 2014; Henderson, Benard, & Sharp-Light, 2007). In this model, the individual or family members experience a crisis that provides a source of stress, and the family interprets or deals with the crisis based on resources available. Families and individuals have **protective factors**, which are characteristics that provide strength and assistance in dealing with crises, and **risk factors**, which are characteristics that promote or contribute to their challenges (Cairns, Yap, Pilkington, et al., 2014). Risk and protective factors can be identified in children, in their families, and in their communities. (See Chapter 17 for further description of the interplay of social and environmental factors with individual characteristics.) A crisis for a young child might be a transfer to a new childcare provider. Protective factors could involve past positive experiences with new people, an "easy" temperament, and the new childcare provider's awareness of adaptation needs of young children to new experiences. Risk factors for a similar child might be repeated moves to new childcare providers, limited close relationships with adults, and a "slow-to-warm-up" temperament.

Once confronted by a stress or crisis, the child and family first experience the **adjustment phase**, characterized by disorganization and unsuccessful attempts at meeting the crisis. In the **adaptation phase**, the child and family meet the challenge and use resources to deal with the crisis. Adaptation may lead to increasing resilience as well when the child and family learn about new resources and inner strengths and develop the ability to deal more effectively with future crises. Components and examples are described in Table 4–8.

NURSING APPLICATION

Nurses gather information about the individual characteristics, prior life experiences, and environmental factors that act as protective and risk factors for children. Table 4–9 lists questions that can be helpful as the nurse gathers information from a child or family members. Nurses then use concepts of resiliency theory in planning interventions for children and families. Nursing strategies can target risk factors, such as encouraging gun safety in families with firearms, and by teaching about use of gun trigger locks and locked gun cabinets. In addition, protective factors can be emphasized, such as encouraging holding and verbalization to parents of infants to provide an environment that allows for trust establishment and speech development.

Influences on Development

Both nature and nurture are important in determining individual patterns of development. The interaction of these two forces can explain differences in time frames for acquisition of developmental skills, personality variations between identical twins, and other unique characteristics of individuals. Genetic

TABLE 4–8 Components of Intervention in the Resiliency Wheel

COMPONENT	EXAMPLE OF INTERVENTIONS
Provide caring and support.	Listen to concerns. Provide information based on developmental level.
Set and communicate high expectations.	Express confidence in child's ability to succeed. Provide youth and families with resources.
Provide opportunities for meaningful participation.	Facilitate the youth's problem solving about ways to improve situations.
Increase prosocial bonding.	Assist youth to work with others on positive, purposeful activities. Facilitate community participation.
Set and communicate high expectations.	Communicate rules and establish routines. Assist families in setting clear expectations for behaviors and consequences.
Teach life skills.	Encourage communication of thoughts and feelings. Facilitate critical thinking and problem solving skills.

Source: Adapted from Resiliency in Action. (2014). *The resiliency wheel*. Retrieved from http://www.resiliency.com/free-articles-resources/crisis-response-and-the-resiliency-wheel/

TABLE 4–9 Assessment Questions to Determine Resilience Capability

CATEGORY	QUESTIONS
To determine risk factors, ask:	• Describe the event that occurred and what it has been like for your family. • What other stressors do you have in your family right now? • Are there financial worries? • Are there things you think and worry about late at night? • Describe your job, your friends. • What is a typical day like? • Describe your neighborhood. • Do you have friends, people to call in emergencies?
To determine protective factors, ask:	• What gives you strength? • How do you deal with this stress? • What do you think you do well in your family? • Who do you call when you need help? • Do you have a computer? Internet access? • Are you religious? Spiritual? • Do you exercise regularly? • How do you spend free time?

and environmental factors interact and contribute to individual differences in rates and outcomes of child development.

Genetic inheritance plays an important part in the child's potential and the unfolding of developmental milestones. See Chapter 3 for a description of chromosomes and genes. Every chromosome carries many genes that determine physical characteristics, intellectual potential, personality type, and other traits. Children are born with the potential for certain features; however, their interaction with the environment influences how and to what extent particular traits are manifested.

Some Asian cultures calculate age from the time of conception. This practice acknowledges the profound influence of the prenatal period. The mother's nutrition and general state of health play a part in pregnancy outcome. Poor nutrition can lead to small infants and infants with compromised neurologic performance, slow development, or impaired immune status with resultant high disease rates. Low maternal stores of iron can result in anemia in the infant (American Academy of Pediatrics, 2013). Maternal smoking is associated with low-birth-weight infants. Ingestion of alcoholic beverages, including beer and wine, during pregnancy may lead to fetal alcohol syndrome (Figure 4–4). Illicit drug use by the mother may result in neonatal addiction, convulsions, hyperirritability, poor social responsiveness, and other neurologic disturbances.

Even prescription or over-the-counter drugs may adversely affect the fetus. This was brought to general attention with the drug thalidomide, which was commonly used in Europe to treat nausea during the 1950s. This drug resulted in the birth of infants with limb abnormalities to women who used the drug during pregnancy. Differences in physiology related to gastric emptying, renal clearance, drug distribution, and other factors contribute to variations in pharmacokinetics during pregnancy. Drugs can cause teratogenesis (abnormal development of the fetus) or mutagenesis (permanent changes in the fetus's genetic material). Certain drugs can cause bleeding, stained teeth, impaired hearing, or other developmental effects. The U.S. Food and Drug Administration (FDA) has established risk categories for drugs in pregnancy.

Some maternal illnesses are harmful to the developing fetus. An example is rubella (German measles), which is rarely a serious disease for adults but can cause deafness, vision defects, heart defects, and intellectual disability in the fetus if it is acquired by a pregnant woman. A fetus can also acquire diseases such as acquired immunodeficiency syndrome (AIDS)/human immunodeficiency virus (HIV) infection or hepatitis B from the mother.

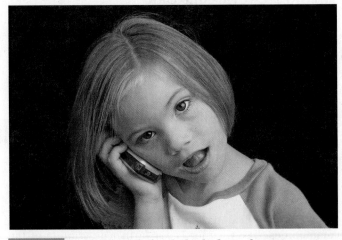

Figure 4–4 **A child with fetal alcohol syndrome.**

SOURCE: Rick's Photography/Shutterstock.

Radiation, chemicals, and other environmental hazards may adversely affect a fetus when the mother is exposed to any of these influences during her pregnancy. The best outcomes for infants occur when mothers eat well; exercise regularly; seek early prenatal care; refrain from use of drugs, alcohol, tobacco, and excessive caffeine; and follow general principles of good health.

As we have seen, both nature and nurture are important in determining individual patterns of development. These two forces interact in unique ways in each individual, explaining differences in time frames for acquisition of developmental skills among children, personality variations between identical twins, and other unique characteristics of individuals. An environmental factor that is extremely important in the development of children is the profile of family characteristics. The family is an important component in the lives of all children and plays an essential role in fostering the development of youth. A significant concept in families is that of parenting. How children are parented interacts with their individual characteristics to influence risk and protective factors, personality characteristics, and developmental outcomes. The families into which children are born influence them profoundly. Children are supported in different ways and acquire different worldviews depending on such factors as whether one or both parents work, how many siblings are present, and whether an extended family is close by. Note should be made of variations in family structure such as single parent, homosexual parents, extended family, and stepparents. Foster parenting and movement of children into a number of foster homes during childhood influences children's self-esteem and the ability to perform at potential. How might a nontraditional "family" setting, such as an adoptive or foster home, influence a child's development?

Professionalism in Practice Foster Care

On a given day, about 400,000 U.S. children are in foster care, with the average time in such care being nearly 2 years (U.S. Department of Health and Human Services, 2013). Each state is responsible for establishing the standards of education, environmental provision, and other factors of foster homes. The Office of Data, Analysis, Research and Evaluation of the Administration on Children, Youth and Families (ACYF) maintains information about foster care in the United States through the Adoption and Foster Care Analysis and Reporting System (AFCARS). The Foster Care Independence Act of 1999 fosters youth who are becoming too old for the foster care system to achieve self-sufficiency. The U.S. Education and Training Voucher Program helps youth to obtain college or vocational training at a free or reduced cost.

Nurses should recognize that children who are in foster care may have experienced family situations that were challenging or traumatic, and can be dealing with new living situations. Carefully assess the stress, adaptation, and risk and protective factors in children who are living in foster homes. Evaluate proximity to siblings and other family members as well as expectations for return to the primary family or adoption options. Support foster families so that they can provide the care needed for their foster children.

Another factor that influences child development is that of culture. The traditional customs of the many cultural groups represented in North American society influence the development of the children in these groups. Foods commonly eaten vary among people with different cultural backgrounds and influence the incidence of health problems such as cardiovascular disease in these groups. The Native American practice of carrying infants on boards often delays walking when measured against the norm for walking on some developmental tests. Children who are carried by straddling the mother's hips or back for extended periods have a low incidence of developmental dysplasia of the hip since this keeps their hips in an abducted position. It is important for nurses to take cultural practices into account when performing developmental screening; some tests may not be culturally sensitive and can inaccurately label a child as delayed when the pattern of development is simply different in the group, perhaps due to childrearing practices in the family. In addition, certain ethnic or racial groups are more prone to develop certain diseases due to genetic variations. Examples include Hispanics, who have a high incidence of diabetes; African Americans, who more commonly have sickle cell disease; and Northern European Americans, who have a higher incidence of phenylketonuria.

All cultural groups have rules regarding patterns of social interaction. Schedules of language acquisition are determined by the number of languages spoken and the amount of speech in the home. The particular social roles assumed by men and women in the culture affect school activities and ultimately career choices. Attitudes toward touching and other methods of encouraging developmental skills vary among cultures. Chapter 10 includes further descriptions of other factors that influence child development such as school and child care, community services, and additional community and family factors.

Infant (Birth to 1 Year)

Imagine the experience of tripling body weight in 1 year, or becoming proficient in understanding fundamental words in a new language and even speaking a few. These and many more accomplishments take place in the first year of life. Starting the year as a mainly reflexive creature, the infant can walk and communicate by the year's end. Never again in life is development so rapid and profound.

Physical Growth and Development

The first year of life is one of rapid change for the infant. The birth weight usually doubles by about 5 months and triples by the end of the first year (Figure 4–5). Height increases by about a foot during this year. Teeth begin to erupt at about 6 months, and by the end of the first year, the infant has six to eight deciduous teeth (see Chapter 5). Physical growth is closely associated with type and quality of feeding. (See Chapter 14 for a discussion of nutrition in infancy.)

Body organs and systems, although not fully mature at age 1 year, function differently from what they did at birth. Kidney and liver maturation helps the 1-year-old excrete drugs or other toxic substances more readily than in the first weeks of life. The changing body proportions mirror changes in developing internal organs. Maturation of the nervous system is demonstrated by increased control over body movements with growing differentiation from general to specific skills, thus enabling the infant to sit, stand, and walk. Sensory function also increases as the infant begins to discriminate visual images, sounds, and tastes (Table 4–10).

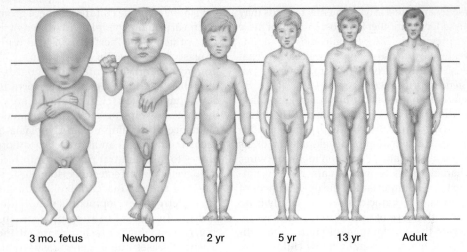

3 mo. fetus	Newborn	2 yr	5 yr	13 yr	Adult

Figure 4–5 **Body proportions at various ages.**

Cognitive Development

The brain continues to increase in complexity during the first year. Most of the growth involves maturation of cells, with only a small increase in number of cells. This growth of the brain is accompanied by development of its functions. One only has to compare the behavior of an infant shortly after birth with that of a 1-year-old to understand the incredible maturation of brain function. The newborn's eyes widen in response to sound; the 1-year-old turns to the sound and recognizes its significance. The 2-month-old cries and coos; the 1-year-old says a few words and understands many more. The 6-week-old grasps a rattle for the first time; the 1-year-old reaches for toys and feeds self.

The infant's behaviors provide clues about thought processes. Piaget's work outlines the infant's actions in a set of

TABLE 4–10 Physical Growth and Development Milestones During Infancy

AGE	PHYSICAL GROWTH	FINE MOTOR ABILITY	GROSS MOTOR ABILITY	SENSORY ABILITY
Birth to 1 month	Gains 140–200 g (5–7 oz)/week Grows 1.5 cm (1/2 in.) in first month Head circumference increases 1.5 cm (1/2 in.)/month	Holds hand in fist (*A*) Draws arms and legs to body when crying	Inborn reflexes such as startle and rooting are predominant activity May lift head briefly if prone (*B*) Alerts to high-pitched voices Comforts with touch (*C*)	Prefers to look at faces and black-and-white geometric designs Follows objects in line of vision (*D*)

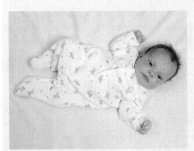

A Holds hand in fist

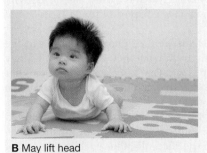

B May lift head

Kenishirotie/Shutterstock

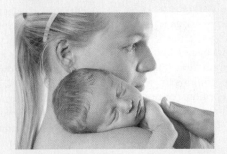

C Comforts with touch

Dora Zett/Shutterstock

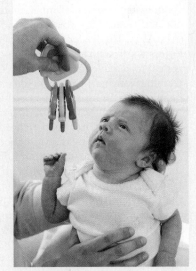

D Follows objects

Vanessa Davis/DK Images

AGE	PHYSICAL GROWTH	FINE MOTOR ABILITY	GROSS MOTOR ABILITY	SENSORY ABILITY
2–4 months	Gains 140–200 g (5–7 oz)/week Grows 1.5 cm (1/2 in.)/month Head circumference increases 1.5 cm (1/2 in.)/month Posterior fontanelle closes Ingests 120 mL/kg/24 hr (2 oz/lb/24 hr)	Holds rattle and other objects when placed in hand (*E*) Looks at and plays with own fingers Brings hands to midline	Moro reflex fading in strength Can turn from side to back and then return (*F*) Decrease in head lag when pulled to sitting position; sits with head held in midline with some bobbing When prone, holds head and supports weight on forearms (*G*)	Follows objects 180 degrees Turns head to look for voices and sounds

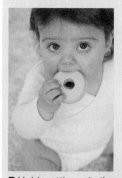

E Holds rattle and other objects

Vanessa Davis/DK Images

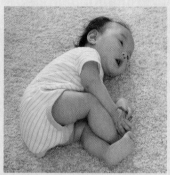

F Can turn from side to back

Vanessa Davis/DK Images

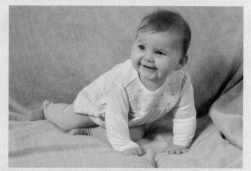

G Holds head up and supports weight with arms

4–6 months	Gains 140–200 g (5–7 oz)/week Doubles birth weight at 5–6 months Grows 1.5 cm (1/2 in.)/month Head circumference increases 1.5 cm (1/2 in.)/month Teeth may begin erupting by 6 months Ingests 100 mL/kg/24 hr (1 1/2 oz/lb/24 hr)	Grasps rattles and other objects at will; drops them to pick up another offered object (*H*) Mouths objects Holds feet and pulls to mouth Holds bottle Grasps with whole hand (palmar grasp) Manipulates objects (*I*)	Head held steady when sitting No head lag when pulled to sitting Turns from abdomen to back by 4 months and then back to abdomen by 6 months When held standing supports much of own weight (*J*)	Examines complex visual images Watches the course of a falling object

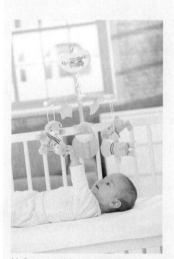

H Grasps objects at will

StockLite/Shutterstock

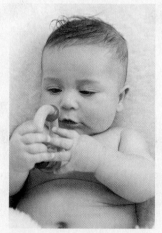

I Manipulates objects

Vanessa Davis/DK Images

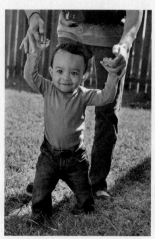

J Supports most of weight when held standing

(continued)

TABLE 4–10 Physical Growth and Development Milestones During Infancy *(continued)*

AGE	PHYSICAL GROWTH	FINE MOTOR ABILITY	GROSS MOTOR ABILITY	SENSORY ABILITY
6–8 months	Gains 85–140 g (3–5 oz)/week Grows 1 cm (3/8 in.)/month Growth rate slower than first 6 months	Bangs objects held in hands Transfers objects from one hand to the other Beginning pincer grasp at times	Most inborn reflexes extinguished Sits alone steadily without support by 8 months (*K*) Likes to bounce on legs when held in standing position	Responds readily to sounds Recognizes own name and responds by looking and smiling Enjoys small and complex objects at play

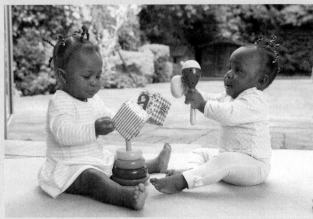

K Sits alone without support

Ruth Jenkinson/DK Images

AGE	PHYSICAL GROWTH	FINE MOTOR ABILITY	GROSS MOTOR ABILITY	SENSORY ABILITY
8–10 months	Gains 85–140 g (3–5 oz)/week Grows 1 cm (3/8 in.)/month	Picks up small objects (*L*) Uses pincer grasp well (*M*)	Crawls or pulls whole body along floor by arms (*N*) Creeps by using hands and knees to keep trunk off floor Pulls self to standing and sitting by 10 months Recovers balance when sitting	Understands words such as "no" and "cracker" May say one word in addition to "mama" and "dada"

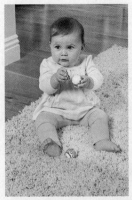

L Picks up small objects

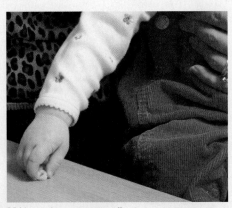

M Uses pincer grasp well

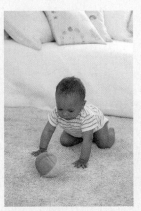

N Crawls or pulls body by arms

Vanessa Davis/DK Images

AGE	PHYSICAL GROWTH	FINE MOTOR ABILITY	GROSS MOTOR ABILITY	SENSORY ABILITY
10–12 months	Gains 85–140 g (3–5 oz)/week Grows 1 cm (3/8 in.)/month Head circumference equals chest circumference Triples birth weight by 1 year	May hold crayon or pencil and make mark on paper Places objects into containers through holes (O)	Stands alone (P) Walks holding onto furniture Sits down from standing (Q)	Plays peek-a-boo and patty cake

O Places objects in container through holes

Vanessa Davis/DK Images

P Stands alone

Q Sits down from standing

Victoria Blackie/DK Images

rapidly progressing changes in the first year of life. The infant receives stimulation through sight, sound, and feeling, which the maturing brain interprets. This input from the environment interacts with internal cognitive abilities to enhance cognitive functioning.

Psychosocial Development

PLAY

An 8-month-old infant is sitting on the floor, grasping blocks and banging them on the floor. Infants spend much of their time engaging in **solitary play**, or playing by themselves. When a parent walks by, the infant laughs and waves hands and feet wildly. Physical capabilities enable the infant to move toward and reach out for objects of interest. Cognitive ability is reflected in manipulation of blocks to create different sounds. Social interaction enhances play. The presence of a parent or other person increases interest in surroundings and teaches the infant different ways to play.

The play of infants begins in a reflexive manner. When an infant moves extremities or grasps objects, the foundations of play are established. The feel and sound of these activities give pleasure to the infant, who gradually performs them purposefully. For example, when a parent places a rattle in the hand of a 6-week-old infant, the infant grasps it reflexively. As the hands move randomly, the rattle makes an enjoyable sound. The infant learns to move the rattle to create the sound and then finally to grasp the rattle at will to play with it.

The next phase of infant play focuses on manipulative behavior. The infant examines toys closely, looking at them, touching them, and placing them in the mouth. The infant learns a great deal about texture, qualities of objects, and all aspects of the surroundings. At the same time, interaction with others becomes an important part of play. The social nature of play is obvious as the infant plays with other children and adults.

Toward the end of the first year, the infant's ability to move in space enlarges the sphere of play (Table 4–11). The infant who has begun crawling or walking can get to new places, find new toys, discover forgotten objects, or seek out other people for interaction. Play is a reflection of every aspect of development, as well as a method for enhancing learning and maturation.

PERSONALITY AND TEMPERAMENT

Why does one infant frequently awaken at night crying while another sleeps for 8 to 10 hours undisturbed? Why does one infant smile much of the time and react positively to interactions while another is withdrawn with unfamiliar people and frequently frowns and cries? Such differences in responses to the environment are believed to be inborn characteristics of temperament. Infants are born with a tendency to react in certain ways to noise and to interact differently with people. They may display varying degrees of regularity in activities of eating and sleeping, and manifest a capacity for concentrating on tasks for different amounts of time.

Nursing assessment identifies personality characteristics of the infant that the nurse can share with the parents. With this information the parents can appreciate more fully the uniqueness of their infant and design experiences to meet the infant's needs. Parents can learn to modify the environment to promote adaptation. For example, an infant who does not adapt easily to new situations may cry, withdraw, or develop another way of coping when adjusting to new people or places. Parents might be advised to use one or two babysitters rather than engaging new sitters frequently. If the infant is easily distracted when eating, parents can feed the infant in a quiet setting to encourage a focus on eating. Although the infant's temperament is unchanged, the ability to fit with the environment is enhanced. See Chapter 7 for further application of this information to health promotion of the infant.

TABLE 4–11 Psychosocial Development During Infancy

AGE	PLAY AND TOYS	COMMUNICATION
Birth–3 months	Prefers visual stimuli of mobiles, black-and-white patterns, mirrors Auditory stimuli are music boxes, tape players, soft voices Responds to rocking and cuddling Moves legs and arms while adult sings and talks Likes varying stimuli—different rooms, sounds, visual images	Coos Babbles Cries
3–6 months	Prefers noise-making objects that are easily grasped like rattles Enjoys stuffed animals and soft toys with contrasting colors	Vocalizes during play and with familiar people Laughs
6–9 months	Likes teething toys Increasingly desires social interaction with adults and other children Soft toys that can be manipulated and mouthed are favorites	Cries less Squeals and makes pleasure sounds Babbles multisyllabically (mamamamama) Increases vowel and consonant sounds Links syllables together Uses speechlike rhythm when vocalizing with others
9–12 months	Enjoys large blocks, toys that pop apart and go back together, nesting cups and other objects Laughs at surprise toys like jack-in-the-box Plays interactive games like peek-a-boo Uses push-and-pull toys	Understands "no" and other simple commands Says "dada" and "mama" to identify parents Learns one or two other words Receptive speech surpasses expressive speech

COMMUNICATION

Even at a few weeks of age, infants communicate and engage in two-way interaction. Comfort is expressed by soft sounds, cuddling, and eye contact. The infant displays discomfort by thrashing the extremities, arching the back, and crying vigorously. From these rudimentary skills, communication ability continues to develop until the infant speaks several words at the end of the first year of life (Table 4–11).

Nurses assess communication to identify possible abnormalities or developmental delays. Infants understand (receptive speech) more words than they can speak (expressive speech). Abnormalities may be caused by a hearing deficit, developmental delay, or lack of verbal stimulation from caretakers. Children in families with multiple languages speak in each language.

Nursing interventions focus on providing a stimulating environment. Encourage parents to speak to infants and teach words. Hospital nurses should include the infant's known words when providing care.

Growth and Development

Strategies for communicating with infants include the following:

- Hold for feedings.
- Hold, rock, and talk to infant often.
- Talk and sing frequently during care.
- Tell names of objects.
- Use high-pitched voice with newborns.
- When the infant is upset, swaddle and hold securely.

Toddler (1 to 3 Years)

Toddlerhood is sometimes called the first adolescence. An infant only months before, the child from 1 to 3 years is now displaying independence and negativism. Pride in newfound accomplishments emerges.

Physical Growth and Development

The rate of growth slows during the second year of life. Parents may become concerned because the child has a limited food intake. They may need reassurance that this is normal. (See Chapter 14 for further discussion of nutrition in toddlerhood.) By age 2 years,

the birth weight has usually quadrupled and the child is about one half of the adult height. Body proportions begin to change, with the legs longer and the head smaller in proportion to body size than during infancy (see Figure 4–5). The toddler has a pot-bellied appearance and stands with feet apart to provide a wide base of support. By approximately 33 months, eruption of deciduous teeth is complete, with 20 teeth being present.

Gross motor activity develops rapidly (Table 4–12) as the toddler progresses from walking to running, kicking, and riding a Big Wheel tricycle (Figure 4–6). As physical maturation occurs, the toddler develops the ability to control elimination patterns (see *Growth and Development* and *Developing Cultural Competence: Childrearing Practices*).

TABLE 4–12 Physical Growth and Development Milestones During Toddlerhood

AGE	PHYSICAL GROWTH	FINE MOTOR ABILITY	GROSS MOTOR ABILITY	SENSORY ABILITY
1–2 years	Gains 227 g (8 oz) or more per month Grows 9–12 cm (3.5–5 in.) during this year Anterior fontanelle closes	By end of second year, builds a tower of four blocks (A) Scribbles on paper (B) Can undress self (C) Throws a ball	Runs Shows growing ability to walk and finally walks with ease Walks up and down stairs a few months after learning to walk with ease (E) Likes push-and-pull toys (F)	Visual acuity 20/50
2–3 years	Gains 1.4–2.3 kg (3–5 lb)/year Grows 5–6.5 cm (2–2.5 in.)/year	Draws a circle and other rudimentary forms Learns to pour Learning to dress self (D)	Jumps Kicks ball Throws ball overhand	

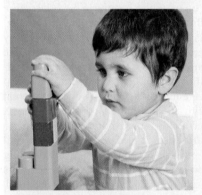

A Builds tower of four blocks

Fernando Cortes/Shutterstock

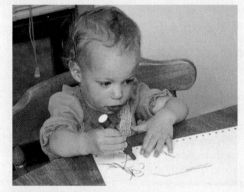

B Scribbles on paper

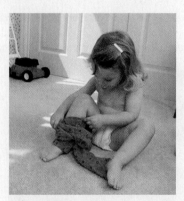

C Can undress self

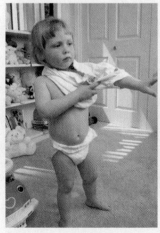

D Learning to dress self

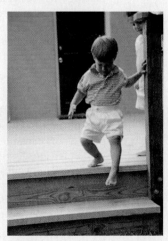

E Walks up and down stairs

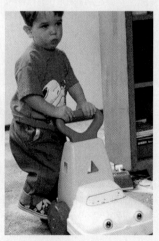

F Likes push-and-pull toys

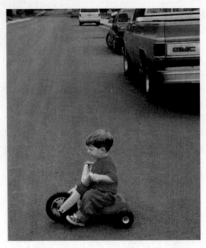

Figure 4–6 **Gross motor activity. This toddler has learned to ride a Big Wheel, which he is doing right into the street. Toddlers must be closely watched to prevent injury.**

Growth and Development

Strategies for toilet training include the following:

- When are children ready to learn toileting?
- Are parents responsible for the differences in ages at which toilet training is accomplished?
- Does toilet training provide clues to a child's intellectual ability?

We know that children are not ready for toilet training until several developmental capabilities exist: to stand and walk well, to pull pants up and down, to recognize the need to eliminate and then to

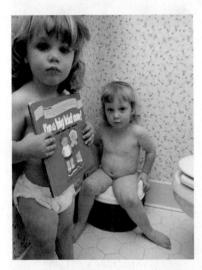

be able to wait until they are in the bathroom. Once this readiness is apparent, the child can be given a small potty chair and the procedure explained.

Children often prefer their own chairs on the floor to using a large toilet. The child should be placed on the chair at regular intervals for a few moments and can be given a reward or praise for successes. If the child seems not to understand or does not wish to cooperate, it is best to wait a few weeks and then try again. Just as all of development is subject to individual timetables, toilet training occurs with considerable variability from one child to another. Identify for parents the developmental characteristics of their child and encourage them to appreciate without anxiety the unfolding of skills. These timetables are not predictive of future development.

The child who is ill or hospitalized or has other stress often regresses in toilet-training activities. It is best to quietly reinstitute attempts at training after the trauma. Potty chairs should be available on pediatric units and toileting habits identified during initial assessment so that regular routines can be followed and the child's usual words for elimination can be used.

Developing Cultural Competence Childrearing Practices

In traditional Native American families, children are allowed to unfold and develop naturally at their own pace. Children thus wean and toilet train themselves with little interference or pressure from parents. In other groups, toilet training is accomplished at an early age. The nurse should be sensitive to the childrearing practices of the family and support them in these culturally accepted practices, rather than imposing a more structured approach to toilet training.

Cognitive Development

During the toddler years, the child moves from the sensorimotor to the preoperational stage of development. The early use of language awakens in the 1-year-old the ability to think about objects or people when they are absent. Object permanence is well developed.

At about 2 years of age, the increasing use of words as symbols enables the toddler to use preoperational thought. Rudimentary problem solving, creative thought, and an understanding of cause-and-effect relationships are now possible.

Psychosocial Development

PLAY

Many changes in play patterns occur between infancy and toddlerhood. For example, developing motor skills enable toddlers to bang pegs into a pounding board with a hammer. The social nature of toddler play is also readily seen. Toddlers find the company of other children pleasurable, even though socially interactive play may not occur. Two toddlers tend to play with similar objects side by side, occasionally trading toys and words. This is called **parallel play**. This playtime with other children helps toddlers develop social skills. Toddlers engage in play activities they have seen at home, such as pounding with a hammer and talking on the phone. This imitative behavior teaches them new actions and skills.

Physical skills are manifested in play as toddlers push and pull objects, climb in and out and up and down, run, ride a Big Wheel, turn the pages of books, and scribble with a pen. Both gross motor and fine motor abilities are enhanced during this age period.

Cognitive understanding enables the toddler to manipulate objects and learn about their qualities. Stacking blocks and placing rings on a building tower teach spatial relationships and other lessons that provide a foundation for future learning. Various kinds of play objects should be provided for the toddler to meet play needs. These play needs can easily be met whether the child is hospitalized or at home (Table 4–13).

PERSONALITY AND TEMPERAMENT

The toddler retains most of the temperamental characteristics identified during infancy but may demonstrate some changes. The normal developmental progression of toddlerhood also plays a part in responses. For example, the infant who previously responded positively to stimuli, such as a new babysitter, may appear more negative in toddlerhood. The increasing independence characteristic of this age is shown by the toddler's use of the word "no." The parent and child constantly adapt their responses to each other and learn anew how to communicate with each other.

COMMUNICATION

Because of the phenomenal growth of language skills during the toddler period, adults should communicate frequently with

TABLE 4–13 Psychosocial Development During Toddlerhood

AGE	PLAY AND TOYS	COMMUNICATION
1–3 years	Refines fine motor skills by use of cloth books, large pencil and paper, wooden puzzles Facilitates imitative behavior by playing kitchen, grocery shopping, toy telephone Learns gross motor activities by riding Big Wheel tricycle, playing with soft ball and bat, molding water and sand, tossing ball or bean bag Cognitive skills develop with exposure to educational television shows, music, stories, and books	Increasingly enjoys talking Exponential growth of vocabulary, especially when spoken and read to Needs to release stress by pounding board, frequent gross motor activities, and occasional temper tantrums Likes contact with other children and learns interpersonal skills

children in this age group. Toddlers imitate words and speech intonations, as well as the social interactions they observe.

At the beginning of toddlerhood, the child may use four to six words in addition to "mama" and "dada." Receptive speech (the ability to understand words) far outpaces expressive speech. By the end of toddlerhood, however, the 3-year-old has a vocabulary of almost 1000 words and uses short sentences.

Communication occurs in many ways, some of which are nonverbal. Toddler communication includes pointing, pulling an adult over to a room or object, and speaking in expressive jargon. **Expressive jargon** is using unintelligible words with normal speech intonations as if truly communicating in words. Another communication method occurs when the toddler cries, pounds feet, displays a temper tantrum, or uses other means to illustrate dismay. These powerful communication methods can upset parents, who often need suggestions for handling them. It is best to verbalize the feelings shown by the toddler, for example, by saying, "You must be very upset that you cannot have that candy. When you stop crying you can come out of your room," and then ignore further negative behavior. The toddler's search for autonomy and independence creates a need for such behavior. Sometimes an upset toddler responds well to holding, rocking, and stroking.

Growth and Development

Strategies for communicating with toddlers include the following:

- Give short, clear instructions.
- Do not give choices if none exist. For example, do not ask "Do you want to take your medicine now?" but rather say "What juice do you want after you take your medicine—apple or orange?"
- Offer a choice of two alternatives when possible.
- Approach positively and slowly, allowing time for the toddler to adjust.
- Tell the toddler what you are doing, and say the names of objects.

Parents and nurses can promote a toddler's communication by speaking frequently, naming objects, explaining procedures in simple terms, expressing feelings that the toddler seems to be displaying, and encouraging speech. The toddler from a bilingual home is at an optimal age to learn two languages. If the parents do not speak English, the toddler will benefit from a daycare experience in which the providers do, so that the child can learn both languages.

The nurse who understands the communication skills of toddlers is able to assess expressive and receptive language and communicate effectively, thereby promoting positive healthcare experiences for these children (Table 4–14).

TABLE 4–14 Communicating With a Toddler

Procedures such as drawing blood can be frightening for a toddler. Effective communication minimizes the trauma caused by such procedures:

- Avoid telling toddlers about the procedure too far in advance. They do not have an understanding of time and can become quite anxious.
- Use simple terminology. "We need to get a little blood from your arm. It will help us find out if you are getting better." If the parent is willing, say, "Your mom will hold your arm still so we can do it quickly."
- Allow the toddler to cry. Acknowledge that it must be frightening and that you understand.
- Perform the procedure in a treatment room so that the toddler's bed and room are a safe haven.
- Be sure the toddler is restrained, with the joints above and below the procedure immobilized.
- Use a Band-Aid to cover up the site. This can reassure the toddler that the body is still intact.
- Allow the toddler to choose a reward such as a sticker after the procedure.
- Praise the toddler for cooperation and acknowledge that you know this was difficult.
- Comfort the toddler by rocking, offering a favorite drink, playing music, and holding. If parents are present, they can offer the comfort needed.

Preschool Child (3 to 6 Years)

The preschool years are a time of new initiative and independence. Most children are in a childcare center or school for part of the day and learn a great deal from this social contact. Language skills are well developed, and the child is able to understand and speak clearly. Endless projects characterize the world of busy preschoolers. They may work with play dough to form animals, then cut out and paste paper, then draw and color.

Physical Growth and Development

Preschoolers grow slowly and steadily, with most growth taking place in the long bones of the arms and legs. The short, chubby toddler gradually gives way to a slender, long-legged preschooler (Table 4–15).

TABLE 4–15 Physical Growth and Development Milestones During the Preschool Years

PHYSICAL GROWTH

Gains 1.5–2.5 kg (3–5 lb)/year   Grows 4–6 cm (1 1/2–2 1/2 in.)/year

FINE MOTOR ABILITY

Uses scissors (A)

Draws circle, square, cross (B)

Draws at least a six-part person

Enjoys art projects such as pasting, stringing beads, using clay

Learns to tie shoes at end of preschool years (C)

Buttons clothes (D)

Brushes teeth (E)

Uses spoon, fork, knife

Eats three meals with snacks

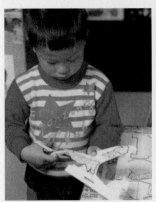

A Uses scissors

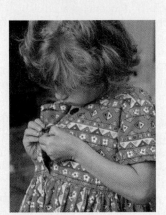

B Draws circle, square, cross

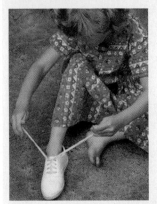

C Ties shoes

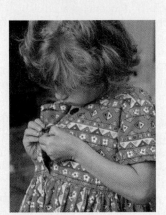

D Buttons clothes

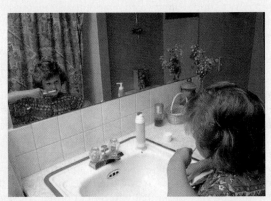

E Brushes teeth

GROSS MOTOR ABILITY

Throws a ball overhand

Climbs well (F)

Rides bicycle (G)

SENSORY ABILITY

Visual acuity continues to improve

Can focus on and learn letters and numbers (H)

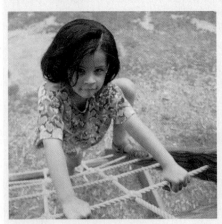

F Climbs well

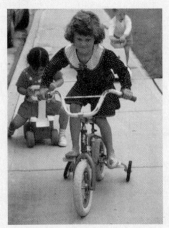

G Rides bicycle or bicycle with training wheels

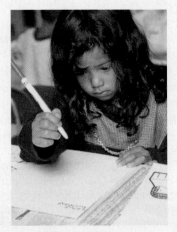

H Learns letters and numbers

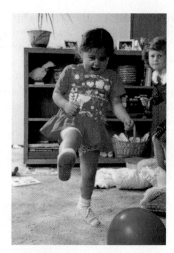

Figure 4–7 Development of physical skills in preschoolers. Preschoolers continue to develop advanced skills such as kicking a ball without falling down.

Physical skills continue to develop (Figure 4–7). The preschooler runs with ease, holds a bat, and throws balls of various types. Writing ability increases, and the preschooler enjoys drawing and learning to write a few letters.

The preschool period is a good time to encourage good dental habits. Children can begin to brush their own teeth with parental supervision and help to reach all tooth surfaces. Parents should floss children's teeth, give fluoride as prescribed if the water supply is not fluoridated, and schedule the first dental visit so the child can become accustomed to the routine of periodic dental care.

Cognitive Development

The preschooler exhibits characteristics of preoperational thought. Symbols or words are used to represent objects and people, enabling the young child to think about them. This is a milestone in intellectual development; however, the preschooler still has some limitations in thought (Table 4–16).

Psychosocial Development

PLAY

The preschooler has begun playing in a new way. Toddlers simply play side by side with friends, engaging in their own activities, but preschoolers interact with others during play. For example, one child cuts out colored paper while her friend glues it on paper in a design. This new type of interaction is called **associative play** (Figure 4–8). The child-life therapist in hospital settings recognizes the therapeutic value of play in planning activities for children that enable them to work through feelings about procedures and separation, as well as facilitating the normal developmental need for interaction with other children.

In addition to this social dimension of play, other aspects of play also differ. The preschooler enjoys large motor activities such as swinging, riding a tricycle, and throwing a ball. Increasing manual dexterity is demonstrated in greater complexity of drawings and manipulation of blocks and modeling. These changes necessitate planning of playtime to include appropriate activities. Preschool programs and child-life departments in hospitals help meet this important need.

Materials provided for play can be simple but should guide activities in which the child engages. Since fine motor activities are popular, paper, pens, scissors, glue, and a variety of other such objects should be available. The child can use them to create important images such as pictures of people, hospital beds, or friends. A collection of dolls, furniture, and clothing can be manipulated to represent parents and children, nurses and physicians, teachers, or other significant people. Because fantasy life

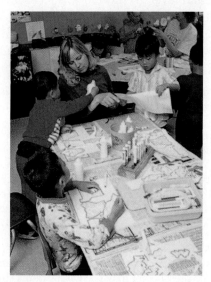

Figure 4–8 These preschoolers are participating in associative play, which means they can interact. One child is cutting out shapes, and the other is gluing them in place.

TABLE 4–16 Characteristics of Preoperational Thought

CHARACTERISTIC	DEFINITION	EXAMPLE
Egocentrism	Ability to see things only from one's own point of view	The child who cannot understand why parents may need to leave the hospital for work when the child wishes them to be present
Transductive reasoning	Connecting two events in a cause-and-effect relationship simply because they occur together in time	A child who, awakening after surgery and feeling pain, notices the intravenous infusion and believes that it is causing the pain
Centration	Focusing on only one particular aspect of a situation	The child who is concerned about breathing through an anesthesia mask and will not listen to any other aspects of preoperative teaching
Animism	Giving lifelike qualities to nonliving things	The child who views a monitoring machine as alive because it beeps

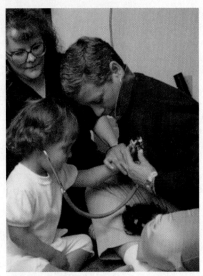

Figure 4–9 Jasmine is participating in dramatic play with a nurse while her mother looks on. In dramatic play, the child uses props to play out the drama of human life. It can be an excellent way for a nurse to assess the developmental level of children while talking to them. Notice that the child and the nurse are on the floor at the same level and the atmosphere is informal. Why is it important to be at the same level as the child?

is so powerful at this age, the preschooler readily uses props to engage in **dramatic play**—that is, the living out of the drama of human life (Figure 4–9).

The nurse can use playtime to assess the preschool child's developmental level, knowledge about health care, and emotions related to healthcare experiences. Observations about objects chosen for play, content of dramatic play, and pictures drawn can provide important assessment data. The nurse can also use play periods to teach the child about healthcare procedures and offer an outlet for expression of emotions (Table 4–17).

PERSONALITY AND TEMPERAMENT

Characteristics of personality observed in infancy tend to persist over time. The preschooler may need assistance as these characteristics are expressed in the new situations of preschool or nursery school. An excessively active child, for example, will need gentle, consistent handling to adjust to the structure of a classroom. Encourage parents to visit preschool programs to choose the one that would best foster growth in their child. Some preschoolers enjoy the structured learning of a program that focuses on cognitive skills, whereas others are happier and more open to learning in a small group that provides much time for free play. Nurses can help parents identify their child's personality or temperament characteristics and find the best environment for growth.

COMMUNICATION

Language skills blossom during the preschool years. The vocabulary grows to over 2000 words, and children speak in complete sentences of several words and use all parts of speech. They practice these newfound language skills by endlessly talking and asking questions.

Growth and Development

Strategies for communicating with preschoolers include the following:

- Allow time for child to integrate explanations.
- Verbalize frequently to the child.
- Use drawings and stories to explain care.
- Use accurate names for body functions.
- Allow choices.

The sophisticated speech of preschoolers mirrors the development occurring in their minds and helps them to learn about the world around them. However, this speech can be quite deceptive. Although preschoolers use many words, their grasp of meaning is usually literal and may not match that of adults. These literal interpretations have important implications for healthcare providers. For example, the preschooler who is told she will be "put to sleep" for surgery may think of a pet recently euthanized; the child who is told that a dye will be injected for a diagnostic test may think he is going to die; mention of "a little stick" in the arm can cause images of tree branches rather than of a simple immunization.

The child may also have difficulty focusing on the content of a conversation. The preschooler is egocentric and may be unable to move from individual thoughts to those the nurse is proposing in a teaching situation.

TABLE 4–17 Psychosocial Development During the Preschool Years

AGE	PLAY AND TOYS	COMMUNICATION
3–6 years	Associative play is facilitated by simple games, puzzles, nursery rhymes, songs	All parts of speech are developed and used, occasionally incorrectly
	Dramatic play is fostered by dolls and doll clothes, play houses and hospitals, dress-up clothes, puppets	Communicates with a widening array of people
	Stress is relieved by pens, paper, glue, scissors	Play with other children is a favorite activity
	Cognitive growth is fostered by educational television shows, music, stories, and books	Health professionals can:
		• Verbalize and explain procedures to children
		• Use drawings and stories to explain care
		• Use accurate names for body functions
		• Allow the child to talk, ask questions, and make choices

Concrete visual aids such as pictures of a child undergoing the same procedure or a book to read together enhance teaching by meeting the child's developmental needs. Handling medical equipment such as intravenous bags and stethoscopes increases interest and helps the child to focus. Teaching may have to be done in several short sessions rather than one long session.

School-Age Child (6 to 12 Years)

Errol, 10 years old, arrives home from school shortly after 3 P.M. each day. He immediately calls his friends and goes to visit one of them. They are building models of cars and collecting baseball cards. Endless hours are spent on these projects and on discussions of events at school that day (Figure 4–10).

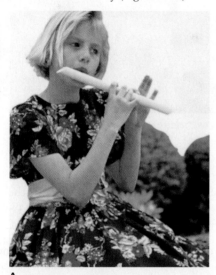

A

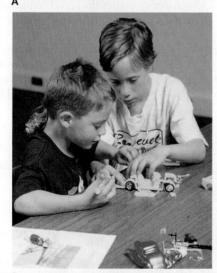

B

Figure 4–10 *A*, School-age children may take part in activities that require practice. This is a consideration when children are hospitalized and unable to practice or perform. Why? *B*, School-age children enjoy spending time with others the same age on projects and discussing the activities of the day. This is an important consideration when they are in an acute care setting. When you are in the clinical setting, look for examples of this type of interaction taking place.

Nine-year-old Karen practices soccer two afternoons a week and plays in games each weekend. She also is learning to play the flute and spends her free time at home practicing. Although practice time is not her favorite part of music, Karen enjoys the performances and wants to play well in front of her friends and teacher. Her parents now allow her to ride her bike unaccompanied to the store or to a friend's house.

These two school-age children demonstrate common characteristics of their age group. They are in a stage of industry in which it is important to the child to perform useful work. Meaningful activities take on great importance and are usually carried out in the company of peers. A sense of achievement in these activities is important in developing self-esteem and preventing a sense of inferiority or poor self-worth.

Physical Growth and Development

School age is the last period in which girls and boys are close in size and body proportions. As the long bones continue to grow, leg length increases (see Figure 4–5). Fat gives way to muscle, and the child appears leaner. Jaw proportions change as the first deciduous tooth is lost at 6 years and permanent teeth begin to erupt. Body organs and the immune system mature, resulting in fewer illnesses among school-age children. Medications are less likely to cause serious side effects, since they can be metabolized more easily. The urinary system can adjust to changes in fluid status. Physical skills are also refined as children begin to play sports, and fine motor skills are well developed through school activities (Table 4–18 and Figure 4–11).

Although it is commonly believed that the start of adolescence (age 12 years) heralds a growth spurt, the rapid increases in size commonly occur during the school-age period. Girls may begin a growth spurt by 9 or 10 years and boys a year or so later. Nutritional needs increase dramatically with this spurt.

The loss of the first deciduous teeth and the eruption of permanent teeth usually occur at about age 6 years, or at the beginning of the school-age period. Of the 30 permanent teeth, 22 to 26 erupt by age 12 years and the remaining molars follow during the teenage years. The school-age child should be closely monitored to ensure that brushing and flossing are adequate, that fluoride is taken if the water supply is not fluoridated, that dental care is obtained to provide for examination of teeth and alignment, and that loose teeth are identified before surgery or other events that may lead to loss of a tooth.

Cognitive Development

The child enters the stage of concrete operational thought at about age 7 years. This stage enables school-age children to consider alternative solutions and solve problems. However, school-age children continue to rely on concrete experiences and materials to form their thought content.

During the school-age years, the child learns the concept of **conservation** (that matter is not changed when its form is altered). At earlier ages a child believes that when water is poured from a short, wide glass into a tall, thin glass, there is more water in the taller glass. The school-age child recognizes that although it may look like the taller glass holds more water, the quantity is the same. The concept of conservation is helpful when the nurse explains medical treatments. The school-age child understands that an incision will heal, that a cast will be removed, and that an arm will look the same as before once the intravenous infusion is removed.

TABLE 4–18 Physical Growth and Development Milestones During the School-Age Years

PHYSICAL GROWTH	FINE MOTOR ABILITY	GROSS MOTOR ABILITY	SENSORY ABILITY
Gains 1.4–2.2 kg (3–5 lb)/year Grows 4–6 cm (1 1/2–2 1/2 in.)/year	Enjoys craft projects Plays card and board games	Rides two-wheeler (A) Jumps rope (B) Roller skates or ice skates	Can read Able to concentrate for longer periods on activities by filtering out surrounding sounds (C)

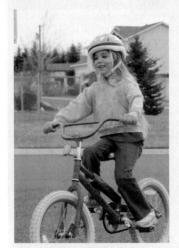

A Rides two-wheeler

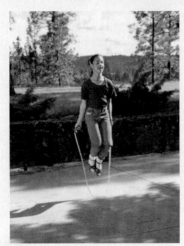

B Jumps rope

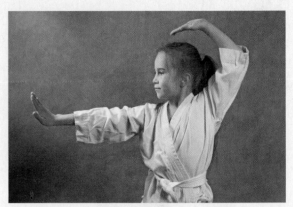

C Concentrates on activities for longer periods

Shutterstock

Psychosocial Development

PLAY

When the preschool teacher tries to organize a game of baseball, both the teacher and the children become frustrated. Not only are the children physically unable to hold a bat and hit a ball, but they seem to have no understanding of the rules of the game and do not want to wait for their turn at bat. By 6 years of age, however, children have acquired the physical ability to hold the bat properly and may occasionally hit the ball. School-age children also understand that everyone has a role—the pitcher, the catcher, the batter, the outfielders. They cooperate with one another to form a team, are eager to learn the rules of the game, and want to ensure that these rules are followed exactly (Table 4–19).

The characteristics of play exhibited by the school-age child are cooperation with others and the ability to play a part in order to contribute to a unified whole. This type of play is called **cooperative play**. The concrete nature of cognitive thought leads to a reliance on rules to provide structure and security. Children have an increasing desire to spend much of playtime with friends, which demonstrates the social component of play. Play is an extremely important method of learning and living for the school-age child. Active physical play has decreased in recent years as television viewing and playing of computer games have increased, leading to poor nutritional status and a high rate of overweight among children. See Chapters 14 and 17 for further discussion of nutrition and physical activity in children.

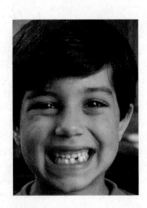

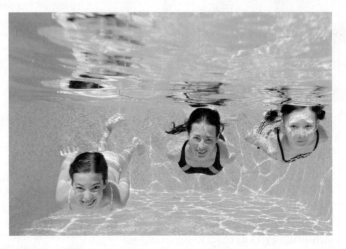

Figure 4–11 **School-age children's physical development. Left, Front teeth are lost around age 6 years. The family may have rituals associated with the loss of teeth that could affect the child's behavior if he loses a tooth while in the hospital. Right, School-age girls and boys enjoy participating in sports. They begin to lose fat while developing their muscles, so they appear leaner than at earlier ages.**

TABLE 4–19 Psychosocial Development During the School-Age Years

AGE	ACTIVITIES	COMMUNICATION
6–12 years 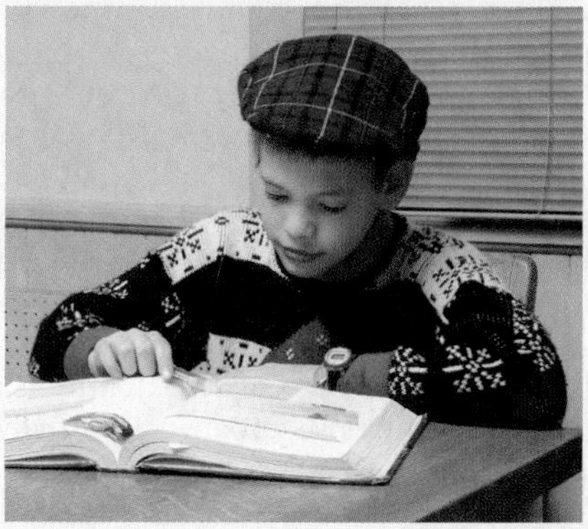	Gross motor development is fostered by ball sports, skating, dance lessons, water and snow skiing/boarding, biking A sense of industry is fostered by playing a musical instrument, gathering collections, starting hobbies, playing board and video games Cognitive growth is facilitated by reading, crafts, word puzzles, schoolwork	Mature use of language Ability to converse and discuss topics for increasing lengths of time Spends many hours at school and with friends in sports or other activities Health professionals can: • Assess child's knowledge before teaching • Allow the child to select rewards following procedures • Teach techniques such as counting or visualization to manage difficult situations • Include both parent and child in health-care decisions

When a child is hospitalized, the separation from playmates can lead to feelings of sadness and purposelessness. School-age children often feel better when placed in multibed units with other children. Games can be devised even when children are wheelchair bound (Figure 4–12). Normal, rewarding parts of play should be integrated into care. Friends should be encouraged to visit or call a hospitalized child. Discharge planning for the child who has had a cast or brace applied should address the activities the child can engage in and those the child must avoid. Reinforce the importance of playing games with friends.

PERSONALITY AND TEMPERAMENT

The enduring aspects of temperament continue to be manifested during the school years. The child classified as "difficult" at an earlier age may now have trouble in the classroom. Advise parents to provide a quiet setting for homework and to reward the child for concentration. For example, after homework is completed, the child can watch a television show. Creative efforts

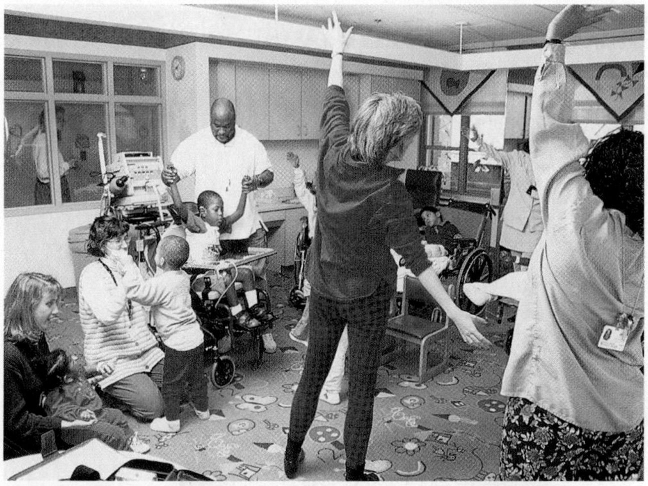

Figure 4–12 **The nurse can help the hospitalized school-age child and family accept and adjust to new circumstances. Encouraging the child in a wheelchair to participate in group activities can help build confidence in physical skills. Good self-esteem, goal attainment, personal satisfaction, and general health are the continued benefits.**

and alternative methods of learning should be valued. Encourage parents to see their children as individuals who may not all learn in the same way. The "slow-to-warm-up" child may need encouragement to try new activities and to share experiences with others, while the "easy" child will readily adapt to new schools, people, and experiences.

COMMUNICATION

During the school-age years, the child should learn how to correct any lingering pronunciation or grammatical errors. Vocabulary increases, and the child is taught about parts of speech in school. School-age children enjoy writing and can be encouraged to keep a journal of their experiences while in the hospital as a method of dealing with anxiety. It is uncommon for school-age children to understand words as literally as preschoolers.

Growth and Development

Strategies for communicating with school-age children include the following:

• Provide concrete examples of pictures or materials to accompany verbal descriptions.

• Assess knowledge before planning teaching.

• Allow child to select rewards following procedures.

• Teach techniques such as counting or visualization to manage difficult situations.

• Include child in discussions and history with parent.

• Be honest in explanations and all communications.

SEXUALITY

Children become aware of sexual differences between genders during preschool years, but they deal much more consciously with sexuality as school-age children. As children mature physically, they need information about their body changes so that they can develop a healthy self-image and an understanding of the relationships between their bodies and sexuality. Children become interested in sexual issues and are often exposed to erroneous information on television shows, in magazines, or from friends and siblings. Schools and families need to find opportunities to teach school-age children factual information about sex and to foster healthy concepts of self and others. It is advisable to ask occasional questions about sexual issues to learn how much the child knows and to provide correct information when answers demonstrate confusion. Both friends and the media are common sources of erroneous ideas. Appropriate and inappropriate touch should be discussed, with lists of trusted people who can be approached (teachers, clergy, school counselors, family members, neighbors) to discuss any episodes with which the child feels uncomfortable. Even these trusted people can be implicated in inappropriate episodes, so encourage the child to go to more than one person, an important approach if the child is uncomfortable about a relationship with any individual.

Adolescent (12 to 18 Years)

Adolescence is a time of passage signaling the end of childhood and the beginning of adulthood. Although adolescents differ in behaviors and accomplishments, they are in a period of identity formation. If a healthy identity and sense of self-worth are not developed in this period, role confusion and purposeless struggling will ensue. The adolescents encountered in nursing practice represent various degrees of identity formation, and each will offer unique challenges.

Physical Growth and Development

The physical changes ending in **puberty**, or sexual maturity, begin near the end of the school-age period. The prepubescent period is marked by a growth spurt at an average age of 10 years for girls and 13 years for boys. The increase in height and weight is generally remarkable and is completed in 2 to 3 years (Table 4–20). The growth spurt in girls is accompanied by an increase in breast size and growth of pubic hair. Menstruation occurs last and signals achievement of puberty. In boys, the growth spurt is accompanied by growth in size of the penis and testes and by growth of pubic hair. Deepening of the voice and growth of facial hair occur later, at the time of puberty. See Chapter 5 for a description of the pubertal stages.

During adolescence children grow stronger and more muscular and establish characteristic male and female patterns of fat distribution. The apocrine and eccrine glands mature, leading to increased sweating and a distinct odor to perspiration. All body organs are now fully mature, enabling the adolescent to take adult doses of medications.

The adolescent must adapt to a rapidly changing body for several years. Height, weight, and body proportions increase. Such changes occur with great variability so an adolescent may be at different points of maturation than peers. These physical changes, hormonal variations, and differences in timing offer challenges to identity formation. The adolescent must incorporate the new body, its functions, and retain a healthy sense of self in relationship to peers. The formation of self-identity is a psychologic process but is necessarily closely connected with the bodily changes occurring.

Cognitive Development

Adolescence marks the beginning of Piaget's last stage of cognitive development, the stage of formal operational thought. The adolescent no longer depends on concrete experiences as the basis of thought but develops the ability to reason abstractly. Such concepts as justice, truth, beauty, and power can be understood. The adolescent revels in this newfound ability and spends a great deal of time thinking, reading, and talking about abstract concepts.

The ability to think and act independently leads many adolescents to rebel against parental authority and experiment with risky behaviors. Through these actions, adolescents seek to establish their own identity and values.

Psychosocial Development

ACTIVITIES

Maturity leads to new activities. Adolescents may drive, ride buses, or bike independently. They are less dependent on parents for transportation and spend more time with friends.

TABLE 4–20 Physical Growth and Development Milestones During Adolescence

PHYSICAL GROWTH	FINE MOTOR ABILITY	GROSS MOTOR ABILITY	SENSORY ABILITY
Variation in age of growth spurt During growth spurt, girls gain 7–25 kg (15–55 lb) and grow 2.5–20 cm (2–8 in.); boys gain approximately 7–29.5 kg (15–65 lb) and grow 11–30 cm (4 1/2–12 in.)	Skills are well developed (A)	New sports activities attempted and muscle development continues (B) Some lack of coordination common during growth spurt	Fully developed

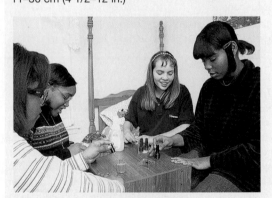

A Fine motor skills are well developed

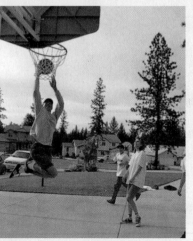

B New sports activities attempted

TABLE 4–21 Psychosocial Development During Adolescence

AGE	ACTIVITIES	COMMUNICATION
12–18 years 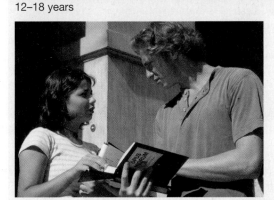	Sports—ball games, gymnastics, water and snow skiing/boarding, swimming, school sports School activities—drama, yearbook, class office, club participation Quiet activities—reading, schoolwork, television, computer, video games, music	Increasing communication and time with peer group—movies, dances, driving, eating out, attending sports events Applying abstract thought and analysis in conversations at home and school

Activities include participation in sports and extracurricular school activities, as well as "hanging out" and attending movies or concerts with friends (Table 4–21). The peer group becomes the focus of activities (Figure 4–13), regardless of the teen's interests. Peers are important in establishing identity and

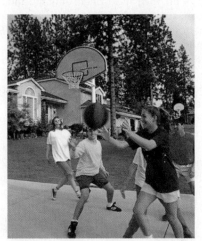

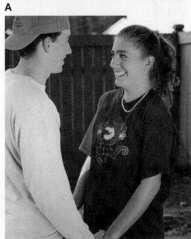

Figure 4–13 Peer group activities in adolescence. Social interaction between children of same and opposite sex is as important inside the acute care setting as it is outside. *A,* Teenagers enjoy playing together. *B,* Emotional relationships form during adolescence.

providing meaning. Although same-sex interactions dominate, boy–girl relationships are more common than at earlier stages. Adolescents thus participate in and learn from social interactions fundamental to adult relationships.

PERSONALITY AND TEMPERAMENT

Characteristics of temperament manifested during childhood usually remain stable in the teenage years. For instance, the adolescent who was a calm, scheduled infant and child often demonstrates initiative to regulate study times and other routines. Similarly, the adolescent who was an easily stimulated infant may now have a messy room, a harried schedule with assignments always completed late, and an interest in many activities. It is also common for an adolescent who was an easy child to become more difficult because of the psychologic changes of adolescence and the need to assert independence.

As during the child's earlier ages, the nurse's role may be to inform parents of different personality types and to help them support the teen's uniqueness while providing necessary structure and feedback. Nurses can help parents understand their teen's personality type and work with the adolescent to meet expectations set by teachers and others in authority.

COMMUNICATION

The adolescent uses and understands all parts of speech. Colloquialisms and slang are commonly used with the peer group. The adolescent often studies a foreign language in school, having the ability to understand and analyze grammar and sentence structure.

The adolescent increasingly leaves the home base and establishes close ties with peers. These relationships become the basis for identity formation. There is generally a period of stress or crisis before a strong identity can emerge. The adolescent may try out new roles by learning a new sport or other skills, experimenting with drugs or alcohol, wearing different styles of clothing, or trying other activities. It is important to provide positive role models and a variety of experiences to help the adolescent make wise choices.

Adolescents also have a need to leave the past, to be different, and to change from former patterns to establish their own identities. Rules that are repeated constantly and dogmatically will probably be broken in the adolescent's quest for self-identity. This poses difficulties when the adolescent has a health problem, such as diabetes, or a heart problem that requires ongoing care. Introducing the adolescent to other teens who manage the same problem appropriately is usually more successful than telling the adolescent what to do.

Ensure privacy during the taking of health histories or interventions with teens. Even if a parent is present for part of a history or examination, the adolescent should be given the opportunity to relay information or ask questions alone with the healthcare provider. Give the adolescent a choice of whether to have a parent present during an examination or while care is provided. Most information shared by an adolescent is confidential. Some states mandate disclosure of certain information to parents, such as an adolescent's desire for an abortion. In these cases, the adolescent should be informed of what will be disclosed to the parent.

Setting up teen rooms (recreation rooms for use only by adolescents) or separate adolescent units in hospitals can provide necessary peer support during hospitalization. Most adolescents are not pleased when placed on a unit or in a room with young children. Choices should be allowed whenever possible. These might include preference for evening or morning bathing, the type of clothes to wear while hospitalized, timing of treatments, and who should be allowed to visit and for how long. Use of negotiations and agreements with adolescents may increase compliance. Firmness, gentleness, choices, and respect must all be balanced during care of adolescent clients.

Growth and Development

Strategies for communicating with adolescents include the following:

- Provide written as well as verbal explanations.
- Direct history and explanations to teen alone; then include parent.
- Allow for safe exploration of topics by suggesting that the teen is similar to other teens. ("Many teens with diabetes have questions about how to eat foods they and their friends like and still stay within their diet needs. How about you?")
- Arrange meetings for discussions with other teens.

SEXUALITY

With maturation of the body and increased secretion of hormones, the adolescent achieves sexual maturity. This complex process involves a growing interest in sexuality and romantic or sexual relationships, an interplay of the forces of society and family, and identity formation. The early adolescent progresses from dances and other social events with members of the opposite sex; the late adolescent is mature sexually and may have regular sexual encounters. Nearly one half of all high-school students in the United States have had intercourse, and 34% had intercourse in the previous 3 months. However, 59% of youth did not use a condom at their last sexual encounter, putting this age group at high risk of acquiring sexually transmitted infections (Kann et al., 2014).

Teenagers need information about their bodies and emerging sexuality. To make informed decisions about their behavior, teenagers should understand the interests and forces they experience. Including sex education in school classes and healthcare encounters is important. Information on how to prevent sexually transmitted infections (STIs) is given, with most school districts now providing some teaching on AIDS. Far more common risks to teens, however, are diseases such as gonorrhea and herpes. Health histories should include questions on sexual activity, STIs, and birth control use and understanding. Most hospitals routinely perform pregnancy screening on adolescent girls before elective procedures.

Adolescents benefit from clear information about sexuality, an opportunity to develop relationships with adolescents in various settings, an open atmosphere at home and school where problems and issues can be discussed, and previous experience in problem solving and self-decision making. Sexual issues should be among topics that adolescents can discuss openly in a variety of settings. Alternatives and support for their decisions should be available.

Some adolescents identify with a sexual minority group such as lesbian, gay, bisexual, or transgender. They are at particular risk of being stigmatized and harassed by other youth or adults. They are more likely to suffer a variety of problems, such as isolation, rejection by family and friends, violence, and suicide, and to take sexual risks (Steever, Francis, Gordon, et al., 2014). Nurses are instrumental in helping these youth by providing information for them and their parents, integrating sexual minority content into school sexual curricula, and providing referrals for health care and social care when needed. See Chapter 17 for further information about the health issues related to homosexuality and other sexual minority practices.

Chapter Highlights

- Development unfolds in a predictable pattern, but at different rates dependent on the particular characteristics and experiences of each child.
- Major theories of development encompass the psychosexual (Freud), psychosocial (Erikson), cognitive (Piaget), moral (Kohlberg), social learning (Bandura), and behavioral (Skinner and Watson) components of individuals.
- The ecologic theory of Bronfenbrenner and the temperament theory of Chess and Thomas emphasize the interactions of the individual with the environment.

- Resiliency theory examines risk and protective factors that hinder or help children and families when dealing with developmental and life crises.
- The newborn period begins at birth and ends at about 1 month of age and is characterized by adaptation to extrauterine life. Infancy spans 1 month to 1 year and is marked by rapid physical growth, mastery of basic fine and gross motor skills, and emerging cognitive and language skills.
- Toddlers range in age from 1 to 3 years and become increasingly mobile and communicative. Preschool years range from

ages 3 to 6 and are marked by increasing social skills, coordination, and language mastery.

- School age spans the years from ages 6 to 12, and puberty occurs from ages 9 to 12 years, marked by a growth spurt and sexual maturation. Adolescence begins at 12 years of age and

lasts through the teen years, with physical, emotional, cognitive, and social maturation.

- The nurse assesses development at each stage and provides anticipatory guidance and other interventions to foster optimal development.

Clinical Reasoning in Action

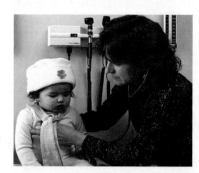

You encounter a 12-month-old child, Julia, while working in the developmental clinic. Her mother tells you that their family practice physician had concerns that Julia might have a developmental delay. She was a full-term baby and there were no complications throughout her mother's pregnancy or delivery. Julia's mother tells you that Julia has a generally shy and slow-to-warm-up temperament. She makes little

eye contact with you and prefers to sit on her mother's lap and cling to her arms if a stranger gets close. She is able to pick up small objects, babble, crawl, and use her pincer grasp. She is not able to walk, hold a crayon, or speak any words. Julia clearly has a developmental delay.

1. What are some examples of toys you can suggest to Julia's parents based on her developmental level (not based on her age)?

2. What are some examples of hazards you can advise Julia's parents about avoiding based on her developmental level?

3. What is a suggestion you can give the parents about dealing with a child like Julia who has a shy or slow-to-warm-up temperament?

References

American Academy of Pediatrics. (2013). *Pediatric nutrition handbook* (7th ed.). Elk Grove Village, IL: Author.

Bandura, A. (1986). *Social foundations of thought and actions: A social cognitive theory.* Englewood Cliffs, NJ: Prentice Hall.

Bandura, A. (1997a). *Self efficacy in changing societies.* New York, NY: Cambridge University Press.

Bandura, A. (1997b). *Self efficacy: The exercise of control.* New York, NY: Freeman.

Benard, B. (2014). *The foundations of the resiliency framework.* Retrieved from http://www.resiliency.com/free-articles-resources/the-foundations-of-the-resiliency-framework/

Bronfenbrenner, U. (1986). Ecology of the family as a context for human development: Research perspectives. *Developmental Psychology, 22,* 723–742.

Bronfenbrenner, U. (Ed.). (2005). *Making human beings human: Bioecological perspectives on human development.* Thousand Oaks, CA: Sage.

Bronfenbrenner, U., McClelland, P. D., Ceci, S. J., Moen, P., & Wethington, E. (1996). *The state of Americans.* New York, NY: Free Press.

Cairns, K. E., Yap, M. B., Pilkington, D., & Jorm, A. F. (2014). Risk and protective factors for depression that adolescents can modify: A systematic review and meta-analysis of longitudinal studies. *Journal of Affective Disorders, 169C,* 61–75. doi:10.1016/j.jad.2014.08.006

The Center for Parenting Education. (2014). *Temperament: Understanding "goodness of fit."* Retrieved from http://centerforparentingeducation.

org/library-of-articles/child-development/unique-child-equation/temperament/understanding-goodness-of-fit/

Chess, S., & Thomas, A. (1995). *Temperament in clinical practice.* New York, NY: Guilford Press.

Chess, S., & Thomas, A. (1996). *Temperament: Theory and practice.* Philadelphia, PA: Brunner/Mazel, Publishers.

Chess, S., & Thomas, A. (1999). *Goodness of fit: Clinical applications from infancy through adult life.* Philadelphia, PA: Brunner/Mazel, Publishers.

Children's Hospital of Philadelphia. (2012). *International adoption health program.* Retrieved from http://www.chop.edu/service/adoption/health-considerations

Davies, J. A., Terhorts, L., Nakonechny, A. J., Skukla, N., & Saadawi, G. E. (2014). The development and effectiveness of a health information website designed to improve parents' self-efficacy in managing risk for obesity in preschoolers. *Journal for Specialists in Pediatric Nursing.* doi:10.1111/jspn.12086

Dunn, W. L., & Craig, G. J. (2013). *Understanding human development* (3rd ed.). Upper Saddle River, NJ: Pearson Education.

Erikson, E. (1963). *Childhood and society.* New York, NY: Norton.

Erikson, E. (1968). *Identity: Youth and crisis.* New York, NY: Norton.

Ginsberg, H., & Opper, S. (1988). *Piaget's theory of intellectual development* (3rd ed.). Paramus, NJ: Prentice Hall.

Henderson, N., Benard, B., & Sharp-Light, M. (2007). *Resiliency in action.* Ojai, CA: Resiliency in Action.

Joshi, A., Trout, K. E., Aguirre, T., & Wilhelm. S. (2014). Exploration of factors influencing initiation and continuation of breastfeeding among Hispanic women living in rural settings: A multi-methods study. *Rural Remote Health, 14,* 2955.

Kann, L., Kinchen, S., Shanklin, S. L., Flint, K. H., Hawkins, J., Harris, W. A., . . . Zaza, S. (2014). Youth Risk Behavior Surveillance—2013. *Morbidity and Mortality Weekly Report SS, 63*(4), 1–172.

Piaget, J. (1972). *The child's conception of the world.* Totowa, NJ: Littlefield, Adams.

Resiliency in Action. (2014). *The resiliency wheel.* Retrieved from http://www.resiliency.com/free-articles-resources/crisis-response-and-the-resiliency-wheel/

Salmon, J., Jorna, M., Hume, C., Arundell, L., Dhahine, J., Tienstra, J., & Crawford, C. (2011). A translational research intervention to reduce screen behaviours and promote physical activity among children: Switch-2-Activity. *Health Promotion International, 26,* 311–321.

Santrock, J. (2012). *Life-span development* (14th ed.). Boston, MA: McGraw-Hill.

Steever, J., Francis, J., Gordon, L. P., & Lee, J. (2014). Sexual minority youth. *Primary Care, 42,* 651–669.

U.S. Department of Health and Human Services. (2013). *Recent demographic trends in foster care. Data brief 2013-1.* Retrieved from http://www.acf.hhs.gov/sites/default/files/cb/data_brief_foster_care_trends1.pdf

U.S. Department of State. (2015). *Intercountry adoption.* Retrieved from http://travel.state.gov/content/adoptionsabroad/en/about-us/statistics.html

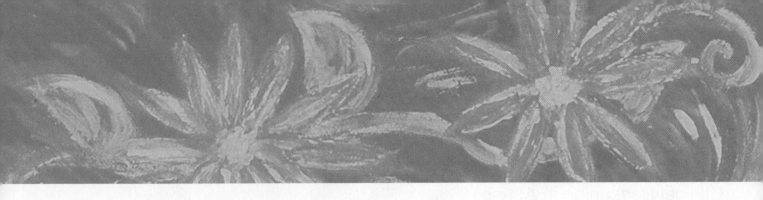

Chapter 5
Pediatric Assessment

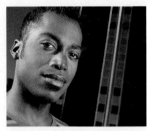

I was scared when we brought Colby to the hospital. He looked helpless, afraid, and sick. The nurses and doctors took over when we got to the hospital, and I felt better because they seemed to know what to do.

—Father of Colby, age 6 months

Ryan McVay/Getty Images

∨ Learning Outcomes

5.1 Describe the elements of a health history for infants and children of different ages.

5.2 Apply communication strategies to improve the quality of historical data collected.

5.3 Demonstrate strategies to gain cooperation of a young child for assessment.

5.4 Describe the differences in sequence of the physical assessment for infants, children, and adolescents.

5.5 Modify physical assessment techniques for the age and developmental stage of the child.

5.6 List five normal variations in pediatric physical findings (such as breast budding in a girl) found during a physical assessment.

5.7 Evaluate the growth pattern of an infant or child.

5.8 Distinguish between expected and unexpected physical signs to identify at least five signs that require urgent nursing intervention.

How do examination techniques vary by the age of the child? How does the nurse encourage infants and toddlers to cooperate with the examination? This chapter provides an overview of pediatric assessment, including history taking and examination techniques geared to the unique needs of pediatric clients. Strategies for obtaining the child's history are presented first. The remainder of the chapter then outlines a systematic process for physical examination of children and adolescents.

Anatomic and Physiologic Characteristics of Infants and Children

Children and infants are not only smaller than adults; they also have very different physiology. Knowledge of pediatric anatomic and physiologic differences will aid in recognizing normal

variations found during the physical examination. It also assists with understanding the different physiologic responses children have to illness and injury. The illustration in *As Children Grow: Children Are Not Just Small Adults* provides an overview of important anatomic and physiologic differences between children and adults.

Obtaining the Child's History
Communication Strategies

The health history interview is a very personal conversation with a parent, caregiver, or adolescent during which private concerns and feelings are shared. Try to ensure that both parties clearly understand the information exchange and use effective communication with the parent or the child. Effective communication is difficult to accomplish because parents and children may not always correctly interpret what the nurse says, just as the nurse

As Children Grow: **Children Are Not Just Small Adults**

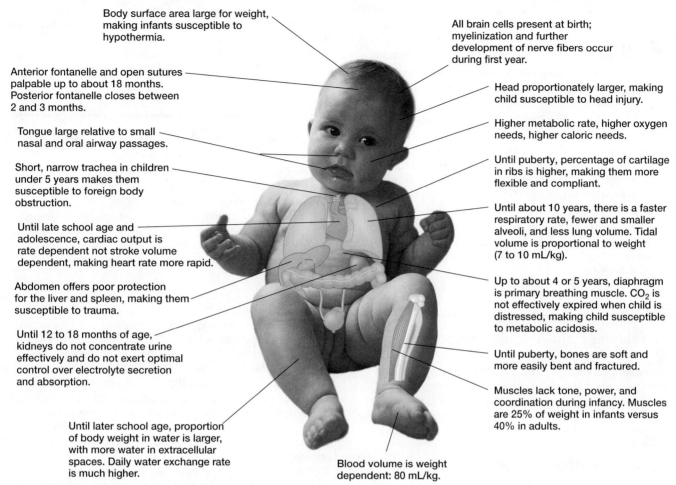

Body surface area large for weight, making infants susceptible to hypothermia.

Anterior fontanelle and open sutures palpable up to about 18 months. Posterior fontanelle closes between 2 and 3 months.

Tongue large relative to small nasal and oral airway passages.

Short, narrow trachea in children under 5 years makes them susceptible to foreign body obstruction.

Until late school age and adolescence, cardiac output is rate dependent not stroke volume dependent, making heart rate more rapid.

Abdomen offers poor protection for the liver and spleen, making them susceptible to trauma.

Until 12 to 18 months of age, kidneys do not concentrate urine effectively and do not exert optimal control over electrolyte secretion and absorption.

Until later school age, proportion of body weight in water is larger, with more water in extracellular spaces. Daily water exchange rate is much higher.

All brain cells present at birth; myelinization and further development of nerve fibers occur during first year.

Head proportionately larger, making child susceptible to head injury.

Higher metabolic rate, higher oxygen needs, higher caloric needs.

Until puberty, percentage of cartilage in ribs is higher, making them more flexible and compliant.

Until about 10 years, there is a faster respiratory rate, fewer and smaller alveoli, and less lung volume. Tidal volume is proportional to weight (7 to 10 mL/kg).

Up to about 4 or 5 years, diaphragm is primary breathing muscle. CO_2 is not effectively expired when child is distressed, making child susceptible to metabolic acidosis.

Until puberty, bones are soft and more easily bent and fractured.

Muscles lack tone, power, and coordination during infancy. Muscles are 25% of weight in infants versus 40% in adults.

Blood volume is weight dependent: 80 mL/kg.

Children are not just small adults. There are important anatomic and physiologic differences between children and adults that will change based on a child's growth and development.

---

may not understand completely what the parent or child says. People's interpretation of information is based on their life experiences, culture, and education.

STRATEGIES TO BUILD RAPPORT WITH THE FAMILY

When obtaining the client history, make sure the parents understand the purpose of the interview and how the information will be used for the child's benefit. To develop rapport, demonstrate interest in and concern for the child and family during the interview. This rapport forms the foundation for the collaborative relationship between the nurse and parent that will lead to the best nursing care for the child. The following strategies help to establish rapport with the child's family during the nursing history:

- *Introduce yourself* (name, title or position, and role in caring for the child). To demonstrate respect, ask all family members present what name they prefer you to use when talking with them.

- *Explain the purpose of the interview* and why the nursing history is different from the information collected by other health professionals. For example, "Nurses use this information to plan nursing care best suited for your child."

- *Provide privacy* and remove as many distractions as possible during the interview. If the client's room does not offer privacy, attempt to find a vacant room or lounge to interview the child and family. Assure the parents and the child that the information provided is protected under the Health Insurance Portability and Accountability Act (HIPAA), a federal law that requires written consent before personal health information can be shared with healthcare providers outside the facility.

- *Direct the focus of the interview* with open-ended questions. Open-ended questions are useful to initiate the interview, develop rapport, and understand the parents' perceptions of the child's problem. For example, "What problems led to Roberto's admission to the hospital?" Use close-ended questions or directing statements to clarify information or to obtain detailed information. For example, "How high was Tommy's fever this morning?"

- *Ask one question at a time* so that the parent or child understands what piece of information is desired and so that it is clear which question the parent is answering. "Does any member of your family have diabetes, heart disease, or sickle cell disease?" is a multiple question. Ask about each disease separately to ensure the most accurate response.

- *Involve the child in the interview* by asking age-appropriate questions. Young children can be asked, "What is your doll's name?" or "Where does it hurt?" Demonstrating an interest in the child initiates development of rapport with both child and parents. Ask older children and teens questions about their illness or injury. Offer them an opportunity to discuss their major concerns privately without parents present.

- *Be honest with the child* when answering questions or when giving information about what will happen. Children need to learn that they can trust their nurse.

- *Choose the language style best understood by the parent and child.* Commonly used phrases or medical terms may have different meanings to different people. To improve communication, ask the parents or child questions to ensure that their understanding of a phrase or term is correct. For example, "You used the term *hyperactivity*. Tell me what this behavior means to you."

- *Use an interpreter to improve communication when not fluent in the family's primary language.* Avoid using a family member or friend for history taking to ensure client and family confidentiality.

Developing Cultural Competence Phrasing Your Questions

Some cultural groups, particularly Asians, try to anticipate the answers you want to hear, or say yes even if they do not understand the question. This is done in an effort to please you or as an expression of politeness. Remember to use open-ended questions or phrase your questions in a neutral manner.

CAREFUL LISTENING

Complete attention is necessary to "hear" and accurately interpret information the parents and child give during the nursing history. While carefully listening to the information provided, pay attention to how it is expressed, and observe behavior during the interaction.

- Does the parent hesitate or avoid answering certain questions?

- Pay attention to the parent's attitude or tone of voice when the child's problems are discussed. Determine if it is consistent with the seriousness of the child's problem. The tone of voice can reveal anxiety, anger, or lack of concern.

- Be alert to any underlying themes. For example, the parent who talks about the child's diagnosis, but repeatedly refers to the impact of the illness on the family's finances or on meeting the needs of other family members, is requesting that these issues be addressed.

- Observe the parent's *nonverbal* behavior (posture, gestures, body movements, eye contact, and facial expression) for consistency with the words and tone of voice used. Is the parent interested in and appropriately concerned about the child's condition? Behaviors such as sitting up straight, making eye contact, and appearing apprehensive reflect appropriate concern for the child. Physical withdrawal, failure to make eye contact, or a happy expression could be inconsistent with the child's serious condition.

Subtle nonverbal and verbal cues may indicate that the parent has not provided complete information about the child's problem. Observe for behaviors such as avoiding eye contact, change in voice pitch, or hesitation when responding to a question. Be supportive and ask clarifying questions to encourage further description or the expression of information that is difficult for the parent or child to share. For example, "It sounds like that was a very difficult experience. How did Lily react?"

Developing Cultural Competence Interaction Patterns

Prolonged eye contact may be avoided by some cultural groups, such as persons of Native American, African American, Hindu, Japanese, and Chinese heritage, because it is considered impolite, aggressive, or a sign of disrespect. Other cultures, such as persons of Arabic, European, and Russian heritage, seek eye contact, and some may look for a response or impact regarding what is said (Purnell, 2014).

Encourage parents to share information, even if it is private or sensitive, especially when it influences nursing care planning. Often parents avoid sharing some information because they want to make a good impression, or they do not understand the value of the missing information. If parents hesitate to share information, briefly explain why the question was asked—for example, to make their child's hospital experience more pleasant or to begin planning for the child's discharge and home care. Silence is common in some Asian and Native American groups as they attempt to form responses to questions.

In some cases, the parent may become too agitated, upset, or angry to continue responding to questions. When the information is not needed immediately, move on to another portion of the history to determine whether the parent is able to respond to other questions. Depending on the emotional status of the parent, it may be appropriate to collect the remaining information later.

Data to Be Collected

Nurses collect and organize health, medical, and personal-social history to plan a child's nursing care. The health status, psychosocial, and developmental data are organized to help develop the nursing diagnoses and the nursing care plan.

CLIENT INFORMATION

Obtain the child's name and nickname, age, sex, and ethnic origin. The child's birth date, race, religion, address, and phone number can be obtained from the admission form. Ask the parent for an emergency contact address and phone number, as well as a work phone number. Record the name of the person providing the client history and that person's relationship to the child.

PHYSIOLOGIC DATA

Collect information about the child's health problems and diseases chronologically using categories specified by the electronic health record, such as the following.

Chief Concern. Identify the child's primary problem or reason for hospital admission or visit to a healthcare setting, and document it using the parent's or child's exact words.

TABLE 5–1 History of Present Illness or Injury

CHARACTERISTIC	DEFINING VARIABLES
Onset	Sudden or gradual, previous episodes, date and time began
Type of symptom	Pain, itching, cough, vomiting, runny nose, diarrhea, rash, etc.
Location	Generalized or localized—be anatomically precise
Duration	Continuous or episodic symptoms, length of episodes
Severity	Effect on daily activities (e.g., interrupted sleep, decreased appetite, unable to attend school)
Influencing factors	What relieves or worsens symptoms, what precipitated the problem, recent exposure to infection or allergen
Past evaluation for the problem	Laboratory studies and diagnostic procedures, physician's office or hospital where done, results of past examinations
Previous and current treatment	Prescribed and over-the-counter drugs used, complementary therapies (e.g., heat, ice, rest), response to treatments

Present Illness or Injury. Obtain a detailed description of the current health problem that includes the characteristics in Table 5–1. Each problem is described separately.

Past History. This more detailed description of the child's prior health problems includes all major past illnesses and injuries. Identify all major illnesses, including common communicable diseases. Identify major injuries, their cause or mechanism, and their severity. Obtain information about each prior surgery, its purpose, and if the surgery required overnight hospitalization. For all hospitalizations, identify the reason and length of stay. Identify the circumstances for any prior transfusion, its type (blood, blood products, or immune globulin), and any reaction. Obtain information about each specific diagnosis, treatment, outcome, complication or residual problem, and the child's reaction to the event. Use the guidelines in Table 5–2 to obtain a *birth history* when the child's present problem may be related to problems during the pregnancy, birth, and newborn care.

Current Health Status. Obtain a detailed description of each aspect of the child's typical health status.

- *Health maintenance*—child's primary healthcare provider, dentist, and other specialty healthcare providers, timing of last visit to each.
- *Medications*—prescribed and over-the-counter medications (oral, topical, injectable) used daily or frequently for fever, colds, coughs, and rashes. Ask about the use of herbs, plants, teas, or other complementary therapies.
- *Allergies*—to food, medication, animals, insect bites, or other exposures, and the type of reaction (e.g., respiratory difficulty, rash, hives, itching).
- *Immunizations*—review dates immunizations were received. Ask about any unexpected reactions. Inquire about the reason if not up-to-date. (See Chapter 16 for the recommended immunization schedule.)

TABLE 5–2 Birth History

Prenatal condition	• Mother's age, health during pregnancy, prenatal care, weight gained, special diet, use of alcohol or drugs, expected date of birth • Details of illnesses, radiograph or sonogram findings, hospitalizations, medications, complications, and their timing during pregnancy • Prior obstetric history
Intrapartum—description of birth	• Site of birth (hospital, home, birthing center) • Labor induced or spontaneous, time of rupture of membranes, length of labor, color of amniotic fluid, complications • Vaginal or cesarean birth, forceps or suction used, vertex or breech position • Length of pregnancy (weeks), single or multiple birth
Condition of baby at birth	• Birth weight, Apgar score, cried immediately • Need for incubator, resuscitation, oxygen, ventilator • Any abnormalities detected, meconium staining
Postnatal condition	• Difficulties in the nursery—feeding, respiratory problems, jaundice, cyanosis, rashes, seizures • Length of hospital stay, special nursery, home with mother • Breastfed or bottlefed, weight lost/gained in hospital • Medical care needed in first week—readmission to hospital

- *Safety measures used*—car restraint system, window guards, medication storage, sports protective gear, smoke detectors, bicycle helmet, firearm storage, water safety, and others.
- *Activities and exercise*—usual play and/or sports activities; physical mobility and limitations, adaptive equipment used.
- *Nutrition*—formula-fed or breastfed; if breastfed, for how long, type and amount of daily formula and other liquid intake; when solid foods were introduced; enrollment in the Special Supplemental Nutrition Program for Women, Infants, and Children (WIC). Contrast the child's food intake to the appropriate amount for age and weight (see Chapter 14).
- *Sleep*—infant sleep position, length and timing of naps and nighttime sleep; nightmares or night terrors, snoring, other sleep disturbances; where the child sleeps; bedtime rituals.

TABLE 5–3 Familial or Hereditary Diseases

Infectious diseases	Tuberculosis, HIV, hepatitis, herpes
Heart disease	Heart defects, myocardial infarctions, hypertension, dyslipidemia, sudden childhood deaths
Allergic disorders	Eczema, hay fever
Eye disorders	Glaucoma, cataracts, vision loss
Ear disorders	Hearing loss, unusual shape or position of ears
Hematologic disorders	Sickle cell disease, thalassemia, glucose-6-phosphate dehydrogenase (G6PD) deficiency, hemophilia
Respiratory disorders	Cystic fibrosis, asthma
Cancer	Retinoblastoma, cancer with early age of onset
Endocrine disorders	Diabetes mellitus types 1 and 2, hypothyroidism, hyperthyroidism, Turner syndrome
Brain disorders	Intellectual disability, epilepsy, psychiatric disorders
Musculoskeletal disorders	Muscular dystrophy, scoliosis, spina bifida
Gastrointestinal disorders	Pyloric stenosis, ulcers, colitis, celiac disease, polycystic kidneys
Metabolic disorders	Phenylketonuria, galactosemia, maple syrup urine disease, Tay-Sachs disease, Gaucher disease
Problem pregnancies	Repeated miscarriages, stillbirths
Learning problems	Attention deficit disorder, Down syndrome, fragile X syndrome

Familial and Hereditary Diseases.   Collect data about hereditary diseases and other significant health conditions for three generations of family members, including the parents, grandparents, aunts, uncles, cousins, child, and siblings, using information listed in Table 5–3. Collect information about the health status of each parent. Record information in either a family genogram or pedigree (see Chapter 3) or a narrative format.

Review of Systems.   Collect a comprehensive overview of the child's health during the review of systems using the guidelines from Table 5–4. Additional signs and symptoms associated with the child's condition may be identified, as well as other problems with no direct relationship to the child's health problem that could potentially impact nursing care or home care. For example, asking about allergies may reveal a latex allergy that requires the use of nonlatex supplies and preparation for allergic reactions. For each problem, obtain the treatment, outcomes, residual problems, and age at time of onset.

PSYCHOSOCIAL DATA
Obtain information about family composition to establish a socioeconomic and sociologic context for planning the child's care in the hospital, community, and at home.

- *Family composition*—family members living in the home, their relationship to the child, marital status of parents or other family structure, and people helping to care for the child
- *Financial resources*—household members employed, family income, healthcare resources (e.g., private insurance, Medicaid, Child Health Insurance Program [CHIP]), and other resources (Supplemental Nutrition Assistance Program [SNAP], Temporary Assistance for Needy Families [TANF], or WIC)
- *Home environment*—housing description (condition, potential lead exposure, safe play area); city or well water; sanitation; and availability of electricity, heat, and refrigeration
- *Community environment*—neighborhood description; safety, playgrounds, transportation, and access to shopping; school or childcare arrangements
- *Family or lifestyle changes*—for example, recent unemployment, relocations, or divorce; how the child and family members have coped

Newborns.   The psychosocial history for parents of newborns should focus on readiness to care for the newborn at home. Inquire about support for the parent in the initial postpartum period, safe transport, and a home environment that provides heat, refrigeration, and safe water supplies.

Children.   Information about the child's daily routines, psychosocial data, and other living patterns should focus on issues that have an impact on the quality of daily living (Table 5–5).

Adolescents.   The psychosocial history for adolescents should focus on critical areas in their lives that may contribute to a less than optimal environment for normal growth and development. Key topics that should be addressed are included in the HEEADSSS screening tool (Brown, 2011):

- **H**ome environment
- **E**ducation and employment
- **E**ating
- **A**ctivities
- **D**rugs (substance abuse)
- **S**exuality
- **S**uicidal thoughts
- **S**afety, savagery (exposure to violence)

DEVELOPMENTAL STATUS
Information about the child's motor, cognitive, language, and social development will help to plan nursing care. Ask the parent about the child's developmental milestones and current fine and gross motor skills. Obtain the age at which the child first used words appropriately and the current words used or language ability. Actual assessment of the child with a parent questionnaire may also be used to collect this information. For children in school, ask about academic performance to assess cognitive development. Ask the parent about the child's manner of interaction with other children, family members, and strangers. For adolescents, ask about school performance and activities indicating development of independence and autonomy. (See Chapter 4 for developmental assessment guidelines.)

TABLE 5–4 Review of Systems

BODY SYSTEMS	SAMPLES OF ISSUES TO IDENTIFY
General	General growth pattern, overall health status, ability to keep up with other children or tires easily with feeding or activity, fever, sleep patterns Allergies, type of reaction (hives, rash, respiratory difficulty, swelling, nausea), seasonal or with each exposure
Skin and lymph	Rashes, dry skin, itching, changes in skin color or texture, new lesions, tendency for bruising, swollen or tender lymph glands
Hair and nails	Hair loss, changes in color or texture, use of dye or chemicals on hair Abnormalities of nail growth or color
Head	Headaches, concern about size of head
Eyes	Vision problems, squinting, crossed eyes, lazy eye, wears glasses; eye infections, redness, tearing, burning, rubbing, swelling eyelids
Ears	Ear infections, frequent discharge from ears, or tubes in ears Hearing loss (no response to loud noises or questions, inattentiveness, date of last hearing test), hearing aids, or cochlear implant
Nose and sinuses	Nosebleeds, nasal congestion, colds with runny nose, seasonal symptoms, sinus pain or infections Nasal obstruction, difficulty breathing, snoring at night
Mouth and throat	Mouth breathing, difficulty swallowing, lesions, sore throats, streptococcal infections, mouth odor Tooth eruption, cavities, braces, orthodontic devices Voice change, hoarseness, speech problems
Cardiac and hematologic	Heart murmur, anemia, hypertension, cyanosis, edema, rheumatic fever, chest pain, bruises easily, easily tires with exercise
Chest and respiratory	Trouble breathing, choking episodes, cough, wheezing, cyanosis; exposure to tuberculosis, bronchiolitis, bronchitis, other infections
Gastrointestinal	Bowel movements, frequency, color, consistency, discomfort; constipation or diarrhea; abdominal pain; bleeding from rectum; flatulence Usual appetite, nausea or vomiting
Urinary	Frequency, urgency, dysuria, foul-smelling urine, dribbling, strength of urinary stream, undescended testicles Toilet trained—age when day and night dryness attained, enuresis

Reproductive
  Female
  Male
  Both
	For pubescent children
	    Menses onset, amount, duration, frequency, discomfort, problems; vaginal discharge, breast development
	    Puberty onset, emissions, erections, pain or discharge from penis, swelling or pain in testicles
	    Sexual activity, use of contraception, sexually transmitted infections

Musculoskeletal	Weakness, clumsiness, poor coordination, balance, tremors, abnormal gait, painful muscles or joints, swelling or redness of joints, fractures
Neurologic	Seizures, fainting spells, dizziness, numbness, brain injury or concussion; problems with articulation Memory or learning problems, attention span, hyperactivity

Developmental Approach to the Examination

The sequence and approach to the examination vary by age, but the techniques are the same for all ages (Table 5–6). Provide a comfortable atmosphere for the examination with privacy so that modesty is respected. Explain the procedures as you begin to perform them. In young children, a foot-to-head sequence is often used so that the least distressing parts of the examination are completed first. In older cooperative children,

the head-to-toe approach is generally used. Experienced examiners often vary the sequence, such as by auscultating the lungs, heart, and abdomen when an infant or toddler is asleep or quiet.

NEWBORNS AND INFANTS UNDER 6 MONTHS OF AGE

Infants are among the easiest children to examine because they do not resist the examination procedure. Keep the parent present

TABLE 5–5 Daily Living Patterns

Role relationships	• Family relationships/alterations in family process • Social and peer relationships and interactions, child care, preschool, school, clubs, sports groups
Self-perception/self-concept	• Personal identity and role identity • Self-esteem, body image, presence of nonvisible disorder such as a brain injury
Coping/stress tolerance	• Temperament, coping behaviors • Discipline methods used • Any substance abuse
Values and beliefs	• Part of a spiritual group or faith community • Any foods, drinks, or medical interventions prohibited according to spiritual beliefs, special food preparation • Personal values/beliefs
Home care provided for child's condition	• Resources needed/available, respite care available • Knowledge and skills of parents, other family members
Sensory/perceptual problems	• Adaptations to daily living for any sensory loss (vision, hearing, cognitive, or motor)

TABLE 5–6 Examination Techniques

TECHNIQUE	DESCRIPTION
Inspection	Purposeful observation of the child's physical features and behaviors during the entire physical examination. Physical feature characteristics include size, shape, color, movement, position, and location. Adequate lighting is essential. Detection of odors is also a part of the inspection.
Palpation	Use of touch to identify characteristics of the skin, internal organs, and masses. Characteristics include texture, moistness, tenderness, temperature, position, shape, consistency, and mobility of masses and organs. The palmar surface of the fingers and the fingertip pads are used for determining position, size, consistency, and masses. The ulnar surface of the hand is best for detecting vibrations.
Auscultation	Listening to sounds produced by the airway, lungs, stomach, heart, and blood vessels to identify their characteristics. Auscultation is usually performed with a stethoscope to enhance the sounds heard in the chest and abdomen. Speech is also assessed during auscultation.
Percussion	Striking the surface of the body, either directly or indirectly, to set up vibrations that reveal the density of underlying tissues and borders of internal organs in the chest and abdomen. As the density of the tissue increases, the percussion tone becomes quieter. The tone over air is the loudest, and the tone over solid areas is soft.

Note: Standard precautions are used during the physical examination. Perform good hand hygiene before contact with the child and wear gloves for any contact with mucous membranes and body fluids.

to provide comfort and security for the infant during the examination by feeding, using a pacifier, cuddling, or changing the diaper to keep the infant calm and quiet. Distraction such as rocking or clicking noises may help when the infant begins to get distressed. Observe the infant for general level of activity, overall mood, and responsiveness to handling.

Be flexible with the sequence of the examination, taking advantage of times when the infant is quiet or asleep to auscultate lung, heart, and abdominal sounds. If the infant continues to be quiet or can be quieted with a pacifier, palpate the abdomen while the muscles are relaxed. The remainder of the examination can proceed in a head-to-toe sequence. Portions of the examination that may disturb the infant, such as the examination of the hips, should be performed last.

INFANTS OVER 6 MONTHS OF AGE

Because of developing separation and stranger anxiety, it is often best to examine the infant and toddler on the parent's lap and then held against the parent's chest for some steps, such as the ear examination (Figure 5–1). The infant will not object to having clothing removed, but make sure the room is warm for the infant's comfort. Observe the infant's general level of activity, mood, and responsiveness to handling by the parent.

Smile and talk soothingly to the infant during the procedure. Use toys to distract the older infant. Use a pacifier or bottle to quiet the child when necessary. Because the infant may be fearful of being touched by a stranger, begin with the feet and hands

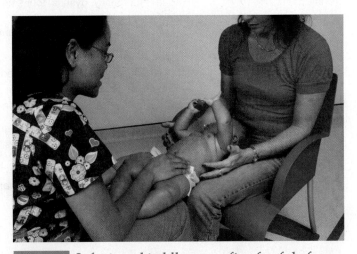

Figure 5–1 **Infants and toddlers are often fearful of separation from the parent. With the legs of the nurse and mother put together knee-to-knee, this infant has a surface to lie on that facilitates cooperation for the abdominal examination.**

before moving to the trunk. However, take advantage of opportunities to listen to heart, lung, and abdominal sounds when the infant is sleeping or quiet.

TODDLERS

Toddlers may be active, curious, shy, cautious, or slow to warm up. Because of stranger anxiety, keep toddlers with their parents, often examining them on the parent's lap. For invasive procedures (ear and mouth examination) the parent can hold the child close to the chest with legs between the parent's legs. Attempt to reduce the child's anxiety by demonstrating the use of instruments on the parent or security object. The cranial nerve assessment or developmental assessment can be used as a method to gain cooperation for other procedures.

Avoid asking the child if you can perform a part of the examination because the typical response will be "No." Rather, tell the child what you will do at each step of the examination, using a confident voice that expects cooperation. When a choice is possible, let the child have some control. For example, let the toddler choose which ear to examine first or to stand or sit for a certain part of the examination. Much of the neurologic and musculoskeletal assessment is performed by observing the child play and walk around in the examining room. Begin the examination by touching the feet and then moving gradually toward the body and head. Use instruments to examine the ears, eyes, and mouth last as they often cause anxiety.

PRESCHOOLERS

Assess the willingness of the child to be separated from the parent. Younger children may prefer to be examined on the parent's lap, whereas older children will be comfortable on the examining table with the parent close by. Most children are willing to undress, but leave the underpants on until conducting the genital examination. Most preschoolers are cooperative during the physical examination. Some children will prefer to have the head, eyes, ears, and mouth examined first while others will prefer to postpone them to the end.

Allow the child to touch and play with the equipment. Give simple explanations about the assessment procedures, and offer choice when there is one during the examination. Use distraction to gain cooperation during the examination, such as asking the child to count, name colors, or talk about a favorite activity. Give positive feedback when the child cooperates.

SCHOOL-AGE CHILDREN

School-age children willingly cooperate and want to be helpful during the examination, so have them sit on the examining table. Anticipate the development of modesty in school-age children and offer a gown to cover the underwear. Let the older school-age child determine if the examination will be conducted in privacy or with the parent or siblings present.

A head-to-toe sequence can be used in this age group. Demonstrate how the instruments are used and let the child handle them if they wish. During the examination, explain what you are doing and why. Offer as many choices as possible to help the child feel empowered. The examination is a good opportunity to teach the child about how the body works, such as letting the child listen to heart and breath sounds.

ADOLESCENTS

Protect the adolescent's modesty by providing a private place to undress and put on the gown, and then during the examination by covering the parts of the body not being assessed. Examine the adolescent in the head-to-toe sequence as used for adults. Perform the examination without parent or siblings unless the adolescent specifically requests the parent's presence, but provide a chaperone (preferably the same gender as the client) when the parent or accompanying adult is not present. See *Professionalism in Practice: Using Chaperones to Examine Adolescents.*

Adolescents often have a lot of concerns regarding their developing bodies. When appropriate, provide reassurance about the normal progression of secondary sexual characteristic development and what further changes to expect.

Professionalism in Practice **Using Chaperones to Examine Adolescents**

A chaperone (same gender as the client), such as a nurse or patient-care technician rather than a family member, should be provided when examining a female adolescent's breasts and during the anorectal and genital examination of both boys and girls. However, the use of a chaperone should be a shared decision between the examiner and the adolescent client (American Academy of Pediatrics Committee on Practice and Ambulatory Medicine, 2011). Hospitals and health clinics often have policies regarding the use of chaperones for physical examinations as well as diagnostic or treatment procedures to guide nurses on when a chaperone should be used and how this should be documented.

General Appraisal

The examination begins upon first meeting the child. Observe the child's general appearance and behavior. The child should appear well nourished and well developed. Infants and young children are often fearful and seek reassurance from their parents. Is the child encouraged to speak? Is the child appropriately reassured or supported by the parent? The child should feel secure with the parent and perceive permission to interact with the nurse.

Measure the infant's weight, length, and head circumference. (See the *Clinical Skills Manual* SKILLS .) After the child is 2 years of age and can stand, measure the child's height rather than length. Accurate measurement is important as medication dosages and fluids are based on weight. Growth measurements are then plotted on growth charts throughout childhood to assure health or to identify the impact of disease on the child. (See the growth charts for all ages of boys and girls in Appendix A.)

Once the weight and height of children have been measured, calculate the body mass index (BMI) (see Chapter 14). The BMI is a formula used to assess total body fat and nutritional status. For children, it helps determine if their height and weight are proportional for their age. Visit the Centers for Disease Control and Prevention website and enter the child's height and weight for an automatic calculation of the BMI. A BMI for age under the 5th percentile indicates the child is underweight. The child is at risk for overweight when the BMI for age is greater than the 85th percentile, and the child is overweight when the BMI is greater than the 95th percentile.

Take the child's temperature, heart rate, respiratory rate, and blood pressure (see the *Clinical Skills Manual* SKILLS .)

Assessing Skin and Hair Characteristics

Examination of the skin requires good lighting to detect variations in skin color and to identify lesions. Daylight is preferred when available. Rather than inspecting the entire skin surface of the child at one time, examine the skin simultaneously with other body systems as each region of the body is exposed. Follow standard precautions by wearing gloves when palpating mucous membranes, open wounds, and lesions.

Inspection of the Skin

SKIN COLOR

The color of the child's skin usually has an even distribution. Check for color variations—such as increased or decreased pigmentation, pallor, mottling, bruises, erythema, cyanosis, or jaundice—that may be associated with local or generalized conditions. Some variations in skin color are common and normal, such as freckles found in the White population and hyperpigmented patches (Mongolian spots) usually found on the sacral region in infants with dark skin (Figure 5–2).

Ecchymosis or bruising is common on the forehead, knees, shins, and lower arms as children stumble and fall. Bruises are uncommon in infants who are not yet walking, unless they have a bleeding disorder condition (Anderst, Carpenter, Abshire, et al., 2013). Bruises found on other parts of the child's body, especially in various stages of healing, should raise a suspicion of child abuse (see Chapter 17). Bruises go through several skin color changes (red, purple, black, blue, yellow, green, and brown) as the body breaks down hemoglobin and blood cells over several days before returning to normal skin color. Note any tattoos or body piercings.

Developing Cultural Competence Skin Tone Differences

The palms of the hands and soles of the feet are often lighter than the rest of the skin surface in children with darker skin. In addition, their lips may appear slightly bluish.

Hyperpigmented patch (Mongolian spot)

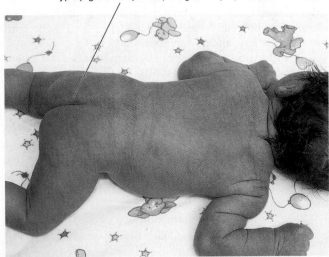

Figure 5–2 **Hyperpigmented patches are bluish-colored skin with an irregular shape often seen over the buttocks and back. They are a normal occurrence in a large majority of Native American, Asian, Black, and Hispanic infants. These patches usually fade during the first few years of life and disappear by puberty.**

When a skin color abnormality is suspected, inspect the buccal mucosa and tongue to confirm the color change. This is important in darker-skinned children because the mucous membranes are usually pink, regardless of skin color. Press the gums lightly for 1 to 2 seconds. Any residual color, such as that seen in jaundice or cyanosis, is more easily detected in blanched skin. Generalized cyanosis is associated with respiratory and cardiac disorders. Jaundice is associated with liver disorders.

Palpation of the Skin

Lightly touch or stroke the skin surface to palpate the skin and to evaluate the following characteristics:

- *Temperature*—normally feels cool to the touch when the wrist or dorsum of the hand is placed against the child's skin. Excessively warm skin may indicate the presence of fever or inflammation, whereas abnormally cool skin may be a sign of shock or cold exposure.

- *Texture*—expect soft, smooth skin over the entire body. Identify any areas of roughness, thickening, or **induration** (area of extra firmness with a distinct border). Abnormalities in texture are associated with endocrine disorders, chronic irritation, and inflammation.

- *Moistness*—normally dry to the touch, but may feel slightly damp when the child has been exercising or crying. Excessive sweating without exertion is associated with a fever or with an uncorrected congenital heart defect.

- *Resilience*—taut, elastic, and mobile because of the balanced distribution of intracellular and extracellular fluids. To evaluate skin turgor, pinch a small amount of skin on the abdomen between the thumb and forefinger, release the skin, and watch the speed of recoil (Figure 5–3). Skin that is elastic rapidly returns to its previous contour and is expected. Skin that tents or feels doughy takes longer to resume its original contour and is commonly associated with dehydration.

If **edema**, an accumulation of excess fluid in the interstitial spaces, is present, the skin feels doughy or boggy. To test for the degree of edema present, press for 5 seconds against a bone beneath the area of puffy skin, release the pressure, and observe how rapidly the indentation disappears. If the indentation disappears rapidly, the edema is "nonpitting." Slow disappearance of

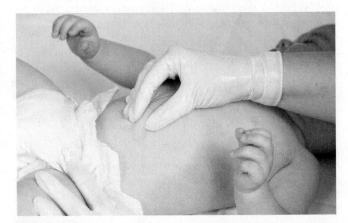

Figure 5–3 **Tenting of the skin is associated with poor skin turgor. Assess skin turgor on the abdomen, forearm, or thigh. Skin with elasticity and normal turgor will return to a flat position quickly.**

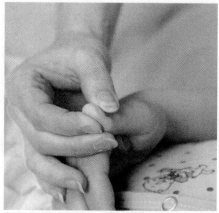

A

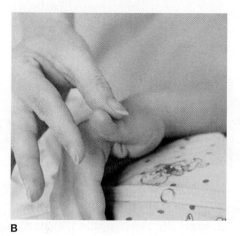

B

Figure 5–4 Capillary refill technique. *A,* Press against the palmar tip of a finger, toe, or over a bony surface (e.g., jaw) for 2 to 3 seconds until the skin is blanched. *B,* Quickly release the pressure and count the number of seconds it takes for the color or blood to return to the veins. A capillary refill time of greater than 2 seconds could be related to dehydration, shock, or constriction around a limb such as a tight bandage or cast.

the indentation indicates "pitting" edema, which is commonly associated with kidney or heart disorders.

Capillary Refill Time

One technique to evaluate the adequacy of tissue *perfusion* (oxygen circulating to the tissues) is the capillary refill time (Figure 5–4*A* and Figure 5–4*B*). The capillary refill time is normally less than 2 seconds. When the time is prolonged, assess the child for dehydration, hypovolemic shock, or a physical constriction such as a cast or bandage that is too tight.

Skin Lesions

Skin lesions usually indicate an abnormal skin condition. Characteristics such as location, size, type of lesion, pattern, and discharge, if present, provide clues about the cause of the condition. Inspect and palpate the isolated or generalized skin color abnormalities, elevations, lesions, or injuries to describe all characteristics present.

Primary lesions (such as macules, papules, and vesicles) are often the skin's initial response to injury or infection.

Hyperpigmented patches (Mongolian spots) and freckles are normal findings also classified as primary lesions (see the illustrations in *Pathophysiology Illustrated: Common Primary Skin Lesions and Associated Conditions*). Secondary lesions (such as scars, ulcers, and fissures) are the result of irritation, infection, and delayed healing of primary lesions (see Table 31–1).

Primary lesions often appear in common patterns that help distinguish between lesions.

- *Annular*—circular, begins in center and spreads to periphery (e.g., ringworm); when annular lesions run together they are polycyclic
- *Linear*—in a row or stripe (e.g., poison ivy)
- *Herpetiform*—grouped or clustered (e.g., herpes, chickenpox)
- *Reticulated*—networked or lacelike (e.g., parvovirus B19)

Inspection of the Hair

Inspect the scalp hair for color, distribution, and cleanliness. The hair shafts should be evenly colored, shiny, and either curly or straight. Variation in hair color not caused by bleaching or coloring may be associated with a nutritional deficiency. Normally, hair is distributed evenly over the scalp. Investigate areas of hair loss. Hair loss in a child may result from tight braids or skin lesions such as ringworm. (See Chapter 31 for information about fungal infections.) Notice any unusual hair growth patterns. An unusually low hairline on the neck or forehead may be associated with a congenital disorder such as hypothyroidism.

Children are frequently exposed to head lice. Inspect the individual hair shafts for small nits (lice eggs) that adhere to the hair (see Chapter 31). None should be present.

Observe the distribution of body hair as other skin surfaces are exposed during examination. Fine hair covers most areas of the body. Body hair in unexpected places should be noted. For example, a tuft of hair at the base of the spine often indicates a spinal defect.

Note the age at which pubic and axillary hair develops in the child. Pubic hair begins to develop in children between 8 and 12 years of age, and axillary hair develops about 6 months later (see Figures 5–29 and 5–30). Facial hair is noted in boys shortly after axillary hair develops. Development at an unusually young age is associated with precocious puberty.

Palpation of the Hair

Palpate the hair shafts for texture. Hair should feel soft or silky with fine or thick shafts. Endocrine conditions such as hypothyroidism may result in coarse, brittle hair. Part the hair in various spots over the head to inspect and palpate the scalp for crusting or other lesions. If lesions are present, describe them using the characteristics presented in *Pathophysiology Illustrated*.

Developing Cultural Competence Hair **Characteristics**

Hair varies by genetic origin. Children of African origin often have curly, wavy, or coiled hair that breaks easily. Children of Asian origin have hair that is coarse and straight. White children have hair with fine to medium coarseness that is straight or wavy.

Pathophysiology Illustrated: Common Primary Skin Lesions and Associated Conditions

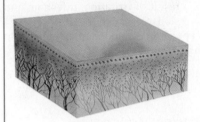

Lesion name: Macule

Description: Flat, nonpalpable, diameter less than 1 cm (½ in.)

Example: Freckle, rubella, rubeola, petechiae

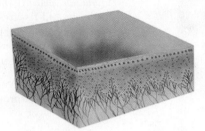

Lesion name: Patch

Description: Macule, diameter greater than 1 cm (½ in.)

Example: Vitiligo, hyperpigmented patch (Mongolian spot)

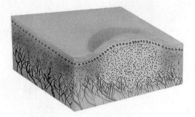

Lesion name: Papule

Description: Elevated, firm, diameter less than1 cm (½ in.)

Example: Warts, pigmented nevi

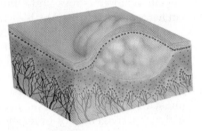

Lesion name: Tumor

Description: Elevated, solid, diameter greater than 2 cm (1 in.)

Example: Neoplasm, hemangioma

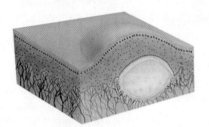

Lesion name: Nodule

Description: Elevated, firm, deeper in dermis than papule, diameter 1 to 2 cm (½ to 1in.)

Example: Erythema nodosum

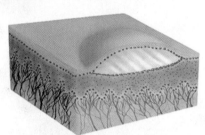

Lesion name: Vesicle

Description: Elevated, filled with fluid, diameter less than 1 cm (½ in.)

Example: Early chickenpox, herpes simplex

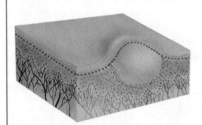

Lesion name: Pustule

Description: Vesicle filled with purulent fluid

Example: Impetigo, acne

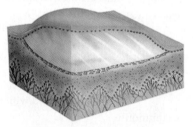

Lesion name: Bulla

Description: Vesicle diameter greater than 1 cm (½ in.)

Example: Burn blister

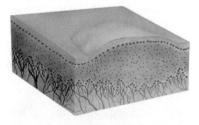

Lesion name: Wheal

Description: Irregular elevated solid area of edematous skin

Example: Urticaria, insect bite

Assessing the Head for Skull Characteristics and Facial Features

Inspection of the Head and Face

During early childhood the skull's sutures expand to allow for brain growth. Infants and young children normally have a rounded skull with a prominent occipital area. The shape of the head changes during childhood, and the occipital area becomes less prominent. An abnormal skull shape can result from premature closure of the sutures.

Clinical Tip

Children who were low-birth-weight infants often have a flat, elongated skull because the soft skull bones were flattened by the weight of the head early in infancy. Head flattening is also associated with the back-lying sleep positions in infants.

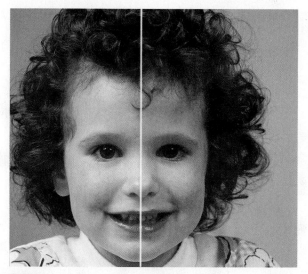

Figure 5–5 To inspect the face for symmetry, draw an imaginary line down the middle of the face over the nose and compare the features on each side. Significant asymmetry may be caused by paralysis of cranial nerve V or VII, in utero positioning, or swelling from infection, allergy, or trauma.

The head circumference of infants and young children is routinely measured until 2 years of age to ensure that adequate growth for brain development has occurred. The *Clinical Skills Manual* **SKILLS** describes the proper technique. A larger-than-normal head is associated with hydrocephalus, and a smaller-than-normal head suggests microcephaly.

Inspect the child's face for symmetry when the child is resting, smiling, talking, and crying (Figure 5–5). Significant asymmetry may result from paralysis of trigeminal or facial nerves (cranial nerves V or VII), in utero positioning, and swelling from infection, allergy, or trauma.

Next inspect the face for unusual facial features such as coarseness, wide eye spacing, or disproportionate size. Tremors, tics, and twitching of facial muscles are often associated with seizures.

Palpation of the Skull

Palpate the skull in infants and young children to assess the sutures and fontanelles and to detect soft bones (see *As Children Grow: Sutures*).

SUTURES

Use your fingerpads to palpate each suture line. The edge of each bone in the suture line can be felt, but normally there is no separation of the two bones. If additional bone edges are felt, a skull fracture may be present.

FONTANELLES

At the intersection of the sutures, palpate the anterior and posterior fontanelles. The fontanelle should feel flat and firm inside the bony edges. The anterior fontanelle is normally smaller than 5 cm (2 in.) in diameter at 6 months of age and then becomes progressively smaller. It closes between 12 and 18 months of age. The posterior fontanelle closes between 2 and 3 months of age.

A tense fontanelle, bulging above the margin of the skull when the child is sitting quietly, is an indication of increased

As Children Grow: **Sutures**

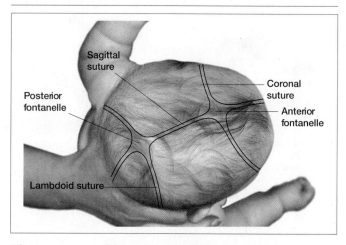

The sutures are fibrous connections between bones of the skull that have not yet ossified. The fontanelles are formed at the intersection of these sutures where bone has not yet formed. Fontanelles are covered by tough membranous tissue that protects the brain. The posterior fontanelle closes between 2 and 3 months. The anterior fontanelle and sutures are palpable up to the age of 18 months. The suture lines of the skull are seldom palpated after 2 years of age. After that time the sutures rarely separate.

> ### Developing Cultural Competence Touching the Head
> The head is a sacred part of the body to some Southeast Asians. Ask for permission before touching the infant's head to palpate the sutures and fontanelles (Purnell, 2014, p. 412). When a Hispanic child is examined, however, many families consider not touching the head bad luck.

intracranial pressure. A soft fontanelle, sunken below the margin of the skull, is associated with dehydration.

Assessing Eye Structures, Function, and Vision

Equipment needed for this examination includes an ophthalmoscope, vision chart, penlight, small toy, and an index card or paper cup.

Inspection of the External Eye Structures

Inspect the external eye structures, including the eyeballs, eyelids, and eye muscles. Test the function of cranial nerves II, III, IV, and VI, which innervate the eye structures.

EYE SIZE AND SPACING

Inspect the eyes and surrounding tissues simultaneously when examining facial features (Figure 5–6). The eyes should be the same size but not unusually large or small. Observe for eye

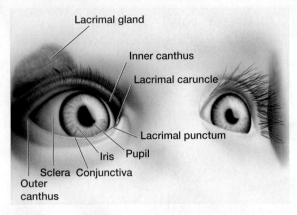

Figure 5–6 External structures of the eye. Notice that the light reflex is at the same location on each eye.

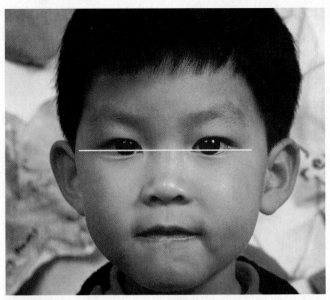

Figure 5–7 To identify the palpebral slant, draw an imaginary line across the medial canthi and extend it to each side of the face. When the imaginary line crosses the lateral canthi, the palpebral fissures are horizontal and no slant is present. When the lateral canthi fall above the line, the eyes have an upward slant. A downward slant is present when the lateral canthi fall below the line. Look at Figures 5–6, 5–8, and 5–10. Which type of eye slant do these children have? Are epicanthal folds present?

bulging, which can be identified by retracted eyelids, or for a sunken appearance. Bulging may be associated with a tumor, and a sunken appearance may reflect dehydration.

Next inspect the eyes to see if they are appropriately distanced from each other. The distance between the inner canthi of the eyes should equal the distance between the inner and outer canthi of the child's eye (Hummel, 2011). **Hypertelorism**, or widely spaced eyes, can be a normal variation in children.

EYELIDS AND EYELASHES

Inspect the eyelids for color, size, position, mobility, and condition of the eyelashes. Eyelids should be the same color as surrounding facial skin and free of swelling or inflammation along the edges. Sebaceous glands that look like yellow striations are often present near the hair follicles. Eyelashes curl away from the eye to prevent irritation of the conjunctivae.

Inspect the conjunctivae lining the eyelids by pulling down the lower lid. Everting (rolling upward) the upper lid is rarely required. The conjunctivae should be pink and glossy. No redness or excess tearing should be present.

When the eyes are open, inspect the level at which the upper and lower lids cross the eye. Each lid normally covers part of the iris but not any portion of the pupil. The lids should also close completely over the iris and cornea. *Ptosis*, drooping of the lid over the pupil, is often associated with injury to the oculomotor nerve, cranial nerve III. *Sunset sign*, in which the sclera is seen persistently between the upper lid and the iris, may indicate hydrocephalus or increased intracranial pressure.

Inspect the eyes for the palpebral slant (Figure 5–7). The eyelids of most people open horizontally. An upward slant is a normal finding in Asian children; however, children with Down syndrome also often have an upward slant (Figure 5–8). A downward slant is seen in some children as a normal variation. Children of Asian descent often have an extra fold of skin, known as the **epicanthal fold**, covering all or part of the lacrimal caruncle on the nasal side of the eye.

EYE COLOR

Inspect the color of each sclera, iris, and bulbar conjunctiva. The sclera is normally white or ivory in darker-skinned children. Sclerae of another color suggest the presence of an underlying disease. For example, yellow sclerae indicate jaundice. Typically, the iris is blue or light colored at birth and becomes pigmented within 6 months. Different colored irises are rare and may be associated with a tumor, injury, or genetic syndrome

(Olitsky, Hug, Plummer, et al., 2016). Inspect the iris for the presence of *Brushfield spots,* white specks in a linear pattern around the iris circumference, which are often associated with Down syndrome. The bulbar conjunctivae, which cover the

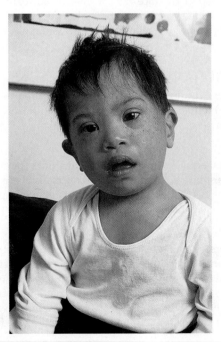

Figure 5–8 The eyes of this boy with Down syndrome show an upward slant.

sclera to the edge of the cornea, are normally clear. Redness can indicate eyestrain, allergies, or irritation.

PUPILS

Inspect the size and shape of the pupils. Normally, the pupils are round, clear, and equal in size. Some children have a **coloboma**, which is a keyhole-shaped pupil caused by a notch in the iris. This sign can indicate that the child has other congenital anomalies.

To test the pupillary response to light, shine a bright light into one eye. A brisk constriction of both the pupil exposed to direct light and the other pupil (consensual response) is a normal finding.

To test pupillary response to accommodation, ask the child to look first at a near object (e.g., a toy) and then at a distant object (e.g., a picture on the wall). The expected response is pupil constriction with near objects and pupil dilation with distant objects. These procedures test cranial nerve II.

ASSESSMENT OF THE EYE MUSCLES

It is important to detect *strabismus*, a muscle imbalance that makes the eyes look crossed, which can cause vision impairment if uncorrected. Use the following procedures to detect a muscle imbalance:

- *Extraocular movements.* Seat the child at eye level to evaluate the extraocular movements. Hold a toy or penlight 30 cm (12 in.) from the child's eyes and move it through the six cardinal fields of gaze. Make sure the child's eyes move rather than the head. Both eyes should move together, tracking the object. This procedure tests the oculomotor, trochlear, and abducens nerves (cranial nerves III, IV, and VI, respectively) (Figure 5–9).
- *Corneal light reflex.* To test the corneal light reflex, shine a light on the child's nose, midway between the eyes. Identify the location where the light is reflected on the cornea of each eye. The light reflection is normally symmetric, at the

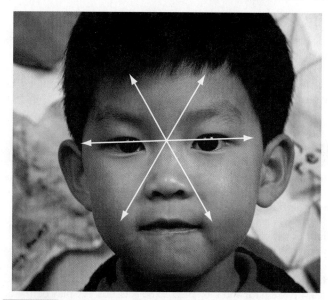

Figure 5–9 To assess extraocular movements have the child sit at your eye level. Hold a toy or penlight about 30 cm (12 in.) from the child's eyes and move it through the six cardinal fields of gaze. Both eyes should move together, tracking the object. This procedure tests cranial nerves III, IV, and VI.

same spot on each cornea (see Figure 5–6). An asymmetric corneal light reflex after 6 months of age indicates a muscle imbalance.

- *Cover–uncover test.* This test can be used only for older, cooperative children, starting at about 5 years of age. See Figure 5–10 for the technique. Perform the procedure for both eyes. Because the eyes work together, no obvious movement of either eye is expected. Eye movement indicates a muscle imbalance.

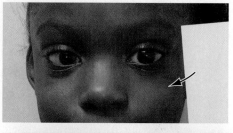

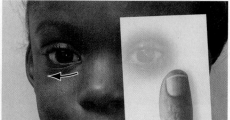

A Right, uncovered eye is weaker.

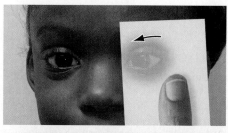

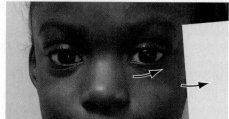

B Left, covered eye is weaker.

Figure 5–10 Cover–uncover test. With the child at your eye level, ask the child to look at a picture on the wall. *A,* Cover one eye with an index card or paper cup and simultaneously watch for any movement of the uncovered eye. If the uncovered eye jumps to fixate on the picture, it has a muscle weakness. *B,* Remove the cover from the eye and simultaneously watch the eye that was covered for any movement to fixate on the picture. If the eye has a muscle weakness, it drifts to a relaxed position once covered.

Vision Assessment

Because vision is such an important sense for learning, assessment is essential to detect any serious problems. Vision is evaluated using an age-appropriate vision test, but no simple method exists. Photo screening or an autorefractor may be used to assess vision in some preschool and school-age children. See the *Clinical Skills Manual* SKILLS.

INFANTS AND TODDLERS

When the infant's eyes are open, test the blink reflex by moving your hand quickly toward the infant's eyes. A quick blink is the normal response. An absent blink reflex can indicate that the infant is blind.

To test an infant's ability to visually track an object, hold a light or toy about 15 cm (6 in.) from the infant's eyes. When the infant has fixated on or is staring at the object, move it slowly to each side. Refer the infant who does not follow the object with the eyes and by moving the head. Once an infant has developed skills to reach for and then pick up objects, observe play behavior to evaluate vision. Children under 3 years of age should be able to easily find and pick up small pieces of food.

STANDARDIZED VISION CHARTS

Standardized vision charts can be used to test vision when the child can understand directions and cooperate, usually at about 3 or 4 years of age. The HOTV, Snellen E, and Picture charts are used to test visual acuity of preschool-age children just as the Snellen Letter chart is used for school-age children and adolescents. For all screening tools used to test far vision, make sure the child is the appropriate distance from the chart, usually 10 or 20 feet. Cover one eye so each eye is evaluated separately before testing them together. See the *Clinical Skills Manual* SKILLS for the use of these charts. Vision develops during early childhood. Refer children who fail photoscreening and those who do not correctly identify most images with each eye on the standardized vision chart 20/50 line for 3-year-olds, 20/40 line for 4-year-olds, and 20/32 line for 5-year-olds (American Association for Pediatric Ophthalmology and Strabismus, 2014).

Inspection of the Internal Eye Structures

The funduscopic examination with an ophthalmoscope allows the structures of the internal eye—the retina, optic disc, arteries and veins, and macula—to be examined. This examination is most often performed by experienced examiners. To assist the examiner, darken the room so the child's pupils dilate. Encourage cooperation by explaining the procedure to the child. Have a picture on the wall or have the parent or assistant hold a toy for the child to stare at so that the child's eye will remain open.

RED REFLEX

A penlight or the light of an ophthalmoscope can be used to assess the **red reflex**, the orange-red glow of the vascular retina as the light travels through the cornea, aqueous humor, lens, and vitreous humor to the retina. Shine the light at both eyes from a distance of 45 cm (18 in.). The red reflexes should be an orange-red glow that is symmetric and uniform in shape and color. Black spots or opacities within the red reflex are abnormal and may indicate congenital cataracts, hemorrhage, or corneal scars. A white reflex is associated with a tumor or retinoblastoma (see Chapter 24).

Assessing the Ear Structures and Hearing

Equipment needed for this examination includes an otoscope, noisemakers (bell, rattle, tissue paper), and a 500- to 1000-Hz tuning fork.

Inspection of the External Ear Structures

The position and characteristics of the *pinna*, the external ear, are inspected as a continuation of the head and eye examination. See Figure 5–11 to determine if the pinna is considered "low set," which is often associated with congenital renal disorders.

Inspect the pinna for any malformation. The pinna should be completely formed, with an open auditory canal. Next, inspect the tissue around the pinna for abnormalities. A pit or hole in front of the auditory canal may indicate the presence of a sinus. If the one pinna protrudes outward, there may be swelling behind the ear, a sign of infection in the mastoid process of the temporal bone of the skull.

Inspect the external auditory canal for any discharge. A foul-smelling, purulent discharge may indicate the presence of a foreign body or an infection in the external canal. Clear fluid or a blood-tinged discharge may indicate a cerebrospinal fluid leak associated with a basilar skull fracture.

Inspection of the Tympanic Membrane

Examination of the tympanic membrane is important in infants and young children because they are prone to otitis media, a middle ear infection. To examine the auditory canal and tympanic membrane, use an otoscope, an instrument with a magnifying lens, bright light, and speculum. Choose the largest ear speculum that fits into the auditory canal to form a seal for testing the movement of the tympanic membrane and to reduce the risk for injury to the auditory canal if the child moves suddenly.

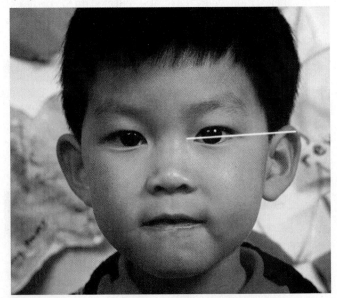

Figure 5–11 To evaluate the placement of the external ears, draw an imaginary line through the medial and lateral canthi of the eye toward the ear. This line normally passes through the upper portion of the pinna. The pinna is considered "low set" when the top lies completely below the imaginary line. Low-set ears are often associated with renal disorders.

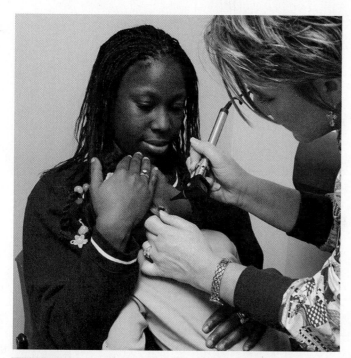

Figure 5–12 Inspecting the tympanic membrane. To restrain an uncooperative child, place the child on the parent's lap with the child's head and chest held firmly against the parent's chest. Keep your hands free to hold the otoscope and position the external ear.

Toddlers and young children often resist having their ears inspected with the otoscope because of past painful experiences, so postpone this until the end of the assessment for this age group. Use simple explanations to prepare the child. Let the child play with the otoscope or demonstrate how it is used on the parent or a doll. Figure 5–12 illustrates one method of human restraint for an uncooperative toddler or preschool child. See the *Clinical Skills Manual* SKILLS .

To begin using the otoscope, hold the handle in the palm of your hand closest to the child's face. If using a pneumatic squeeze bulb, hold it between your index finger and the otoscope handle. When the child is cooperative, rest the back of your hand holding the otoscope against the child's head to stabilize it. Your other hand is used to pull the pinna back and either up or down, whichever position straightens the auditory canal and provides the best view of the tympanic membrane (Figure 5–13).

Slowly insert the speculum into the auditory canal, inspecting the walls for signs of irritation, discharge, or a foreign body. The walls of the auditory canal are normally pink, and some cerumen is present. Children often put beads, peas, or other small objects into their ears. If the auditory canal is obstructed by cerumen or a foreign body, warm water irrigation can be used to clean the canal.

SAFETY ALERT!
Never irrigate the ear canal if any discharge is present in the auditory canal, as the tympanic membrane may be ruptured. Water could enter the middle ear and potentially worsen the infection.

The tympanic membrane, which separates the outer ear from the middle ear, is usually pearly gray and translucent. It reflects light, and the bones (ossicles) in the middle ear are normally visible (Figure 5–14). When the auditory canal is sealed and the pneumatic attachment is squeezed and released, the

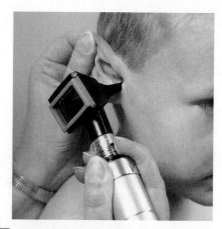

Figure 5–13 To straighten the auditory canal, pull the pinna back and up for children over 3 years of age. Pull the pinna down and back for children under 3 years of age.

tympanic membrane normally moves in and out in response to the positive and negative pressure applied. Table 5–7 lists the abnormal findings during examination of the tympanic membranes. See Figures 19–4 and 19–5 for the tympanic membrane appearance when acute otitis media and otitis media with effusion are present.

Hearing Assessment

Hearing evaluation is important in children of all ages because hearing is essential for normal speech development and learning. Hearing loss may occur at any time during early childhood as the result of birth trauma, frequent otitis media, meningitis, or antibiotics that damage cranial nerve VIII. Hearing loss may also be associated with congenital anomalies and genetic syndromes. The hearing of newborns is evaluated at birth and periodically throughout childhood.

Evaluate hearing by observing the child's responses to various auditory stimuli using age-appropriate methods. Use hearing and speech articulation milestones as an initial hearing screen.

When a hearing deficiency is suspected as a result of screening, refer the child for audiometry or tympanometry. *Audiometry* is a screening procedure using air conduction that measures hearing for pure-tone frequencies and loudness. The high- and low-pitch sounds are presented through earphones and are used to test different sound frequencies and the loudness needed to hear each sound. Hearing loss is determined when the child needs

---

Growth and Development **Indicators of Hearing Loss**

Infant:

- No startle reaction to loud noises.
- Does not turn toward sounds by 4 months of age.
- Babbles as a young infant but does not keep babbling or develop speech sounds after 6 months of age.

Young child:

- No speech by 2 years of age.
- Inability to follow age-appropriate directions, such as "Bring me the block."
- Speech sounds are not distinct at appropriate ages.

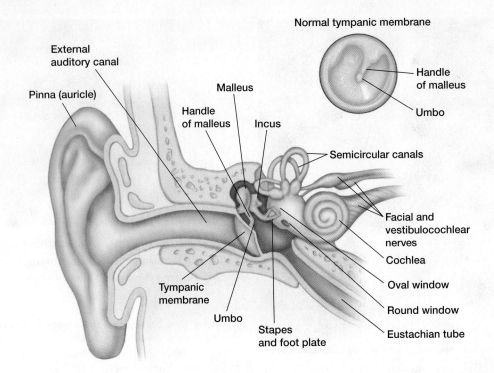

Normal tympanic membrane

Figure 5–14 The tympanic membrane normally has a triangular light reflex with the base on the nasal side pointing toward the center. The bony landmarks, the umbo and handle of malleus, are seen through the tympanic membrane.

higher-than-normal decibels (louder sound) to hear a tone. *Tympanometry* is a test to estimate the pressure in the middle ear, and it is an indirect measure of tympanic membrane movement. See the *Clinical Skills Manual* SKILLS .

INFANTS AND TODDLERS

Select noisemakers with different frequencies that will attract the child's attention, such as a rattle, bell, and tissue paper. Ask the parent or an assistant to entertain the infant with a quiet toy, such as a teddy bear. Stand behind the infant, about 60 cm (2 feet) away from the infant's ear but outside the infant's field of vision, and make a soft sound with the noisemaker. Have the parent or assistant observe the child for any of the following responses when the noisemaker is used: widening the eyes, briefly stopping all activity to listen, or turning the head toward the sound. Repeat the test in the other ear and with the other noisemakers.

PRESCHOOL AND OLDER CHILDREN

Use whispered words to evaluate the hearing of children over 3 years of age. Position your head about 30 cm (12 in.) away from the child's ear, but out of the range of vision so the child cannot read your lips. Use words easily recognized by the child, such as *Mickey Mouse*, *hot dog*, and *popsicle*, and ask the child to repeat the words. Repeat the test with different words in the opposite ear. The child should correctly repeat the whispered words. If the child will not repeat the whispered words, use a whisper to ask the child to point to different body parts or objects. Remember to stay out of the child's line of sight so lip reading is not possible. The child should point to the correct body part each time.

BONE AND AIR CONDUCTION OF SOUND

A tuning fork may be used to evaluate the hearing of school-age children who can follow directions. Hold the stem and lightly tap

TABLE 5–7 Unexpected Findings on Examination of the Tympanic Membrane and Their Associated Conditions

CHARACTERISTICS	TYMPANIC MEMBRANE UNEXPECTED FINDINGS	ASSOCIATED CONDITIONS
Color	Redness	Infection in middle ear
	Slight redness	Prolonged crying
	Amber	Serous fluid in middle ear
	Deep red or blue	Blood in middle ear
Light reflex	Absent	Bulging tympanic membrane, infection in middle ear
	Distorted, loss of triangular shape	Retracted tympanic membrane, serous fluid in middle ear
Bony landmarks	Extra prominent	Retracted tympanic membrane, serous fluid in middle ear
Movement	No movement	Infection or fluid in middle ear
	Excessive movement	Healed perforation

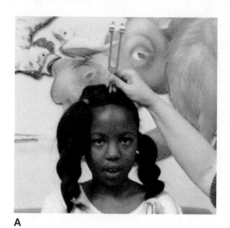
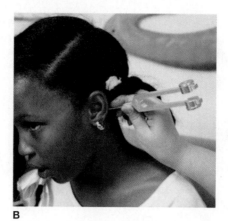
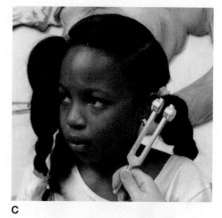

A   B   C

Figure 5–15 Testing bone and air conduction. *A*, Weber test. Place vibrating tuning fork on midline of the child's head. *B*, Rinne test, step 1. Place vibrating tuning fork on mastoid process. *C*, Rinne test, step 2. Reposition still vibrating tines between 2.5 and 5.0 cm (1 and 2 in.) from ear.

the tines of the tuning fork to begin the vibration. Avoid touching the vibrating tines, which will dampen the sound. Test bone conduction by placing the handle of the tuning fork on the child's skull. Test air conduction by holding the vibrating tines close to the child's ear (Figure 5–15).

- *Weber test:* Place the vibrating tuning fork on top of the child's skull in the midline. Ask the child if the sound is heard better in one ear or in both ears equally. The sound should be heard equally in both ears. If the sound is heard better in one ear (lateralized to affected ear), conductive hearing loss may be present.
- *Rinne test:* Place the vibrating tuning fork handle on the mastoid process behind an ear. Ask the child to say when the sound is no longer heard. Immediately move the tuning fork, holding the vibrating tines about 2.5 to 5 cm (1 to 2 in.) from the same ear. Again, ask the child to say when the sound is no longer heard. The child normally hears the air-conducted sound twice as long as the bone-conducted sound. Repeat the Rinne test on the other ear. When the sound is heard longer by bone conduction than air conduction, the affected ear may have conductive hearing loss. When sound is heard longer by air conduction than bone conduction, but less than twice as long, the affected ear may have sensorineural hearing loss.

Assessing the Nose and Sinuses for Airway Patency and Discharge

An otoscope with a nasal speculum or a penlight is needed for this examination.

Inspection of the External Nose

Examine the external nose characteristics and placement on the face during the assessment of the facial features. Inspect the external nose for size, shape, symmetry, midline placement on the face, and for the presence of unusual characteristics. For example, a crease across the nose between the cartilage and bone is often caused when an allergic child uses a hand to rub an itchy nose upward. **Nasal flaring**, widening

of the nares with breathing, is a sign of respiratory distress and should not be present.

The nose should be proportional in size to other facial features, have symmetric nasolabial folds, and be positioned in the middle of the face. Asymmetry of the nasolabial folds may be associated with injury to the facial nerve (cranial nerve VII). A flattened nasal bridge is the expected finding in Asian and Black children but may also be seen in children with Down syndrome. A saddle-shaped nose is associated with congenital defects such as cleft palate.

Palpation of the External Nose

When a deformity is noted, gently palpate the nose to detect any pain or break in contour. No tenderness or masses are expected. Pain and a contour deviation are usually the result of trauma.

NASAL PATENCY
The child's airway must be patent to ensure adequate oxygenation. To test for nasal patency, occlude one nostril and observe the child's effort to breathe through the open nostril with the mouth closed. Repeat on the other nostril. Breathing should be noiseless and effortless.

If the child struggles to breathe, a nasal obstruction may be present. Nasal obstruction may be caused by a foreign body, congenital defect, dry mucus, discharge, polyp, or trauma. Young children commonly place objects up their noses, and unilateral nasal flaring is a sign of such an obstruction.

Growth and Development

Newborns and infants under 6 months of age will not automatically open their mouths to breathe when their nose is occluded, such as by mucus.

Assessment of Smell

The olfactory nerve (cranial nerve I) can be tested in school-age children and adolescents, but it is rarely done. When testing smell, choose scents the child will easily recognize such as orange, chocolate, peanut butter, and mint. When the child's eyes are closed, occlude one nostril and hold the scent under the nose. Ask the child to take a deep sniff and identify the

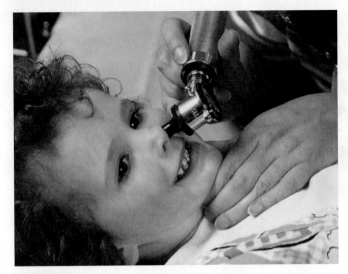

Figure 5–16 Technique for examining the nose. For infants and young children, push the tip of the nose upward and shine the light at the end of the nose. The nasal speculum of the otoscope can be used in older children. Avoid touching the septum of the nose with the speculum to prevent injury.

scent. Alternate odors between the nares. The child can normally identify common scents.

Inspection of the Internal Nose

Inspect the internal nose for color of the mucous membranes and the presence of any discharge, swelling, lesions, or other abnormalities. Use a bright light, such as an otoscope light or penlight. See Figure 5–16.

TABLE 5–8 Nasal Discharge Characteristics and Associated Conditions

DISCHARGE DESCRIPTION	ASSOCIATED CONDITION
Watery	
Clear, bilateral	Allergy
Serous, unilateral	Spinal fluid from a basilar skull fracture
Mucoid or purulent	
Bilateral	Upper respiratory infection
Unilateral	Foreign body
Bloody	Nosebleed, trauma

MUCOUS MEMBRANES AND NASAL SEPTUM

The mucous membranes should be dark pink and glistening. A film of clear discharge may also be present. Turbinates, if visible, should be the same color as the mucous membranes and have a firm consistency. When the turbinates are pale or bluish gray, the child may have allergies. A polyp, a rounded mass projecting from the turbinate, is also associated with allergies.

The nasal septum should be straight without perforations, bleeding, or crusting. Crusting will be noted over the site of a nosebleed.

DISCHARGE

Observe for the presence of nasal discharge, noting if it is unilateral or bilateral. Nasal discharge is not a normal finding unless the child is crying. Discharge may be watery, mucoid, purulent, or bloody. Table 5–8 lists conditions associated with nasal discharge.

Inspection of the Sinuses

The sinuses are air-filled spaces that develop during childhood. See the illustration in *As Children Grow: Sinus Development*.

As Children Grow: **Sinus Development**

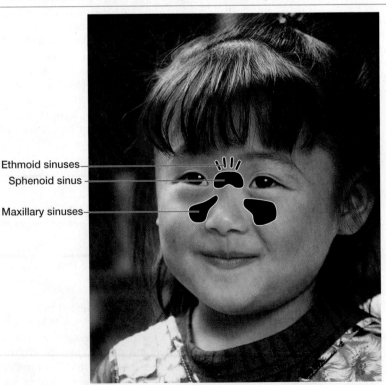

Ethmoid sinuses
Sphenoid sinus
Maxillary sinuses

The ethmoid sinuses are present at birth and air filled. The maxillary sinuses are present at birth and become air filled by 4 years of age. The sphenoid sinuses are present by 5 years of age. The frontal sinuses form at about 7 to 8 years of age and are completely developed by adolescence (Pappas & Hendly, 2016).

Inspect the face for any puffiness and swelling around one or both eyes; normally, neither is present. To palpate over the maxillary sinuses, press up under both zygomatic arches with the thumbs. To palpate the ethmoid sinuses, press up against the bone above both eyes with the thumbs. No swelling or tenderness is expected. Tenderness may indicate sinusitis. Sinus infections can occasionally occur in young children.

Assessing the Mouth and Throat for Color, Function, and Signs of Abnormal Conditions

Equipment needed to examine the mouth and throat includes a tongue blade and penlight. Wear gloves when examining the mouth.

Inspection of the Mouth

Young children often need coaxing and simple explanations before they will cooperate with the mouth and throat examination. Most children readily show their teeth. If the child resists by clenching the teeth, gently separate them with a tongue blade. Mouth structures for inspection are illustrated in Figure 5–17.

LIPS

Inspect the lips for color, shape, symmetry, moisture, and lesions. The lips are normally symmetric without drying, cracking, or other lesions. Lip color is normally pink in White children and more bluish in darker-skinned children. Pale, cyanotic, or cherry-red lips indicate poor tissue perfusion caused by various conditions. Note any clefts or edema.

SAFETY ALERT!
Avoid examining the mouth if there are signs of respiratory distress, high fever, drooling, and intense apprehension. These may be signs of epiglottitis. Inspecting the mouth may trigger a total airway obstruction. (See Table 20–3 for more information.)

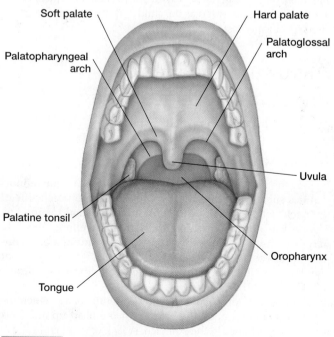

Figure 5–17 **The structures of the mouth.**

Soft palate • Hard palate • Palatoglossal arch • Palatopharyngeal arch • Uvula • Palatine tonsil • Oropharynx • Tongue

TEETH

Inspect and count the child's teeth. The timing of tooth eruption is often genetically determined, but it occurs in a regular sequence. See Figure 5–18 for the typical sequence of tooth eruption for both deciduous and permanent teeth.

Inspect the condition of the teeth, look for loose teeth, and note any spaces where teeth are missing. Note any dental care, braces, or orthodontic appliances. Compare empty tooth spaces with the child's developmental stage of tooth eruption. Once the permanent teeth have erupted, none should be missing. Teeth are normally white, without a flattened, mottled, or pitted appearance. Discolorations on the crown of a tooth may indicate caries. Discolorations on the tooth surface may be associated with some medications or excessive fluoride intake.

MOUTH ODORS

During inspection of the teeth, be alert to any abnormal odors that may indicate problems such as diabetic ketoacidosis, infection, or poor hygiene. Be alert for alcohol odors in older children that could signal substance abuse.

GUMS AND BUCCAL MUCOSA

Inspect the gums for color and adherence to the teeth. The gums are normally pink, with a stippled or dotted appearance. Use a tongue blade to help visualize the gums around the upper and lower molars. No raised or receding gum areas should be apparent around the teeth. When inflammation, swelling, or bleeding is observed, palpate the gums to detect tenderness. Inflammation and tenderness are associated with infection and poor nutrition. Hyperplasia may be associated with some medications, such as phenytoin.

Inspect the mucous membrane lining of the cheeks for color and moisture. The mucous membrane is usually pink, but patches of hyperpigmentation are commonly seen in darker-skinned children. The *Stensen duct*, the parotid gland opening, is opposite the upper second molar bilaterally. Normally pink, the duct opening becomes red when the child is infected with mumps. Small pink sucking pads can be present in infants. No areas of redness, swelling, or ulcerative lesions should be present.

TONGUE

Inspect the tongue for color, moistness, size, tremors, and lesions. The child's tongue is normally pink and moist, without a coating, and it fits easily into the mouth. A protuberant tongue is associated with various genetic conditions, such as Down syndrome. A pattern of gray, irregular borders that form a design (geographic tongue) is often normal, but it may be associated with fever, allergies, or drug reactions. Tremors are abnormal. A white adherent coating on an infant's tongue may be caused by thrush, a *Candida* infection (see Chapter 31).

Observe the mobility of the tongue by asking the child to touch the gums above the upper teeth with the tongue. This tongue movement is adequate to enunciate all speech sounds clearly. Ask the child to stick out the tongue and lift it so the underside of the tongue and the floor of the mouth can be inspected.

PALATE

Inspect the hard and soft palates to detect any clefts or masses or an unusually high arch. The palate is normally pink, dome shaped, and has no cleft. The uvula hangs freely from the soft palate. A high-arched palate can be associated with sucking difficulties in young infants.

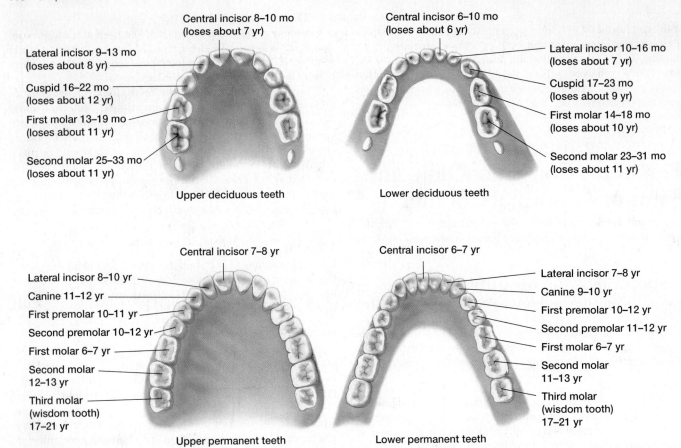

Central incisor 8–10 mo
(loses about 7 yr)

Lateral incisor 9–13 mo
(loses about 8 yr)

Cuspid 16–22 mo
(loses about 12 yr)

First molar 13–19 mo
(loses about 11 yr)

Second molar 25–33 mo
(loses about 11 yr)

Upper deciduous teeth

Central incisor 6–10 mo
(loses about 6 yr)

Lateral incisor 10–16 mo
(loses about 7 yr)

Cuspid 17–23 mo
(loses about 9 yr)

First molar 14–18 mo
(loses about 10 yr)

Second molar 23–31 mo
(loses about 11 yr)

Lower deciduous teeth

Central incisor 7–8 yr

Lateral incisor 8–10 yr

Canine 11–12 yr

First premolar 10–11 yr

Second premolar 10–12 yr

First molar 6–7 yr

Second molar
12–13 yr

Third molar
(wisdom tooth)
17–21 yr

Upper permanent teeth

Central incisor 6–7 yr

Lateral incisor 7–8 yr

Canine 9–10 yr

First premolar 10–12 yr

Second premolar 11–12 yr

First molar 6–7 yr

Second molar
11–13 yr

Third molar
(wisdom tooth)
17–21 yr

Lower permanent teeth

Figure 5–18 Usual ages and sequence of tooth eruption for both deciduous and permanent teeth. The bottom deciduous teeth are shed before upper teeth, and bottom permanent teeth erupt first as well.

Palpation of the Mouth Structures

Using gloves, palpate any masses seen in the mouth to determine their characteristics, such as size, shape, firmness, and tenderness. No masses should be found.

To assess the tongue's strength, while simultaneously testing the hypoglossal nerve (cranial nerve XII), place your index finger against the child's cheek and ask the child to push against your finger with the tongue. Some pressure against the finger is normally felt.

To palpate the palate, insert your gloved little finger, with the finger pad upward, into the mouth. While the infant sucks against your finger, palpate the entire palate. This procedure also tests the strength of the sucking reflex, innervated by the hypoglossal nerve (cranial nerve XII). No clefts should be palpated.

Inspection of the Throat

Use a flashlight to inspect the throat for color, swelling, lesions, and the condition of the tonsils. Ask the child to open the mouth wide and stick out the tongue. Use a tongue blade, if needed, to visualize the posterior pharynx. Moistening the tongue blade may decrease the child's tendency to gag. The throat is normally pink without lesions, drainage, or swelling. The epiglottis lies behind the tongue and is normally pink like the rest of the buccal mucosa. Swelling or bulging in the posterior pharynx may be associated with a peritonsillar abscess (see Chapter 19).

During childhood the tonsils are large in proportion to the size of the pharynx because lymphoid tissue grows fastest in early childhood. The tonsils should be pink without exudate, but crypts (fissures) may be present as a result of prior infections. The size of the tonsils can be graded as indicated in the *Pathophysiology Illustrated: Tonsil Size With Infection* diagram.

When using a tongue blade to see the throat and tonsils, the gag reflex may be triggered. A symmetric rising movement of the uvula should be observed as the child gags. The gag reflex is not often specifically tested in children.

Assessing the Neck for Characteristics, Range of Motion, and Lymph Nodes

Inspection of the Neck

Inspect the neck for size, symmetry, swelling, and any abnormalities such as *webbing*, an extra fold of skin on each side of the neck. A short neck with skinfolds is normal for infants. The neck is normally symmetric without swelling. Swelling may be caused by local infections such as mumps or a congenital defect. The neck lengthens between 3 and 4 years of age. Webbing is commonly associated with Turner syndrome (see Chapter 30).

Infants develop head control by 2 months of age when the infant has enough neck strength to lift the head up and look around when lying on the stomach. A lack of head control can result from neurologic injury, such as an anoxic episode.

Pathophysiology Illustrated: **Tonsil Size With Infection**

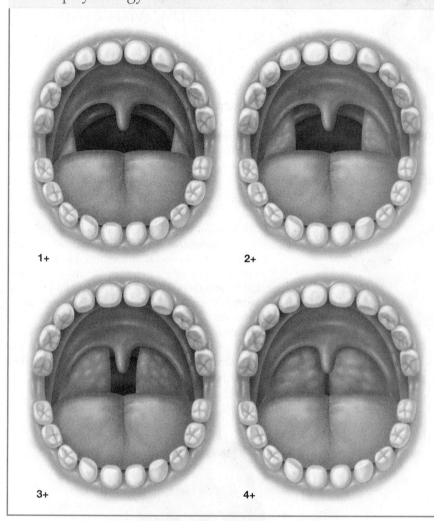

1+

2+

3+

4+

Tonsil size can be graded from 1+ to 4+ in relation to how much of the airway is obstructed. Tonsil size of 1+ and 2+ is normal. Tonsil size of 3+ is common with infections such as strep throat. Tonsils that "kiss" or nearly touch each other (4+) significantly reduce the size of the airway.

Palpation of the Neck

Face the child and use your finger pads to simultaneously palpate both sides of the neck for lymph nodes, as well as the trachea and thyroid.

LYMPH NODES

To palpate the lymph nodes, slide your finger pads gently over the lymph node chains in the head and neck. One sequence is to palpate the lymph nodes in the occipital area, around the ears, under the jaw, and then the cervical chain in the neck (Figure 5–19). Firm, clearly defined, nontender, movable lymph nodes up to 1 cm (½ in.) in diameter are common in young children. Enlarged, firm, warm, tender lymph nodes indicate a local infection.

TRACHEA

To palpate the trachea, place your thumb and forefinger on each side of the trachea near the chin and slowly slide down the trachea to determine its position and to detect the presence of any masses. The trachea is normally in the midline of the neck. It is difficult to palpate in children less than 3 years of age because of their short necks. Any shift to the right or left of midline may indicate a tumor or a collapsed lung.

THYROID

As the fingers slide over the trachea in the lower neck, attempt to feel the isthmus of the thyroid, a band of glandular tissue crossing over the trachea. The lobes of the thyroid wrap behind the trachea and are normally covered by the sternocleidomastoid muscle. Because of the anatomic position of the thyroid, its lobes are not usually palpable in the child unless they are enlarged.

Range of Motion Assessment

To test the neck's range of motion, ask the child to touch the chin to each shoulder and to the chest and then to look at the ceiling. Move a light or toy in all four directions when assessing infants. Children should freely move the neck and head in all four directions without pain.

When the child is unable to move the head voluntarily in all directions, passively move the child's neck through the expected range of motion. Limited horizontal range of motion may be a sign of **torticollis**, persistent head tilting. Torticollis results from a birth injury to the sternocleidomastoid muscle or from unilateral vision or hearing impairment. Pain with flexion of the neck toward the chest (Brudzinski sign) may indicate meningitis (see Chapter 27).

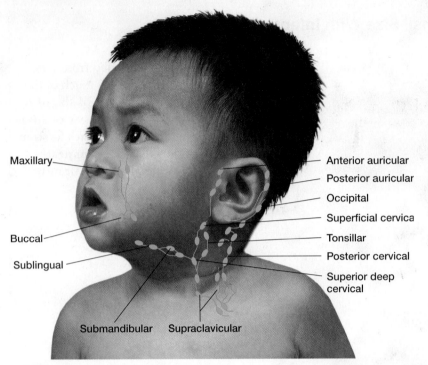

Figure 5-19 Palpate for enlarged lymph nodes in front of and behind the ears, under the jaw, in the occipital area, and in the cervical chain of the neck.

Assessing the Chest for Shape, Movement, Respiratory Effort, and Lung Function

Examination of the chest includes the following procedures: inspecting the size and shape of the chest, palpating chest movement that occurs during respiration, observing the effort of breathing, and auscultating breath sounds. A stethoscope is needed.

Inspection of the Chest

The chest skeleton provides most of the landmarks used to describe the location of findings during examination of the chest, lungs, and heart. The intercostal spaces are the horizontal markers. The sternum and spine are the vertical landmarks. When both a horizontal and a vertical landmark are used, the location of findings can be precisely described on the right or left side of the child's chest (Figures 5-20 and 5-21). The distance between the finding and the center of the sternum (midsternal line) or the midspinal line can be measured with a ruler.

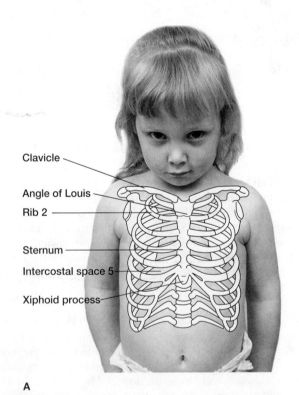

A

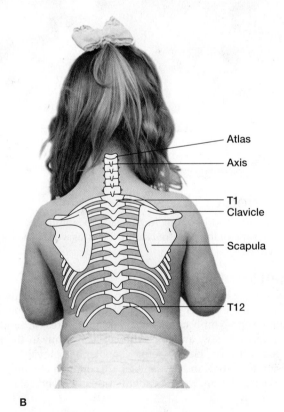

B

Figure 5-20 Ribs and intercostal spaces are the horizontal landmarks used to describe the location of chest findings. *A*, To determine the rib number on the anterior chest, palpate down from the top of the sternum until a horizontal ridge, the angle of Louis, is felt. Directly to the right and left of that ridge is the second rib. The second intercostal space is immediately below the second rib. Ribs 3–12 and the corresponding intercostal spaces can be counted as the fingers move toward the abdomen. *B*, To determine the rib number on the posterior chest, find the protruding spinal process of the seventh cervical vertebra at the shoulder level. The next spinal process belongs to the first thoracic vertebra, which attaches to the first rib.

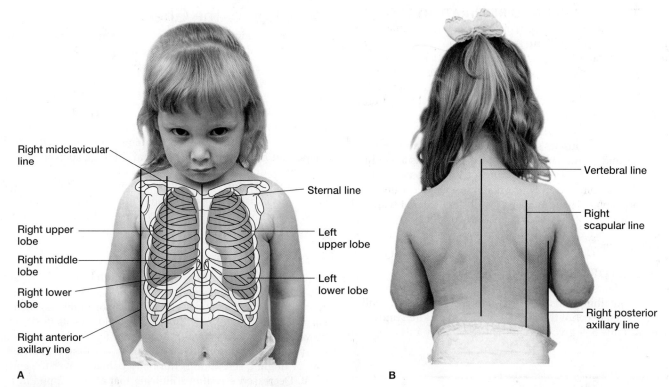

Right midclavicular line

Sternal line

Right upper lobe

Left upper lobe

Right middle lobe

Right lower lobe

Left lower lobe

Right anterior axillary line

A

Vertebral line

Right scapular line

Right posterior axillary line

B

Figure 5–21 The sternum and spine are the vertical landmarks used to describe the anatomic location of findings. Imaginary vertical lines, parallel to the midsternal and spinal lines, are used to further describe the location of findings. The midclavicular line is through the middle of the clavicle. The midaxillary line is through the middle of the axilla. The scapular line is through the bottom angle of the scapula. *A,* Anterior vertical landmarks. *B,* Posterior vertical landmarks.

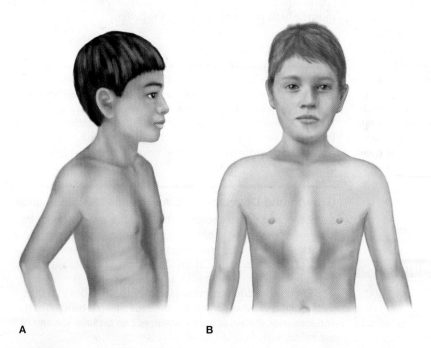

A

B

Figure 5–22 Abnormal chest shape. *A,* Pectus carinatum (funnel chest) in which the lower portion of the sternum is depressed, decreasing the anteroposterior diameter. *B,* Pectus excavatum (pigeon chest) in which the sternum protrudes, increasing the anteroposterior diameter.

Position the child on the parent's lap or on the examining table with all clothing above the waist removed to inspect the chest. The thoracic muscles and subcutaneous tissue are less developed in children than in adolescents and adults, so the chest wall is thinner and the rib cage is more prominent unless obesity is present.

SHAPE OF THE CHEST

Inspect the chest for any irregularities in shape. In infants, the chest is rounded with the anteroposterior diameter approximately equal to the lateral diameter. By 2 years of age, the chest becomes more oval with growth, and the lateral diameter is greater than the anteroposterior diameter. If a child over 2 years of age has a rounded chest, a chronic obstructive lung condition such as asthma or cystic fibrosis may be present.

An abnormal chest shape may result from structural deformities, such as pectus carinatum and pectus excavatum (Figure 5–22). Scoliosis, curvature of the spine, causes a lateral deviation of the chest (see Chapter 29). A shield-shaped chest, unusually broad with widely spaced nipples, may be associated with Turner syndrome (see Chapter 30).

CHEST MOVEMENT AND RESPIRATORY EFFORT

The diaphragm is the primary muscle used for ventilation by infants and young children. As the thoracic muscles develop, they become the primary ventilation muscles. Chest movement with breathing is normally symmetric bilaterally. On inspiration, the chest and abdomen should rise simultaneously and fall on expiration. The chest movement of infants and young children is less pronounced than the abdominal movement. Asymmetric chest rise is associated with a collapsed lung.

The thoracic muscles serve as accessory respiratory muscles in infants and young children. When the child has a condition that causes a partial airway obstruction, the accessory muscles are used for inspiration and retractions are seen. **Retractions**, visible depression of tissue between the ribs of the chest wall with each inspiration, indicate an increased work of breathing and often respiratory distress (see *Pathophysiology Illustrated: Retraction Sites* in Chapter 20).

RESPIRATORY RATE

Because infants and young children use the diaphragm as the primary breathing muscle, observe or feel the rise and fall of the abdomen to count the respiratory rate in children under age 6 years. Table 5–9 gives the normal respiratory rates for each age group.

Growth and Development Respiratory Rate

Infants and children have a faster respiratory rate than adults because of their higher metabolic rate and oxygen requirement. Young children are also unable to increase the depth of respirations because the intercostal muscles are inadequately developed to lift the chest wall and increase intrathoracic volume (Chameides, Samson, Schexnayder, et al., 2011, p. 42).

To get the most accurate reading of a young infant's respiratory rate, wait until the baby is sleeping or resting quietly. Use the stethoscope to auscultate the rate or place your hand on the abdomen. Count the number of breaths for an entire minute because newborns and young infants can have irregular respirations.

Tachypnea, an increased respiratory rate, occurs in response to excitement, fear, respiratory distress, fever, and other conditions that increase oxygen needs. A sustained respiratory rate higher than normal for age is an important sign of respiratory distress. The child is at risk for developing hypoxemia if treatment is not started. An abnormally slow respiratory rate occurs in response to respiratory failure.

TABLE 5–9 Normal Respiratory Rate Ranges by Age

AGE	RESPIRATORY RATE PER MINUTE
Newborn	30–55
1 year	25–40
3 years	20–30
6 years	16–22
10 years	16–20
17 years	12–20

Palpation of the Chest

Palpation is used to evaluate chest movement, respiratory effort, deformities of the chest wall, and tactile fremitus.

CHEST WALL

To palpate the chest motion with respiration, place your palms and outspread fingers on each side of the child's chest. Confirm the bilateral symmetry of chest motion. Use your finger pads to palpate any depressions, bulges, or unusual chest wall shape that might indicate abnormal findings such as tenderness, cysts, other growths, crepitus, or fractures. None should be found. **Crepitus**, a crinkly sensation palpated on the chest surface, is caused by air escaping into the subcutaneous tissues. It often indicates a serious injury to the upper or lower airway.

TACTILE FREMITUS

To palpate **tactile fremitus**, vibrations produced by crying and talking, place the palms of your hands on each side of the chest. Ask the child to repeat a series of words or numbers, such as *puppy dog*, *kitty cat*, or *ice cream*. As the child repeats the words, move your hands systematically over the anterior and posterior chest, comparing the quality of vibrations side to side. The vibration or tingling sensation is normally palpated over the entire chest. Decreased sensations indicate that air is trapped in the lungs, as occurs with asthma.

Auscultation of the Chest

Auscultate the chest with a stethoscope to assess the quality and characteristics of breath sounds, to identify abnormal breath sounds, and to evaluate vocal resonance. Use an infant or pediatric stethoscope when available to help localize any unexpected breath sounds. Use the stethoscope diaphragm because it transmits the high-pitched breath sounds better.

BREATH SOUNDS

Evaluate the quality and characteristics of breath sounds over the entire chest, comparing sounds between the sides. Select a routine sequence for auscultating the entire chest so assessment of all lobes of the lungs will be consistently performed. Figure 5–23 shows one suggested chest auscultation sequence. Listen to an entire inspiratory and expiratory phase at each spot on the chest before moving to the next site.

Growth and Development Auscultating Breath Sounds

Auscultation of breath sounds is difficult when an infant is crying. If the infant continues to cry after giving a pacifier, bottle, or toy, all is not lost. At the end of each cry the infant takes a deep breath, which you can use to assess breath sounds, vocal resonance, and tactile fremitus.

Encourage toddlers and preschoolers to take deep breaths by blowing a pinwheel or a piece of tissue off your hand. This may enhance auscultation of subtle wheezes that occur at the end of expiration.

When trying to encourage the child to breathe normally while auscultating the chest, use suggestive language to increase cooperation: "You certainly are good at breathing slowly. Have you been practicing?" The child will often deepen and slow the breathing pattern as you praise the effort.

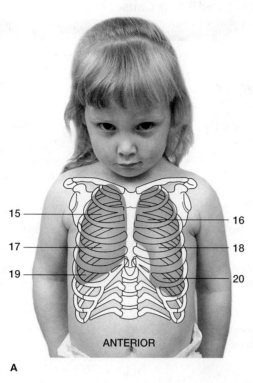

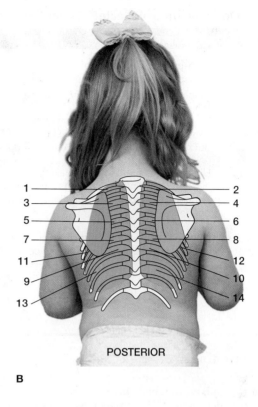

Figure 5–23 One sequence for auscultation of the chest.

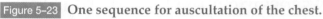

Three types of normal breath sounds are usually heard when the chest is auscultated.

- *Vesicular breath sounds* are low-pitched, swishing, soft, short expiratory sounds usually heard in older children but not in infants and young children.
- *Bronchovesicular breath sounds* are medium-pitched, hollow, blowing sounds heard equally on inspiration and expiration in all age groups.
- *Bronchial/tracheal breath sounds* are hollow and higher pitched than vesicular breath sounds.

Breath sounds normally have equal intensity, pitch, and rhythm bilaterally. Absent or diminished breath sounds may indicate a pneumothorax or airway obstruction.

Clinical Tip

Infants and young children have a thin chest wall because of immature muscle development. The breath sounds of one lung are heard over the entire chest. It takes practice to accurately identify absent or diminished breath sounds in infants and young children. Because the distance between the lungs is greatest at the apices and midaxillary areas in young children, these sites are best for identifying absent or diminished breath sounds. Carefully auscultate, comparing the quality of breath sounds heard bilaterally.

VOCAL RESONANCE

Auscultate to evaluate **vocal resonance**, the transmission of voice sounds through the chest. Have the child repeat a series of words, such as *apple*, *banana*, and *cereal*. Use the stethoscope to auscultate the chest, comparing the quality of sounds from side to side and over the entire chest. Voice sounds, with words and syllables muffled and indistinct, are normally heard throughout the chest.

If voice sounds are absent or more muffled than usual, an airway obstruction condition such as asthma may be present. If voice sounds are more distinct, louder, or clearer, a lung consolidation condition such as pneumonia may be present.

ABNORMAL BREATH SOUNDS

Abnormal breath sounds, also called adventitious sounds, generally indicate disease. Examples of abnormal breath sounds are crackles, rhonchi (sonorous wheezing), and sibilant **wheezing** (a noise resulting from the passage of air through mucus or fluids in a narrowed lower airway). To further assess abnormal breath sounds, identify the following:

- Location—for example, side of body and lung lobe(s)
- Presence during part or entire phase of inspiration or expiration
- Change in character or disappearance when the child coughs or changes position

It takes practice to routinely identify these adventitious sounds. Table 5–10 describes adventitious sounds.

ABNORMAL VOICE SOUNDS

Observe the quality of the voice and other audible sounds. A cough is a reflexive clearing of the airway associated with a respiratory infection. Hoarseness is associated with inflammation of the larynx.

Percussion of the Chest

Percussion of the chest may be performed by an experienced examiner to assess the resonance of the lungs and size of underlying organs, such as the heart. Radiographic examination is commonly used for this evaluation.

TABLE 5–10 Description of Selected Adventitious Sounds and Their Cause

TYPE	DESCRIPTION	CAUSE
Fine crackles	High-pitched, discrete, noncontinuous sound heard at end of inspiration; does not clear with coughing *(Rub pieces of hair together beside your ear to duplicate the sound.)*	Air passing through watery secretions in the smaller airways (alveoli and bronchioles)
Coarse crackles	Loud, lower pitched, more moist or bubbly sound heard during inspiration; does not clear by coughing	Air passing through thicker secretions in the airway
Sibilant wheezing	Higher pitched, musical, squeaking, or hissing noise usually heard continuously during inspiration or expiration, but generally louder on expiration; does not clear with coughing	Air passing through mucus or fluids in a narrowed lower airway (bronchioles) as with asthma
Rhonchi (sonorous wheezing)	Coarse, low-pitched sound like a snore, heard during inspiration or expiration; may clear with coughing	Air passing through thick secretions that partially obstruct the larger bronchi and trachea
Stridor	High-pitched, piercing sound most often heard during inspiration without a stethoscope	Whistling sound as air passes through a narrowed trachea and larynx, associated with croup

---

Clinical Reasoning Assessing a Child With Bronchiolitis

Aliyah, 6 months old, is brought by her mother and father to the emergency department. She is an emergency admission from the local pediatrician's office with a diagnosis of bronchiolitis. As Aliyah's nurse, you are responsible for assessing her condition after she arrives on the pediatric nursing unit.

What procedures are used to perform a physical examination on a 6-month-old? Identify all the components of the physical assessment used to detect signs of respiratory difficulty.

Assessing the Breasts

Inspection of the Breasts

The nipples of prepubertal boys and girls are symmetrically located near the midclavicular line at the fourth to sixth ribs. The areolae are normally round and more darkly pigmented than the surrounding skin. Inspect the anterior chest for other dark spots that may indicate *supernumerary nipples,* small, undeveloped nipples and areolae that may be mistaken for moles. Their presence may be associated with congenital renal or cardiac anomalies.

See the section later in this chapter for a discussion of breast development with puberty.

Palpation of the Breasts

Boys and girls have no palpable breast tissue before puberty. Palpate the developing breasts of female adolescents for abnormal masses or hard nodules. With the girl lying down, use a concentric or vertical stripe pattern covering all areas of each breast, including the axilla, areola, and the nipple. Gently squeeze the nipples for discharge. Breast tissue normally feels dense, firm, and elastic. Any mass needs further evaluation.

During adolescence, the majority of boys have *gynecomastia,* unilateral or bilateral breast enlargement. It is often most noticeable around 14 years of age and commonly disappears by the time of full sexual maturity. Palpate the tissue to differentiate actual breast tissue from fatty tissue in the pectoral area, and to detect any masses.

Assessing the Heart for Heart Sounds and Function

A stethoscope and sphygmomanometer are needed to assess the heart.

Inspection of the Precordium

Begin the heart examination by inspecting the anterior chest (precordium). Place the child in a reclining or semi-Fowler position, either on the parent's lap or on the examining table. Inspect the shape and symmetry of the anterior chest from the front and side views. Asymmetry and bulging of the left side of the chest wall may indicate an enlarged heart. Observe for any chest movement associated with the heart's contraction. A *heave,* an obvious lifting of the chest wall during contraction, may indicate an enlarged heart.

Palpation of the Precordium

Lightly place the surface of your fingers together on the chest wall to systematically palpate the precordium for any pulsations, heaves, or vibrations. Palpating with minimal pressure increases the chance of detecting abnormal findings.

The **apical impulse**, the point of maximum intensity, is located where the left ventricle taps the chest wall during contraction. The apical impulse is sometimes seen on the anterior chest wall of thin children, but it is normally felt as a slight tap against one fingertip. Use the topographic landmarks of the chest to describe its location (see Figures 5–20 and 5–21).

Growth and Development

The location of the apical impulse changes as the child's rib cage grows. In children under 7 years old, it is located in the fourth intercostal space just medial to the left midclavicular line. In children over 7 years old, it is located in the fifth intercostal space at the left midclavicular line.

TABLE 5–11 Normal Heart Rates for Children of Different Ages

AGE	HEART RATE RANGE (BEATS/MIN)	AVERAGE HEART RATE (BEATS/MIN)
Newborns	100–170	120
Infants to 2 years	80–130	110
2–6 years	70–120	100
6–10 years	70–110	90
10–16 years	60–100	85

Any other sensation palpated is usually abnormal. A *lift* is the sensation of the heart lifting up against the chest wall. It may be associated with an enlarged heart or a heart contracting with extra force. A **thrill** is a vibration that may feel like a cat's purr. It is caused by turbulent blood flow from a defective heart valve and a heart murmur. If present, the thrill is palpated in the right or left second intercostal space. To describe the thrill location, use the topographic landmarks of the chest (see Figures 5–20 and 5–21) and estimate the diameter of the thrill palpated.

Heart Rate and Rhythm

The apical heart rate can be counted at the site of the apical impulse either by palpation or by auscultation. Count the apical rate for 1 minute in infants and in children who have an irregular rhythm. The brachial or radial pulse rate should be the same as the auscultated apical heart rate. Table 5–11 gives normal heart rates in children of different ages.

Clinical Tip
The child's heart rate varies with age, decreasing as the child grows older. The heart rate increases in response to exercise, excitement, anxiety, and fever. Such stresses increase the child's metabolic rate, creating a simultaneous need for more oxygen. Children respond to the need for more oxygen by increasing their heart rate, a response called *sinus tachycardia.*

Listen carefully to the heart rate rhythm. Children often have a normal cycle of irregular rhythm associated with respiration called *sinus arrhythmia* in which the child's heart rate is faster on inspiration and slower on expiration. When any rhythm irregularity is detected, ask the child to take a breath and hold it while you listen to the heart rate. The rhythm should become regular during inspiration and expiration. Other rhythm irregularities are abnormal (see Chapter 21).

Auscultation of the Heart

Auscultation is also used to assess the characteristics of the heart sounds and to detect abnormal heart sounds. Use the bell of the stethoscope to detect these lower-pitched sounds.

Auscultate the heart with the child first when sitting and then reclining. This will help detect differences in heart sounds caused by a change in the child's position or by a change in the position of the heart near the chest wall. If differences in heart sounds are detected with a position change, place the child in the left lateral recumbent position and auscultate again.

IDENTIFYING HEART SOUNDS
Heart sounds result from the closure of the valves and any vibration or turbulence of blood produced by that valve closure.

Two primary sounds, S_1 and S_2, are heard when the chest is auscultated.

- S_1, the first heart sound, is produced by closure of the tricuspid and mitral valves at the beginning of ventricular contraction. The two valves close almost simultaneously to prevent the back flow of blood into the atria.
- S_2, the second heart sound, is produced by the closure of the aortic and pulmonic valves. Once blood has reached the pulmonic and aortic arteries, the valves close to prevent back flow into the ventricles.

Clinical Tip
To distinguish between S_1 and S_2 heart sounds in each listening area, palpate the carotid pulse while auscultating the heart. The heart sound heard simultaneously with the pulsation is S_1.

Sound is easily transmitted in liquid, and it travels best in the direction of blood flow. Auscultate heart sounds at specific areas on the chest wall in the direction of blood flow, just beyond the valve (Figure 5–24). The sounds produced by the heart valves or blood turbulence are heard throughout the chest in thin infants and children. Both S_1 and S_2 can be heard in all listening areas.

Auscultate heart sounds for quality (distinct versus muffled) and intensity (loud versus soft). First, distinguish between S_1 and S_2 in each listening area. Heart sounds are usually distinct and crisp in children because of their thin chest wall. Muffled or indistinct sounds may indicate a heart defect or congestive heart failure. Document the area where heart sounds are heard the best. Table 5–12 and Figure 5–24 review the location where each sound is normally best heard for assessment of quality and intensity. If an extra heart sound is heard (e.g., a murmur), auscultate the heart in the sitting, reclining, and left lateral recumbent positions to detect any differences associated with position change.

SPLITTING OF THE HEART SOUNDS
After distinguishing the first and second heart sounds, try to detect a split S_2. When the child takes a deep breath more blood returns to the right ventricle than the left ventricle, causing the pulmonic valve to close a fraction of a second later than the aortic valve; this is called *physiologic splitting*. Auscultate over the pulmonic area while the child breathes normally and then while the child takes a deep breath. The S_2 splitting may be heard after a deep breath, and then with regular breathing, it is heard as a

TABLE 5–12 Listening Sites for Auscultation of the Quality and Intensity of Heart Sounds

HEART SOUND	SITES WHERE BEST HEARD	SITES WHERE HEARD SOFTLY
S_1	Apex of the heart	Base of the heart
	Tricuspid area	Aortic area
	Mitral area	Pulmonic area
S_2	Base of the heart	Apex of the heart
	Aortic area	Tricuspid area
	Pulmonic area	Mitral area
Physiologic splitting	Pulmonic area	
S_3	Mitral area	

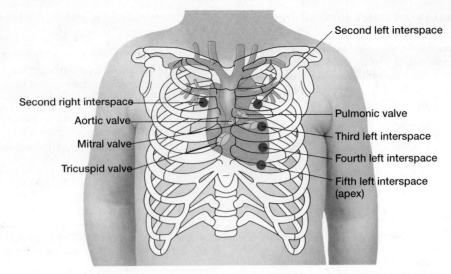

Figure 5–24 Remember that sound travels in the direction of blood flow when auscultating heart sounds. Rather than listen for heart sounds over each heart valve, auscultate heart sounds at specific areas on the chest wall away from the valve itself. These areas are named for the valve producing the sound. *Aortic*: second right intercostal space near the sternum. *Pulmonic*: second left intercostal space near the sternum. *Tricuspid*: fifth right or left intercostal space near the sternum. *Mitral* (apical): in infants—third or fourth intercostal space, just left of the left midclavicular line; in children—fifth intercostal space at the left midclavicular line.

single sound. If S_2 splitting does not vary with normal and deep respirations, it is called *fixed splitting*, which is an abnormal finding associated with an atrial septal defect in the heart.

EXTRA HEART SOUNDS

A third heart sound, S_3, is occasionally heard in children as a normal finding. The S_3 heart sound is caused when blood rushes through the mitral valve and splashes into the left ventricle. It is heard in diastole, just after S_2. It is distinguished from a split S_2 because it is louder in the mitral area than in the pulmonic area.

Murmurs, or abnormal heart sounds, are sometimes auscultated. These sounds are produced by blood passing through a defective valve, great vessel, or other heart structure. Some murmurs are benign or innocent, whereas others may indicate a congenital heart defect. Consult an experienced examiner to distinguish between murmurs.

It takes practice to hear murmurs in children. Often, murmurs must be very loud to be detected. For softer murmurs, normal heart sounds must be distinguished before an extra sound is recognized. When a murmur is detected, define the characteristics of the extra sound, including:

- *Intensity.* How loud is it? Can a thrill also be palpated? (See *Clinical Tip*.)
- *Location.* Where is the murmur the loudest? Identify the listening area and precise topographic landmarks. Is the child sitting or lying down? Do the murmur characteristics change when the child changes position?
- *Radiation or transmission.* Is the sound transmitted over a larger than expected area of the chest, to the axilla, or to the back?
- *Timing.* Is the murmur heard best after S_1 or S_2? Is it heard during the entire phase between S_1 and S_2?
- *Quality.* Describe what the murmur sounds like—for example, machine-like, musical, or blowing.

Clinical Tip

Following are guidelines for grading the intensity of a murmur:

Intensity	Description
Grade I	Barely heard in a quiet room
Grade II	Quiet, but clearly heard
Grade III	Moderately loud; no thrill palpated
Grade IV	Loud; a thrill is usually palpated
Grade V	Very loud, heard when the stethoscope is barely on the chest wall; a thrill is easily palpated
Grade VI	Heard without the stethoscope in direct contact with the chest wall; a thrill is palpated

VENOUS HUM

A venous hum is caused by turbulent blood flow in the internal jugular veins. Auscultate over the supraclavicular fossa above the middle of the clavicle or over the upper anterior chest with the bell of the stethoscope. A venous hum is heard as a continuous low-pitched hum throughout the cardiac cycle. It is heard louder during diastole and does not change with respirations. It may be quieted when the child turns the neck, lies down, or when the jugular vein is occluded. A venous hum may be associated with anemia, but it has no pathologic significance.

Completing the Heart Examination

A complete assessment of heart function also includes palpating the pulses, measuring the blood pressure, and evaluating signs from other systems.

PALPATION OF THE PULSES

Palpate the characteristics of the pulses in the extremities to assess the circulation. The technique and sites for palpating the pulse are the same as those used for adults. Evaluate the pulsation for rate, regularity of rhythm, and strength in each extremity and compare your findings bilaterally. Palpate the femoral pulses, which should be as strong as the brachial pulsations. A weaker femoral pulse is associated with coarctation of the aorta.

Growth and Development

Infants have a low systolic blood pressure, and detecting the distal pulses is often difficult. Use the brachial artery in the arms and the popliteal or femoral artery in the legs to evaluate the pulses. The radial and distal tibial pulses are normally palpated easily in older children.

BLOOD PRESSURE

To assess the blood pressure, wait until the child has been seated and quiet for 3 to 5 minutes. To obtain the most accurate reading, select an appropriately sized cuff for the extremity selected. Use the right arm when possible, as this arm was used for development of blood pressure standards. See the *Clinical Skills Manual* SKILLS for the technique for obtaining the blood pressure in children.

With the cuff snugly wrapped around the arm, hold the arm with the antecubital fossa at the level of the heart. Use the bell of the stethoscope to hear softer Korotkoff sounds. The systolic reading is the onset of Korotkoff sounds. The diastolic reading is the fifth Korotkoff sound (Lande, 2016).

Measure the blood pressure twice and average the two readings. Compare the systolic and diastolic readings with the standard blood pressure values by age, gender, and height percentile in Appendix B. A blood pressure value at the 50th percentile for the child's age, gender, and height percentile is considered the midpoint of the normal blood pressure range. A systolic or diastolic reading at or above the 95th percentile indicates hypertension.

For any child with a potential heart condition, obtain a blood pressure reading in both an arm and a leg and compare the readings. The blood pressure in the leg should be 10 to 20 mmHg higher than the arm reading (Bernstein, 2016). If the reading in the leg is lower than that in the arm, coarctation of the aorta may be present.

OTHER SIGNS

Skin color, capillary refill, and respiratory effort are additional elements of a complete heart examination. Cyanosis is most commonly associated with a congenital heart defect in children. A capillary refill time of greater than 2 seconds indicates poor perfusion of the tissues. Signs of respiratory distress (tachypnea, flaring, and retractions) may be associated with the child's attempts to compensate for hypoxemia caused by a congenital heart defect.

Assessing the Abdomen for Shape, Bowel Sounds, and Underlying Organs

The location of underlying organs and structures of the abdomen must be considered when the abdomen is examined. The abdomen is commonly divided by imaginary lines into quadrants for the purpose of identifying underlying structures (Figure 5–25). A stethoscope is needed to examine the abdomen. Perform inspection and auscultation before palpation and percussion because touching the abdomen may change the characteristics of bowel sounds.

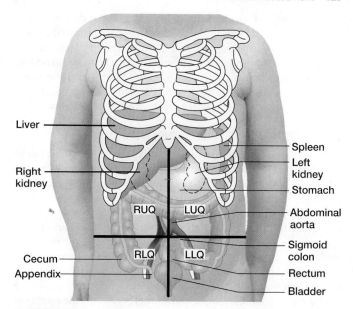

Figure 5–25 Topographic landmarks of the abdomen. The abdomen is commonly divided by imaginary lines into quadrants for the purpose of identifying underlying structures.

Inspection of the Abdomen

Begin the examination of the abdomen by inspecting the shape and contour, condition of the umbilicus and rectus muscle, and abdominal movement. Inspect the shape of the abdomen from the front and side with good lighting to identify an abnormal contour. The child's abdomen is normally symmetric and rounded or flat when the child is supine. A scaphoid or sunken abdomen is abnormal and may indicate dehydration.

After a newborn's umbilical stump falls off, inspect the umbilicus for continued drainage, which may indicate an infection or a granuloma. Inspect the umbilicus in infants and toddlers because these children often have an *umbilical hernia*, a protrusion of abdominal contents through an open umbilical muscle ring.

Inspect the abdominal wall for any depression or bulging at midline above or below the umbilicus, indicating separation of the rectus abdominis muscles. The depression may be up to 5 cm (2 in.) wide. Measure the width of the separation to monitor change over time. As abdominal muscle strength develops, the separation usually becomes less prominent. However, the splitting may persist if congenital muscle weakness is present.

ABDOMINAL MOVEMENT

Infants and children up to 6 years of age breathe with the diaphragm. The abdomen rises simultaneously with the chest during inspiration and falls with expiration. Other abdominal movements such as peristaltic waves are abnormal. **Peristaltic waves** are visible rhythmic contractions of the intestinal wall smooth muscle, which moves food through the digestive tract. Their presence generally indicates an intestinal obstruction, such as pyloric stenosis (see Chapter 25).

Auscultation of the Abdomen

To evaluate bowel sounds, auscultate the abdomen with the diaphragm of the stethoscope. Bowel sounds normally occur every 10 to 30 seconds. They have a high-pitched, tinkling, metallic quality. Loud gurgling (borborygmi) is heard when the child is hungry. Listen in each quadrant long enough to hear at least one bowel sound. Before determining that bowel sounds are absent, auscultate at least 5 minutes in each quadrant. Absence of bowel sounds may indicate peritonitis or a paralytic ileus. Hyperactive bowel sounds may indicate gastroenteritis or a bowel obstruction.

Next, auscultate over the abdominal aorta and the renal arteries for a vascular hum or murmur. No murmur should be heard. A murmur may indicate a narrowed or defective artery.

Percussion of the Abdomen

Indirect percussion is often used by experienced examiners to evaluate borders and sizes of abdominal organs and masses while the child is supine. To perform indirect percussion, lay the middle finger of your nondominant hand on the child's abdomen, keeping your other fingers off the abdomen. With a springlike motion, use the fingertip from your other hand to tap the finger resting on the abdomen. Listen for the tone to detect underlying structures. Dullness is found over the liver, spleen, and full bladder. Tympany is found over the stomach or the intestines when an obstruction is present. Tympany may be found over areas beyond the stomach in infants because of air swallowing. A resonant tone may be heard over other areas.

Palpation of the Abdomen

Both light and deep palpation are used to examine the abdominal organs and to detect any masses. *Light palpation* is used to evaluate the tenseness of the abdomen (how soft or hard it is), the liver, the presence of any tenderness or masses, and any defects in the abdominal wall. *Deep palpation* is used to detect masses, define their shape and consistency, and identify abdominal tenderness.

Perform the abdominal examination when the child is calm and cooperative to get the best assessment. To begin palpation, position the child supine with knees flexed. Stand beside the child and place your warmed fingertips across the child's abdomen. Organs and other masses are more easily palpated when the abdominal wall is relaxed. Watch the child's face during palpation for signs of pain (e.g., a grimace or constriction of the pupils).

Growth and Development **Abdominal Assessment**

Infants and toddlers often feel more secure for the abdominal assessment when lying supine across both the parent's and the examiner's laps. A bottle, pacifier, or toy may distract the child and improve cooperation for the examination.

When examining the child, use suggestive words to help the child relax the abdomen. "How soft will your tummy get when my hand feels it? Does it get softer than this? Yes. See, it softens as you breathe out. Will it also be softer here?" The child learns to relax the abdomen and is challenged to do it better.

When a child is ticklish, use a firm touch and do not pretend to tickle the child at any point in the examination. Alternatively, put the child's hand on the abdomen and place your hand over the child's. Let your fingertips slide over to touch the abdomen. The child has a sense of being in control, and you may be able to palpate directly.

Older children may need distraction, especially when abdominal tenderness and guarding are present. Have the child perform a task that requires some concentration, such as pressing the hands together or pulling locked hands apart.

LIGHT PALPATION

For light palpation, use a superficial, gentle touch that slightly depresses the abdomen. Usually, the abdomen feels soft and no tenderness is detected. Palpate any bulging along the abdominal wall, especially along the rectus muscle and umbilical ring, which could indicate a hernia. If an umbilical hernia is present, measure the diameter of the muscular ring rather than the protrusion. The muscle ring normally becomes smaller and closes by 4 years of age.

Locate and lightly palpate the lower liver edge. Place the fingerpads in the right midclavicular line at the level of the umbilicus and move the fingers closer to the costal margin with each expiration. As the liver edge descends with inspiration, a flat, narrow ridge is usually felt. The liver edge is normally palpated 2 to 3 cm (about 1 in.) below the right costal margin in infants and toddlers, but it may not be palpated in older children. If the liver edge is more than 3 cm (a little over 1 in.) below the right costal margin, the liver is enlarged, possibly due to congestive heart failure or hepatic disease.

DEEP PALPATION

To perform deep palpation, press the fingers of one hand (for small children) or two hands (for older children) more deeply into the abdomen. Because the abdominal muscles are most relaxed when the child takes a deep breath, ask the child to take regular deep breaths when palpating each area of the abdomen.

The spleen tip may be felt at the left costal margin in the midclavicular line when the child takes a deep breath. The spleen is enlarged if it is easily palpated below the left costal margin. The kidneys are in a deep layer of abdominal muscles and intestines, and they are rarely palpated except in newborns. A tubular mass commonly palpated in the lower left or right quadrant is often an intestine filled with feces. A distended bladder is often palpated as a firm, central, dome-shaped mass above the symphysis pubis in young children.

SAFETY ALERT!

If an enlarged kidney or unexpected mass is detected during abdominal palpation, do not continue to palpate the kidney. Notify the primary healthcare provider immediately. The mass could be a Wilms tumor.

Assessment of the Inguinal Area

The inguinal area is inspected and palpated during the abdominal examination to detect enlarged lymph nodes or masses. The femoral pulse, a part of the heart examination, may be assessed simultaneously with the abdominal examination.

Inspect the inguinal area for any change in contour, comparing sides. A small bulging noted over the femoral canal in girls may be associated with a femoral hernia. A bulging in the inguinal area in boys may be associated with an inguinal hernia.

Palpate the inguinal area for lymph nodes and other masses. Small lymph nodes, less than 1 cm (½ in.) in diameter, are often present in the inguinal area because of minor injuries on the legs. Any tenderness, heat, or inflammation in these palpated lymph nodes could be associated with a local infection.

Assessing the Genital and Perineal Areas for External Structural Abnormalities

Nurses may perform an external genital examination or assist another healthcare provider. In younger children, the genital and perineal examination is performed immediately after assessment of the abdomen. Gloves, lubricant, and a penlight are needed for the examination.

Examination of the genitalia and perineal area can cause stress in children because they sense invasion of their privacy. To make young children feel more secure, position them on the parent's lap with their legs spread apart. Children can also be positioned on the examining table with their knees flexed and the legs spread apart like a frog.

Clinical Tip

Preschool-age children are often taught that strangers are not permitted to touch their "private parts." When a child this age actively resists examination of the genital area, ask the parent to tell the child you have permission to look at and touch these parts of the body. You may wish to reinforce the teaching by saying the nurse or doctor can look only when the parent is in the room.

Some children develop modesty during the preschool period. Briefly explain what you need to examine and why. Then calmly and efficiently examine the child.

Inspection of the Female External Genitalia

Inspect the external genitalia of girls for color, size, and symmetry of the mons pubis, labia, urethra, and vaginal opening (Figure 5–26). Simultaneously look for any abnormal findings such as swelling, inflammation, masses, lacerations, or discharge.

Inspect the mons pubis for pubic hair and its characteristics. See Figure 5–29 (shown later in the chapter) for guidelines to assess the stage of pubic hair development.

The labia minora are usually thin and pale in preadolescent girls but become dark pink and moist after puberty. In young infants, the labia minora may be fused and cover the structures in the vestibule. If fused, the adhesions should be separated by another health professional.

Use the thumb and forefinger of one gloved hand to separate the labia minora to inspect the structures in the vestibule. No lesions or signs of inflammation are expected around the urethral or vaginal opening. Redness and **excoriation** (scratches and

abrasions of the skin) are often associated with an irritant such as bubble bath. The hymen is just inside the vaginal opening. In preadolescents, it is usually a thin membrane with a crescent-shaped opening. The vaginal opening is usually about 1 cm (½ in.) in adolescents when the hymen is intact. Sexually active adolescents may have a vaginal opening with irregular edges.

Preadolescent girls do not normally have a vaginal discharge. Adolescents often have a clear discharge without a foul odor. Menses generally begin approximately 2 years after breast bud development. A foul-smelling discharge in preschool-age children may be associated with a foreign body. Various organisms may cause a vaginal infection in older children.

An internal vaginal examination and palpation of the female genitalia by an experienced health professional is indicated when abnormal findings such as a vaginal discharge or trauma to the external structures is noted.

SAFETY ALERT!

Signs of sexual abuse in young children include bruising or swelling of the vulva, foul-smelling vaginal discharge, enlarged opening of the vagina, and rash or sores in the perineal area (see Chapter 17).

Inspection of the Male Genitalia

Inspect the male genitalia for the structural and pubertal development of the penis, scrotum, and testicles. Have boys sit with their legs crossed in front of them. This position puts pressure on the abdominal wall to push the testicles into the scrotum. See Figure 5–30 (shown later in the chapter) for guidelines to assess the staging of pubic hair and external genital development.

PENIS

Inspect the penis for size, foreskin, hygiene, and position of the urethral meatus. The length of the nonerect penis in the newborn is normally 2 to 3 cm (about 1 in.). The penis enlarges in length and breadth during childhood and puberty. The penis is normally straight. A downward bowing of the penis may be caused by a **chordee**, a fibrous band of tissue associated with hypospadias.

When the penis is circumcised, the glans penis is exposed, and it is normally clean and smooth without inflammation or ulceration. The urethral meatus is a slit-shaped opening near the tip of the glans. No discharge should be present. If the penis is not circumcised, a foreskin opening large enough for a good urinary stream is normal even when the foreskin does not fully retract, which is a common finding in boys between 3 and 6 years of age. To inspect the glans penis of an uncircumcised boy, the foreskin is gently retracted by the child, parent, or examiner. Avoid forcible retraction of the foreskin to prevent damage to the tissues and the formation of adhesions between the foreskin and glans. Evaluate the degree of foreskin retraction and the meatal location and size. It is usually possible to visualize the meatus.

Location of the urethral meatus at another site on the penis is abnormal, indicating hypospadias or epispadias (see Chapter 26). A round, pinpoint urethral meatus may indicate meatal stenosis. *Phimosis* is the presence of an abnormal ring of tissue distal to the glans that prevents retraction of the foreskin to allow visualization of the meatus. Erythema and edema of the glans (*balanitis*) may result from an infection or trauma.

Inspect the urinary stream. The stream is normally strong without dribbling.

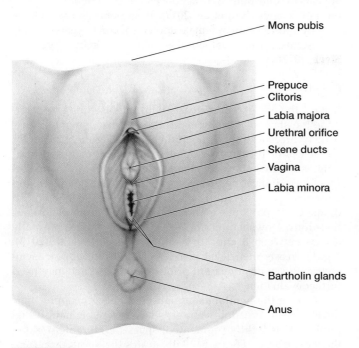

Mons pubis

Prepuce
Clitoris

Labia majora

Urethral orifice

Skene ducts

Vagina

Labia minora

Bartholin glands

Anus

Figure 5–26 **Anatomic structures of the female genital and perineal area.**

SCROTUM

Inspect the scrotum for size, symmetry, presence of the testicles, and any abnormalities. The scrotum is normally loose and pendulous with *rugae* (wrinkles). The scrotum of infants often appears large in comparison to the penis. A small, undeveloped scrotum that has no rugae indicates undescended testicles. Enlargement or swelling of the scrotum is abnormal. It may indicate an inguinal hernia, hydrocele, torsion of the spermatic cord, or testicular inflammation. A deep cleft in the scrotum may indicate ambiguous genitalia.

Palpation of the Male Genitalia

Palpate the shaft of the penis for nodules and masses. None should be present.

Palpate the scrotum for the presence of the testicles. Make sure your hands are warm to avoid stimulating the cremasteric reflex that causes the testicles to retract. Place your index finger and thumb over the inguinal canal on the side palpated. This keeps the testicle from retracting into the abdomen (Figure 5–27). Gently palpate each testicle. The testicles are normally smooth and equal in size. They are approximately 1 to 1.5 cm (½ in.) in diameter until puberty, when they increase in size. A hard, enlarged, painless testicle may indicate a tumor.

If a testicle is not palpated in the scrotum, an experienced examiner palpates the inguinal canal for the presence of the testicle and may try to move the testicle to the scrotum to palpate its size and shape. The testicle is descendable when it can be moved into the scrotum. An undescended testicle is one that will not move out of the inguinal canal or one that cannot be palpated. An experienced examiner also palpates the length of the spermatic cord between the thumb and forefinger from the testicle to the inguinal canal. It normally feels solid and smooth. No tenderness is expected.

When bulging or swelling of the scrotum is present, an experienced examiner palpates the scrotum to identify the characteristics of the mass and whether it is unilateral or bilateral. If the mass pushes back through the external inguinal

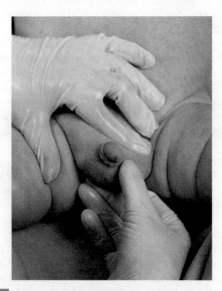

Figure 5–27 When palpating the scrotum for descended testicles and spermatic cords, place the index finger over the inguinal canal to keep the testicle in the scrotum. Gently palpate the testicle with only enough pressure to detect the size and shape.

ring, it is a reducible inguinal hernia rather than incarcerated. A bright penlight under the scrotum is used to see if a red glow is seen (transillumination), indicating a hydrocele rather than a hernia.

Anus and Rectum

When the child is supine or prone, inspect the anus for sphincter control and any abnormal findings such as inflammation, fissures, or lesions. The external sphincter is usually closed. Inflammation and scratch marks around the anus may be associated with pinworms. A protrusion from the rectum may be associated with a rectal wall prolapse or a hemorrhoid.

Lightly touching the anal opening should stimulate an anal contraction or "wink." Absence of a contraction may indicate the presence of a lower spinal cord lesion. Passage of meconium by newborns indicates a patent anus.

Only an experienced examiner should perform a rectal examination. It is indicated for symptoms of intra-abdominal, rectal, bowel, or stool abnormalities. To assist the examiner and to reduce the child's anxiety, distract the child with an age-appropriate toy or discussion. Let the child know that the lubricant might feel cold. As the examiner's finger is positioned, help the child to relax the sphincter by "pushing out the poop."

Assessing Pubertal Development and Sexual Maturation

The age when secondary sexual characteristics appear can vary with race and ethnicity, environmental conditions, geographic location, and nutrition. For example, in the United States, Black girls and boys have an earlier onset of secondary sexual characteristics than non-Hispanic White and Hispanic girls and boys (Herman-Giddens et al., 2012). A higher body mass index appears to contribute to earlier development of puberty in girls, but not in boys (Biro et al., 2013). If no pubertal changes are seen by age 13 years in female adolescents or 14 years in male adolescents, further evaluation is needed (Loomba-Albrecht & Styne, 2012).

Girls

Inspect the adolescent's breasts while she is sitting to determine the stage of development. Breast development in girls usually precedes other pubertal changes. Figure 5–28 shows the stages of breast development. *Thelarche,* or breast budding, is the first stage of pubertal development in the majority of girls, indicating breast stage 2. Breast tissue is seen and palpated below a slightly enlarging areola (1 cm [½ in.] in diameter of palpable glandular tissue) (Herman-Giddens, Bourdony, Dowshen, et al., 2011). Breast budding normally occurs between 8 and 10 years of age (Biro et al., 2013). A girl's breasts often develop at different rates and appear asymmetric. Breast development prior to 6 years of age may need further evaluation.

During the genital examination, observe for pubic hair development. Preadolescent girls have no pubic hair. Initial pubic hair is lightly pigmented, sparse, and straight along the labia majora. Figure 5–29 illustrates the normal stages of female pubic hair development. Breast development usually precedes pubic hair development. The presence of pubic hair

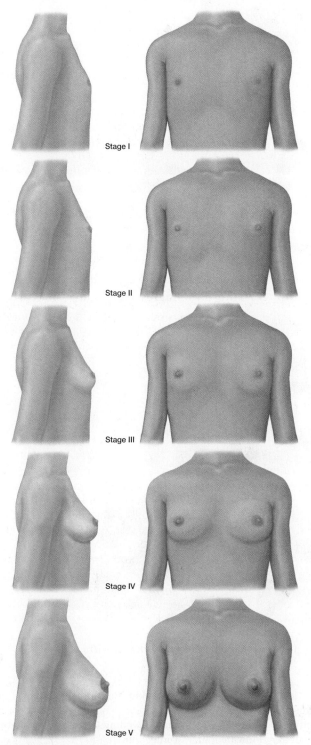

Stage I

Stage II

Stage III

Stage IV

Stage V

Figure 5–28 **Normal stages of breast development.**

later in genitalia Tanner stage 3 (Herman-Giddens et al., 2012). The pubic hair becomes darker, dense, and curly, extending over the pubic area in a diamond pattern by the completion of puberty. The mean age for completing pubertal development for male adolescents (stage 5) in the United States is 15 years of age (Herman-Giddens et al., 2012). Stages of pubic hair and external genital development follow a standard pattern, as seen in Figure 5–30.

Sexual Maturity Timeline

The sexual maturity rating (SMR) is an average of the breast and pubic hair development stages in girls and of the genital and pubic hair stages in boys. The rating is a number between 2 and 5, as stage 1 is prepubertal. The SMR is then related to other physiologic events that happen during puberty. Compare the stage of the child's secondary sexual characteristics with information in Table 5–13.

TABLE 5–13 Sexual Maturity Timeline

GENDER AND DEVELOPMENT CATEGORIES	TIME SPAN AND PHYSIOLOGIC CHANGES
Girls	
Breast development	Over 4 to 4.5 years, proceeding from stages 2 to 5
Pubic hair development	Over 4 to 4.5 years, usually initiated after breast development
Onset of menstruation	At about breast stage 4 (see Figure 5–28), 1 year after peak height velocity
Growth spurt	Height velocity begins increasing about 6 months before breast budding. Peak height velocity occurs between breast and pubic hair stages 3 and 4 (see Figures 5–28 and 5–29)
Boys	
Genital (penis and testes) development	Over 4.5 years, proceeding from stages 2 to 5; testicular development precedes growth of the penis (see Figure 5–30)
Pubic hair development	Over 3.5 years
Facial and axillary hair	Begins about 2 years after pubic hair development begins
Voice change	Greatest change between genital stages 3 and 4
Onset of ejaculation	At about genital stage 3
Growth spurt	Over 4 to 5 years, greatest height velocity is in the first 2 to 3 years with peak height velocity between genital and pubic hair stages 3 and 4 (see Figure 5–30)

Source: Data from Herman-Giddens, M. E., Bourdony, C. J., Dowshen, S. A., & Reiter, E. O. (2011). *Assessment of sexual maturity stages in girls and boys.* Elk Grove Village, IL: American Academy of Pediatrics; Susman, E. J., Houts, R. M., Steinberg, L., Belsky, J., Cauffman, E., De Hart, G., . . . Eunice Kennedy Shriver NICHD Early Child Care Research Network. (2010). Longitudinal development of secondary sexual characteristics in girls and boys between ages 9½ and 15½ years. *Archives of Pediatric and Adolescent Medicine, 164*(2), 166–173; Hochberg, Z., & Belsky, J. (2013). Evo-devo of human adolescence: Beyond disease models of early puberty. *BMC Medicine, 11,* 113. doi:10.1186/1741-7015–11–113.

before 8 years of age is unusual and may indicate premature pubertal development. The progression of puberty changes often takes 5 years to reach maturity.

Boys

Initial signs of pubertal development in boys are enlargement of the testicles and thinning of the scrotum at a mean age of 9 to 10 years of age, depending on ethnicity. Straight, downy pubic hair first appears at the base of the penis at a mean age of 10 to 11.5 years, depending on ethnicity. Penis enlargement generally follows testicular enlargement about 2 years

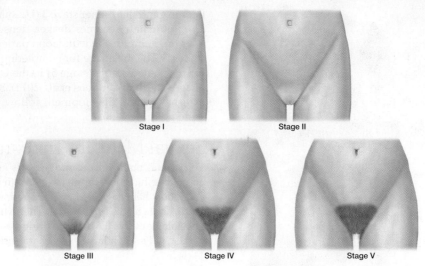

Figure 5–29 The stages of female pubic hair development with sexual maturation. In stage 2, soft downy hair along the labia majora is an indication that sexual maturation is beginning. Hair grows progressively coarse and curly as development proceeds.

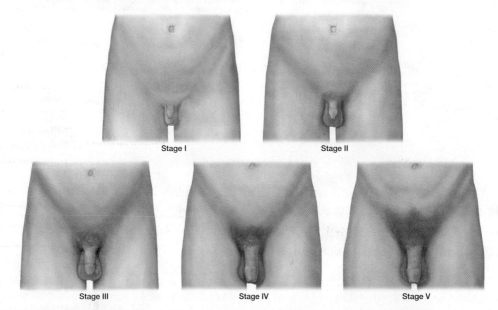

Figure 5–30 The stages of male pubic hair and external genital development with sexual maturation.

Assessing the Musculoskeletal System for Bone and Joint Structure, Movement, and Muscle Strength

Inspection of the Bones, Muscles, and Joints

Inspect and compare the arms and then the legs for differences in alignment, contour, skinfolds, length, and deformities. The extremities normally have equal length, circumference, and numbers of skinfolds bilaterally. Extra skinfolds and a larger circumference may indicate a shorter extremity.

Inspect and compare the joints bilaterally for size, discoloration, and ease of voluntary movement. Joints are normally the same color as surrounding skin, with no sign of swelling. Children should voluntarily flex and extend joints during normal activities without pain. Redness, swelling, and pain with movement may indicate injury or infection.

Palpation of the Bones, Muscles, and Joints

Palpate the bones and muscles in each extremity for muscle tone, masses, or tenderness. Muscles normally feel firm, and bony masses are not normally present. Doughy muscles may indicate poor muscle tone. Rigid muscles, or hypertonia, may be associated with an active seizure or cerebral palsy. A mass over a long bone may indicate a recent fracture or a bone tumor.

Palpate each joint and surrounding muscles to detect any swelling, masses, heat, or tenderness. None is expected when the joint is palpated. Tenderness, heat, swelling, and redness can result from injury or a chronic joint inflammation such as juvenile idiopathic arthritis.

Range of Motion and Muscle Strength Assessment

RANGE OF MOTION

Observe the child during typical play activities, such as reaching for objects, climbing, and walking, to assess range of motion of all major joints. Children spontaneously move their joints through the full normal range of motion with play activities when no pain is present. Limited range of motion may indicate injury, inflammation of a joint, or a muscle abnormality.

When a joint is suspected of having limited active range of motion, perform passive range of motion. Flex and extend, abduct and adduct, or rotate the affected joint cautiously to avoid causing extra pain. Full range of motion without pain is normal. Limitations in movement may indicate injury, inflammation, or malformation. Increased passive range of motion may indicate muscle weakness.

MUSCLE STRENGTH

Observe the child's ability to climb onto an examining table, throw a ball, clap hands together, or move around on the bed. The child's ability to perform age-appropriate play activities indicates good muscle tone and strength. Attainment of age-appropriate motor development is another indicator of good muscle strength (Table 5–14).

To assess the strength of specific muscles in the extremities, engage the child in some games. Compare muscle strength bilaterally to identify muscle weakness. For example, the child squeezes the examiner's fingers tightly with each hand; pushes against and pulls the examiner's hands with the hands, lower legs, and feet; and resists extension of a flexed elbow or knee. Children normally have good muscle strength bilaterally. Unilateral muscle weakness may be associated with a nerve injury. Bilateral muscle weakness may result from a congenital disorder such as Down syndrome. Asymmetric weakness may be associated with conditions such as cerebral palsy.

When generalized muscle weakness is suspected in a preschool- or school-age child, ask the child to stand up from the supine position. Children are normally able to rise to a standing position without using their arms as levers. Children who push their body upright using their arms and hands may have generalized muscle weakness, known as a positive *Gowers sign*. This may indicate muscular dystrophy (see Chapter 29).

TABLE 5–14 Selected Gross Motor Milestones for Age

GROSS MOTOR MILESTONES	AVERAGE AGE ATTAINED (MONTHS)
If prone, pushes up on elbows	4
Rolls over in both directions	6
Gets to sitting position and sits without support	9
Creeps or crawls	9
Pulls self to standing position	12
Takes a few steps walking alone	12
May walk up steps	18
Climbs on furniture without help	24
Rides tricycle	36

Source: Data from Centers for Disease Control and Prevention. (2014). *Developmental milestones*. Retrieved from http://www.cdc.gov/ncbddd/actearly/milestones/index.html

TABLE 5–15 Normal Development of Posture and Spinal Curves

AGE	POSTURE AND SPINAL CURVES
2–3 months	Holds head erect when held upright; thoracic kyphosis when sitting
6–8 months	Sits without support; spine is straight
10–15 months	Walks independently; straight spine
Toddler	Protruding abdomen; lumbar lordosis
School-age child	Height of shoulders and hips is level; balanced thoracic convex and lumbar concave curves

Posture and Spinal Alignment

POSTURE

Inspect the child's posture when standing from a front, side, and back view. The shoulders and hips are normally level. The head is held erect without a tilt, and the shoulder contour is symmetric. After beginning to walk, young children often have a pot-bellied stance because of lumbar lordosis. The spine has normal thoracic convex and lumbar concave curves after 6 years of age. Table 5–15 describes normal posture and spinal curvature development.

SPINAL ALIGNMENT

Assess the school-age child and adolescent for **scoliosis**, a lateral spine curvature. Stand behind the child, observing the height of the shoulders and hips (Figure 5–31). Ask the child to bend forward slowly at the waist, with the head and arms toward the floor. No lateral curve should be present in either position. The ribs normally stay flat bilaterally. The lumbar concave curve

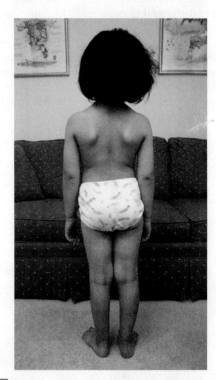

Figure 5–31 When evaluating spinal alignment, look at the level of the iliac crests and shoulders to see if they are level. Are creases at the waist similar or more prominent on one side? What signs does this child have? This child may have scoliosis.

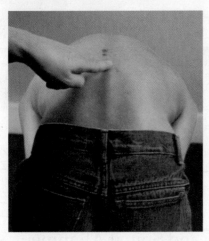

Figure 5–32 To inspect the spine for scoliosis ask the child to slowly bend forward at the waist with arms extended toward the floor. Run your forefinger down the spinal processes, palpating each vertebra for a change in alignment. A lateral curve to the spine or a one-sided rib hump is an indication of scoliosis.

should flatten with forward flexion (Figure 5–32). A lateral curve to the spine or a one-sided rib hump is an indication of scoliosis (see Chapter 29).

Inspection of the Upper Extremities

The alignment of the arms is normally straight, with a minimal angle at the elbows, where the bones articulate.

Count the fingers. Extra finger digits (*polydactyly*) or webbed fingers (*syndactyly*) are abnormal. Inspect the creases on the palmar surface of each hand (Figure 5–33). Multiple creases across the palm are normal.

Inspect the nails for size, shape, and color. Nails are normally convex, smooth, and pink. **Clubbing**, widening of the nail bed with an increased angle between the proximal nail fold and nail, is abnormal (see Figure 21–3 in Chapter 21). Clubbing is associated with chronic respiratory and cardiac conditions.

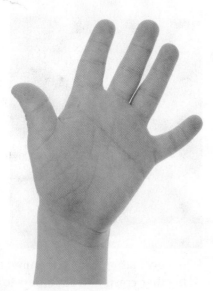

Figure 5–33 Transverse crease on palmar surface of the hand is associated with Down syndrome.

SOURCE: EVAfotografie/Getty Images.

Inspection of the Lower Extremities

Assess the hips of newborns and young infants for dislocation or subluxation. First inspect and compare the number of skinfolds on the upper legs. If the number of skinfolds is unequal, a hip dislocation or difference in leg length may be present. The Ortolani and Barlow maneuvers are used to assess an infant's hips for dislocation or subluxation during the first year (Figure 5–34). Then check for the Allis sign, a difference in knee height symmetry (Figure 5–35).

View the child from behind and observe as the child stands on one leg and then the other. The iliac crests should stay level. If the iliac crest on the lifted leg appears lower, the hip abductor muscles on the weight-bearing side are weak, known as the *Trendelenburg sign*.

LEGS AND FEET

Inspect the alignment of the legs with the child standing. After a child is 4 years of age, the alignment of the long bones is expected to be straight at the knees and ankles. The alignment of the lower extremities in infants and toddlers changes as bones straighten with weight bearing. To evaluate the toddler with bowlegs, have the child stand on a firm surface. Measure the distance between the knees when the child's ankles are together. No more than 1.5 in. (3.5 cm) between the knees is normal. See Figure 5–36 for assessment of knock-knees.

Growth and Development **Leg Alignment**

Infants are often born with a twisting of the tibia caused by positioning in utero (tibial torsion). The infant's toes turn in as a result of the tibial torsion. Toddlers go through a skeletal alignment sequence of bowlegs (genu varum) and knock-knees (genu valgum) before the legs assume a straight alignment.

Inspect the feet for alignment, the presence of all toes, and any deformities. The weight-bearing line of the feet is usually in alignment with the legs. Many newborns have a flexible forefoot inversion (*metatarsus adductus*) that results from uterine positioning. Any fixed deformity is abnormal.

Inspect the feet for the presence of an arch when the child is standing. Children up to 3 years of age normally have a fat pad over the arch, giving the appearance of flat feet. Older children normally have a longitudinal arch. The arch is usually seen when the child stands on tiptoe or is sitting. Inspect the nails of the feet as for the hands.

Assessing the Nervous System

The nervous system is assessed for cognitive function, balance, coordination, cranial nerve function, sensation, and reflexes. Equipment needed for this examination includes a reflex hammer, cotton balls, a penlight, and tongue blades.

Clinical Tip

The neurologic examination provides an opportunity to develop rapport with the child. Many of the procedures can be presented as games that young children enjoy. You can assess cognitive function by how well the child follows directions for tests of strength and coordination. As the assessment proceeds, the child develops trust and may be more cooperative with examination of other body systems.

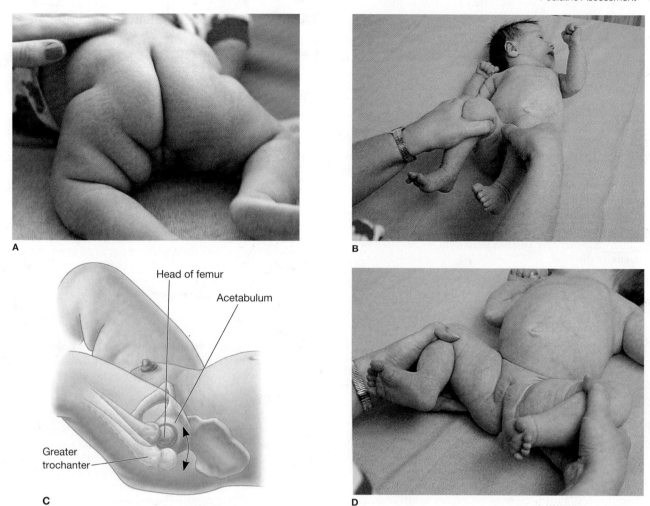

A
B
C
D

Figure 5–34 *A*, The asymmetry of the gluteal and thigh fat folds seen in infant with left developmental dysplasia of the hip. *B*, For the Barlow (dislocation) maneuver grasp adduct the infant's femur and apply gentle downward pressure. *C*, Dislocation is palpable as the femoral head slips out of the acetabulum. *D*, For the Ortolani maneuver place downward pressure on the hip and then inward rotation. If the hip is dislocated, this maneuver will force the femoral head back into the acetabulum with a noticeable "clunk."

Head of femur
Acetabulum
Greater trochanter

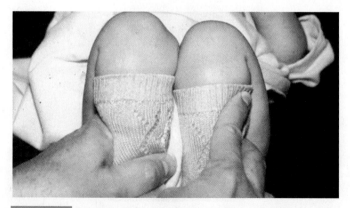

Figure 5–35 To check knee height symmetry flex the infant's hips and knees so the heels are as close to the buttocks as possible. Place the feet flat on the examining table. The knees are usually the same height. A difference in knee height (Allis sign), as seen here, is an indicator of hip dislocation.

SOURCE: International Hip Dysplasia Institute.

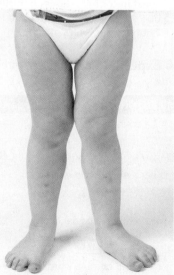

Figure 5–36 To evaluate the child with knock-knees, have the child stand on a firm surface. Measure the distance between the ankles when the child stands with the knees together. The normal distance is not more than 2 in. (5 cm) between the ankles.

Cognitive Function

Observe the child's behavior, facial expressions, gestures, communication skills, activity level, and level of consciousness to assess cognitive functioning. Match the neurologic examination to the child's stage of development. For example, cognitive function is evaluated much differently in infants than in older children because infants cannot use words to communicate.

BEHAVIOR

The alertness of infants and children is indicated by their behavior. Infants and toddlers are curious but seek the security of the parent either by clinging or by making frequent eye contact. Older children are often anxious and watch the examiner's actions. Lack of interest in assessment or treatment procedures may indicate a serious illness. Excessive activity or an unusually short attention span may be associated with an attention deficit hyperactivity disorder.

COMMUNICATION SKILLS

Speech, language development, and social skills provide good clues to cognitive functioning. Listen to speech articulation and words used, comparing the child's performance with standards of social development and expected language development for age (Table 5–16). Toddlers can normally follow simple directions such as, "Show me your mouth." By 3 years of age, the child's speech should be easily understood. Delay in language and social skill development may be associated with cognitive disability or hearing loss.

MEMORY

Immediate, recent, and remote memory can be tested in children starting at approximately 4 years of age. Immediate memory can be tested by asking the child to repeat a series of words or numbers, such as the names of favorite characters from a book, television show, or movie. Children can remember more words or numbers with age: three words or numbers at age 4 years, four words or numbers at age 5 years, and five words or numbers at age 6 years.

To evaluate recent memory, ask the child to repeat and then remember a special name or object (e.g., Cinderella or hamburger). Then 5 to 10 minutes later during the examination, have the child recall the name or object. To evaluate remote memory, ask the child to repeat his or her address or birth date or a nursery rhyme. By 5 or 6 years of age, children are normally able to recall this information without difficulty.

TABLE 5–16 Expected Language Development for Age

LANGUAGE MILESTONES	AGE ATTAINED
Babbles speechlike sounds, including *p*, *b*, and *m*	4–6 months
Has 1–2 words like *mama*, *dada*, *bye-bye*	12 months
Increases words each month; two-word combinations (e.g., "Where baby?" and "Want cookie")	1–2 years
Two- to three-word sentences to ask for things or talk about things; large vocabulary; speech understood by family members	2–3 years
Sentences may have four or more words; speech understood by most people	3–4 years
Says most sounds correctly except a few like *l*, *s*, *r*, *v*, *z*, *ch*, *sh*, *th*; tells stories and uses same grammar as rest of family	4–5 years

Source: Data from American Speech and Language Association. (2014). *How does your child hear and talk?* Retrieved from http://www.asha.org/public/speech/development/chart.htm

TABLE 5–17 Expected Balance Development for Age

BALANCE MILESTONES	AGE ATTAINED
Stands without support briefly	12 months
Walks alone well	15 months
Walks backwards	2 years
Balances on 1 foot momentarily	3 years
Hops on 1 foot	4 years

LEVEL OF CONSCIOUSNESS

When approaching infants or children, observe their level of consciousness and activity, including facial expressions, gestures, and interaction. Children are normally alert, and sleeping children arouse easily. The child who cannot be awakened is unconscious. A lowered level of consciousness may be associated with a number of neurologic conditions such as a brain injury, seizure, infection, or brain tumor.

Cerebellar Function

Observe the young child at play to assess coordination and balance. Development of fine motor skills in infants and preschool children provides clues to cerebellar function.

BALANCE

Observe the child's balance during play activities such as walking, standing on one foot, and hopping. See Table 5–17 for expected balance milestones for age. The Romberg procedure can also be used to test balance in children over 3 years of age (Figure 5–37). Once balance and other motor skills are

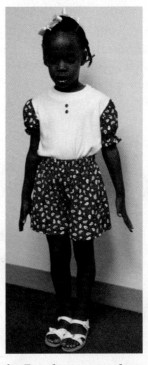

Figure 5–37 Use the Romberg procedure to evaluate balance. Ask the child to stand with feet together and eyes closed. Protect the child from falling by standing close. Preschool-age children may extend their arms to maintain balance, but older children can normally stand with their arms at their sides.

attained, children do not normally stumble or fall when tested. Poor balance may indicate cerebellar dysfunction or an inner ear disturbance.

COORDINATION

Tests of coordination assess the smoothness and accuracy of movement. Development of fine motor skills can be used to assess coordination in young children (Table 5–18). After 6 years of age, the tests for adults (finger-to-nose, finger-to-finger, heel-to-shin, and alternating motion) can be used (Figure 5–38). Jerky movements or inaccurate pointing (past pointing) indicate poor coordination, which can be associated with delayed development or a cerebellar lesion.

GAIT

A normal gait requires intact bones and joints, muscle strength, coordination, and balance. Inspect the walking child from both the front and rear views. The iliac crests are normally level during walking, and no limp is expected. Toddlers beginning to walk have a wide-based gait and limited balance, and eventually gain more balance and a more narrow-based gait.

A limp may indicate injury or joint disease. Staggering or falling may indicate cerebellar ataxia. *Scissoring*, in which

TABLE 5–18 Expected Fine Motor Development for Age

FINE MOTOR MILESTONES	AVERAGE AGE ATTAINED (MONTHS)
Reaches for a toy with one hand	4
Transfers objects between hands, brings objects to mouth	6
Thumb finger grasp to pick up small objects	9
Bangs items together, releases toy without help	12
Uses spoon to feed self	18
Builds tower of four or more blocks	24

Source: Data from Centers for Disease Control and Prevention. (2014). *Developmental milestones.* Retrieved from http://www.cdc.gov/ncbddd/actearly/milestones/index.html

the thighs tend to cross forward over each other with each step, may be associated with cerebral palsy or other spastic conditions.

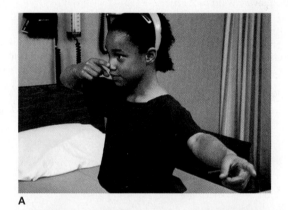

A

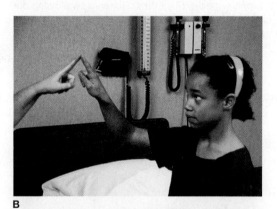

B

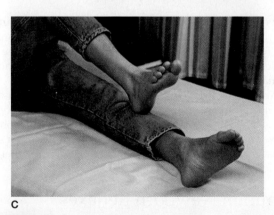

C

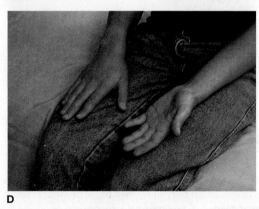

D

Figure 5–38 Tests of coordination. *A, Finger-to-nose test.* Ask the child to close the eyes and touch the nose, alternating the index fingers of the hands. *B, Finger-to-finger test.* Ask the child to alternately touch his or her nose and your index finger with his index finger. Move your hand to several positions within the child's reach to test pointing accuracy. Repeat the test with the child's other hand. *C, Heel-to-shin test.* Ask the child to rub his or her leg from the knee to the ankle with the heel of the other foot. Repeat the test with the other foot. This test is normally performed without hesitation or inappropriate placement of the foot. *D, Rapid alternating motion test.* Ask the child to rapidly rotate his or her wrist so the palm and dorsum of the hand alternately pat the thigh. Repeat the test with the other hand. Hesitating movements are abnormal. Mirroring movements of the hand not being tested indicate a delay in coordination skill refinement.

TABLE 5–19 Age-Specific Procedures for Assessment of Cranial Nerves in Infants and Children

CRANIAL NERVE[a]	ASSESSMENT PROCEDURE AND NORMAL FINDINGS[b]
I Olfactory	Infant: Not tested. Child: Not routinely tested. Give familiar odors to child to sniff, one naris at a time. *Identifies odors such as orange, peanut butter, and chocolate.*
II Optic	Infant: Shine a bright light in eyes. *A quick blink reflex and dorsal head flexion indicate light perception.* Child: Test vision and visual fields if cooperative. *Visual acuity appropriate for age.*
(III Oculomotor) (IV Trochlear) (VI Abducens)	Infant: Shine a penlight at the eyes and move it side to side. *Focuses on and tracks the light to each side.* Child: Move an object through the six cardinal points of gaze. *Tracks object through all fields of gaze.* All ages: Inspect eyelids for drooping. Inspect pupillary response to light. *Eyelids do not droop and pupils are equal size and briskly respond to light.*
V Trigeminal	Infant: Stimulate the rooting and sucking reflex. *Turns head toward stimulation at side of mouth and sucking has good strength and pattern.* Child: Observe the child chewing a cracker. Touch forehead and cheeks with cotton ball when eyes are closed. *Bilateral jaw strength is good. Child points to location touched by cotton ball.*
VII Facial	All ages: Observe facial expressions when crying, smiling, frowning, etc. *Facial features stay symmetric bilaterally.*
VIII Acoustic	Infant: Produce a loud sound near the head. *Blinks in response to sound, moves head toward sound or freezes position.* Child: Whisper words and ask for them to be repeated. *Repeats words correctly.*
(IX Glossopharyngeal) (X Vagus)	Infant: Observe swallowing during feeding. *Good swallowing pattern.* All ages: Elicit gag reflex. *Gags with stimulation.*
XI Spinal accessory	Infant: Not tested. Child: Ask child to raise the shoulders and turn the head side to side against resistance. *Good strength in neck and shoulders.*
XII Hypoglossal	Infant: Observe feeding. *Sucking and swallowing are coordinated.* Child: Tell the child to stick out the tongue. Listen to speech. *Tongue is midline with no tremors. Words are clearly articulated.*

[a] Bracketed nerves are tested together.

[b] Italic text indicates normal findings.

Cranial Nerve Function

To assess the cranial nerves in infants and young children, modify the procedures used to assess school-age children and adults (Table 5–19). Abnormalities of cranial nerves may be associated with compression due to an injury, tumor, or infection in the brain.

Sensory Function

To assess sensory function, compare the responses of the body to various types of stimulation. Bilateral equal responses are normal. Loss of sensation may indicate a brain or spinal cord lesion. Withdrawal responses to painful procedures indicate normal sensory function in an infant.

To test *superficial tactile sensation*, stroke the skin on the lower leg or arm with a cotton ball or a finger while the child's eyes are closed. Cooperative children over 2 years of age can normally point to the location touched.

To test *superficial pain sensation*, ask the child to close the eyes, and touch the child in various places on each arm and leg. Alternate the sharp and dull ends of a broken tongue blade or a paper clip. Children over 4 years of age can normally distinguish between a sharp and dull sensation each time. To improve the child's accuracy with the test, let the child practice describing the difference between the sharp and dull stimulations.

An inability to identify superficial touch and pain sensations may indicate sensory loss. Identify the extent of sensory loss, such as all areas below the knee. Other sensory function tests (temperature, vibratory, deep pressure pain, and position sense) are performed when sensory loss is found. Refer to other texts for a description of these procedures.

Common Newborn Reflexes

Evaluate the movement and posture of newborns and young infants by the Moro, palmar grasp, plantar grasp, placing, stepping, and tonic neck newborn reflexes. These reflexes appear and disappear at expected intervals in the first few months of life as the central nervous system develops. Movements are normally equal bilaterally. An asymmetric response may indicate a serious neurologic problem on the less responsive side (Table 5–20).

TABLE 5–20 Common Newborn Reflexes

Tonic neck reflex (fencer position). Elicited when the newborn is supine and the head is turned to one side. In response, the extremities on the same side straighten, whereas on the opposite side they flex. This reflex may not be seen during the early newborn period, but once it appears, it persists until about the third month.

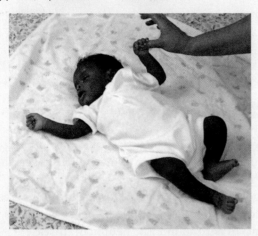

Moro reflex. Elicited when the newborn is startled by a loud noise or lifted slightly above the crib and then suddenly lowered. In response the newborn straightens arms and hands outward while the knees flex. Slowly the arms return to the chest, as in an embrace. The fingers spread, forming a C, and the newborn may cry. This reflex may persist until about 6 months of age.

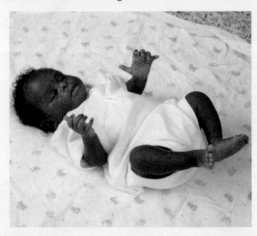

Stepping reflex. When held upright with one foot touching a flat surface the newborn puts one foot in front of the other and "walks." This reflex is more pronounced at birth and lost in 4 to 8 weeks.

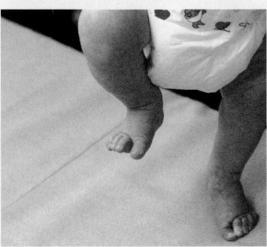

Palmar grasp reflex. Elicited by stimulating the newborn's palm with a finger or object; the newborn grasps and holds the object or finger firmly enough to be lifted momentarily from the crib.

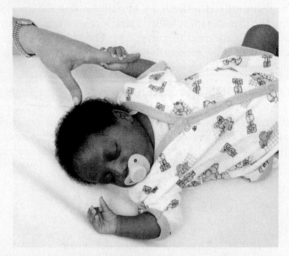

Rooting reflex. Elicited when the side of the newborn's mouth or cheek is touched. In response, the newborn turns toward that side and opens the lips to suck (if not fed recently).

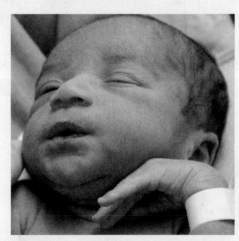

Source: Michele Davidson

Sucking reflex. Elicited when an object is placed in the newborn's mouth or anything touches the lips. Newborns suck even when sleeping; this is called nonnutritive sucking, and it can have a quieting effect on the baby. Disappears by 12 months.

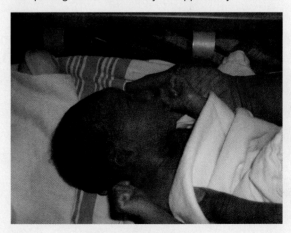

Superficial and Deep Tendon Reflexes

Evaluate the superficial and deep tendon reflexes to assess the function of specific segments of the spine.

SUPERFICIAL REFLEXES

Assess superficial reflexes by stroking a specific area of the body. The plantar reflex, testing spine levels L4 to S2, is routinely evaluated in children (Figure 5–39). The cremasteric reflex is assessed in boys by stroking the inner thigh of each leg. The testicle and scrotum on the stroked side normally rise.

DEEP TENDON REFLEXES

To assess the deep tendon reflexes, tap a tendon near specific joints with a reflex hammer (or with the index finger for infants), comparing responses bilaterally. Inspect for movement in the associated joint and palpate the strength of the expected muscle contraction. The numeric scoring of deep tendon reflexes is as follows:

Grade	Response Interpretation
0	No response
1+	Slow, minimal response
2+	Expected response, active
3+	More active or pronounced than expected
4+	Hyperactive, clonus may be present

Table 5–21 provides guidelines for assessment of the biceps, triceps, brachioradialis, patellar, and Achilles deep tendon

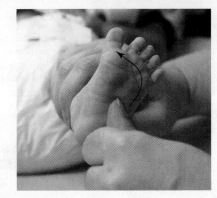

Figure 5–39 To assess the plantar reflex, stroke the bottom of the infant's or child's foot in the direction of the arrow. Watch the toes for plantar flexion or the *Babinski response*, fanning, and dorsiflexion of the big toe (as seen here). The Babinski response is normal in children under 2 years of age. Plantar flexion of the toes is the normal response in older children. A Babinski response in children over 2 years of age can indicate neurologic disease.

reflexes. The best response to deep tendon reflex testing is achieved when the child is relaxed or distracted. Making the child focus on another set of muscles may provide a more accurate response. When testing the reflexes on the lower legs, have the child press the hands together or try to pull them apart when

TABLE 5–21 Assessment of Deep Tendon Reflexes and the Associated Spinal Segment Tested

DEEP TENDON REFLEX	TECHNIQUE AND NORMAL FINDINGS*	SPINE SEGMENT TESTED
Biceps 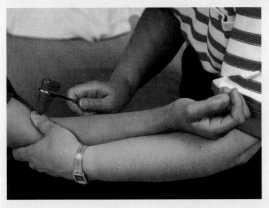	Flex the child's arm at the elbow, and place your thumb over the biceps tendon in the antecubital fossa. Tap your thumb. *Elbow flexes as the biceps muscle contracts.*	C5 and C6
Triceps 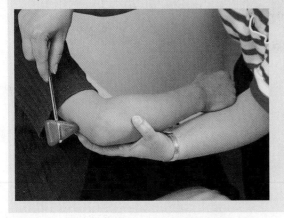	With the child's arm flexed, tap the triceps tendon above the elbow. *Elbow extends as the triceps muscle contracts.*	C6, C7, and C8

TABLE 5–21 Assessment of Deep Tendon Reflexes and the Associated Spinal Segment Tested (*continued*)

DEEP TENDON REFLEX	TECHNIQUE AND NORMAL FINDINGS*	SPINE SEGMENT TESTED
Brachioradialis 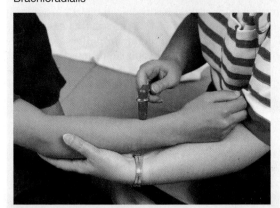	Lay the child's arm with the thumb upright over your arm. Tap the brachioradial tendon 2.5 cm (1 in.) above the wrist. *Forearm pronates (palm facing downward) and elbow flexes.*	C5 and C6
Patellar 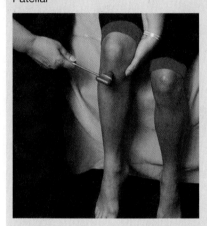	Flex the child's knees, and when the legs are relaxed, tap the patellar tendon just below the knee. *Knee extends (knee jerk) as the quadriceps muscle contracts.*	L2, L3, and L4
Achilles 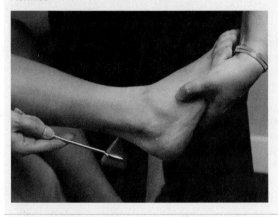	While the child's legs are flexed, support the foot and tap the Achilles tendon. *Plantar flexion (ankle jerk) as the gastrocnemius muscle contracts.*	S1 and S2

* Italic text indicates normal findings.

gripped together. Responses are normally symmetric bilaterally. The absence of a response is associated with decreased muscle tone and strength. Hyperactive responses are associated with muscle spasticity.

Performing an Intermittent Examination

In a hospital setting after a more comprehensive physical examination at time of admission, the nurse performs a focused assessment to monitor the child's status at intervals appropriate for the child's condition. This assessment includes a general health status overview and a more focused review of the body systems or body regions affected by the child's condition. Findings are compared with prior assessments to determine a change that would indicate a need for a more comprehensive assessment.

The general health status overview for all children includes the following:

- Alertness, responsiveness, or ability to interact
- Cardiorespiratory status—color, ease of breathing, vital signs
- Comfort level or pain score
- Movement of extremities

- Behavior—age appropriateness
- Skin—color, temperature, resilience, swelling
- Fluid and food intake
- Bowel function and urinary output
- Focused assessment of the body systems or body regions affected by child's condition and response to treatment (e.g., respiratory infection, surgery, wound)

If findings during this focused assessment reveal differences from a prior assessment, a more thorough assessment is needed.

Analyzing Data From the Physical Examination

Once the physical examination has been completed, group any abnormal findings for each system with those of other systems. Use clinical judgment to identify common patterns of physiologic responses associated with health conditions. Individual abnormal physiologic responses are also the basis of many nursing diagnoses. Be sure to record all findings from the physical assessment legibly, in detail, and in the format approved by your institution.

Chapter Highlights

- The elements of a health history include the chief concern, details about the present illness or injury, past health history, current health status, psychosocial and developmental data, family history, and review of systems. A birth history may be collected for infants.

- Communication strategies that may improve the quality of health information collected include the following: introducing yourself and explaining the purpose of the interview, providing privacy and confidentiality, using open-ended questions, and asking one question at a time. Ask the child questions when appropriate. Seek feedback to confirm your understanding of information provided.

- Several strategies may help improve the cooperation of the young child for the physical examination, such as allowing the child to stay on the parent's lap, providing an opportunity for the child to hold and inspect any equipment before it is used, and making a game out of tests for muscle strength, coordination, and developmental assessment.

- The sequence for performing a physical examination varies by the age of the child.
  - For infants and toddlers, perform procedures in a feet-to-head sequence to postpone the ear and throat examination that cause anxiety until the end. Take advantage of opportunities to listen to the lungs, heart, and abdomen when the infant is quiet or sleeping.
  - A head-to-feet sequence can be used for all other ages; however, the genital examination may be saved to the end.

- Special assessment techniques used for infants and toddlers include measuring the head circumference, palpating the fontanelles, using toys to assess vision and hearing, and keeping the child on the parent's lap.

- Examination modifications for preschoolers include using easily recognized names or words to assess hearing and memory, using play and games to assess muscle strength and coordination, and asking the child to show the teeth to begin assessment of the mouth.

- Adolescents should be asked their preference for having a parent present during the examination, and pubertal development should be assessed.

- Examples of normal variations found when examining children include hyperpigmented patches (Mongolian spots), epicanthal folds of the eyes, sucking pads in the mouth of an infant, breath sounds heard over the entire chest, a rounded chest in infants, abdominal movement with breathing, bowlegs and knock-knees, and pubertal changes.

- Evaluating the growth pattern of a child involves accurate measurements of infant length, child height, weight, and head circumference and then plotting the measurements on the appropriate growth curve for age. The child's percentile of growth for each measurement is then compared to prior measurements. The body mass index is used to determine if the child's weight is appropriate for height.

- Examples of unexpected physical examination findings that require urgent nursing intervention include altered level of consciousness, bradycardia, tachypnea, pain, signs of dehydration, stridor, retractions, and cyanosis.

Clinical Reasoning in Action

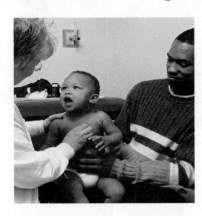

It is a relatively calm night in the children's hospital emergency department when a 6-month-old infant named Colby is brought in by emergency personnel from an automobile crash. Colby was buckled in his infant rear-facing car safety seat, riding with his parents when another car rear-ended them. The parents were not hurt and did not need to go to the hospital. The father immediately called 9-1-1 on his cell phone after the crash. When the ambulance arrived at the emergency department, the EMT gave you this report. Colby was alert and quiet in his father's arms when the ambulance arrived on the scene, and he did not have any obvious signs of injury. Colby and his father were brought to the hospital to make sure Colby did not sustain any injuries from the crash. His vital signs are as follows: temperature—98.9°F, respirations—32, pulse—110, and blood pressure—85/39. Colby is in no apparent distress. His pupils are equal, round, and reactive to light. His anterior fontanelle is flat, and he has equal movements of extremities. His breath sounds are clear and equal bilaterally. His heart sounds have a regular rate and rhythm without murmur. He voided around 2 hours ago, before the accident.

1. The fontanelles are an important body part to examine in infants and toddlers. In the scenario with Colby, it can give an indication of increased intracranial pressure related to a brain injury. Describe the placement of the fontanelles, and when they are expected to close and no longer be palpated. Why is the head more likely to sustain injury in an infant like Colby versus an adult?

2. After reviewing the scenario, what can you tell the parents about Colby's vital signs at this time? What is the difference between adult vital signs and Colby's vital signs?

3. What observations are made to check Colby's mental status?

4. If a heart murmur were to be found on examination of Colby, what would be the five ways to describe it?

References

American Academy of Pediatrics Committee on Practice and Ambulatory Medicine. (2011). Use of chaperones during the physical examination of the pediatric patient. *Pediatrics, 127*(5), 991–993.

American Association for Pediatric Ophthalmology and Strabismus. (2014). *Vision screening recommendations.* Retrieved from http://www.aapos.org/terms/conditions/131

American Speech and Language Association. (2014). *How does your child hear and talk?* Retrieved from http://www.asha.org/public/speech/development/chart.htm

Anderst, J. D., Carpenter, S. L., Abshire, T. C., & the Section on Hematology/Oncology and Committee on Child Abuse and Neglect. (2013). Evaluation for bleeding disorders in suspected child abuse. *Pediatrics, 131*(4), e1314–e1322.

Bernstein, D. (2016). Coarctation of the aorta. In R. M. Kliegman, B. F. Stanton, J. W. St. Geme, & N. F. Schor (Eds.), *Nelson textbook of pediatrics* (20th ed., pp. 2205–2207). Philadelphia, PA: Elsevier.

Biro, F. M., Greenspan, L. C., Galvez, M. P., Pinney, S. M., Teitelbaum, S., Windham, G. C., . . . Wolff, M. S. (2013). Onset of breast development in a longitudinal cohort. *Pediatrics, 132*(5), 1–9.

Brown, N. (2011). Adolescent medicine. In M. M. Tschudy & K. M. Arcara (Eds.), *The Harriet Lane handbook* (19th ed., pp. 118–135). St. Louis, MO: Elsevier.

Centers for Disease Control and Prevention. (2014). *Developmental milestones.* Retrieved from http://www.cdc.gov/ncbddd/actearly/milestones/index.html

Chameides, L., Samson, R. A., Schexnayder, S. M., & Hazinski, M. F. (Eds.). (2011). *Pediatric advanced life support: Provider manual.* Dallas, TX: American Heart Association.

Herman-Giddens, M. E., Bourdony, C. J., Dowshen, S. A., & Reiter, E. O. (2011). *Assessment of sexual maturity stages in girls and boys.* Elk Grove Village, IL: American Academy of Pediatrics.

Herman-Giddens, M. E., Steffes, J., Harris, D., Slora, E., Hussey, M., Dowshen, S. A., . . . Reiter, E. O. (2012). Secondary sexual characteristics in boys: Data from the Pediatric Research in Office Settings Network. *Pediatrics, 130*(5), e1058–e1068.

Hochberg, Z., & Belsky, J. (2013). Evo-devo of human adolescence: beyond disease models of early puberty. *BMC Medicine, 11,* 113. doi:10.1186/1741-7015-11-113

Hummel, P. (2011). Newborn assessment. In E. M. Chiocca (Ed.), *Advanced pediatric assessment* (pp. 199–229). Philadelphia, PA: Wolters Kluwer Lippincott Williams & Wilkins.

Lande, M. B. (2016). Systemic hypertension. In R. M. Kliegman, B. F. Stanton, J. W. St. Geme, & N. F. Schor (Eds.), *Nelson textbook of pediatrics* (20th ed., pp. 2294–2303). Philadelphia, PA: Elsevier.

Loomba-Albrecht, L. A., & Styne, D. M. (2012). The physiology of puberty and its disorders. *Pediatric Annals, 41*(4), e73–e80. doi:10.3928/00904481-20120307-08

Olitsky, S. E., Hug, D., Plummer, L. S., Stahl, E. D., Ariss, M. M., & Lindquist, T. P. (2016). Abnormalities of pupil and iris. In R. M. Kliegman, B. F. Stanton, J. W. St. Geme, & N. F. Schor (Eds.), *Nelson textbook of pediatrics* (20th ed., pp. 3023–3026). Philadelphia, PA: Elsevier.

Pappas, D. E., & Hendly, J. O. (2016). Sinusitis. In R. M. Kliegman, B. F. Stanton, J. W. St. Geme, & N. F. Schor (Eds.), *Nelson textbook of pediatrics* (20th ed., pp. 2014–2017). Philadelphia, PA: Elsevier.

Purnell, L. D. (2014). *Guide to culturally competent care* (3rd ed.). Philadelphia, PA: F. A. Davis.

Susman, E. J., Houts, R. M., Steinberg, L., Belsky, J., Cauffman, E., De Hart, G., . . . Eunice Kennedy Shriver NICHD Early Child Care Research Network. (2010). Longitudinal development of secondary sexual characteristics in girls and boys between ages 9½ and 15½ years. *Archives of Pediatric and Adolescent Medicine, 164*(2), 166–173.

Chapter 6
Introduction to Health Promotion and Maintenance

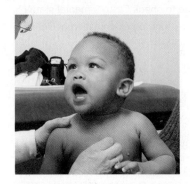

Clarence is so active, and we try to keep up with him, but after working all day we find it hard to have so little quiet time in the evenings. I know we missed his 12-month visit because we were busy with moving.

—Karie, mother of 15-month-old Clarence

Learning Outcomes

6.1 Define health promotion and health maintenance.

6.2 Describe how health promotion and health maintenance are facilitated by partnering with families during health supervision visits.

6.3 Describe the components of a health supervision visit.

6.4 Analyze the nurse's role in providing health promotion and health maintenance for children and families.

6.5 Perform the general observations made of children and their families as they come to the pediatric healthcare home for health supervision visits.

6.6 Synthesize the areas of assessment and intervention for health supervision visits—growth and developmental surveillance, nutrition, physical activity, oral health, mental and spiritual health, family and social relations, disease prevention strategies, and injury prevention strategies.

6.7 Plan health promotion and health maintenance strategies employed during health supervision visits.

6.8 Apply the nursing process in assessment, diagnosis, goal setting, intervention, and evaluation of health promotion and health maintenance activities for children and families.

A major goal of *Healthy People 2020* is to help individuals attain long, healthy lives free of preventable disease, disability, injury, and premature death across all life stages (U.S. Department of Health and Human Services, 2011). The concepts of health promotion and health maintenance provide for nursing interventions that contribute to meeting these goals. Many students in health professions begin their studies with a strong interest in the care of ill individuals. However, as time progresses, students learn that "well" people also require care. They need teaching to improve diet, reduce stress, and obtain immunizations. They may seek information about how to exercise properly or ensure a safe environment for their children. These examples of care and teaching are components of health promotion and health maintenance.

Nursing is a holistic profession that examines and works with all aspects of the lives of individuals, and has a strong focus on family and community as well. Nurses are uniquely positioned to provide health promotion and health maintenance activities, and indeed these activities should be a part of each encounter with families. What is the difference between health promotion and health maintenance? When should nurses engage in activities that focus on health? How are these activities integrated into health supervision visits for the infant and young child? How do nurses partner with other healthcare professionals to offer comprehensive health services in settings accessible to parents and young children? How can nurses help children and their families to maximize length and quality of life? These are some of the questions that will be explored in this chapter, with examples provided for the application of nursing management.

General Concepts

To understand health promotion and health maintenance, it is important to develop a definition of health. The World Health Organization (WHO) defines **health** as a state of complete physical, mental, and social well-being and not merely the absence of disease and infirmity (WHO, 2016). Others view the quality of "complete well-being" as impossible to attain, and therefore have further developed the concept to apply to persons with health challenges as well as those who are "healthy." Health in this expanded view is dynamic, changing, and unfolding; it is the realization of a state of actualization or potential (Pender, Murdaugh, & Parsons, 2015). This basic human right is necessary for the development of societies, so social determinants of health status are increasingly the focus of research and public policy.

Health promotion refers to activities that increase well-being and enhance wellness or health (Pender, Murdaugh, & Parsons, 2015). These activities lead to actualization of positive health potential for all individuals, including those with chronic or acute conditions, as well as persons whose social experiences puts them at risk for poor health. Examples include providing information and resources in order to:

- Enhance good nutrition at each developmental stage
- Integrate physical activity into the child's daily events
- Provide adequate housing
- Promote oral health
- Foster positive personality development

Health promotion is concerned with development of strategies that seek to foster conditions that allow populations to be healthy and to make healthy choices (WHO, 2016). Nurses engage in health promotion by partnering with children and families to promote family strengths in the areas of lifestyles, social development, coping, and family interactions. They also provide **anticipatory guidance** for families because they understand the child's upcoming developmental stages, and they teach families how to provide an environment that helps children achieve the milestones of each stage. This concept is explored more fully later in this chapter. Some nurses become involved in public policy forums in their communities in order to improve the social determinants of health, such as access to care, nutritious foods, and safe environments.

TABLE 6–1 Levels of Preventive Health Maintenance Activities

LEVEL	DESCRIPTION	EXAMPLES OF NURSING ACTIONS
Primary prevention	Activities that decrease opportunity for illness or injury	Giving immunizations Teaching about car safety seats
Secondary prevention	Early identification and treatment of a condition to lessen its severity	Developmental screening Vision and hearing screening
Tertiary prevention	Reduction in the consequences of a disease or condition with aim of restoring optimal function	Rehabilitation activities for child after a car crash

Source: Data from Centers for Disease Control and Prevention (CDC). (2013). *The concept of prevention*. Retrieved from http://www.cdc.gov/arthritis/temp/pilots-201208/pilot1/online/arthritis-challenge/03-Prevention/concept.htm

Health maintenance (or health protection) refers to activities that preserve an individual's present state of health and that prevent disease or injury occurrence. Examples of these activities include conducting developmental screening or surveillance to identify early deviations from normal development, providing immunizations to prevent illnesses, and teaching about common childhood safety hazards. Health maintenance activities are commonly preventive, and terminology common to community or public health nursing explains the levels and aims of preventive actions. Prevention levels are identified as primary prevention, secondary prevention, and tertiary prevention (Table 6–1).

While it is clear that health promotion and health maintenance activities are closely linked and often overlap, there are some differences. Health maintenance focuses on known potential health risks and seeks to prevent them or to identify them early so that intervention can occur. Health promotion looks at the strengths and goals of individuals, families, and populations, and seeks to use them to assist in reaching higher levels of wellness. It involves partnerships with the family as health goals are set, and with other health professionals and resources to provide for meeting a family's goals. Nurses apply both health promotion and health maintenance concepts when providing health care, recognizing that the concepts overlap. Health promotion and health maintenance are integrated into healthcare visits for children, with the care provider applying both knowledge of health maintenance concepts and adding information the family has identified that will assist in increasing health or wellness (health promotion). These activities commonly take place at "well-child" or health supervision visits.

Health supervision for children is the provision of services that focus on disease and injury prevention (health maintenance), growth and developmental surveillance, and health promotion at key intervals during the child's life. What health promotion and health maintenance activities are parts of health supervision visits? How can these activities be integrated into all settings where care is provided for children? What are the recommended times for health visits to occur and what care is provided at certain times? How can health supervision visits be organized to accomplish the goals of the family and health professionals? In this chapter and the following three chapters, we discuss the integration of health supervision in various settings, recommended schedules for health supervision visits, and partnering with families to achieve health goals and promote child development.

All children need a medical home, where accessible, continuous, and coordinated health supervision is provided during the developmental years. *Accessibility* refers to both financial and geographic access; *continuous* indicates that the care is ongoing with consistent care providers; *coordination* refers to the need for communication among health professionals to provide for the needs of the child. A medical home or **pediatric healthcare home** is therefore the site where comprehensive, family-centered, culturally effective, and compassionate health care is provided by a pediatric healthcare professional focused on the overall well-being of children and families (American Academy of Pediatrics, 2014). When a family has an established partnership with a healthcare provider, family-centered health services can be provided based on the family's risks and protective factors. These services may be provided in physicians' offices, community health clinics, the home, schools, childcare centers, shelters, or mobile vans (Figure 6–1). Coordination of care among these entities promotes the concept of a medical neighborhood that includes all components of care, with seamless flow of health information (Taylor, Lake, Nysenbaum, et al., 2011). The U.S. Department of Health and Human Services, the American Academy of Pediatrics (AAP), and the American Medical Association have developed national guidelines for preventive healthcare services for infants, children, and adolescents. The National Association of Pediatric Nurse Practitioners (NAPNAP) supports the list of comprehensive services of a pediatric healthcare home identified by the AAP (AAP, 2014).

Healthy People 2020

(MICH-30.1) Increase the proportion of children who have access to a medical home

- While 57.5% of children under age 18 years had an established medical home in 2007, the objective of 63.3% of children with such access is the present goal (U.S. Department of Health and Human Services, 2011).

The health supervision visit is individualized to the family and child. Standardized screenings and examinations are included, and time is provided for the family's specific concerns and questions about the child's health and development. Nurses play an integral part in these comprehensive visits, and they partner with other healthcare providers to accomplish health supervision.

A tracking system in the pediatric healthcare home site helps to identify appropriate health supervision activities for each child at every visit. Most often, computers are used to list appropriate topics for visits at specific ages. If a child misses a visit, the family can be contacted by phone, text, or e-mail, and encouraged to come in for the recommended care. A family may be called if their child is lacking some immunizations. Recognizing that not all families get into the healthcare home for each recommended visit, every health encounter, including an episodic illness visit or care for a chronic illness, is a potential time to complete health promotion and health maintenance activities. For example, immunizations may sometimes be given during a visit for an acute condition such as otitis media (ear infection) if the child has missed a prior health supervision visit. Even when children are seen in hospitals, emergency departments, or other settings, it is important to ask about their pediatric healthcare home and when the last visit occurred. Identify children who need basic health supervision services and provide them or refer to other settings for meeting these needs at another time.

Nurses play an important role in managing health supervision visits. Depending on the setting, the nurse may provide all services or support other healthcare providers by obtaining an updated health history, screening for diseases and other conditions, conducting a developmental assessment, and providing immunizations, anticipatory guidance, and health education. Nurses in all settings are instrumental in identifying children who need health supervision and are not obtaining recommended care (Figure 6–2).

While health supervision visits can address many health-related topics, there is generally a limited time in which to engage a child or family. The nurse needs to direct the encounters and have some ideas for pertinent agendas. *Bright Futures* booklets

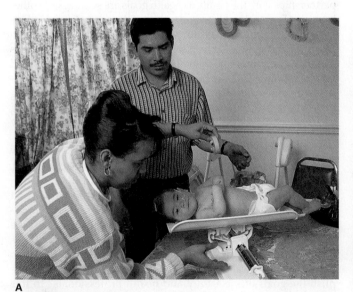

A

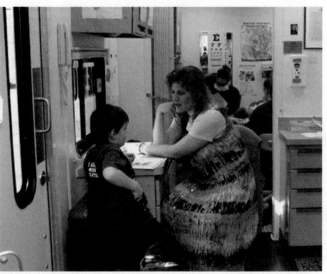

B

Figure 6–1 **Delivery of health promotion services.** *A,* **A nurse is providing a health supervision visit in the child's home after discharge from the hospital for an acute illness.** *B,* **A nurse is providing information to a child visiting a mobile healthcare van.**

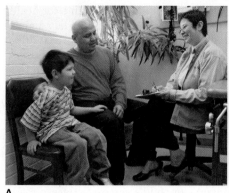
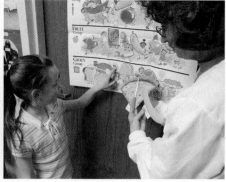
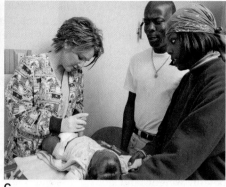

A   B   C

Figure 6–2 Identifying children who need health care. The nurse plays many roles in providing health promotion and health maintenance for children. *A,* Data are collected from the time a nurse calls the child and family to the examination room and during the history-taking phase. The nurse asks questions while observing the child's behaviors and the relationship between parent and child. The nurse also performs screening tests, including blood pressure, tuberculosis, vision and hearing, and developmental screening. *B,* Interventions that include teaching may take place. *C,* A nurse may administer immunizations as parents watch and assist by holding the child. Nurses also play important roles in teaching families information to enhance health.

provide guidance about how the nurse can manage health supervision visits. Six concepts should be integrated into care (Hagan, Shaw, & Duncan, 2008):

1. The healthcare provider *builds effective partnerships* with the family. A **partnership** is a relationship in which participants join together to ensure healthcare delivery in a way that recognizes the critical roles and contributions of each partner in promoting health and preventing illness. The partners in child health include the child, family, health professionals, and the community.

2. The nurse *fosters family-centered communication* by showing interest in the child and family, and effectively conveying information and understanding.

3. The nurse *focuses on health promotion and health maintenance topics during visits*, recognizing that families may not initiate these discussions.

4. The nurse *manages time well* to enable health promotion topics to be addressed during visits. This includes reviewing the child's health record and selecting topics pertinent to the child's age and the family's situation.

5. The nurse *educates the family during "teachable moments."* Large teaching plans are not always needed; children and families often learn best when presented with small bits of information based on the parent's questions or the nurse's observations.

6. The nurse *becomes an advocate for child health issues.* When an issue arises while caring for a child, seek additional data from various sources, talk with others, and strategize how the problem could be solved.

Components of Health Promotion/Health Maintenance Visits

The nurse identifies and addresses pertinent topics for health promotion and health maintenance during health supervision visits. Nurses also apply their knowledge of areas that need to

be addressed with an infant or child of a particular age, and then make general observations of the child and family to identify additional topics for discussion. While categories to consider vary depending on the age of the child, the family's particular needs, and community resources, there are some common topics that generally require attention. Often, nurses start with the topics suggested for the child's age, integrating general observations as the visit progresses and further identifying assessment areas needed in particular situations. The American Academy of Pediatrics and other organizations review and make recommendations for the screening and health assessments to be included at each age.

Professionalism in Practice Schedule for Preventive Health Services

The Recommendations for Preventive Health Care, for the child from the prenatal visit of the mother through age 21 years, were updated in 2016 and published in the journal *Pediatrics* (American Academy of Pediatrics Committee on Practice and Ambulatory Medicine, 2016). The Patient Protection and Affordable Care Act requires the coverage of these recommendations. Some changes in the 2016 schedule include addition of congenital heart disease screening of all newborns; alcohol, drug, and depression screenings; expansion of cholesterol screening; anemia identification; and HIV screening in adolescents.

The nurse should be aware of the screening guidelines and integrate these recommendations into health supervision visits and other child healthcare settings. Screening tools for specific age groups should be readily accessible and provided to the family and primary care providers during visits. Plans should be in place for further evaluation and referral as necessary when screenings result in abnormal findings. The integration of recommended screenings and follow-up should be carefully documented in the child's record.

Pediatric nurses make *general observations* of infants and their families whenever they encounter them. Nurses who are observant during the health supervision visit have many opportunities for assessing the family. These general observations begin when the family is called in and welcomed by the nurse to the facility. They continue as the infant or child is weighed and measured, and throughout the visit. Nurses observe the physical contact between the child and other family members, the developmental tasks displayed by the child, and parental level of stress or ease in conducting childcare activities.

Growth and developmental surveillance provides important clues about the child's condition and environment. The child's height, weight, and body mass index are calculated at each health supervision visit, and results are placed on percentile charts (see Chapters 4 and 14 for more information). Parents are given the information in written form and it is interpreted for them if needed. A thorough physical assessment is performed to ensure the child is growing as expected and has no abnormal or unexplained physical findings (see Chapter 5). **Developmental surveillance** is a flexible, continuous process of skilled observations that provides data about the child's capabilities, allows for early identification of any neurologic problems, and helps verify that the home environment is stimulating. Early development is important to later health, and it must be evaluated consistently and systematically during healthcare visits (Centers for Disease Control and Prevention [CDC], 2014a). Information may be collected from several sources—for instance, a questionnaire that the parent completes, questions asked during the interview, or observation of the child during the visit. Parents can also be interviewed to identify any developmental concerns they may have about the child or adolescent. When talking with parents, review physical, social, and communication milestones for infants, young children, older children, or adolescents. Detailed milestones for each age group are found in Chapter 4. Standardized developmental questionnaires are effective for developmental surveillance of most children, especially when time for health supervision visits is limited. Screening tests should be administered at the 9-, 18-, and the 24- or 30-month visits (CDC, 2014a; Lipkin, 2011). See Tables 6–2 and 6–3. When performing developmental monitoring with standardized screening tools, nurses make sure all directions are followed by:

- Choosing the proper test for the child's age and desired information
- Reading directions thoroughly or using specific training tools available
- Practicing as needed until proficient with the test
- Calculating the infant's or child's age correctly, especially if premature
- Attempting to develop rapport with the infant or child to get the best performance
- Following directions for administration of items; in some cases, parents can be asked if a child demonstrates specific skills at home, especially if the child is not willing to perform an item during testing
- Noting the behavior and cooperativeness of the child during the screening process
- Analyzing the findings using the test instructions to make the correct interpretation

Failure to perform an item on a screening tool does not mean the child has failed the test (see *Developing Cultural Competence: English Language Learners and Developmental Testing*). The child should be reevaluated at a future visit. Schedule the appointment at a time of day when the child is awake and rested. Provide parents with guidance on specific methods for stimulating the child. Failure of multiple items is of greatest concern. Follow the guidelines of the particular developmental screening test for referral to further diagnostic developmental assessment.

TABLE 6–2 Developmental Surveillance Questionnaires

QUESTIONNAIRE	GUIDELINES FOR ADMINISTRATION
Parent's Evaluation of Developmental Status[a] (birth to 8 years)	Consists of 10 questions for parents to answer in interview; based on research about parents' concerns. Requires less than 5 minutes to complete. English and Spanish forms are available.
Prescreening Development Questionnaire (birth to 6 years)	Parents complete an age-specific form. Helps identify children who need Denver II (PDQ and Revised-PDQ)[b] assessment. Requires less than 10 minutes to complete. PDQ is available in English, Spanish, and French versions; R-PDQ in English only.
Ages and Stages Questionnaire[c] (4–48 months)	Questionnaires for 11 specific ages, with 10 to 15 items each in areas of fine motor, gross motor, communication, adaptive, personal, and social skills. Parents try each activity with the child. Requires less than 10 minutes to complete. English and Spanish versions are available.
Child Development Inventories[d] (3–72 months)	Consists of 60 yes–no descriptions for three separate instruments to identify children with developmental difficulties. Requires about 10 minutes to complete.

[a] Frances P. Glascoe, Ellsworth & Vandermeer Press Ltd, P.O. Box 68164, Nashville, TN 37206.
[b] Denver Developmental Material, Inc., P.O. Box 371075, Denver, CO 80237-5075.
[c] Brookes Publishing Co., P.O. Box 10624, Baltimore, MD 21285-0625.
[d] Behavior Science Systems, P.O. Box 580274, Minneapolis, MN 55458.

TABLE 6–3 Developmental Screening Tests for Infants and Young Children

SCREENING TEST	GUIDELINES FOR ADMINISTRATION
Denver II[a] (birth to 6 years)	Consists of observation of the child in four domains: personal social, fine motor-adaptive, language, and gross motor. Requires 30 minutes to complete. A training video is available.
Bayley Infant Neurodevelopmental Screener (BINST)[b] (3–24 months)	Consists of observation of the child with 10 to 13 items for each of six age-specific scales to assess neurologic processes, neurodevelopmental skills, and developmental accomplishments. Requires 10–15 minutes to complete.
McCarthy Scales of Children's Abilities[b] (2.5–8.5 years)	Consists of observation of the child in domains of motor, verbal, perceptual-performance, quantitative, general cognition, and memory. Requires 45 minutes to complete.
Denver Articulation Screening Exam (DASE)[a] (2.5–6 years)	Consists of observation of the child's articulation of 30 sound elements and intelligibility. Requires 5 minutes to complete.
Early Language Milestone Scale—2 (ELM)[c] (birth to 36 months)	Consists of observation of the child to assess auditory expressive, auditory receptive, and visual components of speech. Requires 5–10 minutes to complete.

[a] Denver Development Materials, Inc., P.O. Box 371075, Denver, CO 80237-5075.
[b] Harcourt Assessment: The Psychological Corporation, 19500 Bulverde Rd., San Antonio, TX 78259.
[c] PRO-ED, Inc., 8700 Shoal Creek Blvd., Austin, TX 78758-6897.

Nutrition evaluation is a vital part of each health supervision visit. It makes important contributions to general health and fosters growth and development. Include observations and screening relevant to nutritional intake at each health supervision visit. Eating proper foods for age and activity ensures that children have the energy for proper growth, physical activity, cognition, and immune function. Nutrition is closely linked to both health promotion and health maintenance. See Chapter 14 for detailed nutritional assessments for each age group. Find out what questions parents have about feeding their children. Use the information gathered to provide both health promotion and health maintenance interventions.

Developing Cultural Competence English Language Learners and Developmental Testing

Children who have recently come from other countries and even some born in this country who live in families from minority ethnic groups may have difficulty with some items on developmental screening tests. For example, children who are not skilled in the English language may not understand some instructions or be able to answer questions about definitions of words. When parents do not speak English as a primary language and the examiner uses English, common terms might be misinterpreted. Parents might not understand what is meant if you ask, "Does your baby have a mobile over the crib at home?" or "Is she starting to be afraid of strangers?" How can you be alert for language differences and become sensitive to miscommunication?

Physical activity provides many physical and psychologic health benefits. However, there is a growing disparity between recommendations and reality among most children. Research by the Centers for Disease Control and Prevention (CDC) identified that 15.2% of children from 9th to 12th grades report no free-time physical activity, while 47% had recommended activity 5 days/week and only 27% met the recommendation 7 days/week (CDC, 2014b). When schools do not offer daily physical education, many children have no regular activity. Participation in physical activity declines as youth get older, and females are considerably less active than males (CDC, 2014b). Inquire about activities the child prefers and amount of time for activity during the day. As the child grows older, include questions about sedentary activities such as number of hours spent watching television or playing computer games. Inquire if the child plays sports at school or in the community. Ask about activities in a typical day to measure amount of activity. Once the nurse gathers data about physical activity, interventions are implemented to enhance activity patterns.

Although *oral health* may seem to require the knowledge of a specialist, it has many implications that relate to general health care. Oral health is important because teeth assist in language development, impacted or infected teeth lead to systemic illness, and teeth are related to positive self-image formation. Dental caries is the most common chronic disease of children. Many youth in the United States are affected by tooth decay and pain that interfere with activities of daily living such as eating, sleeping, attending school, and speaking (CDC, 2011a, 2011b). The nurse applies health promotion to dental health by teaching about oral care and access to dental visits. Health maintenance activities relate to prevention of caries and illness related to dental disease.

Mental and spiritual health are important concepts to address in health promotion and health maintenance visits. Parents can be encouraged to keep a record of mental health issues to bring to health supervision visits. This helps them understand that the healthcare professional is willing to partner with them to assist in dealing with mental health. Suggest topics such as child and parental mood, child temperament, stresses and ways that family members manage stress, or sleep patterns. Make notes in the record as a reminder of questions to ask at the next visit.

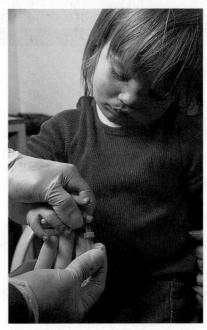

Figure 6–3 Blood screening test. This young child is having a blood screening test to detect iron deficiency anemia. Children are often screened for adequate levels of iron in later infancy and during toddlerhood.

The child and family are both observed for appropriateness of affect and mood. Be alert for signs of depression, stress, anxiety, and child abuse or neglect. The nurse establishes both health promotion and health maintenance goals related to child and family mental health. Health promotion goals relate to adequate resources to meet family challenges and protective factors such as involvement in extended family and the community. Teaching stress reduction techniques such as meditation, relaxation, and imagery is helpful. Resources for yoga or other relaxation techniques can be provided. Health maintenance goals relate to prevention of mental health problems. Examples include providing resources when domestic violence occurs, or referring cases of suspected child abuse or neglect. The **spiritual dimension** is a connection with a greater power than that in the self, and guides a person to strive for life purpose, joy, peace, and fulfillment (Pender, Murdaugh, & Parsons, 2015). For some, spiritual health may be fostered by membership in a faith-based group; for others, it may be feeling part of a society with a purpose of greater good, or setting goals for the future. Ask about the family's meaningful activities. Provide links to faith-based groups as needed.

The *relationships* that a child establishes with others begin at birth. The first and most important set of relationships develops with the family. The mother, father, siblings, and perhaps extended family are the contexts in which the baby learns to relate with others. With growth, the world widens to encompass other children, friends of the family, peers, school, and the larger community network. Analyzing the child's relationships at all ages provides important clues to social interactions. From the moment the family is called in from a waiting area, be alert for clues to family interactions. Likewise, other social interactions are important to evaluate. Does the young infant interact in an age-appropriate manner with the healthcare provider or other children in the area? Ask the parents questions about family and social interactions. Once assessment has taken place, establish goals and interventions related to family and social relationships.

Disease prevention strategies focus mainly on health maintenance, or prevention of disease. Some health disruptions can be detected early and treatment for the condition can begin. **Screening** is a procedure used to detect the possible presence of a health condition before symptoms are apparent. It is usually conducted on large groups of individuals at risk for a condition and represents the secondary level of prevention (Figure 6–3). Most screening tests are not diagnostic by themselves but are followed by further diagnostic tests if the screening result is positive. Once a screening test identifies the existence of a health condition, early intervention can begin, with the goal of reducing the severity or complications of the condition (secondary prevention). Another way to prevent diseases is to immunize children against common communicable diseases (primary prevention). See Chapter 16 for the complete list of childhood immunizations and schedules for administration.

Most childhood mortality and hospitalization is related to injury (CDC, 2012) (see Chapter 1 for more information). Therefore, it is important for the nurse to integrate *injury prevention* strategies in all health supervision visits. The family is constantly challenged to maintain a safe environment as the child grows older, reaches more advanced developmental levels, is exposed to a widening world outside of the family, and has less supervision. Safety teaching should be integrated with developmental progression. Asking parents to bring their questions about safety to each visit can be a good starting point for discussion. The nurse considers knowledge about the age of the child and information from the health supervision visit to plan health maintenance interventions related to injury. Teaching is performed, resources are made available, and parents and children who have experienced injury are invited to present their experiences.

Many other topics might be discussed during health supervision visits. They may relate to either health maintenance activities designed to preserve health, or health promotion activities designed to enhance or improve the state of wellness. Topics include extended family members and their role in the child's life, cultural variations or inclusion, or development of moral values and ethical behaviors.

Nursing Management

Nursing Assessment and Diagnosis

During health supervision visits, a mental portrait of a child and family should be drawn. Observe the parent–child interaction in the waiting room and all throughout the examination. If siblings are present, watch for interactions among all family members. Observe the affect and mood of the child and parents. Nursing assessment of the child and family at each visit for health supervision then focuses on the following:

- Interviewing the family and child to update the health history, asking about the child's developmental or educational progress, and identifying dietary habits, physical activity, and safety practices
- Eliciting questions and concerns that the parent or child may have
- Conducting developmental surveillance assessments, including review of questionnaires completed by the parent in the waiting room
- Performing age-appropriate screening tests
- Performing a physical assessment

Following a thorough assessment, the nurse derives nursing diagnoses that are pertinent for the child's health status and that consider the family's needs. Nursing diagnoses are developed jointly with the family as an essential component of the partnership between nurse and family. Examples of nursing diagnoses for an 18-month-old child for regular health supervision and immunizations may include the following (NANDA-I © 2014):

- *Overweight* related to lack of basic nutritional knowledge
- *Poisoning, Risk for,* related to lack of proper precautions with increased mobility to reach and climb
- *Health Management, Readiness for Enhanced,* related to needed immunizations
- *Parenting, Risk for Impaired,* related to mother's plans to return to full-time work

Planning and Implementation

Nursing management for health supervision visits begins with collaborative planning with the family. They share their concerns and questions, and the nurse also lists procedures and discussion topics to be addressed. (See *Families Want to Know: Health Supervision Visits.*) These may include providing immunizations, offering anticipatory guidance about discipline, educating parents and children about healthy behaviors, addressing health promotion regarding nutrition, suggesting ways to prevent disease and

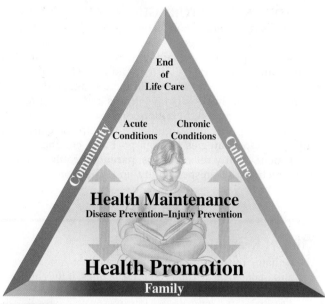

Figure 6–4 Bindler-Ball Healthcare Model. Health promotion and maintenance are foundational to all pediatric health care. They are integrated into every healthcare visit, whether for health supervision or acute and chronic conditions.

injury, and providing referrals for follow-up care. For more information about the recommended schedule for immunizations and the nurse's role in ensuring full immunization status for children, refer to Chapter 16.

Most parents want to know how to contribute to their child's growth and development and need linkages to additional community resources to foster child development. Discussions at the conclusion of the health supervision assessments should focus on building family strengths by promoting the development of competence, confidence, and self-esteem in the growing child. Offering health promotion activities such as these provides a positive ending for the visit. Inquire about the family stresses and strengths to plan with them to provide for the child's health promotion.

Although health supervision most likely takes place in an office or clinic setting, nursing management for health supervision can occur in any setting. The nurse recognizes that health promotion and health maintenance activities are key to any nurse–family relationship. Health promotion and maintenance are constant and foundational aspects of all pediatric care. This approach to health care closely reflects a partnership with families and is essential to every healthcare encounter (Figure 6–4).

Families Want to Know

Health Supervision Visits

Focus groups with parents were conducted to learn parental views about health supervision visits with their children. Parents wanted reassurance about the child's behaviors and wanted an opportunity to discuss health with a professional. An ongoing relationship with one professional was important. Parents requested additional information on development and child behaviors, and additional ways to communicate with healthcare providers (Radecki, Olson, Frintner, et al., 2009). Nurses should:

- Ask what the parent priorities are at each healthcare visit.
- Provide handouts and information on the child's expected developmental achievements.
- Discuss child behaviors such as sleep, discipline, and other parent concerns.
- Integrate communication methods such as phone calls and Internet contact into the care setting.

PROVIDE ANTICIPATORY GUIDANCE

Anticipatory guidance involves prediction of the upcoming developmental tasks or needs of a child and gears teaching to those needs. It provides the family with information on what to expect during the child's current and next stage of development. Topics for each visit should include age-appropriate information about healthy habits, illness and injury prevention, poison prevention, nutrition, oral health, and sexuality. Use health promotional guidance to help the child and family develop strategies that support and enhance social development, family relationships, parental health, community interactions, self-responsibility, and school or vocational achievement.

Clinical Reasoning Health Promotion

The pediatric nurse should apply concepts of health promotion and maintenance in all healthcare settings. If the child is seen in an emergency room for treatment of a fracture, what questions should the nurse ask about immunization status and safety issues? If the nurse sees a child with a chronic disorder of cerebral palsy in the outpatient clinic at an orthopedic hospital, what health promotion and health maintenance services should be integrated?

Because the time for each visit is limited, build on the parents' current knowledge and care practices, and start with a topic about which they express interest. Time can be used to focus on anticipatory guidance to introduce new information, to reinforce what the family is doing well, and to clear up any poorly understood concepts.

Take advantage of other sources of information in the community to enhance the guidance provided. For example, state and local SAFE KIDS coalitions help inform families about injury-prevention strategies. School health programs such as the National Fire Prevention Association's "Risk Watch" may educate children about injury prevention, and other school programs may educate students about smoking and drug avoidance. Keep informed about the types of health education provided in different community settings so it is easier to reinforce the concepts already being taught.

ENCOURAGE HEALTH PROMOTION ACTIVITIES

Families often need health education and counseling to promote healthy behaviors in their own child. Examples of focused health education and counseling may be information about limiting sedentary behaviors, integrating dietary changes to increase fruit and vegetable intake, and increasing daily physical activity.

Patient education and counseling are most effective when the family understands the relationship between a behavior change and the resulting health outcome. When identifying that a family would benefit from a change in health behavior, consider the family members' perceptions about the health change, consider the barriers and benefits to change, and plan interventions to enhance the possibility for change.

Steps in promoting patient education and counseling include (Hagan, Shaw, & Duncan, 2008):

- Clarifying learning needs of child and family
- Setting a limited agenda
- Prioritizing needs with the family
- Selecting a teaching strategy (explaining, showing, providing resources, questioning, practicing, giving feedback)
- Evaluating effectiveness

PERFORM HEALTH SUPERVISION INTERVENTIONS

After all the information from the interviews, physical assessment, and screening tests is collected and analyzed, specific health and developmental achievements should be summarized for the parents and child. Immunizations are provided as appropriate. Anticipatory guidance may be offered at various points during the health supervision visit.

When a child is found to be at risk for a health condition, integrate health maintenance interventions to lessen the possibility of disease or injury. If an actual health problem is detected, follow-up care must be arranged. The child may need to return for another visit to the primary care provider for further evaluation, or referral to another provider may be needed. The nurse needs to learn about all the available community resources to make appropriate referrals. The range of such services may include the following:

- Hospital and community-based healthcare specialists from many disciplines (e.g., dentists, physicians, physical therapists, speech therapists, nutritionists, social workers)
- Community-based programs (e.g., childcare centers, developmental stimulation programs, home visitor programs, early intervention programs, mental health centers, diagnostic and evaluation centers, schools, family support centers, food and nutrition referral centers, public health clinics, churches, and other organizations that support families and children)

Evaluation

Expected outcomes of nursing care include the following:

- The child and family collaborate in a partnership with the healthcare provider in joint problem solving and decision making regarding the management of the child's healthcare needs after appropriate education and counseling.
- The child and family prepare for future health supervision visits by identifying questions or concerns they want to discuss.

Chapter Highlights

- Health is a dynamic state of physical, mental, and social well-being and is the objective of health promotion and health maintenance activities.

- Health supervision visits are healthcare encounters designed to provide assessment, screening, developmental surveillance, immunizations, and health information.

- Health supervision visits include general observations, as well as growth and development, nutrition, physical activity, oral health, mental health, spiritual, and relationship surveillance.

- Partners in providing health supervision are the child, family, health professionals, and community.

- Health promotion and health maintenance interventions are essential components of all child health care, even during periods of acute or chronic illness.

Clinical Reasoning in Action

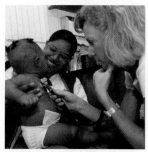

SOURCE: Steven Rubin/The Image Works

Sahil is a 6–month-old boy who is brought to the clinic by his mother, Clarisse, and his grandmother, who just moved into the home to help Clarisse. Sahil's father recently needed to leave the country on a prolonged work assignment. Clarisse is very nervous about being the main adult responsible for Sahil since her husband's departure. As you assess Sahil, you find that he is smiling readily, is able to sit on his own with little support, and has length and weight at the 50th percentiles. His mother told you that she is breastfeeding and has been feeding Sahil some table food such as rice and tofu. She has returned to work so the grandmother will provide care during the day while Clarisse is at work. You review the immunization record and find that several immunizations are due at today's visit.

1. As Clarisse returns to work, Sahil will likely be consuming less breast milk and have more table foods and formula added to the diet. What questions will you ask Clarisse and Sahil's grandmother to evaluate their knowledge of dietary recommendations for infants? Compose a teaching plan that is appropriate for integration of increasing types of food into the diet of a 6-month-old child.

2. What immunizations are generally needed for 6-month-old infants? When should Sahil return for his next immunizations?

3. You have identified that Clarisse needs support and socialization with other young mothers. How will you locate community resources that are helpful to young families? Decide what parenting information would be helpful to build Clarisse's confidence in caring for Sahil without her husband present. Suggest some ways that she, Sahil, and the father can communicate with each other regularly.

4. The major health problem for infants is related to safety hazards. Sahil is becoming more mobile and curious. Write a teaching plan that includes topics and specific teaching requirements at his age.

References

American Academy of Pediatrics (AAP). (2014). *Agenda for children: Medical home.* Retrieved from http://www .aap.org/en-us/about-the-aap/aap-facts/AAP-Agenda -for-Children-Strategic-Plan/Pages/AAP-Agenda-for -Children-Strategic-Plan-Medical-Home.aspx

American Academy of Pediatrics (AAP) Committee on Practice and Ambulatory Medicine. (2016). 2016 Recommendations for preventive pediatric health care. *Pediatrics, 137*(1), e20153908. doi:10.1542/ peds.2015-3908.

Centers for Disease Control and Prevention (CDC). (2011a). *Caries experience and untreated tooth decay.* Retrieved from http://apps.nccd.cdc.gov/ nohss/IndicatorV.asp?Indicator=2,3

Centers for Disease Control and Prevention (CDC). (2011b). *Oral health.* Retrieved from http://www .cdc.gov/chronicdisease/resources/publications/AAG/ doh.htm

Centers for Disease Control and Prevention (CDC). (2012). *Causes of death by age group.* Retrieved from http:// www.cdc.gov/injury/wisqars/pdf/leading_causes_of_ death_by_age_group_2011-a.pdf and http://www .cdc.gov/injury/wisqars/pdf/leading_causes_of_ nonfatal_injury_2012-a.pdf

Centers for Disease Control and Prevention (CDC). (2013). *The concept of prevention.* Retrieved from http:// www.cdc.gov/arthritis/temp/pilots-201208/pilot1/ online/arthritis-challenge/03-Prevention/concept.htm

Centers for Disease Control and Prevention (CDC). (2014a). *Developmental monitoring and screening.* Retrieved from http://www.cdc.gov/ncbddd/ childdevelopment/screening.html

Centers for Disease Control and Prevention (CDC). (2014b). Youth risk behavior surveillance—United States, 2013. *Morbidity and Mortality Weekly Report, 63*(SS-4), 1–172.

Child Trends. (2013). *Unmet dental needs.* Retrieved from http://www.childtrends .org/?indicators=unmet-dental-needs

Hagan, J. G., Shaw, J. S., & Duncan, P. M. (Eds.). (2008). *Bright futures: Guidelines for health supervision of infants, children, and adolescents* (3rd ed.). Elk Grove Village, IL: American Academy of Pediatrics.

Lipkin, P. H. (2011). Developmental and behavioral surveillance and screening within the medical home. In R. G. Voight (Ed.), *Developmental and behavioral pediatrics* (pp. 69–92). Elk Grove Village, IL: American Academy of Pediatrics.

Pender, N. J., Murdaugh, C. L., & Parsons, M. A. (2015). *Health promotion in nursing practice* (7th ed.). Upper Saddle River, NJ: Pearson Prentice Hall.

Radecki, L., Olson, L. M., Frintner, M. P., Tanner, J. L., & Stein, M. T. (2009). What do families want from well-child care: Including parents in the rethinking discussion. *Pediatrics, 124*, 858–865.

Taylor, E. F., Lake, T., Nysenbaum, J., Peterson, G., & Meyers, D. (2011). *Coordinating care in the medical neighborhood: Critical components and available mechanisms.* White Paper (Prepared by Mathematica Policy Research under Contract No. HHSA290200900019I TO2). AHRQ Publication No. 11-0064. Rockville, MD: Agency for Healthcare Research and Quality.

U.S. Department of Health and Human Services. (2011). *Healthy People 2020: The vision, mission, and goals of Healthy People 2020.* Retrieved from http://www.healthypeople.gov/2020/Consortium/ HP2020Framework.pdf

World Health Organization (WHO). (2016). *Health promotion.* Retrieved from http://www.who.int/topics/ health_promotion/en

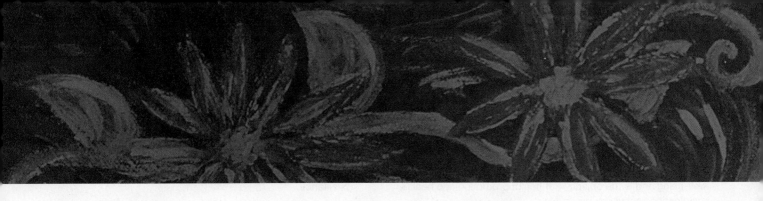

Chapter 7
Health Promotion and Maintenance for the Newborn and Infant

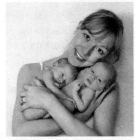

I knew having twins would be a challenge, but so far it has worked well. I am just concerned that as they continue to grow we will have trouble getting them both to sleep and eat on the same schedule.

—Mother of Sheridan and Cyrus, twin 10-day-old boys

Anneka/Shutterstock

⌄ Learning Outcomes

7.1 Synthesize the areas of assessment and intervention for health supervision visits of newborns and infants: growth and developmental surveillance, nutrition, physical activity, oral health, mental and spiritual health, family and social relations, disease prevention strategies, and injury prevention strategies.

7.2 Plan health promotion and health maintenance strategies employed during health supervision visits of newborns and infants.

7.3 Recognize the importance of family in newborn and infant health care, and include family assessment in each health supervision visit.

7.4 Integrate pertinent mental health care into health supervision visits for newborns and infants.

7.5 Evaluate data about the family and other social relationships to promote and maintain health of newborns and infants.

Health Promotion and Maintenance for the Newborn and Infant

The month following delivery is a time of huge transition for the new mother and her family. Not only is the mother coping with hormonal shifts and a **postpartum** (after giving birth) body, but roles and relationships are also changing. The role of the nurse is to assess knowledge about self-care and newborn care, teach health promotion and maintenance activities, promote parental confidence in newborn caregiving, and facilitate a partnership among healthcare professionals and the family.

Infancy is a major life transition for the baby and parents. The infant accomplishes phenomenal physical growth and many developmental milestones while the family adapts to the addition of a new member and establishes new goals for each of its existing members. Infant health supervision visits are very important to support the health of the baby and the family unit. These visits begin after the newborn period, at about 1 month of age. This is the time when parents establish an ongoing partnership with a healthcare provider. A "medical home" or "pediatric healthcare home" is identified to serve the baby's health needs. The goals of health supervision visits are to identify and address the health promotion and health maintenance needs of the infant.

Facilitating breastfeeding, helping parents understand their newborn's/infant's temperament, and employing strategies to ensure adequate sleep by the baby and parents are examples of health promotion activities. Health maintenance activities focus on disease and injury prevention. Some examples of these interventions include administering immunizations and teaching about infant car seats.

An established relationship with a healthcare provider and agency is important so that trust develops and the family will feel comfortable about turning to the professionals for information and guidance as the baby grows. Nurses play a vital role in welcoming new families into office and clinic settings, establishing rapport, and applying principles of communication so that trust and positive partnerships develop between providers and families. Infancy is a time when the child grows in physical, psychologic, and cognitive ways; health supervision visits play a key role in fostering healthy growth and development. When should the infant be seen for health supervision visits? What are key components of these visits? How can the nurse best assess and intervene to ensure the infant's health and safety? These are some of the questions that will be answered in the chapter.

Early Contacts With the Family

Most obstetric healthcare providers encourage the expectant mother to choose her newborn's healthcare provider prior to the baby's birth (see *Clinical Reasoning: Choosing the Newborn's Healthcare Provider*). Pediatric healthcare providers usually welcome a short office visit, sometimes at no charge, to allow the expectant mother and healthcare provider to assess their compatibility prior to initiating the healthcare provider relationship. Many pediatric healthcare providers provide written information to expectant parents, explaining their professional philosophy of care as well as information about services.

Clinical Reasoning Choosing the Newborn's Healthcare Provider

Parents are encouraged to visit the pediatric healthcare home before the baby is born. This will help the parents decide if the healthcare provider offers the type of care they want for their infant. Prepare a list of questions that parents could ask during a visit to the provider they are interested in interviewing. Be sure this list addresses the availability of healthcare providers, frequency of well-child supervision, cost and insurance information, and other pertinent topics.

Health promotion and maintenance for the newborn begin during the stay in the hospital or birthing center. On discharge, referral may be indicated to a lactation consultant or follow-up healthcare visit. The hospital length of stay for a healthy mother and newborn after term delivery is short, approximately 48 hours for a vaginal birth and 72 to 96 hours for an uncomplicated cesarean birth. Discharge of the mother and baby should occur only after appropriate growth is confirmed and a thorough physical examination shows normal results. There should be time to identify any problems and to make certain that the family can care for the newborn at home, and ideally the mother and newborn should be discharged together (AAP, 2011a; AAP, n.d.). For newborns discharged between 48 and 72 hours of age, the first

follow-up healthcare visit should occur by 5 days of age. The purpose of this visit is to ensure that the newborn is continuing to progress normally and that no previously undiscovered problems have surfaced. At this initial contact, the nurse promotes maternal confidence in caregiving and offers education and anticipatory guidance. Careful assessments are made for hyperbilirubinemia, feeding problems, or other abnormalities. Further visits are established as needed from 5 days to 1 month; the first scheduled health supervision of infancy is at 1 month of age.

Health promotion and maintenance for infancy occur in a series of health supervision visits during the first year of life. Schedules vary among facilities, but a common pattern includes visits at about 1 month, 2 months, 4 months, 6 months, 9 months, and 1 year of age. In addition, most children have some episodic illnesses such as gastrointestinal illness or otitis media and visit the facility at other times for treatment of these illnesses. A few children have chronic or serious healthcare problems during the first year, and have extensive contact with the healthcare home and other services.

During these first visits, assess the family for protective factors and risks. Protective factors might include knowledge level of infant needs, support from family and friends, and the mother's good health and nutritional state during pregnancy. Risk factors could include limited financial resources, lack of preparation for the baby, and illness or other stress among family members. Ask about how the family traveled to the visit, and if convenient times and transportation are available. Lack of access during times the family is not at work and other health system barriers sometimes interfere with attendance at health supervision visits. Knowledge of risk factors will shape the nursing interventions during the first health supervision in infancy. The nurse applies health promotion principles by building on strengths and fosters health maintenance by intervening to minimize risks.

General Observations

When the family comes to the clinic or office for care with a newborn or infant, general observations should begin at first contact (Figure 7–1). Welcome the family warmly to the facility and

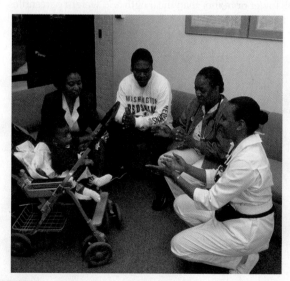

Figure 7–1 **General observations. The nurse begins assessment of the infant's family when they are seen in the waiting room and called in for care. What observations can you make of the infant's general appearance? Developmental accomplishments? Interaction of parents with the baby?**

comment on the baby. Ask how the family is doing with the baby and how the adjustment is going. Be alert for signs of fatigue or depression in the parents, as these can occur when caring for an infant and can interfere with bonding and positive transition. Look for clues about cultural orientation. The nurse gathers information in order to assess the needs of the family, to invite discussion, to validate positive parenting efforts, and to promote partnership between the family and the healthcare team. When entering the examination room, it is helpful to explain the plans for the visit, such as:

> I will weigh and measure Sarah now and show you how she is growing. Then I'll ask a few questions about her eating, sleeping, and other things. Then the nurse practitioner will be in to do Sarah's physical examination. Do you have any questions as we start? Will you undress Sarah now so we can weigh her accurately?

Growth and Developmental Surveillance

Assessment of growth and development begins at birth and continues in newborn and infant health promotion and maintenance visits. (See Chapter 4 for important background/theoretical information about growth and development.) Note the posture, flexion, reflexes, and physical attributes that help evaluate gestational age. Physical growth and meeting of developmental milestones provide important information about infants. The baby is measured for accurate length, weight, and head circumference (Figure 7–2). (See the *Clinical Skills Manual* SKILLS and Chapter 5 for detailed information about the physical examination.) The measurements should be placed on growth grids and interpreted. Parents enjoy seeing how the baby is progressing and are usually eager to learn about the child's weight gain and growth percentiles. Be alert for an infant who demonstrates a change in percentile range. For example, if the baby was in the 75th percentile for length and weight at birth, but has fallen to below the 50th percentile for weight, additional assessment of the baby's feedings is needed. Likewise, if the head circumference is much lower or higher than the length and weight percentiles, further neurologic and developmental assessment should be done.

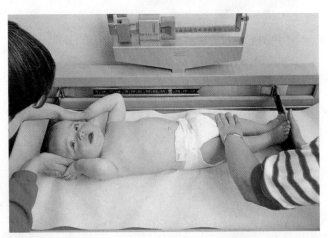

Figure 7–2 Measuring physical growth. Weighing and measuring length during health supervision visits provides important information about the child's nutrition and general development. This young infant was measured and then while the parents dressed the child the nurse placed the findings on the growth grid.

Growth measurement is followed by a physical assessment. The nurse may complete parts of the assessment, with the remainder performed by the physician, nurse practitioner, or other primary care provider. The assessment evaluates each body system, with particular attention being paid to the heart, skin, musculoskeletal system, abdomen, and neurologic status. See Chapter 5 for assessment of the newborn and a thorough discussion of physical assessment throughout infancy and childhood.

Developmental surveillance is integrated into each infant healthcare visit by observing developmental milestones in the infant. (See Chapter 4 for a summary of milestones expected at different ages.) When there is no opportunity to observe a skill directly, ask parents about whether the infant performs the skill (see *Developing Cultural Competence: Cultural Influences on Developmental Tests*). In addition to direct observation, parents are usually requested to fill in a form that asks questions about common developmental tasks. Review the results and determine if additional questions should be asked. Signs of **developmental delay**—a delay in mastering functions, such as motor coordination and behavioral skills—in a full-term infant usually merit immediate investigation by a pediatrician, pediatric developmental specialist, pediatric neurologist, or a multidisciplinary team of professionals. Parents require additional emotional support, clear and honest communication, and resources to cope with the stress of this situation.

Developing Cultural Competence Cultural Influences on Developmental Tests

Be alert for differences in cultural practices and beliefs that may influence developmental milestones. For example, if a child is kept on a cradleboard for much of the time, the baby may be slow in learning to crawl. This baby may progress directly to standing by furniture without demonstrating as much creeping or crawling as other infants. If an item such as "waves good-bye" or "plays patty-cake" represents a practice not common in another culture, the child may not have had exposure to the skill. Be alert for cultural variations, allow the child time to learn a developmental skill, and retest during future healthcare visits.

The nurse establishes health promotion and maintenance interventions related to growth and development assessment data. Anticipatory guidance related to development is a major component of health promotion. The nurse anticipates the next milestones the infant will be meeting, and recommends ways for the parents to support the infant in progression. Some health promotion activities include:

- Teach about introducing foods that will foster growth.
- Encourage use of toys and activities that will assist in meeting the next developmental milestones.
- Demonstrate gross and fine motor skills that the infant has achieved.
- Demonstrate to parents how the child will focus on their faces and mimic their vocal sounds.

Other interventions are focused on health maintenance or disease and injury prevention. Safety hazards and ways to avoid them are discussed, and parents are given brochures, website addresses, or videotapes to enhance injury prevention information. Can you outline additional health promotion and health maintenance interventions that relate to the newborn's/infant's growth and development?

Nutrition

The importance of nutrition during the newborn period and the first year of life cannot be overemphasized. Babies will triple their birth weight by 1 year of age and therefore have a great need for nutritional balance. From the first sips of breast milk or formula as a newborn, to eating the family meal at 1 year of age, the fast progression of nutritional intake patterns is obvious. See Chapter 14 for details about the importance of breastfeeding and a thorough description of nutritional needs for the infant.

During each visit the nurse seeks to learn what the baby is eating, and whether the family has any questions or concerns related to intake (Holt, Wooldridge, Story, et al., 2011). Open-ended questions are a good way to begin, with more specific questions inserted after the parent's perceptions are known. Breastfeeding is encouraged and supported during the newborn and infancy periods, and information about safe formula feeding is provided when the family has chosen that method of feeding. Once the baby is in the second half of the first year, food patterns of the family become more important. Consider childcare settings as well.

Observations from other portions of the visit can provide clues about additional questions to ask. If an infant has not gained weight as expected and has fallen into a lower weight percentile, more specific analysis of intake is needed. Ask for a recall of the baby's intake in the previous day. When the baby does not meet developmental milestones on schedule or is lethargic, intake may be inadequate for age. In these cases, support may be needed to ensure adequate intake; a thorough description of feeding may be the first step in analyzing the problem and planning interventions. When the child's ability to take in nutrients or the parent's ability to feed the baby is questioned, an observation of a feeding might take place, either at the healthcare setting or during a home visit.

Additional nutritional assessment measures are used at certain points in the first year. A hematocrit or hemoglobin is generally performed between 9 and 12 months of age. Lead screening may be needed in certain population groups (see Chapter 17 for more information). Food security screening can be used when appropriate (see Chapter 14) (AAP Committee on Nutrition, 2013). Each visit includes nutritional teaching about important items. The topics for discussion vary according to age group. See Table 7–1 for suggested teaching topics at specific ages. Desired outcomes for nutrition in infancy include adequate growth, normal nutritional assessment findings, and knowledge by parents of the nutritional needs of the infant.

Physical Activity

Muscle development begins early in fetal life. The flexed position of the newborn demonstrates development of the flexor muscles and relaxation of the extensor muscles. This flexed position protects the newborn, conserves energy by reducing movement, and reduces heat loss. During the first month of life, the newborn gradually "unfolds" and the body straightens. Movements begin to change from reflexive to purposeful.

TABLE 7–1 Nutrition Teaching for Health Promotion and Health Maintenance Visits

AGE	NUTRITION TEACHING	
Newborn	Support breastfeeding efforts. Teach correct formula types and preparation if used. Teach burping and rate of feeding information.	Encourage families to view feedings as social interactions; emphasize importance of holding the newborn and not propping bottles.
1 month	Continue teaching listed above. Offer support for breastfeeding and reinforce that breast milk is the only intake needed by infants at this age.	
2 months	Continue teaching listed above. Review fluid needs of infants. Reinforce food safety for partially used bottles of breast milk or formula. Use warm water for heating bottles rather than microwave to avoid burning.	Warn against feeding honey in the first year of life due to risk of botulism. Begin daily cleaning of infant gums. Provide information about any supplements needed (e.g., iron for premature infant; continuation of 400 International Units/day of vitamin D for all infants).
4 months	Continue teaching listed above. Discuss introduction of first foods between 4 and 6 months, and surveillance for symptoms of allergy or intolerance.	Discuss changing food patterns such as increasing amounts and decreasing numbers of daily milk feedings.
6 months	Continue teaching listed above. Reinforce proper introduction of new foods, to include rice cereal, vegetables, and fruits. Discuss any unusual food reactions observed. Introduce cup for drinking. Introduce soft finger foods.	Serve juice only in a cup and limit to no more than 6 oz daily. Caution about common choking foods and items. Provide information about fluoride supplement if water supply is not fluoridated.
9 months	Continue teaching listed above. If mother does not continue to breastfeed, teach family to use iron-fortified formula for the first year of life. Encourage self-feeding of finger foods, integrating common foods for the family.	Introduce source of protein such as tofu, cheese, mashed beans, and slivers of meats.
12 months	Continue teaching listed above. Support mother who wishes to continue breastfeeding beyond 1 year of age.	Encourage cups for all feedings other than breast.

TABLE 7–2 Risk and Protective Factors Regarding Physical Activity in the Newborn and Infancy Periods

RISK FACTORS	PROTECTIVE FACTORS
• Premature birth • Delayed developmental milestones • Limited stimulation by family or other care providers • Lack of knowledge by family about infant's physical activity needs • Limited community resources for families with infants	• Meets developmental milestones at expected ages • Has contact with parents, siblings, and others for significant time each day • A supportive environment with room to play safely; stimulating surroundings • Physically active family • Family knowledge about infant's physical activity needs • Community programs that promote physical activity in infants and information for families

Source: Data from Hagan, J. F., Shaw, J. S., & Duncan, P. M. (Eds.). (2008). *Bright futures: Guidelines for health supervision of infants, children, and adolescents* (3rd ed.). Elk Grove Village, IL: American Academy of Pediatrics.

Physical activity is needed for adequate development of fine and gross motor skills in infancy. Unlike other times of life, the focus is on providing only the opportunities for activity, without a need to focus on motivation. As long as infants are meeting developmental milestones and have a stimulating environment that provides opportunity for fine and gross motor activity, they will use their motor skills, thus enhancing their performance. Time should be provided each day for the infant to reach for objects, freely exercise legs and arms, and increasingly use head control.

Playing with parents or others and being surrounded by toys and other stimulating items will encourage motor behavior in all body parts. Ask the parents for a description of the infant's typical day and listen for these types of play periods. Infants should sleep on their backs, but they also need supervised play periods when they are awake that are spent on their stomachs. This encourages developmental skills and lessens flattening of the back of the head from excessive positioning on back (Kadey & Roane, 2012). Observe the physical skills of the infant (see Chapter 4) for motor developmental norms, ask questions about play periods provided, and compose a list of the family protective factors and risk factors in this area. Table 7–2 lists some risk and protective factors related to physical activity of newborns and infants.

Based on the results of assessment and using the concept of anticipatory guidance, the nurse plans appropriate teaching for health promotion. Health maintenance deals with prevention of physical development delays. Examples of nursing activities are teaching parents to allow the arms and legs of infants to be outside of covers for some period each day to enhance movement, and suggesting toys that encourage attention and movement, such as mobiles and music boxes. The nurse evaluates the success of interventions by the child's progression in physical activity milestones at each health supervision visit. Adequate parental understanding of the importance of physical activity and the means of supporting the child's activities is an important outcome of care.

Oral Health

The first teeth begin to erupt about midway during infancy. Two front teeth are common at about 6 months of age. However, even before this, parents lay the foundation for good oral health. The mother's intake during pregnancy and breastfeeding is essential to ensuring adequate availability of calcium and other nutrients that will be used as the infant's teeth develop. The nurse in child health supervision settings ensures that the infant has adequate intake of these nutrients via breastfeeding and other foods. A dietary recall of the mother's intake, as well as the infant's, is one way of assessing for nutrients. When the water supply is not fluoridated, inquire about use of fluoride drops.

Help the family establish healthy dental habits. The parents should wipe the infant's gums with soft moist gauze once or twice daily. This helps to clean residues of food from the gums and gets the infant accustomed to having something wiping the gums, a practice that may assist when toothbrushing begins. Families are also cautioned to avoid having the infant breastfeed when sleeping, to avoid use of bottles in bed, and not to allow the infant to drink at will from a bottle during the day. These practices are linked to **early childhood caries** (see Chapter 14) and can lead to tooth decay. Nurses assess for the presence of teeth and whether patterns are similar to those expected (see Chapter 5 for additional information). It is wise to ask if the infant has had any difficulty with teeth eruption. Many infants have increased crying and disrupted sleep when teething. Suggest comfort measures such as offering cool beverages and safe "teething toys" for the infant. The American Academy of Pediatric Dentistry (AAPD) recommends an oral examination within 6 months of the eruption of the first tooth and no later than 12 months of age. They recommend that the parents establish a "dental home" by that time to ensure ongoing oral care for the child (AAPD, 2013).

Mental and Spiritual Health

The infant's mental health is related to early experiences, inborn characteristics such as temperament and resilience, and relationships with caregivers. The first year of life provides many opportunities for the infant to develop positive mental health; interventions during this important period can enhance the child's future mental status.

One way to evaluate mental health is to look carefully at the growth and development surveillance data that were described earlier. Children who feel secure and have nurturing environments usually grow as expected and perform milestones at usual times. Slow growth and delayed development are sometimes related to feeding disorders of infancy and early childhood (see Chapter 14). In these cases, a disturbed relationship with the primary caregiver influences the psychologic state of the infant and results in decreased food intake. Another way to assess mental health is to observe the child and parent interacting. Does the parent hold the newborn securely and does the infant cuddle and settle into the parent's arms? (See Figure 7–3.) Is there eye contact between parent and infant? Does the parent appear comfortable in holding and comforting the newborn? These interactions indicate bonding or positive attachment.

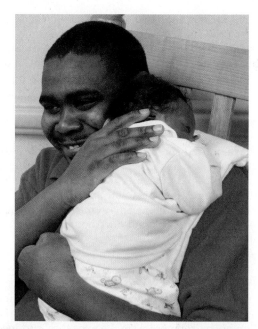

Figure 7–3 **Assessing mental health. Interactions between the parent and infant provide clues to mental health. Do the adult and child appear comfortable with each other? Is eye contact and vocalization present? Are their bodies soft and relaxed or tense?**

During the first year, the infant learns to identify the primary caregivers; beginning at about 6 months of age, infants may cry or protest when a person other than a familiar caregiver holds them. This is called **stranger anxiety** and indicates expected attachment to parents. Similarly, infants in the second half of the first year of life may exhibit **separation anxiety** by inconsolable crying and other signs of distress when parents are not present.

These behaviors are normal, demonstrate healthy attachment to primary caregivers, and indicate mental health. Help parents to recognize them as expected occurrences. Provide ideas of how to deal with this behavior. The parents can remain in sight and talk to the baby during health supervision examinations. They should be encouraged to hold and comfort the baby after painful procedures like immunizations. Once the infant has experienced that the parent leaves and returns, security in the care of others can emerge.

Another important indication of infant mental health is the ability to comfort oneself. **Self-regulation** is the process of dealing with feelings, learning to soothe self, and focusing on activities for increasing periods of time. Newborns learn how to comfort and calm themselves. Ask parents if the newborn or infant sucks a finger, softly rocks, or otherwise comforts self when distressed. Some infants prefer to be alone and quiet when tired or distressed; others calm better when held, rocked, or placed in an infant swing. Help the parents identify and reinforce the baby's methods of self-soothing, and teach swaddling and rocking techniques. Self-regulation is needed by the baby when learning to go to sleep while tired and agitated. Nurses use health promotion principles to teach about sleep patterns in infants, and implement health maintenance when partnering with families to deal with problem sleep behaviors that lead to infant and parent fatigue (see *As Children Grow: Infant Sleep Patterns* and *Evidence-Based Practice: Infant Sleep*).

The newborn enters a family with spiritual strengths and limitations. The nurse assesses the family and provides additional resources when needed. Although the infant is not mature enough to understand the family's spiritual framework, the atmosphere in the family that relates to nurturing, valuing children, providing a safe and secure environment, and recognizing mental balance is conveyed readily to the infant. The infant's social and psychologic health are closely related to these factors. Assess the family's meaningful activities and engagement in faith-based practices. Ask if they have needs or desires for

EVIDENCE-BASED PRACTICE | Infant Sleep

Clinical Question
Many babies have limited sleeping periods during the night, and their night awakenings disturb parents' sleep. Parents may have busy days and be unable to nap and, hence, possibly not be able to perform at a safe and productive level during the day. Parental stress and depression are associated with frequent child awakenings. What strategies are needed to assist them in supporting the infant's sleep?

The Evidence
Sleep of the infant is an important concern for many parents, but there is little research-based evidence about what strategies really improve infant sleep. A study of 314 twin pairs found that most sleep disturbances in early childhood are linked to environmental factors, and thus behavioral interventions with parents are suggested for altering infant sleep patterns (Brescianini, Volzone, Fagnani, et al., 2011). Consistent with these findings, a study evaluating 170 parents for knowledge of child sleep found that most parents could not answer the majority of questions correctly. The researchers suggested that evaluating parental knowledge and teaching about developmental progression of sleep patterns should occur during health visits

(Schreck & Richdale, 2011). A cross-cultural study found that parents from predominantly Asian countries were more likely to identify sleep disturbance in their children than those from countries with a majority of White parents. These findings suggest that information is needed about cultural differences in sleep expectations of parents (Sadeh, Mindell, & Rivera, 2011).

Best Practice
This evidence-based practice provides implications for nursing care. Ask parents of young newborns to record the infant sleep patterns. As the infant nears 3 to 4 months of age, patterns should demonstrate few night wakenings and feedings. Teach parents about how to minimize stimulation and interaction at night. Provide opportunities to review results at future health supervision visits, or offer telephone or other support to parents.

Clinical Reasoning
What reasons might working parents have for responding eagerly and interacting with an infant who awakens at night? Do you think there are other reasons why infants awake at night? What clues help you to decide if an infant sleep problem exists?

As Children Grow: Infant Sleep Patterns

- In the first 6 months, infants sleep from 14 to 18 hours each day.
- The number of night awakenings varies for infants and may even vary from night to night.
- Nurses can teach parents that variability in sleep patterns is common, and not usually the result of changes in the infant's daily schedule.
- From 6 to 12 months, infants generally sleep 12 to 14 hours daily, with longer sleep periods at night and accompanied by one to three naps daily.
- Parents can be encouraged to settle on a nighttime routine for the infant, such as a short quiet playtime, bath, breastfeeding, or bottlefeeding with decreased lighting and soothing music.

Source: Data from Middlemiss, W., Yuare, R., & Huey, E. L. (2014). Translating evidence-based knowledge about sleep into practice. *Journal of the American Association of Nurse Practitioners.* doi:10.1002/2327–6924.12159

referrals in the community such as to an organized religious body or other meaningful activities.

Many of the nurse's interventions are aimed at healthy mental health development in the infant. Health promotion activities focus on teaching parents the needs of infants for security and interaction. Suggest healthy sleep patterns starting with the newborn visit and explain how they can be achieved. Teach self-regulation skills so that the parents can help the infant become quiet and calm. Health maintenance seeks to identify infants with disruptions in mental health status, often manifested by growth or interaction abnormalities. When the infant has disturbed sleep patterns or difficulty calming self when upset, or the parents do not interpret infant cues related to hunger or discomfort, the nurse plans interventions to help prevent further problems. An expected outcome for these activities is the reestablishment of expected growth and development and age-appropriate interactions of the infant with others.

Relationships

Family adaptation to a new baby begins in pregnancy, and evidence of initial family adaptation to pregnancy may be predictive of future parental coping (Hagan, Shaw, & Duncan, 2008). The family is the primary site where the infant learns to interact with other people. Therefore, family dynamics must be examined during health supervision visits. Strengths and needs of the family are identified during psychosocial screening. Some factors in the mental health of the parents directly affect the atmosphere in the home, and the resulting health of the newborn and infant. Depression in parents or other family members is an important condition that has the potential to influence the infant's health. Interactions with parents who are depressed will be altered; caretaking, both physical and emotional, can be impaired. Another challenge to the mental health of families and the infants in these families is that of domestic violence, a situation in which parents or adult care providers commit violent acts toward one another. Child abuse or maltreatment is another risk that occurs in some families with infants. This problem is a serious issue that causes disturbed mental status in the baby. See Chapter 17 for a detailed description of child abuse and its effect on infants and older children. Suspected child abuse must be reported to legal authorities in order to protect children.

The infant's social interactions both within and outside the family display unbelievable growth in the first year. The role of the nurse related to infant social interactions in health supervision visits is to evaluate the social skills of the infant, learn what parents have noticed about the baby's temperament and how it fits with their lives, and make suggestions for positive social development. Desired outcomes for the infant include establishment of close relationships with parents and other family members, a stimulating home environment that is responsive to the baby's temperament, and developmental progression in social interactions.

Disease Prevention Strategies

Disease prevention in the newborn period includes metabolic screening, hearing screening, eye examination, immunization, prevention of environmental smoke exposure, sudden infant death syndrome (SIDS) risk reduction, formula safety, minimizing exposure to disease, and hand hygiene for the family.

Infants are prone to many infectious diseases, especially once passive immunity from the mother wanes at about 6 months of age (see Chapters 16 and 22). Recommended immunizations are administered on schedule to provide protection from some diseases. Recommended immunizations for newborns and infants are listed in Table 7–3. Further details on immunizations can be found in Chapter 16. Instruct parents about upcoming immunizations and when the infant should be seen again. Be sure the parent understands the risks and benefits of each immunization. Answer their questions truthfully, and have resources on hand such as brochures and videotapes for interested parents.

TABLE 7–3 Routine Immunizations Recommended During Newborn and Infancy Periods

IMMUNIZATION	AGE RECOMMENDED
Hepatitis B	At birth (1st dose) 1–2 months (2nd dose) 6–18 months (3rd dose)
Hepatitis A	12 months (1st dose) 18 months or at least 6 months after 1st dose (2nd dose)
Diphtheria, tetanus, pertussis	2, 4, and 6 months (3 doses)
Rotavirus	2 and 4 months (2 doses) **OR** 2, 4, and 6 months (3 doses) (The requirement of 2 or 3 doses is related to which of the two available vaccines is used.)
Haemophilus influenza type b	2, 4, and 6 months (3 doses; 3rd dose is not needed if PRP-OMP [Pedvax HIB or Comvax] is used for primary series)
Inactivated poliovirus	2, 4, and 6–18 months (3 doses)
Pneumococcal	2, 4, and 6 months (3 doses)
Influenza	Annually from 6 months

Families Want to Know
When to Contact the Healthcare Provider

Instruct parents to contact a healthcare provider if the child has:

- Axillary temperature ≥99.3°F (37.4°C) (Identify for the provider the technique used for temperature measurement, such as axillary, forehead, oral, rectal, or ear, so adequate evaluation can be made.)
- Seizure
- Skin rash, purplish spots, petechiae
- Change in activity or behavior that makes the parent uncomfortable
- Unusual irritability, lethargy
- Failure to eat
- Vomiting
- Diarrhea
- Dehydration
- Cough

Source: Data from Hagan, J. G., Shaw, J. S., & Duncan, P. M. (Eds.). (2008). *Bright futures: Guidelines for health supervision of infants, children, and adolescents* (3rd ed.). Elk Grove Village, IL: American Academy of Pediatrics.

During each health supervision visit in infancy, the nurse performs recommended screenings and counsels the parents about why such screenings are important. Vision and hearing screenings are consistently performed. Screenings for anemia and lead poisoning are added at particular times or with certain groups. Families with certain genetic diseases such as sickle cell disease or cystic fibrosis may choose to have screening for the infant so that supportive care can begin early if the child has the disease. Parents benefit from learning about common diseases and conditions of young children and measures for their prevention. Ask about secondhand smoke (environmental tobacco smoke) and encourage smoking parents to quit. Teach parents to put infants to sleep on their backs to assist in lowering the chance of SIDS (see Chapter 20 for a thorough discussion of SIDS). Be sure parents have a phone number to call when they have questions about conditions or whether the baby should be seen by the healthcare provider (see *Families Want to Know: When to Contact the Healthcare Provider*). Evaluate the family's ability to understand verbal and written instructions. Desired outcomes for disease prevention strategies include adequate management of health problems, integration of immunization and other preventive measures into care of the infant, and family understanding of preventive measures recommended for infants.

Injury Prevention Strategies

New parents are sometimes unaware of sources of potential injury for the newborn. Some aspects of injury prevention are pertinent to the newborn's immediate care and other topics promote discussion and provide opportunities for anticipatory guidance during all of infancy. In the immediate newborn period, the nurse should assess the parents' knowledge of injury prevention strategies, and promote healthy and safe behaviors. Injury prevention strategies include proper and consistent use of an infant car seat and strategies to prevent falls, burns, choking, drowning, and suffocation.

During the first year of life, injury becomes an increasingly common cause of mortality. Strategies must be included in every health supervision visit to lower the risk of injury. Nurses should never assume that parents understand how to insert an infant car seat correctly or what types of toys and foods can lead to choking. Know the most common hazards at each age and teach parents methods of avoiding them (Tables 7–4 and 7–5).

Begin the conversation by asking parents what safety hazards they are aware of in the child's environment. Use this information as the starting point for discussion. Give positive feedback for their awareness of hazards and measures they have taken to prevent them. Consider using a home assessment survey that assists parents in identifying hazards that may be present in their homes. When infants visit friends, relatives, or neighbors, they may be exposed to other hazardous situations. Grandparents may not have a home that is "baby-proofed" and the infant could have access to electrical cords, machinery, medicines, or other hazards. Help the parents to evaluate the childcare home or center. Focus on car safety since this is a frequent cause of injury for infants. Provide brochures and other types of information about recommendations. Refer every family for a car seat examination at a certified examination center. Provide resources for car seats if the family is not able to afford one. Discuss other possible safety hazards such as extensions on the parent's bicycle and use of baby strollers in areas where cars are present.

Nursing Management

For the Health Promotion and Maintenance of the Newborn and Infant

Nursing Assessment and Diagnosis

The nurse working in clinics, offices, and other settings that offer primary care for newborns and infants should be skillful in assessing health promotion and health maintenance. The infant's growth, developmental level, general physical health, and mental/social health are assessed. Family interactions and other settings where the infant spends time are evaluated for risks and protective factors that influence the child's development. Assess the health of siblings and patterns of integrating the infant into the rest of the family. Particular attention is directed at assessment of risk for diseases and injuries. The data-gathering phase always provides parents with the opportunity to ask questions and relay concerns. Further assessment may need to be directed at these areas.

TABLE 7–4 Injury Prevention in Infancy

HAZARD	DEVELOPMENTAL CHARACTERISTICS	PREVENTIVE MEASURES
Falls	Mobility increases in first year of life, progressing from squirming movements to crawling, rolling, and standing.	Do not leave the newborn or infant unsecured in infant seat, even in newborn period. Do not place on high surfaces such as tables or beds unless holding child. *(A)* Once mobile by crawling, keep doors to stairways closed or use gates. Standing walkers have led to many injuries and are not recommended.
Burns	Infant is dependent on caretakers for environmental control. The second half of the first year is marked by crawling and increased mobility. Objects are explored by touching and placing in mouth.	Check temperature of bath water and food/liquids for drinking. Cover electrical outlets. Supervise infant so that play with electrical cords cannot occur.
Motor vehicle crashes	Infant is dependent on caretakers for placement in car. On impact with another motor vehicle, an infant held on a lap acts as a missile.	Use only approved restraint systems (according to federal motor vehicle safety standards). The seat must be used for every trip, even if very short. The seat must be properly buckled to the car's lap belt system. *(B)*
Drowning	Infant cannot swim and is unable to lift head.	Never leave a newborn or infant alone in a bath of even 2.5 cm (1 in.) of water. Supervise when in water even when a life preserver is worn. Supervision should be provided by adults, not older children. Flotation devices such as arm inflatables are not certified life preservers.
Poisoning	Newborns and infants are dependent on caretakers to keep harmful substances out of reach.	Keep medicines out of reach. Teach proper dosage and administration of medicines to parents. Cleaning products and other harmful substances should not be stored where the infant can reach them. Remove plants from play areas. Have poison control center number by telephone.
Choking	The second half of infancy is marked by exploratory reaching and mouthing of objects. Infant explores objects by placing them in the mouth. *(C)*	Avoid foods that commonly cause choking. Keep small toys away from infants, especially toys labeled "not intended for use by those under 3 years."
Suffocation	The newborn and young infant have minimal head control and may be unable to move if vomiting or having difficulty breathing.	Position newborn and infant on back for sleep. *(D)* Do not place pillows, stuffed toys, bumpers, blankets, or other objects in the crib (AAP, 2011b). Do not use plastic in crib. Avoid latex balloons. Co-sleeping with the parent is discouraged because of the danger of suffocation. Sleep with the baby near but not in the parental bed.
Strangulation	Infant is able to get head into railings or crib slats but cannot remove it.	Be sure older cribs have slats spaced no more than 6 cm (2⅜ in.) apart. The mattress must fit tightly against the crib rails.

A Never leave infant unsecured or on high surface.

B Always use approved restraint system. Place infant in rear-facing seat in back seat of car.

C Explores objects with mouth.

D Place infant on back for sleeping; keep toys clear.

TABLE 7–5 Injury Prevention Topics by Age

AGE	INJURY PREVENTION	TEACHING TOPICS
Birth–1 month	Use car safety seat approved for the newborn or infant; install as directed in rear-facing direction in the back seat. Put baby to sleep on back. Avoid loose bedding and toys in crib; avoid clothes and blankets with loose strings and do not tie a pacifier around the neck. Avoid tobacco use in the environment. Provide adult supervision of the baby at all times by trusted individuals. Test bath water temperature and never leave the baby alone in the bath.	Never place baby on high object such as counter, table, or bed; always keep one hand on the baby during activities like diaper changes to prevent falling. Wash hands correctly and often. Avoid contact with persons with communicable diseases. Have smoke alarms and avoid fire hazards. Learn infant CPR and airway obstruction removal. Never shake the baby. Have plans for emergency care.
2 months	Follow the above. Use only recommended playpens or cribs and keep sides up. Avoid moldy environments. Keep baby toys cleaned.	Avoid exposure to direct sunlight for the baby. Keep sharp and small objects out of baby's environment. Keep hot water heater lower than 120°F (49°C). Review emergency plan with all care providers.
4 months	Follow the above. Get all poisonous substances out of baby's view and reach; install locks to keep them inaccessible.	Do not use latex balloons or plastic bags near the baby.
6 months	Follow the above. Use only a car seat approved for the weight of the child and always use the seat in rear-facing position in the back seat. Empty containers of water immediately after use; be sure pools or other bodies of water are locked and not accessible to baby. Use sunscreen, hat, and long sleeves when baby is in the sun. Keep heavy and sharp objects out of reach; check that all poisons are locked away including in homes visited; keep pet food and cosmetics out of reach.	Do not drink hot liquids or eat soup while holding the baby. Have poison control number by phones and programmed into cell phones. Be alert for dangers of hot curling irons and other appliances. Have electrical cords out of reach and not hanging down. Have home and environment checked for lead hazards. Lower infant crib mattress if still in upper position. Install gates and guards on stairs and windows. Never use an infant walker.
9 months	Follow the above. Crawl on the floor and look for hazards at baby's eye level. Pad sharp corners on tables and other furniture.	Watch for tables, chairs, and other devices the baby may use for climbing to unsafe places.
12 months	Follow the above. Keep the infant in a rear-facing car seat until 2 years of age; place in back seat and never in front seat with a passenger air bag; have installation checked for safety. Start teaching the child to wash hands frequently, demonstrating and washing with the child. Provide own personal items such as clothing and blankets to childcare providers; wash often. Change batteries in home smoke alarms and check system.	Turn handles to back of stove; use back rather than front burners; watch for hot liquids. Check care provider setting for safety hazards. Remember that responsible adults should always supervise your infant, not other children. Peruse home once again for hazards now that the child is more active, climbing, and walking. Check playgrounds for hazards and always supervise the child in a playground.

Source: Data from Hagan, J. G., Shaw, J. S., & Duncan, P. M. (Eds.). (2008). *Bright futures: Guidelines for health supervision of infants, children, and adolescents* (3rd ed.). Elk Grove Village, IL: American Academy of Pediatrics.

Based on the assessment data, the nurse establishes nursing diagnoses that become the basis for nursing interventions. Both areas of strength and need are included; often the family's strengths can be used to further promote health. Nursing diagnoses established during a health supervision visit of an infant might include the following (NANDA-I © 2014):

- *Breastfeeding, Readiness for Enhanced,* related to the mother's confidence and knowledge

- *Breastfeeding, Interrupted,* related to the mother's resumption of employment outside the home
- *Coping: Family, Compromised,* related to recent role changes
- *Attachment, Risk for Impaired (Parent/Child),* related to anxiety associated with parenting role
- *Sleep Pattern, Disturbed (Infant),* related to frequently changing sleep routines and cycles

- *Skin Integrity, Impaired (Infant),* related to developmental factors
- *Infection, Risk for (Infant),* related to inadequate acquired immunity
- *Injury, Risk for (Infant),* related to design of environment
- *Development: Delayed, Risk for,* related to parental substance abuse

Planning and Implementation

The nurse plays a vital role in successful health promotion and health maintenance activities. The newborn period is essential for building a relationship between parents and healthcare professionals that sets the stage for the months and years to come. Explain to the parents what procedures are being performed and their purpose. Encourage them to ask questions and share their perceptions of the infant's personality, development, and other traits. This will enhance their understanding that health care involves a partnership between them and the care providers. It will lead to trust that promotes their ability to share concerns honestly. The first year of the baby's life is a key time for establishing a trusting relationship with health professionals.

Recognize the importance of data provided by simple assessments such as length and weight. Analyze all findings to learn if the child is developing as expected. Much of the visit is spent in teaching parents about topics such as safety measures, providing anticipatory guidance related to development, assisting with integration of the newborn into the family, and relaying resources for support of the family in the community, on the Internet, or in other areas. Parenting classes, childcare facilities, and family planning resources are examples of common parental needs. Perform recommended physical and developmental assessment, administer screening tests, and give immunizations. Be sure parents understand the need for tests and treatments, and relay the results of tests to them.

Nurses who work in hospitals, emergency services, and other facilities are an important link in health supervision. Ask where and how often the child is seen for care. Check immunization schedules to be sure they are up-to-date. When the child is not being seen regularly, find out if the family does not know the importance of these visits or lacks resources to obtain the necessary care. Refer them to resources as needed so that they can identify a pediatric healthcare home. Some agencies that provide health supervision are equipped to perform home visits on a regular basis or in case of special need. When nurses make regular home visits to families with many risk factors, health outcomes are improved. Seeing the family in the natural setting enables the nurse to tailor interventions to the specific situation. Nutrition, safety, and other teaching is more effective when it matches the family's needs. For example, showing how to set up a stimulating environment with safe materials, even if toys are limited, is an effective nursing strategy. Ensure that home visits are performed whenever appropriate and available either through the pediatric healthcare home or other community agency.

Before the family leaves the facility, be sure they have the next appointment scheduled. Summarize content of the present visit, emphasizing the family's strengths and the baby's newly acquired developmental skills. Sensitively list any areas that require work in the coming weeks, such as baby-proofing the home or encouraging the infant to reach for objects. Provide a journal or notebook in which the parents can record the infant's development and write down questions to ask during future visits. Suggest possible topics for the parents to think about, and provide books, brochures, and other printed material.

Evaluation

Expected outcomes of nursing care for the infant and family in health promotion and health maintenance include the following:

- Parents state common safety hazards at the infant's present and upcoming ages.
- The newborn and infant demonstrate normal patterns of growth and progression in developmental milestones.
- The newborn and infant remain free of disease and injury.
- The newborn and infant are well adjusted, showing positive response to the environment and interactions with significant others.

Chapter Highlights

- The first contact between the infant's pediatric healthcare home and the parents should ideally occur prior to birth.
- A trusting relationship between the family and the healthcare provider fosters a partnership that is influential in promoting the development of the newborn or infant.
- The nurse establishes diagnoses based on a thorough assessment of the child and family during healthcare visits.
- The nurse and family collaboratively establish goals for the newborn or infant, and the nurse plans interventions to meet these goals.

Clinical Reasoning in Action

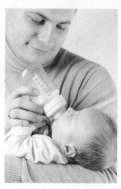

Lipik/Shutterstock

Chad and Jeremy are parents of an adopted newborn. They are eager to learn as much as possible about newborn development, nutrition, and general care. Chad will remain home from work for about 3 months to provide childcare, and both parents will be present on evenings and weekends. They live in a small community and both have supportive family members close. The newborn, Barry, was born after 38 weeks' gestation to a healthy teen mother who allowed the new adoptive fathers to be present soon after birth to meet the baby.

1. Barry is feeding every 2 to 3 hours, and the parents want to know if this is normal. What information about feeding patterns of infants can you provide?
2. Chad and Jeremy are eager to learn as much as possible. What community resources can you explore that provide information to new parents? Does their child's pediatric healthcare home provide educational resources?
3. The birth mother has requested periodic updates and photos about Barry's progress but will not meet him in person. What information is likely to be helpful to her as the baby grows?
4. What questions will you ask to evaluate the parents' knowledge of safety concerns for the newborn?

References

American Academy of Pediatric Dentistry (AAPD). (2013). *Policy on the dental home* (pp. 24–25). AAPD Reference Manual. Chicago, IL: Author.

American Academy of Pediatrics (AAP). (2011a). *Where we stand: Newborn discharge from hospital.* Retrieved from http://www.healthychildren.org/English/ages-stages/prenatal/delivery-beyond/pages

American Academy of Pediatrics (AAP). (2011b). SIDS and other sleep-related infant deaths: Expansion of recommendations for a safe infant sleeping environment. *Pediatrics, 128,* e1341–e1367.

American Academy of Pediatrics (AAP). (n.d.). *Appropriate newborn hospital stays.* Retrieved from http://www.aap.org/en-us/about-the-aap/aap-press-room/aap-press-room-media-center/Pages/Appropriate-Newborn-Hospital-Stays.aspx

American Academy of Pediatrics (AAP) Committee on Nutrition. (2013). *Pediatric nutrition handbook* (7th ed.). Elk Grove Village, IL: Author.

Brescianini, S., Volzone, A., Fagnani, C., Patriarca, B., Grimaldi, V., Lanni, R., . . . Stazi, J. A. (2011). Genetic and environmental factors shape infant sleep patterns: A study of 18-month-old twins. *Pediatrics, 127,* e1296. doi:10.1542/peds.2010-0858

Hagan, J. G., Shaw, J. S., & Duncan, P. M. (Eds.). (2008). *Bright futures: Guidelines for health supervision of infants, children, and adolescents* (3rd ed.). Elk Grove Village, IL: American Academy of Pediatrics.

Holt, K., Wooldridge, N., Story, M., & Sofka, D. (Eds.). (2011). *Bright futures: Nutrition* (3rd ed.). Elk Grove Village, IL: American Academy of Pediatrics.

Kadey, H. J., & Roane, H. S. (2012). Effects of access to a stimulating object on infant behavior during tummy time. *Journal of Applied Behavior Analysis, 45,* 395–399.

Middlemiss, W., Yuare, R., & Huey, E. L. (2014). Translating evidence-based knowledge about sleep into practice. *Journal of the American Association of Nurse Practitioners.* doi:10.1002/2327–6924.12159

Sadeh, A., Mindell, J., & Rivera, L. (2011). "My child has a sleep problem": A cross-cultural comparison of parental definitions. *Sleep Medicine, 12*(5), 478–482.

Schreck, K. A., & Richdale, A. L. (2011). Knowledge of childhood sleep: A possible variable in under or misdiagnosis of childhood sleep problems. *Journal of Sleep Research, 20,* 589–597. doi:10.1111/j.1365-2869.2011.00922.x

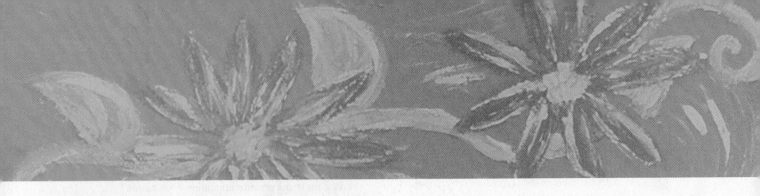

Chapter 8
Health Promotion and Maintenance for the Toddler and Preschooler

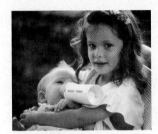

Mommy was really glad to go see the nurse today. She brought our baby and me. Grandma said that they would give us a card that would help us buy food. I'm glad because I'm tired of eating peanut butter. Mommy said we could get some milk and juice, and even some chicken.

—Melody, age 4, sister of 7-month-old Amanda

∨ Learning Outcomes

8.1 Describe the areas of assessment and intervention for health supervision visits for toddler and preschool children: growth and developmental surveillance, nutrition, physical activity, oral health, mental and spiritual health, family and social relations, disease prevention strategies, and injury prevention strategies.

8.2 State components of self-concept for preschool children.

8.3 Plan health promotion and health maintenance strategies employed during

health supervision visits of toddlers and preschoolers.

8.4 Discuss the importance of family in child health care, and include family assessment in each health supervision visit.

8.5 Integrate pertinent mental health care into health supervision visits for toddlers and preschoolers.

8.6 Examine data about the family and other social relationships to prioritize interventions and to maintain health of toddlers and preschoolers.

Health Promotion and Maintenance for the Toddler and Preschooler

The years following infancy are challenging for parents as the child grows and acquires new developmental skills. The child progresses from the first tentative steps and words at 1 year of age through the "terrible twos" of toddlerhood and into preschool age when over half of children attend some type of education program, have developed effective verbal

communication, and acquire many gross and fine motor skills (Child Trends, 2012). Toddler and preschool ages are often grouped as "young childhood" since the family remains the primary system within which the child interacts. Healthcare providers address common health concerns such as nutrition, sleep, and growing independence. Facing consistent changes in development, parents rely on the "pediatric healthcare home" ("medical home") for advice and information (see Chapter 6). Regular health visits are recommended at 12, 15, 18, 24, and 30 months and at about 3, 4, and 5 years of age. The Recommendations for Preventive Pediatric Health Care (American Academy of Pediatrics Committee on Practice and Ambulatory Medicine, 2016) provide guidance for the screenings to perform during the toddler and preschool ages. Nurses apply concepts of anticipatory guidance during visits for health promotion and health maintenance to assist parents in the transitions they face. The child should have an established "dental home" as well. Dental visits are generally recommended twice annually.

Health supervision of young children applies to the following:

1. *Assessment*, including screening tests, evaluations, and observations
2. *Education*, including anticipatory guidance about coming developmental tasks
3. *Intervention*, including parent counseling, home visits when appropriate, and scheduling of future visits
4. *Care coordination* among resources serving the family

General Observations

The relationship with the family should be established as a partnership in care of the child. If, however, the family is new to this healthcare home, reach out to welcome family members warmly and express interest in them as individuals and parents. Families may feel uncomfortable in healthcare settings, and it is important to establish positive rapport so they will be able to ask questions and bring up concerns about the child.

While calling the toddler in from the waiting room, it is amazing that this young child is now able to walk in, even if needing some parental guidance. Watch for the child's desire for independence or signs of continuing reliance on the parent. By preschool age, the child is totally independent in walking and usually engages in conversations easily. After welcoming the preschool child warmly, assess the child's social skills and motor activities. Direct greetings or questions to the child to evaluate stranger anxiety and ability to understand simple commands or questions. What verbal skills are observed? Observe the child's general appearance, nutrition, and state of health.

Health supervision visits are adapted for older toddlers and preschoolers to include observations of parental discipline and interaction style. Does the parent respond to the child's questions? Were age-appropriate toys or activities brought to the visit to help occupy the child while waiting? Is the child alert and observant of the environment?

Growth and Developmental Surveillance

An essential assessment integrated into the visit is measurement of growth. Weight and length are measured and compared to expected patterns of growth. When the child can stand upright to be measured, sometime between 2 and 3 years of age, charts for standing height rather than recumbent length are used. Body mass index (BMI) is first calculated at 2 years of age and provides information about the relationship of height and weight (see Chapter 14 for additional information). Head circumference is usually measured until 2 years of age. (Consult growth grids in Appendix A.)

Growth continues to be a primary way of evaluating the child's nutritional status. It may also provide clues about conditions that have not yet been evaluated such as endocrine, cardiac, or other disorders. Depending on the results of growth measurements, the nurse may gather additional data. For a child under the 5th percentile for weight or BMI, detailed

recording of nutritional intake should begin. Laboratory studies such as hematocrit and hemoglobin can be performed. Patterns of family growth can be examined. What size are the parents and siblings? Ask if the child has had any illness or hospitalization. For children above the 85th percentile for BMI, detailed dietary intake and physical activity history should be taken.

The physical assessment is performed, with some parts conducted by the nurse and others by the primary care provider such as a physician or nurse practitioner. See Chapter 5 for a thorough discussion of physical examination. The order of the examination and the approaches to the child are particularly important at this age. Leave intrusive procedures such as ear and eye examinations and visualization of genitalia until the end of the examination. Integrate techniques such as allowing the child to play with the stethoscope, asking the child to "blow out" the light from the otoscope, or having the child make a game of pushing the legs against the examiner to measure symmetry of strength (Figure 8–1). Preschoolers are generally interested in their bodies, and teaching about parts of the examination is helpful. During the physical examination, ask the parents pertinent questions. Consider the young child's expected developmental milestones (see information in Chapter 4) and ask questions related to these milestones. Recommended screenings include blood pressure, vision and hearing, autism (at 18 and 24 months; see Chapters 5, 19, and 28), and, for the child at risk, hematocrit, hemoglobin, and lead screening (see Chapters 17 and 23).

Nurses generally have in-depth knowledge of child development through growth and development courses and pediatric nursing curricula, and are thus well positioned to address parental concerns related to child development. Development is the key organizing principle of early childhood health care. Developmental screening and services should be integrated within health care, child care, and school settings to include the multiple sites common for young children. (Refer to Chapter 4 for expected milestones at each stage.) Developmental surveillance is integrated throughout the healthcare visit as you observe the child's fine motor, gross motor, language, and social/emotional skills. Developmental screening or testing is also performed; inquire if the child has had developmental testing done at a childcare agency or another site. Ideal screening tools include input from the family in addition to observations by the healthcare provider. Screening tools currently recommended for young children are listed in Table 8–1. See *Evidence-Based Practice: Fetal Alcohol Spectrum Disorders*.

TABLE 8–1 Developmental Screening Tools for Young Children

TOOL	UPPER AGE
Ages and Stages Questionnaire	66 months
Brigance Screens	1st grade
Developmental Assessment of Young Children, 2nd edition	5 years
Early Screening Profiles	7 years
FirstSTEP	6 years
Parents' Evaluation of Developmental Status	8 years
Survey of Well-Being of Young Children	5 years

Source: Adapted from Child Trends. (2014). *Early childhood developmental screening: A compendium of measures for children ages birth to five.* Retrieved from http://www.acf.hhs.gov/programs/ecd/watch-me-thrive

EVIDENCE-BASED PRACTICE | Fetal Alcohol Spectrum Disorders

Clinical Question

Alcohol ingestion by the pregnant woman can result in birth defects called *fetal alcohol spectrum disorders (FASD)*, ranging from fetal alcohol syndrome to fetal alcohol effects. Children may have characteristic facial and other physical abnormalities, or they may appear normal but have learning and behavioral difficulties. Early identification of these disorders can prevent one of the primary causes of developmental delay in children. (See Chapter 28 for further information.) What is the nursing role in prevention of FASD, evaluation of young children for the problem, and becoming knowledgeable about community resources for families when a child exhibits FASD?

The Evidence

In a study of First Steps program (designed to provide pregnancy guidance for women at high risk), retrospective analysis of participants demonstrated significant improvement in alcohol abstinence by participants (Rasmussen et al., 2012). However, in spite of prevention efforts, alcohol exposure during pregnancy occurs and can result in serious consequences for young children. A recent meta-analysis found that prenatal alcohol exposure of the fetus was significantly associated with gross motor deficits in children, particularly in balance, coordination, and ball skills (Lucas et al., 2014). Therefore, motor coordination evaluation is critical in young children so that early identification of problems associated with FASD can result in treatment. In a study with practicing nurses and student nurses, student nurses were found to lack knowledge

related to binge drinking, facial abnormalities associated with FASD, and diagnosis of the disorder (Zoorob, Durkin, Gonzalez, et al., 2014).

Best Practice

Preventive programs with women at high risk of alcohol ingestion during pregnancy can be helpful to decrease consumption and therefore lower risk of FASD occurrence. In addition, when working with toddlers and preschoolers, the nurse must integrate physical assessment for physical signs of fetal alcohol exposure, as well as developmental screening and, particularly, gross motor performance. Children who have difficulty in this area should be referred for further developmental testing. Student nurses should become familiar with both the physical features present in some children with FASD and the developmental/social behavioral components (see Chapter 28). This is an example of the importance of thorough knowledge of development and comprehensive observations and screening during the physical examination.

Clinical Reasoning

How can you ask questions sensitively to determine use of alcohol and knowledge of FASD among pregnant women? Describe the gross motor skills you expect to see in toddlers and preschoolers and areas that might concern you about their abilities. What resources are present in your community to support the toddler or preschooler who manifests fetal alcohol syndrome disorder?

Topics pertinent for inquiry and anticipatory guidance at health supervision visits of young children include sleep patterns, discipline techniques, toilet training, learning and reading practices, communication, and parental issues and questions. Many children, especially by preschool age, are attending a childcare center (Child Trends, 2012). Ask about the experience and whether developmental skills are a focus of activity. Ask if the parent is pleased with the childcare experience or needs further resources. Guidelines for evaluating childcare settings are available through the National Resource Center for Health and Safety in Child Care and Early Education (2013).

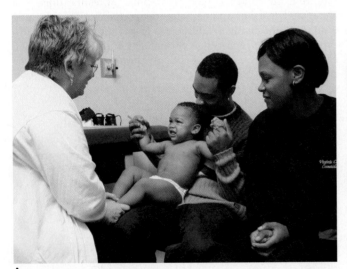
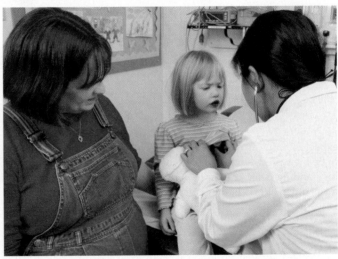

A   **B**

Figure 8–1 **Examining the toddler or preschooler. The approach to examination of the toddler or preschooler is important in order to elicit cooperation.** *A,* **The toddler may accept parts of the examination best when seated on the parent's lap as shown in this photo of a boy with his father.** *B,* **The preschooler likes the opportunity to touch and become comfortable with equipment used or, in this case, holds a doll that receives the same examinations as the child.**

TABLE 8–2 Nutrition Teaching for Health Promotion and Health Maintenance Visits

AGE (YEARS)	NUTRITION TEACHING	
1	Support mother who continues to breastfeed.	Provide food and water safety guidelines (see Chapter 14).
	Wean child from bottle by substituting cup.	Be sure all major food groups have been introduced.
	If beginning to use cow's milk, use whole milk (may change to 2% at 2 years of age).	Limit high-fat and high-sugar foods.
	Limit juice to 4–6 oz daily; offer water several times daily; use plain water and avoid flavored water or sugared/electrolyte drinks.	Review amounts of food commonly consumed and frequency of feedings.
	Encourage safety measures—use high chair with strap, secure child and use caution in grocery carts, do not allow foods to be eaten in car.	Review use of fluoride if water supply is not fluoridated.
	Provide information on choking and airway obstruction removal training.	Educate parents to inquire about water sources in case of lead contamination due to older plumbing systems where pipes could potentially be corroded.
2	Ask if the mother is still breastfeeding and support the decision to continue or to wean child, as she desires.	Teach parents methods for dealing with temper tantrums over food—make food available at meal and snack times only, do not force intake, offer a variety of foods.
	Encourage total removal of bottle if still in use.	Teach that child may have days of very low intake due to slowing growth rate.
	Ensure that all foods common to family have been offered.	
	Offer child-sized eating utensils.	
	Child can change to low-fat or skim milk if family desires.	
	Limit milk to 2–3 servings daily.	
3	Most children are weaned from breastfeeding and drink 1% or 2% milk.	Recognize importance of social nature of eating; expect child to sit for a short period at meals with family.
	Teach normal intake and decreasing number of snacks.	Meals and snacks should not be eaten while watching television.
	Engage child in food preparation and pouring liquids from small pitcher.	
	Recognize that food jags (periods when only 1 or 2 foods are eaten) are common.	
4	Encourage involving child in snack selection and preparation.	Alter intake as appropriate depending on weight and BMI.
	Start to teach food groups and importance of nutrition for the body.	Dairy products consumed should all be low or reduced fat.

Health promotion growth and development issues for toddlers and preschoolers are addressed at each visit. Some common examples include:

- Explaining growth patterns and what is expected in the months ahead

- Providing toys that encourage development of the coming developmental milestones

- Showing parents the child's developmental progression on a screening tool

Likewise, health maintenance activities are included in health supervision visits, with the primary purpose being prevention of disease and injury. Specific examples are included throughout the chapter, but some general areas addressed are:

- Connecting developmental skills with risks for injury such as drowning and motor vehicle crashes

- Recognizing the possibility of exposure to infectious diseases as the child begins a childcare experience and addressing recognition of and treatments for common diseases

Expected outcomes for the child include normal growth and development patterns for motor, language, and social/emotional skills; parental knowledge of stimulating activities for the child; awareness of the family about risks to growth and development; and healthy body systems for the child.

Nutrition

The child's nutritional status continues to play an important part in promoting health and preventing health disruptions during toddler and preschooler years. Good nutrition fosters normal growth patterns, promotes developmental progression, and helps prevent disorders such as anemia, tooth decay, and immune dysfunction. Eating takes on an increasingly social dimension during early childhood as children interact more with adults and other children at mealtimes. See Chapter 14 for further information about nutritional needs and challenges.

For toddlers, questions for the family focus on introduction of foods, the child's eating patterns, and transition from breast or bottle to other liquids. The toddler often consumes small amounts of foods, and parents consequently worry about the change in appetite. Showing them that the child is growing normally can help allay their anxiety about this common developmental variation. Preschoolers interact with others during food preparation and meal consumption. Questions from the nurse should focus on the child's likes and dislikes for particular foods, behavior at the table, and establishment of healthy family eating patterns. Ask how often the family eats out, especially at fast-food restaurants. When parents are busy and older siblings are in activities, both toddlers and preschoolers may be eating foods such as french fries or milk shakes several times weekly. Suggest alternative approaches to the busy lifestyle, such as bringing fresh fruit slices along when an older sibling is at a sporting event, keeping a cooler in the car to maintain cool items, and limiting fast-food meals to no more than one or two weekly. Obtain nutritional information about common fast-food options in your community and share these with parents. Assist them to make healthy choices when eating out. Encourage the family to set times when they all eat together, even if only a few times weekly. If children help with preparations for this family meal, and then eat together, nutritional knowledge and intake can be positively enhanced. When the child is in a childcare center or home, encourage the parents to find out what food is provided for the child in that setting.

During the toddler and preschool years, children are gaining much more independence about food choices and patterns of eating. At the same time, their eating patterns depend mainly on the family, so assessment should involve the entire family unit (see *Developing Cultural Competence: Family Nutrition*). Parents can benefit from receiving information about nutrition for young children (Table 8–2).

Developing Cultural Competence **Family Nutrition**

Each family integrates their own cultural backgrounds and past experiences into food preparation and choices. Ask what foods are common in the child's cultural group and help the family learn when to introduce each food. For example, rice may be a first food for an Asian baby rather than rice cereal. Be sure the child also takes in adequate iron sources in the first foods offered. Tofu or bean paste may be a common protein source in some diets. A Native American child may eat fish or wild game, along with berries and roots. Ask and learn about each family's cultural patterns. Learn what you can about cultural groups in your community. Encourage the family to offer the young child their usual foods, as long as they meet needs for requirements, are prepared with minimal salt and seasoning, and are soft enough to avoid choking. Perform diet recalls and analyses to check for any specific teaching needs in all families.

Health promotion interventions include actions such as supporting breastfeeding for young toddlers and being sure preschoolers have a role in selecting foods for healthy snacks. Parental education is influential in shaping their young child's diet and should be integrated into all visits (Holt, Wooldridge, Story, et al., 2011). Important health promotion teaching includes the concept of "5 a day," or ensuring five servings of fruits and vegetables in the daily diet (American Academy of Pediatrics [AAP] Committee on Nutrition, 2013). Likewise, "3 a day of dairy" encourages families to provide at least three servings of dairy for children every day. Nurses and parents partner together to ensure that the young child establishes healthy eating habits at home and in other daily settings. Health maintenance activities focus primarily on disease and injury prevention, with examples of feeding practices that do not include common choking foods, and limiting daily fruit juice intake to prevent dental caries and excessive caloric intake. Desired outcomes related to nutrition include meeting normal growth and development milestones, maintaining a recommended weight, expanding understanding of healthy food patterns, and preventing nutrition-related disorders.

Physical Activity

The toddler and preschooler consistently show gains in fine and gross motor abilities. They walk and run independently and often engage in physical activity in school and other settings. They commonly visit parks, swim, attend childcare centers, and help with some household tasks. These activities are important, both because they assist the child in continuing to develop motor skills and because they limit the amount of time spent in sedentary behavior. The toddler and preschool years are an important time for setting the habits for physical activity during all of childhood.

During toddler years the main emphasis is on providing experiences that encourage further motor development. The child needs to walk, run, hop, push and pull objects, and throw balls. Motor activity is a major component in all playtimes, and activities should engage the child's large and small muscle groups. The National Association for Sport and Physical Education (NASPE) has established recommendations for toddlers and preschoolers: a minimum of 60 minutes per day of unstructured physical activity, a minimum of 60 minutes per day of structured physical activity, and a maximum of 60 minutes of sedentary behavior at any one time exclusive of sleep (Beets, Bornstein, Dowda, et al., 2011; Centers for Disease Control and Prevention [CDC], 2011) (Figure 8–2).

By the preschool years, coordination develops quickly. Physical activity is important for all children, including those with developmental disabilities. The preschooler learns to balance, walk on one foot, skip, and throw and catch with greater accuracy. **Kinesthesia**, or the sense of one's body position and movement, develops during these years. Eye–hand coordination improves at the same time that visual acuity matures. The social component plays an important role as children learn to engage in games and activities cooperatively with others.

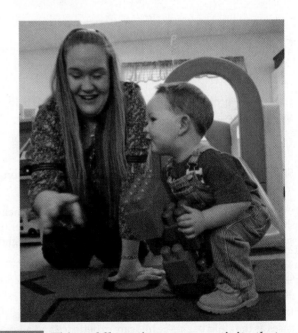

Figure 8–2 This toddler enjoys motor activity that uses large muscle groups. The preschooler spends much of playtime in activities that lead to coordination of both small and large muscle mass. List several physical activities that you can suggest for the parents of children in each of these age groups.

TABLE 8–3 Risk and Protective Factors Regarding Physical Activity in Toddlerhood and Preschool

RISK FACTORS	PROTECTIVE FACTORS
• Developmental delay • Slow development of social skills	• Expected developmental progression
• Limited stimulation by family or other care providers • Limited social time with other children • Long work hours by parents	• Easily engages socially with others • Regular contact with other young children
• Reluctance to try new physical activity • Limited access to balls, slides, balance beams, tricycles, and other materials that foster physical activity • Adequate safety gear for activities is not available	• Eagerness to try new physical activity • Access to balls, slides, balance beams, tricycles, and other materials that foster physical activity • Adequate safety gear that properly fits child is available
• Parents who have little physical activity on a daily basis • Lack of knowledge by family about child's physical activity needs	• Family members engage in daily physical activity • Family members spend time in physical activity with child • Family understands motor developmental milestones and importance of physical activity in childhood
• Television or other screen activities are engaged in for more than 2 hr daily	• Television and other screen activities are limited to no more than 2 hr daily
• Limited community resources for child care and physical activity • Unsafe neighborhood and lack of lawns, parks, and other facilities	• Neighborhood contains access to child care that integrates physical activity • Neighborhood is safe, and contains lawns, parks, and other facilities

The nurse applies the concept of resilience by identifying both risk and protective factors related to physical activity (Table 8–3). The assessment becomes the basis for nursing interventions, both to reinforce positive physical activity and to make recommendations for changes where needed.

Children and adults are commonly overweight and sedentary in today's society, so emphasis on physical activity should be a part of each health supervision visit. Nurses and parents are partners in planning activities for the young child; patterns set in motion at this early age will continue into the rest of childhood and into adulthood (Simmonds et al., 2015). Suggestions for the family may include setting guidelines to limit television and other screen activities to a maximum of 2 hours daily in order to facilitate adequate physical activity time. Children should not have television and computers in their bedrooms because use of such media can disturb sleep, and children learn best from play rather than media exposure (AAP Council on Communications and Media, 2013). Health promotion teaching imparts to parents the benefits of activity, such as a healthy immune and cardiovascular system, positive self-concept of the child, and the child's learning of important motor skills. Health maintenance teaching focuses on disease prevention, such as avoidance of overweight, and injury prevention, with use of protective gear for sports.

Expected outcomes of health promotion and health supervision related to physical activity are daily inclusion of at least 60 minutes of activity into life patterns, normal developmental progression of the musculoskeletal system, growth in coordination, and appropriate balance between dietary intake and physical activity so that normal weight is maintained.

Oral Health

The early childhood years play an important part in the child's future oral health, and yet dental care remains one of the most preventable and common unmet healthcare needs for children in developed countries. About 28% of children from 2 to 5 years have had dental caries, and 21% have untreated dental caries (National Institute of Dental and Craniofacial Research, 2014). **Early childhood caries (ECC)** is defined as one or more decayed, missing, or filled tooth surfaces in a child 71 months of age or younger (AAP Committee on Nutrition, 2013; Colak, Dulgergil, Dalli, et al., 2013). This condition is promoted by inadequate preventive care, which can include diet, brushing, feeding habits, and lack of dental care. ECC is serious because young children with the condition are more likely to have continuing dental problems that can influence speech, cause pain, and delay development. Teaching prevention at an early age is key to preventing the problem.

The nurse assists the family to ensure oral health for the young child. By 1 year of age, the child should have made a first visit to the dentist. The child should have an established dental home for regular care and recommendations (American Academy of Pediatric Dentistry [AAPD] Council on Clinical Affairs, 2013). By about 2 years of age, the toddler has a full set of 20 primary teeth, called **deciduous teeth**, that will be lost during childhood, beginning at about 6 years. Evaluate these teeth for condition and number. They help maintain space for the permanent teeth, foster positive eating habits, and are needed for language development. Inquire about how the family cleans the teeth and, if the child has any dental decay, ask them to demonstrate their daily care. At the end of preschool, the first of the deciduous teeth are lost, an important developmental event for most children.

By 2 to 4 years of age, young children have discontinued using pacifiers and thumbsucking. These habits are harmful when permanent teeth begin erupting at about age 6 years (American Dental Association [ADA], 2011). Parents should be instructed gradually to remove the pacifier by 1 to 2 years of age. Many young children continue to thumbsuck, which is a comforting and reassuring habit. Usually, the child who is 2 to 4 years old is ready to discontinue thumbsucking, and parents can promote this process by praising the child for not sucking, helping the child find alternative sources of comfort such as rubbing a blanket, putting a sock on the hand at nap or nighttime to serve as a reminder not to suck, and working with the preschooler to identify the reward when no thumbsucking is seen for a week or more (ADA, 2011).

Based on the results of the assessment of the child's teeth, observation of language skills, and answers to questions directed at parents, plan interventions that will foster maintenance of oral health, thus preventing dental disease. (See Chapter 19 for emergency treatment of dental injury.) These may include referral to low-cost dental clinics, provision of toothbrush and toothpaste, demonstration to the parents and young child about proper brushing technique, and teaching about limiting sweet snacks and drinks. A dental visit will assist in identifying children at moderate or high risk of dental caries; for these children, a "smear" of fluoridated toothpaste should be used for brushing, and in 2- to 5-year-olds, a pea-size amount of fluoridated toothpaste can be used. For other children, nonfluoridated toothpaste is used (American Academy of Pediatric Dentistry [AAPD], 2014). Remember to positively reinforce health promotion practices such as good oral hygiene for toddlers and preschoolers who brush, visit the dentist, and are careful to limit intake of sweets. Desired outcomes for oral health are eruption of a normal set of deciduous teeth, regular dental care, nutrition and hygiene practices that foster dental health, and knowledge of child and parent about oral health.

Mental and Spiritual Health

The family plays a key role in fostering a positive self-image and setting the stage for the young child's mental health. As the family is called in for the visit, begin an assessment of the family's methods of influencing mental health. Observe communication and interactions in the family and the child's ability to interact with healthcare providers. Ask for a description of a typical day or what the child has recently begun to do. The child's sense of self and mental status are related to new accomplishments. Inquire about toilet training, tooth brushing, choosing clothes and getting dressed, using crayons, or other developmental tasks.

Toddlers and preschoolers use **self-regulation** (the ability to soothe and comfort the self) to control anger, excessive desires for objects or foods, and other nonsocial behaviors. To assist the child in developing the ability to control and regulate self, parents often use discipline techniques. Ask about how the parent deals with the child who is having a temper tantrum or showing other undesirable behaviors. Reinforce positive ways of helping the child set limits for self and make suggestions when parents need assistance (*Families Want to Know: Positive Discipline*). The goal of discipline is to help the child develop a sense of right and wrong, and to learn acceptable ways of dealing with other people.

Adequate sleep and rest are needed for children to master self-regulation. Most toddlers have established regular sleeping patterns with occasional night awakenings. They sleep about 10 to 12 hours at night with one or two daytime naps. Parents have usually learned to establish clear routines such as reading a story, back rubbing, and then leaving the child alone. Occasionally, parents who work during the day may feel guilty about putting the child to sleep. Help them alleviate guilt by suggesting that they spend quality time with the child after arriving home, and then establish clear sleeping expectations. Transitional objects such as blankets or toys are important for the toddler and can be used during childcare experiences to provide comfort and help

Families Want to Know

Positive Discipline

First, provide structure that enhances the possibility of desirable behaviors:

- Limit rules to those that are essential. It will be easier to enforce a few important rules than many that are nonessential.

- Provide an environment where the child is mainly free to explore safely in order to avoid constant cautions. For example, have adequate play space for toddlers with limited fragile glassware in the usual daily environment. It is easier for the toddler to learn not to touch a few objects when adequate objects are provided for play.

- Spend time interacting with the child several times each day. Praise positive behaviors frequently. Preschoolers often like to have charts with stars to record picking up toys, helping a parent, and other positive behaviors. Once a certain number of stars is reached, a reward, such as stickers or an outing with the parent, is earned.

When the child shows undesirable behaviors:

- Use distraction as the first approach and praise the child for selecting the new activity suggested by the parent.

- Tell the child one time that the behavior is unsatisfactory and what will happen if the behavior persists.

- Separate the child from a setting in which behavior is undesirable. Place the child in "time-out," a separate place that is safe. Toddlers can be placed in a playpen or crib, while preschoolers are told to sit on a chair. One minute of time-out per year of age is a good length of time. Once time-out is over, provide a positive activity and move the child directly toward the activity.

When undesirable behaviors include other people, such as biting or hitting:

- Tell the child clearly that it is not okay to hurt another person. Encourage and role model proper language to explain feelings.

- Separate the child immediately from the situation and use time-out.

- If there are repeated episodes, be sure the child is getting adequate sleep and food, has opportunities for active play that releases energy, and has positive attention from many people in the environment. Be sensitive to stresses such as a recent trauma or a new sibling.

- Encourage the child to "use words" instead of hitting or biting. Until able to do so on their own, parents can model this behavior. "You feel like saying, 'I am really upset that you took my toy away.' Let's use words instead of hitting so your sister knows that."

maintain normal routines. Some families prefer to have children sleep in the bed with parents. Advise against this pattern, but if this is the parents' decision, be sure they are aware of safety hazards such as suffocation in excessive bedding, injury related to falling between headboard and frame, parental smoking that could lead to a fire, or parental deep sleeping or alcohol and drug use that can lead to such sound sleep that it is possible to roll onto and suffocate the child.

The preschooler sleeps about 9 to 11 hours and may have one or no naps each day. Some quiet playtime can be beneficial even for the preschooler who does not nap. At this age, some children begin to awaken at night and may need some assistance in falling back to sleep. **Nightmares** are frightening dreams that awaken the child, who is often crying and upset. Parents can reassure the child, rub the child's back, provide some repeat of a bedtime routine such as reading a story, and then allow the child to settle into sleep again. It is not advisable to bring children to the parental bed since they may start to awaken at night in order to continue this practice. **Night terrors** (or sleep terrors) are characterized by a child who cries out, appears frightened, and has tachycardia and tachypnea. However, in contrast to nightmares, the child having a night terror is not fully awake and may appear disoriented (Mayo Clinic, 2014). Parents should quietly talk to and comfort the child, allowing the child to return to sleep. The child has no recollection of these events the next morning.

The toddler gains more independence in many aspects of life such as mobility and speech. The control over toileting is another milestone that signals greater independence and can lead to a sense of self-control. Ask parents if the toddler has shown interest in toilet training and how they intend to work with the child to attain control over bowel and bladder. (See Chapter 4 for further discussion about toilet training.) Preschoolers are generally well trained for bowel and bladder with only occasional accidents. These should be treated with understanding rather than blame in order for healthy self-concept to develop.

Preschoolers have a growing awareness of gender and sexuality issues. They may ask questions about kissing, love, or their genitals. These questions should be truthfully answered, leaving the child with a positive sense of sexuality. Some exploration of genitals may occur, and children should be told simply that it is something that should occur in private, and then be offered other activities to engage them when with other people.

The family's spiritual orientation takes on additional meaning for the toddler and preschooler. They can participate in the family's faith-based practices, which enlarge their microsystem influences to include that of the religious group, thus reinforcing the child's learning about right and wrong. The nurse assesses the family's faith-based or spiritual beliefs and provides support for the family's approach, whether it is in established religious organizations or in the family's other meaningful activities (Pender, Murdaugh, & Parsons, 2015).

Health promotion activities focus on development of a healthy self-concept in the toddler and young child by helping parents set up successful play experiences, praise the child for successes, use effective limit-setting techniques, and realize and appreciate the child's unique characteristics. Health maintenance seeks to avoid the poor self-image that can occur with constant criticism or expectations not in alignment with the toddler's or preschooler's developmental capabilities. Further examples of the family interactions that can influence the child's self-concept are provided in the following section on relationships.

Desired outcomes for the child related to mental and spiritual health include emergence of a positive self-esteem, ability to self-regulate behaviors, emergence of methods to handle daily stressors, and normal developmental progression in tasks such as toilet training and sleep.

Relationships

Family members are part of the microsystem for the toddler and preschooler and, as such, form a vital part of the child's environment. Families with members who handle stress well and have healthy lifestyle patterns offer security for the young child. When parents are stressed or depressed, the mental status of all family members can be affected. Ask how things are going for the family in general. Inquire about siblings and whether there are any issues of concern that might influence the toddler or preschooler. Illness or behavior problems in a sibling can decrease the parent's ability to deal with other children. The focus on a sibling in need can be confusing to a toddler or preschooler. Be alert for signs of child abuse and for substance abuse in family members (refer to Chapter 17). Have the parents become separated or divorced? Is there a new stepparent?

During questions and observations, the nurse identifies family risk and protective factors. Reinforce strengths and provide services and referrals to deal with risks. Some strengths include the following:

- The family spends time together each day.
- Parents are proud of the child's accomplishments and knowledgeable about developmental progression.
- Childcare center personnel and family members interact regularly to plan consistent approaches for the toddler and preschooler.
- The teen mother of a toddler is enrolled in a high school continuation program with a childcare component.

Examples of risks to mental health include the following:

- Mother has been diagnosed with depression.
- Family member in home uses street drugs.
- Child awakens with night terrors.
- Child was recently in a serious motor vehicle crash.
- Teen mother is estranged from own family and has few goals and resources.

Toddlers continue to grow in social abilities, while preschoolers demonstrate large strides in socializing with others. Expect that most toddlers will enjoy playing with other children, although they play "side by side" in a parallel manner and not cooperatively. They also engage in play with adults for short periods, such as throwing a ball. However, preschoolers begin to engage in activities that involve other children directly in cooperative play. They play "house" where one child plays the mother and another plays the child. They engage in simple games where each plays a separate role. Their interactions with adults display similar maturity as they take on tasks such as setting the table for dinner or picking up books from the floor. Social skills involve getting along with others. Young children exhibit maturing skill in language development, a primary medium for social exchange. From just a few words at age 1 year, the child has progressed to stating three-word sentences by 3 years of age. Although all parts of speech are not in place, young children certainly have the ability to make needs and thoughts known. Assessment of language skills provides a mirror into this important means of socializing.

Successful social skills involve separating from the parent at times. During toddlerhood, most children spend some time away from parents. Initially they may be fearful and display crying, but gradually they learn to adapt to the new person and place. Preschoolers need to begin developing relationships with other adults and children in order to adapt to the school setting at about 5 years of age. Ask how many people the child has contact with each week and how they manage separation from the parent. Encourage parents to see separation as a skill the child is learning rather than something that is guilt producing for them. When they leave the child in a secure setting, they should hug, provide a favorite object, and leave. Short periods initially will teach the child that the parent can be trusted to return.

Expected outcomes of health promotion and health maintenance activities with young children include appropriate social skills with parents, siblings, and other children and adults; successful management of temperament characteristics; adjustment to time away from the home; and improving language/communication skills.

Disease Prevention Strategies

Toddlers and preschoolers commonly have 6 to 10 upper respiratory infections annually, so teaching good hygiene is a helpful preventive measure (Lucille Packard Children's Hospital, 2012). Some immunizations are given during this age period in order to complete a basic series. For the child who has not had all immunizations, extra visits to catch them

TABLE 8–4 Routine Immunizations Recommended During Toddlerhood and Preschool Age

IMMUNIZATION	AGE RECOMMENDED
Hepatitis B	6–18 months: Administer dose #3 if series not completed during infancy (usually doses #1 and #2 are administered in early infancy, with dose #3 given from 6–18 months of age)
Hepatitis A	Series of 2 doses with first at 12 months and second at least 6 months later
Diphtheria, tetanus, acellular pertussis (DTaP)	15–18 months (#4) (first 3 administered in infancy) 4–6 years (#5)
Haemophilus influenzae type b	12–15 months (#4 or will be #3 for PRP-OMP type that requires only 3 doses for whole series) (first doses administered in infancy)
Inactivated poliovirus	4–6 years (#4) (first 3 doses administered in infancy)
Measles, mumps, rubella	12–15 months (#1)
Varicella	12–18 months (#1) 4–6 years (#2)
Pneumococcal	12–15 months (#4)
Influenza	Annually

Note: Schedule may need to be adapted if child did not receive all recommended immunizations during infancy. See Chapter 16 and the CDC and AAP websites for further information.

up to recommended levels might be needed. At the end of the preschool period, a complete review of the immunization record is done so that any needed immunizations are administered before school entry. See Table 8–4 for immunizations recommended during toddlerhood and preschool (additional immunizations may be needed for children at high risk for certain diseases). Toddlers and preschoolers should be screened for health problems during health supervision visits, such as asthma, obesity, or other issues manifested by a review of body systems. Earlier visits may have failed to identify a problem on account of the child's young age, so areas such as vision, hearing, and developmental milestones are always included.

Recognize that the environment is a powerful influence on the health of children. Ask if parents or others in the home smoke. Discourage this practice and describe the health implications for the child. Is the neighborhood generally safe? Is there toxicity exposure from air, water, or other mediums? Ask about lead exposure in the home (see Chapter 17 for more information). How much television and other screen time is common in the home? Older siblings who allow the preschooler to play violent video games or watch many hours of inappropriate television can affect the mental health of the young child. Do parents watch the evening news, even when it involves violence, in front of young children? Do they discuss television shows with the child?

Ask if the child has had any diseases, whether common ones such as a middle ear infection, or less common ones such as a serious respiratory infection. Has the child been diagnosed with a chronic disorder such as cystic fibrosis or hemophilia? How has that affected the child's general health and family functioning?

Desired outcomes for disease prevention include integration of a healthy lifestyle into the family's daily life, prompt treatment of acute diseases, and individualization of all health supervision topics for the child with a chronic condition or special healthcare need.

Injury Prevention Strategies

Injuries remain a common healthcare problem for children during the toddler and preschooler years. Toddlers' and preschoolers' mobility, physical skills, and lack of understanding of the presence of hazards put them at particular risk. In addition, children are sometimes left to play alone for short periods, and toddlers and preschoolers can quickly get into dangerous situations. Every healthcare visit needs to include an assessment of risks and teaching to prevent injuries. Tables 8–5 and 8–6 list injury hazards and prevention measures to take during these age periods.

Ask parents what they think the most common hazards are for the age of the child, and add other hazards to their awareness. Car safety always needs reinforcing as the types of seats recommended change as the child matures. Children should be in a rear-facing car seat in the back seat until at least age 2 years, and preferably until 4 years or when the child has reached the top height or weight limit allowed by the car seat manufacturer. When the child has reached the highest height and weight allowed by the rear-facing seat, a forward-facing car seat with a harness should be placed in the back seat. Then, when the child has outgrown the recommendations for height and weight for the forward-facing car seat, a booster seat in the back seat is recommended (AAP, 2014).

TABLE 8–5 Injury Prevention in Toddlerhood

	HAZARD	DEVELOPMENTAL CHARACTERISTICS	PREVENTIVE MEASURES
	Falls	Gross motor skills improve: Toddler is able to move chairs to counters and can climb up ladders.	Supervise toddler closely. Provide safe climbing toys. Begin to teach acceptable places for climbing.
	Poisoning	Gross motor skills enable toddler to climb onto chairs and then cabinets. Medicines, cosmetics, and other poisonous substances are easily reached.	Keep medicines and other poisonous material locked away. Use child-resistant containers and cupboard closures. Post the Poison Control Center number (1-800-222-1222) by telephone and tape it on cell phones and program the cell phone with the number.
	Burns	Toddler is tall enough to reach stove top. Toddler can walk to fireplace and may reach into fire. Electrical cords may be placed in mouth.	Keep pot handles turned inward on stove. Do not burn fires without close supervision. Use a fire screen in fireplaces. Supervise child during play and keep electrical cords, power strips, and other hazards out of reach or covered securely.
	Drowning	Toddler can walk onto docks or pool decks. Toddler may stand on or climb seats on boat. Toddler may fall into buckets, toilets, and fish tanks and be unable to get top of body out.	Supervise any child near water. Swimming classes do not protect a toddler from drowning. Use child-resistant pool covers. Use approved child life jackets near water and on boats. Empty buckets when not in use.
	Motor vehicle crashes	Toddler may be able to undo seat belt, may resist using car seat, demonstrating characteristic negativism and autonomy.	Use approved safety seat only; toddler is not large enough to use car seat belts. Insist on safety seat use for all trips and position seat in rear seat of car. Verify that child is belted in properly before starting car. Keep the child in a rear-facing seat until at least 2 years of age and preferably longer, until achieving the highest weight or height recommended for the seat by the manufacturer; then a forward-facing car seat with harness should be used in the back seat.

TABLE 8–6 Injury Prevention in the Preschool Years

	HAZARD	DEVELOPMENTAL CHARACTERISTICS	PREVENTIVE MEASURES

Ruth Jenkinson/DK Images | Motor vehicle crashes | By about 4–5 years, the child independently gets into car and puts on seat belt. Child may forget to belt up or may do so incorrectly. | Verify that child is belted in properly before starting car. Keep the child in a rear-facing seat secured in the back seat until at least 2 years of age and preferably longer, until achieving the highest weight or height recommended for the seat by the manufacturer. Forward-facing seats with harness placed in the back seat are used next. Once the child has outgrown the car seat, a booster seat is used in the back seat. |
	Motor vehicle and pedestrian accidents	Preschooler may play outside alone or with friends. Preschooler is unable to judge speed of moving car and assumes driver knows that he or she is present.	Teach child never to go into road. A safe, preferably enclosed, play yard is recommended. The child should be supervised by adults at all times.
	Drowning	Preschooler who has had swimming lessons may choose to go into a lake or pool.	Teach child never to go into water without an adult. Provide supervision whenever child is near water.
	Burns	Preschooler can understand the hazards of fire.	Teach child to stop, drop, and roll if clothes are on fire. Practice escapes from home are useful. A visit to a fire station can reinforce learning. Teach child how to call 9-1-1.
	Needlesticks in hospital and home	Preschooler can ambulate and is interested in new objects.	Keep needles out of reach. Remove from hospital unit immediately after use. Instruct families on safe disposal if a family member uses needles at home (e.g., a family member with diabetes).
	Electrical injury in hospital and home	Preschooler is mobile and may trip over cords and equipment or may choose to examine them.	Avoid use of electrical cords if possible. Keep equipment out of major traffic areas. Cover any electrical outlets not being used for equipment. Monitor child closely.

Recommend that parents have their child's car seat checked by a child safety seat inspector (Figure 8–3). Give them the addresses of the closest inspection stations. These can be located by going through the National Highway Traffic Safety Administration (2014) (www.nhtsa.dot.gov). Check your particular state laws regulating car safety seats for children.

Other common and serious safety hazards are falls and drowning. In addition to providing general guidelines about safety, these most common injuries should be directly addressed. Children often fall down stairs, from counters where they have been placed or crawled, and from grocery carts. Drowning episodes occur when toddlers and preschoolers are not watched every moment while in the bathtub, near a pool or spa, at a lake or ocean, or when they fall from boats without personal flotation devices on. All young children should begin to take swimming lessons, but this does not guarantee their safety around water.

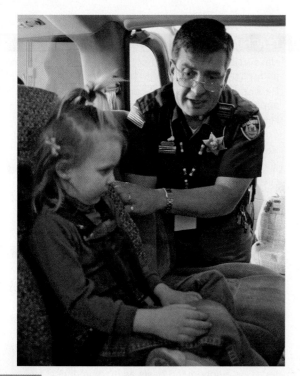

Figure 8–3 This police officer is certified to examine car seats for children and make recommendations for parents. He is examining a preschooler in a car seat for proper fit, alignment, and installation. Many car seats are improperly installed or not the proper type for a specific age/size of child, so centers that check seats provide an important service.

The AAP (2013) recommends swimming lessons for all children by age 4 years and for children from 1 to 4 years if lessons are available and the parents believe the child is ready for lessons. Children also play with balls, and may follow them as they roll or are thrown into the street. Nursing interventions concentrate on relaying to parents the severity of the risk of falls, drowning, and other hazards for children. Teach them to be aware of the dangers and to avoid them, both at home and in other settings. Refer them to classes on first aid and cardiopulmonary resuscitation.

The child spends more time away from the parent than during earlier developmental stages. Childcare situations should provide the same supervision the child receives at home. Help parents to ask questions and feel confident in safety at other settings. For example, while parents may be cautious about gun safety at home, few of them inquire if a home the child is visiting has guns and how they are stored.

Preschool is a time when teaching can become directed both to the parents and to their children. Preschoolers are receptive to practicing street crossing and tricycle/bicycle riding skills. It may be helpful to have a place in the clinic or office where they can be taught basic skills such as hand washing or street crossing. Consider the time of year, climate, and geographic location and teach appropriately. Spring is often a good time to teach bicycle and water safety, while winter hazards may include teaching about the hazards of wood stoves or other heating devices. See Table 8–7 for further information about toddler and preschooler hazards and safety teaching needed.

Desired outcomes for the child are integration of safe practices into car restraints and other daily activities, progression through toddlerhood and preschool with no serious injuries, prompt care for minor injuries, and understanding by child, parent, and other care providers of the common safety hazards at this age.

Nursing Management
For the Health Promotion and Maintenance of the Toddler and Preschooler

Nursing Assessment and Diagnosis

Nurses partner with other healthcare professionals such as physicians, nurse practitioners, and speech therapists to assess health promotion and health maintenance status of young children. The toddler and preschool years are characterized by much developmental progression, and strategies need to be constantly adapted to meet the particular needs of the child and family. It is important to realize that the parents are partners in the care of the child and that every health supervision visit should address their questions and concerns. Their observations of the child are an invaluable part of the process. As preschoolers become more verbal, they become partners with others in the healthcare team. Ask preschoolers what they want to learn, what questions they have about staying well, and other pertinent questions.

Toddlers and preschoolers are examined for growth, physical health status, and mental/social characteristics. Development is an area that many pediatricians feel ill prepared to address but which parents commonly want addressed. Additionally, developmental surveillance must occur at every healthcare visit, with standardized screening at 9, 18, and 24 to 30 months. Nurses are adept at describing normal developmental milestones, evaluating the progression of children, and using anticipatory guidance to address parental developmental concerns.

Based on a thorough assessment, the nurse will establish nursing diagnoses that are appropriate for the young child and family. Potential nursing diagnoses established during a health supervision of a toddler or preschooler might include the following (NANDA-I © 2014):

- *Anxiety* related to change of environment (new care provider)
- *Role Conflict, Parental,* related to lack of support from significant others
- *Development: Delayed, Risk for,* related to lead exposure
- *Sleep Deprivation* related to nightmares and night terrors
- *Knowledge, Readiness for Enhanced,* related to parental desire for safety information
- *Skin Integrity, Impaired,* related to hyperthermia (sunburn)

TABLE 8–7 Disease and Injury Prevention Topics by Age

AGE	INJURY PREVENTION	TEACHING TOPICS
15 months	Wash adult and toddler hands frequently. Clean toys with soap and water regularly. Provide child's own bedding for childcare setting and wash weekly. Use forward-facing car safety seat if child is 20 lb; install correctly and have installation checked; place in back seat and never in front seat with a passenger air bag. Empty containers of water immediately after use; be sure pools or other bodies of water are locked and not accessible. Use sunscreen, hat, and long sleeves in the sun. Keep heavy and sharp objects out of reach; check that all poisons are locked away including in homes visited; keep pet food and cosmetics out of reach.	Have poison control number by phones and taped onto and programmed into cell phones. Be alert for dangers of hot curling irons and other appliances. Have electrical cords out of reach and not hanging down. Keep water temperature no higher than 120°–125°F (49°–52°C). Have home environment checked for lead hazards; arrange for blood lead level testing when appropriate (see Chapter 17). Secure the child in shopping carts. Do not let child have access to alcoholic drinks. Remember that responsible adults—not other children—should always supervise your child. Know CPR, airway obstruction removal, and other first aid.
18 months	Follow the above. Bolt heavy objects securely to the wall to prevent them from being pulled down (such as bookcases and televisions). Be cautious of the toddler near machinery in the yard, such as lawn mowers and farm equipment.	Use a helmet on the child when taking the child on the back of a bicycle. Check batteries in home smoke alarms, CO or radon monitors, and check system monthly; change batteries on a scheduled basis as recommended by manufacturer. Ask care providers about discipline methods; do not allow corporal punishment.
2–3 years	Follow the above. When the child is 40 lb, switch to a belt-positioning booster seat, using vehicle lap and shoulder belt; continue to place booster seat in rear seat of the car. Teach hand hygiene after toileting and other activities. Clean potty chair thoroughly. Keep guns unloaded and locked away in a different locked place than ammunition; have trigger locks installed.	Teach how to cross streets. Provide a helmet for riding tricycles. Check playgrounds for safety hazards and hard surfaces under equipment; ensure cushioned surface.
3–4 years	Follow the above. Do not let child play unsupervised.	Know CPR, airway obstruction removal, and other first aid for the child who has become a preschooler.
4–5 years	Follow the above. Continue teaching safety skills to the child. Continue supervising when near streets or water sources.	Teach safety around strangers (never go with a stranger; find a trusted person such as a parent or police).

Source: Data from Hagan, J. F., Shaw, J. S., & Duncan, P. M. (Eds.). (2008). *Bright futures: Guidelines for health supervision of infants, children, and adolescents* (3rd ed.). Elk Grove Village, IL: American Academy of Pediatrics.

Planning and Implementation

Based on the nursing diagnoses, the nurse works with other partners to plan strategies to meet the needs of the family. Explain that assessment questions are asked to provide a picture of the child that can be helpful in partnering with parents to plan health care. Reinforce the importance of the family coming to health supervision visits with their own list of issues. See *Clinical Reasoning: Families Who Miss Scheduled Healthcare Visits*. Work with other healthcare professionals to be sure all needs of a particular child and family are addressed.

Some teaching takes place as the examination occurs. Explain the height and weight measurements and their meaning. Relate them to questions about dietary intake and family food patterns. During the physical examination, insert information about common infections such as otitis media (middle ear infection) and share immunization information.

Clinical Reasoning Families Who Miss Scheduled Healthcare Visits

Clarence is being seen at 15 months of age. He missed his 12-month visit and was last seen at 9 months. How can you ask the parents about the reasons they may have missed the 12-month visit? What immunizations must be "caught up" now that some were missed? (See Chapter 16 for immunization schedules.) What components of developmental surveillance are particularly important for you to perform at this visit?

If the family has been reluctant to ask questions, reflect on the child's development. "Many children have trouble sleeping through the night; is that the case for Cassandra? What helps her to sleep? What is it like at her bedtime?" Developmental areas such as sleep, discipline, toilet training, and expected developmental milestones should be addressed. If the parents were provided in an earlier visit with a journal to record observations and questions, ask if they have brought it with them.

Health promotion activities are emphasized during the visit. Health promotion related to physical activity includes teaching about toys that encourage activity, such as balls, music, push toys, and tricycles. Review nutritional intake and encourage introduction of new foods, healthy snack and meal choices, and positive eating for busy families. Emphasize the importance of play to healthy child development. Provide ideas for incorporating free playtime each day. Apply concepts of anticipatory guidance as you address the child's approaching developmental progression. If the child will soon be toilet trained, provide information about possible approaches. If the child is learning to swim or has access to water, reinforce safety precautions near water. For the child going to a new childcare center, provide the parents with a list of questions they can ask the care provider, and tips to assist in the transition to a new setting.

Health maintenance activities are added to the visit as you give immunizations and screen for tuberculosis, lead screening, or problems with language, vision, or hearing. Provide instruction on use of nonprescription medications, including use of acetaminophen after immunizations. Precautions, safe dosing, and checking with the healthcare provider should be addressed. The focus of these activities is to prevent disease or to find it early before serious consequences arise. Whenever you find information that may indicate a problem, be sure to refer the child to the primary care provider, such as the physician or nurse practitioner. You may even recommend that another specialist, such as a speech pathologist or dentist, see the child. Other health maintenance activities that must be part of each visit with a toddler or preschooler involve teaching about common hazards and how to avoid them. Emergency care in case of injury is also helpful

information for parents, so first aid classes can be recommended. Ask about daycare, preschool, or kindergarten attendance or future plans.

Healthy People 2020

(V-1) Increase the proportion of preschool children aged 5 years and under who receive vision screening

- While only 40% of preschool children receive vision screening presently, a goal of 44% has been set. Nurses should ensure that all preschool children receive vision screening in childcare centers and at health supervision visits.

(V-2) Reduce blindness and visual impairment in children and adolescents aged 17 years and under

- While 28% of children are blind or visually impaired, when more children are screened in their early years, fewer than 25% of children should experience visual impairment.

SAFETY ALERT!

Nearly 2000 children are injured annually by falls related to baby gates. Those under 2 years more commonly push over an expandable gate and fall down stairs with the gate. Children older than 2 years may climb the gate or open it and thus fall down stairs, often sustaining soft tissue injuries. Ask parents if their homes have stairs. If so, what type of protection is available for the child? Is an expandable gate used? If so, would the parents be able to change to one that is installed into the wall studs? Can a preschooler climb the gate? If so, it is safer to remove the gate and supervise the child more closely (Cheng, Fletcher, Roberts, et al., 2014).

Conclude the visit with some words of praise about both the parent's and child's accomplishments. Schedule the date for the next visit. List any resources helpful to the family, including the clinic/office contact information and emergency services.

Families Want to Know

Toy and Playground Safety

Play is essential to the physical and cognitive growth of toddlers and preschoolers. However, toys can present hazards for young children, and parents need guidelines to follow when selecting toys. These include (Safe Kids, 2011b):

- Select toys intended for the age of the child, as indicated on the label. Some toys have small parts or can break into small parts, and should not be given to children younger than 3 years. They should not be too heavy for the child to manipulate them appropriately. Toys with strings, straps, or cords longer than 7 in. pose strangulation hazards.
- Assemble toys as directed and check them frequently for breakage; remove all packing materials before providing toys for the child.
- Do not use older repainted toys unless the parent is certain that paint used contained no lead.
- Select cloth toys that are nonflammable, flame resistant, or flame retardant. Avoid electrical and battery-powered toys in children younger than 8 years.
- Do not allow latex balloons and especially noninflated balloons to be used as toys.

Playgrounds provide a location for healthy development of children, but can also be responsible for child injuries. Home playgrounds are the sites of most playground injuries. Falls, strangulation, and head impacts are examples of frequent playground injuries. Some tips can be provided to parents (Safe Kids, 2011a):

- Surfaces should be composed of soft and loose material such as mulch or fine sand. The surface should be 12 in. deep and extend 6 ft around equipment.
- Equipment should not allow the child to be more than 5 ft off the surface.
- Strangulation poses a high risk so be sure to remove ties, ribbons, drawstrings, and other hanging items from clothing and play areas.
- Ensure that the equipment is intended for the age of the child. Separate playgrounds for young and older children are recommended.
- Consult the U.S. Consumer Product Safety Commission for playground equipment standards. Inspect equipment regularly.
- Always supervise the young child on a playground at all times.

Evaluation

Parents should be asked occasionally to evaluate the care they are receiving at the health promotion and health maintenance site. Use these comments to monitor and adjust procedures as needed. The expected outcomes for nursing care of the toddler and preschooler include the following:

- The child demonstrates normal patterns of growth and progression in developmental milestones.
- The child remains free of disease and injury.
- Parents relay satisfaction with the pediatric healthcare home.
- The child manifests positive physical, social, and emotional adjustment.

Chapter Highlights

- General observations of physical ability and social interactions are made as the toddler and preschooler appear for the healthcare visit.
- Questions about growth and information related to physical health are integrated during the physical examination.
- The examination should include all areas on the American Academy of Pediatrics Recommendations for Preventive Pediatric Heath Care, with the approaches adapted to the young child.
- Developmental surveillance is integrated within each health promotion/health maintenance visit, and an appropriate developmental screening test is used.

- Toddlers and preschoolers gradually take on mature eating patterns; assessment of nutritional status involves growth, oral health and teeth, foods eaten, and family food patterns.
- Physical ability progresses steadily in young children; opportunities for daily active periods are necessary for healthy growth.
- Early years are essential to development of a positive sense of self, positive social interactions with others, and healthy lifestyle behaviors.
- Immunizations are administered to prevent infectious disease, and safety hazards are addressed at each healthcare visit, with suggestions provided to avoid disease and injury.

Clinical Reasoning in Action

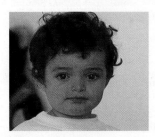

Quinton and his mother have come into the office for his 2-year-old well-child checkup. During the visit you learn that his mother stays home with him during the day and his father often works overtime. His only significant medical history incident was when he had stitches placed in his forehead for falling on the edge of a table when he was 15 months old. There is a family history of attention deficit disorder and Crohn disease. Quinton's height is in the 75th percentile, weight is in the 50th percentile, and body mass index is between the 25th and 50th percentiles. His temperature is 98.9°F (37°C) and his pulse is 80. He is described by his parents as a picky eater and tends to eat the same foods frequently. They also say he tends to eat well on some days and other days will hardly eat anything. On the days he is not eating well, his mother will often resort to giving him soda or a sugary snack just so he is "getting something." Quinton sleeps about 7 hours per night, and his mother usually ends up sleeping with him because he continues to fight going to sleep after being put to bed. He does not have a regular bedtime or rest routine and he usually naps in the car during the day. His mother tells you that her only break during the day when she is at home with Quinton is when he is watching television in his bedroom, so he often watches 2 to 4 hours per day. Quinton has a soft stool every day and has not shown any

interest in potty training at this time. He is developmentally able to go up and down stairs, kick a ball, scribble on paper, and is able to speak in 3- to 4-word sentences. During the visit at the office, it is obvious Quinton's parents have difficulty controlling him and frequently make threats and offer bribes to get him to behave properly. He starts screaming and kicking when his parents set limits on his behavior in the office, and his parents say they are frequently exhausted and do not know what to do about his high energy level. They also are concerned because they feel like the discipline methods they have been using are not working, and he is getting into so many things in the home that they are concerned he may hurt himself. They have used spanking and time-outs, but these methods do not seem to improve his behavior. The parents think their child may have some type of medical condition like attention deficit disorder considering it does run in their family.

1. At 2 years of age, a consistent routine will help a toddler behave more appropriately. What are some of the things you can tell Quinton's parents regarding his sleep and nutrition habits to help establish a better routine?

2. How can you advise Quinton's parents about positive approaches to disciplining him?

3. How can you advise Quinton's parents about disciplining him when it is needed?

4. What are some suggestions you can give Quinton's parents about handling his temper tantrums?

References

American Academy of Pediatric Dentistry (AAPD). (2014). *Guideline on infant oral health care (2012)*. Retrieved from http://www.aapd.org/assets/1/7/G_InfantOral-HealthCare.pdf#xml=http://pr-http://www.aapd.org/media/Policies_Guidelines/G_InfantOralHealthCare.pdf

American Academy of Pediatric Dentistry (AAPD) Council on Clinical Affairs. (2013). *Policy on the dental home* (pp. 24–25). AAPD Reference Manual. Chicago, IL: Author.

American Academy of Pediatrics (AAP). (2013). *Water safety and young children*. Retrieved from http://www.healthychildren.org/English/safety-prevention/at-play/Pages/Water-Safety-And-Young-Children.aspx

American Academy of Pediatrics (AAP). (2014). *Car seats: Information for families for 2014*. Retrieved from http://www.healthychildren.org/English/safety-prevention/on-the-go/Pages/Car-Safety-Seats-Information-for-Families.aspx

American Academy of Pediatrics (AAP) Committee on Nutrition. (2013). *Pediatric nutrition handbook* (7th ed.). Elk Grove Village, IL: Author.

American Academy of Pediatrics (AAP) Committee on Practice and Ambulatory Medicine. (2016). 2016 Recommendations for preventive pediatric health care. *Pediatrics, 137*(1), e20153908. doi:10.1542/peds.2015-3908.

American Academy of Pediatrics (AAP) Council on Communications and Media. (2013). Children, adolescents, and the media. *Pediatrics, 132*, 958–961.

American Dental Association (ADA). (2011). *Thumbsucking*. Retrieved from http://www.ada.org/2977.aspx

Beets, M. W., Bornstein, D., Dowda, M., & Pate, R. R. (2011). Compliance with national guidelines for physical activity in U.S. preschoolers: Measurement and interpretation. *Pediatrics, 127*(4), 658–664.

Centers for Disease Control and Prevention (CDC). (2011). *How much physical activity do children need?* Retrieved from http://www.cdc.gov/physicalactivity/everyone/guidelines/children/html

Cheng, Y. W., Fletcher, E. N., Roberts, K. J., & McKenzie, L. B. (2014). Baby gate-related injuries among children in the United States, 1990–2010. *Academic Pediatrics, 14*, 256–261.

Child Trends. (2012). *Early childhood program enrollment*. Retrieved from http://www.childtrendsdatabank.org/?q=node/280

Child Trends. (2014). *Early childhood developmental screening: A compendium of measures for children ages birth to five*. Retrieved from http://www.acf.hhs.gov/programs/ecd/watch-me-thrive

Colak, H., Dulgergil, C. T., Dalli, M., & Hamidi, M. M. (2013). Early childhood caries updates: A review of causes, diagnoses, and treatments. *Journal of Natural Science, Biology and Medicine, 4*, 29–38.

Hagan, J. F., Shaw, J. S., & Duncan, P. M. (2008). *Bright futures: Guidelines for health supervision of infants, children, and adolescents* (3rd ed.). Elk Grove Village, IL: American Academy of Pediatrics.

Holt, K., Wooldridge, N., Story, M., & Sofka, D. (2011). *Bright futures: Nutrition* (3rd ed.). Elk Grove Village, IL: American Academy of Pediatrics.

Lucas, B. R., Latimer, J., Pinto, R. Z., Ferreira, M. L., Doney, R. Lau, M., . . . Elliot, E. J. (2014). Gross motor deficits in children prenatally exposed to alcohol: A meta-analysis. *Pediatrics, 134*, e192–e209.

Lucille Packard Children's Hospital. (2012). *Upper respiratory infection*. Retrieved from http://www.lpch.org/DiseaseHealthInfo/HealthLibrary/respire/uricold.html

Mayo Clinic. (2014). *Sleep terrors (night terrors)*. Retrieved from http://www.mayoclinic.org/diseases-conditions/night-terrors/basics/risk-factors/con-20032552

National Highway Traffic Safety Administration. (2014). *How to find the right car seat*. Retrieved from http://www.safercar.gov/parents/Car-Seat-Safety.htm

National Institute of Dental and Craniofacial Research. (2014). *Dental caries (tooth decay) in children (age 2 to 11)*. Retrieved from http://www.nidcr.nih.gov/DataStatistics/FindDataByTopic/DentalCaries/DentalCariesChildren2to11.htm

National Resource Center for Health and Safety in Child Care and Early Education. (2013). *Stepping stones* (3rd ed.). Retrieved from http://nrckids.org/CFOC3/index.html

Pender, N. J., Murdaugh, C. L., & Parsons, M. A. (2015). *Health promotion in nursing practice* (7th ed.). Upper Saddle River, NJ: Pearson Prentice Hall.

Rasmussen, C., Kully-Martens, K., Denys, K., Badry, D., Henneveld, D., Wyper, K., & Grant T. (2012). The effectiveness of a community-based intervention program for women at-risk for giving birth to a child with Fetal Alcohol Spectrum Disorder (FASD). *Community Mental Health Journal, 48*, 12–21.

Safe Kids. (2011a). *Playground safety fact sheet*. Retrieved from http://www.safekids.org/our-work/research/fact-sheets/playground-safety-fact-sheet.html

Safe Kids. (2011b). *Preventing injuries: At home, at play, and on the way*. Retrieved from http://www.safekids.org/our-work/research/fact-sheets/toy-safety-fact-sheet.html

Safe Kids. (2014). *Heatstroke*. Retrieved from http://www.safekids.org/heatstroke

Simmonds, M., Burch, J., Llewellyn, A., Griffiths, C., Yang, H., Owen, C., . . . Woolacott, N. (2015). The use of measures of obesity in childhood for predicting obesity and the development of obesity-related disease in adulthood: A systematic review and meta-analysis. *Health Technology Assessment, 19*, 1–336.

U.S. Department of Health and Human Services. (2011). *Healthy People 2020*. Retrieved from http://healthypeople.gov/2020/topicsobjectives2020/pdfs/nutritionandweight.pdf

Zoorob, R. J., Durkin, K. M., Gonzalez, S. J., & Adams, S. (2014). Training nurses and nursing students about prevention, diagnosis, and treatment of fetal alcohol spectrum disorders. *Nurse Education in Practice, 14*, 338–344

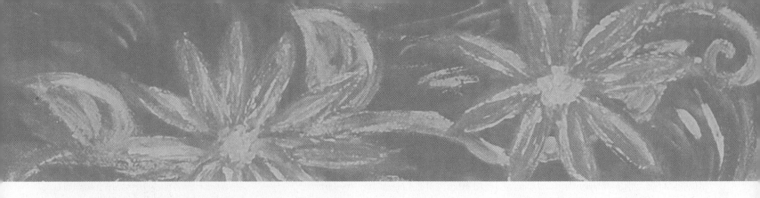

Chapter 9
Health Promotion and Maintenance for the School-Age Child and Adolescent

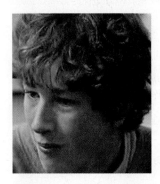

I know I should not be using chewing tobacco, but a lot of my friends use it, and I want to fit in with them. I would like to quit, but I really don't know how.

—Jeremy, 16 years old

⌄ Learning Outcomes

9.1 Identify the major health concerns of the school-age and adolescent years.

9.2 Describe the general observations made of school-age children, adolescents, and families as they come to the "pediatric healthcare home" for health supervision visits.

9.3 Apply communication skills in interactions with school-age children and adolescents.

9.4 Apply assessment skills to plan data-gathering methods for nutrition, physical activity, oral health, and mental health status of youth.

9.5 Synthesize data from history and examination of the school-age child and adolescent with knowledge of development to plan interventions appropriate during health supervision visits.

9.6 Plan with school-age children and adolescents to help them integrate activities to promote health and to prevent disease and injury.

Health Promotion and Maintenance for the School-Age Child

The older childhood years span the time when most children enter kindergarten at about 5 years of age and progress until adolescence begins at about 12 to 13 years of age. Even though health promotion and health maintenance remain important during this time, less frequent visits to the pediatric healthcare home are recommended. In addition, most children are relatively healthy and need few immunizations, which may lead to only sporadic visits for care. Whenever older school-age children are seen in health care, even for illness or emergency care, it is wise to ask when the last "well-child" or health supervision visit was scheduled. Encourage the parents to make an appointment if the child is due for a visit. Visits are generally recommended at about 5 years of age, when most children are going to kindergarten, and then at 6, 7, 8, 9, 10, 11, and 12 years of age. The visits during this time will focus on monitoring physical and developmental changes, establishing good health habits related to important issues such as nutrition, physical activity, and mental health; learning the importance of avoiding tobacco, alcohol, and drugs; ensuring success in school, family, and extracurricular activities; and fostering good decision-making and problem-solving skills.

General Observations

The first school-age health supervision visit usually occurs just before entry into kindergarten. During this visit the child has a thorough examination to be certain that physical development is normal, developmental milestones have been met for fine and gross motor skills, school readiness is displayed in social skills and language, and final sets of basic immunizations are completed. The child is often excited about the visit because it is associated with beginning school; some anxiety is often felt, as it may be the first time the child is aware of getting "shots." As with earlier visits, the nurse's observations begin as the child is called in for the visit. It is wise to speak to the child first, introducing yourself and welcoming the child and parents to the office or clinic. Many children of this age actively participate in conversations, making teaching and gathering data easy. For children who are quiet or look to the parents, allow more time for them to get to know the healthcare provider, directing most initial questions to parents. This may be the first visit where the child is old enough to be a partner in the healthcare visit. Establishing positive rapport with the child will be more likely to enhance efforts designed to teach about health. At the same time, family-centered care, or a partnership to include decision making jointly by the family and the healthcare provider, is important for school-age health (Kuo et al., 2011).

Notice whether the child brought a book, toy, or some other object to the visit. How are the parents interacting with the child? What types of speech tones are used? Is there mutual respect or are parents and child ignoring each other or having disagreements? The child should walk with symmetry and ease of movement, follow instructions about where to go and taking off shoes for weighing, and demonstrate clear language skills with parent or healthcare personnel.

By the time children come for visits at age 6 to 8 years, they are expected to be increasingly active in sports, school activities, music, or other interests. Look for clues about their interests as they arrive. Did they bring books or an electronic device? What are the reading topics or favorite types of music? Ask what they are doing during the summer or about their two favorite after-school activities. Have them describe a typical day to obtain clues about their life.

Some children do not commonly come to clinics, offices, or other settings for health supervision visits. School nurses or nurse practitioners in school-based clinics sometimes offer health promotion/health maintenance activities in the school setting. A major focus of school nurses is making the environment conducive to health for groups of children. School nurses may:

- Offer some parts of examination to individual children, such as growth and developmental surveillance.
- Conduct health screenings, such as vision, hearing, lipids, or scoliosis.

- Work with food service personnel and administration to improve meal and snack quality and minimize unhealthy choices in vending machines.
- Work with teachers to integrate concepts such as physical activity and self-esteem into classroom activities.

The nurse often links children with healthcare needs to other community services.

During health supervision visits, watch the parents' responses as children answer questions. Be alert for the parent who interrupts the child or constantly "corrects" what is said. Comments by the parent should involve praise of the child or looking to the child for opinions on certain topics. This indicates that a partnership is developing in the family and that family members work together and value each other. Also direct some questions to the parents. Ask if they came with specific questions or concerns that should be addressed. If the child has an individualized education or health plan (see Chapter 10), ask if the parent brought a copy, if the plan is still appropriate, or if it needs updating; facilitate a meeting with the school district about the plan if indicated. Allow the parent an opportunity to meet with the physician, nurse practitioner, or other professional in a private place and without the child present if desired. Be alert for family dynamics that can influence mental health status. Ask if there have been any important changes in the family and how they have influenced the child. During conversations, be alert for reports of separation; divorce; remarriages; ill parents, siblings, or grandparents; recent or upcoming moves; parent job changes; substance abuse; incarceration of family members; custody disputes; or other issues. Integrate a family history of diseases into the examination. Such topics can be followed up with further questions, as described later in the mental health section, to learn how they influence the child.

Growth and Developmental Surveillance

When the child first comes into the health supervision site, take height and weight measurements. Be sure to have the child remove shoes and coats. Ask the child and parents if they know the child's current height and weight, and if they have any questions. Plot the percentiles for these measurements, calculate body mass index (BMI) and its percentile, and explain the meaning of these findings later in the visit. Recognize that children do not grow uniformly; they have periods of slow growth followed by fast spurts. Similar to earlier ages, watch for children who have changed channels on a growth grid, and for those above the 85th percentile or below the 5th percentile for BMI, and gather additional nutritional data in these cases (see Chapter 14).

School-age children have begun to learn about their bodies, and so they should be active participants in the physical examination. Explain what you are doing and why. Carry out a head-to-toe examination, paying particular attention to systems and skills that influence performance in school, such as vision, hearing, muscular strength, and coordination. See Chapter 5 for detailed information about the physical examination. Remember to provide feedback about the findings; families appreciate knowing that the child's vision is normal and strength is well developed. Tell them what findings are normal as well as areas that may need more assessment or intervention. Inquire about the child's sleep patterns. During the examination, ask for a description of any illnesses the child has had. Children of school age are generally healthy, with only a few upper respiratory infections or other minor illnesses annually. Unusual complaints may indicate a need for further testing, as discussed in the disease prevention section later in this chapter. Specific screenings for school-age visits include vision, hearing, hematocrit/hemoglobin, and lipid screening (10-year visit recommended for lipids) (American Academy of Pediatrics Committee on Practice and Ambulatory Medicine, 2014).

School-age children frequently have minor injuries. These might include falls from bicycles, skin rashes from exposure to plants on a hiking trip, bruises from a ball sport, and other minor mishaps. Be alert for more serious problems that may indicate a need for additional detailed data gathering and teaching (see *Injury Prevention Strategies* later in this chapter for examples).

Developmental surveillance continues to be an important part of the examination for school-age children. Some milestones can be observed during the visit, while other information is obtained by report of parent and child. This information is combined with reports about school and other activities in order to establish that the child is developing as expected.

Desired outcomes for growth and developmental surveillance include normal progression with developmental tasks, absence of physical and psychosocial abnormalities or trauma, and integration of safe practices into daily life.

Nutrition

Key concepts related to nutrition in school-age children are independence and formation of habits that influence the future. First, children are increasingly independent in food choices. They usually have strong likes and dislikes for certain foods. They may arrive home from school each day to an empty house and prepare their own snacks. During school, they choose what to eat from the school lunch, or the sack lunch sent by family. They may have access to vending machines or sales of snacks during school hours. While independence in food choices is growing, the child is greatly influenced in those choices by friends and the media. Foods that may be rejected often include fresh vegetables and fruits, since they get little media attention, and friends may not prefer them.

At a time when the child chooses many of the foods in the daily diet, habits are being formed that will affect nutrition and health in general in the years to come. Good choices will help promote health—to maintain weight at a recommended level, provide nutrients for adequate growth and activity, and prevent onset of some chronic diseases. Conversely, poor choices can lead to overweight and its accompanying problems, lack of adequate calcium and resultant osteoporosis, eating disorders, or lack of energy for brain growth and optimal performance in school. The patterns established during this period are often influential in later nutritional status. Knowledge about foods, family participation in good nutritional practices, and access to healthy foods can all be enhanced by nursing intervention during this critical formative period.

Continue to perform height and weight measurements, body mass index calculations, and examination of percentiles for growth grid measurements. Slow, steady growth is the norm during the early school-age years; it will be followed by a growth spurt when the child nears puberty.

During the visit, observations provide information about nutritional status. What is the condition of the nails, skin, and hair? What is the energy level and reported physical activity? Does the child look lean or overweight? As the child nears puberty, there may be an increase in fat stores as a preparation for

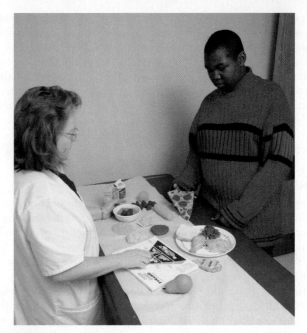

Figure 9–1 This school-age child is receiving teaching from the nurse about food choices. What benefit do the food models provide in this situation? What other teaching techniques can you suggest?

the pubertal growth spurt. Integrate some questions for the parent and child into the visit that provide clues about diet. While observing the child and family and asking dietary questions, list risks and protective factors related to nutrition. Examples of protective factors include adequate access to nutritious foods, a family garden, and weight and height within normal limits; risk factors may include inadequate access to nutritious foods, excess intake of calories during television viewing, and lack of vegetables in the daily diet. Reinforce the positive practices of the family and inform the child of how food choices relate to energy level, school performance, and general health. Risk factors become the basis for teaching and planning with the family for necessary change. It is difficult to tackle several nutritional changes at one time, so concentrate on those most needing attention, and on those the family agrees are important. Provide information about healthy snacks to keep at home, ways to improve calcium intake, the importance of getting at least five fruit/vegetable servings daily, limitation of soft drinks to one serving daily, and the importance of family meals (Figure 9–1). Desired outcomes for health maintenance include absence of overweight and other potential chronic diseases, adequate intake of all nutrients, and increasing child and family knowledge about nutrition.

Physical Activity

Just as food choices during the school-age years are likely to influence the child's future nutrition, physical activity during these years is often crucial to development of lifelong exercise habits. During these years, the child who is physically active continues to refine skills such as eye–hand coordination, muscular strength, agility, and speed. Some children become skilled at ball sports such as basketball, football, soccer, or baseball. Others focus on gymnastics, wrestling, horseback riding, or hockey (Figure 9–2). Some do not like team or organized sports but choose rollerblading, skateboarding, skiing, or biking. Whatever the interest, it is important that children identify some physical

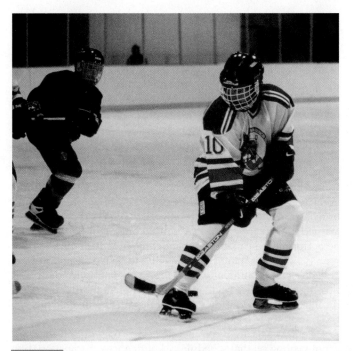

Figure 9–2 Everyone needs to be physically active. Some children participate in school sports. Others, such as these boys playing hockey, choose a sport that is available in the community. Other children prefer to walk, ride a bike, or engage in other more solitary activities. Determine what is enjoyable for a particular child and provide assistance in integrating desired activity into daily routines.

SOURCE: Ruth Bindler.

activity and continue to develop motor skills. The benefits include socialization, positive sense of accomplishment and self-esteem, weight control, and increasing physical ability (Figure 9–3). Children who do not have an activity of importance often fall behind their peers in agility and skill, making future attempts at an activity very difficult and less likely to be successful.

As in earlier periods in life, the nurse lists risk and protective factors related to school-age physical activity (Table 9–1). Families are often significant in promoting physical activity for children. Find out what the parents do for physical activity and how often. Do they attend a sports club after work or does the child see them engaging in exercise? Most families can include some walking, yard work, or other activity that is done together in order to engage the child. Do they walk to a neighbor's house or a nearby store rather than drive? Do they always take elevators, or choose the stairs in buildings? What is the activity level of siblings? When older siblings are involved in sports, the younger child often is encouraged to develop skills in the same sport.

The child spends much of the day in school, and so this setting is important to consider. In an effort to conserve financial resources, some schools have decreased physical education (PE) programs. Children may not have regular PE classes, and there may be few standards of performance. In addition, many states and provinces have established tests and standards for performance in certain cognitive areas. In an attempt to increase teaching time to meet standards, some schools have cut out recess and other breaks. Some schools are located in unsafe areas and outside recreation is not advisable.

It is unrealistic to expect children to sit for long periods without physical activity, and such practice reinforces the poor habits of inadequate exercise among children. Schools that offer a

TABLE 9–1 Risk and Protective Factors Regarding Physical Activity in School-Age Children

RISK FACTORS	PROTECTIVE FACTORS
• Developmental delay and special needs	• Expected developmental skill level
• Limited role modeling of daily physical activity by parents and other family members	• Parents exercise daily and exercise with the child some of this time in a setting the child can see • Parents set expectation that everyone in the family will choose a physical activity and engage in it regularly
• Limited facilities in the neighborhood to encourage activity, such as parks, skateboard facilities, rinks, ball courts	• Neighborhood provides access to parks, skateboard facilities, rinks, ball courts, and other facilities
• Inadequate financial resources to join clubs or pay for organized sports	• Family has adequate financial resources to pay for health club or organized sports
• Safety gear for activities chosen is not available due to cost, or child is reluctant to use the gear	• Recommended safety gear that properly fits child is available • The child understands importance of safety gear and accepts using such equipment
• School cuts to physical education programs and recess	• Schools provide physical education each day with a variety of offerings; student gets to choose and set goals for some activities • Schools schedule recess or physical activity breaks twice daily
• School tryouts for sports that eliminate all but the best players in certain sports	• Sports teams are leveled so that all students desiring to play a particular sport, such as soccer, are able to do so
• Reluctance to try new activity	• Willing to try new activities
• Worry about competence and physical appearance	• Feels self-confident in ability and physical appearance • Sets goals for learning physical skills
• Television viewing or other screen activities for more than 2 hr daily	• Television viewing and other screen activities are limited to no more than 2 hr daily

Source: Data from Hagan, J. F., Shaw, J. S., & Duncan, P. M. (Eds.). (2008). *Bright futures: Guidelines for health supervision of infants, children, and adolescents* (3rd ed.). Elk Grove Village, IL: American Academy of Pediatrics.

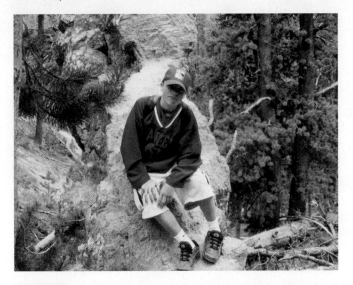

Figure 9–3 **Benefits of physical activity. School-age children often enjoy hikes with family, clubs, or other groups. What are the physical and mental health benefits from this activity?**

SOURCE: Ruth Bindler

variety of activities, including intramural (rather than only organized competitive) sports, are more likely to encourage a wide variety of children to be active. At least half of the recommended 60 minutes of daily vigorous physical activity should be provided in school, along with an adequate amount of unstructured playtime during recess (Centers for Disease Control and Prevention [CDC], 2011a). Nurses are influential members of school committees and can encourage the integration of activity in the school day. They may be able to serve on a school or community committee, informing other committee members of the benefits of exercise to enhance cognitive performance and general health. Teachers and school administrators can be supplied with models of successful school activity programs. Nurses can often be influential in finding community volunteers to work with teams of students. Student nurses, physical education students, senior citizens, and others in the community may be able to help young children play baseball, tennis, or soccer. Other volunteers may teach stretching or warm-up activities. Community partners such as businesses may provide protective gear or uniforms for school sports, especially if the business name can be displayed. In addition, schools can offer alternative activities that some children might prefer to traditional organized sports.

It is essential to consider physical activity for the child who has special healthcare needs. It may be difficult for schools to plan an activity for the child with cerebral palsy, visual impairment, or developmental delay. Search for other community resources and help the family access them. There may be programs for children to ride horses, swim, ski, and engage in other physical activities. Learn about the Special Olympics for children with disabilities. Imagine the thrill that awaits a child who has rarely moved quickly when riding a sled or sliding on skis.

To summarize, health promotion activities for the nurse include teaching about activities that parents can do with their children, becoming active in fostering physical education programs in schools, acting as a positive role model, and helping interested children to partner with community resources for activity. Health maintenance outcomes include encouragement for use of safety gear and correct techniques to prevent injury from sport participation.

Oral Health

Many changes occur in the mouth during the school-age years, necessitating periodic examination. At about 6 years of age, most children lose a tooth, usually in the front. Following that, all 20 of the deciduous or primary teeth will be lost, and the permanent teeth will simultaneously begin to erupt. See Chapter 5 for the schedule of deciduous tooth loss and permanent tooth eruption. In addition, the jaw line elongates and teeth move into new positions. Periodic dental visits focus on both the placement of teeth and oral hygiene.

During the health promotion visit, examine the teeth. Look to see how many deciduous and permanent teeth are present. Describe the child's oral hygiene. Ask how often the child brushes, flosses, and visits the dentist. The child should have learned how to brush and floss during preschool years and now be performing the skills independently. If dental caries or poor oral hygiene is apparent, ask the child to demonstrate brushing and flossing. Reinforce the need for brushing twice daily and flossing once daily. Provide toothpaste and toothbrushes as gifts during health supervision visits. Local dentists will often provide these supplies to encourage oral hygiene.

Dental visits are recommended every 6 months. If the child is not visiting on that schedule, ask if finances or transportation is an issue, if the family needs a referral to a dentist, or if there is some other reason. If caries or malocclusion is present, stress the need for a dental appointment soon. Inquire about use of fluoride if the water supply is not fluoridated. Ask if the child has had sealants applied to the permanent teeth; most dentists believe these will help to prevent future caries (American Academy of Pediatric Dentistry [AAPD], 2012). Offer to help parents locate resources to assist with dental care expenses if needed. State and community programs are often available to assist families, and nurses should search out resources in their own communities and regions.

Many children have a high intake of sugared foods and snacks. If this is apparent from the nutritional assessment, discuss the importance of limiting these foods and brushing after their consumption. Frequent brushing is needed when the child has braces. Ask how they are caring for the braces and what the orthodontist has recommended.

The nurse's health promotion activities include positive reinforcement of good hygiene habits, and health maintenance involves teaching about the need for improved care and limiting food that furthers the formation of caries. Desired outcomes include recommended oral hygiene, attendance at recommended dental visits, and absence of dental caries.

Clinical Reasoning Dental Health

The family of 7-year-old Mario just moved to your city. You learn in a healthcare visit that Mario has never been to a dentist. You notice that several of his teeth are decayed. He has started to lose his primary teeth and has two permanent teeth in place. A dietary recall demonstrates that he drinks two to three sweetened beverages daily and likes to eat candy whenever possible.

Describe the daily dental hygiene that Mario should be practicing. Plan a teaching session for Mario and his parents. What other cues will you look for in his dietary recall in order to identify risk and protective factors for oral health? How will you locate resources in the community to recommend for the family so that Mario can receive dental care?

Mental and Spiritual Health

SELF-ESTEEM AND SELF-CONCEPT

The school-age years are marked by the emergence of new cognitive skills and the development of self-esteem. **Self-esteem** reflects feelings of self-worth or value. **Self-concept** refers to evaluations of the self in certain specific areas, such as those related to academic achievement, athletic ability, physical appearance, and social interactions (Santrock, 2012). A child with a positive self-concept feels competent, is able to meet challenges, and applies lessons from successes and failures. Specific facets of self-concept include **body image**, the idea that one forms about one's body, and **sexuality**, the person's view of self as a sexual being. Together, self-concept and self-esteem include all of the cognitive, emotional, spiritual, sexual, and physical aspects of the individual.

The child who believes in his or her ability to face good times and bad has a lowered chance of mental illness such as depression, eating disorder, and anxiety. Parents are encouraged to evaluate and help to build the child's sense of self-esteem (see *Families Want to Know: Evaluating and Fostering Self-Esteem*).

Many of the areas discussed already in this chapter provide clues to the child's self-concept. Does the child take part in sports or other physical activities? Such activity may reflect a positive self-concept and body image. However, if the child is forced to do these sports by parents and feels inadequate in their performance, these activities may promote a negative self-concept and body image. Ask about children's activities and how they feel about them. Do they enjoy them? How do they rate their performance?

Is the child increasingly independent and responsible for self? Success in achieving developmental milestones leads to a positive sense of self-esteem in the child. Parents are encouraged to evaluate and help to build the child's sense of self-esteem. A low sense of self-esteem is noted when the child states a disinterest in exercise, school clubs, and family activities. This can lead to loneliness, depression, and mental health problems such as eating disorders. When these feelings are noted during a health supervision visit, the nurse should recommend that the child see a counselor at school or another setting, and should recommend that parents be included in the sessions so that they can best help the child.

It is obvious that the family plays a critical part in the child's developing self-esteem and mental health. To understand the child, it is necessary to ask questions about and explore dynamics in the family. Several protective factors have been identified for families (U.S. Department of Health and Human Services, 2011):

- Nurturing bonds and attachment are formed.
- Parents have knowledge about parenting skills and child development.
- Parents demonstrate resilience by recognizing their own stress and enhancing their problem-solving abilities.
- Parents have a wide array of support systems to provide social connections.
- Caregivers are available who provide resources to meet basic needs, such as finances, housing, and food.

School-age children continue to develop their abilities to self-regulate activities and responses to situations. At this age, the abilities to solve problems and assume more responsibility for self are important. Encourage parents to discuss issues with the child and to seek solutions together when appropriate. The child assumes more responsibility for assisting with meal preparation and home chores, coming home alone after school, and caring for younger siblings. Encourage the parents to praise the child for assuming more family responsibilities and recognize that the child will need some guidance when taking on new tasks.

Families Want to Know

Evaluating and Fostering Self-Esteem

Parents play an important part in fostering a child's self-esteem. The nurse can ask parents to evaluate the child and provide suggestions about positive actions.

Evaluation Questions	Positive Actions
What does your child do well?	Build on the child's strengths and talents; affectionately point out the child's abilities.
How does your child respond to failure?	Assist children to assess their own performance; help them to see lessons that mistakes can teach.
Does your child have close friends?	Arrange structured playtimes such as going to a movie or cooking with a friend.
How does your child respond to new challenges?	Give the child responsibilities at home; encourage your child to try new experiences; help the child feel a sense of control over outcomes.
How does your own personality compare to your child's?	Recognize differences in style; appreciate the unique qualities of each child; tailor expectations to the child and not to self or other children.
Are you setting reasonable and attainable expectations for your child?	Be a positive role model; establish goals for behaviors together.

Source: Data from KidsHealth. (2011). *Developing your child's self-esteem.* Retrieved from http://kidshealth.org/parent/emotions/feelings/self_esteem.html

Ask about and observe the family's relationships. Evaluate the effect of family interactions on the child. Model respectful interchanges by listening carefully to the child, as well as the parent. Gently speak directly to the child if parents answer for the child or seem to put the child down. Provide brochures and examples of ways to show children their importance. Encourage both parents to come to child healthcare visits and support the involvement of both parents in childrearing. Ask about family stressors such as job changes, financial concerns, illness, substance abuse, and domestic violence. About one half of marriages end in divorce, so be prepared to offer suggestions to deal with this situation. Ask about and identify risk factors and protective factors. The child's strengths are used to assist the family functioning and will, in turn, give the child a sense of accomplishment. Some examples include the following:

- A child who is able to act independently can be given responsibility for parts of the home or family function, such as planning the menu for dinner two evenings weekly, caring for a family pet, or completing household chores.

- A creative child can be given the task of planning book readings and other activities for a younger sibling.

- A child with a talent for design can be asked to set the table for dinner guests.

SEXUALITY AND SEXUALITY EDUCATION

The school-age child is developing a sense of body image and sexuality. Be aware of the child's appearance and dress. Some children may have poor posture, display a sense of insecurity, and seem uncomfortable with themselves. Others may dress as if they were much older, seem sophisticated, and are clearly assuming the role identification with their gender group. Ask the parents in a private setting what observations they have about the child's body image and sexuality. Inquire about friends in whom the child seems romantically or sexually interested, and whether the parent has concerns.

Questions related to sexuality will emerge during school years. They should be answered truthfully and fully. Even children who do not ask questions usually need information related to sexuality education. They may get information in school beginning in about fourth grade, but often still have misconceptions about the bodies of men and women, sexual intercourse, how babies are born, and other topics. Suggest that parents read books with their children that deal with these issues at a level that children understand. If books are available at home, children will be likely to look at them and ask questions. They should be in the home from third grade on since many young girls have body changes as early as 9 or 10 years of age (see Chapter 5). This can often put both the parent and child at ease and open the door to discussion. Parents should be advised to talk with teachers to learn what is presented in school and be able to supplement and clarify this information. Having discussions at a young age will help lead to further discussion as the child gets older. Nurses often perform sexuality education in schools or work with school districts in establishing policies regarding sexuality education plans. Help the parents plan to discuss appropriate and inappropriate touch so that the child understands and states those who can help in situations that lead to discomfort. (See Chapter 17 for a thorough discussion of child abuse.)

Suggest to parents that computers and other media provide information that can confuse children. Encourage them to watch movies with their children, engage in frank discussions related to sexuality observed, and answer questions truthfully. Children generally learn about topics such as sexual intercourse, homosexuality, and childbirth from school discussions and the media. It is better to learn from parents than from friends or the media. A few moments alone with parents and the child separately at healthcare visits may help to identify the concerns of each related to sexuality.

By approximately 9 to 12 years (fourth to sixth grades), most girls have started to have prepubertal body changes and have had their first menses. This is another opening for discussions about mature bodies of men and women and the transformation from childhood to greater maturity. Boys mature about 2 years later than girls. Without an event such as menstruation, parents may be less likely to start discussions with male children. Suggest that parents consciously begin conversations with boys periodically to explain changes they see in themselves and their peers. See Chapter 5 for further discussion of the body changes seen in the prepubertal period and during puberty.

SLEEP

Sleep is important for children because it helps provide the energy they will need to perform well in school and other activities. They generally take charge of bedtime routines with reminders about the time to go to sleep, and they sleep through the night. Sleep time varies from 8 to 12 hours, depending on the child and activity level. Busy schedules may interrupt this pattern, leading to irritability, lack of concentration, or even hyperactive behavior. Help children and families plan for healthy practices of **sleep hygiene**, or behaviors that foster a regular and sufficient sleep pattern, as well as daytime alertness (Mayo Clinic, 2013).

Sleepwalking and sleep talking sometimes occur at this age, but usually decrease as the child nears adolescence. Children who have stress at home, such as parental fighting, ill family members, or inadequate food or shelter, may not get enough sleep and fall asleep at school. Ask children if they fall asleep in class, and seek additional information about family stressors. This can lead to interventions such as recommending family counseling or referring to resources to obtain better housing or more stable food sources.

SCHOOL

School is a major microsystem that influences the lives of children and plays a role in self-concept and mental health formation. The child is usually ready for kindergarten when (Hagan, Shaw, & Duncan, 2008):

- Communication and cognitive skills are sufficient to support learning.

- The child can successfully separate from parents.

- Experiences with other children show ability to make friends and regulate own behavior.

- The child can follow rules and directions.

Help parents learn ways that they can facilitate a healthy transition to school, such as ensuring good sleep and eating routines, reading with the child, showing interest in school activities, and finding a space in the home for the child's school-related work.

When examining a school-age child, ask for a description of a best friend. If the child is unable to provide this, isolation may be occurring. Inquire about what the three best and three worst things are about school. Children with low self-concepts often have trouble talking about and evaluating school. Find out where

Families Want to Know

Sleep Hygiene

Nurses should inquire about the sleep patterns and amount of sleep that children receive. Ask if they are frequently tired or have trouble sleeping. Some simple behaviors help promote sleep and are referred to as *sleep hygiene.* They include (Mayo Clinic, 2013):

- Go to bed and get up at approximately the same time each day, including weekends.
- Follow a bedtime routine to prepare for sleep.
- Recognize that we do not "make up" sleep that is "lost" by sleeping in.
- Avoid caffeine, including tea, coffee, and carbonated beverages, for several hours before sleep.
- Gradually slow down activity about an hour or two before bedtime.
- Do not watch television, play games, text on the phone, or conduct other activities in the sleep location.
- Avoid naps in the late afternoon or evening.
- Darken the room for sleep.

the child attends school, if the area is generally safe, and how the child gets to school. Encourage the parents to meet the child's teachers, to become active in school activities, and to be available to solve problems with school personnel when needed. Partner with the parents and child when interventions are needed. An office nurse may contact a school nurse when the child needs support in the school environment. This may occur if the child has become ill and missed school, has family stressors, does not get along well with a teacher, or has a condition such as attention deficit disorder. Identify the risk and protective factors in the school environment and plan interventions to support the child when risks are present.

EVALUATING MENTAL HEALTH AND SPIRITUAL HEALTH

Certain mental health disorders are commonly seen during the school years. One example is anxiety problems that result in worries, fears, physical symptoms, stress, and sleep disorders without significantly impairing daily functioning. However, some anxiety disorders affect functioning and have more striking characteristics such as clinging, abdominal pain and headache, and refusal to attend school. Posttraumatic stress syndrome and depression may also be seen. See Chapter 28 for further description of these disorders. Anxiety disorder, posttraumatic stress, and depression should be referred to a mental health specialist for treatment. However, all children worry at times, and this type of anxiety can be helped by learning coping skills and relaxation techniques.

Spiritual health is the ability to develop a spiritual nature, including awareness of a life purpose or meaning, a sustaining power during times of stress, a feeling of harmony with the universe, and a sense of fulfillment (Pender, Murdaugh, & Parsons, 2015). School age is a time when children learn more about the people and the world around them, and begin to find their place in that world. Connection with faith-based groups assists some children and families in defining the purpose of life, while others may do so through social activity or a strong moral sense of responsibility. Ask children what brings happiness, how they help other people, or if they are members of a church, synagogue, or mosque. If families seem to have little purpose, parents are withdrawn or depressed, or the child has difficulty answering questions about meaningful activities, suggest methods of engagement in the community. Strategies might include providing contacts at local religious events, posting flyers about community events designed to bring unity to various cultural groups, or suggesting services needing volunteers

in the community. Families who spend time together and find meaning in supporting each other nurture the spiritual health of their members. Suggest that every family plan a "family night" weekly when they play games, talk, eat, or engage in other activities together.

The nurse has an important role in fostering the mental and spiritual health of school-age children. Health promotion fosters the strengths of families and children, leading to healthy self-concept and positive self-esteem. Health maintenance seeks to prevent mental health disruptions. Be alert for risk factors in families since they represent the need for intervention. Expected outcomes for health promotion and health maintenance activities with school-age children include formation of a positive sense of self-esteem and healthy body image, use of coping skills to deal with stress, sleep patterns that meet needs for rest, and a growing purpose and meaning in life.

Relationships

Although the school-age child is gradually moving away from the family as the center of life, the family remains an important anchor. Ask about siblings, grandparents, and other extended family members. Sometimes these persons assist in the child's formation of a self-concept. Peers are increasingly important to the school-age child's self-identity. School age is a time of cooperative engagement with others. All children need to learn how to make and maintain friendships and work with others on projects and in recreation.

Inquire about the child's friends and activities at school. In private, ask parents if they are comfortable with the child's selection of friends. Find out if the parents facilitate friendships by allowing other children to come to the home and providing transportation as needed. When the child experiences a risk factor such as a move to a new town or school, role-play how to meet new children and how to make friends. If the child feels like an outcast or outsider among peers at school, explore how the family can create a safe and secure place for the child through extracurricular activities with children who have similar interests. When children are home schooled, the family should encourage social events and contacts after usual school hours.

Since peers are important to the school-age child, the child may feel pressure to appear like others, to fit in, and to do what others encourage. Although such pressures are often associated with teen years, they usually begin earlier, at least by 8 or 9 years of age. Ask children what kinds of things their friends try to get them to do that they know they should not do, or if friends have tried to get them to smoke. Middle school years are the most common age for beginning to smoke, so always ask if the child has tried smoking, being careful to do this when the parent is not present and the child is more likely to be honest. When parents are not in the room they may also tell you about other activities, such as playing with guns, trying alcohol or other substances, or other risky behavior. It is best to ask children what they do in these situations, what they want to do, and who they can talk to about these events. Offer information about the risks connected with behaviors that are described, and suggest people such as parents, teachers, counselors, or clergy who are possible resources. If the child's health is at risk, be sure to report the activity to the physician or other healthcare provider so that it can be pursued and the child's safety can be assured. Activities such as playing with firearms or visiting a friend whose parents are making methamphetamine, for example, place children in extreme danger.

Parents often need guidance to help them in setting limits for their school-age children. The child is becoming more independent but unacceptable behaviors must still be managed by successful discipline techniques. Some guidelines that can help families include talking calmly about behaviors that are unacceptable, using techniques such as natural consequences or withholding privileges, modeling, and suggesting stress relief such as physical activity (American Academy of Pediatrics [AAP], 2011a).

School age is often a time when children first experience violence in relationships with others. Some children are bullied, while others are the bullies. Anger and aggression can occur, and children may engage in violence with each other. Ask children to describe when they last had a disagreement with someone and how the problem was solved. Suggest people who can help, such as school nurses, teachers, and counselors, and be sure that children feel safe in schools, neighborhoods, and homes. Ask parents how they resolve arguments between children at home and what help they need to help children learn problem-solving skills. Find out what policies the local schools have to assist in decreasing harassment of and by children. Become active on school committees that help children learn how to solve problems peacefully and how to respond to episodes of violence. See Chapter 17 for further discussion of violence in children and a detailed discussion of bullying.

The child's temperament (see Chapter 4) still plays a part in response to situations and the ability to self-regulate. The "difficult" child may have trouble getting to sleep or being quiet in the classroom. Have parents plan more physical activity for this child. Teach the child that bedtime routines are helpful and that sitting near the front of the class can help with concentration. The "slow to warm up" child may need ideas about what to say when meeting new people. Parents can help the child prepare for a new school by visiting the school with the child, talking about it, and meeting with the teacher so that a warm welcome can occur. The "easy" child is usually adaptable in most situations and is regular in activities. However, this child may object when other children interrupt, fail to take turns, or otherwise "break the rules" of behavior. They might need help in understanding differences in temperament in order to be more tolerant of classmates and their behaviors. Often nurses in schools address the issue of individual differences by speaking with classes or small groups of children.

The nurse takes an active role in promoting the child's health by anticipating developmental issues and preparing the parents and child to deal with them. Health maintenance outcomes include prevention of problems such as bullying.

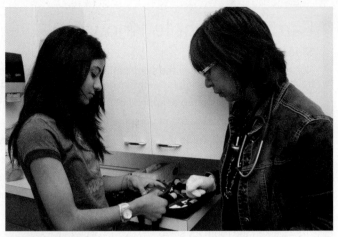

Figure 9–4 School nurse's role in managing health problems. A student with diabetes is showing the school nurse how she programs her insulin pump. The nurse has partnered with nurses in the endocrinology office to learn about the type of pump the student is using. Such collaboration contributes to the monitoring and management of diabetes.

Disease Prevention Strategies

School-age children are generally healthy. The immune system is mature (see Chapter 22), personal hygiene practices are more developed than at earlier ages, and immunizations are usually complete. Engage school-age children in active pursuit of their own health. Teach strategies that can enhance the prevention of diseases. Nurses in offices and schools can teach children how to wash hands effectively, how respiratory infections are transmitted, what can cause gastrointestinal illness, and how to best manage their own health problems (Figure 9–4). Ask children in your settings what topics are of most interest to them and be prepared to suggest common areas of concern such as safety, skin care, athletics, and illnesses. Children can understand the connection between eating well and avoiding illness, maintaining normal weight and preventing type 2 diabetes, avoiding smoking to prevent cancer and other respiratory diseases, maintaining oral hygiene to promote oral health, and exercising to prevent hypertension.

School-age children are in the concrete stage of intellectual development, according to Piaget (see Chapter 4). This means that teaching is most effective when opportunities are provided to touch, feel, and otherwise become actively engaged in learning. When teaching about smoking, provide models of lungs and have the students breathe through a straw to demonstrate the effects of airway narrowing. These concrete activities will teach them concepts better than simple lecture or reading (Figure 9–5). Concepts of health promotion tend to be abstract since they deal with supporting one's highest potential for wellness. Thus it becomes even more important to provide concrete methods of learning.

Immunizations are generally up-to-date for school-age children. However, some children may have missed earlier doses because of illness or missed healthcare visits. Evaluate the immunization record to be sure it meets all recommendations. The most common immunization needs at this time include the following:

- Hepatitis B (whole series or a missed third dose)
- Hepatitis A (two doses if not previously administered)

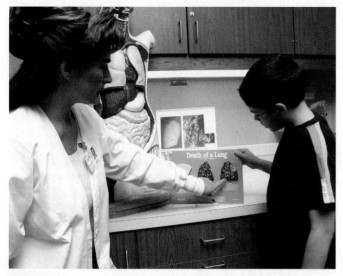

Figure 9–5 Concrete experiences for health teaching. This boy is learning about the effects of smoking on the body through the concrete experience of examining a model of the lungs. Why does this type of hands-on technique help school-age children to learn concepts?

- Poliomyelitis, and measles-mumps-rubella (if booster doses of each were not given prior to school entry)
- Tetanus-diphtheria-acellular pertussis (Tdap) at the 11- to 12-year visit
- Varicella if not given earlier and the child has not had the disease
- Human papillomavirus (HPV) three-dose series at 9 years or older
- Meningococcal conjugate vaccine at 11 years with booster at 16 years
- Influenza annually
- Certain vaccines for children at high risk, such as meningo-coccal and pneumococcal (see Chapter 16 for further infor-mation on immunizations)

Screenings for health risks should occur during the visit. These include hearing and vision screening, blood pressure monitoring, tuberculin skin test, and, in some cases, screening for hyperlipidemia and lead exposure (American Academy of Pediatrics Committee on Practice and Ambulatory Medicine, 2016). Unusual complaints may indicate a need for further test-ing. Examples include the following:

- Pain other than brief discomfort after an injury
- Headaches
- Bruising
- Lack of coordination
- Repeated infections
- Decreasing vision or hearing
- Problems or changes in school performance or behavior

Children who have an identified health problem or devel-opmental disability may have additional needs for screening and for interventions to assist with health maintenance. For example, the child with cystic fibrosis will need information to reduce the risk of respiratory infection, and the child with diabetes may need additional blood studies. The child who has difficulty reading will need alternative approaches to teaching correct hand hygiene; demonstration with explanation may be the best approach.

Inquire about any medications the child takes, including vitamins, fluoride, and nonprescription medications. Some families use complementary therapy for common conditions such as respiratory infections or gastrointestinal complaints. Complementary therapy is quite common in families where children have chronic conditions such as attention deficit hyperactivity disorder, autism, and skin conditions (Ben-Arye et al., 2011).

Parents should receive explanations about the screening tests performed and the results obtained. Inform them about vision and hearing results. Send home or call about results of blood tests when available. Be sure they understand the find-ings and have resources to assist in preventing or treating the specific disease in their children. Have them call with questions about health problems the child develops, and provide informa-tion about lowering risks of diseases. Be sure that families know when to keep children home from school (elevated temperature, active vomiting or diarrhea, coughing up brown or green mucus). Assist schools in setting guidelines for management of infectious diseases in that setting. Contact the local county and state health department for infectious disease guidelines for schools. Desired outcomes for the school-age child include prevention of infec-tious diseases, prompt treatment for acute infections, and careful management of existing health conditions in order to maximize health potential.

Injury Prevention Strategies

Injuries are a common cause of morbidity and mortality among school-age children, and each health maintenance encounter should include injury prevention strategies. Children of this age have more independence and may be harmed by activities they engage in without adults present, such as playing with fire or firearms. They participate in many sports and other physical activities and may sustain related injuries. Some children unfor-tunately suffer from harm due to physical abuse or other forms of violence (see Chapter 17).

Many common injuries are preventable with simple use of protective gear and the following safety guidelines. About 7% to 8% of youth rarely or never wear seat belts in automobiles, and in some states, up to 16% do not use seat belts (CDC, 2014). Certain groups of children are more at risk than others of not taking protective measures. Many children ride bicycles, but only a fraction of them use helmets. Strategies to make helmet use more attractive and to ensure correct wearing of helmets are needed (see *Evidence-Based Practice: Bicycle Helmet Effective-ness and Use*).

Identify youth engaging in risky activities and teach them safe practices. Join with schools and community groups to estab-lish education programs. Provide information about adequate conditioning for sports in order to decrease chance of overuse injury. Each visit should contain basic history questions related to injury prevention. Pursue topics that appear to indicate prob-lems. After information has been collected during the visit, plan two or three health maintenance topics that seem most important for injury prevention in the family. When there is a history of injury in the child, partner with the family to plan ways to avoid repeated harm. Table 9–2 lists some common injury hazards dur-ing the school years, and Table 9–3 offers suggestions for injury prevention teaching.

EVIDENCE-BASED PRACTICE | Bicycle Helmet Effectiveness and Use

Clinical Question

About 800 people die of bicycle-related injuries annually in the United States and there are over 500,000 emergency room visits for bicycle injuries, 60% of which involve children. Youth from 15 to 24 years old have the highest rate of bicycle injuries (CDC, 2013). Although helmets can reduce injury, many times they are not worn or are worn incorrectly. What are the factors that foster helmet use, and how can nurses contribute to efforts for use of bicycle helmets?

The Evidence

Wearing bicycle helmets is associated with higher household incomes, living in a state with a bicycle helmet law, younger ages, and having health insurance (Devoe, Tillotson, Wallace, et al., 2012). Bicycle helmets are often the wrong size or incorrectly adjusted so that they fit children improperly (Thai, McIntosh, & Pang, 2014).

Best Practice

Nurses should provide information about helmet use for bicycles and other vehicles. Engage children at community events and in schools. Inquire about helmet use at every healthcare visit. Reinforce proper fit and maintenance of helmets.

Clinical Reasoning

Where will you find information about helmet safety? What educational programs are available in your schools and communities? Are helmets made available for families that might not be able to buy them? How do you determine if a child is wearing a helmet correctly? Plan educational materials and programs for children who bicycle, ride skateboards, or use scooters.

TABLE 9–2 Injury Prevention in the School-Age Years

	HAZARD	DEVELOPMENTAL CHARACTERISTICS	PREVENTIVE MEASURES
	Motor vehicle/pedestrian/biking crashes	Child plays outside; may follow ball into road; rides two-wheeler.	Teach child safe outside play, especially near streets. Reinforce use of bike helmet. Teach biking safety rules and provide safe places for riding.
	Firearms	Child may have been shown location of guns; is interested in showing them to friends.	Teach child never to touch guns without parent present. Guns should be kept unloaded and locked away. Guns and ammunition should be stored in different locations. Be sure guns have trigger locks.
	Burns	Child may perform experiments with flames or toxic substances.	Teach child what to do in case of fire or if toxic substances touch skin or eyes. Reinforce teaching about 9–1-1.
	Assault	Child may be left alone after school and may walk, bike, or take public transportation alone.	Provide telephone numbers of people to contact in case of an emergency or if child feels lonely. Leave child alone for brief periods initially, and evaluate child's success in managing time. Teach child not to accept rides from, talk to, or open doors to strangers. Teach child how to answer the phone.

TABLE 9–3 Injury Prevention Topics by Age

AGE (YEARS)	INJURY PREVENTION	TEACHING TOPICS
5–8	Use a booster seat, properly positioned in the back seat of the car; when the child is large enough for the vehicle seat belt, use both lap and shoulder belts. Never place a child in the front seat of a car with a passenger air bag. Restrain all children younger than 13 years in the rear seat. Be sure the child knows how to swim and works on these skills regularly. Protect the child with sunscreen when outside. Check smoke alarms and keep them functioning properly. Have an escape plan in case of fire in the home. Keep poisons, electrical appliances, and fire starters locked. Keep firearms unloaded and locked; store ammunition in a separate locked location; have trigger locks installed on guns; keep dangerous knives locked. Provide protective gear for bicycling and other activities and insist that it be worn. Teach safety precautions for bicycling and other activities.	Teach safety with strangers. Provide a list of people a child can approach if feeling threatened by touch or other experience. Choose care providers carefully; occasionally pick up child earlier than expected; ask about policies regarding discipline and do not leave child with someone who uses corporal punishment. Be sure the child knows emergency numbers, names, and plans. Review carefully any hazardous event that has occurred with the child and summarize what was done correctly and how response could be improved. Limit screen time to 2 hr daily; do not allow violent games or viewing. Review behavior with strangers regularly such as not getting in cars and not engaging in phone or Internet conversations.
8–10	Use car booster seat until child sits upright against back seat with bent knees over edge of seat; insist on use of lap and shoulder belts. Do not place child in front seat of car with a passenger air bag.	Do not allow child to operate power tools or machinery. Continue to reinforce other teaching described above, include child more fully, and expand responsibility to the child with increasing age.
10–12	Continue to reinforce teaching described above. Parents and child should attend class on cardiopulmonary resuscitation and airway obstruction removal.	Avoid high noise levels such as when listening to music through earphones.

Source: Data from Hagan, J. F., Shaw, J. S., & Duncan, P. M. (Eds.). (2008). *Bright futures: Guidelines for health supervision of infants, children, and adolescents* (3rd ed.). Elk Grove Village, IL: American Academy of Pediatrics.

Developing Cultural Competence Use of Safety Protection

There are marked differences in behaviors that influence unintentional injuries. Although about 8% of children rarely or never wear a seat belt in the car, Black males are most at risk, with almost 12% not using seat belts. In addition, 88% of youth who ride bicycles rarely or never wear a bicycle helmet, but the rates vary, with 94% of Black and 92% of Hispanic youth not wearing helmets, while 86% of White youth do not wear bicycle helmets (CDC, 2013, 2014). How will you inquire about seat belt and bicycle helmet use in an open-ended manner during health promotion visits? Consider asking these questions:

- Where do you sit when you ride in the car?
- Who do you usually ride with?
- Do you drive? If so, how often do you text or hold and talk on your phone while you drive?
- Are there seat belts? How often do you use them?
- Do you ride a bike?
- Do you have a bicycle helmet? How often do you wear the helmet?

Plan strategies to include all children and families, especially those at high risk of not using seat belts or bicycle helmets.

Nursing Management

For the Health Promotion and Maintenance of the School-Age Child

Nursing Assessment and Diagnosis

Assessment of health promotion and health maintenance topics occurs in many settings with school-age children. They may be seen in offices, clinics, or other settings designed to provide such care. They may come for episodic care for a fracture or infection when health promotion and health maintenance can be easily integrated. They may be seen in the home or neighborhood center, and are frequently encountered by nurses in schools. Opportunities for assessment and intervention should be used whenever they occur. The individual child is examined, and the family, friends, school, and community are addressed. In addition, these visits provide an opportunity to identify early and intervene for health-related problems that emerge or become apparent in school age.

Assessment can be considered on two levels with school-age children. Individual children may be assessed for height and weight, for immunization status, and for use of protective gear during sports. Populations of children may also be assessed since school age is the first time that large numbers of children are together in certain settings. The findings from such assessments will become the basis of an **individualized approach** or a **population-based approach** to health promotion and health maintenance. For example, nurses commonly measure height and weight, calculate body mass index (BMI) for *individual* children seen in a clinic, share results with the family, and address appropriate teaching about weight control and nutritious intake. In other settings, nurses may measure a *classroom* of children and use the collective data to plan appropriate interventions. If 40% of children in a school are classified as overweight by BMI percentile, much emphasis should be placed on teaching about dietary intake, physical activity, and the relationship of recommended weight levels to chronic disease risk. However, if only a small number of children are overweight, interventions may not be as extensive about this topic.

Nurses perform assessment of growth in school-age children, look for achievement of developmental tasks, assess physical and mental health, and assess social characteristics. Based on the assessment of the individual child or populations of children, nursing diagnoses for children and families are established. Possible nursing diagnoses include the following (NANDA-I © 2014):

- *Development: Delayed, Risk for,* related to abuse
- *Parenting, Impaired,* related to lack of knowledge about child health maintenance
- *Sleep Deprivation* related to sleep terrors
- *Violence: Other-Directed, Risk for,* related to history of witnessing family violence
- *Loneliness, Risk for,* related to long periods alone after school

Planning and Implementation

The nurse is instrumental in planning interventions to promote and maintain health in school-age children. These interventions may take place in offices, homes, or clinics with an individual child, or in schools and other community settings with groups of children.

When working with individuals, summarize the strengths and needs identified during the visit, and ask the child and family if they concur. Plan together with them to provide the needed information for topics developed during the visit. Be sure to emphasize those areas where the family excels. For example, positively reinforce use of car seat belts (see *Families Want to Know: Car Safety for the School-Age Child*), use of protective sports gear, and being current with immunizations. Summarize the next expected developmental tasks, such as increasing independence and growing self-responsibility for choosing snacks and television shows. Then provide anticipatory guidance to assist with the child's growing independence. As peers are becoming more

important, always focus some discussion on maintaining healthy social relationships through school peers, religious or community events, and sibling contacts.

Most families welcome a combination of discussion and reading material or pertinent websites for later exploration. Provide telephone numbers of resources for questions and community contacts. Tell the parents when the next health promotion/maintenance visit is recommended. If working with school children for episodic care, ask when the last health maintenance visit occurred. If a child is seen for health care after a bicycling accident, the family may be receptive to teaching about safety precautions. When the child is exposed to skin injuries, a review of the last tetanus booster may reevaluate health maintenance needs. Use every opportunity to work with individual children and insert appropriate health promotion/health maintenance topics.

When working with groups of children, health promotion focuses on known needs, interests, and risk areas. Nurses in school settings have used a variety of creative approaches to promote the health of youth. Nurses in schools can set up a program to train students in health topics; these students then become peer coaches or health advocates in working with other students. Another activity is evaluating the components of school health programs and making recommendations for additions as needed. In school settings, nurses have used a variety of creative approaches to promote the health of youth. Nurses in this setting can establish programs to train students in health topics; these students then become coaches or health advocates who can work with other students, especially those of younger ages. Nurses may also evaluate components of school health programs and offer recommendations for additions as needed. Bulletin boards, community newspapers, television, and community group membership may all be as effective as teaching in school classrooms. Stress reduction teaching should be provided on group and individual levels. Nurses can teach or assist in development of progressive relaxation, deep breathing, biofeedback, yoga, or meditation. Interventions will be most effective if they begin with an understanding of the population served.

Evaluation

Seek evaluation from parents during visits for care. Were their questions answered? Do they know where to turn for advice? Do they know when the child should be seen again for health promotion/maintenance?

Families Want to Know

Car Safety for the School-Age Child

Even though parents may have been diligent about car seat and seat belt use when children were younger, guidelines change and they need teaching about current requirements for the school-age child. Recommendations include the following:

- The child should be kept in a rear-facing seat as long as possible. Generally, by 4 years of age, the child has outgrown the rear-facing seat and should be in a forward-facing car seat with a harness in the back seat. This type of seat is recommended for children 4–7 years of age.

- Once the child outgrows the largest height and weight recommended by the manufacturer for the forward-facing seat (usually by 8 years of age), a booster seat is used in the back seat.

- Once the child is large enough for the regular seat belt, the lap belt must lie snugly across the upper thighs and the shoulder belt should be snug across the shoulder and chest.

- Keep all children in the back seat until 13 years of age; this is the safest location for them in the car (American Academy of Pediatrics, 2011b, 2014; National Highway Traffic Safety Administration, 2012).

The expected outcomes for nursing care of individual school-age children include the following:

- The child demonstrates normal patterns of growth and development.
- The child, family, and community provide a supportive and nurturing environment for the child.
- The child shows growing independence in directing own health promotion activities.

Expected outcomes of nursing care for groups of children include the following:

- The children identify lifestyle decisions that influence their health status.
- The school and community offer resources that help to lessen risk factors related to health and disease/injury prevention.

Health Promotion and Maintenance for the Adolescent

Adolescents are often seen only sporadically for health care, even though visits are recommended annually. They are usually healthy, may not need immunizations, and consequently do not often come for health care, although annual visits are recommended (American Academy of Pediatrics Committee on Practice and Ambulatory Medicine, 2016). If adolescents seek care for a minor illness, birth control, or a sports examination, the visit should be viewed as a health supervision opportunity.

Professionalism in Practice Adolescent Healthcare International Guidelines

The World Health Organization (WHO) realizes that adolescents are neither young children, nor young adults, and therefore have unique healthcare needs. The WHO made several recommendations for adolescent health care (WHO, 2014):

- Adolescent care should evolve from being "adolescent friendly" to "adolescent responsive" in order to be meaningful to youth.
- Universal healthcare coverage should be available for all adolescents.
- E-health, m-health (electronic and mobile, respectively), and in-school delivery of care should be offered for adolescents.
- An adolescent-competent workforce should be trained.

Nurses play a role in establishing adolescent-responsive health care in schools, community centers, and via electronic venues. A full range of services can be developed, with input from adolescents themselves about their needs and delivery choices. All nurses working with adolescents must have a thorough understanding of development, best approaches, and common healthcare needs.

While all components of the usual visit may not be performed, at least those parts most important are inserted into care. If time is limited, the nurse has to decide which topics to address during a healthcare visit. It is advisable to start with the topic of most interest to the teen and then to include injury prevention teaching, since injury is the greatest risk to teens. Health promotion topics such as dietary and exercise habits could be discussed.

Lifestyle behaviors are responsible for most of the preventable diseases, and all typically have origins in adolescent years, including sedentary lifestyle, unhealthy diet, tobacco and other substance use, and risk taking. Mental health assessment and teaching are other areas of prime importance. If the teen is at immediate risk, such as considering suicide in response to depression, this must be dealt with immediately by collaborating with a mental health specialist.

What general principles can guide programs to promote health in adolescents? Some researchers have analyzed theory application and approaches of programs, and others have suggested key elements of programs (see *Clinical Reasoning: Applying Theory to Plan for Adolescent Health*). Programs assist adolescents in taking on health promotion behaviors by fostering a sense of competence, promoting decision making, and increasing motivation for change toward healthy behaviors (Pender et al., 2015). When establishing youth programs, whether with individual adolescents or with groups, the nurse includes evaluation of the effectiveness of the plan, and uses methods to expand and sustain successful approaches.

Clinical Reasoning Applying Theory to Plan for Adolescent Health

Several theories guide healthcare professionals in establishing health promotion programs for adolescents. These theories provide an organized approach to planning and suggest the strategies that will be most successful, based on the person's motivation and developmental age (Pender et al., 2015). One such theory that is commonly used in adolescent care is the social cognitive theory.

This theory was developed by Albert Bandura, whose work is described in Chapter 4, and is frequently used in health research (Bandura, 1986, 1997a, 1997b; Connor, George, Gullo, et al., 2011; Davies, Terhorst, Nakonechny, et al., 2014). The key components of his theory involve **self-efficacy** (the person's belief in the ability to perform a behavior) and **outcome expectancy** (what the person expects to get from performing a certain behavior). Learning a new behavior occurs through **modeling**, or imitating the behavior of someone else. Bandura believes that individuals make decisions about health behaviors based on thoughts about the consequences and outcomes of those behaviors. The person's characteristics, such as self-efficacy and outcome expectancy, interact with the external environment and the behavioral choices available. All of these components together determine health behaviors, and all can be influenced to promote health.

When seeking to promote physical activity behaviors in youth, essential components include the following:

- Encourage the youth to believe they can perform the activity (self-efficacy).
- Point out the positive aspects of the behavior (outcome expectancy).
- Show the youth how to do the activity (modeling).
- Provide a physical setting and opportunity for performing the behavior (environment).
- Allow trial and error, choice in time, and extent of activity (behavioral choices).

Compose a teaching plan to encourage increased physical activity for a teen, using all components of the social cognitive theory. List the outcome measures or goals for the teaching, the interventions, and methods of evaluation.

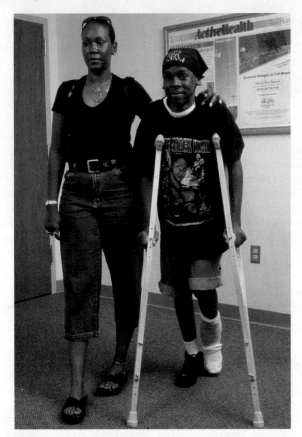

Figure 9–6 **Healthcare visit with a teen. Parents often accompany teens with a healthcare problem when they come in for the examination. Provide an opportunity to see both the teen and parent privately and integrate general health promotion and health maintenance into the visit. What questions can you ask this teen? What teaching might be needed?**

General Observations

The beginning of the visit with an adolescent can be an important time to gather information, just as it is with younger children. However, the observations you make will relate to the adolescent's more advanced stage of development.

Ideally the facility has a waiting area that is designed for adolescents. Teens often dislike waiting for health care with either young children or older adults. Teen waiting areas are popular because they provide a special place, thereby relaying that the adolescent is important, and can use video kiosks and other contemporary methods to impart health information while the teen waits (Figure 9–6). As you call the adolescent back for care, observe if parents or friends are present, or if the teen is alone. Young adolescents often come with parents to the facility, and parents often then wait in the waiting room during the examination. If the young adolescent comes in for a special problem, such as a skin lesion or other health concern, the parent may accompany the adolescent into the examination room. If someone comes with the teen, it may be necessary to provide some private time by asking the other person to wait outside for a moment. Reassure parents that there will be time to talk with them about any of their concerns and questions, and provide them with an opportunity to ask questions and obtain information.

Some teens are comfortable in healthcare settings and actively engage in conversation, while others are nervous and will need more explanations and reassurance during the first steps of measurement and blood pressure. By adolescence, boys and girls should be assuming more of a partnership role in their own health care. As the visit begins, greet adolescents warmly, ask what concerns and questions they have, and ask for their opinions and reactions throughout the visit. This will show that their thoughts are important and that they play an important role in guiding the healthcare visits. When adolescents are visiting the same office or clinic that they came to during childhood, they usually know and feel comfortable with the care providers. If the setting is new to them, explain procedures and introduce personnel so they feel more at ease.

Growth and Developmental Surveillance

Adolescence spans several years, and growth and developmental issues vary throughout the period. For young adolescents, or those from about 12 to 13 years of age, growth measurement remains important. These youth are still growing, and use of percentile grids continues to be an important part of care. Growth should remain in the same percentile channel as during childhood, with girls reaching nearly adult height at this age, and boys still continuing to grow. As always, be alert for youth who have either increased or decreased percentiles, or are above the 85th percentile or below the 5th percentile for body mass index. They will need additional assessment of nutritional intake and physical activity.

By middle (14 to 16 years) and late adolescence (17 to 19 years), adult growth is nearly achieved, earlier for girls than boys. While measurement continues to be performed, nurses assess the BMI carefully to be sure the height and weight indicate appropriate intake and exercise. Overweight at this age is likely to continue into adulthood, particularly if parents are overweight, so early intervention will be needed to decrease this potential. Other youth may have eating disorders and should be referred to a specialist for care. Children from homes without sufficient financial resources may be hungry and lack adequate food of high quality (known as *food insecurity*). Parents who were eligible for the Special Supplemental Nutrition Program for Women, Infants, and Children (WIC) services when children were younger may not receive them once the child is an adolescent, so the increasing dietary intake needs of their teens cannot be met. If an adolescent is thin and has little energy, consider administering a food security questionnaire such as the one provided by the U.S. Department of Agriculture (www.ers.usda.gov). Even the child who is overweight may live in a family with insufficient resources since foods with high fat and caloric content are often less expensive than those with greater nutrient value. For example, a "dollar menu" at a fast-food restaurant meets hunger needs faster and with less expense than a home-prepared meal of fresh fruits, vegetables, and grains. In addition, people who have experienced periods of hunger from inadequate food resources may overeat when food is available, a pattern that promotes weight gain (see Chapter 14).

Few options exist for measuring the developmental competence of adolescents, but observations and questions during care provide information about the meeting of developmental milestones. Key tasks for adolescents involve separating from the parents and establishing positive relationships with peers. The young teen may come to an appointment with a parent and still rely on that parent to answer some questions during the examination. However, middle and late teens should be increasingly able to come alone, answer questions themselves, and assume responsibility for healthcare decisions. Offer older teens the option of coming into the room alone, stating, "Your mom can wait here and we can come and get her later. Does that sound all right?" During time with the adolescent, ask questions to learn about peer interactions and activities.

The adolescent may receive a physical examination from a nurse practitioner or a physician. See Chapter 5 for components of the examination. Some particular parts of the examination to include for teens are scoliosis screening, sexual maturity rating (Tanner stages), breast examination, testicular examination, testing for sexually transmitted infections (among those sexually active), pelvic examination, and Pap smear (for sexually active females), hematocrit/hemoglobin for anemia when risk assessment warrants, hearing and vision screening when needed, annual blood pressure, lipid screening for those with family history of early heart disease or other risk factors, and tuberculosis screening for those in high-risk areas (American Academy of Pediatrics Committee on Practice and Ambulatory Medicine, 2016).

Most adolescents do not want their parents present during the examination, but occasionally will want a parent present for something like a first pelvic examination or a blood draw. Ask them their wishes in a confidential setting so they can freely make the choice. They also may choose to have a same-gender healthcare provider complete the genitourinary examination. Expected outcomes of care include screening and early identification for common health problems, normal patterns of growth, and meeting of developmental milestones.

Nutrition

The young adolescent needs a well-balanced diet to support the growth of this period, and the late adolescent requires intake that supports physical activity and provides nutrients for metabolism and to promote the immune system. While nutritional intake is important, teens often do not eat well. They may be busy and do not want to plan meals, they like to eat foods that are popular with other teens (so high fat and sugar intake can be common), they may be dieting to achieve weight loss, and some do not have enough financial resources to access healthy foods.

Combine the information from measurement of the adolescent with the answers to questions about diet to identify possible areas for intervention. Find out what questions the teen has about foods, diet, maintaining desired weight, and topics such as vegetarianism or supplements to enhance athletic performance. See Chapter 14 for further detail about these special nutritional topics. Health promotion plans focus on practices that lead to healthy growth and development. They may include teaching about:

- Getting five fruits and vegetables daily
- Including whole-grain products to replace refined products whenever possible
- The importance of eating three meals each day, including breakfast and lunch
- Eating together as a family several times weekly, which enhances quality food intake
- How to plan menus and prepare foods for balanced intake

Health maintenance plans center on those practices that prevent disease, including:

- Limiting refined sugar and high-fat intake (such as soft drinks and fried foods) to maintain weight at recommended level

- Including two to three servings of dairy products daily to enhance bone formation and decrease chance of osteoporosis as an adult
- Using resources for treatment of eating disorders if they are identified

While much of nutrition teaching should be aimed directly at the adolescent, parents are also included. They can be effective contributors to healthy intake by providing plenty of fruits and vegetables for snacks, having foods attractively prepared and ready for consumption when the teen is hungry, planning several meals together as a family each week, encouraging milk or other forms of calcium intake, and setting a good example for food intake. Help parents identify the youth with an eating disorder and provide resources for intervention in these cases. Consider as well the teen with a baby. The adolescent who is pregnant or breastfeeding has even more need for nutritional teaching and may need financial resources to access sufficient food. How can the nurse combine in the teaching plan the growth and developmental needs of an adolescent with those of her new baby?

Physical Activity

Many adolescents suffer from the effects of inadequate physical activity. As children get older and enter the teenage years, physical activity decreases, particularly in girls. Sixty minutes daily of moderate or vigorous activity is recommended for teens, but 15% do not get this level of exercise even 1 day a week, and 53% do not achieve this activity 5 out of 7 days of the week (CDC, 2014). The percentage is lower among some groups, such as females, Blacks, and Hispanics, with wide state variation (CDC, 2014). At a time when teens are not very active as a group, physical education requirements in school are also decreasing. Only 24% of 12th-grade male and 16% of 12th-grade female students regularly attend a physical education class (CDC, 2014). Physical activity levels must therefore be assessed at each health supervision visit or in other contacts with adolescents. Apply resilience theory as discussed in Chapter 4, and assess youth, family, and community for risk and protective factors regarding physical activity (Table 9–4).

Some youth have established regular physical activity programs, and their behaviors should be encouraged (Figure 9–7). Be alert for adolescents who exercise but have other health problems. Some athletes try to eat very little to remain a certain weight for wrestling, running, or other sports. Integrate nutritional teaching that includes the importance of adequate intake for sports performance. Other athletes use nutritional supplements to enhance performance. While most are not harmful, few have proven benefits and their cost is not warranted. Some may actually be harmful to adolescents, such as prolonged use of creatinine and any use of steroids.

Some youth have very little physical activity and feel incompetent in performing many sports. Work with them to find at least one thing they can do on a daily basis—walking their dog in the neighborhood, riding a bike to the store, using stairs instead of elevators when possible, parking on the far side of the school lot and walking farther, swimming at a club their parents belong to or at a local YMCA or YWCA, or saving money to take lessons for something they have always dreamed of doing, such as horseback riding or golf. The community health nurse can form interest groups at schools and community centers that provide an outlet for adolescents who cannot "make the team" for school sports. Encourage parents and adolescents to set goals together to integrate some physical activity daily.

TABLE 9–4 Risk and Protective Factors Regarding Physical Activity in Adolescence

RISK FACTORS	PROTECTIVE FACTORS
• Lives in rural or other isolated setting with little opportunity for contact with other teens • Lives in urban area that is unsafe or provides little opportunity for outside physical activity • Presence of neighborhood hazards and unsafe areas • Lack of neighborhood programs for physical activity promotion	• Has opportunities for participation in physical activity at home, at school, and in the community • School provides daily physical education classes • Neighborhood and community provide physical activity options • Has many friends living close who participate in physical activity • Public policies maintain parks, green spaces, biking trails, playgrounds
• Has a developmental disability that impairs physical movement	• Programs are available for adolescents with developmental disabilities or other healthcare needs
• Does not like physical activity • Has a pattern and history of low activity levels • Is overweight • Does not feel competent in most sports	• Likes physical activity • Has exercised during all of childhood, often with parents
• Limited financial resources to pay registration fees or buy protective gear for sports	• Availability of financial and other resources for sports gear and protective equipment
• Family members who have little physical activity • Parents who are not active in school sports and committees • Parents who do not like physical activity and have had low levels while their teen was growing up • Parents who have little time or facilities for exercise, or always exercise at a club—out of view of their family	• Parents participate in regular physical activity and encourage the adolescent to do so also • Youth and parents agree to a limit of 2 hours daily of screen time
• Lack of youth and parent knowledge about physical activity needs and benefits	• Knowledgeable about benefits of activity; committed to maintaining exercise patterns

Source: Data from Hagan, J. F., Shaw, J. S., & Duncan, P. M. (Eds.). (2008). *Bright futures: Guidelines for health supervision of infants, children, and adolescents* (3rd ed.). Elk Grove Village, IL: American Academy of Pediatrics.

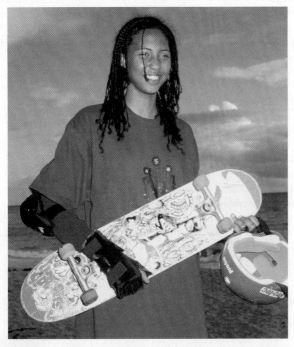

Figure 9–7 **Teen use of safety measures. This teen girl is an avid "skater." How can you encourage and praise her for this activity? What clues do you have that she is using adequate safety measures?**

What risk and protective factors for physical activity exist in your community? Go to www.activelivingbydesign.org to examine the positive effect community planning can have on its members' exercise levels.

The nurse's activities for health promotion concentrate on teaching the health and mental benefits of physical activity such as increased energy, weight control, and a feeling of control and success. Health maintenance focuses on viewing physical activity as a method to prevent disease such as cardiovascular disease and diabetes. Youth who have family members with these diseases or meet adults who have them are more likely to understand the importance of their own activity. Desired outcomes include maintenance of weight within recommended level, daily exercise of 60 minutes, and establishment of lifetime exercise routines.

Oral Health

Continued dental care during the adolescent years can ensure oral health. The recommendations remain the same as those for young children. The adolescent should floss daily, brush twice daily with a small amount of fluoridated toothpaste, and visit a dental care provider every 6 months. By about 14 years of age, those adolescents who do not have fluoridated water and have been taking fluoride can stop this supplement. Even the molars have been formed by that age so fluoride tablets are no longer needed. Continue to examine the condition of the teeth and the number of erupted permanent teeth present. Be alert for any unusual growths and ulcers in the mouth and refer for care as needed.

Unavailability of dental insurance for the adolescent is a potential concern. The teen whose family does not have dental insurance needs referrals for care to affordable resources. Dental specialists clean off plaque that has formed, apply sealants to erupting molars, examine the teeth for caries, and perform restorative care. Certain groups are more at risk for inadequate dental care (see *Developing Cultural Competence: Dental Care*).

When working with these populations, nurses can question access to care and make recommendations that foster regular checkups.

Developing Cultural Competence Dental Care

Analysis of several national surveys, such as the National Center for Health Statistics and the National Health Interview Survey, shows marked disparity in oral health. The major factor in disparity of dental care is lack of dental insurance. While 42% of youth from families without insurance did not have a dental visit in the previous year and 27% of them had unmet dental needs, only 11% of youth from families with insurance lacked a previous year visit and only 4% had unmet dental needs. Poverty and immigrant status are two risk factors associated with lack of dental insurance (Child Trends, 2013).

When working with adolescent populations from groups at high risk for lack of dental coverage or high incidence of caries, include dental assessment in health supervision visits, and have resources for care readily available to carry out referrals as needed. The Affordable Care Act provides for two dental visits annually, so assist families to participate in their state or employment healthcare plan.

Evaluate risk factors for threats to oral health such as tobacco use, particularly chewing tobacco (see quote from Jeremy in the chapter-opening scenario). A risk for oral injury exists with engagement in certain sports. Ask about physical activity and recommend that a mouth guard be worn if the youth engages in hockey, football, or some other sports. Some teens may wish to whiten the teeth or obtain orthodontia to improve appearance. The nurse can help the youth and parents to find resources for needed care.

Expected outcomes for oral health include dental visits twice annually; daily positive oral health habits; absence of risk factors for poor oral health, injury, or tobacco use; and obtaining recommended follow-up care for problems.

Mental and Spiritual Health

Adolescents have many challenges to their mental health and need support to emerge from adolescence with mental and spiritual strengths. Mental health topics must be addressed at each health supervision opportunity to promote mental health among teens. Mental health is closely linked to developmental tasks such as growing independence, formation of close relationships with peers, becoming confident in accomplishments, and setting goals for the future. Some chronic mental health disorders such as schizophrenia can emerge during adolescence, so mental health screening is important to perform with this age group.

As during other developmental stages, the self-concept continues to evolve, influencing how the adolescent reacts to the environment. Self-regulation—making decisions to govern oneself—becomes critically important. Self-esteem, or a positive feeling about the self, is key to meeting life's challenges. Ask what the teen is proud of and has accomplished and what disappointments have occurred as well. Provide resources to deal with disappointments and praise the teen's accomplishments.

The adolescent's self-esteem is connected to perception of body image. Factors such as early or late maturation, overweight or underweight, or the role of the media can influence the teen's body image. A healthy image includes the realization that the body has positive and less positive attributes and that the individual can influence the body by healthy eating and physical activity. Be alert for the teen whose wish for a different body leads to eating disorders and excessive exercise or intake of nutritional supplements.

Sexuality involves both body changes that signal mature sexual development, and the mental concept of oneself as a sexual being. Body changes and mental concepts do not necessarily mature at the same time, and adolescents may not be ready for sexual maturity; decisions about sexual behavior are not necessarily equivalent to achieving sexual maturation. Most young adolescent girls have begun menstruating, and by early to middle adolescence, boys are having nocturnal emissions and ejaculations. Ask teens if they have received information about puberty, body changes, and sexuality. Tell young adolescents that most teens have questions and that they may ask about any areas of interest, including contraception and sexually transmitted infections. Ask older adolescents directly if they have had sexual intercourse and if so, what they are doing to protect against pregnancy and sexually transmitted infections. Provide support for adolescents who have decided not to have sexual intercourse, encouraging them to continue this plan, telling them that sexual feelings are normal, but that decisions about sexual intercourse are their right and privilege. Ask if the adolescent has ever experienced unwanted pressure for intercourse and if there has been help and support to deal with the situation. Intimate partner violence, date rape, and other trauma signal a need for referral to a mental health specialist. See Chapter 17 for further information.

Ask if teens have confusion about their sexuality. If teens have self-identified as being gay, let them know they are welcome and ask about decisions regarding sexual practices, reinforcing the need for protection against sexually transmitted infections. Provide community resources to support gay or lesbian teens so that they can develop a social group in which they feel comfortable. Some adolescents are seen for health care at the time they become sexually active. Use this opportunity to reinforce and correct prior knowledge about the body and protection against pregnancy and sexually transmitted infections.

Clinical Tip

The nurse who works with adolescents dealing with sexuality issues may find that the values of some teens are very different from one's personal values. How do you react when a teen decides to have sexual intercourse or has become pregnant? Can you help teens make wise decisions without telling them what they should do?

It is important for adolescents to learn the significance of sexual intercourse and the meaning of close relationships. Teaching them early about this will enable them to respect others at the time they do have intimate relations. Respect is also the key to working with teens. Nurses should treat them with respect, expecting them to consider options and make wise decisions. Nurses who cannot work with certain groups of teens because of moral values differing from their own have the obligation to refer the teens for care to resources where they can receive the information and services they are requesting.

Most adolescents still need discipline or guidance from parents at certain times. Rather than a constant battle over daily events, it is best if there are just a few important rules that parents have to enforce only rarely. When working with parents, nurses can assist them to set useful boundaries for teens and offer resources such as parenting groups and websites for assistance.

Sleep is necessary for anyone to function safely and at a level of one's potential. Unfortunately, many youth do not get the sleep needed for healthy functioning. Teens have an increased need for sleep due to their growth rates and activity levels. At the same time, their internal clocks change, making it more difficult to get to sleep at the usual time. It is thought that a decrease in secretion of melatonin occurs, so the teen does not feel tired in the late evening. However, they often do not have the number of hours of sleep needed by the time they wake up for school or work. The problem may be worsened if the student participates in sports or other activities. They may need to get to school before normal starting hours for music, sports, or other activities, or perhaps stay late into the evening for practices. Some adolescents work weekends or evenings as well. And of course social activities usually fill much of their time. Although about 9 hours of sleep is needed, most adolescents get about 6 hours (Mayo Clinic, 2013). The effects of sleep deprivation can be serious. Teens cannot perform to their potential in school or at work. Many parents state that adolescents are moody and difficult to communicate with when they are tired. There may be a connection between lack of sleep and substance abuse, and teens commonly use caffeinated beverages to stay awake. Some people tend to eat more when they are tired, and get less physical activity. Perhaps one of the most serious consequences deals with the danger of driving while sleepy; this is a common cause of accidents. Ask adolescents about what time they go to bed, when they awaken, and whether they are frequently tired. Provide suggestions for regular sleep schedules, avoiding caffeine products in the evening, making screen technology unavailable during sleep time, and planning a day of relaxation into every week.

Healthy People 2020

(SH-3) Increase the proportion of students in grades 9 through 12 who get sufficient sleep on school nights

- Less than 31% of adolescents have 8 hours of sleep on school nights. *Healthy People 2020* has set a modest goal to increase this percentage to 33% who achieve at least 8 hours of sleep on school nights.

School plays an increasingly important role in adolescent mental health. School provides peer support, meaningful activities, and a forum for learning time management and other skills. At the same time, some youth become stressed because of inability to fit in, worry about grades and their futures, and violent or unsupportive school situations. Discuss the elements of school that adolescents like and those they do not like. Determine what support is available in the schools. Ask the adolescent about future plans and how those are influencing choices for courses and friends in school.

Temperament or personality characteristics continue into adolescence and generally do not change from earlier years. For example, the active infant and young child is usually an active teenager. The slow-to-warm-up baby may be the adolescent who needs more time to adjust to a new school or teachers. If the adolescent or parent has trouble with personality characteristics, it may be helpful to talk about these traits, help them establish a positive sense about the attributes, and discuss ways to adapt the environment as needed. For example, parents should not expect a slow-to-warm-up teen to be interested in running for a class office. Someone with irregular sleep and eating habits will find

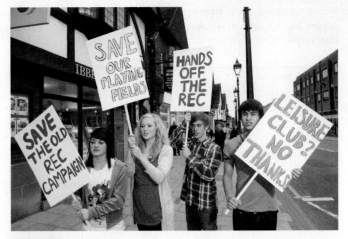

Figure 9–8 Spiritual health for teens. Teens often become associated with causes. This helps them to feel part of a social group and also provides opportunities for examining belief systems and making decisions about meaningful activities.

it difficult to have a job at a set time and will need to set alarms and other reminders.

Spirituality offers comfort and support for the adolescent. Being a member of a teen group in a faith-based home can offer a peer group with similar values and bring meaning to life. Some adolescents reject the faith of their parents and seek a different group; others seek to leave religious practices totally, while others become more committed to them. Ask them if they have the resources they need to bring meaning to their lives; provide them if needed. Realize that participation in community food kitchens, raising money for causes, and other activities also provide meaning for many adolescents (Figure 9–8).

The nurse actively promotes the mental health of youth by understanding their developmental needs and providing information and resources. Gentle guidance and active partnership with youth help to provide the resources to ensure healthy self-concept, sexuality, and personality development. While most teenagers have many protective factors that can be identified and fostered, a few have risks that can harm mental health. It is important to identify the risks, and to use health maintenance techniques to lessen the risk factors. Depression and substance use are two common risks to mental health. Depression is discussed in Chapter 28, and substance abuse is discussed in Chapter 17. See the quick checklists in Table 9–5 to help in identifying these problems during health supervision visits.

Although health promotion and health maintenance activities commonly occur in office or clinic settings, there are many other settings where nurses work with adolescents, and mental health activities are often integrated into these settings. Consider offering health promotion/maintenance wherever students might be found. Some nontraditional settings include correctional facilities, school-based health centers, and programs for pregnant teens. Adolescents in these facilities can benefit from services to improve diet, physical activity, and lifestyle behaviors that influence mental health.

The desired outcomes for mental and spiritual health promotion and maintenance include meaningful activities in the adolescent's life, emerging independence, good choices about lifestyle behaviors, and development of successful coping skills.

TABLE 9–5 Signs of Depression and Substance Abuse

DEPRESSION	SUBSTANCE ABUSE
Changes in appetite and weight	Changes in school performance, sleep, and appetite
Changes in sleep schedules and patterns	Unusual behavior, such as getting into trouble at school
Changes in school performance	Accidents and other unexplained events
Physical complaints	Lack of responsibility for actions
Loss of interest and pleasure in usual activities and friends	Increased mood changes
Depression, irritability, poor concentration	Inability to set goals
Feelings of worthlessness, helplessness	A variety of physical changes depending on the substance used
Thoughts of death or suicide	

Source: Adapted from Tanski, S., Garfunkel, L. C., Duncan, P. M., & Weitzman, M. (2011). *Performing preventive services*. Elk Grove Village, Il: American Academy of Pediatrics.

Relationships

Adolescents form stronger bonds with friends than at any time earlier in development; at the same time, they need their parents for guidance and reassurance as they become more independent. As teenagers strive for independence, they frequently strike out at parents, test limits, and have conflicts with parents. Interactions in the family provide consistent and important ties at the same time that social interactions become a central part of life. Health promotion helps teens to form strong friendships with peers and to continue to value and participate in the family. It helps parents to understand the developmental needs and their role in establishing a new type of relationship with the emerging young adult in the family. Partnerships with healthcare providers are important to help families work together to achieve these outcomes.

When adolescents are seen for healthcare visits, assess relationships with others. Provide time alone with both the adolescent and the parents (if they are present) so that everyone has time to talk freely and to ask questions. Some areas already discussed, such as school performance and activities, provide information about the adolescent's friends and how time is spent. Ask teens to describe their best friends and what they do together. Ask parents their opinions of the youth's friends. Inquire about the youth's roles in the family. Does the teen have jobs and responsibilities? What freedom is allowed? What are relationships like with siblings and extended family members such as grandparents and cousins? What activities are done together as a family? Are there differences in the teen's and the parents' answers to these questions? What are the teen's and parents' desires for how the family unit functions?

Provide an opportunity to talk with the teen alone about issues such as domestic violence. Is the youth abused or is there violence between adults in the family? Are there stressors such as lack of sufficient finances, an ill parent, or a lost job? How have these occurrences affected the adolescent? Minor adjustments can be helped by discussion, whereas some major problems will need referral to mental health specialists.

In their relationships with peers, adolescents often have many of the same issues that emerge with parents. They may have disagreements with friends or feel hurt by things that are said or done. Ask teens about how things are going with friends and what problems they have. Talk about negotiating, joining groups to form new friendships, and the importance of respecting and not making fun of others. Give them strategies for living up to their own standards even when friends are enticing them to do other things. Suggest that having friends one can trust and who have the same ideals can be very supportive and fun in adolescent years. Expected outcomes are the formation of strong relationships both within and outside of the family, along with independence in decision making.

Disease Prevention Strategies

Teenagers typically do not have many diseases and most are minor illnesses like respiratory and gastrointestinal illness. However, there are some diseases that occur and nurses must always be aware of signs of potential disease. Some common health issues that are described throughout this book include the following:

- Acne and skin infections (see Chapter 31)
- Body piercing and tattooing (see Chapter 17)
- Sports overuse injuries (see Chapter 29)
- Constipation and diarrhea (see Chapter 25)

Other observations may signal more serious health concerns and need to be referred for further evaluation. Examples include the following:

- Scoliosis (see Chapter 29)
- Anemia (see Chapter 23)
- Excessive tiredness (see Chapter 24)
- Bruising (see Chapter 23)
- Depression, suicidal thoughts, other mental health issues (see Chapter 28)
- Sexually transmitted infections (see Chapter 26)
- Eating disorders (see Chapter 14)
- Abuse or severe bullying (see Chapter 17)

Several screening tests should be performed during health supervision visits with adolescents, including vision, hearing, smoking, depression, stress, alcohol or other substance use, blood pressure, urinalysis, sexually transmitted infection risk, and, in some cases, Pap smears and breast examinations. Screening tests with abnormal results require follow-up and intervention. For example, if the adolescent is anemic, iron tablets may be needed and teaching about high-iron foods should be done. Vision impairment requires referral to an eye specialist. Presence of sexually transmitted infections requires teaching and medication treatment. History of sexual activity will guide the nurse to tests that should be included in the examination (see *Clinical Tip*).

Sexually active teens should be screened annually for the following:

- Chlamydial infection
- Gonorrhea
- Trichomoniasis
- Human papillomavirus
- Herpes simplex virus
- Bacterial vaginosis
- Human immunodeficiency virus

Individuals should be screened for syphilis and HIV/AIDS if requesting testing or meeting any of these criteria:

- History of sexually transmitted infection
- More than one sexual partner in past 6 months
- Intravenous drug use
- Sexual intercourse with a partner at risk
- Sex in exchange for drugs or money
- Homelessness
- Males—sex with other males
- Syphilis—residence in areas where disease is prevalent

See Chapter 26 for further information on screening procedures.

Source: Data from Hagan, J. F., Shaw, J. S., & Duncan, P. M. (2008). *Bright futures: Guidelines for health supervision of infants, children, and adolescents* (3rd ed.). Elk Grove Village, IL: American Academy of Pediatrics.

The adolescent should receive extensive information about ways to protect health and prevent disease. The hazardous outcomes of smoking are discussed, and smoking cessation programs are encouraged for smokers. Unprotected sexual activity is presented as a serious health threat. Use of sunscreens to prevent burns and future skin cancer is encouraged. Females are taught breast self-examination, and males are taught testicular examination. For youth who are overweight and sedentary, the possible outcomes such as type 2 diabetes and cardiovascular disease are mentioned. While it would not be advisable to threaten or frighten an adolescent with descriptions of diseases, an understanding of the potential serious outcomes can be motivators for behavior change.

In addition to teaching to prevent disease, the nurse also administers any needed immunizations. Many adolescents have not had immunizations since about school entry time, so their record should be carefully reviewed (see Chapter 16). When checking the adolescent's record, consider the following questions about some common immunizations that are needed:

- *When was the last tetanus-diphtheria (Td) booster?* It is recommended every 10 years if no wounds have required an update in the interim. If the child received it at age 5 years, a booster is needed at 15 years. A Tdap (tetanus-diphtheria-acellular pertussis) booster is given, with the preferred age of 11 to 12 years.
- *Was a second measles-mumps-rubella administered?* A second dose may not have been routine when teens were younger so they may need it now.
- *Is hepatitis A common in your state?* If so, the teen needs to get that vaccine.

- *Has the youth had hepatitis B vaccine?* This is important for all youth, and some may not have received it as infants.
- *Did the youth have a documented history of varicella disease?* If not, two doses of the vaccine are needed.
- *Has the youth received meningococcal vaccine?* Meningococcal vaccine is now recommended for all youth.
- *Have the adolescent female and male received the human papillomavirus vaccine?* Human papillomavirus vaccine (three-dose series) is recommended for females and males from 11 to 12 years, or for those 13 to 26 years not previously immunized. The vaccine can be given as early as 9 years of age.
- *Has the youth received the annual influenza vaccine?* Annual influenza vaccine is now recommended for all children and adolescents.

The results of health screening are shared with the teen and with the parent as appropriate. Teaching and other interventions for disease prevention are examples of health maintenance activities. Expected outcomes are increasing knowledge of common diseases and methods of prevention among teen and parent, use of screening tests by the healthcare provider, and use of the healthcare home by the adolescent for treatment of diseases.

Injury Prevention Strategies

Injury is the greatest health hazard for adolescents, so injury prevention must be integrated into every health contact with youth. The major hazard is automobile crashes (see Chapter 1). Many teens learn to drive and have a license by 16 years of age. They often transport friends, get distracted by social interactions in the car, have little experience about what to do if a car slides or has mechanical problems, may drink and drive, talk or text on cell phones while driving, and are often tired when driving (Figure 9–9). Many states have instituted graduated driving licensing to help decrease some risks. Know the graduated driver license laws in your state and reinforce them with youth

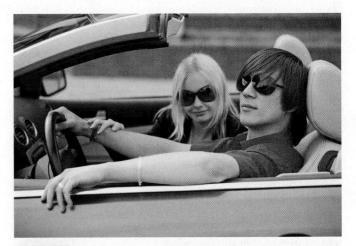

Figure 9–9 **Injury prevention for teens. Adolescents often drive motorized vehicles and may be at risk for injury if not properly prepared or protected. What teaching and experience do these youth need for safe enjoyment of the experience of driving and riding with friends? Do schools in your area offer driver education classes? What are the state requirements for youth driver licensure?**

SOURCE: wrangler/Shutterstock

and families. Driving should always be presented as a privilege and a responsibility. Suggest that parents consider enforcing serious consequences such as losing the ability to drive for a time after any infraction. Because of the great risk of injury and death from motor vehicle crashes, ask at each health visit if the teen drives, rides with other teens, what rules parents have established about driving, and whether the teen ever drinks and drives or rides with someone who does. Reinforce the need to wear a lap and shoulder belt at all times and to never drink and drive.

SAFETY ALERT!

Major risk factors for teen drivers include inexperience (especially vulnerable time is the first 6 months of driving), transporting other teens, night driving, non-use of seat belt, and distractions such as texting and playing music. Graduated driver licensing is an approach used to decrease motor vehicle crashes among novice teen drivers. The CDC recommends that no learners' permits be allowed before 16 years of age, that permits must be held for at least 6 months, that driving from 10 p.m. to 5 a.m. not be allowed except with adult chaperone, that other youth not be transported, and that regular licenses (without youth restrictions) not be allowed until 18 years of age. Zero-tolerance policies for drinking, texting or cell phone use, and non-use of seat belts should be enforced (CDC, 2011b). How can nurses be active in political discussions to promote graduated driver licensing and support parents of novice teen drivers?

Youth are at risk for injury with other motorized vehicles. Motorcycles, four-wheelers, boats, jet skis, farm machinery, and tools are other sources of injury. Ask about the youth's exposure to various machines and teach about avoiding alcohol and drug use and safety gear and precautions to be used. Every health visit should include other questions that help identify a wide variety of injury hazards. Be sure to discuss and provide written material to perform injury prevention teaching. Such measures are important health maintenance activities (Tables 9–6 and 9–7). Desired outcomes for nursing care include absence of serious injury, the ability to state sources of risk for injury, and emergency plans for assistance when engaging in any risky activities.

Nursing Management

For the Health Promotion and Maintenance of the Adolescent

Nursing Assessment and Diagnosis

Nurses assess adolescents in a variety of settings, including offices, clinics, schools, homes, correctional facilities, extended care facilities, sports-related facilities, and family planning clinics. A wide array of health concerns should be included in these assessments:

- Measurement of growth
- Presence of any unusual findings on physical examination
- Lifestyle choices related to dietary intake, physical activity, and oral hygiene
- Assessment of mental status, family interactions, and social connections with peers

- Any risky behaviors the adolescent engages in such as smoking, unprotected sexual relations, alcohol or drug use, or unsafe driving practices

The people and organizations around the adolescent such as family, school, and neighborhood are all assessed. Remember to list both risks and protective factors. The protective factors can be used during implementation to enhance the youth's resilience.

Based on a thorough assessment, you will establish nursing diagnoses that are appropriate for the adolescent and family. Some possible nursing diagnoses might include the following (NANDA-I © 2014):

- *Rape-Trauma Syndrome* related to date rape
- *Dentition, Impaired,* related to ineffective oral hygiene
- *Obesity* related to lack of basic nutritional knowledge and obesity in both parents
- *Nutrition, Readiness for Enhanced,* related to increasing interest in nutritional knowledge
- *Sleep Pattern, Disturbed,* related to frequently changing sleep—wake schedule
- *Self-Esteem, Situational Low,* related to situational crisis of friends making fun of adolescent
- *Injury, Risk for,* related to psychomotor and cognitive factors

Planning and Implementation

Whatever the setting, the nurse partners with the adolescent, the parents, and other persons such as teachers or school counselors to plan appropriate goals and related interventions. Nurses work with individual adolescents in offices, schools, and other settings, and often work with groups of adolescents to perform teaching. Apply communication skills that are effective with teens, such as listening to concerns, allowing for discussion, and bringing in peers who have had experiences related to the topic being discussed.

Many nursing interventions involve teaching, so it is wise to develop a number of resources for working with teens. Consult the resources on this textbook's companion website, and visit agencies in your community to gather appropriate materials. Teaching topics should be directed both at health promotion (providing information to enhance the adolescent's state of health) and health maintenance (sharing tips about how to avoid disease and injury). A good starting point is to have the adolescent identify a personal health goal and begin teaching there. In addition to teaching, direct care is provided when administering immunizations, performing vision screening, and examining the spine and posture for scoliosis.

One of the challenges during health supervision for adolescents is including the right mix of teen and parent decision making and involvement. It is again important to apply communication skills by tactfully allowing time for both parent and adolescent to be seen alone. Realize that health supervision provides support and information for parents, such as useful discipline techniques, recognition of common parental feelings about teens, and the need for growing independence by their youth. When providing teaching to groups of teens in schools, there may be policies about what needs to be sent home to parents. For topics such as sexually transmitted infections or substance use, some schools require that an outline be sent home for parents to read. Parents may call with

TABLE 9–6 Injury Prevention in Adolescence

	HAZARD	DEVELOPMENTAL CHARACTERISTICS	PREVENTIVE MEASURES
	Motor vehicle crashes	Adolescents learn to drive, enjoy new independence, and often feel invulnerable.	Insist on driver's education classes. Enforce rules about safe driving. Seat belts should be used for every trip. Discourage drug and alcohol use. Get treatment for teenagers who are known substance abusers.
	Sporting injuries	Adolescents may participate in physically challenging sports such as soccer, gymnastics, or football. They may be allowed to drive motorboats.	Encourage use of protective sporting gear. Teach safe boating practices. Perform teaching related to hazards of drug and alcohol use, especially when using motorized equipment.
	Drowning	Adolescents overestimate endurance when swimming. They take risks diving.	Encourage swimming only with friends. Reinforce rules and teach them about risks.

questions about content and approach, or some may choose to attend the presentation. To create an effective presentation, the nurse must partner with the school administration, teachers, parents, and others. The ability to collaborate successfully with many individuals and agencies is an important skill for the nurse.

Wherever adolescents are seen, whether in offices or other private settings, schools, correction facilities, or other places with groups present, it is important to leave information about how to contact the nurse or another care provider. Provide brochures, referral numbers, names, and e-mails related to the topics discussed. Encourage annual visits for health supervision and suggest a variety of places to obtain this care. For example, if a youth will soon graduate from high school, find out if the youth will be working or attending college and provide links to health insurance or care providers in the new location.

Evaluation

Expected outcomes for care of adolescents and their families during health promotion and health maintenance include the following:

- Normal growth patterns and healthy weight are maintained.
- The adolescent is physically active for 60 minutes daily.
- Debris and plaque are absent on dental surfaces.
- The adolescent establishes a positive self-concept.
- The adolescent establishes positive relationships with peers, family members, teachers, and others.
- Healthy lifestyle habits are maintained that promote prevention of disease and injury.

TABLE 9–7 Injury Prevention Topics for Adolescents

TOPIC	INJURY PREVENTION TEACHING
Driving	Always wear seat and shoulder belts. Do not drink alcohol or take drugs and drive or ride with others who do. Do not talk or text on a cell phone as you drive. Do not drive when you are tired. Drive with parents or other adults for several months in winter driving conditions if you live where there is snow, ice, or heavy rains. Keep your car in good repair.
Sun	Wear sunscreen. Limit direct exposure to the sun, especially early in the summer when the skin is most sensitive to burns. This can be achieved by wearing sunscreen, hats, and clothing that prevent sunburns.
Machinery	Learn how to use power tools correctly. Always have someone near when you use tools or machinery. Follow guidelines for agricultural safety (CDC, 2011c).
Emergency care	Learn first aid, CPR, and airway obstruction removal.
Water safety	Learn to swim well. If you supervise younger children near water, never leave them alone, even for a minute.
Fires	Do not play with fire. Follow guidelines to avoid igniting gasoline. Test smoke alarms in your house every 6 months and change batteries annually.
Firearms	Know and follow rules to keep firearms locked, with ammunition locked in a separate place. Never take out a gun to show a friend unless your parent is also present. Take firearm safety classes if you hunt or target shoot.
Hearing	Avoid loud music especially for long periods and through earphones.
Sports	Wear protective gear recommended for your sport.
Abuse	Report any abuse to an adult you trust. Date with other couples whenever possible and report date rape. Do not drink or take drugs.

Source: Data from Hagan, J. F., Shaw, J. S., & Duncan, P. M. (2008). *Bright futures: Guidelines for health supervision of infants, children, and adolescents* (3rd ed.). Elk Grove Village, IL: American Academy of Pediatrics.

Chapter Highlights

- Health promotion visits are recommended annually and should take place in any setting where the child is seen, even for episodic or emergency care.

- Developmental surveillance, growth measurement, and physical examination provide the basis for establishing risk and protective factors for each child and adolescent.

- School-age children and adolescents are increasingly independent in making choices about nutrition and physical activity, while peer influence continues to grow.

- Establishment of affirmative self-esteem is important for school-age children and adolescents in order to develop positive mental health.

- Injury and disease prevention for school-age children and adolescents focuses on common causes of morbidity and mortality, such as firearms, abuse, motor vehicle crashes, alcohol and substance use, lack of immunizations, and sports-related injuries.

- The nurse integrates information from the health supervision visit to plan appropriate interventions for school-age children, adolescents, and their families.

Clinical Reasoning in Action

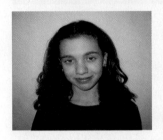

Tammy is a 13-year-old coming into the office for her yearly checkup and she has never been in the hospital or had surgery. She is a good student and is excited to start seventh grade next year. She has not had any immunizations since going into kindergarten. Tammy arrives with her mother, with whom she lives; she has no contact with her biologic father. Her mother decides to stay in the waiting room, but did note on the written history form that there is a family history of high cholesterol and heart disease in family members under 50 years old. Tammy's mother is a single parent working full time with two other children at home. Tammy's body mass index is in the 85th percentile and she passed her hearing and vision tests. Her blood pressure is 115/70 and her urinalysis shows blood, but Tammy has her menses today. Tammy has a period every month and menarche started at 10 years old. Her menses lasts 5 to 7 days and she denies experiencing cramping or excessively heavy menses. Tammy enjoys being a member of the volleyball team and is involved in a church youth group. She does not get to spend much time with her friends because she watches her two younger siblings in the afternoons while her mother is at work. When her mother is away, she admits to sitting and playing video games or watching TV most of the day. Tammy says she has had a boyfriend, but denies sexual activity. She also denies any experimentation with substance use.

1. What vaccines is Tammy due for at this age if she has not already had them?
2. A dietary assessment demonstrates that Tammy frequently skips meals and eats fast food almost daily. What are some of the suggestions you can give Tammy to improve her nutritional status?
3. What are some of the injury prevention topics you can discuss with Tammy?
4. Based on the additional information you collected about Tammy, what are some of the areas of recommended health teaching?
5. Develop a concept map for Tammy that includes all of the health promotion areas important to all youth, such as nutrition, oral health, physical activity, social interactions, family relationships, and disease/injury prevention. How can her development be enhanced to draw on strengths and improve areas of need? What part does the healthcare provider play in promoting her health?

References

American Academy of Pediatric Dentistry (AAPD). (2012). *Policy on third-party reimbursement of fees related to dental sealants.* Retrieved from http://www.aapd.org/media/Policies_Guidelines/P_3rdPartSealants.pdf\#xml=http://pr-dtsearch001.americaneagle.com/service/search.asp?cmd=pdfhits&DocId=330&Index=F%3a%5cdtSearch%5caapd%2eorg&HitCount=16&hits=18+46+57+11f+149+155+162+18e+1b6+1d2+207+228+246+269+2a8+2ca+&hc=314&req=sealants

American Academy of Pediatrics (AAP). (2011a). *Discipline.* Retrieved from http://www.healthychildren.org

American Academy of Pediatrics (AAP). (2011b). *Car safety seats.* Retrieved from http://www.healthychildren.org

American Academy of Pediatrics (AAP). (2014). *Car seats: Information for families for 2014.* Retrieved from http://www.healthychildren.org/English/safety-prevention/on-the-go/Pages/Car-Safety-Seats-Information-for-Families.aspx

American Academy of Pediatrics (AAP) Committee on Practice and Ambulatory Medicine. (2016). 2016 Recommendations for preventive pediatric health care. *Pediatrics, 137*(1), e20153908. doi:10.1542/peds.2015-3908.

Bandura, A. (1986). *Social foundations of thought and actions: A social cognitive theory.* Englewood Cliffs, NJ: Prentice Hall.

Bandura, A. (1997a). *Self-efficacy in changing societies.* New York, NY: Cambridge University.

Bandura, A. (1997b). *Self-efficacy: The exercise of control.* New York, NY: Freeman.

Ben-Arye, E., Traube, Z., Schachter, L., Jaimi, M., Levy, M., Schiff, E., & Lev, E. (2011). Integrative pediatric care: Parents/attitudes toward communication of physicians and CAM practitioners. *Pediatrics, 127*(1), 384–395.

Centers for Disease Control and Prevention (CDC). (2011a). *How much physical activity do children need?* Retrieved from http://www.cdc.gov/physicalactivity/everyone/guidelines/children/html

Centers for Disease Control and Prevention (CDC). (2011b). *Policy impact: Teen driver safety.* Retrieved from http://www.cdc.gov/Motorvehiclesafety/teenbrief/

Centers for Disease Control and Prevention (CDC). (2011c). *Agricultural safety.* Retrieved from http://www.cdc.gov/niosh/topics/aginjury

Centers for Disease Control and Prevention (CDC). (2013). *Bicycle-related injuries.* Retrieved from http://www.cdc.gov/HomeandRecreationalSafety/Bicycle/

Centers for Disease Control and Prevention (CDC). (2014). Youth risk behavior surveillance—United States, 2013. *Morbidity and Mortality Weekly Report, 63*(SS04), 1–172.

Child Trends. (2013). *Health care services.* Retrieved from http://www.childtrends.org/wp-content/uploads/2013/10/2013-10HealthCareServices.pdf

Connor, J. P., George, S. M., Gullo, M. J., Kelly, A. B., & Young, R. M. (2011). A prospective study of alcohol expectancies and self-efficacy as predictors of young adolescent alcohol misuse. *Alcohol and Alcoholism, 46*(2), 161–169.

Davies, M. A., Terhorst, L., Nakonechny, A. J., Skukla, N., & ElSaadawi, G. (2014). The development and effectiveness of a health information website designed to improve parents' self-efficacy in managing risk for obesity in preschoolers. *Journal for Specialists in Pediatric Nursing.* doi:10.1111/jsph.12086

Devoe, J. E., Tillotson, C. J., Wallace, L. S., Lesko, S. E., & Pandhi, H. (2012). Is health insurance enough? A usual source of care may be more important to ensure a child receives preventive health counseling. *Maternal and Child Health Journal, 16,* 306–315.

Hagan, J. F., Shaw, J. S., & Duncan, P. M. (Eds.). (2008). *Bright futures: Guidelines for health supervision of infants, children, and adolescents* (3rd ed.). Elk Grove Village, IL: American Academy of Pediatrics.

KidsHealth. (2011). *Developing your child's self-esteem.* Retrieved from http://kidshealth.org/parent/emotions/feelings/self_esteem.html

Kuo, D. Z., Houtrow, A. J., Arango, P., Kuhlthau, K. A., Simmons, J. M., & Neff, J. M. (2011). Family-centered care: Current applications and future directions in pediatric health care. *Maternal Child Health Journal, 16*(2), 297–305.

Mayo Clinic. (2013). *Teen sleep: Why is your teen so tired?* Retrieved from http://www.mayoclinic.org/healthy-living/tween-and-teen-health/in-depth/teens-health/art-20046157

National Highway Traffic Safety Administration. (2012). *Car seats and booster basics.* Retrieved from http://www.safercar.gov/parents/RightSeat.htm

Pender, N. J., Murdaugh, C. L., & Parsons, M. A. (2015). *Health promotion in nursing practice* (7th ed.). Upper Saddle River, NJ: Pearson Prentice Hall.

Santrock, J. W. (2012). *Child development* (12th ed.). Boston, MA: McGraw-Hill.

Tanski, S., Garfunkel, L. C., Duncan, P. M., & Weitzman, M. (2011). *Performing preventive services.* Elk Grove Village, IL: American Academy of Pediatrics.

Thai, K. T., McIntosh, A. S., & Pang, T. Y. (2014). Bicycle helmet size, adjustment and stability. *Traffic Injury Prevention*, June 20.

U.S. Department of Health and Human Services. (2011). *Strengthening families and communities.* Washington, DC: Author.

World Health Organization (WHO). (2014). *Adolescent responsive health systems.* Retrieved from http://www.who.int/maternal_child_adolescent/topics/adolescence/health_services/en/

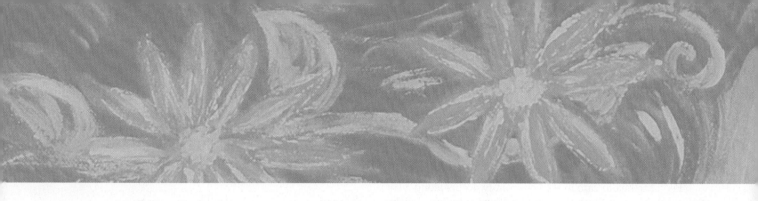

Chapter 10
Nursing Considerations for the Child in the Community

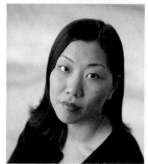

Sometimes Lani's asthma attacks really frighten me because she struggles so hard to breathe. She has a lot of trouble with asthma in the summertime with all the heat. I'm afraid to let her play outside with her friends for fear that she will have another attack. I'd really like to know how to keep Lani's asthma under control.

—Mother of Lani, 8 years old

Ryan McVay/Getty Images

∨ Learning Outcomes

10.1 Discuss the community healthcare settings where nurses provide health services to children.

10.2 Compare the roles of the nurse in each identified community healthcare setting.

10.3 Assemble a list of family support services that might be available in a community.

10.4 Develop a nursing care plan for a child in the school setting who has short-term mobility limitations.

10.5 Examine five ways in which nurses assist families in the home care setting.

10.6 Summarize the special developmental needs of children to consider in disaster preparedness planning.

Children receive most of their health care in community settings. Depending on the community, healthcare resources, and age of the child, nurses have an important role related to the care provided in each of these settings. When providing health care to the child and family, it is important for the nurse to assess the family's strengths, be aware of community resources, help families manage the complex health care that is often provided in the home, and prepare for emergencies and disasters.

Community-Based Health Care

Health plans and healthcare providers continue to explore options to provide safe, high-quality care in the community with fewer hospitalizations or shorter stays when hospitalization is needed. Patterns of healthcare delivery have changed due to

technologic developments and efforts to reduce healthcare costs. For example:

- Surgery and invasive diagnostic procedures are performed in ambulatory settings.

- Short-stay or observation units in hospital settings reduce the number of hospital admissions.

- Long-term intravenous antibiotic therapy can be provided in the home.

- Pediatric hospice and palliative care services occur in the home setting.

The trend in out-of-hospital care continues to increase for children with chronic health conditions and advanced disease states. Families are often willing to care for their child who is

medically fragile (having complex chronic health conditions that require skilled nursing and often technology support for vital functions) in the home because of their desire to have the child integrated into the family and community (Spratling, 2012). Technologic advances, such as portable medical equipment, enable families to provide complex healthcare services in the home and other community settings, and such care in the community is less costly. Home care services and other support services have been developed to support these families.

Pediatric health care in the community occurs along a continuum that covers the entire child healthcare system. This continuum is reflected in the Bindler-Ball Continuum of Pediatric Health, including health promotion and health maintenance services, care for chronic conditions, acute illnesses and injuries, and end-of-life care (see Chapter 1 for this model). Health care for individual children is improved when there is continuity of care and communication between healthcare settings.

The nurse working with families in a community setting uses knowledge of how the larger environment influences the child's health and development and the family's functioning, and integrates that information into the nursing care plan. To work effectively in the community, the nurse needs to gain experience and skills in:

- Conducting a child and family assessment and collaborating with the family to plan, implement, and evaluate healthcare strategies that fit the family's economic, cultural, and social situation
- Working with community agencies (schools, faith-based groups, military-based groups, and other community-based resources) to assess, plan strategies, and implement and evaluate approaches addressed to the healthcare needs of the community's children

Community Healthcare Settings

Children receive most of their health care (health promotion and episodic health care for acute illnesses and injuries) in community settings. Depending on the community, healthcare resources, and age of the child, care may be received in all or only a few of the following settings:

- A healthcare center or a physician's office is the usual site for health promotion, health maintenance, episodic acute care, and health management of children with chronic conditions.
- A public health clinic may provide health promotion and health maintenance services as well as treatment for specific health conditions. A homeless shelter may also have the capacity to offer such services.
- A hospital outpatient center may provide specialized services to children with chronic conditions or the full range of services offered in a healthcare center.
- Schools usually provide health promotion and health maintenance services, plus first aid and emergency care as needed. School-based healthcare centers exist in some schools to provide health care, counseling, health education, and care for acute conditions. Some school settings also offer preschool and after-school childcare services.
- Childcare centers provide first aid for emergencies and some health promotion services.
- The home is where the family provides care for minor illnesses and injuries and for chronic and complex health conditions, including end-of-life care when the child's family is supported by home health services.

A nurse may serve as a community health nurse, home health nurse, school nurse, pediatric nurse in an office setting, and nurse practitioner or advanced practice nurse in these settings. The nurse in any of the above settings has an important role in promoting the health and safety of the child, being a leader in setting policies in the healthcare center, and using the nursing process to help families meet the healthcare needs of their children. The nurse may assume the role of direct care provider, educator, advocate, or planner.

Nursing Roles in the Office or Healthcare Center Setting

The nursing process is used when providing care for children in the healthcare center. The range of assessment responsibilities may vary by setting as well as the nurse's preparation and experience (Figure 10–1). Specific functions of the pediatric nurse in this setting include the following:

- Identifying children in need of urgent care or isolation
- Performing nursing assessments, including the health history, vital signs, growth and development, nutritional status, immunization status, family strengths and challenges
- Conducting physical examinations
- Performing age-appropriate screening tests to detect health problems such as vision or hearing loss, anemia, and lead poisoning to ensure that the child has access to all needed health services
- Assisting with health examinations, diagnostic tests, and procedures
- Developing nursing diagnoses and implementing a plan of care
- Providing immunizations
- Providing information about procedures and offering reassurance
- Providing family and client education for health promotion or management of the health condition
- Linking families with community resources

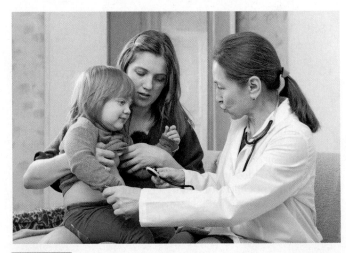

Figure 10–1 Nurses carefully assess children in the office setting who present with an acute care illness to identify how serious the child's illness is. Monitor the child for symptom changes during the visit. Gather information about the child's illness, and identify the education needed for the family to care for the child at home.

- Ensuring a safe healthcare setting and adherence to infection control guidelines (See the *Clinical Skills Manual* SKILLS for infection control methods.)
- Participating in the healthcare center's performance improvement program to identify ways to enhance services provided to children and their families

An important goal is to develop a positive relationship with the child and family so that optimal health care is provided. This relationship is strengthened during future healthcare visits.

Clinical Tip

Developing a relationship with the child and family in a community setting is equally as important as it is in the hospital. The initial interaction often sets the stage for a long-term relationship with the family that returns to the same setting for health care over many years. Remember to put aside the stressors you may be feeling before you approach the child and family. Take a few moments to play with the infant or child and to comment on a positive attribute of the child to the parents. This should help reduce the parents', and perhaps the child's, stress level, which helps set the stage for a long-term partnership with the child and family.

EDUCATING THE CHILD AND FAMILY

Family and client education regarding injury prevention, growth and development, nutrition, healthy lifestyles, and the home care of episodic illnesses and injuries are important nursing roles. The nurse may be responsible for selecting client education materials for the waiting area and those specifically used to teach families about various conditions. Knowledge of the community and population served by the healthcare center enables the nurse to select appropriate education materials for the culture and literacy level served.

Nurses teach families to provide the condition-specific care for the child at home. Examples of information provided include:

- Signs that the condition is not improving as expected and when to return to the healthcare provider
- How and when to administer prescribed medications and their potential side effects
- Recommended diet and activity
- Other supportive care for the child's condition
- Education to help the child and family recognize when to initiate care for a new episode of a chronic condition (e.g., asthma and sickle cell disease) to avoid a healthcare visit or reduce the episode severity

IDENTIFYING SEVERELY ILL AND INJURED CHILDREN

Each child with an episodic illness or injury presenting to the healthcare center must be assessed on arrival to determine the urgency of care needed. Quickly assess for changes in mental status, airway patency, labored breathing, or poor circulation to identify a child who needs immediate medical attention. The child with an urgent condition must be monitored frequently to detect any worsening of condition and need for emergency care.

EMERGENCY RESPONSE PLANNING

The nurse collaborates with all health professionals and the office manager to develop an emergency response plan for the healthcare center. The nurse teaches office staff to recognize a child needing immediate assessment by the nurse. The nurse is often responsible for ensuring that all emergency care equipment, supplies, and medications are organized and readily available in a central treatment room. The nurse may also coordinate mock drills so that all health professionals and support staff know and perform their designated role when a true emergency occurs.

SAFETY ALERT!

Required emergency equipment for managing a pediatric emergency in a healthcare center includes the following in various pediatric sizes (Wright & Krug, 2016):

- Oxygen delivery system (bag-valve masks in 450- and 1000-mL sizes, clear oxygen face masks with and without reservoir)
- Airway equipment (oral and nasopharyngeal airways, Magill forceps, suction devices, laryngoscope handle and blades, endotracheal tubes and stylet, end-tidal CO_2 detector, nasogastric tubes)
- Pulse oximeter, automated external defibrillator with pediatric capabilities
- Intravenous (IV) and intraosseous needles, IV tubing and microdrip, and 500 mL bags of normal saline, lactated Ringer, and 5% dextrose 0.45 normal saline IV solution
- A length-based resuscitation tape and preprinted drug dosage chart to quickly identify equipment sizes and drug dosages by the length or weight of the child
- Essential drugs, including oxygen, epinephrine 1:1000, and albuterol for inhalation; suggested drugs, including activated charcoal, naloxone, 25% dextrose, diphenhydramine, antibiotics, oral and parenteral corticosteroids, atropine, and sodium bicarbonate

Locate the emergency equipment in every clinical setting where you have assignments so that you can quickly take the child to it or bring the equipment to the child if an emergency occurs.

IDENTIFYING COMMUNITY RESOURCES

Nurses are often involved in identifying community resources needed by the child and family to help promote the child's health. Compiling a manual of community resources and regularly updating names, phone numbers, and websites of contacts will make it easier to provide information efficiently. Examples of community resources that might be included are early intervention programs, support groups, translation services, food banks, lead paint abatement services, social services, and mental health services.

ENSURING A SAFE ENVIRONMENT FOR CHILDREN

The healthcare center has many potential hazards such as equipment, cleaning supplies, sharps, medications, and laboratory chemicals and supplies from which the child needs to be protected. The child must be attended at all times when in the examination area. Develop and implement infection control guidelines to reduce the transmission of infectious diseases among child patients and among the healthcare providers and children.

Nursing Roles in the Specialty Healthcare Setting

Pediatric nurses also provide care for children with acute and chronic conditions within hospital outpatient or specialty care ambulatory settings. Children may be referred to physician specialists for diagnostic workups or for the long-term management

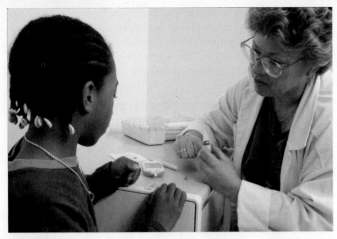

Figure 10–2 **Nurses often assume a larger role in working with children and families with a chronic health condition in the hospital ambulatory setting. Developing a plan of care and educating the family to manage type 1 diabetes is an important role of this pediatric nurse who is also a nationally certified diabetic educator.**

of their chronic conditions. In some cases, health promotion, health maintenance, and episodic illness care are provided to children with chronic conditions in these settings. With experience, pediatric nurses working in a hospital ambulatory setting develop specialized knowledge and skill to meet the specific needs of the children cared for in that setting (Figure 10–2). The roles for nurses in these settings are similar to those described for the healthcare center.

Nursing Roles in the School Setting

School nursing is a specialized practice of professional nursing in the education setting that advances the well-being, academic success, and lifelong achievement of students. School nurses care for children and youth with a wide range of physical and mental health challenges. They advocate for the children as policies are developed for the school community, such as nutritious school breakfasts and lunches or recess and physical education classes for all students. Because of their role in the education system, they are able to educate teachers and administrators about how health conditions affect student functioning and ways to integrate children with special healthcare needs into the school setting (Taras, 2014).

Healthy People 2020

(EMC-4) Increase the proportion of elementary, middle, and senior high schools that require school health education

(NWS-2) Increase the percentage of schools with a school breakfast program and offer nutritious foods and beverages outside of school meals

---

In 2013, 61.7 million children and adolescents attended public and private elementary and secondary schools in the United States. An estimated 12.9% of the enrolled children had a known medical condition or disability for which they received Individuals with Disabilities Education Act services (U.S. Department of Education, National Center for Education Statistics, 2014).

Approximately 11% to 13% of children and adolescents require daily medication administered at school for at least 3 months for conditions such as asthma, diabetes, and seizures. Additional children need medications for a shorter interval for an acute health problem (Center for Health and Healthcare in Schools, 2013). Children who have complex health conditions (e.g., dependent on medical technology, such as peritoneal dialysis, tracheostomies, and ventilators) need school nurses to develop and coordinate the plan for their care during school. These include children who are medically fragile. (See Chapter 12 for a discussion of children with chronic conditions and planning for their care in the school setting.)

The breadth of school health issues addressed by school nurses is illustrated in national health objectives published in *Healthy People 2020*. Additional examples of objectives addressing children and youth in the school setting include (U.S. Department of Health and Human Services, 2015):

- (ECBP-2) Increase the proportion of elementary, middle, and senior high schools that provide comprehensive school health education to prevent health problems in the following areas: unintentional injury, violence, suicide, tobacco use and addiction, alcohol or other drug use, unintended pregnancy, HIV/AIDS and sexually transmitted infections, unhealthy dietary patterns, and inadequate physical activity

- (PA-4) Increase the proportion of the nation's public and private schools that require daily physical education for all students

- (IVP-27) Increase the proportion of public and private schools that require students to wear appropriate protective gear when engaged in school-sponsored physical activities

- (DH-14) Increase the proportion of children and youth with disabilities who spend at least 80% of their time in regular education programs

- (ECBP-5) Increase the proportion of elementary, middle, and senior high schools that have a full-time registered school nurse-to-student ratio of at least 1:750

The school nurse plans, develops, manages, and evaluates healthcare services to all children in the educational setting. Other roles of the nurse in the school setting include the following: maintaining infection control, participating on teams to develop student individualized education plans (IEPs) and individualized health plans (IHPs), updating health records, collecting data on services provided to students, consulting with health teachers about educational topics, investigating environmental safety hazards, developing an emergency preparedness plan, and planning for crisis intervention and support services. The traditional tasks of screening, first aid, and monitoring immunization status are still performed (Figure 10–3). In many cases, the nurse works with families of the students to ensure that needed care is provided. See Chapter 12 for more information on IEPs and IHPs.

Collaboration with the other health professionals in the community is also important to promote health in the school setting, as the following examples illustrate:

- Partnering with the school physician consultant to discuss and update standing orders for the care of children. These standing orders usually address urgent and emergency care potentially needed by students and the variety of student healthcare problems that may occur.

- Working with the parent–teacher association and other community organizations to organize health fairs and injury prevention programs for students.

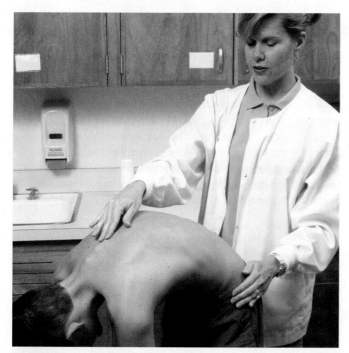

Figure 10–3 **The school is often the setting for screening tests of large groups of students to identify those who may have a health problem that could interfere with learning. Screening tests are often organized so all children in a particular grade are assessed, such as scoliosis screening for children in fifth grade.**

- Communicating with the child's primary healthcare provider or pediatric specialist about a child's specific health condition that needs to be effectively managed in the school setting. Obtain the parent's permission to request confidential client information. The school nurse has regular opportunities to monitor the child's health status and to provide information that may help the primary healthcare providers with the child's ongoing management.

In some communities, school-based healthcare centers provide comprehensive physical, dental, reproductive, and mental health services plus health education to students. They provide service coordination and collaboration to address the health needs of youth with health problems or poor access to healthcare services, especially those not readily available in the community (American Academy of Pediatrics [AAP], 2012). A multidisciplinary team of nurse practitioners, physicians, physician assistants, mental health providers, and other supporting staff often provides care.

PREPARATION FOR EMERGENCIES

Because children spend so much of their day in school, this setting is a common location of injury and acute illnesses. The school nurse often works with school administrators, the physician consultant, and the local emergency medical services (EMS) agency to develop a response plan for true emergencies. School personnel (administrators, secretaries, and health aides) also need training to identify an emergency that requires activation of the local EMS system and to provide emergency care until the EMS providers arrive.

Other potential emergencies can occur during school hours, such as natural and man-made disasters, and behavioral crises (e.g., school shootings). Nurses may participate in

planning committees to develop an **emergency preparedness plan**, a community-based coordinated response plan for the incident (see information later in the chapter). Children experiencing a traumatic event may need psychologic support (see Chapter 17).

Clinical Reasoning Acute Asthma Episode at School

Lani, 8 years old, is at school and is getting anxious because she is having more trouble breathing than usual. Her teacher notices her breathing difficulty and sends Lani to the school nurse for treatment. Lani has a rescue inhaler at school, and this treatment often relieves her symptoms and allows her to return to classes. In this case, Lani's acute asthma episode does not respond to the treatment, so the school contacts her mother. Because it will take Lani's mother at least 45 minutes to reach the school, the school nurse and mother decide that 9-1-1 should be called to get Lani to the emergency department more quickly.

What special arrangements are needed to permit a child to receive care for asthma or another chronic condition while at school? See Chapter 20 and *Evidence-Based Practice: Improving Asthma Management at School* for more information about asthma management.

FACILITATING A CHILD'S RETURN TO SCHOOL

The school nurse also helps the child return to the classroom following an acute illness or injury. Examples include making environmental adaptations, creating an IHP when a new health condition is diagnosed, or revising the IHP when a significant change in the status of the child's chronic condition has occurred (see Chapter 12). The child's parents or the pediatric nurse in the hospital or community setting may initiate the request to coordinate the child's return to school. Educational materials about the child's condition can be recommended to educate students, faculty, and staff. The school nurse then begins to work with the family to prepare teachers and school administrators for the child's special needs, such as limited mobility or medications. The child's teacher and classmates can be prepared for the child's physical changes if appropriate. Sometimes the teacher's expectations of the child need to be modified, such as a child with a mild brain injury who may have decreased ability to concentrate for several weeks during recovery.

Nursing Roles in the Childcare Setting

An estimated 12.5 million children under 5 years of age receive care in out-of-home childcare settings while parents are at work (U.S. Census Bureau, 2011). Many types of childcare arrangements exist, such as in-home care by a family member or nanny, a babysitter cooperative, a licensed childcare family home setting for up to five children, or a licensed childcare center for six or more children.

States establish minimum licensure requirements and guidelines for the safe operation of childcare settings that address the staff qualifications, staff-to-child ratio, staff training requirements, safe food handling, safe health practices, and environmental safety. Guidelines for the safe operation of childcare centers are available through the National Resource Center for Health and Safety in Child Care.

EVIDENCE-BASED PRACTICE | Improving Asthma Management at School

Clinical Question

Because of the potential for frequent absences and the need to manage their condition at school, what are some strategies for helping children with asthma to decrease their episodes during the school day?

The Evidence

A study recruited 530 children with persistent asthma, ages 3 to 10 years, from 67 schools for a randomized controlled trial with school daily-observed therapy compared to parent-administered therapy. Families of all children received a diary to track the child's symptoms, which were retrieved by a monthly telephone interview. Children in the school treatment group had more symptom-free days, significantly fewer nights with symptoms, fewer days with activity limitations, and fewer school absences than the children in the control group. Children in the school treatment group were also less likely to have an asthma episode requiring oral prednisone treatment (Halterman et al., 2011).

A subsequent study recruited 100 children with persistent asthma, ages 3 to 10 years, from 19 schools to participate in a pilot study to compare a web-based screening process and school daily-administered therapy to parent-administered therapy. Parents were expected to administer therapy on nonschool days for children in the intervention group. The web-based screening tool integrated national guidelines for assessment of asthma severity, selected prescribed medications for severity level, and sent information to the child's primary care provider. At the end of the school year, children in the school treatment group had fewer school absences related to asthma, fewer nighttime symptoms, and fewer days needing rescue medications compared to the comparison group. Primary care providers and school nurses reported support for the school-observed therapy program after learning study outcomes (Halterman et al., 2012).

A questionnaire was used to investigate the knowledge of 38 elementary school teachers from two schools about the care of children with asthma. More than 50% of teachers missed questions about characteristics of children with severe asthma, signs that asthma is under good control, signs of a life-threatening asthma episode, proper technique for medication administration, and the common symptoms after rescue inhaler medication (Lucas, Anderson, & Hill, 2012).

Best Practice

Children with persistent asthma are often unable to perform their best in school. Teachers also need increased awareness of asthma symptoms to help identify children who need rescue medications during the school day. School health programs can offer effective strategies to help manage asthma, such as identifying children needing daily asthma medications, offering supervised medication administration, and educating children to manage their asthma. Prior research revealed a relationship between how well the children self-manage their asthma and the children's asthmatic symptoms and morbidity (Kaul, 2011).

Clinical Reasoning

During a school clinical experience, identify the number of children with asthma and how many children report to the school nurse with asthma episodes in a month. What strategies has the school nurse used to work with children who have persistent asthma (e.g., educating students about self-management, providing medication at school, or seeking an asthma action plan)? Have those strategies helped to reduce the number of asthma episodes?

Healthy People 2020

(NWS-1) Increase the number of States with nutrition standards for foods and beverages provided to preschool-aged children in child care

(PA-9) Increase the number of States with licensing regulations for physical activity provided in child care

---

Nurses can assume an important consultant role in the establishment of a childcare center's policies for healthcare practices, teaching staff about safe healthcare practices, and monitoring and promoting healthcare practices in the setting. The nurse consultant can also teach staff to identify children with illnesses and to provide first aid for injured children. Nurses may provide health screening and direct care in childcare centers that care for ill children.

REDUCING DISEASE TRANSMISSION

Children attending childcare centers are at increased risk for infectious diseases. Children are close together in large numbers, put things in their mouths, may be contagious before symptoms occur, and are susceptible to most infectious agents. The nurse can educate and work with the childcare center manager and staff to reduce disease transmission in the following ways (American Academy of Pediatrics, American Public Health Association, & National Resource Center for Health and Safety in Child Care, 2013):

- Teach staff when and how to perform hand hygiene, manage a child's secretions, sanitize toys and surfaces, and treat a child's cuts and scrapes.

- Develop guidelines for diapering infants and toddlers to reduce disease transmission.

- Check each child's health daily for signs of acute illness (e.g., behavior changes, rashes, fever, vomiting, diarrhea, or eye drainage). Isolate and care for ill children until they return home.

- Monitor the immunization status of children and plan for the exclusion of unimmunized children and children with immune deficiencies and disorders when a vaccine-preventable disease occurs in a child attending the facility (see Chapter 16).

- Develop and follow guidelines for safe food preparation and handling.

HEALTH PROMOTION AND HEALTH MAINTENANCE

Health promotion activities within a childcare center promote the child's highest level of functioning and development, such as activities to stimulate physical, cognitive, and emotional development, and nutritious food to foster growth. Health maintenance activities are those that prevent injury or disease, such as immunization monitoring, infection control, and practices like putting infants on their backs to sleep. See the *Sudden Infant Death Syndrome* section in Chapter 20 for additional information.

Health Promotion

Nurses working with a childcare center can design and offer health education programs for the children (such as toothbrushing, hand hygiene, blowing the nose into a tissue, and coughing or sneezing into the elbow or shirt sleeve if a tissue is not available) to promote healthy habits.

Growth and Development   Childcare Outcomes

When children receive quality child care that addresses their health and developmental needs, there are numerous benefits in cognitive development, language, math proficiency, social skills, interpersonal relationships, and self-regulation of behavior. These benefits lead to improved school readiness (Hillemeier, Morgan, Farkas, et al., 2013).

ENVIRONMENTAL SAFETY

To prevent child abduction, ensure that the childcare center maintains a current list of family members who may take a child from the facility and has guidelines for verifying identity when necessary.

The nurse should inspect the childcare environment to identify hazards that could cause injury to the children. Cleaning supplies and other toxins must be stored in a locked cabinet to prevent exposure. Inspect toys used by children to ensure that there are no sharp edges or points, small parts, or pinching parts. Check the safety of playground equipment (Figure 10–4).

EMERGENCY CARE PLANNING

As in the school setting, guidelines for assessing and identifying the child with an emergency health condition and the development of an emergency care plan for an acutely ill or injured child is essential. This plan should include giving first aid, calling EMS to transport the child to the emergency department, notifying the parent, and accompanying the child to the emergency department until the parent arrives.

Nursing Roles in the Home Healthcare Setting

Home health care is a component of the continuum of comprehensive health care provided to children and families. Children with episodic or long-term health conditions can benefit from home healthcare services to promote their optimal function and participation in the family. Home healthcare services may be provided to children with complex health conditions, short-term acute care conditions, and even for hospice care.

Pediatric in-home healthcare services for children with complex healthcare conditions or who are medically fragile have increased because of the increased survival of preterm infants, infants with complex congenital conditions, children with severe trauma, and children with life-limiting or life-threatening

conditions (Mendes, 2013). Technologies now used in the home include ventilators, suction, peritoneal dialysis, enteral feeding tubes, pumps for feeding tubes, intravenous fluids, and medications.

The home environment is believed to improve the long-term care of these children by integrating them into the family, promoting their growth and development, and minimizing the number of hospitalizations. The family may feel as if some control over family life is achieved by having the child in the home. However, the health and well-being of parents is affected by limited sleep, chronic distress, and less time to engage in social and personal health-oriented activities (Murphy, Carbone, & the Council on Children with Disabilities, 2011). Many families feel like they were offered no choice about assuming responsibility for the nursing and technologic care of their child who is medically fragile (Mendes, 2013). This causes stress as the family attempts to balance the child's constant care requirements and needs of the entire family. Healthcare providers and insurers are challenged to simultaneously address the child's illness and developmental needs while supporting families when these children are transitioned to care at home.

Home health care is considered by health payers to be a cost-effective alternative to hospital inpatient care. Many different options for health insurance payment exist, such as family health insurance, the Child Health Insurance Program (CHIP), Social Security, and state Medicaid programs. The family also has a financial burden because of paying some costs out of pocket—for medications, supplies, and transportation. A parent may need to give up employment to care for the child and to qualify for Medicaid.

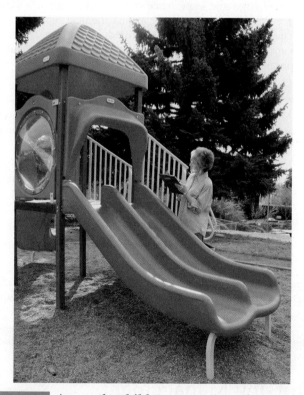

Figure 10–4 **Assess the childcare center's environment for safety hazards. Check the area around playground equipment, making sure there are wood chips or cushioned tiles under the equipment. Inspect the playground equipment for protruding screws, loose nuts and bolts, and instability at least monthly.**

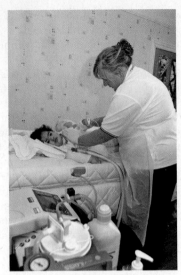

Figure 10–5 Nurses provide both short-term and long-term services to families in the home setting. In some cases, families need support for a short time after the child is discharged from the hospital following an acute illness. In other cases, families need assistance with complex nursing care for the child assisted by technology.

SOURCE: Paula Solloway/Alamy

Nurses need a variety of skills, knowledge, and experience to work in the pediatric home care setting, such as:

- Knowledge and experience in pediatric assessment and acute care practice using various medical technologies. These skills enable nurses to provide direct care, teach the family and child self-care practices, and monitor the child's progress.
- The ability to adapt, be creative, and be prepared to deal with the unexpected, such as equipment malfunctions.
- An understanding of community resources, financing mechanisms, and multiagency collaboration; and good communication skills.
- Knowledge of the community's health resources to help families obtain services that match the child's and family's needs.
- An understanding of the community's cultural diversity and the cultural values of the families served.
- Skill in collaborating with other healthcare team members.

Home care nursing is focused on assisting a family to gain a greater ability to more independently manage the child's care related to a chronic condition or an acute condition following hospital discharge. Nurses also work with the family in the home care setting to promote or restore the child's health while attempting to minimize the effects of the disability and illness, including life-limiting illness (Figure 10–5).

Nursing Management
For the Child in the Home Healthcare Setting

Nursing Assessment and Diagnosis

Home health nurses assess the home, the child, and the family during intermittent skilled nursing visits. Assessment of the home is focused on environmental safety, adapting the environment for the child's care, and identifying needed resources. When working with the hospital discharge planner or case manager to initiate home health services, the following aspects of the home are assessed:

- Home readiness (safe sleeping arrangements, adequate supplies, ability to meet nutritional and fluid needs, telephone access, heat, electricity, refrigeration, lack of any communicable diseases in the home, and safe access into and out of the home)
- Potential hazards related to the child's age, condition, and requirements for technology-assisted care (e.g., extension cords used to plug equipment into electrical outlets and inadequate space for a wheelchair or walker)
- Features of the home environment that could cause an acute illness (e.g., use of a woodstove or fireplace for heating that could cause respiratory distress, active renovation of a house releasing lead dust, and family members who smoke)

Assessment of the child is focused on the current health status, growth, developmental progress, and social interaction with family members and healthcare providers. The potential for abuse and neglect is assessed in children with complex health conditions who are at higher risk.

Family strengths and coping abilities are evaluated along with parenting methods. Parents' skills in giving the child needed medications, performing care procedures, and detecting signs of an urgent change in the child's health status are assessed. The presence of siblings, their developmental and physical status, and their needs should also be assessed.

Developing Cultural Competence **Assessment**
When assessing the child and family in the home, recognize when any potential conflicts might exist between recommended medical care and the family's preferences. Identify which family member is most influential in decisions about the child's care. Use open-ended questions to talk with families and understand the issue from their point of view. Ask family members to identify the issue, why it is a concern, and the impact on their lives. Information gained can be used to educate the family, communicate with healthcare providers about potential alternate care options, and develop a nursing care plan that integrates the family's preferences.

Examples of nursing diagnoses that could apply to the family as the child transitions from the hospital to home setting include the following (NANDA-I © 2014):

- *Home Maintenance, Impaired,* related to insufficient family organization and planning
- *Coping: Family, Compromised,* related to multiple stressors in caring for a child with a complex health condition
- *Health Management, Family, Ineffective,* related to complexity of medical interventions
- *Social Interaction, Impaired,* related to therapeutic isolation

Planning and Implementation

Nursing care should focus on promoting an environment within the home for the child to develop, learn social skills, and gain a sense of identity based on family values. Nurses help families in the home setting in the following ways:

- Ensuring that the child will be safe at home
- Providing competent nursing care to the child
- Educating parents about the child's condition and signs that may indicate an urgent change in health status
- Educating family members to safely administer medications and feedings, and perform medical procedures
- Demonstrating methods to promote the child's development
- Linking families to community resources, including support groups, respite care, and therapeutic recreation
- Assisting families in time management skills
- Advocating for increased health insurance coverage or locating other sources of financial assistance

COLLABORATING WITH THE FAMILY

The nurse works in partnership with the family in the home to promote the health of the child and of the family unit. The nurse must develop a respectful and trusting relationship with the family, remembering that the family maintains control in the home care setting. Open communication is essential so the nurse can learn what is important to the child and family, and then modify the nursing care plan when appropriate.

Role expectations of the nurse, especially when in the home for extended hours, must be clearly understood to reduce stress in the family. House rules for such things as parking, private areas in the home, door to use, where to store belongings, and routines need to be negotiated, and then those rules need to be followed. The success of home care is also based on effective cultural communication. For example, some Jewish families follow strict dietary guidelines that do not permit dairy products and meat to be served together in the same dishes or during the same meal. The nurse needs to abide by the dietary guidelines and observe the family's food preparation practices.

The range of nursing care that may be included in a child's home care plan may include sensory stimulation, routines of daily living, positioning and skin care with gentle handling, respiratory care, nutrition and elimination, medications, and other supportive therapies. Other providers, such as physical therapists, speech-language therapists, occupational therapists, and social workers, may provide other healthcare services in collaboration with the home health nurse.

A parent or guardian should be present when nurses provide home care. Informed consent is needed for invasive treatments and decisions for provision of needed emergency care to prevent serious consequences. A plan for communication about key client-care information (e.g., daily notes written by both the family members and nurse) and scheduled meetings with family members are important to ensure that needed information is shared. This also helps the family members evaluate how well the nurse meets their expectations for care of the child.

SUPPORTING THE FAMILY

When home health nursing is episodic, parents of children with complex conditions often feel stressed by the constant care demands. They may be sleep deprived when caring for the child 24 hours a day and need some assistance in identifying alternative care options, such as **respite care**, short-term home care to relieve the primary caregiver and allow time away from home (see Chapter 12 for more information). Families often need support in identifying and advocating for potential services that may be of value to their child and financial resources for which they may be eligible.

EMERGENCY PREPAREDNESS

The nurse should help the family develop an emergency care plan for any child whose condition could worsen rapidly and become life threatening (e.g., severe congenital heart defect, tracheostomy, or apnea), or be more than the parents or home health nurse can provide with resources available. The plan should provide guidelines for when to call 9-1-1. The emergency care plan should include an essential medical history that provides the emergency care providers with enough information to understand the child's health condition, to prevent delays in disease-specific treatment, and to minimize unnecessary interventions until the child's personal physician can be consulted. Refer to the American Academy of Pediatrics website for an emergency information form.

Families should develop a plan for safe evacuation of the home in case of fire or other emergency. This is very challenging when the child cannot mobilize independently and requires equipment for continued survival or quality of life. See *Families Want to Know: Home Evacuation Plan* for information to help families develop a plan for safe evacuation of the home.

Families Want to Know

Home Evacuation Plan

Developing a home evacuation plan is important when the family has one or more children with special healthcare needs. Important steps to have families take in developing the plan include:

- Have working smoke and carbon monoxide detectors in the home and teach children what the alarm means. Make sure batteries are changed twice a year.
- Draw a diagram of your house. Mark all windows and doors. Plan two routes out of every room. Think about an escape plan if the fire starts in the kitchen, bedroom, or basement.
- Figure out the best way to get infants and young children out of the house. Will you carry them? Is there more than one small child, and if so, how will you get all the small children out if you are the only adult?
- Teach preschool and school-age children to follow the escape plan by crawling, touching doors, and going to the window if the door is hot. Show children how to cover their nose and mouth to reduce smoke inhalation.
- Prepare an alternate fire escape plan in case you are alone with the child when the fire begins.
- Keep home exits clear of toys and debris.
- Select a safe meeting place outside the home. Teach children not to go back inside the burning home.

When the child is dependent on technology, the family should notify the power company so that the home is on the high-priority list for service after power outages. Backup generators may be needed if electrical power for life-sustaining equipment is essential. The child should also be registered for a disaster shelter that can accommodate the healthcare needs of the child and at least one caregiver when major power outages occur.

Evaluation

Expected outcomes of nursing care include the following:

- Care of the child's medical needs is integrated into the family's routines when possible.
- The family has an emergency care plan for the child in the event of a disaster, a weather emergency, or if the child's condition suddenly worsens.
- The home health nurse and family work in partnership to promote the child's health and growth and development.

Assessment of Community Needs and Resources

Community Assessment

Community assessment is a process of compiling data about a community's health status and resources to develop a public health plan to address the priority health needs of a target population within that community. For example, the target population could be all children, a specific age group, or even a special group of children (such as those with a chronic condition). The assessment process involves community partners but follows the nursing process format. Analysis of information gained about the number of individuals with the health need and existing resources helps healthcare professionals determine if additional programs or resources are needed. An overview of the community assessment process is described, but additional resources such as a community health nursing textbook are needed to complete a full assessment.

Community assessments may be conducted for the following reasons:

- A request is made by interested community advocates or the local health department.
- Justification is needed to fund a new or expanded healthcare program.
- Evaluation of responses to healthcare programs or interventions (such as immunizations, injury prevention programs, or services targeted to new immigrants in the community) may provide the data to determine if the children with the greatest needs have been appropriately targeted and are benefiting equally from the intervention.

The focus of a community assessment is on the target population. For example, the focus might be on ensuring that all children in the community, regardless of socioeconomic status and racial group, are considered when trying to ensure access to care or specific interventions—such as injury prevention programs, immunizations, school health services, or suicide prevention programs.

A community assessment is often initiated because one or more individuals (i.e., concerned parents, school nurse, or community leader) are concerned about a health or social issue, such as a child who is severely injured in a pedestrian crossing on the way to school. The concerned individuals partner with other **stakeholders** (all community residents, policy makers, health providers, and funders concerned with the outcome of the assessment) to investigate if this is an isolated event, or if similar incidents have happened at other locations and to identify ways to protect other children. Community partners for this investigation and community assessment may include nurses, family members, local organizations (e.g., Kiwanis, Safe Kids, parent-teacher association), the faith community, the local trauma center, an epidemiologist, elected officials, and health department representatives.

Developing Cultural Competence Integrating Cultural Groups Into Community Assessments

Community assessment leaders should invite community members representing different cultural groups to participate in the process. They help provide an important perspective of the community's needs and help identify culturally appropriate and acceptable strategies to address the health problem.

Family members, a pediatric nurse, and a school nurse are important members of the group when pediatric health issues are being addressed.

The first step in beginning a community assessment is to clearly define its purpose and scope to keep the process focused. The purpose is often associated with a specific problem that an advocate or community leader would like to have addressed by the community. Example issues could be one of the following:

- Several child pedestrians and bicyclists have been injured or killed by motor vehicles over the past 3 months in the same neighborhood.
- Two children drowned at the local lake in a boating incident.
- Three teens from a local high school have committed suicide in the past 2 months.
- The number of children who are fully immunized on school entry has decreased in the last year.

Once the purpose and scope of the assessment are determined, various factors that influence the health of a community should be considered when collecting assessment data (Clark, 2015, pp. 356–370), such as the following:

- Demographic characteristics such as age composition of the community, birth statistics, age-specific and cause-specific mortality rates, racial composition, and **morbidity** (incidence and prevalence of certain diseases), as well as the immunization status of children
- Community prospects for continuing growth or economic challenges, cohesion of the community in dealing with past health problems or crises, existing tensions between various community groups, adequacy of personal safety services, communication networks, stresses in the community, and incidence of crime, homicide, and suicide
- Type of community (rural, urban, suburban), size, climate, topographical features, housing adequacy, water supply, waste disposal, and potential hazards that could lead to a disaster
- Sociocultural characteristics such as local government and community leadership, transportation, income and education levels, employment rates, occupations, family composition, faith communities, cultural groups represented, language barriers to health care, number of homeless families and children, recreation, shopping, and social service agencies

- Behavioral characteristics such as nutrition and specific dietary patterns, use of harmful substances, exercise and recreational opportunities, and population use of safety practices
- Health services available to children in the community covered by health insurance, Medicaid, or the State Children's Health Insurance Program (SCHIP); services available to uninsured children; and barriers to healthcare access

Stakeholders next make plans for data collection (types of data to be gathered, sources of data, and methods for obtaining the data) and data analysis. Some of the best data to use are those calculated as rates, such as the following:

- Birth rate $= \dfrac{\text{number of births in a state in a year}}{\text{total state population (same year)}} \times 1000$

- Mortality rate $= \dfrac{\substack{\text{number of deaths in a state} \\ \text{in a year}}}{\substack{\text{total state population} \\ \text{(same year)}}} \times 100,000$

- Age-specific mortality rate $= \dfrac{\substack{\text{number of deaths in children} \\ \text{aged (e.g., 1 to 4 years)} \\ \text{in a year}}}{\substack{\text{total population of children} \\ \text{aged 1 to 4 years} \\ \text{(same year)}}} \times 10,000$

- Cause-specific mortality rate $= \dfrac{\substack{\text{number of deaths due to} \\ \text{(e.g., injury) in a year}}}{\substack{\text{total state population} \\ \text{(same year)}}} \times 100,000$

- Incidence rate $= \dfrac{\substack{\text{number of new cases} \\ \text{of a disease (e.g., type 2} \\ \text{diabetes) in a year}}}{\substack{\text{total population at risk} \\ \text{at the midyear}}} \times 1000$

- Prevalence rate $= \dfrac{\substack{\text{number of children with} \\ \text{a disease (e.g., asthma)} \\ \text{in a year}}}{\substack{\text{total population at risk} \\ \text{at the midyear}}} \times 1000$

National, neighboring state, and state data can be compared with community data using rates to determine how similar or different the community statistics are for the health problem.

Data may be collected from many sources. For example, the Centers for Disease Control and Prevention collects state data and calculates birth rates and death rates for all types of conditions. Population data are available on the Internet from the U.S. Census. Other potential sources of data include a state or local trauma registry; an immunization registry; community surveys; a telephone book for numbers of healthcare providers and faith communities; and local health agencies for such information as the number of child abuse incidents, trauma centers for injuries requiring hospitalization, clinics for specific services, and infants served by the WIC program. Law enforcement agencies may provide information on motor vehicle crashes, assaults, or homicides. In many cases databases include specific locations of where events occurred with geographic information systems (GIS) coding. Focus groups or interviews with key community representatives may provide information on perceptions of health needs.

An **epidemiologist**, a specialist with training in the study of patterns of diseases or health risks in a population, is often responsible for analyzing the data. Data trends are analyzed over several years to determine if the identified problem is a cluster of events that is part of a larger significant pattern. For example, the timing and clustering of events, such as the number of child pedestrians and bicyclists killed or injured, provide a clue to explore recent changes in the community. Have traffic patterns changed because of construction? Does this happen every year as school sessions begin? Is it related to children enjoying spring weather after school? Once the data are collected and analyzed, the community group can then develop a plan to address the problem and have baseline data for evaluation of the planned community intervention.

Key community assets should also be identified during the data collection stage. A **windshield survey**, a walking or driving tour around a neighborhood or community for the purpose of identifying resources and characteristics of the community, often provides important information needed to plan interventions. What could be collected during a windshield survey to study child pedestrian injuries and deaths?

A community assets map can be developed to help identify the presence of some community resources such as its healthcare facilities, local library, grocery stores, recreation facilities, schools, and so on.

Planning and Evaluation

An intervention is planned and implemented after the collected data have been analyzed and the community health problem is more clearly described. The planning involves a collaborative effort with all the stakeholders contributing ideas, developing strategies, considering funding sources, and ultimately promoting and advertising the plan in the community. The collaboration often includes persons with specific skill sets who can take leadership roles with different aspects of the interventions. The planning group's knowledge of the cultural beliefs, primary language, income levels, reading level, sources of community health education, and potential community partners is valuable in designing the intervention. Knowledge about potential community funding resources or barriers helps in determining potential strategies that may be approved and endorsed by community decision makers.

The plan and interventions for the health problem need to be evaluated. Data collected before the intervention can serve as one comparison for the evaluation. Evaluation should also focus on the intervention and how well the target population received it, as well as the outcome, such as reduced injuries and deaths.

Preparation for Disasters

Disasters are serious and massive events that impact many people in a community and cause extensive damage, hardship, deaths, injuries, and psychologic trauma. Natural disasters include floods, ice storms, hurricanes, earthquakes, volcanic eruptions, tornados, and wild fires. Trains or trucks carrying toxic chemicals and nuclear waste that crash or explode may also cause a disaster. Terrorism is another potential cause of disasters and may involve the use of bombs, infectious organisms, toxic chemicals, or radioactive agents. (See Chapter 16 for information about infectious agents used for bioterrorism.) Disasters may cause death, injury, physical damage, psychologic trauma, and economic disruption.

State and federal agencies, hospitals, and health professionals are participating in **disaster preparedness**, community planning for responses to natural and man-made disasters that involve multiple casualties. Special planning for the needs of infants, children, and adolescents must be integrated into these efforts. Health services are needed to treat injuries and potential illnesses caused by contaminated water and other exposures.

Children have special vulnerabilities during a disaster. Disasters are very traumatic for the children involved, and there may be immediate and delayed responses. Disbelief, fright, and grief reactions are among immediate responses (Jones & Schmidt, 2013). Children may lose their homes and personal possessions. They may be separated from their families. Friends, pets, and family members may be injured or dead. They may also have problems expressing their feelings about the disaster.

Growth and Development

Developmental considerations must be considered during disaster planning because young children may be unable to do the following (AAP, 2013a):

- Walk or mobilize to escape danger.
- Understand what is happening.
- Understand the need to flee or take evasive action.
- Follow the instructions regarding evacuation or safe actions.
- Tell others they need help.
- Distinguish between reality and fantasy.

As Children Grow: **Response to Terrorism Agents**

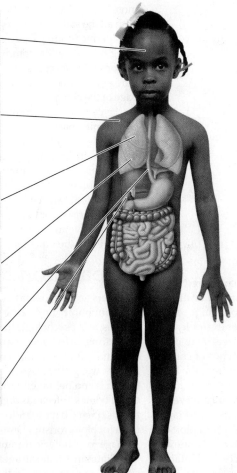

Children's developmental abilities and cognitive levels may interfere with their ability to escape danger.

Children's skin is thinner, so toxic agents falling on the skin can be absorbed more rapidly. Their increased body surface area means greater exposure to toxic agents falling on the skin.

Children breathe faster and inhale more air per weight than adults, meaning a greater exposure to aerosol toxins.

Children are shorter and have greater exposure to heavier aerosol agents that fall to the ground.

Children drink more fluids per kilogram than adults, so there is greater exposure to contaminants in water or other fluids such as milk.

Children also differ in their ability to detoxify and excrete toxic substances.

The child's size, physiology, and cognitive vulnerabilities lead to special considerations when the child is exposed to chemical, radiologic, or biologic agents of terrorism.

Clinical Manifestations

Injuries caused by explosions or falling debris may affect any part of the body. Exposures to various chemicals and toxins may cause burning sensations in the respiratory tract, increased secretions, coughing, respiratory distress, tearing, blurred vision, eye pain, sweating, nausea and vomiting, bradycardia or tachycardia, seizures, muscle weakness, and burns to the skin. Few signs of radiation exposure are seen initially, but nausea, vomiting, and immunosuppression may develop.

Fear, anxiety, sadness, and confusion are some common initial responses to a disaster, whether it is natural or man-made. The responses of children may be even greater if parents are also anxious or overwhelmed. Developmental stage, prior life experience, and the ability of the primary caregiver to meet safety and security needs will determine a child's response to disaster. Support for early responses to the disaster include the following (Jones & Schmidt, 2013):

- *Infants:* Disrupted routine such as changes in sleeping and eating patterns, crying, and irritability associated with family responses to the disaster. Support involves providing a consistent caregiver and maintaining normal routines as much as possible.

- *Toddlers:* Disrupted sleep, nightmares, night terrors, regressive behaviors such as clinging behaviors, withdrawal, and temper tantrums. Support involves reestablishing routines for sleep, meals, and play as much as possible as well as a comfort item and storytelling.

- *Preschoolers:* Similar to toddlers, regressive behaviors (bed wetting, thumb sucking, fear of the dark), disrupted sleep, anxiety, and complaints of stomachaches or headache. Support involves reestablishing routines, allowing regression during stress, and promoting play and storytelling to express feelings.

- *School-age children:* Preoccupation with the disaster details and anxiety about consequences, fear of more harm for themselves and their family. Support involves restricting media exposure, explanations of the event in age-appropriate terms, opportunities to express their feelings, and play therapies.

- *Adolescents:* More awareness of the disaster's severity and its significance that may complicate responses, anxiety, unrealistic fears, anger, changes in mood, stomachaches, and headaches. Support involves engaging adolescents in disaster response efforts when it is safe, encouraging them to talk with peers and teachers about their feelings, relaxation techniques, exercise, and journal writing.

Clinical Therapy

Children have different physiologic responses to emergencies because of their smaller anatomy and developing organ systems. As a result they require special management considerations when exposed to chemical or radiologic agents used by terrorists or to toxins released during another type of exposure, such as a train crash (see *As Children Grow* for more information).

The initial response to the scene of a disaster is to get victims to fresh air and to quickly identify the level of injury or illness severity of all individuals. Emergency care and transportation to facilities that can provide needed care are initiated. Clinical therapy is focused on determining the type of exposure and providing immediate care to reduce the agent's effects.

Decontamination, the removal of chemicals and nerve agents from the skin, should be performed as soon as possible. Clothing is removed, and the child is washed with soap and water. Eye irrigation may be needed to reduce pain and eye damage. Decontamination reduces the child's exposure to the toxin and helps protect medical personnel who will care for the child.

Some children need fresh air, oxygen supplementation, a secured airway with an endotracheal tube, eye irrigation, fluids, and other symptomatic care. Burns and other injuries are cleaned and treated. Antidotes may be administered, such as potassium iodide for radiation exposure or atropine for nerve agent exposure.

Nursing Management

DISASTER PREPARATION

Pediatric nurses in schools and other community settings play an important role in preparing families for a disaster. They can guide families to developmentally appropriate resources for talking with their children about disaster planning and disasters that occur. Families who discuss disaster planning with health professionals are more likely to follow disaster preparedness recommendations, and children may cope better if involved in the family's disaster planning (Jones & Schmidt, 2013). Children need to know what to do in case of a disaster and that police officers, firefighters, and emergency medical personnel are available to help them. They should be taught areas that are safest in the home, how to respond to smoke detector alarms and community alerts, when to call the emergency number, and how to contact the family members when separated (AAP, 2013b).

Help the family develop a disaster plan for staying at home or for evacuation. Families must prepare to manage for 72 hours within their own home following a major disaster or epidemic. The family needs a 3-day supply of nonperishable food and bottled water, flashlights and batteries, a battery-powered radio, over-the-counter medications, and many other resources. Remember to have formula, diapers, bottles, powdered milk, moist towelettes, and diaper rash ointment for infants and children if needed. A plan for family pets should also be made. Refer to the Federal Emergency Management Agency (FEMA) website for the most current recommendations for family supplies to have on hand.

Parents should also carry phone numbers of out-of-town contacts, schools, and neighbors at all times. Developing a list of each family member's medications, clothing, food, water, and other essentials is important so the family can quickly pack and respond to an evacuation order.

Advance planning is needed to ensure that children assisted by technology have the resources needed in the event of a disaster. Help the family register with the designated community shelter caring for individuals needing electrical power for their medical equipment. Batteries for medical equipment should be fully charged at all times. Additionally, parents need to arrange for a durable power of attorney so that consent for emergency medical care can be available should the child and parents become separated during a disaster.

Professionalism in Practice Pediatric Nursing Role in Disaster Planning

Pediatric nurses have an important role in helping community organizations plan and implement emergency preparedness plans for disasters. Each of the community settings where nurses work should have a disaster plan in which pediatric nurses advocate for children and their families. Children and their families may experience adverse outcomes if emergency preparedness plans do not integrate the special needs of children (Society of Pediatric Nurses, 2014).

EMERGENCY RESPONSE

Nurses are important first responders during disasters. They provide emergency health care for rescued victims and first aid for the walking wounded, work in disaster shelters, and perform general public health interventions (e.g., vaccines, sanitation, food and water). Nurses can provide a safe place for children, away from media and unfolding traumatic events, such as the rescue of dead and injured. Do not allow children to leave a scene unaccompanied by a parent or other responsible adult. Assess for panic reactions, unexpected behaviors, and changing conditions.

Clinical Tip

A 12-volt inverter is an inexpensive device that can be plugged into a car's cigarette lighter and delivers 110 to 120 volts of alternating-current power. This device can be powered with the car's battery or by turning on the engine and can be used to keep a patient's life-support device working.

PSYCHOLOGIC SUPPORT

Nurses with knowledge of child and adolescent development can meet the psychologic needs of youth after a disaster. Respond to families in a compassionate and supportive manner, comfort and console children, and provide information and some guidelines for positive coping.

Once the initial disaster is managed and children return to home or other settings, children may need extra time with their parents. Parents should attempt to reestablish daily routines for school, meals, play, and rest as soon as possible. Encourage parents to listen and answer the child's questions about the disaster honestly and in language the child can understand. If they cannot answer a question, it is better to be honest and say so. Reassure the child that they are trying to do everything to keep the child safe. Encourage older children and adolescents to discuss the disaster with family members and peers if desired.

Because disasters may cause disruption for extended periods, the child may have prolonged periods of emotional distress. Identify children and families who do not return to normal life patterns. Worrisome signs include persistently reliving the event in dreams or memories, hypervigilance, difficulty sleeping, irritability, difficulty concentrating, and avoiding stimuli associated with the event. Children who may be more vulnerable to posttraumatic stress reactions (PTSD) include those who change schools, witness destruction, lose a parent or a sibling, lose a home, or remain in a shelter (Jones & Schmidt, 2013). (See Chapter 28 for a discussion of PTSD.) Use these signs to identify children for whom more psychologic help is needed and to promote access to those services.

Chapter Highlights

- Pediatric care in the community occurs in many settings such as physician offices, mobile vans, healthcare centers, hospital outpatient clinics, schools, childcare centers, the home, and disaster shelters.

- Working with the child and family in the community setting requires an understanding of how the larger environment influences the child's health and development.

- Nurses working in many community healthcare settings develop a long-term relationship with the child and family over time that helps promote the provision of optimal health care.

- Examples of community family support services include Head Start education programs, before- and after-school programs, peer support groups, faith community social service programs, crisis care, and respite care programs.

- Pediatric nurses in community settings assist with diagnostic workups and management of children with chronic health problems, including family and client assessment, health education, health promotion, and linking families with community resources.

- School nursing focuses on removing or minimizing health barriers to learning so children can perform academically. Services include prevention, health promotion, health education, emergency care, and managing chronic health problems.

- Nurse consultants to childcare settings assist the administrators in the establishment of the childcare center's policies for healthcare practices, teach staff about safe healthcare practices, and monitor healthcare practices.

- Home care nursing goals include promoting or restoring the health of the child while attempting to minimize the effects of the disability and illness.

- Pediatric nurses help families prepare for a disaster by helping them develop a disaster plan, use developmentally appropriate information to talk with children about what to do when disasters occur, provide direct care in a disaster shelter, and provide psychosocial support to families and children.

Clinical Reasoning in Action

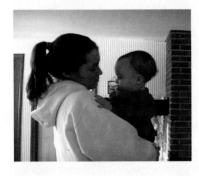

Gavin is a 1-year-old coming into the clinic for his well-child checkup. The clinic is set up to see teen mothers and their babies for well-child visits and immunizations. Tanika, his mother, has been bringing him there since he was born. Gavin qualifies for healthcare coverage through the Medicaid system in his state. He was born full term and has never been in the hospital or had surgery. Tanika is still attending high school and plans to graduate this year. She and Gavin are living with her boyfriend's (Gavin's father) parents until they can raise enough money to live on their own. Gavin's father does not come to the well-baby visits. Gavin attends child care while his mother is at school. He is up-to-date on immunizations so far and there is no significant family medical history, but there is smoking in the home. Gavin has been walking since he was 9 months old. He is able to point, wave, clap, and speak two words. He is able to drink from a cup and put objects into a cup. He has been growing and thriving at an appropriate pace. Tanika describes him as a good eater and tells you that he is currently on whole milk. He has soft stools daily and five to six wet diapers per day. He sleeps through the night and takes two naps per day. Tanika describes him as an extremely active child and has worked on childproofing everything in the house.

1. What is the role of the nurse in caring for Gavin and his parents in the clinic?

2. What data does the nurse collect to perform a family assessment?

3. What strengths and stressors are likely to be present in this family?

4. What information should the nurse provide to help Tanika prepare for evacuation with Gavin since springtime flooding is anticipated?

References

American Academy of Pediatrics (AAP). (2012). School-based health centers and pediatric practice. *Pediatrics, 129*(2), 387–393.

American Academy of Pediatrics (AAP). (2013a). *Pediatric preparedness resource kit.* Retrieved from http://www.aap.org/en-us/advocacy-and-policy/aap-health-initiatives/Children-and-Disasters/Documents/PedPreparednessKit.pdf

American Academy of Pediatrics (AAP). (2013b). *Safety and prevention: Getting your family prepared for disasters.* Retrieved from http://www.healthychildren.org/English/safety-prevention/at-home/Pages/Getting-Your-Family-Prepared-for-a-Disaster.aspx

American Academy of Pediatrics, American Public Health Association, & National Resource Center for Health and Safety in Child Care. (2013). *Stepping stones to caring for our children: National health and safety performance standards; Guidelines for early care and education programs* (3rd ed.). Retrieved from http://www.cfoc.nrckids.org/

Caldwell, B. M., & Bradley, R. H. (1984). *The home observation for measurement of the environment.* Little Rock, AR: University of Arkansas.

Center for Health and Healthcare in Schools. (2013). *Medication management*. Retrieved from http://www .healthinschools.org/Health-in-Schools/Health -Services/School-Health-Services/School -Health-Issues/Medication-Management.aspx

Clark, M. J. (2015). *Population and community health nursing* (6th ed.). Hoboken, NJ: Pearson.

Hackman, D. A., Betancourt, L. M., Brodsky, N. L., Kobrin, L., Hurt, H., & Farah, M. J. (2013). Selective impact of early parental responsivity on adolescent stress reactivity. *PLOS One, 8*(3), e58250.

Halterman, J. S., Fagnano, M., Montes, G., Fisher, S., Tremblay, P., Tajan, R., . . . Butz, A. (2012). The school-based preventive asthma care trial: Results of a pilot study. *Journal of Pediatrics, 161*(6), 1109–1015.

Halterman, J. S., Szilagyi, P. G., Fisher, S. G., Fagnano, M., Tremblay, P., Conn, K. M., . . . Borrelli, B. (2011). Randomized controlled trial to improve care for urban children with asthma. *Archives of Pediatric and Adolescent Medicine, 165*(3), 262–268.

Herrman, H., Stewart, D. E., Diaz-Granados, N., Berger, E. L., Jackson, B., & Yuen, T. (2011). What is resilience? *Canadian Journal of Psychiatry, 56*(5), 258–265.

Hillemeier, M. M., Morgan, P. L., Farkas, G., & Maczuga, S. A. (2013). Quality disparities in child care for at-risk children: Comparing Head Start and non-Head Start settings. *Maternal and Child Health Journal, 17*, 180–188.

Jones, S. L., & Schmidt, C. K. (2013). Psychosocial effects of disaster in children and adolescents: Significance and management. *Nursing Clinics of North America, 48*, 229–239.

Kaul, T. (2011). Helping African American children self-manage asthma: The importance of self-efficacy. *Journal of School Health, 81*(1), 29–33.

Lester, P., Stein, J. A., Saltzman, W., Woodward, K., McDermid, S. W., Milburn, N., . . . Beardslee, W. (2013). Psychological health of military children: Longitudinal evaluation of a family-centered prevention program to enhance family resilience. *Military Medicine, 178*(8), 838–845.

Lucas, T., Anderson, M. A., & Hill, P. D. (2012). What level of knowledge do elementary school teachers possess concerning the care of children with asthma? A pilot study. *Journal of Pediatric Nursing, 27*, 523–527.

Mendes, M. A. (2013). Parents' descriptions of ideal home nursing care for their technology-dependent children. *Pediatric Nursing, 39*(2), 91–96.

Murphy, N. A., Carbone, P. S., & the Council on Children with Disabilities. (2011). Parent-provider-community partnerships: Optimizing outcomes for children with disabilities. *Pediatrics, 128*(4), 795–802.

Ramisch, J. (2012). Marriage and family therapists working with couples who have children with autism. *Journal of Marital and Family Therapy, 38*(2), 305–316.

Sarsour, K., Sheridan, M., Jutte, D., Nuru-Jeter, A., Hinshaw, S., & Boyce, W. T. (2011). Family socioeconomic status and child executive functions: The roles of language, home environment, and single parenthood. *Journal of the International Neuropsychological Society, 17*, 120–132.

Society of Pediatric Nurses. (2014). *Disaster management for children and families*. Retrieved from http://www .pedsnurses.org/p/cm/ld/fid=57&tid=28&sid=50

Spratling, R. (2012). Recruitment of medically fragile children and adolescents: Lessons learned from qualitative research. *Journal of Pediatric Health Care, 27*(1), 62–65.

Taras, H. L. (2014). School nursing: Beyond medications and procedures. *JAMA Pediatrics, 168*(7), 604–606.

U.S. Census Bureau. (2011). *Child care: An important part of life*. Retrieved from https://www.census.gov/how/ pdf/childcare.pdf

U.S. Census Bureau. (2013). *Current population survey (CPS)—Definitions and explanations*. Retrieved from http://www.census.gov/cps/about/cpsdef.html

U.S. Department of Education, National Center for Education Statistics. (2014). *Digest of education statistics, 2013* (NCES 2011-015). Retrieved from http://nces .ed.gov/programs/digest

U.S. Department of Health and Human Services. (2015). *Healthy People 2020*. Retrieved from http://www .healthypeople.gov/2020/topicsobjectives2020/ default.aspx

Wright, J. L., & Krug, S. E. (2016). Emergency medical services for children. In R. M. Kliegman, B. F. Stanton, J. W. St. Geme, & N. F. Schor (Eds.), *Nelson textbook of pediatrics* (20th ed., p. 478). Philadelphia, PA: Elsevier.

Wright, L., & Leahey, M. (2013). *Nurses and families: A guide to family assessment and intervention* (6th ed.). Philadelphia, PA: F. A. Davis.

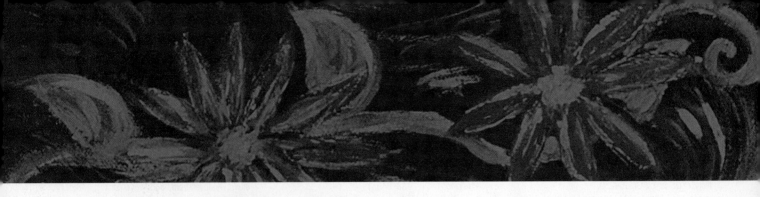

Chapter 11
Nursing Considerations for the Hospitalized Child

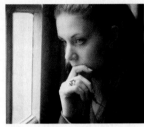

Mel Curtis/Getty Images

We live 50 miles from the hospital and have three other children. We were worried about how we were going to be able to stay with Sabrina. She's only 4, and it's her first time in the hospital. Fortunately, they have beds for parents, so one of us can always be by her side throughout her procedure and recuperation.

—Mother of Sabrina, 4 years old

∨ Learning Outcomes

11.1 Compare and contrast the child's understanding of health and illness according to the child's developmental level.

11.2 Explain the effect of hospitalization on the child and family.

11.3 Describe the child's and family's adaption to hospitalization.

11.4 Apply family-centered care principles to the hospital setting.

11.5 Identify nursing strategies to minimize the stressors related to hospitalization.

11.6 Integrate the concept of family presence during procedures and nursing strategies used to prepare the family.

11.7 Summarize strategies for preparing children and families for discharge from the hospital setting.

Hospitalization, whether it is elective, planned in advance, or the result of an emergency or trauma, is stressful for children of all ages and their families. Because most pediatric conditions can be managed within the home and community, hospitalization is not always required to manage the child with an illness. Additionally, many pediatric surgical procedures are being performed on an outpatient basis. However, for children who are hospitalized, the illness acuity is frequently high. Because of advances in medical technology in recent years, children with complex medical conditions have improved survival rates, resulting in an increase in the rate of chronically ill children who require frequent and sometimes long-term hospitalization (LeGrow, Hodnett, Stremler, et al., 2014).

Hospitalized children experience a variety of emotions because they are in an unknown environment, surrounded by strangers, unfamiliar equipment, and frightening sights and sounds. These children are subjected to unfamiliar procedures, some of which are invasive or painful and may even require surgery. For both children and families, routines are disrupted and normal coping strategies are tested.

Nurses today are challenged to provide individualized care for the hospitalized child with complex medical conditions, acute illnesses, or injury. As a key aspect of that role, nurses must address the psychosocial and developmental concerns that accompany hospitalization. (Developmental theorists and stages are presented in Chapter 4.) To minimize the stress of hospitalization, nurses provide support and education to children and their families before, during, and after hospitalization.

During hospitalization, nurses use a family-centered approach and work collaboratively with parents to implement various strategies that promote coping and adaptation and to prepare children for necessary procedures. Nurses also collaborate with members of a multidisciplinary team and partner with families to prepare them for discharge home or transfer to a long-term care or rehabilitation facility.

Effects of Hospitalization on Children and Their Families

Children's Understanding of Health and Illness

Can you remember as a child thinking that yelling at your mother caused your strep throat? Young children have limited knowledge about the body and its relation to health and illness. They do not understand what causes them to get sick. Their understanding is based primarily on their cognitive ability at various developmental stages and on previous experiences with healthcare professionals. As children become older, they develop a more accurate understanding of illness. For example, perhaps as an adolescent you believed that you would never become ill or have an accident; or maybe you feared being in a car crash similar to that of a friend. Knowledge of a child's understanding of health and illness is essential in assisting a child to adapt to the hospital experience.

Hospitalization and the accompanying medical procedures are very stressful for children, especially very young children such as toddlers and preschoolers. The child's attempts to deal with these stressors impact both the psychologic and physiologic well-being of the child. Infants, toddlers, and preschoolers lack the cognitive skills to understand hospitalization and are the age groups most likely to exhibit regressive behaviors. Young children have fears and anxieties related to things such as the dark, strangers, and monsters. A hospital's unfamiliar environment can exacerbate those anxieties. Significant stressors for hospitalized children include:

- Separation from parents, the primary caretaker, or peers
- Loss of self-control, autonomy, and privacy
- Painful and/or invasive procedures
- Fear of bodily injury and disfigurement

Nursing care of the hospitalized child focuses on minimizing the child's fears, anxieties, and disruption of the child's usual routine, and supporting the family through the stressful experience. Strategies include minimizing separation anxiety, loss of control, pain related to procedures, and fear. Table 11–1 highlights key stressors of hospitalization for children at each developmental stage.

INFANT

By about 6 months of age, infants have developed an awareness of themselves as separate from their mothers or fathers. They are able to identify primary caretakers and to feel anxious when in contact with strangers. Hospitalization can be a traumatic time for an infant, particularly if the parents are not staying with the child. Infants can sense the anxiety their parents are experiencing during a hospitalization.

Common stressors to the infant include painful procedures, immobilization of extremities, and the sleep deprivation caused by the disruption of the infant's normal sleep patterns and routines. However, the most common stressor of hospitalization for the infant is separation from parents, which is manifested by **separation anxiety**. Characteristic behaviors of children in the

three phases of separation anxiety are listed in Table 11–2. Infants and toddlers between 6 and 19 months of age who are hospitalized often display some of these behaviors, particularly if parents are unable to remain with the child. In addition to separation anxiety, children between 6 and 18 months of age may display **stranger anxiety** (wariness of strangers) when confronted with unfamiliar healthcare professionals. See *Evidence-Based Practice: Anxiety and Fears in Children Related to Hospitalization and Surgery.*

Encourage family members to be active participants in the care of the hospitalized infant through touch, sight, and sound. Infants get satisfaction from meeting their oral needs, so parents and nurses should provide sources for oral stimulation, such as pacifiers and age-appropriate teething toys. The infant should be rocked and touched with light stroking to provide tactile stimulation for developmental growth. However, minimize excessive noise and prolonged stimuli to allow the infant periods of rest.

Encourage parents to stay with the hospitalized infant. If family members are unable to remain at the hospital, encourage them to visit their infant as often as possible. Explain and emphasize the importance of parent–newborn attachment and bonding to the parents.

Clinical Tip

Children encounter many members of the healthcare team, in addition to other hospital personnel, when hospitalized. Children ages 6 to 18 months perceive these people as strangers and may cry when someone new enters the room. As the child sees a person over and over again, the stranger anxiety for that person subsides. Providing consistent nursing staff as much as possible will limit the number of "strangers" that the child encounters while hospitalized.

TODDLER

Toddlers are the group most at risk for a stressful experience as a result of illness and hospitalization. This age group is old enough to understand that their routine has been disrupted, but they do not understand why. Separation from parents is the major stressor, and toddlers protest vigorously when their parents depart. When one or both parents cannot be present, they can leave mementos to comfort the child. These might include an object belonging to a parent, a picture, or an audiotape or videotape with messages from the parents.

Disruption of routine also causes stress for the toddler. The nurse encourages parents to remain present as much as possible for important rituals such as toileting, carrying out bedtime routines, and singing favorite nursery rhymes. Autonomy is the developmental task of the toddler (see Chapter 4). Having their activities limited and being confined especially threaten children in this age group. When possible, maintain the toddler's normal home routines for bathing and other activities. Offer the toddler choices when possible, such as choosing the color of Jell-O or which gown/pajamas to wear.

Clinical Tip

Toddlers may challenge a nurse by refusing to cooperate with treatments and procedures, including physical assessments. To diffuse such confrontations, encourage cooperation by offering the toddler some sense of control. For example, a nurse might let the child handle the stethoscope first before listening to the child's heart.

TABLE 11–1 Stressors of Hospitalization for Children at Various Developmental Stages

DEVELOPMENTAL STAGES AND STRESSORS	RESPONSES	NURSING MANAGEMENT
INFANT		
Separation anxiety Stranger anxiety Painful, invasive procedures Immobilization Sleep deprivation, sensory overload	Sleep–wake cycle disrupted Feeding routines disrupted Displays excessive irritability	Encourage parental presence. Adhere to infant's home routine as much as possible. Utilize topical anesthetics or preprocedural sedation as prescribed (see Chapter 15). Promote a quiet environment and reduce excess stimuli.
TODDLER		
Separation anxiety Loss of self-control Immobilization Painful, invasive procedures Bodily injury or mutilation Fear of the dark	Cries if parents leave the bedside Is frightened if forced to lie supine Wonders why parents do not come to the rescue Associates pain with punishment	Encourage parental presence. Allow parents to hold child in their lap for examinations and procedures when possible. Allow choices when possible. Utilize topical anesthetics or preprocedural sedation as prescribed. Explain all procedures using simple developmentally appropriate language. Provide a night-light.
PRESCHOOLER		
Separation anxiety and fear of abandonment Loss of self-control Bodily injury or mutilation Painful, invasive procedures Fear of the dark and monsters	Displays difficulty separating reality from fantasy Fears ghosts and monsters Fears body parts will leak out when skin is not intact Fears that tubes are permanent Demonstrates withdrawal, projection, aggression, regression	Encourage parental presence. Allow choices when possible. Utilize topical anesthetics or preprocedural sedation as prescribed. Explain all procedures. Provide a night-light or flashlight.
SCHOOL-AGE CHILD		
Loss of control Loss of privacy and control over bodily functions Bodily injury Separation from family and friends Painful, invasive procedures Fear of death	Displays increased sensitivity to the environment Demonstrates detailed recall of events to self and other patients	Encourage parental participation. Allow the child choices when possible. Explain all procedures and offer reassurance. Utilize topical anesthetics or preprocedural sedation as prescribed. Encourage peer interaction via Internet, phone calls, and other methods of communication.
ADOLESCENT		
Loss of control Fear of altered body image, disfigurement, disability, and death Separation from peer group Loss of privacy and identity	Displays denial, regression, withdrawal, intellectualization, projection, displacement	Include the adolescent in the plan of care. Encourage discussion of fears and anxieties. Explain all procedures. Ask the adolescent about the desire for parental involvement. Encourage peer interaction.

TABLE 11–2 Stages of Separation Anxiety

PROTEST	DESPAIR	DENIAL (DETACHMENT)
Screaming, crying Clinging to parents May resist attempts by other adults to comfort them	Sadness Quiet, appear to have "settled in" Withdrawal or compliant behavior Crying when parents return	Lack of protest when parents leave Appearance of being happy and content with everyone Show interest in surroundings Close relationships not established

EVIDENCE-BASED PRACTICE | Anxiety and Fears in Children Related to Hospitalization and Surgery

Clinical Question

What fears do children experience related to hospitalization and surgery, and how do they best express them?

The Evidence

In the past several years, many research studies have focused on the child's response to procedures and hospitalization and how best to prepare children of different ages. Recent studies have focused specifically on the child's fears related to this experience, how they express those fears, and how nurses can provide support.

A study by Salmela, Aronen, and Salanterä (2011) examined how children experience fears related to the hospital in 90 children ages 4 to 6. The children were interviewed in either a kindergarten classroom or hospital setting. Interviews were semistructured and accompanied by pictures of a fairy-tale figure in a hospital setting. The main fears identified were those related to nursing interventions and pain, separation from parents and being alone, lack of information, and equipment and instruments. The children described their fears in a variety of ways, including verbally expressing the fear, shouting, crying, fooling around, downplaying the fear, or expressing the fear in a picture or in their surroundings. The meanings of the hospital-related fears were grouped into four categories: insecurity, being injured, helplessness, and rejection.

Researchers explored the views of 93 children ages 5 to 9 related to hospitalization (Wilson, Megel, Enenbach, et al., 2010). Both hospitalized and never-hospitalized children were included in the study. The Barton Hospital Picture Test, a tool consisting of eight drawings related to situations that occur in the hospital, was shown to the children. The children were asked to tell a story about the pictures. The main theme that emerged from the stories was fear of being alone. Other feelings included being scared, mad, sad, bored, and lonely. The stories also indicated that the children wanted to be protected from uncertainty and scary things, and they wanted companions because they were not at home.

Karlsson, Rydström, Enskär, and Carlson (2014) discussed fears of children related to needle-related medical procedures and described the experience of nurses providing support during these procedures. The study utilized video-recorded observations of 20 needle-related medical procedures with follow-up interviews with a nurse. Fourteen different nurses took part in the study, which was conducted in both inpatient and outpatient settings. The interviewers asked the nurses about their experiences supporting children during needle-related medical procedures. Findings of the study indicated that children experience needle-related medical procedures in a variety of ways, and that it is essential to assess each child's ability to cope, taking into account age, developmental level, and previous experiences.

Six components of supportive actions were identified in the study, including developing relationships through conversation with both the parent and the child and being sensitive to the body language expressed by the child and the parents. Another component was identified as balancing between tact and use of restraint. This sometimes involved the use of preparation and play to distract the child, but at times, the child needed to be restrained in order to complete the procedure. Being an advocate for the child was an additional supportive action identified. Although parents are generally the primary advocate for children during procedures, the nurse may take on this primary role if the parent is unable to do so. Adjusting time is a component that refers to the need for nurses to give the child the right amount of time for the procedure, including time for the child to become familiar with the environment. The final component of support identified in the study was maintaining belief, which referred to giving hope and courage prior to the procedure and praising the child afterwards. This might entail the use of the words *brave* and *good* and the opportunity for the child to look in a gift box prior to the procedure.

Best Practice

Research demonstrates that children have fears related to health care and hospitalization. These fears vary among children of different ages and those in well settings versus the hospital setting. Children fear medical staff, equipment, instruments, pain, procedures, and needles, and they fear being left alone. Policies that provide open visitation for parents and include them in the care of the child will decrease fears related to being alone. Therapeutic nursing interventions that provide developmentally psychosocial care and education to hospitalized children is essential to decrease fear and anxiety related to staff and procedures.

Clinical Reasoning

How can children in school settings be prepared for future encounters with health care? Describe policies that promote parental presence for hospitalized children. How can fears related to medical staff, equipment, instruments, pain, procedures, and needles be reduced in hospitalized children?

PRESCHOOLER

The greatest stressors for preschoolers are their fears: fear of being alone, fear of being in the dark, fear of abandonment, fear of loss of self-control related to the body and emotions, and fear of bodily injury or mutilation. Preschoolers may also feel guilty about being sick, or they may view illness and hospitalization as punishment.

Similar to the toddler, preschoolers desire a normal routine, and the nurse can partner with the family to maintain routines as much as possible. Developmentally, preschoolers exhibit a sense of initiative (see Chapter 4) as they explore the world around them. To promote that initiative, the nurse can encourage the preschool child's independence by offering choices such as, "Do you want to take the red medicine or the purple medicine first?"

Parents should be encouraged to stay with the child if possible. For those who cannot stay, preschoolers need to know when to expect their parents to return to the hospital. Because most preschoolers lack a conception of time measurements like "2 hours," "half-past 4," or "3 o'clock," respond with simpler statements of time, such as "after supper" or "before breakfast." Encourage parents to make telephone calls to the preschooler if possible. Some parents are able to make calls from work. Preschoolers get a sense of security from hearing their parent's voice confirming that the parent will return to the hospital.

Parents often believe it is better to leave the hospital room after their child has fallen asleep, as their departure will not stress the child. In fact, the opposite is true. If a child awakens to find the parent gone unexpectedly, the child may become anxious and may develop a lack of trust. Instead, encourage parents to tell their child when they need to leave and why (e.g., has to go to work or go home). By providing honest information to the child, parents or caregivers demonstrate that they can be trusted.

SCHOOL-AGE CHILD

The school-age child relies on parents and others for support and understanding during stressful events and procedures. Although school-age children attempt to maintain their composure during painful or invasive procedures, generally they still require a great deal of support. Major sources of stress for hospitalized school-age children include:

- Loss of control related to bodily functions
- Privacy issues
- Fear of bodily injury, pain, and concerns related to death
- Separation anxiety from family and friends

School-age children understand concepts, so parents who cannot remain at the bedside are encouraged to tell the child what time they will return and to let the child know if the time changes. Parents are encouraged to be available for telephone calls to provide support and comfort to their child. Stressful procedures can lead to regression or other behavioral changes, although this is less likely than with younger patients. Inform the parents that this behavior is normal during stressful situations.

Developmentally, school-age children exhibit a sense of industry (see Chapter 4), taking pride in their achievements at home, at school, and in sports. To foster that sense of industry, allow children to participate in their care as much as possible. Encourage them to continue with schoolwork and engage in creative outlets such as art or crafts.

Growth and Development

School-age children between the ages of 5 and 8 years believe that the internal body consists mainly of a heart and bones. They view the digestive system as having two parts, the mouth and the stomach. Showing them how parts of the body are related can be helpful to enhance their understanding. However, young adolescents, ages 11 to 13 years, can describe the location and function of major body parts such as the brain, nose, eyes, heart, and stomach. However, they usually have gaps in understanding and may have misconceptions, so evaluating their knowledge is a part of the nursing plan in order to plan teaching to meet their knowledge needs.

ADOLESCENT

Preoccupation with appearance and body image are paramount in this age group. By offering education and explanations that focus on these issues, nurses can provide significant reassurance to the adolescent. Nevertheless, adolescents often try to maintain independence and rigid self-control when undergoing painful and invasive procedures. Because hospitalization may increase dependence on their parents, adolescents may respond with frustration and anger. The nurse who respects the adolescent's desire for privacy and independence is often successful in establishing a trusting relationship and assisting the adolescent to cope with the

hospitalization and illness. Encourage the adolescent to discuss thoughts and feelings about experiences. Careful listening by the nurse is essential for establishing a positive rapport.

Major stressors for hospitalized adolescents include:

- Loss of independence, control, and privacy
- Fear of bodily injury or changes in body image
- Fear of disability, pain, and even death
- Separation from peers, home, and school

Adolescents are in the process of establishing their identity and becoming independent of their parents' influence, so control over aspects of their care is important. Partner with the family and multidisciplinary team to ensure that the adolescent is an active participant in decisions and the plan of care. Privacy and modesty are major concerns, as adolescents' physical characteristics are rapidly changing. To demonstrate respect for their feelings, knock on the door before entering and ask permission before conducting assessments or other procedures. By allowing choices in clothing, hair, and music, the nurse can acknowledge the importance of the adolescent's self-image.

The peer group is a major influence in adolescents' lives. Allowing flexible visiting hours for friends helps teens maintain their social network and provides needed support. When friends are not able to visit, providing teens with Internet access provides a means of accessing their friends for support. Encouraging participation in recreation and teen lounge facilities available during hospitalization provides the adolescent with additional peer group support opportunities.

Family Responses to Hospitalization

The hospitalization of a child disrupts a family's usual routines. Parental roles change when the child is hospitalized and care is being provided by nursing staff. Roles may be altered as one parent stays at the hospital with the child while the other parent or siblings take on additional tasks at home. Family members may experience anxiety and fear, especially when the outcome is unknown or a potentially serious health condition prompted the hospitalization.

Family members' ability to cope can be challenged by a serious emergency, lengthy illness, chronic condition, poor prognosis, lack of family support, and lack of financial or community services. The stress on parents can be compounded by the burden of missed work, additional expenses, and concerns about feeding and caring for children at home. (See Chapter 13 for a description of nursing support for the child with life-threatening illness or injury.) Stress interferes with the parents' ability to provide support to the hospitalized child (Agazio & Buckley, 2012).

It is essential that nurses assess parental needs and attend to those needs in order to establish a trusting relationship. Parents who have support from nursing staff have less anxiety and more self-confidence, and are better equipped to make decisions and participate in their child's care.

Nurses also need to be alert to family members' cultural views about health, illness, and the causation of illness, which can influence their response to hospitalization and the family's management of the experience. Cultural influences may also determine which family member is the decision maker regarding healthcare practices, and provide guidelines for acceptable treatments.

The siblings of a hospitalized child may receive little attention from the parents who are overwhelmed and anxious about their hospitalized child's health. How siblings respond depends on their developmental level and ability to understand what is going on. Younger siblings who do not understand the causes of illness and hospitalization may feel guilty about fighting with or being mean to their brother or sister in the past. Some siblings may fear becoming ill themselves. Some may believe that they played a role in the child's illness or injury and need reassurance that they did not cause it. If the sibling did in some way contribute to the illness or injury, help that child cope with the guilt by providing an opportunity to discuss these feelings. Siblings often have nightmares about the illness or injury their brother or sister has sustained and about the ill child dying (see Chapter 13).

As hospitalization causes family roles and routines to change, siblings may feel insecure and anxious. Education and support for siblings of hospitalized children promotes coping and adaptation to a sibling's illness.

As appropriate, encourage siblings to visit. Such a visit is especially encouraged if the child could potentially die, as it allows the sibling the opportunity to say good-bye. (See Chapter 13 for further discussion of the dying child.) These visits often help improve the mood of the hospitalized child and assist the sibling in overcoming misconceptions or negative emotions. Because children's fantasies are often worse than reality, unfounded fears may be relieved by a visit.

Before the visit, prepare the siblings by explaining what they will likely encounter. Describe the hospital environment, including equipment, sounds, and smells. Describe how the ill brother or sister will appear. If the hospitalized child acts, moves, talks, or appears differently than before the hospitalization, provide an explanation beforehand. A child-life specialist may be involved with this preparation (see specific information related to this role later in the chapter). Consider using a doll, drawing pictures, or showing an actual photograph of the hospitalized child to help prepare the siblings. (See *Families Want to Know: Strategies for Working With the Sibling of a Hospitalized Child*.)

During the visit, demonstrate how to talk to and touch the ill child and encourage the siblings to do the same. After the visit, discuss with siblings what they saw and felt, and answer any questions they may have. When a sibling cannot visit, contact with the hospitalized child can be maintained by sending pictures, drawings, cards, and messages recorded on iPods or other electronic devices, and through e-mail, instant messaging, or webcam. Partner with the family to determine the most appropriate and effective method of communicating if the sibling is unable to visit. If parents are staying at the hospital with the hospitalized child, partner with them to help establish communication routines for the well siblings. For example, encourage the parents to call the siblings at home at a regular time each night. Allowing the siblings at home the opportunity to share their day, and to receive an update on the hospitalized child, provides a feeling of connectedness and may minimize feelings of worry and resentment. The phone call offers siblings a consistent link to the parent and the reassurance that they are important and loved.

Family Assessment

To support the hospitalized child and provide family-centered care, nurses develop an understanding of the family dynamics and individualize the nursing care according to the needs of the child and family. To develop a plan of care that involves all family members, the nurse assesses the impact of the child's illness or hospitalization on the family. Table 11–3 provides a list of questions to guide the nurse in determining the roles of family, knowledge of family, support systems, and effects on siblings. (See Chapter 2 for further discussion of family assessment.)

Collaborate with the family to determine their resources, such as:

- Coping strategies of family members
- Financial resources
- Access to health care
- Availability of community services

One family with limited financial support may manage quite well because they have effective coping strategies, whereas another family with greater financial resources may have difficulty if their coping strategies are ineffective. Staying with a hospitalized child can be a financial drain for parents if one or both must take a leave of absence from work, miss scheduled workdays, or travel to the hospital. Additional expenses may include hotel rooms, meals, parking fees, and child care for other children. Assess the family's ability to manage these additional expenses. To evaluate the burden of hospitalization, use a multidisciplinary approach, which may lead to increased access to community resources and support for families.

Assess the family dynamics by evaluating:

- The quality of communication
- Methods of coping with stress
- Risk factors
- Sources of strength

Families Want to Know
Strategies for Working With the Sibling of a Hospitalized Child

The nurse working with siblings of a hospitalized child can implement the following strategies to assist the siblings in understanding what is happening to their brother or sister:

- *Be truthful.* Explain why the child is hospitalized, what the treatment involves, and how long the hospitalization is expected to last.
- *Assure siblings that they did not cause the illness and that the hospitalized child did nothing wrong.* If a sibling had some involvement in or responsibility for the health crisis, referral for mental health counseling may be needed.
- *Allow siblings to ask questions and discuss fears and other feelings.*
- *Encourage siblings to visit if possible.* Cover tubes and wires with a sheet. Wash off blood or cover bloody bandages if possible. Prepare the siblings for any equipment, dressing, and procedures they might see and any sounds they might hear.
- *Warn siblings if the hospitalized child is not speaking.* Say something like, "John can't talk now. He seems to be sleeping deeply. He may be able to hear, though, so you can touch him and talk to him."
- *Encourage siblings to express their feelings related to the disruptive effect of the child's hospitalization on family life.*

TABLE 11–3 Family Assessment

FAMILY ROLES

- What changes will the child's illness create in the family?
- Will household tasks need to be reallocated?
- What specific burdens will be placed on family members?
- Will one parent stay with the child or spend a great deal of time in the hospital?
- Will one parent or guardian be primarily responsible for communicating with other family members?

KNOWLEDGE

- What knowledge does the family have about the child's condition and treatment? Does the family need further information?
- How quickly can discharge planning and teaching begin?

SUPPORT SYSTEMS

- Does the child or family have health insurance? What percentage of costs will it cover? Will other financial support be needed? Will costs continue for ongoing care after hospitalization? If so, will existing health insurance cover those costs?
- Are close friends or family available to provide care for other children, assist with family tasks, or help in other ways?
- Are there community services such as support groups, camps for children with disabilities, education sessions, or equipment and financial resources to which the nurses can refer the family?

SIBLINGS

- Have siblings been informed of the ill child's condition and the expected outcome?
- Have they been reassured that they did not cause the illness?
- Do they understand the change in roles and family routines?
- Are they able to visit the ill child?
- Have their teachers been informed of the family stress?
- If the hospitalized child's life is threatened, are the siblings involved in a plan to promote coping?

Common sources of strength and support include friends and relatives, religious leaders, hospital chaplains, and social workers.

Examine how the family has dealt with the health needs of the child if the child has been hospitalized or required home care in the past. (See *Developing Cultural Competence: Supporting Alternative Health Practices*.) Determine the family members' level of understanding related to the child's hospitalization and anticipated therapy. Collaborate with family members to determine their desired role in the child's care. Assess the family's needs for referral to family service agencies or other community organizations that may be required. Evaluate the need for support groups or agencies that provide medical equipment or other assistance.

Developing Cultural Competence Supporting Alternative Health Practices

Many cultural groups, such as Asians, African Americans, Europeans, Hispanics, and American Indians, may continue to use their traditional healthcare practices (Spector, 2013). They may not share this information with nurses or healthcare providers, both out of respect and in fear that they will be told not to use these methods. Recognizing and supporting use of traditional practices along with Western medicine can promote health and provide comfort for children and families. Ask the families about the use of traditional, complementary, or alternative therapies. Examples include herbal remedies, healers, acupuncture, prayer, and hot and cold foods.

Teaching the child and family, providing support, and referring them to community resources are key elements in providing family-centered care. Additional resources available for the child and family include social workers, child and family mental health professionals, and advanced practice nurses. Additionally, hospital programs and parent support groups are available to assist families in coping with a child's illness.

Nurse's Role in the Child's Adaptation to Hospitalization

Hospitalization of the child may be planned or unexpected. A child may be hospitalized for any of the following reasons:

- The child develops an acute illness or exacerbation of chronic illness.
- The child requires diagnostic or treatment procedures or requires elective surgery.
- The child who was previously healthy suffers an injury, necessitating unexpected hospitalization.

Planned Hospitalization

When hospitalization is planned, children and their parents have time to prepare for the experience. Assess the family's knowledge and expectations and then provide information about likely experiences. A variety of approaches can be used to provide information and allay fears:

- Tours of the hospital unit or surgical area are helpful. This activity assists the child and family to become familiar with the environment they will encounter. During tours, preschoolers and school-age children can see and handle items

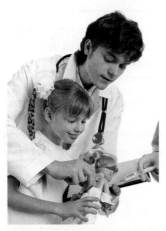

Figure 11–1 **The child's anxiety and fear often will be reduced if the nurse explains what is going to happen and demonstrates how the procedure will be done by using a doll. Based on your experience, can you list five things you can do to prepare a school-age child for hospitalization?**

SOURCE: Poznyakov/Shutterstock

with which they will come in contact. If a tour is not possible, photographs or a DVD can be used to demonstrate the medical setting and procedures.

- The surgical team's attire is less frightening if the child has a chance to try it on and engage in play while wearing the attire.

- Medical equipment is not as frightening when the child learns what it does and observes how it is used—for example, through demonstration on a doll (Figure 11–1).

- Puppets and skits can be used to help explain procedures to children.

- Offer health fairs, as many hospitals do, to explain healthcare procedures to children. During a tour, while hospitalized, or at home, the child can be exposed to books or media that explain in age-appropriate terms what to expect during various procedures.

- Reinforce teaching through coloring books or other educational materials.

Different approaches may be more effective in helping adolescents prepare for hospitalization. In addition to written materials, models, and DVDs, adolescents also learn from talking with peers who have had similar experiences. To demonstrate respect for their sense of independence and privacy, offer adolescents an opportunity to ask questions without their parents present.

Include the family in preparing the child of any age for hospitalization. Parents can be instrumental in preparing a child for hospitalization by reviewing material presented, being available to answer questions, and being truthful and supportive (Tables 11–4 and 11–5).

Unexpected Hospitalization

An unanticipated admission places the child at emotional risk for several reasons, including:

- Lack of preparation for the experience
- Uncertainty and unpredictability of events that follow

TABLE 11–4 Parental Preparation of Children for Hospitalization

The nurse can assist the parents in preparing the child for hospitalization by suggesting the following interventions:

- Read stories to the child about the experience. Numerous books and pamphlets are available (see Table 11–5).
- Talk about going to the hospital and what it will be like. Talk about coming home.
- Encourage the child to ask questions about the hospital and surgery.
- Encourage the child to draw pictures of what the hospital will be like.
- Visit the hospital unit before hospitalization if possible.
- Let the child touch or see equipment if possible.
- Provide a doctor or nurse kit for the child to play with.
- Provide clothing so the child can dress up like a nurse or healthcare provider if desired.
- Plan for support via parents' presence, telephone calls, and special items belonging to the parents that child can keep during the stay.
- Be honest.

- Unfamiliarity of the environment
- Heightened anxiety of the child's parents

An admission for exacerbation of a disease, such as cystic fibrosis or leukemia, can provoke feelings of depression or hopelessness. See Chapter 12 for information related to coping with chronic illness.

Assist the child and family who are not prepared for hospital admission to adapt to the experience by orienting them to the environment, providing an opportunity for questions, offering truthful responses, and explaining all procedures and expectations. Discuss the anticipated plan of care for the child and involve the family in the child's care. Give the family an opportunity to express their fears and concerns. Refer to social services and/or parent support groups if additional support is needed.

TABLE 11–5 Examples of Children's Books Regarding Hospitalization

The Berenstain Bears Go to the Doctor, by S. Berenstain & B. Berenstain

Clifford Visits the Hospital, by N. Bridwell

Corduroy Goes to the Doctor, by D. Freeman & L. McCue

Curious George Goes to the Hospital, by M. Rey & H. A. Rey

Do I Have to Go to the Hospital? A First Look at Going to the Hospital, by P. Thomas

Franklin Goes to the Hospital, by P. Bourgeois & B. Clark

Going to the Hospital, First Experiences, by M. Bates

Lions Aren't Scared of Shots: A Story for Children About Visiting the Doctor, by H. J. Bennett & M. S. Weber

Nursing Care of the Hospitalized Child

Family-centered nursing care of the hospitalized child focuses on promoting the child's and family's coping strategies to deal with the stressors of hospitalization, promoting optimal development and safety and minimizing disruption of the child's usual routine as much as possible.

Special Units and Types of Care

Children admitted to a hospital may be cared for in one or more of the following units: general pediatric unit, short-stay unit, outpatient unit, ambulatory surgical unit, emergency department, or pediatric intensive care unit. Hospitalized children may require surgical treatment involving preoperative and postoperative care. Children with infectious diseases require isolation precautions. Other children may need rehabilitative care to achieve or restore maximum potential.

GENERAL PEDIATRIC CARE UNIT

Smaller facilities typically incorporate all pediatric care specialties in one unit or area, whereas larger medical centers and children's hospitals have separate medical units for different specialties. Specialized units may include medical and/or surgical units, orthopedic units, oncology units, mental health units, and units specific to developmental levels (e.g., adolescent unit). Admission to a specialized unit may be the result of an acute condition, such as pneumonia or trauma, or the result of an exacerbation of a chronic condition, such as asthma. Other causes for admission include surgical procedures requiring longer than a 24-hour stay and the need for inpatient treatments and services. Nursing care for regular hospital admission includes orienting the child and family to the unit and procedures, adhering to the child's normal routine as much as possible, including both the child and the family in the decision-making process, providing direct care to the child, promoting a safe environment for the child, and promoting the child's growth and developmental needs.

SHORT-STAY, OUTPATIENT, AND AMBULATORY SURGICAL UNITS

Hospital stays for children have generally become short, with many procedures being performed in outpatient units such as minor surgery (in ambulatory surgical centers), diagnostic tests (such as cardiac catheterizations), radiology studies requiring sedation, and treatments (such as chemotherapy). The child may be admitted in the morning and discharged that afternoon. In addition, children who have potentially serious illnesses may be placed on a short-stay or observation unit for monitoring or limited treatment, after which medical staff decide either to hospitalize the child for additional treatment or, if improvement occurs, to discharge the child. These short stays are considered beneficial primarily because they cause minimal disruption of family patterns and are cost effective for the institution, health insurance company, and family. Nurses assist parents to prepare the child properly for planned admissions, monitor the child during the procedures, encourage family participation in care, and keep families well informed (Table 11–6).

Nursing care of the child in short-stay, outpatient, and ambulatory surgical units is the same as for regular hospital admission. However, time for teaching is compressed, requiring the nurse to implement teaching methods in a minimal amount of time to ensure the family understands discharge instructions.

TABLE 11–6 Nursing Considerations When Preparing Parents and Child for Planned Short-Stay Admission

- Are there special requirements prior to arrival, such as not being permitted food or drink or needing extra fluid intake?
- At what time and where must the child arrive?
- Are any special forms, insurance numbers, or previous records needed?
- How long will the child stay in the hospital?
- Can the child bring something familiar from home such as a blanket or stuffed animal?
- Are parents expected or encouraged to be with the child or stay in the health facility?
- Is there a chance the child may need to remain longer than expected?
- What will the child's condition be for discharge home?
- Will special equipment or care be needed?
- What symptoms can indicate problems?
- Where can the family go or whom can they call in case of problems or questions?

Effective teaching methods on this accelerated schedule include demonstration, videos, pamphlets with verbal review, and informal teaching sessions.

EMERGENCY CARE

When a child is brought to an emergency department, the parents are usually frightened and insecure and may even be in a state of shock. The fast pace and critical nature of the unit creates an atmosphere in which parents are hesitant to ask questions and are anxious about the outcome. Many factors can contribute to the parents' anxiety and stress (see Chapter 13), including the unexpected nature of the situation; uncertainties in the emergency

---

Clinical Reasoning Preparing Children for Hospitalization or Short-Stay Surgery

Six-year-old Kate has had several nosebleeds and fainting spells recently. After examination by her healthcare provider and a number of diagnostic studies, such as chest x-ray examination, echocardiography, and electrocardiography, coarctation of the aorta is diagnosed. Kate will come in this week for a cardiac catheterization. She is scheduled to have open heart surgery in 2 weeks.

Kate has had few health problems, and her experiences with healthcare professionals are limited. Her parents, who are anxious about the heart surgery, are concerned about how their daughter will adapt to hospitalization.

How should you prepare Kate for the cardiac catheterization and later for the surgery? Include knowledge of her developmental stages and cognitive understanding in your planned intervention approaches. How far in advance should teaching take place? What teaching aids are helpful? How can Kate's parents be involved in and reinforce the teaching? What kind of support do her parents, siblings, and friends need during hospitalization?

The Emergency Nurses Association (ENA) (2012) recommends that family members be allowed to be at the
bedside during invasive procedures and resuscitation
following the written policy of the institution. The clinical
practice guideline developed by the ENA recommends
that a healthcare professional be designated for explanations and support for the family. During development of
the guideline, research by the ENA concluded that family
presence during invasive procedures and resuscitation is
not detrimental to the patient, family, or healthcare professionals. The ENA also concluded that development of a
written policy can provide some structure and support for
the healthcare team.

Parents who wish to remain with a child even during
invasive procedures or resuscitation efforts should be
allowed to do so. The nurse collaborates with the family
members to determine their desired presence in critical
situations and keeps them informed about the health care
provided.

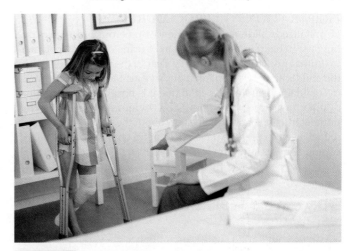

Figure 11–2 **Rehabilitation units provide an opportunity
for the child to relearn tasks such as walking and
climbing stairs. They provide an important transition
from hospital to home community.**

SOURCE: CandyBox Images/Shutterstock

environment; the necessity for quick decision making; the need
for numerous procedures, tests, and treatments; and fear of pain.
The nurse keeps both the child and the family informed about
what is being done and when more news may be available. The
parents and child are encouraged to remain together as much as
possible (see Chapter 13).

INTENSIVE CARE UNIT

Intensive care units provide nursing care to infants and children, including children with life-threatening illnesses and
injuries, acute exacerbations of chronic illness (such as severe
or life-threatening asthma exacerbation), or any other condition
requiring advanced support and continuous monitoring (see
Chapter 13). Parents of a critically ill or injured child admitted
to the pediatric intensive care unit (PICU) experience high levels
of stress (Ames, Rennick, & Baillargeon, 2011). They are likely to
be anxious, particularly since the child's condition may be severe
and the prognosis may be guarded. The unfamiliar equipment
may create an atmosphere of fear or anxiety. Numerous healthcare professionals work in the intensive care environment, and
without effective and open communication, parents may not
know whom to question or even what questions to ask. Partner
with the family and encourage them to write down their questions and direct them to the appropriate source if you are unable
to answer the question.

ISOLATION

Children who require isolation to prevent spread of infection
may experience lack of stimulation due to limited contact with
other children and visitors. Frequent family visits are important
and should be encouraged. Family members may be reluctant to
wear protective garments either out of fear of using them incorrectly or because they believe they are unnecessary. The nurse
ensures that the family understands the reason for isolation and
any special procedures. Having contact with and holding the
child are encouraged when possible.

REHABILITATION

Rehabilitation is the process of assisting a child with physical
or mental challenges to reach full potential through therapy and

education. Rehabilitation units provide children with ongoing
care and support to continue recovery beyond the initial period
of illness or injury (Figure 11–2). These may be separate units
within a hospital or independent centers. The objective of rehabilitation is to assist children with physical, psychosocial, or educational challenges to reach their fullest potential and to promote
achievement of developmentally appropriate skills. Collaboration with a multidisciplinary team including parental involvement is essential.

Parental Involvement and Parental Presence

Family members are essential to the child's care during illness. Integrity of the family unit is fostered through parental
involvement during the child's hospital stay. Involvement
provides parents with control and a feeling that they are
active participants in their child's progress, and it also prepares the family for care that will be required when the child
goes home. The child benefits greatly from parental presence
and participation and experiences less emotional distress
and anxiety if the parents are present (see *Developing Cultural
Competence: Support Systems*). If the parent–child attachment
remains uninterrupted, the child experiences fewer behavioral
maladjustments.

A positive relationship between the parents and the
healthcare team is an essential component of family-centered
care. Parental satisfaction is enhanced when parents' questions
about their child's care and condition are answered; when the
healthcare team is kind, caring, and takes experiences of parents seriously; and when prompt and consistent care is provided (Fisher & Broome, 2011). Parents need to feel valued.
Romaniuk, O'Mara, and Akhtar-Danesh (2014) found a significant difference in parents' desires to participate in their child's
care and their actual level of participation. Parents indicated
that they wanted to be more involved in the care of their child,
especially in activities related to being an advocate for their
child. The nurse should partner with the family to determine the extent to which parents desire to be involved in the
child's care.

PREPARATION FOR PROCEDURES

Hospitalized children may experience numerous procedures during hospitalization, from collection of urine or blood specimens to lumbar punctures and surgery. Fear of the unknown increases the child's anxiety. Maintain a positive attitude when preparing the child and reassure the child that it is normal to be frightened of unknown experiences. Special techniques can help the child understand and cope with feelings about these procedures. Techniques used to prepare the child depend on developmental age, coping abilities, and previous experience.

Developing Cultural Competence Support Systems

Culture can have a significant influence on health beliefs and practices. For example, Mexican Americans view family as a strong support. Extended family may want to be with a hospitalized child. The father of the child is often the spokesperson, and mothers commonly are influential in decisions regarding child health care. The nurse should incorporate all the people the family wishes to have present in the hospital and include them in explanations about health care.

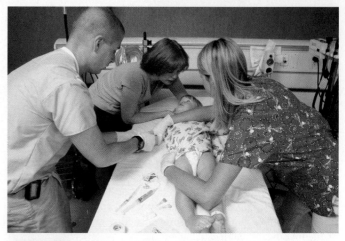

Figure 11–3 Health facility policies that permit parents to be present during a procedure performed on their child are an example of a family-centered care policy. The parent plays an important role in providing security and comfort to this child who is having blood drawn.

PSYCHOLOGIC PREPARATION

Preparation may begin a few moments to several days before the procedure, depending on the child's age and developmental level. In providing sensitive care to the child, nurses assume that a procedure can potentially be traumatic for the child. Even providing urine in a specimen cup or undergoing radiologic examination can be frightening if the child does not understand the reason for the procedure or know what to expect. Administration of medication can also make the child frustrated or anxious. When preparing the child for medication administration using techniques appropriate to the developmental level of the child, the nurse ensures that the medication is safely given (see Table 11–7).

Use developmentally appropriate techniques to assess the child's knowledge and feelings about an upcoming procedure. For example, with a school-age child, the nurse might explain the procedure using drawings, stories, body outline dolls, anatomically correct dolls, and conversation. When assessing the child's perception about procedures, the nurse should consider the following:

• Does the child know the purpose of the procedure?

• Has the child experienced this procedure before? If so, was the experience painful, frightening, or reassuring?

• What does the child think will happen? Are the child's beliefs accurate?

• Is the procedure painful?

• What techniques does the child use to gain control in challenging situations?

• Will the parents or other caregiver be present to provide support?

When explaining a procedure and its purpose, use words that the child understands. Older children require explanations geared to their cognitive level and previous experiences. They will want to know what is happening, why, and what they can do to cope during the procedure (see Table 11–8).

For adolescents, provide written information, DVDs, and other available media. Schedule time for questions and discussions. Allow adolescents to make choices about their own health care when possible. For example, ask them to make those choices with questions such as, "Do you want your hand numbed for the IV start?" Maintain a positive attitude when preparing adolescents and reassure them that it is normal to be frightened of unknown experiences.

Parental presence can provide comfort and support to the child during procedures. Parents should be allowed to choose whether they want to stay for the procedure (Figure 11–3). Some parents may feel that they will be too upset to support the child; many choose to stay. Some adolescents want their parents to be involved in their care; others prefer to minimize their parents' roles. Partner with the adolescents to ensure that their wishes are known regarding parental presence.

PHYSICAL PREPARATION

Physical preparation depends on the age of the child and the procedure. Preprocedural sedation may be required. If sedation is required, the child will not be able to have anything by mouth (NPO) for a period of time. Young infants might be provided sucrose for procedures (see Chapter 15 for pain management). Procedural checklists are often utilized.

Performing the Procedure

Procedures on young children are generally performed in a **treatment room** (a room designated for performing treatments such as intravenous starts, blood draws, and lumbar punctures) to promote the children's sense of security that their own room is a "safe" and relatively pain-free site unless this is contraindicated, such as in the presence of skeletal traction or isolation. Older children can be given the option of having a procedure performed in the treatment room or in their own hospital room. Older school-age children and adolescents may prefer to remain in their room for the procedure.

Perform the procedure as quickly and efficiently as possible. If the parents wish to participate, ask them to hold the child's

TABLE 11–7   Variations in Medication Administration to Children

ROUTE	DEVELOPMENTAL CONSIDERATIONS	TECHNIQUES
Oral	Children under 5 years cannot generally swallow pills and capsules. Children may not want to take medicine.	• Medications are usually given in liquid form (e.g., elixir, syrup, or suspension). • Sometimes tablets are crushed or capsules are opened and mixed with a small amount of food. Check with pharmacy to be sure this does not inactivate the drug. Never crush enteric-coated or timed-release medicine. • When choosing a vehicle for crushed tablets, use only 1 spoonful of applesauce, pudding, jelly, or similar food or 1–2 mL of liquid so that it is easier to ensure that the entire dose will be taken. • Use an oral syringe to increase accuracy when administering a liquid medication. • Position young children upright to avoid choking and aspiration. • Give liquid medicines slowly by oral syringe (for infants) aimed at the inside of the cheek or by medicine cup (for toddlers and preschoolers) for drinking. • Communicate with the child that you expect that the medicine will be taken. Let children choose the type of fluid to drink after, but do not ask if they will take their medicine now.
Rectal	Colon is small in size.	• Lubricate the tip of the suppository before placement. • Place the suppository at the rectal opening and advance past the sphincter. • For children younger than 3 years, the nurse's gloved fifth finger is used for insertion. After this age, the index finger can usually be used.
Ophthalmic and otic	Young children may be fearful of medicines placed in the eyes or ears.	• Adequate immobilization is needed to avoid injury. • The nurse's hand can be stabilized by resting the wrist on the child's head. • Explanations and therapeutic play can be used with children old enough to explain the process of administration. • Have medication at room temperature.
Topical	Skin of infants is thin and fragile.	• Only prescribed doses and medicines appropriate for young children should be used on the skin. • Covering the area or keeping the child's hands occupied may be necessary to ensure adequate contact of medication with the skin.
Intramuscular	Anatomy and physiology of children differ from those of adults.	• The gluteus maximus muscle (dorsal gluteal site) is not recommended in children because of danger of injury to the sciatic nerve (Engorn & Flerlage, 2015). • The vastus lateralis site is preferred for children. • The deltoid muscle is rarely used in young children except for the small amounts injected in some vaccines. • Amounts to be administered should be limited to no more than 1–2 mL for ventrogluteal and vastus lateralis sites and 0.5 mL for deltoid depending on muscle size. Refer to the *Clinical Skills Manual* SKILLS for illustrations. • Z-track technique (retracting tissue to the side and releasing it after injection to prevent seepage into tissue) is often used.
Intravenous	Veins are small and fragile. Fluid balance is critical.	• Careful maintenance of sites is needed. • Common infusion sites include hands and feet, although scalp veins are sometimes used in infants. • Infusion pumps require frequent monitoring. • Syringe pumps are often used to administer medications when minimal fluid is to be given. • Central lines are commonly used for long-term intravenous medication therapy.

Note: See *Clinical Skills Manual for Maternity and Pediatric Nursing, Fifth Edition,* for further medication administration techniques. See Appendix F for information related to how drug dosages are determined for children.

Source: Bindler, R. C., Ball, J. W., London, M. L., & Davidson, M. R. (2017). *Clinical skills manual for maternity and pediatric nursing* (5th ed., p. 106). Hoboken, NJ: Pearson.

hand or stand close by for comfort. Utilize nursing staff instead of parents to immobilize the child as needed. The parents, or another nurse, can be designated to support the child by means of a gentle touch, talking, singing, giving reassurance, or illustrating stress-reduction techniques.

After the procedure, no matter how the child responded, the child should be praised. A choice of reward often soothes the young child. If the procedure is performed in a treatment room, the child is returned to the room for comfort and reassurance.

TABLE 11–8 Assisting Children Through Procedures

DEVELOPMENTAL STAGE	BEFORE PROCEDURE	DURING PROCEDURE
Infant	None for infant. Explain to parents the procedure, the reason for it, and their role. Allow parents the option of being present for procedures. Parents may be able to touch a foot, rub a cheek, and talk soothingly to the infant.	• Nursing staff should immobilize the infant securely and gently. Parents should not be asked to hold the child down. • Perform procedure quickly. Use touch, voice, pacifier, and bottle as distractions. • Ask parent to hold, rock, and sing to infant after procedure.
Toddler	Give explanation just before procedure, since toddler's concept of time is limited. Explain that child did nothing wrong; the procedure is simply necessary.	• Perform in treatment room. • Nursing staff should immobilize the child securely. • Give short explanations and directions in a positive manner. • Avoid giving choices when none is available. For example, "We are going to do this now" is better than "Is it okay to do this now?" • Allow child to cry or scream. • Comfort child after procedure. Give child a choice of favorite drink, if allowed, or special sticker.
Preschool child	Give simple explanations of procedure. Basic drawings may be useful. While providing supervision, allow the child to touch and play with equipment to be used, if possible. Since any entry into the body is viewed as a threat, state that the child's body will remain the same, and use adhesive bandages to reassure the child that the body is intact and parts will not "fall out."	• Perform in treatment room. Nursing staff should immobilize the child securely. • Give short explanations and directions in a positive manner. Encourage control by having the child count to 10 or spell name. • Allow child to cry. Give positive feedback for cooperation and getting through procedure. • Encourage the child to draw afterward to explore the experience.
School-age child	Clear, thorough explanations are helpful. Use drawings, pictures, books, and contact with equipment. Teach stress-reduction techniques such as deep breathing and visualization. Offer a choice of reward after procedure is completed.	• Be ready to immobilize the child if needed. Allow child to remain in position by self if child is able to be still. • Explain throughout procedure what is happening. • Facilitate use of stress-control techniques. • Praise cooperative efforts.
Adolescent	Give clear explanations orally and in writing. Teach stress-reduction techniques. Explore fear of certain procedures, such as staple removal or venipuncture.	• Assist adolescent in self-control. Assist with use of stress-control techniques. • Explain expected outcome and tell when results of test will be completed.

Refer to Chapter 15 for discussion of pain management and sedation for procedures.

Preparation for Surgery

A child's surgical experience may be elective, planned in advance, or the result of an emergency or trauma. How a child responds to the experience is related to the psychologic and physical preparation the child receives. Preoperative preparation, including familiarization with the environment and equipment and explaining surgical procedure, can decrease anxiety in both the child and the parent (Healy, 2013). The accompanying nursing care plan provides information related to care of the child undergoing surgery. Additional nursing diagnoses include (NANDA-I © 2014):

- *Infection, Risk for,* related to exposure to hospital-acquired infection

- *Injury, Risk for,* related to exposure to hospital-acquired infection and use of preoperative medication

- *Skin Integrity, Impaired,* related to disruption of skin surface and limited mobility after surgery

- *Constipation, Risk for,* related to surgical procedure and anesthetics

- *Fluid Volume: Imbalanced, Risk for,* related to intravenous infusion and NPO status

- *Gas Exchange, Impaired,* related to anesthetics and pain

Nursing Care Plan: The Child Undergoing Surgery

1. Nursing Diagnosis: *Knowledge, Deficient,* related to preoperative and postoperative events (NANDA-I © 2014)

GOAL: The child and family will acquire knowledge related to the operation.

INTERVENTION	RATIONALE
• Ask questions of the parent and child about surgery.	• Prior knowledge and understanding can be reinforced and used to guide your presentation.
• Teach about preoperative and postoperative events using appropriate developmental methods such as dolls, drawings, stories, and tours.	• Developmental level determines the cognitive approach that works best for teaching.
• Reinforce information the family has received about the purpose of surgery.	• The healthcare provider may have explained operation.
• Have the children demonstrate postoperative events that pertain to their care such as deep breathing, putting bandage on doll, taping intravenous line on doll, and pressing patient-controlled analgesia button.	• Concrete experience promotes learning.
• Allow the parents and child to ask questions.	• Learners must have opportunity to ask questions.

EXPECTED OUTCOME: Child and family will be able to verbalize details about expected preoperative and postoperative events. They will ask questions that demonstrate understanding. Child will demonstrate skills needed in the postoperative period.

2. Nursing Diagnosis: *Anxiety* related to planned surgery (NANDA-I © 2014)

GOAL: The child and family will show decreased behavior indicating anxiety.

INTERVENTION	RATIONALE
• Question the child about expectations of hospitalization and previous experiences.	• Previous experiences can influence present anxiety level.
• Orient the child to the hospital setting, routines, staff, and other patients.	• Familiarity with the setting and people can decrease anxiety by removing unknown factors.
• Institute age-appropriate play and interactions with the child.	• Play can increase trust level and decrease anxiety.
• Explain procedures and prepare for those that might cause trauma. Encourage parents to support the child.	• The child is more likely to trust healthcare providers if they are truthful and if parents are present.
• Allow the parents and child to ask questions.	• Questioning provides an opportunity to explain the unknown, which decreases anxiety.

EXPECTED OUTCOME: Child and family will demonstrate less anxiety. They will verbalize understanding and comfort in hospital routines. Parents will support the child during traumatic procedures.

3. Nursing Diagnosis: *Pain, Acute,* related to surgical procedure (NANDA-I © 2014)

GOAL: The child will maintain an adequate comfort level.

INTERVENTION	RATIONALE
• Assess behavioral cues (e.g., crying, movement, guarding ability to participate in activities of daily living).	• Behavior of preverbal children provides clues to pain experience.
• Use an appropriate pain assessment tool for verbal and nonverbal children.	• An age-appropriate pain assessment tool allows verbal children to quantify the amount of pain. Pain assessment tools designed for nonverbal children allow the nurse to quantify the amount of pain when the child cannot provide a self-report. (See Chapter 15 for descriptions of a variety of pain assessment tools.)
• Administer prescribed pain medications around the clock.	• Narcotics and nonnarcotic analgesics alter pain perception.
• Use age-appropriate nonpharmacologic methods of pain control (e.g., distraction, repositioning, massage).	• Nonpharmacologic interventions interfere with pain perception and may decrease the child's anxiety.

(continued)

Nursing Care Plan: The Child Undergoing Surgery (*continued*)

EXPECTED OUTCOME: Child's pain will be controlled as demonstrated by a low number on the pain assessment tool (behavioral or verbal).

4. Nursing Diagnosis: *Knowledge, Deficient*, related to care at home (NANDA-I © 2014)

GOAL: The child and family will verbalize self-care required at home.

INTERVENTION	RATIONALE
• Provide oral and written home care instructions regarding surgical wound care, medications, activities, and diet.	• Teaching regarding home care is necessary early in hospitalization.
• Provide a number to call for questions or concerns. Instruct on follow-up visits.	• Parents need to know emergency information and that follow-up care is required.

EXPECTED OUTCOME: Child and family will demonstrate skills needed for home care following discharge. They will verbalize plans for future care.

PREOPERATIVE CARE

Preoperative care of the child includes both psychosocial and physical preparation for surgery. The goal of preoperative teaching is to reduce the fear associated with the unknown and decrease stress and anxiety associated with surgery.

Psychosocial Preparation.   Preoperative teaching is geared to the child's developmental level. If child-life specialists are available, they can play an important role in preparing the child for surgery. When the child will be transferred to an intensive care unit or recovery room after surgery, a visit to the area before surgery can reduce the fear and anxiety associated with waking up in a strange environment filled with frightening sights, sounds, and smells. The use of DVDs, body outline dolls, anatomically correct puppets and dolls, drawings, and models is encouraged to teach the child about the surgical procedure (Figure 11–4). Playing with stethoscopes, gowns, masks, and syringes without needles also helps the child feel more in control (see discussion about dramatic play later in this chapter). Children are reassured that their parents can accompany them to the operating room floor and will be waiting when they awaken from surgery. Parents should be allowed to carry infants and young toddlers to the pediatric

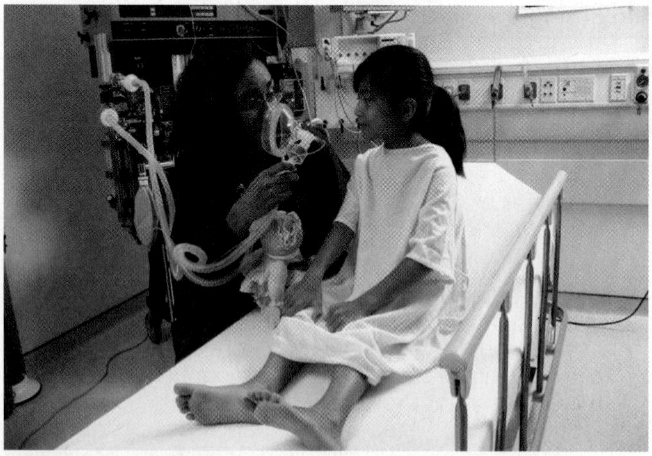

Figure 11–4 **Showing young school-age children equipment that will be used in surgery will help to decrease anxiety related to the unknown. What are other methods the nurse can use to teach young school-age children about surgery?**

holding area or have them ride in one parent's lap in a wheelchair. Older toddlers and preschoolers should be allowed to ride in a special wagon if possible. Special teddy bears and blankets are generally allowed in the preoperative holding area and provide comfort to the child. The nurse should make sure that the item is labeled with the child's name. Prepare family members for what to anticipate and what is expected of them. Explain the purpose of special equipment such as intravenous setups and monitoring devices. In some hospitals, only one or two immediate family members are allowed to visit the child at one time. Visitors may be required to wear special gowns, shoes, or hats, and they may be restricted to certain areas.

Parental Presence During Anesthesia Induction.   Many hospitals now allow parents to be present with their child during anesthesia induction and again in the postanesthesia recovery area. Parents often want to support their child before and immediately after a surgical procedure, and their presence offers reassurance and comfort to the child. The decision to allow parents to be present during anesthesia induction must be made on an individual basis. The nurse explains expectations, such as surgical gown, cap, shoe covers, and the parent's role during induction. The nurse offers the parents an opportunity to ask questions and voice concerns.

Physical Preparation.   Preparation for surgery may occur in designated preoperative areas. Procedures generally conducted in preoperative areas include premedication, intravenous start (if not performed following general anesthesia), and preparation of the surgical site. If urinary catheterization is necessary, it is usually not performed until the child has been anesthetized.

Preoperative procedures and guidelines vary among hospitals and outpatient surgical centers. Preoperative checklists, such as the sample shown in Table 11–9, are used in ambulatory and acute care settings to ensure proper physical preparation of patients for surgery. Weigh the preoperative child accurately, measure vital signs, and ask about last fluid intake amount and type. Monitor urinary output. NPO status in an infant and young child is distressing to both the child and the parents. Reinforce teaching regarding necessary NPO status and provide support to the family as needed.

Nursing management during the preoperative period includes establishing accurate baseline data, administering prescribed fluids, and performing assessments of fluid status. When an intravenous infusion is prescribed, start the infusion (see the *Clinical Skills Manual* **SKILLS**), ensuring that the type of fluid and flow rate match those that are ordered and that would be expected for the weight of the child.

TABLE 11–9 Preoperative Checklist

_____	Check that consent forms are witnessed and signed and in the patient's chart.
_____	Be sure the child's name band is in place.
_____	Be sure any allergies are prominently noted in the child's chart and on a special name band.
_____	Remove any prosthetic devices, including orthodontic appliances and body piercings.
_____	Check the child's mouth for loose teeth and tongue piercings.
_____	Remove eyeglasses, jewelry, and nail polish.
_____	Bathe and cleanse the operative site if ordered.
_____	Put the child in a hospital gown, allowing the child to wear underwear.
_____	Check that all special tests have been completed and the results are in the child's chart.
_____	Have the child void before surgery.
_____	Keep the child NPO before surgery.
_____	Give the child prescribed medications.
_____	Check vital signs and record on chart.
_____	Transport the child safely to the operating room.

Of necessity, the young child who undergoes surgery usually is restricted from consuming oral foods and fluids just before, during, and for a period after surgery, thus creating a risk of fluid imbalance. The length of time the child is kept without oral intake before surgery varies. Recommendations from the American Society of Anesthesiologists indicate that clear liquids may be given up until 2 hours before surgery, breast milk until 4 hours before surgery, and infant formula 6 hours before. Milk and a light meal may be consumed up until 6 hours before surgery (American Society of Anesthesiologists, Committee on Standards and Practice Parameters, 2011).

Infants will generally have very specific orders related to what time they should be made NPO for breast milk, formula, and clear liquids. This time will depend on what time the infant is scheduled for surgery. Because children beyond infancy do not usually eat or drink during the night, orders are usually written for NPO after midnight. However, if surgery is not scheduled for the morning, more specific orders should be written, especially for the toddler and preschool-age child, who will not be as tolerant of an extended NPO status. The ultimate decision on how long the child is NPO lies with the anesthesiologist. Sometimes, because of emergencies, planned surgeries for infants and young children may be postponed for several hours. These children are NPO and generally do not have IV access. What action should the nurse take in this case?

POSTOPERATIVE CARE

Postoperative care of the child includes both physical and psychologic care. In the immediate postoperative period, the nurse should perform baseline monitoring of vital signs according to hospital protocol, maintain effective airway clearance and monitor for evidence of respiratory depression or distress (see Chapter 20), evaluate the child's level of consciousness, evaluate

the surgical site for evidence of drainage or bleeding, and record urine output and output from drainage tubes. The nurse should also examine the postoperative orders and ensure that the child receives the correct type and amount of intravenous fluid prescribed. In addition, the nurse should provide comfort and pain relief (see Chapter 15).

Resumption of oral intake depends on the surgical procedure, the child's condition, and surgeon protocol. Once oral fluids are resumed, the nurse should monitor for emesis. When the child is consuming adequate fluids, the rate of intravenous fluids should be decreased or discontinued according to healthcare provider orders.

Parents are encouraged to visit with the child as soon after surgery as possible (Figure 11–5). In some facilities, children are brought to postoperative anesthesia care units (PACUs) after surgery, where they recover from anesthesia. Depending on the child's condition, the child may be discharged home directly from an outpatient surgical procedure or admitted to a short-stay, general pediatric, or intensive care unit.

POSTOPERATIVE HOME CARE INSTRUCTIONS

Routine postoperative instructions for the family of the child undergoing outpatient or 1-day-stay surgical procedures include monitoring for signs of infection such as drainage, redness, or swelling of the surgical incision, fever, and change in behavior. Instructions for follow-up visit, medications, other treatments, wound care, and signs and symptoms that require medical attention are also provided. Additional instructions are tailored according to the surgical procedure and the child's condition. The nurse ensures the family understands home care instructions through their return demonstration statement of understanding.

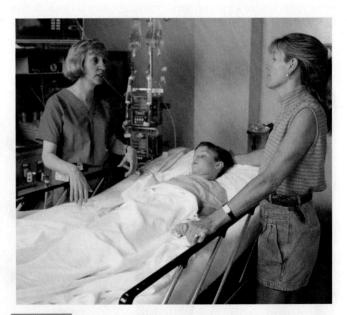

Figure 11–5 This child has just undergone surgery and is in the postanesthesia care unit. Although the child's physical care is immediate and important, remember that both the child and the family have strong psychosocial needs that must be addressed concurrently. It is important to reunite the family as soon as possible after surgery.

Strategies to Promote Coping and Normal Development of the Hospitalized Child

During hospitalization, care of the child focuses not only on meeting physiologic needs, but also on meeting psychosocial and developmental needs. Nurses can employ several strategies to help children adapt to the hospital environment, promote effective coping, and provide developmentally appropriate activities, such as rooming in, child-life programs, therapeutic play, and therapeutic recreation.

Rooming In

The practice of **rooming in** involves a parent staying in the child's hospital room during the course of the child's hospitalization. Some hospitals provide cots, others have special built-in beds on pediatric units, and, in some institutions, a parent is provided a separate room on the unit. Parents who stay at the bedside usually want to help care for their child to some degree. Most parents are comfortable providing basic care to their child, such as feeding and diapering, while parents of chronically ill children might be comfortable participating in more technical aspects of care (Romaniuk et al., 2014). Communication between the nurse and family is important so that the parents' desire for involvement is understood and supported.

Rooming in provides the child with the comfort and security of parental presence. Some parents may feel more comfortable staying with their child and participating in care, others may experience more stress if they are missing work and are away from home and other children. Partner with the parent to assist them in establishing a rooming-in plan that is beneficial to both the child and family. For example, in longer hospital stays, parents may alternate turns staying with the child. Grandparents, aunts and uncles, and grown siblings may be included in the plan.

Some facilities offer free or reduced-cost meals to the parent rooming in. The parent who does not receive these meals may often skip many meals because of the financial impact on an already overburdened budget related to illness and hospitalization. The nurse should be alert to the parent who never leaves the bedside and should make sure parents are eating. Emphasize the importance of the child's need for a healthy parent. Social services or other departments may be able to assist the family in obtaining meals while rooming in with the hospitalized child.

Parents rooming in with their child for an extended hospitalization can be encouraged to take advantage of facilities such as the Ronald McDonald House or other housing available for parents, at some point during the stay, as a respite for a few hours. This break will provide them with an opportunity for needed rest and privacy.

Child-Life Programs

Many hospitals have child-life programs that focus on the psychosocial needs of hospitalized children. Professional child-life specialists, paraprofessionals, and volunteers staff these departments (Figure 11–6). A **child-life specialist** plans activities to provide age-appropriate playtime for children either in the child's room or in a specialized playroom. Some of the planned activities are designed to assist children in working through feelings about illness. Examples include playing with medical equipment, acting out procedures or treatments on dolls, using games to act out feelings, or drawing pictures about hospital treatments.

Therapeutic Play

Play is a significant component of childhood, and the stress of illness and hospitalization increases the value of play. Yet, because of the need to contain costs, hospitals may minimize their play programs. Therefore, nurses should document the need for and

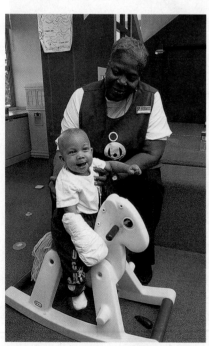

A

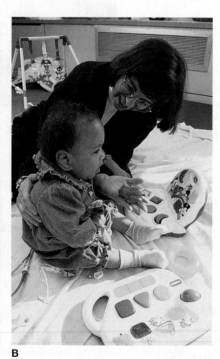

B

Figure 11–6 *A*, Volunteers such as this grandmother can provide stimulation and nurturing to help young children adapt to lengthy hospitalizations. *B*, Child-life specialists plan activities for young children in the hospital to facilitate play and stress reduction.

benefits of play. Beyond facilitating normal development, play sessions can provide a means for the child to:

- Learn about health care
- Express anxieties
- Work through feelings
- Achieve a sense of mastery or control over frightening or little-understood situations

Play that presents an opportunity to deal with the fears, concerns, and stressors of health experiences is called **therapeutic play**. Therapeutic play has many benefits for both the child and the health professional. It allows the child an opportunity to relive, understand, and integrate fearful healthcare experiences. The child can achieve a sense of mastery by being in control of the occurrences during play. This helps lower the child's stress and anxiety about the events. In addition, the healthcare professional can observe the child's play to learn more about the type of events that cause anxiety to the child. The child's coping methods can be observed and additional techniques offered to the child. *Play therapy* is a mental health technique used to treat children with mental health problems rather than normal life events that have caused anxiety. This technique is discussed in Chapter 28.

Through therapeutic play, children's knowledge of their illnesses or injuries can be assessed. A common technique involves using an outline drawing of the body (Figure 11–7) or having the child draw a picture about the hospitalization. Drawings can be used to determine what the child knows and understands about the hospitalization. In addition to assessment, drawing can be used as a nursing intervention. Demonstrate to the child on a drawing what will occur during surgery or a treatment. Children's drawings of healthcare experiences allow them to express fears and gain mastery over the situation.

Dramatic play, in which medical situations encountered are reenacted by the child, often helps the child cope with painful

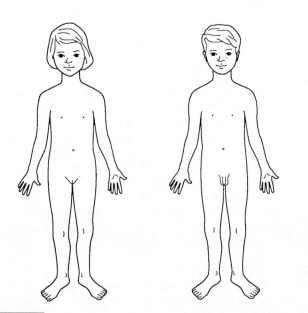

Figure 11–7 The nurse can use a simple gender-specific outline drawing of a child's body to encourage children to draw what they think about their medical problem. Such drawings reveal a child's interpretation, which the nurse can work with to provide appropriate care.

treatments and intrusive procedures. Play using safe medical equipment, such as bandages and syringes without needles, and providing scrubs and uniforms for dress-up are effective materials for encouraging dramatic play. Dramatic play offers an outlet for anxiety in children who are trying to deal with stressful and confusing situations. At the same time, these activities allow the nurse to observe and assess the child's perception of the illness and procedures. The nurse is then able to clarify any of the child's misconceptions.

A variety of techniques may be used to promote therapeutic and dramatic play (Table 11–10), depending on the child's developmental stage. The nurse can ensure that a selection of age-appropriate toys, distraction materials (stress balls, bubbles, music), and "prizes" are available.

Many hospitals, particularly children's hospitals, provide playrooms on each of the units to allow children a place to play and socialize with same-age peers. These rooms are generally brightly decorated in children's themes, and provide numerous opportunities for play, such as board games, video games, supplies for painting or drawing, and age-appropriate toys for each developmental level. For younger children, families may be encouraged to bring the child's favorite age-appropriate toys from home. For older children, there may be options for computer communication with children in other hospitals. Portable electronic gaming equipment may be available to children in isolation or those unable to come to the playroom or teen lounge. Specific interventions according to developmental level are discussed next.

INFANT

Infants require external stimuli for growth. The use of mobiles, music, mirrors, and other methods promotes stimulation and offers comfort to the newborn or infant. Parents and family are encouraged to cuddle or rock the infant and sing lullabies. Talking to the infant encourages interaction and play.

TODDLER

Approach toddlers slowly and make the initial approach in their parents' presence, if possible, to decrease feelings of stranger anxiety. Playing a variation of peek-a-boo or hide-and-seek using the curtain surrounding the toddler's crib or bed helps promote the realization that objects out of sight, such as parents, do return. Transitional objects, such as a familiar blanket or stuffed animal, can temporarily substitute for the security of parents. The toddler can be read familiar stories. Repetition of stories promotes a sense of stability in the unfamiliar hospital environment.

A doll is a familiar toy that can be used to re-create a stressful environment, thereby providing an opportunity for the child to express and work through feelings. Children's hospitals may have condition-specific and anatomically correct dolls for this purpose. Other developmentally appropriate toys for toddlers include familiar objects from home such as measuring cups or spoons, wooden puzzles, building blocks, and push-and-pull toys. Playing with safe hospital equipment helps toddlers overcome the anxiety associated with these items. Supervise these play sessions and remove hospital equipment when you leave.

PRESCHOOLER

The nurse can intervene to reduce the stress produced by preschoolers' fears through the use of some kinds of play. A simple outline of the body or a doll can be used to address the child's

TABLE 11–10 Therapeutic Play Techniques

TECHNIQUE	ASSESSMENT	INTERVENTIONS
Stories	Have the child make up a story about a picture. Analyze content and emotional clues in the story. Have the child tell a story about an important experience in a group of other children.	Read or make up stories to explain illness, hospitalization, or other specific aspects of health care. Emotions such as fear can be included.
Drawings	Ask the child to draw a picture about being in the hospital. Consider subject matter, size, and placement of items in drawings, colors used, presence or absence of physical barriers, and general emotional feeling.	Use the child's drawings or outlines of the body to explain care, procedures, or conditions. Provide an opportunity for children to draw pictures of their choice or directed topics such as a picture of the child's family or healthcare encounter. Ask the child: "Tell me about your picture." Be alert to the child's emotions: "This child must be frightened by the big x-ray machine."
Music	Observe types of music chosen and effects of played music on behavior.	Encourage parents and children to bring favorite music to the hospital for stress relief. Have music playing during tests and procedures. Parents can tape their voices to play for infants and young children during separations. During longer hospitalizations children can tape messages for siblings or classmates, who are then encouraged to retape their responses. Playtime can include the opportunity to play instruments and sing.
Puppets	The puppets can ask questions of young children, who are often more likely to answer the puppet than a person.	Perform short skits to teach children necessary healthcare information. Include emotional content when appropriate.
Dramatic play	Provide dolls and medical equipment, and analyze the roles assigned to dolls by the child, the behavior demonstrated by the dolls in the child's play, and the apparent emotions. Dolls with health problems like those of the child are especially helpful.	Provide dolls and equipment for play sessions. To ensure safety, supervise closely when actual equipment is used. Respond to emotions and behavior shown. Use dolls and equipment such as casts, nebulizer, intravenous apparatus, and stethoscope to explain care. Use dolls with problems or handicaps similar to those of the child when available. Provide toys that foster expression of emotion, such as a pounding board and indoor darts.
Pets	Provide animal-assisted therapy. Watch the interaction between child and animal.	Respond to emotions the child shows. Facilitate touch and stroking of animals.

Note: Additional techniques, such as sand or water play, may be appropriate in specific situations.

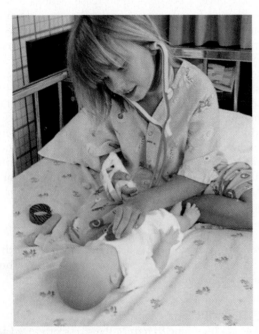

Figure 11–8 Age-appropriate play will help the child adjust to hospitalization and care.

fantasies and fears of bodily harm. Playing with safe hospital equipment may help preschoolers to work through feelings such as aggression (Figure 11–8).

Preschoolers prefer crayons and coloring books, puppets, felt and magnetic boards, play dough, books, and recorded stories. Preschoolers and older children often enjoy animal-assisted therapy. Some hospitals and units may have scheduled visits from pets, most commonly dogs. **Animal-assisted therapy (AAT)** is goal directed and individualized for each child while animal-assisted activity (AAA) may include visits to several children without specific goals. Both of these have positive benefits for hospitalized children (Goddard & Gilmer, 2015) (Figure 11–9).

SCHOOL-AGE CHILD

Although play begins to lose its importance in the school-age years, the nurse can still use some techniques of therapeutic play to help the hospitalized child deal with stress. School-age children often regress developmentally during hospitalization, demonstrating behaviors characteristic of an earlier state, such as separation anxiety and fear of body injury. Outlines of the body and anatomically correct dolls or condition-specific dolls can be used to illustrate the cause and treatment of the child's

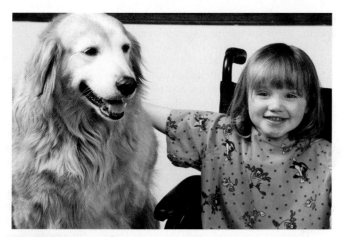

Figure 11–9 Hospitals may have animal-assisted therapy from specially trained animals to provide comfort and distraction during health care. Both the child and the dog seem to be smiling.

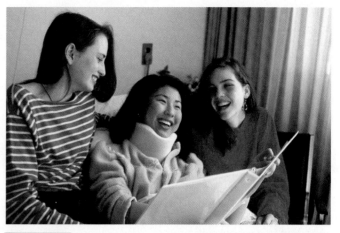

Figure 11–11 Having interaction with other hospitalized adolescents and maintaining contact with friends outside the hospital are very important so that the teenager does not feel isolated and alone.

SOURCE: Cusp/Superstock.

illness (Figure 11–10). Use terms for body parts that are suitable for older children. Drawings provide an outlet for expression of fears and anger.

School-age children enjoy collecting and organizing objects and often ask to keep disposable equipment that has been used in their care. They may use these items later to relive the experience with their friends. Games, books, puzzles, schoolwork, crafts, tape recordings, and computers provide an outlet for aggression and increase self-esteem in the school-age child. The type of play used should promote a sense of mastery and achievement.

Therapeutic Recreation

Many of the special play techniques used with younger children are not suitable for adolescents, but adolescents do need a planned recreation program to help them meet developmental needs during hospitalization. Peers are important, and the isolation

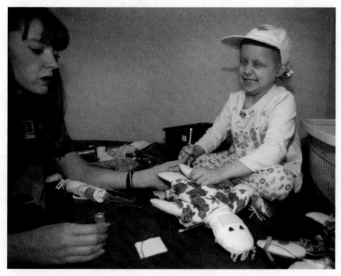

Figure 11–10 Having the child play with specialty dolls will help the child adjust. Such play helps the child realize what activities are possible.

SOURCE: John F. Rhodes/Newscom.

of hospitalization can be difficult. Telephone contact with other teenagers and visits from friends should be encouraged. Interactions with other teenagers at a pizza party, video game, or movie night or during other activities can help adolescents feel normal (Figure 11–11). Physical activities that provide an outlet for stress are recommended. Even adolescents on bed rest or in wheelchairs can play a modified form of basketball. Some hospitals provide a teen room or teen lounge with age-appropriate activities such as a pool table, video games, and computers.

The independence of adolescence is interrupted by illness. Nurses can provide choices for teenagers to assist them in regaining control. Providing adolescents options and encouraging them to choose an evening recreational activity can promote their feelings of independence.

Strategies to Meet Educational Needs

Some hospitalizations are so brief that the absence of the child or adolescent from school and peers is of minimal concern. However, if hospitalization is expected to last longer than a few days or if the child's condition changes so that the child needs special school arrangements, the nurse should assess the effects of hospitalization on the child's education.

When an elective procedure occurs, encourage families to assist in the arrangement of the extended school absence with teachers. The child can then be provided with schoolwork to complete in the hospital or at home when capable. This minimizes educational deficits and future problems for the child. Pencils, paper, comfortable work areas, computers, and quiet work times are provided to meet the child's educational needs. Telephone calls, Internet connections, and live video conferencing with teachers can be arranged as needed.

Hospitals or rehabilitation units may have classrooms, teachers, and facilities to promote learning. The hospital teachers collaborate with the child's school teachers to ensure the child is meeting the educational objectives to avoid deficits upon return to school. Many school districts provide tutors or computer connections for students who are hospitalized or receiving home care for extended periods. Teachers can visit children at the hospital or at home. Parents are often pivotal in making arrangements to meet the child's educational needs, since they interact with the child, the school, and the healthcare team.

Nurses should also consider the social aspects of school and peers. Peers can be encouraged to visit a hospitalized classmate, send cards and letters, call on the phone, or communicate via the Internet. Classmates may even videotape a class session, allowing everyone the opportunity to send messages to the hospitalized child. When the child returns to school, information may be shared about the child's special needs. Maintain the child's and family's privacy by discussing with them the information needed by others, and obtaining written permission before disclosing any information. The hospital and school nurse often collaborate with each other, as well as the child and family, to plan for the child's needs. The child with chronic health problems or who requires long-term hospitalization has additional needs with regard to school. See Chapter 12 for information related to the child with a chronic condition in a school setting.

Growth and Development

For children who are given the opportunity to hear, touch, see a model or equipment, read, look at pictures, or even smell things like alcohol swabs, learning is more complete. This is particularly important for the school-age child in the stage of concrete operational thought, who must be able to manipulate material in order to learn.

CHILD AND FAMILY TEACHING

Teaching is an essential part of the nurse's role in care of hospitalized children and their families and begins with the initial contact between the family and healthcare providers. Teaching may be informal, as when the nurse integrates an explanation during routine care, or structured, as when the nurse plans and implements a formal teaching program.

Nurses emphasize to the family that most teaching will occur in informal sessions rather than in formalized programs. The family should be aware of the teaching process to encourage active listening and participation. Actively involve the family in the learning process to ensure their understanding. The nurse and family partner together to identify the family's learning needs and appropriate teaching method to best convey the information. Recall that family members may be at various cognitive and anxiety levels and therefore have needs for different types of teaching. Develop a plan with both the family and other healthcare professionals to facilitate learning among the child and family members.

Prior to implementing teaching for the child, it is essential to assess the child's developmental level. Teaching directed at parents must also be geared to their level of understanding. If English is not spoken or is the parents' second language, an interpreter may be necessary. If interpreters are needed to facilitate understanding, be sure they are contacted and are available for teaching sessions.

Depending on the information to be presented, teaching may use the cognitive, psychomotor, or affective domains of learning. Teaching that includes all three domains is more effective. Explanations or reading materials, including pamphlets, booklets, DVDs, and models, are tailored to a level the parent can understand. The choice of tools used varies depending on the child's diagnosis and available materials.

Timing is a critical factor in teaching. Parents and children are less receptive to teaching when they are preoccupied with stress or activities. Collaborating with the parents in scheduling specific times for teaching sessions may be helpful.

TEACHING PLANS

A teaching plan is a written plan that includes goals and expected outcomes, interventions needed to achieve the specified goals, and a method and time for evaluation of the expected outcomes. The teaching plan may also specify teaching methods and types of materials to be used. By developing a teaching plan, a nurse helps to ensure that all the necessary information is included and taught efficiently. Additionally, this written documentation of teaching allows for continuity of care between nurses and other disciplines. Multidisciplinary teaching plans provide clear communication for all healthcare team members in the teaching process.

The child's primary caretaker should be an active participant in the development and implementation of the teaching plan. The primary caretaker is most often a parent but may be a close family member (uncle, aunt, or grandparent). Before establishing a teaching plan, the nurse should assess the child's or parent's knowledge, skills, and feelings by considering the following questions:

- What does the parent/caretaker or child know about the health issue?
- What are the expectations of the child and family?
- What is the cognitive level or ability to learn?
- Is there a desire to learn?
- What previous experiences affect the learning experience, either positively or negatively?
- What previous interventions have been the most useful for the child and family?
- What resources are available to the parents, child, and nurse that enhance understanding of the health condition?
- Are there feelings or beliefs that might interfere with the learning process?
- What complementary care does the family use, and how does this relate to the teaching plan?

The second step involves deciding what knowledge, skill, or change in attitude is desired. Outcome criteria or objectives are established with the parent and child. Possible teaching methods and a range of approaches are explored. A variety of resources, including written materials (books, pamphlets, handouts, and stories), computer software, audiovisual presentations, dolls, and body models are available to encourage interest from the child and family. Refer to Chapter 1 for information on reading level of patient education materials. In some settings, audiovisual and computer resources may be limited. Small group teaching sessions (e.g., for children with recently diagnosed diabetes) may be another option and provide the child with an opportunity to interact and learn from peers experiencing the same condition. Gathering two or three parents together on a unit to learn and share experiences may also be helpful. For some conditions, standardized teaching plans are available in books and from healthcare agencies. These plans can serve as a guide in developing an individualized teaching plan.

TEACHING FOR CHILDREN WITH SPECIAL HEALTHCARE NEEDS

Children who have disabilities may have special learning needs. If the child has a visual impairment or perceptual difficulty, material is presented in auditory and tactile ways. Children who have hearing deficits require visual and tactile presentations. Children who have learning disabilities may require more frequent reinforcement and shorter teaching sessions. These children are evaluated often for comprehension in order to adjust teaching as necessary.

Children who have chronic conditions or special healthcare needs may have been hospitalized numerous times and have received other health care at home and in the community. They usually have adapted coping mechanisms that help them deal with their illness. Nurses can talk with the child to determine what has helped in the past, provide information about what to expect during the current hospitalization, assign staff members who are familiar when possible, and follow each child's lead in assisting the child in coping. Do not assume that the child with a history of numerous hospitalizations understands all activities, for each hospitalization is different. Even the most routine activities should be explained. Regularly review the updated plan of care with the parents and child. Provide the child with opportunities to ask questions and express concerns and fears. Assess the child's individual learning needs. Older children can be asked how they best like to learn. Determine the necessity for special equipment or teaching methods.

Preparation for Home Care

Nurses play an important role in preparing the child and family for discharge home; this preparation starts early during the hospitalization. The nurse works with the social service department, home care agencies, and the family to plan for equipment, procedures, and other home care needs. Home care nurses collaborate with the hospital nurse and assist families to meet the child's healthcare needs.

Assessing the Child and Family in Preparation for Discharge

Preparations for the discharge process are best started upon admission to the hospital. The healthcare team, including the primary healthcare provider, nurse, social worker, and discharge planner partner with the family to ensure a smooth transition. Assess the family's ability to manage the child's care and if any special adaptation to the home environment is necessary.

When a child who has been hospitalized for an extended time is to be discharged home, the school district is contacted by the hospital school teacher (if available) or social worker, and plans for education or reentry into school are made. This involves an assessment of the child by the school district and formulation of an individualized education plan (IEP). The IEP may include home tutors, specialized services from persons such as physical or speech therapists, or arrangements for transport of the child with a disability to the school and provisions for special medical care as needed. An individualized health plan (IHP) may also be required. See Chapter 12 for definitions and a detailed discussion on IEPs and IHPs. Some common problems that interfere with successful discharge planning include financial concerns, the family's unavailability for teaching and planning, lack of equipment, and lack of teamwork among involved healthcare disciplines. Nurses who assess for these potential problems from the initial contact with the child and family can intervene and assist the family to resolve them as soon as possible.

Preparing the Family for Home Care

The family may need to learn physical and rehabilitative procedures for the child's care. Short-term care may be necessary until the child regains full function. In other situations, care may be required throughout the child's life. This may involve measuring vital signs or assessing blood glucose levels.

For the child requiring complex long-term care, parents may need to learn about intravenous lines, medications, oxygen administration, or ventilators (Figure 11–12). See Chapter 12 for discussion of the child with a chronic condition.

Parents need to be taught how to use the equipment needed for the child's care and must show that they can use it correctly. They must be able to identify symptoms of distress and report them immediately to the healthcare provider. The education provided and the parents' ability to perform care are discussed with a visiting nurse or individual who manages the home care program. Parents should be encouraged to learn cardiopulmonary resuscitation (see the *Clinical Skills Manual* SKILLS). Help parents explore options for respite care. If they cannot provide daily care or need a break, they should be able to rely on others for a short period. Some agencies are available to provide respite care. Ongoing assistance may be needed to help families deal with finances, time, and other challenges. If parents must take a leave of absence from work to provide care for the child, inform them about the coverage provided by the Family Medical Leave Act (U.S. Department of Labor, 2012).

Preparing Parents to Act as Case Managers

The family is an integral part of the plan of care for an ill or hospitalized child. The child with a chronic illness or an injury requiring long-term care will probably require the services of numerous healthcare personnel or healthcare agencies. One person needs to be identified as a **case manager** to coordinate health care and to prevent gaps and overlaps. In some hospitals, nurses act as case managers. They may organize a patient care conference while the child with a chronic condition is hospitalized. Management goals are set and decisions are made about which healthcare provider or agency is responsible for helping the child meet each goal.

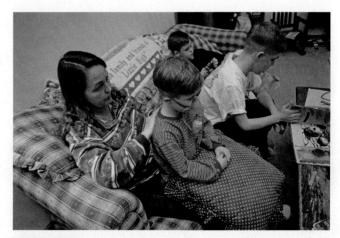

Figure 11–12 **This child with chronic medical problems is being cared for at home. Are there any legal implications for the hospital and the nurse associated with the preparation of the child and family for home care?**

SOURCE: Karen Kasmauski/Corbis.

Parents can also be case managers. The parent as case manager coordinates medical care, hospital stays, and visits to specialists; meets with school district representatives to plan the individualized education program for the child; finds equipment, personnel, and other services for home care; and manages the child's overall care.

Nurses should strongly encourage parents who want to take over case management to do so. Help them learn the management skills required. Many community agencies such as social service or home health agencies hold workshops for parents managing the complex care of their children.

Chapter Highlights

- Hospitalization is a stressful event for all children and their families and affects families in a variety of ways, including disruption of usual routines, anxiety and fear related to the unknown, sibling concerns, financial difficulties, and parental anxiety over changing roles.

- The understanding of children about their illnesses and hospitalizations is based on cognitive and psychosocial stage/level and on previous healthcare experiences.

- Nurses assess the impact of the child's illness or hospitalization on the family unit and provide individualized family-centered care. Supporting rooming in by parents or other family members, promoting development and safety, minimizing disruption of routines, and orientation to special units and expectations are specific strategies that can be implemented.

- Families are always disrupted by a child's hospitalization, and various approaches can help them understand the process and cope more successfully. Specific examples include promoting parental involvement in care; orienting the child and family to the hospital setting, routines, and staff; age-appropriate explanations of procedures; and encouraging parents to support the child.

- When hospitalization is planned, both the child and family can prepare for the experience. Nurses assist this process by teaching them what to expect. Preparation may include tours, therapeutic play, books, and developmentally appropriate explanations.

- When hospitalization is unplanned, nurses can prepare the child and family by orienting them to the environment and use of developmentally appropriate explanations of procedures and equipment.

- A teaching plan includes goals and expected outcomes, interventions needed to achieve the specified goals, and a method and time for evaluation of the expected outcomes. How the teaching plan is implemented depends on the unique characteristics of the child/family to be taught.

- The child is prepared for procedures using a variety of techniques, taking into consideration the child's developmental age, coping abilities, and previous experience.

- Strategies such as child-life programs, rooming in, therapeutic play, and therapeutic recreation help meet the psychosocial needs of the hospitalized child.

- The nurse assists the family in planning for the child's long-term healthcare needs and home care issues. Culturally competent care is integrated throughout all provisions of care.

Clinical Reasoning in Action

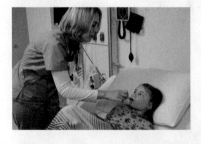

Five-year-old Tiona has a history of frequent tonsillitis and was scheduled for a tonsillectomy and adenoidectomy (T&A). Following the operation, Tiona refused to drink liquids because she was afraid it would hurt when she swallowed. After receiving intravenous pain medication, Tiona realized that she could swallow without too much pain and began to eat popsicles and drink liquids. She was then switched to oral pain medication. Later in the day, Tiona was drinking liquids well enough to be discharged home.

1. What information should the nurse include in the discharge teaching plan for Tiona's mother?
2. As Tiona and her mother are preparing to leave the hospital, Tiona states, "I am going to be good so I do not have to come to the hospital anymore!" How should the nurse respond?
3. Tiona's mother states that she is worried that her daughter will not drink enough at home. What can the nurse suggest to Tiona's mother to encourage her to drink fluids? What are the symptoms of dehydration that Tiona's mother should watch for over the next few days?
4. Children Tiona's age have many fears and stressors related to hospital and surgery. How can Tiona's mother assist her daughter to express her feelings about the hospital experience once she is home?

References

Agazio, J. G., & Buckley, K. M. (2012). Revision of a parental stress scale for use on a pediatric general care unit. *Pediatric Nursing, 38*(2), 82–87.

Ames, K. E., Rennick, J. E., & Baillargeon, S. (2011). A qualitative interpretive study exploring parents' perception of the parental role in the paediatric intensive care unit. *Intensive and Critical Care Nursing, 27*, 143–150.

American Society of Anesthesiologists, Committee on Standards and Practice Parameters. (2011). Practice guidelines for preoperative fasting and the use of pharmacologic agents to reduce the risk of pulmonary aspiration: Application to healthy patients undergoing elective procedures. *Anesthesiology, 114*(3), 495–511.

Bindler, R. C., Ball, J. W., London, M. L., & Davidson, M. R. (2017). *Clinical skills manual for maternity and pediatric nursing* (5th ed., p. 106). Hoboken, NJ: Pearson.

Emergency Nurses Association. (2012). *Emergency nursing resource: Family presence during invasive procedures and resuscitation in the emergency department.* Retrieved from http://www.ena.org/practice-research/research/CPG/Documents/FamilyPresenceCPG.pdf

Engorn, B., & Flerlage, J. (2015). *The Harriet Lane handbook* (20th ed.). St. Louis, MO: Elsevier Mosby.

Fisher, M. J., & Broome, M. E. (2011). Parent–provider communication during hospitalization. *Journal of Pediatric Nursing, 26*(1), 58–69.

Goddard, A. T., & Gilmer, M. J. (2015). The role and impact of animals with pediatric patients. *Pediatric Nursing, 41*(2), 65–71.

Healy, K. (2013). A descriptive survey of the information needs of parents of children admitted for same day surgery. *Journal of Pediatric Nursing, 28*, 179–185.

Karlsson, K., Rydström, I., Enskär, K., & Englund, A. D. (2014). Nurses' perspectives on supporting children during needle-related medical procedures. *International Journal of Qualitative Studies on Health and Well-Being, 9*. Retrieved from http://dx.doi.org/10.3402/qhw.v9.23063

LeGrow, K., Hodnett, E., Stremler, R., & Cohen, E. (2014). Evaluating the feasibility of a parent-briefing intervention in a pediatric acute care setting. *Journal for Specialists in Pediatric Nursing, 19*, 219–228.

Romaniuk, D., O'Mara, L., & Akhtar-Danesh, N. (2014). Are parents doing what they want to do? Congruency between parents' actual and desired participation in the care of their hospitalized child. *Issues in Comprehensive Pediatric Nursing, 37*(2), 103–121.

Salmela, M., Aronen, E. T., & Salanterä, S. (2011). The experience of hospital-related fears of 4- to 6-year-old children. *Child: Care, Health and Development, 37*(5), 719–726.

Spector, R. E. (2013). *Cultural diversity in health and illness* (8th ed.). Upper Saddle River, NJ: Pearson.

U.S. Department of Labor. (2012). *Fact sheet #28: The Family and Medical Leave Act of 1993.* Retrieved from http://www.dol.gov/whd/regs/compliance/whdfs28.pdf

Wilson, M. E., Megel, M. E., Enenbach, L., & Carlson, K. L. (2010). The voices of children: Stories about hospitalization. *Journal of Pediatric Health Care, 24*(2), 95–100.

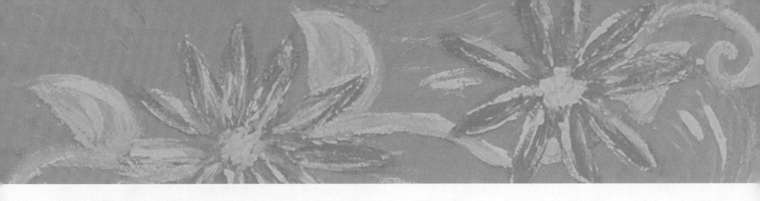

Chapter 12
The Child With a Chronic Condition

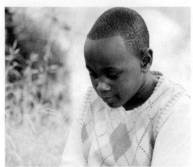

I'm nervous about going to school for the first time since my diabetes was diagnosed. I'm worried that my friends will make fun of me because I have to check my blood and give myself a shot at lunchtime. I wish this would just go away, but I know it's something I will have for the rest of my life. My mom and dad were really upset, but they are getting used to the idea now and will do anything to make sure I am doing okay.

—Mark, 10 years old

Ethno Images, Inc./Alamy

⌄ Learning Outcomes

12.1 Explain the causes of chronic conditions in children.

12.2 Identify the categories of chronic conditions in children.

12.3 Describe the nurse's role in caring for a child with a chronic condition.

12.4 Assess the family of a child with a chronic condition.

12.5 Prepare the family of a child with a chronic condition to effectively care for the child in the home.

12.6 Summarize nursing management for the child with a chronic condition to support transition to school and adult living.

12.7 Discuss the family's role in care coordination.

Overview of Chronic Conditions

A **chronic condition** is generally thought of as one that is expected to last at least 3 months (Kennedy, 2011). An estimated, 14.6 million children under the age of 18 in the United States have special healthcare needs related to some type of chronic condition (Data Resource Center for Child & Adolescent Health, 2012). Chronic conditions vary in etiology, manifestations, severity, and their effect on the child's physical, psychosocial, and cognitive development. Chronic conditions develop from multiple causes:

- Genetic or inheritable conditions may manifest as a chronic condition. Examples include muscular dystrophy, hemophilia, sickle cell disease, and cystic fibrosis.

- Conditions may result from a congenital defect or insult to the infant during fetal development, such as neural tube defect, maternal substance abuse, cleft palate, and cerebral palsy.

- Insult or injury may be associated with birth and care following birth (sepsis, prematurity, intraventricular hemorrhage) that lead to conditions such as bronchopulmonary dysplasia, attention deficit disorder, and vision or hearing impairment.

- Conditions can be acquired through injury or acute medical condition such as brain injury, cancer, HIV infection, drowning, and mental health problems. These and additional chronic illnesses are discussed in the systems chapters later in this text.

In most cases, these chronic conditions become lifelong disorders, but the impact on the affected child varies according to the severity of the condition, the stage of growth and development when the condition occurs, and the child's and family's responses to the condition. Whereas some conditions require intense monitoring and technologic support for survival, other conditions cause few limitations and have a minimal effect on quality of life (Figure 12–1).

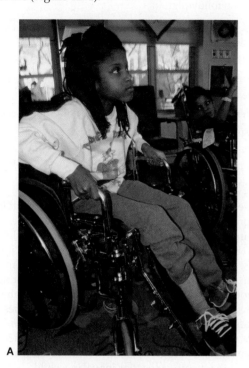

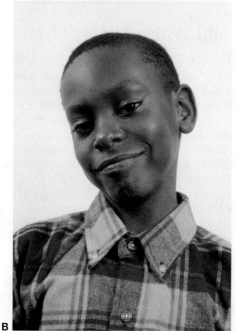

Figure 12–1 **Children with chronic conditions may have a visible or nonvisible health condition, or nonvisible until an acute episode of their condition makes the condition visible.** *A,* The child in a wheelchair has a visible disability. *B,* The child with a seizure disorder may have no visible signs of the condition unless a seizure is witnessed.

TABLE 12–1 Examples of Conditions by Special Healthcare Need Category

SPECIAL HEALTHCARE NEED CATEGORY	CHRONIC HEALTH CONDITION EXAMPLES
Dependent on medications or special diet	Diabetes mellitus, asthma, seizures, phenylketonuria, organ transplantation, cystic fibrosis, celiac disease
Dependent on medical technology	Renal failure, bronchopulmonary dysplasia
Increased use of healthcare services	Cancer, sickle cell disease, cystic fibrosis
Functional limitations	Down syndrome, brain injury, autism, myelodysplasia, cerebral palsy

Categories of chronic conditions may include functional limitations, developmental disorders, behavioral issues, anatomical problems, and limb dysfunction (Goodman, Posner, Huang, et al., 2013). The condition may also be further defined based on the amount of care that is needed, such as special medications, special diet, or medical technology. Children with chronic conditions require more care than healthy children require.

See Table 12–1 for examples of chronic conditions that may fall into a specific category. Many children with chronic conditions have special healthcare needs that fall into several of these areas. In the majority of cases, the more severe the chronic condition, the greater the number of categories of special healthcare needs. Many children with a chronic condition and children dependent on technology require specialized health care. The term **children with special healthcare needs (CSHCN)** is applied to "those who have one or more chronic physical, developmental, behavioral, or emotional conditions for which they require an above routine type or amount of health and related services" (U.S. Department of Health and Human Services, Health Resources and Services Administration [USDHHS/HRSA], 2011).

Many of these children have a **disability**, a limitation that interferes with a child's ability to fully participate in society, which can be related to medical impairment (chronic health condition), functional limitation (mobility, self-care, communication, or learning behavior impairment), or a mental condition that interferes with social interactions.

Data show that 19.8% of children in the United States have a special healthcare need (Data Resource Center for Child & Adolescent Health, 2012). Although these children represent a small percentage of the nation's children, they require significantly more healthcare resources than those without special healthcare needs, including more visits to clinics and emergency departments, dental visits, inpatient hospital days, and prescription medications. Efforts to reduce health costs have resulted in fewer hospitalizations and more care in the community for children with special healthcare needs.

The child with a life-threatening illness or a chronic condition as the result of a complex illness, prematurity, or a congenital defect may be considered **medically fragile** (Miles, Holditch-Davis, Burchinal, et al., 2011). Some of these children are **technology assisted**, dependent on a medical device that is required to sustain life or to maintain health status (mechanical ventilators, intravenous nutrition or drugs, tracheostomy, suctioning, oxygen, or nutritional support with tube feedings) (Figure 12–2). Other children depend on medical devices that compensate for vital body functions and require nursing care management such as renal dialysis, urinary catheters, and colostomies.

Children assisted by technology can be cared for at home because compact portable equipment is available. Home-based equipment used for the child with a chronic condition may include ventilators, enteral feeding tubes, intravenous catheters, infusion pumps, dialysis equipment, and oxygen. With the support of home health services, parents can learn to manage the child's care. The benefit of home health services to the child is support of physical, emotional, and cognitive growth and development within the normal environment of the home.

All families with children experiencing a chronic condition need to make lifestyle adjustments, ensuring a baseline of care that helps maintain the child's health status and promotes growth and development. In many cases, the child has a baseline level of home management with episodic exacerbations that require the family to make sudden adjustments in family routines, such as may occur with the child who has seizures or an infection. These exacerbations often cause stress and disrupt family routines. In other cases, the chronic condition requires the family to learn and provide care that is complex and time intensive, such as cystic fibrosis, diabetes mellitus, bronchopulmonary dysplasia, and significant cognitive impairment. These more severe chronic conditions often impact the child's physical and psychologic development. Table 12–2 outlines healthcare

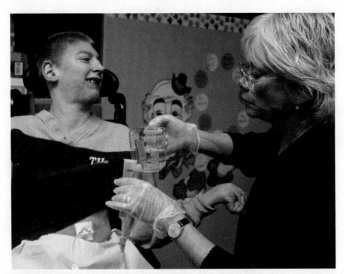

Figure 12–2 **This child needs a gastrostomy tube to ensure adequate nutrition is obtained to support growth and promote resistance to infection.**

needs of these children and families and the nursing implications related to planning health services delivery to children and their families.

Role of the Nurse

The nurse's role in caring for the child with a chronic condition includes the following:

- Providing health supervision from infancy to transition into adulthood
- Collaborating with the multidisciplinary healthcare team
- Partnering with parents or caregivers to manage the child's care at home
- Referring the family to appropriate community services
- Assisting with planning for education services
- Promoting positive parenting behaviors and psychosocial adaptation and well-being of the child and family
- Promoting growth and development of siblings

Assess each family member's level of understanding of the condition, treatment, and anticipated outcome of the condition. Determine the family's stage of acceptance of the child's chronic illness, and how well the child's care is integrated into family routines. Evaluate the child's home care environment to determine the potential for abuse, lack of adequate care, or neglect, or for opportunities to enhance care provided. Assess the family's strengths, stressors, risk factors, and coping strategies. Provide information related to community resources. See *Nursing Care Plan: The Child With a Chronic Condition*. See Chapter 13 for stages that a family might progress through when faced with a diagnosis of a life-threatening illness or injury in a child.

The Child With a Newly Diagnosed Chronic Condition

Informing the child of a newly acquired chronic condition is individualized and is based on the child's developmental level and age. See *Growth and Development: Developmental Considerations for the Child With a Chronic Condition*. Questions the child may ask vary, but often focus on the cause of the condition, how to make it better, and how it will affect daily life. Provide information tailored to the child's level of understanding and answer questions honestly. The nurse should also address the fears and concerns of the family. Provide condition-specific education to help prepare the family for care at home and begin discharge planning. See *Families Want to Know: Discussing a Child's Condition* and *Families Want to Know: Informing Parents of Their Child's Chronic Illness or Disability*. The parents' heightened anxiety level may reduce the comprehension of information heard. See *Developing Cultural Competence: Cultural Sensitivity in Healthcare Providers for Children With Special Healthcare Needs*.

Most children with chronic conditions live at home, which causes other family members, including siblings, to be affected as well (Nielsen et al., 2012). Siblings of children with a chronic condition are affected in a variety of ways. These children experience some degree of disruption in their lives and demonstrate a variety of emotional responses (Fleary & Heffer, 2013). They may feel powerless and may receive less attention from their parents than the ill child. Siblings may have feelings of jealousy, anger, depression, guilt, resentment, worry, and anxiety (Fleary & Heffer, 2013; Vermaes, van Susante, & van Bakel, 2012). Siblings may fear that they themselves will have the same disease or condition as the affected child.

TABLE 12–2 Healthcare Needs of Children With Chronic Conditions

HEALTHCARE NEED	DEFINITION	NURSING ACTIONS
Access to care	Care includes the availability and accessibility of providers with knowledge as well as ancillary services needed by children and their families.	Assist the family in obtaining transportation assistance if required. Assist the family in identifying healthcare providers who provide health promotion and other services to address the child's specific healthcare needs.
Appropriateness of care	Services and care are delivered by individuals with expertise and experience and are developmentally and culturally appropriate for the child and family.	Support the family by outlining educational and health services needed when developing an individualized education plan (IEP) and individualized health plan (IHP).
Comprehensiveness of care	Care includes coverage of the preventive, primary, and tertiary care needs of children, and linkages with other service systems, such as education, social services, and family support systems.	Provide the family with resource contacts such as social services, family support groups, and other systems to help the family manage the child's condition. Assist the family in identifying a care coordinator or developing the skills to take on the care coordination role themselves.
Coordination of care	Families are linked to medical care, financial health resources, and educational and community-based services; information is centralized.	Assist the family to identify a care coordinator or to develop the skills to become the care coordinator. See additional information in this chapter related to care coordination. Provide guidance and resources if the family decides to assume the role of care coordinator. Encourage the family to partner with the healthcare team to ensure continuity of care.
Continuity of care	Care is provided through a medical home or pediatric healthcare home; linkages between primary, specialty, therapeutic, and home care exist throughout childhood.	Facilitate communication between all the child's healthcare providers. Include the family and older child in all decision making.
Degree to which family-centered services are provided	The importance of the family is reflected in the way services are planned and delivered, building on individual and family strengths, and respecting the diversity of each family.	Determine the needs of the child and the family to ensure they are being addressed. Assist the family in identifying local and specialized healthcare providers. Recognize and respect the culture and cultural practices of the child and family.

Developing Cultural Competence Cultural Sensitivity in Healthcare Providers for Children With Special Healthcare Needs

The 2009/2010 National Survey of Children with Special Health Care Needs found that the majority of physicians and other healthcare providers were sensitive to family values and customs. Specific results indicated that 69.6% of physicians or other healthcare providers were always sensitive to family values and customs, 19.3% were usually sensitive, and 11.1% were sometimes or never sensitive (Child and Adolescent Health Measurement Initiative, 2012). It is essential for all healthcare providers to be sensitive to family values and customs of children with special healthcare needs.

Siblings may also have positive responses related to growing up with a chronically ill sibling, including an increased awareness of illness, maturity, family bonding and support, and an increased appreciation for life (Fleary & Heffer, 2013). See Chapter 11 for siblings' responses to the child experiencing an illness.

Discharge Planning and Home Care Teaching

As the child with a newly diagnosed chronic condition transitions to the home, parents often feel overwhelmed with preparations for home care, the anxiety of caring for a child with special healthcare needs, and supporting the child's growth and development needs. Work with the parents to ensure a smooth transition from hospital to the home environment. Assist the family in the initial discussions with the multidisciplinary team that participates in developing the child's care plan. Ensure that the family understands the role of each care provider. Provide contact numbers for parents to call should any issues arise at home.

Education to provide care of the child at home may be initiated by the hospital nursing staff, and then transitioned to special nurse educators or the home health nurses. Care is taken to ensure that all aspects of management are discussed with the family and that they demonstrate an understanding of and ability to perform the care required.

During discharge planning it may be helpful to identify a parent peer or peer support group to provide support to the family. Parent peers who have had similar experiences may be very helpful in identifying strategies for the initial care transition in

Nursing Care Plan: The Child With a Chronic Condition

1. Nursing Diagnosis: *Knowledge, Deficient (Child),* related to learning self-care skills (NANDA-I © 2014)

GOAL: The child will acquire self-care skills for lifetime management.

INTERVENTION	RATIONALE
• Assess the child's developmental level and select an educational approach and self-care activities to match.	• Learning goals for the child must match knowledge and skill expectations appropriate for developmental stage.
• Review with the child all steps involved in the self-care skill and how to perform the skill.	• The child may have watched the routine used by parents many times, and asking the child to list each step helps the nurse identify extra training needed.
• Use demonstration/return demonstration until the child is comfortable with procedures.	• Evaluation permits positive reinforcement and guidance for modification of techniques.
• Help parents develop a planned sequence of self-care skills to teach the child.	• Parents need guidance to identify appropriate self-care skills that the child is developmentally ready to learn.
• Discuss a plan for increased responsibility for self-care with the child and parents.	• Parents often need encouragement to transition responsibility to the child, becoming a supervisor rather than the person controlling care.

EXPECTED OUTCOME: Child will demonstrate the proper technique in the self-care skill and be able to assume responsibility for that skill with supervision by the parent. Responsibility for self-care increases as new skills are learned.

2. Nursing Diagnosis: *Family Processes, Interrupted,* related to management of chronic disease (NANDA-I © 2014)

GOAL: The child and family will manage the required treatments, monitoring, and medication regimen for the child's condition while maintaining family routines and functioning.

INTERVENTION	RATIONALE
• Assess the child's and family's lifestyle and attempt to fit the child's care needs into those schedules.	• Fitting the child's care to the child's and family's lifestyle promotes adherence to regimen and healthier family processes.
• Discuss the family's routines for special occasions and vacations and any activities important to the child. Identify ways to modify the child's management for these occasions and activities.	• It is important for the child to participate in special events with the family and peers as a normal child to promote psychologic development.

EXPECTED OUTCOME: Child and family will maintain important family routines and successfully manage the child's condition.

3. Nursing Diagnosis: *Coping: Readiness for Enhanced* related to self-care management of chronic condition (NANDA-I © 2014)

GOAL: The child will develop a support system network.

INTERVENTION	RATIONALE
• Talk with the child about how to tell friends, teachers, and other important people about the chronic condition.	• These important people can assist the child in an emergency if they have enough information to assess the problem.
• Discuss ways to explain the condition to important people and how to answer questions.	• Having an opportunity to plan and role-play the conversation will reduce the child's anxiety about condition disclosure.
• Role-play ways to talk about the condition with friends and teachers.	• Sharing information about the condition helps others understand changes in lifestyle needed by the child.
• Encourage the child to attend peer support groups or camps specific to the child's condition.	• Learning and support networks developed at camp can promote development of problem-solving skills that increase coping abilities.

EXPECTED OUTCOME: Child will identify the friends, teachers, and other important persons informed about the chronic condition who can provide support when needed.

Growth and Development Developmental Considerations for the Child With a Chronic Condition

Newborns and Infants

- Newborns and infants who are medically fragile are at risk for chronic conditions related to brain injury, oxygen deprivation, and respiratory problems.
- Newborns cared for in the NICU are exposed to an environment of bright lights and high-pitched noises that can negatively affect their development (Aita, Johnston, Goulet, et al., 2013).
- Promote development and parent–infant bonding by encouraging the parents to spend time with the infant and engage in face-to-face interaction. When the newborn is stable, provide opportunities for parents to touch, soothe, and care for the infant.
- Provide sensory stimuli such as mobiles, soft music, and different textures for the infant to touch.

Toddlers

- Chronic illness can interfere with the achievement of autonomy and development of self-control. Some parents are overprotective and may do simple tasks they feel the child is incapable of accomplishing, rather than encouraging the child to try to do things independently. The child can lose independence and lack opportunities to meet developmental tasks.
- Nurses can promote the development of toddlers with chronic conditions by offering the child choices when possible, such as which color gown to wear or which food to eat first.
- Help parents recognize the toddler's capabilities, and allow the child to take the time to practice and learn a skill. Identify the next most appropriate developmental tasks for the child to learn and give the parents some strategies they can use to offer learning opportunities.

Preschoolers

- Preschool children recognize the association between body parts and problems associated with the chronic condition. The preschooler engages in magical thinking during this stage, and the child may believe that his or her thoughts or behaviors caused the condition. The child may also think the condition is a form of punishment.
- Hospitalization or implementation of a treatment plan, such as a new medication, may interfere with the preschool-age child's developing independence (University of Michigan Health System, 2014).
- Nurses can promote development by explaining the purpose of treatments and procedures in terms the preschooler can understand, and by emphasizing that treatments and procedures are not punishment for any wrongdoing.
- Look for ways to use play so the child can learn an aspect of self-care, perform an activity, and feel a sense of accomplishment. Encourage social interactions with other children when possible. Give positive feedback to the child for appropriate efforts and successes.

School-Age Children

- Early school-age children have an increased understanding of their condition and are capable of participating in certain aspects of monitoring and care. Older school-age children begin to understand about managing their condition and the long-term needs associated with their condition. They can assume more responsibility for their care such as serum glucose monitoring, intermittent self-catheterization, or monitoring the condition of skin under braces.

- Some children with chronic conditions have learning difficulties and other limitations that interfere with education and social competence. The child needs to gain social skills, interact with peers, master new information, learn to cope with stress, and acquire skills that lead to self-sufficiency in order to develop a sense of industry.
- The school-age child senses that he or she is different from peers and may feel left out, especially if functional limitations affect his or her ability to participate in extracurricular activities. It is important that children with chronic health conditions be allowed to participate in activities as much as their condition allows and their physician approves (University of Michigan Health System, 2014).
- Nurses can promote development of school-age children by encouraging their interaction with children in the same age group. When possible, this should occur with children who have the same type of chronic condition. Link the child to a peer support group to promote social interaction and to help the child recognize that others also have the same condition. When the child has an extended absence from school because of the chronic condition, encourage contact from school peers and friends through cards and computer messages, as well as the completion of school assignments.
- Begin to identify aspects of the child's care that the child can learn to assume under the parents' supervision. Inform families of the benefit of special camps for children with the chronic condition (when available) to promote recreation, social interaction, and learning skills of self-care.

Adolescents

- The adolescent with a chronic condition has numerous challenges with the rapid changes in growth and sexual maturation; ongoing development of identity, body image, and self-concept; and the need to plan for vocational and healthcare transitions. Cognitive development and abstract thinking skills are achieved during this stage, allowing the adolescent to develop an understanding of the short-term and long-term consequences related to the condition.
- The adolescent becomes more aware of differences between self and peers. Some adolescents are unable to cope with the recognizable differences between themselves and healthy peers, and they withdraw from social activities and relationships. Others may engage in risky behavior (e.g., alcohol, sexual activity, eating foods that interfere with therapy) that may be harmful to themselves or to management of their condition, just to be accepted by peers.
- Nursing actions to promote development of the adolescent include client education to help the adolescent learn about the chronic condition, care needed to manage or control the condition, and problem solving and specific skills for integrating self-care management into daily life. Parents need to be coached to transition care over to the adolescent and to support the adolescent to make healthy decisions regarding care.
- Encourage the adolescent to build a safety net of friends who know enough about the chronic condition to assist if a problem occurs, such as a seizure, asthma episode, or insulin reaction.
- Discuss sexual maturation and the importance of protected sexual activity, and discourage risky behaviors by the adolescent.
- Provide adolescents with an opportunity to express concerns regarding self-management, vocational planning, and future independent living. Refer them to their local vocational rehabilitation services.

Families Want to Know
Informing Parents of Their Child's Chronic Illness or Disability

The following guidelines may be considered when informing parents of the diagnosis of a chronic illness or disability in their child:

1. Inform parents of their child's diagnosis in person, in a private setting, and free from interruptions. Tell both parents together. Offer parents the opportunity to have a relative or friend as a support person during the discussion.

2. Present information in small amounts at a time and at the level of the parents' understanding.

3. Plan and organize the information to be provided. Use simple, direct language without medical jargon. Individualize the pace of the interview and approaches taken to present the explanation, taking into consideration a family's culture and the family's response to the information.

4. Share accurate, up-to-date information about the diagnosis, treatment options, specialty referrals, and community resources.

5. Talk about the strengths and positive attributes of the child, as well as the child's limitations and characteristics due to the illness or disability.

6. Evaluate the discussion to assess whether the family's needs were met and to determine the type of support and/or additional information that should be provided.

7. Plan a follow-up discussion to repeat and clarify the information provided, and to give the parents a chance to get additional questions answered.

Families Want to Know
Discussing a Child's Condition

When discussing a child's chronic condition with the family, use the child's name. Avoid labeling the child with a condition, such as "diabetic child"; instead, refer to the situation as "the child with diabetes." This places the emphasis on the child rather than the condition.

---

the home and additional issues that arise over time. If the family has a computer that family members frequently use, Internet resources for information and family support should be provided.

Collaborate with the family and healthcare team to ensure that the child has a medical or healthcare home in the local community to provide health promotion and maintenance and to assist with the coordination of local community resources. Promote communication and joint planning of care between the specialty care provider and local healthcare provider. Nurses working in hospital specialty clinics and other community settings can help ensure that children with chronic conditions receive multidisciplinary referrals and have appointments scheduled. Social services may be called to assist the family with identifying financial resources and other community resources for home management. Ongoing assistance may be required to help families deal with financial issues, time management, and other challenges.

Coordination of Care

Care coordination is the process of planning and integrating healthcare services among providers in an effort to achieve and promote good health in the child. Care coordination in a medical home facilitates transition from a pediatric healthcare provider to an adult healthcare provider (American Academy of Pediatrics, 2012). Care coordination also improves the quality and safety of client care (Taylor et al., 2012). See *Evidence-Based Practice: Care Coordination for Children With Special Healthcare Needs*. A **case manager**, often a nurse or social worker, may be given responsibility to help the family with care coordination. Case managers are often paid by a healthcare insurer to reduce healthcare costs by coordinating the healthcare team, determining family needs,

identifying financial and local support resources, and arranging for needed healthcare services.

Care coordination may help families who have children with special healthcare needs (Lawson, Bloom, Sadof, et al., 2011; Taylor et al., 2012). It may include helping the family modify the home to support required technology, such as mechanical ventilation or wheelchair use. Assistance may be required in purchasing or leasing ventilators, infusion pumps, or other specialized equipment. The coordination plan also includes determining the potential need for home health nursing, physical therapy, or other home health services. See *Developing Cultural Competence: Disparities in Care Coordination*.

Developing Cultural Competence Disparities in Care Coordination

Research by Toomey, Chien, Elliott, et al. (2013) found that children with special healthcare needs (CSHCN) were more likely to have inadequate care coordination than children without special healthcare needs. The study also found that Black and Latino children were more likely to have unmet care coordination needs than White children. Effective care coordination is essential for all CSHCN.

Families become very well educated about their child's condition and the services that would make managing the condition easier. After management goals are established by the multidisciplinary team, the case manager partners with the family to help in the decision-making process regarding how goals will be met. An important role is helping the family determine cost-effective

EVIDENCE-BASED PRACTICE | Care Coordination for Children With Special Healthcare Needs

Clinical Question

How can care coordination enhance the care that children with special healthcare needs (CSHCN) and their families receive?

The Evidence

Taylor et al. (2012) evaluated the effectiveness of a care coordination program for CSHCN. The goal of the program was to assist families in achieving competency in care coordination and to support healthcare providers in the care coordination process. This study evaluated the effectiveness of a care coordination counselor implemented at a children's hospital with 430 beds and 50 outpatient care sites. The care coordination counselor was a BSN-prepared nurse who was made available to clients and families with complex needs. Additional tools provided to the families included a care binder, Care Coordination Network Committee, and the Community Resources for Families database. A survey was used to compare responses from families who received services from the care coordination counselor and those who received only a care binder. Twenty-five families who received services from the care coordination counselor and 50 families who received only the care binder completed the survey. Eighty-three percent of those receiving services responded positively overall to the survey, compared with 55% of those receiving only the binder. Additionally, 67% of those receiving services stated that care coordination for their child had improved over the past 6 months, compared to 47% of those who received only the care binder.

Looman et al. (2013) examined the importance of the role of the advanced practice nurse in relationship-based care coordination of children with complex special healthcare needs. Outcomes were measured using the Tele-Families study, a 4-year randomized controlled study whose goal is to evaluate the effectiveness of an enhanced interactive telehealth program and care coordination by the advanced practice nurse for children with complex special healthcare needs. Preliminary findings based on qualitative data from 94 families receiving telenursing interventions from an advanced practice nurse indicate increased parent satisfaction with having one person to coordinate care. Parents also expressed satisfaction with decreased time needed to have forms and prescriptions updated.

Petitgout, Pelzer, McConkey, et al. (2013) described the development of a hospital-based care coordination program for CSHCN. The program includes inpatients and outpatients and utilizes a family-centered approach to provide care coordination and a medical home. Over the past 10 years, improved client outcomes have been noted and include a decrease in length of stay, high family satisfaction, and decreased cost. In this program, the pediatric nurse practitioners collaborate with other healthcare providers and services to provide care coordination.

Best Practice

Care coordination is essential when working with CSHCN and their families. Care coordination in which nurses work with families to facilitate coordination of services is effective and leads to greater satisfaction with care and improved client outcomes. The nurse assists families to identify needed programs and services and is in an excellent position to serve as a liaison between these programs and the family to decrease the risk for fragmentation of care.

Clinical Reasoning

Why is care coordination a vital aspect of care for CSHCN? Provide an example of coordination of services for CSHCN. How do nurses play a role in care coordination for CSHCN?

---

strategies to meet healthcare goals and to delay the time when the child reaches the cap on health insurance benefits.

Some families assume the role of care coordinator for their child. It is essential for the family to understand that care coordination is time consuming and requires ongoing assessment and evaluation of the child's status and anticipated outcomes. Support family members in their decision to lead the care coordination process by helping the parents to become knowledgeable about the child's condition and treatment regimen. Encourage the parents to take an active role in the treatment planning and decision-making process so that they gain confidence in their abilities. Many hospitals have workshops for parents who are managing the complex care of their children. Parent-to-parent support groups can provide advice, support, and suggestions for referrals. Review the care coordination to ensure that the child has access to the most appropriate care and resources. Provide positive feedback to the parents as their advocacy skills increase.

Suggest that the family maintain a log of the healthcare team members, their roles, when the child was seen and any interventions, the results of interventions, and future planned interventions or treatments. The family can use this information when communicating with the healthcare providers, particularly in an emergency, and it may also help eliminate unnecessary duplication of procedures.

Community Sites of Care

Most children with chronic conditions are cared for in the home with or without home nursing or other health services. The healthcare provider for children with chronic conditions varies by the type of condition, type of health insurance coverage, preferences of the family, and availability of pediatric specialty resources.

Office or Health Center

Every child should have a "healthcare home" or "medical home," a consistent, continuous, comprehensive, family-centered, and compassionate source of primary health care. A healthcare home or medical home for these children is especially important because children with chronic conditions need regular preventive health care just as healthy children do. Health promotion, disease prevention, and anticipatory guidance have greater significance for the child with special healthcare needs. These children already have a condition that places them at higher risk for additional problems, such as infectious diseases, injury, or developmental delay. Information about community resources that may help the child and family is usually more extensive when the child's healthcare home is in the local community. The goal is for the child to have as normal a childhood as possible.

Ideally, this healthcare provider is located in the community where the family resides, making it more convenient for the family to obtain routine health care as well as care for episodic illnesses. Having a regular healthcare provider has many advantages for the family:

- Because the child and family are seen more frequently, a trusting, family-centered relationship can develop. The healthcare provider learns about the family's strengths and coping abilities.

- The healthcare provider sees the child and family when things are going well and during exacerbations. This may enable the healthcare provider to identify strategies that help the family to better coordinate the child's care.

- When the provider is based in the same community as the child, it is likely that information about community resources is known; this will reduce the efforts that families must make to identify appropriate services needed by the child.

Specialty Referral Centers

An optimal healthcare arrangement for the child with a chronic condition exists when the medical or healthcare home provider collaborates with a pediatric team or specialist that specializes in the care of children with a specific chronic condition. Pediatric specialists, advanced practice nurses, and other healthcare providers (e.g., physical therapists, social workers, and nutritionists) often function as a team, providing coordinated care to the family and child with a chronic condition, such as spina bifida, cystic fibrosis, or diabetes. These specialty teams are often found in major medical centers, requiring travel to the facility. When communication flows from the team to the child's healthcare provider and back to the team, new treatments can be monitored by the child's physician, and consultation can be sought if the child's health status changes (Figure 12–3).

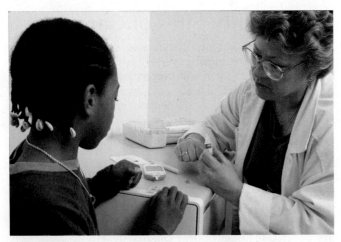

Figure 12–3 **Nurses often assume a larger role in working with children and families with a chronic health condition in the ambulatory setting. Developing a care plan and educating the child and family to manage type 1 diabetes is an important role of this pediatric nurse, who is also a certified diabetes educator.**

Nurses working in hospital specialty clinics and other community settings can help ensure that these children receive the appropriate health promotion services. The nurse in a tertiary care facility needs to identify appropriate resources and to help the family connect with local community resources. This is a greater challenge if the child and family have traveled a distance to obtain the specialty services, supporting the need for a primary care provider in the home community to provide regular care and to help coordinate local community resources.

Schools

All children, including those with chronic conditions and special healthcare needs, are entitled by federal law to a free education that is matched to their developmental and functional capabilities (Individuals with Disabilities Education Act [IDEA] and Section 504 of the Rehabilitation Act of 1973). **Early intervention** provides special services for infants and toddlers up to age 3 years who have a developmental delay or are at risk for a developmental delay. Early intervention programs are federal programs administered by the states. Children are evaluated at age 3 to determine continued eligibility in preschool (Caley, 2012; Pacer Center, 2012). IDEA has led to support of communities that are developing early childhood education programs and to schools with students who are blind, deaf, or have autism or traumatic brain injury. Provisions for adolescent transitional planning for adult living, including vocational training and independent living, are also included in the Individuals with Disabilities Education Act (U.S. Department of Education [USDOE], 2011).

Attending school is an important transition for children with chronic conditions and their families. Sending the child to school has several benefits for the child and family, including opportunities for socialization with children and adults outside of the family. School attendance promotes a feeling of normalcy in the family and provides a break for the primary care provider. Integration into the school system requires collaboration of family, school personnel, the nurse, and other members of the healthcare team.

EDUCATIONAL SYSTEM PLANNING

Careful planning is needed when a child with special needs attends school or receives other education services. Many children have chronic medical conditions that require management during the day in the school environment, such as asthma, diabetes, and attention deficit disorder. Some children simply need medications administered regularly or episodically. Other children require more extensive interventions integrated into the school day, such as blood glucose monitoring or intermittent self-catheterization. The education system is obligated to provide reasonable accommodations to ensure that the child's medical needs are met during the school day. The education system's obligation is negotiated with the family in formalized plans. The school nurse is an active participant on the team that collaborates with the family to develop these formalized plans.

- An **individualized family service plan (IFSP)** is developed for the early intervention process for infants with special healthcare needs and their families. The IFSP contains information about the services required to support a child's development and enhance the family's capacity to facilitate the child's development. The family and education service providers work as a team to plan, implement, and evaluate services specific to the family's unique concerns, priorities, and resources.

Clinical Tip

Federal laws for providing education services for children with special healthcare needs include:

- The Rehabilitation Act, PL 93-112, of 1973 prohibited discrimination against people with a disability. Section 504 specifies that each student who has a disability is entitled to **accommodations**—services or special assistance provided in the school setting to ensure that a student with a physical or mental impairment has access to an appropriate education and is able to participate as fully as possible in school activities. Examples of accommodations might include allowing additional time to take a test, using strategies that decrease exposure to peanuts in a child who has an allergy to peanuts, or allowing a child to test his or her blood glucose level. Students with disabilities must be provided with educational services to meet their needs just as services are provided to those without disabilities. See Chapter 10 for further discussion on the nurse's role in the school setting.

- The Education for All Handicapped Children Act, PL 94-142, of 1975 mandated that all children, even those with disabilities, be provided with free public education and related services. Safeguards were put into place to ensure that the rights of children with disabilities and their parents are protected. Additional purposes of this legislation were to assist states to provide education to children with disabilities and to evaluate the effectiveness of efforts to educate children with disabilities.

- The Education for All Handicapped Children Amendments, PL 99-457, of 1986 expanded the scope of PL 94-142 to include appropriate services for infants and toddlers with disabilities and their families.

- The Individuals with Disabilities Education Act (IDEA), PL 105-17, of 1997 and the Individuals with Disabilities Education Act of 2004, PL 108-446, with final regulations published in 2006 (reauthorization of the 1997 legislation), ensure that all children with disabilities have available to them a free and appropriate public education that emphasizes special education and related services designed to meet their unique needs and prepare them for employment and independent living. Every child with a disability must have a written individualized education plan (IEP), and parents have the right to question placement decisions and to due process when settling differences. In addition, the 2004 legislation focused more on state and local accountability to educate children with disabilities. This legislation also added a requirement that the child be invited to the IEP meeting.

Source: Data from Kim, D., & Samples, E. (2013). Comparing individual healthcare plans and Section 504 plans: School districts' obligation to determine eligibility for students with health related conditions. *Urban Lawyer, 45*(1), 263–279; Project Ideal. (2013). *Special education public policy.* Retrieved from http://www.projectidealonline.org/v/special-education-public-policy/; Yell, M. L., Conroy, T., Katsiyannis, A., & Conroy, T. (2013). Individualized education programs and special education programming for students with disabilities in urban schools. *Fordham Urban Law Journal, 41*(2), 669–714.

- An **individualized education plan (IEP)** is developed for a child with cognitive, motor, social, and communication impairments who needs special education services. The IEP is jointly planned with the school administrator, teacher, parents, and other special support professionals as appropriate for the child's condition. The child is also included in the process when possible. The plan is developed after an assessment of the child's abilities and specific functional limitations.

- An **individualized health plan (IHP)** is developed for the child with medical conditions that need to be managed

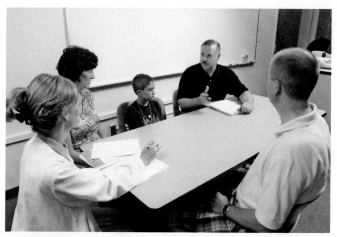

Figure 12–4 **Because some children need medications or other therapies during school hours, the parents and child, school nurse, teacher, and school administrators develop a plan to manage the child's condition during school hours. The resulting document is the child's individualized health plan.**

within the school setting. An IHP may be developed simultaneously with the IEP for the child with a health problem and a coexisting functional impairment. Some children need an IHP only for management of their chronic medical condition at school, such as daily medication administration or for glucose monitoring and insulin injection. An order from a licensed healthcare provider is required for medication administration and special treatments. Learning may be challenged when the child has frequent acute illness episodes that result in missed days of school, and the IHP often integrates methods to prevent the child from being penalized for those absences (Figure 12–4).

- An Individualized Section 504 Accommodation Plan may be used rather than an IHP for children with physical or mental impairments. The same process is used for development of the plan.

- An **individualized transition plan (ITP)** is included in the development of an IEP for each child with a chronic disability who is 14 years or older. The ITP focuses on helping individuals receive vocational training and in moving successfully from the home into other community living settings as they grow older.

Parents have an important role in advocating for their child to ensure that the child receives the most appropriate educational services. School systems must provide a full range of educational services for the children with special healthcare needs, including services that support cognitive development, self-care skills, mobility, improved communication, and social skills. Because each child's severity and combination of impairments is unique, identifying and matching the specific services for each child requires discussion and negotiation. Parents should make an effort to learn about the different types of educational services that address a child's specific disability in preparation for the IEP meeting. Parents often need a mentor or experienced parent to help with the development of the IEP the first few times. In this way, the parents are better prepared to participate in the educational planning and development of the child's IEP. School nurses are employees of the school system and may be limited in their

Clinical Tip

The elements of an IEP are as follows:

- Student's name
- Date of meeting to develop or review the IEP
- Statement of transition service needs of student beginning at age 14 years
- Present level of assessments and education performance, including how the child's disability affects the child's involvement and progress in a general curriculum or participation in appropriate activities
- Measurable annual goals that include short-term objectives in meeting the child's needs that enable the child to be involved in or progress in the general curriculum or participate in appropriate activities
- Special education and related services, supplementary aids and services, and program modifications or supports for school personnel needed to enable the child to make advancements toward attaining annual goals
- Explanation of the extent to which the child will or will not participate with nondisabled children
- Any specific modification in the administration of state or districtwide assessments of achievement that are needed for the child to participate in the assessment, or reasons for excluding the child from assessment
- How the child's progress toward annual goals will be measured
- How the child's parents will be regularly informed of the child's progress toward annual goals and the extent to which the child's progress is sufficient to meet goals by the end of the year

Source: Data from U.S. Department of Education (USDOE). (2000). *A guide to the individualized education program*. Retrieved from http://www.ed.gov/parents/needs/speced/iepguide/index.htm; U.S. Department of Education. (2006). *Individualized education programs*. Retrieved from http://idea.ed.gov/explore/view/p/%2Croot%2Cdynamic%2CTopicalBrief%2C10%2C; Yell, M. L., Conroy, T., Katsiyannis, A., & Conroy, T. (2013). Individualized education programs and special education programming for students with disabilities in urban schools. *Fordham Urban Law Journal, 41*(2), 669–714.

advocacy role on behalf of individual students. However, school nurses are in a good position to educate the IEP team about specific interventions needed by children with medical conditions and ways to integrate those interventions into the school day.

Teachers will need to learn to identify specific health problems, such as increased respiratory effort in a child with asthma or sweating, and pallor and loss of concentration in a child with diabetes. The child's teachers become part of the child's safety net for rapid access to needed healthcare intervention. With support from the school administration and school nurse, teachers can learn about the child's condition and special care that may be needed during the school day, such as a snack for the child with diabetes, management of the child who has a seizure, and ways to reduce the spread of infection within the classroom.

THE CHILD'S RESPONSE TO ENTERING SCHOOL

Children with chronic conditions—whether the conditions cause minimal interference in the child's daily life or significant interference, such as dependence on technology—face certain challenges in the school setting. They may for the first time recognize differences between themselves and other children, such as appearance, abilities, social skills, or special treatment needs. Limitations in abilities may cause the child to be shy or embarrassed. Affected children may also be teased or bullied by other children because of their disability (Vessey & O'Neill, 2011).

Some children, particularly adolescents, may attempt to hide their condition or fail to adhere to necessary recommendations, such as dietary restrictions, to appear like their peers.

EDUCATION FOR CHILDREN WHO ARE MEDICALLY FRAGILE

Children who are medically fragile or technology assisted are also entitled to education and education services in the school setting. The parents and the school system must carefully consider the child's need for skilled supportive nursing care. Parents are often anxious about how well the child will be cared for by others during the school day. Risks for the child in the school setting include safety issues related to ventilators, tracheostomy, and medication therapy, as well as exposure to infectious diseases. The school administration must provide the personnel resources and equipment needed to ensure that care and a care provider are consistently available. Modifications to the school setting for the child, such as wheelchair ramps or an elevator, may be needed. Sometimes the child is placed in a classroom with healthy children, and the teacher is expected to monitor the child with a chronic condition and provide care as needed. Health aides may be assigned to provide care for one or more children with school nurse supervision. Some children are placed in classes composed of children with special healthcare needs where health aides are more available to provide needed care.

Nurses play a key role in assisting the family to understand that a teacher's primary responsibility is to teach, not to provide health care. The teacher is responsible for the health and safety of all children in the classroom. Parents need to have realistic expectations about the level of skilled support services that can be provided to a child who is medically fragile in a classroom. The need to balance the obligations for a child's special education services with the needs of all other children in a classroom can be a challenge for teachers and education leaders.

HOME SCHOOLING

The family of a child who is medically fragile or technology dependent may choose the option of home schooling the child, with resources provided through the school system. Home schooling may be used for all of the child's education or for periods when the child is experiencing exacerbations or more complications from the condition. The benefits of home schooling include continuity of education when the child would otherwise be unable to attend school and reductions in the child's stress and fatigue levels. Potential negative effects of home schooling include lack of peer and social interaction and decreased opportunity to develop social skills. The family that chooses home schooling needs to establish a routine for the education process.

TRANSITION TO ADULTHOOD

The number of adolescents with special healthcare needs transitioning to adulthood has increased as medical advances have increased life expectancy for many people with disabilities and chronic healthcare conditions (Oswald et al., 2013). Effective transition from pediatric-focused to adult-focused healthcare systems is essential in adolescents with these chronic health conditions (Huang et al., 2014). When their chronic condition could affect their future ability to work and live independently, customized transition planning is needed in preparation for adulthood and self-determination. A transition plan is developed in collaboration with the family based on the needs that have been identified in relation to the adolescent's goals for health care, employment, and community living. The plan should be individualized with psychosocial support provided to the adolescent during the transition planning and process (Oswald et al., 2013). Healthy & Ready to Work services may be particularly helpful to adolescents and families in planning for transition to adulthood (HRTW National Resource Center, 2014).

Home Care

Many families become the primary caregiver for the child with a chronic condition, assuming responsibility for assessment and treatment despite the level of skill and complexity involved in that care. The numerous benefits of home care include the promotion of health, well-being, and development for the child, decreased financial costs to health insurance companies and the healthcare system, and a sense of satisfaction to families when they are able to care for their child at home. The family faces numerous challenges for home care, including modification of the home. Management of the condition involves technologic support, medications, and treatment regimens, all potential necessities to maintain the child in the home. Family members must decide who has responsibility for different aspects of the child's care. Many families must also decide whether both spouses will continue to work or if one parent will stay home to care for the child. Home health nursing care may be needed if both parents continue to work or to cover the night shift so parents can sleep.

Moving the child who is chronically ill, or a technology-assisted child, to the home setting is a life-changing decision for the family and it must be done with collaboration between the family and the healthcare team. Preparation for the child's transition to the home requires that the family receive extensive training and instructions on the child's care. Management of the condition involves technologic support, medications and treatment regimens, and all potential necessities to maintain the child in the home.

This transition is often challenging and intimidating for the family who now must assume the role of independent caregiver for a child who may have been hospitalized for several months. Family members often feel unprepared to handle the complex situation of the chronic condition and/or technologic supports. They are at risk to develop **caregiver burden**, the unrelenting

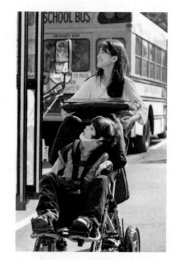

Figure 12–5 Daily caregiving demands of the child who is medically fragile continue 24 hours a day, 7 days a week. Parents need to identify ways to share the care of the child and other family care management. When the child lives with a single parent, additional healthcare resources are needed so the parent can sleep.

Source: Jaren Jai Wicklund/Shutterstock

pressure and anxiety related to providing daily care to a child with disabilities while meeting other family obligations. The family needs to be highly motivated and possess strength and resiliency factors to overcome the obstacles that will arise. These characteristics will help them be successful in assuming management responsibility for the child's care (Figure 12–5).

RESPITE CARE

Respite care is an important support service that involves caring for the child with a chronic condition while the parents take a short break away from the daily care. Whiting (2014) identified respite care as the greatest unmet need of parents of children with complex healthcare needs. Respite care may be provided by extended family, friends, or an agency, and may take place in the home or an area outside of the home. An example of respite might be skilled nursing care in a facility or the home so the family can have a weekend away. Assist the family in identifying respite care that meets the individual family's needs from the services available in the community. Many states have passed legislation for in-home family support services that include respite care. Because many respite services charge for their assistance, the family may require help in identifying respite waiver subsidies available to them. Reliable childcare and enrollment in school are other mechanisms for families to obtain respite care.

EMERGENCY PREPAREDNESS

Advance planning is needed to ensure that medically fragile children who require technology for survival or have the potential for life-threatening episodes have the necessary resources in the event of a disaster. The designated shelter for such children, with health professionals and electrical power for the needed equipment, should be identified and known to the family. In the meantime, battery packs for power backup should be available at all times. Additionally, parents need to arrange for durable power of attorney so that consent for emergency medical care can be available as needed. The child and parents may become separated during the disaster, or the parents may become injured and unable to care for the child. Refer to Chapter 10 for more information related to emergency preparedness.

Chapter Highlights

- A chronic condition is a long-term, ongoing condition that is expected to last 3 months or more and may involve functional limitations, developmental disorders, behavioral issues, anatomic problems, and limb dysfunction or require special medications, a special diet, or more healthcare services than a healthy child would require.

- Approximately 14.6 million children in the United States have special healthcare needs related to a chronic condition.

- Chronic conditions can occur as a result of a genetic condition, congenital anomaly, injury during fetal development or at birth, complication of care after birth, serious infection, or significant injury.

- Children who are medically fragile are dependent on a medical device for survival or prevention of further disability.

- A developmental delay results when there is failure to achieve anticipated milestones during specific developmental stages.

- Families with children experiencing a chronic condition need to make lifestyle adjustments, ensuring a baseline of care that helps maintain the child's health status and promotes growth and development.

- Siblings of the child with a chronic illness may have feelings of jealousy, anger, depression, guilt, resentment, worry, and anxiety.

- The time of diagnosis is one of the most stressful times for families of children with chronic conditions as the parents wait anxiously for the outcome of diagnostic procedures. Other times associated with significant stressors for the family include developmental milestones, school entry, adolescence, and planning for the transition to adult health and vocational services.

- Moving the child with a chronic illness who is dependent on technology to the home setting is a life-changing decision for the family, and it must be done with collaboration between the family and the healthcare team.

- Caregiver burden is the unrelenting pressure and anxiety related to providing daily care to a child with disabilities while meeting other family obligations.

- The financial burden of caring for a child with special healthcare needs is significant even when the family has health insurance.

- Sending the child to school has several benefits for the child and family, including socialization for the child beyond the immediate family and respite for parents.

- An individualized education plan (IEP) is developed for a child with cognitive, motor, social, or communication impairments who needs special education services in the school setting. An individualized health plan (IHP) is developed for the child with medical conditions that need to be managed within the school setting.

- All children, including those with chronic conditions and special healthcare needs, are entitled by federal law to a free education that is matched to their developmental and functional capabilities.

- An individualized transition plan (ITP) is developed for adolescents with a chronic condition in collaboration with the family to assist in identifying appropriate support programs, living arrangements, and employment for adult life.

- Children with chronic health conditions require regular health promotion, health screening, and health maintenance care, as well as specialized health services to assist the child and family in management of the condition.

- The role of the nurse in caring for the child with a chronic condition includes providing health supervision from infancy to transition into adulthood, collaborating with the multidisciplinary healthcare team, partnering with the family to manage the child's care at home, referring the family to appropriate community services, assisting with planning for education services, promoting positive parenting behaviors and psychosocial adaptation and well-being of the child and family, and promoting growth and development of siblings.

- Nurses who specialize in caring for children with complex chronic conditions may experience compassion fatigue as they continue their efforts to meet the ongoing needs of these families.

Clinical Reasoning in Action

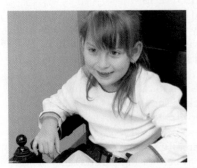

Haley is an 8-year-old child with cerebral palsy who will be attending school for the first time. Her mother had initially preferred home schooling for Haley and now wants to support her social development with other children. A case manager is asked to assist with facilitating Haley's entry into school. The case manager coordinates a multidisciplinary meeting of the clinic nurse, physical therapist, physician, and Haley's family to review her health status and to discuss the transition to school. They also discuss potential accommodations needed for Haley's mobility limitations. The multidisciplinary team assists the parents in developing a plan for Haley's transition to school.

1. What role will the clinic nurse and case manager have in helping develop Haley's IEP and IHP?

2. What role will the school nurse have with the child, caregivers, teacher, and classmates during the facilitation of school entry?

3. What actions will the mother need to take in preparing the school personnel for Haley's health needs?

4. Haley's 10-year-old sister attends the same school. What effects of Haley's entry into school might the sibling experience?

References

Aita, M., Johnston, C., Goulet, C., Oberlander, T. F., & Snider, L. (2013). Intervention minimizing preterm infants' exposure to NICU light and noise. *Clinical Nursing Research, 22*(3), 337–358.

American Academy of Pediatrics. (2012). *Care delivery management*. Retrieved from http://www.medical-homeinfo.org/how/care_delivery/

Caley, L. (2012). Risk and protective factors associated with stress in mothers whose children are enrolled in early intervention services. *Journal of Pediatric Health Care, 26*(5), 346–355.

Child and Adolescent Health Measurement Initiative. (2012). *National survey of children with special health care needs* (NS-CSHCN 2009/10). Retrieved from http://www.childhealthdata.org

Data Resource Center for Child & Adolescent Health. (2012). *Who are children with special health care needs?* Retrieved from http://childhealthdata.org/docs/nsch-docs/whoarecshcn_revised_07b-pdf.pdf

Fleary, S. A., & Heffer, R. W. (2013). Impact of growing up with a chronically ill sibling on well siblings' late adolescent functioning. *ISRN Family Medicine, 2013*, 1–8.

Goodman, R. A., Posner, S. F., Huang, E. S., Parekh, A. K., & Kokh, H. K. (2013). Defining and measuring chronic conditions: Imperatives for research, policy, program, and practice. *Preventing Chronic Disease, 10*(April 25). doi:http://dx.doi.org/10.5888/pcd10.120239

HRTW National Resource Center. (2014). *Systems and services*. Retrieved from http://www.syntiro.org/hrtw/systems/index.html

Huang, J. S., Terrones, L., Tompane, T., Dillon, G., Pian, M., Gottschalk, M., . . . Bartholomew, K. (2014). Preparing adolescents with chronic disease for transition to adult care: A technology program. *Pediatrics, 133*(6), e1639–e1646.

Kennedy, A. P. (2011). Systematic ethnography of school-age children with bleeding disorders and other chronic illnesses: Exploring children's perceptions of partnership roles in family-centred care of their chronic illness. *Child: Care, Health & Development, 38*(6), 863–869.

Kim, D., & Samples, E. (2013). Comparing individual healthcare plans and Section 504 plans: School districts' obligation to determine eligibility for students with health related conditions. *Urban Lawyer, 45*(1), 263–279.

Lawson, K. A., Bloom, S. R., Sadof, M., Stille, C., & Perrin, J. M. (2011). Care coordination for children with special health care needs: Evaluation of a state experiment. *Maternal Child Health Journal, 15*, 993–1000.

Looman, W. S., Presler, E., Erickson, M. M., Garwick, A. W, Cady, R. G., Kelly, A. M., & Finkelstein, S. M. (2013). Care coordination for children with complex special health care needs: The value of the advanced practice nurse's enhanced scope of knowledge and practice. *Journal of Pediatric Health Care, 27*(4), 293–303.

Miles, M. S., Holditch-Davis, D., Burchinal, M. R., & Brunssen, S. (2011). Maternal role attainment with medically fragile infants: Part 1. Measurement and correlates during the first year of life. *Research in Nursing and Health, 34*, 20–34.

Nielsen, K. M., Mandleco, B., Roper, S. O., Cox, A., Dyches, T., & Marshall, E. S. (2012). Parental perceptions of sibling relationships in families rearing a child with a chronic condition. *Journal of Pediatric Nursing, 27*(1), 34–43.

Oswald, D. P., Gilles, D. L., Cannady, M. S., Wenzel, D. B., Willis, J. H., & Bodurtha, J. N. (2013). Youth with special health care needs: Transition to adult health care services. *Maternal Child Health Journal, 17*, 1744–1752.

Pacer Center. (2012). *Preparing for transition from early intervention to an individualized education program*. Retrieved from http://www.pacer.org/parent/php/php-c158.pdf

Petitgout, J. M., Pelzer, D. E., McConkey, S. A., & Hanrahan, K. (2013). Development of a hospital-based care coordination program for children with special health care needs. *Journal of Pediatric Health Care, 27*(6), 419–425.

Project Ideal. (2013). *Special education public policy*. Retrieved from http://www.projectidealonline.org/v/special-education-public-policy/

Slive, L., & Cramer, R. (2012). Health reform and the preservation of confidential health care for young adults. *Journal of Law, Medicine & Ethics, 40*(2), 383–390.

Sorrell, J. (2012). Ethics: The Patient Protection and Affordable Care Act: Ethical perspectives in 21st century health care. *OJIN: The Online Journal of Issues in Nursing, 18*(1). Retrieved from http://www.nursingworld.org/MainMenuCategories/ANAMarketplace/ANAPeriodicals/OJIN/Columns/Ethics/Patient-Protection-and-Affordable-Care-Act-Ethical-Perspectives.html

Taylor, A., Lizzi, M., Marx, A., Chilkatowsky, M., Trachtenberg, S. W., & Ogle, S. (2012). Implementing a care coordination program for children with special healthcare needs: Partnering with families and providers. *Journal for Healthcare Quality, 35*(5), 70–77.

Toomey, S. L., Chien, A. T., Elliott, M. N., Ratner, J., & Schuster, M. A. (2013). Disparities in unmet need for care coordination: The National Survey of Children's Health. *Pediatrics, 131*(2), 217–223.

U.S. Department of Education (USDOE). (2000). *A guide to the individualized education program*. Retrieved from http://www.ed.gov/parents/needs/speced/iepguide/index.htm

U.S. Department of Education (USDOE). (2006). *Individualized education programs*. Retrieved from http://idea.ed.gov/explore/view/p/%2Croot%2Cdynamic%2CTopicalBrief%2C10%2C

U.S. Department of Education (USDOE). (2011). *Q and A: Questions and answers on secondary transition*. Retrieved from http://idea.ed.gov/explore/view/p/%2Croot%2Cdynamic%2CQaCorner%2C10%2C

U.S. Department of Health and Human Services (USDHHS). (2015). *Healthy People 2020*. Retrieved from http://idea.ed.gov/explore/view/p/%2Croot%2Cdynamic%2CQaCorner%2C10%2C

U.S. Department of Health and Human Services (USDHHS). (2015). *Healthy People 2020*. Retrieved from http://www.healthypeople.gov/2020/topicsobjectives2020/default.aspx

U.S. Department of Health and Human Services, Health Resources and Services Administration (USDHHS/HRSA). (2011). *Children with special health care needs in context: A portrait of states and the nation 2007*. Rockville, MD: Author.

University of Michigan Health System. (2014). *Children with chronic conditions*. Retrieved from http://www.med.umich.edu/yourchild/topics/chronic.htm

Vermaes, P. R, van Susante, A. M. J., & van Bakel, H. J. A. (2012). Psychological functioning of siblings in families of children with chronic health conditions. *Journal of Pediatric Psychology, 37*(2), 166–184.

Vessey, J. A., & O'Neill, K. M. (2011). Helping students with disabilities better address teasing and bullying situations: A MASNRN study. *The Journal of School Nursing, 27*(2), 139–148.

Whiting, M. (2014). Support requirements of parents caring for a child with disability and complex health needs. *Nursing Children and Young People, 26*(4), 24–27.

Yell, M. L., Conroy, T., Katsiyannis, A., & Conroy, T. (2013). Individualized education programs and special education programming for students with disabilities in urban schools. *Fordham Urban Law Journal, 41*(2), 669–714.

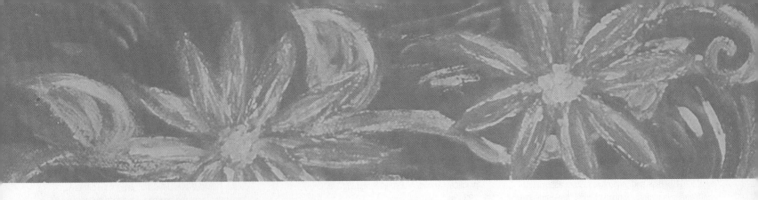

Chapter 13
The Child With a Life-Threatening Condition and End-of-Life Care

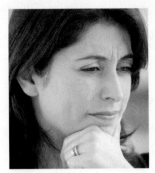

It all happened so fast. No one saw the car coming. Next thing I knew, we were in the emergency room talking about abdominal and head injuries. Now Alexa is in the intensive care unit, and I'm worried because she is still unconscious and on a ventilator. It was helpful for the nurse to tell me that even though Alexa couldn't respond, it was good to talk to her, because she will probably hear me and be comforted.

—Mother of Alexa, 6 years old

Michael Matisse/Getty Images

Learning Outcomes

13.1 Summarize the effects of a life-threatening illness or injury on children.

13.2 Examine the family's experience and reactions to having a child with a life-threatening illness or injury.

13.3 Identify the coping mechanisms used by the child and family in response to stress.

13.4 Develop a nursing care plan for the child with a life-threatening illness or injury.

13.5 Apply assessment skills to identify the physiologic changes that occur in the dying child.

13.6 Develop a nursing care plan to provide family-centered care for the dying child and family.

13.7 Plan bereavement support for the parents and siblings after the death of a child.

13.8 Evaluate strategies to support nurses who care for children who die.

The intense emotional and physical demands placed on the critically ill or injured child present a challenge to nurses' attempts to provide developmentally appropriate care. The child's parents and siblings are confronted with a stressful situation. A family-centered model of nursing practice offers a framework for performing interventions that help minimize stress and enhance coping by the ill or injured child, parents, and siblings.

Life-Threatening Illness or Injury

A **life-threatening condition** is one in which there is a likelihood that the child will die prematurely (Randall, Cervenka, Arday, et al., 2011). A threat to a child's life may be expected, as in a chronic illness or progressive disabling disease. More often, the death is unexpected as a result of an unintentional injury, the leading cause of death in children, or an acute illness. How children, parents, and siblings cope with the threat will depend on the anticipated or unanticipated nature of the event and the conditions surrounding the child's admission to the hospital.

When death results from a chronic disease or terminal illness, the child and family have time to adjust to episodes of life-threatening crises and impending death. Although the child could die unexpectedly during treatment, parents have some knowledge of the condition, the hospital setting, and the healthcare team and have had an opportunity to become involved in the child's therapy as integral members of this team. Emergency admission for an acute illness or unintentional injury, in contrast, brings with it sudden stressors as the child and family are thrust into an unfamiliar environment, confronted with frightening or invasive procedures, and faced with an uncertain outcome.

Nursing care of children and families coping with specific chronic diseases or terminal illnesses such as cancer, cystic fibrosis, or muscular dystrophy is discussed elsewhere in this text. The following discussion focuses on care of children with life-threatening illnesses or injuries and care of the dying child.

Child's Experience

Admission to the hospital, emergency department, or pediatric intensive care unit (PICU) is one of the most frightening experiences a child can have. Critically ill children may appear extremely anxious and fearful, or withdrawn, solemn, and preoccupied with their own physical condition. The illness or injury often brings pain, decreased energy, and changes to the affected child's level of consciousness.

Young children admitted to the PICU may be unable to understand what is happening to them. The PICU environment appears overwhelming, fast paced, and frightening, secondary to the numerous machines, noises, people, and procedures the child encounters. The child's normal sleep patterns can be disrupted because of the lack of day–night patterns in many intensive care units (Figure 13–1). Being cared for by strangers contributes to the child's anxiety. The child's limited ability to move intensifies feelings of powerlessness and vulnerability.

Children's responses to stress are influenced by their developmental levels, past experiences, types of illness, coping mechanisms, and available emotional support. Nurses must consider how their developmental level and coping skills will influence their ability to deal with the emergency department or PICU experience. Successful coping can provide these children with the skills to handle difficult situations in the future.

An unanticipated admission places the child at emotional risk because of the lack of preparation for the experience, the uncertainty and unpredictability of events that follow, the unfamiliarity of the environment, and the heightened anxiety of parents. An admission for an acute exacerbation of a disease such as cystic fibrosis or leukemia can provoke feelings of depression or hopelessness. Chapter 11 describes the stressors and responses to hospitalization of children by age group.

The child cared for in the PICU will experience the same stressors as any child who is hospitalized. However, the PICU environment is more intense and is very stressful for children. Treatment, disease, and/or environmental-related stressors place these children at risk for posttraumatic stress disorder. They are exposed to strangers, unfamiliar equipment, other sick children, and noises from alarms, phones, and pagers (Dow, Kenardy, Long, et al., 2012).

Coping Mechanisms

Coping refers to the cognitive and behavioral responses that help a person manage specific internal and external demands that exceed personal resources, enabling the person to solve problems and to respond appropriately. The child may mirror the parents' behaviors and responses, which may help or hinder the child's response to stress. The child's temperament, previous coping experiences, and availability of **support systems** (extended network of family, friends, and religious and community contacts that provide nurturance, emotional support, and direct assistance to parents) all combine to influence the child's ability to cope with the current experience.

The nature and severity of the illness and an emergency admission to the hospital stress a child's coping capabilities. Defense mechanisms displayed by children in these situations include **regression**, or return to an earlier behavior (a common reaction to stress), denial, **repression** (involuntary forgetting), postponement, and bargaining.

Nursing Management
For the Child With a Life-Threatening Illness or Injury

Nursing care of the child with a life-threatening illness or injury and the child's family includes assessing the child's physical and psychosocial needs, assessing the family's psychosocial needs, providing physical and psychosocial care for the child, and providing support for parental physical and emotional needs.

Nursing Assessment and Diagnosis

Nursing assessment involves physiologic parameters, plus skilled observation of the child's psychosocial and emotional needs. An understanding of normal psychosocial and cognitive development is necessary to plan developmentally appropriate interventions. Assessment should include the child's response to illness, the environment, coping strategies, and the need for information and support.

The accompanying *Nursing Care Plan* includes common nursing diagnoses for the child with a life-threatening illness or injury. The following nursing diagnoses may also be appropriate (NANDA-I © 2014):

- *Communication: Verbal, Impaired,* related to the effects of endotracheal intubation and mechanical ventilation
- *Spiritual Distress* related to the crisis of illness or suffering
- *Sleep Pattern, Disturbed,* related to circadian asynchrony, excessive stimulation, pain, and anxiety caused by the critical care unit environment
- *Activity, Deficient Diversional,* related to forced inactivity

Planning and Implementation

Nursing care focuses on promoting a sense of trust, providing education about the illness or injury, preparing the child for

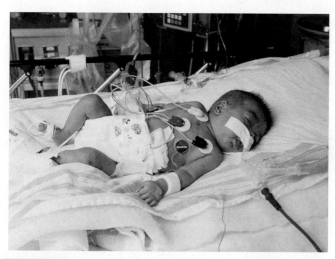

Figure 13–1 **Jooti feels pain, hears noises, has her sleep disrupted, and has limited mobility because of all the equipment attached to her.**

Clinical Reasoning PICU Stressors

The PICU receives a call from a community hospital requesting transport for an unstable 12-year-old boy, Gavin, who is in status epilepticus. Gavin has a seizure disorder controlled with medications, but several days ago he decided to stop taking his medications. After receiving several medications in the community hospital emergency department to stop the seizures, Gavin experienced some respiratory depression. He has been intubated to maintain his airway until the medications wear off.

The transport team is in the air within minutes and arrives at the rural community hospital 25 minutes later. The team stabilizes Gavin, receives reports from the medical and nursing teams, meets briefly with his parents, answers a few questions, and is back in the air.

Gavin is admitted directly to the PICU and connected to cardiorespiratory and noninvasive blood pressure monitors. His existing intravenous lines and endotracheal tube are evaluated for patency as team members quickly complete a head-to-toe assessment. When Gavin's parents arrive, his nurse meets them and prepares them for what they will see.

What stressors do children like Gavin face after sudden admission to the PICU? What stressors will parents face during the initial period when you work with them?

procedures, facilitating the use of play, and promoting a sense of control. Physiologic care for the child in the PICU may include the following: frequent physiologic assessment, pain and sedation management, nutritional support, medication administration, management of multiple IV lines and pumps, maintenance of ventilatory and hemodynamic monitoring equipment, and wound care.

PROVIDE PSYCHOSOCIAL CARE FOR THE CHILD

Children admitted to a PICU need support for the stressful experience. They often feel and hear, even when unconscious, so touch and talking to the child are important. Nurses play a key role in providing developmentally appropriate support to the child. Nursing interventions are directed at building a trusting relationship, minimizing the stressors experienced by the child, and promoting coping. Ongoing reassessment of progress in meeting the child's needs is critical.

PROMOTE A SENSE OF SECURITY

For children of all ages, feeling secure depends on a sense of physical and psychologic safety. A sense of physical security is difficult to attain within the PICU because frequent procedures are part of the child's treatment plan. Parental presence at the bedside is one of the best ways to decrease anxiety and promote a sense of security. Including parents as partners in the child's care provides comfort and reassurance to the child. Children whose parents have high anxiety levels pick up their parents' emotional cues and become more anxious. Consistency of staff is

---

Nursing Care Plan: The Child Coping With a Life-Threatening Illness or Injury

1. Nursing Diagnosis: *Anxiety (Child)* related to separation from parents, unfamiliar environment, strangers as caretakers, invasive procedures (NANDA-I © 2014)

GOAL: The child will exhibit or express an increased sense of security.

INTERVENTION	RATIONALE
• Encourage parents to remain at the bedside (open visitation) and to participate in the child's care by touching, talking to, reading to, and singing to the child.	• Presence of the parents is comforting to the child.
• Talk with the child. Avoid discussions at bedside that the child should not overhear.	• The child may overhear and remember, even if unconscious.
• Offer to arrange a visit from the chaplain or other spiritual support.	• Spiritual support often provides comfort and sustenance in a time of crisis.
• Provide the child with developmentally appropriate explanations when possible. Encourage the child to ask questions and express concerns.	• Information reduces anxiety and builds trust.
• Make the child's bedside more personal and familiar by encouraging parents to bring in security objects, family photos, and favorite toys from home.	• Security objects decrease foreignness of hospital environment. The child derives comfort from presence of personal items.
• Involve the child in play appropriate to developmental age (see Chapter 4).	• Play provides familiarity, decreases fantasy, and provides motor activity.
• Provide care using a primary nursing care model.	• Consistency in healthcare givers helps to build the child's trust. Healthcare giver learns child's cues.

EXPECTED OUTCOME: Child will appear more relaxed and acknowledge parents' presence. Behavioral manifestations of anxiety will be absent. Restful periods of sleep will be noted.

2. Nursing Diagnosis: *Powerlessness* related to inability to communicate and control relinquished to the healthcare team (NANDA-I © 2014)

GOAL: The child or adolescent will have an increased sense of control over the situation.

INTERVENTION	RATIONALE
• Provide opportunities for choices when possible. Encourage participation in self-care.	• Such opportunities provide sense of control and autonomy through decision making.
• Prepare the child or adolescent in advance (timing dependent on developmental level) for procedures. Describe the sensations that will be experienced. Allow some choice in timing or method of pain relief.	• Providing information to children or adolescents lets them know what to expect. Allowing choices gives them a sense of involvement and lets them know their input is important.
• Provide routines for the child both within a 24-hour period and for scheduled care. Tell the child before the procedure (timing dependent on developmental level), repeat explanation of why procedure is necessary, complete procedure in a consistent manner, and offer praise or a special story when completed. When possible, incorporate rituals from home.	• Routines and rituals provide a sense of continuity and comfort for the child.
• Provide other means of communication to the intubated child (e.g., a word board or finger board).	• Fostering communication by some means helps the child maintain some sense of control.
• For the child requiring restraints or immobilizers, use as seldom as possible, provide appropriate explanations, and release at regular intervals. Wrapping IV lines well can help maintain lines and avoid the need for restraints.	• Release from restraints or immobilizers helps diminish the sense of powerlessness that accompanies their use.

EXPECTED OUTCOME: Child or adolescent will express satisfaction over ability to control some elements of situation. Child or adolescent will participate in self-care and decision making.

3. Nursing Diagnosis: *Pain, Acute,* related to injuries, invasive procedures, surgery (NANDA-I © 2014)

GOAL: The child will experience reduced pain and improved comfort.

INTERVENTION	RATIONALE
• Assess the child's pain location, intensity, and what makes it better or worse.	• Assessment provides baseline information from which a plan of care can be developed.
• If appropriate, use a pain assessment scale (see Chapter 15).	• Use of a scale provides continuity and consistency in monitoring of the child's pain.
• Provide optimal pain relief with prescribed analgesics. Provide comfort measures such as position changes and back rubs. Provide diversional activities as appropriate or possible. Incorporate the family in pain-relief modality.	• Physiologic and psychologic methods of pain control can be used in combination to maximally improve outcomes.

EXPECTED OUTCOME: Child will experience a perceived or actual improvement in comfort level.

invaluable in developing familiarity and a trusting relationship with the child.

Personalizing the child's bedside can promote comfort and a sense of security. Pictures from home, a favorite blanket or toy, music tapes, or posters can make the environment friendlier and more familiar to the child (Figure 13–2). Religious or spiritual symbols may also provide psychologic support.

PROVIDE EDUCATION AND PREPARE THE CHILD FOR PROCEDURES

The ability of children to understand the cause of their illness and its therapy depends on their cognitive abilities. Help younger children to understand that illness and hospitalization are not a punishment.

Preparation for procedures is important at all ages, even for the unconscious or sedated child. Toddlers will benefit from being talked to, soothed, and touched during and after the procedure. Provide preschoolers, school-age children, and adolescents with an explanation of the sensations they can expect to experience (temperature, vibrations, sounds, smells, tastes, sight). (See Chapter 11.)

FACILITATE THE USE OF PLAY

Play can be used to alleviate stress and to help prepare children for procedures. The nurse can also use play to assess the child's developmental level. Even within the PICU, therapeutic play diminishes negative fantasies, provides motor activity, and helps the child cope with stressors (see Chapter 11). Children with limited

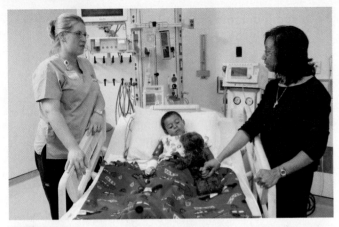

Figure 13–2 By their very nature, PICUs are ominous and sterile. To lessen this effect, it can help to personalize the child's space. Being there with the child and parent, answering questions, or just talking can be a comfort to both.

mobility due to tubes and immobilizers can still feel a sense of accomplishment, for example, by completing a puzzle, even if the nurse points and moves each piece as the child responds through nods and gestures to indicate where the puzzle piece should be placed. Play can help children work through a painful situation, making it more tolerable. The child-life specialist may also be able to facilitate coping by assisting in preparation for procedures and providing distraction during procedures. See a discussion of the role of the child-life specialist in Chapter 11.

PROMOTE A SENSE OF CONTROL

Children between toddlerhood and adolescence experience a loss of control during a life-threatening illness. This loss of control may be related to the body, emotions, normal routines, or privacy. Nursing interventions should promote a sense of control over these areas.

Children hospitalized in an intensive care unit experience a heightened sense of loss of control secondary to the many machines, noises, and limits on mobility. These children often self-remove or threaten to self-remove technologic equipment or devices employed in their care such as an endotracheal tube, peripheral IV line or central line, nasogastric tube, or arterial line. Physical immobilizers are sometimes used in children with altered levels of consciousness to prevent them from pulling out tubes and lines. Although immobilizers are sometimes necessary, they contribute to the child's sense of powerlessness. Nurses should position these devices in a way that maintains comfort as much as possible.

Enhance the child's coping skills by teaching the child and family a combination of relaxation, visual imagery, or distraction techniques, and comforting self-talk phrases, such as "This will be over soon," "If I stay calm, it will be all right," and "It will be over fast so I can do something fun." Help the parents become the child's coping coaches.

Evaluation

Expected outcomes of nursing care include the following:

- A trusting relationship is developed with the child and family.
- The child is given preparation and support for procedures.
- The child's coping is promoted by family presence and therapeutic play.

Parents' Experience of a Child's Life-Threatening Illness or Injury

The uncertainty and unpredictability of a child's life-threatening illness or injury challenge a family's coping and stability. Admission of a child to the pediatric intensive care unit is one of the most stressful events that a parent can experience (Jee et al., 2012). The sudden loss of the parenting role with the child's emergency admission causes stress. Families display many different responses and coping mechanisms such as crying, emotional outbursts, fear, and demanding information. Parents are at risk for long-term psychologic effects, including the development of posttraumatic stress disorder (PTSD), when the child is hospitalized in an intensive care unit (Jee et al., 2012). Parents may find it difficult to support the child if their own needs are not met. They may also transmit their anxiety to the child, who then becomes even more anxious. Family-centered care must be provided to meet the needs of parents with a variety of personalities, coping mechanisms, and responses to the crisis. Clear, concise communication is imperative.

The Family in Crisis

The critical care environment and the implications of a child's life-threatening illness or injury are far removed from the everyday experiences of most families. The unfamiliarity of the environment and the uncertainty and seriousness of the illness or injury create a **family crisis**, which occurs when the family encounters a problem that seems insurmountable and usual coping skills are not effective.

Since families have little time to prepare for the experience, a sudden admission threatens family integrity, causing enormous stress and separation from loved ones. The interruption of the unique parent–child relationship can be more stressful to parents than the physical PICU environment. Siblings are also affected. See the section titled *The Siblings' Experience* later in this chapter. In addition, extended family members such as grandparents must be considered. Stresses are further intensified in the case of divorce, separation, and stepparenting. Financial problems, a long distance from home to hospital, or another ill or injured family member can compound the crisis.

Parental Reactions to Life-Threatening Illness or Injury

When faced with a threat to their child's life, parents typically progress through stages that might include shock and disbelief, anger and guilt, deprivation and loss, anticipatory waiting, and readjustment or mourning. Some families progress through these stages in a linear fashion, whereas others go back and forth between stages, especially if the child's condition improves and then worsens.

SHOCK AND DISBELIEF

The universal reaction to a child's life-threatening condition is shock and disbelief. As the familiar is disrupted, parents experience a loss of control, an inability to regain their bearings, and feelings of immobility. The hospital environment, emergency department, or PICU may seem unreal. The emotions parents experience initially are intensified by the physical appearance of their child (particularly after a major injury); the presence of monitors, tubing, and equipment; and the actual injury or illness.

Shock and disbelief begin in the first few moments after hearing the "news" and can last for days. The shock helps postpone the full impact of the crisis. During this period, parents search for answers and explanations about the illness or injury. Information must be repeated many times to parents, since in this stage they are often unable to assimilate information easily.

ANGER AND GUILT

Anger and guilt surface as parents become more aware of their child's illness or injury. Their anger may be directed toward themselves or each other because they could not protect the child. Other individuals may be blamed, such as the driver of a motor vehicle who injured the child. Parents may also be angry with their child. This anger may be a result of injuries the child sustained when breaking known rules, such as drinking and driving, playing with matches, or riding a bike without a helmet. Last, the anger may not be directed at anyone specifically. Injuries caused by natural disasters such as an earthquake, flood, or hurricane provoke just as much anger as those that result from the actions of people, and they may pose a challenge to the parents' spiritual beliefs.

Parents typically react to their child's illness or injury with some degree of guilt. This reaction may be magnified in the PICU environment. The fact that the guilt usually has no basis in real events does not lessen the feeling. A question parents frequently ask at this stage is, "Why not me instead of my child?" Parents' feelings of guilt may be related to the following:

1. They may feel responsible for causing the illness or injury. A statement such as "If only I hadn't sent him to the store on his bike, this wouldn't have happened" reflects feelings of guilt for causing or failing to prevent the injury.

2. They may feel guilty about not noticing the onset of an illness or disregarding earlier illness symptoms. The mother of a 1-year-old with meningitis might repeatedly say, "I shouldn't have waited so long to take her to the doctor!"

DEPRIVATION AND LOSS

As the shock associated with the child's life-threatening condition slowly recedes, new stressors emerge. Within minutes or hours, parents are deprived of their familiar role as the parent of a healthy child and find themselves in an unexpected and unfamiliar role as the parent of a critically ill child.

The difficulty and ambivalence parents feel in releasing a part of their responsibility as the child's primary caretakers can threaten their self-esteem and self-control. If parents cannot participate in the child's care, they may feel helpless or worthless.

ANTICIPATORY WAITING

When the child's condition is stabilized and survival seems likely, parents often move into a period of anticipatory waiting. This stage is characterized as "life suspended in time." Parents spend a great deal of time waiting: for test results, for explanations, for their child to become conscious, or for surgery to be over. Parents may fear leaving the area because they may miss an important procedure, healthcare provider visit, or decisions or changes in treatment. Lack of mobility decreases the parents' use of typical coping mechanisms, so anxiety and the sense of powerlessness may increase. If the parents have a cell phone, write down the number and ensure them that they will be called for any change in the child's condition. This allows parents to feel like they can leave at least for a few minutes. If the parents do not have a cell phone, provide a pager if available.

Parents may have a preoccupation with medical details. During this period, they may ask questions about the long-term effects of the illness or injury on the child, about the potential for brain damage, or about the need for additional surgeries. Parents may place demands on staff and be frustrated when the child's progress is slow.

READJUSTMENT OR MOURNING

The last stage that parents experience is readjustment or mourning. Readjustment is experienced as the child recovers, improves steadily, and prepares for transfer and discharge. In contrast, parents of the child who dies reenter the cycle of emotions characteristic of grief. Parents also mourn when the child remains seriously ill or unresponsive, when the outcome remains uncertain for an extended period, or when long-term care is required.

Table 13–1 lists the most important needs of parents when a child is hospitalized with a life-threatening illness or injury.

Nursing Management

For the Parents of a Child With a Life-Threatening Illness or Injury

Nursing care of the family includes assessing the family's psychosocial needs and providing support for parental physical and emotional needs.

Nursing Assessment and Diagnosis

Nurses who work with families of critically ill children have a unique opportunity to help them adapt and to promote family functioning. Begin by assessing the family's reaction to the illness, coping skills, stressors, and needs. (See Chapter 12.) This initial assessment provides a baseline of information for developing a care plan and strategies to meet the psychosocial as well as physiologic needs of families.

Several nursing diagnoses may apply to parents who are dealing with their child's life-threatening condition. Examples include the following (NANDA-I © 2014):

- *Family Processes, Interrupted,* related to the impact of a critically ill child on the family system
- *Spiritual Distress* related to the child's life-threatening condition, suffering, or death
- *Fatigue* related to extreme stress, sleep deprivation, and crisis

TABLE 13–1 Nursing Interventions to Meet Parental Needs When a Child Is Hospitalized With a Life-Threatening Illness or Injury

PARENTAL NEEDS	NURSING INTERVENTIONS
Information	• Provide information and frequent updates about the child's condition using terminology that parents can understand. • Repeat the information and provide other materials frequently because parents forget or cannot concentrate on details with all the stress they are under. • Explain the child's condition, equipment being used, and procedures of care. • Facilitate a discussion with the healthcare provider at least daily. • Provide general information about unit policies, team members, and phone numbers.
Proximity to their child	• Provide permission for the parents to remain at the bedside. • Encourage parents to touch and speak with the child and demonstrate ways if parents are hesitant. • Work within the unit to provide open, flexible visiting hours.
Reestablishment of their parental role and control	• Implement family-centered care so parents feel recognized as important to their child's recovery and as the decision maker for the child's treatment options.
Participation in their child's care	• Encourage parents to participate in care (e.g., bathing and hair care, diaper changes, feeding, range-of-motion exercises, massages). • Encourage parents to help with diversional activities (e.g., reading, singing, telling stories). • Encourage parents to explain equipment and procedures to the child to reduce the child's fears.
Confidence in the treatment plan and caregivers	• Try to maintain continuity in staffing and healthcare contacts. • Demonstrate caring for the child. • Provide assurance that the child is receiving appropriate treatment and pain management.
Psychologic support	• Acknowledge that the situation is difficult. • Help parents focus on the positive or unchanged aspects of the child's appearance. • Encourage parents to get rest and nutrition to help them maintain physical resources necessary for coping. • Provide space and privacy as needed. • Give hope if realistic—an essential component of coping. • Offer the choice of other family members to be present. • Discuss the possible responses of siblings and the long-term emotional responses of the patient.

• *Hopelessness* in parents related to the child's deteriorating physical condition

• *Grieving* related to potential death of the child or loss of body functions

• *Coping: Family, Compromised,* related to the severity of the illness or injury in the child

Planning and Implementation

Nursing care focuses on providing family-centered care to help meet the needs of families, minimize stress, and enhance family coping (see Table 1–1). Nurses are challenged to blend and balance technology with caring.

PROVIDE INFORMATION AND BUILD TRUST

Orienting parents to the hospital, as well as to the unit routines, helps them adapt to their surroundings. Parents will gain a sense of control and independence if they know where to get supplies and how to find the lounge, cafeteria, and restrooms.

Provide frequent and accurate information. Deliver information on the child's illness, condition, and plan of care in

a manner and language readily understandable to parents. Upon admission, provide the parents with an idea of what to expect in the days ahead and to be prepared for special procedures or major changes in therapy. Parents also need to be prepared before they see the child the first time. Explain the tubes and monitors that are present and how the child will look and react.

Honesty in discussions is extremely important. If parents feel misled or that information is being withheld, a trusting relationship will be impossible. However, informed parents will feel that they are active participants in decision making and care planning for their child. Trust is facilitated when parents believe that the staff truly cares about the child and sees the child as a special individual. Trust is especially important when difficult decisions must be made, such as withdrawal of life support, or to reduce the risk for conflict.

Parents also need a sense of hope regarding their child's condition to help them cope. Focus on the positives as the child progresses through the different phases of the life-threatening condition.

Explain to the child and parents, in easy-to-understand terms, the purpose of equipment that is being used. Answer alarms quickly regardless of the reason for the alarm. Follow with an explanation of why alarms sound, including the fact that many times monitor alarms will sound when the child moves, if the monitor becomes disconnected, or if the monitor patches are loose.

FACILITATE POSITIVE STAFF–PARENT RELATIONSHIPS AND COMMUNICATION

Given the intensity of the parents' experience when their child is critically ill, it is easy to see how problems can arise between staff and parents. Each healthcare team member must be aware of the child's current status so that parents receive consistent information from all staff. A consistent message can instill confidence. Provide explanations geared to the parents' level of understanding, using language the parents can understand.

Introduce the parents to the nurse and the intensive care physician who have overall responsibility for the child's care. This is especially important in teaching hospitals that have rotating interns and residents. The attending physician with the overall responsibility should meet with parents as often as necessary to talk about changes in the child's condition or treatment plan and to allow time for parents to ask questions (Figure 13–3). Encourage parents to keep a daily log or notebook to record information on the child's care, progress, and needs, as well as questions they want to ask. Family care conferences can be helpful when a large number of team members provide care. Arrange for daily visits by an interpreter if the family does not speak or understand English. Have information about the child's condition and care summarized for communication at that time.

PROMOTE PARENTAL INVOLVEMENT

An important role of nurses is to encourage and support parents in their parenting role. The parents' place when possible is at the bedside. Parents can provide comfort to their child and

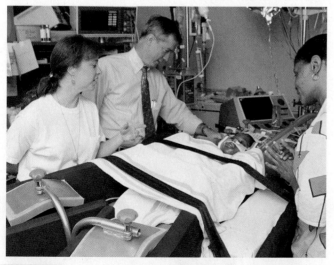

Figure 13–3 In times of crisis, everyone likes to know that someone is in charge and who that person is. The parents should meet and talk with the healthcare provider in charge and the nurses as often as possible. Parents need to know that someone is responsible, even if different people are providing care.

can assist in explanations that offer reassurance to their child. They may also be able to assist with basic care needs such as bathing and changing diapers (Ames, Rennick, & Baillargeon, 2011). Parents provide continuity and may notice subtle condition changes that an assigned nurse may miss. Throughout the child's hospitalization, parents will continue to need reassurance and encouragement.

Participation in care of the child is an integral aspect of family-centered care and enhances the family's ability to cope with the child's illness or injury. Open communication with the family about the child's treatments and plan of care is essential. Parents need to know how their child is doing, understand the care being provided to their child, and know what to expect next (Ames et al., 2011). Parents who do not remain at the child's bedside may feel that they are not an important team member. When parents are unable to remain at the bedside, they should be allowed to call the unit at any time to check on their child.

FAMILY PRESENCE DURING RESUSCITATION AND INVASIVE PROCEDURES

Many hospitals are implementing policies that permit families to be present during resuscitation and invasive procedures. Healthcare professionals have expressed concern that parents who are allowed to witness resuscitation efforts might lose control and interfere. Another concern is that medical staff, especially those in training, might feel uncomfortable, and that there is an increased risk for litigation. However, reports related to family presence during resuscitation have failed to demonstrate any increase in litigation (Jabre et al., 2013). Families have reported that they felt being present during resuscitation and invasive procedures helped their child and helped them (Meert, Clark, & Eggly, 2013). In addition, studies have failed to show that family presence interrupts care or interferes with the healthcare providers' ability to intervene in the care of the child (Emergency Nurses Association [ENA], 2012).

The Emergency Nurses Association supports the option of family presence during invasive procedures and resuscitation (ENA, 2012). Parents and other family members (e.g., grandparents) may wish to be present during invasive procedures (such as lumbar puncture) or resuscitation of the child. The nurse partners with the family to determine their needs at the time. To better facilitate the needs of the family, the following should be determined:

- Who desires to be present during resuscitation or invasive procedures?
- What role will they play during the procedure (e.g., snuggle child for comfort)?

Healthcare agencies should have an established policy for family presence during invasive procedures or resuscitation (ENA, 2012). Care must be family centered and individualized to each situation according to the child's and family's needs. A designated healthcare professional should be available to stay with family members during resuscitation and provide comfort and explanations as needed (ENA, 2012).

If parents choose not to witness the resuscitation, regular updates (5- to 10-minute intervals) should be provided to the parents as they wait in a private area. A hospital chaplain or other family support team member should support the parents while they wait.

PROVIDE FOR PARENTAL PHYSICAL AND EMOTIONAL NEEDS

The experience of having a child with a life-threatening condition drains the parents' physical and emotional reserves. Parents often need encouragement to take care of themselves and to periodically take a break. A statement such as "It is important for you to eat and rest because Alexa is really going to need you when she wakes up" helps parents realize that becoming exhausted benefits neither them nor the child.

Many communities have a residence for families of hospitalized children. This is often an inexpensive but warm and supportive environment for families. The Ronald McDonald Children's Charities supports many of these residences. A Ronald McDonald Family Room may be found in some hospitals and is provided as a comfortable setting where families of hospitalized children can get away from the high-tech hospital atmosphere while remaining close to the child. Computer resources in one of these locations or in a Family Resource Center may make it possible for parents to stay in contact with concerned family and friends. When financial burdens are a consideration, parents may need family support and social service referrals.

Parents are often at different levels of coping during a crisis. The severity of the child's illness or injury may foster cohesion between the parents and build a stronger relationship. Unfortunately, the reverse may also be true—differences in styles or levels of coping may foster a sense of isolation, placing a strain on the couple's relationship. Nurses should be alert to family dynamics and refer the family for counseling or therapy if indicated.

MAINTAIN OR STRENGTHEN FAMILY SUPPORT SYSTEMS

Support systems enable parents to cope with overwhelming problems and crises. Most parents indicate that having family or friends nearby is crucial as a support system. Some families seek support through prayer and from religious or faith-based leaders.

Extended family, especially grandparents and friends, frequently offer the family assistance, but parents may need to be reassured that it is all right to ask for help as well. Some parents are uncomfortable asking for help, instead attempting to handle multiple responsibilities themselves, often to the point of exhaustion. Some parents are so overwhelmed that they are unable to respond to offers of help because it requires too great a mental effort on their part. The nurse should assist the parents in responding to these offers for assistance.

Nurses may need to intervene on parents' behalf when they have inadequate support. Parents may be frustrated by people who come to visit unannounced, stay too long, or visit too often. They may find it difficult to tell well-meaning but insensitive friends that they cannot deal with visitors right now. In these situations, it may be helpful for the nurse to offer to serve as a gatekeeper. Suggest that parents inform family and friends about specific times for visits or phone calls to allow for rest periods. An extended family member may be given the responsibility of relaying information to others.

Families of children with a life-threatening illness or injury often have emotional needs beyond the support capabilities of the nurse caring for the child. Referrals to family and support services or pastoral care may be beneficial in these instances.

Evaluation

Expected outcomes of nursing care include the following:

- The nurse establishes a trusting relationship and effective communication with the family.
- Parents participate in their child's care as much as desired.
- Parents and extended family members receive emotional support and nurturance needed to sustain them through the child's illness.

The Siblings' Experience

As the parents' focus shifts to the critically ill child, they may need support in dealing with the healthy siblings. Siblings of a critically ill child may experience stress related to parental absence, being cared for by others, changes in routine, and lack of information about their ill sibling (Meert et al., 2013). Nurses should recognize that siblings may fear becoming ill themselves or believe that they played a role in the child's illness. Siblings often have nightmares about the illness or injury their brother or sister has sustained and about the ill child dying. Inform siblings about their brother's or sister's condition using language and concepts appropriate to their ages and developmental levels. Being allowed to visit the sick child may help siblings to cope (Meert et al., 2013).

Before the visit, talk with the siblings about what to expect and describe how their brother or sister will look. If the ill child acts, moves, talks, or looks different than usual, provide an explanation beforehand. Describe the hospital environment, including equipment, sounds, and smells. Use a doll, draw pictures, or show an actual picture of the child to prepare the siblings. See *Families Want to Know: Strategies for Working With the Sibling of a Hospitalized Child* in Chapter 11. The child-life specialist may also be able to assist in preparing siblings for a visit to the intensive care unit (see Chapter 11).

During the visit the nurse should demonstrate how to talk to and touch the ill child and encourage the siblings to do the same (Figure 13–4). The length of the visit should be relatively short

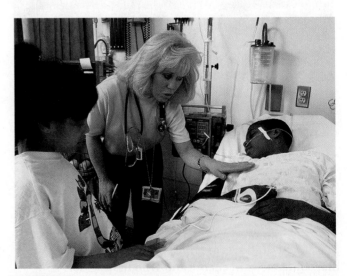

Figure 13–4 During the sibling's visit to the ill child, it is important to talk with the sibling and answer any questions in an honest manner at a level the child can understand.

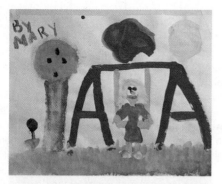

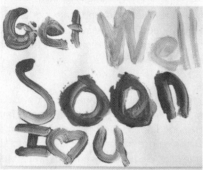

Figure 13–5 It is important that parents and siblings feel comfortable communicating with the seriously ill child. If siblings cannot visit, they should be encouraged to paint or record messages. They need to be able to express themselves and to feel that they are helping.

and based on the child's developmental age. After the visit, the nurse should talk with siblings about what they saw and felt, and answer their questions. When a sibling cannot visit, contact with the ill child can be maintained by sending pictures, drawings, cards, and messages recorded on audiotapes or cell phones if allowed (Figure 13–5).

If parents are staying at the hospital with the ill child, encourage them to call the siblings at home daily. This allows the siblings at home to feel connected by the opportunity to share their day and to receive an update on the ill child. The phone call offers siblings a consistent link to the parents and the reassurance that they are important and loved. Internet contact or text messaging may be another way to communicate with older siblings. Arrange for parents to access a computer, if possible, for families who might find this contact supportive.

Evaluation

Expected outcomes of nursing care include:

- Siblings are prepared for visits to the child with a life-threatening illness or injury.
- Siblings receive emotional support and assistance to cope with the unfamiliar environment.

End-of-Life Care

When the family is faced with end-of-life decision making and care because of a child's chronic condition or multiple acute care episodes, the family needs honest information about various treatment options and potential outcomes. Depending on cognitive abilities, developmental stage, physical and mental status,

and prior experiences with health care, the child may also participate in the decision-making process. The family may need to consider issues such as palliative care, hospice care, do-not-resuscitate requests, continuation of schooling, organ/tissue donation, and autopsy.

Palliative and Hospice Care

Pediatric **palliative care** is a multidisciplinary care approach for children with life-shortening disorders and their families. It is intended to relieve suffering of all types (physical, psychologic, spiritual, and social); to enhance quality of life for patients and their families; to facilitate informed decision making by the patient, family, and healthcare professionals; and to improve care coordination (American Academy of Pediatrics [AAP] Section on Hospice and Palliative Medicine and Committee on Hospital Care, 2013). Palliative care may be provided along with curative care, life-prolonging care, or as the main focus of care. Palliative care may be seen as the holistic care provided to a child until the family decides to view dying as a natural process and stops curative care (Trotzuk & Gray, 2012). Children may require these services for many years.

Hospice is a form of palliative care that is provided by licensed agencies. For children it is most often provided in the home but may also be provided in special centers or the hospital. Federal regulations outline the required bundle of services that include nursing, healthcare provider, psychosocial, and spiritual services; medications; durable medical equipment; and a range of diagnostic tests and therapeutic interventions (AAP, 2013). Hospice care is provided to the child near the end of life, and it is focused on supporting the family and ensuring that the remaining time for the child is lived as comfortably and as fully as possible.

About 75% of all children who die each year in a hospital, often in an intensive care unit from a life-threatening condition, do not have palliative or hospice care management (Keim-Malpass, Hart, & Miller, 2013). It is estimated that 5000 children in the United States on any day are within the last 6 months of dying and could benefit from palliative or hospice services (Crozier & Hancock, 2012). These services are also an option for neonates on the edge of viability.

When a child receives hospice care, the family and healthcare providers collaborate to determine which treatments are appropriate to continue with the child's end-of-life care, such as IV fluids, gastrostomy feedings, and certain medications. The child is maintained as alert and comfortable as possible. Hospice also provides grief counseling and support to parents for 1 year following the death of the child. See *Evidence-Based Practice: Responding to the Needs of the Family.*

Ethical Issues Surrounding a Child's Death

Because the death of a child is so emotionally charged, misunderstandings and conflicts can develop between families and healthcare providers. The more common ethical issues that need to be addressed include withdrawing or withholding treatment, parental treatment refusal, and do-not-resuscitate orders.

Brain Death Criteria

A commonly accepted definition of death in the United States is **brain death**, the irreversible cessation of all functions of the brain. Specific medical protocols are used to declare brain death before

EVIDENCE-BASED PRACTICE | Responding to the Needs of the Family

Clinical Question

The families of children with life-limiting conditions often have difficulty expressing their needs for support. What are some of the most important focus areas for nursing support in palliative care programs for children and their families?

The Evidence

A survey of 50 parents whose child died as a result of advanced heart disease in the intensive care unit setting was conducted to gain information about the care provided at the child's end of life. The majority of parents (66%) believed they had little or no preparation for the way their child died or about the child's medical problems in the last month of life. Many (40%) reported receiving conflicting information from the child's healthcare team about expectations of the child's end of life. Parents (66%) reported that the child's quality of life was poor to fair during the final month, and half of children experienced suffering. Most did not realize their child would not survive until death was imminent, indicating a gap in understanding the child's prognosis (Blume et al., 2014).

A pilot study explored a method to promote advance care planning for 30 adolescents (with a mean age of 16 years) with cancer and a parent. Dyads were randomly assigned to the intervention group or control group. The control group received a brochure about advance care planning and no additional information. Six different end-of-life scenarios with possible care options for additional medical interventions or limiting treatment were provided by the research team during education and data collection sessions. Intervention adolescents were encouraged to write five wishes for their own care if a bad outcome were to occur in the future. Adolescents in the intervention group were significantly better informed about advance care planning, and adolescent–parent dyads were more likely to agree about when to limit treatment than control dyads. The intervention adolescents

(100%) wanted their parents to select the best option at the time compared to control adolescents (60%) (Lyon, Jacobs, Briggs, et al., 2013).

A focus group qualitative research process was used to help plan a legacy-making project. Eight children (7 to 12 years old) with cancer and their parents were asked to provide feedback to the legacy-making project and the questions that would guide children when they shared their story. Children wanted to participate, and said they wanted to leave a story in which others would know or remember their personal characteristics, things they like to do, and the important people in their lives. Based on feedback, questions were revised to help guide the script for a customized digital story that a child could develop (Akard et al., 2013).

Best Practice

Palliative care professionals continue to seek evidence-based care interventions to support children and families with life-limiting conditions. The previously mentioned studies reveal challenges in care and strategies to support patients and families. Each of these topics was consistent with major themes found in systematic analysis of 21 qualitative and survey-based studies about patient and family needs. These included accurate and clear information about the child's illness, treatments, and prognosis; spiritual needs and ways to remember the child after death; and decision making with regard to treatment decisions (Stevenson, Achille, & Lugasi, 2013).

Clinical Reasoning

When in a clinical setting where children with life-limiting conditions receive treatment, seek information about the resources and strategies used by the palliative care team to meet the needs of children and their families. What additional resources would be helpful for nursing support in this population?

---

withdrawal of life support or when organ transplantation is planned. To declare brain death, the child must be unresponsive in an irreversible coma from a known cause and have absence of brainstem reflexes, and apnea testing must reveal hypercarbia. Before an evaluation for brain death is performed, it is confirmed that the child does not have hypothermia, conditions, or medications that could contribute to brain death findings. The two required examinations by different healthcare providers for brain death to be declared are separated by 24 hours for newborns and 12 hours for infants and children (Nakagawa, Ashwal, Mathur, et al., 2011).

Withdrawal of or Withholding Treatment

The decision to withdraw or withhold life-sustaining treatments, such as mechanical ventilation or dialysis, from the dying child is very difficult and emotional for parents. Parents may feel that agreeing to withdraw treatment is a form of abandonment. When treatments are withdrawn, reassure parents the child will receive comfort measures, including pain medication. Reinforce the fact that the underlying disease process is

causing the child to die rather than withdrawing life-sustaining treatments.

Medically provided nutrition and hydration (through nasogastric or gastrostomy tubes and IV catheters) support a child's existence at the end of life, but research has not demonstrated an association with survival or improved quality of care (Rapoport, Shaheed, Newman, et al., 2013). Food and fluids may be withheld when they would be of no benefit to the child, but this is a difficult decision for parents because food and fluid are associated with nurturing and love.

Conflicted opinions often develop if parents and the healthcare provider are unable to discontinue aggressive therapies that may also cause discomfort. The nurse may experience moral distress, believing that the child's suffering is being extended without much hope for improvement. Consultation with a member of the hospital ethics committee can help clarify the issues involved and reduce the emotions of healthcare professionals associated with the conflict. During the consultation an unbiased professional collects facts about the child's condition, clarifies the beliefs and values of parents and healthcare professionals, and improves communication while investigating options for compromise. Families are often invited to a meeting in which the ethical dilemmas regarding their child's care are discussed so they are better informed to make decisions.

Developing Cultural Competence End-of-Life Care

Discussing the option with parents about withholding or withdrawing therapy is challenging as they are struggling to accept that no further curative care is possible for their child. The focus becomes what is best for the child within the context of the culture, faith, and values of the family. Latino families may believe that all care and every effort should be provided to their child. African American families with a strong Christian belief may want all efforts continued in the hope of divine intervention. Palliative care with a focus on reducing suffering, promoting comfort, and providing information about end-of-life care planning may not be viewed by these families as the best care (Wiener, McConnell, Latella, et al., 2013).

Professionalism in Practice DNAR Order in the School Setting

The National Association of School Nurses' position statement on Do Not Attempt Resuscitation (DNAR) provides guidelines for the development of a plan for students who have such an order. The school nurse should work with the family, school administrators, the child's healthcare team, local emergency medical services providers, and others such as a local funeral director to develop plans for the supportive response when a child has an arrest. This plan is spelled out in the child's individualized health plan. The nurse must also educate school personnel about the planned response and their role, permitting discussion about their feelings concerning a child's death in the school setting. Keep in mind that a plan for bereavement support of faculty, staff, and students should also be developed for implementation when a child dies (National Association of School Nurses, 2014).

Do-Not-Resuscitate Orders

Parents faced with a child's end-stage, irreversible life-limiting condition may be asked to consider a do-not-resuscitate (DNR) order. Terms becoming more common are **"allow natural death" (AND)** and comfort care, which involve the continuation of ongoing care, managing pain, and choosing not to initiate cardiopulmonary resuscitation if the child stops breathing or the heart stops beating. Medical care is not discontinued; rather the DNR order is part of the child's management plan. Palliative care is provided, and, in some cases, curative care continues for these children.

A DNR order is part of advance care planning. A recent survey of healthcare providers and nurses revealed that advance care planning discussions often occur later in the child's care than they should, either during an acute illness or when death is imminent rather than during a period of stability (Sanderson, Zurakowski, & Wolfe, 2013). This planning process is becoming more important in pediatrics because of the increasing number of children with complex health conditions that have a variable but prolonged disease trajectory that leads to death. Honest and compassionate discussions between healthcare professionals and families, including adolescents, should occur. The family should be informed about significant condition changes and what to expect. Time should be provided for the family and adolescent to consider what is important to them at the end of life. Families can participate in planning the child's end-of-life care with healthcare providers.

The Americans with Disabilities Act of 1990 and the Education for All Handicapped Children Act mandate that all children with disabilities—including those with complex chronic conditions and terminal illnesses—are entitled to the same education as other students. It is estimated that in the United States nearly 4000 children and adolescents attend school and may be within 6 months of dying from their chronic condition (National Association of School Nurses, 2014). These children may be at higher risk of dying while at school, and many school districts have established policies and protocols for dealing with a student's DNR order. Advance planning with an individualized health plan and emergency care plan are needed for the school setting.

Care of the Dying Child

Caring for a dying child is challenging and requires the utmost sensitivity and compassion. Children as young as 5 years of age can sense when they are seriously ill. Their awareness of death develops more rapidly when they are experiencing the progression of a disease and ongoing medical treatment. Children with life-limiting illnesses often learn about death and their own illness from exposure to other seriously ill and dying children during hospitalization or clinic visits.

Awareness of Dying by Developmental Age

Infants and toddlers are not actually aware of death, but they are aware of and react to changes in normal routines and the behavior of parents. Toddlers know they feel tired and sick, but they do not understand that their physical symptoms are associated with impending death (Figure 13–6).

Preschool children can see their bodies deteriorate and feel the effects of medications used during disease progression and treatment. Changes in self-concept occur as they perceive these body changes. They often describe their illness in terms of mutilation to their body. These physical changes may make them realize that they are dying.

School-age children also have subtle fears about body integrity and anxieties about the seriousness of their illness. This greater preoccupation with illness is considered by many professionals as the child's version of **death anxiety**, a feeling of apprehension or fear of death. Children may express death anxiety as a concern with treatments that invade the body or interfere with normal body functions.

Adolescents have a mature understanding of death, but the normal developmental milestones of adolescence add to their problems in facing a terminal illness. They are struggling to establish their own identity and plans for the future. At a time when body image is extremely important, they may be faced with the possibility of mutilation and disfigurement. Dying adolescents are often isolated from their peers during a period when peers are the most essential social group. Adolescents nearing the end of life may be angry because they recognize that their loss is occurring at a time when the whole world is opening up to them.

Do not expect adolescents to handle feelings in the same way that adults do. They often avoid expressing anger against the family, seeking to control and direct these feelings elsewhere. Adolescents may become angry at changes in treatment procedures, lack of explanations, and threats to their independence. As death nears, the adolescent may permit comforting and support and may accept care from warm and loving family members, as long as it is not given in a condescending manner.

Nursing Management

For the Dying Child

Nursing care of the dying child and family focuses on providing family-centered support for their physical and psychosocial needs.

Nursing Assessment and Diagnosis

Assess the child's physiologic status and comfort level. Physiologic changes in the dying child may be directly related to the child's disease process or injury. Signs and symptoms of approaching death are provided in Table 13–2.

Assess the child's awareness of impending death. Examples of questions the child may ask include: "What will death be like? Will it hurt? What happens to me when I die? Will I be with [a deceased person whom the child was close to] again? Will my parents be all right? Will you remember me?" Assess the ability of the parents to talk with the child about dying.

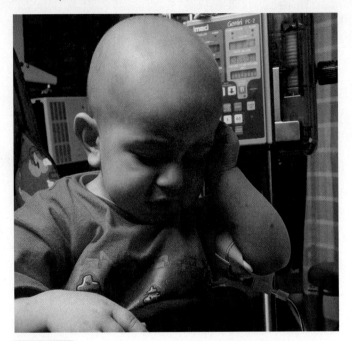

Figure 13–6 The toddler with a life-limiting condition recognizes that he feels sick and that routines are different. His anxiety may increase because of the concern and feelings of sadness exhibited by his parents.

TABLE 13–2 Clinical Manifestations of the Dying Child

SYSTEM	CLINICAL MANIFESTATIONS
Cardiovascular system (decreased cardiac output and peripheral circulation)	• The heart rate may initially increase as hypoxia develops; then the heart rate and blood pressure decrease. • A change in pulse pressure and a decrease in the volume of Korotkoff sounds indicate imminent death. • Diaphoresis, clammy cool skin, and changes in skin coloring (mottled to cyanotic). Mottling is a sign of imminent death.
Respiratory system (pulmonary congestion due to impaired cardiac function)	• Tachypnea, diminished breath sounds, and hypoxia. • Dyspnea; **air hunger**, the most severe form of dyspnea, may cause the child to look panicked, gasp for breath, and sit upright; it may not be relieved by oxygen. • Cheyne-Stokes breathing (periods of shallow breathing alternating with apnea) is a sign of imminent death. • As muscles relax, secretions accumulate in the oropharynx and bronchi causing noisy breathing as air passes through the secretions. • Moaning or grunting with breathing is common.
Neurologic system (neurologic dysfunction due to decreased cerebral perfusion, metabolic acidosis, and accumulated toxins from renal and liver failure)	• Hypoxemia. • Agitation or restlessness, withdrawal, increasing drowsiness, confusion. • May be unconscious during final hours. • May speak of visions (persons or objects) not visible to others. • Deterioration of hearing and vision acuity. Remember that hearing is one of the last senses to diminish before death.
Musculoskeletal system	• Extreme muscle weakness and fatigue. • May be unable to reposition self or toilet self. • Difficulty swallowing; may be unable to cough effectively and clear secretions.
Renal system (decreased renal function)	• Decreased urine production. • Sphincters relax and incontinence can occur.
Gastrointestinal system	• Decreased oral fluid intake and anorexia are common. • Sphincters relax and bowel incontinence can occur.

Assess the family for coping skills and need for social supports. Identify any cultural or spiritual traditions, rituals, and beliefs related to loss and grieving that may provide comfort to the family.

Examples of nursing diagnoses that apply to the dying child and family include the following (NANDA-I © 2014):

- *Fear (Child)* related to unanswered questions and concerns of abandonment
- *Anxiety, Death (Child),* related to own impending death
- *Grieving (Parents)* related to imminent death of child
- *Hopelessness (Parents)* related to failure of therapies to prolong life

Planning and Implementation

Nursing care for the dying child and the family includes providing comfort, assisting the child in a peaceful death, assisting the child and family with coping strategies, and facilitating grief.

PHYSIOLOGIC CARE

A major goal in care of the dying child is to promote comfort and keep the child pain free. Opioids may be prescribed to promote optimal pain relief. Oral, transdermal, or rectal analgesia is available for families who choose to withhold IV fluids. Complementary therapies for comfort and pain management can be used by the nurse and family members (see Chapter 15).

If dyspnea, or air hunger, occurs, position the child to maintain the airway and promote breathing. Open a window or use a circulating fan to ease the child's distress. An opioid may be prescribed for air hunger or tachypnea as its action dilates the pulmonary vessels, reduces oxygen consumption, and decreases pulmonary congestion.

Other physiologic care includes keeping the airway clear of secretions, bathing and keeping the skin dry and intact, changing the child's position frequently, and encouraging favorite foods and liquids as tolerated. Decrease excessive stimulation and reduce unnecessary activities. Involve the parents in physical care and encourage them to hold and comfort the child.

COMMUNICATING WITH THE CHILD ABOUT HIS OR HER IMPENDING DEATH

The dying child may be aware of impending death before being told, and parents may not understand this. When the child has no opportunity to talk about death, the child may feel isolated and distressed. The child may believe that initiating the conversation about an awareness of death and related fears will add to the family's emotional burden.

Some parents wish to protect the child from bad news and avoid talking to the child about the child's serious illness and potential death. Parents often do not know how to talk with their child about dying. Some parents feel emotionally unable to answer the child's questions about dying. They may fear that talking about the impending death will take away the child's hope. A professional who has special training in bereavement counseling can assist children and families with the discussion. When the family is ready to talk with the child about the child's death, suggest some developmentally appropriate words to use. Emphasize to the parents that the child may actually need to hear the word *dying* in order to understand. Strategies for talking with a dying child are described in Table 13–3. Families who have talked with their child about dying report they have rarely regretted having the discussion (Gaab, Owens, & MacLeod, 2013).

Provide the child with opportunities for fantasy play, drawing, and storytelling, without emphasizing or reinforcing death themes. Listen to what children tell you about themselves and their lives. **Death imagery**, references to death or death-related topics (going away, separation, funerals), may be a theme of their stories.

Some dying children want to leave a legacy so they will be remembered or to express their good-byes through photography, journals, poetry, writing letters, or music. Some children choose to make crafts or a memory box for others, or to give away special possessions.

When caring for adolescents, outbursts of frustration and anger are common, but these are not personally directed at the nurse. Provide activities to help adolescents channel their feelings. Continue providing support in spite of their behavior. This approach may encourage adolescents to accept comforting without losing face. Be available to listen when the adolescent wants to talk and express feelings and frustrations. Promote friendships with other adolescents who have similar interests or problems.

FAMILY SUPPORT

Parents need to be present when possible as the child is dying, a pivotal event in their parent–child relationship. Work closely with the family when the child's death is imminent; they will remember the experience and words spoken for the rest of their lives. Prepare the family for changes in the child's appearance and behavior. Providing the parents with a room to be alone with the child ensures privacy at this extremely personal time.

TABLE 13–3 Strategies for Communicating With Dying Children

- Be receptive when dying children initiate a conversation, or look for opportunities to talk with them, such as when their physical health or behavior is changing.
- Ask dying children what they know. Correct any misunderstood information with language appropriate for their age. Ask what they want to know. Be honest when answering questions, but do not provide more information than requested.
- Encourage dying children to talk about what worries them. Allow them to express their feelings and to be upset. Empathize with these children's feelings.
- Ask dying children what is most important to them with the time they have left.
- Offer opportunities for nonverbal expression of feelings, such as art, music, and writing. Ask what the art represents.
- Let dying children know they will not be abandoned and that any suffering they may have will be treated.
- Let dying children know they will always be loved and remembered.

Source: Data from Evan, E. E., & Cohen, H. J. (2011). Child relationships. In J. Wolfe, P. S. Hinds, & B. M. Sourkes (Eds.), *Textbook of interdisciplinary pediatric palliative care* (pp. 125–134). Philadelphia, PA: Elsevier Saunders; You, J. J., Fowler, R. A., & Heyland, D. K. (2014). Just ask: Discussing goals of care with patients in hospital with serious illness. *Canadian Medical Association Journal, 186*(6), 425–432; MacPherson, C. F. (2013). The final chapter. *Clinical Journal of Oncology Nursing, 16*(5), e190–e191.

Ask the family what is important to them in the final moments and hours of the child's life and what will be important to them in the grief process. Each culture has its own way of defining, addressing, and acknowledging death. Customs, ceremonies, religious laws, and beliefs are strongly connected with dying (see Table 13–4 for rituals regarding dying and after death). Accommodate desired spiritual or cultural practices when possible. Holding the child is a universal request and should be permitted, along with touching, stroking, kissing, and talking soothingly.

Many families find that saying good-bye as a group is helpful. Families need to cry together and to tell each other how much they will miss each other. Assure them that the vigil with the child prevents the child from feeling isolated or abandoned as death approaches. The dying child should never be left alone when dying is imminent.

TABLE 13–4 Spiritual Traditions Regarding Dying and After-Death Rites

RELIGIOUS GROUP	RITUALS YOU MIGHT OBSERVE
American Indians	• Beliefs and practices vary widely among tribes • Autopsy is generally acceptable
Buddhism	• Family presence is important • Last-rite chanting at bedside • Cremation is common
Catholicism	• Sacrament of the sick, baptism of newborn • Obligated to take ordinary but not extraordinary means to prolong life • Burial is common
Christian Science	• No medical help is sought to prolong life • No donation of body parts; disposal of body and parts decided by family
Hinduism	• Family presence with chanting, prayers, and singing • Final rites by a religious leader; a thread tied around neck or wrist signifies a blessing; do not remove • Autopsy if required by law; organ donation may be acceptable • Cremation is common.
Islam	• Deathbed should be turned to face Mecca, reading from the Qur'an stressing hope and acceptance • Body is washed 3 times, only by Muslim of the same gender • Autopsy only for medical or legal reasons; organ donation is acceptable • Burial as soon as possible
Jehovah's Witness	• Prayer and reading the Bible • Organ donation is forbidden • Autopsy acceptable for legal reasons • Burial determined by family preference
Judaism	• Autopsy if required by law and organ donation in some cases • Prefer natural death rather than technologic support • Body ritually washed, and a living person is always with the body after death • Burial occurs as soon as possible; all body parts buried together • Seven-day mourning period
Mormonism	• If death inevitable, promote a peaceful and dignified death; laying on of hands, anointing with oil • Organ donation is an individual choice • Burial in "temple clothes"
Protestantism	• Variable rituals, laying on of hands, anointing with oil, communion, final blessing • Organ donation, autopsy, and burial or cremation are individual decisions • Means to prolong life is individual decision
Seventh Day Adventist	• Prayer, anointing with oil • Prefer prolonging life • Organ donation and autopsy are individual decisions • Disposal of body and burial are individual decisions

Source: Adapted from Spector, R. E. (2013). *Cultural diversity in health and illness* (8th ed., pp. 151–152). Upper Saddle River, NJ: Prentice Hall Health; Purnell, L. D. (2014). *Guide to culturally competent health care* (3rd ed.). Philadelphia, PA: F. A. Davis; Wiener, L., McConnell, D. G., Latella, L., & Ludi, E. (2013). Cultural and religious considerations in pediatric palliative care. *Palliative and Supportive Care, 11*, 47–67.

Developing Cultural Competence Diverse Perspectives on Death

Consider cultural differences when working with families who are dealing with the death of a loved one, for example (Evans & Ume, 2012; Purnell, 2014; Weiner et al., 2013):

- African Americans often place great importance on the presence and involvement of their families in their care. They embrace religion and spirituality. They may be less likely to request medications for pain and other symptoms because of an expectation to suffer. They may seek more aggressive care.

- Some Asian families desire to protect the terminally ill from knowledge of their condition, so their final days will be peaceful. Decision making is often collectively decided by the family, and a spokesperson for the family is often the oldest male or head of household. Some families may believe that making plans for the child's death could cause the child's premature death or having a visit by the chaplain may signify an impending death.

- Hispanics generally believe the entire family makes important decisions. They see death as a natural part of life, and they do not want to be a burden for their families. Cultural customs related to grief and loss vary. Crying openly is seen as appropriate. Faith is very important in times of death. The anniversary of a loved one's death is celebrated every year.

TISSUE AND ORGAN DONATION

Healthcare professionals are obligated to ask families about making an anatomic gift. Become familiar with national guidelines for organ collection and donation so you will be better prepared to serve the family of the dying child and potential organ recipients. An organ procurement coordinator collaborates with the healthcare team to help explain the organ donation process to the family, and to assure family members that the organ donation process is totally separate from decisions regarding their child's care. Organ donation costs are paid by the organ procurement organization, but recipients pay transplantation costs.

NEED FOR AUTOPSY

When the exact cause of death is unclear, an autopsy may be suggested. An autopsy may be required by state law for an unnatural or unexpected death, such as suicide, homicide, child abuse, or sudden infant death syndrome. When parents have a choice, they may be hesitant to consent to autopsy because it further invades the child's body. Support the family during the decision-making process by explaining that the autopsy will likely reveal the cause of death or inevitability of death.

POSTMORTEM CARE AND FAMILY SUPPORT

Offer ongoing support after the child dies. Questions like the following may help begin the conversation: "I am sorry for your loss. How can I help?" "What are your traditions when an infant or child dies?" "Is there someone I can call for you?" Nurses should feel free to express their sorrow and grief for the child and family. Crying with families is recognized as an expression of caring and empathy.

Identify the family's wishes for postmortem care before performing any care. Ask before removing any jewelry or other item from the child because cultural and spiritual practices may specify that the article remain on the child after death. Follow the healthcare facility's guidelines for postmortem care. Position the child according to guidelines or cultural/religious practices, clean the room, and remove medical equipment.

After the child's death, allow the family to spend as much time as they need with the child's body. Never rush family members who are saying good-bye to the child. Save all of the child's personal items—especially in the case of an infant. A lock of hair, hand- or footprints, the infant's identification band, the child's weight and height, or a picture of the infant can be sources of comfort and remembrance for families. Ask for permission before cutting a lock of hair, as some cultural and religious groups prohibit it. Seal the last clothes or patient gown used by the child, or the infant's blanket, in a plastic bag to retain the child's scent. Use a special remembrance box or container for this purpose. If parents refuse to take the items, give them to another family member or retain them. Document the collection of the mementos and who received them in case parents ask for them at a later time.

Clinical Tip

When a sudden violence-related death of a child or adolescent occurs, steps to preserve forensic evidence are taken. Removal of medical equipment is not permitted. Follow facility guidelines for evidence collection (e.g., child's clothing, sheet used during resuscitation) and the chain of possession prior to giving evidence to law enforcement authorities. The child may be swaddled in a clean sheet for family member access. Depending on the injuries and circumstances, the family may not be permitted to have physical contact with the child's body (O'Malley et al., 2014).

When a newborn or young infant has died, wrap the baby in a blanket and offer the mother and other family members the opportunity to hold the baby. Parents may want to bathe and dress the infant. The family experiencing the death of a newborn may appreciate an offer to take pictures of the baby and family together, if picture taking is not prohibited by religious or cultural traditions. Some families may feel uncomfortable taking pictures and refuse the offer. The nurse should question the family about baptism or other ritual requests for the newborn, and facilitate arrangements for a religious or spiritual leader at the family's request. Ensure that the mother experiencing the death of a newborn receives information about lactation suppression or milk donation options if she has been breastfeeding.

A bereavement folder should be provided to parents with information that includes resources available to help with a memorial service or funeral and potential sibling responses. Include grief counseling resources and support groups and encourage the family to use these resources for the first year after the child's death. Inform parents that certain dates, such as the day of the week the child died, the child's birthday, or family holidays, will be difficult and may trigger intense sadness. Parents may benefit from keeping a journal of their thoughts and memories, or writing letters or poems to or about their child. Follow-up phone calls from healthcare providers are appreciated by families.

Evaluation

Expected outcomes of caring for the dying child and family may include the following:

- The child is pain free and comfortable, and the child's physiologic needs are met.
- The cultural and spiritual needs of the dying child and family are met.
- The dying child and family receive support during the dying process.
- The family receives continued support after the child's death.

Bereavement

Parents' Reactions

The death of one's child is likely the most traumatic event a parent will experience. Grief, an individual's feelings and behaviors in response to death or loss, is painful, individualized, and exhausting. Many factors influence the parents' grief responses, including their perception of whether the death could be prevented, the suddenness and other circumstances of the death, the nature of their attachment to the child, previous losses, spiritual or religious orientation, and culture.

Sudden Death of a Child

An estimated 25% of child and adolescent deaths each year are related to complex chronic conditions (Klein & Saroyan, 2011). The majority of child and adolescent deaths are sudden and unexpected, such as from sudden infant death syndrome, injury, illness, suicide, or violence. Parents need additional support to deal with the sudden and unexpected death of their child and with their surviving children.

Death of a Newborn or Young Infant

In 2013, in the United States, 29,138 infants died shortly after birth or during their first year of life (Centers for Disease Control, National Center for Health Statistics, 2015). The death of a newborn forces the parents to experience their child's entire life cycle in a short period of time, and they are faced with overwhelming grief at a time when they anticipated the experience of joy. Refer parents to a perinatal bereavement program or support group.

Grief and Bereavement

Although parents progress through distinct stages of grief, as described previously in this chapter, the timeline and nature of the grief process differ for each individual. The intense pain and shock initially felt by parents gradually give way to feelings of anger, guilt, depression, and loneliness. Very slowly, and with much support, energy returns and parents again begin to enjoy life experiences. Parents may experience friction due to differing intensities of grief and coping processes. Additional support may be needed to prevent a sense of loneliness and isolation.

Let parents know that caring for themselves physically and mentally is important, even though the period surrounding their child's death is difficult. Refer parents to local support groups for bereaved parents and siblings (e.g., Compassionate Friends, First Candle, and SHARE Pregnancy and Infant Loss Support), and provide books and articles for later use. Some facilities and most palliative care programs have formal follow-up programs for bereaved parents to encourage a healthy progression through the grieving process.

Siblings' Reactions

Siblings experiencing the death of a brother or sister grieve and require supportive and compassionate care. Siblings anticipating the addition of a new baby to the family will also feel the loss. The siblings may have received less attention from parents during the child's illness. Depending on their development, they may fear that they caused their brother's or sister's illness or injury, or worry that their bad thoughts caused the illness. Table 13–5 highlights children's understanding of death at different developmental stages, some of the possible behavioral responses, and nursing considerations for family education.

Clinical Tip

The following strategies can assist the nurse in working with parents whose child dies suddenly and who are not present during the resuscitation:

- Identify a spokesperson for the medical team to keep the family informed during resuscitation efforts. Call support resources (e.g., chaplain service, social worker, or interpreter).
- Create time for families to assimilate the child's worsening status by providing two to three updates during the resuscitation. Prepare them for what is to come.
- Ensure that the right family members are present for discussions after the death, or have a family support member for a single parent. Provide a private space with telephone access.
- Turn off your phone and beeper, sit close, and make eye contact. If the family arrived after resuscitation ended, ask them what they know about what happened. Prepare them by saying you are sorry to give them this bad news. Verify that the child (use the child's name) has died. Let the family know that everything possible was done to save the child, but the injuries or illness complications were too severe to survive.
- Allow the family time to absorb the information. Accept whatever emotions family members express. Let the family be first to talk. Answer any questions asked. Be prepared to repeat information.
- Offer to telephone family or friends.
- After the death, prepare the body for viewing in a private place, covering disfiguring wounds. Escort the family to the body and explain any tubes or lines that must remain in place. Allow them time to say goodbye.
- Convey information to the family about the cause of death, autopsy, funeral preparations, and the normal grief process. Provide contact information for the family in case of questions.
- Arrange for family follow-up to see how they are responding to the child's loss and to review autopsy findings.

Source: Data from Shoenberger, J. M., Yeghiazarian, S., Rios, C., & Henderson, S. O. (2013). Death notification in the emergency department: Survivors and physicians. *Western Journal of Emergency Medicine, 14*(2), 181–185; O'Malley, P. J., Barata, I., Snow, S., American Academy of Pediatrics Committee on Pediatric Emergency Medicine, American College of Emergency Physicians Pediatric Emergency Medicine Committee, & Emergency Nurses Association Pediatric Committee. (2014). Death of a child in the emergency department. *Pediatrics, 134*(1), e313–e330; Old, J. L. (2011). Communicating bad news to your patient. *Family Practice Management.* Retrieved from http://www.aafp.org/fpm/2011/1100/p31.html

TABLE 13–5 Children's Understanding of Death, Their Potential Behaviors, and Nursing Management

UNDERSTANDING OF DEATH	POTENTIAL BEHAVIORS	NURSING MANAGEMENT
Infant		
Cognitive stage: Sensorimotor Senses emotions of caregivers and altered routines Senses separation	Resists cuddling and eats less May have feeding problems Cries excessively, clingy Sleeps more than usual	Provide a sense of security by holding and hugging and a soothing voice by a caring person if the parent is too distraught. Try to return to usual routines.
Toddler		
Cognitive stage: Preoperational No understanding of true concept of death Aware someone is missing—separation anxiety Unable to distinguish death from temporary separation or abandonment	Regresses to younger stage of development Clingy; does not want to let parent out of sight Whiney, irritable, may show distress by biting, hitting, tears Problems eating and sleeping Sleep disturbances Fearfulness	Encourage parents to hold and cuddle the toddler to help reduce the fear of separation. Follow familiar routines. Be tolerant of regressive behaviors. Use distraction (toys, games, videos) when the child is fussy or clingy.
Preschooler		
Cognitive stage: Preoperational Believes death is temporary and the dead person will return Experiences magical thinking (believes own thoughts or actions potentially caused the death) Confuses death with being away or asleep Has beginning experience with death of animals and plants	Regression to earlier developmental stage, problems with bowel and bladder control, tantrums, may withdraw from activities, disobedience May fear going to sleep, has nightmares, afraid of the dark, separation anxiety Crying spells Seems morbidly fascinated with death Asks when deceased will return Asks many questions Complaints of abdominal pain	Provide honest and consistent responses to the child's questions; say the person is not coming back. Try to follow usual routines. Be tolerant of regressive behaviors; provide play activities. Keep memories alive with pictures and items that remind the child of the loved one. Participate in rituals, e.g., going to the cemetery, releasing helium balloons, and planting flowers.
School-Age Child		
Cognitive stage: Concrete operations Understands difference between temporary separation and death By 6 years, knows death is permanent. By 9–10 years, understanding of death is same as adult May have guilt or assume blame for the death May not realize that death can occur at any age	Crying, moody, may become more withdrawn and distant, may have angry outbursts or disruptive behaviors, may dwell on absence of loved one Decreased concentration for schoolwork, may refuse to go to school Psychosomatic complaints—stomachache or headache May try to comfort parents by taking over tasks May fear another loved person will die	Listen to the child and answer questions honestly. Return to usual routines and activities. Have the parent let the child know when parents will return and a how to contact them. Keep memories alive through activities such as art, music, creating a memory book, sewing a quilt, and planting a garden. Share Internet resources; suggest coping support groups. Encourage the family to seek faith-based support.
Adolescent		
Cognitive stage: Formal operations Intellectually capable of understanding death Recognizes all people and self will die Understands the association between illness and death Sense of invincibility conflicts with fear of death Able to recognize effect of death on others	May have severe depression, mood swings, withdrawal from friends, may feel angry or guilty Girls may seek comfort from friends Eating and sleeping problems May act-out or display risk-taking behaviors May assume responsibility for family well-being Uses abstract and philosophical reasoning to try to make sense of life	Be available and encourage open communication. Share your own grief and feelings with the adolescent. Keep memories alive with pictures and items that remind the teen of the loved one. Access counseling and support groups; share Internet resources. Encourage the child to seek support from the family's faith group.

Source: Data from Evan, E. E., & Cohen, H. J. (2011). Child relationships. In J. Wolfe, P. S. Hinds, & B. M. Sourkes, Textbook of interdisciplinary pediatric palliative care (pp. 125–134). Philadelphia, PA: Elsevier Saunders; You, J. J., Fowler, R. A., & Heyland, D. K. (2014). Just ask: Discussing goals of care with patients in hospital with serious illness. Canadian Medical Association Journal, 186(6), 425–432; MacPherson, C. F. (2013). The final chapter. Clinical Journal of Oncology Nursing, 16(5), e190–e191.

When possible, siblings should have the opportunity to visit when the child is dying so that they feel nothing was hidden from them. Memories about the death process are part of the grieving process (Lancaster, 2011). Nurses and other support personnel can assist the surviving children to adapt to their parents' distraction, grief, and increased protectiveness of them. The siblings need to hear that the parents' grief in no way diminishes the love felt for them.

When talking to the siblings of a child who has died, be honest and answer questions truthfully. Provide information about the child's death in a manner they can understand. Use developmentally appropriate terms, such as, "Adam's heart will never beat again," "He will never get cold or hungry," and "He will never come home again." Reassure siblings that they did not cause their brother or sister to die (unless they did contribute to the child's death) and that death was not a punishment for wrongdoing. Allow the siblings to ask questions and acknowledge the emotions they are feeling. Emphasize that it is okay for them to be sad, angry, frightened, or tearful. Use the same amount of energy and concern to acknowledge the sibling's and the adult's grief.

Encourage the parents, if appropriate, to allow siblings to participate in planning the child's memorial or funeral service. A funeral service director can be supportive to provide family time for the sibling to say good-bye. Attending the service assists the sibling to grieve, and being able to grieve as a family provides a sense of connectedness to parents and security at a vulnerable time. When siblings attend the funeral, they should be prepared for what to expect, such as an open casket and the behaviors of mourners. Suggest that parents designate a family member or close friend to monitor the siblings' needs while the parents attend to other matters. Keep the family together as much as possible.

As with parental bereavement, sibling bereavement is intense and a lifelong process. Sad feelings may return repeatedly as understanding about death increases. Be open and available when children wish to talk about a dead sibling to support their grieving. Encourage parents to make sure other caregivers and teachers know about the sibling's loss. Books for the family that might help children with grief include *Tell Me, Papa: Answers to Questions Children Ask About Death and Dying* by M. Johnson, J. Johnson, and A. C. Blake; *What Happens When Someone Dies: A Child's Guide to Death and Funerals* by M. Mundy and R. W. Alley; and *A Complete Book About Death for Kids* by E. Grollman and J. Johnson.

Staff Reactions to the Death of a Child

Caring for dying children is especially stressful and demanding for healthcare professionals. Some nurses cope by distancing themselves socially from the dying child and family to maintain composure and a professional demeanor. Nurses with young children may have more difficulty caring for the dying child. They tend to identify with the child, making it more difficult to recognize the dying child's anxiety and fears because of their own personal defenses against a sense of helplessness to alter the course of the child's disease.

When the child dies, the bond that was developed with the child and family is lost, and feelings of helplessness or powerlessness may be related to failed efforts to relieve suffering (Duvall, 2011). Nurses may feel extreme sadness and helplessness in association with a child patient's death and the grief observed among the child's family members. Nurses may alternate between dealing with their grief and suppressing it, which permits them to avoid becoming consumed by the loss.

Nurses who work with terminally ill children and their families need special preparation to care for children and families and to manage personal stress simultaneously. Mentoring by experienced hospice nurses, as well as additional educational experiences, may be helpful. Nurses must learn to cope effectively with grief and develop empathy, competence, and confidence in their ability to provide more humane and effective nursing care. Nurses should feel free to express their sorrow and grief for the child and family. Some nurses attend funeral and memorial services when invited by the patient's family.

Nurses working in emergency departments caring for children who die suddenly or in hospice settings and hospital units that care for terminally ill children need support systems to help balance the stresses of working with dying children. An important support system often gives an opportunity to discuss the experience with a supportive peer (Figure 13–7). Many facilities offer debriefing group sessions with mental healthcare professionals to discuss feelings and concerns, as well as resources to help nurses learn about self-care activities, relaxation techniques, and how to maintain a balance between their work and personal lives.

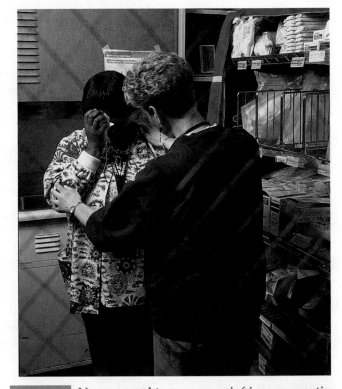

Figure 13–7 Nurses need to express grief in a supportive environment after a child's death. Sharing the sadness and grief or futility of resuscitation efforts with colleagues can often help nurses continue to provide supportive care to the next families who need compassionate care.

Chapter Highlights

- A life-threatening illness or injury places intense emotional and physical demands on the child and family due to the unfamiliar environment of the emergency department or intensive care unit, frightening or invasive procedures, and an uncertain outcome.

- Defense mechanisms displayed by children in stressful situations such as a life-threatening illness or injury include regression (return to an earlier behavior), denial, repression (involuntary forgetting), postponement, and bargaining.

- Nursing interventions to promote a child's psychologic health include permitting parents to be present, preparing children for procedures, using play to help the child manage anxiety, and allowing the child some choices to gain a sense of control.

- Parents typically progress through the stages of shock and disbelief, anger and guilt, deprivation and loss, anticipatory waiting, and readjustment or mourning when their child has a life-threatening illness or injury.

- A family-centered approach will help meet the needs of families, minimize stress, and enhance family coping. Appropriate nursing care includes providing information and building trust, promoting family involvement (including presence during invasive procedures and resuscitation if desired), encouraging parents to meet physical and emotional needs, facilitating effective communication, and maintaining family support systems.

- The nurse should ensure siblings receive information about their critically ill or injured brother or sister in preparation for a visit, and they should support the parents to provide regular messages to help them control feelings of jealousy, guilt, fear, and insecurity. Allowing the siblings to visit the child may help them cope.

- Palliative care is a service for persons with life-limiting conditions that provides therapies to reduce suffering, to improve the quality of remaining life, to facilitate decision making regarding end of life, and to coordinate care. Hospice is one category of palliative care.

- The families of dying children face many decision-making issues such as when to begin palliative and/or hospice care, advance care planning, the withholding or withdrawal of treatments, and DNR requests.

- One commonly accepted definition of death in the United States is brain death, or the irreversible cessation of all functions of the brain, including the cerebral cortex and brainstem.

- Children with life-threatening illnesses often learn about death and their own illness through exposure to other ill and dying children. Children recognize that their condition is worsening when receiving extra treatments, feeling ill, and noticing cues from their parents, even if they are not told they are dying.

- It is essential to work closely with the family when a child's death is imminent, helping to provide the support and services most important to them in the last moments or hours of their child's life.

- The nurse caring for the dying child and family offers physiologic and psychosocial support during end-of-life care.

- Bereavement support must be provided to the family, making sure that siblings are not overlooked. Allow siblings to participate in planning the memorial service. Encourage parents to allow siblings to express their emotions.

- Caring for a dying child is difficult, and nurses need special preparation to meet the needs of the child and family, and to manage their own responses when a child they cared for dies.

Clinical Reasoning in Action

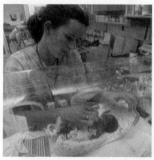

Kelly is a premature baby weighing 500 g (1.1 lb) when born at 24 weeks' gestation after her mother had premature rupture of membranes. Her parents, Shawn and Lori, are of Navajo Indian descent. Kelly's condition is extremely critical and she is on life support. You know that any amount of touch can be extremely stressful for newborns this small and in critical condition. The mother has been pumping and freezing breast milk for future use. The parents are encouraged to assist the nurse in any way they can, but they are not able to touch Kelly. Although the parents know how critical Kelly's condition is and have learned about the machines and medications being used, they are still confused and uncertain about the situation. They have not left the hospital at all. The grandparents have been helping care for Roseanne, Kelly's 7-year-old sister,

and she has visited her sister once. On her third day of life, Kelly gained weight and started to show an increase in activity. The parents thought this could be a positive sign, but the nurse explained that swelling caused the weight gain and the increased activity was from agitation as Kelly struggled to breathe. When the parents were at the bedside, Kelly started to become cyanotic and her oxygen saturation level dropped to the 60s. The healthcare team tried to save her but were unsuccessful. This was a devastating loss for the family and all the medical personnel involved.

1. What are some of the stressors Kelly experienced while in the hospital?

2. What are the stages of grief Kelly's family is likely to experience?

3. What are some strategies that can be used to help Roseanne deal with the loss of her sister?

4. What are some of the strategies for supporting Kelly's parents?

References

Akard, T. F., Gilmer, M. J., Friedman, D. L., Given, B., Hendricks-Ferguson, V. L., & Hinds, P. S. (2013). From qualitative work to intervention development in pediatric oncology palliative care research. *Journal of Pediatric Oncology Nursing, 30*(3), 153–160.

American Academy of Pediatrics (AAP) Section on Hospice and Palliative Medicine and Committee on Hospital Care. (2013). Pediatric palliative care and hospice care: Commitments, guidelines, and recommendations. *Pediatrics, 132*(5), 966–972.

Ames, K. E., Rennick, J. E., & Baillargeon, S. (2011). A qualitative interpretive study exploring parents'perception of the parental role in the paediatric intensive care unit. *Intensive and Critical Care Nursing, 27*, 143–150.

Blume, E. D., Balkin, E. M., Aiyagari, R., Ziniel, S., Beke, D. M., Thiagarajan, R., . . . Wolfe, J. (2014). Parental perspectives on suffering and quality of life at end-of-life in children with advanced heart disease: An exploratory study. *Pediatric Critical Care Medicine, 15*(4), 336–342.

Centers for Disease Control and Prevention, National Center for Health Statistics. (2015). *Underlying Cause of Death 1999–2013 on CDC WONDER Online Database.* Retrieved from http://wonder.cdc.gov/ucd-icd10.html

Crozier, F., & Hancock, L. E. (2012). Pediatric palliative care: Beyond the end of life. *Pediatric Nursing, 38*(4), 198–203, 227.

DeFrancis Sun, B., & Richards, J. T. (Eds.) (2011). *The grieving child: Helping children cope with grief when an infant dies* (2nd ed.). Retrieved from http://www.mchlibrary.info/suid-sids/documents/SIDRC/HelpingChildrenCope.pdf

Dow, B., Kenardy, J., Long, D., & Le Brocque, R. (2012). Children's post-traumatic stress and the role of memory following admission to intensive care: A review. *Clinical Psychologist, 16*, 1–14.

Duvall, A. (2011). Care of the caretaker: Managing the grief process of health care professionals. *Pediatric Annals, 40*(5), 266–273.

Emergency Nurses Association (ENA). (2012). *Emergency nursing resource: Family presence during invasive procedures and resuscitation in the emergency department.* Retrieved from http://www.ena.org/practice-research/research/CPG/Documents/FamilyPresenceCPG.pdf

Evan, E. E., & Cohen, H. J. (2011). Child relationships. In J. Wolfe, P. S. Hinds, & B. M. Sourkes (Eds.),

Textbook of interdisciplinary pediatric palliative care (pp. 125–134). Philadelphia, PA: Elsevier Saunders.

Evans, B., & Ume, E. (2012). Psychosocial, cultural, and spiritual health disparities in end-of-life and palliative care: Where we are and where we need to go. *Nursing Outlook, 60*, 370–375.

Gaab, E. M., Owens, G., & MacLeod, R. D. (2013). Primary caregivers' decisions around communicating about death with children involved in pediatric palliative care. *Journal of Hospice and Palliative Nursing, 15*(6), 322–329.

Jabre, P., Belpomme, V., Azoulay, E., Jacob, L., Bertrand, L., Lapostolle, F., . . . Adnet, F. (2013). Family presence during cardiopulmonary resuscitation. *The New England Journal of Medicine, 368*(11), 1008–1018.

Jee, R. A., Shepherd, J. R., Boyles, C. E., Marsh, M. J., Thomas, P. W., & Ross, O. C. (2012). Evaluation and comparison of parental needs, stressors, and coping strategies in a pediatric intensive care unit. *Pediatric Critical Care Medicine, 13*(3), e166–e172.

Keim-Malpass, J., Hart, T. G., & Miller, J. R. (2013). Coverage of palliative and hospice care for pediatric patients with a life-limiting illness: A policy brief. *Journal of Pediatric Health Care, 27*(6), 511–516.

Klein, S. M., & Saroyan, J. M. (2011). Treating a child with a life-threatening condition. *Pediatric Annals, 40*(5), 259–265.

Lancaster, J. (2011). Developmental stages, grief, and a child's response to death. *Pediatric Annals, 40*(5), 277–281.

Lyon, M. E., Jacobs, S., Briggs, B., Cheng, Y. I., & Wang, J. (2013). Family-centered advance care planning for teens with cancer. *JAMA Pediatrics, 167*(5), 460–467.

Machajewski, V., & Kronk, R. (2013). Childhood grief related to death of a sibling. *Journal of Nurse Practitioners, 9*(7), 443–448.

MacPherson, C. F. (2013). The final chapter. *Clinical Journal of Oncology Nursing, 16*(5), e190–e191.

Meert, K. L., Clark, J., & Eggly, S. (2013). Family-centered care in the pediatric intensive care unit. *Pediatric Clinics of North America, 60*(3), 761–772.

Nakagawa, T. A., Ashwal, S., Mathur, M., Mysore, M., & the Society of Critical Care Medicine, Section on Critical Care and Section on Neurology of the American Academy of Pediatrics, and the Child Neurology Society. (2011). Guidelines for the determination of brain death in infants and children: An update of the 1987 task force recommendations. *Pediatrics, 128*(3), e720–e740.

National Association of School Nurses. (2014). *Do not attempt resuscitation (DNAR)—The role of the school nurse.* Retrieved from http://www.nasn.org/Portals/0/positions/2014psdnr.pdf

Old, J. L. (2011). Communicating bad news to your patient. *Family Practice Management.* Retrieved from http://www.aafp.org/fpm/2011/1100/p31.html

O'Malley, P. J., Barata, I., Snow, S., American Academy of Pediatrics Committee on Pediatric Emergency Medicine, American College of Emergency Physicians Pediatric Emergency Medicine Committee, & Emergency Nurses Association Pediatric Committee. (2014). Death of a child in the emergency department. *Pediatrics, 134*(1), e313–e330.

Purnell, L. D. (2014). *Guide to culturally competent health care* (3rd ed.). Philadelphia, PA: F. A. Davis.

Randall, V., Cervenka, J., Arday, J., Hooper, T., & Hanson, J. (2011). Prevalence of life-threatening conditions in children. *American Journal of Hospice and Palliative Care, 28*, 310–315.

Rapoport, A., Shaheed, J., Newman, C., Rugg, M., & Steele, R. (2013). Parental perceptions of forgoing artificial nutrition and hydration during end of life care. *Pediatrics, 131*(5), 861–869.

Sanderson, A., Zurakowski, D., & Wolfe, J. (2013). Clinician perspectives regarding the do-not-resuscitate order. *JAMA Pediatrics, 167*(10), 954–958.

Shoenberger, J. M., Yeghiazarian, S., Rios, C., & Henderson, S. O. (2013). Death notification in the emergency department: Survivors and physicians. *Western Journal of Emergency Medicine, 14*(2), 181–185.

Spector, R. E. (2013). *Cultural diversity in health and illness* (8th ed., pp. 151–152). Upper Saddle River, NJ: Prentice Hall Health.

Stevenson, S., Achille, M., & Lugasi, T. (2013). Pediatric palliative care in Canada and the United States: A qualitative metasummary of the needs of patients and families. *Journal of Palliative Medicine, 16*(5), 566–577.

Trotzuk, C., & Gray, B. (2012). Parents' dilemma: Decisions concerning end-of-life care for their child. *Journal of Pediatric Health Care, 26*(1), 57–61.

Wiener, L., McConnell, D. G., Latella, L., & Ludi, E. (2013). Cultural and religious considerations in pediatric palliative care. *Palliative and Supportive Care, 11*, 47–67.

You, J. J., Fowler, R. A., & Heyland, D. K. (2014). Just ask: Discussing goals of care with patients in hospital with serious illness. *Canadian Medical Association Journal, 186*(6), 425–432.

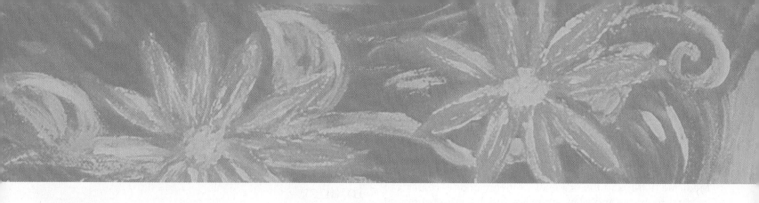

Chapter 14
Infant, Child, and Adolescent Nutrition

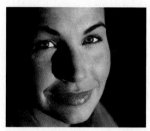

It is exciting to see Joey progressing into the school setting. Being with children his age will really help him develop in many ways. We're just worried because he needs to get only foods he can chew and swallow so he does not choke. He also needs his tube feedings during school to be sure he gets enough energy to do well.

—Mother of Joey, 11 years old

Ryan McVay/Getty Images

Learning Outcomes

14.1 Discuss major nutritional concepts pertaining to the growth and development of children.

14.2 Describe and plan nursing interventions to meet nutritional needs for all age groups from infancy through adolescence.

14.3 Integrate methods of nutritional assessment into nursing care of infants, children, and adolescents.

14.4 Identify and explain common nutritional problems of children.

14.5 Develop nursing interventions for children with nutritional disorders.

Adequate nutrition is an essential component of growth and development. The child's nutritional status begins before birth and is related to the mother's nutritional state. All children must be assessed for nutritional status, followed by teaching or other interventions to enhance health. Nurses are instrumental in giving parents information about normal nutritional needs of infants, children, and adolescents. Common techniques to assess nutrition, such as measuring growth and monitoring hematocrit, provide needed information about whether intake of nutrients is adequate.

All children and their parents can benefit from information about nutritional needs, but some children have additional concerns that must be considered. The nurse recognizes the special requirements of children with conditions such as feeding disorders, food allergies, cystic fibrosis, cerebral palsy, or diabetes. Nutrition monitoring is provided throughout childhood so that dietary counseling can be integrated with other teaching to promote development. How can the nurse bridge the various settings in which children's nutritional needs are met? These might include the home, childcare settings, schools,

and hospitals. How can the nurse help the family prepare for meeting the nutritional needs of a child who has special needs during car or plane travel?

Some children have unique nutritional needs due to their social environments. Parents may not be knowledgeable about the nutritional requirements of children. Perhaps the family is vegetarian and needs extra help to ensure intake of essential nutrients. If finances are limited, the family may need resources such as food stamps, food banks, or budget planning. The nurse considers the high rate of childhood obesity and common nutritional deficits when applying concepts of health promotion with families. Whatever the nurse's setting, knowledge of nutrition must be integrated within nursing care.

General Nutrition Concepts

Nutrition refers to taking in food and assimilating it metabolically for use by the body. It is an essential component of life and therefore an important body of knowledge to consider in discussions of child growth and development. The body

281

requires a wide array of nutrients. **Macronutrients**, or the major building blocks of the body, are carbohydrates, protein, and fat. Vitamins and minerals are **micronutrients**, or substances needed in small quantities for healthy body functioning. The need for nutrients is dependent on activity level, state of health, and the presence of disease or other stress-related and age-related requirements.

The **Dietary Reference Intakes (DRIs)** are a set of values established by the Food and Nutrition Board of the Institute of Medicine (IOM) and the National Academy of Science that can be used to assess and plan intake for individuals of different ages (Institute of Medicine, 2011). They commonly include the Estimated Average Requirement, or EAR (intake needed to meet requirements of 50% of the population); Recommended Dietary Allowance, or RDA (intake needed to meet requirements of 97% to 98% of the population); Adequate Intake, or AI (used when data to support EAR are not available); and Upper Intake, or UI (maximum level unlikely to pose health risk). Although the DRI approach is used in the United States, other countries have developed their own approaches to dietary standards. For example, Canada uses Adequate Intake and Reference Nutrient Intake, while the United Kingdom uses Recommended Daily Nutrient Intakes. The aims of these standards are to provide a method to evaluate individual and population diets and to plan nutrition programs and education. DRIs are generally specific to males and females in several age categories. See Appendix C for a list of DRIs for children and adolescents.

Although the DRIs provide useful information when evaluating diets, their use can be time consuming. What "quick check" can provide feedback about the daily diets of children? The nurse should be familiar with the U.S. MyPlate food guide and hang posters that illustrate its healthy choices in schools, clinics, and hospitals. It is a fast way to examine children's intakes for 1 day and evaluate whether they meet most requirements. Instead of calculating amounts of nutrients ingested, the MyPlate program focuses on categories of foods, which readily reflects the actual intake. The numbers of servings from various categories stay constant throughout childhood, while the serving sizes increase as the child gets older. See Figure 14–1 for MyPlate, and consult the U.S. Department of Agriculture (USDA) website for ethnic/cultural food guides for vegetarians and those from various ethnic groups, such as Hispanic and Native American.

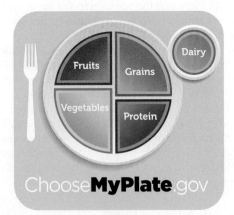

Figure 14–1 The U.S. MyPlate food guide is used to provide teaching about amounts of foods recommended for daily intake.

SOURCE: From U.S. Department of Agriculture and U.S. Department of Health and Human Services. (2011). Retrieved from http://www.choosemyplate.gov

Nutritional Needs

Nutritional needs evolve during all of infancy and childhood. They support growth and development and influence the progression of the child along the developmental path. Nutritional intake helps maintain the health of the child and fosters a state of maximal potential or health promotion. Specific needs during each developmental stage are discussed in this section.

Infancy

FLUID AND MACRONUTRIENTS

Fluid requirements during the neonatal period are high (140 to 160 mL/kg/day) because of the newborn's decreased ability to concentrate urine and increased overall metabolic rate. Although the infant's total body water content is high (75% to 80%) compared with that of an adult (60%), the infant has an increased surface area to mass ratio and decreased renal absorptive capacity that makes the infant more susceptible to dehydration from insufficient fluid intake or increased fluid loss caused by diarrhea, vomiting, or another source of fluid loss. Parents and caretakers should be aware of the signs of dehydration. See Chapter 18 for further information about fluid needs in infancy.

The basal metabolic rate (BMR) refers to the energy needed for thermoregulation, cardiorespiratory function, cellular activity, and growth. A newborn requires 100 to 115 kcal/kg/day at age 1 month. In breast milk, the primary carbohydrate is lactose. In addition to providing energy, lactose also functions to enhance the absorption of calcium, magnesium, and zinc. Human milk also contains other carbohydrates such as glucosamines and nitrogen-containing oligosaccharides. Glucosamines are one of the building blocks for connective tissues. Oligosaccharides promote the growth of *Lactobacillus bifidus*, which promotes an intestinal acidic environment that is hostile to harmful bacteria, making it difficult for them to thrive (Lawrence & Lawrence, 2011).

Infants receive approximately 50% of their calories from fat. Fats also help the body absorb the fat-soluble vitamins A, D, E, and K. Fats are a precursor of prostaglandins and other hormones. Fatty acids are a key component to brain development. Their derivatives, docosahexaenoic acid (DHA) and arachidonic acid (ARA), are long-chain polyunsaturated fatty acids (LCPUFAs) needed for myelination of the spinal cord and other nerves, and for development of visual acuity and cognitive and behavioral functions (Cloherty, Eichenwald, & Stark, 2012).

Approximately 98% of human milk fat is in the form of triglycerides, and a small amount is from cholesterol. Cholesterol levels in breast milk may also stimulate the production of enzymes that lead to more efficient metabolism of cholesterol, thereby reducing its harmful long-term effects on the cardiovascular system.

Fat content is the most variable component in breast milk, ranging from 30 to 50 g/L. It is influenced by maternal parity, duration of pregnancy, the stage of lactation, diurnal regulation, and changes in fat content even during a single feeding. Multiparous mothers produce milk with a lower content of fatty acids than primiparous women. Mothers of preterm infants have a greater concentration of LCPUFAs in their milk compared with mothers of term infants. By receiving this preterm breast milk, preterm infants receive the increased concentrations of DHA and ARA intended for their growth (Lawrence & Lawrence, 2011).

Phospholipids and cholesterol levels are higher in colostrum compared with mature milk, although overall fat content is higher in mature breast milk compared with colostrum. Fat content is generally higher in the evening and lower in the early morning. Within a single feeding session, an infant initially receives the low-fat foremilk before receiving the higher calorie, high-fat hindmilk. Finally, the fat content of breast milk is also affected by maternal diet and maternal fat stores. Mothers on low-fat diets have increased production of medium-chain fatty acids (C6–C10), and mothers with high levels of body fat produce breast milk with a higher fat content (Lawrence & Lawrence, 2011).

The fats in milk-based formulas are modified in an attempt to parallel the fat profile of breast milk by removing the butterfat from cow's milk and adding vegetable oils. The different blends of fats all provide a fatty acid profile that is similar to breast milk in terms of amount of saturated, monounsaturated, and polyunsaturated fats present. Since 2002, infant formulas have been supplemented with DHA and ARA. However, breast milk also contains 167 other fatty acids of uncertain function that are absent from formula (Cloherty et al., 2012).

Proteins are the building blocks for muscle and organ structure. They are key to the body's metabolic processes including energy metabolism, cell signaling, growth, and immune function. Milk proteins are often grouped into casein and whey proteins. Whey protein is the predominant dietary protein in human milk. During digestion this type of protein creates soft curds that are easily and quickly broken down. Because of this, breastfeeding babies digest their meals in 90 minutes and need to feed often, receiving about 8 to 12 feedings per day. Casein is the major phosphoprotein found in milk. Cow's milk contains a high amount of casein (a low ratio of whey to casein—approximately 20:80) compared with mature human milk (60:40 whey:casein). Because of its tendency to form curds, milk with high amounts of casein is less easily digested. Cow's milk–based formulas are usually modified to get closer to the whey:casein ratio of human milk.

MICRONUTRIENTS

The fat-soluble vitamins (vitamins A, D, E, and K) are found in both cow's milk–based formula and breast milk. After absorption via the lymphatic system, vitamins enter the blood and are transported to the various tissues. Excessive amounts of fat-soluble vitamins may result in toxicity, and there is general agreement that no routine fat-soluble vitamin supplementation is needed with the exception of vitamin D. See *Families Want to Know: Supplements for Breastfed Babies* for recommendations regarding vitamin D and other nutrients.

The vitamin B complex and vitamin C are water-soluble vitamins that pass readily from serum to breast milk. However, mothers who follow a strict vegetarian or macrobiotic diet may have insufficient vitamin B_{12} in their milk. In that case, the exclusively breastfed infant should receive vitamin B_{12} supplementation. Formula is fortified with adequate amounts of the water-soluble vitamins to meet the DRIs. Unlike fat-soluble vitamins, any

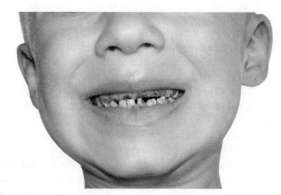

Figure 14–2 **Early childhood caries. This child has had major tooth decay related to sleeping as an infant and toddler while sucking bottles of juice and milk.**

SOURCE: Everst/Alamy.

excess water-soluble vitamins ingested are simply excreted and the threat of toxicity is low (Lawrence & Lawrence, 2011).

Both human milk and infant formulas contain several major and trace minerals to satisfy the needs of the growing infant. The mineral content of breast milk does not appear to be influenced by maternal diet.

DENTAL HEALTH

Early childhood caries, the presence of one or more decayed, lost, or filled tooth surfaces in a primary tooth from birth to 6 years of age, can occur when a young child is allowed to breastfeed or drink from a bottle for long periods, especially when sleeping (AAP Committee on Nutrition, 2013; Colak, Dulgergil, Dalli, et al., 2013) (Figure 14–2). The milk, juice, or other fluid pools around the upper anterior teeth, salivary flow decreases, and acid buffering is decreased, resulting in tooth decay. Nurses should teach parents to avoid putting the child to bed with a bottle and encourage pacifier use or a bottle of water instead. The child should not walk around with a bottle during the day. Mothers who breastfeed should also be cautioned to limit feeding to specific times rather than letting the infant breastfeed every few minutes (sometimes done when infant and mother co-sleep) so that milk will not pool in the mouth during sleep. When sleepy, the infant does not swallow well and the milk is in constant contact with the teeth where milk sugars can decay erupting teeth.

Parents can be taught beginning dental care for the infant, which includes wiping the teeth off daily once they erupt with a piece of moist gauze or a small infant toothbrush. Some pediatric dentists like to see the child for a first dental visit at about 1 year of age; others wait until the child is older. The nurse should encourage the parents to select and establish contact with a dental provider when the child is nearing the end of infancy.

Families Want to Know
Supplements for Breastfed Babies

1. Each baby receives a vitamin K injection after birth to promote adequate blood clotting. After that, no further vitamin K is needed since children manufacture this vitamin in the gut once they begin eating.

2. Vitamin D is recommended at a minimum of 400 International Units/day for all infants (American Academy of Pediatrics [AAP] Section on Breastfeeding, 2012).

3. Iron is not needed unless the infant is not eating food containing iron by 4 to 6 months of age. The baby may need an iron source earlier if the mother was anemic during pregnancy or while breastfeeding.

4. Fluoride 0.25 mg is given after 6 months of age if water is not fluoridated to a level of 0.6 part per million (ppm), or if the baby is not drinking any water (American Association of Pediatric Dentistry, 2014).

WEANING

Weaning is the term used when infants stop breastfeeding or bottlefeeding and obtain most liquids by cup. At about age 8 to 9 months, a cup should be offered to the infant with assistance being provided so that learning about drinking from a cup can begin. By about 1 year of age, infants are usually able to drink most liquids from a cup with a lid, so bottles can be slowly withdrawn and replaced by cups.

The decision to wean the baby from the breast may be made for a variety of reasons, including family or cultural pressures, changes in the home situation, pressure from the woman's partner, or a personal opinion about when weaning should occur. Some infants wean themselves spontaneously despite the wishes of the mother. For the woman who is comfortable with breastfeeding and well informed about the process, the appropriate time to wean her infant will become evident if she is sensitive to the child's cues, such as increased interest in other foods and decreased frequency of feeding (Centers for Disease Control and Prevention [CDC], 2011a). The infant who is weaned before age 12 months should be given iron-fortified infant formula rather than cow's milk.

Healthy People 2020

(MICH-21) Increase the proportion of infants who are breastfed

- Ever: target 81.9%
- At 6 months: target 60.6%
- Exclusively through 3 months: target 46.2%
- Exclusively through 6 months: target 25.5%

If weaning is timed to respond to the child's cues, and if the mother is comfortable with the timing, it can be accomplished with less difficulty than if the process begins before mother and child are ready emotionally. Nevertheless, weaning is a time of emotional separation for mother and baby; it may be difficult for them to give up the closeness of their nursing sessions. The nurse who understands this possibility can help the mother see that her infant is growing up and plan other comforting, consoling, and play activities to replace breastfeeding. A gradual approach is the easiest and most comforting way to wean the child from breastfeeding.

During weaning, the mother should substitute one cup feeding or bottlefeeding for one breastfeeding session over a few days to a week so that her breasts gradually produce less milk. Eliminating the breastfeedings associated with meals first facilitates the mother's ability to wean the infant because satiation with food lessens the desire for milk. Over a period of several weeks she can substitute more cup feedings or bottlefeedings for breastfeedings. The slow method of weaning prevents breast engorgement, allows infants to alter their eating methods at their own rates, and provides time for psychologic adjustment.

INTRODUCTION OF COMPLEMENTARY FOODS

When should other foods be added to the infant's diet? Although some parents add other foods when the infant is only days or weeks old, and such practices are often culturally derived, it is best to take cues from the infant's developmental milestones. The American Academy of Pediatrics recommends introducing complementary foods at about age 6 months (AAP, 2014a). At this age, the extrusion reflex (or tongue thrust) decreases and the infant can sit well with support. The infant is also developing the ability to appreciate texture and swallow nonliquid foods

TABLE 14–1 Introduction of Solid Foods in Infancy

RECOMMENDATION	RATIONALE
Introduce rice or other single-grain baby cereal at about age 6 months.	Single grains are easy to digest and have low allergenic potential, and baby preparations contain iron.
Introduce fruits or vegetables at 6–8 months of age. Some health-care providers recommend vegetable introduction before fruits.	Fruits and vegetables provide needed vitamins. Vegetables are not as sweet as fruits; introducing them first may enhance acceptability to the infant.
Introduce meats at age 8–10 months.	Meats are harder to digest, have high protein load, and should not be fed until close to 1 year of age.
Use single-food prepared baby foods rather than combination meals.	Combination meals usually contain more sugar, salt, and fillers.
Introduce one new food at a time, waiting at least 3–4 days to introduce another. Delay feeding eggs, strawberries, wheat, corn, and fish until close to 2–3 years of age. Consult a pediatrician or an immunologist about the best timing to introduce peanut and other nut products.	If a food allergy or intolerance develops, it will be easy to identify. The foods listed are those most commonly associated with food allergies.
Avoid carrots, beets, squash, beans, and spinach (especially if prepared at home) before 6 months of age. Have well water evaluated for nitrates (the recommended level is less than 10 mg/L).	Nitrates in these foods and in water near agricultural runoff can be converted to nitrite by young infants, causing methemoglobinemia. Commercial baby foods are adjusted for nitrates, so levels are lower than in foods prepared in the home.
Infants can be fed mashed portions of table foods such as peas, corn, rice, and potatoes.	This is a less expensive alternative to jars of commercially prepared baby food; it allows parents of various cultural groups to feed ethnic foods to infants.
Avoid adding sugar, salt, and spices when preparing baby foods at home.	Infants need not become accustomed to these flavors; they may get too much sodium from salt or develop gastric distress from some spices.
Avoid honey until at least 1 year of age.	Infants cannot detoxify *Clostridium botulinum* spores sometimes present in honey and can develop botulism.

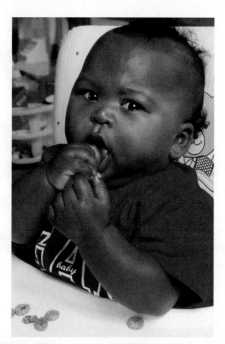

Figure 14-3 **Introducing finger foods. The baby who has developed the ability to grasp with thumb and forefinger should receive some foods that can be held in the hand.**

and can indicate desire for food or turn away when full. At 6 to 12 months, complementary foods are offered in addition to the intake of breast milk or formula rather than replacing that essential nutrient (AAP, 2014a) (see Table 14–1).

The first complementary food added to the infant's diet is often rice or other single-grain cereal. The advantages of introducing cereal first is that it provides iron at an age when the infant's prenatal iron stores begin to decrease, it seldom causes allergy, and it is easy to digest. A tablespoon or two is fed to the infant once or twice daily just before formula or breastfeeding. The infant may appear to spit out food at first because of normal back-and-forth tongue movement. Parents should not interpret this early feeding behavior as indicating dislike for the food. With a little practice the infant becomes adept at spoon feeding.

Once the infant eats 1/4 cup of food twice daily, usually at 6 to 8 months of age, vegetables or fruits can be introduced, at a rate of one new food every several days (Table 14–1). By 8 to 10 months of age, most fruits and vegetables have been introduced and strained meats or other protein (e.g., tofu, cheese, mashed cooked beans) can be added to the infant's diet. Finger foods are introduced during the second half of the first year as the infant's palmar and then finger grasp develops and as teeth begin to erupt (Figure 14–3). Infants enjoy toast, O-shaped cereal, finely sliced meats, cheese, yogurt, tofu, and small pieces of cooked, softened vegetables. Certain foods are associated with choking and should be avoided.

SAFETY ALERT!

Advise parents to use caution when providing finger foods to the infant. Hard foods and some soft and malleable ones slip easily into the throat and may cause choking. Avoid hot dogs, hard vegetables, candy, and chunks of peanut butter. Infants and other young children should always be supervised while eating. Be sure parents are familiar with techniques for airway obstruction removal and have emergency numbers clearly listed on their phones.

TABLE 14–2 Infant Nutritional Patterns

AGE	PATTERN
Birth–1 month	• Eats every 2–3 h, breast or bottle • 2–3 oz (60–90 mL) per feeding
2–4 months	• Has coordinated suck–swallow • Eats every 3–4 h • 3–4 oz (90–120 mL) per feeding
4–6 months	• Begins baby food, usually rice cereal, 2–3 T, twice daily • Consumes breast milk or formula 4 or more times daily • 4–5 oz (100–150 mL) per feeding
6–8 months	• Eats baby food such as rice cereal, fruits, and vegetables, 2–5 T, 3 times daily • Consumes breast milk or formula 4 times daily • 6–8 oz (160–225 mL) per feeding
8–10 months	• Enjoys soft finger foods 3 times daily • Consumes breast milk or formula 4 times daily • 6 oz (160 mL) per feeding • Uses cup with lid
10–12 months	• Eats most soft table foods with family 3 times daily • Uses cup with or without lid • Attempts to feed self with spoon though spills often • Consumes breast milk or formula 4 times daily • 6–8 oz (160–225 mL) per feeding

Certain foods are more commonly associated with development of food allergies, and avoiding them in infancy may decrease allergy incidence. Typically, recommendations for infants at risk due to family history of allergy are to delay feeding of cow's milk until age 1 year, eggs until age 2 years, and peanuts, nuts, fish, and shellfish until age 3 years (AAP, 2014a). However, a recent study found that children at risk of peanut allergy due to manifestation of food allergy in infancy or a family history of allergy have a lowered risk of having peanut allergy at age 5 years if they consume peanuts frequently within the first year of life (Du Toit et al., 2015). When infants have allergies to some foods or have a family history of allergy, refer them for current management to a pediatrician and/or an immunologist.

As food and juice intake increase, formula-feedings or breastfeedings decrease in amount and frequency (Table 14–2). If breastfeeding is not chosen, or if supplemental feedings are provided, only iron-fortified infant formula should be used during the first year of life. Cow's milk (including evaporated milk) can lead to bleeding and anemia (see sections on iron and anemia in this chapter), can interfere with absorption of some nutrients, and has a high solute load, which immature kidneys can have difficulty excreting. Iron-fortified formula should always be used when the infant under 12 months old drinks formula. When breastfed babies are not eating foods with iron by age 6 months, supplemental iron may need to be added. Careful dietary assessment and discussion of intake by the nurse at health visits helps the practitioner decide if supplemental iron is needed.

Parents who want to make baby foods at home can be encouraged and instructed to do so. Some commercially prepared foods have unnecessary additives such as salt, sugar, and food starch, and they may be costly for some families. Parents can easily blend fruits and vegetables the family is eating without adding salt, sugar, or seasoning. Prepared foods should be used promptly and stored in the refrigerator between feedings. Foods can also be placed into ice cube trays and frozen; a cube or two can be defrosted at mealtime. Nurses should caution parents to avoid certain home-prepared vegetables and not to use honey in foods for infants as it can lead to infant botulism because infants cannot detoxify the *Clostridium botulinum* spores sometimes present in honey (see Table 14–1). If foods or fluids are microwaved, they should be shaken, stirred, and checked for temperature so that hot areas in the food do not burn the infant.

Toddlerhood

Why do parents of toddlers frequently become concerned about the small amount of food their children eat? Why do toddlers seem to survive and even thrive with minimal food intake? The toddler often displays the phenomenon of **physiologic anorexia**, which occurs when the extremely high metabolic demands of infancy slow to keep pace with the more moderate growth rate of toddlerhood. Although it can appear that the toddler eats nothing at times, intake over days or a week is generally sufficient and balanced enough to meet the body's demands for nutrients and energy.

Parents often need knowledge about the types of foods that constitute a healthy diet. The nurse can offer fresh food alternatives with lower sodium content to replace hot dogs, microwave meals, or fast foods by providing information about easy preparation of sliced meats, cheese, tofu, fruits, and vegetables. Healthy snacks for young children include yogurt, cheese, milk, slices of bread with peanut butter, thinly sliced fruits, and soft vegetables.

Healthy People 2020

(NWS-19) Reduce consumption of sodium in the population aged 2 years and older

---

Parents should be advised to offer a variety of nutritious foods several times daily (three meals and two snacks) and let the toddler make choices from the foods offered. They should offer foods only at mealtimes and have the child sit in a high chair or on a special seat at the table to eat (Figure 14–4). Small portions are most appealing to the toddler. A general guideline for food quantity at a meal is one tablespoon of each food per year of age.

The toddler should drink 16 to 24 oz (1/2 to 3/4 L) of milk daily; whole milk is recommended from age 1 to 2 years, and after 2 years of age 2% is appropriate. Parents should be cautioned against giving the toddler more than a quart (1 L) of milk daily since this interferes with the desire to eat other foods, leading to dietary deficiencies. Recall that the child should not be put to bed with a bottle or allowed to carry a bottle of milk or juice around during the day on account of the risk of early childhood caries (see earlier discussion). In addition, parents should be advised to use only 100% fruit juice and to limit consumption of this juice to 4 to 6 oz daily for children ages 1 to 6 years to decrease the likelihood of becoming overweight, developing dental caries, or experiencing abdominal discomfort (AAP, 2011). Unpasteurized juice should never be used since it may contain pathogens particularly harmful to young children. Drinking water and eating whole fruits, which provide fiber, are healthier alternatives. Avoid more than one meal weekly from a fast-food restaurant because such meals generally are high in fat and sugar and low in fiber.

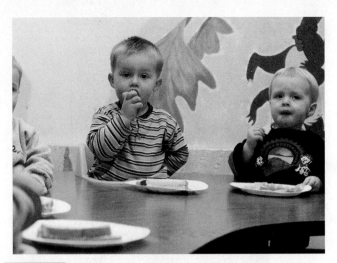

Figure 14–4 **Fostering healthy eating habits. Toddlers should sit at a table or in a high chair to eat to minimize the chance of choking and to foster positive eating patterns.**

Growth and Development

Toddlers generally eat three meals and two to three snacks daily. Toddlers can drink 2% milk or "follow-up" formula, starting at 2 years of age. Follow-up formula contains less fat than infant formula, and some parents prefer its convenience, although it is not necessary; 2% milk is appropriate to use at that age. Cups are recommended, and bottle use should be discontinued. Drinks should be consumed at mealtimes and for snacks while sitting at a table; carrying cups during the day while playing or at other activities is not recommended. The child is learning to use utensils but may prefer fingers, and still needs small serving sizes.

Learning how to eat with others is an important task of toddlerhood. The toddler displays characteristic autonomy or independence during mealtime. Advise parents to provide opportunities for self-feeding of food with fingers and utensils and to allow some simple choices, such as type of liquid or cup to use. Young children should eat at a table with others, not be allowed to run and play while eating, and eat at specified meal and snack times. Toddlers should be taught to brush teeth after each meal, and care providers should offer assistance and supervision. A dental visit should occur during toddlerhood.

Because social skills are developing, the hospitalized toddler may eat better if allowed to have meals with parents or other hospitalized children. See Chapter 11 for further suggestions about management of nutrition in hospitalized children.

Preschool

The diet of the preschooler is similar to that of the toddler, but mealtime is now a more social event. Preschoolers like the company of others while they eat, and they enjoy helping with food preparation and table setting (Figure 14–5). Involving them in these tasks can provide a forum for teaching about nutritious foods and principles of preparation, such as the need for refrigeration, safety around stoves, and cleanliness. Visits to fast-food restaurants should be limited to about once weekly, and parents can use the opportunity to assist the child in making wise choices of nutritionally adequate foods in that setting.

Although the rate of growth is slow and steady during the preschool years, the child may have periods of **food jags**

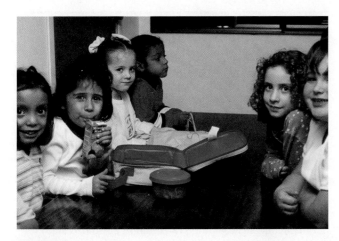 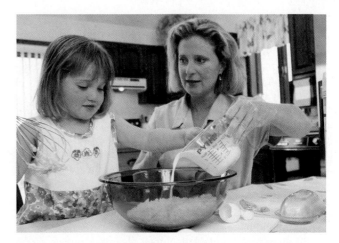

Figure 14–5 **Preschoolers learn food habits by eating with others. Engaging them in food preparation enhances knowledge of food and promotes intake at meals.**

(eating only a few foods for several days or weeks) and greater or lesser intake. Parents should be advised to assess food intake over a 1- or 2-week period rather than at each meal to obtain a more accurate impression of total intake. Food jags can be handled by providing the desired food along with other foods to foster choice. The child who chooses not to eat at snack time or mealtime should not be given other foods in between. The child will become hungry and get accustomed to eating when food is provided. Three meals and two or three snacks daily are the norm. Fruit juice should be limited to 8 to 12 oz daily, and begin teaching the "5-a-day" program that supports having five servings of fruits/vegetables each day.

The preschool period is a good time to continue encouraging good dental habits. Children can begin to brush their own teeth with parental supervision and help to reach all tooth surfaces. Fluoride supplements should be used when the water supply is not fluoridated (fluoride concentration below 0.7 mg/L) (U.S. Department of Health and Human Services [USDHHS], 2015). If the child has not yet visited a dentist, the first dental visit should be scheduled so the child can become accustomed to the routine of dental care.

School Age

The school-age years are a period of gradual growth when energy requirements remain at a steady level, although at some point during these years most children experience a preadolescent growth spurt. Girls may begin a growth spurt by 10 or 11 years, and boys a year or so later. Nutritional needs increase dramatically with this spurt, with large numbers of calories and increased amounts of other nutrients being required (see Appendix C for Dietary Reference Intakes).

School-age children are increasingly responsible for preparing snacks, lunches, and even some other meals. These years are a good time to teach children how to choose nutritious foods and plan a well-balanced meal. Because school-age children operate at the concrete level of cognitive thought, nutrition teaching is best presented by using pictures, samples of foods, videos, handouts, and hands-on experience.

Generally, school-age children prefer the types of food eaten at home and may be resistant to new food items. A hospitalized child may refuse to eat, slowing the recuperative process. Nurses should encourage family members to bring favorite foods from home that meet nutritional requirements. This can be especially helpful when the hospital serves food only from the dominant

cultural group. A child accustomed to a diet of rice, tofu, and vegetables may not enjoy a hospital meal of hamburger and fries. By school-age, food has become strongly associated with social interaction, so it is beneficial to have children eat together or to invite family members to take the child off the unit to eat or to bring in food from home and eat with the child. Many hospitals allow children to plan a pizza night or sponsor other events to encourage eating in a social atmosphere.

Most children consume at least one meal daily in school. While children may bring lunches to school, most participate in school lunch programs and perhaps school breakfast programs. Nurses should become familiar with the policies of school districts in their areas for providing foods, snacks, and reduced-price food to students in need. During the past decade, many school systems in the United States have allowed vending machines for carbonated sweetened beverages and snacks to be installed in public schools. Part of the profits from these machines has enabled revenue-strapped school districts to enhance their incomes. Today, however, schools are increasingly challenged about the presence of the machines, especially in light of the growing problem of overweight among youth. Some school districts have now limited the number of machines or the hours during which they can be used by students, and some have removed all sweetened beverages from vending machines. Nurses are able to provide information for districts about the problems of obesity and the need for healthy foods for youth. Nurses are also involved in planning for nutritional maintenance when children have special needs in the school setting, such as diet or tube feedings.

Healthy People 2020

(NWS-14) Increase the contribution of fruits to the diets of the population aged 2 years and older

(NWS-15) Increase the variety and contribution of vegetables to the diets of the population aged 2 years and older

---

The loss of the first deciduous teeth and the eruption of permanent teeth usually occur at about 6 years, or at the beginning of the school-age period. Of the 32 permanent teeth, 22 to 26 erupt by age 12 years, and the remaining molars follow in the teenage years. See Chapter 5 for the typical sequence of tooth eruption and Chapters 8 and 9 for dental care needs during childhood. The school-age child should be closely monitored to

Professionalism in Practice The National School Lunch Program

The National School Lunch Program is a federally assisted meal program operating in over 100,000 public and non-profit private schools and residential childcare institutions. It provides nutritionally balanced lunches to more than 31 million children on each school day at free or reduced cost. Recently, increased access to fruits, vegetables, and whole grains, along with decreased foods high in sodium content, have been mandated. Specific nutritional and caloric requirements are in place for grades K to 5, 6 to 8, and 9 to 12 (U.S. Department of Agriculture [USDA], 2013b). Nurses can ensure that parents are aware of the program and have assistance to translate or complete the application forms if needed. Nurses also work with school administrators for seamless integration of all children into the school food program so that no student is aware of those who are eligible for this service.

Clinical Reasoning The Child With Special Nutritional Needs

The opening quote in this chapter is from the mother of Joey, a young boy with cerebral palsy who has a gastrostomy feeding tube to assist him in ingestion of adequate nutrients (see the *Clinical Skills Manual* SKILLS for the process of gastrostomy feeding). Joey is attending school and the teacher has been taught to administer his tube feedings. Nurses often assist families who have children with special needs to integrate them into the school environment. How might the nurse plan for Joey to participate in school lunchtime with peers? Since he can eat some soft foods by mouth, what types of foods are commonly available at school that he might be able to enjoy?

ensure that brushing and flossing are adequate, that fluoride is taken if the fluoride concentration in the water supply is below 0.7 mg/L, that dental care is obtained to provide for examination of teeth and alignment, and that loose teeth are identified before surgery or sports participation.

Adolescence

Most adolescents need well over 2000 calories daily to support the growth spurt, and some adolescent boys require nearly 3000 or more calories daily. When teenagers are active in a variety of sports, these requirements increase further. Because adolescents prepare much of their own food and often eat with friends, they need to be taught about good nutrition. Developing a diet that includes a large number of calories, meets vitamin and mineral requirements, and is acceptable to the teen may be a challenge.

The pregnant adolescent has even more challenging nutrient requirements. Increased need of calories, calcium, iron, folic acid, and other nutrients may provide challenges for the adolescent who is pregnant. An adolescent who is hospitalized and does not like the hospital lunch might ask a friend who visits to bring a soft drink and chips; however, the teen may be receptive to offers of juice and pizza, a more nutritious meal. Small improvements should be viewed positively because they may lead to further changes. See *Evidence-Based Practice: Adolescents and Nutritional Choices.*

EVIDENCE-BASED PRACTICE | Adolescents and Nutritional Choices

Clinical Question

Adolescents are largely independent in their food choices. They often eat "on the run" and are influenced by peers and the media. At the same time, rates of obesity are on an escalating upward trajectory. How can nurses understand and apply evidence-based practices for influencing eating behaviors in adolescents?

The Evidence

The HEALTHY study found that a middle school–based intervention program resulted in significant positive changes in students' fruit and water intake (Siega-Riz et al., 2011). Another middle school program with young adolescents, the TEAMS study, asked parents, youth, and school officials to identify barriers to health as well as solutions for healthier environments. Students had knowledge deficits but identified low access to healthy foods and busy schedules as barriers, while teachers tended to believe parents frequently did not provide healthy food options and parents identified teens' preferences for unhealthy foods as an important barrier (Bindler et al., 2012). School boards are instrumental in establishing school wellness policies (USDA, 2014). Achieving healthy weight by adolescents should include nutrition and activity teaching, technology-based approaches, and peer modeling. The community can be engaged in healthy weight goals by introducing measures to monitor weight, nutrition, and activity at all health visits. One tool called Passport to Health was developed and implemented successfully by nurse practitioners in a pediatric practice setting (Vaczy, Seaman, Peterson-Sweeney, et al., 2011).

Best Practice

Child and adolescent eating patterns set an important example for life. Family eating patterns, school setting, and community influences must all be examined to identify risk and protective factors in the adolescent diet. Barriers to adolescent healthy eating include lack of accurate information, availability of "junk food" snacks, lack of parental involvement in the lives of teens, peer influence, and media messages about food consumption.

Clinical Reasoning

1. What developmental stages of the adolescent provide both challenges to healthy eating and ability to make wise food choices?
2. Construct a list of questions about family food patterns that will help you identify risk and protective factors of the family.
3. Visit a local high school and then travel 1/2 mile in each direction from the school. Record the number of fast-food restaurants, billboards about foods, and any other food-related resources or media. Watch 2 hours of television at 3 to 5 p.m., the time at which adolescents frequently arrive home. Record the number of food-related messages, what types of foods are advertised, and other observations.
4. How can you integrate knowledge about adolescent nutrition into your potential role as a school nurse at a high school?

Fast food represents a significant intake for many adolescents. It is commonly high in fat, calories, and sodium while being low in essential nutrients such as calcium, folic acid, riboflavin, vitamins A and C, and fiber. Many schools are redesigning cafeterias and food programs to entice more teens to eat at school rather than nearby fast-food restaurants. Adding fruits and salads and allowing choices can enhance the quality of food intake. School nurses play a vital role in helping to tailor a healthy school nutrition program and teaching teens about the healthiest choices at their favorite fast-food restaurants.

Peer group influence is important to teens, so group sessions in which adolescents eat lunch together can provide a forum for influencing food habits. What other methods might encourage positive nutritional habits among teens?

Nutritional Assessment

What is the best indication that a child's nutrition is adequate? Which data collection methods provide the most accurate information about a child's dietary intake? The nurse plays an important role in assessing the diets of children and in seeking additional evaluation from dietitians and nutritionists in complex situations.

Physical and Behavioral Measurement

GROWTH MEASUREMENT

A common method of evaluating the adequacy of diet is measurement of growth. **Anthropometric measurement** is the term used to refer to assessment of various parts of the body. Anthropometry of young children commonly includes weight, length, and head circumference. Standing height is substituted for length once the child can stand. Head circumference, also known as *occipital-frontal circumference (OFC)*, is measured during infancy and into early years when there are growth concerns. Additional measurements that may be included in special circumstances include chest circumference, mid–upper arm circumference, and skinfold measurement at sites such as triceps, abdomen, and subscapular regions. Grids are available for each measurement and assist in providing a thorough nutritional assessment when weight and height are abnormally high or low. The accompanying *Clinical Skills Manual* SKILLS presents techniques for accurate measurement of weight, length, height, chest circumference, and head circumference.

After collecting the measurements, the nurse plots them on the appropriate standardized growth curves for weight, length to height, head circumference, and body mass index (Figure 14–6). **Body mass index (BMI)** is a calculation based on the child's

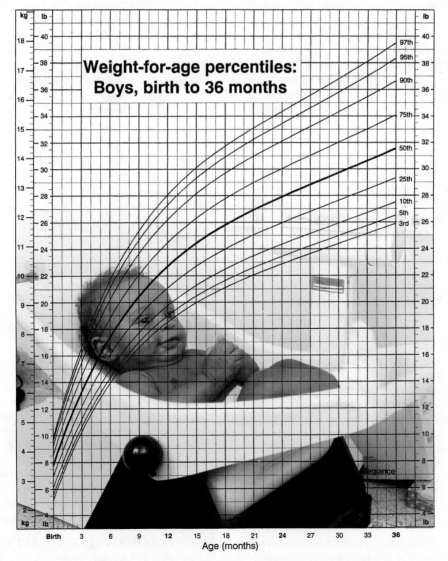

Figure 14–6 **Plotting measurements on the growth curve. The nurse accurately measures the child and then places height and weight on appropriate growth grids for the child's age and gender.**

weight and height, or length, and is calculated as kilograms of weight per square meter of height. This is a useful calculation for determining if the child's height and weight are in proportion and identifies which percentile the child falls in for each measurement. Children normally fall between the 10th and 90th percentiles. A measurement below the 10th percentile, especially for BMI, may indicate undernutrition, and one over the 90th percentile can indicate overnutrition. However, it is important to look at the differences between measurements. An infant in the 90th percentile for length, weight, and head circumference is proportional and may be a naturally large baby. On the other hand, a child who is consistently in the 10th percentile for all measurements, but is growing steadily and is at a normal development level, may simply be a small child. Much cultural and individual variation exists in size. See Appendix A for standardized growth curves by gender and age for infants, children, and adolescents. Visit the Centers for Disease Control and Prevention (CDC) website (www.cdc.gov) to find specialized growth grids for children with conditions such as Down syndrome.

Developing Cultural Competence Growth Patterns Among Immigrant Children

The revised growth grids now in use were standardized using a cross section of the U.S. population. However, children from some other countries or cultures may fall outside of these curves. For example, new immigrants or adoptees may be in lower percentiles and may "catch up" over several months or years. Children of immigrants from developing countries tend to be larger than their parents. Even when children are small, they should follow normal growth patterns.

The nurse should plot measurements on the same growth curve with earlier percentiles for the child. When measurements follow the same percentile over time, growth is generally normal for the child and nutrition is likely adequate. However, a sudden or sustained change in percentile may indicate a chronic disorder, emotional difficulty, or a nutritional intake problem. Further assessment of physical status and dietary intake will be needed.

ADDITIONAL PHYSICAL MEASUREMENTS

Many observations from the physical assessment provide clues to nutritional status. Dietary intake can affect every body system, and a combination of certain symptoms may suggest specific nutritional problems. Some common physical manifestations of nutritional status are outlined in Table 14–3.

Laboratory measurements can provide useful information when nutritional status is questionable. Some common studies include hematocrit and hemoglobin, serum glucose and fasting insulin, lipids and lipoproteins, and liver and renal function studies. Adding some further measurements such as chest circumference and skinfolds (measurement of fat at certain body sites such as triceps, scapular, and abdominal areas) may also be useful (Lee & Nieman, 2013).

Dietary Intake

The nurse should obtain detailed information about the child's dietary intake when there is a potential for nutritional deficiency due to disease, knowledge deficit, or socioeconomic status. The mother's dietary intake during pregnancy may

TABLE 14–3 Clinical Manifestations of Dietary Deficiencies/Excesses

NUTRIENT	DEFICIENCY MANIFESTATION	EXCESS MANIFESTATION
Vitamin A	Night blindness Skin dryness and scaling	Headache Drowsiness Hepatomegaly Vomiting and diarrhea
Vitamin C	Abnormal hair (coiled shape) Skin abnormalities (dermatitis and lesions) Purpura Bleeding gums Joint tenderness Sudden heart failure	Usually none—excess is excreted in urine
Vitamin D	Rib deformity Bowed legs Bone and joint pain Muscle weakness Periodontal disease Increased rates of respiratory and skin infections/irritation	Drowsiness
B vitamins	Weakness Decreased deep tendon reflexes Dermatitis	Usually none—excess is excreted in urine
Protein	Hepatomegaly Edema Scant, depigmented hair	Kidney failure
Carbohydrate	Emaciation Decreased energy Retarded growth and development	Overweight
Iron	Lethargy Slowed growth and developmental progression Pallor	Vomiting, diarrhea, abdominal pain Pallor Cyanosis Drowsiness Shock

provide information about the child's nutritional state and it can be assessed for pertinent information. After the information is collected, the dietary intake should be compared to the recommended levels for a child of that age and gender (see Figure 14–1 for the U.S. MyPlate food guide; see Appendix C for Recommended Dietary Allowances). The 24-hour recall of intake, a food frequency questionnaire, and a dietary screening history (Tables 14–4 and 14–5) provide a good overview of the infant's or child's intake and eating patterns. A food diary provides precise information about the child's food intake.

TWENTY-FOUR–HOUR RECALL OF FOOD INTAKE

The 24-hour diet recall is frequently used to assess the adequacy of the diet. People can generally remember their intake in the past day, so results are fairly accurate, it is easy to gather the

TABLE 14–4 Dietary Screening History for Infants

Overview Questions

What was the infant's birth weight?

At what age did the birth weight double and triple?

Was the infant premature?

Does the infant have any feeding problems such as difficulty sucking and swallowing, spitting up, fatigue, or fussiness?

If Infant Is Breastfed

How long does the baby nurse at each breast?

What is the usual schedule for breastfeeding?

Does the baby also take any milk or formula? Amount and frequency? What type?

If Infant Is Formula-Fed

What formula is used? Is it iron fortified?

How is it prepared?

Do you hold or prop the bottle for feedings?

How much formula is taken at each feeding?

How many bottles are taken each day?

Does the baby take a bottle to bed for naps or nighttime? What is in the bottle?

If Infant Is Fed Other Foods

At what age did the baby start eating other foods?

Cereal	Finger foods
Fruit/juices	Meats
Vegetables	Other protein sources

Do you use commercial baby food or make your own?

Does the baby eat any table foods?

How often does the baby take solid foods?

How is the baby's appetite?

Do you have any concerns about the baby's feeding habits?

Does the baby take a vitamin supplement? Fluoride?

Have there been any allergic reactions to foods? Which ones?

Does the baby spit up frequently?

Have there been any rashes?

What types of stools does the baby have? Frequency? Consistency?

TABLE 14–5 Dietary Screening History for Children

What types of food or beverage does the child especially like?

What foods or beverages does the child dislike?

What is the child's typical eating schedule? Meals and snacks?

Does the child eat with the family or at separate times?

Where does the child eat each meal?

Who prepares the food for the family?

What methods of cooking are used? Baking? Frying? Broiling? Grilling?

What ethnic foods are commonly eaten?

Does the family eat in a restaurant frequently? What type?

What type of food does the child usually order?

Is the child on a special diet?

Does the child need to be fed, feed himself or herself, need assistance eating, or need any adaptive devices for eating?

What is the child's appetite like?

Does the child take any vitamin supplements (iron, fluoride)?

Does the child have any allergies? What types of symptoms?

What types of regular exercise does the child get?

Are there any concerns about the child's eating habits?

- Additives used, such as condiments, table salt, spices, milk to mix formula
- Food preparation methods, including adding fats to cook, removal or retention of fats on meats
- Vitamins and supplements, types and doses
- Whether the intake is typical (in situations such as illness or vacation, intake may be different than usual)

Once the 24-hour recall is obtained, the nurse needs to analyze the intake by first doing a quick check to compare servings of various food types with the U.S. MyPlate food guide, as described earlier (see also Figure 14–1). Next the nurse should do a detailed analysis to compute calories, carbohydrate, protein, and fat intake and compare them to recommended amounts. All major vitamins and minerals are also computed and comparisons made to the DRIs. This computation may be done by hand,

data and analyze results, and only a few minutes are needed. The nurse should ask the parent or child to list all foods eaten during the past 24 hours (Figure 14–7). It is usually helpful to ask for a description of activities in the last day, then start with the most recent event and move backwards, integrating food intake into the daily schedule. For example, the nurse might begin by saying, "You mentioned you got up early to come to the clinic today. What did Sam eat at home before you left? Did he have a snack as you traveled here or after you arrived?" While asking about the foods eaten, the nurse should inquire specifically about the following:

- All meals and snacks
- Amounts of each food item consumed (having various size measuring cups, bowls, and plates available so accurate amounts can be indicated is helpful)
- Types of specific foods used, such as whole milk versus nonfat or 2%, brand names of cereals, specific types of margarine or butter

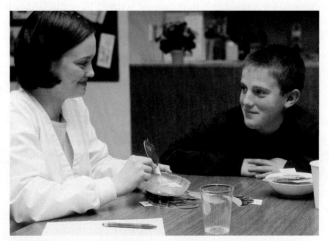

Figure 14–7 The 24-hour diet recall. The nurse is interviewing a child about foods eaten in the last day. Note the models of food and dishes for accurate assessment of serving sizes.

using a book of nutrients in common foods, or it may be done on the computer. Several computer programs are available, and the federal government has a website that provides intake levels and comparisons to the RDAs. It may be useful to compute a personal 24-hour recall or that of a child in the clinical setting with the Healthy Eating Index.

FOOD FREQUENCY QUESTIONNAIRE

Food frequency questionnaires are available that can be easily administered to parents or children. Usually, they ask about how often certain types of foods are eaten in a specified period such as a week. Long questionnaires can evaluate a total diet, while short ones focus on specific items such as fruit and vegetable intake. A short questionnaire about milk intake or fruit and vegetable intake may be helpful before planning a teaching project on nutrition to a class of school-age children. Knowing their usual intake of a food item can provide helpful information for planning the project.

DIETARY SCREENING HISTORY

The nurse should ask the parent about the infant's or child's eating habits using the questions listed in Tables 14–4 and 14–5. Responses provide information about the family's eating habits and food beliefs beyond that collected on a 24-hour dietary recall or food frequency questionnaire.

FOOD DIARY

Parents are asked to keep a food diary when the child has a nutrition problem or disorder that requires dietary management, such as malnutrition, obesity, or diabetes. All meals and snacks, with food preparation method and quantities eaten over a 1- to 7-day period, are recorded. Eating patterns change significantly for holidays or family gatherings, so parents should be asked to select typical days for the food diary or to record specific events affecting food intake. Including 1 weekday and 1 weekend day may be helpful. Parents need to be reminded of all the places children might have eaten, such as the childcare center, school, or friends' or neighbors' homes. Food diaries can provide a great deal of helpful information, but they take time and motivation to complete well (Lee & Nieman, 2013). The nurse should be sure instructions are complete and that the form has a place to record amounts, preparation, events occurring, and where food was eaten. The nurse or parent may need to obtain the school lunch menu and talk with the school lunch personnel to add accurate school intake. The nurse completes the nutritional assessment indicated for a child and may consult with or refer the family to a dietitian or nutritionist for additional assessment and teaching.

Developing Cultural Competence Dietary Intake Varies Among Cultures

Each culture has eating practices that influence dietary intake. It is important to understand the foods commonly eaten by each cultural group and their contribution to the total nutrition of the child. Depending on the populations nurses work with, they may need to ask about intake of freshly caught fish or wild game such as pheasant and elk. Home-prepared sausages and cheese may be part of diets. Berries and garden produce might be eaten. Foods from ethnic markets may include spices, dried mushrooms, and other products. Some groups do not eat meat or specific types of meats. Using open-ended questions when gathering data will increase the likelihood of obtaining an accurate evaluation of diet.

TABLE 14–6 Food Insecurity Screening

1. Does your household ever run out of money to buy food to make a meal?
2. Do you or members of your household ever eat less than you feel you should because there is not enough money for food?
3. Do you or members of your household ever cut the size of meals or skip meals because there is not enough money for food?
4. Do your children ever eat less than you feel they should because there is not enough money for food?
5. Do you ever cut the size of your children's meals or do they skip meals because there is not enough money for food?
6. Do your children ever say they are hungry because there is not enough food in the house?
7. Do you ever rely on a limited number of foods to feed your children because you are running out of money to buy foods for a meal?
8. Do any of your children ever go to bed hungry because there is not enough money to buy food?

Scoring: 5–8 yes responses = hungry; 1–4 yes responses = risk of hunger. From Washington State Department of Health.

Common Nutritional Concerns

Childhood Hunger

Although most Americans live in a land of plenty, significant numbers of children periodically experience hunger. **Food security** is access at all times to enough nourishment for an active, healthy life. In contrast, **food insecurity** indicates an inability to acquire or consume adequate quality or quantity of foods in socially acceptable ways, or the uncertainty that one will be able to do so; at least 10% of U.S. children live in households that periodically experience food insecurity (USDA, 2013a).

The major cause of hunger in children is poverty, and since, on average, more than one in five children are poor, their families may be unable to provide sustainable nutrition at all times (Children's Defense Fund, 2014). Many single-income families have a head of household moving into the workforce, so incomes are often not sufficient to provide for family food needs (see Chapter 1 for a description of Temporary Assistance for Needy Families). Families may be ineligible for food assistance programs even though they cannot afford enough food for all their members. Children with special nutritional needs are at particular risk since it may be more costly to buy and prepare formula or foods for a child with allergies, diabetes, or an immune disorder.

Children with insufficient dietary intake are at risk for a wide array of health problems. They may become anemic; have a high rate of infectious disease due to a lowered immune response; have slowed developmental maturation, delayed or stunted physical growth, and learning disorders; and be at greater risk of overweight, cardiovascular disease, and diabetes in adulthood (Children's Defense Fund, 2014). Subsequently, the national and individual cost of childhood hunger is great.

Nurses are well positioned to evaluate families for food insecurity in a variety of hospital, clinic, school, and home settings. In addition to the assessment of the individual child's nutritional status, further questions can determine families with potential problems. Nurses should administer a screening tool to identify risk in families (Table 14–6). Most parents go

Families Want to Know
Community Resources for Food

Supplemental Nutrition Assistance Program (SNAP)—Eligibility based on household size and income; refer students and those with low incomes, especially when they have young children; education services often available

Child Nutrition Programs—School lunch, breakfast, and milk programs; free and lowered cost meals in schools; assist parents to apply

Special Child Programs—Summer programs, Head Start, childcare centers, and homeless children programs may provide nutritional support in some communities

Special Supplementary Food Program for Women, Infants, and Children (WIC)—Supplemental foods and nutrition education to pregnant, breastfeeding, and postpartum women and to their young children; assessment of child growth often included

Nutrition Education and Training Program—Nutrition education for teachers and school food service personnel

Community Services—May include food banks, field gleaning (collecting produce from farmers' fields that will not be sold due to excess or small blemishes), community gardens, and other programs

Find out what services are available to provide food and nutrition education in your community. Make a list to use in clinical settings with families.

without food themselves in order to feed their children, so food insecurity may not have directly affected all children. However, anxiety over providing food can be very stressful for families, and diet quality deteriorates as insecurity increases. If families have experienced food insecurity or may be likely to at some time, nurses should be sure to provide them with access to community agencies and programs that can help. What resources are available locally to help families with food insecurity?

Overweight and Obesity

The current incidence of overweight children in the United States is epidemic and is associated with a wide array of health problems, such as type 2 diabetes, stroke, gallbladder disease, arthritis, cardiovascular disease, sleep disturbances, hypertension, dyslipidemia, respiratory problems, certain cancers, interference with physical activity, social stigma, discrimination, depression, and low self-esteem (CDC, 2014a). A historic high of 17% of children and adolescents are at or above the 95th percentile for BMI (obese) and about the same amount fall from the 85th to 94th percentiles for BMI (overweight), designating about one third of U.S. youth as being overweight or obese (CDC, 2014a).

Many reasons are cited for the increase in overweight children. The number of calories consumed is not increasing, but children tend to exercise less, particularly in daily life. They infrequently walk or ride bikes either because of the convenience of driving or because of unsafe neighborhoods. Television viewing is very high among youth; movies, Internet, computer games, social networking, and cell phones are further examples of media commonly used by youth. U.S. children spend, on average, over 7 hours daily on such media (National Heart, Lung and Blood Institute, 2013). Inactive pursuits do not require high caloric energy, leading to an imbalance in intake and demand for calories. Additionally, television viewing is often accompanied by ingestion of high-calorie foods and subjects children to food marketing of unhealthy foods.

The percentage of calories from fat consumed in the United States is among the highest in the world. Although no more than 25% to 35% of calories should come from total dietary fat, and no more than 10% from saturated fat, about 35% of calories consumed in the United States are supplied by fat and over 11% by saturated fat (USDHHS, 2011). Most fats should be supplied from polyunsaturated and monounsaturated fatty acids, but current diets contain low amounts of those fats and high amounts of trans-fatty acids (USDHHS, 2011). The high rate of dietary fat is related to the amount of fast food consumed, and influenced by snacking as well.

Goals of nursing management are to prevent new cases of overweight, identify children who are overweight, and to support youth and families to establish healthy lifestyles that promote weight loss and maintenance of recommended weight. Perform assessment of height, weight, and BMI. Measure blood pressure and determine whether it is within normal limits. Evaluate amount of screen/social activities, sedentary behavior, and physical activity levels. When prevention and behavioral changes have not been successful, some adolescents will have bariatric surgery. Guidelines have been established for adolescents that consider age, physical maturity, BMI, and comorbidities (Brei & Mudd, 2014).

Nurses can help parents and children build good nutritional and exercise habits throughout life, thus decreasing the incidence of overweight and its attendant health risks. Children under 2 years of age should have no exposure to screen activities. Parents should be advised that screen activities by children older than age 2 should be limited to a maximum of 2 hours daily, and that a television, video games, or other screens should not be placed in children's bedrooms (AAP, 2014b). Daily exercise routines of 30 to 60 minutes can be included in the schedules of most families. Aim to meet the current recommendation of 60 minutes daily for children with some activity including muscle strengthening and flexibility. Also, nurses should teach about the MyPlate food guide and its integration into a healthy life. Healthy snacks include fruits, vegetables, grains, and nuts. "Super-sizing" fast foods and eating out often should be avoided.

Risks for poor health often cluster together in individuals and families. Nurses need to be alert for situations in which parents are overweight and children have elevated blood pressure, exercise infrequently, or are in upper percentiles for weight, BMI, or skinfold measurements. Be alert for early menarche, which can help identify overweight girls who need intervention for obesity prevention. The presence of risk factors necessitates further dietary and risk assessment so that a management plan can be implemented. See resources such as "Helping Your Overweight Child" and "Take Charge of Your Health: A Teenager's Guide to Better Health" (http://win.niddk.nih.gov/publications).

Consult the *Nursing Care Plan* in this chapter for further interventions appropriate for the child who is overweight.

Nursing Care Plan: The Child Who Is Overweight

1. Nursing Diagnosis: *Overweight* related to excessive intake in comparison to metabolic needs (NANDA-I © 2014)

GOAL: The child will demonstrate adequate intake of all nutrients without excessive energy intake.

INTERVENTION	RATIONALE
• Perform thorough nutritional assessment of child.	• Assessment assists in identification of dietary risks and strengths as well as health conditions related to nutrition.
• Share results of assessment with child and family by showing weight, height, and body mass index grids.	• Many families do not consider their child overweight. Concrete information about the child's size in comparison with recommendations assists in establishing the importance of weight management.
• Assess access to sufficient nutritious foods for the family at all times.	• Food insecurity promotes inadequate intake alternating with excess intake of high-calorie foods.
• Identify with the child and family 2–3 target areas to begin weight management. Examples might include: • Having fast food only once weekly • Switching to low-fat dairy products • Keeping two more fresh fruits and vegetables in the house and two less snack foods	• Changing dietary patterns drastically is difficult and may lead to giving up the attempt at weight management. Partnering with the family to set goals enhances chances of success.
• Integrate nutrition information into each visit. Examples of topics include: • Dietary requirements for age group • Effects of simple sugar and fat intake on weight • Beneficial effects of fruits, vegetables, whole grains, and nonfat dairy • Reading food labels • Healthy choices in fast-food restaurants • Calculation of fat content of foods	• Nutrition information is best learned in an ongoing program.
• Use growth grids to help child and family establish a weight reduction or maintenance goal.	• Goals motivate families to achieve desired health behaviors. The goal for a young child may be weight maintenance so that as the child grows in height, the correct proportion is reached, while weight reduction may be needed for older children or youth who are very obese.

EXPECTED OUTCOME: Child meets all dietary requirements while achieving weight and body mass index goal.

2. Nursing Diagnosis: *Coping: Family, Readiness for Enhanced,* related to need to foster health of family member (NANDA-I © 2014)

GOAL: The family will assist child to manage stressors and to develop new strategies to support weight control goals.

INTERVENTION	RATIONALE
• Include key family members in some of the counseling sessions with the child who is overweight.	• Key members of the family are those who purchase foods, provide support for the child, and participate in decisions about health.
• Encourage the family to eat together at least once daily if possible or to increase number of meals eaten together weekly.	• The family is an important support system in weight loss programs. Eating as a family or in a social situation can provide a chance to promote healthy foods; intake is generally lower fat and calorie than when eating alone.
• Seek a resource for the child to be monitored about twice monthly; this may be a healthcare provider office, nutritionist, school nurse, or other person.	• The resource provides opportunity to monitor the child's progress and to offer support, additional information, and problem-solving techniques.

EXPECTED OUTCOME: Child expresses satisfaction with family understanding and support of weight.

3. Nursing Diagnosis: *Activity Intolerance* **related to sedentary lifestyle (NANDA-I © 2014)**

GOAL: The child will demonstrate activity tolerance by adequate oxygenation, respiratory effort, and ability to speak during brisk walking, biking, or other activity.

INTERVENTION	RATIONALE
• Establish daily exercise routine beginning with 15–30 minutes daily of walking.	• Starting with brief amounts of exercise makes the child feel comfortable and enhances potential for success.
• Gradually increase activity over 1–2 months until 60 minutes of daily exercise is maintained.	• Gradual increase as the cardiovascular and respiratory systems adapt is generally comfortable for children; 60 minutes of moderate activity daily is recommended for children.
• Use activities enjoyed by the child and suggest options as necessary; refer the family to community resources such as swimming pools, organized sports, and biking groups.	• Activities the child enjoys will be more likely to remain in usual activity patterns; exercising with others in groups increases motivation.
• Have families plan at least 1–2 activities they can do together weekly.	• This fosters family relationships and provides support and motivation for the child.
• Limit screen activities to a maximum of 2 hours daily.	• Increased use of screen activities is related to poor dietary habits and increased sedentary behaviors and excess weight.
• Have child keep a log of hours of television, video games, computer, and other similar activities. Tell child never to snack while doing screen activities.	
• Ask about use of tobacco in children in fifth grade or higher.	• Most adults who smoke began the habit in childhood; middle school years are the most common age for smoking initiation.
• Inquire about exposure to environmental tobacco smoke at all ages.	• Smoking by others in the household can be harmful to children.
• Perform teaching to discourage tobacco use or offer cessation programs as needed.	• Smoking decreases respiratory reserves and worsens several cardiovascular disease risks.

EXPECTED OUTCOME: Child demonstrates ability to engage in moderate activity for 60 minutes with minimal respiratory discomfort.

4. Nursing Diagnosis: *Self-Esteem, Chronic Low,* **related to weight (NANDA-I © 2014)**

GOAL: The child expresses positive perception of self-worth and confidence in ability to deal with issues related to weight.

INTERVENTION	RATIONALE
• Facilitate development of a positive outlook by exposing child to others who have been successful with weight loss.	• Increases motivation and feelings of self-efficacy.
• Praise child for weight loss, weight maintenance, increased physical activity, and other achievements.	• Enhances judgment of self-worth and pride in accomplishments.
• Help the child establish rewards for meeting goals, such as purchase of new clothing.	
• Partner with parents so that they understand the value of praise and never label the child using derogatory words such as "fat."	• Family members are usually the most intimate support system for the child.

EXPECTED OUTCOME: Child speaks positively about accomplishments in weight control management.

Developing Cultural Competence Overweight Causes Health Disparities Among Certain Groups

Overweight is more common among some ethnic and socioeconomic groups. Lack of knowledge about foods and physical activity, limited access to fresh produce and safe places to exercise, and easy access to increasing numbers of fast foods may all constitute risk factors. Lower income, and Hispanic, African American, or Native American ethnic identity are all associated with higher incidence of overweight, especially among women. National goals to eliminate health disparities in income and ethnic groups have been set (USDHHS, 2011).

Food Safety

In the United States, about 48 million people (1 in 6) contract foodborne illnesses every year. Some cases are quite mild, whereas others can be very severe. About 128,000 people are hospitalized, and about 3000 die from these illnesses (CDC, 2014b). Children are at greater risk of severe illness and death from food and water because of their immature gastrointestinal and immune systems. Children who are immunocompromised are at even greater risk. Among the most common pathogens are *Campylobacter, Salmonella, Vibrio, Shigella, Cryptosporidium, Listeria, Yersinia,* and *Escherichia coli* (CDC, 2011b, 2014c). Worldwide, over 3 million people die of illness related to unsafe drinking water each year, and most of those deaths are among children.

Families Want to Know

Food Safety Guidelines

Teach clients to follow these four key food safety practices:

1. *Clean:* Wash hands and surfaces often.
2. *Separate:* Do not cross-contaminate.
3. *Cook:* Cook to proper temperature.
4. *Chill:* Refrigerate promptly.

Source: From Partnership for Food Safety Education. (2011). *Safe food handling.* Retrieved from http://www.fightbac.org/safe-food-handling

Foodborne illness transmission is associated with food preparation and storage practices, lack of adequate training of retail employees about foods and hygiene, and increasing amounts and types of foods being imported from other countries. Some examples of contaminated foods in the past few years include undercooked hamburger meat, cross-contamination of salad bar items from meats, unpasteurized apple cider, green onions, raw spinach, prepackaged salad and delicatessen meat, berries, and sprouts. While most infected persons experience acute diarrhea, some can develop complications such as hemolytic uremic syndrome (Chapter 26) or thrombocytic purpura (Chapter 23). Health personnel should integrate teaching regularly so that families can decrease risks of foodborne illness. Recommend that families avoid consumption of unpasteurized milk, raw or undercooked oysters, raw or undercooked eggs, raw or undercooked ground beef, and undercooked poultry (CDC, 2011b). Check the information regarding outbreaks at www.foodsafety.org.

Food may carry products other than microorganisms that can be harmful. An example is mercury, which may be concentrated in certain types of fish. This metal can cause harm to the developing nervous system of fetuses, infants, and young children when consumed regularly. The U.S. Food and Drug Administration (FDA) and Environmental Protection Agency (EPA) note that fish are an important part of a healthy diet, but that certain recommendations should be followed to lower the risk of experiencing mercury's detrimental effects. Women who may become pregnant, are pregnant or breastfeeding, and young children should:

- Eliminate shellfish, shark, swordfish, king mackerel, and tilefish from the diet.
- Eat 8 to 12 oz (two average meals) a week of a variety of low-mercury fish, such as shrimp, canned light tuna, salmon, pollock, and catfish. Albacore or white tuna has more mercury than light tuna, so limit white tuna to one meal weekly. (Children should have two to three servings per week of low-mercury fish in amounts appropriate for their age and caloric needs.)

Check for local advisories about the safety of fish caught in local waters (U.S. Food and Drug Administration, 2014).

Common Dietary Deficiencies

Dietary deficiencies can occur in children and some are common in selected populations. Children can have deficits in nearly any nutrient, but a number of nutrient deficits are more common in childhood. Limitations in the food supply or patterns of dietary intake cause most deficiencies, while children with certain disease processes, such as metabolic diseases, may have difficulty absorbing or using nutrients ingested. (See Chapter 30 for a discussion of inborn errors of metabolism.) The nutrient deficiencies of a population are a result of genetic factors, characteristics of the food supply, and intake patterns of particular groups.

Developing Cultural Competence　Vitamin A Deficiency

Vitamin A deficiency is common in developing countries. The vitamin is found in liver, dairy products, and fish. Provitamin A sources are yellow and dark green vegetables. The vitamin is fat soluble and stored in the liver. When deficient, children develop night blindness, vision loss, and high rates of infection. Public health efforts have been directed at identifying populations of children with low vitamin A status and providing the vitamin in capsule form or in commonly ingested foods.

IRON

Newborns have a store of iron obtained from their mothers in the uterus if the maternal nutritional state was satisfactory and the baby was of normal gestational age. Breast milk contains little iron, but the iron it does contain has high bioavailability. However, by 4 to 6 months of age, the baby's iron stores begin to decrease and a dietary source of iron must be added for the infant. Enriched rice cereal is commonly used to meet these initial iron needs. In babies who do not have adequate stores or do not take in enough iron, **anemia**, or a reduction in the number of red blood cells, can result (Figure 14–8). Feeding cow's milk during infancy can also cause anemia by irritating the gut and leading to small but consistent loss of blood from the gastrointestinal tract; cow's milk should not be fed in the first year of life. When formulas are used, they should be iron fortified to help avoid

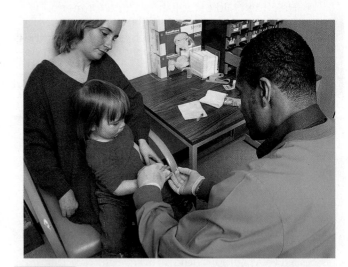

Figure 14–8 Screening for anemia. Most Head Start centers participate in screening programs to identify children at risk for anemia.

iron-deficiency anemia. Iron-fortified infant cereals are a good source of the mineral.

Adolescent females comprise another group commonly deficient in iron. Their deficiency is related to loss of blood in menses, metabolic need of the growth spurt, and poor dietary balance due to sporadic dieting. Further discussion of the symptoms and treatment of iron-deficiency anemia can be found in Chapter 23. Encourage intake of good iron sources such as meats, eggs, dried fruits, and iron-fortified cereal. Instruct families on safe iron administration, and ensure follow-up evaluations of iron levels when nutritional supplements are administered.

CALCIUM

Calcium is an essential nutrient for bone development during childhood and adolescence. An increased intake of soft drinks and fruit juices is related to a decrease in calcium intake, especially among adolescents. During the adolescent growth spurt, almost 40% of the adult bone mass is accumulated, and by age 18 years for females and age 20 years for males, 90% of peak bone mass is achieved (National Institute of Arthritis and Musculoskeletal and Skin Diseases, 2012). Inadequate intake puts the person at risk for osteoporosis later in life since it is not possible to make up for earlier deficits. Although genetic variables account for some of the influence on adult bone mass, increasing calcium intake has been shown to promote bone formation. While the recommended daily intake for adolescents is 1300 mg, but the average intake for young males is 870 to 1260 mg and for females is only 750 to 960 mg (only half of the recommended level) (National Institutes of Health, 2013). Nurses should encourage foods such as milk and milk products, egg yolks, grains, legumes, nuts, and fruit juice with added calcium.

Adolescents at highest risk for impaired bone development include female athletes and others who diet excessively to maintain slimness. Teens who exercise excessively may manifest the "female athlete triad" of disordered eating that leads to excessive thinness, excessive exercise, and amenorrhea. A high rate of fractures and osteomalacia can result, in addition to an extreme risk of osteoporosis in adulthood (Ackerman & Misra, 2011). Asking about menstrual patterns as well as exercise and diet can be combined with physical measurements of height and weight to obtain pertinent information about the teen athlete. See the discussion of the eating disorders anorexia nervosa and bulimia nervosa later in this chapter.

VITAMIN D

Vitamin D is needed for bone mineralization. Vitamin D deficiencies were once believed to be rare; however, an increase in cases of vitamin D–deficient rickets has recently been observed. Although vitamin D can be synthesized in the skin when exposed to sunlight, the amount of sunlight needed for manufacture is variable and determined by the amount of skin exposed, the color of the skin, the latitude, and time of the year (Wagner, Greer, Section on Breastfeeding, et al., 2008). Because of this variability and the small amount of vitamin D in breast milk, it is now recommended that all infants from birth to 6 months old receive a minimum intake of 400 International Units daily. All persons 6 months and older should receive 600 International Units daily (Ross, Taylor, Yaktine, et al., 2011). This vitamin is needed to enhance absorption of calcium, so a lack of vitamin D can contribute to calcium deficiency as well. When rickets is suspected, laboratory studies should include 25-OH vitamin D (20–29 ng/mL indicates insufficiency of vitamin D, and below 20 ng/mL is a deficiency state), serum calcium, phosphorus, alkaline phosphatase, creatinine, electrolytes, parathyroid hormone, and hematocrit. Radiographs of extremities should be taken (American Association for Clinical Chemistry, 2014). Encourage parents to discuss vitamin D intake with the healthcare provider at health promotion visits so proper intake can be ensured.

FOLIC ACID

Epidemiologic evidence has linked increasing maternal folic acid (the most common form of folate in the human body) intake with decreased incidence of neural tube defects such as spina bifida in offspring. Folate levels are low among adolescents, putting them at particular risk of birth defects when they have babies (AAP Committee on Nutrition, 2013). The FDA approved fortification of cereals and breads with folate to decrease the population risk of related congenital anomalies. All women ages 15 to 45 years should consume 0.4 mg of folic acid daily, and pregnant women should consume 0.6 mg. In addition to cereals and breads, other good sources of folate include spinach, avocado, green leafy vegetables, beans and peas, liver, and fruits such as oranges and grapefruits.

PROTEIN-ENERGY MALNUTRITION

Although the micronutrient deficiencies described previously are the most common problems in developed countries, macronutrient deficiencies are the most common nutritional problems worldwide. Kwashiorkor indicates protein deficiency and marasmus is a lack of energy-producing calories, but both deficiencies often occur together and are referred to as protein-energy malnutrition (PEM). Protein deficiency manifests with edema, leading to the large abdomens and rounded faces seen in severely malnourished children. Other symptoms include scant, depigmented hair, skin changes, and decreased serum proteins. It can occur following severe diarrhea or other infection in susceptible children. Caloric deficiency results in emaciation, decreased energy levels, and retarded development (see Table 14–3). PEM may occur when a child is weaned in order for the mother to provide breast milk to a new baby. Adoptees and immigrants to developed countries sometimes manifest with at least mild PEM, so careful nutritional assessment is needed to provide adequate nutrition.

Celiac Disease

Celiac disease, or gluten-sensitive enteropathy, is a chronic malabsorption syndrome. About 1 in 133 persons have celiac disease. It is more common among members of the same family and in children with Down syndrome or Turner syndrome (National Institute of Diabetes and Digestive and Kidney Disease [NIDDK], 2012).

Celiac disease is an immunologic disorder characterized by intolerance for gluten, a protein found in wheat, barley, rye, and oats. Inability to digest glutenin and gliadin (protein fractions) results in the accumulation of the amino acid glutamine, which is toxic to mucosal cells in the intestine. Damage to the villi ultimately impairs the absorptive process in the small intestine.

In the early stages, celiac disease affects fat absorption, resulting in excretion of large quantities of fat in the stools (steatorrhea). Stools are greasy, foul smelling, frothy, and excessive. As changes in the villi continue, the absorption of protein, carbohydrates, calcium, iron, folate, and vitamins A, D, E, K, and B_{12} becomes impaired.

Symptoms usually occur when solid foods containing gluten are introduced to the child's diet (generally between 6 months to 2 years of age), although celiac disease is sometimes first diagnosed in adulthood. The classic features of celiac disease in infancy include chronic diarrhea, growth impairment, and abdominal distention. The child also demonstrates poor appetite, lack of energy, and muscle wasting with hypotonia. Atypical features are present in children diagnosed with delayed-onset celiac disease around 5 to 7 years of age. Symptoms include nausea, vomiting, recurrent abdominal pain, bloating, tooth enamel defects, and aphthous ulcers (Rashid, Zarkadas, Anca, et al., 2011). Other symptoms may include delayed growth, iron deficiency, and abnormal liver function tests.

Diagnosis is confirmed through measurement of fecal fat content, duodenal biopsy, and improvement with removal of gluten products from the diet. Serum screening tests for immunoglobulin (IgA) antiendomysial antibodies and IgA antitissue transglutaminase antibodies are commonly used in the diagnosis of celiac disease (Garcia-Manzanares & Lucendo, 2011; NIDDK, 2012).

Management of celiac disease involves total exclusion of gluten from the diet. This gluten-free diet is a lifetime treatment. Barley, wheat, and rye are completely eliminated; oat products are sometimes tolerated. Symptoms generally improve within a few days to weeks. Supplementation with fat-soluble vitamins, vitamin B_{12}, folic acid, calcium, and iron may be needed depending on the results of serum testing (Daitch & Epperson, 2011).

The intestinal villi return to normal in about 6 months. Growth should improve steadily, and height and weight should reach normal range within 1 year.

Nursing Management

Nursing care focuses on supporting the parents in maintaining a gluten-free diet for the child. Thoroughly explain the disease process to the parents. Emphasize the necessity of following a gluten-free diet. Help parents to understand that celiac disease requires lifelong dietary modifications that should not be discontinued when the child is symptom-free. Discontinuation of the diet places the child at risk for growth retardation and the development of gastrointestinal cancers in adulthood. All children with celiac disease should be seen by a dietitian several times during childhood. Nutritional assessment and continued teaching to maintain a gluten-free diet take place at these visits. Dietary management is made difficult by hidden gluten in many prepared foods, such as chocolate candy, prepared meats, ice cream, soups, condiments, and food starch.

An infant or toddler's diet is easily monitored at home. When the child enters school, however, ensuring adherence to dietary restrictions becomes more difficult. In addition to easily identified gluten-based foods, such as bread, cake, doughnuts, cookies, and crackers, the child must also avoid processed foods that contain gluten as a filler. School-age children and adolescents are often tempted to eat these foods, especially when among peers. Emphasize the need for compliance while meeting the child's developmental needs.

The child's special dietary needs can place a financial burden on the family. Parents need to purchase prepared rice or corn flour products or make their own bread and bakery products. Advise parents that getting a dietary prescription enables them to deduct the cost of these ingredients and commercially prepared products as a medical expense.

Because the entire family must adapt to the diet, parents and siblings need support and management skills. For information and support, refer parents and children to several organizations, including the American Celiac Society, the Celiac Sprue Association/United States of America, and the Gluten Intolerance Group.

Expected outcomes of nursing care include the following:

- The child maintains adequate nutrition to support growth and development needs.
- The child achieves growth and developmental milestones appropriate for age.
- The child and family understand the dietary restrictions and appropriately plan meals.

Feeding and Eating Disorders

Deficiencies in food intake related to available nutrients and safety of the food supply were discussed in the previous section. In addition to these issues of availability, nutrient intake is affected by psychologic issues of individuals as well. Disorders of food intake span the entire developmental spectrum and can affect pregnant women, young children, and adolescents. Some of the most common feeding and eating disorders are discussed in the following sections.

COLIC

Colic is a feeding disorder of infants characterized by paroxysmal abdominal pain and severe crying. The crying generally lasts at least 3 hours and occurs on at least 3 days per week. Crying episodes peak around 6 weeks of age and generally resolve by 3 to 4 months of age (Holt, Wooldridge, Story, et al., 2011). The etiology of colic is unknown. Proposed causes include feeding too rapidly and swallowing large amounts of air.

Characteristically, the infant cries loudly and continuously, often for several hours. The infant's face may become flushed. The abdomen is distended and tense. Often the infant draws up the legs and clenches the hands. Episodes occur at the same time each day, usually in the late afternoon or early evening. Crying may stop only when the child is completely exhausted or after passage of flatus or stool.

The symptoms initially may resemble intestinal obstruction or peritoneal infection. These conditions must be ruled out along with sensitivity to formula. Treatment is supportive; no general medical consensus exists on effective treatments or interventions for colic. Some healthcare providers recommend medications such as simethicone (Mylicon) drops. Some recommend formula change to a soy formula or an elemental formula such as Pregestimil.

Nursing care requires a thorough history of the infant's diet and daily schedule and the events surrounding episodes of colicky behavior. Assessment of the infant's feeding patterns and diet includes type, frequency, and amount of feeding (if breastfeeding, maternal diet history) and frequency of burping. Inquire about onset, duration, and characteristics of cry during colic episodes. Ask the parents what measures are used to relieve crying and their effectiveness.

When possible, observe the feeding method. Parents of infants with colic are often tired and frustrated. They require frequent reassurance that they are not to blame for the infant's condition. Suggest ways of alleviating some of the infant's symptoms and discomfort. These include using a front-carrying sling, swaddling, playing soothing music, using a pacifier, or giving a warm bath or massage of the abdomen. The breastfeeding mother should avoid gas-producing foods and the infant should be burped frequently during feedings. An important consideration is the significant impact of colic on families. Colic can place extreme stress and fatigue on the family, so active support and counseling for the mother and other family members is important.

PICA

Pica is an eating disorder characterized by ingestion of nonfood items or food items consumed in abnormal quantities or forms. Examples of ingested items include starch, peeling paint, paper, soil components, flour, and coffee grounds. Clinical manifestations include zinc and iron deficiencies as well as symptoms of lead or other heavy metal poisoning (see Chapter 17) if these substances are contained in peeling paint or other ingested material. Pica most commonly manifests in pregnancy when women have abnormal cravings for nonfood products, and this can seriously impair the developing fetus. Some children also ingest abnormal amounts of nonfood items and fail to take in adequate nutrients from food. Treatment for children involves removing access to the substances, ensuring an adequate and nutritious diet, and treating any dietary deficiencies noted.

AVOIDANT/RESTRICTIVE FOOD INTAKE DISORDER (FORMERLY CALLED FEEDING DISORDER OF INFANCY AND EARLY CHILDHOOD OR FAILURE TO THRIVE)

Avoidant/restrictive food intake disorder describes a syndrome in which infants or young children fail to eat enough food to meet requirements for nutrition or energy (American Psychiatric Association [APA], 2013). This disorder accounts for 5% to 10% of pediatric hospitalizations in children under 1 year of age, and many more children are managed in community settings (Kliegman, Stanton, St. Geme, et al., 2011).

Etiology and Pathophysiology.   Some disease states can contribute to poor intake, such as congenital AIDS (see Chapter 22), inborn errors of metabolism (see Chapter 30), congenital heart defect (see Chapter 21), neurologic disease (see Chapter 27), and esophageal reflux (see Chapter 25). However, avoidant/restrictive food intake disorder is not attributable to a medical or mental disorder (APA, 2013).

Infants and children whose parents or caretakers experience poverty, depression, substance abuse, intellectual disability, or psychosis are at risk for this disorder. Parents may be socially and emotionally isolated, or may lack knowledge of infant nutritional and nurturing needs. A reciprocal interaction pattern may exist in which the parent does not offer enough food or is not responsive to the infant's hunger cues, and the infant is irritable, not soothed, and does not give clear cues about hunger. Parental neglect is a contributor to the condition. Preterm and small-for-gestational-age babies more commonly have eating disorders (Kliegman et al., 2011).

Clinical Manifestations.   The characteristics of this food intake disorder are persistent failure to eat adequately with no weight gain or with weight loss in an infant or child that is not associated with other medical conditions or mental disorders, and is not caused by lack of or unavailability of food. Weight is generally below the 5th percentile, and weight-for-length is less than 80% of ideal weight (Kliegman et al., 2011). Infants with food intake disorder refuse food, may have erratic sleep patterns, are irritable and difficult to soothe, and are often developmentally delayed (Figure 14–9).

Clinical Therapy.   A thorough history and physical examination are needed to rule out any chronic physical illness. The infant or child may be hospitalized so that healthcare providers can establish a routine for feeding and sleeping. The goals of treatment are to provide adequate caloric and nutritional intake, promote normal growth and development, and assist parents in developing feeding routines and responding to the infant's cues of physical and psychologic hunger. Interprofessional teams that include nutrition teaching, home visits, parenting skills information, and other support are most successful (Cole & Lanham, 2011).

Nursing Management

For the Child With Avoidant/Restrictive Food Intake Disorder

Nursing Assessment and Diagnosis

Nursing assessment of the child is essential for establishing the best intervention plan for a child with food intake disorder. Documenting accurate weight and height each time any child is seen for health care provides an important record of growth patterns over time. This helps identify the child with an eating food intake disorder. The child's activity level, developmental milestones, and interaction patterns provide important information. When feeding the child, observe how the child indicates hunger or satiety, the ability of the child to be soothed, and general interaction patterns such as eye contact, touch, and "cuddliness."

Ask parents about stresses in their lives; these may prevent appropriate interaction with the child. Asking about the pregnancy and birth can elicit information about early disturbances in the child–parent relationship. Are there other children in the family, and, if so, do they have eating problems? Observe the child and parent behaviors while they feed the child; cues given by each person and interactional modes such as rocking, singing, talking, and body postures are important.

Some of the nursing diagnoses pertinent for the young child with an eating food intake disorder include the following (NANDA-I © 2014):

- *Nutrition, Imbalanced: Less than Body Requirements,* related to inability to ingest proper amounts of food
- *Development: Delayed, Risk for,* related to inadequate food intake
- *Growth: Disproportionate, Risk for,* related to inadequate food intake
- *Parenting, Risk for Impaired,* related to lack of knowledge about the child's nutritional needs
- *Fatigue* related to malnutrition

Planning and Implementation

Nursing care focuses on performing a thorough history and physical assessment, observing parent–child interactions during feeding times, and providing necessary teaching to enable parents to respond appropriately to their child's needs. The child is often hospitalized initially and evaluated for potential organic causes while staff members feed the child. Tube feedings may be

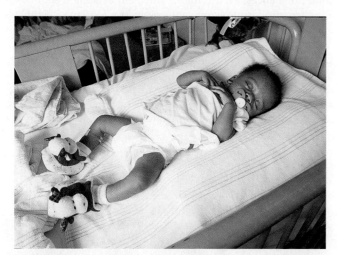

Figure 14–9   Avoidant/restrictive food intake disorder (formerly feeding disorder of infancy and childhood or failure to thrive). Infants with food intake disorder may not look severely malnourished, but they fall well below the expected weight and height norms for their age. This infant, who appears to be about 4 months old, is actually 8 months old. He has been hospitalized for food intake disorder.

needed temporarily until normal intake can be ensured. Accurate weights, nutritional assessments, and developmental evaluation should be done to see if the child grows more normally. Additional diagnostic tests may be carried out at this time to rule out organic causes of poor growth.

Once a diagnosis of nonorganic food intake disorder is confirmed, parents become involved in feeding the child. Observations of feeding and continued careful physical assessments are needed. Carefully record the child's intake at each meal or feeding. Teach parents how to understand and respond to the child's cues of hunger and satiety. Teach them to hold, rock, and touch the infant during feedings and establish eye contact with infants and older children.

Developing Cultural Competence Height and Weight Growth Standards

Each child should maintain a height and weight growth pattern similar to the population standard. Asian American children may normally be below the 5th percentile on growth charts and not have an eating food intake disorder. Suspect a food intake disorder when the infant or child falls 1 standard deviation below the prior achieved growth curve and either fails to gain weight or loses weight over several months.

Upon discharge, referral to an agency that can continue monitoring of the home situation is needed. This provides an opportunity to observe feeding during a home visit and evaluate stresses and behavior patterns among family members. Frequent growth measurement and development must be ensured so the child is adequately nourished. Parents may need referral to community resources to help them manage stressful situations in their lives and to enhance their parenting skills.

Evaluation

Expected outcomes of nursing care include the following:

- Adequate growth and normal development of the infant is achieved.
- An improved parent–child relationship is established.

ANOREXIA NERVOSA

Anorexia nervosa is a potentially life-threatening eating disorder that occurs primarily in teenage girls and young women. An estimated 3% of adolescents in the United States are affected by anorexia nervosa or a related eating disorder, with females affected nearly three times more than males (National Institute of Mental Health [NIMH], 2011). The typical client is White and from a middle-class to upper-middle-class family. Age at onset varies from 8 years onward, with 19 years as the most common age at onset (NIMH, 2011).

Etiology and Pathophysiology. Many causes are believed to contribute to the onset of anorexia. Cultural overemphasis on thinness may contribute to the excessive concern with dieting, body image, and fear of becoming fat that is experienced by many adolescents. Chemical changes have been found in the brain and blood of individuals with anorexia, leading to theories about a biologic cause. Often a significant life stress, loss, or change precedes the onset of anorexia. Stress hormones are commonly elevated in adolescents with anorexia, and immune system function may be disturbed.

Many experts view family issues as contributory to anorexia. Intrafamilial conflicts and dysfunctional family patterns may occur when parents are overly controlling and perfectionistic. The adolescent's eating behaviors may be an attempt to exercise independence and resolve internal psychologic conflicts.

The adolescent may engage in lengthy and vigorous exercise (up to 4 hours daily) to prevent weight gain. Laxatives or diuretics may be used to induce weight loss. As the disorder progresses, the adolescent perceives the ever-thinner body as becoming more beautiful. Youths may share weight loss techniques with friends who are anorectic and search out Internet sites that are positive about anorexia. The body responds to the abnormal eating behaviors as if starvation were occurring. Leukopenia, electrolyte imbalance, and hypoglycemia develop as a result of PEM. Once the body mass decreases below a critical level, menstruation ceases.

The adolescent who has anorexia and becomes pregnant is at risk for disturbances in prenatal care and outcomes as well as potential harm to the baby.

Clinical Manifestations. Adolescents with anorexia are characterized by extreme weight loss accompanied by a preoccupation with weight and food, excessive compulsive exercising, peculiar patterns of eating and handling food, and distorted body image. They may prepare elaborate meals for others but eat only low-calorie foods. Characteristically, the fear of becoming fat does not decrease with continued weight loss. Accompanying signs and symptoms of depression, crying spells, feelings of isolation and loneliness, and suicidal thoughts and feelings are common. The disorder is often associated with mental illness such as obsessive-compulsive disorder, anxiety disorders (see Chapter 28), and history of abuse.

Physical findings include cold intolerance, dizziness, constipation, abdominal discomfort, bloating, irregular menses, and malnutrition (Figure 14–10). Hypothalamic suppression can lead to disturbances of gynecologic function, osteoporosis, decreased bone density, and fractures. Lanugo (fine, downy body hair) may be present. Fluid and electrolyte imbalances, especially potassium imbalances, are common. The child or adolescent is usually energetic despite significant weight loss. Extreme weight loss often leads to cardiac arrhythmias (bradycardia).

Clinical Therapy. Diagnosis is based on a comprehensive history, physical examination revealing characteristic clinical manifestations, and the criteria listed in Table 14–7. Diagnostic tests commonly include hematocrit and hemoglobin, serum electrolytes, and serum vitamins and vitamin precursors.

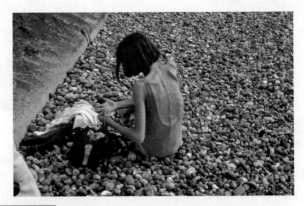

Figure 14–10 Anorexia nervosa. Note the loss of subcutaneous tissue in the back, arms, and pelvis.
SOURCE: Sally and Richard Greenhill/Alamy.

TABLE 14–7 *DSM-5* Diagnostic Criteria for Anorexia Nervosa

A. Restriction of energy intake relative to requirements, leading to a significantly low body weight in the context of age, sex, developmental trajectory, and physical health. *Significantly low weight* is defined as a weight that is less than minimally normal or, for children and adolescents, less than that minimally expected.

B. Intense fear of gaining weight or of becoming fat, or persistent behavior that interferes with weight gain, even though at a significantly low weight.

C. Disturbance in the way in which one's body weight or shape is experienced, undue influence of body weight or shape on self-evaluation, or persistent lack of recognition of the seriousness of the current low body weight.

Specify whether:

- *Restricting type:* During the last 3 months, the individual has not engaged in recurrent episodes of binge eating or purging behavior (i.e., self-induced vomiting or the misuse of laxatives, diuretics, or enemas). This subtype describes presentations in which weight loss is accomplished primarily through dieting, fasting, and/or excessive exercise.
- *Binge-eating/purging type:* During the last 3 months, the individual has engaged in recurrent episodes of binge eating or purging behavior (i.e., self-induced vomiting or the misuse of laxatives, diuretics, or enemas).

Specify if:

- *In partial remission:* After full criteria for anorexia nervosa were previously met, Criterion A (low body weight) has not been met for a sustained period, but either Criterion B (intense fear of gaining weight or becoming fat or behavior that interferes with weight gain) or Criterion C (disturbances in self-perception of weight and shape) is still met.
- *In full remission:* After full criteria for anorexia nervosa were previously met, none of the criteria have been met for a sustained period of time.

Specify current severity:

The minimum level of severity is based, for adults, on current body mass index (BMI) (see below) or, for children and adolescents, on BMI percentile. The ranges below are derived from World Health Organization categories for thinness in adults; for children and adolescents, corresponding BMI percentiles should be used. The level of severity may be increased to reflect clinical symptoms, the degree of functional disability, and the need for supervision.

- *Mild:* BMI $\geq$ 17 kg/m^2
- *Moderate:* BMI 16–16.99 kg/m^2
- *Severe:* BMI 15–15.99 kg/m^2
- *Extreme:* BMI < 15 kg/m^2

Source: Used with permission from American Psychiatric Association. (2013). *The diagnostic and statistical manual of mental disorders* (5th ed.). Washington, DC: Author. Copyright © 2013 American Psychiatric Association.

Bone density examination for females with lengthy amenorrhea is recommended (Mehler, Cleary, & Gaudiani, 2011).

The goals of treatment are to restore a healthy weight, address the psychologic issues associated with the condition, and reduce behaviors that lead to inadequate intake and relapse (NIMH, 2011). A firm focus is placed on reaching a targeted weight with a gradual weight gain of 2 to 3 lb/week in those hospitalized or 0.5 to 1 lb/week in outpatient care (Agency for Healthcare Research and Quality, 2014). Enteral feedings or total parenteral nutrition (TPN) may be necessary to replace lost fluid, protein, and nutrients, although the adolescent often perceives these feedings as a punitive measure.

Individual treatment and family therapy are used to address dysfunctional family patterns and assist the family to accept and deal with the adolescent as an independent and less-than-perfect individual (Brewerton & Costin, 2011; Lock, 2011). Family involvement is crucial to effect a lasting change in the adolescent. Nurses, psychologists, family therapists, and dietitians commonly partner to plan and implement therapy.

Long-term outpatient treatment, in either an individual or a group setting, is frequently necessary. Counseling that engages self-help techniques may be continued for 2 to 3 years to ensure that weight gain and self-image are maintained. Antidepressant drugs such as imipramine (Tofranil) or desipramine (Norpramin) may be prescribed for coexisting conditions such as depression, anxiety, or obsessive-compulsive disorders. However, they are not generally useful in the primary treatment of the disorder (Flament, Bissada, & Spettique, 2011).

Indications for hospitalization include loss of 25% to 30% of body weight or being at 85% or less of healthy weight, fluid and electrolyte imbalances, cardiac arrhythmias, hypotension, or the need to provide a more intense period of therapy if outpatient treatment fails to produce improvement. Behavior modification techniques are used extensively in combination with counseling and other methods in the care of the hospitalized adolescent with anorexia.

Nursing Management

For the Child With Anorexia Nervosa

Nursing Assessment and Diagnosis

Obtain a thorough individual and family history. Ask about usual eating patterns, daily caloric intake, exercise patterns, and menstrual history. Ask about medication use; include prescription, nonprescription, and herbal products. Is there a family history of eating disorders? Assess for signs of malnutrition. Obtain height and weight measurements and compare with norms for the general population. Because the client with anorexia often wears layers of clothes when being weighed, strive to obtain an accurate measurement. Mid–upper arm circumference, skinfold thickness, waist-to-hip ratio, and body composition measurement may all be obtained (Mattar, Godart, Melchior, et al., 2011).

Nursing diagnoses for the adolescent with anorexia nervosa include the following (NANDA-I © 2014):

- *Nutrition, Imbalanced: Less than Body Requirements,* related to inadequate food intake
- *Fluid Volume: Deficient, Risk for,* related to inadequate fluid intake or fluid volume loss from overuse of laxatives and diuretics
- *Body Temperature, Imbalanced, Risk for,* related to excessive weight loss and absence of subcutaneous fat
- *Constipation* related to inadequate food intake and overuse of laxatives
- *Body Image, Disturbed,* related to distorted perception of body size and shape
- *Self-Esteem, Chronic Low,* related to dysfunctional family dynamics
- *Coping: Family, Compromised,* related to parental tendency to be overly controlling and perfectionistic

Planning and Implementation

Nursing care focuses on meeting nutritional and fluid needs, preventing complications, administering medications, supporting psychologic interventions, and providing referral to appropriate resources. Specific treatment measures vary depending on physical complications, length and degree of illness, emotional symptoms accompanying the disorder, and family dynamics. Resistance to treatment is common, and nurses who care for adolescents with anorexia must deal with their own feelings of frustration and anger.

PROVIDE PSYCHOLOGIC SUPPORT

Care for the adolescent with anorexia necessarily includes psychologic support as an important component. The nurse will refer the family to a specialist who can counsel and recommend further treatment. Families of a youth with anorexia should be involved in support groups and should also receive information about the condition and the youth's plan of care. The adolescent is often treated with individual counseling and encouragement to participate is needed. Interventions that improve self-concept and lead to a realistic body image are needed. They may include encouragement for participation in sports, praise for participation in the treatment plan, and immediate referral for relapses as treatment progresses.

MEET NUTRITIONAL AND FLUID NEEDS

Monitor nutritional and fluid intake, encourage consumption of food, and observe eating behaviors at mealtime. Elimination patterns may be altered as a result of increased intake during hospitalization. Monitor for possible problems, including abdominal distention, constipation, or diarrhea. Daily monitoring of serum electrolytes is necessary.

If TPN is administered, watch for complications such as circulatory overload, hyperglycemia, or hypoglycemia. Use strict aseptic technique when changing tubing or dressings.

ADMINISTER MEDICATIONS

Monitor vital signs if the adolescent is receiving antidepressants. Watch for signs of hypertension and tachycardia. Administer medications after meals because it helps to prevent gastric irritation. Be alert for substance abuse. People with anorexia often use excessive laxatives or products such as ephedra (also known as *ma huang*) to induce weight loss. Changes in the central nervous system, vital signs, and other findings may indicate over-the-counter or herbal drug use.

PROVIDE REFERRAL TO APPROPRIATE RESOURCES

Refer parents and other family members to the American Anorexia and Bulimia Association, National Eating Disorders Organization, and National Association of Anorexia Nervosa & Associated Disorders for further information about the disorder and a list of support groups in their area.

Evaluation

Expected outcomes for nursing care include recommended level of weight gain, maintenance of adequate fluid volume and balanced electrolytes, maintenance of normal blood pressure and heart rhythm, beginning of positive sense of self-esteem, intake of nutritionally balanced diet, and use of psychologic counseling to understand the disorder.

BULIMIA NERVOSA

Bulimia nervosa is an eating disorder characterized by **binge eating** (a compulsion to consume large quantities of food in a short period of time). Usually the episodes of bingeing are followed by various methods of weight control (purging), such as self-induced vomiting, large doses of laxatives or diuretics, or a combination of methods. Persons are overly concerned with body shape and weight (APA, 2013). Bulimia affects 1% of the general population, with prevalence in young women about 3 times that in men (NIMH, 2011). Like anorexia, it affects adolescent and young adult females more commonly than males. The disorder usually begins in middle to late adolescence at an average age of 20 years.

Etiology and Pathophysiology. Causes of bulimia nervosa are similar to those of anorexia nervosa: sensitivity to social pressure for thinness, body image difficulties, and long-standing dysfunctional family patterns. Families may be chaotic and distant rather than overinvolved as seen in the person with anorexia. Many individuals with bulimia experience depression. It is not clear whether the depression is a cause or a result of the individual's inability to control the bingeing and purging cycles. An adolescent with bulimia often binges after any stressful event.

Bingeing usually occurs in secret for several hours until the individual is stopped by abdominal discomfort, by another person, or by vomiting. At first, the episodes of binge eating are pleasurable. Immediately following the binge episode, however, feelings of guilt, shame, anger, depression, and fear of loss of control and weight gain arise. As these feelings intensify, the adolescent with bulimia becomes increasingly anxious. This usually initiates the purge behaviors.

Purging eliminates the discomfort from bloating and also prevents weight gain. This relieves the feelings of depression and guilt, but only temporarily. Adolescents with bulimia commonly practice the binge–purge cycle many times a day, losing their ability to respond to normal cues of hunger and satiety.

Clinical Manifestations. Bulimia is often called a "silent" disorder since it is easily concealed from healthcare providers and families. Only about 6% of those with the condition are believed to receive treatment. Adolescents with bulimia are preoccupied with body shape, size, and weight. They may appear overweight or thin and usually report a wide range of average body weight over the years. Physical findings depend on the degree of purging, starvation, dehydration, and electrolyte disturbance. Erosion of tooth enamel, increased dental caries, and gum recession, which result from vomiting of gastric acids, are common findings. Vomiting-induced calluses may be seen on the back of an affected individual's hand. Abdominal distention is often seen. Esophageal tears and esophagitis may also occur.

Clinical Therapy. A comprehensive history is necessary because most adolescents with bulimia appear normal in weight or only slightly underweight. Diagnostic tests include hematocrit, hemoglobin, and serum electrolytes; they may identify signs of altered electrolyte and hematologic status. Lowered potassium levels are related to repetitive vomiting since gastric contents have a high potassium level. The diagnosis is confirmed by the presence of specific criteria (Table 14–8).

Treatment includes management of physiologic problems and cognitive-behavior therapy. Medications, such as fluoxetine 60 mg/day for adolescents, may be prescribed (Hay & Claudino, 2011). Management involves a variety of healthcare providers such as physicians, nurses, and therapists. Behavior modification focuses on modifying the dysfunctional eating patterns and restoring normal patterns. Until the episodes of bingeing and purging are under control, feelings of discouragement and hopelessness prevail. Thus the focus early in treatment is on initiating

TABLE 14–8 *DSM-5* Diagnostic Criteria for Bulimia Nervosa

A. Recurrent episodes of binge eating. An episode of binge eating is characterized by both of the following:
- Eating, in a discrete period of time (e.g., within any 2-hour period), an amount of food that is definitely larger than what most individuals would eat in a similar period of time under similar circumstances.
- A sense of lack of control over eating during the episode (e.g., a feeling that one cannot stop eating or control what or how much one is eating).

B. Recurrent inappropriate compensatory behaviors in order to prevent weight gain, such as self-induced vomiting; misuse of laxatives, diuretics, or other medications; fasting; or excessive exercise.

C. The binge eating and inappropriate compensatory behaviors both occur, on average, at least once a week for 3 months.

D. Self-evaluation is unduly influenced by body shape and weight.

E. The disturbance does not occur exclusively during episodes of anorexia nervosa.

Specify if:
- *In partial remission:* After full criteria for bulimia nervosa were previously met, some, but not all, of the criteria have been met for a sustained period of time.
- *In full remission:* After full criteria for bulimia nervosa were previously met, none of the criteria have been met for a sustained period of time.

Specify current severity:

The minimum level of severity is based on the frequency of inappropriate compensatory behaviors (see below). The level of severity may be increased to reflect other symptoms and the degree of functional disability.
- *Mild:* An average of 1–3 episodes of inappropriate compensatory behaviors per week.
- *Moderate:* An average of 4–7 episodes of inappropriate compensatory behaviors per week.
- *Severe:* An average of 8–13 episodes of inappropriate compensatory behaviors per week.
- *Extreme:* An average of 14 or more episodes of inappropriate compensatory behaviors per week.

Source: Used with permission from American Psychiatric Association. (2013). *The diagnostic and statistical manual of mental disorders* (5th ed.). Washington, DC: Author. Copyright © 2013 American Psychiatric Association.

an immediate behavioral change. Once initial interventions have been successful, group therapy sessions work well for people with anorexia or bulimia. Specific treatment measures may include the following:

- Educating the adolescent about good nutrition (including food choices and caloric content)
- Encouraging the adolescent to keep a log or food journal and assisting the adolescent to make connections between emotional states, stress, and the impulse to binge or purge
- Setting up a daily dietary routine of three meals and three snacks a day (using the same foods for each meal and snack every day to change misconceptions about the weight-gaining potential of certain foods and to decrease anxiety about what food must be eaten at the next meal)

Once these initial measures have been taken, the underlying psychosocial issues are explored. The goals of therapy are to

provide the adolescent with bulimia with adaptive coping skills and to improve self-esteem.

Most adolescents with bulimia do not require hospitalization. Serious abnormalities in fluid and electrolyte levels caused by uncontrollable cycles of bingeing and vomiting, accompanied by depression or suicidal activity, are indications of the need for hospitalization. The prognosis is good with long-term therapy.

Nursing Management
For the Child With Bulimia Nervosa

Nursing Assessment and Diagnosis

Obtain a thorough individual and family history, including daily dietary intake and weight fluctuations. Inquire about problems such as abdominal pain or distention, which may indicate an abnormal eating or elimination pattern. Assess the oral mucosa for signs of damage to tooth enamel caused by purging; examine hands for evidence of vomiting-induced calluses.

Following are nursing diagnoses that may be appropriate for the adolescent with bulimia nervosa (NANDA-I © 2014):

- ***Nutrition, Imbalanced: Less than Body Requirements,*** related to disordered food intake
- ***Fluid Volume, Deficient, Risk for,*** related to fluid volume loss
- ***Tissue Integrity, Impaired,*** related to chemical effects of vomited gastric acids on mucous membranes
- ***Knowledge, Deficient (Adolescent),*** related to health risks of excessive use of laxatives and diuretics
- ***Anxiety*** related to discomfort with weight and eating patterns
- ***Self-Esteem, Chronic Low,*** related to dysfunctional family dynamics
- ***Coping, Ineffective,*** related to life stressors

Planning and Implementation

Nursing care includes monitoring nutritional intake and elimination patterns, preventing complications, and providing appropriate referrals.

During hospitalization the client should keep a food diary. Be alert to the adolescent who hides, gives away, or discards food from the tray or who exits to use the bathroom after meals. The adolescent should be monitored for at least 30 minutes after meals by remaining in a central area in the company of the nurse or other responsible individuals. Withdrawal from laxatives and diuretics is managed with careful observation for alterations in fluid and electrolyte status. Cardiac monitoring may be necessary if potassium levels are seriously altered. Esophageal tearing or esophagitis is treated to promote mucosal healing. Medications such as antidepressants may be administered. Encourage continuation of group and other therapy sessions.

Adolescents with bulimia and their families can be referred to organizations such as those listed earlier in the section on anorexia for assistance and information about the disorder.

Evaluation

Expected outcomes for nursing care for the adolescent with bulimia include healthy mucous membranes and skin, adequate intake of fluids and food, balanced food intake, maintenance of normal weight, adequate support and healthy psychologic balance, and absence of bingeing and purging.

Food Reactions

Food reaction encompasses any adverse reaction to foods or substances ingested in foods. The most common food reaction is **food intolerance**, an abnormal physiologic response to a food that is not immunoglobulin E (IgE)–mediated. Examples include indigestion or flatulence when eating certain foods, a sweating reaction to some spices, rhinitis, and hives with urticaria (Mansoor & Sharma, 2011). See the discussion of lactose intolerance that follows. Milk and grain products are common causes of food intolerance. Chemical additives, antibiotics, preservatives, and food colorings also can cause food-sensitivity reactions.

The most serious type of reaction is **food allergy**, an IgE-mediated reaction that is potentially systemic, characteristically rapid in onset, and may be manifested as swelling of the lips, mouth, uvula or glottis, generalized urticaria, and in severe reactions, anaphylaxis. Food allergies are the most common cause of anaphylaxis and are more prevalent in children with a family history of allergic reactions to various substances and foods (**atopy**). The foods that most commonly cause allergy are fish, shellfish, peanuts, tree nuts, eggs, soy, wheat, corn, strawberries, and cow's milk products. About 0.6% of children have an allergy to peanuts, and the incidence has increased in the past two decades (National Institute of Allergy and Infectious Diseases [NIAID], 2011). A majority of the 150 deaths from food allergies that occur annually in the United States are due to peanut allergy.

Children who have both food allergy and asthma are most at risk of death from anaphylaxis due to a food allergy. Allergic individuals need to be aware of hidden substances in prepared foods. For example, the child allergic to nuts will experience a reaction to a food if nut extracts are used in its preparation. Note that certain foods can cause either allergy or intolerance so accurate diagnosis is needed. An example is cow's milk, which can cause an allergy with IgE-mediated systemic reaction, or an intolerance from gastrointestinal response to milk proteins (diarrhea, vomiting, abdominal pain) as a result of lack of the enzyme lactase in the gastrointestinal tract.

Delayed hypersensitivity reactions are attributed to digestive products of food and require a thorough diet history over several days to identify the offending food. These reactions are more difficult to diagnose, since the reaction can occur up to 24 hours after ingestion of the food. There may also be biphasic reactions that occur 1 to 30 hours after an initial anaphylaxis. Such reactions can be severe and life threatening. Therefore, every child with a food allergy who ingests the allergen should be promptly treated with epinephrine and transported to an emergency facility for further management and monitoring.

Diagnostic tests to identify suspected food allergies include measurement of serum IgE levels, scratch tests, and the **radioallergosorbent test (RAST)**, in which radioimmunoassay measures IgE antibodies to specific allergens. (See Chapter 22 for further information about these tests.) In cases of past allergic response, the food is absolutely avoided. In food intolerance, a diet diary is kept, noting date, type of foods eaten, and reaction, if any. Foods should be eaten singly for several days to determine whether they cause a reaction.

Treatment consists of eliminating the offending foods from the child's diet. Collaborative care involving the child, parents, school, and healthcare providers is needed to ensure that the child with food allergies does not get exposed to the offending allergen, and that all children with food reactions can avoid contact with foods to which they are allergic or intolerant. When the child is exposed to the food, epinephrine should be administered and transport to a treatment center should be immediate. Treatment in the hospital may include additional measures as needed such as bronchodilators, antihistamines, and oxygen therapy (NIAID, 2011).

Nursing Management

Prevention is the first step. Instruct parents of infants to introduce new foods at a rate of not more than one new food every 3 to 5 days. If food intolerance is noted, the causative food can be easily identified. Discuss any changes in diet or preparation of formula. Reassure parents that the child's symptoms will disappear when the offending foods are removed from the diet.

Be alert for skin, respiratory, and other characteristic manifestations of food allergy in children. Immediately call 9-1-1 for care. All such cases should be referred to an allergist for diagnosis. If an allergy is identified, help the family identify and remove the offending foods. Emphasize the importance of reading food labels for hidden foods that can trigger an allergic response. The child, family, school, and other settings should be prepared at all times for immediate response to food allergy.

SAFETY ALERT!

Children with food allergies should wear an alert bracelet and carry emergency medication such as an EpiPen. Nurses in schools and offices must instruct families, schoolteachers, and others about the child's allergy and what to do in case of accidental ingestion of the food product. Assist them to set up prevention and emergency treatment plans.

Refer the family to the Food Allergy Network. Recognize that food allergies can be stressful for children and families, as they worry about exposure in daily life.

The child with food intolerance needs to avoid the food to ensure comfort and an absence of the annoying symptoms associated with it. Although, unlike with an allergic reaction, intolerance is not life threatening, the family needs to learn about hidden sources of the food product so that it can be avoided and alternative foods can be suggested for their use.

Lactose Intolerance

Lactose intolerance is the inability to digest lactose, a disaccharide found in milk and other dairy products. It results from a congenital or acquired deficiency of the enzyme lactase. Congenital lactase deficiency of infancy is a rare disorder. Lactose intolerance is considered a biologic norm, occurring in 50% to 100% of African Americans, Native Americans, Asian Americans, and Hispanics, and only 15% of White Americans (National Dairy Council, 2011).

Abdominal pain, flatulence, and diarrhea occur shortly after birth when the infant is unable to hydrolyze lactose. Diarrhea develops rapidly after the child ingests milk and milk products. Some children are able to tolerate small ingestions of lactose but have symptoms when larger amounts are consumed. Incidence of lactose intolerance increases with advancing age throughout childhood.

Diagnosis is based on a thorough history and a hydrogen breath test, which measures the amount of hydrogen left after fermentation of unabsorbed carbohydrates. Implementing a lactose-free diet for a period of time may eliminate the symptoms, thus confirming the diagnosis. Treatment for infants includes switching to lactose-free formula. For older children, eliminating lactose-containing foods is recommended. Lactase enzyme tablets can be added to milk or sprinkled on foods to aid digestion.

Nursing Management

Nursing care is primarily supportive. Carefully explain dietary modifications to parents and discuss alternative sources of calcium. Discuss the need for supplementation of calcium and vitamin D to prevent deficiencies. Teach families how to read food labels to find hidden sources of lactose. For example, milk solids may be found in breads, cakes, candies, salad dressings, margarine, and processed food. Suggest lactase tablets for children who want to eat some dairy products.

Nutritional Support

Sports Nutrition and Ergogenic Agents

Regular physical activity should be encouraged for all children, with at least 60 minutes of activity recommended daily. However, during vigorous or prolonged exercise, or during hot weather, child and adolescent athletes may have special nutritional needs. A well-balanced diet, reflective of recommended foods, is needed. A wide variety of fresh fruits and vegetables, grains, and complex carbohydrates usually provides for adequate caloric intake. When the child is hungry, extra calories should come from the food groups listed here rather than from increased intake of fat. When the child or teen is very active, sports bars or drinks can provide the additional needed calories in a nutritionally balanced manner. As always, the height, weight, and BMI percentiles are the best assurance that the child is growing adequately over time. Adequate energy to perform the sport as well as be attentive and productive at school and for other activities should also be considered.

Water should be increased during activity both to minimize chance of dehydration and also to maximize performance. About 1 hour before vigorous exercise, the child should drink 1 to 2 glasses (8 to 16 oz) of water and should repeat the same amount of fluid just before the exercise begins. Young children may not feel thirsty and should be encouraged to drink 13 mL/kg during activity and exercise with rest periods every 15 to 20 minutes (Rowland, 2011). Water is usually the best replacement, but during extended exercise, sports drinks may be a good alternative for some of the fluid intake. Frequent or excessive intake of caloric sports drinks and those with caffeine should be discouraged (AAP Committee on Nutrition and the Council on Sports Medicine and Fitness, 2011). Additional water is needed for the first 2 hours after activity. Weight loss of 1 lb indicates a loss of about 1/2 quart of fluid, and weight loss of 1% of body weight can influence performance. The nurse should be sure the child takes in fluid to replace all losses.

Some common nutrients that may be deficient in all teens, but even more often in the athlete, are calcium and iron. The increased blood volume common in the well-conditioned person necessitates greater intake. Calcium-rich foods such as milk products and dark green vegetables, and iron-rich foods such as meats and grains, can guard against deficiencies. While many adolescents believe that they need extra protein during athletic season, most Americans eat adequate protein to meet even the increased needs of sports. On the other hand, the vegetarian child or adolescent may need help to plan a diet with adequate protein.

Many teens take a wide variety of dietary supplements, believing that they act as **ergogenic aids**, or products that enhance performance during sports by influencing energy, alertness, or body composition. Most of the claims of these products are unproven, and their safety has not usually been investigated, especially in the young. Effects on youth whose bodies are still developing are particularly unknown and the risks are high for permanent interference with some normal growth patterns. Offer guidance and help the family and teen investigate claims before choosing to use a product. If youth use supplements, they should be instructed about doses, desired effects, and potential side effects. Some sports and coaches may encourage small size and dieting, or encourage use of dietary supplements to increase weight and muscle. Children and adolescents in activities such as ballet, wrestling, track or running, and horse racing may have health risks associated with inconsistent or inadequate intake.

Approximately 3.2% of U.S. high school students (4.0% of males and 2.2% of females) report taking illegal anabolic steroids; up to 8.8% in some communities report use (CDC, 2014d). These products can have a wide array of side effects. They may stop growth of long bones, lead to endocrine imbalance, and cause increased tendon rupture. They are also illegal in sporting events. Andro and DHEA are steroidal hormones used by some athletes. They can cause masculinization of females, disruption of glucose balance, insulin sensitivity, dyslipidemia, decrease in potential height, bone and joint abnormalities, and aggressive behavior (O'Malley, 2013).

Some common amino acid nutritional supplements include creatine, carnitine, and glutamine. Although the side effects of these substances are minimal, their possible enhancement of performance is temporary and outcomes of long-term use are unknown. Increasing protein intake to meet needs during periods of high activity is a better alternative. Creatine has been studied more than most supplements; it is made by the body and is present in many protein sources. Supplemental creatine increases the creatine level in muscle and may help to increase performance in short bursts of activity, while not affecting endurance sports. The increase in muscle mass that can occur is actually due to water and is lost quickly when the supplement is discontinued.

Minerals such as chromium, iron, and calcium are used by some youths. Ask about the athlete's social group and whether ergogenic aids are used; this is a strong predictor of their adoption and is reason for additional counseling. The nurse should ask careful and sensitive questions such as, "Many athletes take supplements to aid in performance in sports. What supplements do you take or are you considering?" Information should be provided to enhance the youth's understanding of nutrition and sports performance. Generally, a balanced diet with adequate carbohydrate, protein, and fat will meet the needs of most athletes and lead to maximal sport performance. School nurses can work with physical education teachers and coaches to plan appropriate programs for youth to prevent use of ergogenic aids.

Herbs, Probiotics, and Prebiotics

Many families use food products to promote health and treat diseases. These include herbal products that may be acquired from health food stores or the Internet. Herbs are not tested nor regulated by the government, so amounts of ingredients are often not known. Ask families about what herbal products they use regularly or to treat disease. Learn about the herbs and any research that has been conducted with children.

Another type of food product is a **probiotic**, a food supplement containing a live microorganism that alters the balance of gut microflora, thereby providing a health benefit. Common probiotics include *Lactobacillus* and *Bifidobacterium*, which are commonly found in the human gastrointestinal tract, are enhanced by eating yogurt with live cultures, and may be helpful in treating diarrhea or atopic dermatitis. Daily intake of pasteurized yogurt with live cultures can safely be encouraged for children.

A **prebiotic** is a nondigestible food ingredient that can stimulate growth or activity of probiotic bacteria (Mitsuoka, 2014). For example, oligosaccharides enhance proliferation of the beneficial *Bifidobacterium*.

Inquire about the family's treatment of common childhood disorders. Include questions about food and nutritional supplements at all well-child visits. Provide information for the family as needed.

Health-Related Conditions

Many health conditions influence the child's nutritional state. Conversely, the child's nutritional state can influence the state of health. See *Pathophysiology Illustrated* for examples of some common conditions that influence nutritional needs. These conditions are discussed in various chapters throughout the text. Discuss with classmates how to adjust normal nutritional assessment and teaching due to the presence of a healthcare concern. Which conditions influence absorption of nutrients? Which cause changes in nutritional intake requirements? Some children benefit from special dietary aids, such as eating utensils and cups that are easy to grasp. Therapists can evaluate and make recommendations about devices that can assist the child at meals.

Vegetarianism

Some families choose to eat vegetarian diets and can be helped and encouraged in their endeavors. Several variations in intake occur. **Vegetarians** eat no poultry, meat, or fish. **Lacto-ovovegetarians** eat eggs and dairy products, whereas **lactovegetarians** eat dairy products but not eggs. In contrast, **vegans** are strict vegetarians and eat no animal products. When someone says he or she is vegetarian, it is best if the nurse asks specific questions about what the individual will and will not eat.

The vegetarian diet is healthy, easy to follow, and may even provide extra health benefits (Academy of Nutrition and Dietetics, 2013). Some deficiencies may exist; assessment and planning can ensure that they do not develop. Vegans should be sure to include adequate dietary vitamins D and B_{12}, zinc, iron, calories, protein, and fat. Completing a 24-hour diet recall for pregnant or lactating women and vegetarian children, with analysis for RDAs, can be helpful. The nurse should be sure to routinely assess growth and other nutritional measures, as well as provide

ideas of various foods to meet nutritional needs and perform other general nutritional teaching. When a vegetarian child is hospitalized, the nurse should plan with the nutrition department and the child's family to meet intake needs.

Growth and Development

When a pregnant teen follows a vegetarian diet, she needs additional help to encourage adequate nutrition. A 24-hour or 2-day diet diary helps identify nutritional needs. Consider additional pregnancy needs for energy, protein, omega-3 fatty acids, iron, vitamin D, and calcium; note that vitamin B_{12} is recommended as a supplement. Use the vegetarian food guide available through the Academy of Nutrition and Dietetics.

Enteral Therapy

Enteral therapy is a form of nutritional support provided when a child cannot take in enough food orally to sustain health. Since it is the closest form of nutritional support to the natural method of eating, it has the least untoward effects and greatest rate of success. Some children who use enteral therapy are those with cerebral palsy or other neurologic conditions that lead to weakness of the throat and mouth, those with neoplasm or immune dysfunction, and those in acute states of recovery from accidents or illness (Figure 14–11).

Although a tube can be inserted into the nasal opening and placed through the esophagus into the stomach (nasogastric tube),

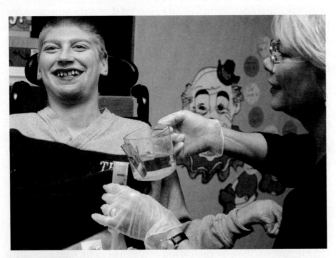

Figure 14–11 Enteral therapy. This child has returned to school following surgery. He has difficulty chewing and swallowing food due to cerebral palsy. The school nurse has taught his teacher how to safely administer some enteral feedings during school hours.

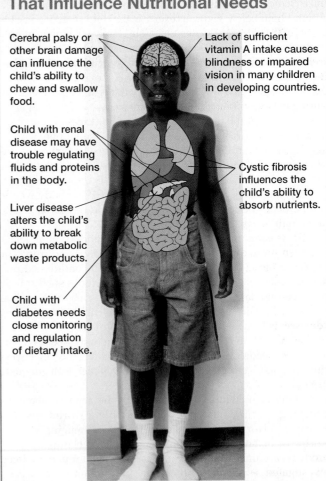

Pathophysiology Illustrated: Conditions That Influence Nutritional Needs

Cerebral palsy or other brain damage can influence the child's ability to chew and swallow food.

Lack of sufficient vitamin A intake causes blindness or impaired vision in many children in developing countries.

Child with renal disease may have trouble regulating fluids and proteins in the body.

Cystic fibrosis influences the child's ability to absorb nutrients.

Liver disease alters the child's ability to break down metabolic waste products.

Child with diabetes needs close monitoring and regulation of dietary intake.

a tube surgically placed into the stomach through an abdominal opening, a jejunal or gastric tube, is preferred for long-term use. As long as the child can absorb and use nutrients, enteral therapy can be successful in providing calories and essential nutrients. Commercially prepared formulas are available, and specially formulated solutions can be adapted for children with specific dietary needs. Nursing care includes care of the gastrostomy tube and entry site to prevent infection and skin breakdown. Ensure that a nasogastric tube is correctly placed before each tube feeding. For both nasogastric and gastric feedings, an empty syringe is often used to check residuals or the amount of fluid not absorbed since the previous feeding. Teach families enteral feeding techniques when they will perform the process at home and arrange for periodic evaluation of technique. Perform regular nutritional assessments. See Chapter 25 for suggestions on management of nursing care during tube feedings. See the accompanying *Clinical Skills Manual* SKILLS.

Total Parenteral Nutrition (TPN)

Total parenteral nutrition (TPN) makes it possible to provide intravenous nutritional support for people who cannot eat or are unable to absorb nutrients from the intestinal tract in a normal manner and are at risk of severe malnutrition. Examples of children who benefit from this method of nutrition are those with congenital malformation of the gastrointestinal tract, brain injury, or severe burns; it may also be used for support after bone marrow transplant, sepsis, or other critical conditions.

A catheter is inserted so that a sterile nutrition solution is infused directly into the bloodstream. A central venous catheter is used to promote safe infusion. Fluids usually contain glucose; electrolytes such as sodium, potassium, calcium, magnesium, phosphate, and chloride; vitamins; and proteins. Lipid emulsions are another type of TPN used in some children. Meticulous care is needed, whether in the hospital or at home, to ensure safe TPN infusion and treatment. The nurse performs initial assessment, ongoing evaluation, and monitoring of treatment; verifies the solution type and rate of administration; ensures that solution storage recommendations are followed; and administers the solutions in the hospital or other settings. See the *Clinical Skills Manual* SKILLS for the protocols for TPN management.

Clinical Reasoning   The Child With Special Nutritional Needs

Joey was diagnosed with cerebral palsy early in life. He is now 11 years old and has recently been enrolled in school. Part of the healthcare plan being implemented in the school involves fostering a positive nutritional state. Joey has limited ability to swallow, related to muscle weakness of cerebral palsy, and is therefore unable to ingest enough calories by mouth to ensure his optimal growth and development. Joey had a feeding tube inserted into his stomach at an early age and receives some of his nutrition by this method.

The school nurse has met with Joey's parents and his home health nurse to learn about the amount and type of tube feedings he receives, as well as the texture of oral feedings he can manage. The nurse will plan the feeding schedule at school to facilitate adequate nutrition in that setting. In addition, careful ongoing nutritional assessment will be needed to evaluate if Joey is getting the calories and other nutrients he needs for growth and development. The school nurse is also educating the classroom teachers and other school personnel about Joey's unique nutritional requirements.

How will you organize Joey's care and educate teachers and other staff if you are the case manager for his integration within the school system?

Chapter Highlights

- Adequate nutritional intake is necessary for the normal growth and development of children.

- Children with medical or psychosocial conditions require additional nutritional support.

- Dietary intake patterns vary throughout childhood. As the child grows, the child is able to metabolize different types of food and gain greater gross and fine motor control.

- Nutritional assessment is an essential part of nursing care and may involve approaches such as growth measurement and intake records.

- Common nutrition concerns in childhood include hunger, overweight, foodborne illness, celiac disease, and dietary deficiencies.

- The child with avoidant/restrictive food intake disorder requires comprehensive assessment and ongoing management to foster parent–child interaction and adequate nutritional intake.

- The most common eating disorders of adolescents are anorexia nervosa and bulimia nervosa.

- A combination of behavioral management, counseling, and medication is often used in treatment programs for eating disorders.

- Food allergy represents a life-threatening condition for children, whereas food intolerance can lead to uncomfortable but non-life-threatening symptoms.

- Children engaging in sports, and those who eat vegetarian diets, may need guidance to meet nutrition needs.

- Some children require alternative feeding methods, such as enteral and parenteral feedings.

Clinical Reasoning in Action

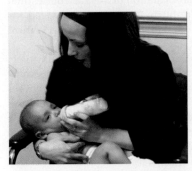

A mother is seeing the pediatric nurse practitioner you are working with for her son Jonathan's 3-month, well-baby checkup at the local community health clinic. The baby is in the 90th percentile for weight and in the 50th percentile for length and is fed Similac formula with iron. According to the medical history, Jonathan had respiratory syncytial virus (RSV) when he was 1 month old and there are smokers in the house (see Chapter 20 for more information on RSV). The nurse practitioner has asked you to educate the mother about feeding her 3-month-old baby. The mother has raised concerns that the baby is not sleeping through the night, and the baby's grandmother has suggested adding cereal to his bottle at night to help him sleep. Jonathan has met all developmental milestones and has not yet developed teeth.

1. What type of advice can you give the mother about adding cereal to the bottle?

2. Why is rice cereal recommended as the first food to introduce when Jonathan is able to start solid foods?

3. What is the reason only iron-fortified formula or breast milk is recommended the entire first year of life for Jonathan rather than cow's milk?

4. Based on Jonathan's length and weight percentiles on the growth chart, his mother wonders if he should be put on a "diet." What would be the appropriate response to her concern?

References

Academy of Nutrition and Dietetics. (2013). *Vegetarianism: The facts*. Retrieved from http://www.eatright.org/Public/content.aspx?id=6442478107&terms=vegetarian%20diet

Ackerman, K. E., & Misra, M. (2011). Bone health and the female athlete triad in adolescent athletes. *Physician Sportsmedicine, 39*, 131–141.

Agency for Healthcare Research and Quality. (2014). *Practice guideline for treatment of persons with eating disorders*. Retrieved from http://www.guideline.gov/content.aspx?id=9318

American Academy of Pediatrics (AAP). (2011). *Fruit juice and your child's diet*. Retrieved from http://www.healthychildren.org

American Academy of Pediatrics (AAP). (2014a). *Switching to solid foods*. Retrieved from http://www.healthychildren.org/English/ages-stages/baby/feeding-nutrition/Pages/Switching-To-Solid-Foods.aspx

American Academy of Pediatrics (AAP). (2014b). *Where we stand: TV viewing time*. Retrieved from http://www.healthychildren.org/English/family-life/Media/Pages/Where-We-Stand-TV-Viewing-Time.aspx

American Academy of Pediatrics (AAP) Committee on Nutrition. (2013). *Pediatric nutrition handbook* (7th ed.). Elk Grove Village, IL: American Academy of Pediatrics.

American Academy of Pediatrics (AAP) Committee on Nutrition and the Council on Sports Medicine and Fitness. (2011). Clinical report—Sports drink and energy drinks for children and adolescents: Are they appropriate? *Pediatrics*. doi:10.1542/peds.2011-0965

American Academy of Pediatrics (AAP) Section on Breastfeeding. (2012). Breastfeeding and the use of human milk. *Pediatrics, 129*, e827–e841.

American Association for Clinical Chemistry. (2014). *The ABC's of pediatric laboratory medicine—R is for Rickets*. Retrieved from https://www.aacc.org/members/divisions/pediatrics/Newsletter/2013/summer2013/Pages/story3.aspx\#

American Association of Pediatric Dentistry. (2014). *Guidelines for fluoride therapy*. Retrieved from http://www.aapd.org/media/PoliciesGuidelines/Gfluoride-therapy.pdf

American Psychiatric Association (APA). (2013). *The diagnostic and statistical manual of mental disorders* (5th ed.) (*DSM-5*). Washington, DC: Author.

Bindler, R. C., Goetz, S., Butkus, S. N., Power, T. G., Ullrich-French, S., & Steele, M. (2012). The process of curriculum development and implementation for an adolescent health project in middle schools. *Journal of School Nursing, 28*, 13–23.

Brei, M. N., & Mudd, S. (2014). Current guidelines for weight loss surgery in adolescents. *Journal of Pediatric Health Care, 28*, 288–294.

Brewerton, T. D., & Costin, C. (2011). Long-term outcome of residential treatment for anorexia nervosa and bulimia nervosa. *Eating Disorders, 19*, 132–144.

Centers for Disease Control and Prevention (CDC). (2011a). *Breastfeeding among U.S. children born 1999–2007* (CDC National Immunization Survey). Retrieved from http://www.cdc.ov/breastfeeding/data/NISdata

Centers for Disease Control and Prevention (CDC). (2011b). *2011 estimates of foodborne illness in the United States*. Retrieved from http://www.cdc.gov/Features/dsFoodborneEstimates

Centers for Disease Control and Prevention (CDC). (2014a). *Childhood obesity facts*. Retrieved from http://www.cdc.gov/obesity/data/childhood.html

Centers for Disease Control and Prevention (CDC). (2014b). *Estimates of foodborne illness in the United States*. Retrieved from http://www.cdc.gov/foodborneburden/index.html

Centers for Disease Control and Prevention (CDC). (2014c). *Trends in foodborne illness in the United States*. Retrieved from http://www.cdc.gov/foodborneburden/trends-in-foodborne-illness.html

Centers for Disease Control and Prevention (CDC). (2014d). Youth risk behavior surveillance—United States, 2013. *Morbidity and Mortality Weekly Report, 63*(SS-4), 1–172.

Children's Defense Fund. (2014). *The state of America's children*. Washington, DC: Author. Retrieved from www.childrensdefense.org/child-research-data-publications/state-of-americas-children/

Cloherty, J. P., Eichenwald, E. C., & Stark, A. R. (2012). *Manual for neonatal care* (7th ed.). Philadelphia, PA: Lippincott Williams & Wilkins.

Colak, H., Dulgergil, C. T., Dalli, M., & Hamidi, M. M. (2013). Early childhood caries updates: A review of causes, diagnoses, and treatments. *Journal of Natural Science, Biology and Medicine, 4*, 29–38.

Cole, S. Z., & Lanham, J. S. (2011). Failure to thrive: An update. *American Family Physician, 83*, 829–834.

Daitch, L., & Epperson, J. N. (2011). Celiac disease. *Clinician Reviews, 21*(4), 49–55.

Du Toit, G., Roberts, G., Sayre, P. H., Bahnson, H. T., Radulovic, S., Santos, A. F., . . . LEAP Study Team. (2015). Randomized trial of peanut consumption in infants at risk for peanut allergy. *New England Journal of Medicine, 372*, 803–813.

Flament, M. F., Bissada, H., & Spettique, W. (2011). Evidence-based pharmacotherapy of eating disorders. *International Journal of Neuropsychopharmacology, 15*, 189–207.

Garcia-Manzanares, A., & Lucendo, A. J. (2011). Nutritional and dietary aspects of celiac disease. *Nutrition in Clinical Practice, 26*, 163–173.

Hay, P. J., & Claudino, A. M. (2011). Clinical psychopharmacology of eating disorders: A research update. *International Journal of Neuropsychopharmacology, 15*, 209–222.

Holt, K., Wooldridge, N., Story, M., & Sofka, D. (2011). *Bright futures nutrition* (3rd ed.). Elk Grove Village, IL: American Academy of Pediatrics.

Institute of Medicine. (2011). *Dietary reference intakes: Calcium and vitamin D*. Washington, DC: National Academies Press.

Kliegman, R. M., Stanton, B., St. Geme, J., Schor, N., & Behrman, R. E. (2011). *Nelson's textbook of pediatrics* (19th ed.). Philadelphia, PA: Elsevier Saunders.

Lawrence, R. A., & Lawrence, R. M. (2011). *Breastfeeding: A guide for the medical profession* (7th ed.). Philadelphia, PA: Mosby.

Lee, R. D., & Nieman, D. C. (2013). *Nutrition assessment* (6th ed.). Boston, MA: McGraw-Hill.

Lock, J. (2011). Evaluation of family treatment models for eating disorders. *Current Opinion in Psychiatry, 24*, 274–279.

Mansoor, D. K., & Sharma, H. P. (2011). Clinical presentations of food allergy. *Pediatric Clinics of North America, 58*, 315–326.

Mattar, L., Godart, N., Melchior, J. C., & Pichard, C. (2011). Anorexia nervosa and nutrition assessment: Contribution of body composition measurements. *Nutrition Research Reviews, 24*, 39–45.

Mehler, P. S., Cleary, B. S., & Gaudiani, J. L. (2011). Osteoporosis in anorexia nervosa. *Eating Disorders, 19*, 194–202.

Mitsuoka, T. (2014). Development of functional foods. *Bioscience of Microbiota, Food and Health, 33*, 117–128.

National Dairy Council. (2011). *Lactose intolerance among different ethnic groups*. Retrieved from http://www.nationaldairycouncil.org/SiteCollectionDocuments/LI%20and%20MinoritesFINALIZED.pdf

National Heart, Lung and Blood Institute. (2013). *Reduce screen time*. Retrieved from http://www.nhlbi.nih.gov/health/educational/wecan/reduce-screen-time/

National Institute of Allergy and Infectious Diseases (NIAID). (2011). *Guidelines for diagnosis and management of food allergy in the United States*. Washington, DC: U.S. Department of Health and Human Services.

National Institute of Arthritis and Musculoskeletal and Skin Diseases. (2012). *Osteoporosis: Peak bone mass in women*. Retrieved from http://www.niams.nih.gov/HealthInfo/Bone/Osteoporosis/bonemass.asp

National Institute of Diabetes and Digestive and Kidney Diseases (NIDDK). (2012). *Celiac disease*. Retrieved from http://digestive.niddk.nih.gov/ddiseases/pubs/celiac

National Institute of Mental Health (NIMH). (2011). *What are eating disorders?* Retrieved from http://www.nimh.nih.gov/health/publications/eating-disorders/index.shtml

National Institutes of Health. (2013). *Calcium*. Retrieved from http://ods.od.nih.gov/factsheets/Calcium-HealthProfessional/

O'Malley, P. A. (2013). The drive to win and never grow old: the risks of anabolic steroid abuse and update for the clinical nurse specialist. *Clinical Nurse Specialist, 27*, 117–120.

Rashid, M., Zarkadas, M., Anca, A., & Limeback, H. (2011). Oral manifestations of celiac disease: A clinical guide for dentists. *Journal of the Canadian Dental Association, 77*, b39.

Ross, A. C., Taylor, C. L., Yaktine, A. L., & Del Valle, H. B. (Eds.). (2011). *Dietary reference intakes for calcium and vitamin D*. Washington, DC: Institute of Medicine.

Rowland, T. (2011). Fluid replacement requirements for child athletes. *Sports Medicine, 41*, 279–288.

Siega-Riz, A. M., El Ghormli, L., Mobley, C., Gillis, B., Stadler, D., Hartstein, J., . . . HEALTHY Study Group. (2011). The effects of the HEALTHY study intervention on middle school student dietary intakes. *International Journal of Behavioral Nutrition and Physical Activity, 8*, 7.

U.S. Department of Agriculture (USDA). (2013a). *Household food security in the United States in 2012*.

Retrieved from www.ers.usda.gov/media/1183204/err-155-report-summary.pdf

U.S. Department of Agriculture (USDA). (2013b). *National school lunch program*. Retrieved from http://www.fns.usda.gov/sites/default/files/NSLP-FactSheet.pdf

U.S. Department of Agriculture (USDA). (2014). *Local school wellness policy*. Retrieved from http://www.fns.usda.gov/tn/local-school-wellness-policy

U.S. Department of Health and Human Services (USDHHS). (2011). *Healthy People 2020*. Retrieved from http://healthypeople.gov/2020/topicsobjectives2020/pdfs/nutritionandweight.pdf

U.S. Department of Health and Human Services (USDHHS). (2015). *U.S. public health service recommendation for fluoride concentration in drinking water for the prevention of dental caries*. Retrieved from http://www.publichealthreports.org/documents/PHS-2015FluorideGuidelines.pdf

U.S. Food and Drug Administration. (2014). *Fish: What pregnant women and parents should know*. Retrieved from http://www.fda.gov/food/foodborneillnesscontaminants/metals/ucm393070.htm

Vaczy, E., Seaman, B., Peterson-Sweeney, K., & Hondorf, C. (2011). Passport to health: An innovative tool to enhance healthy lifestyle choices. *Journal of Pediatric Health Care, 25*, 31–37.

Wagner, C. L., Greer, F. R., Section on Breastfeeding, & Committee on Nutrition (2008). Prevention of rickets and vitamin D deficiency in infants, children, and adolescents. *Pediatrics, 122*, 1142–1152.

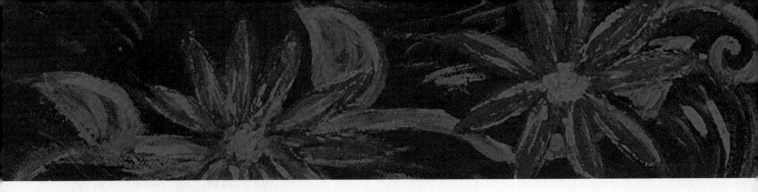

Chapter 15
Pain Assessment and Management in Children

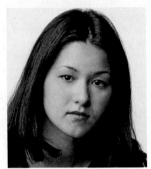

Kevin Peterson/Getty Images

Felicia must be in pain so soon after her surgery. I know I would have pain if it were me. Can she get pain medicine without getting another needle?

—Mother of Felicia, 5 years old

⌄ Learning Outcomes

15.1 Summarize the physiologic and behavioral consequences of pain in infants and children.

15.2 Analyze the behaviors of an infant or a child to assess for pain.

15.3 Assess the developmental abilities of children to perform a self-assessment of pain intensity.

15.4 Plan the nursing care for a child receiving an opioid analgesic.

15.5 Examine the role of nonpharmacologic (complementary) interventions in effective pain management.

15.6 Plan nursing care for a child in acute pain that integrates pharmacologic interventions and developmentally appropriate nonpharmacologic (complementary) therapies.

15.7 Develop a nursing care plan for the child with a chronic painful condition.

15.8 Develop a nursing care plan for assessing and monitoring the child having sedation and analgesia for a medical procedure.

Every child has an individual perception of pain. A neurologic response to tissue injury, **pain** is an unpleasant sensory and emotional experience associated with actual or potential tissue damage. Much of the acute pain infants and children feel associated with medical conditions and procedures can be prevented or greatly relieved. Effective pain management is every child's right.

Pain

Pain may be either acute or chronic. **Acute pain** is sudden, of short duration, and may be associated with a single event, such as surgery, injury, or an acute exacerbation of a condition such as a sickle cell crisis. An immediate pain response occurs at the time of tissue damage, and the inflammatory response that follows causes a sustained pain response that decreases as healing occurs.

Chronic pain is persistent, lasting longer than 3 months, and generally associated with a prolonged disease process such as juvenile idiopathic arthritis or cancer. Chronic pain affects the entire central nervous system, and the child has increased neuron responsiveness to painful and nonpainful stimuli (American Pain Society [APS], 2012). Chronic pain may be nociceptive or neuropathic. **Nociceptive pain** is the normal processing of pain stimuli caused by tissue injury or damage. **Neuropathic pain** is an abnormal processing of pain stimuli by the peripheral or central nervous system. It may be initiated or caused by a primary lesion or dysfunction of the nervous system. Chronic pain is discussed more fully later in this chapter.

Pain transmission to the brain occurs through specialized nerve fibers (see *Pathophysiology Illustrated: Pain Perception*). The pain signal may be modified depending on the presence of other stimuli, either from the brain or from the periphery.

If pain is untreated or poorly treated, neurons become hyperexcited by the N-methyl-D-aspartic acid receptor system, which sensitizes the central nervous system. This leads to initiation of a pain memory and potentially to permanent alterations in pain pathways of young infants that may result in chronic pain syndromes (Rosen & Dower, 2011; Tobias, 2014a).

Misconceptions About Pain in Children

Healthcare professionals once believed that children feel less pain than adults. Undertreatment of pain was based on these attitudes about pain and the difficulty and complexity of pain assessment in children. Healthcare professionals now recognize that infants and children of all ages feel pain, just as adults do. For a review of past myths and the contrasting reality, see Table 15–1.

Developmental Aspects of Pain Perception, Memory, and Response

Although every infant and child perceives pain, their understanding, response to pain, and memory of painful events change as they develop. A number of factors influence the pain perceived by the child, including maturation of the nervous system, the child's developmental stage, and previous pain experiences.

Pathophysiology Illustrated: **Pain Perception**

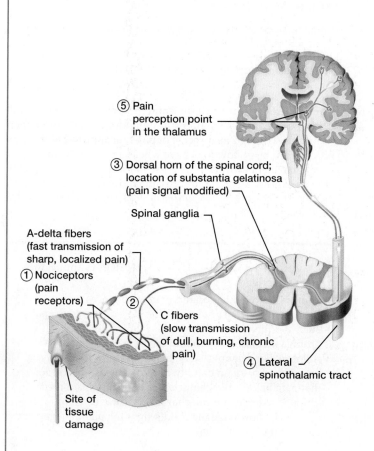

1. Nociceptors (free nerve endings at the site of tissue damage that are able to detect and respond to chemical, mechanical, and thermal stimuli) transmit information via specialized nerve fibers to the spinal cord.

2. Unmyelinated C fibers slowly transmit dull, burning, diffuse pain as well as chronic pain. Large, myelinated A-delta fibers quickly transmit sharp, well-localized pain. Inflammatory mediators (e.g., bradykinin, prostaglandins, leukotrienes, serotonin, and substance P) are produced in response to tissue damage. These substances help move the pain impulse from the nerve endings to the spinal cord.

3. After the sensory information reaches the substantia gelatinosa in the dorsal horn of the spinal cord, the pain signal may be modified depending on the presence of other stimuli. Nonpainful touch, vibration, or pressure at the periphery and endogenous opioids from the brain can interfere with and reduce the transmission of pain to the brain.

4. The pain signal is then transmitted through the lateral spinothalamic tract to the thalamus of the brain where perception occurs.

5. Once the sensation reaches the brain, interpretation of pain occurs, and emotional responses may increase or decrease the intensity of the pain perceived.

Figure labels:
⑤ Pain perception point in the thalamus
③ Dorsal horn of the spinal cord; location of substantia gelatinosa (pain signal modified)
Spinal ganglia
A-delta fibers (fast transmission of sharp, localized pain)
① Nociceptors (pain receptors)
②
C fibers (slow transmission of dull, burning, chronic pain)
④ Lateral spinothalamic tract
Site of tissue damage

TABLE 15–1 Misconceptions About Pain in Infants and Children

MYTH	REALITY
Newborns and infants are incapable of feeling pain. Children do not feel pain with the same intensity as adults because a child's nervous system is immature.	The anatomic, physiologic, and neurochemical structures for pain transmission are well developed at birth, even in preterm infants (Huether, 2014, p. 495). Children feel a similar amount of pain as adults postoperatively (Tobias, 2014a).
Infants are incapable of expressing pain.	Infants express pain with both behavioral and physiologic cues that can be assessed.
Infants and children have no memory of pain.	Children remember painful episodes, fear procedures that cause pain, and may have increased pain responses during future procedures (Fein, Zempsky, Cravero, et al., 2012).
Parents exaggerate or aggravate their child's pain.	Parents know their child and are able to identify behaviors associated with pain.
Children are not in pain if they can be distracted or if they are sleeping.	Children use distraction to cope with pain, but they soon become exhausted when coping with pain and fall asleep.
Repeated experience with pain teaches the child to be more tolerant of pain and cope with it better.	Children who have more experience with pain respond more vigorously to pain. Experience with pain teaches how severe the pain can become.
Children recover more quickly than adults from painful experiences such as surgery.	Children heal quickly from surgery, but they have the same amount of tissue injury and pain from surgery as an adult.
Children tell you if they are in pain. They do not need medication unless they appear to be in pain.	Children may be too young to express pain or afraid to tell anyone other than a parent about the pain. The child may fear treatment for pain will be worse than the pain itself.
Children without obvious physical reasons for pain are not likely to have pain.	The cause of pain cannot always be determined. The feeling of pain is subjective and should be accepted.
Children run the risk of becoming addicted to pain medication when used for pain management.	Children may develop physical dependence and tolerance after prolonged use of opioids for a serious injury, but addiction is uncommon (Galinkin, Koh, & Committee on Drugs and Section on Anesthesiology and Pain Management, 2014).

See Table 15–2 to learn more about the child's understanding of pain as well as the behavioral and verbal responses to pain at each age.

Children's responses to acute or chronic pain are influenced by factors such as memory of a past painful experience, their temperament, their ability to control what will happen, their use of a pain-coping mechanism, and emotions such as fear or anxiety. Pain may be expressed as anger, anxiety, feeding problems, and sleep disturbances (Rosen & Dower, 2011).

Depending on their developmental stage, children use different coping strategies to deal with pain, such as escape, postponement or avoidance, diversion, and imagery. Children may not complain of pain for several reasons:

- Young children cannot give a description of their pain because of a limited vocabulary or few pain experiences.
- Some children believe they need to be brave and not worry their parents.
- Preschoolers and adolescents may assume the nurse knows they have pain.
- Some children are afraid it will hurt more to have the pain treated.

learning greatly influence the child's expression of pain. Children observe family members in pain and try to imitate their responses. Through the process of parental approval and disapproval, they learn how to behave when in pain, how much pain should be tolerated, how much discomfort justifies a complaint, how to express a complaint of pain, and who to approach for pain relief. See *Developing Cultural Competence: Examine Your Own Experience.*

Developing Cultural Competence Examine Your Own Experience

Think about your childhood pain experiences and how your family encouraged you to be stoic or to express pain. Such childhood experiences often contribute to a health professional's attitudes about the pain experienced by children. For example, some healthcare providers may believe that being in pain for a little while is not so bad, that pain helps build character, or that using pain medication is a sign of a weak character. However, all nurses need to acknowledge the child's right to pain management because it is the standard of care.

Cultural Influences on Pain

Pain sensitivity is believed to vary by race and ethnicity, with evidence that Blacks and Latinos perceive greater pain than Whites (Sadhasivam et al., 2012). In addition, culture and social

Many ethnic groups, such as Irish, Japanese, Russian, Amish, and Appalachian, encourage a stoic response with a diminished expression of pain. Other ethnic groups, such as people of Puerto

TABLE 15–2 The Child's Understanding of Pain, Behavioral Responses, and Verbal Descriptions by Developmental Stage

AGE GROUP	UNDERSTANDING OF PAIN	BEHAVIORAL RESPONSE	VERBAL DESCRIPTION
INFANT			
0–6 months	Has no understanding of pain; is responsive to parental anxiety	Generalized body movements, chin quivering, facial grimacing, poor feeding	Cries
6–12 months	Has a pain memory; responsive to parental anxiety	Reflex withdrawal to stimulus, facial grimacing, disturbed sleep, irritability, restlessness	Cries
TODDLER			
1–3 years	Lacks understanding of what causes pain and why it might be experienced	Demonstrates fear of painful situations; may resist with entire body or localized withdrawal; aggressive behavior, disturbed sleep	Cries or wails, cannot describe intensity or type of pain Uses common words for pain such as *owie* and *boo-boo*
PRESCHOOLER			
3–6 years (preoperational)	Pain is a *hurt* Does not relate pain to illness; may relate pain to an injury Often believes pain is punishment or someone else is responsible for the pain Unable to understand why a painful procedure will help them feel better	Active physical resistance, directed aggressive behavior, strikes out physically and verbally when hurt, easily frustrated	Has the language skills to express pain on a sensory level Can identify location and intensity of pain, may deny pain, may believe their pain is obvious to others
SCHOOL-AGE CHILD			
7–9 years (concrete operations)	Understands simple relationships between pain and disease Understands the need for painful procedures to monitor or treat disease May associate pain with feeling bad or angry May recognize psychologic pain related to grief and hurt feelings	Passive resistance, clenches fists, holds body rigidly still, suffers emotional withdrawal, engages in plea bargaining	Can specify location and intensity of pain; can describe physical characteristics of pain in relation to body parts
10–12 years (transitional)	Better understanding of the relationship between an event and pain Has a more complex awareness of physical and psychologic pain, such as moral dilemmas and mental pain	May pretend comfort to project bravery, may regress with stress and anxiety	Able to describe intensity and location with more characteristics, able to describe psychologic pain
ADOLESCENT			
13–18 years (formal operations)	Has a capacity for sophisticated and complex understanding of the causes of physical and mental pain Recognizes that pain has both qualitative and quantitative characteristics Can relate to the pain experienced by others	Wants to behave in a socially acceptable manner, shows a controlled behavioral response May immerse self in an activity as a pain distraction May not complain about pain if given cues that nurses and other healthcare providers believe it should be tolerated	More sophisticated descriptions as experience is gained; may think nurses are in tune with their thoughts, so they do not need to tell the nurse about their pain

TABLE 15–3 Physiologic Consequences of Unrelieved Pain in Children

RESPONSES TO PAIN	POTENTIAL PHYSIOLOGIC CONSEQUENCES
RESPIRATORY CHANGES	
Rapid shallow breathing	Alkalosis
Inadequate lung expansion	Decreased oxygen saturation, atelectasis
Inadequate cough	Retention of secretions, pneumonia
NEUROLOGIC CHANGES	
Increased sympathetic nervous system activity and release of catecholamines	Tachycardia, elevated blood pressure, vasoconstriction, and decreased tissue oxygenation
	Increased intracranial pressure, change in sleep patterns, irritability
METABOLIC CHANGES	
Increased metabolic rate with stress response, increased release of hormones, suppressed release of insulin	Increased fluid and electrolyte losses
	Altered nutritional intake, hyperglycemia
IMMUNE SYSTEM CHANGES	
Depressed immune and inflammatory responses	Increased risk of infection, delayed wound healing
GASTROINTESTINAL CHANGES	
Decreased gastric acid secretions and intestinal motility	Impaired gastrointestinal functioning, nausea, poor nutritional intake, ileus
ALTERED PAIN RESPONSE	
Increased pain sensitivity	Hyperalgesia, decreased pain threshold, exaggerated memory of painful experiences

Source: Data from Greenwald, M. (2010). Analgesia for the pediatric trauma patient: Primum non nocere? *Clinical Pediatric Emergency Medicine, 11*(1), 28–40; Huether, S. E. (2014). Pain, temperature regulation, sleep, and sensory function. In K. L. McCance, S. E. Huether, V. L. Brashers, & N. S. Rote (Eds.), *Pathophysiology: The biologic basis for disease in adults and children* (7th ed.,pp. 481–524). St. Louis, MO: Mosby Elsevier; Clark, L. (2011). Pain management in the pediatric population. *Critical Care Nursing Clinics of North America, 23*, 291–301; Tobias, J. D. (2014a). Acute pain management in infants and children—Part 1: Pain pathways, pain assessment, and outpatient pain management. *Pediatric Annals, 43*(7), e163–e168.

Rican, Jewish, and Arabic heritage, are more likely to use both verbal and nonverbal methods (moans and groans) to express pain freely (Purnell, 2014). However, not all members of a cultural group will demonstrate the same pain response. Children will have individualized responses to pain based on past experiences, and younger children have had less time to acquire culturally learned behaviors.

Consequences of Pain

Unrelieved pain is stressful and has many undesirable physiologic consequences (Table 15–3). For example, the child with acute postoperative pain takes shallow breaths and suppresses coughing to avoid more pain. These self-protective actions increase the potential for respiratory complications. Unrelieved pain may also delay the return of normal gastric and bowel functions and cause a stress ulcer. Anorexia associated with pain may delay the healing process. Pain drains the body of energy resources needed for healing and growth.

Pain Assessment

The goal of pain assessment is to provide accurate information about the location and intensity of pain and its effects on the child's functioning.

Pain History

Parents can provide a great deal of information about the child's response to pain, such as the following:

- How the child typically expresses pain. Children and parents use similar terms to describe pain. Knowing the appropriate word to use makes communicating with the child easier. See *Growth and Development*.

- The child's previous experiences with painful situations and reactions.

- How the child copes with and manages pain. The child with several past pain experiences may not exhibit the same types of stressful behaviors as the child with few pain experiences.

- What works best to reduce the child's pain?

- The parent's and child's preferences for analgesic use and other pain interventions.

Growth and Development

Children slowly acquire words for pain over the first 6 years of life. Toddlers and preschoolers use *ouch, pinch,* and *hurt* to describe pain. Other pain words include *owie, boo-boo, ache, stinging, cutting, burning, itching, hot,* and *tight.* Expressions of pain intensity by young children may include "hurts a lot" or "a really bad hurt" (Rashotte et al., 2013).

Ask older children to give a history of painful procedures. Keep in mind that children may modify their pain descriptions depending on the type of questions asked and what they expect will happen as a result of their response. Examples of questions to ask include the following:

- What kinds of things caused hurt in the past? What made it feel better?

- What do you tell your mother or caregiver when you hurt or are in pain? What do you, your caregiver, or your mother do for the pain?

- What would you like the nurse to do for the hurt? What should the nurse or other caregiver do for your pain?

- Where do you hurt? What does it feel like? What do you think is causing the pain?

Pain Assessment Tools

Various scales and tools are used to assess pain in children. After a pain assessment tool is designed, it must be evaluated for **validity** (accurately measures the concept it was designed to measure) and **reliability** (consistent results are obtained when measured by the same rater or other raters). All of the following pain assessment tools have validity and reliability established.

PAIN BEHAVIOR SCALES FOR NONVERBAL CHILDREN

Physical and behavioral indicators are used to quantify pain in infants and nonverbal children. For example, the Neonatal Infant Pain Scale (NIPS) and the Faces, Legs, Activity, Cry, and Consolability (FLACC) Observational Tool rely on the nurse's observation of the child's behavior (expression, positioning, movement, and crying).

Neonatal Infant Pain Scale (NIPS). The NIPS is designed to measure procedural pain in preterm and full-term newborns up to 6 weeks after birth. The newborn facial expression, cry quality, breathing patterns, arm and leg position, and state of arousal are observed. See Table 15–4.

The Faces, Legs, Activity, Cry, and Consolability (FLACC) Observational Tool. The FLACC scale is designed to measure acute pain in infants and young children following surgery, and it can be used until the child is able to self-report pain with another pain scale. The tool has validity and reliability for evaluation of postoperative pain. See Table 15–5.

Pain Location. Young children (3 years and older) can localize pain if given an outline of the front and back of the body. The child can mark where the pain is located or color the area of pain with crayons. The child should use one color for the place where it hurts the most, and another color for areas with less pain.

ASSESSING CHILDREN WITH INTELLECTUAL DISABILITY

Assessing the pain of a child with severe intellectual disability is challenging. Many children with intellectual disability are able to use simple self-report pain tools. In other cases, behavioral pain assessment tools are appropriate.

The FLACC scale with some modifications can be successfully used by parents and nurses to assess postoperative pain in children with intellectual disability. Before surgery the parent identifies pain behaviors the child displays, such as a specific facial expression, body posture, leg position, and vocalizations to help guide the assessment. These behaviors are added to the descriptors for the scores in each of the FLACC scale categories. This tool has shown good validity and inter-rater reliability for use in this population (Ely et al., 2012).

SELF-REPORT PAIN SCALES

Self-report assessment tools of pain intensity are considered to be the best method of assessing pain in children and adolescents who can use such tools (see the *Clinical Skills Manual* SKILLS). Examples of self-report tools developed for children include the Faces Pain Rating Scale, the Oucher Scale, and the Poker Chip Tool.

TABLE 15–4 Neonatal Infant Pain Scale (NIPS)

CHARACTERISTIC	SCORING CRITERIA
FACIAL EXPRESSION	
0 = Relaxed muscles	• Restful face with neutral expression
1 = Grimace	• Tight facial muscles; furrowed brow, chin, and jaw (*Note:* At low gestational ages, infants may have no facial expression.)
CRY	
0 = No cry	• Quiet, not crying
1 = Whimper	• Mild moaning, intermittent cry
2 = Vigorous cry	• Loud screaming, rising, shrill, and continuous (*Note:* Silent cry may be scored if infant is intubated, as indicated by obvious facial movements.)
BREATHING PATTERNS	
0 = Relaxed	• Relaxed, usual breathing pattern maintained
1 = Change in breathing	• Change in drawing breath; irregular, faster than usual, gagging, or holding breath
ARM MOVEMENTS	
0 = Relaxed/restrained (with soft restraints)	• Relaxed, no muscle rigidity, random movements of arms
1 = Flexed/extended	• Tense, straight arms; rigid; or rapid extension and flexion
LEG MOVEMENTS	
0 = Relaxed/restrained (with soft restraints)	• Relaxed, no muscle rigidity, occasional random movements of legs
1 = Flexed/extended	• Tense, straight legs; rigid; or rapid extension and flexion
STATE OF AROUSAL	
0 = Sleeping/awake	• Quiet, peaceful, sleeping; or alert and settled
1 = Fussy	• Alert and restless or thrashing; fussy

Source: From Lawrence, J., Alcock, D., McGrath, D. P., Kay, J., MacMurray, S. B., & Dulberg, C. (1993). The development of a tool to assess neonatal pain. *Neonatal Network, 12*(6), 61; Taddio, A., Hogan, M. E., Moyer, P., Girgis, A., Gerges, S., Wang, L., & Ipp, M. (2011). Evaluation of the reliability, validity and practicality of 3 measures of acute pain in infants undergoing immunization injections. *Vaccine, 29,* 1390–1394.

TABLE 15–5 FLACC Behavioral Pain Assessment Scale

	SCORING		
CATEGORIES	**0**	**1**	**2**
Face	No particular expression or smile	Occasional grimace or frown; withdrawn, disinterested	Frequent to constant frown, clenched jaw, quivering chin
Legs	Normal position or relaxed	Uneasy, restless, tense	Kicking or legs drawn up
Activity	Lying quietly, normal position, moves easily	Squirming, shifting back and forth, tense	Arched, rigid, or jerking
Cry	No cry (awake or asleep)	Moans or whimpers, occasional complaint	Crying steadily, screams or sobs; frequent complaints
Consolability	Content, relaxed	Reassured by occasional touching, hugging, or being talked to; distractible	Difficult to console or comfort

Instructions: Observe the child for 5 minutes or longer. Observe the legs and body uncovered. Reposition the child or observe activity. Assess body for tenseness and tone. Initiate consoling interventions if needed. Each of the five categories is scored from 0 to 2, resulting in a total score between 0 and 10. A total score of 0 = relaxed and comfortable; 1–3 = mild discomfort; 4–6 = moderate pain; 7–10 = severe discomfort or pain.

Source: Used with permission from Merkel, S. I., Voepel-Lewis, T., Shayevitz, J. R., & Malviya, S. (1997). The FLACC: A behavioral scale for scoring post-operative pain in young children. *Pediatric Nursing,* 23(3), 293–297; Gomez, R. J., Barrowman, N., Elia, S., Manias, E., Royle, J., & Harrison, D. (2013). Establishing intra- and inter-relater agreement of the Faces, Legs, Activity, Cry, Consolability scale for evaluating pain in toddlers during immunization. *Pain Research & Management, 18*(6), e124–e128.

To use pain scales, the child must understand the concept of a little or a lot of pain well enough to tell the nurse and to follow simple directions. Children 2 to 3 years of age can usually understand the concept of "more or less." Only three choices should be offered these children when assessing pain (none, some, a lot). Most children at ages 4 to 5 years can distinguish a larger number from a smaller number or correctly put different sized blocks in largest to smallest order. These children can use a self-report pain rating tool.

Faces Pain Rating Scale. This scale has a series of six or seven cartoonlike faces with expressions from smiling (or neutral) to tearful, depending on the model selected. The Wong-Baker scale is commonly used for children from 3 years through adolescence (Figure 15–1). After explanations about the meaning for each face, the child selects the face that is the closest match to the pain felt. The nurse should not use the tool to compare with the child's facial expression to determine pain level. Older children can use the words associated with the tool to provide a pain rating. The Faces Pain Rating Scale has good validity and reliability for measuring pain intensity (Wood et al., 2011).

Oucher Scale. The Oucher Scale presents a series of six photographs of a child expressing increasing pain intensity in combination with a vertical Visual Analog Scale (Figure 15–2). The tool

has been developed and tested in four cultural groups: White, African American, Hispanic, and Asian.

Poker Chip Tool. This tool uses four checkers or poker chips to quantify acute procedural pain. The child is asked to pick the number of chips that best match the pain felt, with one chip being a little pain and four being the most pain one could have.

School-age children and adolescents have better number concepts and language skills, so additional tools can be used to assess their pain. The nurse should ask the child to describe the pain and give its location. Providing some words such as *sharp, dull, aching, pounding, cold, hot, burning, throbbing, stinging, tingling,* or *cutting* can help children describe their pain.

Numeric Pain Scale. This tool, also called the Visual Analog Scale, is a single 10-cm horizontal or vertical line that has descriptors of pain at each end (no pain, worst possible pain). Marks and numbers are placed at each centimeter on the line. The child marks the amount of pain felt, and the numbers on the line are used to score the pain. Younger school-age children often have less understanding of numbers and directions to use this tool.

Word-Graphic Rating Scale. This tool has words rather than numbers describing increasing pain intensity across a

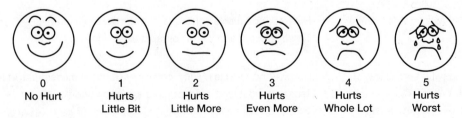

0	1	2	3	4	5
No Hurt	Hurts Little Bit	Hurts Little More	Hurts Even More	Hurts Whole Lot	Hurts Worst

Figure 15–1 Teach the child to use the Faces Pain Rating Scale by pointing to each face and using the words under the picture to describe the amount of pain felt. Then ask the child to select the face that comes closest to the amount of pain felt. Use the number under the selected face to score the pain.

SOURCE: Used with permission from Wong, D. L., & Baker, C. M. (1988). Pain in children: Comparison of assessment scales. *Pediatric Nursing, 14,* 9–16.

10-cm Visual Analog Scale without numbers. The child marks the line that is closest to the level of pain felt. A millimeter ruler can be used to quantify the pain and record the pain score (Figure 15–3).

Adolescent Pediatric Pain Tool. This tool includes a human figure drawing, the Word-Graphic Rating Scale, and a choice of descriptive words—for example, *burning, ache, sharp,* and *dull.* Adolescents indicate pain sites on the human figure

outline, use the Word-Graphic Rating Scale as described, and use the word choices to characterize the pain felt. This tool may be used to assess acute and chronic pain.

Acute Pain

Children experience acute pain related to a variety of illnesses and injuries, surgery, and invasive procedures. Just as with adults, children must have their pain assessed and managed.

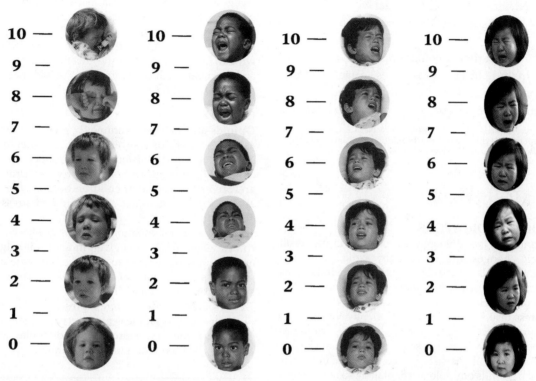

Figure 15–2 Use the Oucher Scale with the best match for the child's ethnicity. Teach the child to use the scale. Point to each photograph and explain that the bottom picture is "no hurt," the second picture is a "little hurt," the third picture is "a little more hurt," and so on until the sixth picture which is the "biggest or most hurt you could ever have." The young child selects a face that matches the level of pain. The numbers beside the photos are used to score the amount of pain the child reports. The older child can select a pain intensity number between 0 and 10. The nurse should not compare the photos with the child's expression to determine a pain level. See http://www.oucher.org for more information.

SOURCE: The White version of the Oucher Scale used with permission from Judith E. Beyer, RN, PhD, 1983. The African American version of the Oucher Scale used with permission from Mary J. Denyes, RN, PhD, and Antonia M. Villarruel, RN, PhD, 1990. The Hispanic version of the Oucher Scale used with permission from Antonia M. Villarruel, RN, PhD, 1990. The Asian version of the Oucher Scale used with permission from C. H. Yeh, RN, PhD, and C. H. Wang, BSN, 2003.

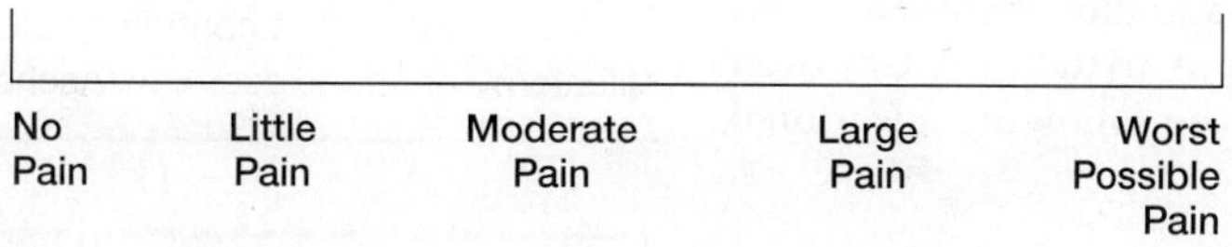

| No Pain | Little Pain | Moderate Pain | Large Pain | Worst Possible Pain |

Figure 15–3 The Word-Graphic Rating Scale has words rather than numbers under the line. Teach the child to use the tool by pointing to the side of the line that is no pain and then to the side that is the worst possible pain. Ask the child to make a mark along the line that matches the amount of pain felt. Use a millimeter ruler to measure from the "no pain" end of the line to the marked location to identify the pain score. Make sure the line is 10 cm each time pain is assessed so comparisons can be made.

SOURCE: Reprinted from Pediatric Nursing, 1997, Volume 23, Number 1, pp. 31–34. Reprinted with permission of the publisher, Jannetti Publications, Inc., East Holly Avenue/Box 56, Pitman, NJ 08071-0056; (856) 256-2300; FAX (856) 589-7463; Website: www.pediatricnursing.net ; For a sample copy of the journal, please contact the publisher.

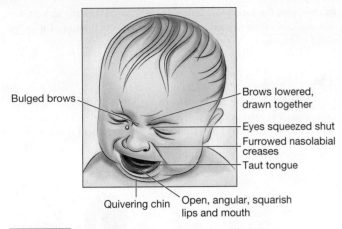

Bulged brows

Brows lowered, drawn together

Eyes squeezed shut

Furrowed nasolabial creases

Taut tongue

Quivering chin

Open, angular, squarish lips and mouth

Figure 15–4 **Characteristic neonatal pain facial expressions include bulged brow, eyes squeezed shut, furrowed nasolabial creases, open lips, pursed lips, stretched mouth, taut tongue, and a quivering chin.**

SOURCE: Adapted from Carlson, K. L., Clement, B. A., & Nash, P. (1996). Neonatal pain: From concept to research questions and the role of the advanced practice nurse. *Journal of Perinatal Neonatal Nursing, 10*(1), 64–71.

Clinical Manifestations

PHYSIOLOGIC INDICATORS

Acute pain stimulates the adrenergic nervous system and results in physiologic changes, including tachycardia, tachypnea, hypertension, pupil dilation, pallor, increased perspiration, and increased secretion of stress hormones such as the catecholamines and cortisol (Huether, 2014). These signs demonstrate a complex stress response. The body adapts physiologically to acute pain; after several minutes, the vital signs return to near normal and perspiration decreases, so these signs cannot be used for monitoring acute pain. Persistent or continuous chronic pain of long duration permits physiologic adaptation, so normal heart rate, respiratory rate, and blood pressure levels are often seen (Huether, 2014).

BEHAVIORAL INDICATORS

Newborns and infants demonstrate knitted brows, squinted eyes with cheeks raised, eyes closed, crying, jerky or flailing movements, and stiff posture in response to pain. See Figure 15–4. A preterm or sick newborn may have a weaker cry, a less expressive face, or not have the energy to make as many body movements as the well infant (Badr, 2013).

Children in acute pain are often distressed and anxious, especially if they have experienced pain previously. Behaviors that could indicate pain or anxiety in infants and toddlers include crying, restlessness or agitation, hyperalertness or vigilance, sleep disturbances, and irritability. Children and adolescents may demonstrate the following additional behaviors:

- Short attention span (child is easily distracted)
- Posturing (guarding a painful joint by avoiding movement), remaining immobile, or protecting the painful area
- Drawing up knees, flexing limbs, massaging affected area
- Lethargy, remaining quiet, or withdrawal
- Sleep disturbances
- Depression and/or aggressive behavior, especially for those who fear that the discomfort will worsen

Clinical Therapy

Acute pain management includes both drug and nondrug measures. Children need adequate pain medication, but complementary therapies can enhance pain management and ultimately reduce the amount of pain medication needed.

ACETAMINOPHEN AND NONSTEROIDAL ANTI-INFLAMMATORY DRUGS

Nonsteroidal anti-inflammatory drugs (NSAIDs) such as ibuprofen, primarily given orally, are effective for the relief of mild to moderate pain and chronic pain. Acetaminophen is a nonnarcotic analgesic and antipyretic that is used like an NSAID; however, it does not have a systemic anti-inflammatory action. NSAIDs are most commonly used for bone, inflammatory, and connective tissue conditions. An NSAID may be prescribed in combination with an opioid to increase the effectiveness of the opioid drug, and potentially reduce the amount of opioids needed. See *Medications Used to Treat: Pain*.

OPIOIDS

Opioids are analgesics commonly given for severe pain, such as after surgery or a severe injury. Opioids (e.g., morphine) are commonly administered by oral, subcutaneous, intramuscular (IM), and intravenous (IV) routes. Oral and IV routes are preferred for use in children because the intramuscular and subcutaneous routes cause pain and stress at the time of administration.

Oral administration of opioids is as effective as IM and IV routes when the drug is given in an **equianalgesic dose** (the amount of drug needed to produce the same analgesic effect regardless of the route used). The optimal analgesic dose is not specific for age or ethnicity of clients. See *Medications Used to Treat: Pain*. Meperidine is rarely prescribed for children because of adverse effects on the central nervous system, including seizures, agitation, and depressed mood (Tobias, 2014b). Codeine must also be used with caution in children.

SAFETY ALERT!
Codeine acquires its analgesic properties with its conversion to morphine by the liver, and it requires metabolism by the CYP2D6 enzyme. About 10% of White people and varying frequencies in other ethnic groups are poor metabolizers and therefore do not receive adequate pain relief from codeine (Pasero & McCaffery, 2011, p. 330). Children of North African, Ethiopian, and Saudi heritage are more likely to be ultrarapid metabolizers and risk a life-threatening overdose, even at recommended dosages (Watt & Arnstein, 2013). Genetic testing is not currently recommended.

After reports of several pediatric deaths and overdoses associated with codeine, the U.S. Food and Drug Administration issued a boxed warning that contraindicates the use of codeine after tonsillectomy or adenoidectomy (Aschenbrenner, 2013).

Clinical Tip
Analgesics were often withheld from children with acute abdominal pain until surgeons could complete an assessment, as it was believed that analgesia would interfere with diagnosis. Studies involving children with appendicitis revealed that giving morphine did not delay the diagnosis or cause complications associated with opioid use (Fein et al., 2012). Be an advocate for pain management in these children.

Medications Used to Treat: Pain

MEDICATION AND ACTION	NURSING MANAGEMENT

Nonopioid Analgesic

Acetaminophen (Tylenol), *Oral, Rectal, IV*

Inhibits prostaglandin synthesis in the central nervous system (CNS) and blocks pain impulse generation in the periphery

- Use for mild or moderate pain.
- Ensure that families avoid liver toxicity by using appropriate dosing.
- Avoid using other medications with acetaminophen as an ingredient.
- Give with food to decrease gastrointestinal (GI) upset.
- Give no more than 5 doses in 24 hours.

Nonsteroidal Anti-Inflammatory Drugs (NSAIDS)

Acetylsalicylic Acid (Aspirin), *Oral, Rectal*

Inhibits prostaglandin synthesis involved in pain synthesis in periphery

Ibuprofen (Motrin), *Oral*

Cyclooxygenases 1 and 2 (COX-1 and COX-2) NSAID inhibitors that block prostaglandin synthesis

Naproxen (Naprosyn, Aleve), *Oral*

Inhibits prostaglandin synthesis by inhibiting COX-1 and COX-2 isoenzymes

Ketorolac (Toradol), *IV, IM*

Inhibits prostaglandin synthesis by decreasing activity of the COX enzyme, which decreases prostaglandin precursors

- Use for short-term management of mild or moderate pain.
- Do not use aspirin in children recovering from chickenpox or influenza because of concern about Reye syndrome.
- Give with food to decrease GI upset.
- Monitor for prolonged bleeding time with extended use.
- Run periodic lab tests for blood counts with differential, serum electrolytes, liver function tests with extended use.
- Monitor for hypersensitivity reaction, especially if child is allergic to aspirin.
- Educate parents about signs of GI bleeding if prescribed for extended use.

Opioids

Morphine Sulfate, *IV, IM, Subq, Oral*

Agonist that binds with mu receptors in the brain and spinal cord to provide analgesia; gold standard for comparison of other analgesics

Hydromorphone (Dilaudid)

Opiate receptor agonist in central nervous system (CNS) leading to changes in pain perception

Levorphanol (Levo-Dromoran)

Synthetic morphine derivative with opiate receptor agonist activity, more potent and longer duration of action than morphine

Methadone (Dolophine), *Oral, IV*

Synthetic narcotic that has increased duration of action with repeated doses

- Use for moderate to severe pain.
- Carefully calculate the dosage to be administered and verify with another nurse.
- Obtain baseline vital signs before administration for future comparison.
- Assess pain regularly for pain relief and duration.
- Carefully monitor for signs of respiratory depression, especially during drug-specific peak action time.
- Anticipate and provide preventive treatment for constipation.
- Monitor for other adverse effects and notify healthcare provider.
- For severe pain, administer every 4 hours or continuously to avoid pain breakthrough.

Fentanyl, *IV, Intranasal, Transmucosal, Transdermal*

Synthetic and potent narcotic agonist that causes analgesia and sedation, short action time

- May be used for sedation and analgesia for painful procedures.
- Monitor vital signs.
- Observe the child for thoracic and skeletal muscle rigidity and weakness that may depress respirations.
- Respiratory depression effect may last 4 hours longer than analgesic effect; be prepared to support ventilations and give naloxone.

(continued)

Medications Used to Treat: Pain (continued)

Oxycodone (Roxicodone), *Oral*

Semisynthetic derivative of an opium agonist that binds with receptors in the CNS to alter the perception of pain and emotional response to pain

- Use for moderate pain.
- Monitor respiratory status for respiratory depression.
- Note adverse effects such as nausea, dizziness, and sedation.
- Determine child's continued need for medication, as the potential for drug abuse is high.

Codeine, *Oral*

Opiate receptor agonist in CNS leading to changes in pain perception

- Use for mild or moderate pain.
- Assess pain regularly for pain relief and duration.
- Observe for nausea, a common side effect.
- See *Safety Alert!*

Source: Data from Taketomo, C. K., Hodding, J. H., & Kraus, D. M. (2014). *Pediatric dosage handbook* (21st ed.). Hudson, OH: American Pharmacists Association; Barnes, S. (2014). Analgesia and sedation. In B. Engorn, & J. Flerlage (Eds.), *The Harriet Lane handbook* (20th ed.). Philadelphia, PA: Elsevier; Wilson, B. A., Shannon, M. T., & Shields, K. M. (2016). *Nurse's drug guide 2016*. Hoboken, NJ: Pearson Education.

Common opioid side effects include sedation, nausea, vomiting, constipation, urinary retention, and itching. These may be treated by rotating the opioids used or with specific therapies as follows:

- *Sedation*—supplement lower opioid dose with nonsedating analgesia or psychostimulant such as methylphenidate (Pasero & McCaffery, 2011, p. 512; Rosen & Dower, 2011)
- *Nausea and vomiting*—antiemetic medication, alternate opioid
- *Constipation*—prophylactic stool softener, a stimulating laxative, and increased fluids and dietary fiber
- *Urinary retention*—place child in bathtub, run water, intermittent catheterization
- *Pruritus*—antihistamine, alternate opioids, or naloxone 0.1 to 0.2 mcg/kg/hr continuous IV infusion (given simultaneously with opioid) (Pasero & McCaffery, 2011, p. 500)

The major life-threatening complication of opioid administration is **respiratory depression** (unresponsiveness and progressively decreasing respiratory rate that may progress to respiratory arrest). Clinical signs that indicate the development of respiratory depression include sleepiness, small pupils, and shallow breathing. Children at higher risk for opioid-induced respiratory depression have an altered level of consciousness, an unstable circulatory status, a history of apnea, a known airway problem such as obstructive sleep apnea, or are receiving another medication that potentiates the CNS effect of the opioid (e.g., benzodiazepines or barbiturates). Starting opioid dosages for these children may be 50% of the recommended dose (Tobias, 2014b). Frequent

visual assessments and cardiorespiratory monitoring or pulse oximetry are important safety guidelines when the infant or child is at increased risk for respiratory depression.

SAFETY ALERT!

Respiratory depression is most likely to occur when the child is sleeping and the tongue may obstruct the airway. Carefully monitor the child's vital signs during the drug-specific peak action time to detect respiratory depression. Monitor the respiratory rate because pulse oximetry does not measure ventilation.

If respiratory depression occurs, naloxone is administered at a rate of 1 to 2 mcg/kg every 1 to 2 minutes to gradually reduce the opioid effects without losing analgesia effects (Tobias, 2014b). Continue to monitor the child for respiratory depression because the half-life of naloxone is shorter than the opioid's half-life.

When given opioids over an extended period of time, children develop **physical dependence**, the physiologic adaptation to an analgesic or sedative drug by the peripheral and central nervous systems that may lead to **withdrawal**, the physical signs and symptoms that occur when a sedative or pain drug is stopped suddenly. Physical dependence is not addiction. **Tolerance** is an adaptation to an opioid dosage that results in a shorter duration of drug effectiveness over time. An increasing dosage is needed to produce the same level of pain relief. For example, a child might develop physical dependence or tolerance after being in an intensive care setting long term with pain management for life-threatening injuries, multiple surgeries, and invasive procedures. See Table 15–6 for signs and symptoms of withdrawal. The child is weaned off

TABLE 15–6 Clinical Manifestations of Opioid or Sedative Withdrawal

SYSTEM	SIGNS AND SYMPTOMS
Central nervous system	Anxiety, irritability, increased wakefulness, tremors, increased muscle tone, inability to concentrate, frequent yawning, sneezing, delirium, visual or auditory hallucinations
Gastrointestinal system	Decreased appetite, nausea, vomiting, diarrhea, uncoordinated suck and swallow
Sympathetic nervous system	Tachycardia, tachypnea, increased blood pressure, nasal stuffiness, lacrimation, sweating, fever, increased salivation

Source: Data from Pasero, C., & McCaffery, M. (2011). *Pain assessment and pharmacologic management*. St. Louis, MO: Mosby Elsevier; Suddaby, E. C., & Josephson, K. (2013). Satisfaction of nurses with the Withdrawal Assessment Tool-1 (WAT-1). *Pediatric Nursing, 39*(5), 238–242, 259; Galinkin, J., Koh, J. L., & Committee on Drugs and Section on Anesthesia and Pain Management. (2014). Recognition and management of iatrogenically induced opioid dependence and withdrawal in children. *Pediatrics, 133*(1), 152–155.

opioids over 2 to 4 weeks to prevent withdrawal symptoms. One plan is to switch the child to oral opioids and reduce the daily dose by 10% over several days. The longer the child has been taking the opioids, the longer the tapering should take.

DRUG ADMINISTRATION

Pain from surgery, major trauma, acute episodes such as vaso-occlusive crisis, or cancer is present for predictable periods because of the effects of tissue damage. Pain relief should be provided around the clock. Every effort should be made to give the child analgesics without causing more pain. The preferred routes of administration are intravenous, local nerve block, and oral.

Continuous infusion analgesia is recommended for children with persistent severe pain, as it keeps blood levels constant. Analgesics may also be given intravenously on a scheduled basis (e.g., every 3 to 4 hours). Delays in analgesia administration increase the chances of **breakthrough pain** (pain that emerges as the pain medication wears off, resulting in the loss of pain control) and the subsequent anticipation of pain. Giving analgesics on an as-needed (PRN) basis for acute pain results in the loss of pain control. More medication is often needed to restore pain control than would have been required with continuous infusion analgesia.

Patient-Controlled Analgesia.

Patient-controlled analgesia (PCA) is a method of administering an intravenous analgesic, such as morphine, using a computerized pump programmed by the health-care professional and controlled by the child (see the *Clinical Skills Manual* SKILLS). After pain control has been achieved with a continuous IV infusion of morphine (basal dose) by the nurse, the child presses a button to receive a smaller analgesic dose (bolus dose) for episodic pain relief. This method of pain management is especially useful for pain control in the first 48 hours after surgery or until oral pain management is possible. Safety features to prevent overdoses include the ability to set the maximum number of bolus infusions per hour and the maximum amount of drug received in a specific time period. Once oral analgesics can be taken, PCA is discontinued.

Pain-controlled analgesia is prescribed mostly for children age 6 years and older, but may be offered to children as young as 5 years. The child should be able to self-report pain with a pain scale and understand that pushing the button will give them medication to relieve pain. See *Families Want to Know: Patient-Controlled Analgesia (PCA)*. Nurse-controlled analgesia, with the nurse taking responsibility for bolus infusions, is sometimes provided for younger children or those with cognitive impairments.

The nurse must assess pain before pushing the device button to reduce risks for adverse events.

SAFETY ALERT!

Pain-controlled analgesia by proxy, such as giving a parent permission to push the PCA button, has been used for some children with disabilities or too young to be responsible. Many facilities no longer permit parents to administer PCA to their child. If permitted, parents must be taught to follow guidelines for pain assessment and PCA use, and adherence to guidelines must be monitored to reduce the risk for an adverse event associated with too much medication.

REGIONAL PAIN MANAGEMENT

Epidural pain control provides selective analgesia for a body region, and it has become more common for postoperative pain management. A catheter is inserted into the epidural space during general anesthesia through which anesthetics and opioids may be administered in small doses. Analgesia may be administered by intermittent bolus, continuous infusion by a small pump, or PCA to maintain pain control for the first 24 to 48 hours after surgery. Urinary retention may be a complication and a urinary catheter may be required for the duration of epidural pain management. Monitor vital signs, pain level, and degree of motor and sensory block.

Regional nerve blocks, such as a popliteal or femoral for the lower extremity, or interscalene (in a muscle of the cervical vertebrae) for the upper extremity, are used for anesthesia and to control pain after surgery. A subcutaneous catheter is inserted into the local area for infusion of the medications. The single dose administered during surgery may last up to 15 hours postoperatively (Guarin, 2013). A continuous infusion may also be given using a pump.

Clinical Tip

Assess the extremity receiving the local nerve block for color, temperature, and capillary refill. Assess motor function by asking children if they can move their legs, wiggle their toes, and lift their buttocks off the bed. Ensure proper positioning of the extremity to prevent nerve damage. Protect the extremity from injury because the child has reduced feeling in the limb. Monitor the child every 2 hours for tingling felt in the fingers or toes of the affected extremity, the first sign that the nerve block is receding. Effective oral analgesia should be initiated to maintain pain control when the nerve block begins to recede.

Families Want to Know

Patient-Controlled Analgesia (PCA)

- What is PCA? *Analgesia* means pain relief: You get to control the amount of medicine you receive by using the PCA machine.

- The machine gives the medicine by passing it through the tube that is connected to your IV line. When you push the button, the machine pumps pain medicine into the IV line to make you feel better.

- The machine limits the amount of medicine you can get to what the healthcare provider prescribes. You can get any amount up to the maximum hourly limit by pushing the button at times during the hour. The push button will not let you make a mistake if you drop it or roll on it.

- Whenever you feel pain, hurt, or discomfort, push the button to get more medicine. You should be the only one to push the button. Do not let another family member push the button.

- No needles for pain shots are needed as long as the IV line is in place.

- The PCA may not relieve all your pain, but it should make you feel comfortable. Let the nurse know if you think your PCA is not working.

- The PCA will be used until you can take pain medicine by mouth.

Nonpharmacologic Methods of Pain Management

Complementary therapies are nonpharmacologic methods used for pain management that can enhance the effect of analgesics and potentially reduce the amount of analgesics needed. One or more of these methods may provide adequate pain relief when the child has low levels of pain.

DISTRACTION

Distraction involves engaging a child in a pleasant activity to help focus attention on something other than pain and the anxiety. Teach the parent to be a distraction coach and suggest developmentally appropriate distraction activities to use. Examples of distraction activities are provided in *Growth and Development: Distraction Activities* later in the chapter. Note that children in severe pain cannot be distracted; do not assume that pain is gone if a child can be distracted.

GUIDED IMAGERY

Imagery is a cognitive behavioral process that encourages the child to relax (often with progressive muscle relaxation techniques) and focus on vivid mental images as if they were real, and to ignore things, such as a painful procedure. For example, help the child visualize and explore a favorite place, do a fun activity, remember a funny story, or be a superhero. Ask the child to think about all the sights, sounds, smells, tastes, and feelings that will enhance the image and experience. Imagery has been used successfully by school-age children to reduce the pain associated with sickle cell disease (Dobson & Byrne, 2014).

RELAXATION TECHNIQUES

Progressive muscle relaxation is used to reduce muscle tension that may worsen pain. Teach children to tense and relax different muscle groups, starting with the hands and feet, and then moving to more central muscles. Ask the child to tense a muscle group for 10 seconds and notice how it feels, and then ask the child to relax the muscle group for 10 seconds and compare the feelings. With practice, the child should be able to detect the difference between tense and relaxed muscles and then to reduce the tension. Relaxation techniques may be combined with rhythmic breathing.

BREATHING TECHNIQUES

Rhythmic deep breaths can be used with distraction or muscle relaxation during a painful procedure or as a mechanism to reduce stress. Ask the child or adolescent to take a deep breath, hold it for 5 seconds, and blow out through the mouth, as if to push the tension out or the needle away. Another breathing technique is patterned, shallow breathing. The young child is encouraged to take shallow breaths in through the nose and blow out through the mouth while thinking of a particular image. For example, the short breaths could be the "toot, toot" of a train horn.

CUTANEOUS STIMULATION

Gently rub the painful area, massage the skin gently, and hold or rock the child. Touching competes with the pain stimuli that are transmitted from the peripheral nerves to the spinal cord and brain and may reduce the pain felt by the child. Swaddling and skin-to-skin contact are methods to reduce neonatal pain responses.

HYPNOSIS

Hypnosis is an altered state of awareness facilitating heightened concentration, decreased awareness of external stimuli, increased relaxation, and increased suggestibility. The hypnotic or positive therapeutic suggestion often uses muscle relaxation and guided imagery, and posthypnotic suggestions are given for the relief of anxiety, tension, and pain. Children more easily respond to hypnosis than adults because of their imaginative powers for fun and fantasy. Hypnosis has been successful in helping children and adolescents manage the stress and pain associated with invasive medical procedures and chronic pain such as daily headaches and surgery (Kohen, 2011; Martin, Smith, Newcomb, et al., 2014).

SUCROSE SOLUTION

A sucrose solution (2 mL of 24% solution) is effective for pain relief during painful procedures (venipuncture, heel sticks, cannulation) in preterm and term newborns up to 1 month of age (Cooper & Petty, 2012). The sweet taste is believed to activate the endogenous opioid pathways, leading to the release of endogenous opioids. The effectiveness of sucrose solution beyond 4 weeks of age for immunizations has not been consistently demonstrated in research (Wilson, Bremmer, Mathews, et al., 2013). Give the solution 2 minutes before the procedure, and the analgesic effect of sucrose lasts approximately 3 to 5 minutes. Allow the infant to continue sucking on a pacifier or to breastfeed during the procedure to enhance the effect of sucrose.

APPLICATION OF HEAT AND COLD

Heat application promotes dilation of blood vessels. The increased blood circulation permits the removal of cell breakdown debris from the site. Heat also promotes muscle relaxation, breaking the pain–spasm–pain cycle. To reduce edema, do not apply heat in the first 24 hours after an injury.

The application of cold is believed to slow the ability of pain fibers to transmit pain impulses to help control pain. Apply ice for 20 to 30 minutes and then remove for about 10 minutes before continuing therapy. Assess the skin for redness or signs of irritation. Discontinue cold applications immediately if the skin alternately blanches and reddens afterwards.

ELECTROANALGESIA

Also known as transcutaneous electrical nerve stimulation (TENS), **electroanalgesia** delivers small amounts of electrical stimulation to the skin by electrodes. This electronic stimulation is stronger than the pain impulses and is thought to interfere with the transmission of pain impulses from the peripheral nerves to the spinal cord and brain. TENS may be used for both acute and chronic pain management. The only known side effect is skin irritation at the electrode site.

ACUPUNCTURE

A traditional Chinese treatment for pain relief, acupuncture has been gaining greater acceptance in Western medicine. Acupuncture is based on the theory that energy, or *chi*, flows along channels through the body (meridians) that are connected by acupuncture points. Placement of acupuncture needles at specific pain points interferes with the transmission of pain impulses to the brain, and it also stimulates the release of endogenous opioids (Chon & Lee, 2013). Limited research has been conducted about the use and effectiveness of acupuncture in children.

Nursing Management

For the Child With Acute Pain

Nursing Assessment and Diagnosis

Nurses have an ethical obligation to relieve a child's suffering. Unrelieved pain has consequences, and appropriate pain management may have benefits such as earlier mobilization, shortened hospital stays, and reduced costs. Anticipate the presence of pain and recognize the child's right to pain control.

Professionalism in Practice Pain Management

In 2001, the Joint Commission introduced standards for the assessment and management of pain in clients treated in healthcare facilities. Nurses have a responsibility to assess a child's pain during their initial assessment and as appropriate during subsequent care. Pain management should be provided, and children and parents should be educated about managing pain (Joint Commission, 2014).

When assessing pain in children, keep the following questions in mind:

- What is happening in tissues that might cause pain? Assume that children who have had surgery, injury, a vaso-occlusive episode, or illness are experiencing pain since these events also cause pain in adults.
- What external factors could be causing pain? For example, is the cast too tight or is the child poorly positioned in bed?
- Are there any indicators of pain, either physiologic or behavioral?
- How is the child responding emotionally?
- How does the child or parent rate the pain?

Physiologic symptoms such as nausea, fatigue, dyspnea, bladder and bowel distention, and fever may influence the intensity of pain felt by a child. The child's behavior or responses to pain stimuli may also be affected by fear, anxiety, separation from parents, anger, culture, age, or a previous pain experience.

When working with an infant or child, determine which pain scale is the most appropriate for the circumstance and developmental stage. When using a self-report pain assessment tool, *use the same tool each time* you assess for pain or for the evaluation of pain management. This makes comparison of assessment results possible. A chronologic record of the child's pain assessments must be documented along with actions taken to relieve pain in addition to the follow-up assessments to determine the effectiveness of those actions.

Remember that surgery and trauma can result in multiple sites of pain (incision or laceration, cut or bruised muscles, interrupted blood supply, nasogastric tube placement, insertion sites of IV lines). Attempt to evaluate the intensity of pain at each site.

Examples of nursing diagnoses for children in pain include the following (NANDA-I © 2014):

- *Pain, Acute,* related to injury and femur fracture
- *Anxiety* related to anticipation of pain from an invasive procedure
- *Mobility: Physical, Impaired,* related to pain
- *Nausea* related to opioids used for pain medication

Other nursing diagnoses are included in *Nursing Care Plan: The Child With Postoperative Pain.*

Planning and Implementation

Nursing management involves the following actions to increase and maintain client comfort: pharmacologic intervention; complementary therapy; monitoring, evaluating, and documenting the

---

Nursing Care Plan: The Child With Postoperative Pain

1. Nursing Diagnosis: *Pain, Acute (severe abdominal),* related to surgery and injury (NANDA-I © 2014)

GOAL: The child will report relief.

INTERVENTION	RATIONALE
• Have the child select a pain scale and rate the amount of pain perceived before and 30–60 minutes after analgesia is given to ensure pain relief.	• The child's pain rating is the best indicator of pain. Maintenance of pain control requires less analgesia than treating each acute pain episode.
• Assess pain control each hour to ensure that the child's pain is relieved.	• Frequent monitoring identifies inadequate pain control before it becomes significant.
• Reposition the child every 2 hours to maintain good body alignment.	• New positions decrease muscle cramping and skin pressure.
• Provide therapeutic touch or massage. Encourage the parents to read a story or play favorite music.	• Complementary therapy reduces stress and enhances the analgesic action.

EXPECTED OUTCOME: Child will report pain relief after administration of analgesia, respositioning, and complementary therapy, as indicated by a lower level on the pain scale.

2. Nursing Diagnosis: *Sleep Pattern, Disturbed,* related to inadequate pain control (NANDA-I © 2014)

GOAL: The child will experience fewer disruptions of sleep by pain.

INTERVENTION	RATIONALE
• Give analgesia by continuous infusion or every 3–4 hours around the clock.	• Pain breakthrough occurs even during sleep and disturbs its healing effects.

EXPECTED OUTCOME: Child will sleep for age-appropriate number of hours per day, undisturbed by pain.

(continued)

Nursing Care Plan: The Child With Postoperative Pain (*continued*)

3. Nursing Diagnosis: *Health Management, Readiness for Enhanced,* **related to self-management of pain control and use of nonpharmacologic pain-control measures (NANDA-I © 2014)**

GOAL: The child and family will effectively use patient-controlled analgesia (PCA) and complementary therapy pain-control measures.

INTERVENTION	RATIONALE
• Teach the child how the PCA works and when to push the button.	• The child must know that pain can be relieved by pushing the PCA button and how the button works.
• Teach the family and the child how to use age-appropriate complementary therapies for pain management.	• Complementary therapy pain-control measures may reduce the amount of analgesia needed.

EXPECTED OUTCOME: Child's pain rating will stay low. Child and family will independently use complementary therapies for pain control.

GOAL: The child and family will use appropriate analgesia after discharge.

INTERVENTION	RATIONALE
• Explain why managing pain is helpful for the child's healing.	• The family and child may not know the benefits of relieving pain.
• Discuss how to assess the child's pain and ways to manage it at home after discharge.	• The family and child may be anxious about pain management at home.

EXPECTED OUTCOME: Family will understand pain assessment and pain-relief measures and state appropriate dose and frequency for pain medication use at home.

4. Nursing Diagnosis: *Breathing Pattern, Ineffective,* **related to opioid overdose (NANDA-I © 2014)**

GOAL: The child will maintain adequate ventilations.

INTERVENTION	RATIONALE
• Verify that correct opioid dose is given for the child's weight.	• Respiratory depression is a significant complication when too much opioid medication is given.
• Monitor vital signs and depth of respirations before analgesic is administered and at time of peak drug action. Withhold opioid if vital signs fall within parameters set by the healthcare provider or policy.	• A respiratory depression episode must be identified before it progresses to respiratory arrest. All opioids act on brainstem center, which decreases responsiveness to CO_2 tension.
• Calculate agonist dose prescribed by healthcare provider to be sure it will reverse respiratory depression, but not counteract effect of analgesia.	• Valuable time will be saved if agonist is needed to treat respiratory depression. Complete reversal of analgesia will cause the child to have significant pain.

EXPECTED OUTCOME: Child will not have episodes of respiratory depression associated with analgesia.

5. Nursing Diagnosis: *Constipation, Risk for,* **related to opioid administration and decreased motility of gastrointestinal tract (NANDA-I © 2014)**

GOAL: The child will have minimal constipation.

INTERVENTION	RATIONALE
• Assess bowel sounds and abdominal distention, and palpate the abdomen.	• Signs of constipation must be anticipated and identified.
• Request healthcare provider order for stimulating laxative and stool softener.	• Opioids increase the transit time of feces and interfere with bile enzymes needed for evacuation.
• Provide fluids of choice to increase fluid intake when IV fluids are decreased.	• Extra fluids will counteract opioid action of increasing the absorption of water from the large intestine.
• Inform family and child that constipation is a side effect of pain medication.	• Parents can become partners in increasing fluid intake and monitoring bowel movements.

EXPECTED OUTCOME: Child will have bowel movements at least every 2 days while on opioid pain control.

EVIDENCE-BASED PRACTICE | Challenges to Adequate Pain Management

Clinical Question

Why does adequate management of children with acute pain continue to be a problem despite the increased knowledge about children's needs for pain relief?

The Evidence

A children's hospital committed to pain management conducted a survey of nurses ($n = 272$) to rate 18 potential barriers to optimal pain management. The five leading barriers identified were inadequate healthcare provider orders, insufficient premedication orders before procedures, insufficient time allowed to premedicate before procedures, low priority given to pain management by medical staff, and parents' reluctance to have children receive medication (Czarnecki et al., 2011).

After implementation of some quality improvement projects related to the identified barriers to optimal pain management, a follow-up survey using the same questions was conducted with nurses ($n = 442$) in the same hospital. Consistency in barriers perceived by nurses was found for four of the five leading barriers. Insufficient time allowed to premedicate before procedures was less of a barrier, perhaps due to development of a hospitalwide procedure guideline. A significant decrease in perceptions related to the barriers of inadequate healthcare provider orders and insufficient premedication orders before procedures was found, both also having been the focus of quality improvement efforts. A new barrier was identified related to the time taken to process and deliver pain medications from pharmacy (Czarnecki, Salamon, Thompson, et al., 2014). Findings revealed that more work is needed.

Thirty nurses working in a general hospital participated in focus groups to identify their perceptions about barriers and facilitators to pediatric pain management and the effectiveness of the facility's 3-year-old pediatric pain practice guideline. One nursing barrier related to knowledge deficiencies about pain management and analgesics and the potential of overdosing a child. The nurses expressed an expectation that parents and children inform them when in pain rather than being proactive in assessing for pain, and they were concerned about parents requesting pain medication when the child's behavior did not reflect pain. It was not evident that all nurses knew about or used the pain practice guideline since participating nurses requested pediatric pain assessment tools and a pain medication flow chart that was part of the practice guideline (Twycross & Collins, 2013).

Best Practice

Pain management is a complex process that requires the nurse to assess the child and make clinical judgments about treatment. The expectations that children must display pain behaviors to have their pain believed or that pain assessment and management is a low nursing priority are ongoing concerns. The facility's structure and culture also have an important influence on pain management. The Czarnecki studies focused on organizational contributors to pain management and efforts to change the system. Findings revealed some improvements but illustrate the challenges of making systemwide improvements, even in a pediatric hospital. System changes to improve pain management require collaboration among healthcare providers and the development of practice guidelines. Hospitals then need to educate healthcare providers about the care expectations in the practice guidelines and evaluate how well they are implemented. Nurses must take responsibility for learning and consistently using the guidelines.

Clinical Reasoning

In the clinical setting, identify the infrastructure supports to promote pain management of children, such as pain assessment tools, pain flow sheets, pain management policies and guidelines, education, and resources for complementary therapies. Identify additional supports that would help you as an inexperienced nurse to gain competence in pediatric pain management.

---

effectiveness of pain-control measures to provide optimal comfort; and client education. See *Evidence-Based Practice: Challenges to Adequate Pain Management.*

PHARMACOLOGIC INTERVENTION

Give analgesics as ordered by the healthcare provider, ensuring that the dose is appropriate for the child's weight. When administering an opioid by intravenous infusion or PCA, monitor the flow rate and the site for infiltration. Follow facility guidelines for monitoring vital signs, and use a pulse oximeter or cardiorespiratory monitor with audible alarm for children at risk for respiratory depression. Vital signs (heart rate and blood pressure) may not change in response to effective analgesia when infection, trauma, or other stressors keep them elevated. Make sure that naloxone is available in case adverse effects develop. The dose should be precalculated and the medication immediately available when an opioid is used.

Check for the presence of other side effects of analgesics, such as sedation, nausea, vomiting, itching, urinary retention, and constipation. An alternative opioid or medications to treat the side effects may be prescribed when analgesia is needed long term.

Oral NSAIDs, sometimes in combination with an opioid, are generally ordered for less severe pain or chronic pain. These drugs may mask fever. Be alert to the potential complication of gastrointestinal hemorrhage in critically ill children who have increased gastric acids as a physiologic stress response to pain.

Assess the child for pain using a behavioral or self-report pain scale 15 to 30 minutes following intravenous pain medication and 1 hour after oral pain medication to determine if adequate pain control was achieved. Evaluate the child's level of pain frequently to identify any increase in pain intensity. Use information collected from the child and parent. Dramatic reductions in pain should occur, although not all pain may disappear. Be certain to record results of pain-control measures to guide future nursing actions. Use a flow sheet to document assessments, medication administration, complementary therapies, and other comfort measures during the postoperative period.

Many children sleep after receiving an analgesic. This sleep is not a side effect of the drug or a sign of an overdose, but the result of pain relief. Pain interrupts sleep, and once pain is relieved, the child can sleep comfortably. However, sleep does not always indicate pain control. A child in pain may fall asleep in exhaustion. Look for other symptoms of pain, such as excess movement or moaning.

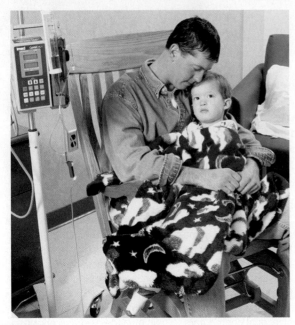

Figure 15–5 **The presence of the parent is an important part of pain management. Children often feel more secure telling their parents about their pain and anxiety.**

Become an advocate for the child when the dose or type of analgesic ordered is inadequate. When the child with severe pain has been taking opioids for several days, tolerance may occur and an increasing amount of the opioid may be needed to produce or maintain the same level of pain relief. The duration of effective analgesia becomes shorter than expected, and breakthrough pain occurs. Review the child's record to verify that the opioid was given at the appropriate dose and frequency before asking the healthcare provider to modify the child's pain medication.

COMPLEMENTARY THERAPY

Complementary therapies can be implemented for all children with discomfort and pain, with or without pain medication. Parents are one of the most powerful nonpharmacologic methods of pain relief available to children (Figure 15–5). When parents are actively participating in the child's care during hospitalization,

---

Growth and Development Distraction Activities

Children of all ages feel more secure and may have less pain and anxiety when parents are present. Parents can actively participate during their child's care with selection of age-appropriate distraction strategies, such as the following:

- *Infants:* holding, rocking, pacifier, mobiles, music, soft toys, massage
- *Toddlers:* massage, pinwheels, stories, bubbles, touch, holding, rocking, music
- *Preschoolers:* puzzles, action figures and other toys, being a superhero, kaleidoscopes, books, videos
- *School-age children:* rhythmic breathing, muscle relaxation, guided imagery, talking about pleasant experiences, playing games, watching a video, video games
- *Adolescents:* rhythmic breathing, muscle relaxation, guided imagery, having visitors, video games, watching videos, listening to CD player or iPod

---

Clinical Reasoning Determining When a Child Is in Pain

Felicia, who is 5 years old, was struck by a car. Six hours ago, she had surgery to repair a liver laceration, but she also has numerous bruises and abrasions on her body. After spending 3 hours in the postanesthesia unit, she was moved to the pediatric inpatient unit. She has an intravenous line in place, as well as a nasogastric tube attached to low suction. Her abdominal dressing is clean and dry. Felicia has orders for morphine IV every 3 hours around the clock for the first 24 hours.

Felicia's mother is rooming in with her during her hospital stay. Twelve hours after surgery, Felicia is dozing but is responsive to verbal stimuli. Her most recent IV morphine was given 2 hours ago. The nurse attempts to determine how well Felicia's pain is managed. Her facial expression indicates that she is not in pain. Felicia's mother feels that she is resting comfortably.

How do you know whether Felicia is in pain? Can you expect her to tell you if she feels pain? What other pain-relief measures could reduce or help to control her pain in the first 24 hours? What is the appropriate dose of IV morphine for Felicia, who weighs 25 kg? What is the timing of assessments of the response to pain medication and potential side effects? What signs of respiratory distress indicate a need for naloxone administration?

---

provide suggestions for some age-appropriate interventions to improve comfort (see *Growth and Development: Distraction Activities*).

MEASURES TO INCREASE COMFORT DURING PAINFUL PROCEDURES

Make every effort to increase the child's comfort during painful procedures, including the use of complementary therapies. Topical anesthetics can be used to reduce the pain associated with an immunization, other injection, intravenous insertion, venipuncture, heel lance, or the first needlestick of another procedure. Give time for the medication to become effective. Mechanisms for administration of topical anesthetics include the following:

- Vapocoolant sprays can be used for injections. Spray the site or soak a cotton ball and apply to intact skin for about a minute.
- EMLA (eutectic mixture of local anesthetics) cream, an emulsion of 2.5% lidocaine and 2.5% prilocaine, is effective if applied 60 minutes before a needlestick, venipuncture, or circumcision procedure on intact skin in infants and children (Barnes, 2014). The depth of penetration deepens if left on longer.
- L-M-X4, 4%, liposomal lidocaine (formerly called ELA-MAX), is effective if applied 30 minutes before a needlestick. It is available without a prescription. See Figure 15–6.
- The Synera anesthetic patch, containing 70 mg of lidocaine and 70 mg of tetracaine, can be applied to intact skin for 20 to 30 minutes prior to a procedure. It becomes heated on application and results in more rapid anesthesia.
- Buzzy for Shots is a device that has a cold pad placed against the skin and a buzzing bee that vibrates. Buzzy is placed over the site of a needlestick for 30 seconds and then moved and placed proximally during the needlestick. The cold and vibration stimulation interferes with pain

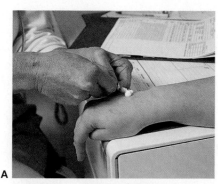

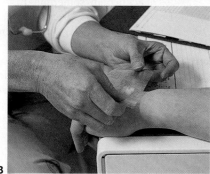

Figure 15-6 Anesthetizing cream (e.g., L-M-X4 or EMLA) may be prescribed for use prior to a painful needlestick. *A*, Apply a thin layer on selected sites and wait 30 seconds, and then apply a thick layer of cream over intact skin. *B*, Cover the cream with plastic wrap or a transparent adhesive dressing to keep the cream in place and to prevent ingestion. Depending on the cream used, the dermal surface is anesthetized in 30 to 60 minutes.

transmission, and it also provides distraction for the child (Buzzy, 2014). See Figure 15–7.

- A needle-free powder lidocaine delivery system (J-Tip) produces rapid analgesia (within 1 to 3 minutes) for IV starts and venipuncture. The system has a sterile, single-use, prefilled, and disposable cartridge that is pressed against the skin. Pressurized carbon dioxide gas ruptures the cartridge and forces lidocaine particles to penetrate the skin. Prepare the child for the small pop sound when it is used.

- LET (lidocaine, epinephrine, and tetracaine) is a topical anesthetic for laceration repair. The LET liquid is applied to a cotton ball and the skin, or LET gel is applied to the skin and covered with an occlusive dressing. The anesthetic works in 30 minutes (Barnes, 2014).

A local anesthetic such as lidocaine buffered by sodium bicarbonate or bupivacaine is often injected subcutaneously to provide analgesia for emergent invasive procedures.

Assemble a pain management kit to promote distraction, imagery, and relaxation in children. Include items such as magic wands, pinwheels, bubble liquid, a Slinky spring toy, a foam ball, party noisemakers, and pop-up books. It may also be helpful to include items for therapeutic play such as syringes, adhesive bandages, alcohol swabs, and other supplies from a medical kit. The pain management kit may be especially helpful for distracting children who are being prepared for medical procedures.

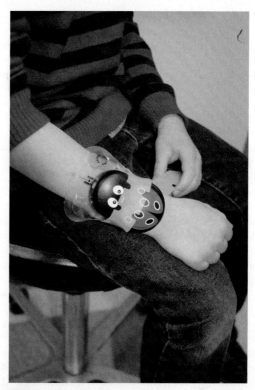

Figure 15–7 Buzzy for Shots is a device that uses cold and vibration stimulation to interrupt and reduce pain transmission due to immunization and venipuncture needlesticks. The vibration and colorful bee distract the child. Start by attaching the cold pack to Buzzy and placing this on the target area. Turn the buzzer on for 30 seconds. Then move Buzzy to an area proximal to the planned needle site, turn on the buzzer, and keep in place during the needlestick. This child is being prepared for an IV start on his arm.

SOURCE: Photo courtesy of Jane Ball, RN, DrPH.

Clinical Tip

Teach parents about the use of anesthetic cream (e.g., L-M-X4 or EMLA) or other pain management tool when the child is scheduled for an immunization or venipuncture. Anesthetic cream can be applied to the skin before departing for the healthcare visit. Provide directions regarding the correct placement of the cream on the arm or leg. Have the parents follow the directions from the package regarding the amount to use and how to cover the site with plastic wrap during the trip to the health center.

DISCHARGE PLANNING AND HOME CARE TEACHING

Children are frequently discharged from the hospital with oral analgesics following surgery, injury, or treatment of acute medical conditions. The child usually leaves the hospital or surgical center pain free, and the parents may not anticipate pain. Provide information about the child's need for pain medication around the clock for the first 1 to 2 days to prevent the child from feeling pain, and the benefits of pain management in promoting the child's healing.

Provide guidance to help parents assess their child's pain, and for school-age children and adolescents to assess their own pain. Teach parents and children about the dosage and frequency of administration and the side effects of the analgesic ordered. Consider providing a calendar or recommended schedule for daily pain medication and other medications for at least a week. Parents can post this on the refrigerator and check off doses as administered. This strategy may improve adherence with recommendations. Review complementary therapies and encourage children and parents to use the techniques that work best for them.

SAFETY ALERT!

Parents may make common dosing errors when using teaspoons or tablespoons to measure medications such as liquid acetaminophen or ibuprofen for their children, especially if abbreviations (tsp or tbs) are used on the label instructions. For example, use of a tablespoon rather than the recommended teaspoon dose leads to 3 times the appropriate dose. Additionally, the size of tableware spoons varies, which can also affect dose accuracy. Use of dosing devices measured in millimeters (mL) (e.g., oral syringe, dosing spoon, or measuring cup) is an effective way to reduce medication errors that can lead to adverse effects associated with medications prescribed for pain. Educate parents about the correct milliliter dose when labels specify medication volume by teaspoon or tablespoon. The American Academy of Pediatrics (AAP) now recommends that all oral liquid medications be prescribed using metric units or milliliters (AAP Committee on Drugs, 2015).

Remember that many common health problems (otitis media, pharyngitis, and urinary tract infection) have pain as one of the presenting symptoms. Often the only medication prescribed is an antibiotic to clear the infection. The child may be in pain for 48 to 72 hours until the antibiotic controls the infection. Give parents recommendations for pain control and comfort measures during this period. Review the dose, dosing device, and formulation of acetaminophen or ibuprofen used by parents to identify any risk for overdose. Avoid using any leftover pain medications prescribed for other conditions. See Chapter 16.

SAFETY ALERT!

Warn parents who are sent home with a prescription for an opioid for their child about the need to dispose of the remaining medication or to lock it up after it is no longer needed. Adolescents may share unprotected tablets with friends leading to and supporting substance abuse. The rate of poisoning death due to prescription drug misuse has increased dramatically in recent years (see the *Healthy People 2020* objective). Check with local law enforcement or the pharmacy about the availability of medication disposal sites or options.

Healthy People 2020

(SA-19) Reduce the past-year nonmedical use of prescription drugs

---

Evaluation

Expected outcomes of nursing care include the following:

- The child's pain level is assessed frequently and pain management is effective in improving the child's comfort.

- The child successfully uses a PCA pump to control acute pain.
- Age-appropriate complementary therapies enhance the comfort provided by medications.
- Parents maintain the child's pain management after discharge.

Chronic Pain

Some children have medical conditions that cause chronic pain or recurrent episodes of acute pain, sometimes in more than one body system. Medical conditions such as juvenile idiopathic arthritis, sickle cell disease, cancer, headaches, recurrent abdominal pain, and HIV infection all cause chronic and recurrent pain. Approximately 20% to 35% of children and adolescents are estimated to have chronic pain (APS, 2012). These children and adolescents often have functional limitations related to school, social activities and relationships, physical activity, and family responsibilities. Chronic pain has social and emotional consequences for the child and family.

Clinical Manifestations

Behavioral indicators of chronic pain may include fatigue, inactivity, posturing, difficulty concentrating and sleeping, withdrawal from activities, and mood disturbances. Persistent or continuous chronic pain permits physiologic adaptation so the elevated heart rate, respiratory rate, and blood pressure levels associated with the initial response to acute pain are rarely seen (Huether, 2014). However, the child with intermittent acute painful episodes may have initial vital sign changes. Varying levels of disability may also exist.

Clinical Therapy

An interdisciplinary team that collaborates on addressing the factors that stimulate and contribute to the child's pain in an individualized treatment plan should focus on improving function and comfort. Cognitive behavioral therapies are used to address the connection between thoughts, feelings, and behaviors; reduce stress; and promote coping. Physical and occupational therapy may help restore function. Treatment for sleep disturbances and strategies for school functioning are addressed. Complementary therapies such as relaxation strategies, ice, or heat should be used when appropriate (APS, 2012). Analgesics rarely include opioids except for acute painful episodes. NSAIDs or acetaminophen may be prescribed. Complete pain relief may not be possible. A tricyclic antidepressant may be prescribed for its analgesic properties and because depression may be a coexisting condition.

Health Promotion

Children with chronic pain should learn a cognitive behavioral therapy (e.g., hypnosis, guided imagery) that helps the child to reduce stress, cope with pain, and enhance pain management. Use of relaxation techniques with guided imagery that includes positive suggestions for comfort has helped many children with a chronic painful condition reduce their pain. Improved quality of life scores have been noted (Gottsegen, 2011).

Nursing Management

When assessing chronic pain in the child, approach pain as if it were the primary problem for attention. Consider the physical, behavioral, and psychologic signs and symptoms together. Focus on the following topics to assess and evaluate chronic pain in children (APS, 2012):

- Obtain the history of pain onset, its development over time, intensity, duration, variability, location, and what worsens or relieves it. Ask what the family and child believe causes the pain. Identify past pain problems in the family.

- Learn about the impact of the pain on the child's daily life (sleep, appetite, school, activity, and social interactions). Identify how much distress the child and family experience with pain.

- Identify the child's methods for coping with pain. How does the pain impact the child's emotional function?

- Ask about the current treatment methods, including complementary therapies.

- Observe the child's appearance, posture, gait, and emotional and cognitive state. Perform a complete neurologic examination. Assess muscle spasms, trigger points, and areas sensitive to light touch.

Encourage older school-age children and adolescents with chronic pain or recurrent episodes of acute pain to keep a pain diary to describe the pain intensity, characteristics, timing, activities, and potential triggers of their pain, as well as their response to pain treatment measures. A pain assessment scale should be used to rate the pain intensity before and after medications and other pain-control measures are used. This record can help improve pain management when shared with healthcare providers.

Monitor pain intensity at each office visit and frequently during hospitalizations. Believe the child who reports chronic pain or recurrent episodes of pain, and use pharmacologic and nonpharmacologic methods to reduce or relieve the child's pain. Remember the child may have increased pain sensitivity in anticipation of and during needlesticks and other procedures.

Work with the pain management team to individualize the pain management plan to meet the child's needs, family's beliefs and values, and their cultural preferences for care. Develop a care plan for acute painful episodes associated with the condition. Assist the child and family in identifying age-appropriate and acceptable complementary therapies to help cope with discomfort. Encourage daily exercise to promote function.

Sedation and Analgesia for Medical Procedures

Children undergo a wide variety of painful diagnostic and treatment procedures in the hospital and in outpatient settings. Procedures such as chest tube insertion, arterial puncture, lumbar puncture, bone marrow aspiration, fracture reduction, laceration repair, insertion of a central or peripheral intravenous line, and burn debridement cause significant pain in children. The anticipation of these procedures causes anxiety and emotional distress that can lead to greater pain intensity. For example, children with prior painful cancer treatment procedures may express greater pain during later procedures, even when provided with adequate analgesia (Rosen & Dower, 2011).

Sedation is a medically controlled state of depressed consciousness (light to deep) used for painful diagnostic and therapeutic procedures. **Moderate sedation** (formerly called *conscious sedation*) occurs with lower doses of sedatives and enables the child to maintain protective reflexes independently, continuously maintain a patent airway, and respond to tactile and verbal stimuli. **Deep sedation** is a controlled state of depressed consciousness or unconsciousness in which protective airway reflexes are lost. See Table 15–7 for characteristics of different sedation levels.

Drugs used for sedation include the following:

- Benzodiazepines: midazolam (Versed), diazepam (Valium), and lorazepam (Ativan); antagonist agent is flumazenil

- Hypnotics or barbiturates: methohexital

- Ketamine

- Propofol (Diprivan) or Etomidate

- Chloral hydrate

- Analgesics: fentanyl, alfentanil; antagonist agents are naloxone and nalmefene

Every healthcare facility should have guidelines for the use of sedation to ensure safe healthcare practices. Healthcare providers monitoring the child should have specific qualifications, such as training in pediatric advanced life support. Potential complications of sedation include respiratory depression, a compromised airway, delayed awakening, agitation, nausea and vomiting, and tachycardia or bradycardia (Krauss & Green, 2013).

TABLE 15–7 Clinical Manifestations of Light, Moderate, and Deep Sedation

ASSESSMENT FACTORS	LIGHT SEDATION	MODERATE SEDATION	DEEP SEDATION
Airway	Maintains airway independently and continuously	Maintains airway independently and continuously	Airway may not be maintained, may need ventilation assistance
Cough and gag reflexes	Reflexes intact	Reflexes intact	Partial or complete loss of reflexes
Level of consciousness	Responds normally to verbal stimuli	Purposeful response to verbal or gentle tactile stimuli	Difficult to arouse, purposeful response after repeated or painful stimuli

Source: Data from Jest, A. D., & Tonge, A. (2011). Using a learning needs assessment to identify knowledge deficits regarding procedural sedation for pediatric patients. *AORN Journal, 94*(6), 567–574; Barnes, S. (2014). Analgesia and sedation. In B. Engorn, & J. Flerlage (Eds.), *The Harriet Lane handbook* (20th ed.). Philadelphia, PA: Elsevier Mosby; Krauss, B., & Green, S. M. (2014). Systemic analgesia and sedation for procedures. In J. R. Roberts, & C. B. Custalow (Eds.), *Roberts and Hedges' clinical procedures in emergency medicine* (6th ed.,pp. 586–610). Philadelphia, PA: Elsevier Saunders.

SAFETY ALERT!

Sedation is a continuum, and the child may move from one level of sedation to another. The child must be carefully monitored for respiratory depression and signs of deep sedation, so the airway can be protected and ventilatory support can be provided if needed. A pediatric code cart, resuscitation bag-valve-mask and drugs, oxygen, and suction must be available, along with antagonist agents (naloxone and flumazenil) for opioids and benzodiazepines, when the effects of sedation and respiratory depression must be reversed.

Nursing Management

When the child receives sedation, continuously assess the child's status to include visual confirmation of respiratory effort, chest wall movement, color, vital signs, level of consciousness, and oxygen saturation. Document vital signs every 5 minutes (Jest & Tonge, 2011). A cardiorespiratory monitor, pulse oximeter, and expiratory CO_2 monitor should be used, but the equipment must not replace visual assessment. Be prepared to suction emesis or excessive salivation that could obstruct the airway. After the procedure, check vital signs every 15 minutes until the child regains full consciousness and level of functioning, usually within 30 minutes.

Criteria for discharging the child after sedation include the following (Krauss & Green, 2013):

- Stable vital signs, airway patency, and intact protective reflexes are evident.
- The child sits up without assistance; the infant holds head up.
- Discharge status is the same as admission status.
- Fluid intake is not essential as some sedation medications stimulate vomiting in children.

Inform parents that the child may have mild adverse effects from sedation, such as crying, lethargy, and vomiting. Avoid food and fluids for 2 hours if the child has nausea. For the next 12 hours, do not permit activities such as bicycle riding or gymnastics that require coordination, and do not leave the child unattended in the bathtub or pool.

Chapter Highlights

- Pain is an unpleasant sensation that is either acute or chronic. It is perceived in response to tissue damage that increases the stress in children of all ages. Neuropathic pain is one form of chronic pain.

- Unrelieved pain causes many undesirable physiologic consequences on body systems, such as inadequate lung expansion and coughing, increased metabolic rate, increased sympathetic nervous system activity, decreased gastric acids and intestinal motility, depressed inflammatory responses, and increased pain sensitivity.

- A child's responses to and understanding of pain depend on age, stage of development, culture, and prior painful experiences.

- Assessment of acute and chronic pain should include physical, behavioral, and emotional factors to obtain the most accurate information about the location and intensity of the child's pain and how the child responds to it.

- Pain assessment should include the use of a valid and reliable pain assessment tool that is appropriate for the child's age, cognitive development, and condition.

- Every infant, child, and adolescent has the right to adequate pain control.

- Pharmacologic interventions for pain control include opioids, nonsteroidal anti-inflammatory drugs (NSAIDs), and acetaminophen.

- Analgesia for continuous or severe pain should be given around the clock to maintain pain control.

- Complementary therapies for pain management include the following: parental presence, distraction, cutaneous stimulation, sucrose solution, electroanalgesia, guided imagery, breathing techniques, progressive muscle relaxation techniques, hypnosis, application of heat and cold, biofeedback, and acupuncture.

- Methods to reduce pain associated with needlesticks include vapocoolant spray, LMX-4 cream, Synera patch, Buzzy for Shots, and needle-free lidocaine delivery system.

- Epidural and regional nerve blocks are pain-control methods used more frequently for postsurgical pain management because they have fewer side effects than systemic medications.

- Parents need education and preparation to provide pain management for children who are discharged home following surgery and injuries.

- Children with recurrent and chronic painful conditions need an individualized pain management plan that includes cognitive behavioral therapies, physical and occupational therapy, and other measures to improve function, quality of life, and comfort.

- The child receiving sedation should be continuously and visually monitored for respiratory effort, vital signs, color, level of responsiveness, vomiting, and excessive salivation.

Clinical Reasoning in Action

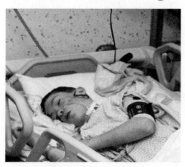

A 12-year-old boy, Kevin, is recovering at a local children's hospital from a four-wheeler all-terrain vehicle (ATV) crash. He was riding the ATV unsupervised and without permission while his parents were at work. He suffered three broken bones, several lacerations, and an abdominal injury that required surgery. His parents are very worried about his injuries and at the same time angry with him for not following the rules. Kevin appears expressionless in his hospital bed, but cries and grimaces at any slight movement. When asked on a scale of 1 to 10 (10 being the most pain) how much pain he is feeling, he says a 10. His parents are reluctant to let him have any pain medications because they fear he may become dependent on the medication. His father states that Kevin should be a man and

tolerate the pain, and he thinks enduring the pain will teach him a lesson about responsibility. The nurse explains that pain management is necessary to improve Kevin's healing, help him mobilize sooner, and potentially shorten his hospital stay. She explains the physiologic consequences of ineffective pain management and discusses how the medication will help him sleep and rest. She explains that some of the pain medications can be addicting, but the chances of Kevin becoming addicted to pain medications for this injury are extremely rare. She also reviews the nonpharmacologic methods of relieving pain. The parents are still reluctant to allow the medications, but agree to conform to the healthcare provider's orders.

1. What are some of the potential physiologic consequences of letting Kevin suffer pain?
2. What are some examples of opioid analgesics appropriate for Kevin?
3. What are some examples of NSAIDs available to Kevin?
4. What are the signs of tolerance to the prescribed opioid?

References

American Academy of Pediatrics (AAP) Committee on Drugs. (2015). Metric units and the preferred dosing of orally administered medications. *Pediatrics, 135*(4), 784–787.

American Pain Society (APS). (2012). *Assessment and management of children with chronic pain.* Retrieved from http://www.americanpainsociety.org/uploads/pdfs/aps12-pcp.pdf

Aschenbrenner, D. S. (2013). Drug watch. *American Journal of Nursing, 113*(6), 23–24.

Badr, L. K. (2013). Pain in premature infants: What is conclusive evidence and what is not? *Newborn & Infant Nursing Reviews, 13*, 82–86.

Barnes, S. (2014). Analgesia and sedation. In B. Engorn & J. Flerlage (Eds.), *The Harriet Lane handbook* (20th ed., pp. 111–126). Philadelphia, PA: Elsevier Mosby.

Buzzy. (2014). *Buzzy drug free pain relief.* Retrieved from http://buzzy4shots.com/

Chon, T. Y., & Lee, M. C. (2013). Accupuncture. *Mayo Clinic Proceedings, 88*(10), 1141–1146.

Clark, L. (2011). Pain management in the pediatric population. *Critical Care Nursing Clinics of North America, 23*, 291–301.

Cooper, S., & Petty, J. (2012). Promoting the use of sucrose as analgesia for procedural pain management in neonates: A review of the current literature. *Journal of Neonatal Nursing, 18*, 121–128.

Czarnecki, M. L., Simon, K., Thompson, J. J., Armus, C. L., Hanson, T. C., Berg, K. A., . . . Malin, S. (2011). Barriers to pediatric pain management: A nursing perspective. *Pain Management Nursing, 12*(3), 154–162.

Czarnecki, M. L., Salamon, K., Thompson, J. J., & Hainsworth, K. R. (2014). Do barriers to pediatric pain management as perceived by nurses change over time? *Pain Management Nursing, 15*(1), 292–305.

Dobson, C. E., & Byrne, M. W. (2014). Using guided imagery to manage pain in young children with sickle cell disease. *American Journal of Nursing, 114*(4), 26–36.

Ely, E., Chen-Lim, M. L., Zarnowsy, C., Green, R., Shaffer, S., & Holtzer, B. (2012). Finding the evidence to change practice for assessing pain in children who are cognitively impaired. *Journal of Pediatric Nursing, 27*, 402–410.

Fein, J. A., Zempsky, W. T., Cravero, J. P., & The Committee on Pediatric Emergency Medicine and the Section on Anesthesiology and Pain. (2012). Relief of pain and anxiety in pediatric patients in emergency medical systems. *Pediatrics, 130*(5), e1391–e1405.

Galinkin, Koh, & Committee on Drugs and Section on Anesthesiology and Pain Management. (2014). Recognition and management of iatrogenically induced opioid dependence and withdrawal in children. *Pediatrics, 133*(1), 152–155.

Gomez, R. J., Barrowman, N., Elia, S., Manias, E., Royle, J., & Harrison, D. (2013). Establishing intra- and inter-relater agreement of the Faces, Legs, Activity, Cry, Consolability scale for evaluating pain in toddlers during immunization. *Pain Research & Management, 18*(6), e124–e128.

Gottsegen, D. (2011). Hypnosis for functional abdominal pain. *American Journal of Clinical Hypnosis, 54*(1), 56–69.

Greenwald, M. (2010). Analgesia for the pediatric trauma patient: Primum non nocere? *Clinical Pediatric Emergency Medicine, 11*(1), 28–40.

Guarin, P. L. B. (2013). How effective are nerve blocks after orthopedic surgery? A quality improvement study. *Nursing 2013, 43*(6), 63–66.

Huether, S. E. (2014). Pain, temperature regulation, sleep, and sensory function. In K. L. McCance, S. E. Huether, V. L. Brashers, & N. S. Rote (Eds.), *Pathophysiology: The biologic basis for disease in adults and children* (7th ed., pp. 481–524). St. Louis, MO: Mosby Elsevier.

Jest, A. D., & Tonge, A. (2011). Using a learning needs assessment to identify knowledge deficits regarding procedural sedation for pediatric patients. *AORN Journal, 94*(6), 567–574.

Joint Commission. (2014). *Facts about pain management.* Retrieved from http://www.jointcommission.org/pain_management

Kohen, D. P. (2011). Chronic daily headache: Helping adolescents help themselves with self-hypnosis. *American Journal of Clinical Hypnosis, 54*, 32–46.

Krauss, B., & Green, S. M. (2014). Systemic analgesia and sedation for procedures. In J. R. Roberts & C. B. Custalow (Eds.), *Roberts and Hedges' clinical procedures in emergency medicine* (6th ed., pp. 586–610). Philadelphia, PA: Elsevier Saunders.

Lawrence, J., Alcock, D., McGrath, D. P., Kay, J., MacMurray, S. B., & Dulberg, C. (1993). The development of a tool to assess neonatal pain. *Neonatal Network, 12*(6), 61.

Martin, S., Smith, A. B., Newcomb, P., & Miller, J. (2014). Effects of therapeutic suggestion under anesthesia on outcomes in children post tonsillectomy. *Journal of Perianesthesia Nursing, 29*(2), 94–106.

Merkel, S. I., Voepel-Lewis, T., Shayevitz, J. R., & Malviya, S. (1997). The FLACC: A behavioral scale for scoring post-operative pain in young children. *Pediatric Nursing, 23*(3), 293–297.

Pasero, C., & McCaffery, M. (2011). *Pain assessment and pharmacologic management.* St. Louis, MO: Elsevier Mosby.

Purnell, L. D. (2014). *Guide to culturally competent care* (3rd ed.). Philadelphia, PA: F. A. Davis.

Rashotte, J., Coburn, G., Harrison, D., Stevens, B. J., Yamada, J. Abbott, L. K., & CIHR Team on Children's Pain. (2013). Healthcare professionals' pain narratives in hospitalized children's medical records: Part 1, Pain descriptors. *Pain Research and Management, 18*(5), e75–e83.

Rosen, D. A., & Dower, J. (2011). Pediatric pain management. *Pediatric Annals, 40*(5), 243–252.

Sadhasivam, S., Chidambaran, V., Ngamprasertwong, P., Esslinger, H. R., Prows, C., Zhang, X., . . . McAuliffe,

J. (2012). Race and unequal burden of perioperative pain and opioid related adverse effects in children. *Pediatrics, 129*(5), 832–838.

Suddaby, E. C., & Josephson, K. (2013). Satisfaction of nurses with the Withdrawal Assessment Tool-1 (WAT-1). *Pediatric Nursing, 39*(5), 238–242, 259.

Taddio, A., Hogan, M. E., Moyer, P., Girgis, A., Gerges, S., Wang, L., & Ipp, M. (2011). Evaluation of the reliability, validity and practicality of 3 measures of acute pain in infants undergoing immunization injections. *Vaccine, 29*, 1390–1394.

Taketomo, C. K., Hodding, J. H., & Kraus, D. M. (2014). *Pediatric dosage handbook* (21st ed.). Hudson, OH: American Pharmacists Association..

Tobias, J. D. (2014a). Acute pain management in infants and children—Part 1: Pain pathways, pain assessment, and outpatient pain management. *Pediatric Annals, 43*(7), e163–e168.

Tobias, J. D. (2014b). Acute pain management in infants and children—Part 2: Intravenous opioids, intravenous nonsteroidal anti-inflammatory drugs, and managing adverse events. *Pediatric Annals, 43*(7), e169–e175.

Twycross, A., & Collins, S. (2013). Nurses' views about the barriers and facilitators to effective management of pediatric pain. *Pain Management Nursing, 14*(4), e164–e172.

Watt, L. D., & Arnstein, P. (2013). Codeine for children: Weighing the risks. *Nursing2013, 43*(11), 62–63.

Wilson, B. A., Shannon, M. T., & Shields, K. M. (2016). *Nurse's drug guide 2016*. Hoboken, NJ: Pearson Education.

Wilson, S., Bremmer, A. P., Mathews, J., & Pearson, D. (2013). The use of oral sucrose for procedural pain relief in infants up to six months of age: A randomized controlled trial. *Pain Management Nursing, 14*(4), e95–e105.

Wood, C., von Baeyer, C. L., Falinower, S., Moyse, D., Annequin, D., & Legout, V. (2011). Electronic and paper versions of a faces pain intensity scale: Concordance and preference in hospitalized children. *BMC Pediatrics, 11*, 87–95.

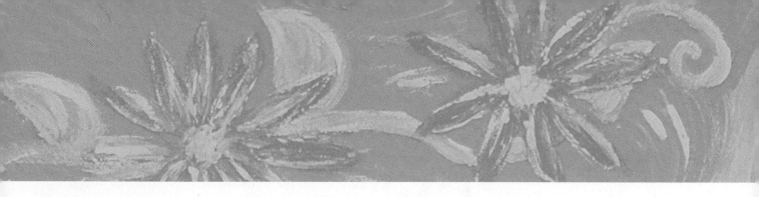

Chapter 16
Immunizations and Communicable Diseases

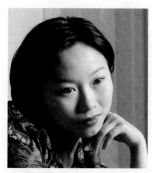

We came in today because Chang has a fever. I know Lian and Chang need immunizations. Lian will be going to kindergarten in the fall, so it's very important for her to get all of the immunizations she needs now.

—Mother of Lian, 5 years old, and Chang, 2 years old

Peter Hendrie/Getty Images

∨ Learning Outcomes

16.1 Compare the vulnerability of young children and adults to communicable diseases.

16.2 Propose strategies to control the spread of infection in healthcare and community settings and the home.

16.3 Examine the role that vaccines play in reducing and eliminating communicable diseases.

16.4 Select the appropriate vaccines to administer to an infant, a toddler, a child entering kindergarten, an older school-age child, and an adolescent.

16.5 Plan the nursing care for children of all ages needing immunizations.

16.6 Outline a plan to maintain the potency of vaccines.

16.7 Create a parent education session that focuses on the care of infants and children with a fever.

16.8 Recognize common infectious and communicable diseases.

16.9 Develop a nursing care plan for the child with a common communicable disease.

A communicable disease is an infection often caused by **direct transmission** (from one person or animal to another by body fluid contact), via **indirect transmission** (to a person by contact with contaminated objects), or by *vectors* (ticks, mosquitoes, other insects). An **infectious disease** is any communicable disease caused by microorganisms transmitted from one person to another or from an animal to a person. Children can develop complications or secondary infections that require health care and can sometimes result in death.

For a communicable disease to occur three factors need to be in place:

1. An infectious agent or pathogen
2. An effective means of transmission
3. Presence of susceptible host (See *Pathophysiology Illustrated: The Chain of Infection Transmission*.)

Special Vulnerability of Infants and Children

Infants and young children are often susceptible hosts. Newborns are more susceptible because the immune system is not fully mature at birth and disease protection from vaccines

Pathophysiology Illustrated: **The Chain of Infection Transmission**

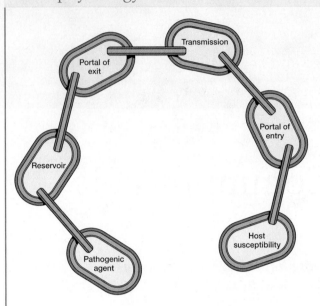

An effective chain of infection transmission requires a suitable habitat or reservoir for the pathogen. To prevent or control the spread of infection, one of the links in the chain must be broken, such as eliminating one or more of the habitats or reservoirs (e.g., insecticide spraying to kill mosquitoes that carry malaria). Isolating an infected individual interferes with disease transmission, and killing the pathogen eliminates the causal agent.

is incomplete. Maternal **antibodies** (proteins capable of responding to specific infectious agents) transferred through the placenta and breast milk provide **passive immunity** to the newborn. Passive immunity may also be provided with immune globulin. These antibodies provide limited protection for some infections, and this protection decreases over several months after birth. Immunodeficiency and poor health may also increase a child's risk for a communicable disease.

Infants and children develop **active immunity**, antibody development for specific infections through immunization or exposure to the natural disease. Exposure to infectious agents leads children to naturally develop antibodies that prevent or reduce the response to future exposure to the same infectious agent (Figure 16–1). (Refer to the section titled *Anatomy and Physiology of Pediatric Differences* in Chapter 22.)

The poor hygiene behaviors of young children promote transmission of communicable diseases in environments where

children are in close contact. The fecal–oral and respiratory routes are the most common sources of transmission in children. Children do not wash their hands after toileting unless closely supervised. They then put their hands in their mouth and rub their nose and eyes. Diapers may leak stool and provide the fecal exposure to organisms. In some cases, the child may be contagious before disease symptoms occur (e.g., varicella and parvovirus B-19) and before the child can be isolated. See Table 16–5 later in this chapter for more information about these and other communicable diseases.

Public Health and Communicable Diseases

Reducing the number of preventable childhood illnesses is a national goal of *Healthy People 2020*. Approximately 300 children in the United States die each year from vaccine-preventable diseases. Routine immunization, with all recommended vaccines administered to children beginning at birth, is estimated to save 33,000 lives, prevent 14 million cases of disease, and reduce direct healthcare costs by $9.9 billion (U.S. Department of Health and Human Services, 2015).

Healthy People 2020

(IID-1) Reduce, eliminate, or maintain elimination of cases of vaccine-preventable diseases

(IID-3) Reduce meningococcal disease

(IID-4) Reduce invasive pneumococcal infections

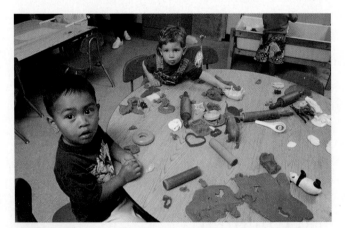

Figure 16–1 Infectious diseases are easily transmitted in settings such as childcare centers where multiple children handle common objects that have been sneezed, coughed, or drooled upon.

Nurses have an important health promotion role in reducing the transmission of infectious diseases by immunization and in educating families to interrupt the transmission of infection. Preventing the spread of infectious diseases involves several strategies that must be well coordinated. Nurses have a significant

Families Want to Know

Reducing the Transmission of Infection

Teach families how to reduce the spread of infection among family members with the following practices:

- Wash hands thoroughly with soap and water or cleansing gels after all contact with the child's diaper, used tissues, runny nose, and mucous membranes.

- Use disposable tissues and discard immediately after use.

- Teach children to cough or sneeze into their elbow rather than their hands.

- Teach children to wash their hands with soap and water after toileting and before eating.

- Do not allow children to share dishes and utensils.

- Wash hands before preparing food and again several times during food preparation. Follow guidelines for safe food preparation and storage. Use warm soapy water to wash dishes and cutting boards.

- Wipe counters and surfaces that are used for diaper changes or that the child touches with a disinfectant such as bleach solution, Lysol, or isopropyl alcohol. Make sure the diaper-changing area is well away from food preparation areas.

- Dispose of diapers in closed containers.

---

role in this process and are responsible for implementing several infection-control strategies:

- Use proper hand hygiene. Wash hands with soap and water when visibly dirty, when contaminated by blood or other body fluids, when in contact with a contaminated surface, and after using the toilet (Centers for Disease Control, 2014a). Use alcohol-based hand sanitizer to clean the hands in all other routine clinical situations.

- Use standard and transmission-based precautions (see the *Clinical Skills Manual* SKILLS for more information).

- Promote and provide immunizations.

- Separate and quarantine ill children from well children. Separate children at high risk for infection from those with infections in all clinical settings.

- Eliminate the habitat or reservoir of the host (e.g., eliminate standing water where mosquitoes breed).

- Kill the pathogen (e.g., sanitize toys and surfaces exposed to organisms).

- Educate parents and caregivers to reduce the transmission of infectious diseases. (See *Families Want to Know: Reducing the Transmission of Infection*.)

Professionalism in Practice Infection Control in Schools

School nurses have an important leadership role in targeting communicable diseases because of their professional knowledge and public health perspective (National Association of School Nurses, 2011). School nurses document the student immunization records and encourage families to have their children fully immunized. Students with communicable diseases are identified so they can be sent home for care, reducing exposure to other students. It is important for school nurses to stay informed about communicable disease outbreaks in the community and then to be vigilant about monitoring illness patterns among students and faculty. When a communicable disease outbreak occurs in the school setting, the school nurse reports the outbreak to local health officials so that communitywide infection-control information can be shared. They also develop programs and teach students how to reduce the spread of infection.

Immunization

The development and wide use of vaccines is one of the great achievements of modern medicine. A vaccine introduces an **antigen** (a foreign substance that triggers an immune system response) into the body, and the vaccinated person produces antibodies that provide active immunity to a disease without having the clinical disease.

When a child needs antibodies faster than the body can develop them, passive immunity may be provided by giving the child antibodies produced by another human or animal host (e.g., immune globulin). This approach is used with children at risk for a disease to prevent the disease from occurring or to reduce its severity after an exposure. For example, if an unimmunized toddler receiving chemotherapy for cancer is exposed to chickenpox, the child needs immediate protection (passive immunity). Varicella immune globulin is given to reduce the child's risk for developing chickenpox, a potentially fatal infection for this child. Passive immunity does not last long, so the child needs to receive the varicella vaccine at a later time in order to develop active immunity.

Since the first vaccines were developed in the late 1800s, the incidence of many diseases has decreased dramatically. The average infant born in 2016 receives vaccines for 14 childhood diseases by age 6 years. Vaccines have also been developed for older children, adolescents, and adults to protect against pertussis, meningococcus, human papillomavirus, pneumococcus, and herpes zoster. Vaccines improve the health of children and reduce the parents' burden of caring for ill children.

The following lists the types of vaccines against childhood illnesses used in the United States:

- **Killed virus vaccine.** A microorganism has been killed but is still capable of causing the human body to produce antibodies. Example: inactivated poliovirus.

- **Toxoid.** A toxin has been treated (by heat or chemical) to weaken its toxic effects but retain effective antigens. Example: tetanus toxoid.

- **Live virus vaccine.** A microorganism is in a live but attenuated, or weakened, form. Example: measles and varicella vaccines.

- **Recombinant forms.** A genetically altered organism is used in vaccines. Examples: hepatitis B and **acellular pertussis vaccine** (a vaccine that uses pertussis proteins rather than the whole cell to stimulate active immunity).

• **Conjugated forms.** An altered organism is joined with another substance to increase the immune response. Examples: The *Haemophilus influenzae* type b (Hib) vaccine is conjugated with a protein-carrier like tetanus toxoid. No immunity to tetanus develops with this vaccine.

Today's vaccines are often produced synthetically with recombinant DNA technology or genetic engineering to improve vaccine safety and efficacy and to reduce their side effects. See Table 16–1 for recommended pediatric vaccines.

TABLE 16–1 Pediatric Vaccines

VACCINE TYPE	SIDE EFFECTS	CONTRAINDICATIONS	NURSING CONSIDERATIONS
Diphtheria, Pertussis (Whooping Cough), and Tetanus Toxoid (DTaP, Tdap)			
Type: Inactivated *Dosage:* 0.5 mL, IM *Age(s) given:* 2, 4, 6, 15–18 months; 4–6 years (5 doses); 11–12 years (Tdap) *Caution:* For a prior serious reaction to the pertussis component of DTaP vaccine, use DT (children less than 7 years) and Td (children 7 years and older) vaccines. *Storage:* Refrigerate, do not freeze. Tripedia and Infanrix vial stopper contains latex.	*Common:* Redness, pain, swelling, nodule at injection site; fever up to 38.3°C (101.0°F); drowsiness, irritability, fussiness; anorexia within 2 days of injection Increase in frequency and magnitude of local reactions with fourth and fifth doses (e.g., entire limb swelling) *Serious:* Allergic reaction, anaphylaxis; shock or collapse (an episode with sudden loss of muscle tone, pallor, fever, and unresponsiveness), fever above 40.5°C (104.8°F); febrile seizure; persistent inconsolable crying	Gelatin allergy (do not use Tripedia) Serious side effects after a prior dose: e.g., anaphylaxis, encephalopathy within 7 days of vaccine dosage ***Precautions and temporary deferral for DTaP and Tdap administration:*** • Infants under age 1 year with evolving neurologic disorder • Guillain-Barré syndrome less than 6 weeks after previous dose • Moderate to severe febrile illness • Older children with a progressive neurologic condition	• Use same brand for all doses if possible. • Ask about previous vaccine reactions. • Shake vaccine before withdrawing. Solution will be cloudy. Do not use if it contains clumps that do not resuspend. • If a child has a history of seizures with or without fever, give acetaminophen at the time of vaccine and then every 4 hr for 24 hr. • Inform parents about an increased potential reaction to the fourth and fifth doses. • A tetanus booster may be given for a contaminated wound or burn, if 5 or more years since the last dose (AAP, 2015, p. 775).
Haemophilus influenzae Type B (Hib)			
Type: Inactivated *Dosage:* 0.5 mL, IM *Age(s) given:* 2, 4, 6, 12–15 months; (4 doses for PRP-T [ActHIB]) *or* 2, 4, 12–15 months (3 doses for PRP-OMP [PedvaxHIB]) *Storage:* Refrigerate, loss of potency if frozen. Vial stopper with Pentacel and MenHibRix contains no latex.	*Common:* Pain, redness, or swelling at site *Serious:* Anaphylaxis (extremely rare); fever	Prior anaphylactic reaction Comvax is contraindicated if yeast allergy exists. *Precautions:* Moderate or severe acute illness with or without fever Ask if child is immunosuppressed. Some children benefit from additional doses (AAP, 2015, p. 373).	• Solution is clear and colorless. • Since different product preparations (e.g., single and combination vaccines) affect the immunization schedule, read package inserts carefully. • Follow directions for reconstituting, refrigerating, and discarding unused reconstituted vaccine.
Hepatitis A (HepA)			
Type: Inactivated *Dosage:* 0.5 mL (1.0 mL over age 19 years), IM *Age(s) given:* 12–23 months; second dose 6–12 months after first dose *Storage:* Refrigerate, loss of potency if frozen.	*Common:* Pain and induration at injection site; fever *Serious:* Anaphylaxis reactions are rare.	Known hypersensitivity to any component of vaccine, including neomycin Anaphylactic reaction to prior vaccine dose *Precautions:* Pregnancy	• Shake well, slightly opaque white suspension. No reconstitution is needed. • Some Havrix and all Vaqta vials have a latex stopper. • Can be given for postexposure prophylaxis against hepatitis A (AAP, 2015, p. 398). • Immune globulin and vaccine can be given at the same time in different sites.

VACCINE TYPE	SIDE EFFECTS	CONTRAINDICATIONS	NURSING CONSIDERATIONS
Hepatitis B (HB) *Type:* Inactivated *Dosage:* 0.5 mL (1.0 mL at 20 years), IM *Age(s) given:* Birth, 1–2 months, 6–18 months; 3 doses; a 3-dose series can be started at any age. *Storage:* Refrigerate, do not freeze. Vaccine brands can be interchanged for 3-dose series. Use the monovalent (single vaccine) preparation for newborns up to 6 weeks of age.	*Common:* Pain or redness at injection site *Serious:* Anaphylaxis is uncommon.	Anaphylaxis reaction to prior dose Serious hypersensitivity reaction to prior dose related to vaccine component (e.g., yeast) *Precautions:* Newborn weighing less than 2000 g (4.4 lb) may receive dose at birth, but receive 3 additional doses starting at 1 month of age Moderate or severe acute illness with or without fever	• Check status of mother's hepatitis B test. If mother has HBsAg+ or unknown status, give vaccine to newborn within 12 hr of birth along with hepatitis B immune globulin in another site. • Shake vaccine before withdrawing. Solution will appear cloudy. • Formulations (pediatric, adult, dialysis) and combination vaccines are available. Read package insert carefully and follow directions for the product used. • Check the anti-HBs and HBsAg levels in infants of HBsAg+ mothers at age 9–18 months, after series completion (AAP, 2015, p. 421).
Human Papillomavirus (HPV4 or HPV2) *Type:* Recombinant *Dosage:* 0.5 mL, IM *Age(s) given:* 11–12 years, second dose 2 months later, third dose 6 months after the first dose. May be administered to males and females between 9 and 26 years of age. HPV2 is not licensed for males (Markowitz et al., 2014). *Storage:* Refrigerate, do not freeze. Light exposure reduces vaccine potency.	*Common:* Pain, swelling, erythema at the injection site, headache, nausea, pruritus, and fever *Potential serious reactions:* Guillain-Barré syndrome, blood clot, bronchospasm, asthma, arthritis	Severe allergic reaction to prior dose or hypersensitivity to a vaccine component (e.g., yeast) Pregnancy *Precautions and deferral:* Moderate to severe acute illness with or without fever. Can be given when mild acute illness is present.	• Use same brand for each dose if possible. • Shake well before use. Solution is a white cloudy liquid. No dilution or reconstitution. • Observe adolescent for 15 min when seated because of risk of fainting and syncope. • Administer vaccine before onset of sexual activity. • Educate adolescents that this vaccine prevents only one sexually transmitted infection.
Influenza (IIV or LAIV) *Type:* Inactivated (IIV), or live attenuated (LAIV) for intranasal (IN) use *Route:* IM (all ages), IN (2 years and older) *Dosage:* 0.25 mL in infants 6–35 months, 0.5 mL starting at 3 years for IIV; 0.2 mL for LAIV *Age(s) given:* Annually in the fall, beginning at 6 months of age; then annually. Children under age 9 years receiving IIV or LAIV for the first time should receive a second dose 4 weeks later (AAP, 2015, p. 483). *Storage:* *IIV:* Refrigerate, do not use if frozen. *LAIV:* Keep frozen. May thaw and refrigerate for 24 hr before use.	*Common after IIV:* Soreness at injection site, fever, aches *Common after LAIV:* Runny nose or nasal congestion, decreased appetite, irritability, sore throat, fever	*IIV and LAIV:* Severe allergic reaction to eggs or prior vaccine dose, such as anaphylaxis *LAIV:* Contraindicated in children less than 2 years old with immunosuppression, asthma or wheezing episode in prior 12 months, or receiving an aspirin-containing product. *Precautions:* *LAIV:* Postpone vaccine when child has nasal congestion. *IIV:* May be given with minor illness, with or without fever. Give IIV if close contact with a severely immunocompromised person.	• Thawed LAIV is pale yellow, clear to slightly cloudy. • Split LAIV dose with a dose divider clip. Administer while child is sitting upright. Insert the tip of the sprayer inside each nostril and depress the plunger. • Reimmunize with 1 dose each year as immunity wanes, and vaccines are modified to include the new season's viruses. • If the child has received at least 2 doses of IIV since July 2010, only 1 annual dose is needed (Grohskopf et al., 2014).

(continued)

TABLE 16–1 Pediatric Vaccines (*continued*)

VACCINE TYPE	SIDE EFFECTS	CONTRAINDICATIONS	NURSING CONSIDERATIONS
Measles, Mumps, Rubella (MMR)			
Type: Live attenuated **Dosage:** 0.5 mL, subcutaneously (SQ) **Age(s) given:** 12–15 months; 4–6 years (2 doses) Give MMR and varicella vaccines on the same day or at least 4 weeks apart. **Storage:** Freeze or refrigerate vaccine before reconstitution. When reconstituted, keep refrigerated and away from light; discard if unused within 8 hr. Diluent is stored at room temperature or in a refrigerator; do not freeze.	**Common:** Fever 6–12 days after immunization; redness or pain at injection site; noncontagious rash; joint pain **Serious:** Allergic reaction or anaphylaxis; febrile seizure; meningitis (usually mild); encephalopathy; thrombocytopenia purpura; and rare cases of coma and permanent brain damage Children, ages 12–23 months, receiving the combined MMR and varicella vaccine have an increased risk of febrile seizures compared to children receiving MMR as separate vaccines (CDC, 2014g).	Prior anaphylactic reaction to neomycin Severe allergic reaction to prior vaccine dose or vaccine component Pregnancy Severe immunodeficiency due to malignancy, congenital immunodeficiency disease, long-term immunosuppressive therapy, or child with HIV infection **Precautions and deferral:** Receipt of immune globulin or blood product in last 3–11 months. History of thrombocytopenia or thrombocytopenic purpura Moderate or severe acute illness with or without fever Personal or family history of seizures may increase risk of febrile seizures after immunization (McLean, Fiebelkorn, Temte, et al., 2013).	• Ask about immune suppression. • Reconstituted vaccine is a clear, yellow solution. • Give entire contents of reconstituted vial even if more than 0.5 mL. • May give to a child with an egg allergy (AAP, 2015, p. 541). • Give to children with HIV unless severely immunocompromised. • Give tuberculosis (TB) test at same time as MMR or 4–6 weeks later. • Educate adolescent girls to avoid pregnancy for 28 days after immunization.
Meningococcal Tetravalent Conjugate (MenACWY-D, MenACWY-CRM)			
Type: Conjugate **Dosage:** 0.5 mL, IM **Age(s) given:** 11–12 years, and booster dose 16–18 years MenACWY-CRM may be given to high-risk children (2 months and older). Infants under 7 months get 4 doses (2, 4, 6, and 12 months); older children get 2 doses, with second dose 3 months later or after 12 months of age (MacNeil et al., 2014). **Storage:** Refrigerate until used, do not freeze.	**Common:** Swelling and pain at injection site, irritability, headache, fatigue, anorexia, and diarrhea	Severe allergic reaction (e.g., anaphylaxis) after prior dose or to a vaccine component (e.g., diphtheria toxoid) **Precautions:** Previous history of Guillain-Barré syndrome, unless at high risk for meningococcal disease	• Protect vaccine from light. • Verify that correct vaccine licensed for infants and children less than 24 months of age is used. • Give a booster dose to children 2–6 years old with immunosuppression 3 years after first dose for children 2–6 years and then every 5 years. • Give a booster dose to children 7 years and older with immunosuppression 5 years after first dose and then every 5 years (AAP, 2015, p. 555).
Pneumococcal Conjugate (PCV13)			
Type: Conjugate **Dosage:** 0.5 mL, IM **Age(s) given:** 2, 4, 6, 12–15 months **Storage:** Refrigerate, do not freeze.	**Common:** Pain, redness, swelling, induration at injection site; fever; irritability, decreased appetite, increased or decreased sleep **Severe:** Allergic reaction or anaphylaxis	Severe allergic reaction (e.g., anaphylaxis) after a prior dose of PCV7, PCV13, or vaccine containing diphtheria toxoid, or a component of one of the listed vaccines **Precautions and deferral:** Moderate or severe acute illness with or without fever	• Clear, colorless, or slightly opalescent liquid. • Give a supplemental dose using PCV13 if a child 6–18 years is at risk for invasive pneumococcal disease who also received PPSV23 (AAP, 2015, p. 635).

VACCINE TYPE	SIDE EFFECTS	CONTRAINDICATIONS	NURSING CONSIDERATIONS
Poliovirus Vaccine (IPV) **Type:** Inactivated **Dosage:** 0.5 mL, subcutaneously or IM, follow guidance for brand used **Age(s) given:** 2, 4, 12–18 months; 4–6 years (4 doses) **Storage:** Refrigerate, do not freeze.	**Common:** Swelling and tenderness, irritability, tiredness **Serious:** Allergic reaction or anaphylaxis	Severe allergic reaction, e.g., anaphylaxis, after prior dose or to vaccine components (neomycin, streptomycin, polymyxin B) **Precautions and deferral:** Pregnancy Moderate or severe acute illness with or without fever	• Ask about an allergy to the antibiotic contained in the specific IPV product available. • Clear, colorless suspension. Do not use if it contains particulate matter, becomes cloudy, or changes color.
Rotavirus Vaccine (RV1, RV5) **Type:** Live **Dosage:** 1 mL or 2 mL, oral **Age(s) given:** RV1 at 2 and 4 months (2 doses); RV5 at 2, 4, and 6 months (3 doses); all 3 doses of vaccine should be completed by 8 months of age. Complete the series with the same vaccine. **Storage:** Refrigerate, do not freeze.	**Common:** Irritability, cough, runny nose, loss of appetite, vomiting **Severe:** Potential increased risk for intussusception	Severe allergic reaction to a previous dose or to a vaccine component Severe combined immunodeficiency disease Uncorrected gastrointestinal malformation that puts infant at risk for intussusception History of intussusception **Precautions and deferral:** Altered immunosuppression Moderate or severe acute illness with or without fever, including diarrhea and vomiting Preexisting chronic gastrointestinal disease Spina bifida or bladder exstrophy	• Pale yellow clear liquid. Protect vaccine from light. • Ask about contacts that might have immunodeficiency; viral shedding is known to occur. • Squeeze the liquid into the infant's mouth toward the inner cheek until the dosing tube is empty. • RV1 applicator has latex; RV5 applicator is latex-free. • Do not repeat the dose if the infant spits out, vomits, or regurgitates during or after the dose. • There are no food or liquid restrictions before or after vaccine.
Varicella Virus Vaccine **Type:** Live attenuated **Dosage:** 0.5 mL, subcutaneously **Age(s) given:** 12–18 months, 4–6 years May be given in combined vaccine with MMR. **Storage:** Keep frozen at 5°F (–15°C) or colder. May be stored for up to 72 hr in refrigerator prior to reconstitution. Diluents kept at room temperature. Once reconstituted, use vaccine within 30 min or discard.	**Common:** Pain or redness at injection site; fever; a vaccine-related rash (2–5 maculopapular or vesicular lesions may occur 5–26 days after injection). **Severe:** Allergic reaction or anaphylaxis; rare cases of encephalitis, pneumonia, erythema multiforme, Stevens-Johnson syndrome, thrombocytopenia, seizure, and Guillain-Barré syndrome	Severe allergic reaction (e.g., anaphylaxis) after a prior dose or to a vaccine component (e.g., neomycin or gelatin). Known severe immunodeficiency due to malignancy, chemotherapy, congenital immunodeficiency disorder, long-term immunosuppressive therapy, or clients with HIV infection who are severely immunocompromised Pregnancy Active untreated tuberculosis **Precautions and deferral:** Receipt of blood products or immune globulin within past 3–11 months Moderate or severe acute illness with or without fever	• Ask if child is immunodeficient or has an allergy to a vaccine component. • Clear, colorless to pale yellow liquid when reconstituted. • Give the entire contents of the vial even if more than 0.5 mL. • Instruct adolescent girls of childbearing age to avoid pregnancy for 3 months after immunization. • Antiviral agents should not be used 1 day before or for 21 days after vaccine. • Avoid exposure to immunodeficient persons for 6 weeks after vaccinated.

Source: Data from American Academy of Pediatrics. (2015). *Red Book: Report of the Committee on Infectious Disease* (30th ed.). Elk Grove Village, IL; McLean, H. Q., Fiebelkorn, A. P., Temte, J. L., & Wallace, G. S. (2013). Prevention of measles, rubella, congenital rubella syndrome, and mumps, 2013: Summary recommendations of the Advisory Committee on Immunization Practices. *Morbidity and Mortality Weekly Report, 62*(4), 1–34; Markowitz, L. E., Dunne, E. F., Saraiya, M., Chesson, H. W., Curtis, C. R., Gee, J., . . . Unger, E. R. (2014). Human papillomavirus vaccination: Recommendations of the Advisory Committee on Immunization Practices. *Morbidity and Mortality Weekly Report, 63*(5), 1–30; Grohskopf, L. A., Olsen, S. J., Sokolow, L. Z., Bresee, J. S., Cox, N. J., Broder, K. R., . . . Walter, E. B. (2014). Prevention and control of seasonal influenza with vaccines: Recommendations of the Advisory Committee on Immunization Practices (ACIP)—United States, 2014–15 influenza season. *Morbidity and Mortality Weekly Report, 63*(32), 691–697; MacNeil, J. R., Rubin, L., McNamara, L., Briere, E. C., Clark, T. A., & Cohn, A. C. (2014). Use of MenACWY-CRM vaccine in children aged 2 through 23 months at increased risk for meningococcal disease: Recommendations of the Advisory Committee on Immunization Practices, 2013. *Morbidity and Mortality Weekly Report, 63*(24), 527–530.

Clinical Manifestations

Children have a variety of reactions to the antigens in different vaccines, and those reactions occur because of the child's immune system response. Common local reactions at the injection site include erythema, swelling, pain, and induration. Systemic reactions such as fever, fussiness or irritability, malaise, and anorexia may occur. A rash or arthralgia may occur with some vaccines. Highly anxious adolescents may have syncope or a vasovagal reaction within 15 minutes of immunization, leading to fall-related injuries (American Academy of Pediatrics [AAP] Committee on Infectious Disease, 2015, p. 26–27).

Allergic reactions to vaccines occur occasionally, such as a wheal and urticaria, within minutes to hours after the injection. A severe local allergic reaction is manifested by warmth, erythema, edema, petechiae, or ulceration occurring 2 to 8 hours after vaccination. A non–life-threatening systemic allergic reaction, such as generalized urticaria or transient petechiae, may occur within minutes. Anaphylaxis, a life-threatening reaction manifested by hypotension, generalized urticaria, angioedema, and laryngeal edema, rarely occurs with any vaccine. Allergic reactions are most often associated with vaccine components such as eggs, gelatin, yeast, and neomycin (AAP, 2015, pp. 54–56). See Table 16–1 for potential vaccine allergies.

Collaborative Care

Vaccines are recommended for administration at specific ages and intervals. Timing for first immunizations is determined by the age at which **transplacental immunity** (passive immunity transferred from mother to infant) decreases or disappears, and the infant or child develops the ability to make antibodies in response to the vaccine. Scientists continue to study the duration of protection from vaccines. Many vaccines are repeated at a later age to boost immunity.

Clinical Tip

Make every effort to stay current on immunization guidelines and information about vaccines, safe administration, adverse effects, and so on. Major resources provide more extensive information about immunization schedules and specific vaccines, as well as infectious and communicable diseases. The American Academy of Pediatrics' *Red Book: Report of the Committee on Infectious Diseases* is updated about every 3 years. Another resource is *Epidemiology and Prevention of Vaccine-Preventable Diseases*, commonly called the *Pink Book*, published by the Public Health Foundation, which has comprehensive information on communicable diseases and vaccines. The revised immunization schedule is published each January in several pediatric medical and nursing journals. The Centers for Disease Control and Prevention (CDC) maintains a website with detailed information about immunizations, the recommended vaccine schedule, and infectious and communicable diseases.

IMMUNIZATION SCHEDULES

The recommended immunization schedule is updated at least annually to reflect new vaccine information. The Advisory Committee on Immunization Practices (ACIP) of the Centers for Disease Control and Prevention (CDC), the American Academy of Pediatrics (AAP), and the American Academy of Family Practitioners (AAFP) collaborate to provide a uniform recommended schedule. See Figure 16–2 for the 2016 recommendations for vaccines that all children should receive. Schedules and recommendations vary for children who begin immunizations later in childhood or need catch-up doses.

Children with **asplenia** (loss of the spleen due to surgery or nonfunctioning due to sickle cell disease) are at higher risk for invasive pneumococcal and meningococcal infections. After completion of the PCV13 series, these children should receive pneumococcal polysaccharide vaccine (PPSV23) beginning at age 24 months. A second dose is given 5 years later. Some children who are American Indians or Alaska Natives living in areas of increased incidence of invasive pneumococcal disease may also be given PPSV23 (AAP, 2015, p. 92). See Table 16–1 for MCV4 guidelines.

Healthy People 2020

(IID-7) Achieve and maintain effective vaccination coverage levels for universally recommended vaccines among young children

(IID-10) Maintain vaccination coverage levels for children in kindergarten

(IID-11) Increase routine vaccination coverage levels for adolescents

---

IMPROVING IMMUNIZATION RATES

The effort to increase the numbers of children protected from vaccine-preventable diseases and to monitor immunization status is a national public health initiative.

For children between 19 and 35 months of age in 2014, the *Healthy People 2020* goal of 90% of children in this age group immunized with these vaccines—three IPV, one MMR, three HepB, and one varicella—was achieved. The goal was not achieved for full immunization of DTap, Hib, PCV, rotavirus, and HepA. Less than 1% of children received no vaccines. Variations were found by racial and ethnic groups and family income level (Hill, Elam-Evans, Yankey, et al., 2015). In 2014, adolescents between 13 and 17 years of age were found to have the following rates of immunization for recommended vaccines: one Tdap (87.9%), one MCV4 (79.3%), second MMR (90.7%), three HB (91.4%), second varicella or disease (85.0%), and three HPV (in females, 39.7%, and in males, 21.6%) (Reagan-Steiner, Yankey, Jeyarajah, et al., 2015). Increasing the immunization rate of adolescents has many challenges.

Lower immunization rates are often associated with economic factors, limited access to health care, lack of primary care at hours convenient for working parents, inadequate education about the importance of immunization, and cultural or religious prohibitions. The federal Vaccines for Children program provides free vaccines for qualified children and adolescents less than 19 years of age and has resolved some of the economic factors associated with vaccine coverage. However, the cost of vaccines, approximately $2575 for all approved vaccines for fully immunizing a child through the adolescent years in 2015, may be a barrier for children with private health insurance whose parents must co-pay (CDC, 2015a).

An increasing number of parents are choosing not to immunize their children for philosophical, religious, or other reasons, such as (Hendrix et al., 2014):

- Belief that vaccine-preventable diseases are not dangerous, and they occur rarely today
- Concerns that the frequency and number of vaccines to be administered cause pain and may overwhelm an infant's immune system

A. Recommended immunization schedule for persons aged 0 through 18 years – United States, 2016.

(FOR THOSE WHO FALL BEHIND OR START LATE, SEE THE CATCH-UP SCHEDULE [FIGURE 2]).

These recommendations must be read with the footnotes that follow. For those who fall behind or start late, provide catch-up vaccination at the earliest opportunity as indicated by the green bars in Figure 1. To determine minimum intervals between doses, see the catch-up schedule (Figure 2). School entry and adolescent vaccine age groups are shaded.

Vaccine	Birth	1 mo	2 mos	4 mos	6 mos	9 mos	12 mos	15 mos	18 mos	19–23 mos	2–3 yrs	4–6 yrs	7–10 yrs	11–12 yrs	13–15 yrs	16–18 yrs
Hepatitis B[1] (HepB)	1st dose	◄----- 2nd dose -----►			◄--------------------------- 3rd dose ---------------------------►											
Rotavirus[2] (RV) RV1 (2-dose series); RV5 (3-dose series)			1st dose	2nd dose	See footnote 2											
Diphtheria, tetanus, & acellular pertussis[3] (DTaP: <7 yrs)			1st dose	2nd dose	3rd dose		◄----- 4th dose -----►					5th dose				
Haemophilus influenzae type b[4] (Hib)			1st dose	2nd dose	See footnote 4		◄ 3rd or 4th dose, ► See footnote 4									
Pneumococcal conjugate[5] (PCV13)			1st dose	2nd dose	3rd dose		◄----- 4th dose -----►									
Inactivated poliovirus[6] (IPV: <18 yrs)			1st dose	2nd dose	◄--------------------------- 3rd dose ---------------------------►							4th dose				
Influenza[7] (IIV; LAIV)					◄------------ Annual vaccination (IIV only) 1 or 2 doses ------------►					Annual vaccination (LAIV or IIV) 1 or 2 doses		Annual vaccination (LAIV or IIV) 1 dose only				
Measles, mumps, rubella[8] (MMR)					See footnote 8		◄----- 1st dose -----►					2nd dose				
Varicella[9] (VAR)							◄----- 1st dose -----►					2nd dose				
Hepatitis A[10] (HepA)							◄------- 2-dose series, See footnote 10 -------►									
Meningococcal[11] (Hib-MenCY ≥ 6 weeks; MenACWY-D ≥9 mos; MenACWY-CRM ≥ 2 mos)							See footnote 11							1st dose		Booster
Tetanus, diphtheria, & acellular pertussis[12] (Tdap: ≥7 yrs)														(Tdap)		
Human papillomavirus[13] (2vHPV: females only; 4vHPV, 9vHPV: males and females)														(3-dose series)		
Meningococcal B[11]															See footnote 11	
Pneumococcal polysaccharide[5] (PPSV23)											See footnote 5					

▢ Range of recommended ages for all children	▢ Range of recommended ages for catch-up immunization	▢ Range of recommended ages for certain high-risk groups	▢ Range of recommended ages for non-high-risk groups that may receive vaccine, subject to individual clinical decision making	▢ No recommendation

This schedule includes recommendations in effect as of January 1, 2016. Any dose not administered at the recommended age should be administered at a subsequent visit, when indicated and feasible. The use of a combination vaccine generally is preferred over separate injections of its equivalent component vaccines. Vaccination providers should consult the relevant Advisory Committee on Immunization Practices (ACIP) statement for detailed recommendations, available online at http://www.cdc.gov/vaccines/hcp/acip-recs/index.html. Clinically significant adverse events that follow vaccination should be reported to the Vaccine Adverse Event Reporting System (VAERS) online (http://www.vaers.hhs.gov) or by telephone (800-822-7967). Suspected cases of vaccine-preventable diseases should be reported to the state or local health department. Additional information, including precautions and contraindications for vaccination, is available from CDC online (http://www.cdc.gov/vaccines/recs/vac-admin/contraindications.htm) or by telephone (800-CDC-INFO [800-232-4636]).

This schedule is approved by the Advisory Committee on Immunization Practices (http://www.cdc.gov/vaccines/acip), the American Academy of Pediatrics (http://www.aap.org), the American Academy of Family Physicians (http://www.aafp.org), and the American College of Obstetricians and Gynecologists (http://www.acog.org).

NOTE: The above recommendations must be read along with the footnotes of this schedule. See http://www.cdc.gov/vaccines/schedules/index.html.

Figure 16–2 *A,* Recommended immunization schedule for children 0 to 18 years, United States, 2016. For further guidance on the vaccines listed see http://www.cdc.gov/vaccines/hcp/acip-recs/index.html.

- A vaccine's potential harm to the child because of the amount of its chemical and biologic content and its side effects
- Concerns that vaccines are related to autism
- Mistrust in healthcare provider recommendations

Other parents are selecting an alternate immunization schedule to delay or space out vaccines, such as the Sears Alternative Vaccine Schedule. However, this approach is not supported by evidence or public health officials.

See Table 16–2 for common misconceptions some parents have about vaccines and vaccine safety information. Increasing immunization rates of children whose parents are hesitant is a challenge. See *Evidence-Based Practice: Immunization Challenges.*

VACCINE INJURY COMPENSATION

Vaccines are tested for safety before being licensed by the U.S. Food and Drug Administration; however, serious vaccine reactions occur in rare instances. When a link between a child's immunization and a serious adverse reaction is identified, the National Vaccine Injury Compensation Program provides compensation for the family. The Vaccine Adverse Event Reporting System (VAERS) was established in 1988 to track serious vaccine reactions. See Table 16–3 for the serious reactions specific to each vaccine that are eligible for compensation.

Nursing Management

For the Child Receiving Immunizations

Nursing Assessment and Diagnosis

Nurses are responsible for reviewing a child's health record to determine whether the child needs vaccines. Identify any potential contraindications to vaccines by asking the following:

- Has the child had a serious reaction to any vaccine? Has the child had any vaccines in the last 4 weeks?
- Are there allergies to any vaccine components (e.g., eggs, neomycin, gelatin, or yeast) or latex?
- Does the child have a serious medical condition (seizures, cancer, HIV infection, immune diseases, blood disorder, asthma) or wheezing in the past 12 months?
- Has the child received any blood products, immune globulin, or any antiviral drugs in the past year?

B. Catch-up immunization schedule for persons aged 4 months through 18 years who start late or who are more than 1 month behind — United States, 2016.

The figure below provides catch-up schedules and minimum intervals between doses for children whose vaccinations have been delayed. A vaccine series does not need to be restarted, regardless of the time that has elapsed between doses. Use the section appropriate for the child's age. Always use this table in conjunction with Figure 1 and the footnotes that follow.

Vaccine	Minimum Age for Dose 1	Minimum Interval Between Doses			
		Dose 1 to Dose 2	Dose 2 to Dose 3	Dose 3 to Dose 4	Dose 4 to Dose 5
Children age 4 months through 6 years					
Hepatitis B[1]	Birth	4 weeks	8 weeks *and* at least 16 weeks after first dose. Minimum age for the final dose is 24 weeks.		
Rotavirus[2]	6 weeks	4 weeks	4 weeks[2]		
Diphtheria, tetanus, and acellular pertussis[3]	6 weeks	4 weeks	4 weeks	6 months	6 months[3]
Haemophilus influenzae type b[4]	6 weeks	4 weeks if first dose was administered before the 1st birthday. 8 weeks (as final dose) if first dose was administered at age 12 through 14 months. No further doses needed if first dose was administered at age 15 months or older.	4 weeks[4] if current age is younger than 12 months **and** first dose was administered at younger than age 7 months, **and** at least 1 previous dose was PRP-T (ActHib, Pentacel) or unknown. 8 weeks *and* age 12 through 59 months (as final dose)[4] • if current age is younger than 12 months **and** first dose was administered at age 7 through 11 months (wait until at least 12 months old); OR • if current age is 12 through 59 months **and** first dose was administered before the 1st birthday, **and** second dose administered at younger than 15 months; OR • if both doses were PRP-OMP (PedvaxHIB; Comvax) **and** were administered before the 1st birthday (wait until at least 12 months old). No further doses needed if previous dose was administered at age 15 months or older.	8 weeks (as final dose) This dose only necessary for children age 12 through 59 months who received 3 doses before the 1st birthday.	
Pneumococcal[5]	6 weeks	4 weeks if first dose administered before the 1st birthday. 8 weeks (as final dose for healthy children) if first dose was administered at the 1st birthday or after. No further doses needed for healthy children if first dose administered at age 24 months or older.	4 weeks if current age is younger than 12 months and previous dose given at <7months old. 8 weeks (as final dose for healthy children) if previous dose given between 7-11 months (wait until at least 12 months old); OR if current age is 12 months or older and at least 1 dose was given before age 12 months. No further doses needed for healthy children if previous dose administered at age 24 months or older.	8 weeks (as final dose) This dose only necessary for children aged 12 through 59 months who received 3 doses before age 12 months or for children at high risk who received 3 doses at any age.	
Inactivated poliovirus[6]	6 weeks	4 weeks[6]	4 weeks[6]	6 months[6] (minimum age 4 years for final dose).	
Measles, mumps, rubella[8]	12 months	4 weeks			
Varicella[9]	12 months	3 months			
Hepatitis A[10]	12 months	6 months			
Meningococcal[11] (Hib-MenCY ≥ 6 weeks; MenACWY-D ≥9 mos; MenACWY-CRM ≥ 2 mos)	6 weeks	8 weeks[11]	See footnote 11	See footnote 11	
Children and adolescents age 7 through 18 years					
Meningococcal[11] (Hib-MenCY ≥ 6 weeks; MenACWY-D ≥9 mos; MenACWY-CRM ≥ 2 mos)	Not Applicable (N/A)	8 weeks[11]			
Tetanus, diphtheria; tetanus, diphtheria, and acellular pertussis[12]	7 years[12]	4 weeks	4 weeks if first dose of DTaP/DT was administered before the 1st birthday. 6 months (as final dose) if first dose of DTaP/DT or Tdap/Td was administered at or after the 1st birthday.	6 months if first dose of DTaP/DT was administered before the 1st birthday.	
Human papillomavirus[13]	9 years	Routine dosing intervals are recommended.[13]			
Hepatitis A[10]	N/A	6 months			
Hepatitis B[1]	N/A	4 weeks	8 weeks **and** at least 16 weeks after first dose.		
Inactivated poliovirus[6]	N/A	4 weeks	4 weeks[6]	6 months[6]	
Measles, mumps, rubella[8]	N/A	4 weeks			
Varicella[9]	N/A	3 months if younger than age 13 years. 4 weeks if age 13 years or older.			

NOTE: The above recommendations must be read along with the footnotes of this schedule. See http://www.cdc.gov/vaccines/schedules/index.html.

Figure 16–2 *(Continued)* B, Catch-up immunization schedule for children 4 months to 18 years, United States, 2016. For further guidance on the vaccines listed see http://www.cdc.gov/vaccines/hcp/acip-recs/index.html

SOURCE: Centers for Disease Control (CDC)

- Has the child taken cortisone, prednisone, other steroids, or anticancer drugs or had radiation treatments in the past 3 months?
- Is the female adolescent possibly pregnant now, or will she be in the next month?

Healthcare providers miss many opportunities to immunize children. Assess the immunization status of children (and siblings present) during all healthcare visits and hospitalizations and in schools. Use the most current immunization schedule to identify needed vaccines. When a child needs immunizations, determine the best combination of vaccines to give at this visit to better protect the child. However, make sure the appropriate interval has occurred between vaccine dosages, using the catch-up vaccine schedule. Ways to reduce the number of missed opportunities for full immunization of children include the following:

- Place a reminder in the child's health record to alert health professionals about the child's need for immunizations. Establish a system to send parents a reminder when the child's immunizations are due or overdue.

SAFETY ALERT!

Immune globulin, blood products, and immunosuppressive agents inhibit the child's response to live virus vaccines (MMR, varicella), so ask parents about any recent administration of these products. When possible, administer inactivated vaccines 2 or more weeks before and live virus vaccines 4 or more weeks before immunosuppressive therapy is begun (Rubin et al., 2013). Refer to the most current guidelines from the Centers for Disease Control and Prevention's Advisory Committee on Immunization Practices (ACIP) to identify the correct interval (3 to 11 months) between the administration of the blood product, immune globulin, or completion of immunosuppression therapy and administration of a live virus vaccine (Kroger, Sumaya, Pickering, et al., 2011.

If immune globulin or blood products were given 14 days before or up to several months following a vaccine, readminister the vaccine after the period specified by the CDC, unless serologic testing determines that the child developed adequate serum antibodies (AAP, 2015, pp. 38–39).

Text continues on page 345

TABLE 16–2 Common Misconceptions About Vaccines and Correct Information

COMMON MISCONCEPTIONS	CORRECT VACCINE INFORMATION
Vaccine-preventable diseases have been eliminated.	The incidence of vaccine-preventable diseases is low in the United States, but these diseases occur elsewhere in the world. Unvaccinated travelers have reintroduced diseases from a country or a U.S. community where the disease exists. Recent outbreaks of measles have been linked to unimmunized travelers who became infected in one of 18 countries (Gastañaduy et al., 2014). Children with lowered immune status (e.g., treatment for cancer) are at higher risk for exposure to infection because of lowered herd immunity. **Herd immunity** is the protection provided by a large group of persons who have immunity to a disease and indirectly protect others without immunity by reducing the risk for exposure and infection.
Immunization weakens the immune system. Multiple vaccines overload the immune system and cause harmful effects.	Vaccines use the body's immune system to prevent a future infection. Infants are capable of developing protective immune responses to multiple vaccines simultaneously. The number of antigens in these vaccines is substantially fewer than the immune challenges associated with daily environmental exposures (DeStefano, Price, & Weintraub, 2013).
Thimerosal use in vaccines may cause mercury poisoning.	Thimerosal, a bacteriostatic agent that contains ethyl mercury, previously was used to sterilize vaccines in multidose vials. Because of concerns about mercury poisoning and related nerve and brain damage, thimerosal has been eliminated from all but the influenza vaccine. A thimerosal-free influenza vaccine is available for children (AAP, 2015, p. 18).
It would be better to let the child get the disease than get immunized.	Most parents have never seen these diseases and do not understand how dangerous they may be, sometimes leading to hospitalization, disability, and even death. Infected children can spread the infection to pregnant women, exposing the fetus, and to infants and children with serious medical conditions.
Vaccines do not work; children still get the disease.	No vaccine is 100% effective, and immunity does wane over time, leading to the need for a booster dose.

EVIDENCE-BASED PRACTICE | Immunization Challenges

Clinical Question

What strategies are needed to increase acceptance of vaccines in hesitant parents?

The Evidence

A randomized trial study using web-based interactions with 1759 parents investigated the effectiveness of public health messages about the safety of the MMR vaccine or the danger of measles, mumps, and rubella diseases. The four messages integrated CDC vaccine language and included (1) corrected misinformation that vaccines cause autism, (2) presented information on disease risks, (3) a story about a child hospitalized with measles, and (4) photographs of infected children to emphasize the disease risks. The outcome measure was parent intention to give the MMR vaccine to a future child. None of the messages increased parents' intent to immunize a future child with the MMR vaccine. Provaccine messages were least effective in parents with negative attitudes about vaccines. In some cases, messages increased beliefs about MMR side effects (Nyhan, Reifler, Richey, et al., 2014).

A randomized trial survey of 802 parents of infants less than 12 months of age were presented four vaccine messages to identify which one increased a parent's intent to immunize their child with the MMR vaccine. The Vaccine Information Sheet (VIS) was the control message. The other three messages included the VIS plus (1) the benefits of the vaccine to the child, (2) the benefits of immunizing the child to society, and (3) the benefits of the vaccine to the child plus society. Parents had a significantly higher intent to immunize their infant when the benefits of the vaccine to the child or the benefits to the child plus society messages were used when compared to the control message (Hendrix et al., 2014).

A study using data from the National Immunization Survey for Teens focused on reasons parents gave for adolescents who were not up-to-date on Tdap/Td, MCV4, and HPV as not receiving the vaccines. The reasons given for Tdap/Td and MCV4 were the same: not recommended by a healthcare provider, not needed, lack of knowledge, or don't know. The HPV vaccine was not accepted more commonly for these reasons: not sexually active, not needed or not necessary, and vaccine safety concerns (Darden et al., 2013).

Best Practice

With the increased trend in undervaccination of children, efforts have shifted to finding messages that will increase a parent's acceptance of vaccines. One study identified that a higher acceptance occurred when the discussion with the parent about a vaccine focused on the benefit for their child rather than societal benefits. Exposure to viruses and bacteria causing vaccine-preventable diseases is unpredictable, so vaccines are given before an exposure. For adolescents, it is important to emphasize the reduced risk of cervical cancer that may occur 20 to 40 years after exposure to HPV. Since the virus is acquired during sexual activity, it is important for adolescents to receive the vaccine before sexual activity begins.

Clinical Reasoning

Think about some specific benefits to a child for each of the vaccines administered (e.g., no discomfort due to the disease, fewer days of school missed, fewer days the parents have to miss work because of a sick child). When in a clinical setting, identify and include the specific benefits for the child for each vaccine in the education provided to parents when seeking consent for vaccine administration.

TABLE 16–3 National Vaccine Injury Act—Vaccine Injury Table

VACCINE	ILLNESS, DISABILITY, INJURY, OR CONDITION COVERED	TIME PERIOD FOR FIRST SYMPTOM OR MANIFESTATION OF ONSET OR OF SIGNIFICANT AGGRAVATION AFTER VACCINE ADMINISTRATION
Vaccines containing tetanus toxoid (e.g., DTaP, Tdap, DTP-Hib, DT, Td, or TT)	Anaphylaxis or anaphylactic shock	4 hr
	Bacterial neuritis	2–28 days
	Any acute complication or sequela (including death) of above events occurring in the specified time period	Not applicable
Vaccines containing whole cell pertussis bacteria, extracted or partial cell pertussis bacteria, or specific pertussis antigen(s) (e.g., DTaP, Tdap, DTP, P, DTP-Hib)	Anaphylaxis or anaphylactic shock	4 hr
	Encephalopathy (or encephalitis)	72 hr
	Any acute complication or sequela (including death) of above events occurring within the specified time period	Not applicable
Measles, mumps, rubella vaccine or any of its components (e.g., MMR, MR, M, R)	Anaphylaxis or anaphylactic shock	4 hr
	Encephalopathy (or encephalitis)	5–15 days
	Any acute complication or sequela (including death) of above events occurring within the specified time period	Not applicable
Vaccines containing rubella virus (e.g., MMR, MR, R)	Chronic arthritis	7–42 days
	Any acute complication or sequela (including death) of above events occurring within the specified time period	Not applicable
Vaccines containing measles virus (e.g., MMR, MR, M)	Thrombocytopenic purpura	7–30 days
	Vaccine strain measles viral infection in an immunodeficient recipient	6 months
	Any acute complication or sequela (including death) of above events occurring within the specified time period	Not applicable
Vaccines containing polio live virus (OPV)	Paralytic polio	
	• in a nonimmunodeficient recipient	30 days
	• in an immunodeficient recipient	6 months
	• in a vaccine-associated community case	Not applicable
	Vaccine-strain polio viral infection	
	• in a nonimmunodeficient recipient	30 days
	• in an immunodeficient recipient	6 months
	• in a vaccine-associated community case	Not applicable
	Any acute complication or sequela (including death) of above events	Not applicable
Vaccines containing polio inactivated virus (IPV)	Anaphylaxis or anaphylactic shock	4 hr
	Any acute complication or sequela (including death) of above events occurring within the specified time period	Not applicable
Hepatitis B vaccines	Anaphylaxis or anaphylactic shock	4 hr
	Any acute complication or sequela (including death) of above events occurring within the specified time period	No limit
Haemophilus influenzae type b polysaccharide conjugate vaccines	No condition specified	Not applicable
Hepatitis A vaccines	No condition specified	Not applicable
Varicella vaccine	No condition specified	Not applicable
Rotavirus vaccine	No condition specified	Not applicable
Pneumococcal conjugate vaccines	No condition specified	Not applicable
Meningococcal vaccines	No condition specified	Not applicable
Trivalent influenza vaccines	No condition specified	Not applicable
Human papillomavirus (HPV) vaccines	No condition specified	Not applicable
Any new vaccine recommended by the CDC for routine administration to children after publication by the Secretary of the Department of Health and Human Services of notice of coverage	No condition specified	Not applicable

Effective date: November 12, 2013. For guidance in further interpretation of this table, visit the website below.

Source: From Health Resources and Services Administration. (2013). *Vaccine injury table*. Retrieved from http://www.hrsa.gov/vaccinecompensation/vaccineinjurytable.pdf

- Give vaccines when the child has a minor illness, even with a low-grade fever and antibiotic treatment, or has a recent exposure to an infectious disease.
- Use combination vaccines (e.g., DTaP-HepB-IPV) to reduce the number of injections from 20 to 13 in the first 2 years (see Table 16–4).
- Give multiple vaccines at the same time, using separate syringes and injecting in separate sites. If using the same extremity, separate injection sites by an inch (AAP, 2015, p. 36).
- Give medically stable low–birth-weight infants all vaccines appropriate for chronologic age as full-term infants. Use the full dose (AAP, 2015, pp. 68–69).
- Give the vaccine even when a prior dose caused a local reaction or a family member had an adverse response.

The accompanying *Nursing Care Plan* explores two potential nursing diagnoses that apply to the child needing immunizations. Additional nursing diagnoses may include the following (NANDA-I © 2014):

- *Skin Integrity, Risk for Impaired,* related to vaccine response
- *Health Maintenance, Ineffective,* related to philosophical beliefs regarding routine immunization
- *Anxiety* related to fear of needles

Planning and Implementation

Nursing management focuses on protecting the potency of vaccines, being a strong advocate for immunization, educating parents about immunizations and possible side effects, addressing their fears about possible reactions, obtaining consent, and reporting adverse reactions.

PROTECT VACCINE POTENCY

Take special care to ensure vaccine potency, so all children develop adequate immune response (CDC, 2014b).

- Store vaccines properly in the refrigerator or freezer (i.e., separate doors for refrigerator and freezer, storage conditions should be adequate: Refrigeration: 35°F to 46°F [2°C to 8°C]; Freezer: 5°F [–15°C] or lower as stated in vaccine package inserts).
- Keep jugs of water in the refrigerator and trays of ice in the freezer to help maintain a consistent temperature.
- Store the vaccines on the middle shelves of the units, 2 to 3 in. away from the walls, with space for air to circulate between boxes; place older vaccines in the front.
- Check the refrigerator and freezer temperatures twice daily and record the temperatures on a log or use an automatic temperature measurement system.
- Make an emergency plan for safe storage of vaccines in case of a power outage or natural disaster.

TABLE 16–4 Combination Vaccines

VACCINE NAME	VACCINE COMPONENTS	AGES USED
Comvax	Hib and HepB	2, 4, and 12–15 months of age, 3 doses
TriHIBit	DTaP and Hib	15–18 months, fourth dose of Hib and DTaP series
Twinrix	HepA and HepB	18 years and older
Pediarix	DTaP, HepB, and IPV	2, 4, and 6 months of age, 3 doses
ProQuad	MMR and Varicella	12–15 months of age, and 4–6 years of age
Kinrix	DTaP and IPV	4–6 years, fifth dose of DTaP and fourth dose of IPV
Pentacel	DTaP, IPV, and Hib	2, 4, 6, and 15–18 months of age, 4 doses
MenHibrix	Hib, Meningococcal CY serotypes	2, 4, 6, and 12–15 months of age

Source: Adapted from Kroger, A. T., Sumaya, C. V., Pickering, L. K., & Atkinson, W. L. (2011). General recommendations on immunization: Recommendations of the Advisory Committee on Immunization Practices (ACIP). *Morbidity and Mortality Weekly Report, 60*(2), 37; MacNeil, J. R., Rubin, L., McNamara, L., Briere, E. C., Clark, T. A., & Cohn, A. C. (2014). Use of MenACWY-CRM vaccine in children aged 2 through 23 months at increased risk for meningococcal disease: Recommendations of the Advisory Committee on Immunization Practices, 2013. *Morbidity and Mortality Weekly Report, 63*(24), 527–530.

OBTAIN CONSENT

Federal legislation requires written consent before administering a vaccine. The nurse often has the responsibility to inform the child's parents or legal guardian, and supply the most current Vaccine Information Statement (VIS) for each vaccine to be given, a requirement of the National Vaccine Injury Act.

Explain the risks and benefits of each vaccine and common local reactions. Answer all the parents' questions. Parents may have heard sensational stories about vaccines, and correct information is needed to help them make informed decisions.

Developing Cultural Competence Vaccine Information Statements (VIS)

Consider literacy and reading level when giving a VIS to a parent. The VIS is written at a sixth-grade level, but parents may have poor literacy. The VIS has been translated into 40 languages, and these are available through the CDC website. Ask rather than assume the parent can read the preferred spoken language. It is acceptable to read the VIS to parents and make sure that they understand the information.

Nursing Care Plan: The Child Needing Immunizations

1. Nursing Diagnosis: *Infection, Risk for,* related to incomplete immunizations for age (NANDA-I © 2014)

GOAL: The child will become adequately protected from disease-preventable illnesses.

INTERVENTION	RATIONALE
• Review the child's immunization record for needed vaccines at each healthcare visit.	• Children who need vaccines can be identified.
• Identify all due vaccines that can be provided simultaneously.	• Multiple vaccines given at the same visit more adequately protect the child.
• Identify potential contraindications to needed vaccines. Review past reactions to vaccines.	• Identifying contraindications and past reactions reduces the risk for adverse reactions to vaccines.

EXPECTED OUTCOME: Child will be adequately protected for age from vaccine-preventable illnesses.

2. Nursing Diagnosis: *Health Management, Readiness for Enhanced* (NANDA-I © 2014)

GOAL: Parents will sign consent for vaccines to be given.

INTERVENTION	RATIONALE
• Educate the parents and adolescents about the need for specific vaccines and the risk if not given. Obtain signed consent before giving vaccines.	• Informed consent is required for all treatments.

EXPECTED OUTCOME: Parent(s) will complete the consent forms, which are placed in the child's file.

GOAL: Parents and adolescents will state the side effects of vaccines given.

INTERVENTION	RATIONALE
• Review past reactions to vaccines and describe common potential reactions and why they occur.	• Parents should expect common reactions and know they indicate the child's body is building protection to the illness.
• Describe serious side effects that should be reported to the healthcare provider.	• Parents need to be prepared for potential serious side effects so they can obtain care if needed.

EXPECTED OUTCOME: Parents will report all serious side effects to the healthcare provider.

GOAL: Parents will manage common side effects of vaccines.

INTERVENTION	RATIONALE
• Teach parents general comfort measures for common side effects, for example:	• Parents will know how to make the child more comfortable during the 24–48 hr after the vaccine is given.
• Cool pack to tender leg	
• Acetaminophen or ibuprofen for fever and discomfort	
• Rocking and holding the infant	
• Gentle movement of affected extremity	

EXPECTED OUTCOME: Child will be given comfort measures after vaccine administration.

Families Want to Know

Care of the Child After Immunizations

When a child receives an immunization, educate parents to observe for any reactions that might occur and call the child's healthcare provider if there is concern about any of the symptoms listed.

- Local pain, redness, and swelling are common. Use ice on the injection site to help reduce swelling and pain. Acetaminophen or ibuprofen may be given to reduce a fever and pain. The symptoms should disappear in a day or two.

- The child may have a fever, joint pain, muscle aches, or fatigue within hours to days after the vaccine is given. Give acetaminophen or ibuprofen for pain.

- With a mild allergic reaction to the vaccine, a few hives may be noted around the injection site.

- A severe allergic reaction is indicated by a flushed face; swelling of the face, mouth, or throat; wheezing or other difficulty breathing; shock (confusion, lack of movement or response, or unconsciousness); and abdominal cramping. Call 9-1-1 for emergency treatment. Have the child lie down with the legs raised higher than the level of the heart until the ambulance arrives to promote blood return to the vital organs.

When a parent refuses to accept a particular vaccine, have the parent sign an informed refusal document. If a disease outbreak occurs, the unimmunized child must be kept out of school or child care. See the section on fever, later in this chapter, for guidance on home care of the child with an infectious disease.

For each vaccine administered, the nurse is required to record the (1) month, day, and year of administration, (2) vaccine given, (3) manufacturer, (4) lot number and expiration date of the immunization given, (5) site and route of administration, and (6) name, title, and address of the person who administers the vaccine. Provide parents with a record of the child's immunizations, and enter the information on vaccines administered into the healthcare agency's official records.

Provide guidance for managing expected mild reactions at home (see *Families Want to Know: Care of the Child After Immunizations*). Provide information about the proper dose of acetaminophen or ibuprofen to give the child.

ADMINISTER VACCINES

Check the expiration of vaccines before use. Follow the manufacturer's directions for reconstituting vaccines and use the solution provided. Write the date and time on the bottle if it is a multidose vial. Reconstitute vaccines immediately before use as some have a short shelf life.

Use 1-in. needles rather than 5/8 in. (25 mm rather than 16 mm) for infants for IM injections to give the vaccine deep in the muscle mass. Stretch the skin to decrease the amount of subcutaneous tissue the needle must go through. Follow facility needle length guidelines for children of other ages. For vaccines given subcutaneously, select a 5/8-in. 23- to 25-gauge needle. Use the upper thigh in infants less than 12 months of age, and the upper outer triceps region for older children (Kroger et al., 2011).

SAFETY ALERT!

Adolescents who are extremely fearful of getting an injection are at a greater risk for fainting, syncope, or vasovagal response after a vaccine injection. Provide the injection when the adolescent is sitting or lying down. Observe the adolescent while sitting or lying down for 15 minutes to prevent secondary injury in case of syncope.

REDUCE PAIN AND ANXIETY

Make an effort to reduce the pain associated with vaccine injections, especially since infants and children must return for more injections. Give the appropriate immunizations to the child as

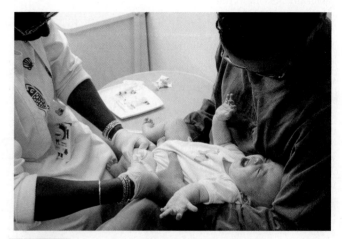

Figure 16–3 Give immunizations quickly and efficiently. Do not prolong the wait and let fear grow. The child will be anxious, especially if more than one injection must be given.

efficiently as possible, while providing support to the child (Figure 16–3). Suggestions for pain management include the following techniques:

- Coach the parent to hold and talk with the child during the injections. Funny faces, a toy, or age-appropriate distraction might also help. Encourage parents to give comfort measures after the injection.

- Give infants up to 4 months of age 24% sucrose water to drink (e.g., Sweetease or mix 1 packet of table sugar with 10 mL of tap water) prior to the injection (see Chapter 15). Then allow the infant to suck on a pacifier or breastfeed during the injections.

- Apply pressure at the site for 10 seconds before the injection.

- Provide information about obtaining L-M-X4 (a topical anesthetic available without a prescription) prior to the next visit. Instruct parents how to apply L-M-X4 cream to one or more sites prior to the child's appointment. See Chapter 15 for information regarding use of L-M-X4.

- Spray the planned injection site with vapocoolant spray immediately before the injection, or spray it on a cotton ball and hold that against the skin.

- Have two providers each give an injection simultaneously in different extremities.

- Do not prolong the process of giving immunizations. Give the child honest answers that the needles will cause some pain.
- Let the child select the arm or leg for the injection and forms of distraction to promote coping.

PREPARE FOR EMERGENCIES

Be prepared for potential vaccine anaphylaxis even though it is a rare event. Keep epinephrine and resuscitation equipment immediately available. The dose for epinephrine (aqueous 1:1000) is 0.01 mL/kg per dose (maximum dose is 0.5 mL) intramuscularly. The dose can be repeated every 5 to 15 minutes in order to control symptoms and maintain blood pressure. When the child is stable, oral antihistamines and corticosteroids may be prescribed for an additional 24 to 48 hours (AAP, 2015, pp. 66–68).

Remember to report anaphylaxis and other severe reactions following immunization to the Vaccine Compensation Injury Program. See Table 16–3.

Evaluation

Expected outcomes of nursing care include the following:

- Parents are fully informed and give consent for immunizations.
- All vaccines appropriate for the child's age are given at each health visit.
- The parents are prepared to identify serious vaccine reactions and manage mild reactions at home.

Clinical Reasoning Immunizations

A 5-year-old girl, Lian, has accompanied her mother and 2-year-old brother Chang to the pediatric clinic. Lian's mother is concerned because Chang has had a fever of 38.3°C (101.0°F) for the past 3 days. Although Chang has visited this clinic several times in the past few months for health care, this is the first time Lian has come along.

When asked, Lian's mother says Lian had a healthcare visit about 2 years ago, but she does not know if she had all of her shots. In checking Lian's health records, the nurse notes that she needs DTaP, IPV, PCV13, MMR, varicella, and HepA vaccines. Chang needs MMR, varicella, HepA, and PCV13 vaccines.

Should Lian receive any of these vaccines today, even though her brother is ill? Which vaccines could be given during one visit? Should Chang receive any vaccines today?

Communicable Diseases in Children

Communicable diseases cause acute illnesses resulting from bacterial, viral, protozoan, or fungal organisms. Infants and children are more susceptible and develop communicable diseases more frequently than adults do. Active immunity to microorganisms does not occur until there is natural exposure or immunization that leads to antibody production.

The epidemiology, clinical manifestations, treatment, prevention, and nursing care of selected communicable diseases of childhood are described in Table 16–5. Infectious diseases transmitted by animal vectors are detailed in Table 16–6. See Chapter 26 for information on sexually transmitted infections, Chapter 19 for information about conjunctivitis, Chapter 20 for information on tuberculosis, and Chapter 25 for information on hepatitis and parasites.

Clinical Manifestations

The child with an infectious or communicable disease has a cluster of symptoms specific to the disease that appear at the end of the **incubation period**, the time interval between exposure and development of symptoms. Some diseases have a **prodrome**, the phase of early manifestations of the infection until the development of the overt clinical syndrome. Fever is the most common sign of communicable disease in infants and children. Other nonspecific signs are related to the specific disease and may include fatigue, malaise, weakness, decreased responsiveness or inability to concentrate, skin rash, poor appetite, vomiting, diarrhea, and body aches.

Developing Cultural Competence Disease Causation

In some cultures, infectious diseases are seen as punishment or the result of curses or evil spirits. For example, American Indians (e.g., Navajo) traditionally view illnesses as the result of disharmony or displeasing the spirits. They may not believe in the germ theory of disease causation (Purnell, 2014).

FEVER

Fever is an increased body temperature of 38.0°C (100.4°F) or higher taken by rectal or tympanic route, and 37.8°C (100.0°F) or higher by the oral or temporal route. The hypothalamus is the body's thermostat or control center for the regulation of body temperature (see *Pathophysiology Illustrated: Fever*). As blood circulates through the hypothalamus, the body is directed to conserve or release heat, depending on the temperature of the blood.

FEVER MANAGEMENT

A fever can be a beneficial physiologic response to infection, helping to slow the growth and reproduction of organisms that thrive at lower body temperatures. A fever decreases the serum levels of zinc, iron, and copper needed by bacteria for reproduction. It also encourages the body to shift to a metabolism that burns fat and proteins rather than glucose, which deprives bacteria of a food source (Huether, 2014). Fever is not inherently harmful until it reaches 41.0°C (105.9°F). Medical management may include postponing treatment of low-grade fevers (under 38.9°C [102.0°F]) to promote the body's natural defenses against an infection.

Fevers are often treated if they cause discomfort with acetaminophen or ibuprofen. Aspirin is no longer recommended for children because of its association with Reye syndrome (see Chapter 27). Antipyretics inhibit prostaglandin synthesis, which results in lowering of the body's temperature set point and reducing the fever.

Developing Cultural Competence Hot and Cold Therapy

Many Latino and Asian cultures subscribe to the hot and cold theory of disease causation. Fever, a hot condition, is treated by giving the ill person cold substances (either foods or medicines). Cold foods include dairy products, fresh vegetables, fruits, chicken, goat meat, and fish. Cold medicines include orange flower water, linden, and sage (Purnell, 2013). See Table 2–2, *Hot and Cold Conditions and Foods*.

Text continues on page 361

TABLE 16–5 Selected Infectious and Communicable Diseases in Children

DISEASE	CLINICAL MANIFESTATIONS	CLINICAL THERAPY	NURSING MANAGEMENT
CHICKENPOX (VARICELLA)[a,b] **Causal agent:** Varicella-zoster, human herpesvirus 3. **Epidemiology:** Humans are the source of infection. Peak occurrence is in the late fall, winter, and spring. Maternal antibodies disappear 2–3 months after birth. **Transmission:** Direct contact of the virus to the mucous membranes or conjunctiva primarily through airborne secretions and sometimes with lesion contact. **Incubation period:** 14–21 days. **Period of communicability:** Most contagious 1–2 days before the rash to shortly after onset of rash. Contagious until all lesions are crusted over. Contagious state may be prolonged after passive immunization or in immunodeficient children. 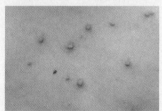 Kasiap/Shutterstock	Acute onset of mild fever, malaise, anorexia, headache, mild abdominal pain, and irritability occurs before and with eruption. Begins as a macular rash that progresses to a papule, then clear fluid-filled vesicle before crusting. Rash erupts for 1–5 days, and up to 250–500 lesions of all stages may be present at any one time. Crusts may remain for 1–3 weeks. Lesions begin on the trunk, scalp, and face, and spread to the rest of the body. Mucous membranes may have ulcerative lesions. Mouth lesions may lead to decreased fluid intake. **Complications:** Complications are rare but can include secondary infection (cellulitis, local abscesses, sepsis, meningitis, encephalitis, pneumonia), thrombocytopenia, and Reye syndrome. Chickenpox can be fatal in newborns of infected mothers and immunocompromised children. Carefully monitor children undergoing chemotherapy, steroid treatment, or transplant therapy after exposure to the disease.	**Diagnostic testing:** Polymerase chain reaction or direct fluorescent antibody testing of fluid from vesicle or scab. **Medical management:** Supportive care. IV acyclovir is used for immunocompromised clients and those on high-dose corticosteroids (AAP, 2015, p. 851). Give varicella-zoster immune globulin as soon as possible (within 10 days) to newborns of infected mothers, hospitalized premature neonates, and immunocompromised, unimmunized children (Marin, Bialek, & Seward, 2013). **Prognosis:** Most children recover fully. Children who are immunocompromised must be treated aggressively. **Prevention:** Varicella is vaccine preventable (see Table 16–1). The vaccine may be given within 72 hr after exposure to prevent or to significantly modify the disease. Wild virus (varicella strain not covered in the vaccine) cases occur in vaccinated children.	• Use airborne and contact precautions. • Isolate all hospitalized children with a recent exposure to varicella to protect newborns and immunocompromised clients. Nurses caring for the child should have documented immunity. • At home, isolate the child from susceptible individuals (medically fragile and immunocompromised children or adults, and women early in pregnancy). Notify the school or childcare facility of the child's illness. • Secondary cases are often more severe than the primary case. The child with atopic eczema or sunburn may have a more severe rash. • Give acetaminophen or ibuprofen to control fever. • Control itching with oral antihistamines, soothing oatmeal and Aveeno baths, or Caladryl lotion. • Keep the child's fingernails trimmed and clean. Place soft cotton mittens over the hands of young children when itching cannot be controlled. • Change bed linens frequently. • Reassure the child that the lesions are temporary and will go away. • Monitor for signs of complications (e.g., drowsiness, meningeal signs, respiratory distress, and dehydration). Disorientation and restlessness may indicate viral encephalitis. • Monitor for acyclovir side effects. Monitor renal function if the child has renal insufficiency.

(continued)

TABLE 16–5 Selected Infectious and Communicable Diseases in Children (*continued*)

DISEASE	CLINICAL MANIFESTATIONS	CLINICAL THERAPY	NURSING MANAGEMENT
DIPHTHERIA[a],[b] **Causal agent:** *Corynebacterium diphtheriae.* **Epidemiology:** Occurs mostly in colder months in unimmunized and inadequately immunized children. Cases of cutaneous and wound diphtheria occur sporadically in the tropics. The disease is endemic in parts of Africa, Latin America, Asia, the Middle East, and states of the former Soviet Union. **Transmission:** Contact with respiratory droplets, nasal or eye discharge, or skin lesion; less commonly by indirect contact with contaminated items; or unpasteurized milk. **Incubation period:** 2–7 days or longer. **Period of communicability:** Usually 2–4 weeks or until 4 days after antibiotics are started.	The characteristic lesion is an adherent grayish pharyngeal membrane that in severe cases may extend into the trachea or cause airway obstruction. Attempts to remove the membrane result in bleeding. Symptoms can be mild or severe with a gradual onset over 1–2 days. A sore throat and enlarged tender cervical lymph nodes are present. The child may have a swollen neck. **Complications:** The organism produces an endotoxin that causes myocarditis and peripheral neuropathy (diplopia, slurred speech, difficulty swallowing, or paralysis of the palate) or ascending paralysis that may be confused with Guillain-Barré syndrome.	**Diagnostic testing:** Culture from any mucosal or cutaneous lesion. **Medical management:** IV equine antitoxin (for respiratory diphtheria) is given after the child is tested for sensitivity. Antibiotic therapy is prescribed for 14 days with IV or IM penicillin G, changing to oral erythromycin when the child can swallow. **Prognosis:** Respiratory diphtheria may be complicated by life-threatening airway obstruction. **Prevention:** Diphtheria is a vaccine-preventable disease (see Table 16–1). This is a reportable disease.	• Use transmission-based precautions and isolate the child. • Monitor closely for signs of increasing respiratory distress, as well as cardiac and neurologic complications. • Have emergency airway equipment available. Provide humidified oxygen as necessary. • Administer antitoxin and antibiotics as prescribed. Give no medications containing caffeine or other stimulants. • Use oral suction gently as necessary. • Allow children to use mouthwash if desired. Gargling is not permitted because it can irritate the pharyngeal surfaces. • Encourage liquids as tolerated. Intravenous fluids may be necessary. • Provide emotional support to the family. • Initiate the search for client contacts to give antibiotics and immunization boosters.
ENTEROVIRUSES **Causal agent:** Group A and B coxsackieviruses, human enteroviruses. **Epidemiology:** Occurs worldwide, most commonly in summer and early fall. More common in settings with poor hygiene and overcrowding. Immunity to specific virus probably occurs after infection, but duration is unknown. **Transmission:** Fecal–oral and respiratory routes. **Incubation period:** 3–6 days. **Period of communicability:** Viral shedding may occur for weeks or months after infection.	Irritability, fever, anorexia, malaise, rash, and a sore throat. Each virus causes additional manifestations. **Herpangina:** Small, grayish papulovesicular ulcerative pharyngeal lesions that gradually increase in size. **Hand, foot, and mouth disease:** Diffuse lesions on the mucous membranes of the mouth; papulovesicular lesions on the hands and feet last for 7–10 days. **Enterovirus D-68:** Severe respiratory illness in children with history of asthma or wheezing (Midgley et al., 2014). **Complications:** Children with immune deficiency may have more severe manifestations.	**Diagnostic testing:** Polymerase chain reaction or culture of stool, throat, or other primary site may be obtained. **Medical management:** Supportive care. IV immune globulin may be used in life-threatening neonatal infections and in immunodeficient children with chronic meningoencephalitis (AAP, 2015, p. 336). **Prognosis:** Recovery is generally good with supportive care. **Prevention:** Avoid contact with infected persons early in the disease.	• Use standard and contact precautions if the child is hospitalized. • Use good hand hygiene. • Apply topical lotions and give systemic medications as ordered to lessen the pain and relieve the irritation. • Offer cool drinks and soft, bland foods (no citrus, salty, or spicy foods). Swallowing may be painful. Observe for dehydration. • Offer warm saline mouth rinses. • Provide reassurance and support to parents. • Give acetaminophen or ibuprofen for fever. • Keep the child out of school or child care while febrile.

[a]Indicates that a vaccine or antitoxin is available for use in high-risk or as-needed situations.

[b]Indicates that the disease has a safe and effective vaccine.

DISEASE	CLINICAL MANIFESTATIONS	CLINICAL THERAPY	NURSING MANAGEMENT

ERYTHEMA INFECTIOSUM (FIFTH DISEASE)

Causal agent: Human parvovirus B19.

Epidemiology: Occurs worldwide, most often in winter and spring. Also occurs in epidemics, with peak activity every 3–4 years (CDC, 2012). The incidence is highest in children between the ages of 5 and 14 years.

Transmission: Respiratory secretions and blood.

Incubation period: 4–20 days.

Period of communicability: No longer contagious once rash appears.

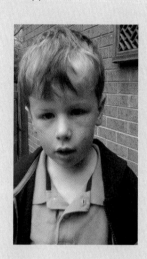

Stage 1: Begins as a mild illness (fever, headache, chills, malaise, nausea, body ache) lasting 2–3 days, followed by a symptom-free period of 1–7 days.

Stage 2: Fiery-red rash on the cheeks giving a "slapped face" appearance (see figure); circumoral pallor. In 1–4 days a lacelike symmetric, erythematous, maculopapular rash appears on the trunk and spreads to the extremities; spares the palms and soles. The rash may last 7–10 days or longer.

Stage 3: Over 1–3 weeks the rash fades, but can reappear if the skin is irritated or exposed to sunlight.

Complications: Children with hemolytic conditions may have transient aplastic crisis. Polyarthropathy is rare in children.

Diagnostic testing: Diagnosis by physical signs or positive serum immunoglobulin (Ig) M parvovirus B19-specific antibody (important when exposure to a pregnant woman is likely).

Medical management: Supportive care usually leads to spontaneous recovery. Children with hemolytic conditions may need blood transfusions if an aplastic crisis occurs. Administer IV immune globulin to immunodeficient clients who develop a chronic infection (AAP, 2015, p. 595).

Prognosis: Fetal infection may occur resulting in fetal hydrops, anemia, or spontaneous abortion.

Prevention: Avoid contact with infected persons. Exposed pregnant women should seek prompt medical attention.

- Use standard and droplet precautions. Isolation is needed only for children hospitalized with aplastic crisis or when immunosuppressed.
- Give acetaminophen or ibuprofen to control fever.
- Use soothing oatmeal or Aveeno baths if the rash is pruritic. Antipruritics may also help to relieve itching.
- Encourage rest and offer frequent fluids.
- Keep children out of direct sunlight if possible. Provide protective, light, loose clothing if exposure to sunlight cannot be avoided.
- Provide quiet diversionary activity.
- Allow the child to return to school or child care once the rash appears (AAP, 2015, p. 596).
- Explain the three stages of rash development to parents.

HAEMOPHILUS INFLUENZAE, TYPE B[b]

Causal agent: Coccobacilli *H. influenzae* bacteria (several serotypes, encapsulated or nonencapsulated).

Epidemiology: Occurs most often in the spring and summer. Unimmunized and inadequately immunized infants and young children are most commonly affected. Neonates may acquire the organism by aspirating amniotic fluid or contact with vaginal secretions.

Transmission: Direct contact or respiratory droplet inhalation. Asymptomatic colonization in the nose and throat is common.

Incubation period: Unknown, but may be a few days.

Period of communicability: 3 days from onset of symptoms.

Begins with a viral upper respiratory infection. The organism passes through the mucosal barrier to directly invade the bloodstream. It can cause severe invasive illnesses, including meningitis, epiglottitis, pneumonia, infectious arthritis, and cellulitis. It may cause sepsis in infants. Other illnesses caused by the organism include sinusitis, otitis media, bronchitis, and pericarditis. Each disease has specific clinical manifestations.

Invasive disease has decreased 99% since introduction of the vaccine (AAP, 2015, p. 369).

Complications: Responds to antibiotic therapy. If untreated, severe sequelae and death can occur from conditions such as meningitis, epiglottitis, sinusitis, pneumonitis, and cellulitis, especially in young infants.

Diagnostic testing: Culture of blood, cerebrospinal fluid, or middle ear aspirate may be obtained.

Medical management: Treatment for invasive disease is IV antibiotics for 10 days. Dexamethasone may be given to reduce the neurologic sequelae of meningitis. Infections such as otitis media can be managed with oral antibiotics.

Rifampin may be given to unprotected household contacts if another child 4 years or younger has not had the vaccine series.

Prognosis: With rapid diagnosis and treatment, recovery is good. When treatment is delayed, disability may occur.

Prevention: *H. influenzae* type b is a vaccine-preventable disease (see Table 16–1).

- Use droplet precautions until 24 hr after the initiation of antibiotics.
- Identify potential contacts and review their immunization status. Determine the need for rifampin. Inform parents to seek health care rapidly if the exposed child becomes ill.
- Administer acetaminophen or ibuprofen to increase the child's comfort.
- Closely monitor IV sites for patency and infiltration.
- Perform nursing care measures specific to the illness.
- Inform family members that rifampin turns urine and other body fluids orange, and it will cause stains.

(continued)

TABLE 16–5 Selected Infectious and Communicable Diseases in Children (*continued*)

DISEASE	CLINICAL MANIFESTATIONS	CLINICAL THERAPY	NURSING MANAGEMENT

INFLUENZA[b]

Causal agent: Orthomyxoviruses, types A, B, and C. Type A can be subtyped based on surface proteins: hemagglutinin (H) and neuraminidase (N).

Epidemiology: Prevalent in the United States from October to March, but the virus is active in other parts of the world year-round. The influenza A virus mutates each season. The number of infections peak in about 3 weeks from the initial case and continue for about 3 months. Incidence of infection is often greater in young children who have fewer prior influenza infections and antibodies.

Transmission: Spreads by aerosolized particles and direct contact with respiratory secretions.

Incubation period: 1–4 days.

Period of communicability: 1 day before symptoms to 5–7 days after symptom onset.

Abrupt onset of fever 100.4–104.0°F (38–40°C), chills, cough, runny nose, sore throat, malaise, aches, headache, and anorexia. Children may have nausea and vomiting, diarrhea, and abdominal pain. Recovery usually occurs in 3–5 days.

Complications: Pneumonia, otitis media, asthma exacerbations, tracheitis, myocarditis, myositis, febrile seizures, sinusitis, and neurologic conditions such as meningitis, encephalitis, encephalopathy, or Guillain-Barré syndrome. Children with chronic pulmonary, hematologic, metabolic, and cardiovascular conditions are at greater risk for severe infection.

In the 2013–2014 influenza season, 924 children aged 0–17 years were hospitalized, and 50 children died due to influenza (Arriola et al., 2014).

Diagnostic testing: Rapid antigen testing from throat swabs, nasopharyngeal washings, and sputum detects antigens of influenza A and B. Viral cultures, direct fluorescent antibody, or indirect immunofluorescent antibody staining.

Medical management: Treatment is supportive. Antiviral therapy may be used to treat symptomatic children or for prevention. Oseltamivir (Tamiflu), amantadine (Symmetrel), zanamivir (Relenza), and rimantadine (Flumadine) are approved for children with specific age guidelines. Antiviral therapy should be started within 48 hr of symptoms for best results (AAP, 2015, p. 481).

Prognosis: Most children recover.

Prevention: Annual influenza immunization beginning at age 6 months (see Table 16–1).

- Use droplet and contact precautions for hospitalized infants and children.
- For home care, encourage parents to wash hands frequently and to isolate the child from other family members.
- Provide fluids to keep nasal secretions moist and to prevent dehydration.
- Provide acetaminophen or ibuprofen for fever management and mild pain.
- If antiviral medications are given, be alert for nausea and vomiting. Zanamivir can exacerbate asthma.
- Provide rest and quiet diversional activities.
- Children should be kept home until 24 hr after fever is gone.
- Teach parents to be alert to signs of complications from the viral infection.
- Become familiar with community pandemic infection plans.

MEASLES (RUBEOLA)[a,b]

Causal agent: Morbillivirus, a member of the paramyxovirus group.

Epidemiology: Occurrence peaks in the late winter and early spring. In 2014, 592 cases and 18 outbreaks occurred in the United States, mostly in unimmunized children. Most outbreaks were linked to cases imported from other countries (CDC, 2014c).

Transmission: Direct contact with respiratory droplets and airborne spread.

Incubation period: About 8–12 days.

Period of communicability: From 4 days before the rash until 4 days after its appearance.

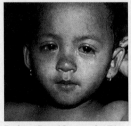

Barbara Rice/Centers for Disease Control and Prevention

Prodromal stage: High fever (up to 105.0°F [40.5°C]), malaise, cough, coryza, conjunctivitis. Koplik spots (1–3 mm gray or blue-gray spots on an erythematous base) appear opposite the second molars on the buccal mucosa. They slough before or during the onset of the rash. This stage lasts 1–3 days.

Stage 2: Maculopapular rash (dark red to purple), reaching a peak in 2–4 days when it becomes confluent. The mildly pruritic rash begins on the face and spreads to the trunk and extremities.

Other symptoms include fatigue, photophobia, and generalized lymphadenopathy.

Complications: About 30% of cases develop pneumonia, otitis media, diarrhea, or encephalitis (CDC, 2014c). Complications and death occur most often in children who are malnourished or immunocompromised.

Diagnostic testing: Serologic test for immunoglobulin (Ig) M measles antibody.

Medical management: Supportive care. No antiviral therapy is available. Antibiotics are used for secondary bacterial infections.

MMR vaccine within 72 hr of exposure or immune globulin within 6 days of exposure may help prevent or reduce disease severity.

Prognosis: Increased risk of death in children under age 5 years and immunocompromised persons (AAP, 2015, p. 535).

Prevention: Measles is a vaccine-preventable disease (see Table 16–1). This is a reportable disease.

- Maintain airborne precautions when the child is hospitalized.
- Use a cool-mist vaporizer to help clear respiratory passages. Suction nose and oral cavity gently if needed.
- Give nonaspirin antipyretics for fever and antipruritics for itching. Cough medication may be prescribed.
- Teach parents to observe for complications and to seek care as needed.
- Keep lights dim, and cover windows if the child has photophobia.
- Keep skin clean and dry. Avoid using soap.
- Offer cool liquids frequently in small amounts. Blended, pureed, and mashed foods are most easily tolerated.
- Maintain bed rest. Visitors should be immune to measles. Provide diversional activities.

[a]Indicates that a vaccine or antitoxin is available for use in high-risk or as-needed situations.

[b]Indicates that the disease has a safe and effective vaccine.

DISEASE	CLINICAL MANIFESTATIONS	CLINICAL THERAPY	NURSING MANAGEMENT
MENINGOCOCCUS *Causal agent: Neisseria meningitidis,* a gram-negative diplococcus. *Epidemiology:* Often occurs in winter or early spring. Serogroups B, C, and Y cause the most disease in the United States. Highest rates occur in infants under 1 year of age and adolescents 16–21 years. Outbreaks have occurred in childcare centers, college dormitories, and military recruit camps. There are fewer than 1000 cases annually in the United States (CDC, 2014e). *Transmission:* Spread by direct contact with respiratory secretions from human carriers. *Incubation period:* 3–7 days. *Period of communicability:* Until 24 hr of treatment with an effective antibiotic. 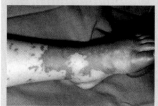 Medical-on-Line/Alamy	**Meningitis:** Most common invasive disease. Abrupt onset of flulike symptoms of fever, malaise, stiff neck, nausea, vomiting, decreased mental status, seizures, and coma. *Meningococcemia* (sepsis caused by meningococcus): Fatigue; vomiting; cold hands and feet; chills; severe aches and pains in muscles, joints, chest, and abdomen; rapid breathing; diarrhea. An urticarial, maculopapular or petechial rash appears that may progress to purpura (see figure) and severe septic shock. *Complications:* Approximately 11%–19% of survivors have serious sequelae (CDC, 2014d). Survivors of meningitis may develop hearing loss or neurologic disability. Survivors of meningococcemia may have permanent disabilities from digit or limb amputations, and scarring from skin grafts.	*Diagnostic testing:* Cultures of the blood and cerebrospinal fluid, and a Gram stain of petechial skin scrapings. *Medical management:* IV antibiotics with penicillin G, cefotaxime, ceftriaxone, or ampicillin; chloramphenicol for children allergic to penicillin. The child is treated in the ICU for shock with IV fluids and vasopressors, and with respiratory support. Blood products are used to treat disseminated intravascular coagulation. Several surgeries may be needed for removal of necrotic tissue. *Prognosis:* Even with antibiotic treatment about 10%–15% of clients die (CDC, 2013e). *Prevention:* Several serotypes are vaccine preventable (see Table 16–1). Close contacts receive an antibiotic. Community contacts should also receive the meningococcal vaccine to prevent an outbreak (AAP, 2015, p. 557). This is a reportable disease.	• Use standard and droplet precautions until an effective antibiotic has been administered for 24 hr. • Be alert for development of shock and respiratory compromise as the disease progresses quickly. Have emergency equipment available. • Avoid overloading the child with IV fluids and blood products. Administer medications as prescribed. • Monitor the child with meningitis for signs of increased intracranial pressure. • Help the family mobilize its support system, and keep the family informed of the child's status and treatment as the disease progresses. • Help identify contacts who should receive prophylactic antibiotics. Educate them about the expected side effects (i.e., orange urine with rifampin). • Teach contacts to be observant for signs of illness and to seek health care promptly if they occur. • The surviving child will often need rehabilitation for limb amputations or hearing loss. Work with the social worker to transition the child to long-term care.
MONONUCLEOSIS *Causal agent:* Epstein-Barr virus (EBV), human herpesvirus type 4. *Epidemiology:* The virus infects the oral mucosa and salivary glands. Occurs worldwide in no seasonal pattern. Infection is common in adolescents and young adults in the United States. *Transmission:* Direct contact with saliva or exposure to body fluids (e.g., blood or semen). *Incubation period:* Estimated to be 4–6 weeks.	Young children may have a mild infection with no distinguishing clinical signs. Symptoms include fever, malaise, headache, anorexia, abdominal pain, a painful sore throat (exudative pharyngotonsillitis), and enlarged cervical lymph nodes. An enlarged spleen and liver may occur. The syndrome typically lasts 2–4 weeks, but fatigue may continue for weeks. *Complications:* Peritonsillar abscess, sinusitis, mastoiditis.	*Diagnostic testing:* A heterophil antibody response test. Greater than 10% atypical lymphocytes and a positive heterophil antibody response test are diagnostic (AAP, 2015, pp. 337–338). *Medical management:* Supportive care. Corticosteroids may be used for tonsillar swelling and impending airway obstruction, massive splenomegaly, myocarditis, or hemolytic anemia. Antibiotics (ampicillin and amoxicillin) are not used because a nonallergic rash often develops (AAP, 2015, p. 339).	• Use standard precautions if the child is hospitalized. • Give antipyretics and analgesics for fever and sore throat. Offer warm salt water for gargling. Offer soft foods and encourage fluids. • Maintain bed rest during acute phase. • Educate the teen to avoid intimate contact and not to share food and beverages until recovered.

(continued)

TABLE 16–5 Selected Infectious and Communicable Diseases in Children (*continued*)

DISEASE	CLINICAL MANIFESTATIONS	CLINICAL THERAPY	NURSING MANAGEMENT
MONONUCLEOSIS (*continued*) ***Period of communicability:*** May be weeks before symptoms occur, and becomes latent after infection. Contagious if reactivation occurs (CDC, 2014e).	Rare conditions include neurologic disorders (e.g., meningitis, encephalitis, and Guillain-Barré syndrome), hematologic disorders (lymphocytosis), and immune disorders. Those with immune disorders have more severe disease.	***Prognosis:*** Rarely fatal. After recovery, the virus becomes latent in the lymphoid system and can reactivate during periods of immunosuppression. ***Prevention:*** No known prevention.	• Return to contact sports and strenuous activity (e.g., weight lifting) is approved by the healthcare provider when the liver and spleen are normal size, usually in about 4 weeks. • If splenomegaly is present, alcohol should be avoided for 3 months after liver function test results return to normal.
MUMPS (PAROTITIS) [b] ***Causal agent:*** *Rubulavirus* in the Paramyxoviridae family. ***Epidemiology:*** Occurs worldwide in unvaccinated children, most often in winter and spring. Infection and vaccination induce lifelong immunity. ***Transmission:*** Inhalation of respiratory secretion droplets. ***Incubation period:*** 12–25 days. ***Period of communicability:*** Up to 5 days before and after parotid swelling onset. 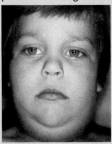 Centers for Disease Control and Prevention	Acute onset of malaise, fever, muscle aches, and swelling of one or more salivary glands (parotid, sublingual, or submaxillary) are the classic signs. Other signs include earache, headache, pain with chewing, and decreased appetite and activity. May be asymptomatic in some children. ***Complications:*** **Orchitis** (inflammation of the testicles) that rarely leads to fertility problems, encephalitis, oophoritis (inflammation of ovaries), temporary or permanent deafness. Viral meningitis occurs in less than 10% of cases (AAP, 2015, p. 564).	***Diagnostic testing:*** Viral culture from a throat washing, urine, or cerebrospinal fluid. A serologic test for mumps-specific IgM antibodies may be performed. ***Medical management:*** Supportive care focused on symptom relief. ***Prognosis:*** Mumps is usually self-limiting. ***Prevention:*** Mumps is a vaccine-preventable disease. See Table 16–1. This is a reportable disease.	• Use standard and droplet precautions for hospitalized children while contagious. • Children are cared for at home. They may be uncomfortable but rarely very ill. Provide diversion. • Avoid exposure to immunocompromised or susceptible individuals. • Give acetaminophen or ibuprofen to control fever and pain. • Encourage fluid intake. Offer soft and blended foods as chewing and swallowing may be painful. Avoid foods and beverages that increase salivary flow and cause pain (e.g., citrus, spices, and candies). • Be alert for signs of complications. • Keep children out of school or child care until 5 days after parotid swelling occurs.
PERTUSSIS (WHOOPING COUGH)[b] ***Causal agent:*** *Bordetella pertussis.* ***Epidemiology:*** Occurs worldwide and year-round. Rates have increased because of waning immunity with 28,639 cases in 2013 (CDC, 2013a). Children with waning immunity can spread the disease to unimmunized young infants at greatest risk for death from the infection. ***Transmission:*** Inhalation or direct contact with respiratory droplets. ***Incubation period:*** 5–10 days.	***Catarrhal stage:*** The onset is insidious with cold symptoms, a runny nose, mild cough, and fever, lasting about 1–2 weeks. ***Paroxysmal stage:*** A series of rapid coughs followed by a forceful inspiration through a narrowed glottis causes stridor, or the "whoop." The child has cyanosis, vomiting, and exhaustion associated with coughing paroxysms. Infants under 6 months of age may have gagging, gasping, or apnea rather than whooping. Sucking on a bottle may trigger coughing, leading to poor oral intake and dehydration. The "whoop" may be absent in immunized children.	***Diagnostic testing:*** Nasopharyngeal culture, polymerase chain reaction (PCR) testing, and serology. ***Medical management:*** Supportive care. Macrolide antibiotics (erythromycin, clarithromycin, azithromycin, and trimethroprim-sulfamethoxazole). Symptoms are reduced only if initiated in the catarrhal stage (CDC, 2013a). ***Prognosis:*** The disease is most severe in infants younger than 6 months, of which 1.6% will die (CDC, 2013a).	• Use droplet precautions until 5 days after effective antibiotic is initiated. • Monitor respirations and oxygen saturation with a cardiac monitor and pulse oximetry. The smaller the infant, the greater the risk for apnea. • Meet infant needs promptly to reduce crying, which can precipitate coughing. Remain with the child during coughing spells, when hypoxic and apneic episodes are most likely. Give oxygen if ordered. Have emergency equipment available.

[a]Indicates that a vaccine or antitoxin is available for use in high-risk or as-needed situations.

[b]Indicates that the disease has a safe and effective vaccine.

DISEASE	CLINICAL MANIFESTATIONS	CLINICAL THERAPY	NURSING MANAGEMENT
Period of communicability: Most contagious prior to the paroxysmal cough stage and for 2 weeks after cough onset if untreated. Communicable for 5 days after beginning effective antibiotic.	**Convalescent stage:** Up to 6–10 weeks later paroxysms gradually subside. **Complications:** Among infants: pneumonia, seizures, apnea, encephalopathy, and death. In adolescents: sleep disturbance, incontinence, syncope, rib fractures, and pneumonia (CDC, 2013a).	**Prevention:** Pertussis is a vaccine-preventable disease (see Table 16–1). The vaccine protection wanes over time. All adults should receive a Tdap booster every 10 years. Pregnant women should be immunized to protect their newborns from pertussis during the third trimester. The father and family members who will have close contact with the newborn should receive a Tdap booster prior to the newborn's birth (CDC, 2015b). Close contacts should receive macrolide antibiotic prophylaxis.	• Provide humidification. Gentle suctioning may be necessary. • Give nonaspirin antipyretics as needed for fever. • Encourage frequent rest periods. • Provide small frequent feeding of desired foods. Encourage fluids. The child may need IV hydration if oral intake is not tolerated. • Provide emotional support to parents. • Teach parents to watch for signs of respiratory failure and dehydration if the child is managed at home.

PNEUMOCOCCAL INFECTION[b]

Causative agent: *Streptococcus pneumoniae*, a gram-positive diplococcus, many serotypes.

Epidemiology: Found in the pharynx of healthy people. Outbreaks occur in winter and spring in temperate climates, and only a few of the 90 serotypes account for most of the invasive pediatric infections.

Transmission: Direct contact with respiratory secretions, and droplets and self-innoculation.

Incubation period: 1–3 days.

Period of communicability: Unknown. Probably within 24 hr after effective antibiotic therapy is initiated.

Causes invasive disease with signs and symptoms are related to the focal area of infection.

Otitis media—upper respiratory infection, fever, ear pain, and decreased appetite.

Bacteremia—unexplained fever, reduced responsiveness, and no localized infection site.

Pneumonia—fever, chills, chest pain, dyspnea, malaise, and a productive cough.

Meningitis—inconsolable crying, increased irritability, lethargy, refusal to eat, nausea, vomiting, diarrhea, myalgia, photophobia, and seizures.

The organism also causes sinusitis, pharyngitis, cellulitis, and laryngotracheobronchitis.

Children under age 2 years, or having immunodeficiency (e.g., asplenia, malignancy, sickle cell disease, HIV infection, and nephrotic syndrome) and cochlear implants are at higher risk of invasive disease.

Complications: Hearing loss or developmental delay from meningitis, empyema or pericarditis from pneumonia, and death.

Diagnostic testing: Bacterial culture from the site of infection.

Medical management: Symptomatic care. Antibiotic selection is based upon culture sensitivity. Many pneumococcal strains are resistant to penicillin, cefotaxime, and ceftriaxone. Vancomycin may be required. Dexamethasone may be an adjunctive therapy for meningitis.

Prognosis: An estimated 200 children die annually from pneumococcal disease (CDC, 2013b). Pneumococcal meningitis is associated with neurologic sequelae (e.g., hearing loss, motor deficits).

Prevention: Many serotypes are vaccine preventable (see Table 16–1). Pneumococcal vaccine with 23 serotypes (PPSV23) is used for children at high risk of pneumococcal invasive disease.

• Maintain standard precautions.
• Provide nonaspirin antipyretics for control of fever and comfort.
• Encourage fluids, and monitor intake and output.
• Monitor vital signs and level of consciousness to identify signs of worsening condition.
• Educate parents about the need for the vaccine. The unimmunized child can become infected repeatedly with different serotypes.
• Many children with mild disease will be treated at home. Educate parents about signs indicating a need to seek urgent medical care, medication administration, and comfort measures for the child.

(continued)

TABLE 16–5 Selected Infectious and Communicable Diseases in Children (*continued*)

DISEASE	CLINICAL MANIFESTATIONS	CLINICAL THERAPY	NURSING MANAGEMENT
POLIOMYELITIS[b]			
Causal agent: Poliovirus is an enterovirus with three serotypes. **Epidemiology:** Global eradication efforts have interrupted the transmission of polio in all but three countries—Afghanistan, Nigeria, and Pakistan (CDC, 2013c). Imported and wild polio is a threat to inadequately immunized children. **Transmission:** Direct contact with respiratory secretions and body fluids. **Incubation period:** Usually 7–10 days (range 3–36 days). **Period of communicability:** Greatest shortly before and with onset of clinical symptoms. The virus is excreted in the feces for 3–6 weeks.	More than 90% of infections are asymptomatic. **Mild illness:** A low-grade fever and sore throat. This minor illness may be followed by aseptic meningitis and paresthesias. **Serious illness:** Asymmetric flaccid paralysis may occur acutely in up to 1% of cases. Site of paralysis is commonly the legs, but it may affect the respiratory muscles. Residual paralysis may occur in more than half of those affected (AAP, 2015, p. 644). **Complications:** Permanent motor paralysis, respiratory arrest, postpolio syndrome, and death.	**Diagnostic testing:** Cell culture from stool or throat swabs. **Medical management:** Supportive therapy. No effective chemotherapeutic agents exist. **Prognosis:** Respiratory paralysis may lead to death. Motor paralysis may result in long-term disability. **Prevention:** Poliomyelitis is a vaccine-preventable disease (see Table 16–1). The vaccine is believed to confer lifelong immunity. This is a reportable disease.	• Use standard and droplet precautions. • Monitor for respiratory paralysis (ineffective cough, talking with frequent pauses, shallow and rapid respiratory rate). Have emergency equipment at bedside. Assist ventilations as needed until mechanical ventilation is set up. • Use moist hot packs, which may relieve discomfort. • Encourage fluids. • Keep the child on bed rest. Position the child to promote body alignment. • Perform range of motion exercises to prevent contractures after the acute phase. • Provide emotional support. Keep the child and family informed about the illness and therapies. • Help coordinate rehabilitation, such as long-term physical therapy when needed.
ROSEOLA (EXANTHEM SUBITUM, SIXTH DISEASE)			
Causal agent: Human herpesvirus type 6 (HHV-6). **Epidemiology:** Occurs worldwide year-round with no seasonal pattern. Occurs primarily in children 6–24 months of age (as maternal antibodies decline). Nearly all children are infected by 3 years of age. Congenital infection is also possible (AAP, 2015, p. 451). **Transmission:** Contact with saliva or respiratory secretions. **Incubation period:** Appears to be 9–10 days. **Period of communicability:** Healthy persons shed the virus (AAP, 2015, p. 450).	**Prodromal stage:** Sudden fever greater than 103.0°F (39.5°C) for 3–7 days, during which the child has a normal appetite and behavior, no rash or specific disease signs. **Rash stage:** A characteristic pale pink, discrete, maculopapular rash starts on the trunk and spreads to the face, neck, and extremities, lasting hours to days. The child may have characteristic postoccipital lymphadenopathy, tympanic membrane redness, and respiratory and gastrointestinal signs. **Complications:** Febrile seizures are common; encephalopathy or encephalitis may occur.	**Diagnostic testing:** Polymerase chain reaction (PCR) testing for HHV-6 in the blood or cerebrospinal fluid. **Medical management:** Supportive treatment for this self-limiting condition. **Prognosis:** Full recovery is usual. **Prevention:** No preventive measures.	• Use standard precautions if the child is hospitalized. • Give nonaspirin antipyretics to control fever. • Observe closely for any seizure activity, especially during the acute febrile periods. • Encourage fluids to maintain hydration. • Reassure parents that the rash will disappear in a few days.
ROTAVIRUS[b]			
Causal agent: RNA viruses of the Reoviridae family. Groups A, B, and C infect humans.	Acute onset of fever and vomiting followed by watery diarrhea 1–2 days later. Up to 10–20 diarrheal stools a day. Symptoms last 3–8 days.	**Diagnostic testing:** Enzyme immunoassay or latex agglutination assay of a stool specimen.	• Use standard and contact precautions. • Use good hand hygiene with soap and water or gel cleansers.

[a]Indicates that a vaccine or antitoxin is available for use in high-risk or as-needed situations.

[b]Indicates that the disease has a safe and effective vaccine.

DISEASE	CLINICAL MANIFESTATIONS	CLINICAL THERAPY	NURSING MANAGEMENT
Epidemiology: Occurs more often in cool periods, peaking in the spring in the United States. A common cause of severe diarrhea in children less than age 5 years. *Transmission:* Fecal–oral route, direct contact with contaminated objects. *Incubation:* 1–3 days. *Period of communicability:* Virus may persist in stool when child is immunocompromised.	*Complications:* Dehydration and electrolyte disturbances. Immunocompromised children may develop persistent infection and diarrhea (AAP, 2015, p. 684).	*Medical management:* Treatment involves adequate amounts of fluid and electrolyte replacement with oral rehydration solution. Antimotility drugs should not be used. If severely dehydrated, IV fluid resuscitation is performed. No antiviral therapy is available. *Prevention:* Vaccine prevents several common viral groups (see Table 16–1).	• Clean and disinfect contaminated surfaces. • Assess hydration status frequently. • Breastfeeding is continued during oral rehydration therapy, but wait up to 24 hr before giving formula. • Feed older children complex carbohydrates and lean meats, yogurt, fruits, and vegetables 12–24 hr after starting oral rehydration therapy.

RUBELLA (GERMAN MEASLES)[b]

Causal agent: An RNA virus, member of the family Togaviridae, genus *Rubivirus*. *Epidemiology:* Occurs worldwide. Most prevalent in winter and spring. No longer endemic in the United States (AAP, 2015, p. 689). Most U.S. cases occur among persons from other countries and those underimmunized. Congenital rubella syndrome occurs between 12 weeks of gestation to the end of the second trimester. *Transmission:* Droplet spread, direct contact with nasal secretions. *Incubation period:* 14–21 days. *Period of communicability:* 7 days before until 7 days after rash onset. Infants with congenital rubella may shed the virus for 1 year or longer after birth.	*Prodromal stage:* Asymptomatic or low-grade fever, malaise, coryza, and sore throat, 1–5 days before the rash. Forschheimer spots (discrete, erythematous pinpoint or larger lesions on the soft palate) are seen. Posterior auricular and suboccipital lymphadenopathy may precede the rash. *Rash stage:* 1–5 days later a pink, maculopapular rash appears on the face and neck. The rash spreads to the trunk and legs, and fades in the same sequence. *Complications:* Transient arthralgia in adolescents; encephalitis. Pregnant females infected during the first trimester may have a fetus with congenital rubella syndrome birth defects (e.g., cataracts, heart defects, hearing impairment, thrombocytopenia, and purpuric skin lesions that give a "blueberry muffin" appearance) (see figure).	*Diagnostic testing:* Cell culture from a nasal swab, and detection of IgM or IgG antibodies. *Medical management:* Supportive treatment. Rubella is self-limiting in children. *Prognosis:* Full recovery is expected. Congenital rubella syndrome may result in death or congenital anomalies. *Prevention:* Rubella is a vaccine-preventable disease (see Table 16–1). 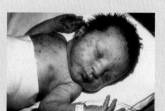 Centers for Disease Control and Prevention	• Maintain standard and droplet precautions. • Maintain contact precautions for infants with congenital rubella syndrome until 1 year of age unless nasopharyngeal and urine cultures are repeatedly negative after 3 months of age (AAP, 2015, p. 691). • Children are usually treated at home. Provide quiet activities. • Isolate the child from pregnant women. • Give nonaspirin analgesics and antipyretics for any pain and fever. • Encourage the child to consume preferred fluids and food. • Exclude children from child care or school for 7 days after onset of rash. Notify the school or childcare facilities of the child's illness.

STREPTOCOCCUS A

Causal agent: Group A streptococci (GAS), numerous serotypes. *Epidemiology:* Pharyngeal infections tend to occur more in late fall, winter, and spring when closer person-to-person contact occurs. Pyodermal infections more often occur in warmer seasons with minor skin trauma and insect bites. Different serotypes are associated with pharyngeal and pyodermal infections, rheumatic fever, and acute glomerulonephritis (AAP, 2015, p. 733).	*Pharyngeal:* Abrupt onset with a sore throat, dysphagia, tender cervical lymph nodes, malaise, high fever, chills, headache, abdominal pain, anorexia, and vomiting. The pharynx is beefy red with exudates, and palatal petechiae may be seen. *GAS respiratory tract infection:* Children younger than 3 years may have serous rhinitis, moderate fever, irritability, and anorexia rather than pharyngitis.	*Diagnostic testing:* Rapid strep test or a culture of secretions from the pharynx and tonsils, blood culture for invasive disease. Cultures of skin lesions do not reveal primary organism (AAP, 2015, p. 737). *Medical management:* Prompt oral antibiotic therapy with penicillin V or amoxicillin or IM penicillin G benzathine. Clindamycin or oral macrolide may be used if the child is allergic to penicillin.	• Use standard and droplet precautions for pharyngeal infections and contact precautions for skin infections. • Promote bed rest during the febrile stage. • Give nonaspirin antipyretics to control fever. Teach parents important signs of a worsening condition. • For pharyngeal infections, offer warm salt water for gargling and nonacidic beverages. Encourage cool, clear liquids and a soft diet. Swallowing may be difficult.

(continued)

TABLE 16–5 Selected Infectious and Communicable Diseases in Children (*continued*)

DISEASE	CLINICAL MANIFESTATIONS	CLINICAL THERAPY	NURSING MANAGEMENT
STREPTOCOCCUS A (*continued*)			

STREPTOCOCCUS A (*continued*)

Transmission: Contact with respiratory secretions for pharyngitis or skin lesions for pyoderma.

Incubation period: Pharyngeal: usually 2–5 days. Pyodermal: usually 7–10 days.

Period of communicability: For weeks in untreated pharyngeal infections; not contagious within 24 hr of starting antibiotics.

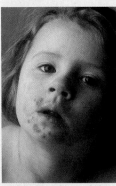

Bubbles Photolibrary/Alamy

Scarlet fever: A characteristic erythematous, confluent, sandpaper rash, starting on the neck and spreading to the trunk and extremities. The rash blanches with pressure, concentrates in flexor skin creases, and spares the circumoral area. In 3–4 days, the rash begins to fade and the tips of the toes and fingers peel. The classic strawberry tongue is seen on days 4–5. Most often occurs after pharyngeal symptoms.

Pyodermal: Lesions (impetigo) are honey-colored crusts at the site of open lesions (see figure).

Complications: If untreated, acute otitis media, sinusitis, peritonsillar or retropharyngeal abscess, cervical lymphadenitis, acute rheumatic fever, and acute glomerulonephritis. Invasive disease with toxic shock syndrome, bacteremia, necrotizing fasciitis, or myositis can be fatal.

Uncomplicated impetigo is treated with mupirocin or retapamulin ointment. See Chapter 31 for more information about bacterial skin infections and toxic shock syndrome. See Chapter 21 for treatment of acute rheumatic fever.

Prognosis: Recovery is usually good with antibiotic therapy. Children can become long-term carriers of streptococcus A in their pharynx.

Prevention: None.

- Explain to parents the importance of giving the full course of antibiotics.
- Encourage other family members with sore throats to have throat cultures taken.
- For impetigo, encourage good hand hygiene. Teach the parents to wash the skin, remove crusts, and apply antibiotic ointment.
- Replace the child's toothbrush after treatment to prevent reinfection.

TETANUS[a,b]

Causal agent: *Clostridium tetani,* an anaerobic gram-positive bacillus.

Epidemiology: Bacillus is common and exists as a spore in soil, dust, and manure. The organism produces an endotoxin that affects the central nervous system.

Transmission: Wounds (e.g., superficial, puncture, burns, crush injuries) exposed to contaminated soil or objects.

Incubation period: 3–21 days (average 10 days).

Period of communicability: No direct person-to-person contact.

Fever, diaphoresis, headache, and neck and jaw stiffness with painful facial spasms and difficulty chewing and swallowing, seizures, painful muscle stiffness, hypertension, tachycardia. Facial muscle spasms may produce a grinning expression (risus sardonicus).

Eventual rigidity of the abdomen and trunk produce **opisthotonos** (rigid hyperextension of the entire body). Respiratory muscles may be affected and cause airway obstruction and suffocation.

Newborns have increasing difficulty with sucking, irritability, and neck stiffness.

Complications: Laryngospasm, respiratory distress, death.

Diagnostic testing: Based on clinical signs; cultures often ineffective.

Medical management: IM human tetanus immune globulin with some injected into the wound site.

The wound is cleaned and debrided. Antibiotics and medications to relieve muscle spasms are administered. Intensive care is provided with assisted ventilation, nutrition, and supportive care. Complete recovery may take weeks.

Prognosis: Fatality rates are 10%–20%, depending on quality of supportive care (CDC, 2013d).

Prevention: Tetanus is a vaccine-preventable disease (see Table 16–1). A tetanus booster is needed every 10 years, or, if a contaminated wound occurs, in 5 years.

- Use standard precautions.
- Assist with wound debridement.
- Monitor the child's condition. Handle as little as possible. Reduce stimulation by placing the child in a quiet, darkened room.
- Offer skin and respiratory care. The child may need an endotracheal tube, suctioning, and supplemental oxygen for airway support.
- Provide feedings via total parenteral nutrition or feeding tube.
- Maintain hydration with IV fluids and electrolytes.
- Try to reduce the child's anxiety, as mental status may be unaffected by disease process.
- Prepare the family for a possible poor prognosis.

[a]Indicates that a vaccine or antitoxin is available for use in high-risk or as-needed situations.

[b]Indicates that the disease has a safe and effective vaccine.

TABLE 16–6 Selected Infectious Diseases Transmitted by Insect or Animal Hosts (Zoonosis)

DISEASE	CLINICAL MANIFESTATIONS	CLINICAL THERAPY	NURSING MANAGEMENT

LYME DISEASE

Causal agent: Borrelia burgdorferi, a spirochete transmitted by ixodid ticks.

Epidemiology: It occurs in most U.S. states, with greatest number of cases in the Northeastern, Mid-Atlantic, and North Central states. Exposure occurs in any outdoor setting where ticks are endemic. Most cases occur between May and November, with the highest rate in the summer.

Among children, the highest incidence in the United States is in 5- to 9-year-olds (AAP, 2015, p. 518).

Transmission: The tick is attached for 36–48 hr before the infection is transmitted (CDC, 2014f). Lyme disease is the most common vectorborne illness in North America.

Incubation period: 1–32 days after an infected tick bite.

Period of communicability: The infection is not communicable from person to person.

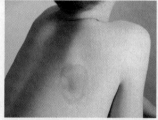

Kevin Shields/Alamy

Localized disease (LD): Erythema migrans, a painless annular red rash that expands over days or weeks to 5–30 cm (2–12 in.) in diameter (see figure). It may have partial central clearing (bull's eye) or look like a bruise in clients with dark skin. It occurs in about 70%–80% of cases, an average of 7 days after the tick bite (CDC, 2014f). The client may only have fever, chills, fatigue, body aches, malaise, and swollen lymph nodes. Some clients have both the rash and illness.

Early disseminated disease (EDD): In 3–10 weeks after the tick bite, multiple smaller erythema migrans lesions, generalized lymphadenopathy, and fatigue. Meningitis, facial nerve palsy, carditis, and migratory muscle and joint pain may occur.

Late disseminated disease (LDD): In 2–12 months, Lyme arthritis develops, commonly in the large joints such as the knee. Joint swelling, pain, and tenderness are seen.

Complications: Left untreated, Lyme disease progresses to LDD with cranial nerve palsies, carditis, encephalitis, or meningitis.

Diagnostic testing: Enzyme-linked immunosorbent assay (ELISA) plus the Western blot test.

Medical management: Oral amoxicillin, cefuroxime axetil, or doxycycline for 14–21 days for LD, 21–28 days for EDD, and up to 28 days for LDD. Intravenous antibiotics may be administered for up to 28 days for persistent arthritis, carditis, meningitis, or encephalitis.

Prognosis: Treatment during LD or EDD rarely progresses to LDD. May result in significant morbidity when chronic Lyme disease develops.

Prevention: No vaccine is available. There is no acquired immunity, so reinfection may occur.

Avoid areas that are heavily tick infested, and wear protective clothing. Check for ticks (especially hidden in hair) after every outing. Check pets that may carry home ticks that can transfer to the child. Remove ticks as soon as possible.

- Use standard precautions if the child is hospitalized.
- Educate parents about the importance of giving the full course of antibiotics.
- Have the child avoid sun exposure when taking doxycycline.
- Provide nonaspirin analgesics and antipyretics for relief of fever, headache, and muscle or joint aches.
- Children with Lyme disease may tire easily. Promote rest and avoid vigorous activities.
- Teach parents to safely remove ticks. Grasp the tick gently but firmly with fine-point tweezers where the mouthparts are attached. Pull gently until the tick releases. Clean the area with soap and water.

MALARIA

Causal agent: Plasmodium, four species (*P. falciparum, P. vivax, P. ovale, P. malariae*)

Epidemiology: Occurs in tropical and subtropical regions on four continents (Africa, Americas, Asia, and Oceana). Children have the highest mortality. The disease is acquired during travel to an endemic area, most often among immigrants visiting their home country who did not take preventive measures. *P. falciparum* causes the most serious disease. In 2011, 1947 cases were reported in the United States; 15% of all reported cases occurred in children 18 years old and younger (Cullen & Arguin, 2013).

Malaria begins with nonspecific signs such as high fever alternating with chills, profuse diaphoresis, and fatigue. Periods of symptomatic improvement may be seen between cycles lasting 48 or 72 hr depending upon type of infection.

Children may also have fever, anorexia, vomiting, jaundice, splenomegaly, and anemia. Additional symptoms include nausea, vomiting, diarrhea, cough, tachypnea, arthralgia, and body aches.

Attacks may recur over the course of the year after infection, but the parasites die out gradually if no reinfection.

Diagnostic testing: Blood smears for parasites, or a PCR assay. A rapid malaria test is available. Blood tests may show anemia and thrombocytopenia.

Medical management: The child is hospitalized for fluid replacement, anemia management, and antipyretics. The blood is regularly monitored for parasite density.

IV or oral antimalarial medication (e.g., chloroquine, quinine sulfate, doxycycline, mefloquine, and atovaquone-proguanil) is selected based on region visited and resistance of species to the medication. Hypoglycemia may result from quinine treatment or because parasites consume large quantities of glucose.

- Use standard precautions.
- Maintain fluid intake. Monitor intake and output.
- Monitor the hematocrit and hemoglobin, as well as the blood glucose level.
- Observe for signs of increasing illness severity such as confusion, seizures, and shock. Be prepared to protect the child from injury and provide emergency support with airways and oxygen until the child can be transferred to the ICU.
- Administer antipyretics to control the fever and promote comfort.

(continued)

TABLE 16–6 Selected Infectious Diseases Transmitted by Insect or Animal Hosts (Zoonosis) (continued)

DISEASE	CLINICAL MANIFESTATIONS	CLINICAL THERAPY	NURSING MANAGEMENT
MALARIA (continued) **Transmission:** An infected female mosquito introduces the parasite through a bite. The parasite infects hepatic cells and reproduces leading to hepatic cell rupture. Parasites are released and infect the red blood cells. Transmission can occur by blood transfusion or transplacentally **Incubation period:** Varies by type, generally 8–25 days after a mosquito bite, but may be up to 1 year. **Period of communicability:** Communicable by blood, blood product transfusion, or organ transplant from an infected person.	Children who live in endemic areas and survive the first 5 years of life develop immunity to the severe effects of the disease as long as they have frequent reexposure to the infection. **Complications:** Severe anemia and cerebral malaria in young children. Pulmonary edema, respiratory failure, renal failure, spontaneous bleeding, and shock in older children and adolescents. Children with asplenia are at high risk for death.	Children may need blood transfusions. Primaquine may be prescribed to prevent relapse. **Prognosis:** Certain species have dormant liver-stage parasites, which can reactivate several months or years after initial infection. **Prevention:** While traveling in endemic areas, use DEET insect repellent, screened rooms, DEET-treated mosquito netting, and cover the body with light-colored clothing. Antimalarial chemoprophylaxis may be prescribed when traveling in an endemic region. A vaccine is being tested in children. This is a reportable disease.	• Educate families traveling to endemic areas about the need for and correct administration of antimalarial drugs, despite the nausea and vomiting side effects. • Discuss protecting children during mosquitoes' nocturnal feeding times with protective clothing, mosquito repellent, and mosquito netting around the bed.
RABIES (HYDROPHOBIA) **Causal agent:** *Lyssavirus* in the Rhabdoviridae family, two types (urban, in dogs; wild, in wildlife). **Epidemiology:** Occurs worldwide. Urban rabies is generally controlled by vaccination of dogs and cats. The most common carriers of rabies are raccoons, bats, skunks, and foxes (CDC, 2013e). **Transmission:** Infected saliva from the bite of a rabid animal introduces the virus into the wound. The virus travels along the nerves to the brain where it multiplies and migrates along the efferent nerves to the salivary glands. Rare cases of human-to-human transmission through exposure to mucous membranes, aerosol droplets, and organ transplant. **Incubation period:** Highly variable but usually 1–3 months.	No signs during the long incubation period. **Prodromal stage:** Over 2–10 days the child has fever, headache, malaise, apprehension, and paresthesia at the site of the bite. **Neurologic stage:** Cerebral signs of agitation, anxiety, confusion followed by abnormal behavior, delirium, hallucinations, and insomnia. The child progresses to coma and respiratory failure. **Complications:** Usually results in death.	**Diagnostic testing:** Confirmed by direct fluorescent antibody staining of the dead animal's brain tissue or detection of the virus in the client's saliva or cerebrospinal fluid. **Medical management:** Immediately wash animal bites thoroughly with soap and water and irrigate well with a virucidal agent such as povidone-iodine. Antibiotics and wound suturing are determined for individual cases. Postexposure prophylaxis—1 dose of human rabies immune globulin (HRIG) and human diploid cell rabies vaccine (HDCV) is given IM the day of the bite when the animal may be rabid. HRIG is infiltrated locally around the bite with remaining volume given IM at a site distant from the vaccine. HDCV is repeated on days 3, 7, and 14 after the bite (4 doses) (CDC, 2013e). The vaccine is of no value once rabies symptoms are present. **Prognosis:** Usually fatal. **Prevention:** Immunize all domestic animals against rabies.	• Alert the local animal control to find and quarantine the unimmunized animal for observation. • Administer human rabies immunoglobulin (HRIG) and human diploid cell vaccine (HDCV) as ordered. Inject vaccine into the muscle to prevent vaccine failure. • Support the family while reinforcing the urgency for the vaccine and series of injections. • Educate parents about the vaccine side effects—irritation and itching at the injection site, headache, muscle aches, nausea, and dizziness. • If the child acquires rabies, the child will be hospitalized. Use standard and contact precautions. • Make the child as comfortable as possible. • Keep liquids out of sight of the hydrophobic child. • Provide emotional support to the family of the dying child. • Teach children to avoid contact with all unknown animals, dead or alive. • Participate in local education about rabies and safe interactions with dogs. See Chapter 31.

DISEASE	CLINICAL MANIFESTATIONS	CLINICAL THERAPY	NURSING MANAGEMENT

ROCKY MOUNTAIN SPOTTED FEVER (TICKBORNE TYPHUS FEVER, SAO PAULO TYPHUS)

DISEASE	CLINICAL MANIFESTATIONS	CLINICAL THERAPY	NURSING MANAGEMENT
Causal agent: *Rickettsia rickettsii*, a gram-negative coccobacillus. **Epidemiology:** Occurs throughout the United States, southern Canada, and Central and South America. In the United States, 60% of cases occur in North Carolina, Oklahoma, Arkansas, Tennessee, and Missouri (CDC, 2013f). Most infections generally occur between April and September. **Transmission:** Transmitted by bites of ticks, principally dog and wood ticks. **Incubation period:** 2–14 days (most commonly 7 days) after bite of an infected tick. **Period of communicability:** There is no evidence of person-to-person transmission. 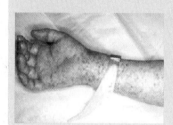 Science Source	Onset may be gradual or rapid with vague signs that mimic other diseases. Early symptoms are fever, malaise, headache, muscle aches, anorexia, nausea, vomiting, and diarrhea. The red maculopapular rash that blanches generally occurs 2–5 days after the fever. It appears first on the wrist, forearms, and ankles and then spreads to trunk and sometimes the palms and soles (see figure). The rash may be difficult to see on children with dark skin. A petechial rash appearing about day 6 is a sign of progression to severe disease. **Complications:** Vasculitis resulting in bleeding, disseminated intravascular coagulation (DIC), reduced circulation resulting in gangrene of digits or extremities, and neurologic deficits.	**Diagnostic testing:** Immunofluorescent antibody testing; direct immunofluorescence or immune-peroxidase tests may be performed on skin biopsies. Blood test may reveal thrombocytopenia. **Medical management:** Doxycycline regardless of client's age for 7–14 days (at least 3 days after fever subsides). The client with severe disease needs IV antibiotics. **Prognosis:** Delay in treatment can cause severe disease. A mortality rate of 1% is associated with delayed treatment (CDC, 2013f). **Prevention:** Avoid areas that are heavily tick infested, and wear protective clothing. Check children for ticks and remove promptly if found.	• Use standard precautions. • The child may require care in the ICU. Have hemodynamic monitoring equipment and emergency supplies readily available. • Administer antibiotics as ordered. • Observe for any purpura development or abnormal bleeding. • Make the child as comfortable as possible. • Provide quiet diversion activities. • Provide emotional support, and keep parents informed about the child's condition. • Educate parents about prevention and the appropriate technique for tick removal.

ANTIBIOTIC USE

Antibiotics are often prescribed to treat bacterial infectious diseases; however, strains of bacteria have developed resistance to many antibiotics. Examples are community-acquired methicillin-resistant *Staphylococcus aureus* and drug-resistant strains of tuberculosis. Children with chronic conditions may be more susceptible to infection by drug-resistant pathogens. Many specialty organizations and medical centers have developed best practice guidelines for the use of antibiotics in treating common infections, such as acute otitis media.

Antiviral medications may be prescribed for viral infections, such as chickenpox and influenza. When the child is immunocompromised, antiviral medication should be started early to minimize the potential life-threatening consequences of the infection.

Cases of many communicable diseases must be reported to the state health department, using standardized state forms or on a designated website.

Nursing Management

For the Child With a Communicable Disease

Nursing Assessment and Diagnosis

Assess the child's hydration status and fluid intake, vital signs, comfort level, and appetite. Observe for seizures and for a **toxic appearance** (lethargy, poor perfusion, hypoventilation or hyperventilation, and cyanosis). The child with a fever may be irritable and restless, sleep fitfully, and have nonspecific muscular pain. Identify febrile children who may be at higher risk for a serious illness, in particular:

- Infants and children having a toxic appearance.
- Newborns less than 28 days of age with a temperature over 38.0°C (100.4°F).
- Children less than 4 years of age with a temperature over 41.0°C (105.8°F).
- Children with conditions such as a congenital heart disease, ventriculoperitoneal shunt, asplenia, and sickle cell disease.

Observe the child for other signs of infection, such as a rash, nausea and vomiting, or diarrhea, as well as generalized symptoms of a poor appetite, muscle aches, and malaise.

The following nursing diagnoses may be appropriate for children with communicable diseases (NANDA-I © 2014):

- *Hyperthermia* related to infectious disease process
- *Skin Integrity, Impaired,* related to skin lesions and scratching
- *Mucous Membrane: Oral, Impaired,* related to infectious disease process
- *Fluid Volume: Deficient* related to repeated episodes of vomiting and diarrhea
- *Health Management, Family, Ineffective,* related to complexity of care required by child

Pathophysiology Illustrated: **Fever**

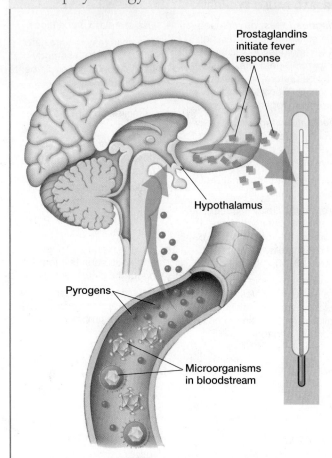

Prostaglandins initiate fever response

Hypothalamus

Pyrogens

Microorganisms in bloodstream

The hypothalamus functions as the body's thermostat, directing the body to conserve or dissipate heat. When microorganisms invade the body, **endogenous pyrogens** (interleukins, interferons, and tumor necrosis factor) are released by macrophages into the bloodstream. These substances travel to the hypothalamus where they trigger the production and release of prostaglandins, resulting in the fever response. A rise in the hypothalamus's set point leads to heat generation with shivering and chills, vasoconstriction, and decreased peripheral perfusion. Blood is diverted from the extremities to more central vessels to decrease heat loss. Shivering increases both metabolic action and heat production. The hypothalamus then maintains the temperature at the new set point. When the temperature is elevated, the heart rate, respiratory rate, and metabolic rate increase. Vasodilation occurs and the skin flushes, becoming warm to the touch.

Planning and Implementation

Most children with communicable diseases are cared for at home; however, infected children are seen in all healthcare settings. Nursing care includes collecting cultures, providing supportive care, administering antibiotics on schedule, monitoring antibiotic blood levels if indicated to ensure appropriate results, promoting the child's comfort, and educating parents.

PREVENT DISEASE TRANSMISSION

Nursing care of children with communicable diseases in healthcare settings focuses on preventing the spread of infection. Isolate children with suspicious rashes and respiratory infections. Cover draining wounds and dispose of dressings appropriately. All items with which the infected child comes into contact are considered contaminated (e.g., linens, toys, medical equipment). Use standard precautions and good hand hygiene. Recall that the fecal–oral and respiratory routes are the most common routes of transmission in children. Wipe down hard surfaces in the examining room with an antiseptic solution before another child uses the room. If possible, wipe down toys in the waiting room daily with a nontoxic antiseptic solution. Dispose of linens in appropriately marked linen bags. Ensure that all healthcare providers are fully immunized or that unimmunized or pregnant healthcare providers are not exposed to children with certain infections (e.g., pertussis, rubella, or varicella). See *Families Want to Know: Reducing the Transmission of Infection* earlier in this chapter.

Children with severe infections are often admitted to the hospital for treatment. In addition, countless numbers of **nosocomial** (hospital-acquired) **infections** occur each year. Follow the facility's standard and transmission-based precautions to reduce the spread of infectious diseases to staff and other children. Discuss any concerns with the hospital's infection control nurse. (See the *Protective Methods* chapter in the *Clinical Skills Manual* SKILLS for more detailed information.)

FEVER MANAGEMENT

Nursing care for treatment of fever includes removing unnecessary clothing, encouraging increased fluid intake, and administering nonaspirin antipyretics. Identify clear fluids the child prefers to drink to encourage greater intake. Parents often fear a fever, believing it is a disease rather than a symptom of an illness. Provide information and reassurance. Help them to recognize signs that the child's condition is worsening. See *Families Want to Know: Guidelines for Evaluating and Treating Fever in Children*.

EDUCATING THE FAMILY

Teach parents to care for their child at home. This includes how and when to give antipyretics and antibiotics if ordered, when over-the-counter medications may be used, appropriate fluids and foods to provide, and the care of rashes and other symptoms.

Teach parents to give all the antibiotic doses for the full number of days prescribed. Help develop a schedule that matches the family's routines. Make sure family members know whether to give the antibiotic by mouth with or without food or apply topically. Inform them to discard the antibiotic when all doses have been given, and not to share the antibiotic with any other family member. These efforts will help fully treat the infection and reduce the chance that the infectious organism develops resistance to the antibiotic.

Families Want to Know

Guidelines for Evaluating and Treating Fever in Children

Facts about fevers:

- A fever is not a disease; it is the body's response to an infection. It means the child's body is using natural defenses to fight an infection.
- If the child has a fever and does not look sick, it may be better to let the child use natural defenses to fight off the virus or bacteria causing the fever.

Treating the fever:

- Use a thermometer to check the child's temperature every 4 to 6 hours, or more often if the fever returns.
- Use acetaminophen or ibuprofen (do not use aspirin) to lower the temperature. Use the correct dose and preparation for the child's weight, and mark down when the medication is given. Do not exceed the number of doses per day listed on the bottle to prevent an overdose. If the child is taking a cold medication with acetaminophen, call the healthcare provider for advice about acetaminophen dosage.
- Remove all but a light layer of the child's clothing.
- Monitor the child's behavior and response to fever medication. The medication will reduce the child's temperature. The temperature may rise again in 4 to 6 hours after the medicine has worn off. Check the temperature and give another dose of medication. The temperature will return to normal when the child is recovering from the illness.
- Sponging the child is not recommended. The lukewarm water may increase shivering and discomfort. Do not use alcohol for sponge baths.
- Give the child lots of fluids to drink and allow the child to rest.

Contact your healthcare provider immediately if:

- The infant is under 2 months old and has a fever over 38.0°C (100.4°F).
- The child has a fever over 40.1°C (104.2°F) and any of the following symptoms:
  - The child acts or looks very sick.
  - Inconsolable crying or whimpering. The child cries when moved or otherwise touched by the parent or other family members.
  - Difficult to awaken.
  - A stiff neck.
  - Purple spots on the skin.
  - Difficulty breathing that does not improve after the nose is cleared.
  - Unable to swallow and drooling saliva.
  - The child has a seizure.

Call your healthcare provider within 24 hours if:

- The child is 2 to 4 months old (unless fever occurs within 48 hours of a DTaP shot and the infant has no other serious symptoms).
- The child's fever is higher than 40.1°C (104.2°F), especially if the child is younger than age 3 years.
- The child complains of burning or pain with urination.
- The fever has been present more than 24 hours without an obvious cause or location of infection.
- The fever went away for more than 24 hours and then returned, or the fever has been present for more than 72 hours.

SAFETY ALERT!

Acetaminophen and ibuprofen preparations are available as infant drops, liquid syrup, chewable tablets, and adult-strength tablets or capsules. Identify the preparation used in the home to recommend the correct dosage for the child. The dose of acetaminophen is 10–15 mg/kg/dose and of ibuprofen is 4–10 mg/kg/dose. Alert parents that many over-the-counter medications also contain acetaminophen or ibuprofen; they should not be used at the same time as the antipyretic for fever to prevent an overdose.

ACETAMINOPHEN	IBUPROFEN
Infant drops—160 mg/5 mL using package dispenser	Infant drops—50 mg/1.25 mL using package dispenser
Children's liquid—160 mg/5 mL	Children's liquid—100 mg/5 mL
Chewable tablets—80 mg and 160 mg	Chewable and junior tablets—50 mg and 100 mg
Adult tablets or caplets—325 mg and 500 mg	Adult tablets or caplets—200 mg

Educate parents about methods to reduce disease transmission in the home. Encourage parents to limit the exposure of elderly family members, those with impaired immunity, infants, and visitors to the ill child. Make sure that the ill child's dishes and utensils are washed in hot soapy water or sanitized in a dishwasher. Place dressings with drainage in a plastic bag for disposal to prevent contact by other family members.

Encourage children to rest. Provide quiet diversional activities such as board games, computer games, DVDs, and music. Promote fluid intake and provide foods that the child prefers and do not cause discomfort. Reduce itching of rashes with lukewarm baths with Aveeno or oatmeal and topical lotions. Keep the child's hands clean and nails trimmed. Cover the hands with clean socks or mittens if scratching cannot be controlled.

Evaluation

Expected outcomes of nursing care include the following:

- Opportunities for spread of infection between clients and family members are minimized.
- The child's fever is effectively managed with antipyretics.
- The full treatment with antibiotics, if ordered, is completed.

Sepsis and Septic Shock

Sepsis or septicemia is a systemic inflammatory response syndrome (SIRS) in the presence of infection, such as bacteria invading the bloodstream. Infants and children who are at high risk include those with a chronic condition, burns, multiple invasive procedures, invasive catheters, a compromised immune system, or those on long-term antibiotics. Severe sepsis that progresses to septic shock is a significant health problem with an estimated in-hospital mortality rate of up to 10% (Hazinski, Mondozzi, & Baker, 2014).

Sepsis is caused by the effects of the infectious agent and its toxins. At least one of these significant events leads to the development of sepsis: an infectious agent causes severe tissue injuries that result in multiple system organ failure, the child's excessive inflammatory response triggers a secondary response, or counterregulatory mechanisms are ineffective (Roberts & Coffin, 2013). Septic shock results from a disrupted balance between proinflammatory mediators and anti-inflammatory mediators. The disrupted inflammatory mediators lead to greater tissue injury, abnormalities in coagulation and fibrinloysis, disseminated intravascular coagulation (DIC), vasodilation, major organ dysfunction, and increased susceptibility to other infections (see Chapter 23 for more information on DIC). Fibrin deposits in the microcirculation disrupt the blood flow and the delivery of oxygen and nutrients to the tissues. Cellular hypoxia and major multiple organ system dysfunction result.

Early signs of SIRS in children include fever or hypothermia, tachycardia, and tachypnea. Signs of septic shock include fever, tachycardia, tachypnea, and inadequate perfusion (altered responsiveness, prolonged capillary refill time, either diminished or bounding pulses, mottled cool extremities, and decreased urine output). Hypotension may be present despite adequate fluid resuscitation.

Diagnosis is often suspected from clinical signs and symptoms. Cultures of the blood, urine, cerebrospinal fluid, and skin lesions are obtained, as well as a complete blood count with differential. The white blood cell count may be elevated or low for age. Clinical therapy focuses on preserving vital organ function with oxygen, IV fluid resuscitation, vasopressor medications, and antibiotics. The treatment plan focuses on restoring the blood pressure, returning the heart rate and capillary refill rate to more normal levels, maintaining the cardiac output, and increasing oxygen delivery to the tissues and vital organs. Acid–base, glucose, and electrolyte level imbalances are managed. Enteral or parenteral nutritional support may be initiated early. Septic shock may progress to cardiac arrest if interventions are unsuccessful.

Nursing Management

Nursing care of the infant or child with sepsis occurs in the neonatal or pediatric intensive care unit. Nursing care of children with sepsis involves careful assessment and management of the child's vital signs, fluid and electrolyte balance, perfusion, hemodynamic stability, and response to clinical therapy. Families need extensive support for this life-threatening infection. Encourage the parents to participate in the child's care as much as possible. Observe for signs that the condition is worsening or resolving.

Emerging Infection Control Threats

Public health officials are conducting disease surveillance to identify emerging infections, such as **pandemic flu**, a worldwide influenza epidemic, or other epidemics such as Ebola and Zika virus. Some infectious agents have the potential to be weapons of terrorists (anthrax, smallpox, plague, botulism, hemorrhagic fever, or tularemia). Early recognition and reporting of clusters of patients with similar symptoms is essential to initiate public health measures that will reduce disease transmission. Additionally, confirmation of an epidemic triggers the mass casualty response needed to care for large numbers of ill adults and children. See Table 16–5 for influenza information.

Nursing Management

Maintain a high level of suspicion when greater than the expected number of individuals with similar signs and symptoms come to school or seek care in any healthcare facility. Initiating airborne and contact precautions and instituting isolation before a definitive diagnosis is appropriate when the level of suspicion is high. Assess children and provide supportive nursing care for the identified infection.

Chapter Highlights

- Reducing the number of preventable childhood illnesses is a major national public health goal.

- A communicable disease is an illness caused by microorganisms that are commonly transmitted from one host (animal or human) to another.

- Newborns and infants are especially vulnerable to infectious diseases because their immune systems are immature, their passively acquired maternal antibodies provide limited protection, and disease protection through immunization is not yet complete.

- For a child to acquire a communicable disease, an infectious agent or pathogen, an effective means of transmission, and a susceptible host need to be present.

- Infection control measures caregivers can take include the following: good hand hygiene with soap and water or alcohol-based gels, disinfecting hard surfaces touched by the child or the child's body fluids, disinfecting toys, and making sure all children are fully immunized.

- The average infant born in 2016 will receive immunizations for 16 communicable diseases by 18 years of age.

- The Vaccines for Children program provides free immunizations for low-income children to ensure that finances are not a barrier to full immunization of those children.

- When parents resist immunizations for religious or philosophical reasons, the nurse should provide them with accurate information and help them understand how their child may benefit from immunization. If they still resist, inform them that their child may be at a significant risk for an infection and will need to be held out of school if an outbreak occurs.

- The potency of vaccines must be protected with storage in the refrigerator or freezer at the appropriate temperature.

- The National Vaccine Injury Acts of 1986 and 1993 provide compensation if a link between immunization and a serious adverse effect is found. The Vaccine Adverse Event Reporting System has been established to track serious vaccine reactions.

- Immunization information is updated frequently. It is the nurse's responsibility to regularly obtain current information about vaccines, immunization schedule, and important information to share with parents and adolescents.

- Infectious and communicable diseases are caused by bacterial, viral, protozoan, or fungal organisms.

- Fever is often a sign of infectious disease in children. When pathogens invade the body, endogenous pyrogens travel to the hypothalamus, where they trigger the production and release of prostaglandins, which initiate the fever response.

- The child with a toxic or septic appearance has the following signs: lethargy, poor perfusion, tachypnea or bradypnea, and pallor or cyanosis.

- The appropriate use and administration of antibiotics to help reduce the development of antibiotic-resistant bacteria includes the following: Give antibiotic dosages as prescribed for the full number of days ordered, do not share with other family members who might be ill, and discard when all doses have been given.

- Sepsis is a systemic response to infection that has a high mortality rate.

- The public health system conducts disease surveillance to detect the emergence of rare infections, an epidemic, or the presence of infectious disease potentially caused by terrorists.

Clinical Reasoning in Action

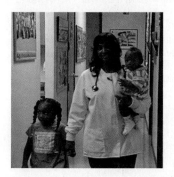

Keisha, 7 years old, and Brandon, 6 months old, are brought to the pediatric clinic, needing immunizations. Even though Brandon is sick today, their mother would still like Keisha to have her vaccines, and she would also like both children to have a complete checkup before their vaccines to make sure they are healthy.

You examine Keisha's vital signs as: 80th percentile in height, 40th percentile in weight, temperature 98.9°F, blood pressure 105/62 mmHg, urinalysis with a trace of leukocytes, and she passes her hearing and vision screening. She seems extremely anxious about having to get a needle. There is evidence of eczema and allergic rhinitis.

You examine Brandon as a sick visit while he clings to his mother. His vital signs are: temperature 102°F, respiratory rate of 30 breaths per minute, and heart rate of 90 beats per minute.

In Brandon's mouth, grayish, papulovesicular, ulcerative lesions are observed, evidence of an enterovirus. This type of illness does not respond to antibiotics. You advise the mother to avoid exposing Brandon to other persons because it is contagious and to offer cool drinks and bland foods. You also suggest that warm saline mouth rinses may be helpful if Keisha develops the illness. You advise the mother to observe for dehydration, and to give ibuprofen or acetaminophen as needed.

1. Since Brandon has been in to the office several times for various infections, what education can be given to his mother to reduce the chances of future infections?

2. Keisha has eczema and allergic rhinitis. Would this be a contraindication to giving vaccines?

3. What are questions the nurse should ask the mother before administering vaccines to Keisha to make sure there are no contraindications to giving them?

4. What should the mother be told about caring for Keisha after her vaccines?

5. How should the mother be told to manage Brandon's fever?

References

American Academy of Pediatrics (AAP) Committee on Infectious Disease. (2015). *Red book: Report of the Committee on Infectious Disease* (30th ed.). Elk Grove Village, IL: Author.

Arriola, C. S., Brammer, L., Epperson, S., Blanton, L., Kniss, K., Mustaquim, D., . . . Jhung, M. (2014). Update: Influenza activity—United States, September 29, 2013–February 8, 2014. *Morbidity and Mortality Weekly Report, 63*(07), 148–154.

Centers for Disease Control and Prevention (CDC). (2012). *Fifth disease.* Retrieved from http://www.cdc.gov/parvovirusB19/fifth-disease.html

Centers for Disease Control and Prevention (CDC). (2013a). *Pertussis.* Retrieved from http://www.cdc.gov/pertussis/index.html

Centers for Disease Control and Prevention (CDC). (2013b). *Pneumoccocal disease.* Retrieved from http://www.cdc.gov/pneumococcal/about/index.html

Centers for Disease Control and Prevention (CDC). (2013c). *Polio.* Retrieved from http://www.cdc.gov/polio/about/index.htm

Centers for Disease Control and Prevention (CDC). (2013d). *Tetanus.* Retrieved from http://www.cdc.gov/tetanus/index.html

Centers for Disease Control and Prevention (CDC). (2013e). *Rabies.* Retrieved from http://www.cdc.gov/rabies/

Centers for Disease Control and Prevention (CDC). (2013f). *Rocky Mountain spotted fever.* Retrieved from http://www.cdc.gov/rmsf/index.html

Centers for Disease Control and Prevention (CDC). (2014a). *Hand hygiene basics.* Retrieved from http://www.cdc.gov/handhygiene/Basics.html

Centers for Disease Control and Prevention (CDC). (2014b). *Vaccine storage and handling.* Retrieved from http://www.cdc.gov/vaccines/recs/storage/default.htm

Centers for Disease Control and Prevention (CDC). (2014c.) *Measles*. Retrieved from http://www.cdc.gov/measles/index.html

Centers for Disease Control and Prevention (CDC). (2014d). *Meningococcal disease*. Retrieved from http://www.cdc.gov/meningococcal/index.html

Centers for Disease Control and Prevention (CDC). (2014e). *Epstein-Barr virus and infectious mononucleosis*. Retrieved from http://www.cdc.gov/epstein-barr/index.html

Centers for Disease Control and Prevention (CDC). (2014f). *Lyme disease*. Retrieved from http://www.cdc.gov/lyme/

Centers for Disease Control and Prevention (CDC). (2014g). *Vaccines and immunizations: Possible side effects from vaccines*. Retrieved from http://www.cdc.gov/vaccines/vac-gen/side-effects.htm

Centers for Disease Control and Prevention (CDC). (2015a). *CDC vaccine price list*. Retrieved from http://www.cdc.gov/vaccines/programs/vfc/awardees/vaccine-management/price-list/#pediatric

Centers for Disease Control and Prevention (CDC). (2015b). *Pregnancy and whooping cough*. Retrieved from www.cdc.gov/pertussis/pregnant/index.html

Cullen, K. A., & Arguin, P. M. (2013). Malaria surveillance—United States, 2011. *Morbidity and Mortality Weekly Report, 62*(5), 1–18.

Darden, P. M., Thompson, D. M., Roberts, J. R., Hale, J. J., Pope, C., Thompson, D. M., . . . Jacobson, R. M. (2013). Reasons for not vaccinating adolescents: National immunization survey of teens, 2008–2010. *Pediatrics, 131*(4), 645–651.

DeStefano, F., Price, C. S., & Weintraub, E. S. (2013). Increasing exposure to antibody-stimulating proteins and polysaccharides in vaccines is not associated with risk of autism. *Journal of Pediatrics, 163*(2), 561–567.

Gastañaduy, P. A., Redd, S. B., Fiebelkorn, A. P., Rota, J. S., Rota, P. A., Bellini, W. J., . . . Wallace, G. S. (2014). Measles—United States, January 1–May 23, 2014. *Morbidity and Mortality Weekly Report, 63*, 1–4.

Grohskopf, L. A., Olsen, S. J., Sokolow, L. Z., Bresee, J. S., Cox, N. J., Broder, K. R., . . . Walter, E. B. (2014). Prevention and control of seasonal influenza with vaccines: Recommendations of the Advisory Committee on Immunization Practices (ACIP)—United States, 2014–15 influenza season. *Morbidty and Mortality Weekly Report, 63*(32), 691–697.

Hazinski, M. F., Mondozzi, M. A., & Baker, R. A. U. (2014). Shock, multiple organ dysfunction syndrome and burns in children. In K. L. McCance, S. E. Huether, V. L. Brashers, & N. S. Rote (Eds.), *Pathophysiology: The biologic basis for disease in adults and children* (7th ed., pp. 1699–1727). St. Louis, MO: Elsevier Mosby.

Health Resources and Services Administration. (2013). *Vaccine Injury Table*. Retrieved from http://www.hrsa.gov/vaccinecompensation/vaccineinjurytable.pdf

Hendrix, K. S., Finnell, M. E., Zimit, G. D., Sturm, L. A., Lane, K. A., & Downs, S. M. (2014). Vaccine message framing and parents' intent to immunize their infants for MMR. *Pediatrics, 134*(3), e675–2683.

Hill, H. A., Elam-Evans, L. D., Yankey, D., Singleton, J., & Kolasa, M. (2015). National, state, and selected local area vaccination coverage among children aged 19–35 months—United States, 2014. *Morbidity and Mortality Weekly Report, 64*(33), 899–896.

Huether, S. E. (2014). Pain, temperature regulation, sleep, and sensory function. In K. L. McCance, S. E. Huether, V. L. Brashers, & N. S. Rote (Eds.), *Pathophysiology: The biologic basis for disease in adults and children* (6th ed., pp. 481–524). St. Louis, MO: Mosby Elsevier.

Kroger, A. T., Sumaya, C. V., Pickering, L. K., & Atkinson, W. L. (2011). General recommendations on immunization: Recommendations of the Advisory Committee on Immunization Practices (ACIP). *Morbidity and Mortality Weekly Report, 60*(2), 1–62.

MacNeil, J. R., Rubin, L., McNamara, L., Briere, E. C., Clark, T. A., & Cohn, A. C. (2014). Use of MenACWY-CRM vaccine in children aged 2 through 23 months at increased risk for meningococcal disease: Recommendations of the Advisory Committee on Immunization Practices, 2013. *Morbidity and Mortality Weekly Report, 63*(24), 527–530.

Marin, M., Bialek, S. R., & Seward, J. F. (2013). Updated recommendations for use of VariZIG—United States, 2013. *Morbidity and Mortality Weekly Report, 62*(28), 574–576.

Markowitz, L. E., Dunne, E. F., Saraiya, M., Chesson, H. W., Curtis, C. R., Gee, J., . . . Unger, E. R. (2014). Human papillomavirus vaccination: Recommendations of the Advisory Committee on Immunization Practices. *Morbidity and Mortality Weekly Report, 63*(5), 1–30.

McLean, H. Q., Fiebelkorn, A. P., Temte, J. L., & Wallace, G. S. (2013). Prevention of measles, rubella, congenital rubella syndrome, and mumps, 2013: Summary recommendations of the Advisory Committee on Immunization Practices. *Morbidity and Mortality Weekly Report, 62*(4), 1–34.

Midgley, C. M., Jackson, M. A., Selvarangan, R., Turabelitze, G., Obringer, E., Johnson, D., . . . Gerber, S. I. (2014). Severe respiratory illness associated with Enterovirus D68—Missouri and Illinois, 2014. *Morbidity and Mortality Weekly Report, 63*(36), 798–799.

National Association of School Nurses. (2011). *Infectious disease management in the school setting*. Retrieved from http://www.nasn.org/PolicyAdvocacy/PositionPapersandReports/NASNPositionStatementsFullView/tabid/462/ArticleId/34/Infectious-Disease-Management-in-the-School-Setting-Revised-2011

Nyhan, B., Reifler, R., Richey, S., & Freed, G. L. (2014). Effective messages in vaccine promotion: A randomized trial. *Pediatrics, 133*(4), e835–e842.

Purnell, L. D. (2013). *Transcultural health care: A culturally competent approach* (4th ed.). Philadelphia, PA: F. A. Davis.

Purnell, L. D. (2014). *Culturally competent health care* (3rd ed., pp. 48–75). Philadelphia, PA: F. A. Davis.

Reagan-Steiner, S., Yankey, D., Jerarajah, J., Elam-Evans, L. D., Singleton, J. A., Curtis, C. R., . . . Stokley, S. (2015). National and state vaccination coverage among adolescents aged 13–17 years—United States, 2014. *Morbidity and Mortality Weekly Report, 64*(29), 784–792.

Roberts, K. E., & Coffin, S. E. (2013). Immunology and infectious disease. In M. F. Hazinski (Ed.), *Nursing care of the critically ill child* (3rd ed., pp. 851–867). St. Louis, MO: Elsevier.

Rubin, L. G., Levin, M. J., Ljungman, P., Davies, E. G., Avery, R., Tomblyn, M., . . . Kang, I. (2013). 2013 IDSA clinical practice guideline for vaccination of the immunocompromised host. *Clinical Infectious Diseases*. doi:10.1093/cid/cit684

U.S. Department of Health and Human Services. (2014). *Healthy People 2020*. Retrieved from http://www.healthypeople.gov/2020/default.aspx

U.S. Department of Health and Human Services. (2015). *Immunizations and infectious diseases*. Retrieved from http://www.healthypeople.gov/2020/topics-objectives/topic/immunization-and-infectious-diseases

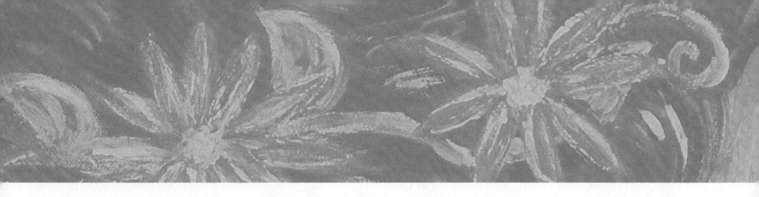

Chapter 17
Social and Environmental Influences on the Child

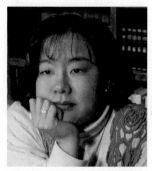

Amy has always been a challenge! She has already left home a couple of times and lived on the streets, which was very hard on us. Lately, she has been more interested in school and is living at home and trying to do well. We want her to succeed and learn the skills she needs in her life. I wish she would not have all of these body piercings, but we don't want to make too big an issue of it as long as she is doing well in school.

—Mother of Amy, 15 years old

Steve Skjold / Alamy

Learning Outcomes

17.1 Identify major social and environmental factors that influence the health of children and adolescents.

17.2 Apply the ecologic model and resiliency theory to assessment of the social and environmental factors in children's lives.

17.3 Examine the effects of substance use, physical activity, and other lifestyle patterns on health.

17.4 Plan nursing interventions for children who experience violence.

17.5 Evaluate the environment for hazards to children, such as exposure to harmful substances and potential for poisoning.

17.6 Explore the nursing role in prevention and treatment of child abuse and neglect and other forms of violence.

17.7 Plan nursing interventions for children related to social and environmental situations.

Many of the major causes of mortality and morbidity in children and adolescents are closely linked with social influences in the child's world. The social contexts for young children growing up today are different from those of even a decade ago. Examining the social contexts in which children live and grow can provide insights into behavior, and present opportunities for nursing interventions. All nurses must examine the social influences and apply the knowledge gained to plan health care that will benefit youth as they grow into adulthood.

Children and adolescents are also influenced by their environments. The physical setting, exposure to chemical agents, and other environmental factors are increasingly identified as being instrumental in determining health. Nurses assess the environment for its risk and protective factors, and then use this information to plan nursing care appropriate to enhance the health status of children and adolescents.

What are the settings where nurses might work with youth in the community? What are the challenges of today's society that children must often face at very young ages? How can nurses help children face these challenges and emerge as healthy and contributing members of society? What roles do nurses play in identifying and using the protective factors and in minimizing the risk factors of youth? This chapter will examine and apply these social and environmental concepts in a variety of nursing settings.

Examine again the major causes of death for children from 1 year of age through adolescence that are presented in Chapter 1. Notice that most morbidity is related to preventable causes linked to present-day lifestyles. Car crashes, fires, drowning, and homicides are a few examples of common causes of death in children and adolescents.

Respiratory conditions and injuries are major causes of hospitalization in children. By the teen years, pregnancy and mental disorders are the most common admitting diagnoses to hospitals (Agency for Healthcare Research and Quality, 2013). All of these conditions are related, at least in part, to the social and environmental settings in which children live. These settings and their influences must be examined to understand how best to intervene with children. Consult other chapters for additional information on related topics. For example, Chapter 4 fully discusses growth and development of children, Chapter 9 addresses health promotion topics of adolescents including homosexuality, Chapter 12 discusses chronic conditions, and Chapter 28 details cognitive variations and mental health issues such as suicide.

Basic Concepts

In this chapter, two main theories provide a framework for examining societal influences on children. The ecologic and resiliency theories are discussed in Chapter 4, and should be reviewed now to assist in evaluating the environmental settings that influence children.

The ecologic theory views the child and the environment as interacting forces, with children influencing systems around them, even while they are influenced by these systems (Bronfenbrenner, 2005). The systems with which the child has daily contact are microsystems (e.g., family, child care, school), but other systems such as parental work and political or cultural environments are also important. Understanding these systems, or the forces in which children function, can provide information that guides healthcare providers. For example, if the parents' employers do not provide healthcare insurance, their children may not get needed health care such as immunizations, treatment for diseases, and growth monitoring.

Resiliency theory examines risk and protective factors in the child's environment and their influence on the child's ability to adapt to stressful events. Such factors can be modified to lead to more productive and healthy outcomes. Resilience is the ability to exhibit healthy responses even when faced with significant stress and adversity (see Chapter 4 for a further description of resiliency theory) (Benard, 2014; Henderson, Bernard, & Sharp-Light, 2007). Families may have protective factors that provide strength and assistance in dealing with crises and risk factors that contribute to healthcare challenges. For example, if a young child is hospitalized for treatment of an acute infectious illness, some **protective factors** might include the ability of one parent to stay with the child at all times, the ability of a grandmother to care for siblings at home during this time, and the child's ability to adapt to new situations and communicate readily with staff members. On the other hand, **risk factors** might include lack of comprehensive health insurance to pay for the hospitalization, lack of an identified healthcare "home" (consistent healthcare provider) for the child, and incomplete immunizations. The concepts of resiliency theory can be applied to Amy's family as described in the chapter-opening quotation. She experienced disruption in family stability. The risk and protective factors interacted with her own personality in ways that resulted in her desire to be an independent person, establishing her identity through body art, and, finally, a desire to return to school.

The National Longitudinal Study of Adolescent Health was conducted with over 100,000 adolescents in the United States, and found that parent–family connectedness, school connectedness, a belief in a higher being, and academic success were predictive of youth having lower health risks. Follow-up interviews are currently being carried out with the participants, who are now young adults; the resulting longitudinal data will show what characteristics and influences persist into adult life (Add Health Study, 2014). Nurses can assist adolescents and their families in establishing a sense of attachment to each other. Encourage families to include adolescents in activities, attend their sports and other school events, have meals together regularly, and attend faith-based activities or other community events as a family.

Theoretical frameworks are discussed in Chapter 4 and are useful when examining social and environmental influences on children because they guide us to examine certain factors that can be altered or understood. They suggest the assessment data to collect and pertinent nursing interventions to use. They also foster partnerships with other care providers who use these and similar theories to plan social, psychologic, and other types of care for children and their families.

Social Influences on Child Health

Poverty

An important risk factor that influences the health of children is poverty. Conversely, basic financial stability is a protective factor that contributes to the general health and well-being of children. Twenty percent (14.7 million) of U.S. children are poor and living in a family earning less than $23,624 annually for a family of four (Federal Interagency Forum on Child and Family Statistics, 2015).

Children who are poor are more likely to have unmet health needs, to have difficulty in school, to become teen parents, and to experience multiple health problems, including stunted growth and lead poisoning. Inadequate or unsafe housing, food insecurity, and poor dietary quality are more common (Federal Interagency Forum on Child and Family Statistics, 2015). What is the face of poverty? Some statistics that may prove surprising include the following:

- Children most likely to be living in poor households are those below 5 years of age.

- About 48% of children living in a single-headed household are poor, whereas only 11% in married-couple households are poor.

- Ethnic variations are startling: 13% of White children, 39% of African American children, and 34% of Hispanic children live in poverty.

- Poverty rates are higher in suburban and rural areas than in central cities.

- Nearly 70% of poor children have at least one parent working full time (Federal Interagency Forum on Child and Family Statistics, 2015).

Poverty leads to homelessness for some children. Families with children are the fastest growing group of homeless people; families experiencing homelessness comprise one third of the total homeless population. Each year, 1 in 30, or 2.5 million, children experience homelessness (National Center on Family Homelessness, 2015). The reasons for homelessness are also common risks for a number of the other challenges to health discussed in this chapter, including poor finances, abuse or other violence, and mental instability.

Children who experience homelessness often have multiple physical and mental health problems, and lack health insurance to provide care for these problems. Some of the common problems faced by homeless children and families include trauma, substance use, respiratory and skin infections, tuberculosis and HIV, and nutritional disorders. Children may have developmental delays, learning problems, or growth disruptions (American Academy of Pediatrics Council on Community Pediatrics, 2013; Kerker et al., 2011). Teens who have been homeless are more likely to engage in risky behavior such as unprotected sex, sex with multiple partners, and substance abuse. They are more likely than other teens to need emergency care, to be depressed or have some other mental illness, and to become pregnant (National Center on Family Homelessness, 2015).

Health problems related to homelessness, and other family characteristics, continue even after finding a place to live. Even after families leave homeless shelters, children frequently become separated from their mothers because of parent stress, lack of access to resources, and inability of parent(s) to provide adequate homes for the children. Complex, ongoing care is needed. This may begin in a shelter for the homeless, but should continue while the family obtains a place to live, accesses other community services, gets the children safely enrolled in school, and has financial and mental stability.

Nursing management for families with children that are poor or homeless focuses on identification of poverty, careful assessment of health risks, and linking the family to resources that can assist with stability and health. There is often no way to identify a poor child from appearance, and they may hide their status when they are in school or come to a healthcare facility. Addresses given may not be accurate, or the address of a shelter might be used. Children living at shelters or in cars and on the street usually do not take the school bus but prefer to walk to avoid stigma. Alternatively, they may be picked up by the bus first, and dropped off last, to reduce embarrassment. Be alert for children who have multiple health problems and repeated infectious diseases. They may be hungry and without adequate nutrition either at times or consistently. Degrees of personal hygiene may vary depending on access to laundry and bathing facilities. See Table 17–1 for examples of nursing care needs for homeless children and families. See *Evidence-Based Practice: Developmental and Health Implications of Homelessness.*

Stress

The adverse effect of stress on adults is well documented and the impact of stress on children has also been recognized. Stress can be acute, such as when a child has an argument with a friend, a test in school, or a family crisis. Stress can also become chronic when the family frequently does not have enough food, when fighting or abuse is frequent, or when the child is overscheduled and feels under constant pressure to perform (Elkind, 2007). Children manifest stress in a variety of ways, including regressive behavior, interrupted sleep, hyperactive behavior, gastrointestinal symptoms, crying, and withdrawal from normal events. Common stressful events for children include moving to a new home or school, marital difficulties in the family, abuse, one or both parents deployed in the military (Figure 17–1), and being expected to achieve at an extremely high level in school or sports. The busy pace of today's lifestyles and the media's encouragement of early development in children may put undue stress on some children and preteens (Elkind, 2007). Adolescents may be stressed by fulfilling many roles, such as student, part-time worker, and active member of a family. They may be in school all day, be in sport or music practice for 2 to 3 hours after school, and then have a job for several additional hours. Lack of adequate sleep is common and adds further to stress, in addition to putting the teen at risk for car crashes and poor school performance. For poor families, commonly reported stressors are related to food, shelter, transportation, medical care, and personal-time needs.

EVIDENCE-BASED PRACTICE | Developmental and Health Implications of Homelessness

Clinical Question
Children are the age group showing the fastest growth in homelessness. Because of their ages, children are vulnerable to developmental delays, mental health problems, poor school achievement, and effects of violence. Mothers are the main support for young children, but when they are homeless, they may not be able to provide the care children need for healthy growth and development. Most nurses have not been homeless and do not understand the experience of homelessness for children. What is the experience of homelessness like for children?

The Evidence
A 15-week nutrition education and physical activity program in a homeless shelter had 162 child participants. The researchers found that the children's past experiences of hunger and food insecurity influenced their present food choices. Their life experiences must be understood to influence changes in nutrition (Rodriguez, Appelbaum, Stephenson-Hunter, et al., 2013). Children from 11 to 14 years in a homeless shelter reported 13 times less suicide ideation following family strengthening approaches to care (Lynn et al., 2014). A report of an undergraduate nursing student experience in a service-learning research project in homeless shelters resulted in many changes in students. These included increased understanding of the needs of homeless people, recognition of mental health disorders, identification of vulnerable populations, and increased advocacy in social justice (August-Brady & Adamshick, 2013).

Best Practice
Youth and families in homeless shelters have multiple healthcare, educational, and social needs. Understanding the backgrounds and offering programs that are most needed can benefit families and children. Developmental screening, identification of health issues, and provision of educational programs are needed.

Clinical Reasoning
Find at least two agencies that provide health care for persons who are homeless in your community. What are some of the common health problems treated? How are youth engaged in care? What explanations are provided? Are mothers of young children offered parenting classes and stress-reduction interventions? What links are available to other community resources? What is the nursing role in the community agencies you located?

TABLE 17–1 Common Health Problems and Nursing Management of Children Who Are Poor and/or Homeless

COMMON HEALTH PROBLEMS	NURSING MANAGEMENT
Lack of immunizations	Check immunization records. Provide immunizations at schools and in homeless shelters.
Common infectious diseases	Facilitate free clinics in shelters, schools, community settings. Teach hygiene measures. Provide information about resources for bathing and hygiene. Provide resources for disease management. Arrange for medications when needed.
Sleep deficits	Inform parents about respite facilities. Arrange for children to have quiet sleep time in school if possible.
Vision and hearing deficits	Perform screening for deficits. Provide resources for eyeglasses, hearing aids, care for ear infections. (Service organizations such as the Lion's Club are good options.)
Nutritional deficits	Perform height and weight checks and a nutritional assessment. Evaluate the family for food security (see Chapter 14). Be sure the child is registered for school breakfast and lunch programs if available. Ensure that children are linked to summer food programs at the end of the academic year. Link to the Special Supplemental Nutrition Program for Women, Infants and Children (WIC). Inform about resources for meals and field gleaning (collecting unused farm produce) in the community.
Dental care problems	Teach oral hygiene. Provide toothbrushes and toothpaste. Provide bottled water if the child lives in a car or on the street. Perform oral assessment. Refer to dental programs for people with low incomes.
Injuries	Teach basic safety precautions. Visit the living situation if possible to assess for safety hazards. Provide helmets, car seats, or other gear as needed. Teach "street safe" skills. Provide resources for violence prevention and intervention.
Adolescent pregnancy and sexually transmitted infections	Provide sexuality teaching in accordance with state law. Inform about access to family planning services. Assess for child abuse and prostitution.
Mental illness	Assess for depression. Evaluate for suicide potential. Provide links to services. Plan programs to foster self-esteem. Arrange for a Big Brother or Big Sister. Refer to extracurricular activities in the school and community. Arrange for a school bus stop away from a shelter so other students do not stigmatize the homeless child.

The child experiencing stress has more frequent respiratory and gastrointestinal illnesses and is more likely to be the victim of an injury. The negative long-term effects of stress on body organs and systems suggest that children under stress are more likely to develop illnesses such as strokes, hypertension, and heart attacks later in life (Balodis, Wynne-Edwards, & Olmstead, 2010; Slopen, McLaughlin, & Shonkoff, 2014).

Nurses help children manage stress by encouraging good coping strategies (Sapienza & Masten, 2011). Emphasize healthy lifestyles with all children, including good nutrition, exercise, and plenty of sleep. Classes in yoga or martial arts may be stress-reducing for some children. Encourage parents to provide youth with activities that foster self-esteem, and to avoid unrealistic expectations about performance in sports and other activities. Provide resources to help with food acquisition, shelter, transportation, and medical care for families needing them. Adolescents may benefit from various approaches for stress management such as massage, rest, physical activity, and yoga.

Since military deployment can create family stress, partner with military families to assist them as one or both parents are deployed for duty in a remote location. Connect parents with resources for child care, mental health services, and arrangements that need to be made to prepare for the absence. If the

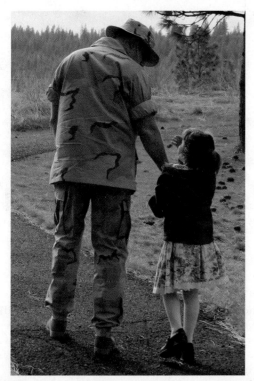

Figure 17-1 Stress from military deployment. The special relationship between a father about to be deployed in the military and his young daughter is clear. This father has two other children and is spending time with each of them, as well as with the family together, before leaving. The cycle of leaving and returning home can be stressful for families. Nurses can assist military families in making plans for health care, finances, and communication while gone and providing resources for emotional support for the entire family.

Clinical Reasoning Demographics and Nursing Care

Nurses should understand the demographics in the areas where they work. What is the poverty rate in your community? What ethnic groups are overrepresented among the poor? Locate needed resources such as food services, health care for the underserved, and enhanced school programs in order to refer poor families. Recognize that health promotion services may not be a high priority when a family does not have adequate housing or food. When children are seen in any setting, such as in school or in an emergency department or hospital for acute care, perform needed assessments and intervention. Measure growth, assess vision and hearing, evaluate dietary intake, and check immunization status. Find out the stresses the family experiences and what resources they need to meet basic necessities. Construct a nursing care plan for a family living in poverty with two young children.

---

family has had frequent moves, they may not be strongly connected to resources in the community. During deployment the remaining parent may return to the home of origin; some family support may then be present. Help families explain to children why and where the parents are going, and how they will keep

in touch during their absence. Children need to know who they will stay with, whether they will attend the same school, and how food and other needs will be provided. Parents need family, mental health, and financial support whether they are being deployed or remaining at home (Allen, Rhoades, Stanley, et al., 2011; Aranda, Middleton, Flake, et al., 2011).

Families

The families into which children are born influence them greatly. Children are supported in different ways and acquire different worldviews depending on such factors as whether one or both parents work, how many siblings are present, and whether an extended family is close by. Examine the family structure such as two parents present, single parent, adolescent parent, same-sex parents, extended family, grandparents raising grandchildren, and stepparents. Financial challenges influence work requirements and lifestyle stability. Resources in the community interact with family structures and can provide support and foster resilience in the face of challenges. All of these factors influence the physical and mental health of children, and can determine their needs for nursing interventions.

One common occurrence in the lives of many children is divorce of parents. The divorce rate in the United States is estimated to be around 50% of all marriages. Each year, an additional 1 million children are affected by divorce (Children and Divorce, 2013). Children are inevitably affected by the parents' divorce, even if the divorce was preceded by many periods of stress and tension in the home.

Many children believe they are at fault for the separation and divorce, that they said or did something to make the parent leave. When one parent leaves, the children may feel abandoned by that parent and may fear being abandoned by the remaining parent. Also, children may become engaged in the disputes of parents, and experience conflicts of loyalty when parents fight for their affection.

In divorces involving conflict and hostility, the children may have increased problems with adjustment. When children must make a series of changes in their lives in addition to the parents' separation (new home, different school), their adjustment is made more difficult as their sense of order is upset. Predictable routines have changed, and children may test limits to see if they still apply; academic and behavior problems may manifest.

The age of the child also influences understanding of and reactions to the divorce. For 3- to 5-year-olds, anxiety, temper tantrums, and other behavioral changes may occur; children ages 6 to 8 years are frequently worried and blame themselves for the divorce; 9- to 10-year-old children are predominantly angry; 11- to 13-year-olds feel lonely and deny the permanence of divorce; 14- to 17-year-olds are angry at parents and may act out frustration by abusing substances or challenging parents (Dunn & Craig, 2013).

A family's risk factors (e.g., recent separation, parental stress, and limited healthcare coverage) and its strengths (e.g., loving relationships, influential grandparents or other extended family members, and general good health) should be identified and used in planning care. Parents who are divorced can be assisted to plan strategies to ensure that the child does not feel responsible for the divorce and is able to form strong relationships with both parents. Encourage the family to ensure that the child has a relationship with both parents, using phone, Internet, and other methods to remain in close contact. See Chapter 2 for a thorough discussion of family factors as they relate to family-centered care and a description of strategies for assessment and intervention with families.

School and Child Care

Once a child is 5 or 6 years of age, several hours daily are spent in a school setting. Children develop physical skills through participation in education and sports. Psychosocial stages are met as the child interacts with children and adults and achieves social interaction patterns and pride in accomplishments. The presentation of concepts that challenge thought processes enhances cognitive development.

Although the primary role of schools is educational, they also perform several health-related functions. School health screening programs identify children with problems such as hearing loss, visual impairment, and scoliosis. Nurses provide assessment, teaching, and clinical management related to some health problems. Some schools have clinics that examine and provide even more complete health care for children. Many schools teach good nutrition, healthful living, safe sexual practices, and other health-related subjects. A school nurse may be present, at least part time, to plan these classes or to work with teachers. Nurses assist school districts in providing plans for emergency health care when needed. With the increase in mainstreaming, school staff now have the responsibility for administering medications, maintaining urinary catheters, and providing respiratory care and other treatments to ensure children's proper growth and development. See Chapter 10 for further discussion of school nurse activities.

Some children spend part or nearly all of their days in childcare settings (Figure 17–2). Over 60% of children under 6 years receive some type of child care regularly. Children spend an average of 33 hours/week in childcare settings (Laughlin, 2013). The closeness of the parent–child relationship, the quality of care, and the length of the childcare day are important in determining childcare effects on children. The mother's sensitivity to her child is the best indicator of child behavior regardless of childcare arrangements (ChildStats, 2011).

Nursing management involves helping parents explore types of daycare options available and to evaluate programs in their communities (Table 17–2). Care options for young school-age children, either before or after school, can also be shared with parents. When available, recommend early intervention programs with at-risk children, such as the Zero to Three Project and Head Start, which contribute to children's health and welfare. Nurses frequently manage the health programs in early intervention, providing screening, doing health evaluations, and establishing early intervention education plans. Nurses assist families in evaluation of childcare centers and share information about accreditation. The National Association for the Education of Young Children (2010) has established childcare criteria.

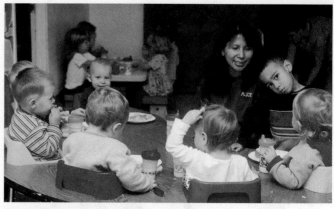

Figure 17–2 Most children will spend time in childcare settings. It is important to explore options and find the best fit for the child's needs.

Community

The community in which a child lives may support the child's development or, conversely, expose the child to hazards. Social programs such as Head Start preschools, sports activities, afterschool programs, and child abuse treatment centers offer valuable services that improve the experience of growing children. On the other hand, an economically depressed community with scant services and a high homicide rate is unsupportive and hazardous for growing children.

The physical environment is supportive when the child has sidewalks on which to walk to school, open spaces in which to learn and play, and clean air to breathe. Children who must walk to school on unsafe roads, have access to contaminated drinking supplies, or live near polluting manufacturing companies or in crowded housing or old structures are at risk for injuries and health problems such as lead poisoning (see discussion of poisoning later in this chapter).

TABLE 17–2 Types of Child Care

TYPE OF CARE/DESCRIPTION	ADVANTAGES	DISADVANTAGES
In home (caretaker comes to home of the child)	Child can remain at home Little exposure to infectious diseases No need for alternative care when child is ill	Limited contact with other children to encourage development Limited ability to rapidly locate alternate when provider is ill Most costly
Family child care (parent brings child to home of a caretaker)	Limited number of children Family-type atmosphere Some exposure to other children and encouragement of development	Little governmental regulation or examination Care provider may be distracted by activities in the home
Parent brings child to a center where many children receive care	A learning curriculum plan is in place Contact with other children can enhance development Subject to regulation and licensing Care providers are focused solely on the children	Exposure to multiple children increases infectious disease risk Demands of multiple children may distract or tire care providers

Families Want to Know

Evaluation of Child Care

The nurse can help parents evaluate childcare options and make decisions about placement for their children. Parents should always be welcomed to visit an agency or home childcare site—this is essential so they can see the routines in action. Some questions they can ask are suggested as follows:

Administration

Is the facility licensed?

Who are the administrators? What is their training and experience?

How many staff are employed? What is their training?

Is there a parent board? What part does it play in administering the center?

Physical Environment, Health, and Safety

What is the neighborhood like? Is transportation to the center convenient?

What is the condition of the lighting, heat, cooling, and ventilation systems; play spaces (inside and out); and the building's general condition?

Is playground equipment safe?

Is there a soft material such as bark, sand, or rubber tiles under climbing equipment?

Are the children always supervised?

Are there emergency medical forms and signed forms for field trips?

Who may pick up children? How are they signed in and out?

What is the immunization policy and how are records examined and maintained?

Are criminal background checks of staff done for potential child abuse and other problems?

What is the policy for children with infectious diseases and other illness?

How are foods prepared? Are the staff licensed in food handling?

What is the state of general cleanliness?

Who changes diapers? Are recommendations for standard precautions to prevent pathogen transfer followed?

What arrangements and routines are made for naps and quiet times?

Developmental Approaches

Is the curriculum appropriate for different age groups?

Are there materials and plans for gross motor, fine motor, language, and social development?

How much time do children spend in structured time? Free time?

How is discipline handled?

Do the children appear occupied and happy?

What reading materials are available?

What type and quantity of field trips are planned?

What is the educational level and longevity of the childcare workers?

Is there a diversity among the children's backgrounds and experiences?

Source: Adapted from the National Association for the Education of Young Children. (2010). *Introduction to the NAEYC early childhood program standards and accreditation criteria: Program standards*. Retrieved from http://www.naeyc.org/accreditation.

Culture

The child's cultural group may influence the use of traditional and contemporary healthcare practices. If the parents or children are recent immigrants, they may still be learning the English language and finding out about healthcare resources. Children and adolescents of immigrants may feel stress as they combine their family's traditional culture with the new culture in which the family now lives. They may also have a great deal of responsibility to interpret for the family since they often can speak two languages and understand practices in the new culture.

Recent immigrants may experience culture shock, a state of crisis related to the difference in values and lifestyle between the two cultures they have experienced. This can lead to stress-related symptoms, and create a need for healthcare intervention. Children whose parents emigrated from another country may feel different from peers and develop conflict with their parents, particularly during adolescence.

All cultural groups have rules about patterns of social interaction. Schedules of language acquisition are determined by the number of languages spoken and the amount of speech in the home. The particular social roles assumed by men and women in the culture affect school activities and ultimately career choices. Attitudes toward touching and other methods of encouraging developmental skills vary among cultures.

Nurses must become aware of common characteristics of the cultural groups they serve so that they can provide culturally competent nursing care. Arrange for interpreters when needed. Be aware that families often accept and use both traditional and westernized health care, and remain nonjudgmental about traditional healing practices. Provide access to foods for a variety of ethnic backgrounds in healthcare facilities. Evaluate youth in immigrant families for conflict between family and societal expectations. Incorporate communication with the school nurse, who often has experience with a diversity of ethnic and racial groups and their cultural practices. See Chapter 2 for further exploration of cultural awareness.

Lifestyle Activities and Their Influence on Child Health

Many patterns of daily life play a part in determining the length and quality of one's life. A child's use of tobacco products and controlled substances influences both physical and mental health. Patterns of exercise and use of protective gear protect against early disabilities. The use of decorative patterns to tattoo or scar the skin and can introduce pathogens is an example of a lifestyle pattern that influences mental health, body image, and the body's physical health.

Tobacco Use

Tobacco use is the most preventable cause of adult death in the United States. It leads to 438,000 premature deaths annually, and will be responsible for the premature death of 5 million of today's youth as they reach adult years (U.S. Department of Health & Human Services [USDHHS], 2011). Major health problems linked to tobacco use include cardiovascular disease, cancer, chronic lung disease, increased prevalence of car crashes, low birth weight, and other maternal problems. Cigarette use is most common; however, chewing tobacco, snuff, cigars, hookahs (water pipe for smoking flavored tobacco), and bidis (small, brown, hand-rolled cigarettes) also pose significant health hazards. Even passive smoking (secondhand smoke) or environmental tobacco smoke (ETS) is linked to increased heart disease, blood pressure, respiratory problems, sudden infant death syndrome (SIDS), middle ear infections, and decreased youth academic performance (U.S. Environmental Protection Agency, 2014). "Thirdhand" tobacco exposure refers to the smoking residues that remain on clothing and room/automobile surfaces.

Clinical Tip

Electronic cigarettes, known as e-cigarettes, provide an aerosol that contains nicotine and other substances. Flavorings such as spices or chocolate are frequently added. In just a 1-year period, from 2011 to 2012, e-cigarette use in 6th to 12th graders doubled, from 3.3% to 6.8%. The effects of e-cigarettes and the additives are unknown at this time, but concerns are warranted. Whether they lead to smoking of traditional cigarettes is a question yet unanswered (Centers for Disease Control and Prevention [CDC], 2013a, 2014a). When inquiring about tobacco use, specifically mention new and popular trends such as e-cigarettes and hookah pipes. Ask about frequency, type, and other details of use.

Many nurses view tobacco use as an adult issue, but each day 3200 youths try their first cigarette, and the usual age for trying tobacco is 9 to 14 years (Figure 17–3). Peer pressure is a powerful incentive for trying some form of tobacco. Nicotine is highly addictive, and most people become addicted to the substance in adolescent years. Early initiation of smoking is an extremely risky behavior because 90% of adult smokers began smoking before 18 years of age (CDC, 2011a, 2013b; 2014a). Although sale of tobacco products to children and advertisements aimed at this age group are forbidden by federal law, many youths obtain and

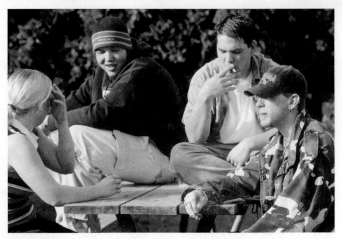

Figure 17–3 **Approximately 70% of children have tried smoking by their high school years. Early intervention can begin with discussions about smoking starting at 9 or 10 years of age.**

use tobacco. About 16% of high school students in the United States have smoked within the past 30 days, and one half of all youth have tried tobacco, making this an important health risk (CDC, 2014a).

Developing Cultural Competence Smoking Rates Among Youth

Among youth in the United States, White youth are significantly more likely to smoke than either Hispanic or African American peers. About 19% of White students reported smoking in the previous month, while 14% of Hispanic and 8% of African American students reported this behavior (CDC, 2014a). American Indian and Alaska Natives also have high smoking rates, while Asian Americans have low rates. Youth smoking rates also vary by state, ranging from 4% to 20% among various states (CDC, 2014a; USDHHS, 2011).

Certain characteristics contribute to the likelihood of tobacco use. They include increasing age, male gender, ethnic group, ease of obtaining tobacco products, and smoking among family members. Low socioeconomic group membership, access to tobacco products, low price of products, advertising, and lack of parental involvement in the lives of youth are associated with tobacco use (USDHHS, 2011). Gender differences may exist for youth who are beginning or seeking to quit tobacco use. For example, girls may be more worried about the smell and effect of tobacco on clothing and appearance, while boys more commonly express concern about smoking's effects on sports or activities (Sullivan, Bottorff, & Reid, 2011).

Several programs have been developed to encourage youth to avoid tobacco use. In addition, smoking cessation programs are available to assist youth who are already regular smokers to successfully achieve the goals of cessation or decrease in tobacco use. Use of counseling, tobacco-free environments, and peer cessation programs have been useful. Aids such as patches, gum, lozenges, nasal spray, and medications have not been adequately tested for safety in adolescents (Broberg & Nield, 2013). Once a teen is identified as a tobacco user, a biologic marker such as urine cotinine (a by-product of tobacco) levels can help to identify the frequency of smoking. This information can be used to make suggestions to the teen about the potential outcomes of the behavior and the cessation program that is most likely to be helpful.

Nursing Management

Tobacco Use

Nursing Assessment and Diagnosis

Nurses are in a unique position to inquire about the incidence of smoking and other tobacco use among youth. Insert questions into all well-child visits, beginning at about 9 to 10 years of age. Inquire about whether family members (especially parents and siblings) smoke or chew, and ask if some of the child's friends have tried smoking. Try to find out the child's knowledge and beliefs about the benefits and risks of tobacco use. As the child gets older, ask more direct and detailed questions. A nonjudgmental and collegial approach will be best to obtain a truthful response. School nurses can make observations about numbers of teens smoking and general attitudes about tobacco use. When children come to hospitals and other health facilities for care, use of tobacco should be part of general admission questions. Include questions about chew and hookah or flavored tobacco exposure.

Some nursing diagnoses that may apply to youth who smoke or show potential for this behavior include the following (NANDA-I © 2014):

- *Activity Intolerance* related to lowered oxygen supply
- *Gas Exchange, Impaired,* related to ventilation-perfusion imbalance
- *Self-Esteem, Chronic Low,* related to negative self-appraisal
- *Knowledge, Deficient,* regarding dangers of tobacco use related to developmental focus on present
- *Nutrition, Imbalanced: Less than Body Requirements,* related to effects of chemical dependence

Planning and Implementation

The roles of nurses in preventing and intervening in youth smoking are to inform youth, identify smokers, and implement programs (Table 17–3). Provide developmentally appropriate information about the hazards of tobacco use in all settings where youth are present. Addicted teens who share their stories

of difficult withdrawal from tobacco and adults who have had cancer of the lungs or larynx may be effective speakers. Offer information on prevention and cessation programs to youths and families in clinics, outpatient surgery centers, community activities, and hospitals. Use opportunities such as adolescent pregnancy and illness to reinforce the hazardous effects of tobacco on the individual and on those around. Adolescent mothers should understand the risks for small-for-gestational age babies when they smoke in pregnancy and the increased risk of sudden infant death syndrome (SIDS) when infants are exposed to secondhand smoke (see Chapter 20). Speak to young athletes about the effects of tobacco on athletic performance. Show youth the ways this product can interfere with meeting life goals. Role-play how to tell other youth "no" when tobacco is offered. Establish programs that increase the sense of self-esteem without tobacco use. Be sure to include parents in the programs so that they see and acknowledge their role in setting an example about tobacco use and in providing guidelines for the child. Provide information on the influence of environmental tobacco smoke (secondhand smoke).

Adopt a nonjudgmental attitude when asking questions about smoking so that youth using tobacco can be identified. Ask questions without parents present and assure youth that the information will not be shared. Encourage youth to cut back and to quit use of tobacco products. Offer assistance to them in these efforts. Encourage positive coping techniques for youth who are engaged in cessation. Such techniques include keeping busy, avoiding smoking situations, using oral stimulation such as a toothpick or gum, exercising, relaxing, and using nicotine replacement approaches (Audrain-McGovern et al., 2011).

Work with the schools and school districts to help establish preventive and cessation programs. There should be clear guidelines about school policies regarding tobacco use on school grounds. Keeping occasional youth tobacco users from becoming regular users should be a goal in order to avoid nicotine addiction. Find out what positive incentives can be offered to youth who are successful in quitting tobacco use. Contract with them to achieve their goals.

Evaluation

Expected outcomes of nursing interventions regarding tobacco use are lowered rates of regular use, delayed initiation of use, and success of cessation programs. *Healthy People 2020* objectives can be used to plan programs.

TABLE 17–3 Nursing Role in Youth Tobacco Use Prevention

INFORM
- Hang posters, provide brochures, and facilitate presentations about tobacco risks in all settings where youth are present. Include contemporary uses such as e-cigarettes and hookahs.
- Target tobacco users with special information about the effects of nicotine on their bodies.

IDENTIFY
- Ask questions about smoking and other tobacco use at every health encounter beginning at about 9 to 10 years of age. Ask if the child's parents, siblings, and/or friends use tobacco.
- For users, ask amount and type of tobacco and nicotine.
- Find resources where youth obtain tobacco in the community and become proactive in stopping sales.

IMPLEMENT
- Encourage youth tobacco users to quit.
- Facilitate referral to cessation programs.
- Arrange positive rewards for youth successful in cessation.

Alcohol Use

Alcohol use by the young is common. An estimated 66.6% have tried alcohol, which is the drug of choice and convenience for youth. By 12th grade, 76.3% of females and 74.9% of males have had alcoholic drinks (CDC, 2014a). Current use is also common with 34% of high school students admitting to drinking within the last month, and 20.8% having engaged in binge drinking, or having five or more drinks within a 2-hour period. Even very young adolescents are affected since 40% of eighth graders have tried alcohol and 11% have had one or more episodes of binge drinking (National Institute on Alcohol Abuse and Alcoholism, n.d.). About 18.6% of high school students report that their first drink was before age 13 (CDC, 2014a).

Many factors influence the child and adolescent who drink alcohol. Patterns in the family, media advertisements, and social environments in high school and college that honor or expect drinking all contribute to the problem. Access to alcohol is easy for most youth because older siblings or classmates often obtain drinks for them. It is a "rite of passage" for many at teen birthday parties or college events. Alcohol is the most common and accepted drug in today's society and, as such, youth are exposed to it. They often experiment with alcohol and experience its effects without understanding or considering the implications of its use. A significant risk factor for initiation of alcohol use is a transition time, such as change from middle to high school, or a major family stress, such as parental separation or divorce.

Drug Use

Substance use occurs in children and adolescents of all socioeconomic levels and is a growing health problem. The use of any drug can pose a serious psychologic and physical risk to children and adolescents.

In addition to alcohol, a variety of other drugs are used by youth. Over 41% of U.S. high school students have used marijuana, and 23% have used it in the last month; 5.5% have used cocaine, with nearly 3% having used it in the last month; 6.6% have used Ecstasy. Inhalant use of glue, paints, or other substances is more common, with nearly 9% reporting use. Approximately 3.2% report methamphetamine use (Figure 17–4), and 2.2% use heroin (CDC, 2014a). Synthetic drugs (commonly referred to as "designer" drugs), such as phencyclidine (PCP), mimic other narcotics, stimulants, and hallucinogens and are also dangerous. "Bath salts" are a contemporary drug that has effects similar to those of amphetamines. These drugs are synthetic versions of cathinone, which occurs naturally in the khat plant (Lehner & Baumann, 2013; McGraw & McGraw, 2012). Common contemporary drugs and street names are listed in Table 17–4. Some youth use these drugs with alcohol, which can lead to deadly consequences.

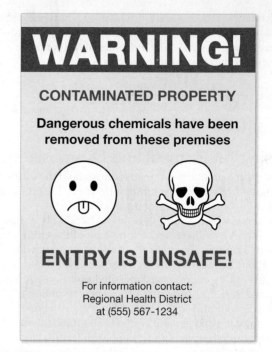

Figure 17–4 Methamphetamine is a popular drug because it can be manufactured with items that are available to the lay public. Manufacture of the substance in homes has become a concern of health departments and communities at large. Children can be harmed by the chemicals produced and may experience neglect and abuse. They may suffer even after the home is found and adults are apprehended as they must be placed in foster homes.

Prescription drugs are sometimes used for nonmedical purposes. For example, methylphenidate (Ritalin) is used for treatment of attention deficit hyperactivity disorder (ADHD) and generally acts as a stimulant. Its unprescribed use among youth has increased dramatically during the past few years. Prescription pain medications are another example of drugs that are easily abused by youth who are treated with them after surgery or other procedures.

Over-the-counter medications are legal, but frequently abused. Easily obtainable at grocery stores and drug stores, these drugs include antihistamines, atropine, bromides, caffeine, ephedrine, pseudoephedrine, phenylpropanolamine, and amphetamine-like substitutes. Volatile inhalants, such as glues, are dangerous substances of abuse, and their use appears to be rising among school-age children and adolescents. Anabolic steroids are the drugs of abuse most commonly used by athletes (see Chapter 14 for further information on enhancing substances).

ETIOLOGY AND PATHOPHYSIOLOGY

In most cases, substance use represents a maladaptive coping response to the stressors of childhood and adolescence. Individual, peer, family, and community risk factors all contribute to increased incidence of use (American Academy of Child and Adolescent Psychiatry [AACAP], 2013). A child may begin using drugs or alcohol to deal with stress because family members or peers do so. Children in families with a history of substance abuse are at higher risk of abusing drugs and alcohol. Other risk factors include rebelliousness, aggressiveness, low self-esteem, dysfunctional parental relationships, lack of

TABLE 17–4 Common Contemporary Club Drugs, Street Names, and Drug Information

DRUG	ACTION	STREET NAMES	ROUTE	TIME OF ACTION
Methylenedioxymethamphetamine (MDMA)	Stimulant; appetite suppressant; increased pulse, BP, temperature; overhydration; hyponatremia; memory loss	Ecstasy, XTC, X, Adam, Clarity, Lover's speed, E	PO (tablets, capsules)	3–6 hr
Cathinone ("bath salts")	Similar to amphetamines: agitation, combative behavior, hallucinations, delusions, hyperthermia, tachycardia, hypertension	Many names such as Bliss, Blue Silk, Charge, Energy-1, Gold Rush, K2, Meph, Mephisto, Ocean Burst, Rave ON, Rush, Special Gold, Spice, Tranquillity, White Knight	PO (capsules), snorted, IV, IM, rectal	2–4 hr but up to 8 hr possible
Gamma-hydroxybutyrate (GHB) (Xyrem)	CNS depressant, euphoria, growth hormone release, hypersalivation, hypotonia	Grievous Bodily Harm, G., Liquid Ecstasy, Georgia Home Boy, date-rape drug	PO (liquid, powder, tablets, capsules)	4 hr
Ketamine	Anesthetic; decreased memory, attention, learning; increased BP; respiratory collapse	Special K, K, Vitamin K, Cat Valiums, Jet	IV, respiratory (injected, snorted, or smoked; liquid or powder)	1 2 hr
Rohypnol (benzodiazepine; flunitrazepam)	Amnesia, sedative; decreased BP, urinary retention; given prior to sexual assault	Roffies, Rophies, Roche, Forget-me Pill	PO, respiratory (snorted; tablets)	8–12 hr
Methamphetamine	Stimulant; highly addictive; memory loss; violence, psychosis; cardiac and neurologic damage	Speed, Ice, Chalk, Meth, Crystal, Crank, Fire, Glass, Tina, Tweak, Yaba (meth and caffeine)	PO, respiratory, IV (smoked, snorted, injected)	Several hours; long-term permanent effects
Lysergic acid diethylamide (LSD)	Hallucinogen; increased pulse, BP, temperature; psychosis, flashbacks	Acid, Boomers, Blotters, Dots, Yellow Sunshines	PO (liquid, tablets, capsules)	1–2 hr; trips last 12 hr; possible flashbacks later

Source: Data from National Institute on Drug Abuse. (2011). *NIDA InfoFacts: Club drugs*. Retrieved from http://www.nida/nih.gov/Infofacts/clubdrugs.html and http://www.drugabuse.gov/drugpages.clubdrugs.html

adequate support systems, academic underachievement, poor judgment, and poor impulse control.

Initial experimentation with alcohol or drugs may be unpleasant. However, with continued use, the adolescent learns to "achieve the high," an illusion of power and well-being. The adolescent wants the high more frequently and actively seeks alcohol or drugs. Tolerance to the substance occurs with continued use, and ever-increasing amounts are required to achieve a pleasurable high. Physical and psychologic dependence ensues as the body's tissues require the substance to function properly. Withdrawal symptoms occur when the child or adolescent is deprived of the substance.

Clinical Tip

Following are common inhalant agents:

AEROSOLS

Cooking spray
Whipped cream
Spray paint
Cosmetic sprays

ADHESIVES

Model glues
Rubber cements

SOLVENTS

Nail polish remover
Paint thinner or cleaner
Lighter fluid
Degreaser

OTHER

Gasoline
Helium

CLINICAL MANIFESTATIONS

Substance abuse in children and adolescents is commonly overlooked and underdiagnosed by healthcare providers, in part because of the wide range of clinical presentations, which vary according to type of drug used, amount, frequency, time of last use, and severity of drug dependence (Table 17–5).

Common physical manifestations include alterations in vital signs, weight loss, chronic fatigue, chronic cough, respiratory congestion, red eyes, and general apathy and malaise. Withdrawal may be shown by anxiety, headache, tremors, nausea and vomiting, malaise, weakness, insomnia, depressed mood or irritability, and hallucinations. The mental status examination (refer to Chapter 5) may reveal alterations in level of consciousness, impaired attention and concentration, impaired thought processes, delusions, and hallucinations. Low self-esteem, feelings of guilt or worthlessness, and suicidal or homicidal thoughts are also common.

Poor school performance and changes in mood, sleep habits, appetite, dress, and social relationships are nonspecific characteristics of the child or adolescent who is using substances.

CLINICAL THERAPY

Multiple psychiatric diagnostic criteria exist for each drug class. Children and adolescents who have other psychosocial disorders commonly use or abuse drugs or alcohol. Treatment should therefore focus not only on the substance use or abuse but also on the issues underlying the problem. Intervention includes the family as well as the substance-abusing child or adolescent.

TABLE 17–5 Clinical Manifestations of Commonly Abused Drugs

DRUG	POTENTIAL FOR DEPENDENCE	CLINICAL MANIFESTATIONS
DEPRESSANTS		
Alcohol, barbiturates (amobarbital, pentobarbital, secobarbital)	Physical and psychologic: high; varies somewhat among drugs	Physical: decreased muscle tone and coordination, tremors Psychologic: impaired speech, memory, and judgment; confusion; decreased attention span; emotional lability
STIMULANTS		
Amphetamines (e.g., Benzedrine), caffeine, cocaine, "bath salts"	Physical: low to moderate Psychologic: high; withdrawal from amphetamines and cocaine can lead to severe depression	Physical: dilated pupils, increased pulse and blood pressure, flushing, nausea, loss of appetite, tremors Psychologic: euphoria; increased alertness, agitation, or irritability; hallucinations; insomnia
OPIATES		
Codeine, heroin, meperidine (Demerol), methadone, morphine, opium, oxycodone (Percodan)	Physical and psychologic: high; varies somewhat among drugs; withdrawal effects are uncomfortable but rarely life threatening	Physical: analgesia, depressed respirations and muscle tone (may lead to coma or death), nausea, constricted pupils Psychologic: changes in mood (usually euphoria), drowsiness, impaired attention or memory, sense of tranquility
HALLUCINOGENS		
Lysergic acid diethylamide (LSD), mescaline, phencyclidine (PCP)	Physical: none Psychologic: unknown	Physical: lack of coordination, dilated pupils, hypertension, elevated temperature; severe PCP intoxication can result in seizures, respiratory depression, coma, and death Psychologic: visual illusions and hallucinations, altered perceptions of time and space, emotional lability, psychosis
VOLATILE INHALANTS		
Glues, typing correction fluid, acrylic paints, spot removers, lighter fluid, gasoline, butane	Physical and psychologic: varies with drug used	Physical: impaired coordination, liver damage (in some cases) Psychologic: impaired judgment, delirium
MARIJUANA		
	Physical: low Psychologic: usually low; occasionally moderate to high	Physical: tachycardia, reddened conjunctiva, dry mouth, increased appetite Psychologic: initial anxiety followed by euphoria; giddiness; impaired attention, judgment, and memory

Families Want to Know

Identifying the Youth Who Is Abusing Substances

Families are often confused about the behavior of adolescents and unsure whether it represents normal development or abuse of substances. Some characteristics of normal development that help to differentiate these occurrences are listed here. When concerned about possible substance use, the parent can confront the child or talk with school nurses or counselors.

- Many youth are periodically distant with parents but remain involved with peers in school sports and other activities. Withdrawal from all activities and friends may indicate substance abuse.

- Adolescents often complain about school, but when teachers report the student meets expectations and is consistently performing in the classroom, this is normal behavior.

- Teens may be weepy on occasion when having a difficult time with friends or not performing as desired. Continued, consistent weepiness is likely to indicate depression or substance abuse.

- Teens like to stay up late and are frequently tired in the morning, whereas abusing teens may "nod off" frequently during the day.

- Many adolescents like to achieve a disheveled look in clothing, but the teen who frequently neglects basic hygiene or does not seem to have the energy to wash and dress may be depressed or be abusing substances.

- All teens get some infections, but teens who are abusing substances may have reddened eyes, oral sores, and constant respiratory discomfort from "snorting" substances.

The primary goal of treatment is to teach the child and other family members to develop and sustain positive coping patterns, and to support them during this process. Most treatment programs offer inpatient and outpatient services, as well as after-care programs. These programs usually consist of peer support that focuses on developing a drug- and alcohol-free lifestyle, healthy family relationships, and positive coping skills. Family involvement is strongly encouraged. Hospitalization is required if the physical dependence is significant and withdrawal places the child at risk for complications such as seizures, depression, or suicidal behavior.

Nursing Management

Alcohol and Drug Use

Nursing Assessment and Diagnosis

Mental health assessment of all older children and adolescents requires screening for alcohol and other substances, including screening for over-the-counter and prescription medication use (American Academy of Pediatrics Committee on Practice and Ambulatory Medicine, 2014; Havens, Young, & Havens, 2011). Maintaining a confidential approach will increase the ability to obtain truthful information about use of substances. Assessment tools provide useful information for the healthcare provider.

Nurses may encounter the substance-abusing child or adolescent in the emergency department or outpatient clinic, in schools and other community settings, or during hospitalization for an injury or other acute problem. Diagnosis includes assessment of both the family and the substance-abusing child or adolescent. Nursing assessment includes taking a thorough history from the parents and child, observing the child's behavior, and performing a physical examination. The history should include the age at which drug use began, pattern of use, length of time the drug has been used, amount of drug used, and psychologic state while on drugs. A history of parental drug use and noninvolvement in parenting the child puts the child at higher risk for substance abuse, reflecting the combined effects of genetic and environmental influences. Environmental factors such as access to the substance, use with other teens or adults, and resources for treatment are important to consider. Evaluate the home, education, alcohol, drugs, smoking, and sex practices of the teen.

PHYSIOLOGIC ASSESSMENT

Look for physical signs and symptoms of substance use, including bloodshot eyes, dilated pupils, slurred speech, and weight loss. Blood and urine levels of substances and metabolite are sometimes measured. The adolescent may appear sleepy or restless, or may show signs of clumsiness or inconsistent behavior. Consider all types of substances, including model glue, gasoline, and other sources. Consider signs of withdrawal as well as current intoxication.

PSYCHOLOGIC ASSESSMENT

Changes in social habits may indicate substance use. Parents may report a drop in the school-age child's or adolescent's grades or decreased interest in school activities. The adolescent does not introduce new friends to parents, and has less contact with parents, teachers, and other adults who were previously important. The youth may appear more energetic than usual, always "on a high," or exhibit weight loss. Note the child's current drug use, potential for violence, and motivation to make changes. Assess the degree of family support available.

FAMILY ASSESSMENT

In families with substance-using adults, children may experience neglect and abuse, as well as exposure to drugs. When family members are substance users, young children may experience periods when adults cannot provide supervision and do not encourage healthy activities, or they may be exposed to potentially unsafe or violent episodes. When parents are manufacturing products such as methamphetamine, young children are exposed to toxic chemicals and run the risk of suffering burns and other sequelae from home laboratory production and explosions. Be alert for unusual injuries, signs of inconsistent parenting, and delays in or disturbed growth and development. Be prepared to refer parents for care and for following protocols for child abuse prevention (see sections on abuse and neglect later in this chapter).

Nursing diagnoses for children and adolescents who abuse drugs or alcohol might include the following (NANDA-I © 2014):

- *Social Interaction, Impaired*, related to altered thought processes
- *Self-Esteem, Chronic Low*, related to dysfunctional family and social relationships
- *Injury, Risk for*, related to altered perceptions and sensorium
- *Violence: Self-Directed or Other-Directed, Risk for*, related to physiologic dependence on drugs, alcohol, and other substances

Planning and Implementation

Care of children and adolescents who abuse drugs, alcohol, and other substances is challenging and often frustrating. Long-term mental health counseling may be necessary to resolve underlying issues and foster lifestyle and behavioral changes.

Prevention is the most desirable intervention. The nurse can play a major role in teaching children and their families about substance abuse. Education should begin in primary school, and continue with intensification during middle school and high school. Nurses also can play a major role in community education. Various prevention programs have been developed by federal and private organizations. Referral to support organizations may be beneficial for the child, parents, and other family members. Self-help groups, available in most communities, include Alcoholics Anonymous, Narcotics Anonymous, Al-Anon, Nar-Anon, and Ala-Teen. Parents may receive support from a group such as Parents Anonymous.

The youth's protective factors can be identified and used in planning appropriate interventions. For example, a child with goals for a future career can be helped to see how substance use will interfere with goal attainment. Identifying a strong role model through a program like Big Brothers or Big Sisters can assist children who lack that strength in their families.

The child who has begun to use and abuse drugs needs an intensive intervention program. Referral to a psychiatric health specialist is needed for diagnosis and intervention. Group programs and those that integrate the family are most effective. Find out what resources are present in your community to treat youth who are using alcohol or other drugs. Nurses are active in treatment programs as well as sustaining treatment effects and avoiding relapse during visits to community agencies once the youth returns to family, school, and other surroundings.

Evaluation

Expected outcomes of nursing interventions include abstention from alcohol and street drugs, successful participation in substance abuse programs, and developmentally appropriate social and cognitive skills.

Physical Inactivity and Sedentary Behavior

In the past few decades, children have become increasingly sedentary. This change is a reflection of lifestyles in which car travel is valued, computers and televisions are part of daily life, neighborhoods are sometimes unsafe places for play, and schools do not routinely require daily physical education classes (Figure 17–5). Children and adolescents spend an astounding amount of time with media (television, computers, games, and phone applications)—an average of 2 hours of television daily for those under 6 years, and 4 hours of television and an additional 2 hours of other media use daily for older youth (KidsHealth, 2014). Excessive screen time influences behavior because there is physical inactivity during viewing, a lack of social interaction and cognition, and a tendency to eat high-fat snacks with high caloric content. While screen time increases, physical activity decreases, with only 25% of youth engaged in the recommended moderate to vigorous physical activity for 60 minutes daily (Fakhouri et al., 2014).

Physical inactivity leads to many health concerns. A primary outcome is overweight or obesity (see Chapter 14 for a definition and further information on obesity). Other outcomes can be an increased rate of type 2 diabetes (see Chapter 30), increased exposure to television/computer game violence and sexual activity at early ages, and early progression of cardiovascular disease (see Chapter 21).

However, patterns of physical activity established in childhood can lead to increased exercise behaviors in adulthood, contributing to lower rates of low back pain, overweight, osteoporosis, heart disease, diabetes, colon cancer, and high blood pressure, and also lead to a more positive self-image.

Although many children demonstrate low levels of physical activity, a profound decrease in vigorous activity is common in grades 9 through 12. Boys more commonly participate in team sports than girls. Although about 48% of students attend physical education (PE) classes at least once a week, only 29% have daily PE classes (CDC, 2014a).

Healthcare providers can integrate assessment of physical activity into all health care, and make recommendations to children and families that will help to increase opportunities for physical activity. Nurses can assess height, weight, and body mass index (BMI) to look for signs of overweight (see Chapter 14). Children should be asked about how they like to spend free time. Community and school activities should be encouraged and rewarded. Examples include fun runs, walks for benefit causes, aerobics classes, team sports, roadside cleanups, fairs, and carnivals. Help parents and children learn what they can do for physical fitness. Work with school physical education personnel to plan activities both in and out of physical education class that promote lifelong exercise routines. Work toward the goal of 60 minutes of daily moderate intensity physical activity for all children (CDC, 2014a). During health promotion visits, help children identify ways to gradually increase physical activity and decrease sedentary time.

Injury and Protective Equipment

In the discussion of causes of childhood and adolescent morbidities and mortalities in Chapter 1, unintentional injuries are listed as a common problem. In fact, a majority of deaths from age 10 years onward result from four causes: motor vehicle crashes, other unintentional injury, homicide, and suicide (National Center for Health Statistics & National Vital Statistics System, 2012). Chapters 7, 8, and 9 discuss the frequent injuries seen in children at different developmental ages, and safety precautions to avoid injuries from car crashes, falls, poisonings, and other developmentally related injuries. Many common injuries are preventable with simple use of protective gear and following of safety guidelines (Figure 17–6). Some sports and activities that require safety gear include rollerblading, skateboarding, roller hockey, ice hockey, football, soccer, baseball, scooters, all-terrain vehicles, and skiing or snowboarding fast or using jumps.

Over 8% of youth rarely or never wear car safety belts in automobiles; 22% have recently ridden with someone who had been drinking alcohol (CDC, 2014a). Emphasize safe automobile

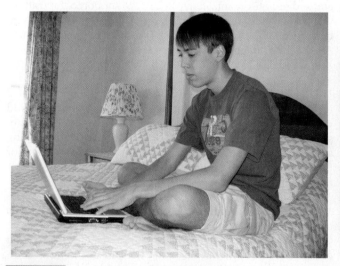
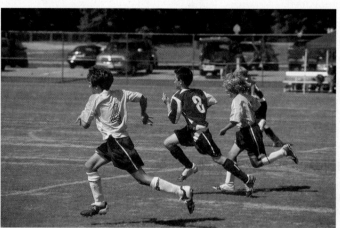

Figure 17–5 **Role of sports in development. Physical inactivity is a growing problem among children and can contribute to poor health. It is important to balance sedentary activities, such as playing computer games, with physical and social activities. Sports are an excellent way for children to develop their psychosocial, cognitive, and motor skills.**

SOURCE: Soccer photo courtesy of Robert Young/Fotolia.

Families Want to Know

Physical Activity Guidelines for Youth

- Engage in moderate to vigorous physical activity (such as bike riding, walking, baseball, and rollerblading) for at least 60 minutes daily.
- Engage in vigorous activity that causes sweating and hard breathing (such as soccer, running, and ice hockey) at least 3 times weekly.
- Engage in muscle strengthening activity at least 3 times weekly.
- Engage in bone strengthening activity at least 3 times weekly.
- Encourage schools to offer physical education to all students, and have students sign up when this is an elective.
- Encourage walking and bike riding to friends' homes and stores whenever safe.
- Plan physical activities together as a family.
- Get a pet and plan to walk the pet together daily.
- Limit television and other similar sedentary activities to no more than 2 hours daily.
- On days home, allow the child to watch television for up to 1 hour, and then insist on 1 hour of reading, 1 hour of physical activity, and 1 hour of socializing with others before returning to more television.

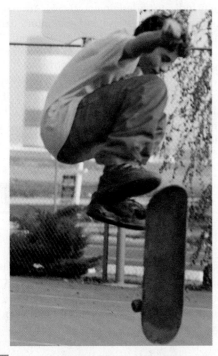

Figure 17–6 Use of protective gear. What protective gear should children use for skateboarding? How would you convince them to use the protection?

and motorcycle behaviors in adolescence, with the recognition that risks increase if driving is combined with use of alcohol and controlled substances. Adolescents sometimes engage in practices that put them at particular risk, and nurses should be alert for such activities in their communities. Examples include car surfing (standing on the trunk, hood, or roof of a moving vehicle), street racing (racing cars down a street at extremely high speed), or "extreme" sports.

About 44 million U.S. children ride bicycles, a beneficial physical activity. However, only about 12% are protected by helmet use, even though bicycling is the most common activity associated with injury (CDC, 2014a). Strategies to make helmet use more attractive to children and adolescents are needed. Nurses can play a major role in programs to educate and reward children for helmet use, and can assist families to find affordable helmets.

Nurses can be active in identifying behaviors in youths in specific communities and working with schools and other community groups to support legislation for helmet use, evaluate proper fits of helmets, and work to locate sources for incentives and low-cost helmets. Efforts should also include adequate conditioning for sports, proper treatment of injuries, and prevention of overuse injuries.

A growing number of children engage in "extreme" sports—those that carry a high degree of risk and have not traditionally been common. Some examples are mountain biking, skateboarding with ramps, motocross racing, three-wheeling, ski racing, snowboarding through trees and on courses with pikes and other challenges, ice climbing, rock climbing, and wakeboarding. While the nurse is probably unable to dissuade youth from engaging in these activities, safety measures should be emphasized. Find out what protective gear the youth wears and what is recommended. Provide examples of stories of youth who have been saved by use of such gear. Encourage the youth to engage in sports activities only when others are present and to have a plan for emergencies, including a working cell phone, leaving information with an adult about plans and expected return, and planning for harsh weather with items such as emergency blankets, gear, and food. Encourage the youth to talk with parents and other adults about the risks and responsibilities of the activities.

Developing Cultural Competence Ethnic Disparity in Unintentional Childhood Injuries

Although the unintentional injury rate in children under age 19 declined 39% from 1987 to 2013, striking ethnic disparity rates exist in the rates of unintentional injury among children. These differences are mainly due to living in impoverished communities rather than any innate biologic variations. The rate of death from unintentional injury ranges from 23.8/100,000 in American Indian/Alaska Native, to 12.8 among African Americans, 11.5 among Whites, and 8.8/100,000 in Hispanics (CDC, 2012a). What are the major causes of unintentional injury in your community and state? What ethnic and age groups are at greatest risk? How can you integrate teaching in your practice that is specific to the findings in your community?

Body Art

Body art in the form of painting, tattooing, and piercing has been used by humans throughout history. In recent years, there has been a resurgence of interest in this decorative art among teens. Many adolescents have multiple body piercings and tattoos, and they may even resort to performing these decorations on themselves or friends.

Approximately 21% of adolescents and young adults have tattoos, and even more have at least one body piercing (Owen, Armstrong, Koch, et al., 2013). In some states, teens must be 18 years of age or have parental permission to obtain body art, but students often report that it is easy to have an adult present who signs and claims to be a parent. Amy, described at the opening of this chapter, had her piercing done by a friend. In some states, tattoo and body piercing businesses must be licensed and comply with certain regulations; other states have no regulations. Amy demonstrates some common characteristics of teens who choose to use body art. It may be seen as a way to establish individualism and independence, and it may help some teens to feel part of a peer group. Multiple tattoos and piercings are common, as is the case with Amy (Figure 17–7).

Body art is a common source of infections with skin pathogens. Infections can range from mild inflammatory reactions to bacterial and viral infections and serious long-term infections. Body piercing is a major method of transmission of hepatitis C, a disease that may not be manifested until years later (see Chapter 25). It can be a source of HIV if proper techniques are not followed. Serious systemic infections such as endocarditis have occurred after some piercings. Piercings in parts of the body such as the mouth or navel are most prone to bacterial infection and continued redness and irritation. The pierced site may not appear infected, but transfer of organisms can lead to serious infection and heart damage. Examples of serious infective agents include *Neisseria, Mycobacterium, Staphylococcus, Pseudomonas, Streptococcus, hepatitis B,* and *hepatitis C* (Juhas & English, 2013). A number of cases of *Mycobacterium chelone* skin infection from contaminated ink were identified across the country in 2012 (CDC, 2012b). When noting signs of systemic infection such as fever, weakness, malaise, and arthralgia (see Chapter 21 for full discussion of endocarditis), gather history about body piercings and refer for care to the primary healthcare provider. Pierced tongues can lead to chipped teeth or even be the cause of choking if the piercing is dislodged from the site.

Another issue that teens should consider is the relationship of the tattoos to future lifestyle changes. Advise teens to avoid tattooing the name of a person or musical group since relationships change and tastes in music evolve. Be sure they know the meaning of phrases, foreign words, or Asian symbols. Consider the visibility of the tattoo and its effect on future employment. Tattoos on the face, neck, or other readily visible places may be a detriment during employment interviews. Tattoos should always be considered permanent. Methods for removal may be costly, painful, and unsuccessful.

Another form of body art that is regarded as disfigurement is *deliberate self-harm* or *nonsuicidal self-injury.* One example is *branding,* or scarification, whereby the skin is burned to result in a scar. Commonly a desired sign, symbol, or word is inscribed. Results are usually not precise and do not adhere to expected designs. This procedure is done on the self or friend, using common household metal implements heated in fires or stoves. Others cut themselves in the form of a desired design, a process called *cutting.* This type of self-harm or self-injury is performed with razor blades, knives, scissors, broken glass, needles, or sharp pencils. These practices can result in infection, often do not yield the desired result, and may indicate underlying problems. Adolescent screenings should ask about cutting or intentional injury to skin. Using a nonjudgmental attitude, the youth involved should be referred for further assessment by primary care providers or counselors (Catledge, Scharer, & Fuller, 2012; Smith, 2011).

Because teens may choose to obtain body art even if parents object and even when there are state laws to prohibit or make it difficult to do so, nursing care must focus on providing information for the teen, assessing sites, identifying infections, and referring if needed. Care is almost always provided in community settings such as clinics or schools. Consider asking teens if they are thinking about body art since they often do not seek advice before obtaining the body art and may not get adequate teaching.

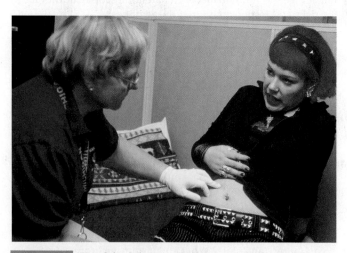

Figure 17–7   **Health risks to adolescents. Talk openly with adolescents about their health and teach them to avoid health risks connected with tattoos and piercing.**

Clinical Reasoning   The Adolescent With Body Piercings

Amy is 15 years old and attends an alternative high school. She recently had an ear piercing and it is painful. She comes to the health room to ask the advice of the school nurse. The area around the piercing is inflamed and mildly edematous. After asking some questions, the nurse learns that Amy's ear was pierced by a friend, using a needle that had been "sterilized" by passing it through a match flame. She has had a slight fever, but otherwise feels fine.

In her home state, adolescents under 18 years of age must have the signature of a parent for body piercings and tattoos, so Amy chose to have the procedure done by a friend. She believes this is safe since her friend has done many piercings on others. She admits that her parents are not very pleased with her body art, but that they allow her to do it as long as she agrees to stay in high school. She had previously run away and spent several weeks living on the streets.

- What healthcare and social needs does Amy have?
- How can you support both Amy and her parents?
- What physical care does Amy need to treat potential infection at her piercing site?
- What systemic infectious diseases is Amy at risk of acquiring due to repeated body piercings using an unsterile technique?

Families Want to Know

Care for Tattoos and Body Piercings

Before the Procedure

- Does the studio look clean?
- Visit several studios to make comparisons of techniques, quality, and cleanliness.
- Ask to watch a tattoo or piercing done on someone else.
- What are the artist's sterilization and hygiene practices?
- Is the artist licensed? Trained?
- Look at pictures of completed art and talk with former clients.
- Insist that new, sterile equipment be opened in front of the person to be decorated.
- Consider if this permanent body decoration is desired for a lifetime.
- Consider what the tattoo or piercing will look like in several years.
- Consider the possible side effects such as infection, future dislike for the art, and allergy to dyes or metals.
- Be sure that hepatitis B vaccination is completed before the procedure.
- Be aware that no immunization is available to protect against the health risks of hepatitis C and HIV.

Care After the Procedure

- Touch the area only after carefully washing your hands.
- Keep the area elevated and use ice for the first 2 days to minimize swelling.
- Avoid contact with another person's body fluids until well healed.
- Turn the piercing jewelry gently several times daily using washed hands.
- Use antibacterial mouthwash or cleaner or ointment as recommended.
- Avoid pressure and rubbing on the site (such as belts on navel piercings).
- Watch carefully for signs of infection and report them to a healthcare provider:
  - Increased redness
  - Swelling
  - Pain
  - Hot feeling
  - Discharge
- Ask the artist how long healing will take. It varies from 2 months in the mouth or up to 6 or 8 months for a navel.
- Metal is dangerous during some medical procedures such as magnetic resonance imaging (MRI) or during surgery. Be sure to tell doctors and nurses about your piercings when you are hospitalized or receiving medical care, especially if they are in a part of the body not readily visible.
- If you decide to remove a piece of jewelry soon after it is placed, the skin may heal with only a slight scar.

Sexual Orientation

Adolescence is a time of identifying emerging sexuality. Most teens establish relationships with members of the opposite sex and learn how to interact in ways guided by their peer group, family, and culture. For some youth, the transition into adult sexuality can be more challenging if they feel an emotional and sexual attraction to people of the same sex (**homosexuality**). The term **gay** is often used for homosexual males and **lesbian** for homosexual females. Other youth are **bisexual**, or attracted to both men and women, and some are **transgendered**, or attracted to dress and act like members of the opposite sex. The abbreviation LGBT is sometimes used to refer to lesbian, gay, bisexual, or transgendered, and LGBT/Q indicates those who are questioning their sexual orientation. About 5% to 12% of persons report an experience with someone of the same sex, and about 3% identify as being LGBT/Q (Chandra, Mosher, Copen, et al., 2011). Data on youth are not often reported; however, the National Survey of Family Growth reports that about 90% of adolescents and young adults report that they are heterosexual, with the remainder reporting that they are homosexual,

bisexual, or not sure (Sexuality Information and Education Council of the United States, n.d.).

Sexual attractions and practices different than the mainstream are not deviant nor symptomatic of a mental disorder but should be viewed as part of a continuum of sexual expression. No known gene, early life experience, or other event causes homosexuality (American Psychiatric Association, 2012).

LGBT/Q youth are at risk for a variety of problems related to emotional and physical health. These include rejection by family members and peers, verbal harassment, sexual abuse and physical assault, a high rate of suicide, substance abuse, a high rate of homelessness, and sexual risks of HIV and other sexually transmitted infections. Their health risks need to be identified and appropriate care provided in welcoming and nonjudgmental healthcare facilities.

Nurses can provide health care for LGBT/Q youth in a variety of settings. School nurses and clinics can display a sign to demonstrate that they are accepting of persons with minority sexual orientation. These signs are rainbows or triangles with several colors shown and can be obtained from local gay or lesbian community groups. Terminology in assessment should be gender free. Ask "Do you have one or more sexual partners?" rather than "Do you have a boyfriend?" When youth identify as LGBT/Q, provide usual care of all kinds. This includes preventive care such as immunizations, sports assessments, and injury prevention teaching. Be alert that youth may have additional health challenges. Ask about peer and parental support; refer to support groups if needed. Provide resources for homelessness and when the teen is depressed or suicidal (see Chapter 28). Perform testing for sexually transmitted infections if the teen is having sexual contact, and teach preventive measures. Foster a positive sense of self-esteem through encouraging positive activities such as sports, music, and friendships with peers.

Effects of Violence

Violence is a threatened or actual use of physical force or power that leads to actual or potential physical or emotional trauma. Violence can be directed at oneself, another person, or against a group or community. Violence can result in injury, death, psychologic harm, disruption of development, or deprivation (Child Trends, 2015). In the past several years, adults and children alike have been shocked by violent episodes in schools. Although these incidents had much media coverage, they are just one type of violence to which children may be regularly exposed. Children can be the recipients of violence during child abuse and homicides, and they themselves can perform acts of violence on others. They may be touched by violence when parents, siblings, or other family members are killed in gang conflicts, in terrorist attacks, or in wars. The effects of violence are far reaching and ongoing; they permeate the victim's entire lifetime. This section explores some types of violence affecting children.

Schools and Communities

At a time when firearm deaths are decreasing overall, unintentional deaths and suicides have increased among children. Many of these deaths are committed with firearms found in the home. Over 4000 youth from 10 to 19 years old die from firearm homicides annually, and another approximately 15,000 die from firearm suicide. Firearm homicide is the second leading cause of injury death for youth, and firearm suicide is the fifth leading cause of injury death for youth (CDC, 2011b). Forty percent of households with children have guns (2 million children live in these homes), and in many of those homes, the firearms are stored loaded or are not secured under lock. Parents often report that children do not know firearm locations when 39% of the children are actually able to state the locations and 22% have handled the guns (Children's Defense Fund, 2014).

Homicide in children has gained attention in the past several years because of several shootings at schools, universities, and other community sites. While homicide is an extreme example, there are other types of violence. Children report being threatened verbally and with guns or knives at home, in schools, and in their neighborhoods. They may be beaten up or bullied or harassed. An estimated 3 to 10 million children are exposed to acts of domestic violence by adults in their homes. They may be subjected to dangerous situations in their neighborhoods or during times of homelessness. Date rape or other sexual violence is reported by up to 10% of teens (CDC, 2014a).

SAFETY ALERT!
When a group of children is attacked or killed in a school shooting, this tragic occurrence has the attention of the media. The tragedy of violence involving children occurs somewhere in the United States daily. A firearm kills about seven children every day in the United States, or about 50 per week. An additional 200 to 300 children suffer from nonfatal firearm injuries (Children's Defense Fund, 2014). Nurses must intervene in this national tragedy. Become familiar with firearm injury statistics in your community. Teach families, children, and youth about the dangers of firearms. Urge safe storage. Help schools establish programs to ensure safety for students.

Internationally, millions of children experience violence annually, and decreasing violence against children has become a focus of the World Health Organization and the United Nations (World Health Organization, 2014). Common forms of violence worldwide are war and terrorism. War affects children in several ways: Parents leave home to fight in wars; children may be forced to take on adult roles in families when parents leave; children become orphans when parents are killed; children may be raped, sexually trafficked, or forced to be sex slaves; and some children are trained and forced to fight in battles, carry messages, or otherwise engage in combat themselves. Children who live through wars or have a parent or sibling die in war can be permanently affected by these events. Depression and other mental health problems are common in youth who have experienced war.

Natural disasters and terrorism also take a large toll on the mental health of children and adolescents. Most children and adolescents who live through terrorism experience profound sadness, cling to adults who provide security, and have a variety of somatic complaints. Interventions should be directed at different phases of violence, such as preevent preparation (emergency preparation and training) and postevent activity (offering special services and resources).

Several resources have been developed to help families and healthcare professionals help children deal with war and violence. See the resources at the National Center for Children Exposed to Violence, Society of Pediatric Nurses, and American Academy of Child and Adolescent Psychiatry websites.

Bullying

One type of violence that frequently occurs in schools is **bullying**, or aggressive behavior that is intended to cause harm, exists in a relationship with imbalance of power, and occurs repeatedly. Bullies are aggressive, impulsive, and need to dominate others. Bullying behaviors include verbal abuse (taunting, teasing), name calling, threats, spreading rumors, social exclusion, and physical abuse (hitting, shoving, kicking, tripping). About 20% of children suffer bullying at school each year, and about 5% did not go to school at least 1 day in the previous month because of safety concerns due to bullying (CDC, 2014a). Although bullying is most commonly reported in schools, it can occur in neighborhoods as children go to and from school, on school buses, on sports teams, and in other settings.

Bullying can also occur through the Internet and is reported by 20% (with a range of 9% to 40% in various studies) of young people (Cyberbullying Research Center, 2011; Schneider, O'Donnell, Stueve, et al., 2012). **Cyberbullying** occurs when a child or adolescent is targeted by another via an Internet posting or other digital technology and threatened, tormented, harassed, humiliated, or embarrassed. Personal information may be disclosed or fabricated, persons are excluded, offensive messages are sent, or harmful messages are sent out under the target person's name. Such attacks are socially aggressive and often anonymous.

Bullies themselves are at risk and are more likely than other youth to abuse substances, be depressed, and carry weapons to school, putting other children at risk. Bullying is associated with future delinquent behavior, depression, low self-esteem, loneliness, suicidal ideation, and suicide attempts (Tsitsika et al., 2014).

Children who are bullied are more commonly socially isolated and anxious. Health problems such as migraines, stomach pains, suicidal thoughts, and other problems can result. Academic performance commonly deteriorates and rates of school absenteeism increase (American Academy of Pediatrics, 2011). Realizing the serious effects of such behaviors, a number of states have now passed legislation that reiterates the rights of all children to attend school in a safe and peaceful manner. Some state education departments mandate school district programs for students about bullying, and clear school policies about dealing with the behavior. See the Health Resources and Services Administration (HRSA) Maternal and Child Health Bureau website at www.stopbullyingnow.hrsa.gov.

Nurses can be active in setting up school policies about bullying and integrating assessment and interventions related to bullying into health promotion visits. School programs should:

- Inform all students that bullying is not tolerated.
- Train teachers and other personnel about signs of bullying.
- Ensure adult supervision in hallways and on playgrounds, sites where bullying is most common.
- Teach children to promptly report bullying that is experienced or observed.
- Set up peer support for those who are bullied.
- Arrange therapeutic treatment through school counselors and other resources for those who bully; involve parents in the treatment plan.
- Measure incidence of bullying, monitor outcomes of policies, and use data to evaluate policies in schools.

Nurses who are in clinics, offices, and other health promotion settings can:

- Be alert for children with behavior changes (irritability, anxiety, poor self-concept).
- Consider bullying as a potential cause when fear or refusal to attend school is reported by child or parents.
- Ask questions during visits, such as "Have you ever been afraid to go to school?," "What are the best and worst things about going to your school?," and "What are the other kids in your neighborhood like?"
- Ask parents what they have done about any situations identified. Partner with the parent to act as liaison to the school or other agency.
- Refer identified bullies and victims of bullying to mental health specialists.

Incarceration

A growing number of children are entering the judicial system, and many are admitted at young ages. About 3.4% of youth in the United States are incarcerated at any given time (Annie E. Casey Foundation, 2011). Children in detention, courts, and other facilities have frequently been victims as well as perpetrators of violence. They often have multiple risks such as substance abuse, early sexual activity, multiple sexual partners, sexual abuse, lack of a healthcare home, and mental health problems. The incarceration facility itself may subject youth to additional violence, abuse, and other maltreatment (Annie E. Casey Foundation, 2011). Nurses work within the juvenile justice system to provide episodic care for children or to partner with others to establish health-related programs within facilities. Youth who are incarcerated need the following:

- Basic physical care such as immunizations, vision, and hearing screening
- Nutrition assessment and teaching
- Skin assessment and hygiene practice teaching
- Information about sexuality, sexual practices, and sexually transmitted infections
- Assessment for substance abuse
- Teaching about hazards of substance use and assistance with quitting
- Mental health services
- Developmental assessment
- Individualized education plans to meet cognitive needs

Hazing

Hazing is an activity that is forced on an individual, causes humiliation, and is required for membership in an organization or group. It can sometimes be harmful and even lead to death. Sports teams, music groups, and Greek sororities and fraternities are examples of groups commonly associated with hazing. Activities might include removing clothes, drinking large amounts of alcohol, using snuff or other substances, being locked in small places, being beaten, and many other behaviors. In spite of its common practice, many students do not know what to do about hazing practices; coaches or other adult leaders may or may not be aware of hazing practices. Youth often believe that they must experience and uphold the traditions of hazing to belong to their group (Allan & Madden, 2011). Ask during health visits if the student has ever had to do something to belong to a group or team. Ask about "scary" things others have had them do. Assist schools and colleges in setting up antihazing policies. Encourage students to report hazing. Be aware of the possibility of hazing when seeing children with traumatic injuries (Hazing Prevention, 2011).

Domestic Violence

Domestic violence occurs between members of a family. The specific type of violence known as *intimate partner abuse* occurs between adult partners in the family. It may involve the parents of a child, or one parent and a significant other. This type of abuse injures the child or adolescent because it is traumatic to witness a close family member or loved one become the recipient of violence. About 3.3 million children annually in the United States are exposed to violence against their mothers or other female care providers; children who live in homes where intimate partner abuse occurs are significantly more likely to be abused themselves (Cross, Matthews, Tonmyr, et al., 2012; Davidov, Nadorff, Jack, et al., 2012). Children may also be the direct victims of domestic violence in a family. See the section on child abuse later in this chapter.

Dating Violence

Dating violence is another type of intimate partner abuse; this type occurs in relationships among youth. Over 10% of adolescent males and females report being victims of dating violence (CDC, 2014a). Such behaviors include being hit, slammed into something, or intentionally injured with an object or weapon. Girls who reported dating violence were also more likely to report other risk behaviors, such as feeling sad, having attempted suicide, or having used substances such as tobacco and drugs. Early sexual activity, having a higher number of sex partners, and being less likely to use birth control are also associated with a higher incidence of dating violence. A risk profile with a cluster of potentially dangerous behaviors may therefore put adolescents more at risk for dating violence.

Date rape is a term used when dating violence takes the form of rape. This can be particularly harmful to females who often do not want to share the event or press charges against the attacker.

Nurses should screen for violence at each health promotion visit, including gynecologic visits and prenatal care. Ask what is going well and not going well in intimate relationships, and whether the person ever feels unsafe or is forced to do things she does not wish to do. Recognize that while not as common, males may even be victims of violence in close relationships. Recognize that alcohol and other drugs are often connected with violence in relationships so ask about their use. Organize peer discussion groups about intimacy in order to help youth develop a sense of self-confidence and self-efficacy that will empower them to refuse participation in activities in which they do not wish to engage.

Nursing Management

Violence

Nursing Assessment and Diagnosis

Nurses are in key positions to identify children at risk of being recipients and victims of violence. The ecologic framework can be used to assess children. Some questions that can be asked are listed in Table 17–6. It is important to detect both the risks that lead to vulnerability and the protective factors that can promote resilience and safety. (Refer to Chapter 4 for explanations of these factors and the systems that influence the child.) Adapt questions to each age group and insert them in every healthcare encounter.

Nursing care for violence is discussed in the *Nursing Care Plan*. The following nursing diagnoses may be appropriate (NANDA-I © 2014):

* *Violence: Self-Directed, Risk for,* related to history of violence
* *Self-Esteem, Chronic Low,* related to history of abuse
* *Family Processes, Dysfunctional,* related to situational crises
* *Development: Delayed, Risk for,* related to environmental deficiencies

Planning and Implementation

Prevention is an important role for the nurse. Interventions such as providing resources for family planning; teaching self-regulation/control techniques; and applying technology such as kiosks in health centers, virtual training for healthcare providers, and

TABLE 17–6 Assessment Questions to Identify Violence Risk and Protective Factors

MICROSYSTEM

* Have you been hurt by your parents or anyone else at home?
* When was the last time you were made fun of or bullied at school? What did you do?
* Have you ever brought a gun or knife or other weapon to school?
* Do you have access to guns and knives at home? At friends' houses?
* What stresses are there in your family now?
* Tell me about school—what you like and don't like.

MESOSYSTEM

* Do your parents attend school meetings? Talk with your teachers?
* Do you participate in any church, synagogue, or mosque services?
* Do you participate in any community activities?

EXOSYSTEM

* What stresses do your parents have at work, in their families, with their health or finances?
* Do you feel like your school helps to keep you safe?
* Are there plans for handling violent episodes at your school if they were to occur?
* Do you feel safe in your neighborhood?
* Where would you go or who would you call if you felt unsafe or were hurt and no one was at home?

positive media messages are all important measures in preventing violence (Child Trends 2015). Nurses intervene with individual children, with families, and in schools and communities to increase safety and decrease violence. Help children and families meet basic needs and access resources to assist with finances, respite care, domestic violence, and other issues. Education is a key element of intervention.

PROVIDING INFORMATION

Teach the family the dangers of firearms and the necessity for using gun locks and locked cabinets, storing guns unloaded, and storing guns and ammunition in separate places. Suggest alternative activities to minimize child exposure to violence in the media. Inform parents about rating systems for television and other media, and about lockout mechanisms for televisions and computers. Discuss the harmful effects of verbal and physical abuse to the child or other family members and explore alternatives.

Present the school-age child and adolescent with information about bullying and strategies for dealing with it. Provide school and community resources where the child can go if there are threats of any kind. Discuss date rape and violence with all teens and encourage them to report it.

COMMUNITY-BASED NURSING CARE

Both in schools and in community settings, nurses can plan peer mentoring to provide assistance to children at high risk of experiencing violence. Nurses can link and coordinate school and community programs for children to provide for parent involvement and child support. Discuss safety issues, both risk factors

Nursing Care Plan: The Child and Violent Behavior

1. Nursing Diagnosis: *Violence: Other-Directed, Risk for,* related to history of family violence (NANDA-I © 2014)

GOAL: The child will demonstrate impulse control.

INTERVENTION	RATIONALE
• Identify violent behaviors in the child.	• Violence in the child usually develops over time.
• Provide a safe place for exploration of feelings by referral to school or other counseling, support groups, and other resources.	• The child needs an opportunity to explore feelings and vulnerability.
• Provide strategies for managing anger and alternative ways for coping with problems.	• Coping strategies can be learned from others and can help in dealing with a stressful home situation.

EXPECTED OUTCOME: Child will express the ability to manage problems in acceptable ways.

GOAL: The child will be secure in a safe environment.

INTERVENTION	RATIONALE
• Perform a thorough assessment of hazards to the physical and emotional state in the child's home, neighborhood, and school.	• Hazards to physical and emotional health promote violence to and from the child.
• Institute actions that will result in removal of child from unsafe situations.	• Removal from family, community, or school may be needed to ensure child safety.
• Use community resources to provide respite care, teaching for families, and safety instructions for the child.	• Stress reduction measures may help to decrease violent behaviors.

EXPECTED OUTCOME: Child will express a sense of physical and emotional safety in daily life.

2. Nursing Diagnosis: *Injury, Risk for,* related to physical or psychologic conditions in the environment (NANDA-I © 2014)

GOAL: Risk for physical and emotional injury to the child is decreased.

INTERVENTION	RATIONALE
• Identify physical and psychologic factors that affect the child's safety.	• Multiple factors in the family can contribute to risk of violence and lack of safety for the child.
• Assist family to deal with issues such as mental status challenges, fatigue, financial concern, substance abuse, and lack of adequate childcare resources.	
• Instruct family on methods of keeping the child safe.	• Families need information about the impact of unsafe settings on the child and methods that can decrease risk of injury.

EXPECTED OUTCOME: Child will not be injured in physical or emotional ways in the home or other immediate settings.

3. Nursing Diagnosis: *Post-Trauma Syndrome* related to physical or psychosocial abuse (NANDA-I © 2014)

GOAL: The child will demonstrate abuse or violence recovery.

INTERVENTION	RATIONALE
• Assess the child's affect and behaviors.	• Disturbed child behaviors can demonstrate a sense of mistrust and insecurity.
• Evaluate social interactions and sense of trust in others.	
• Assist the child in identifying feelings and coping strategies by providing counseling, art therapy, and other strategies.	• Establishment of close interactions with others demonstrates reestablishment of a sense of trust.

EXPECTED OUTCOME: Child will identify feelings related to violent episode(s) and express healing of the self.

and protective actions, in schools and community groups. Report children who are at risk. Work to establish extended programs for children so that they are safe after school. Help children learn behaviors that will help them be safe in their communities and at home. Teach positive problem-solving and conflict-management techniques to children and parents.

Youth with special needs are a special concern of nurses. Jails and detention centers often have a nurse who visits youth on a regular basis or when health problems occur. Health teaching may be provided in some facilities. Halfway houses and homeless shelters are examples of settings where violence prevention and intervention can occur with youth. Mental health centers and other programs have nurses that work with children who are victims of violence (for example, have witnessed domestic violence, have witnessed or had a family member murdered, have been abused at home or school) or perpetrators of violence. See Chapter 28 for a discussion of posttraumatic stress disorder and its effects on the child and adolescent.

Partner with families to assist them in talking to children about war and terrorism. Recognize that youth who have experienced such events themselves are more at risk for mental health disruptions with future events. Answer questions from children honestly but reassure them that many people are trying to make the situation safe. Other suggestions for parents include the following:

- Limit television viewing and other media exposure because of its constant replaying of the events of terrorism or war. Preschoolers may think the events continue to happen, rather than being a one-time occurrence. Watch with children and talk with them about what is happening.
- Continue with structured family events such as meals, recreation, and faith-based activities. Spend time with your child.
- Take cues from the child about how much to discuss. Use words the child or adolescent can understand.
- Partner with the school so teachers know what parents have discussed and parents are aware of how events are discussed at school.
- If youth decide to become active by writing letters or joining campaigns, allow them to participate in this way.
- Be alert for regression in behavior, sleep and eating problems, or other indications of stress. Consider talking with the healthcare provider or a counselor in such situations.
- Expect that even after the child has adjusted, there may be delayed reactions. Anniversaries of events, holidays, and birthdays often bring renewed pain and sadness.
- Realize that adults must care for themselves, obtain stress relief, and talk with others in order to have strength and resources available for children.

Evaluation

The expected outcomes of nursing care for violence prevention include a decrease in incidents of homicides, firearm injuries, abuse, date rape, and other violence among children. Additional outcomes are establishment of programs to decrease violence, and verbalization by all children of what to do if violence occurs and how to solve problems without becoming violent.

Child Abuse

One of the most common types of violence against children is child abuse. Children from all socioeconomic groups and both genders are victims of abuse. This type of violence can have implications for both the physical and mental health of children, and can influence their health status even long after the abuse has occurred. Awareness of the problem of child abuse is increasing. More cases are being reported; however, these are probably only a small percentage of the total.

There are 3.4 million reports of abuse and neglect annually, with 78% of them due to neglect, 18% related to physical abuse, 9% to sexual abuse, and 11% to other types of abuse; about 1640 children die annually (5 children daily) from abuse (CDC, 2014b; Childhelp, 2013). Infants have the highest rate of abuse (21.9 per 1000 children,) with decreasing rates as children get older. Twenty-seven percent of victims are under 3 years of age, and 20% are 3 to 5 years old (CDC, 2014b).

Physical abuse is only one part of a larger problem. The definition of child abuse has expanded during the past decades and includes physical neglect, emotional abuse and neglect, verbal abuse, and sexual abuse, as well as physical abuse. Abuse generally involves an act of commission—that is, actively doing something to a child physically, emotionally, or sexually, such as hitting, belittling, or molesting. Neglect more often involves an act of omission, such as not providing adequate nutrition, emotional contact, or necessary physical care, or abandoning a child. Because the evidence is often not visible, emotional abuse and neglect are more difficult to identify and prove than physical abuse or neglect. Risk factors for abuse and neglect are listed in Table 17–7.

Physical Abuse

Physical abuse is the deliberate maltreatment of another individual that inflicts pain or injury and may result in permanent or temporary disfigurement or even death. Common methods of physical abuse in children are listed in Table 17–8.

TABLE 17–7 Risk Factors for Child Abuse and Neglect

FACTORS INCREASING RISK FOR PHYSICAL ABUSE
Poverty
Violence in the family
Prematurity or low birth weight
Unrelated male primary caretaker
Parents who were abused as children
Age less than 3 years
Child disability or condition that requires a great deal of care (e.g., intellectual disability, attention deficit hyperactivity disorder)
Parental substance abuse or social isolation

FACTORS INCREASING RISK FOR SEXUAL ABUSE
Absence of natural father or having a stepfather
Being female
Mother's employment outside the home
Poor relationship with parent
Parental relationship characterized by conflict
Parental substance abuse or social isolation

TABLE 17–8 Methods of Physical Abuse in Children

Hitting, slapping, kicking, or punching

Whipping with belts, shoes, or electrical cords (**A**)

Inflicting burns with a lit cigarette or lighter (**B**)

Immersing child or body part in scalding water (commonly legs, perineal area, hands, or feet; see Figure 31–16)

Shaking the child violently ("shaken child" syndrome)

Tying the child to a fence, bed, tree, or other object

Throwing the child against a wall, down stairs, or against a window

Choking or gagging the child

Fracturing the legs, arms, ribs, or skull

Deliberately administering excessive doses of prescribed or non-prescribed drugs

Deliberately withholding prescribed medication

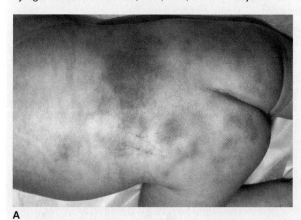

A

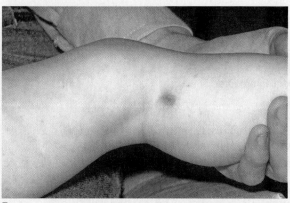

B

SOURCE: *A*, BioPhoto Associates/Science Source; *B*, Mediscan/Alamy.

Physical Neglect

Physical neglect is the deliberate withholding of or failure to provide the necessary and available resources to the child. Behaviors constituting physical neglect include failure to provide for the following basic needs: supervision appropriate for child's age, adequate nutrition and hydration, hygiene (e.g., clean diapers and clothes, bathing and toileting facilities), shelter (e.g., warmth in winter), and appropriate health care (e.g., immunizations, dental care, medications, eyeglasses).

Abandoned Babies

There are no accurate statistics on numbers of babies that are abandoned in dumpsters, on doorsteps, and in other locations. This tragedy has been addressed by Safe Haven laws in some states that allow women to drop unwanted babies at certain locations such as hospitals and fire stations without legal recrimination. In spite of these laws, babies continue to be abandoned, perhaps because mothers do not know about the laws or because they do not believe they will not be found guilty. Young teen mothers may not want others to know they had a baby. In addition, placement of these babies in adoptive homes is difficult because of paternity suits. Nurses should know their state's Safe Haven law details. Inform adolescents and young women about the law and post information in community sites frequented by women. Partner with young pregnant women to link them to resources such as adoption agencies when they might not want to keep a baby.

Emotional Abuse

Emotional abuse usually involves shaming, ridiculing, embarrassing, or insulting the child. It can also include the destruction of a child's personal property, such as tearing up the child's favorite family photographs or letters or harming, killing, or giving away the child's pet. These actions are frequently used as a means of frightening or controlling the child.

Verbal abuse is a common method of emotional abuse. Words can be a violent and volatile weapon against a child, eroding the child's fragile sense of self and destroying self-esteem. Common examples of verbal abuse include yelling obscenities at the child, calling the child names, threatening to "put the child away" or to give away or kill the child's pet, telling the child "I wish you were never born" or "You're worthless," and using words to humiliate, shame, or degrade the child.

Emotional Neglect

Emotional neglect is characterized by the caretaker's emotional unavailability to the child. The usual style of interaction is cold and lacking in sensitive personal attention. The child suffers from a lack of nurturance and failure of the parent or caretaker to meet basic dependency needs. An example of emotional neglect is the parent who is mentally ill, or abusing alcohol or other substances, and cannot respond adequately to the child's developmental needs.

Sexual Abuse

Child sexual abuse is the exploitation of a child for the sexual gratification of an adult. About 1.2 per 1000 children (almost 100,000) children in the United States are sexually abused each year. Approximately 10% of schoolchildren report that they have been sexually abused. Many children who are sexually abused are under the age of 5 years, some as young as 3 months. The perpetrator is often the parent, stepparent, or someone else known to the child such as a friend, neighbor, or babysitter. Methods of sexual abuse may be sexual acts, allowing others to commit sexual abuse, threats, exploitation via video or other means, and a variety of other actions (Childhelp, 2013; National Center for PTSD, 2011). Use of the word *child* in relation to sexual abuse and molestation refers to anyone who has not reached the age of consent, even if a teenager. **Incest** is sexual activity between close family members, so that marriage would be legally or culturally prohibited. Abusers often threaten to harm or kill the child or another family member if the child discloses the abuse. Some abusers are pedophiles, people who have sexual impulses toward preadolescent children. The pedophile is at least 16 years of age and is at least 5 years older than the victim, and the victim is 13 years of age or younger. Another form of sexual abuse is *exhibitionism*, or obtaining sexual arousal by exposing one's genitals to a stranger. Some children are victims of prostitution, forced to offer themselves for money or the pleasures of others, either in person or through videos and Internet sources.

Clinical Tip

Following are common forms of sexual abuse:

- Oral–genital contact
- Fondling and caressing the genitals
- Anal intercourse/sodomy
- Sexual intercourse
- Rape
- Prostitution
- Forced viewing of or participation in pornography such as sexually explicit or nude photographs
- Encouraging nude photos or sexual activity via Internet or video

ETIOLOGY AND PATHOPHYSIOLOGY

Regardless of the type of abuse, the most common abuser is the child's parent or guardian or a male friend of the child's mother. Substance abuse is a major contributor to the problem, with one half of cases related to parental alcohol or drug abuse (Childhelp, 2013). Risk factors associated with abusive behavior in adults include the following:

- Psychopathology, such as drug addiction or alcoholism, low self-esteem, poor impulse control, and other personality disorders
- Poor parenting experiences, such as abuse in the abuser's own childhood, rejection by the abuser's own parent(s), lack of knowledge of alternative methods of discipline, strong belief in or family tradition of harsh discipline, and lack of parental affection
- Marital stressors and problems with partners, such as hostile-dependent, abusive, or nonsupportive relationships, and one-sided decision making
- Environmental stressors, such as legal, financial, medical, or housing problems
- Social isolation, such as few friends and limited use of sitters, family, or other resources
- Inappropriate expectations for the developmental level of the child

CLINICAL MANIFESTATIONS

See Table 17–9 for clinical manifestations of physical abuse in children and adolescents. Behaviors inconsistent with developmental stage may be apparent. For example, the toddler or preschool child may be indiscriminately friendly with unfamiliar adults, including healthcare providers, rather than demonstrating shyness or anxiety. For the infant or young child with shaken baby syndrome or shaken child syndrome, the symptoms are those of central nervous system injury from repeated coup and contrecoup injury (see Chapter 27). These may include vomiting, irritability, fatigue, poor feeding, bradycardia, apnea, enlarged fontanelle, and seizures. Bruises are usually not present, but

TABLE 17–9 Clinical Manifestations of Physical Abuse in Children and Adolescents

- Multiple bruises in various stages of healing
- Scald burns with clear lines of demarcation and in a glove or stocking distribution (see Figure 31–16)
- Rope, belt, or cord marks, usually seen on the mouth, buttocks, back, legs, and arms (see Figure A in Table 17–8)
- Burn scars in various stages of healing
- Multiple fractures in various stages of healing, spiral fractures not explained by accident
- Shortness of breath and distress upon being moved, indicating chest contusions and possible rib fractures
- Sedation from overmedication
- Exacerbation of chronic illness (such as diabetes or asthma) because of withholding of medication
- Cranial and abdominal injuries
- Change in behavior or school performance
- Fear and avoidance of certain people or situations

computerized tomography (CT) is often definitive for the diagnosis with radiographs and MRI used to provide a thorough diagnostic profile (National Center for PTSD, 2011).

Manifestations of physical neglect include undernourishment (evidenced by constantly feeling hungry, hoarding or stealing food, and being underweight), unclean clothes and body, poor dental health (extensive cavities or generally poor condition of teeth), and inappropriate clothing for the season.

Manifestations of emotional abuse, verbal abuse, and emotional neglect include fear, poor physical growth, and failure to meet appropriate developmental milestones. The child may have difficulty relating to adults, impaired communication skills, and developmental delays. Behavioral manifestations include anxiety, fear, shame, aggression, delinquency, and depression.

Children who have been sexually abused may exhibit a variety of physical and behavioral signs and symptoms (Table 17–10). Bruising, bleeding, and laceration of the genital area are obvious signs of trauma (National Center for PTSD, 2011). However, sexual abuse does not always result in apparent injury. Among the many long-term consequences of child sexual abuse are ongoing feelings of shame, guilt, anger, and hostility; decreased self-esteem, which leads to increased self-destructive behavior, risk of suicide, and decreased ability to establish positive relationships in adulthood; recurrence of victimization experiences; substance abuse; and eating disorders. The results can be long lasting, with children experiencing posttraumatic stress disorder (PTSD) or substance abuse in adulthood. Factors associated with greater psychologic harm to the child include (1) a long period of abuse, (2) use of violent force or threat of violence, (3) abuse involving penetration (intercourse or oral–genital sex), and (4) abuse involving family members, especially the father or stepfather.

CLINICAL THERAPY

Diagnosis of abuse is made on the basis of a careful history and thorough physical examination. X-ray, CT, and MRI studies may be ordered to identify signs of recurrent abuse (e.g., healed fractures). Laboratory studies may involve urine culture for signs of infection or screening for sexually transmitted infections; they can also rule out other causes of bleeding such as hemophilia. Genitourinary examination may be performed if sexual abuse

TABLE 17–10 Clinical Manifestations of Sexual Abuse in Children and Adolescents

- Vaginal discharge
- Blood-stained underpants or diaper
- Genital redness, pain, itching, or bruising
- Difficulty walking or sitting
- Urinary tract infection
- Sexually transmitted infection
- Somatic complaints, such as headaches or stomachaches
- Sleeping problems, such as nightmares or night terrors
- Bed-wetting
- Unwillingness to go to babysitter, family member, neighbor, or other person
- New or excessive sexual curiosity or play
- Fear of strangers
- Constant masturbation
- Curling into fetal position
- Phobias about particular places, people, or things
- Abrupt changes in school performance and attendance
- Changes in eating habits
- Abrupt changes in behavior (especially withdrawal)
- Child or adolescent female acts like a wife or mother
- Excessively seductive behavior

is suspected. Some children are admitted directly to the hospital with the diagnosis of suspected abuse or neglect. Less obvious as a victim of abuse is the child admitted with a skull fracture who "fell off a chair."

Clinical Tip

About 8000 to 9000 U.S. children are hospitalized with fractures each year, and it is estimated that 20% to 25% of children under 1 year of age and 6% to 7% of older children experience abuse as the cause of fracture. Current guidelines of the American Academy of Pediatrics recommend skeletal survey in fractures known to be due to abuse, domestic violence, or being hit by a toy, or when there is no history of trauma that caused the fracture. From 12 to 23 months, all fractures must be evaluated by skeletal survey, and in children older than 24 months, the fracture type determines the need for skeletal survey (Wood et al., 2014).

Neglect, which is more difficult to define and identify, frequently requires hospitalization with a comprehensive medical, social, and psychiatric evaluation. Five basic categories must be considered when attempting to diagnose neglect: (1) medical care neglect (lack of necessary medical care), (2) gross safety neglect (lack of appropriate supervision), (3) physical neglect (lack of food and shelter), (4) emotional neglect, and (5) educational neglect.

All 50 states have extensive, complex statutes about reporting child abuse and neglect. A specialist must be consulted, especially if the child's testimony will be used in court.

Children do not routinely make false allegations of abuse. If indeed there is reason to believe the allegations are false, a child and adolescent therapist (psychiatrist, psychologist, psychiatric clinical nurse specialist, or social worker) with special expertise should be consulted to determine the truth. Keep in mind that children who withdraw their accusations may have

been threatened or coerced into doing so. Because children who have been physically, emotionally, or sexually abused are at risk for major depression, they require skilled care by mental healthcare providers who are specially trained in this area. Initially, the treatment goals include prevention of self-destructive or other dangerous acts. Children must be encouraged to express their fears and feelings in a safe and supportive environment. Equally important is the child's need to build coping skills and self-esteem. These children must be reassured and convinced that they are in no way responsible or to blame for what happened.

Professionalism in Practice Laws Regarding Child Abuse Reporting

Every state has a child abuse law specifying the particular behaviors that define every type of abuse. Any professional who works with children and reasonably suspects that a child has been abused is required to report suspicions of abuse or neglect to the local agency for child protective services. Reports made in good faith are not liable to countersuits. However, professionals who suspect abuse and do not report it may be held responsible by the judicial system. In some states, all citizens are mandated to report suspected abuse. Check the law in your state to learn those particular details. See the U.S. Department of Health and Human Services website for state laws (www.childwelfare.gov/systemwide/laws_policies/state/can).

Individual treatment with art therapy is used initially because it is the least threatening method in the early stages of treatment, it can easily be tailored to meet the child's individual needs, and it prepares the child for other forms of treatment such as family and group therapy (Figure 17–8). Family or group therapy may be of benefit in exploring the child's concerns and feelings. Anger is common, especially in children who were abused by a trusted adult such as the father or stepfather.

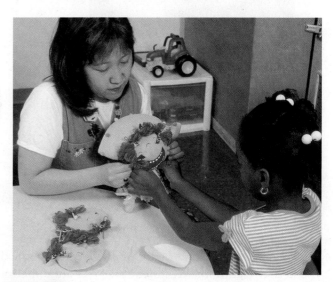

Figure 17–8 **Clinical interventions with children. Therapeutic strategies with young children involve various methods of communication, such as dramatic play and art.**

Nursing Management

Child Abuse and Neglect

Nursing Assessment and Diagnosis

Nursing assessment in instances of suspected child abuse or neglect requires a comprehensive history and physical examination, with documentation of findings. Consultation with social service agencies in the community is important if the family is receiving services.

Obtaining the history can be stressful for both the nurse and the parent. Use of therapeutic communication techniques and a quiet, unhurried environment are helpful. Be open, nonjudgmental, and calm. A statement such as "Hello, Mr. S. My name is Joan T. I'm Jonathan's nurse, and I will be asking you some questions about his overall health" may be a good start. It is important to differentiate true child abuse from cultural variations that might inaccurately be assumed to indicate abuse (Figure 17–9*A* and *B*). Obtaining information about abusive and neglectful behaviors requires a trusting relationship with parents, who are often afraid to trust any healthcare professional.

The health history sequence should include (1) parental concerns, (2) general family history, and (3) specific child history. This sequence begins with nonthreatening topics and allows the nurse to demonstrate concern before asking about abuse-related concerns. Obtain details about how injuries occurred. Document the parents' and child's own words verbatim using quotation marks. Compare reports obtained from each family member for lack of consistency and details that change over time.

It is desirable to interview the parent and child separately as well as together. Parent–child interaction during an intensive history-taking session provides an opportunity to observe the child's behavior and the parent's method of handling and responding to the child.

Data gathered during history taking are particularly important in light of physical findings. Are there discrepancies between the history and physical assessment data? Do the parents give a history of an uncontrollable, inattentive toddler when the nurse observes a child who is attentive throughout a 15-minute examination? Assess the child's general appearance, including dress and behavior during the assessment. How do the child's affect, behavior, and development compare with those of other children the same age? Document all lesions and bruising, including site, size, and color. Be aware of Mongolian spots that can mistakenly be interpreted as a sign of child abuse (see Chapter 5). If there are fractures, follow the guidelines given earlier regarding need for skeletal survey. Be alert for the signs of shaken child syndrome; this most often appears as a subtle neurologic condition. Measure head circumference and perform a neurologic examination (see Chapter 27).

Documentation of findings is important in all situations but is essential in cases of suspected child abuse and neglect. Each person who handles a laboratory specimen or other item (e.g., clothing soiled with semen) in cases of suspected child abuse must be identified in the client's record, and the specimen must never be left unattended. Record physical findings as observed. Use figure diagrams to document skin injuries. Take photographs as directed to document the location, nature, and extent of injuries.

Among the nursing diagnoses that might be appropriate for the physically abused or neglected child are the following (NANDA-I © 2014):

- *Pain, Acute,* related to inflicted injuries
- *Skin Integrity, Impaired,* related to inflicted injuries
- *Development: Delayed, Risk for,* related to lack of supportive parenting and environment
- *Nutrition, Imbalanced: Less than Body Requirements,* related to inadequate caloric intake

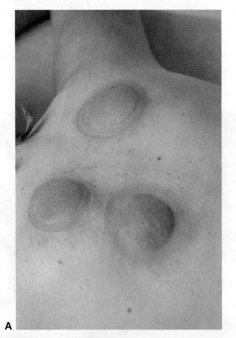

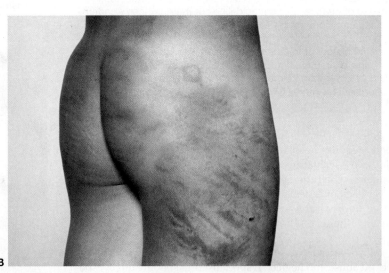

A   **B**

Figure 17–9 It is important to differentiate cultural practices, such as *A*, cupping, and *B*, coining, from signs of child abuse. Traditional treatment practices are sometimes mistaken for signs of physical abuse. Inquire about what treatments have been tried for the child at home. If unfamiliar with the treatment, ask the family members to explain what they have done. When there is lack of clarity, work with other healthcare professionals to decide if child abuse is a potential concern.

SOURCE: *A,* © doc-stock/Alamy; *B,* Biophoto Associates/Science Source.

- *Health Maintenance, Ineffective,* related to lack of parental provision of child's essential needs
- *Fear* related to actual physical harm or repeated risk of injury
- *Injury, Risk for,* related to physical abuse
- *Violence: Other-Directed, Risk for (Parent),* related to inability to manage anger

Additional diagnoses that might apply to the emotionally abused or neglected child include the following (NANDA-I © 2014):

- *Coping, Defensive,* related to psychologic impairment
- *Self-Esteem, Chronic Low,* related to lack of appropriate emotional support from parents
- *Coping: Family, Disabled,* related to dysfunctional family dynamics and pattern of physical abuse

Diagnoses that might apply to the sexually abused child include the following (NANDA I © 2014):

- *Anxiety* related to potential separation from parent
- *Rape-Trauma Syndrome* related to sexual exploitation
- *Role Performance, Ineffective,* related to domestic violence
- *Personal Identity: Disturbed,* related to disturbance of usual activities of childhood

Developing Cultural Competence Cupping and *Cao Gio*

Traditional treatment practices are sometimes mistaken for signs of physical abuse. The Chinese practice of cupping, which involves heating a bamboo cup and placing it on the skin, is a traditional treatment for headaches or abdominal pain. The Vietnamese practice of *cao gio* ("rubbing out the wind"), in which a coin or the fingers are forcefully rubbed on the chest, back, or neck, is used to treat minor ailments. Ask about marks on the skin, how they occurred, and what health practices the family uses.

Planning and Implementation

Nursing care focuses on helping to remove the child from an abusive environment, preventing further injury, providing supportive care, and reinforcing the importance of follow-up care and counseling.

PREVENT FURTHER INJURY

Work with social services and community agencies to assess the child's home environment, individuals living in the home, and the actions surrounding the abuse. Assist in removing the child from the home to temporary custody of the court or foster care of another relative if indicated. Counsel family members about abuse and refer them for appropriate therapy.

PROVIDE SUPPORTIVE CARE

Protect and treat the child's injuries (e.g., fractures, burns). Include parents in the child's treatment plan, and keep them informed about the child's progress. Even if suspected of inflicting injuries to the child, the parent is still the child's primary caretaker. Talk with the parent as you would with any parent. Be supportive of any guilt expressed. Encourage the parent to assist with the child's care. Observe parent–child interactions and

document supportive behaviors and the child's response to the parent versus other healthcare providers.

Interacting nonjudgmentally with a parent suspected of child abuse can be difficult. Nurses should talk with a colleague about any anger they feel toward such a parent or about the child's injuries or specific actions surrounding the abuse. Use team meetings to develop strategies that enable healthcare providers and other professionals to work with the parents and child.

Clinical Tip

When children have been abused, they are often frightened in new situations. Sexually abused children may resist removing clothes and may become very anxious during a physical examination or medical test. They may distrust members of the gender that abused them. When aware of a history of abuse, ask the parents or guardians how to best facilitate the child's health care. Be sensitive to fears and allow the child to wear clothing, have a support person present, or whatever may provide a sense of security. Consistency of nurses assigned to the child and the presence of a counselor may help to increase rapport and trust.

HOME CARE TEACHING

If there is any question about the child returning to a potentially dangerous situation, support the child's removal from the situation. The child may receive supervised care in the home by court order. Day care, home nursing, and social worker visits may be arranged. Parents should be referred to parent effectiveness classes, family therapy, and support groups as necessary. When a neighbor or friend is the abuser, the family may need support and legal advice when a term of incarceration is finished and the perpetrator returns to the community. Some states and communities have sexual offender laws that publicize the presence of an offender on parole within neighborhoods.

Encourage the family to inform other care providers when the child's abuse history may affect a response to care. They should be alert to signs of PTSD so they can seek assistance if the child has continuing problems (see Chapter 28).

Evaluation

Expected outcomes of nursing care for the child who has been abused or neglected include the following:

- The child maintains normal growth and development.
- A positive sense of self-esteem emerges in the child.
- Parents are provided with information and resources for stress relief.
- The child is provided with a nurturing environment.
- The child experiences no further episodes of abuse.

Münchausen Syndrome by Proxy (Factitious Disorder)

Münchausen syndrome by proxy is a potentially deadly form of child abuse that involves the fabrication of signs and symptoms of a health condition in a child. In most cases, the mother creates these fictitious signs in her child (the proxy). The victim is usually less than 6 years old, and commonly less than 1 year of age. Frequently, the child's symptoms of illness are used to gain entry into the medical system to meet the abuser's own psychologic needs for attention. The perpetrator may induce illness by giving the child medications or perform other actions such as adding blood to the child's urine specimen (National Center for Biotechnology Information, 2011).

The issues of abuse are multidimensional. The child is a victim of the feigned illness, repeated hospitalizations, and invasive procedures. Equally disruptive is the deprivation of the child's daily routine caused by the periodic medical crises.

Münchausen syndrome by proxy should be suspected when unexplained, recurrent, or extremely rare conditions occur; illness is unresponsive to treatment; and the history and clinical findings are inconsistent. The most commonly reported signs and symptoms are central nervous system dysfunction, apnea, diarrhea, vomiting, fever, seizures, signs of bleeding (in urine or stool), and rashes. The parent may overdose the child on medications, such as nonprescription drugs and even syrup of ipecac, causing a variety of side effects. The symptoms occur in the presence of the same caretaker and disappear when the child is separated from that caretaker.

The child often appears uncooperative, extremely anxious, fearful, and negative. The caretaker, who in contrast appears very cooperative, competent, and loving, often expresses a desire for the child to recover. The caretaker may even suggest diagnostic procedures to try to determine "what's wrong." Characteristically, the caretaker thrives in the healthcare environment.

The cause of factitious disorder is often complex and rooted in the caretaker's own abusive or neglectful childhood. The disorder occurs in all socioeconomic classes. Often the perpetrator has some type of healthcare background, such as nursing or another allied health profession. The abuser is often young and married, and appears very involved with and interested in the child (National Institutes of Health, 2013).

A suspicion of Münchausen syndrome by proxy requires a coordinated evaluation by a collaborative care team. Members of the team must organize and communicate a strategic plan regarding collection of evidence, confrontation of the abuser, and management of the hospitalized child. The child's safety is the ultimate concern. The case must also be reported to the appropriate child protective services. Remember also that some health conditions are very hard to diagnose and that sometimes unexplained health problems are related to an underlying disease. As one possible example, see mitochondrial disease that is described in Chapter 30.

Nursing Management

Take special care to maintain a trusting relationship with the parent or guardian so that person does not become suspicious and leave the hospital. Often the best person on the team to function in the role of "trusted other" is a member of the psychiatric consultation team.

Careful documentation of parent–child interactions, presence or absence of symptoms, and other pertinent observations is essential. The child must be closely monitored. If blood is present in the child's urine, stool, or vomitus, carefully document whether the nurse was present or whether the sample was provided by the parent. Covert video surveillance may be ordered by the hospital when the syndrome is highly suspected in a particular situation. Expert consultants may be needed to ensure legal requirements for investigation are met. When enough evidence is collected to prove Münchausen syndrome by proxy, the caretaker is confronted by the healthcare provider or a member of the psychiatric team in planning with law enforcement officials.

Environmental Influences on Child Health

Environmental contaminants, poisoning, and accidental respiratory ingestion are discussed in this section. See Chapter 10 for a discussion of the effects of disasters on children and related nursing management.

Environmental Contaminants

Contaminants are **toxins**, harmful or poisonous chemicals produced by metabolism or an organism (e.g., ricin), or **toxicants**, harmful natural or synthetic chemicals not metabolically produced by an organism (Genius, Sears, Schwalfenberg, et al., 2013). These products are commonly produced during industrial manufacture, but could be released as a form of terrorism. Children are generally more vulnerable than adults to such exposures because of their developing bodies. They consume high amounts of food, water, and air per unit of body weight. Consequences to the neurologic system are particularly important to developmental and behavioral outcomes (Magzamen, Van Sickle, Rose, et al., 2011).

Knowledge of environmental contaminants and their effects on children is limited. Environmental contaminants may be found in the air, water, soil, food, complementary therapies, and various objects, such as jewelry. Ground and surface water can be contaminated by manufacturing processes, agricultural and urban runoff into streams, sewage treatment plants, landfills, and particulates in the air. Some toxicants associated with deleterious effects on the child's developing nervous system include phthalates, bisphenol A, brominated flame retardants, polycyclic aromatic hydrocarbons, and gas cooking (Jurewicz, Polanska, & Hanke, 2013).

Contaminants in the environment can influence children in complex ways. Prenatal exposure can affect the developing fetus. Exposure during lactation may bring contaminants to the breastfed baby. Environmental effects may occur as the child grows through skin contact, inhalation, or food and water ingestion. Because children are exposed to many chemicals on a daily basis, harmful exposures are often difficult to identify. One example of a known harmful agent is environmental tobacco smoke (ETS). The mother who smokes or is exposed to ETS runs an increased risk of having a baby that is small for gestational age or who dies of sudden infant death syndrome (SIDS) (see Chapter 20). The child exposed to ETS has an increased risk of occurrence and severity of asthma and other respiratory diseases. The homes of smokers have higher nicotine levels even if adults are not smoking in the house (Kassem et al., 2014).

One to 2 million migrant workers travel from their homes, often in Central or South America, to work in the U.S. farm industry each year (Schmalzried & Fallon, 2012). The children of migrant farm workers constitute a group that is at particular health risk. The farm industry presents many environmental health risks: exposure to pesticides, unsanitary drinking water, overcrowding, insect exposure, equipment hazards, poor transportation, social isolation, and poverty (Shelton et al., 2014). Children living in migrant farm worker families are more likely to have respiratory and ear infections, gastroenteritis, intestinal parasites, skin infections, unmet dental needs, poor nutrition and anemia, delayed development, and occupation injuries (Schmalzried & Fallon, 2012). Families travel frequently; provision of coordinated health care is therefore difficult, leading to low immunization rates and academic challenges. Adolescents may even travel alone, lacking supervision by parents or other adults.

Some potentially harmful environmental exposures across various settings include the following (American Academy of Pediatrics Council on Environmental Health, 2011; Karr, 2012; Meadows-Oliver, 2012):

- Pesticides such as organophosphates, organochlorine, chlorpyrifos, dialkyl phosphates, carbamates, pyrethroids (Children may be exposed through home use, parents who work in pesticide manufacturing, garden/farm/agricultural use, and ingestion through food treated with pesticides.)
- Outdoor air pollution from automobiles, power plants, and other sources (Children spend time outside and therefore have increased exposure.)
- Indoor air pollution from dust mites, molds, lead particles from old housing, wood smoke, and other sources
- Heavy metal exposure, including lead, mercury, arsenic, and chlorine
- Substances such as polychlorinated biphenyls (PCBs) stored in fatty tissues of the mother and causing fetal exposure or in animal fats; also present in electrical wiring
- Phthalates used to make flexible plastic products, such as catheters, intravenous tubing and bags, food packaging, and toys
- Bisphenol A (BPA) used to make hard plastics, such as baby bottles, containers used for microwaving, toys, and linings of food cans (Recent legislation mandates that BPA can no longer be used in baby bottles.)

Nursing Management

Nurses are instrumental in identifying exposure to environmental toxic agents. Inquire about:

- Parental work with harmful substances such as dust and chemicals
- Age of home (homes built before 1978 or renovated in the last 6 months are at risk for contamination with chemicals.)
- Safety items in home such as radon, carbon monoxide, and smoke alarms
- Child and family member with hobby requiring use of toxic materials, such as lead with stained glass work or glue with model building
- Child's consumption of nonfood products

Nurses in public health agencies often coordinate care for migrant farm workers. Evaluating living conditions and hazards through home visits is necessary. Provision of care and electronic and paper records can enhance care with distant sites where the family spends part of the year. Screening for health and developmental progression should be carried out whenever children are evaluated. In some northern U.S. communities, Head Start or other daycare centers open additional facilities during summer months when migrant families need such care while adults work in fields.

For children in all settings, consider the possibility of environmental exposure and refer for blood testing and further evaluation whenever delayed development or behavioral problems are evident. Test blood levels for contaminants such as lead (see later section). Hair, urine, and other testing may be possible as well. Identification of the toxic exposure and its removal from the environment are critical. Removal from the body by drug treatment is possible for some substances. Instruct the family in prevention of further exposure. Perform periodic growth and developmental measurements on the child and ensure return for further blood tests and other monitoring.

Poisoning

Young children are at risk for ingestion of foreign substances because of their characteristic behaviors, which involve exploration of the environment. Poisonings are the second leading cause of unintentional home-injury death and account for nearly one third of all unintentional home injuries. Annually, over 2 million calls are made for human ingestions to poison control centers, 80% for children under 6 years of age. About 130,000 visits to emergency departments occur, and over 800 children die from poisoning (Bronstein, Spyker, Cantilena, et al., 2012; CDC, 2013c).

Infants and toddlers commonly place objects in their mouths. Although most poisons are ingested, other routes of contamination include dermal, inhalation, and ocular. The Poison Prevention Packaging Act of 1970 mandates child protective devices for all potentially toxic substances, such as household cleansers and medications. However, many are still ingested by children.

The most dangerous toxic substances a small child may ingest include iron, antidepressants, hypoglycemic agents, cardiovascular drugs, salicylates, anticonvulsants, and illicit drugs. The five most common classifications of poisons ingested by children less than 5 years of age are cosmetics and personal care products, analgesics, household cleaning products, miscellaneous foreign bodies and toys, and topical preparations (Bronstein et al., 2012). Other common causes of poisoning include vitamins, cold and cough preparations, pesticides, and plants (e.g., Boston ivy, poinsettia, philodendron, lily-of-the-valley, daffodil bulbs, azalea, and rhododendron). Some household items are nontoxic and cause little harm; however, items that contain caustic agents or toxic chemicals can cause irreversible damage or death. Substances most often associated with a fatality in children less than 6 years of age include analgesics, plants, cold and cough preparations, and hydrocarbons (Bronstein et al., 2012).

SAFETY ALERT!
Most of the deaths resulting from poisoning occur in teens and are related to use or abuse of prescription pain medications. Pain relievers, tranquilizers, sedatives, and stimulants are frequently available in homes and pose a risk for young children who take them out of curiosity and teens who may take them in an experimental manner (CDC, 2013c). When youth combine alcohol with prescription medications, the outcomes can be even more serious. Another contemporary exposure involves marijuana; states that have legal medical and personal-use marijuana practices create another potential exposure for children. The median age for children requiring care for marijuana exposure is 1.5 to 2 years (Wang et al., 2014). Nurses should inquire about toxic substances in the homes of all youth and provide safety teaching regarding ways to keep children of all ages from having access to these substances.

CLINICAL MANIFESTATIONS
The manifestations of poisoning depend on the toxin. Some common effects include altered mental status, respiratory or cardiac symptoms, seizures, vital sign changes, and gastrointestinal symptoms. See Table 17–11.

TABLE 17-11 Clinical Manifestations of Commonly Ingested Toxic Agents

TYPE	SOURCES	CLINICAL MANIFESTATIONS	CLINICAL THERAPY
Corrosives (strong acids and alkaline products that cause chemical burns of mucosal surfaces)	Batteries Oven and drain cleaners Clinitest tablets Denture cleaners Bleach Toilet bowl cleaners Hair relaxers	Severe burning pain in mouth, throat, or stomach Swelling of mucous membranes; edema of lips, tongue, and pharynx (respiratory obstruction) Violent vomiting; hemoptysis Drooling; inability to clear secretions Signs of shock Anxiety Agitation	• Do not induce vomiting! • Dilute toxin with water to prevent further damage.
Hydrocarbons (organic compounds that contain carbon and hydrogen; most are distillates of petroleum)	Gasoline Kerosene Furniture polish Lighter fluid Paint thinners	Gagging Choking Coughing Nausea Vomiting Alteration in sensorium (lethargy) Weakness Respiratory symptoms of pulmonary involvement, tachypnea, cyanosis, retractions, grunting	• Do not induce vomiting! (Aspiration of hydrocarbons places the child at high risk for pneumonia.) • Use gastric lavage for highly toxic hydrocarbons. • Provide supportive respiratory care. • Decontaminate skin by removing clothing and cleansing skin.
Acetaminophen	Many over-the-counter products	Nausea Vomiting Sweating Pallor Hepatic involvement (pain in upper right quadrant, jaundice, confusion, stupor, coagulation and bilirubin abnormalities)	• Administer the antidote N-acetylcysteine, which binds with the metabolite, preventing absorption and protecting the liver. • Activated charcoal may be used.
Salicylate	Products containing aspirin	Nausea Disorientation Vomiting Dehydration Diaphoresis Hyperpnea Hyperpyrexia Bleeding tendencies Oliguria Tinnitus Convulsions Coma	• Depends on amount ingested. • Induce vomiting. • Administer intravenous sodium bicarbonate, fluids, and vitamin K.
Mercury	Broken thermometers Chemicals Paints Pesticides Fungicides	Tremors Memory loss Insomnia Weight loss Diarrhea Anorexia Gingivitis	• Similar to that for lead poisoning (see text discussion).

TYPE	SOURCES	CLINICAL MANIFESTATIONS	CLINICAL THERAPY
Iron	Multiple vitamin supplements and therapeutic iron tablets	Vomiting Hematemesis Diarrhea Bloody stools Abdominal pain Metabolic acidosis Shock Seizures Coma	• Activated charcoal may be used. • Administer intravenous fluids and sodium bicarbonate. • Deferoxamine chelation therapy.
Cardiac medications	Calcium channel blockers Beta blockers Digoxin	Bradycardia, arrhythmias, heart block Hypotension Dizziness, unsteady gait Altered mental status, seizures Nausea, vomiting	• Administer IV fluids. • Administer prescribed medications: • Vasopressor therapy • Calcium chloride • Glucagon, or high-dose regular insulin with supplemental glucose to achieve euglycemia • Digoxin immune Fab
Hypoglycemic agent	Sulfonylurea	Hypoglycemia Tachycardia Diaphoresis, clammy skin Mental status changes, coma	• Administer prescribed medications: • Glucagon • Octreotide

Source: Data from O'Donnell, K. A., & Ewald, M. B. (2011). Poisonings. In R. M. Kleigman, R. B. F. Stanton, J. St. Geme, N. F. Schor, & R. E. Behrman (Eds.), *Nelson textbook of pediatrics* (19th ed., pp. 250–270). Philadelphia, PA: Elsevier Saunders; McGregor, T., Parkar, M., & Rao, S. (2009). Evaluation and management of common childhood poisonings. *American Family Physician, 79*(5), 397–403; and Smollin, C. G. (2010). Toxicology: Pearls and pitfalls in the use of antidotes. *Emergency Medical Clinics of North America, 28,* 149–161.

CLINICAL THERAPY

Specific information about the poison is obtained from the parent to guide medical management. Blood and urine toxicology screens, as well as arterial blood gas and electrolyte testing, are performed. Testing of vomitus for the presence of medication or other poisonings may be helpful in determining the amount ingested. Other tests may include serum glucose, an electrocardiogram, serum electrolytes, and arterial blood gases. Testing of vomitus for the presence of medications or poisons may be helpful in determining the amount ingested.

In the emergency department the child's airway, breathing, circulation, and level of consciousness are assessed. The goal of treatment is to prevent further absorption of the poison and to reverse or eliminate its effects. The Poison Control Center is consulted to obtain guidance for treatment. An antidote is prescribed if one is available. Gastric lavage and activated charcoal are no longer routine therapy but may be used in some children if within 1 hour of ingestion. Cathartics or whole bowel irrigation with polyethylene glycol may be used for heavy metals or for long-acting or sustained-release medications. Syrup of ipecac is no longer recommended for treating suspected poisoning. Vomiting is rarely induced because too much of the poison may be absorbed before the agent used to cause vomiting is effective. In addition, vomiting is actually harmful when corrosives have been ingested and must absolutely be avoided in these situations.

Children with severe poisoning are admitted to the intensive care unit to carefully monitor the child and provide supportive care for the toxin's effects (e.g., arrhythmias, depressed respirations, seizures, hypotension, hypoglycemia, and electrolyte abnormalities). Potential complications of poisoning, depending on the type of poison, include respiratory and/or cardiac arrest, hypovolemic shock, liver failure, renal failure, seizures, and esophageal or tracheal burns.

Nursing Management

Poisoning

Nursing care focuses on initial emergent care and stabilization of the child with poisoning, followed by family education to reduce the risk of repeated poisoning.

Nursing Assessment and Diagnosis

Parents who suspect that their child has ingested a poison should immediately call the Poison Control Center (PCC). The PCC will advise parents about treatment to begin at home, and if the child needs treatment in the emergency department. If the child has vomited, the vomitus should be brought to the emergency department. With older children, the possibility of intentional ingestion needs to be considered.

Take a history from the family about the child's suspected ingestion substance, time, amount, and symptoms. Initial assessment focuses on airway, vital signs, and neurologic status. Assess for the following:

• Drooling, diaphoresis, and increased or depressed respirations

• Wheezing, respiratory distress, or stridor

• Decreased responsiveness and seizure activity

• Heart rate, skin color, capillary refill, peripheral and central pulses, and blood pressure

• Pupils (abnormally large or pinpoint pupils may be observed)

- Mouth, lips, and tongue for corrosive burns or edema and breath for unusual odor
- Vomiting and diarrhea (vomitus for presence of medication or other ingested substances)
- Height and weight

Nursing diagnoses for the child with ingestion of a toxic substance may include (NANDA-I © 2014):

- *Airway Clearance, Ineffective,* related to excessive secretion effect of toxic substance
- *Gas Exchange, Impaired,* related to depressed neurologic status
- *Aspiration, Risk for,* related to depressed neurologic status and vomiting
- *Cardiac Output, Decreased,* related to effects of toxic substance
- *Injury, Risk for,* related to repeated occurrence of poisoning
- *Family Processes, Interrupted,* related to poisoning of a family member

Planning and Implementation

Emergency care focuses on airway and hemodynamic stability, removal of toxic agents, and support of the family. The child is attached to pulse oximetry and cardiorespiratory monitors. An intravenous line is started for the administration of fluids and an antidote, if available. When activated charcoal is prescribed, it may be in a ready-to-drink solution in an opaque container, or it may need to be mixed with sorbitol or apple juice to encourage the child to drink it. Cover the cup so the child does not see the black liquid, and provide a straw to prevent spillage. Once immediate care has been provided, nursing care shifts to providing emotional support and preventing recurrence.

PROVIDE EMOTIONAL SUPPORT

Wait until the child is out of immediate danger before questioning parents in detail about the incident. Encourage parents to express feelings of anger, guilt, or fear about the incident.

PREVENT RECURRENCE

Discuss with parents the need to supervise infants and young children at all times. Ask parents how medicines and cleaning agents are stored and whether the house contains any plants. Teach parents proper methods of childproofing the home. Have the PCC number readily available. Suggest measures for preventing recurrence of poisoning. (See *Families Want to Know: Avoiding Childhood Poisoning*.)

The toll-free number for the American Association of Poison Control Centers (AAPCC) is 1-800-222-1222. The number can be accessed from anywhere in the United States and Puerto Rico, and the caller will be connected to the nearest poison control center.

Evaluation

Expected outcomes for nursing care of the child with poisoning include:

- The child maintains an open airway, effective gas exchange, and ventilatory function.
- The child is free from wheezing, coughing, pneumonia, or other signs indicating aspiration.
- The child's heart rate and blood pressure remain stable and appropriate for age.
- Neurologic status is appropriate for age.
- The family and child (if older) verbalize understanding of preventive measures and demonstrate measures to improve home environment safety.

Ingestion of Foreign Objects

There are about 100,000 cases of ingestion of foreign objects by children under 5 years of age annually in the United States. Coins, parts of toys, buttons, batteries, and glass are common objects ingested by young children (Bronstein et al., 2012). Adults often witness infants and young children ingesting foreign bodies, and older children will usually report swallowing a foreign object. Most small, round, smooth objects may not cause any clinical distress. However, if the foreign body is lodged in the esophagus, children may present with substernal pain, drooling, and dysphagia. Some children may exhibit respiratory symptoms including wheezing or coughing.

Serious complications can occur following foreign body ingestion. These complications include perforation of the intestinal tract, the most serious sequela of foreign body ingestion. Sharp objects are associated with a higher perforation rate than dull objects; perforations commonly occur in the region of the ileocecal

---

Families Want to Know

Avoiding Childhood Poisoning

Families with children require instructions for avoiding childhood poisoning. Teach family members these interventions to help avoid childhood poisonings:

- Place household cleaners, medications, vitamins, and other potentially poisonous substances out of the reach of children or in locked cabinets.
- Keep alcohol, marijuana, and prescription medications out of access for all youth, including teens.
- Use warning stickers such as "Mr. Yuk" on all containers.
- Buy products with child-resistant caps.
- Store products in their original containers.
- Never place household cleansers or other products in food or beverage containers.
- Remove all houseplants from the child's play areas.
- Put the Poison Control Center phone number by every phone in the house.
- Use caution when visiting other settings that are not childproofed (e.g., grandparents' homes). Remember that visitors may have pills in their purses or pockets that are easily reached by children.

valve. Development of strictures at the site of a retained foreign body may also occur. Respiratory complications arise if the object becomes lodged in the trachea, bronchi, or lungs. See Chapter 20 for care of the child with a foreign body airway obstruction.

Many ingested foreign bodies in children are radiopaque, so radiographs of the neck, chest, esophagus, and abdomen are useful tools for verifying ingestion and identifying the location of the object. Most foreign bodies pass spontaneously through the gastrointestinal system and are eliminated through stool. However, foreign bodies may become lodged in the esophagus and pose a significant risk to the child. Endoscopic examination and retrieval of the ingested foreign body may be necessary. Potentially harmful objects such as batteries, sharp objects, and magnets are removed surgically.

Nursing Management

Nursing care centers on supporting the child, providing collaborative assistance in the identification and removal of the foreign body, and teaching the child and family measures to reduce reoccurrence. Assess the child for drooling, wheezing, substernal pain, dysphagia, and coughing. Obtain a thorough history from the family. Determine, if possible, what was ingested, when the ingestion occurred, and any symptoms that the child experienced. Assess breath sounds.

Prepare the child for radiologic studies. Explain the procedures and reassure the child and family during the studies. Prepare for endoscopic examination and/or retrieval if necessary. If the foreign object is in the stomach and the child is to be observed for natural excretion of the object, explain monitoring of stools to parents. Suggest the use of tongue blades to examine stools for presence of the foreign body and to report if the object has not been passed within the expected time frame (generally 48 hours). Encourage the family to return for further radiologic examinations to determine the foreign object's progress of passage.

Partner with the family and assist them in establishing a safe home environment for the child. Encourage the family to keep all small items out of the child's reach and to ensure the child is monitored at all times. Expected outcomes for nursing care of the child who has ingested a foreign body include removal of the foreign body, reduction in risk, and family verbalization of preventive measures to reduce risk of ingestion of foreign bodies.

Lead Poisoning

Lead poisoning has been successfully prevented in many areas of the United States, with a substantial decline in lead levels from the mid-1970s. The average blood lead level for children is now 1.9 mcg/dL, down from 15 mcg/dL in 1976. Approximately 450,000 U.S. children (1%) from 1 to 5 years of age have blood lead levels above the recommended upper level of 5 mcg/dL. There is no safe level of lead exposure—even children with blood lead levels lower than 5 mcg/dL have been reported to have a decrease in cognition (CDC, 2012c; AAP Council on Environmental Health, 2016).

Lead in paint is the most common source of lead exposure for preschool children. Children are also exposed to lead when they ingest contaminated food, water, and soil or when they inhale dust contaminated with lead. A recent infiltration of lead into the water supply in Flint, Michigan, and in school water supplies in other communities points out the dangers of aging lead-lined pipes (U.S. Department of Health & Human Services, 2016). Paints on toys and crafts from some foreign countries may contain lead; unless such products are certified safe they should not be used by children.

Children are at greater risk for lead poisoning because they absorb and retain more lead in proportion to their weight than adults do. Lead is particularly harmful to children under the age of 7 years.

CLINICAL MANIFESTATIONS

Lead interferes with normal cell function, primarily of the nervous system, blood cells, and kidneys, and adversely affects the metabolism of vitamin D and calcium. Clinical manifestations depend on the degree of toxicity. Neurologic effects include decreased IQ scores, cognitive deficits, impaired hearing, and growth delays. Impaired mental function can occur with blood levels even lower than 5 mcg/dL. Lead ingestion by a woman during pregnancy can result in fetal malformations, reduced birth weight, and premature birth. Severe lead poisoning, which can result in encephalopathy, coma, and death, is now rare in developed countries.

Once in the body, lead accumulates in the blood, soft tissues (kidney, bone marrow, liver, and brain), bones, and teeth. Lead that is absorbed by the bones and teeth is released slowly; thus exposure to even small doses, over time, can result in dangerously high levels of lead in the body. See Table 17–12.

CLINICAL THERAPY

An environmental history should be obtained for all children. For those with risk of elevated lead (Pb) levels (living in homes completed before 1978, receiving Medicaid, in communities where schools or homes have been shown to have high levels of lead, and/or living in poverty), blood screening should be considered (CDC, 2012c, 2014c; U.S. Department of Health & Human Services, 2016). Follow-up testing is required in 2 to 3 months. Because most children are asymptomatic, careful history and identification of risk factors will guide healthcare providers in identifying children who need blood testing for lead.

TABLE 17–12 Clinical Manifestations of Lead Poisoning

LEVEL	CLINICAL MANIFESTATIONS
Less than 9 mcg/dL	Generally asymptomatic although subtle neurologic effects may be present with any exposure
10–19 mcg/dL	Mild impairment in growth, fine motor skills, and cognition Anemia
20–44 mcg/dL	General fatigue and motor impairment Difficulty concentrating Paresis or paralysis, tremor Headache Diffuse abdominal pain, vomiting, weight loss, constipation Anemia
45–69 mcg/dL	Colic (intermittent, severe abdominal cramps), anorexia, vomiting Hyperirritability Increased lethargy Lead line (blue-black) on gingival tissue
Over 70 mcg/dL	Encephalopathy, which may lead abruptly to seizures, changes in consciousness, coma, and death Ataxia

Source: Adapted from Agency for Toxic Substances & Disease Registry. (2011). *Lead toxicity clinical evaluation*. Atlanta, GA: Author.

Children with elevated Pb levels require a full medical evaluation, including a detailed environmental and behavioral history, physical examination, and tests for iron deficiency. Interventions to remove sources of lead from the child's environment are necessary. Blood screening is performed at ages 12 and 24 months, as well as for children in these groups who are 36 to 72 months old but not previously screened. A venous blood sample is preferred because it reduces the risk of specimen contamination from lead on the skin. Capillary specimens are used in some cases with careful skin preparation. Any elevation in a capillary specimen must be confirmed by a venous sample. A blood Pb level below 5 mcg/dL is considered acceptable, although it may still not screen out all children with impaired development due to lead. *Healthy People 2020* objectives aim at decreasing blood levels of children and the number of children with elevated levels (USDHHS, 2011).

Healthy People 2020

(EH-8.1) Eliminate elevated blood levels in children

(EH-8.2) Reduce the mean blood levels in children from 1 to 5 years to 1.4 mcg/mL

Children with very high blood Pb levels require medical treatment. For levels above 45 mcg/dL, chelation therapy is considered for administration. Children with blood Pb levels greater than 70 mcg/dL are critically ill from lead poisoning and require immediate chelation therapy and interventions to provide a lead-free environment.

Chelation is a reaction in which an organic compound, containing carbonyl (CO) and hydroxyl (OH) groups, coordinates with a metal to form a firmly bound ringlike structure. Chelation therapy for lead poisoning involves the administration of an agent that binds with lead, decreasing its effects and increasing its rate of excretion from the body. Calcium disodium ethylenediamine tetraacetate ($CaNa_2$ EDTA) IM or IV, dimercaprol (BAL) deep IM, penicillamine PO, or succimer (DMSA) PO may be used. Children with blood Pb levels between 25 and 69 mcg/dL receive $CaNa_2$ EDTA for 5 to 7 days, followed by a rest period and then a second chelation treatment. Children with Pb-B levels greater than 70 mcg/dL are given both BAL and $CaNa_2$ EDTA, followed by a rest period and a second chelation treatment using $CaNa_2$ EDTA alone. Chelation therapy has the potential for serious side effects. $CaNa_2$ EDTA can cause tubular necrosis and cardiac arrhythmia; IM administration is painful, so it is generally given IV. BAL can lead to hypertension, tachycardia, headache, fever, or nephrotoxicity. Penicillamine is used only when treatment with other drugs is not effective because of its multisystem side effects. Succimer is associated with GI side effects, rash, headache, and neurologic symptoms. Long-term follow-up of children receiving chelation therapy is essential. The child should never be discharged unless a lead-free home environment has been ensured.

Nursing Management

Nursing care centers on screening, education, and follow-up. Nurses often work with state and local health officials to plan screening for children at high risk of lead exposure. Ask parents about the child's development and eating habits and be alert for risk of lead exposure. Educate parents about sources of lead in the environment and techniques to reduce exposure. Make home visits to evaluate exposure to lead and to perform individualized teaching. Emphasize the importance of housekeeping interventions to reduce exposure to lead dust. These interventions include damp mopping of hard surfaces, floors, window sills, and baseboards; washing the child's hands and face before meals; and frequent washing of toys and pacifiers. Be alert that home renovation can significantly increase the levels of lead in dust.

Teach parents the importance of including foods high in iron and calcium in the child's diet to counteract losses of these minerals associated with lead exposure. The child should eat meals at regular intervals because lead is absorbed more readily on an empty stomach.

Be sure that parents understand the importance of follow-up testing of lead levels. If the child is developmentally delayed, refer the family to an infant stimulation or early intervention program. Referral to social services and either a visiting nurse or home healthcare nurse may also be appropriate.

Nurses who administer chelating drugs are challenged by the complexity of treatment and required care. Chelation should always be managed by experts in such care, and in consultation with the Lead Poisoning Prevention Branch of the National Center for Environmental Health of the CDC. Careful monitoring of liver and kidney function, cardiac, GI, and neurologic systems is needed for all chelating drugs. Administration for some drugs is via IM route and is painful; children will need skilled nursing and child life specialist care.

Expected outcomes of nursing care for the child with lead or other poisoning include the following:

- The child exhibits normal growth and development, including cognition.

- Adequate nutritional intake is ensured for the child.

- Lead or other poisons are removed from the child's environment.

- The family expresses understanding of measures to establish a safe environment for the child.

Chapter Highlights

- Many of the major morbidities and mortalities of childhood and adolescence are related to social and environmental factors.

- The theories of ecologic development and resilience provide frameworks to assess interactions of children and their environments, and to mitigate risk factors.

- Poverty and homelessness are pervasive and influence many health outcomes.

- Substance use, particularly of alcohol and drugs, poses risks to youth and requires screening, prevention, and cessation programs appropriate for developmental age.

- Violence can be directed at children, and children can be the perpetrators of violence. The nurse plans interventions for an array of abusive situations such as child abuse, sexual abuse, and domestic violence.

- Environmental contaminants affect the health of children, from the prenatal period through childhood. Medicines, plants, pesticides, lead, and other household products pose risks at all ages, even though most poisonings occur in children under 5 years of age.

Clinical Reasoning in Action

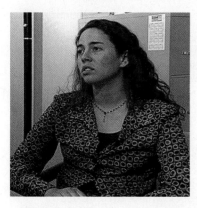

You are working at the inpatient adolescent psychiatric unit where there are approximately 20 teens between the ages of 12 and 17 years old. The teens are admitted for several different diagnoses, including depression, suicide attempts, bipolar disorders, and eating disorders. The nurses are in charge of medication administration, vital signs, unit safety issues, physical assessments, and basic therapeutic interventions. You are working with a client named Cindy, 15 years old, who was admitted because of a suicide attempt and has been given a dual diagnosis of bulimia nervosa and depression. She has had extreme weight loss and gain over the past year and is currently 67 inches tall and weighs 140 lb. She has stated she tried to commit suicide with a knife because she was upset over the loss of her boyfriend. She thought she was fat and was trying to lose weight by using laxatives and vomiting after meals. There is a family history of depression and substance abuse, but Cindy denies any substance use. She lives with her mother and has no contact with her father. She does not feel she has anyone to discuss her feelings with, and states her mother is gone from the house frequently. Cindy admits to often eating fast food and snacking on other junk food and soda. She has been in the hospital for 2 weeks and was resistant to treatment at first, but seems to be improving with therapy and medication. She has lost 3 lb while she has been hospitalized, and her average vital signs are temperature 98.7°F, pulse 70, respirations 12, and blood pressure 110/70 mmHg. (Review the content on bulimia in Chapter 14 to answer the following questions.)

1. What are some of the signs of bulimia Cindy may exhibit?

2. What can you tell the mother about Cindy's vital signs and stability at this time? How can you explain the weight loss?

3. What behavioral signs of bulimia should be part of your nursing assessment of Cindy while she is hospitalized?

4. What are the treatment recommendations for Cindy?

References

Add Health Study. (2014). *Add Health: The National Longitudinal Study of Adolescent Health.* Retrieved from http://www.cpc.unc.edu/projects/addhealth

Agency for Healthcare Research and Quality (AHRQ). (2013). *Most frequent conditions in U.S. hospitals.* Rockville, MD: Author.

Agency for Toxic Substances & Disease Registry. (2011). *Lead toxicity clinical evaluation.* Atlanta, GA: Author.

Allan, E. J., & Madden, M. (2011). The nature and extent of college student hazing. *International Journal of Adolescent Medicine and Health, 24*(1), 83–90.

Allen, E. S., Rhoades, G. K., Stanley, S. M., & Markman, H. J. (2011). On the home front: Stress for recently deployed army couples. *Family Process, 50,* 235–247.

American Academy of Child and Adolescent Psychiatry (AACAP). (2013). *Substance use resource center.* Retrieved from http://www.aacap.org/AACAP/AACAP/ Families_and_Youth/Resource_Centers/Substance_ Use_Resource_Center/Home.aspx

American Academy of Pediatrics. (2011). *Bullies beat down self-esteem.* Retrieved from http://www. healthychildren.org

American Academy of Pediatrics Council on Community Pediatrics. (2013). Providing care for children and adolescents facing homelessness and housing insecurity. *Pediatrics, 131,* 1206–1210.

American Academy of Pediatrics Council on Environmental Health. (2016). Prevention of childhood lead toxicity. *Pediatrics, 138*(1), e20161493.

American Academy of Pediatrics Committee on Practice and Ambulatory Medicine, Bright Futures Periodicity Schedule Workgroup. (2014). 2014 recommendations for pediatric preventive health care. *Pediatrics, 133,* 568–570.

American Academy of Pediatrics Council on Environmental Health. (2011). Chemical-management policy: Prioritizing children's health. *Pediatrics, 127*(5), 983–990.

American Psychiatric Association. (2012). *LGBT—Sexual orientation.* Retrieved from http://www.psychiatry.org/ mental-health/people/lgbt-sexual-orientation

Annie E. Casey Foundation. (2011). *No place for kids: The case for reducing juvenile incarceration.* Baltimore, MD: Author.

Aranda, M. C., Middleton, L. S., Flake, E., & Davis, B. E. (2011). Psychosocial screening in children with wartime-deployed parents. *Military Medicine, 176*, 402–407.

Audrain-McGovern, J., Stevens, S., Murray, P. J., Kinsman, S., Zuckoff, A., Pletcher, J., . . . Wileyto, E. P. (2011). The efficacy of motivational interviewing versus brief advice for adolescent smoking behavior change. *Pediatrics, 128*(1), e101–e111.

August-Brady, M., & Adamshick, P. (2013). Oh, the things you will learn: Taking undergraduate research to the homeless shelter. *Journal of Nursing Education, 52*, 342–345.

Balodis, I. M., Wynne-Edwards, K. E., & Olmstead, M. C. (2010). The other side of the curve: Examining the relationship between pre-stressor physiological responses and stress reactivity. *Psychoneuroendocrinology, 35*, 1363–1373.

Benard, B. (2014). *The foundations of the resiliency framework.* Retrieved from http://www.resiliency.com/free-articles-resources/the-foundations-of-the-resiliency-framework/

Broberg, M. C., & Nield, L. S. (2013). Helping adolescents kick the habit. *Consultant for Pediatrics,* August, 375–377.

Bronfenbrenner, U. (2005). *Making human beings human: Bioecologic perspectives.* Thousand Oaks, CA: Sage.

Bronstein, A. C., Spyker, D. A., Cantilena, L. R., Rumack, B. H., & Dart, R. C. (2012). 2011 annual report of the American Association of Poison Control Centers' National Poisoning Data System (NPDS): 29th annual report. *Clinical Toxicology, 50*, 911–1164.

Catledge, C. B., Scharer, K., & Fuller, S. (2012). Assessment and identification of deliberate self-harm in adolescents and young adults. *The Journal for Nurse Practitioners, 8*, 299–305.

Centers for Disease Control and Prevention (CDC). (2011a). *Youth and tobacco use.* Retrieved from http://www.cdc.gov/tobacco/data_statistics/fact_sheets/youth_data/tobacco_use/index.htm

Centers for Disease Control and Prevention (CDC). (2011b). Violence-related firearm deaths among residents of metropolitan areas and cities—United States, 2006–2007. *Morbidity and Mortality Weekly Report, 60*, 573–578.

Centers for Disease Control and Prevention (CDC). (2012a). Vital signs: Unintentional injury deaths in persons aged 0–19 years—United States, 2000–2009. *Morbidity and Mortality Weekly Report, 61*, 270–276.

Centers for Disease Control and Prevention (CDC). (2012b). Tattoo-associated nontuberculous mycobacterium skin infections, multiple states 2011–2012. *Morbidity and Mortality Weekly Report, 61*, 653–656.

Centers for Disease Control and Prevention (CDC). (2012c). *Low level lead exposure harms children: A renewed call for primary prevention.* Retrieved from http://www.cdc.gov/nceh/lead/acclpp/final_document_030712.pdf

Centers for Disease Control and Prevention (CDC). (2013a). Notes from the field: Electronic cigarette use among middle and high school students—United States, 2011–2012. *Morbidity and Mortality Weekly Report, 62*, 729–730.

Centers for Disease Control and Prevention (CDC). (2013b). *National youth tobacco survey.* Retrieved from http://www.cdc.gov/tobacco/data_statistics/surveys/nyts

Centers for Disease Control and Prevention (CDC). (2013c). *A national action plan for child injury prevention: Reducing poisoning injuries in children.* Retrieved from http://www.cdc.gov/safechild/NAP/overviews/poison.html

Centers for Disease Control and Prevention (CDC). (2014a). Youth risk behavior surveillance—United States, 2013. *Morbidity and Mortality Weekly Report, 63*(SS04), 1–172.

Centers for Disease Control and Prevention (CDC). (2014b). *Child maltreatment.* Retrieved from http://www.cdc.gov/violenceprevention/pdf/childmaltreatment-facts-at-a-glance.pdf

Centers for Disease Control and Prevention (CDC). (2014c). Lead screening and prevalence of blood lead levels in children aged 1–2 years—Child blood lead surveillance system, United States, 2002–2010, and National Health and Nutrition Examination Survey, United States, 1999–2010. *Morbidity and Mortality Weekly Report, 63*(02), 36–42.

Chandra, A., Mosher, W. D., Copen, C., & Sionean, C. (2011). Sexual behavior, sexual attraction, and sexual identity in the United States: Data from the 2006–2008 National Survey of Family Growth. *National Health Statistics Report, 36*, 1–36.

Childhelp. (2013). *Child abuse statistics and facts.* Retrieved from https://www.childhelp.org/child-abuse-statistics/

Child Trends. (2015). *Preventing violence: Understanding and addressing determinants of youth violence in the United States.* Retrieved from http://www.childtrends.org/wp-content/uploads/2015/03/2015-10PreventingViolence21.pdf

Children and Divorce. (2013). *Children divorce statistics.* Retrieved from http://www.children-and-divorce.com/children-divorce-statistics.html

Children's Defense Fund. (2014). *State of America's children 2014.* Retrieved from http://www.childrensdefense.org/child-research-data-publications/data/2014-soac.pdf?utm_source=2014-SOAC-PDF&utm_medium=link&utm_campaign=2014-SOAC

ChildStats. (2011). *Child care.* Retrieved from http://www.childstats.gov/americaschildren09/famsoc3.asp

Cross, T. P., Matthews, B., Tonmyr, L., Scott, D., & Ouimet, C. (2012). Child welfare policy and practice on children's exposure to domestic violence. *Child Abuse and Neglect, 36*(3), 210–216.

Cyberbullying Research Center. (2011). *Research.* Retrieved from http://cyberbullying.us/research.php

Davidov, D. M., Nadorff, M. R., Jack, S. M., Coben, J. H., & NFP IPV Research Team. (2012). Nurse home visitors' perspective of mandatory reporting of children's exposure to intimate partner violence to child protection agencies. *Public Health Nursing, 29*(5), 412–423.

Dunn, W. L., & Craig, G. J. (2013). *Understanding human development* (3rd ed.). Upper Saddle River, NJ: Pearson Education.

Elkind, D. (2007). *The hurried child: 25th anniversary edition.* Cambridge, MA: Da Capo Lifelong Publishing.

Fakhouri, T. H. I., Hughes, J. P., Burt, V. L., Song, M., Fulton, J. E., & Ogden, C. L. (2014). *Physical activity in U.S. youth aged 12–15 years, 2012.* NCHS data brief, no 141. Hyattsville, MD: National Center for Health Statistics.

Federal Interagency Forum on Child and Family Statistics. (2015). *America's children: Key national indicators of well-being.* Washington, DC: U.S. Government Printing Office. Retrieved from http://www.childstats.gov/americaschildren/eco1.asp

Genius, S. J., Sears, M. E., Schwalfenberg, G., Hope, J., & Bernhoft, R. (2013). Clinical detoxification: Elimination of persistent toxicants from the human body. *Scientific World Journal,* June 6, 238–347. doi: 10.0055/2013/238347

Havens, J. R., Young, A. M., & Havens, C. E. (2011). Nonmedical prescription drug use in a nationally representative sample of adolescents: Evidence of greater use among rural adolescents. *Archives of Pediatrics and Adolescent Medicine, 165*, 250–255.

Hazing Prevention. (2011). *Hazing information.* Retrieved from http://www.hazingprevention.org/hazing-information.html

Henderson, N., Bernard, B., & Sharp-Light, N. (2007). *Resiliency in action.* Ojai, CA: Resiliency in Action.

Juhas, E., & English, J. C. (2013). Tattoo-associated complications. *Journal of Pediatric and Adolescent Gynecology, 26*, 125–129.

Jurewicz, J., Polanska, K., & Hanke, W. (2013). Exposure to widespread environmental toxicants and children's cognitive development and behavioral problems. *International Journal of Occupational Medicine and Environmental Health, 26*, 185–204.

Karr, C. (2012). Children's environmental health in agricultural settings. *Journal of Agromedicine, 17*(2), 127–139.

Kassem, N. O., Daffa, R. M., Liles, S., Jackson, S. R., Kassem, N. O., Younis, M. A., . . . Hovell, M. F. (2014). Children's exposure to secondhand and thirdhand smoke carcinogens and toxicants in homes of hookah smokers. *Nicotine and Tobacco Research, 16*, 961–975.

Kerker, B. D., Bainbridge, J., Kennedy, J., Bennani, Y., Agerton, T., Marder, D., . . . Thorpe, L. E. (2011). A population-based assessment of the health of homeless families in New York City, 2001–2003. *American Journal of Public Health, 101*, 546–553.

KidsHealth. (2014). *How TV affects your child.* Retrieved from http://kidshealth.org/parent/positive/family/tv_affects_child.html

Laughlin, L. (2013). *Who's minding the kids? Child care arrangements: Spring 2011.* Retrieved from http://www.census.gov/prod/2013pubs/p70-135.pdf

Lehner, K. R., & Baumann, M. H. (2013). Psychoactive "bathsalts": Compounds, mechanisms, and toxicities. *Neuropsychopharmacology Reviews, 38*, 242–244.

Lynn, C. J., Acri, M. C., Goldstein, L., Bannon, W., Beharie, N., & McKay, M. M. (2014). Improving youth mental health through family-based prevention in family homeless shelters. *Child and Youth Service Review, 44*, 243–248.

Magzamen, S., Van Sickle, D., Rose, L. D., & Cronk, C. (2011). Environmental pediatrics. *Pediatric Annals, 40*(3), 144–151.

McGraw, M., & McGraw, L. (2012). Bath salts: Not as harmless as they sound. *Journal of Emergency Nursing, 38*(6), 582–588.

Meadows-Oliver, M., (2012). Environmental toxicants: Lead and mercury. *Journal of Pediatric Health Care, 26*, 213–215.

National Association for the Education of Young Children. (2010). *Introduction to the NAEYC early childhood program standards and accreditation criteria: Program standards.* Retrieved from http://www.naeyc.org/accreditation

National Center for Biotechnology Information. (2011). *Münchausen syndrome by proxy.* Retrieved from http://www.ncbi.nih.gov/pubmedhealth/PNH0002522/

National Center for Health Statistics & National Vital Statistics System. (2012). *Fatal injury reports, 2008.* Retrieved from http://webapppa.cdc.gov/cgi-bin/broker.exe

National Center for PTSD. (2011). *Child sexual abuse.* Retrieved from http://www.ptsd.va.gov/public/pages/child-sexual-abuse.asp

National Center on Family Homelessness. (2015). *The characteristics and needs of families experiencing homelessness.* Retrieved from http://www.family-homelessness.org

National Institute on Alcohol Abuse and Alcoholism. (n.d.). *Snapshot of underage drinking.* Retrieved from http://www.niaaa.nih.gov

National Institute on Drug Abuse. (2011). *NIDA InfoFacts: Club drugs.* Retrieved from http://www.nida/nih.gov/Infofacts/clubdrugs.html and http://www.drugabuse.gov/drugpages.clubdrugs.html

National Institutes of Health. (2013). *Münchausen syndrome by proxy.* Retrieved from http://www.nlm.nih.gov/medlineplus/ency/article/001555.htm

O'Donnell, K. A., & Ewald, M. B. (2011). Poisonings. In R. M. Kleigman, R. B. F. Stanton, J. St. Geme, N. F. Schor, & R. E. Behrman (Eds.), *Nelson textbook of pediatrics* (19th ed., pp. 250–270). Philadelphia, PA: Elsevier Saunders.

Owen, D. C., Armstrong, M. L., Koch, J. R., & Roberts, A. E. (2013). College students with body art: Well-being or high-risk behavior? *Journal of Psychosocial Nursing and Mental Health Services, 51,* 20–28.

Rodriguez, J., Applebaum, J., Stephenson-Hunter, C., Tinio, A., & Shapiro, A. (2013). Cooking, health eating, fitness and fun (CHEFFs): Qualitative evaluation of a nutrition education program for children living at urban family homeless shelters. *American Journal of Public Health, 103*(Suppl 2), S361–S367.

Sapienza, J. K., & Masten, A. S. (2011). Understanding and promoting resilience in children and youth. *Current Opinion in Psychiatry, 24,* 267–273.

Schmalzried, H. D., & Fallon, L. F. (2012). Reducing barriers associated with delivering health care services to migratory agricultural workers. *Rural and Remote Health, 12*(3), 2088.

Schneider, S. K., O'Donnell, L., Stueve, A., & Coulter, R. W. S. (2012). Cyberbullying, school bullying, and psychological distress: A regional census of high school students. *American Journal of Public Health, 102,* 171–177.

Sexuality Information and Education Council of the United States. (n.d.) *Questions and answers: LGBTQ youth.* Retrieved from http://www.siecus.org/index.cfm?fuseaction=page.viewpage&pageid=605&grandparentID=477&parentID=591

Shelton, J. F., Geraghty, E. M., Tancredi, D. J., Delwiche, L. D., Schmidt, R. J., Ritz, B., . . . Herty-Picciotto, I. (2014) Neurodevelopmental disorders and prenatal residential proximity to agricultural pesticides: The CHARGE study. *Environmental Health Perspectives, 122,* 1103–1109.

Slopen, N., McLaughlin, K. A., & Shonkoff, J. P. (2014). Intervention to improve cortisol regulation in children: A systematic review. *Pediatrics, 133,* 312–326.

Smith, B. D. (2011). Adolescent self-injury: Evaluation, referral, and treatment. *Consultant for Pediatricians, June 2011,* 190–195.

Smollin, C. G. (2010). Toxicology: Pearls and pitfalls in the use of antidotes. *Emergency Medical Clinics of North America, 28,* 149–161.

Sullivan, K. M., Bottorff, J., & Reid, C. (2011). Does mother's smoking influence girls' smoking more than boys' smoking? A 20-year review of the literature using a sex- and gender-based analysis. *Substance Use and Misuse, 46,* 656–668.

Tsitsika, A. K., Barlou, E., Andrie, E., Dimitropoulou, C., Tzavela, E. C., Janidian, M., & Tsolia, M. (2014). Bullying behaviors in children and adolescents: "An ongoing story." *Frontiers in Public Health, 2.* doi: 10.3389/fpubh.2014.00007

U.S. Department of Health and Human Services (USDHHS). (2011). *Healthy People 2020.* Retrieved from http://www.healthypeople.gov/2020

U.S. Department of Health and Human Services (USDHHS). (2016). *Public health emergency: Contaminated water in Flint.* Retrieved from http://www.phe.gov/emergency/events/Flint/Pages/default.aspx

U.S. Environmental Protection Agency. (2014). *Information for child care providers on environmental tobacco smoke.* Retrieved from http://www2.epa.gov/childcare/information-child-care-providers-about-environmental-tobacco-smoke

Wang, G. S., Roosevelt, G., Le Lait, M. C., Martinez, E. M., Bucher-Bartelson, B., Bronstein, A. C., & Heard, K. (2014). Association of unintentional pediatric exposure with decriminalization of marijuana in the United States. *Annals of Emergency Medicine, 63,* 684–689.

Wood, J. N., Fakeye, O., Feudtner, C., Mondestin, V., Localio, R., & Rubin, D. M. (2014). Development of guidelines for skeletal survey in young children with fractures. *Pediatrics, 134,* 45–53.

World Health Organization. (2014). *Global status report on violence prevention.* Geneva, Switzerland: World Health Organization.

Chapter 18
Alterations in Fluid, Electrolyte, and Acid–Base Balance

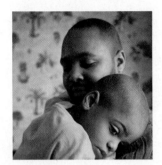

LeShan always likes to eat, so when he won't even drink I know he is sick. We just didn't know how sick he was or that he had gotten dehydrated. I wonder if we should have done something else for him at home.

—Father of LeShan, 18 months old

Iofoto/Shutterstock

∨ Learning Outcomes

18.1 Describe normal fluid and electrolyte status for children at various ages.

18.2 Identify regulatory mechanisms for fluid and electrolyte balance.

18.3 Interpret threats to fluid and electrolyte balance in children.

18.4 Describe acid–base balance and recognize disruptions common in children.

18.5 Analyze assessment findings to recognize fluid-electrolyte problems and acid–base imbalance in children.

18.6 Plan appropriate nursing interventions for children experiencing fluid-electrolyte problems and acid–base imbalance.

A thorough understanding of fluid, electrolyte, and acid–base homeostasis and imbalances is essential when providing nursing care to children like LeShan described in the chapter opener. This chapter presents information about the processes that maintain fluid and electrolyte balance and describes the common imbalances that may occur in children. It also describes how the body regulates acid–base status and explains the management of acid–base imbalances.

Many health conditions cause changes in body fluids that must be regulated and managed. Sometimes management of fluid status in the home or in a short-term ambulatory facility can prevent more serious illness or hospitalization.

FLUID VOLUME IMBALANCES

When fluid excretion and losses are balanced by the proper volume and type of fluid intake, fluid balance will be maintained. However, if fluid output and intake are not matched, fluid imbalance may occur rapidly. The major types of fluid imbalances are:

- Extracellular fluid volume deficit (dehydration)
- Extracellular fluid volume excess
- Interstitial fluid volume excess (edema)

Text continues on page 409

FOCUS ON:
Fluid, Electrolyte, and Acid–Base Balance

Physiology of Fluid and Electrolyte Balance

Fluid in the body is in a dynamic state. In persons of all ages, fluid continuously leaves the body through the skin, in feces and urine, and during respiration. Much of the human body is composed of water. **Body fluid** is body water that has solutes dissolved in it. Some of the solutes are **electrolytes**, or charged particles (ions). Electrolytes such as sodium (Na^+) potassium (K^+) calcium (Ca^{2+}) magnesium (Mg^{2+}) chloride (Cl^-) and inorganic phosphorus (Pi) ions must be present in the proper concentrations for cells to function effectively.

In persons of all ages, body fluid is located in several compartments. The two major fluid compartments contain the **intracellular fluid** (fluid inside the cells) and the **extracellular fluid** (fluid outside the cells). The extracellular fluid is made up of **intravascular fluid** (the fluid within the blood vessels) and **interstitial fluid** (the fluid between the cells and outside the blood and lymphatic vessels). Extracellular fluid accounts for about one third of total body water, and intracellular fluid accounts for about two thirds. The concentrations of electrolytes in the fluid differ depending on the fluid compartment. For example, extracellular fluid is rich in sodium ions; intracellular fluid, by contrast, is low in sodium ions but rich in potassium ions (Table 18–1).

Buffers

The maintenance of hydrogen ions within the normal range relies heavily on buffers. A **buffer** is a compound that binds hydrogen ions when their concentration rises and releases them when their concentration falls (see *Pathophysiology Illustrated: Buffer Responses to Excess Acid or Base*). Several kinds of buffers are present in the body (Table 18–2). Various body fluids have buffers to meet their special needs. The bicarbonate buffer system neutralizes metabolic acids (see *Pathophysiology Illustrated: The Bicarbonate Buffer System*); however, it cannot neutralize carbonic acid.

Fluid moves between the intravascular and interstitial compartments by a process called filtration. Water moves into and out

TABLE 18–1 Electrolyte Concentrations in Body Fluid Compartments

COMPONENTS	EXTRACELLULAR FLUID (ECF)		INTRACELLULAR FLUID (ICF)
	VASCULAR	INTERSTITIAL	
Na^+	High	High	Low
K^+	Low	Low	High
Ca^{2+}	Low	Low	Low (higher than ECF)
Mg^{2+}	Low	Low	High
P_i	Low	Low	High
Cl^-	High	High	Low
Proteins	High	Low	High

TABLE 18–2 Important Buffers

BUFFER	MAJOR LOCATIONS IN THE BODY
Bicarbonate	Plasma; interstitial fluid
Protein	Plasma; inside cells
Hemoglobin	Inside red blood cells
Phosphate	Inside cells; urine

of the cells by the process of osmosis. These processes are discussed later in the chapter. Electrolytes move over cell membranes both by **diffusion** of particles from a location of greater to less concentration and by active transport that is effective even against the concentration gradient.

Pathophysiology Illustrated: **Buffer Responses to Excess Acid or Base**

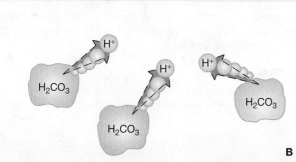

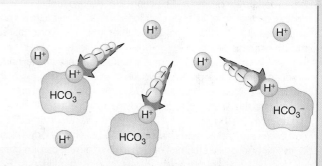

A, **How buffers respond to an excess of base.** If the blood has too much base, the acid portion of a buffer pair (e.g., H_2CO_3 of the bicarbonate buffer system) releases hydrogen ions (H^+) to help return the pH to normal.

B, **How buffers respond to an excess of acid.** If the blood has too much acid, the base portion of a buffer pair (e.g., HCO_3^- of the bicarbonate buffer system) takes up hydrogen ions (H^+) to help return the pH to normal.

(continued)

Pathophysiology Illustrated:
The Bicarbonate Buffer System

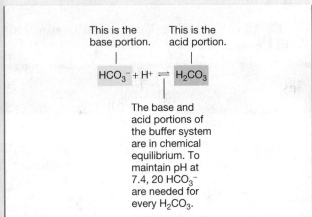

This is the base portion.

This is the acid portion.

$$HCO_3^- + H^+ \rightleftharpoons H_2CO_3$$

The base and acid portions of the buffer system are in chemical equilibrium. To maintain pH at 7.4, 20 HCO_3^- are needed for every H_2CO_3.

Physiology of Acid–Base Balance

Normal acid–base balance is necessary for proper function of the cells and the body. The number of hydrogen ions (H^+) present in a fluid determines its acidity. Increasing the hydrogen ion concentration makes a solution more acidic. Because the hydrogen ion concentration in body fluids is very low, acidity is expressed as **pH** (the negative logarithm of the hydrogen ion concentration) rather than as the hydrogen ion concentration itself. The range of possible pH values is 1 to 14. A pH of 7 is neutral. The lower the pH, the more acidic the solution. A pH above 7 is basic or alkaline. The higher the pH, the more basic the solution. Body fluids are normally slightly basic.

The pH of body fluids is regulated carefully to provide a suitable environment for cell function. The pH of the blood influences the pH inside the cells. **Acidemia** refers to a blood pH below normal levels, whereas **alkalemia** is an increased blood pH. Normal arterial blood pH ranges are 7.36 to 7.42 for infants, 7.37 to 7.43 for children, and 7.35 to 7.41 for adolescents. For the enzymes outside the cells to function optimally, the pH must be in the normal range. If the pH inside the cells becomes too high or too low, then the speed of chemical reactions becomes inappropriate for proper cell function. Cell protein function relies on the correct level of hydrogen ions. Thus, acid–base imbalances result in clinical signs and symptoms. In severe cases, they may cause death.

In the course of their normal function, all cells in the body produce acids. Cells produce two kinds of acids: carbonic acid (H_2CO_3) and metabolic (non-carbonic) acid. These acids are released into the extracellular fluid and must be neutralized or excreted from the body to prevent dangerous accumulation. They can be neutralized to some degree by the buffers in body fluids. Carbonic acid is excreted by the lungs in the form of carbon dioxide and water. Metabolic acids are excreted by the kidneys. Examples of metabolic acids are pyruvic, sulfuric, acetoacetic, lactic, hydrochloric, and beta-hydroxybutyric acids.

All buffer systems have limits. For example, if there are too many metabolic acids, the bicarbonate buffers become depleted. The acids then accumulate in the body until they are excreted by the kidneys. Clinically, this is seen as a decreased serum bicarbonate concentration and decreased blood pH.

Role of the Lungs

The lungs are responsible for excreting excess carbonic acid from the body. A child breathes out carbon dioxide and water, the components of carbonic acid, with each breath. With faster and deeper breaths, more carbonic acid is excreted. Because carbonic acid is converted in the body to carbon dioxide and water by the enzyme carbonic anhydrase, an indirect laboratory measurement of carbonic acid is Pco_2, the partial pressure of carbon dioxide in arterial blood.

Although a child can voluntarily increase or decrease the rate and depth of respirations, they are usually involuntarily controlled. The Po_2 (partial pressure of oxygen in arterial blood), Pco_2, and pH of the blood are monitored by chemoreceptors in the hypothalamus of the brain and in the aorta and carotid arteries. The input from the chemoreceptors is combined with other neural input to change breathing according to needs. Rate and depth increase or decrease according to the amount of carbonic acid that needs to be excreted.

If a child has a condition that decreases the excretion of carbonic acid or causes breathing to be too slow or shallow (such as overmedication following surgery), carbonic acid accumulates in the blood. Clinically, this is seen as an increased blood Pco_2 and is a form of respiratory acidosis. The reverse will also be true in the child breathing excessively or deeply. This leads to decreased Pco_2 and respiratory alkalosis.

Role of the Kidneys

The kidneys regulate metabolic acids from the body in two ways: They reabsorb filtered bicarbonate to prevent its loss in the urine, and they regenerate bicarbonate when needed to restore balance. Bicarbonate is formed when acids and ammonium combine with extra ions. The blood bicarbonate concentration is an indicator of the amount of metabolic acids present, because bicarbonate is used in buffering the acids. When the concentration is normal, metabolic acids are present in usual amounts (see *Pathophysiology Illustrated: The Kidneys and Metabolic Acids*).

In a healthy child, the result of these renal processes is excretion of metabolic acids and maintenance of blood bicarbonate concentration within normal limits. These processes may take several hours to days to be effective in restoring balance when acidosis occurs. In the child whose kidneys are not producing enough urine, metabolic acids may not be effectively excreted. Accumulation of these acids uses up many of the available bicarbonate buffers, resulting in a decreased serum bicarbonate concentration and metabolic acidosis.

Role of the Liver

The liver plays a role in maintaining acid–base balance by metabolizing protein, which produces hydrogen ions. It also synthesizes proteins needed to maintain osmotic pressures in the fluid compartments.

Pediatric Differences

Infants and young children differ physiologically from adults in ways that make them vulnerable to fluid, electrolyte, and acid–base imbalances. The percentage of body weight that is composed of water varies with age (Figure 18–1). The percentage is highest at birth (and higher in premature than in full-term infants) and decreases with age (see *As Children Grow: Fluid and*

Pathophysiology Illustrated: **The Kidneys and Metabolic Acids**

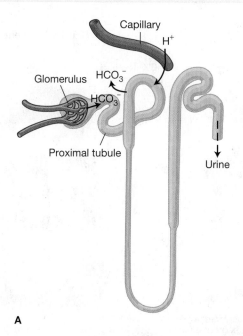

A

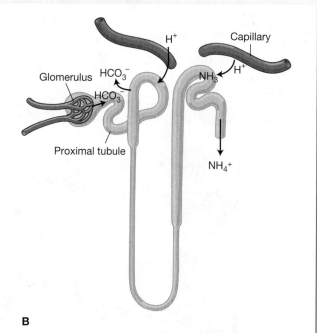

B

A, Recycling of bicarbonate by the kidneys. Bicarbonate ions that are in the blood are filtered into the renal tubules at the glomerulus. In the proximal tubules, bicarbonate ions are reabsorbed into the blood at the same time that hydrogen ions are transported from the blood into the renal tubular fluid.

B, Secretion and buffering of hydrogen ions in the kidneys. If the urine is too acidic, the cells that line the urinary tract could be damaged. To prevent this problem, hydrogen ions secreted into the distal tubules are neutralized by phosphate buffers or bound to ammonia and excreted in the form of ammonium ions.

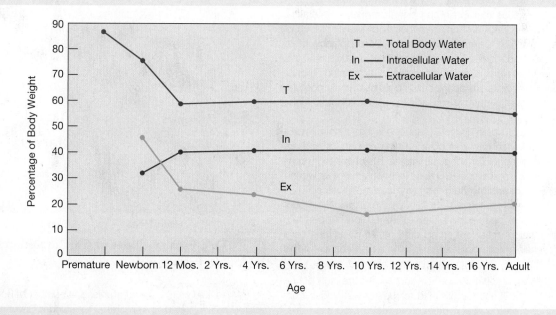

Figure 18–1 The major body fluid compartments. Extracellular fluid is composed mainly of intravascular fluid (fluid in blood vessels) and interstitial fluid (fluid between cells and outside the blood and lymphatic vessels). Intracellular fluid is that within cells.

(continued)

As Children Grow: **Fluid and Electrolyte Differences**

Newborn

75% Total
body water
• ECF 45%
• ICF 30%

Brain and skin occupy
a greater proportion of
body weight and are
high in interstitial fluid

Infant

65% Total
body water
• ECF 25%
• ICF 30–40%

High BSA
promotes fluid loss

Little fluid reserve
in intracellular fluid

5–6x greater fluid
exchange daily

High metabolic rate requires
generous fluid intake

Child/Adolescent

50% Total
body water
• ECF 10–15%
• ICF 40%

Kidneys are immature
until 2 years and unable
to conserve water and
electrolytes or fully assist
in acid–base balance

The newborn and infant have a high percentage of body weight composed of water, especially extracellular fluid, which is lost from the body easily. Note the small stomach size, which limits a newborn's ability to rehydrate quickly.

Electrolyte Differences). Neonates and young infants have a proportionately larger extracellular fluid volume than older children and adults because their brain and skin (both rich in interstitial fluid) occupy a greater proportion of their body weight. Much of our extracellular fluid is exchanged each day. During infancy, there is a high daily fluid requirement with little fluid volume reserve; this makes the infant vulnerable to dehydration. As an infant grows, the proportion of water inside the cells increases, the extracellular amount decreases in comparison, and the risk of fluid imbalance begins to decrease.

Infants and children under 2 years of age lose a greater proportion of fluid each day than older children and adults and are thus more dependent on adequate intake. They have high **sensible fluid loss** (measurable loss such as through urine or wound drainage) and **insensible fluid loss** (immeasurable loss such as through skin and respiratory tract). They have a greater amount of skin surface or body surface area (BSA; relationship between height and weight measured in squared meters) and thus have greater insensible water losses through the skin. Because of this large BSA, they are also at greater risk when burned.

In addition, respiratory and metabolic rates are high during early childhood. These factors lead to greater water loss from the lungs and greater water demand to fuel the body's metabolic processes (Figure 18–2). Because of these factors, the exercising child dehydrates easily and must consume more fluid during physical activity, particularly during hot weather (Mayo Clinic, 2011).

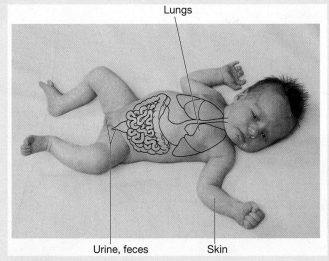

Lungs

Urine, feces   Skin

Figure 18–2 **Normal routes of fluid excretion from infants and children.**

When fluid status is compromised, a number of body mechanisms are activated to help restore balance. Several of these mechanisms occur in the kidneys. The kidneys conserve water and needed electrolytes while excreting waste products and drug metabolites. However, in children under 2 years of age, the glomeruli, tubules, and nephrons of the kidneys are immature. They are thus unable to conserve or excrete water and solutes effectively (see Chapter 26). Because more water is generally excreted, the infant and young child can become dehydrated quickly or develop electrolyte imbalances. In addition, infants have a weaker transport system for ions and bicarbonate, placing them at greater risk for acidosis and acid–base imbalances. Children under 2 years of age also have difficulty regulating electrolytes such as sodium and calcium. Renal response to high solute loads is slower and less developed, with function improving gradually during the first year of life.

Diagnostic and laboratory tests for fluid and electrolyte status include:

- Arterial blood gases
- Serum electrolyte panel
- Urinary specific gravity

See Appendices D and E for more information about diagnostic and laboratory tests.

Use the following guidelines to perform a nursing assessment of fluid and electrolyte status.

ASSESSMENT GUIDE | The Child With a Fluid, Electrolyte, or Acid–Base Alteration

Assessment Focus	Assessment Guidelines
Body weight	- Has weight decreased since the last measurement or weight reported by the family? - If so, how much? What percent of body weight is the weight loss?
Skin and mucous membranes	- What are the temperature, turgor, and moistness of the skin? - Describe moistness of oral mucous membranes. - Describe moistness of the eyes and presence of tears. - Is edema present in any body parts?
Cardiovascular and respiratory systems	- What are pulse and blood pressure? - Test capillary refill and small-vein filling times. - What is the respiratory rate? Is the rate regular?
Gastrointestinal system	- Does the child have nausea, vomiting, or diarrhea? If so, how often and for how long has it continued? - Is the child eating and drinking? How much and what types of foods and fluids?
Urinary system	- What is the child's urinary output? Number of wet diapers/day? - What is the urine specific gravity?
Musculoskeletal system	- Describe muscle tone and symmetry.
Neurologic system	- Describe the child's state of alertness and any changes observed. - What is the level of consciousness? - Is the anterior fontanelle at the skin surface or does it appear sunken?

Extracellular Fluid Volume Imbalances

Extracellular Fluid Volume Deficit (Dehydration)

Extracellular fluid volume deficit occurs when there is not enough fluid in the extracellular compartment (vascular and interstitial). Depending on the cause of dehydration, sodium may be at normal, low, or elevated levels. (Hyponatremia and hypernatremia are described later in the chapter.) The state of body water deficit is called **dehydration**. There are three major types of dehydration:

- **Isotonic dehydration** (or **isonatremic dehydration**) occurs when fluid loss is not balanced by intake, and the loss of water and sodium are in proportion. The serum sodium is therefore within normal limits or slightly low even though the circulating blood volume is lowered. Most of the fluid lost is from the extracellular component. This type of dehydration is commonly manifested in the illnesses of young children such as vomiting and diarrhea.

- **Hypotonic dehydration** (or **hyponatremic dehydration**) occurs when fluid loss is characterized by a proportionately greater loss of sodium than water. Serum sodium is below normal levels. Compensatory fluid shifts occur from the extracellular to intracellular components in an attempt to establish normal proportions, thus leading to even greater extracellular dehydration. Severe and prolonged vomiting and diarrhea, burns, and renal disease can lead to this condition, as well as administration of intravenous fluid without electrolytes in treatment of dehydration.

- **Hypertonic dehydration** (or **hypernatremic dehydration**) occurs when fluid loss is characterized by a proportionately greater loss of water than sodium. Serum sodium is above normal levels. Compensatory fluid shifts occur from the intracellular to extracellular components in an attempt to establish normal proportions. The extracellular component therefore remains fairly normal, delaying the onset of signs and symptoms of dehydration until the condition is quite serious. Neurologic symptoms reflecting intracellular imbalance may occur simultaneously with more common symptoms of dehydration. The condition may be caused by health problems such as diabetes insipidus (see Chapter 30) or administration of intravenous fluid or tube feedings with high electrolyte levels.

The body continuously attempts to compensate for fluid and electrolyte imbalance by shifting fluid and electrolytes from one component to another. Therefore, it is rare for only one type of dehydration to occur; the child's fluid and electrolyte status and symptoms are constantly changing. Ongoing assessment and management are needed.

ETIOLOGY AND PATHOPHYSIOLOGY

Extracellular fluid volume deficit is usually caused by the loss of sodium-containing fluid from the body. Vomiting, diarrhea, nasogastric suction, hemorrhage, and burns most often cause loss of fluid containing sodium. Vomiting and diarrhea are common manifestations of disease in children throughout the world, and each year up to 5 million children die from dehydration related to diarrhea. In the United States, about 300 to 500 die annually from this problem, about 220,000 are hospitalized, and 1.5 million receive outpatient care (Kinlin & Freedman, 2012).

Type 1 diabetes may become a cause of dehydration as the child exhibits polydipsia and polyuria (see Chapter 30 for a detailed description of diabetes). Another cause of extracellular fluid volume deficit in infants is increased water loss in low–birth-weight infants kept under radiant warmers to maintain heat (Figure 18–3). Less frequently, adrenal insufficiency, accumulation of extracellular fluid in a "third space" such as the peritoneal cavity, and overuse of diuretics may be the cause. The latter etiology is most often seen in adolescents with bulimia (see Chapter 14).

Excessive exercise during very hot weather without sufficient fluid replacement can lead to fluid and electrolyte imbalance. Physiologic differences can place children at high risk, especially when they have vigorous outdoor activity in extreme heat with inadequate rest periods. Children may not feel thirsty and therefore may fail to drink adequately even when dehydrated. Additional risk factors include obesity and a combination of high temperature, high humidity, wind, and exposure to radiant heat (American Academy of Pediatrics [AAP] Council on Sports Medicine and Fitness & Council on School Health, 2011).

Burns and gastroenteritis are characterized by initial dehydration in the first 3 days due to a high loss of extracellular fluid. About 80% of the fluid loss is extracellular and only about 20% is intracellular. However, with time, the relationship begins to

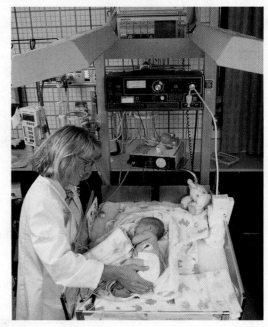

Figure 18–3 Fluid loss from overhead warming. Use of an overhead warmer or phototherapy increases insensible fluid excretion through the skin, thus increasing the fluid intake needed.

change, so that in illnesses over 3 days, about 60% of fluid loss is extracellular while 40% is intracellular (Engorn & Flerlage, 2014). Since the electrolyte composition of extracellular and intracellular fluids differs (see Table 18–1), electrolyte management will need to change for long-term conditions.

CLINICAL MANIFESTATIONS

The signs of dehydration relate to the severity or degree of the body water deficit (Table 18–3). They are a result of both the decreased fluid (e.g., diminished turgor and mucous membrane moisture) and the body's response to the fluid deficit (e.g., pulse and blood pressure changes).

TABLE 18–3 Severity of Clinical Dehydration

	MILD	MODERATE	SEVERE
Percentage of body weight lost	Up to 5% (40–50 mL/kg)	6–9% (60–90 mL/kg)	10% or more (100 mL/kg)
Level of consciousness	Alert, restless, thirsty	Irritable or lethargic (infants and very young children); alert, thirsty, restless (older children and adolescents)	Lethargic to comatose (infants and young children); often conscious, apprehensive (older children and adolescents)
Blood pressure	Normal for age	Normal or low; postural hypotension (older children and adolescents)	Low to undetectable
Pulse	Regular and strong	Rapid	Rapid, weak to nonpalpable
Skin turgor	Immediate	Poor	Very poor
Mucous membranes	Moist	Dry	Parched
Urine	Usual output	Decreased output (<1 mL/kg/hr); dark color; increased specific gravity	Very decreased or absent output
Thirst	Slightly increased	Moderately increased	Greatly increased unless lethargic
Fontanelle	Normal	Sunken	Sunken
Extremities	Warm; rapid capillary refill	Delayed capillary refill (>2 sec)	Cool, discolored; delayed capillary refill (>3–4 sec)
Respirations	Regular, usual rate	Usual or rapid rate	Changing rate and regularity
Eyes	Normal	Slightly sunken, decreased tears	Deeply sunken, absent tears

TABLE 18–4 Clinical Manifestations of Extracellular Fluid Volume Deficit

CLINICAL MANIFESTATIONS	ETIOLOGY
Weight loss	Decreased fluid volume; 1 L of fluid weighs 1 kg
Postural blood pressure drop (older children)	Inadequate circulating blood volume to offset the force of gravity when in upright position
Increased small vein filling time	Decreased vascular volume
Delayed capillary refill time	Decreased vascular volume
Flat neck veins when supine (older children)	Decreased vascular volume
Dizziness, syncope	Inadequate circulation to brain
Oliguria	Inadequate circulation to kidneys
Thready, rapid pulse	Cardiac reflex response to decreased vascular volume
Sunken fontanelle (infants)	Decreased fluid volume
Decreased skin turgor	Decreased interstitial fluid volume

Mild dehydration is hard to detect because children appear alert and have moist mucous membranes. Infants may be irritable and older children are thirsty. In moderate dehydration, the child is often lethargic and sleepy, but there may be periods of restlessness and irritability, especially in infants. Skin turgor is diminished, mucous membranes appear dry, and urine is dark in color and diminished in amount. Pulse rate is usually increased, and blood pressure can be normal or low. Severe dehydration is manifested by increasing lethargy or nonresponsiveness, markedly decreased blood pressure, rapid pulse, nonelastic skin turgor, dry mucous membranes, sunken and dry eyes, and markedly decreased or absent urinary output (Feld & Kaskel, 2012). See Table 18–4.

CLINICAL THERAPY

Diagnosis of dehydration is best accomplished by clinical observations. Medical management depends on accurate identification of the degree of dehydration. In addition to physical signs and symptoms (see Table 18–3), elevated blood urea nitrogen (BUN) (over 17 mg/dL) and low serum bicarbonate (16–17 mEq/L or mmol/L) are useful to identify dehydration from moderate and severe diarrhea (Corbett & Banks, 2013; Dzierba & Abraham, 2011). The treatment of extracellular fluid volume deficit is administration of fluid containing sodium, by oral rehydration therapy or by intravenous fluids.

Oral rehydration is the treatment of choice to treat mild and moderate dehydration in children. The therapy successfully treats the dehydration caused by many gastrointestinal illnesses and prevents hospitalization for many infants and young children (Engorn & Flerlage, 2014; Freedman, Ali, Oleszczuk, et al., 2013; Jablonski, 2012). Commercially available solutions contain water, carbohydrate (sugar), sodium, potassium, chloride, and lactate. Examples include Pedialyte, Infalyte, Rehydralyte, Ricelyte, Resol, Nutrilyte, Hydralyte, and Lytren. Some clinicians allow lactose-free milk, breast milk, or half-strength milk to be given in addition to oral rehydration therapy solution. Oral rehydration may be accompanied by ondansetron to decrease vomiting in the child and its resultant continued dehydration (Freedman et al., 2013). In developing countries, an oral rehydration solution with zinc added has been effective in diarrhea treatment (Frohna, 2011). Prebiotics (oral supplements that stimulate growth of probiotic bacteria to positively alter intestinal flora) have also been found to be effective in decreasing the number of diarrheal stools in children with acute gastrointestinal disease (Frohna, 2011).

When the child is severely dehydrated, electrolytes are measured by laboratory analysis, and isotonic intravenous fluid is given, often accompanied by oral rehydration. The intravenous fluid is commonly lactated Ringers or dilute saline, such as one half or one quarter normal saline (see Table 18–5 for types of intravenous fluids and their uses). The fluid combination replenishes the extracellular fluid volume and adds solutes to return the body fluid back to normal. Note that only isotonic solutions are used for rapid infusion, and D_5W is avoided for this treatment (Carcillo, 2014; Engorn & Flerlage, 2014; Wang, Xu, & Xiao, 2014). The child may be hospitalized or treated with intravenous fluids in a short-stay unit until the dehydration is controlled. Once hydrated, the child resumes an age-appropriate diet.

Growth and Development

Urine specific gravity may increase in older children who are dehydrated, but children under 2 years of age are not able to concentrate urine effectively. A rising specific gravity may not be seen in the younger dehydrated child.

Nursing Management
For the Child With Extracellular Fluid Volume Deficit (Dehydration)

Nursing Assessment and Diagnosis

Weigh the child daily with the same scale and without clothing. Compare to past weights and calculate weight loss. Carefully measure intake and output, urine specific gravity, level of consciousness, pulse rate and quality, skin turgor, mucous membrane moisture, quality and rate of respirations, and blood pressure. For older children and adolescents, the nurse can compare the blood pressure when the child is supine with the pressure when the child is sitting with legs hanging down or standing. If the child is dehydrated, the sitting or standing blood pressure will be lower than the supine blood pressure because blood accumulates in the dependent legs. Obtain samples of urine and blood as needed for dehydration evaluation. Urinalysis can usually be completed on a very small urine sample, such as 1 mL.

The nursing diagnosis *Fluid Volume: Deficient* applies to all children who have an extracellular fluid volume deficit. Other diagnoses depend on the severity of the condition and the age of the child. Several nursing diagnoses that might be

TABLE 18–5 Common Intravenous Solutions, Uses, and Components

IV SOLUTION	USES	CHO (g/100 mL)	PROTEIN (g/100 mL)	CAL/L	Na⁺ (mEq/L)	K⁺ (mEq/L)	Cl⁻ (mEq/L)	HCO₃⁻ (mEq/L)	Ca²⁺ (mEq/L)
					COMPONENTS				
D₅W	Restores water loss, plasma volume, and calories; lowers sodium levels	5	—	170	—	—	—	—	—
Normal saline (0.9% NaCl)	Restores water and sodium loss; maintains sodium and chloride at present levels	—	—	—	154	—	154	—	—
Lactated Ringers solution	Expands intracellular fluid; replaces extracellular losses	0–10	—	0–340	147	4	155.5	—	4
Lactated Ringers solution	Replaces fluid loss from burns, bleeding, and severe diarrhea	0–10	—	0–340	130	4	109	28	3
Albumin 25% (salt-poor albumin)	Restores major plasma protein in blood loss that has been treated with NS (plasma expander)	—	25	1000	100–160	—	<120	—	—

Note: A normal saline (NS) solution is a salt solution that has the same percentage of salt as the human body. This is a 0.9% solution of sodium chloride. The term *normal* indicates that there is the same weight, in grams, of sodium and chloride in the solution. Variations and combinations are available to tailor intake to needs of the child. For example, ½ NS (0.45% NaCl) or ¼ NS (0.225% NaCl) is often used in young children; the lower sodium content helps to avoid inadvertent hypernatremia. D₅ ½ NS and D₅ ¼ NS are combinations of D₅W and NS; they provide both carbohydrate and sodium.

Source: Adapted from Engorn, B., & Flerlage, J. (2014). *The Harriet Lane handbook* (20th ed.) St. Louis, MO: Elsevier Saunders; LeMone, P., Burke, K. M., Bauldoff, G., & Gubrud, P. (2015). *Medical surgical nursing* (6th ed.). Hoboken, NJ: Prentice Hall Health.

appropriate for the mildly to severely dehydrated child are included in the accompanying *Nursing Care Plans*. Additional care of the child with dehydration from gastroenteritis can be found in Chapter 25. Nursing diagnoses might include the following (NANDA-I © 2014):

- *Fluid Volume: Deficient* related to active fluid volume loss or failure of regulatory mechanisms
- *Tissue Perfusion: Peripheral, Risk for Ineffective*, related to hypovolemia
- *Injury, Risk for*, related to postural hypotension

Clinical Reasoning The Dehydrated Child

LeShan is 18 months old. Several days ago he developed vomiting and diarrhea. His parents tried to get him to eat, but he had little appetite. He drank a little water and a few sips of juice, but the next morning he was listless and would not drink anything. The diarrhea continued.

His father has brought him to the urgent care center. LeShan is irritable on arrival, and his father reports that he has been alternately irritable and lethargic. His mucous membranes and tongue appear dry, and his skin turgor over the abdomen is slightly decreased. His father notes that LeShan has had only two wet diapers today and says the urine in his diaper was dark in color. He also reports that LeShan weighed 12 kg (26 lb) at the clinic last week. However, when the nurse weighs him, the scale reads only 11 kg (24.5 lb). What do LeShan's symptoms suggest about his degree of dehydration? What nursing interventions should be planned?

Planning and Implementation

Nursing care of the dehydrated child focuses first on prevention of the problem, and then on providing oral rehydration fluids, teaching parents oral rehydration methods, and, if necessary, administering intravenous fluids to restore fluid balance. The accompanying *Nursing Care Plans* summarize care of the child with mild to severe dehydration.

Clinical Tip

To obtain urine from an infant for testing specific gravity, place two cotton balls in the diaper. When they are wet, push them into a 10-mL syringe and squeeze out the urine with the plunger. Remember to use gloves for this procedure.

PREVENT DEHYDRATION

Nursing care can often prevent dehydration. Carefully monitor temperature probes in radiant warmers and isolettes for newborns to prevent overheating and resulting dehydration. Teach parents proper clothing for infants to prevent overheating. Nurses play an important role in educating parents, youth, school personnel, and coaches about the dangers of heat-related illness. Prevention is essential, so that children can exercise safely. Prior to a new exercise regimen, assessment for risk factors is performed. This includes medical conditions that put the child at high risk, such as cystic fibrosis, diabetes, obesity, or intellectual disability. Prior history of heat-related illness or recent change from a cooler to a hotter environment increases risk. Long exercise periods increase the stress on the body. The major nursing interventions are partnering with families and athletic coaches to prevent problems and to recognize and treat them promptly.

Nursing Care Plan: The Child With Mild or Moderate Dehydration

1. Nursing Diagnosis: *Health Management, Family, Ineffective,* **related to knowledge deficit about diarrhea and vomiting (NANDA-I © 2014)**

GOAL: The parents will describe appropriate home management of fluid replacement for diarrhea and vomiting.

INTERVENTION	RATIONALE
• Explain how to replace body fluid with an oral rehydration solution. Encourage parents to keep the solution at home and begin use with the first sign of diarrhea.	• Use of an oral rehydration solution can enable successful treatment of vomiting and diarrhea at home.
• Teach parents to continue the child's normal diet in addition to providing replacement fluids for diarrhea.	• Diet plus fluid supplementation leads to faster recovery.
• Provide verbal and written instructions to parents at each well-child visit. Teach hand hygiene for general use and during illness.	• Parents are provided with a reference for later use. Hand hygiene is the most effective measure to prevent illness that leads to dehydration.

EXPECTED OUTCOME: Parents will be able to treat successfully the child's diarrhea and vomiting at home.

2. Nursing Diagnosis: *Knowledge, Deficient (Parent),* **related to causes of dehydration (NANDA-I © 2014)**

GOAL: The parents will state common causes of childhood dehydration.

INTERVENTION	RATIONALE
• Teach parents childhood conditions that commonly lead to dehydration.	• If parents recognize situations that can lead to dehydration, they will be more alert to its appearance.

EXPECTED OUTCOME: Parents will recognize conditions of risk for dehydration in children.

3. Nursing Diagnosis: *Fluid Volume: Deficient, Risk for,* **related to worsening of child's condition (NANDA-I © 2014)**

GOAL: The parents will seek health care for the child's worsening condition.

INTERVENTION	RATIONALE
• Teach parents to seek care when the child's vomiting or diarrhea worsens, when urine output via diaper or toilet decreases, or when the child's mental alertness changes.	• Severe dehydration may occur if milder forms are not successfully treated.

EXPECTED OUTCOME: Parents will seek prompt attention for the child's worsening condition, preventing the development of severe dehydration.

Nursing Care Plan: The Child With Severe Dehydration

1. Nursing Diagnosis: *Fluid Volume: Deficient* **related to excess losses and inadequate intake (NANDA-I © 2014)**

GOAL: The child will return to normal hydration status and will not develop hypovolemic shock.

INTERVENTION	RATIONALE
• Monitor weight daily. Assess intake and output every shift. Assess heart rate, postural blood pressure, skin turgor, small vein filling time, capillary refill time, fontanelle (infant), and urine specific gravity every 4 hours or more frequently as indicated.	• Frequent assessment of hydration status facilitates rapid intervention and evaluation of the effectiveness of fluid replacement.
• Administer intravenous fluid as ordered. Monitor for crackles in dependent portions of the lungs.	• Replace fluid lost from the body. Excessive replacement of sodium-containing fluids could cause extracellular fluid volume excess.

EXPECTED OUTCOME: The child will exhibit signs of normal hydration.

Nursing Care Plan: The Child With Severe Dehydration (*continued*)

2. Nursing Diagnosis: *Injury, Risk for,* related to decreased level of consciousness (NANDA-I © 2014)

GOAL: The child will not experience injury.

INTERVENTION	RATIONALE
• Raise the side rails of the bed. Ensure that a small child does not become tangled in bed covers.	• Safety measures protect the child.
• Monitor level of consciousness every 2–4 hr or more often as indicated.	• Frequent assessment provides evidence of the need for safety interventions and of the effectiveness of therapy.
• Monitor serum sodium concentration daily or more often.	• Elevated serum sodium concentration causes brain cell shrinkage and decreased level of consciousness.
• Have the child sit before rising from bed and assist to stand slowly.	• Slow adjustment to upright posture reduces lightheadedness from decreased blood volume.

EXPECTED OUTCOME: Child will not fall or suffer other injuries.

3. Nursing Diagnosis: *Activity Intolerance* related to bed rest immobility (NANDA-I © 2014)

GOAL: The child will engage in normal activity for age.

INTERVENTION	RATIONALE
• Plan activities appropriate for the age of the child that can be done in bed.	• Activities will provide distraction and promote recovery.
• Group nursing interventions to provide time for the child to rest.	• The child will require more rest than usual.
• Provide assistance during meals and other activities as needed.	• Prevention of overexertion will conserve body fluid and promote healing.

EXPECTED OUTCOME: Child will engage in normal developmental activities and receive adequate rest.

PROVIDE ORAL REHYDRATION FLUIDS

In mild or moderate dehydration, oral rehydration fluid is the first intervention. It is given in frequent small amounts; for example, 1 to 3 teaspoons of fluid every 10 to 15 minutes is a useful guideline for starting oral rehydration. For the first 2 to 4 hours of treatment, 50 mL of fluid for each kilogram of the child's weight should be the target intake (Children's Mercy Hospital, 2011). Instruct parents to continue to administer 1 teaspoon every 2 to 3 minutes even if the child vomits, because small amounts of the fluid may still be absorbed. Table 18–6 outlines guidelines for oral rehydration therapy.

TEACH PARENTS ORAL REHYDRATION METHODS

Instruct parents about the types of fluids and amounts to be given. Begin teaching with parents of all newborns and reinforce

TABLE 18–6 Oral Rehydration Therapy Guidelines

CHILD'S CONDITION	RECOMMENDATION
No diarrhea, no dehydration	Continue on age-appropriate diet.
Minimal dehydration	If the child weighs less than 22 lb (10 kg), give 60–120 mL oral rehydration solution (ORS) for each diarrheal stool or vomiting episode; if over 22 lb (10 kg) in weight, give 120–240 mL ORS for each diarrheal stool or vomiting episode. Meanwhile, continue breastfeeding, or resume age-appropriate diet after initial hydration. Start slowly, administering 3–5 mL in a small cup or spoon every few minutes. Increase amounts gradually if no vomiting occurs. Recommend or provide samples of ORS; suggest ready-to-feed or powdered forms to use by parents.
Moderate dehydration	Give 50–100 mL/kg ORS in 3–4 hr in addition to replacing fluids lost as described above.
Severe dehydration	The child is hospitalized and treated with intravenous fluids. When hydrated adequately or concurrently with intravenous rehydration, begin oral rehydration therapy with 100 mL/kg of fluid in 4 hr and stool replacement as described above. Recalculate fluid needs after first 4 hr and adjust as needed.
Rehydration complete	Resume normal diet.

Source: Data from Children's Mercy Hospital. (2011). *Guidelines for oral rehydration.* Retrieved from http://www.childrensmercy.org/Content/view.aspx?id=8130

teaching at each well-child visit. Advise parents to continue the child's normal diet in addition to providing the rehydration solution. Cereal, starches, soup, fruits, and vegetables are all allowed. Tell parents to avoid simple sugars, which can worsen diarrhea because of osmotic effects. This includes soft drinks (if used, they should be diluted with equal parts of water), undiluted juice, Jell-O, and sweetened cereal.

SAFETY ALERT!

Encourage parents to keep an oral rehydration solution in liquid or powder form on hand at all times and to use these solutions rather than juice, soda, or other drinks when the child first develops diarrhea or vomiting.

If an oral rehydration solution is too concentrated, it can make diarrhea worse. Juice, cola, and many sports drinks are very concentrated and should be diluted to half strength if they are the only fluids available to be given to a child who has diarrhea. Sugar facilitates the absorption of sodium in oral rehydration fluids. In addition, tell parents not to give diet beverages for oral rehydration because they contain no sugar and will not be effectively absorbed.

Repeated vomiting of large volumes of fluid, increasing diarrhea, or a worsening of the child's condition can indicate the need for intravenous therapy. Teach parents when to seek further medical care. If the child's condition worsens or does not improve after 4 hours of oral rehydration therapy, parents should contact a healthcare provider. Dizziness or lethargy are symptoms that can be manifestations of dehydration and indicate the need for further health care.

MONITOR INTRAVENOUS FLUID ADMINISTRATION

The hospitalized child usually requires intravenous fluids. Use volume control devices for measuring and monitoring intake. Be sure that the amount of fluid administered corresponds with the diagnosed dehydration state of the child (Table 18–7). Usually, about one half of the 24-hour total maintenance and replacement needs is given in the first 6 to 8 hours, with a slower rate infused for the remainder of the 24 hours. During the first 1 to 3 hours, the infusion rate may be highest to rapidly expand the vascular space. Electrolytes, such as potassium, are not added until the child has voided a sufficient quantity of urine for age in order to avoid hyperkalemia. Rapid infusion of a bolus of isotonic fluid (normal saline or lactated Ringers but *not* D_5W) in the amount of 20 mL/kg over 20 minutes is sometimes used in outpatient settings, followed by oral fluids (Kliegman, Stanton, St. Geme, et al., 2011). Careful monitoring of intake and output is needed to ensure that the intravenous line remains in place until the child is tolerating oral fluids and taking in enough to maintain hydration. Verify that the type of fluid prescribed is being administered. When oral fluids are maintained, the child may be discharged and hospitalization avoided.

Maintain the intravenous line carefully so fluid infusion can be kept on schedule (refer to the *Clinical Skills Manual* SKILLS). Use a pump to prevent inadvertent, rapid infusion, which can lead to fluid overload and electrolyte imbalance (Figure 18–4). Play with the toddler and preschool child frequently and use diversionary methods as necessary to distract the child from the intravenous line. Monitor the child carefully and implement safety precautions as necessary. Once the child begins to tolerate some oral fluids, substitute oral rehydration therapy for intravenous fluids. Frequent administration of appropriate fluids is needed.

TABLE 18–7 Calculation of Intravenous Fluid Needs

STEP	CALCULATION
Calculate the maintenance fluid needs of the child, using guidelines at right.	Usual Weight Maintenance Amount Up to 10 kg 100 mL/kg/24 hr 11–20 kg 1000 mL + (50 mL/kg for weight above 10 kg)/24 hr >20 kg 1500 mL + (20 mL/kg for weight above 20 kg)/24 hr
Calculate replacement fluid for that lost, using formula at right to obtain mL/kg/24 hr required.	Percentage of body weight loss × 10 × normal weight = mL/kg/24 hr required
Calculate continued losses; add them to total of maintenance and replacement needs.	

DISCHARGE PLANNING AND HOME CARE TEACHING

Prior to discharge, parents need instructions about types of fluids and amounts to encourage. Teach the signs of dehydration (see Table 18–3) so that if the child does not take in adequate fluids, parents can seek help immediately. Instruct them to begin the child's normal diet once hydration is completed, determined by adequate urinary output and normal behaviors. Review methods of minimizing the child's chance of acquiring gastrointestinal infections (e.g., avoiding contact with other children who are infected; using careful hand washing and dishwashing procedures when another child in the home is sick). During well-child visits, encourage all parents to keep oral rehydration fluids at home in case they are needed; they are available in most grocery stores and pharmacies. Address the needs for increasing fluids in hot weather and when the child is exercising. See *Evidence-Based Practice: Treatment for Mild and Moderate Dehydration.*

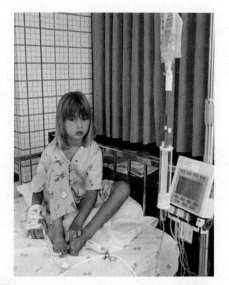

Figure 18–4 The use of a volume control device with an intravenous saline solution is important to prevent a sudden extracellular fluid volume overload.

EVIDENCE-BASED PRACTICE | Treatment for Mild and Moderate Dehydration

Clinical Question

In spite of recommendations that children with mild or moderate dehydration be treated with oral rehydration therapy for gastroenteritis, many healthcare facilities and providers administer intravenous fluids to these children. How can nurses work to improve dehydration treatment to be consistent with current guidelines?

The Evidence

In the United States alone, gastroenteritis leads to 1.5 million healthcare visits annually and 200,000 hospitalizations. Most children can effectively be treated with an oral solution of glucose, electrolytes, and water. Such treatment is less invasive and painful than intravenous therapy for young children and is safe, effective, and easy to administer in the home setting. It is also recommended by the World Health Organization (WHO, 2014) and the American Academy of Pediatrics (AAP, 2013). However, many healthcare providers continue to use intravenous fluid treatment for mild to moderate rehydration (Jablonski, 2012). Even though nasogastric feeding is recommended when oral rehydration fails, all healthcare providers in a study of 113 emergency department personnel bypassed nasogastric feeding and began an intravenous line (Freedman, Keating, Rumatir, et al., 2012). A majority of 75 parents who visited an emergency department with a child who had gastroenteritis and dehydration expected the child to have an intravenous line, even when dehydration was mild or moderate (Nir, Nadir,

Schechter, et al., 2013). A meta-analysis of 19 studies on use of oral rehydration solution found that social marketing, media education, and distribution of product increased parental acceptance and use of oral rehydration therapy (Lenters, Das, & Bhutta, 2013).

Best Practice

Nurses can partner with other healthcare providers to establish clinical pathways for dehydration treatment that follow recommendations for oral or nasogastric feedings. Implementing oral rehydration therapy immediately after assessment of the child assists in effective treatment. Appropriate oral rehydration solutions should be available on pediatric units, in emergency departments, and in all homes with children. Educate parents and healthcare providers about the benefits of oral rehydration for mild or moderate dehydration.

Clinical Reasoning

What questions can you ask a parent and what assessments can you perform to accurately evaluate if the child has mild or moderate dehydration? What oral rehydration solutions can the parent have available in the home setting? How will you inform colleagues of the current recommendations for the treatment of mild or moderate dehydration? How will you teach parents to administer oral rehydration in the home and what symptoms indicate that they need to seek additional care for the child?

Evaluation

Expected outcomes of nursing care include the following:

- Water and electrolytes in intracellular and extracellular compartments show adequate balance.
- The child has normal urinary output.
- The child maintains adequate fluid intake for maintenance needs.
- Vital signs remain within normal limits.

Extracellular Fluid Volume Excess

Extracellular fluid volume excess occurs when there is too much fluid in the vascular and interstitial compartment. This imbalance may also be called saline excess or extracellular volume overload. If this disorder occurs by itself (without saline disturbance), the serum sodium concentration is normal. There is simply too much extracellular fluid, even though it has a normal concentration.

Infants and children who develop an extracellular fluid volume excess have a condition that causes them to retain **saline** (sodium and water) or have been given an overload of sodium-containing isotonic intravenous fluid (Figure 18–5). What conditions cause retention of saline? The hormone aldosterone is secreted by the adrenal cortex. One of its normal functions is to cause the kidneys to retain saline in the body (see *Pathophysiology Illustrated: Aldosterone Effects*). Saline excess can be caused by any condition that results in excessive aldosterone secretion, such as adrenal tumors that secrete aldosterone, congestive heart failure, liver cirrhosis, and chronic renal failure. Most glucocorticoid medications (such as prednisone) have a mild saline-retaining effect when taken

on a long-term basis. Intravenous fluid volume regulation is important, especially in young children. Either inaccurate calculation of needed fluid or inadvertent infusion of excess fluids can cause overload.

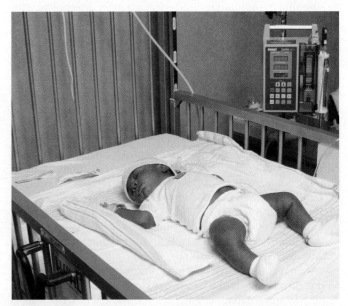

Figure 18–5 **Preventing extracellular fluid volume overload. If isotonic fluid containing sodium is given too rapidly or in too great an amount, an extracellular fluid volume excess will develop. Carefully monitor fluid intake, excretion, and retention in infants and children.**

Pathophysiology Illustrated: **Aldosterone Effects**

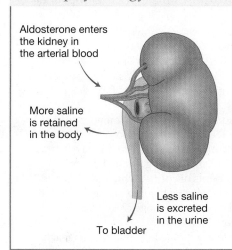

Aldosterone enters the kidney in the arterial blood

More saline is retained in the body

Less saline is excreted in the urine

To bladder

Aldosterone has a saline-retaining effect. Increased aldosterone secretion can be caused by adrenal tumors or congestive heart failure.

Extracellular fluid volume excess is characterized by sudden weight gain. A gain of 0.5 kg (1 lb) in a day is related to fluid, and represents 500 mL of saline. An overload of fluid in the blood vessels and interstitial spaces can cause clinical manifestations such as bounding pulse, distended neck veins in children (not usually evident in infants), periorbital edema, hepatomegaly, dyspnea, orthopnea, and lung crackles. Edema is the sign of overload of the interstitial fluid compartment. In an infant, edema is often generalized (Figure 18–6). Edema in children with extracellular fluid volume excess occurs in the dependent parts of the body—that is, in the parts closest to the ground. Thus, edema is evident in sacral areas in a child supine in bed. Scrotum or labia may be edematous. (Edema that develops from other causes is described in the next section of this chapter.)

The clinical therapy for extracellular fluid volume excess focuses on treating the underlying cause of the disorder. For example, a child who has congestive heart failure is given medications to strengthen the heart's ability to contract. Managing the cause also helps reduce the extracellular fluid volume excess. Diuretics may be given to remove fluid from the body, thus reducing the extracellular fluid volume directly.

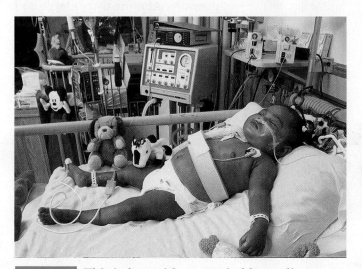

Figure 18–6 This infant with congenital heart disease has signs of generalized edema. Note the fluid retention in the face and abdomen.

Nursing Management

Rapid weight gain is the most sensitive index of extracellular fluid volume excess. Therefore, daily weighing with the same scale and articles of clothing is an important nursing assessment. Measure the child's intake and output. For babies in diapers, a diaper is weighed dry and then wet, with grams of weight increase equal to urine volume in milliliters. When treatment is successful, output is greater than intake. Assess the character of the pulse and observe for neck vein distention when the child is sitting (usually visible only in older children). Monitor for signs of pulmonary edema (an indication of severe imbalance) by listening to lung sounds in the dependent lung fields (crackles) and assessing for respiratory distress (rapid respiratory rate, use of accessory muscles of respiration). Observe for edema.

A child may develop a fluid overload whenever an isotonic intravenous solution containing sodium, such as normal saline or lactated Ringers solution, is administered. Therefore, monitor the infusion rate frequently and carefully and use a volume control device and pump whenever possible to aid in accurate administration. Use only small bags (e.g., 250 or 500 mL) for infants and young children, and check pumps frequently. If an excess of fluid has already developed, administer the medical therapy as prescribed and monitor for any complications of the medical therapy. For example, many diuretics increase potassium excretion in the urine, which may lead to an abnormally low plasma potassium concentration unless potassium intake is increased. (Refer to the discussion of hypokalemia later in this chapter.) It is also important to monitor for the development of extracellular fluid volume deficit as a result of diuretic therapy.

If edema is present, provide careful skin care and protection for edematous areas. Teach parents how to provide skin care and perform position changes at home. See the following section for additional interventions related to edema.

If a child has a long-term condition such as chronic renal failure that predisposes to extracellular fluid volume excess, a dietary fluid and sodium restriction may be prescribed (see Chapter 26 for further details). Teach parents how to manage sodium restriction. Plan low-sodium meals that fit the family's cultural practices. If the child is old enough to participate, incorporate games into the teaching. If a scale is available, teach parents to take and record an accurate daily weight.

Desired outcomes include electrolyte balance, maintenance of intact skin, and dietary intake as prescribed.

Interstitial Fluid Volume Excess (Edema)

Edema is an abnormal increase in the volume of the interstitial fluid. It may be caused by an extracellular fluid volume excess or it may result from other causes.

The causes of edema are best understood in the context of normal capillary dynamics. Fluid moves between the vascular and interstitial compartment by the process of **filtration**. Filtration is the net result of forces that tend to move fluid in opposing directions. The strongest forces determine the direction of fluid movement.

At the capillary level, two forces (blood hydrostatic pressure and interstitial osmotic pressure) tend to move fluid from the capillaries into the interstitial fluid, while two other forces (blood colloid osmotic pressure and interstitial fluid hydrostatic pressure) tend to move fluid in the opposite direction (from the interstitial fluid into the capillaries). The net result of these forces usually moves fluid from the capillaries into the interstitial compartment at the arterial end of the capillaries, and fluid from the interstitial compartment back into the capillaries at the venous end of the capillaries. This process brings oxygen and nutrients to the cells and removes carbon dioxide and other waste products.

Developing Cultural Competence Low-Sodium Diets

To adapt teaching about low-sodium diets to the cultural practices of a family, ask clients what types of food they usually eat. Help them choose low-sodium foods from their diets and avoid high-sodium foods. This approach is more effective than giving the same list of restricted foods to each family.

For example, some Asians may use monosodium glutamate to flavor foods and can be encouraged to add this at the table for family members who can have extra sodium rather than during cooking. Many Hispanic groups use large amounts of cheese, which can provide significant sodium. Encourage them to look for low-sodium cheese and substitute cottage cheese for other types since it is lower in sodium.

Canned foods tend to have high sodium, so teach all families to use fresh or frozen produce rather than canned when possible. Low-sodium milk is available and is a good option for young children. Teach families how to read and interpret food labels to identify salt (sodium) content.

Pathophysiology Illustrated: Capillary Dynamics and Edema

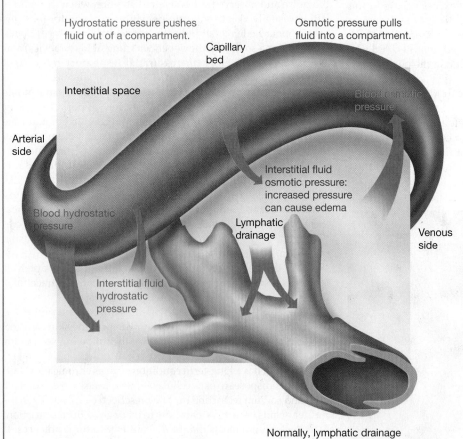

Hydrostatic pressure pushes fluid out of a compartment.

Osmotic pressure pulls fluid into a compartment.

Capillary bed

Interstitial space

Blood osmotic pressure

Arterial side

Blood hydrostatic pressure

Interstitial fluid osmotic pressure: increased pressure can cause edema

Lymphatic drainage

Venous side

Interstitial fluid hydrostatic pressure

Normally, lymphatic drainage removes small proteins and excess interstitial fluid. Blocked lymphatic drainage can cause edema.

With normal capillary dynamics, fluid moves out of the compartment by the force of hydrostatic pressure in the blood vessel and is pulled out by interstitial osmotic pressure. Fluid is forced into the compartment by interstitial hydrostatic pressure and pulled in by compartment osmotic pressure. Abnormal capillary dynamics can cause edema.

TABLE 18–8 Clinical Conditions That Cause Edema

CONDITION	RESULTING HEMODYNAMIC CHANGE	RESULT
Increased blood hydrostatic pressure	Increased capillary blood flow Venous congestion	Inflammation Local infection Extracellular fluid volume excess Right heart failure Venous thrombosis External pressure on vein Muscle paralysis
Decreased blood osmotic pressure	Increased albumin excretion Decreased albumin synthesis	Nephrotic syndrome (albumin leaks into urine) Protein-losing enteropathies (excess albumin in feces) Kwashiorkor (low-protein, high-carbohydrate starvation diet provides too few amino acids for liver to make albumin) Liver cirrhosis (diseased liver unable to make enough albumin)
Increased interstitial fluid osmotic pressure	Increased capillary permeability	Inflammation Toxins Hypersensitivity reactions Burns
Blocked lymphatic drainage	Venous congestion	Tumors Goiter Parasites that obstruct lymph nodes Surgery that removes lymph nodes

Edema occurs if the balance of these four forces is altered so that excess fluid either enters or leaves the interstitial compartment (see *Pathophysiology Illustrated: Capillary Dynamics and Edema*). This may occur through:

1. Increased blood hydrostatic pressure
2. Decreased blood colloid osmotic pressure
3. Increased interstitial fluid osmotic pressure
4. Blocked lymphatic drainage

Many clinical conditions are associated with these altered forces (Table 18–8), as described in the following list:

1. Increased blood hydrostatic pressure. When extracellular fluid volume excess occurs, the increased fluid volume in the vascular compartment congests the veins. The pressure against the sides of the capillary is increased and more fluid then enters the interstitial compartment.

2. Decreased blood colloid osmotic pressure. Much of the osmotic pressure that pulls fluid into the capillaries is a result of the presence of albumin and other plasma proteins made by the liver. The part of the blood osmotic pressure that results from plasma proteins is often called **oncotic pressure**, or blood colloid osmotic pressure. Any condition that decreases plasma proteins will decrease blood colloid osmotic pressure and cause edema. For example, if a clinical condition causes large amounts of albumin to leak into the urine, the liver will not be able to make albumin fast enough to replace it. As a result the plasma protein level will fall, decreasing the blood osmotic pressure. Without this pulling force to return fluid to the capillaries, edema will occur. This is the cause of edema in children who have nephrotic syndrome (see Chapter 26).

3. Increased interstitial fluid osmotic pressure. Ordinarily, only a few small proteins enter the interstitial fluid, and the interstitial fluid osmotic pressure is small. However, if the capillary becomes abnormally permeable to proteins, the influx of large amounts of proteins into the interstitial fluid causes a dramatic increase in interstitial fluid osmotic pressure. The increased pulling force keeps an abnormal amount of fluid in the interstitial compartment. This mechanism plays an important part in the edema caused by a bee sting or a sprained ankle. It occurs to a greater extent in burns, leading to swelling at the same time that there is a great loss of fluid volume through the burned skin (see Chapter 31).

4. Blocked lymphatic drainage. The lymph vessels normally drain small proteins and excess fluid from the interstitial compartment and return them to the blood vessels. If lymph vessels are blocked, fluid accumulates in the interstitial compartment. This may occur when a tumor blocks lymphatic drainage.

Edema causes localized or generalized swelling, which may cause pain and restrict motion. Edema due to extracellular fluid volume excess or right-sided heart failure usually occurs in the dependent portion of the body. In a child who is walking, dependent edema is observed in the ankles; in a bedfast, supine child, it is seen in the sacral area. The skin over an edematous area often appears thin and shiny.

The main focus of clinical therapy for edema is to treat the underlying condition that caused the edema. Such conditions are discussed throughout this book. The edema from inflammation of an injury is initially treated with cold to reduce capillary blood flow and thus reduce blood hydrostatic pressure.

Nursing Management

A child or parent may make comments that alert the nurse to the development of edema. Shoes may become tight by the end of the day (dependent edema); the waistband of pants or a skirt may be "outgrown" suddenly (generalized edema or ascites [accumulation of fluid in the peritoneal cavity]); the eyes may be puffy (periorbital edema); a ring may be too tight; fingers may "feel like sausages." In many cases, visual inspection is sufficient to recognize edema. Observe for **pitting**

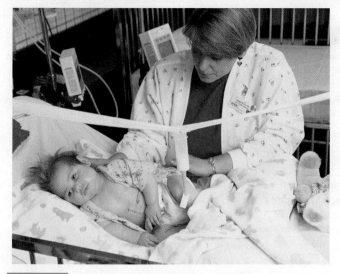

Figure 18–7 **Care of edematous tissue. Edematous tissue is easily damaged. It must be kept clean and dry and free of pressure.**

edema, a "pit" or concave indentation that remains after an edematous area is pressed downward by the examiner's fingers. To detect changes in the amount of swelling, measure around the edematous part. If the edema is caused by extracellular fluid volume excess, daily measurements of weight and intake and output are a necessary part of the daily assessment. Nursing assessment should also focus on the integrity of the skin, presence of pain, restricted motion, and alterations in the child's body image.

Elevation of an area of localized edema helps to reduce the swelling. The skin over an edematous area needs extra care because it is fragile and prone to breakdown (Figure 18–7). Carefully position an infant or child on bed rest and turn frequently to prevent pressure sores. Perform turning carefully to avoid skin abrasion by rubbing against the sheets. Pat the skin dry after cleansing rather than rubbing it. Trim the child's fingernails smooth to prevent scratching. Teach parents skin care for the child at home. Teach older children to inspect their skin carefully to identify areas needing special care.

If restricted mobility is a problem, make specific plans to help the child manage activities. For example, if an edematous finger restricts the motion of a hand, food can be cut into bite-sized portions before the meal is served, so that the child can still eat independently.

Discomfort from edema may require creative nursing interventions. Distraction with toys or activities appropriate to the child's developmental level can be useful. Interventions to treat the underlying problem can also reduce the edema and its accompanying discomfort. Interventions for edema should be added to the nursing management of the underlying condition that causes the edema. Administration of the prescribed medical therapy and observation for the complications of therapy are nursing responsibilities.

Discuss with school-age children and adolescents feelings of embarrassment about the edematous appearance. They need to understand the reason for edema and be able to explain it to peers. Arrange for the child to meet other children with similar concerns.

Desired outcomes of care include maintenance of intact skin, normal respiratory sounds and effort, and normal weight patterns.

ELECTROLYTE IMBALANCES

All body fluids contain electrolytes, although the concentration of those electrolytes varies depending on the type and location of the fluid. When a serum electrolyte value is reported from the laboratory, it provides information about the concentration of that electrolyte in the blood. It may not necessarily reflect the concentration of the electrolyte in other body compartments. Refer to Table 18–1 to see which electrolytes have the highest and lowest concentrations in the blood and other fluid compartments.

Electrolytes are normally gained and lost in relatively equal amounts so that the body remains in balance. However, when a child has an abnormal route of loss, such as vomiting, wound drainage, or nasogastric suction, electrolyte balance can be disturbed. In addition, supplementation with electrolytes via intravenous fluids in proportions different than body fluids can also cause electrolyte imbalance. Children with disease states that interfere with normal mechanisms of electrolyte regulation, such as renal disease, also have disturbance in electrolyte levels. Monitoring for signs of imbalance becomes important in all of these situations.

Sodium Imbalances

The serum sodium concentration reflects the **osmolality** of body fluids—that is, their degree of concentration or dilution. It refers to the number of moles of the substance per kilogram of water in the solution. Serum sodium concentration reflects the proportion of water and sodium in the extracellular compartment. When the osmolality of body fluids becomes abnormal, the cells swell or shrink. These cell size changes are due to **osmosis**, the movement of water across a semipermeable membrane into an area of higher particle concentration. Sodium levels are maintained at high extracellular and low intracellular levels by the sodium-potassium pump, which moves these electrolytes against their expected concentration gradients (Figure 18–8).

Hypernatremia

Hypernatremia is a condition of increased osmolality of the blood. The body fluids are too concentrated, containing excess sodium relative to water. Sodium level generally falls between 132 and 141 mmol/L, and a serum sodium level above 146 mmol/L in children (146 mmol/L in newborns) is diagnostic of hypernatremia (Engorn & Flerlage, 2014; Greenbaum, 2011) (Table 18–9).

Hypernatremia is caused by conditions that cause the body to lose relatively more water than sodium or to gain relatively more sodium than water (Table 18–10). Special circumstances in which a high solute intake may occur without adequate water include an infant formula that is too concentrated or one that is prepared with salt instead of sugar. A breastfed baby not receiving adequate breast milk who has normal water loss may develop hypernatremic dehydration. This is a risk at 2 to 3 days of age, when babies generally have a diuresis, if the baby does not feed well or the mother does not yet produce an adequate amount of breast milk (Bolat et al., 2013).

An infant or child who has hypernatremia is generally thirsty. The urine output is small unless the hypernatremia is caused by diabetes insipidus. A decreased level of consciousness manifested by confusion, lethargy, or coma results from shrinking of the brain cells. Seizures can occur when hypernatremia occurs rapidly or is severe. Severe hypernatremia can be fatal.

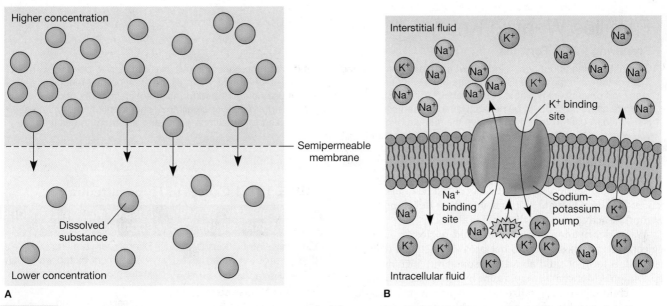

Figure 18–8 The sodium-potassium pump. *A*, Water balance is maintained by the simple passage of molecules from greater to lesser concentration across cell membranes. *B*, Sodium levels are maintained by an active transport system, the sodium-potassium pump, which moves these electrolytes across cell membranes in spite of their concentration.

TABLE 18–9 Normal Serum Values

BLOOD COMPONENT	VALUES
Sodium	Newborn: 131–144 mmol/L
	Children: 134–143 mmol/L
Potassium	Premature infants: 4.5–7.2 mmol/L
	Full-term infants: 3.2–5.7 mmol/L
	Children: 3.7–5.0 mmol/L
Calcium (total)	Premature infants: 1.7–2.3 mmol/L (6.9–9.2 mg/dL)
	Full-term infants: 1.98–2.68 mmol/L (7.9–10.7 mg/dL)
	Children: 2.18–2.68 mmol/L (8.7–10.7 mg/dL)
Magnesium	Infants: 0.65–1.02 mmol/L or 1.6–2.5 mg/dL
	Children: 0.66–0.99 mmol/L or 1.6–2.4 mg/dL
Arterial pH	Infants: 7.18–7.5
	Children: 7.27–7.49
	Adolescents: 7.35–7.41
Arterial Po_2	Infants: 60–70 mmHg (8–9.3 pKa)
	Children: 80–108 mmHg (10.7–14.4 pKa)
	Adolescents: 80–100 mmHg (4.3–6.4 pKa)
Arterial Pco_2	Infants: 27–41 mmHg (3.6–5.5 pKa)
	Children and adolescents: 32–48 mmHg (4.3–6.4 pKa)
Arterial bicarbonate	Infants: 19–24 mmol/L
	Children: 18–25 mmol/L
	Adolescents: 20–29 mmol/L

Note: Laboratories may have slightly different levels for normal depending on assays performed. Always consult the normal values for your particular laboratory.

Source: From Greenbaum, L. A. (2011). Electrolyte and acid–base disorder. In R. M. Kliegman, B. F. Stanton, J. W. St. Geme, N. F. Schor, & R. E. Behrman (Eds.), *Nelson textbook of pediatrics* (19th ed., pp. 212–242). Philadelphia, PA: Saunders; Soldin, S. J., Wong, E. C., Brugnara, C., & Soldin, O. P. (2011). *Pediatric reference ranges* (7th ed.). Washington, DC: American Association for Clinical Chemistry.

TABLE 18–10 Causes of Hypernatremia

LOSS OF RELATIVELY MORE WATER THAN SODIUM	GAIN OF RELATIVELY MORE SODIUM THAN WATER
Inadequate breastfeeding intake with normal output	Inability to communicate thirst
Diabetes insipidus (not enough antidiuretic hormone)	Limited or no access to water
Diarrhea or vomiting without fluid replacement	High solute intake without adequate water (e.g., tube feedings)
Excessive sweating without fluid replacement	Intravenous hypertonic saline
Increased aldosterone	Improper formula preparation leading to excessive concentration

Serum sodium, specific gravity of urine, antidiuretic hormone (ADH), and 24-hour urine are common diagnostic tests. Hypernatremia is treated by intravenous administration of **hypotonic fluid**, or fluid that is more dilute than normal body fluid. This therapy dilutes the body fluids back to normal concentration. If a child is dehydrated, **isotonic fluids** (those with the osmolality of body fluids) may be administered first to replenish the volume, followed by hypotonic fluid to correct the osmolality. The underlying cause of the disorder is also treated.

Nursing Management

Monitor serum sodium level and measure intake and output and urine specific gravity. Normal specific gravity under 2 years is 1.001 to 1.018, while in children over 2 years 1.001 to 1.030 is the normal range (Corbett & Banks, 2013). Specific gravity changes toward normal levels as therapy progresses. Frequently assess responsiveness to monitor the effect of hypernatremia on brain cells. As the concentration of body fluids returns to normal, the child will become more alert and responsive. Watch for rebound hyponatremia while monitoring the fluid replacement.

Families Want to Know

Preparing Infant Formula

Careful teaching about how to mix powdered formula is needed so that it is not too concentrated; this can help to prevent hypernatremia in the infant. Demonstrate the technique so that parents are well informed. Pictures are an important teaching tool if the parents are not able to read labels or instructions. When families use concentrated formula, equal amounts of concentrate and water should be mixed. Caution parents that even if an infant is premature or small, they should mix the formula as instructed. A useful strategy is to have the parents bring the formula being used to a healthcare visit and ask them to mix it as you watch. Any errors in technique can easily be corrected.

Implement safety interventions such as raised bed rails for protection. Ensure adequate rest and introduce developmentally appropriate activities when the child is alert.

Water deprivation is a form of child neglect or abuse. In neglect, the parents simply do not provide adequate water for the child. A form of child abuse that sometimes includes water deprivation is Münchausen syndrome by proxy (see Chapter 17). A small child who is hospitalized with hypernatremia that does not have a detectable cause may be subject to water deprivation. Assess the child's general condition, developmental tasks, the family dynamics, and the parents' understanding of formula preparation and the child's fluid intake needs.

Teaching can prevent many cases of hypernatremia. Be sure the breastfeeding mother has instruction and resources about lactation before discharge after birth. If the newborn is discharged soon after birth, schedule an appointment to check weight within the first few days, and alert the parents to expected output of at least six wet diapers daily. By about 10 days, newborns should have regained the birth weight.

When an infant is sick or developing slowly, parents sometimes want to feed the infant more concentrated formula to make the baby stronger. Parents and caregivers of bottlefed babies should be taught never to give undiluted formula concentrate or evaporated milk. Parents should be cautioned to keep salt out of reach, since eating handfuls of salt has caused hypernatremia. Teach parents to offer extra fluids during hot weather. Teach oral rehydration therapy for use at home during mild vomiting and diarrhea.

Nurses can prevent hypernatremia in hospitalized infants and children by administering water between tube feedings, keeping water available, and offering it frequently. Offering frequent small amounts and using popsicles and other creative interventions can increase children's intake.

Desired outcomes of treatment for hypernatremia include balance of electrolytes and fluid in the intracellular and extracellular compartments and an alert level of consciousness.

Hyponatremia

In hyponatremia, the osmolality of the blood is decreased. The body fluids are too dilute, containing excess water relative to sodium. Hyponatremia is the most common sodium imbalance in children (Kliegman et al., 2011). A serum sodium level below 134 to 135 mmol/L in children (131 mmol/L in newborns) is diagnostic of hyponatremia (Greenbaum, 2011).

ETIOLOGY AND PATHOPHYSIOLOGY

Hyponatremia is caused by conditions that cause gain of relatively more water than sodium or loss of relatively more sodium than water (Table 18–11). Oral intake of water causes hyponatremia in unusual conditions such as forced fluid intake. More commonly, parents feed an infant only water or dilute formula to save money instead of using regular-strength formula or breast milk. Excessive swallowing of swimming pool water by an infant can have the same effect. Infants are vulnerable to the type of

TABLE 18–11 Causes of Hyponatremia

GAIN OF RELATIVELY MORE WATER THAN SODIUM	LOSS OF RELATIVELY MORE SODIUM THAN WATER
Excessive intravenous D_5W (5% dextrose in water)	Diarrhea or vomiting with replacement by tap water only instead of fluid containing sodium
Excessive tap water enemas	
Irrigation of body cavities with distilled water	Excessive sweating
Excessive antidiuretic hormone	Diuretics, especially thiazides
Forced excessive oral intake of tap water	
Congestive heart failure	

hyponatremia caused by water intoxication since they have a poorly developed thirst mechanism and may continue to drink, and then are unable to excrete excess water quickly because of immature kidney function. Forced water intake is another cause and form of child abuse. Exercise-induced hyponatremia can occur when people in prolonged physical activity such as marathon running consume hypotonic fluids in the form of water or sports drinks above the levels lost in respiratory, gastrointestinal, skin, and urinary routes (AAP Council on Sports Medicine and Fitness & Council on School Health, 2011).

CLINICAL MANIFESTATIONS

The child with hyponatremia has a decreased level of consciousness, which results from swelling of brain cells. This can manifest as anorexia, nausea, vomiting, headache, muscle weakness, decreased deep tendon reflexes, agitation, lethargy, or confusion. The condition can progress to respiratory arrest, dilated pupils, decorticate posturing, and coma. If hyponatremia arises rapidly or is extreme, seizures may occur. Hyponatremia is a frequent cause of seizures in infants under 6 months of age. Severe hyponatremia can be fatal.

CLINICAL THERAPY

Laboratory studies are the same as those used to diagnose hypernatremia. In most cases, hyponatremia is treated by restricting the intake of water. This therapy allows the kidneys to correct the imbalance by excreting excess water from the body. If a child is having seizures from hyponatremia, intravenous **hypertonic saline** (more concentrated than body fluid) may be administered. Use of this concentrated fluid rapidly increases body fluid concentration, but the process must be monitored carefully because it can easily cause rebound hypernatremia. For exercise-associated hyponatremia, intravenous access is established at the first-aid site, hypertonic saline is administered, and oxygen is delivered (AAP Council on Sports Medicine and Fitness & Council on School Health, 2011). In cases of diabetes insipidus, treatment for the condition is needed (see Chapter 30).

Nursing Management
For the Child With Hyponatremia

Nursing Assessment and Diagnosis

Hyponatremia should be prevented in hospitalized children receiving intravenous solutions (particularly postoperatively) by administering isotonic rather than hypotonic solutions. Monitor serum sodium level and measure intake and output. If an infant with hyponatremia has normal antidiuretic hormone (ADH) levels, and other causes have been ruled out, carefully question parents about proper preparation of formula and feeding practices. A toddler or school-age child may be subjected to forced fluid intake as a form of child abuse. Sensitive interviewing and a caring manner can help identify such problems in a family.

Because hyponatremia is characterized by a decreased level of consciousness, frequently assess responsiveness to monitor the response to therapy. The child will become more alert and responsive as the concentration of body fluids returns to normal.

The highest priority nursing diagnosis for hyponatremia is *Injury, Risk for,* as it relates to the child's decreased level of consciousness. The following diagnoses might also apply (NANDA-I © 2014):

- *Self-care Deficit: Dressing and Feeding* related to weakness and tiredness
- *Health Maintenance, Impaired,* related to parental misinterpretation about infant formula preparation
- *Breastfeeding, Ineffective,* related to inadequate sucking by infant or inadequate milk production

Planning and Implementation

Nurses can prevent hyponatremia in hospitalized children by using normal saline instead of distilled water for irrigations and by avoiding tap water enemas. Verify intravenous fluid types and amounts and question use of hypotonic fluids in a child with no intake of sodium. Help the child comply with any prescribed fluid restrictions. Allow the child to choose favorite fluids to drink. Teach parents to replace body fluids lost through diarrhea or vomiting with oral electrolyte solutions.

Evaluation

Expected outcomes are maintenance of safety, balance of fluid and electrolytes, and establishment of adequate formula or breastfeeding intake.

Potassium Imbalances

Potassium, an essential electrolyte, performs many necessary functions in the body such as muscle contraction and enzymatic reactions. Potassium intake in healthy children comes from potassium-rich foods such as fruits and vegetables. Potassium is absorbed easily from the intestine. A normal potassium distribution is important for proper function.

A potassium imbalance arises when the serum potassium concentration rises or falls outside the normal range. Potassium imbalances are caused by alterations in potassium intake, distribution, or excretion, or by loss of potassium through an abnormal route such as burns, emesis, or renal failure.

Most potassium ions in the body are found inside the cells. The sodium-potassium pump in cell membranes moves potassium ions into cells to maintain the high intracellular potassium concentration. Potassium ions can be shifted into or out of cells by various physiologic factors (see *Pathophysiology*

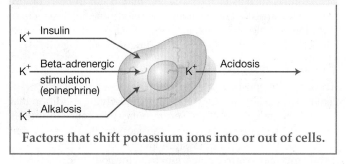

Pathophysiology Illustrated:
Potassium Ions

Factors that shift potassium ions into or out of cells.

Illustrated: Potassium Ions). Potassium is excreted from the body through urine, feces, and sweat. The hormone aldosterone increases potassium excretion in the urine.

Hyperkalemia

Hyperkalemia is an excess of potassium in the blood. Potassium levels generally range from 3.2 to 5.7 mmol/L for newborns, and 3.7 to 5.0 mmol/L for infants and children. Hyperkalemia is reflected by a level above 5.7 mmol/L in newborns or above 5.5 mmol/L in children (see Table 18–9).

ETIOLOGY AND PATHOPHYSIOLOGY

Hyperkalemia is caused by conditions that include increased potassium intake, shift of potassium from cells into the extracellular fluid, and decreased potassium excretion. Renal insufficiency is a primary cause of hyperkalemia. Premature infants commonly have low systemic blood flow and resultant poor renal function, leading to hyperkalemia. Increased potassium intake is frequently due to intravenous potassium overload. Excessive or too rapid intravenous administration of potassium-containing solutions can occur if the potassium requirement is overestimated or if the intravenous infusion runs in too fast.

Blood transfusion is another source of potassium intake that may cause hyperkalemia. Potassium ions leak out of red blood cells that are stored in a blood bank. The longer the blood is stored, the more the potassium leaks out of cells and accumulates in the fluid portion of the transfusion. Hyperkalemia from administration of stored blood arises when multiple units are transfused, as when infants receive exchange transfusions or children receive multiple blood transfusions after a serious injury or during surgery.

Shift of potassium from cells into the extracellular fluid occurs when there is massive cell death, as with a crush injury, in sickle cell disease (hemolytic crisis), or when chemotherapy for a malignancy is rapidly effective (tumor lysis syndrome). In these situations, the dead cells release their high-potassium contents into the extracellular fluid. Potassium ions also shift out of cells in metabolic acidosis caused by diarrhea and in diabetes mellitus when insulin levels are low.

Decreased potassium excretion occurs with acute or chronic oliguria during renal failure, severe hypovolemia, and conditions that decrease the secretion of aldosterone by the adrenal cortex (lead poisoning, Addison disease, hypoaldosteronism). Several medications can cause hyperkalemia, including some cancer chemotherapies, potassium-sparing diuretics, angiotensin-converting enzyme inhibitors, and nonsteroidal anti-inflammatories.

CLINICAL MANIFESTATIONS

The clinical manifestations of hyperkalemia are all related to muscle dysfunction since potassium plays a vital role in muscle activity. Hyperactivity of gastrointestinal smooth muscle causes intestinal cramping and diarrhea in some children. The skeletal muscles become weak, typically beginning with leg weakness and ascending. Weakness can progress to flaccid paralysis. The child is often lethargic. Dysfunction of cardiac muscle causes cardiac arrhythmias such as tachycardia and may result in heart failure and cardiac arrest. Abnormalities in the electrocardiogram include a prolonged QRS complex, a peak in T waves, atrioventricular block, and ventricular dysrhythmia (Engorn & Flerlage, 2014).

CLINICAL THERAPY

The major diagnostic test is the serum potassium level. Hyperkalemia is treated by management of the underlying condition that caused the imbalance. If the serum potassium concentration is very high or is causing dangerous cardiac arrhythmias, treatment to decrease the serum potassium level may be ordered. These treatments may remove potassium from the body or drive it from the extracellular fluid into the cells. Potassium is removed from the body by peritoneal dialysis or hemodialysis, by potassium-wasting diuretics, or with a cation exchange resin (Kayexalate) administered orally or rectally. Medical treatments that drive potassium ions into cells are intravenous sodium bicarbonate, intravenous insulin, glucose, and calcium gluconate.

Nursing Management

For the Child With Hyperkalemia

Nursing Assessment and Diagnosis

Monitor serum potassium levels with prescribed laboratory analysis. Ongoing assessment of muscle strength is important because the muscle weakness may progress to flaccid paralysis. This paralysis is reversible on correction of the potassium imbalance. Diarrhea can occur in infants and children. An older child may complain of intestinal cramping. Monitor the pulse rate carefully.

Nursing diagnoses for a child who has hyperkalemia depend on the severity of the clinical manifestations. The cause of the imbalance may also lead to useful diagnoses that guide teaching for the child and the parents. The following nursing diagnoses may apply (NANDA-I © 2014):

- *Activity Intolerance* related to decreased cardiac output secondary to cardiac arrhythmias
- *Injury, Risk for,* related to muscle weakness
- *Self-care Deficit: Bathing and Dressing* related to neuromuscular impairment
- *Anxiety* related to change in health status
- *Health Maintenance, Ineffective,* related to parental lack of exposure about potassium intake in chronic renal failure
- *Health Management, Family, Ineffective,* related to complexity of therapy

Planning and Implementation

Nursing care includes measures to prevent hyperkalemia from developing in hospitalized children. If hyperkalemia does develop, care shifts to administering intravenous solutions, monitoring cardiopulmonary status, ensuring safety, promoting adequate nutrition, and preparing the child and family for discharge.

PREVENT HYPERKALEMIA

Any child receiving an intravenous infusion that contains potassium is at risk for hyperkalemia. Check that urine output is normal (1 to 2 mL/kg/hr) before administering intravenous potassium solutions. Turn over intravenous solutions to which potassium has been added several times to mix the contents thoroughly before connecting them to the infusion tubing. Double-check the potassium

Growth and Development

The nursing diagnoses for hyperkalemic children will prompt a nurse to provide safety measures appropriate to the child's developmental level and to assist the child with activities that muscle weakness makes difficult. It is important to provide play and diversional activities that take into account the child's degree of muscle strength as well as the appropriate developmental level.

order and intravenous dosage with another nurse. Observe the child closely and perform cardiorespiratory monitoring.

Be sure blood or packed red blood cells are fresh, especially for the child receiving multiple transfusions and for all newborns. Use a cardiac monitor during infusion of these products to watch for arrhythmias.

ADMINISTER INTRAVENOUS SOLUTIONS

Once a child is diagnosed as being hyperkalemic, ensure that any infusions with added potassium are stopped. Several other infusions may need to be managed, including those containing glucose, sodium bicarbonate, and calcium gluconate. Maintain these infusions at the prescribed rates and monitor the child's condition frequently.

MONITOR CARDIOPULMONARY STATUS

Upon diagnosis of hyperkalemia, an electrocardiogram is performed and a cardiac monitor applied. Monitor for any changes in cardiac status and for cardiac arrhythmias. Report abnormal rate and character of pulse as well as shortness of breath.

ENSURE SAFETY

Since the child is weak, raise side rails. Position the child carefully. Assist the child with activities requiring leg muscle strength, such as climbing into bed or pushing up in bed. Encourage quiet activities with frequent rest periods. Document and report any change in muscle weakness.

PROMOTE ADEQUATE NUTRITIONAL INTAKE

Adequate caloric intake is necessary to prevent tissue breakdown and the resultant potassium release from cells. If the child's appetite is decreased, offer nourishing snacks. Restrict potassium-rich foods.

DISCHARGE PLANNING AND HOME CARE TEACHING

If the child has chronic renal failure or another condition that decreases aldosterone secretion, teach parents and children to restrict foods high in potassium. Most oral rehydration solutions, including Pedialyte, contain potassium and should not be used to provide fluid for the child. Instruct the family not to use salt substitutes, which commonly contain potassium. Parents should check with the healthcare provider and pharmacist before giving even over-the-counter products to the child because some of these medications contain potassium. Management of renal failure at home with frequent visits for dialysis and other treatments can be challenging. Refer to Chapter 26 for further suggestions to help parents handle this condition.

Evaluation

Expected outcomes for the child with hyperkalemia include the following:

- The child returns to a state of fluid and electrolyte balance.
- The child's safety is maintained.
- The child has adequate nutritional intake to provide essential potassium.
- The child maintains normal cardiac rate and rhythm.

Hypokalemia

Hypokalemia occurs when the serum potassium concentration is too low. Total body potassium may be decreased, normal, or even increased when the serum level is low, depending on the cause of the imbalance. Serum potassium levels below 3.7 mmol/L in children (3.2 mmol/L for newborns) are diagnostic of hypokalemia.

ETIOLOGY AND PATHOPHYSIOLOGY.

Hypokalemia is caused by increased potassium excretion, decreased potassium intake, shift of potassium from the extracellular fluid into cells, and loss of potassium by an abnormal route.

Increased potassium excretion through the gastrointestinal tract is the major cause of hypokalemia in children. In addition to diuretics and other medications, causes of increased urinary potassium excretion are osmotic diuresis (glucose present in urine), hypomagnesemia, increased aldosterone (hyperaldosteronism, congestive heart failure, nephrotic syndrome, cirrhosis), and increased cortisol (Cushing disease and syndrome) (Engorn & Flerlage, 2014). Eating large amounts of black licorice increases renal excretion of potassium.

Decreased potassium intake will lead to hypokalemia slowly or more rapidly if combined with increased excretion or loss of potassium. Hospitalized children who are placed on NPO status and receive prolonged intravenous therapy should have added potassium. Adolescents concerned about weight loss or those with anorexia nervosa may embark on fad diets low in potassium.

A shift of potassium from the extracellular fluid into cells occurs in alkalosis and hypothermia (unintentional or induced for surgery). Hyperalimentation often causes hypersecretion of insulin, which also shifts potassium into cells.

Vomiting is a route for the loss of potassium; for example, self-induced vomiting in bulimia can cause hypokalemia. Nasogastric suctioning (Figure 18–9) and intestinal decompression can cause potassium loss. Hypokalemia can also be caused by several medications (Crawford & Harris, 2011a) (Table 18–12).

CLINICAL MANIFESTATIONS

Since the ratio of intracellular to extracellular potassium determines the responsiveness of muscle cells to neural stimuli, it is not surprising that the clinical manifestations of hypokalemia involve muscle dysfunction. Gastrointestinal smooth muscle activity is slowed, leading to abdominal distention, constipation, or paralytic ileus. Skeletal muscles are weak and unresponsive to stimuli, and weakness may progress to flaccid paralysis. The respiratory muscles may be impaired. Cardiac arrhythmias

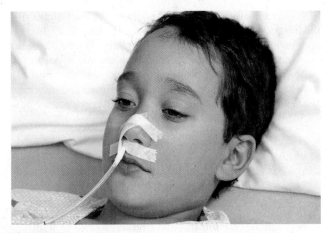

Figure 18–9 Nasogastric tubes and potassium levels. Because this child has a nasogastric tube in place, it is important to monitor his potassium levels.

can occur. Symptoms may range from mild fatigue to flat or absent T waves. Polyuria results from changes in the kidney caused by hypokalemia.

CLINICAL THERAPY

Serum measurement of potassium is the major diagnostic tool, and electrocardiograph may be used. Medical management of hypokalemia focuses on replacement of potassium while treating the cause of the imbalance. Potassium replacement may be given intravenously or orally.

Nursing Management

For the Child With Hypokalemia

Nursing Assessment and Diagnosis

Monitor serum potassium levels. Observe for muscle weakness, which is frequently detected first in the legs. Parents may report that muscle weakness restricts the child's activities and impairs interactions with peers. Skeletal muscle strength can be difficult to assess if the child is lethargic.

Muscle weakness may affect the respiratory muscles. Assess the child frequently to determine the need for assisted ventilation. Cardiac monitoring is important for continued assessment of hypokalemia-associated arrhythmias. Apical pulse rate should be monitored.

TABLE 18–12 Drugs That May Cause Electrolyte Disturbance

HYPERKALEMIA	HYPOKALEMIA	HYPOCALCEMIA	HYPERMAGNESEMIA	HYPOMAGNESEMIA
Potassium-containing medications	Beta-adrenergic agonists	Antacids (if overused)	Magnesium antacids	Magnesium-wasting diuretics
Potassium-sparing diuretics	Insulin	Laxatives (if overused)	Magnesium-containing cathartics	Antineoplastics
Angiotensin-converting enzyme inhibitors	Potassium-wasting diuretics	Oil-based bowel lubricants		Systemic antifungals
Cytotoxic agents	Parenteral penicillins	Anticonvulsants		Aminoglycoside antimicrobials
	Glucocorticoids	Phosphate-containing preparations		Laxatives
	Aminoglycoside antimicrobials	Protein-type plasma expanders during rapid infusion		
	Systemic antifungals	Antineoplastics		
	Antineoplastics			
	Laxatives			

Assess for diminished bowel sounds. Ask the parents if the child has recently been awakening to use the toilet at night or has begun bed-wetting after previously being dry at night. These may be symptoms of polyuria associated with chronic hypokalemia.

The most important nursing diagnoses in the child with severe hypokalemia relate to cardiac arrhythmias and respiratory muscle weakness. The following nursing diagnoses may apply (NANDA-I © 2014):

- *Activity Intolerance, Risk for,* related to decreased cardiac output secondary to cardiac arrhythmia
- *Breathing Pattern, Ineffective,* related to respiratory muscu-loskeletal impairment
- *Injury, Risk for,* related to muscle weakness
- *Self-care Deficit: Bathing and Dressing* related to neuromus-cular impairment
- *Constipation* related to decreased motility
- *Anxiety* related to change in health status
- *Health Maintenance, Ineffective,* related to management of potassium supplements or high-potassium diet
- *Health Management, Family, Ineffective,* related to com-plexity of potassium therapy
- *Nutrition, Imbalanced: Less than Body Requirements,* related to lack of basic nutritional knowledge regarding safe weight-loss diet

Planning and Implementation

Nursing care of the child with hypokalemia focuses on ensuring adequate potassium intake, monitoring cardiopulmonary status, promoting normal bowel function, ensuring safety, providing dietary counseling, and preparing the child and family for discharge.

Growth and Development

Bradycardia occurs at a different level for children of various ages. For infants, a pulse rate below 100 is considered bradycardia. For young children, 80 may be the identified number, whereas for ado-lescents, a pulse below 60 is bradycardia. Look at the child's age and normal pulse range to find changes that indicate bradycardia.

ENSURE ADEQUATE POTASSIUM INTAKE

Since potassium is excreted from the body every day, daily potas-sium intake is necessary to prevent hypokalemia. A hypokalemic child who is able to eat should be given a high-potassium diet. Teach parents (and the child if old enough) which foods are high in potassium and how to incorporate them into the daily diet (Table 18–13).

Children who have no oral intake for a period of time should receive intravenous fluids that contain potassium. Calculate the dosage to be sure it is accurate. Ensure that the infusion runs on schedule. Sometimes the child will complain of burning along the vein when potassium is infused. The infusion may need to be slowed temporarily to allow it to continue. Check serum potas-sium to watch for high or low potassium levels. Monitor urine output. A child with oliguria can develop hyperkalemia when receiving supplements.

MONITOR CARDIOPULMONARY STATUS

Hypokalemia potentiates digitalis toxicity. A hypokalemic child receiving digitalis needs careful surveillance for digitalis toxicity, which is manifested as anorexia, nausea, vomiting, and brady-cardia. Observe for these effects. Take the pulse rate and rhythm regularly. Monitor respirations and ease of breathing to watch for decreased respiratory muscle activity.

PROMOTE NORMAL BOWEL FUNCTION

Ensure adequate fluids and fiber in the diet. Monitor and record the number of stools and report inadequate stools.

ENSURE SAFETY

Keep bed side rails up. Assist the child as needed to move into and out of bed. Reposition the child frequently to preserve skin integrity of limbs that are not moved regularly. Perform passive range of motion if the child is not moving. Use supportive pillows to position the child properly.

PROVIDE DIETARY COUNSELING

The adolescent trying to lose weight and not consuming a nutri-tious diet needs dietary teaching. More intensive treatment will be needed for teens who are anorexic or bulimic (see Chapter 14 for interventions).

DISCHARGE PLANNING AND
HOME CARE TEACHING

Teach parents how to give potassium supplements, if pre-scribed. Liquid or powdered potassium supplements can be mixed with juice or sherbet to improve the bitter taste. The par-ent should call the mixture "medicine" so that the child does not learn to dislike all juices. Teach the parents signs of hypo-kalemia and hyperkalemia and whom to call to report these symptoms. These signs must be reported promptly so medica-tions can be adjusted.

Evaluation

Expected outcomes for the child with potassium imbalance include normal rate and rhythm of heart and respiratory sys-tem, regular bowel movements, maintenance of safety, and knowledge of child and family regarding food sources of potassium.

TABLE 18–13 Food Sources of Electrolytes

POTASSIUM-RICH FOODS		CALCIUM-RICH FOODS		MAGNESIUM-RICH FOODS
Apricots	Orange juice	Milk	Legumes	Whole-grain cereal
Bananas	Peaches	Cheese	Nuts	Dark green vegetables
Cantaloupe	Potatoes	Yogurt	Figs	Soy
Cherries	Prunes	Pudding	Chicken	Almonds
Dates	Raisins	Egg yolks	Salmon (canned with bones)	Peanut butter
Figs	Strawberries	Grains (cream of wheat, farina, bran muffins)	Tofu	Bananas
Molasses	Tomato juice		Fruit drinks with added calcium	Egg yolk
		Sardines (canned)		

Calcium Imbalances

A normal serum calcium concentration is important for many physiologic functions, including muscle and nerve function, secretion of hormones, bone formation and strength, and clotting of the blood. Calcium is the most abundant mineral in the body, with about 98% of it being present in bones (AAP, 2013). There are three forms of calcium in plasma: calcium bound to protein, calcium bound to small organic ions (e.g., citrate), and free ionized calcium (Ca^{2+}), which is physiologically active. A discussion of dietary calcium intake and its importance in bone formation can be found in Chapter 14. (See *Developing Cultural Competence: Calcium Intake and Osteoporosis*.)

Calcium imbalances are caused by alterations in calcium intake, absorption, distribution, or excretion. Calcium absorption requires vitamin D for maximum efficiency and is greatest in the duodenum. Calcium distribution involves calcium entry into and exit from bones and the distribution of different forms of calcium in the plasma. Ionized calcium is the only physiologically active form; additional calcium is bound to protein or ions. Calcium is excreted in urine, feces, and sweat (see *Pathophysiology Illustrated: Calcium Imbalances*).

Parathyroid hormone is the major regulator of the plasma calcium concentration. It increases the plasma calcium concentration by increasing calcium absorption, increasing calcium withdrawal from bones, and decreasing calcium excretion in the urine. The plasma calcium concentration has an important influence on cell membrane permeability and influences the threshold potential of excitable cells. For this reason, calcium imbalances alter neuromuscular irritability.

Hypercalcemia

Hypercalcemia refers to a plasma excess of total calcium (above 2.7 mmol/L in infants and children) (see Table 18–9). Because so much calcium is stored in the bones, however, the serum levels of calcium may not reflect body stores.

ETIOLOGY AND PATHOPHYSIOLOGY

Hypercalcemia is caused by conditions that include increased calcium intake or absorption, shift of calcium from bones into the extracellular fluid, and decreased calcium excretion. Hypercalcemia due to increased calcium intake or absorption may occur if an infant is fed large amounts of chicken liver (source of vitamin A) or is given megadoses of vitamin D or vitamin A, or if a child or adolescent consumes large amounts of calcium-rich foods concurrently with antacids (milk-alkali syndrome). Infants with very low birth weight can develop hypercalcemia if they have inadequate phosphorus intake because bone phosphorus and calcium will be resorbed. Hypercalcemia may also occur when children receiving total parenteral nutrition are given excessive doses of calcium.

Developing Cultural Competence Calcium Intake and Osteoporosis

Ingestion and absorption of calcium are important for the growing child to ensure formation of strong bones. Adolescents who ingest more calcium have less risk of osteoporosis in later life. It has been noted that Black women have less bone loss and fewer fractures than White women. Studies with these two groups of women have demonstrated that Blacks absorb more calcium from the diet and lose less in their urine, leading to increased bone density. However, this has led to an underidentification of osteoporosis in Black women who have relative risks of lactose intolerance and low dairy intake. Assess calcium intake for all and suggest appropriate interventions for your population group and individuals (NIH Osteoporosis and Related Bone Diseases National Resource Center, 2011).

Pathophysiology Illustrated: **Calcium Imbalances**

Some causes of excess calcium in the blood (hypercalcemia)

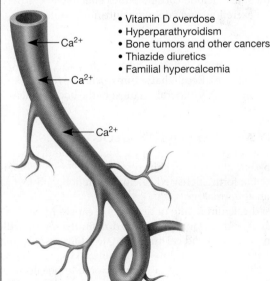

- Vitamin D overdose
- Hyperparathyroidism
- Bone tumors and other cancers
- Thiazide diuretics
- Familial hypercalcemia

Some causes of decreased calcium in the blood (hypocalcemia)

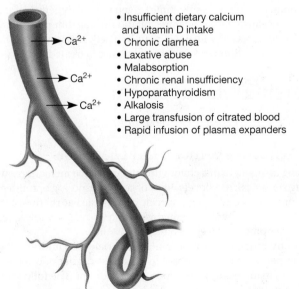

- Insufficient dietary calcium and vitamin D intake
- Chronic diarrhea
- Laxative abuse
- Malabsorption
- Chronic renal insufficiency
- Hypoparathyroidism
- Alkalosis
- Large transfusion of citrated blood
- Rapid infusion of plasma expanders

A variety of conditions can lead to hypercalcemia and hypocalcemia.

Most cases of hypercalcemia in children are due to a shift of calcium from bones into the extracellular fluid. The excessive amounts of parathyroid hormone produced in hyperparathyroidism cause calcium withdrawal from bones. Prolonged immobilization also causes withdrawal of calcium from bones. Often, the excess calcium ions are excreted in the urine. However, if calcium is withdrawn from bones faster than the kidneys can excrete it, hypercalcemia results. Hypercalcemia also occurs with many types of malignancies, such as leukemias. The malignant cells produce substances that circulate in the blood to the bones and cause bone resorption. The calcium from the bones then enters the extracellular fluid, causing hypercalcemia. Bone tumors destroy bone directly, leading to the release of calcium. Familial hypercalcemia and infantile hypercalcemia are rare congenital disorders.

Thiazide diuretics (e.g., thiazide and hydrochlorothiazide) decrease calcium excretion in the urine and may contribute to development of hypercalcemia. Lithium and theophylline can induce hypercalcemia (Ruppe, 2011).

CLINICAL MANIFESTATIONS

Hypercalcemia may have nonspecific symptoms, making diagnosis difficult. Many signs and symptoms of hypercalcemia are manifestations of decreased neuromuscular excitability. Constipation, anorexia, nausea, and vomiting can occur. Fatigue and skeletal muscle weakness dominate. Confusion, lethargy, and decreased attention span are common. Polyuria develops. Severe hypercalcemia may cause cardiac arrhythmias and arrest. Newborns with hypercalcemia have flaccid muscles and exhibit failure to thrive. Hypercalcemia increases sodium and potassium excretion by the kidneys and can lead to polyuria and polydipsia.

CLINICAL THERAPY

Serum calcium is tested although the blood level may not accurately reflect bone stores. Additional laboratory tests include serum albumin, phosphate, magnesium, alkaline phosphate, electrolytes, blood urea nitrogen, creatinine, and parathyroid hormone. Hypercalcemia is treated by increasing fluids and administering the diuretic furosemide (Lasix) to increase excretion of calcium in the urine. Treatment to decrease intestinal absorption of calcium involves effective use of glucocorticoids. Bone resorption can be decreased by administration of glucocorticoids and calcitonin. Phosphate is sometimes given to treat hypercalcemia, but it may cause dangerous precipitation of calcium phosphate salts in body tissues. Dialysis may be used, if necessary. The underlying condition causing the imbalance is treated.

Nursing Management

For the Child With Hypercalcemia

Nursing Assessment and Diagnosis

Nursing assessment of a child with hypercalcemia includes monitoring serum calcium levels, level of consciousness, gastrointestinal function, urine volume, specific gravity, cardiac rhythm, and pH. With chronic hypercalcemia, assessment of activity tolerance and developmental level becomes important.

Many nursing diagnoses are appropriate for children who have hypercalcemia. Diagnoses that address cardiac and neuromuscular manifestation are especially important. The following nursing diagnoses may apply (NANDA-I © 2014):

- *Activity Intolerance, Risk for,* related to decreased cardiac output secondary to cardiac arrhythmia

- *Injury, Risk for,* related to decreased level of consciousness
- *Injury, Risk for,* related to neuromuscular impairment
- *Injury, Risk for,* related to possibility of spontaneous fractures
- *Self-care Deficit: Bathing and Dressing* related to neuromuscular impairment
- *Anxiety* related to change in health status
- *Constipation* related to decreased motility
- *Nutrition, Imbalanced: Less than Body Requirements,* related to anorexia and nausea
- *Urinary Elimination, Impaired,* related to renal calculi

Planning and Intervention

Carefully calculate calcium in total parenteral nutrition and other solutions, administer these solutions with caution, and use cardiac monitoring to prevent hypercalcemia in hospitalized children.

Interventions to increase fluid intake are important for children with hypercalcemia or those who are immobilized. An increased fluid intake, appropriate to the child's age, is necessary to keep the urine dilute and to help reduce constipation (a common symptom of hypercalcemia). An acidic urine helps to keep calcium from forming stones. Because urinary tract infections may cause the urine to be alkaline, institute nursing interventions to prevent urinary tract infection. Thiazide diuretics, which decrease calcium excretion, should not be given to the hypercalcemic child. Provide a high-fiber diet to help reduce constipation.

Increasing mobility through assisted weight bearing helps decrease the withdrawal of calcium from bones that is caused by immobility. If the hypercalcemia is caused by withdrawal of calcium from bones, the child is at risk for fractures with minor trauma and must be handled with special care. See Chapter 29 for further discussion of care following fractures and prolonged casting.

Teach parents to avoid giving calcium-rich foods (such as dairy products) and calcium antacids (e.g., Tums) to children with hypercalcemia. Vitamin D supplements should be avoided as they increase calcium absorption from the gastrointestinal tract.

Evaluation

Expected outcomes include cardiac pump effectiveness, safety, normal bowel excretion, and adequate nutritional status.

Hypocalcemia

Hypocalcemia is a serum deficit of calcium (below 2.1 mmol/L in infants and children). Recall that serum calcium levels may not reflect body stores of this mineral, as most of the body's calcium is stored in bone.

ETIOLOGY AND PATHOPHYSIOLOGY

Hypocalcemia is caused by conditions that include decreased calcium intake or absorption, shift of calcium to a physiologically unavailable form, increased calcium excretion, and loss of calcium by an abnormal route.

Decreased calcium intake or absorption causes hypocalcemia in children with chronic generalized malnutrition or with a diet low in vitamin D and calcium. Female adolescents trying to lose weight or maintain a low weight often decrease foods that contain calcium and may develop chronic hypocalcemia. They may have premature bone loss and inadequate bone. (See Chapter 14 for further discussion of calcium intake during adolescence.) This deficit cannot be made up later in life, increasing the risk of osteoporosis.

Even with a normal calcium intake, hypocalcemia occurs if the mineral is not absorbed. If a child does not have enough vitamin D, calcium is not absorbed efficiently from the duodenum. Sunlight speeds formation of vitamin D in the skin. Children institutionalized without access to sunlight (e.g., severely developmentally delayed children), those with very dark skin, or children kept well covered when outside may become hypocalcemic because of the lack of vitamin D (see Chapter 14). Uremic syndrome is another cause of vitamin D deficiency. It interferes with the kidney's ability to activate vitamin D. High phosphate intake can cause hypocalcemia. Chronic diarrhea and steatorrhea (fatty stools) also reduce calcium absorption from the gastrointestinal tract.

About 40% of calcium is bound to proteins and not available for interactions, 10% is bound to small organic ions such as citrate, and 50% is ionized and physiologically active. Calcium becomes physiologically unavailable when calcium shifts into bone or free ionized calcium in plasma binds to proteins or small organic ions in the plasma. Excessive calcium shifts into bones in various types of hypoparathyroidism, including DiGeorge syndrome (congenital absence of the parathyroid glands). Hypomagnesemia impairs parathyroid hormone function and may cause hypocalcemia. Some types of neonatal hypocalcemia are associated with delayed parathyroid hormone function or hypomagnesemia. Calcium shifts rapidly into bone when rickets is treated. A high plasma phosphate concentration causes plasma calcium to decrease. Ionized hypocalcemia, due to an increased binding of plasma ionized calcium, occurs very rapidly. The ionized hypocalcemia persists until the alkalosis resolves or the citrate is metabolized by the liver. Children who receive liver transplants are hypocalcemic for several days because of impaired citrate metabolism.

Increased calcium excretion occurs in steatorrhea, when calcium secreted into the gastrointestinal fluid binds to the fecal fat in addition to the dietary calcium that is bound in the feces. A similar situation occurs in acute pancreatitis.

Loss of calcium by an abnormal route may contribute to hypocalcemia; calcium is lost through burn or wound drainage or sequestered in acute pancreatitis. Many medications can cause hypocalcemia (see Table 18–12).

CLINICAL MANIFESTATIONS

The signs and symptoms of hypocalcemia are manifestations of increased muscular excitability (tetany). In children, they include twitching and cramping, tingling around the mouth or in the fingers, carpal spasm, and pedal spasm. Laryngospasm, seizures, and cardiac arrhythmias are more severe manifestations of hypocalcemia and may be fatal. Hypocalcemia may cause congestive heart failure, especially in newborns.

Although these symptoms are diagnostic of acute calcium deficiency, a more common state in children and adolescents is chronic low intake of calcium. This may be manifested by spontaneous fractures in infants and in adolescents who exercise excessively.

CLINICAL THERAPY

Laboratory measurement of serum calcium and cardiac monitoring are used for diagnosis. Hypocalcemia is treated by oral or intravenous administration of calcium. The original cause of the imbalance is also treated. If the hypocalcemia is due to hypomagnesemia, the magnesium must be replenished before the calcium replacement can be successful. When the cause is chronic low dietary intake, counseling is needed about high-calcium foods, and perhaps the necessity for vitamin D intake or supplements.

Nursing Management
For the Child With Hypocalcemia

Nursing Assessment and Diagnosis

Carefully assess growth in the young female who is trying to diet. Whenever a female adolescent is very thin, be sure to ask about excessive sports and other activities, and about regularity of menstrual periods. If periods are irregular or not occurring, collect additional dietary information to help determine whether the girl is lacking in intake of calcium, calories, and other nutrients. These assessments are needed even if serum calcium values are normal. Look for signs of inadequate nutrition such as fat and muscle wasting, dry hair, and cold hands and feet. Assess for muscle cramps, stiffness, and clumsiness; grimacing caused by spasms of facial muscles and twitching of arm muscles; and laryngospasm. Increased neuromuscular excitability may be detected by testing for Trousseau sign or Chvostek sign (see Chapter 5). Many healthy newborns have a positive Chvostek sign; however, this assessment should be reserved for children over several months of age. Monitor serum calcium levels and perform cardiac monitoring to observe for cardiac arrhythmias.

Growth and Development

Hypocalcemia in infants is more often seen as tremors, muscle twitches, and brief tonic–clonic seizures. Perform careful neurologic assessments on infants at risk of electrolyte imbalance.

The effects of increased neuromuscular excitability in the child with hypocalcemia are the basis for several nursing diagnoses. These include the following (NANDA-I © 2014):

- *Injury, Risk for,* related to potential for fractures
- *Injury, Risk for,* related to increased neuromuscular excitability
- *Breathing Pattern, Ineffective,* related to laryngospasm
- *Activity Intolerance* related to decreased cardiac output secondary to cardiac arrhythmias
- *Anxiety* related to change in health status
- *Nutrition, Imbalanced: Less than Body Requirements,* related to lack of basic nutritional knowledge of sources and recommended amounts of calcium intake

Planning and Implementation

To correct calcium deficiency in the hospitalized child, give oral or intravenous calcium as prescribed. Monitor for complications of calcium supplementation. Monitor for the side effect of constipation with oral supplements, or for tissue sloughing, elevated serum calcium, or decreased serum phosphate with intravenous supplementation. Verify dosage of calcium gluconate with another nurse, and monitor heart rate and rhythm. Calcium is never given subcutaneously or intramuscularly because it causes tissue necrosis. A 10% calcium gluconate intravenous solution should be readily available for emergency use in severe hypocalcemia.

Take measures to ensure safety for the child who is hospitalized with hypocalcemia. Seizure precautions may be necessary. Explain the cause of muscle cramps to parents and older children.

Counsel the family about dairy products and nondairy foods rich in calcium (see Table 18–13). For the female adolescent whose weight and menstrual patterns show irregularities, total calories and calcium intake should be increased. Teaching may also be needed about proper calcium intake and its importance both to athletic performance and to the prevention of osteoporosis. Encourage three glasses of nonfat milk per day. Teach ways to use milk in the diet. For example, sprinkle nonfat dry milk on cereal and other foods. If the child is lactose intolerant, emphasize nondairy sources of calcium and advise parents to purchase special milk treated with lactase. However, be aware that this milk is more costly, and inadequate family finances may prevent its use. If a child has a health condition leading to chronic diarrhea, encourage increased intake of calcium-rich foods. Calcium supplements in the form of calcium carbonate tablets may be used.

Evaluation

Expected outcomes of nursing care include ingestion of recommended dietary allowances for calcium, absence of discomfort related to calcium imbalance, and freedom from injury.

Magnesium Imbalances

Magnesium is necessary for enzyme function in cells, acetylcholine release, glycolysis, stimulation of ATPases, and bone formation. Since magnesium is a component of chlorophyll, dark green leafy vegetables are a good dietary source of magnesium. Nuts and grains are also good sources of magnesium. Magnesium is absorbed primarily from the terminal ileum. It is distributed among the extracellular fluid (small amounts), the cells (larger amounts), and the bones (large amounts). Magnesium is excreted in urine, feces, and sweat.

Magnesium imbalances are caused by alterations in magnesium intake, distribution, or excretion; by loss of magnesium through an abnormal route; or by a combination of these factors. The plasma magnesium concentration influences the release of acetylcholine at neuromuscular junctions. Thus, magnesium imbalances are characterized by alterations in neuromuscular irritability.

Hypermagnesemia

Hypermagnesemia occurs when the plasma magnesium concentration is too high (above 2.4 mg/dL [0.99 mmol/L]) (see Table 18–9). Keep in mind that the serum levels measured in the laboratory may not reflect body magnesium stores because most magnesium in the body is located in the bones and inside the cells.

Hypermagnesemia is caused by conditions that involve increased magnesium intake and decreased magnesium excretion. Impaired renal function leading to decreased magnesium excretion is the most common cause of hypermagnesemia in children. In both oliguric renal failure and adrenal insufficiency, magnesium ions that cannot be excreted in the urine accumulate in the extracellular fluid.

Less frequently, increased magnesium intake may cause hypermagnesemia. Magnesium sulfate ($MgSO_4$) given to treat eclampsia in the mother before birth causes hypermagnesemia in the newborn. Abnormally high amounts may also be taken in magnesium-containing enemas, laxatives, antacids, and intravenous fluids. Epsom salt is a readily available product that is a nearly pure magnesium sulfate preparation; its use

as an enema has caused death in children (see Table 18–12). Aspiration of seawater, as in near-drowning, is an uncommon but potentially serious source of excessive magnesium intake. Children with Addison disease can have abnormally high magnesium levels.

Clinical manifestations of hypermagnesemia include decreased muscle irritability, hypotension, bradycardia, drowsiness, lethargy, and weak or absent deep tendon reflexes. In severe hypermagnesemia, flaccid muscle paralysis, fatal respiratory depression, cardiac arrhythmias, heart block, and cardiac arrest can occur (Crawford & Harris, 2011b).

Hypermagnesemia is managed primarily by increasing the urinary excretion of magnesium. This is usually accomplished by increasing fluid intake (except in oliguric renal failure) and by the administration of diuretics. Dialysis may sometimes be necessary.

Nursing Management

Monitor serum magnesium levels. Take the child's blood pressure (to watch for hypotension), heart rate and rhythm (to monitor for bradycardia and cardiac arrhythmias), respiratory rate and depth (to observe for respiratory depression), and deep tendon reflexes (to assess muscle tone and paralysis or movement). Keep the side rails of the bed raised. Children with hypermagnesemia or oliguria should not be given magnesium-containing medications or sea salt.

Teach parents of children with chronic renal failure that these children should never be given milk of magnesia, antacids that contain magnesium, or other sources of magnesium. When hypermagnesemia is treated with diuretics, monitor potassium levels to watch for hypokalemia.

Expected outcomes of nursing care include maintenance of electrolyte balance, normal neuromuscular tone, safety, and regular heart rate and rhythm.

Hypomagnesemia

Hypomagnesemia refers to a plasma magnesium concentration that is too low (below 1.6 mg/dL [0.66 mmol/L]). Remember that the serum levels of magnesium may not reflect body stores, since most of the magnesium in the body is found in cells and bones.

Hypomagnesemia is caused by conditions that include decreased magnesium intake or absorption, shift of magnesium to a physiologically unavailable form, increased magnesium excretion, and loss of magnesium by an abnormal route.

Decreased magnesium intake or absorption can occur if a child who is not eating has prolonged intravenous therapy without magnesium. Chronic malnutrition is another cause of decreased magnesium intake. Magnesium absorption is decreased in chronic diarrhea, short bowel syndrome, malabsorption syndromes, and steatorrhea.

Magnesium may shift to a physiologically unavailable form after transfusion of many units of citrated blood products; magnesium bound to the citrate is not physiologically active. Such transfusions cause prolonged hypomagnesemia in liver transplant patients, who have impaired citrate metabolism. Magnesium shifts rapidly into bones that have been deprived of adequate stores.

Increased magnesium excretion in the urine occurs with diuretic therapy, the diuretic phase of acute renal failure, diabetic ketoacidosis, and hyperaldosteronism. Chronic alcoholism, occasionally seen in adolescents, increases urinary magnesium excretion. Magnesium contained in gastrointestinal secretions is bound to fat and excreted in the stool.

Instruct parents of a child with chronic renal failure to read labels to detect magnesium in antacids and cathartics. Encourage them to check with their pharmacist and other healthcare providers before administering any over-the-counter medication to the child.

Loss of magnesium by an abnormal route occurs with prolonged nasogastric suction and through sequestration of magnesium in acute pancreatitis. Several medications may cause hypomagnesemia (see Table 18–12).

Hypomagnesemia is characterized by increased neuromuscular excitability (tetany). The clinical manifestations are hyperactive reflexes, skeletal muscle cramps, twitching, tremors, and cardiac arrhythmias. Seizures can occur with severe hypomagnesemia.

Hypomagnesemia is managed by administering magnesium and treating the underlying cause of the imbalance.

Nursing Management

In addition to monitoring serum magnesium levels, nursing assessment of hypomagnesemia includes monitoring deep tendon reflexes, testing for Trousseau and Chvostek signs, monitoring cardiac function, and observing for muscle twitching. Children who are able to talk may report muscle cramping. Because magnesium levels are not routinely measured in many settings, request the test for any child who has risk factors and early manifestations of hypomagnesemia. When intramuscular or intravenous magnesium is ordered, administer carefully as directed and monitor vital signs. Electrocardiogram and renal studies may precede drug administration. Have resuscitative drugs and equipment readily available during drug administration.

Teach parents of a child with hypomagnesemia or continuing risk factors such as chronic diarrhea to include magnesium-rich foods in the diet (see Table 18–13). Before administering magnesium supplements, verify that the child's urine output is adequate. Monitor deep tendon reflexes if intravenous magnesium is given, and observe for complications of magnesium supplementation. Oral magnesium may lead to diarrhea, and intravenous magnesium can cause flushing, elevated serum magnesium, cardiac arrhythmias, or decreased deep tendon reflexes.

Expected outcomes of nursing care for the child with an imbalance in magnesium are restoration and maintenance of electrolyte balance.

CLINICAL ASSESSMENT OF FLUID AND ELECTROLYTE IMBALANCE

How can a nurse assess children appropriately for fluid and electrolyte imbalance without thinking through the clinical manifestations of every possible disorder one after the other? First, perform a rapid risk factor assessment on each child to see which factors are present (Tables 18–14 and 18–15).

A risk factor assessment may be performed mentally while providing care. Look for factors that alter the intake, retention, and loss of isotonic fluid and water. Use this information to evaluate which fluid imbalance is most likely to occur in a particular child. Next, look for factors that alter electrolyte intake and absorption, distribution between plasma and other electrolyte pools, excretion, and abnormal routes of electrolyte loss. Use this information to evaluate which electrolyte imbalances are most likely to occur in the child. A review of pathophysiology is important to understand the role of the other electrolytes and substances, such as phosphorus, in the body.

After evaluating possible imbalances for the child, perform a clinical assessment. Assess for fluid imbalances by assessing weight changes, vascular volume, interstitial volume, and cerebral function (Table 18–16). Assess for electrolyte imbalances by assessing serum electrolyte levels, skeletal muscle strength, neuromuscular excitability, gastrointestinal tract function, and cardiac rhythm (Table 18–17). Next, check for other manifestations specific to a particular high-risk imbalance (e.g., polyuria in hypokalemia). Evaluate any serum laboratory values available. This method of risk factor assessment followed by clinical assessment provides a rapid yet thorough approach to assessment for fluid and electrolyte imbalances.

TABLE 18–14 Risk Factor Assessment for Fluid Imbalances

TYPE OF FLUID	FACTORS TO ASSESS
Isotonic fluid (extracellular fluid volume imbalances)	Source of increased intake?
	Aldosterone secretion increased or decreased?
	Source of loss from the body?
Water	Source of increased intake?
	Antidiuretic hormone secretion increased or decreased?
	Source of unusual loss from the body?

TABLE 18–15 Risk Factor Assessment for Electrolyte Imbalances

POTENTIAL ELECTROLYTE IMBALANCE	ASSESSMENT FINDING
Electrolyte intake and absorption	Increased?
	Decreased?
Electrolyte shifts	From electrolyte pool to plasma?
	From plasma to electrolyte pool?
Electrolyte excretion	Increased?
	Decreased?
Electrolyte loss by abnormal route	Vomiting?
	Diarrhea?
	Nasogastric suction?
	Wound?
	Burn?
	Excessive sweating?

TABLE 18–16 Summary of Clinical Assessment of Fluid Imbalances

ASSESSMENT CATEGORY	SPECIFIC ASSESSMENTS	CHANGES WITH FLUID IMBALANCES
Rapid changes in weight	Daily weights	Weight gain—extracellular volume excess
		Weight loss—extracellular volume deficit; clinical dehydration
Vascular volume	Small vein filling time	Increased—extracellular volume deficit; clinical dehydration
	Capillary refill time	Increased—extracellular volume deficit; clinical dehydration
	Character of pulse	Bounding—extracellular volume excess
		Thready—extracellular volume deficit; clinical dehydration
	Postural blood pressure measurements	Postural drop—extracellular volume deficit; clinical dehydration
	Lung sounds in dependent portions	Crackles—extracellular volume excess
	Central venous pressure	Increased—extracellular volume excess
		Decreased—extracellular volume deficit; clinical dehydration
	Tenseness of fontanelle (infants)	Bulging—extracellular volume excess
		Sunken—extracellular volume deficit; clinical dehydration
	Neck vein filling (older children)	Full when upright—extracellular volume excess
		Flat when supine—extracellular volume deficit; clinical dehydration
Interstitial volume	Skin turgor	Skin tents—extracellular volume deficit; clinical dehydration
	Presence or absence of edema	Edema—extracellular volume excess
Cerebral function	Level of consciousness	Decreased—clinical dehydration

TABLE 18–17 Summary of Clinical Assessment of Electrolyte Imbalances

ASSESSMENT CATEGORY	SPECIFIC ASSESSMENTS	CHANGES WITH ELECTROLYTE IMBALANCES
Skeletal muscle function	Muscle strength	Weakness, flaccid paralysis—hyperkalemia; hypokalemia
Neuromuscular excitability	Deep tendon reflexes	Depressed—hypercalcemia; hypermagnesemia
		Hyperactive—hypocalcemia; hypomagnesemia
	Chvostek sign (not seen in infants)	Positive—hypocalcemia; hypomagnesemia
	Trousseau's sign	Positive—hypocalcemia; hypomagnesemia
	Paresthesias	Digital or perioral—hypocalcemia
	Muscle cramping or twitching	Present—hypocalcemia; hypomagnesemia
Gastrointestinal tract function	Bowel sounds	Decreased or absent—hypokalemia
	Elimination pattern	Constipation—hypokalemia; hypercalcemia
		Diarrhea—hyperkalemia
Cardiac rhythm	Arrhythmia	Irregular—hyperkalemia; hypokalemia; hypercalcemia; hypocalcemia; hypermagnesemia; hypomagnesemia
	Electrocardiogram	Abnormal—hyperkalemia; hypokalemia; hypercalcemia; hypocalcemia; hypermagnesemia; hypomagnesemia
Cerebral function	Level of consciousness	Decreased—hyponatremia; hypernatremia

ACID–BASE IMBALANCES

There are four acid–base imbalances. Two are the result of processes that cause too much acid in the body and are referred to as **acidosis**. The other two are the result of processes that cause too little acid in the body and are called **alkalosis**. An acid–base disorder caused by too much or too little carbonic acid is called a *respiratory acid–base imbalance*. A disorder caused by too much or too little metabolic acid is called a *metabolic acid–base imbalance*.

Arterial blood gas measurements (ABGs) provide a laboratory evaluation of a child's current acid–base status. In addition, oxygen saturation, or the percentage of hemoglobin saturated with arterial blood, is normally 95% to 100%. Table 18–18 provides a method that can help interpret the pH, P_{CO_2}, and bicarbonate concentrations, the most important acid–base measures. End-tidal CO_2 can provide a continuous noninvasive measurement. (Remember that P_{CO_2} reflects carbonic acid status, and bicarbonate concentration reflects the metabolic acid status.)

Clinical Tip

Acidosis: Relatively too much acid in the body

Respiratory acidosis: Relatively too much carbonic acid

Metabolic acidosis: Relatively too much metabolic acid

Alkalosis: Relatively too little acid in the body

Respiratory alkalosis: Relatively too little carbonic acid

Metabolic alkalosis: Relatively too little metabolic acid

TABLE 18–18 Questions to Ask to Interpret Arterial Blood Gas Measurements

QUESTION TO ASK	CONCLUSION
What is the pH?	• If the pH is normal, the child has no imbalance or has compensated for an imbalance. • If the pH is below normal, the child has acidosis. • If the pH is above normal, the child has alkalosis.
What is the Pco_2?	• If the Pco_2 is normal, the child does not have an acid–base imbalance. • If the Pco_2 is above normal, the child has respiratory acidosis. This may be the primary disorder or may be a compensatory response to metabolic alkalosis. Looking at the bicarbonate concentration helps you decide. • If the Pco_2 is below normal, the child has respiratory alkalosis. Again, this can be the primary disorder or may be a compensatory response to metabolic acidosis.
What is the bicarbonate concentration?	• If the bicarbonate concentration is within normal range, the child does not have a metabolic acid–base imbalance. • If the bicarbonate is above normal, the child has metabolic alkalosis. This can be a primary disorder or a compensatory response to respiratory acidosis. • If bicarbonate is below normal, the child has metabolic acidosis, either as a direct disorder or as a compensatory response to respiratory alkalosis.
What do the results together tell you?	• If the pH is abnormal and either the Pco_2 or bicarbonate concentration is normal, there is an uncompensated acid–base disorder. • If all three values are abnormal, the child has a partially compensated disorder and the pH will provide the definitive answer. • If Pco_2, pH, and bicarbonate are all decreased, then partially compensated metabolic acidosis is most likely. • If pH is normal and Pco_2 and bicarbonate are abnormal, there is a fully compensated acid–base disorder.
What are the child's history and clinical signs?	• Does your interpretation fit with what you know about the child's medical condition and with assessments you are making? • This last step helps you to integrate laboratory data with the clinical picture to strengthen your nursing care of the child with an acid–base imbalance.

Respiratory Acidosis

Respiratory acidosis is caused by an accumulation of carbon dioxide in the blood. Since carbon dioxide and water can be combined into carbonic acid, respiratory acidosis is sometimes called carbonic acid excess. The condition can be acute or chronic. It is controlled by the lungs.

ETIOLOGY AND PATHOPHYSIOLOGY

Any factor that interferes with the ability of the lungs to excrete carbon dioxide can cause respiratory acidosis. These factors may interfere with the gaseous exchange within the lungs, may impair the neuromuscular pump that moves air in and out of the lungs, or may depress the respiratory rate (Table 18–19 and Figure 18–10).

As the Pco_2 begins to increase, the pH of the blood begins to decrease. Compensatory mechanisms begin to act in the form of nonbicarbonate buffers, additional hydrogen ion excretion by the kidneys, and formation and decreased bicarbonate excretion by the kidneys. These compensatory mechanisms take several days to become active so the child manifests a changing clinical situation, depending on the underlying cause and the amount of compensation occurring (Table 18–20).

TABLE 18–19 Causes of Respiratory Acidosis

FACTORS AFFECTING THE LUNGS	FACTORS AFFECTING THE NEUROMUSCULAR PUMP	FACTORS AFFECTING CENTRAL CONTROL OF RESPIRATION
Aspiration	Flail chest	Sedative overdose
Spasm of the airways	Pneumothorax or hemothorax	General anesthesia
Laryngeal edema	Mechanical underventilation	Head injury
Epiglottitis	Hypokalemic muscle weakness	Brain tumor
Croup	High cervical spinal cord injury	Central sleep apnea
Pulmonary edema	Botulism	
Atelectasis	Tetanus	
Severe pneumonia	Kyphoscoliosis	
Cystic fibrosis	Poliomyelitis	
Bronchopulmonary dysplasia	Muscular dystrophy	
Pulmonary embolism	Congenital diaphragmatic hernia	
	Guillain-Barré syndrome	

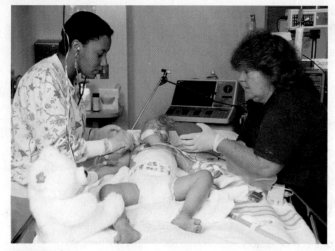

Figure 18–10 **Respiratory acidosis/alkalosis and mechanical ventilation. This child may develop respiratory acidosis or respiratory alkalosis. If the tidal volume is set too low during mechanical ventilation, carbon dioxide (carbonic acid) will accumulate in the body (respiratory acidosis) because it is not being excreted by the lungs. If the tidal volume is set too high, carbon dioxide will be depleted in the body (respiratory alkalosis) because it is being excreted in great quantities.**

CLINICAL MANIFESTATIONS

Acidosis in the brain cells causes central nervous system depression, manifested by confusion, lethargy, headache, increased intracranial pressure, and even coma. Acute respiratory acidosis can lead to tachycardia and cardiac arrhythmias. The child's arterial blood gases always show an increased Pco_2, the laboratory sign of increased carbonic acid. Serum pH can be decreased or normal.

CLINICAL THERAPY

Treatment of respiratory acidosis requires correction of the underlying cause. For example, treatment may include bronchodilators for bronchospasm, mechanical ventilation for neuromuscular defects, decreasing sedative use, or surgery for kyphoscoliosis.

Nursing Management

For the Child With Respiratory Acidosis

Nursing Assessment and Diagnosis

Nursing assessment plays a pivotal role in decisions about interventions for respiratory acidosis. This is especially true in chronic conditions such as cystic fibrosis and kyphoscoliosis. Assess respiratory rate, rhythm, and depth carefully. Take the apical pulse and be alert for tachycardia or arrhythmia. A cardiac monitor may be used. Obtain serial arterial blood gas measurements in acute conditions to evaluate changing status. Assess the level of consciousness and energy. Observe for chronic fatigue, headache, or decreased level of consciousness.

Several nursing diagnoses may apply to the child with respiratory acidosis. The most important addresses the child's *Injury, Risk for.* Other nursing diagnoses depend on the specific clinical manifestation and the particular cause of the acidosis. Examples include the following (NANDA-I © 2014):

- *Injury, Risk for,* related to decreased level of consciousness

TABLE 18–20 Laboratory Values in Uncompensated and Compensated Respiratory Acidosis

TYPE OF RESPIRATORY ACIDOSIS	HCO₃⁻	pH	Pco₂
Uncompensated	Normal	Decreased	Increased
Partially compensated	Increasing	Decreasing but moving toward normal	Increased
Fully compensated	Increased	Normal	Increased

- *Activity Intolerance* related to decreased cardiac output secondary to cardiac dysrhythmias
- *Breathing Pattern, Ineffective (Hypoventilation),* related to neuromuscular impairment
- *Pain (Headache)* related to cerebral vasodilation
- *Health Management, Family, Ineffective,* related to complexity of bronchodilator therapy

Planning and Implementation

COMMUNITY-BASED NURSING CARE

Teach children at risk for respiratory acidosis and their parents preventive measures to use at home. For the child with a chronic condition such as cystic fibrosis, muscular dystrophy, or kyphoscoliosis, demonstrate deep breathing and encourage its use several times each day. Teach the family signs of infection—including fever, increased respiratory secretions, and discomfort with breathing—so that these problems can be treated promptly, preventing further respiratory involvement. Position the child to facilitate chest expansion. Teach parents about proper administration of any necessary medications. For example, the child with cystic fibrosis may receive antibiotics to prevent respiratory infections. Teach parents and older children about home respirator use (Figure 18–11).

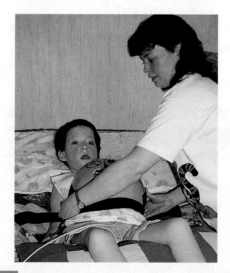

Figure 18–11 **Home respirator use. This child, who has muscular dystrophy, uses a "turtle" respirator at home to assist with breathing. His parents required instructions from the nurse on use of the respirator. The family has a generator to provide electricity for the respirator during power outages.**

HOSPITAL-BASED NURSING CARE

For the hospitalized child, the focus is on ensuring safety. Keep bed side rails raised, and turn and position the child frequently. Evaluate mental status and document and report any changes in alertness. When laboratory values of blood pH and Pco_2 are available, evaluate them promptly and report any changes or abnormalities. Administer medications as ordered. Carefully monitor the doses of sedatives to avoid further respiratory depression. Provide suctioning and encourage deep breathing.

Evaluation

Expected outcomes of nursing care for the child with respiratory acidosis include maintenance of safety, adequate rate and rhythm of respirations, and management of causative disorders.

Growth and Development

It is usually difficult to get a young child to do deep breathing or to use the "blow bottle" that is often given to older children and adults. To make deep breathing fun, use a pinwheel and have the child turn it during play. Alternatively, give a child a straw to blow bubbles in a glass of water or to blow scraps of paper across the bedside table.

Respiratory Alkalosis

Respiratory alkalosis occurs when the blood contains too little carbon dioxide. This condition is sometimes called *carbonic acid deficit*.

Excess carbon dioxide loss is caused by hyperventilation, in which more air than normal is moved into and out of the lungs. Some common causes of hyperventilation are hypoxia due to severe asthma, salicylate poisoning, and sepsis. Other causes are anxiety, fear, pain, meningitis, septicemia, and mechanical overventilation.

In many cases, respiratory alkalosis lasts for several hours only. Renal compensation does not occur because these compensatory mechanisms take several days to begin action. An example is the hyperventilation that occurs with acute anxiety. However, if the condition persists, the kidneys will begin to retain more acid and excrete more bicarbonate. Hydrogen ions will be released from body buffers to decrease plasma bicarbonate. While the imbalance continues, cellular function is thus protected by returning pH to normal levels (Table 18–21).

Arterial blood gas measurements show a decreased Pco_2 in respiratory alkalosis. Blood pH is generally elevated. The lack of carbon dioxide causes neuromuscular irritability and paresthesias in the extremities and around the mouth. Muscle cramping and carpal or pedal spasms can occur. The child may be dizzy or confused.

TABLE 18–21 Laboratory Values in Uncompensated and Compensated Respiratory Alkalosis

TYPE OF RESPIRATORY ALKALOSIS	HCO₃⁻	pH	Pco₂
Uncompensated	Normal	Increased	Decreased
Partially compensated	Decreasing	Increasing but moving toward normal	Decreased
Fully compensated	Decreased	Normal	Decreased

Medical management focuses on correcting the condition that caused the hyperventilation so that the body's compensatory mechanisms can return carbon dioxide levels to normal.

Nursing Management

For the Child With Respiratory Alkalosis

Nursing Assessment and Diagnosis

Assess the child's level of consciousness and ask if the child feels light-headed or has tingling sensations or numbness in the fingers or toes or around the mouth. Assess the rate and depth of respirations. Monitor the hospitalized child's Po_2 with serial arterial blood gas measurements to evaluate changes in status. Make a careful assessment about the cause of hyperventilation. Did an occurrence cause anxiety for the child? Is the child in pain? (See Chapter 15.) Has the child received salicylates in any form? Is the child mechanically ventilated? Is there a central nervous system infection such as meningitis?

Planning and Implementation

Nursing care for the child with respiratory alkalosis centers on teaching stress management techniques, maintaining pain control, promoting respiratory function, ensuring safety, regulating fluid status, and providing health supervision and home care.

SAFETY ALERT!

Check the Po_2 before any therapy for respiratory alkalosis is started because it is dangerous to stop hyperventilation if oxygenation is poor.

TEACH STRESS MANAGEMENT TECHNIQUES

When anxiety is the cause of respiratory alkalosis, instruct the child to breathe slowly; demonstrate the rhythm. Use a calm voice, stuffed toys, and supportive reassurance. Teach stress-control techniques such as relaxation and imagery for situations that cause anxiety.

MAINTAIN PAIN CONTROL

Use medications, imagery, distraction, positioning, massage, and other techniques to decrease pain and maintain pain management. See Chapter 15 for a description of these and other measures to assist with pain control.

PROMOTE RESPIRATORY FUNCTION

Have the child cough, or apply suction as needed. Be certain that mechanical ventilation systems are working properly.

ENSURE SAFETY

Provide a safe environment for the child who has a decreased level of consciousness. Be sure the child is supervised when sitting or standing up. Keep bed rails up.

REGULATE FLUID STATUS

Renal compensation to manage ongoing respiratory alkalosis requires adequate urinary output. Regulate fluid intake to ensure urine output unless fluids are restricted because of a medical condition.

COMMUNITY-BASED NURSING CARE

Teach parents to keep aspirin and other salicylate products out of reach of children, preferably in a locked medicine box. Provide stickers with the number of the Poison Control Center.

Evaluation

Expected outcomes of nursing care for the child with respiratory alkalosis include normal respiratory rate and rhythm, maintenance of safety, and regulation of fluid status.

Metabolic Acidosis

Metabolic acidosis is a condition in which there is an excess of any acid other than carbonic acid. For this reason, it is sometimes called *noncarbonic acid excess.*

ETIOLOGY AND PATHOPHYSIOLOGY

Metabolic acidosis is caused by an imbalance in production and excretion of acid or by excess loss of bicarbonate. Excess accumulation occurs by one of two mechanisms. First, a child can eat or drink acids or substances that are converted to acid in the body. Examples include aspirin, boric acid, and antifreeze. Second, cells can make abnormally high amounts of acid that cannot be excreted. This is the case in ketoacidosis of untreated diabetes mellitus, untreated growth hormone deficiency, bladder construction that uses part of the bowel, or the starvation that can occur in anorexia or bulimia. A disorder of excretion occurs in conditions such as oliguric renal failure (Figure 18–12).

The body can lose bicarbonate through the urine or through excessive loss of intestinal fluid. Diarrhea, fistulas, and ileal drainage are all possible sources. Carbonic anhydrase inhibitors can cause loss of excess bicarbonate in the urine.

Below-normal pH of the blood stimulates the chemoreceptors in the brain and arteries and respiratory compensation begins. The child's rate and depth of breathing increase and carbonic acid is removed from the body. The blood pH shifts to a

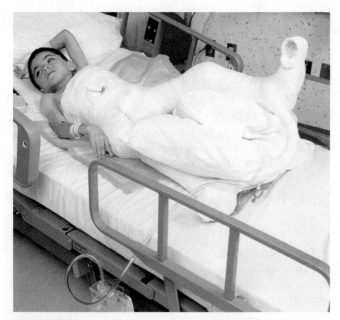

Figure 18–12 Disorders of excretion. With any postoperative or immobilized child, it is important to monitor urine output to detect oliguria. If the kidneys do not produce sufficient urine, the metabolic acids accumulate in the body and cause metabolic acidosis. Inadequate fluid intake in the postoperative or immobilized child can lead to oliguria and, potentially, metabolic acidosis.

TABLE 18–22 Laboratory Values in Uncompensated and Compensated Metabolic Acidosis

TYPE OF METABOLIC ACIDOSIS	HCO_3^-	pH	Pco_2
Uncompensated	Decreased	Decreased	Normal
Partially compensated	Decreased	Decreased but moving toward normal	Decreasing

more normal range even though the cause is not corrected. The underlying condition and the degree of compensation alter the clinical laboratory values observed (Table 18–22).

CLINICAL MANIFESTATIONS

Laboratory values show decreased blood pH and decreased HCO_3^- and Pco_2. An attempt at respiratory compensation causes one of the most important signs of metabolic acidosis, increased rate and depth of respirations (hyperventilation) or **Kussmaul respirations**. Severe acidosis can cause decreased peripheral vascular resistance and resultant cardiac arrhythmias, hypotension, pulmonary edema, and tissue hypoxia. Confusion or drowsiness may result, as well as headache or abdominal pain.

CLINICAL THERAPY

Treatment of metabolic acidosis depends on identification and treatment of the underlying cause. In severe metabolic acidosis, intravenous sodium bicarbonate may be used to increase the pH and to prevent cardiac arrhythmias. This treatment is difficult to manage because renal excretion can cause excess retention of bicarbonate; therefore, intravenous sodium bicarbonate is used only in severe situations, such as prolonged cardiac arrest.

Nursing Management

For the Child With Metabolic Acidosis

Nursing Assessment and Diagnosis

Teach prevention of poisoning at each health promotion visit. For the child admitted with acidosis, assess the rate and depth of respirations. Evaluate the child's level of consciousness frequently. Be alert for signs or complaints of headache and abdominal pain. Serial arterial blood gas measurements will usually be obtained to evaluate changes in status.

Several nursing diagnoses can apply to the child with metabolic acidosis, including the following (NANDA-I © 2014):

- *Injury, Risk for,* related to confusion/drowsiness or decreased responsiveness
- *Cardiac Output, Decreased,* related to cardiac arrhythmias
- *Tissue Perfusion: Cerebral, Risk for Ineffective,* related to tissue hypoxia
- *Health Management, Family, Ineffective,* related to complexity of management of diabetes mellitus

Planning and Implementation

Ensure safety, taking into account the child's level of consciousness and alertness. Change the child's position to prevent pressure on the skin. Limit the child's activities to decrease cardiac workload.

Position the child to facilitate chest expansion. Provide oral care during rapid respirations because the mouth may become dry.

Monitor intravenous solutions and laboratory values indicating acid–base balance. Report changes promptly.

Once the child is stabilized, provide teaching to compensate for knowledge deficits. Teach parents of young children to keep medications and acids locked up and out of reach to prevent poisoning (Figure 18–13). This includes medicines with aspirin as well as substances commonly kept in the garage for car maintenance. Teach about home management of diabetes and about early identification and treatment to avoid diabetic ketoacidosis.

Evaluation

Expected outcomes of nursing care relate to prevention of acidosis and restoration of normal body balance during disease processes.

Metabolic Alkalosis

Metabolic alkalosis occurs when there are too few metabolic acids. It is sometimes called *noncarbonic acid deficit*.

A gain in bicarbonate or a loss of metabolic acid can cause metabolic alkalosis. Bicarbonate is gained through excessive intake of bicarbonate antacids or baking soda or through metabolism of bicarbonate precursors such as the citrate contained in blood transfusions. Increased renal absorption of bicarbonate can occur in profound hypokalemia, primary hyperaldosteronism, or extreme deficit in extracellular fluid volume. Use of enhanced water to constitute powdered formula can be a cause of metabolic alkalosis. Acid can be lost through severe vomiting, such as that seen in infants with pyloric stenosis, and through continued removal of gastric contents through suction.

When the chemoreceptors in the brain and arteries detect the rising pH of metabolic alkalosis and respirations decrease, the body retains carbonic acid. This carbonic acid can neutralize the bicarbonate and return pH toward normal.

Blood pH, bicarbonate, and P_{CO_2} are usually elevated in metabolic alkalosis (Table 18–23). Hypokalemia often occurs simultaneously. Respiratory rate and depth usually decrease.

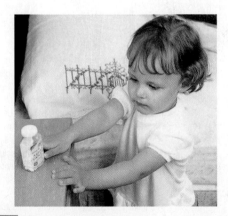

Figure 18–13 **Prevent metabolic acidosis from poisoning. Teaching parents to use safety latches on cabinets to keep aspirin away from small children can help prevent one cause of metabolic acidosis.**

TABLE 18–23 Laboratory Values in Uncompensated and Compensated Metabolic Alkalosis

TYPE OF METABOLIC ALKALOSIS	HCO$_3^-$	pH	P$_{CO_2}$
Acute condition; uncompensated	Increased	Increased	Normal
Partially compensated	Increased	Increased but moving toward normal	Increasing
Fully compensated	The need for oxygen drives respirations and limits full compensation for metabolic alkalosis		

Increased neuromuscular irritability, cramping, paresthesia, tetany, seizures, and excitation can occur. Finally, this state can progress to weakness, confusion, lethargy, and coma.

Clinical therapy is directed at treating the underlying cause of the condition. Increasing the extracellular fluid volume with intravenous normal saline facilitates renal excretion of bicarbonate.

Nursing Management

Assess the child's level of consciousness frequently. Alertness may decrease after an initial period of excitement, so regular assessments are needed. Monitor neuromuscular irritability. Observe for nausea and vomiting. Assess the rate and depth of respirations carefully. Obtain serial arterial blood gas measurements as ordered.

Facilitate ease of respirations. Ensure safety by keeping bed rails elevated and by turning the child frequently. Position the child on the side to avoid aspiration of vomitus.

If antacids or improper formula constitution were the cause of the alkalosis, teach the child and parents about correct use of these medications.

Mixed Acid–Base Imbalances

It is possible for two acid–base imbalances to occur at the same time. For example, a child with cystic fibrosis can develop respiratory acidosis from lung problems and concurrent metabolic alkalosis from vomiting during an illness. Treatment with diuretics may cause concurrent metabolic alkalosis resulting from extracellular volume depletion and hypokalemia in a child with congestive heart failure and chronic respiratory acidosis. In these cases, all underlying causes must be identified and treated. Care of children with mixed acid–base imbalances is often complicated, requiring hospitalization and careful management. On discharge, the nurse can teach parents about signs of imbalance that need to be reported and treated to prevent further complications. Evaluation of care is based on outcomes of adequate respiratory ventilation and metabolic balance.

Chapter Highlights

- Young children are at risk for fluid and electrolyte imbalance due to differences in body fluid compartments and regulation systems.

- Nurses institute health promotion and health maintenance measures to maintain normal body fluids for children who exercise in hot weather and those undergoing surgery.

- Extracellular fluid volume deficit manifests as dehydration.

- Extracellular fluid volume excess is due to an excess of saline in the body. Interstitial fluid volume excess manifests as edema and weight gain. Nurses carefully manage fluid status of young children and teach parents prevention and treatment

of fluid imbalances caused by gastroenteritis and other disease states.

- The most common electrolyte imbalances are hypernatremia and hypokalemia, and thus involve sodium and potassium.

- Normal acid–base balance is necessary for proper function of cells in the body.

- The lungs, kidneys, and liver play a role in maintaining acid–base balance.

- Acid–base imbalance can involve alkalosis or acidosis; either can have a respiratory or metabolic origin.

Clinical Reasoning in Action

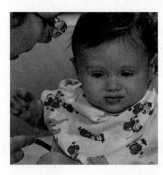

A 10-month-old named Devin comes to the emergency department by ambulance at 3:00 a.m. for respiratory distress. His parents state that he was experiencing a cough for the past week and developed a fever of over 103.0°F (39.4°C) tonight. He woke up crying with a frightening cough and could barely catch his breath; the parents called 9-1-1. Devin's respiratory rate is 50 times per minute with moderate retractions, his temperature is 104.2°F (40.1°C), his heart has a regular rhythm with a rate of 150 beats per minute, and he has stridor while breathing. At the hospital, after a breathing treatment with racemic epinephrine, his respiratory rate decreases to 40 and retractions improve. The arterial blood gas measurements show an increased P_{CO_2}, a decreased pH, and a normal HCO_3^-. A diagnosis of croup syndrome and resultant respiratory acidosis is made. Devin is admitted for monitoring.

1. What are some of the other possible causes of respiratory acidosis in children such as Devin?

2. What are some of the signs and symptoms of respiratory distress and the central nervous system problems associated with Devin's particular acid–base imbalance?

3. Devin's heart rate and rhythm are monitored closely in the hospital. What is the reason for these assessments?

4. What is the treatment for Devin's acid–base imbalance?

5. What are some of the measures taken in the hospital to ensure Devin's safety?

References

American Academy of Pediatrics (AAP). (2013). *Pediatric nutrition handbook* (7th ed.). Elk Grove Village, IL: Author.

American Academy of Pediatrics (AAP) Council on Sports Medicine and Fitness & Council on School Health. (2011). Policy statement—Climatic heat stress and exercising children and adolescents. *Pediatrics, 128,* e741–e747. doi:10.1542/peds.2011-1664

Bolat, F., Oflaz, M. B., Guven, A. S., Ozdemir, G., Alaygut, D., Dogan, M. T., . . . Fultekin, A. (2013). What is the safe approach for neonatal hypernatremic dehydration? A retrospective study from a neonatal intensive care unit. *Pediatric Emergency Care, 29,* 808–813.

Carcillo, J. A. (2014). Intravenous fluid choices in critically ill children. *Current Opinion in Critical Care, 20,* 396–401.

Children's Mercy Hospital. (2011). *Guidelines for oral rehydration.* Retrieved from http://www.childrens-mercy.org/Content/view.aspx?id=8130

Corbett, J. V., & Banks, A. (2013). *Laboratory tests and diagnostic procedures* (8th ed.). Upper Saddle River, NJ: Pearson.

Crawford, A., & Harris, H. (2011a). Balancing act: Sodium and potassium. *Nursing 2011, 41,* 44–50.

Crawford, A., & Harris, H. (2011b). Balancing act: Hypomagnesemia and hypermagnesemia. *Nursing 2011, 41,* 52–55.

Dzierba, A. L., & Abraham, P. (2011). A practical approach to understanding acid-base abnormalities in critical illness. *Journal of Pharmacy Practice, 24,* 17–26.

Engorn, B., & Flerlage, J. (2014). *The Harriet Lane handbook* (20th ed.). St. Louis, MO: Elsevier Saunders.

Feld, L. G., & Kaskel, F. J. (2012). *Fluid and electrolytes in pediatrics.* New York: Humana Press, Springer Publishers.

Freedman, S. B., Ali, S., Oleszczuk, M., Gouin, S., & Hartling, L. (2013). Treatment of acute gastroenteritis

in children: An overview of systematic reviews of interventions commonly used in developed countries. *Evidence Based Child Health, 8,* 1123–1137.

Freedman, S. B., Keating, L. E., Rumatir, M., & Schuh, S. (2012). Health care provider and caregiver preferences regarding nasogastric and intravenous rehydration. *Pediatrics, 130,* e1504–e1511.

Frohna, J. G. (2011). Oral rehydration solution with zinc and prebiotics decreases duration of acute diarrhea in children. *Journal of Pediatrics, 158,* 288–292.

Greenbaum, L. A. (2011). *Electrolyte and acid–base disorder.* In R. M. Kliegman, B. F. Stanton, J. W. St. Geme, N. F. Schor, & R. E. Behrman (Eds.), *Nelson textbook of pediatrics* (19th ed., pp. 212–242). Philadelphia, PA: Saunders.

Jablonski, S. (2012). Oral rehydration of the pediatric patient with mild to moderate dehydration. *Journal of Emergency Nursing, 38,* 185–187.

Kinlin, L. M., & Freedman, S. B. (2012). Evaluation of a clinical dehydration scale in children requiring intravenous rehydration. *Pediatrics, 129*, e1211–e1219.

Kliegman, R. M., Stanton, B. F., St. Geme, J., Schor, N. F., & Behrman, R. E. (Eds.). (2011). *Nelson textbook of pediatrics* (19th ed.). Philadelphia, PA: Saunders.

LeMone, P., Burke, K. M., Bauldoff, G., & Gubrud, P. (2015). *Medical surgical nursing* (6th ed.). Hoboken, NJ: Prentice Hall Health.

Lenters, L. M., Das, J. K., & Bhutta, Z. A. (2013). Systematic review of strategies to increase use of oral rehydration solution at the household level. *BMC Public Health, 13*(Suppl 3), S3–S28.

Mayo Clinic. (2011). *Dehydration and youth sports: Curb the risk*. Retrieved from http://www.mayoclinic.com

NIH Osteoporosis and Related Bone Diseases National Resource Center. (2011). *Osteoporosis and African American women*. Retrieved from http://www.niams.nih.gov/Health_Info/Bone/Osteoporosis/Background/default.asp

Nir, V., Nadir, E., Schechter, Y., & Kline-Kremer, A. (2013). Parents' attitudes toward oral rehydration therapy in children with mild-to-moderate dehydration. *Scientific World Journal,* Nov. 4, doi:10.1155/20

Ruppe, M. D. (2011). Medications that affect calcium. *Endocrine Practice, 17*(Suppl. 1), 26–30.

Soldin, S. J., Wong, E. C., Brugnara, C., & Soldin, O. P. (2011). *Pediatric reference ranges* (7th ed.). Washington, DC: American Association for Clinical Chemistry.

Wang, J., Xu, E., & Xiao, Y. (2014). Isotonic versus hypotonic maintenance IV fluid in hospitalized children: A meta-analysis. *Pediatrics, 133*, 105–113.

World Health Organization (2014). *Oral rehydration solutions*. Retrieved from http://rehydrate.org/solutions/homemade.htm

Chapter 19
Alterations in Eye, Ear, Nose, and Throat Function

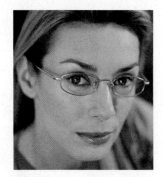

The early intervention program that Raeanne attended to help her deal with her visual impairment prepared her well for preschool. We learned a lot too about how to help her. We are still really nervous about her starting at preschool and being with a lot of other children. We want it to go well for her.

—Mother of Raeanne, 3 years old

Digital Vision/Getty Images

⌄ Learning Outcomes

19.1 Identify anatomy, physiology, and pediatric differences in the eye, ear, nose, and throat of children and adolescents.

19.2 Describe abnormalities of the eyes, ears, nose, throat, and mouth in children.

19.3 Carry out screening programs to identify children with vision and hearing abnormalities.

19.4 Plan nursing care for children with vision or hearing impairments.

19.5 Select and apply latest recommendations when implementing care and teaching for children with abnormalities of eyes, ears, nose, throat, and mouth.

19.6 Integrate preventive and treatment principles when implementing health promotion for children related to eyes, ears, nose, and throat.

The eye, ear, nose, and throat are connected, so a malformation, infection, or other condition in one of these structures may affect them all. Intact sensory structures enable children to reach developmental milestones; thus alterations, especially to the eye and ear, may delay a child's development. Most children with eye, ear, nose, and throat disorders are treated at home or in the community rather than in the hospital. How are conditions of the eye, ear, nose, and throat related? Which conditions have the potential to affect a child's growth, development, and behavior? In what settings do children with eye, ear, nose, and throat conditions receive care? How can parents be helped to foster development in their children when they have a visual or hearing disorder?

Disorders of the Eye

Infectious Conjunctivitis

Conjunctivitis is an inflammation of the conjunctiva, the clear membrane that lines the inside of the lid and sclera. Bacteria, viruses, allergies, trauma, or irritants cause the conjunctiva to become swollen and red with a yellow or white discharge (Figure 19–1). Parents commonly refer to all conjunctivitis as "pink eye."

Conjunctivitis in a newborn or infant under 30 days of age is called *ophthalmia neonatorum*. These infections are usually acquired from the mother during vaginal birth as a result

Text continues on page 444

FOCUS ON:
Eyes, Ears, Nose, and Throat

Anatomy and Physiology

Sight, hearing, taste, and smell depend on proper functioning of receptor organs and interpretation by the brain. Thus, certain cranial nerves are also an integral part of the anatomy and physiology of the eye, ear, nose, throat, and mouth. Children are prone to both inborn and acquired sensory alterations, as well as a wide array of infections and injuries that can affect the eye, ear, nose, throat, mouth, and upper respiratory system. Because these body parts are connected anatomically, conditions in one necessarily affect the others. Other conditions of the respiratory system, including obstructive sleep apnea, are discussed in Chapter 20.

Eye

The eye is a complex structure composed of the eyeball and its supporting structures. The *sclera,* or white part of the eye, is the outermost layer. It is transparent in the anterior eye to form the *cornea*, which allows light to enter. The *iris,* or colored part of the eye, is muscular, allowing it to change the size of the *pupil* and regulate the light that enters the eye. The *lens* is located behind the pupil and focuses light onto the retina. The *anterior chamber,* or the space between the cornea and iris, is filled with a fluid called *aqueous humor.* The *posterior chamber* is located behind the lens and is filled with *vitreous humor.* The innermost, posterior section of the eye is the *retina,* which has an inner layer that receives light impulses and an outer neural layer that transports visual images to the brain by the optic nerve (cranial nerve II). The *rods* in the retina perceive vision in dim light and allow for peripheral vision; the *cones* perceive vision in bright light and are responsible for color discernment. See *As Children Grow: The Eye* for normal structures of the child's eye.

The eye has several supporting structures that assist in the sensation of vision. *Eyebrows*, *eyelids*, and *eyelashes* protect the eye and add touch sensation. The *conjunctiva* lines the cornea and the inside of the eyelids, lubricating the eye and keeping it viable. The lacrimal apparatus and ducts bathe the eye and produce tears. A series of six muscles allow the eye to move to all planes and maintain the shape of the eyeball. They are innervated by the oculomotor, trochlear, and abducens nerves (cranial nerves III, IV, and V).

Ear

The ear is responsible for the sensory ability of hearing and it establishes the sense of equilibrium. The *external ear* contains the *auricle,* which is visible outside the body; the *external canal*; and the *tympanic membrane*. These structures collect sound waves and direct them to the middle and inner ear. The *middle ear* lies behind the tympanic membrane and contains three bones necessary for sound vibrations: the *incus*, *malleus*, and *stapes*. Another part of the middle ear, the *eustachian tube*, connects to the nasopharynx and equalizes ear pressure. The *inner ear* contains the bony labyrinth, which in turn houses the *vestibule, semicircular canals*, and the *cochlea*. The vestibule and semicircular canals are responsible for the sense of equilibrium. The cochlea contains the *organ of Corti,* which contains sensory hair cells that are innervated by the acoustic nerve (cranial nerve VIII).

As Children Grow: **The Eye**

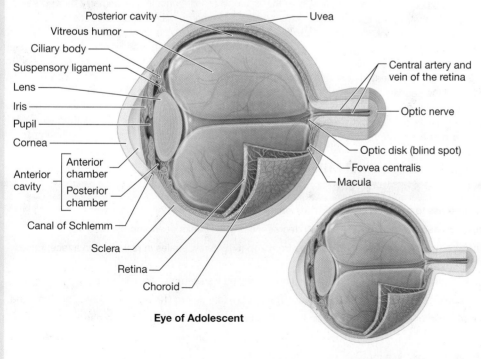

Eye of Adolescent

Eye of Young Child

The eye is well developed at birth, but there are some variations in the visual acuity of the infant and young child. What influence would the young child's visual acuity have on the types of toys and books that should be made available?

(continued)

Nose, Throat, and Mouth

The structures of the nose, throat, and mouth are important to all humans. Mucous membranes bathe these body parts and have a high rate of growth. They help maintain hygiene and protect the body from infectious agents. Salivary apparatus and taste buds are essential parts of the mouth and tongue. The nasal passages contain external nostrils, the sinuses, and the pharynx (or throat). The olfactory, facial, glossopharyngeal, and vagus nerves (cranial nerves I, VII, IX, and X) are responsible for the sense of smell, taste, coordinated swallowing, and the gag reflex, respectively.

Pediatric Differences

Eye

How are the eyes of children different from those of adults? Chapter 5 provides a detailed discussion of the assessment of the eyes and **visual acuity**, the ability to discriminate letters or other objects. The eyes of neonates differ from the eyes of adults in several ways. Visual acuity in neonates ranges between 20/100 and 20/400. The lens is more spherical and cannot accommodate to both near and far objects, which means that the neonate sees best at a distance of about 20 cm (8 in.). Because the optic nerve is not yet completely myelinated, the ability to distinguish color and other details is decreased. If the infant is preterm, especially less than 32 weeks' gestation, retinal vascularization, particularly in the periphery of the retina, may be incomplete (Hou et al., 2011; Wang, Spencer, Leffler, et al., 2012). Pupillary reflex reaction is detected by about 28 to 30 weeks' gestation and so may be sluggish in preterm infants. The rectus muscles that control binocular vision may be somewhat uncoordinated at birth. The eyes should be aligned and movement coordinated by the age of 3 months. Transient nystagmus (involuntary rapid eye movement) and esotropia (momentary turning inward of eyes) are common in neonates but decrease in incidence during the first few months of life. Conjunctival and retinal hemorrhages may be observed in the newborn as a result of the trauma of birth; they usually improve gradually and have no lasting effects. The red reflex is examined in children, because it is a key method for identifying the presence of retinoblastoma (see Chapter 5 for the method to evaluate the red reflex and Chapter 24 for a description of retinoblastoma).

The cornea of the infant and young child occupies a larger portion of the orbit than in the adult; the eyeball is about 3/4 of its adult size. Because the eyeball is relatively unprotected laterally, it is more easily injured. The sclera of the neonate is thin and translucent with a bluish tinge, and the iris is blue or gray. Eye color changes during the first 6 months of life. Infants produce tears to nourish and oxygenate the outer layers of the cornea. However, parents do not see tears when a young infant cries because the infant's lacrimal system drains them efficiently into the nasal cavity.

As infants grow, their eyes mature and their vision improves. The eyeball grows until the third year, when growth slows, until normal adult size is reached by 14 years. By the age of 2 or 3 years, most children have a visual acuity of 20/50, and by the age of 6 or 7 years, it is 20/20. See *As Children Grow: The Eye* for a summary of pediatric differences of the eye. Visual acuity is measured using standardized letter or picture charts (see Chapter 5 and the *Clinical Skills Manual* SKILLS. **Vision** refers to the complex process of acquiring meaning from what is seen, involving the eye, brain, and related neurologic and physiologic structures. Cognitive development interacts with a child's maturing physiologic system to bring increasing meaning to objects in sight (Table 19–1). The first few years of life are considered critical for the formation of normal vision. As acuity improves, the brain learns to interpret messages received from the eyes. Disturbances in vision, even in one eye, can affect the retinal nerve function, muscle function in the eye, or the brain's ability to interpret visual input.

Ear

Why do infants and young children have more ear problems than adults? The eustachian tube, which connects the nasopharynx to the middle ear, is proportionately shorter, wider, and more horizontal in infants than in older children or adults (see *As Children Grow: Eustachian Tube*). During sucking, yawning, and other movements, the tube opens for milliseconds, allowing free passage of air between the nasopharynx and the middle ear. These factors predispose young children to development of otitis media, or middle ear infection.

The fetus can hear at about 20 weeks' gestation. The auditory nerve function is mature at about 5 months of age in the infant. Before 34 weeks' gestation, the external ear is soft with little cartilage apparent. The external ear canal is small at birth, although the internal ear and middle ear are relatively large. As a result, the tympanic membrane is close to the surface and can be easily injured.

Nose, Throat, and Mouth

Up to the age of 6 months, infants are primarily nasal breathers. Edema and nasal discharge may interfere with adequate air intake and feeding. Mucosal swelling and exudate may block the small nasal passages of young children. The immature immune system of young children (see Chapter 22 for further description) and the frequent exposure to other children with illnesses causes a high rate of upper respiratory infections in this population.

The palatine tonsils, which are visible on oral examination, are located on each side of the oropharynx. The method for examining a child's throat is discussed in Chapter 5. Although tonsils

TABLE 19–1 Visually Related Developmental Milestones

AGE	MILESTONE
Term neonate	Demonstrates alertness to light and visual stimulus presented 20–30 cm (8–12 in.) from eyes.
1 month	Follows an object 60 degrees horizontally and 30 degrees vertically; blinks at an approaching object.
2 months	Follows a person or moving object for 180 degrees from 2 m (6 ft) away; smiles in response to a face; raises head 30 degrees from prone.
3 months	Tracks an object through 180 degrees; regards own hand; begins visual–motor coordination.
4–5 months	Social smile; reaches for a cube 30 cm (12 in.) away; notices a raisin 30 cm (12 in.) away; stares at own hand.
7–8 months	Reaches and grasps an object, picks up a raisin by raking, transfers objects from hand to hand.
8–9 months	Pokes at holes in a peg board; well-developed pincer grasp; crawls; uncovers toy after seeing it hidden.
12–14 months	Stacks blocks; places a peg in a round hole; stands and walks.

Source: Data from Rudolph, C., Rudolph, A., Lister, G., First, L., & Gershon, A. (Eds.). (2011). *Rudolph's pediatrics* (22nd ed.). New York, NY: McGraw-Hill; Kliegman, R. M., Stanton, B. F., St. Geme, J., Schor, N. F., & Behrman, R. E. (Eds.). (2015). *Nelson textbook of pediatrics* (20th ed.). Philadelphia, PA: Saunders.

As Children Grow: **Eustachian Tube**

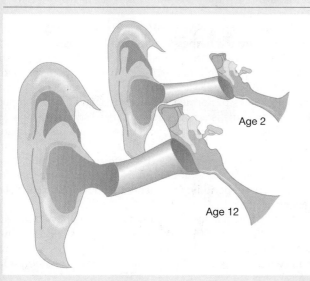

Age 2

Age 12

Position of eustachian tube is at less of an angle in the young child, resulting in decreased drainage (more horizontal).

End of eustachian tube in nasal pharynx opens during sucking.

Eustachian tube equalizes air pressure between the middle ear and the outside environment and allows for drainage of secretions from middle ear mucosa.

Of the three anatomic differences in the eustachian tube between adults and small children (shorter, wider, more horizontal), which do you think could cause more problems for the child and why?

vary in size considerably during childhood, they are normally large, especially in school-age children. The nasopharyngeal tonsils (adenoids) lie in the posterior wall of the nasopharynx, just above the oropharynx. In children, the adenoids may become enlarged, harboring bacteria and interfering with breathing.

The mouth is an important organ for the infant, because strong muscles are needed for sucking and thereby receiving nutrients. Sucking is an important developmental skill that promotes the muscles needed for later speech development. Taste sensation is present before birth, as evidenced by increased swallowing of amniotic fluid that has been sweetened. Taste sensations

increase during childhood. By about 6 months of age the first tooth emerges, and by about 2 years the full set of 20 primary teeth is present. Tooth loss of the primary set begins at about 5–6 years, and gradually the secondary teeth (32 total) erupt during childhood. See Chapter 5 for a further description of teeth eruption.

A variety of diagnostic and laboratory tests are used to evaluate the eye, ear, nose, and throat. See Appendices D and E and Chapter 5 for details about audiologic screening, newborn hearing screening, tympanogram, complete blood count (CBC), and culture/sensitivity test. See *Assessment Guide: The Child With an Alteration of the Eye, Ear, Nose, or Throat.*

ASSESSMENT GUIDE | The Child With an Alteration of the Eye, Ear, Nose, or Throat

Assessment Focus	Assessment Guidelines
Eyes	• Describe eye structures and symmetry.
	• Describe visual acuity using the screening test appropriate for age.
	• Measure extraocular movements to all quadrants. Evaluate corneal light reflex, cover–uncover test, and visual fields.
	• Using the ophthalmoscope, elicit and evaluate the red reflex bilaterally.
	• Observe for and report abnormalities such as eye drainage, cloudiness of lens, or abnormal movement.
Ears	• Describe placement and symmetry of the external ear.
	• Describe auditory acuity using the screening test appropriate for age.
	• Using the otoscope, evaluate the ear canal and tympanic membrane.
	• Ask about pain and discomfort from the ear; observe for drainage.
Nose	• Describe the nose for symmetry and placement. Are the nares bilaterally patent? Are there lesions or drainage?
	• Can the child identify several smells?
	• Are signs of sinus infection present, such as facial edema or pain, headache, and tenderness upon palpation over the sinus areas?
Mouth and throat	• Are the oral mucous membranes intact? Is there an odor?
	• How many primary/secondary/loose teeth are present? Are there visible caries? Are there broken or chipped teeth present?
	• Evaluate the soft and hard palate for intactness.
	• Describe the throat and size/appearance of the tonsils.
	• Palpate cervical lymph nodes, noting size and tenderness.

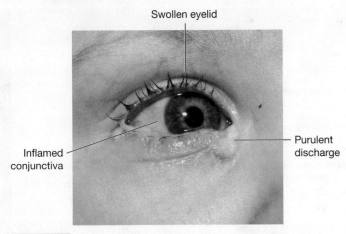

Swollen eyelid

Inflamed
conjunctiva

Purulent
discharge

Figure 19–1 **Acute conjunctivitis. The major difference between bacterial and viral conjunctivitis is that bacterial conjunctivitis has a purulent discharge that may result in crusting, whereas the discharge from viral conjunctivitis is serous (watery). Allergic conjunctivitis produces watery to thick drainage and is characterized by itching.**

SOURCE: Dr. P. Marazzi/Science Source.

of contact with infected vaginal discharge containing organisms such as *Chlamydia trachomatis* and *Neisseria gonorrhoeae*. Newborns occasionally get chemical conjunctivitis in response to prophylactic eye treatment. This may be a cause when the conjunctivitis develops within 24 to 48 hours after instillation of the medication.

Another cause of infection in infants is herpesvirus, which requires prompt and vigorous treatment to prevent eye injury or blindness. Infants with herpesvirus infections of the eye are treated with intravenous acyclovir as well as topical drops.

In infants who have frequent tearing and "mattering" (eyelid discharge that has formed a crust) on awakening, a plugged lacrimal duct may mimic conjunctivitis. Treatment involves massaging the tear duct every 4 hours when the infant is awake. Lacrimal ducts that remain plugged after the age of 1 year may have to be opened surgically.

Bacterial conjunctivitis can occur in children of any age. It is characterized by edema of the eyelid, red conjunctiva, and enlarged preauricular lymph glands. There is usually mucopurulent exudate that causes mattering, making the eyes difficult to open upon awakening. Older children with conjunctivitis complain of itching or burning, mild photophobia, and a feeling of scratching under the lids. Parents may notice increased tearing or a mucoid or mucopurulent discharge, redness and swelling of the conjunctiva, a pink sclera, and crusty eyelids, especially in the morning. There is no change in vision. Common infectious organisms include *Staphylococcus aureus, Haemophilus influenzae, Streptococcus pneumoniae,* and *Moraxella catarrhalis* (Gold, 2011). Most cases are caused by hand-to-eye contact, and the disease can rapidly spread whenever groups of youth spend time together, such as among young children and adolescents in schools and childcare centers, and even among college students in dormitories, sororities, fraternities, and on sports teams. Although bacterial conjunctivitis can be bilateral, it is more commonly unilateral.

Other infections in newborns and children can be caused by viruses. *Viral conjunctivitis* is more often bilateral than unilateral. Adenovirus is a common cause and spreads from respiratory adenovirus infection in hand-to-eye transmission. Signs and symptoms are similar to those of bacterial conjunctivitis, although they are sometimes milder in severity and slower in onset.

Herpes simplex virus (HSV) can also cause infection, either by transfer from a herpes-infected mother to her baby during birth or by contact with an infected person in infants or children of any age. Ophthalmic herpes infection is often accompanied by characteristic vesicular lesions on the skin of the face. A culture of the lesions is performed for diagnosis, and any accompanying conjunctivitis is assumed to be caused by herpesvirus. For the infection caused by HSV, prompt and vigorous treatment is needed to prevent eye injury or blindness, which can occur in children with recurrent herpesvirus infections as a result of antibody reaction to the viral antigen. Herpesvirus infections commonly recur so periodic treatment and sometimes prophylaxis may be needed.

Allergic conjunctivitis is a common cause of eye discomfort (Ortiz, 2013; Steele, 2012). When conjunctivitis is caused by an allergy, the child complains of intense itching. Eyes are red with watery discharge, and the conjunctivae have a "cobblestone" appearance.

In most cases, a diagnosis of the cause of conjunctivitis is made based on the history and symptoms. Cultures can be taken, especially in infants or in cases suspected of being an unusual bacterial illness or herpesvirus infection. A Gram stain of discharge and conjunctival scraping for potential chlamydial infection or herpesvirus infection are performed. Infants and children must be promptly referred to primary healthcare providers or eye specialists for treatment of possible eye infections. When diagnosed in the neonatal intensive care unit, the infant is isolated to prevent spread to other infants.

Antibiotic eye medication is prescribed in droplet or ointment form if a bacterial infection is suspected. Treatment may be started after a laboratory sample is obtained but before the results are known. Fluoroquinolones are now frequently used to treat bacterial conjunctivitis; drops or ointment can be used (O'Brien, 2012). Other drugs used to treat bacterial infections include bacotracom, erythromycin, azithromycin, and aminoglycosides (Granet, 2011; O'Brien, 2012). Newborn gonococcal conjunctivitis is treated with ceftriaxone. Chlamydial infections are treated with oral erythromycin. Careful total evaluation of the newborn with any conjunctivitis is also performed to watch for other signs of infection. Instructions for instilling eye medication are provided in the *Clinical Skills Manual* SKILLS .

Viral conjunctivitis may be treated with comfort measures such as cleaning drainage away with a warm clean cloth and avoiding bright lights and reading to the child. Ophthalmic antibiotics may sometimes be given to prevent bacterial invasion due to frequent rubbing of the eyes. Herpes simplex virus infections of the eye are treated promptly by an ophthalmologist, neonatologist, or others who are trained in this serious disease. Topical drugs are used, and often are combined with a systemic antiviral agent such as acyclovir. Neonatal herpes simplex virus infection is treated vigorously with parenteral acyclovir for 14 days (or longer if central nervous system involvement is found upon lumbar puncture) and with topical ophthalmic medication (trifluridine, iododeoxyuridine, or vidarabine). Recurrent lesions may necessitate suppressive or prophylactic treatment with oral acyclovir, the dosage of which must be adjusted according to the child's age and weight (Liu, Pavan-Langston, & Colby, 2012).

If an allergen is diagnosed as the cause of conjunctivitis, systemic or topical antihistamines may be prescribed. Topical steroids and vasoconstrictors may also be used. Decongestants can be combined with systemic antihistamines for short-term therapy. Mast-cell stabilizers may be used to decrease the activation of mast cells that accompanies allergic reactions; their use is safe in children 3 years of age and older.

Nursing Management

Nurses routinely instill antibiotics into the eyes of newborns after birth. Perform a careful examination so that any cases of ophthalmia neonatorum can be referred promptly to an ophthalmologist. Women infected with gonococcus or chlamydia should be identified so their babies can receive attention and medication at birth to prevent infection. Babies born at home should have ocular examinations soon after birth.

In suspected conjunctivitis, gentle pressure for several seconds with a gloved index finger placed next to the inner corner of the eye may cause a discharge of mucopurulent drainage. Refer for care and report the findings. Since infectious conjunctivitis is extremely contagious, tell parents that children should not return to child care or school until they have been taking an antibiotic for 24 hours. Teach parents the importance of careful hand hygiene and the avoidance of shared towels. Tell parents that children should not rub their eyes. Mittens may help prevent infants from rubbing their eyes. Toddlers may be distracted by activities that keep their hands busy. Teach parents the proper techniques for instilling eye medications. For children with allergies, alert parents to signs of infection so if the child gets an eye infection, they will seek prompt treatment.

Periorbital Cellulitis

Periorbital cellulitis is a bacterial infection of the eyelid and surrounding tissues that is usually caused by *Streptococcus* or *Staphylococcus*. Children present with swollen, tender, red or purple eyelids; restricted, painful movement of the area around the eye; and fever. Periorbital cellulitis should be treated promptly to prevent the spread of the infection to the posterior orbit. Orbital cellulitis is a serious outcome that can lead to bacterial meningitis. Management includes hospitalization for intravenous antibiotics and the application of hot packs. Children usually respond favorably within 48 to 72 hours (Cohen, 2011; Seltz, Smith, Durairaj, et al., 2011).

Visual Disorders

Vision, the complex process of acquiring meaning from what is seen, depends on many factors. The eyes must move quickly and in a coordinated manner. (See Chapter 5 for discussion of eye movement assessment.) They must function together for clear, single vision to occur. If this ability, called **binocularity**, is not present (perhaps because of strabismus or amblyopia), the child may have double vision and the brain cannot make sense of the images it receives. Normally, perceptions of objects seen are integrated with other senses through eye–hand coordination, and with the brain through visual imagery and discrimination of objects seen. Although visual acuity is essential, the child's movements, mental processes, and other senses all interact to give meaning to objects that are viewed. Vision therefore influences learning and school performance (Davidson & Quinn, 2011).

Visual disturbances must be diagnosed and treated promptly to prevent impairment or loss of vision. Most children undergo a simple test for visual acuity during healthcare visits as soon as they can cooperate with the examiner. Once in school, children's visual acuity is screened every 2 to 3 years during the elementary years. Nurses often organize vision screening programs for children. Table 19–2 provides a series of questions that can be used to identify visual disturbances in children. A child who does not pass vision screening is referred to an ophthalmologist or optometrist for more detailed examination of near and far vision, eye structure and movement, and color discrimination.

Families Want to Know

Instilling Eye Medications in Children

It can be challenging to safely instill medication into young children's eyes. Give parents the following suggestions:

- Wash your hands well.
- Be sure the medicine is warmed at least to room temperature.
- Remove any drainage from the eye with a clean or sterile, moist, warm cloth or gauze.
- Wash your hands again.
- Have the child lie on the back with eyes closed.
- Gently pull the lower lid down to form a small pocket.
- Apply a thin string (for ointment) or drops of the medicine.
- Allow the eyelid to return to normal position.
- Have the child keep the eye closed for several seconds.
- Help prevent spread of the infection by keeping the child's hands clean.
- Enhance comfort by keeping the head elevated to decrease swelling and avoid exposure to bright light.

TABLE 19–2 Assessment Questions for Identifying Visual Disturbances in Children

YOUNG CHILD

Ask the parents:

Do your child's eyes follow you as you come into a room?

Are other objects followed with ease?

Do both eyes work together or does one seem to wander off?

At what age did your baby sit, stand, walk?

Does your child have any difficulty picking up objects?

SCHOOL-AGE CHILD

Ask the parents:

Does your child like to look at pictures and read?

Does your child hold toys or books close or sit very close to the television?

Does your child squint or rub the eyes?

Is your child at grade level in all subjects?

Has your child demonstrated any learning difficulties?

Does your child use a computer, watch television, or play computer games?

Does your child play sports and games at the same level of ability as peers?

Some of the common visual disorders in children are:

- *Hyperopia (farsightedness):* Light rays focus posterior to the retina, resulting in an inability to focus on nearby objects. All children have some degree of hyperopia until 9 to 10 years of age. However, their eyes can accommodate sufficiently to enable them to see near objects clearly. Blurring of vision occurs only in children with excessive hyperopia, or a difference in accommodation between the two eyes. *Amblyopia*, or a weakening of the poorer eye, can occur in these children if treatment is not obtained.

- *Myopia (nearsightedness):* Light rays focus anterior to the retina, resulting in an inability to see far-off objects. Although children of any age can manifest myopia, it most commonly develops at about 8 years of age. The child may complain of headaches and often squints to improve distance vision.

- *Astigmatism:* Light rays are refracted differently depending on their place of entry to the eye. The curvature of the cornea or lens is not uniformly spherical, causing blurred images. The child with astigmatism often holds pages very close to the face to obtain the best visual image.

For the description and management of four disorders that can significantly affect vision—strabismus, amblyopia, cataracts, and glaucoma—see Table 19–3.

Compensatory lenses are prescribed for most visual disorders. A significant difference in visual acuity between the eyes is often a result of amblyopia or strabismus, and further treatment may be needed. The visual acuity of a child with compensatory lenses should be reevaluated every 1 to 2 years. More frequent visits to an eye specialist are needed when a child is being treated for amblyopia or strabismus.

Nursing Management

The nurse plays an important role in identifying visual disorders in children and performing careful eye examinations of newborns and children. Observe for symmetry of placement and movement, ability to follow objects with each eye, and any abnormalities in appearance. The light reflex, cover–uncover test, and visual acuity testing are essential tests for every child. See Chapter 5 for a description of eye examination and the *Clinical Skills Manual* for visual acuity tests `SKILLS`.

Nurses in preschools and schools plan and carry out visual acuity screening on children. Generally, certain grades (such as kindergarten, 2, 4, 6, and 8) are screened annually along with any children new to a district. The nurse performs and records the screening results and informs the school and families of any children with abnormal results, who are then referred to an eye specialist for care. An important part of the screening process is following up on referrals to be certain that children receive the diagnostic care they need.

Healthy People 2020

(V-1) Increase the proportion of preschool children aged 5 years and under who receive vision screening

- Currently, only 40% of preschool children receive vision screening, while the goal is for 44% to have such screening by 2020. Clearly, nurses can play a role in increasing the number of young children who have vision screening.

When abnormalities are found on screening, nurses refer families to the care of an eye specialist. When prescriptive lenses are used, the nurse instructs the parent and child on correct wear practices and care. If surgery is required, surgical and postoperative follow-up are needed. This will include pain control, observing for signs of infection (ophthalmic or systemic), and administering needed eye medications. Sterile technique is used postoperatively to provide eye care. Promptly report deviations from normal such as increased pain, redness, discharge, or edema of the eye; increased temperature or pulse, which may indicate infection; increased sensitivity to light; or other abnormalities. Children are usually discharged home with instructions to minimize certain vigorous activities for a certain period of time. Perform postoperative and discharge teaching and emphasize the importance of follow-up visits.

Color Blindness

Color blindness is an X-linked recessive disorder found in 10% of males and very rarely in females; it is more common in White than Black males. The most common form affects the ability to distinguish between the colors red and green; blue-yellow discrimination and other colors can also be involved. Preschool boys are tested for color blindness in some clinics to identify those with the disorder (Adams, Verdon, & Spivey, 2012). Color blindness is not treatable, and management focuses on issues of safety (e.g., problems in distinguishing between red and green traffic signals) and techniques to improve discrimination of colors in the affected color groups.

TABLE 19–3 Clinical Manifestations of Visual Disorders

ETIOLOGY	CLINICAL MANIFESTATIONS	CLINICAL THERAPY
STRABISMUS Can be congenital or acquired. Seen in up to 4% of all children; 30%–50% of children with strabismus develop amblyopia. Most common types: **Esotropia:** inward deviation of eyes ("crossed eyes") **Exotropia:** outward deviation of eyes ("wall-eyes") 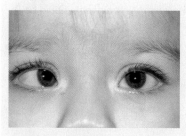 Strabismus. Source: Biophoto Associates/Science Source/Photo Researchers, Inc.	Eyes appear misaligned to observer. May occur only when child is tired. Symptoms include squinting and frowning when reading; closing one eye to see; having trouble picking up objects; dizziness and headache. Corneal light reflex and cover–uncover tests confirm diagnosis. Child may have no other abnormalities but certain conditions such as cerebral palsy, hydrocephalus, Down syndrome, and seizure disorder are more commonly accompanied by strabismus.	Occlusion therapy (patching the fixating or good eye for 1–2 hr daily to force use of the weak eye) Compensatory lenses Surgery of the rectus muscles to correct muscle imbalance Eye drops to cause blurring of the good eye Prisms Vision therapy (eye exercises) If treatment is begun before 24 months of age, amblyopia (reduced vision in one or both eyes) may be prevented.
AMBLYOPIA (LAZY EYE) Reduced vision in one or both eyes; affects up to 4% of children and is the leading cause of vision loss in children. Amblyopia can result from anything that causes visual deprivation to one eye. The most common causes are untreated strabismus, with the child "tuning out" the image in deviating eye, congenital cataract, or uncorrected refractive errors causing visual differences between eyes.	Symptoms are the same as for strabismus. Vision testing can be used to diagnose condition.	Compensatory lenses Occlusion therapy for 2–6 hr daily through patching the eye or eye glass Occasionally, vision therapy (eye exercises) is used in an attempt to improve the weaker eye. Atropine 1% 1 drop/day in unaffected eye. Treatment is discontinued when visual acuity no longer improves; 20/20 acuity rarely attained. Treatment is most successful if received by 5–6 years of age.
CATARACTS Occurs when all or part of lens of eye becomes opaque, which prevents refraction of light rays onto retina. Seen in 1–2/10,000 newborns. 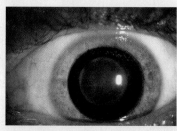 Congenital cataract. Source: Sue Ford/Science Source/Photo Researchers, Inc.	Can affect one or both eyes and may be congenital or acquired. Examples include a variety of genetic syndromes and maternally transmitted intrauterine infections. Clouding of lens indicates presence of cataract; however, cataracts are not always visible to naked eye. Symptoms include distorted red reflex, symptoms of vision loss (see strabismus), white pupil. May be present alone but sometimes associated with other conditions such as fetal alcohol syndrome, Down syndrome, and Turner syndrome.	Must be diagnosed at a young age for successful treatment; many cases are missed. When diagnosed, a thorough examination is warranted because of genetic systemic disorders that are sometimes associated with pediatric cataracts. Specific treatment depends on whether one or both eyes are affected, extent of clouding, and presence of other ocular abnormalities. Surgical removal of lens and corrective lenses; contact lenses frequently used; results of surgery are good; surgery before the age of 2 months is associated with the best results; visual acuity in 55% of children is 20/40 or better. Lens implant may be used. Eye protectors and restraints are used postoperatively to prevent injury; antibiotic or steroid drops may be used for several weeks; treatment for amblyopia may be necessary.

TABLE 19–3 Clinical Manifestations of Visual Disorders (*continued*)

ETIOLOGY	CLINICAL MANIFESTATIONS	CLINICAL THERAPY
GLAUCOMA		
Increased intraocular pressure damages eye and impairs visual function; ciliary body of eye produces aqueous fluid that flows between iris and lens into anterior chamber; if enough fluid accumulates, blindness results; about 1 in 10,000 newborns have glaucoma. May be congenital (occurring in first 3 years of life) or juvenile (occurring from 3–30 years) and affect one or both eyes. Acquired cases can be related to conditions such as eye trauma or neoplasm. Primary glaucoma (50% of cases) is an isolated anomaly of drainage; secondary glaucoma (50% of cases) is associated with other ocular or systemic abnormalities.	Symptoms of congenital glaucoma include tearing, blinking, corneal clouding, eyelid spasms, and progressive enlargement of eye; photophobia (extreme sensitivity to light). Symptoms of juvenile glaucoma include constant bumping into objects in child's periphery (painless visual field loss); seeing halos around objects. Diagnosis is made using a tonometer, which measures intraocular pressure.	Surgery to reduce intraocular pressure is treatment of choice, since medications used to combat glaucoma in adults are not as effective in children. Compensatory lenses are used following surgery. Treatment is not always successful, especially if the child has congenital glaucoma, so parents' feelings regarding care of a child with a visual impairment should be explored.

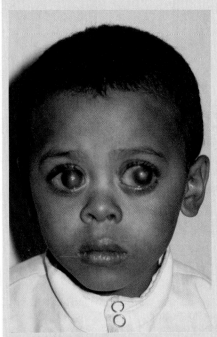

Congenital glaucoma.
Source: Custom Medical Stock Photo/Newscom.

Source: Data from American Association for Pediatric Ophthalmology and Strabismus. (2014). *Strabismus.* Retrieved from http://www.aapos.org/terms/conditions/100; Bradfield, Y. S. (2013). Identification and treatment of amblyopia. *American Family Physician, 87,* 348–352; Yeung, H. H., & Walton, D. S. (2012). Recognizing childhood glaucoma in the primary pediatric setting. *Contemporary Pediatrics, 29*(5), 32–40; Trumler, A. A. (2011). Evaluation of pediatric cataracts and systemic disorders. *Current Opinion in Ophthalmology, 22,* 365–379; Kliegman, R. M., Stanton, B., St. Geme, J., & Schor, N. (Eds.). (2016). *Nelson textbook of pediatrics* (20th ed., pp. 3021–3061). Philadelphia, PA: Saunders.

Retinopathy of Prematurity

Retinopathy of prematurity (ROP) occurs when immature blood vessels in the retina constrict and become necrotic. This condition, which may occur in infants of low birth weight or of short gestation, can heal completely or lead to mild myopia or retinal detachment and blindness.

ETIOLOGY AND PATHOPHYSIOLOGY

Retinopathy of prematurity results from injury to the developing capillaries of the retina. Oxygen therapy is associated with the development of ROP (Figure 19–2), but other factors such as respiratory distress, artificial ventilation, apnea, cerebral palsy, bradycardia, heart disease, multiple blood transfusions, infection, hypoxia, hypercarbia, acidosis, shock, and sepsis have also been linked with the disorder. It is most common in male infants born before 28 weeks of gestation and weighing under 1600 g (3 lb, 8 oz) at birth. A genetic link may be present because White infants are more commonly affected than those of African heritage, and Alaskan Natives have a high rate of the disorder. In developed countries, ROP is the second most common cause of blindness, with increasing prevalence in infants of lesser gestational age (Hartnett et al., 2014; National Eye Institute, 2014).

Pathophysiology Illustrated:
Visual Abnormalities

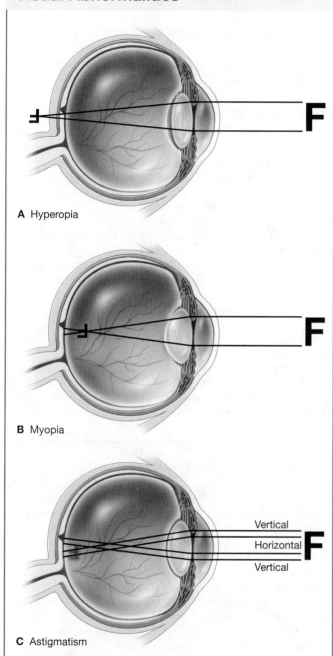

A Hyperopia

B Myopia

C Astigmatism

A, In hyperopia, light rays focus behind the retina, making it difficult to focus on objects at close range. *B,* In myopia, light rays focus in front of the retina, making it difficult to focus on objects that are far away. *C,* In astigmatism, light rays do not uniformly focus on the eye because of abnormal curvature of cornea or lens.

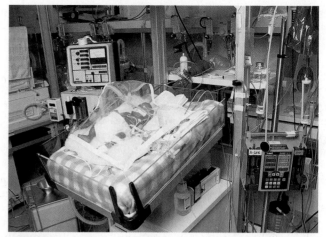

Figure 19–2 **Artificial ventilation and risk for retinopathy of prematurity. This premature infant in the neonatal intensive care unit is receiving artificial ventilation—a risk factor for retinopathy of prematurity. The infant will need careful management of oxygen exposure and periodic eye examinations.**

The retina is normally vascularized by about 8 months' gestation. However, for the premature infant, this process must continue after birth, and the environmental and other conditions listed in the preceding paragraph appear to affect its course. Arteriole constriction, followed by vascular proliferation of abnormal vessels, occurs. In most cases, the abnormal vessels gradually regress and normal vascularization occurs. Sometimes, however, the abnormal vascularization continues into the vitreous cavity, causing abnormalities of the retina, optic disc, and macula. It is not known why the disease progresses in some cases, but progression is directly linked to lower birth weight, greater prematurity, and duration (not necessarily concentration) of oxygen therapy. Raeanne, the child described in the scenario at the beginning of this chapter, developed retinopathy of prematurity after receiving oxygen therapy to aid her underdeveloped lungs.

Although the developing capillaries are lost, in many cases, some degree of revascularization occurs later (National Eye Institute, 2014). The degree of visual loss, varying from slight to total, is determined by the degree of revascularization.

CLINICAL MANIFESTATIONS

Retinopathy of prematurity is characterized by progressive changes in the retinal blood vessels, and in severe disease, by retinal detachment. Premature and low–birth-weight infants at risk for the disease are given frequent ocular examinations to ensure early detection of these changes. For infants who do not receive ophthalmologic examinations, resulting visual impairment may be detected only later in infancy when the child progresses slowly in meeting developmental milestones, fails to reach for objects, and does not follow objects or faces with the eyes. When visual impairment is present, the child usually manifests myopia. Total loss of vision can occur in the child who suffers a retinal detachment.

CLINICAL THERAPY

Diagnosis is made by ophthalmologic examination. A classification system that includes zone (area of retina with abnormal vasculature), stage (severity of disease), and plus disease (vascular dilation and tortuosity in posterior pole near optic nerve) is used to describe the location, extent, and severity of the disease (International Committee for the Classification of Retinopathy of Prematurity, 2005; National Institutes of Health, 2013). All infants at risk—namely, those born before 32 weeks of gestation and under 1500 g (3 lb, 7 oz) or those born after 32 weeks' gestation with birth weight from 1500 to 2000 g (3 lb, 7 oz to 4 lb, 3 oz)—are assessed frequently, using binocular ophthalmoscopy, by an ophthalmologist experienced with the condition. The disease is not manifested before 4 to 6 weeks after birth, so it is important that the infant receive regular eye examinations until the risk is discounted. Eye examinations continue every 1 to 3 weeks, with the frequency being determined by the location of disease, progress of disease, and the infant's degree of immature vascularization. Involvement of blood vessels in the periphery of the retina rarely leads to visual impairment. With involvement in other areas of the retina, risk of visual problems is more common.

Treatment of infants with retinopathy of prematurity may include laser therapy or cryotherapy to stop progression of the disease process. New therapies such as injections are being explored in research protocols. Surgical procedures such as a scleral buckle procedure and vitrectomy have been used in retinal detachments. Prompt treatment of accompanying problems such as strabismus, amblyopia, and myopia can promote maximal development.

Nursing Management

For the Child With Retinopathy of Prematurity

Nursing Assessment and Diagnosis

Assessment of the infant at risk for retinopathy of prematurity begins at birth by identifying infants who may require oxygen therapy or assisted ventilation. Look for risk factors such as prematurity and low birth weight. Assess the infant's breathing efforts and report any changes. Be certain the ventilation equipment is properly set to deliver the correct ventilatory pressure and amount of oxygen, evaluated by pulse oximetry saturation (see the *Clinical Skills Manual* SKILLS). Note the cumulative risks in a particular case and suggest the need for a referral to an ophthalmologist, as necessary.

The following *Nursing Care Plan: The Child With a Visual Impairment Secondary to Retinopathy of Prematurity* outlines several nursing diagnoses. Other nursing diagnoses may be appropriate for an infant with the potential to develop retinopathy of prematurity or a child with resulting visual impairment. They include the following (NANDA-I © 2014):

- *Gas Exchange, Impaired,* related to ventilation-perfusion imbalance
- *Development: Delayed, Risk for,* related to effects of visual impairment
- *Family Processes, Interrupted,* related to a child with a visual impairment

Planning and Implementation

The nurse plays an important role in preventing retinopathy of prematurity. Encourage early and regular prenatal care to prevent unnecessary premature births. Administer oxygen only to newborns who need it, and in the amount specified by the physician to maintain prescribed oxygen saturation. Ensure that the proper ventilatory settings are used. Shield newborns from excessive exposure to light, since that may decrease susceptibility to retinopathy of prematurity. Be alert for infants with multiple risk factors and refer them, when appropriate, for ophthalmologic examination. Parents of infants at risk for retinopathy of prematurity require information about the disorder, as well as support, because the long-term effects on the child's vision are often identified only after subsequent examinations as the child grows.

The accompanying *Nursing Care Plan* summarizes care for the child with a visual impairment resulting from retinopathy of prematurity. The nurse is instrumental in case management for such children. Reinforce to parents the importance of follow-up eye examinations. Teach methods of stimulating development for a child with a visual impairment (refer to the next section).

Clinical Reasoning The Child With ROP

Raeanne, 3 years old, has a severe visual impairment. Born prematurely at 25 weeks of gestation, she received oxygen therapy, which damaged her retinal blood vessels. As a result, Raeanne developed retinopathy of prematurity (ROP). While in the hospital, Raeanne was given frequent ophthalmoscopic examinations. She received cryotherapy to the retinal vessels—a treatment designed to prevent detached retinae and the resulting total vision loss. Although this treatment halted progression of the disorder, Raeanne was left severely myopic (nearsighted).

For the first 3 years of life, Raeanne and her mother attended an early-intervention program, which provided stimulation for Raeanne and helped teach her mother techniques for enhancing her developmental progress. Raeanne will soon begin attending preschool. Her speech is well developed for a 3-year-old; she is socially mature, converses readily, and shows no developmental delays. However, she has had little contact with other children.

As the nurse in the preschool Raeanne will be attending, how will you assist both her parents and the preschool staff in helping Raeanne adapt to the preschool experience?

Nursing Care Plan: The Child With a Visual Impairment Secondary to Retinopathy of Prematurity

1. Nursing Diagnosis: *Communication, Readiness for Enhanced,* related to altered reception, transmission, and integration resulting of visual images (NANDA-I © 2014)

GOAL: The child will receive adequate sensory input.

INTERVENTION	RATIONALE
• Provide kinesthetic, tactile, and auditory stimulation during play and in daily care (e.g., talking and playing). Provide music while bathing an infant, using bells and other noises on each side of infant. Verbally describe to a child all actions being carried out by adult.	• Because visual sensory input is not present, the child needs input from all other senses to compensate and provide adequate sensory stimulation.

EXPECTED OUTCOME: Child will demonstrate minimal signs of sensory deprivation.

2. Nursing Diagnosis: *Injury, Risk for,* related to impaired vision (NANDA-I © 2014)

GOAL: The child will be protected from safety hazards that can lead to injury.

INTERVENTION	RATIONALE
• Evaluate environment for potential safety hazards based on age of child and degree of impairment. Be particularly alert to objects that give visual cues to their dangers (e.g., stairs, stoves, fireplaces, candles). Eliminate safety hazards and protect the child from exposure. Take the child on a tour of new rooms, explaining safety hazards (e.g., schools, hotel room, hospital room).	• The child may be at risk for injury related both to developmental stage and to inability to visualize hazards.

EXPECTED OUTCOME: Child will experience no injuries.

3. Nursing Diagnosis: *Development: Delayed, Risk for,* related to impaired vision (NANDA-I © 2014)

GOAL: The child has experiences necessary to foster normal growth and development.

INTERVENTION	RATIONALE
• Help parents plan early, regular social activities with other children.	• The child with a visual impairment benefits developmentally from contact with other children.
• Provide opportunities and encourage self-feeding activities.	• To obtain adequate nutrients, the child needs to feel comfortable feeding self.
• Provide an environment rich in sensory input.	• Sensory input is needed for normal development to occur.
• Assess growth and development during regular examinations to identify the child's strengths and needs.	• Regular examinations aid in early identification of growth problems or developmental delays, so that appropriate interventions can be planned.

EXPECTED OUTCOME: Child will demonstrate normal growth and development milestones.

4. Nursing Diagnosis: *Family Processes, Interrupted,* related to child's prolonged disability from sensory impairment (NANDA-I © 2014)

GOAL: The family will identify methods for coping with their child with a visual impairment.

INTERVENTION	RATIONALE
• Provide explanation of visual impairment as appropriate.	• The parents may feel guilt about the child's visual impairment, which can be allayed by knowledge of the cause.
• Refer parents to organizations, early intervention programs, and other parents of children with visual impairments.	• The parents will receive needed information and support from others.
• Assist parents to plan for meeting the developmental, educational, and safety needs of their child with a visual impairment. Offer resources for changing home environment to assist child.	• The child may require an enhanced environment in order to foster developmental progress.

EXPECTED OUTCOME: Family will successfully cope with the experience of having a child with a visual impairment.

Evaluation

Expected outcomes of nursing care for the child with retinopathy of prematurity include the following:

- Visual impairment is identified early in life.
- The child achieves normal developmental milestones.
- The family effectively manages the child's visual condition.

Visual Impairment

Visual impairment related to refractive errors, amblyopia, strabismus, and astigmatism occurs in 5% to 10% of young children (Granet & Khayali, 2011). About 500,000 children in the United States have visual impairment and about 60,000 are legally blind (vision 20/200 or worse) (American Foundation for the Blind, 2011).

Many conditions discussed earlier in this chapter lead to temporary or permanent visual impairment. Infants who are premature; whose mothers were infected prenatally with rubella, toxoplasmosis, or other viruses; and who have certain congenital and hereditary conditions have a high risk of visual problems (Table 19–4). Fetal alcohol syndrome (FAS) is a major cause of visual disturbance; 90% of children with FAS have eye abnormalities. See Chapter 28 for further description of FAS.

The signs of visual impairment depend on the cause and degree of the problem and the age of the child (Table 19–5). The child's eyes may appear crossed or watery, and the lids may be crusty. Verbal children may complain of itching, dizziness, headache, or blurred, double, or poor vision.

Diagnostic tests include vision screening, followed by referral to an eye specialist for full examination. Tests that are commonly performed include responses to visual stimuli, symmetry of eye movements, location of corneal light reflex, cover–uncover testing, visual field testing, and funduscopic examination of the retina. The U.S. Preventive Services Task Force (2011) recommends screening to detect amblyopia, strabismus, and defects in visual acuity in children at least once between 3 and 5 years of age. The American Academy of Pediatrics (2011) recommends age-appropriate eye evaluations at health visits from birth through 4 years and age-appropriate visual acuity testing and ophthalmoscopy in children 5 years and older.

Clinical therapy depends on the child's condition and may include surgery, medication, and supportive aids. In the case of a disorder that results in permanent visual impairment, a collaborative care team of specialists works with the child and family. Nurses have an important role in this team to ensure developmental progression for the child and ongoing support for the family.

Growth and Development

Infants with visual impairment use kinesthesia, touch, and language to socialize. They appreciate and use touch more than other children and respond to verbal explanations when others use nonverbal communication. Vision affects both fine and gross motor skills, so skills such as hand-to-mouth coordination and walking may be delayed in children who have visual impairments.

Nursing Management

For the Child With Visual Impairment

Nursing Assessment and Diagnosis

Prevent visual deficits by teaching safety in activities that can injure the eye, engage in activities for early identification of the condition, and enhance the development of children with low vision. Vision screening facilitates early detection and treatment of conditions that can lead to vision loss. Visual testing can be done at any age, including immediately after birth. Developmental milestones that require vision, such as following bright lights, reaching for objects, or looking at pictures in a book, can be used to assess vision. For children over the age of 3 years, visual acuity is most frequently measured by means of an age-appropriate acuity test (see the *Clinical Skills Manual* SKILLS). Vision screening should begin at 3 years of age and take place during annual healthcare visits. See *Evidence-Based Practice: Nursing Role in Vision Screening and Follow-Up*. Most states mandate school screening of vision (see Chapter 5). The photo screener, a device that can be used to take a photo of the child's eyes, is useful for infants, toddlers, and preschoolers. The photo can be used to diagnose refraction errors, eye opacities, and misalignment. Visual fields and the ability to discriminate colors are tested at school age, when children can cooperate.

Children who have a visual impairment may lag in development of cognitive and other skills. Sighted children learn the word *cup* using four senses—sight, touch, hearing, and taste—to obtain the information necessary to connect words with the objects they represent. In contrast, children with visual impairments rely on only three senses—touch, hearing, and taste. They learn concepts through differences in sounds, textures, and shapes.

Many visual disorders are linked with conditions that influence development. Thus a child with cerebral palsy or fetal alcohol syndrome should be assessed frequently to identify a visual disorder, as well as to evaluate normal developmental milestones.

TABLE 19–4 Common Causes of Visual Impairment in Children

CONGENITAL OR HEREDITARY	ACQUIRED
Cataracts	Injury to eye or head
Glaucoma	Infections
Tay-Sachs disease	Rubella
Marfan syndrome	Measles
Down syndrome	Chickenpox
Fetal alcohol syndrome	Brain tumor
Prenatal infections (maternal infection):	Retinopathy of prematurity
Rubella	Cerebral palsy
Toxoplasmosis	
Herpes simplex	
Zika virus	
Retinoblastoma	

TABLE 19–5 Signs of Visual Impairment

INFANTS	TODDLERS AND OLDER CHILDREN
May be unable to follow lights or objects	May rub, shut, or cover eyes
Do not make eye contact	Tilt or thrust head forward
Have a dull, vacant stare	Blink frequently
Do not imitate facial expressions	Hold objects close
	Bump into objects
	Squint

EVIDENCE-BASED PRACTICE | Nursing Role in Vision Screening and Follow-Up

Clinical Question

Screening for visual ability is important to identify children with impairments. The American Academy of Pediatrics recommends that children be screened at every well-child visit, beginning in the newborn period. Screenings should include vision history, vision assessment, external inspection of the eyes and lids, eye movement assessment, pupil examination, and elicitation of red reflex. Once the child can cooperate, usually by about age 3 years, a vision test such as HOTV or tumbling E, along with ophthalmoscopic examination, should be added to the examination (Chou, Dana, & Bougatsos, 2011; U.S. Preventive Services Task Force, 2011). Worldwide, 13 million children are visually impaired because of uncorrected refractive errors, so vision screening is critical as the first step in providing corrective lenses (Sharma, Congdon, Patel, et al., 2012). How can nurses integrate into their practice the completion of vision examinations, provision of training for other screeners, evaluation of results, referral to specialists when abnormalities are found, and provision of follow-up care after diagnosis and treatment?

The Evidence

A study of the outcomes of school vision screening of 2726 children in North Carolina found that 3 children in 100 were identified upon follow-up with a vision problem, such as myopia, hyperopia, and astigmatism (Kemper, Helfrich, Talbot, et al., 2012). This study also found that no follow-up information was obtained on the outcome of referral for a full eye examination for 35% of the children with potential problems. School nurse staffing issues have made vision screening for children in schools a challenge, but innovative programs for

training and supervising screeners such as volunteer parents, nursing students, and others have been successful. Key components of programs are to ensure that the nurse is present during screening for monitoring accuracy and consistency checks, performs the questionable results found by screeners, performs referrals, and conducts follow-up of vision referral results (National Association of School Nurses [NASN], 2012; Sides & Sigmon, 2013).

Best Practice

Nurses play a vital role in ensuring that children receive early, periodic, and regular visual and eye screening. Evidence that suggests the most accurate methods should be closely examined. While identification of problems is important, the nursing roles of training screeners, referral for care, identifying barriers to care, and ensuring that follow-up care has been received are also integral to vision care.

Clinical Reasoning

What vision screening methods are available in the offices, clinics, and schools in your community? How could you perform vision screening in the hospital setting if a child did not demonstrate expected visual ability for age? Design a program to train and supervise nursing students to perform vision screening. What are the essential components of a follow-up program for a school that screens all kindergartners and first graders for visual acuity? What questions will you ask parents during a well-child visit for a 2-year-old to determine if vision is normal? How will you combine your knowledge of developmental milestones with screening for vision?

Nursing diagnoses for the child with impaired vision might include the following (NANDA-I © 2014):

- *Mobility: Physical, Impaired,* related to altered sensory perception
- *Injury, Risk for,* related to poor vision
- *Development: Delayed, Risk for,* related to visual impairment
- *Family Processes, Interrupted,* related to demands of a child with a sensory impairment

Planning and Implementation

Promote safety in sports and other activities to prevent visual impairment when possible. Nursing care for a child with a visual impairment focuses on encouraging the child's use of all senses, promoting socialization, helping parents to meet the child's developmental and educational needs, and providing emotional support to parents. Refer the parents to an early intervention program as soon as the diagnosis is made. Nearly all care occurs in community and home settings.

ENCOURAGE USE OF ALL SENSES

Children who are partially sighted or blind use other senses to a great extent. Encouraging the use of the eyes as much as possible is important even if a child has poor vision (Figure 19–3).

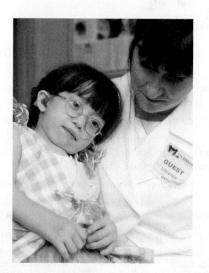

Figure 19–3 Encouraging use of the senses. This child needs ongoing developmental assessment and a comprehensive individualized education plan. Since she has impaired vision, the nurse uses touch and speaks with her throughout procedures to ensure sensory input.

PROMOTE SOCIALIZATION

The child's interactions and socializations should be as normal as possible (similar to those of sighted children of the same age and development).

- Stroke, rock, and hug infants and children who have a visual impairment. Sing and talk to them. These infants do not make eye contact and have rather blank expressions.
- Call the child's name and speak before touching the child. Tell the child when the nurse and others are leaving the room. Describe locations of foods on the plate and tray to orient the child.
- Teach parents to read body language and vocalization as expressions of emotion. Facial expressions give a great deal of information, but infants and children with poor vision do not have the ability to learn by visual imitation. Show parents how to use tactile means to teach appropriate facial expressions. For example, a touch on the arm can be soft and stroking to indicate a smile, but firmer to indicate dismay or frown.
- Describe procedures such as blood pressure, ear examination, or cast application so the child knows what they will feel like. Let the child touch the equipment.
- Explain to parents that discipline and rewards for children with poor vision should be the same as those for other children in the family. The child should be given age-appropriate tasks.
- Encourage contact with peers as the child grows older. Teach children to look directly at persons who are talking to them. Play, sports, and other activities can be modified to give the child with a visual impairment the same social experiences as a sighted child.

COMMUNITY-BASED NURSING CARE

Public laws require that each state provide educational and related services for children with disabilities (see Chapter 1). Parents and healthcare providers should develop an individualized education plan (as discussed in Chapter 12) that maximizes the child's learning ability. If possible, the child with a vision problem should attend child care and preschool with children who have normal visual acuity. What nursing actions are needed to help a child with a visual impairment adjust to child care or school?

- Provide parents with information about educational options before their child reaches school age. Education should take place in a setting that allows the child to have contact with other children and to participate in social activities.
- The child may be mainstreamed with a tutor, be partially mainstreamed in a resource room, attend special classes, or be tutored at home. If the child is to attend public school, suggest to parents that they contact the school well before enrollment to ensure that school personnel understand the child's disability.
- Make sure that equipment such as large-print books, Braille materials, audio equipment, or an Optacon (described in *Families Want to Know: Enhancing Development of the Child With a Visual Impairment*) is available. Ensure that frequent eye examinations are performed and assist with proper use and care of prescribed glasses or contact lenses as necessary. Clean glasses daily with warm water and dry with a clean, soft cloth. Follow the directions that the family provides, which describe the methods they use for cleaning contact lenses.
- Familiarize the child with the new environment.

Growth and Development

Children with visual impairment may take longer to master self-help skills such as feeding and dressing. Perform regular developmental assessments and suggest adaptive ways that parents can help the child learn these skills.

Families Want to Know

Enhancing Development of the Child With a Visual Impairment

- Encourage a toddler or preschooler who has a visual impairment to look at pictures in well-lit settings. Have a school-age child read large-print books. Computers designed for people with visual impairments are also available. The Optacon (a device that raises print so it can be felt by the child) and View Scan (which magnifies print) improve reading capability.
- Expose the infant and child to everyday sounds.
- Encourage the infant to use the sense of touch to explore people and objects. Have the parents purchase toys with sound and texture in mind. Directional concepts can be taught using games. Responding to the infant's and child's vocalizations encourages the use of speech.
- Teach specific techniques for toileting, dressing, bathing, eating, and safety.
- When the child becomes mobile, furniture and other objects in the environment should be kept in the same positions so the child can safely move around independently. Extra care must be taken to prevent injuries when a child does not see.
- Emphasize the child's abilities. Adolescents can use seeing-eye dogs or a white cane to function independently.
- Encourage the child to function independently within normal developmental parameters.
- If the child goes to a hospital or another strange environment, orient the child to the placement of objects and do not rearrange them.
- Teach those around the child to:
  - Announce their presence to the child when approaching.
  - Walk slightly ahead of the child so the child can sense the movement of the accompanying person.
  - Let the child hold the seeing person's arm rather than the reverse.
  - Identify the contents of meals and encourage the child to feed self.

PROVIDE EMOTIONAL SUPPORT

The family often needs help to understand the child's abilities and disabilities. Support them as they learn about their child's visual problems, tell friends and family, and then adjust to supporting the child.

- Encourage habilitation as soon as realistically possible. Make the adjustment easier by providing information about the child's specific type of visual impairment, available community services, and groups or associations for children with similar vision conditions.
- Suggest resources to families of children with visual disorders.
- Be supportive and listen to the family's concerns about the child's visual deficit.
- Make sure the parents meet their own physical and emotional needs so they are better able to care for and provide support to their child.

Evaluation

Expected outcomes of nursing care for the child with a visual impairment include the following:

- The child is protected from injury.
- The child manifests growth and development to maximum potential.
- The child establishes a successful individualized education plan.

Injuries of the Eye

In the United States, eye injuries are common in children of all ages, especially from 11 to 14 years, and particularly in boys. Sports, darts, fireworks, air-powered BB guns, blunt and sharp objects, chemical and thermal burns, physical irritants, and abuse are causes of eye trauma. Sports injuries are most common, with 100,000 occurring annually; they are a common cause of blindness in children (National Eye Institute, n.d.).

Prevention is an important part of health promotion. Protective eyewear should be used by participants in all sports with a risk of eye injury, with extreme caution in those with diminished vision or only one functional eye. Common injuries occur in baseball, basketball, swimming, bicycling, and football so preventive measures should be taken such as proper training and use of protective gear. Chemicals and objects such as scissors and knives should be placed out of reach.

Some injuries can be treated at home but many require emergency care or hospitalization. The nurse will document the history of the injury, perform an assessment of the eye, and measure the visual acuity. If a tetanus booster has not been given in the last 5 years, the child is reimmunized. Table 19–6 summarizes emergency treatment of common eye injuries.

Disorders of the Ear

Otitis Media

Otitis media, or inflammation of the middle ear, is sometimes accompanied by infection. This condition is one of the most common childhood illnesses, with a majority of infants having at least one case of acute otitis media by 3 years of age (Qureishi, Lee, Belfield, et al., 2014). Otitis media occurs more frequently among boys and in children who attend childcare centers, in those with allergies, in children exposed to tobacco smoke, and in those who use pacifiers several hours daily. It is most common during the winter months. Children with conditions such as cleft lip and palate or Down syndrome more often experience otitis media. Breastfeeding appears to be protective against otitis media. In the past decade, an increased number of cases have been observed, and recent changes have been made in recommendations for treatment.

TABLE 19–6 Emergency Treatment of Eye Injuries

INJURY	TREATMENT
Subconjunctival hemorrhage (caused by coughing, mild trauma, or increased physical activity)	Usually heals spontaneously; child should see ophthalmologist if most of sclera is covered or if condition does not clear up in 1–2 weeks.
Periorbital ecchymosis ("black eye")	Apply ice to eye area (both eyes) for 5–15 min every hour for the first 1–2 days after injury (even if only one eye is affected, both eyes may discolor); then apply warm compresses.
Foreign body on conjunctiva	Do not let child rub eye; remove material on surface of eye by closing upper lid over lower lid, irrigating or everting upper lid, visualizing material, and removing it with slightly damp handkerchief; patch eye and transport child to emergency department if foreign body cannot be removed.
Corneal abrasion	Superficial corneal abrasions are diagnosed by touching sterile fluorescein strip to lower conjunctiva; dye remains where corneal epithelial cells are disrupted; most corneal abrasions heal spontaneously, although antibiotic ointment may be prescribed and eyes may be patched in some children.
Burns (alkaline burns readily penetrate cornea and are more serious than acid burns)	For child with chemical burn, irrigate eye for 15–30 min; transport child to emergency department where irrigation should continue (see the *Clinical Skills Manual* SKILLS); pupils are dilated to reduce pain and prevent adhesions; after irrigation is complete, eyes are patched and antibiotics are prescribed.
Penetrating and perforating injuries	Obtain medical assistance immediately; never try to remove an object that has penetrated the child's eye; such objects should be removed by an ophthalmologist; prevent the child from rubbing injured eye; cover both eyes with shield before transportation to emergency department.
Eye injuries caused by severe blows to head and eye (blunt trauma can seriously injure all eye structures, including orbit, which can be fractured)	Transport immediately to ophthalmologist's office or emergency department for evaluation and treatment; retinal hemorrhage is a common presentation of the type of child abuse called "shaken child syndrome."

Growth and Development

Fluid accumulation in the middle ear prevents the efficient transmission of sound and can result in hearing loss over time, potentially delaying speech and language development. These delays may manifest as cognitive deficits or behavior problems. Motor development has been found to be impaired in children with chronic ear infections.

ETIOLOGY AND PATHOPHYSIOLOGY

The specific cause of otitis media is unknown, but it appears to be related to eustachian tube dysfunction. Often, an upper respiratory infection precedes otitis media. This infection causes the mucous membranes of the eustachian tube to become edematous. As a result, air that normally flows to the middle ear is blocked, and the air in the middle ear is reabsorbed into the bloodstream. Fluid is pulled from the mucosal lining into the former air space, providing a medium for the rapid growth of pathogens. The tympanic membrane and fluid behind it become infected. The most common causative organisms are *Streptococcus pneumoniae*, *Haemophilus influenzae*, and *Moraxella catarrhalis* (Harmes et al., 2013).

Conditions such as enlarged adenoids or edema from allergic rhinitis can also obstruct the eustachian tube and lead to otitis media. Pacifier use raises the soft palate and may alter dynamics in the eustachian tube, providing for entry of microorganisms from the nasopharynx. Recurrent otitis media has an increased frequency in children of parents who smoke. Children with multiple siblings and those who attend childcare centers have increased rates of recurrent acute otitis media. Ethnicity appears to be a factor (see *Developing Cultural Competence: Otitis Media*).

Developing Cultural Competence Otitis Media

American Indian, Alaskan Native, and Black children have high rates of otitis media. Recent research is identifying genetic links in this disease, since it is more common in certain families (Rye, Blackwell, & Jamieson, 2012). However, major risk factors for frequent otitis media, such as crowding, exposure to tobacco smoke, and lack of breastfeeding for infants, are the same regardless of ethnicity. Be alert for frequent recurrent otitis media, plan prevention programs, and ensure prompt care and teaching about treatments for families of children affected. What prevention measures would you emphasize with families that have high rates of otitis media among children? See the following *Nursing Management* section for suggestions of preventive approaches.

CLINICAL MANIFESTATIONS

Otitis media is the general term for inflammation of the middle ear. *Acute otitis media (AOM)* is diagnosed when the child has acute onset of ear pain, bulging of the tympanic membrane upon otoscopy, and middle ear effusion (Figure 19–4). *Recurrent acute otitis media* is defined as three or more separate AOM episodes in 6 months, or four or more episodes in 12 months with at least one episode in the past 6 months (Lieberthal et al., 2013). *Otitis media with effusion (OME)* is evidence of fluid in the middle ear without inflammation (Figure 19–5). Sometimes OME becomes chronic in nature (continuing more than 3 months) and is more commonly associated with hearing loss (Williamson, 2011).

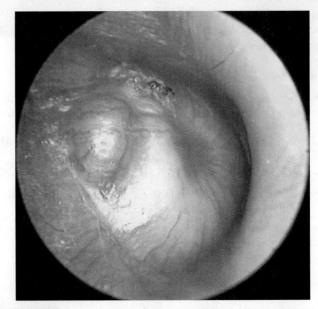

Figure 19–4 Acute otitis media is characterized by pain and a red, bulging, nonmobile tympanic membrane.

SOURCE: Courtesy of Kevin Kavanagh, MD, FACS/Cumberland Otolaryngology Consultants.

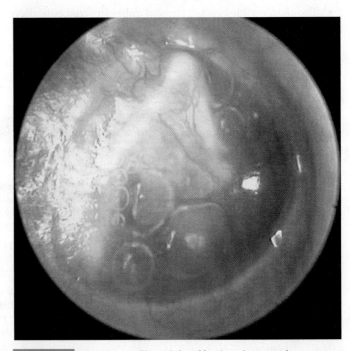

Figure 19–5 Otitis media with effusion is noted on otoscopy by fluid line or air bubbles.

SOURCE: Courtesy of Kevin Kavanagh, MD, FACS/Cumberland Otolaryngology Consultants.

Infants and young children have characteristic behaviors that indicate otitis media may be present. Pulling at the ear is a sign of ear pain (Figure 19–6). Diarrhea, vomiting, and fever are typical of otitis media. Irritability and "acting out" may be signs of a related hearing impairment. The child with otitis media often has night awakenings with crying due to increased pressure when prone or supine. Some children with otitis media are asymptomatic; therefore, an ear examination should be performed at every healthcare visit (see Chapter 5). See Table 19–7.

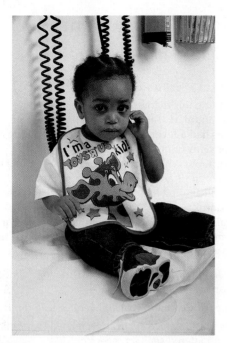

Figure 19–6 This young child is pulling at the ear, an important sign of otitis media. Ask the parents about fussiness, presence of fever, and night awakenings; these are additional signs that are often observed in children with this condition.

CLINICAL THERAPY

Otoscopic examination includes visualization and pneumatic otoscopy. The trained clinician can perform pneumatic otoscopy in which positive air pressure in the external canal is used to measure the movement of the tympanic membrane. Special gradient acoustic reflectometry (SGAR) measures the condition of the middle ear by introducing a sound and measuring the tympanic membrane response. A "flat" tympanogram is also suggestive of otitis media. (The tympanogram is described in a later section on hearing impairment.)

Since otitis media with effusion may only involve fluid in the middle ear, it is best diagnosed by pneumatic otoscopy and tympanometry. Since this type of otitis media is most commonly associated with hearing loss, audiologic testing should be performed in the pediatric healthcare home (medical home) (see Chapter 5) if the effusion persists for 3 months or longer.

Concern has developed about the increasing appearance of drug-resistant microbials as causative agents in otitis media. These organisms may explain the increase in otitis media observed in the past decade. Based on current knowledge, the American Academy of Pediatrics (AAP) established recommendations for diagnosis and management of otitis media in 2004, which were updated in 2013 (Lieberthal et al., 2013). Consistent with current guidelines, for children from 6 months to 23 months with nonsevere unilateral disease, the healthcare provider and parent should consult about whether antibiotic use or observation for 48 to 72 hours is best. If nonsevere bilateral AOM is present or if severe AOM is present (temperature of 39.0°C [102.2°F] with pain for 48 hours) the young child should be treated with antibiotic. For children 24 months and older, nonsevere AOM can be treated with antibiotic or by observation for 48 to 72 ours (Lieberthal et al., 2013). In all cases where 48- to 72-hour observation is implemented, a method for follow-up is needed to ensure that the child has improved. When not improved during the period of watchful waiting, acute otitis media is treated with antibiotic therapy for 10 days in children under 6 years, and 5 to 7 days for children 6 years and over (Hoberman et al., 2011).

When prescribed, the choice of antibiotic depends on the probable organism, ease of administration, cost, previous effectiveness, and any history of allergies. First-line therapy

TABLE 19–7 Clinical Manifestations of Acute Otitis Media and Otitis Media With Effusion

ETIOLOGY	CLINICAL MANIFESTATIONS	CLINICAL THERAPY
Acute otitis media—bacterial infection in the middle ear from pathogens transferred from the nasopharynx; most common infectious agents are *S. pneumoniae, H. influenzae, M. catarrhalis*	*Behavioral*—ear pain, pulling at ear, rapid onset, irritability, malaise, poor feeding *Examination*—bulging tympanic membrane, air or fluid bubbles present behind tympanic membrane; immobile or poorly mobile tympanic membrane, red (or other color change such as white, gray, or yellow as long as bulging is present) tympanic membrane, reduced visibility of tympanic membrane landmarks with displaced light reflex	Treat ear pain with anesthetic ear drops, herbal pain products instilled into the auditory canal, or systemic acetaminophen or ibuprofen. Verify that the tympanic membrane is intact before inserting ear drops. In cases of nonsevere unilateral disease, consult with parents of children under 2 years to decide together on observation or antibiotic treatment. For child 2 years and above with nonsevere disease, observe the child's condition for 48–72 hr and, if not improved, treat with course of antibiotics. Severe and bilateral disease is always treated with antibiotic.
Otitis media with effusion—collection of fluid in the middle ear behind the tympanic membrane, which is not infected with bacteria	*Behavioral*—difficulty hearing or responding as expected to sounds *Examination*—signs of acute inflammation are NOT present; tympanic membrane is retracted or neutral; immobile or partly mobile tympanic membrane; yellow or gray tympanic membrane; opaque or thickened tympanic membrane with visibility of landmarks reduced	Symptomatic treatment and pain relief Careful assessment of hearing acuity over several months Speech assessment if loss of hearing acuity occurs Developmental assessment

Professionalism in Practice Clinical Guidelines

In recent years, the American Academy of Pediatrics and other bodies have established new guidelines for treatment of conditions such as acute otitis media and sinusitis (described later in this chapter). Parents often expect antibiotics for any illness their child may have and do not understand the rationale for guidelines that recommend watchful waiting for a limited time to see if the child improves. Nurses should be familiar with recommendations and guidelines for preventive care (e.g., vision and hearing screening) and treatments (e.g., acute otitis media and sinusitis) so that they can explain the rationale for these approaches to parents. Such explanations can often allay concern and worry, and help build confidence in healthcare providers as partners with parents in care for their children.

is amoxicillin, unless it has been given to the child in the previous 30 days. Amoxicillin with clavulanate and cefuroxime are second-line drugs. If an intramuscular drug is preferred, cefdinir at 14 mg/kg/day, cefpodoxime at 10 mg/kg/day, or cefuroxime at 30 mg/kg/day can be prescribed (Tschudy & Arcara, 2012).

OME is not treated with antibiotics but is evaluated periodically to be sure there is not an additional AOM that needs treatment. Children with OME generally improve within 3 months. Because this type of otitis is more commonly associated with hearing loss and cochlear damage, follow-up with audiology is essential. If hearing is abnormal, speech testing should be performed (Farboud, Skinner, & Pratap, 2011; Williamson, 2011).

Neither decongestants nor antihistamines have been shown to be effective in the treatment of otitis media with or without effusion. If infection recurs in spite of antibiotic treatment, **myringotomy** (surgical incision of the tympanic membrane) may be performed and **tympanostomy tubes** (pressure equalizing tubes) inserted to drain fluid from the middle ear. (See *Families Want to Know: Care of the Child With Tympanostomy Tubes.*)

Nursing Management
For the Child With Otitis Media

Nursing Assessment and Diagnosis

Assess the tympanic membrane for color, transparency, mobility, presence of landmarks, and light reflex. Ask the parents whether the child has had a fever, been fussy, or been pulling at the ears. Observe for signs of impaired hearing.

Inquire about what the family has done at home to treat the ear infection and its associated pain. Some home remedies, such as rocking and singing to the child, are safe. Some other practices may be harmful.

Several nursing diagnoses that may apply are included in *Nursing Care Plan: The Child With Otitis Media.* Additional nursing diagnoses might include the following (NANDA-I © 2014):

- *Body Temperature: Imbalanced, Risk for,* related to infectious process
- *Fatigue (Child and Parent)* related to sleep deprivation
- *Health Maintenance, Ineffective,* related to chronic ear infections and altered sensory reception

Planning and Implementation

Most children with otitis media are not hospitalized; therefore, nursing management centers on care of the child in the home. The child having tympanostomy tubes inserted is generally treated in a day surgery setting. Occasionally, children admitted to the hospital for other problems have a concurrent ear infection. The accompanying *Nursing Care Plan* summarizes nursing care for the child with otitis media.

Emphasize preventive measures. Exposure to secondhand smoke in the home increases the incidence of otitis media in children, so encourage parents who smoke to avoid smoking near the child or in the home. Wood-burning stoves should also be avoided when possible. If young children are in child care with fewer than 10 children, incidence decreases. Breastfeeding provides some protection from the disease. Placing infants or toddlers to sleep with a pacifier may increase incidence and should be avoided in the infant with prior infections. Many cases of otitis

Families Want to Know
Care of the Child With Tympanostomy Tubes

After Surgery

- Encourage the child to drink generous amounts of fluids.
- Reestablish a regular diet as tolerated.
- Give pain medication (acetaminophen) as ordered for discomfort and at bedtime.
- Place drops in child's ears if prescribed.
- Restrict the child to quiet activities.

Following Postoperative Period

- Follow the care provider's instructions regarding swimming and water (some practitioners caution against swimming and other activities that might get water in ears; others do not).
- Ear plugs can be used to prevent water from getting into ears.
- Be alert for tubes becoming dislodged and falling out and alert healthcare provider (they usually fall out within 1 year).
- Report purulent discharge from the ear, which may indicate a new ear infection. Contact the healthcare provider.

Nursing Care Plan: The Child With Otitis Media

1. Nursing Diagnosis: *Pain, Acute,* related to inflammation and pressure on tympanic membrane (NANDA-I © 2014)

GOAL: The child or parent will indicate absence of pain.

INTERVENTION	RATIONALE
• Give analgesic such as acetaminophen. Use analgesic ear drops.	• Analgesics alter perception or response to pain.
• Have the child sit up, raise head on pillows, or lie on unaffected ear.	• Elevation decreases pressure from fluid.
• Apply warmth to the ear.	• Heat increases blood supply and reduces discomfort.
• Have the child blow a pinwheel to relieve pressure in ear.	• Attempts to open the eustachian tube may help aerate the middle ear.

EXPECTED OUTCOME: Verbal child will state that pain is relieved. Nonverbal child will exhibit improved disposition and comfort.

2. Nursing Diagnosis: *Infection, Risk for,* related to presence of pathogens (NANDA-I © 2014)

GOAL: The child will be free of infection.

INTERVENTION	RATIONALE
• Encourage breastfeeding of infants.	• Breastfeeding affords natural immunity to infectious agents.
• Instruct the parents to administer antibiotics exactly as directed and to complete prescribed course of medication.	• Taking antibiotics as prescribed minimizes chance for overgrowth of pathogens.
• Telephone the parents 2 or 3 days after initial examination.	• If symptoms have not improved in 36 hours, treatment should be evaluated.
• Examine ear 3 or 4 days after completion of antibiotic treatment, or if symptoms worsen in child on symptomatic treatment.	• Checkup determines whether treatment is effective.

EXPECTED OUTCOME: Child's temperature will be normal, symptoms will disappear, and tympanic membrane will show no signs of infection.

3. Nursing Diagnosis: *Development: Delayed, Risk for,* related to hearing loss (NANDA-I © 2014)

GOAL: The child will have normal hearing.

INTERVENTION	RATIONALE
• Assess hearing ability frequently.	• Monitoring detects hearing loss early.

EXPECTED OUTCOME: Child's general health and hearing will improve, and incidence of the condition will decrease.

GOAL: The child will have normal motor and language development.

INTERVENTION	RATIONALE
• Assess motor and language development at each healthcare visit.	• Early detection of developmental delays can lead to appropriate intervention.

EXPECTED OUTCOME: Child will have language and motor development within norms for age group.

media are related to microbials such as *H. influenzae* and *Pneumococcus pneumoniae,* so immunization against these pathogens (see Chapter 16) can be effective preventive measures.

Help parents understand why there is a waiting period before prescriptions are given for antibiotics. When antibiotics are prescribed, review administration techniques, side effects, and the need for a repeat appointment when the medication is completed.

Chronic otitis media can create problems for the family. The child's waking at night with ear pain results in lack of sleep and parental fatigue. Since many children with otitis media experience ear pain that can disrupt their sleep and that of family members, anesthetic ear drops have been used for their analgesic effect on the tympanic membrane, and some families might prefer use of natural remedies for ear pain. Herbal extract ear drops (a naturopathic herbal extract of *Allium sativum, Verbascum thapsus, Calendula flores, Hypericum perforatum,* lavender, and vitamin E) with a local anesthetic of amethocaine and phenazone have been used. Parents often become frustrated and disillusioned by the healthcare system's inability to cure the child and may fear a permanent hearing impairment. Reassure parents that as the child grows older, the recurrent infections eventually cease.

Teach them that asking for courses of antibiotics for every infection may not be the best treatment.

Provide pain relief techniques such as teaching correct administration of ear drops, oral administration of acetaminophen, and positioning the baby with the head slightly elevated.

Provide hearing and language examinations at regular intervals, inform parents of results, and refer to an audiology specialist if hearing problems are identified. Make sure parents of children with tympanostomy tubes know how to care for the child and what symptoms to report. For the child with some hearing loss due to otitis media with effusion, a home environment that fosters cognitive skills can overcome the effects of lowered hearing during the time of infection. Focus interventions on helping parents to read and talk with children frequently who have otitis media with effusion.

Evaluation

Expected outcomes of nursing care for the child with otitis media include the following:

- The child returns to normal sleep and feeding patterns.
- The child maintains normal hearing and speech development.
- Pain and temperature are effectively managed.
- Parents demonstrate understanding of the treatment regimen.

Otitis Externa

Otitis externa is an inflammation of the skin and surrounding soft tissue of the ear canal. It is sometimes called "swimmer's ear" because it is common in children who swim frequently, especially during hot and muggy weather. The ear canal can also be injured by use of cotton-tipped applicators, foreign objects, or sprays used near the face. If the tympanic membrane is not intact because of tympanostomy tubes or breakage of the membrane, drainage may be visible in the canal; this drainage may irritate the canal and lead to otitis externa. Any irritation of the canal can become infected with bacteria, virus, or fungi; sometimes it represents an allergic reaction. The child usually complains of pain and itching, and may have intense pain when the examiner presses on the tragus, or skin tab in front of the ear. Sometimes the ear appears swollen, and redness or drainage of the canal may be seen upon otoscopic examination.

Treatment of otitis externa requires removing the dried and flaking epithelium and cerumen. Burrow solutions or normal saline is used to irrigate and clean the canal if the tympanic membrane is intact. Steroid ear drops are used to decrease inflammation, and antibiotic drops are also used if a bacterial infection is suspected. If the child has tympanostomy tubes or a perforated tympanic membrane, nonototoxic ear antibiotic such as quinolone antibiotic ear drops are used. Ibuprofen or acetaminophen may be helpful for pain control. The ear canal should then be kept dry by using ear plugs or a swim cap for swimming and gently blow-drying the canal after bathing. The child should not return to swimming for about 5 days. Cotton-tipped applicators or other objects should not be placed in the ear canal so that the skin in the canal can heal. If hair sprays or other solutions are irritating, they should not be used by the child or adolescent.

Nurses should be aware of the signs of otitis externa such as a painful ear, drainage, and irritated canal. Verify that the tympanic membrane is intact during otoscopic examination. Teach families to avoid the irritants identified such as cotton-tipped applicators, sprays, and frequent swimming. Demonstrate proper instillation of drops (see the *Clinical Skills Manual* SKILLS) and give instructions for use of acetaminophen for pain relief in the acute period.

Hearing Impairment

About 1.6% of newborns do not pass the newborn hearing examination (Centers for Disease Control and Prevention [CDC], 2012). Additional children receive a diagnosis after the newborn period, and approximately 1 million children (2–3 of every 100 births) in the United States have some form of hearing impairment (National Institute of Deafness and Other Communication Disorders, [NIDCD], 2014). Hearing impairment is expressed in terms of **decibels (dB)**, which are units of loudness, and rated according to severity (Table 19–8). Children who have a mild hearing loss (35 to 40 dB) may miss 50% of everyday conversation and are considered at high risk for school failure. Children with a hearing loss of more than 80 dB are considered legally deaf.

Hearing disorders can be classified according to the location of the deficit. **Conductive hearing loss** occurs when conditions in the external auditory canal or tympanic membrane prevent sound from reaching the middle ear. **Sensorineural hearing loss** occurs when the hair cells in the cochlea or along the vestibulo-cochlear (acoustic) nerve (cranial nerve VIII) are damaged. This leads to permanent hearing loss. A **mixed hearing loss** indicates a hearing loss having a combination of conductive and sensorineural causes.

ETIOLOGY AND PATHOPHYSIOLOGY

About 50% of hearing loss is genetically caused, generally in a recessive inheritance pattern with *GJB2* gene abnormalities (American Speech-Language-Hearing Association [ASLHA], 2011). Another 25% is due to environmental causes around the time of birth. Acquired causes are due to injury or disease later in life such as frequent ear infections, infectious diseases, ototoxic drugs, head injury, and noise exposure (ASLHA, 2011). This type of loss is increasing; hearing loss among all populations has doubled in the past 30 years, and now approximately 14.9% of U.S. children have low-frequency or high-frequency hearing loss of at least 16-dB hearing level in one or both ears (ASLHA, 2014). Infants at risk for hearing loss include those with:

- Family history of congenital hearing loss
- Positive titer for TORCH infections (toxoplasmosis, rubella, cytomegalovirus, syphilis, herpes)

TABLE 19–8 Severity of Hearing Loss

TYPE OF LOSS	HEARING ABILITY
Slight/mild (20–40 dB)	Some speech sounds are difficult to perceive, particularly unvoiced consonant sounds.
Moderate (41–60 dB)	Most normal conversational speech sounds are missed.
Severe (61–80 dB)	Speech sounds cannot be heard at a normal conversational level.
Profound (81–90 dB)	No speech sounds can be heard; considered legally deaf.
Deaf (over 90 dB)	No sound at all can be heard.

Source: Data from American Speech-Language-Hearing Association. (2011). *Type, degree, and configuration of hearing loss.* Retrieved from http://www.asha.org/public/hearing/disorders/types.htm

- Craniofacial abnormalities
- Very low birth weight (less than 1500 g [3.3 lb])
- Stay in neonatal intensive care unit of over 5 days, or need for extracorporeal membrane oxygenation (ECMO), assisted ventilation, administration of ototoxic medications (e.g., gentamicin, tobramycin) or loop diuretics (e.g., furosemide), or hyperbilirubinemia that requires exchange transfusion
- Chemotherapy, particularly with aminoglycoside medications over 5 days
- Low Apgar score at 1 or 5 minutes
- Bacterial or viral meningitis
- Head trauma, especially basal skull/temporal bone fractures requiring hospitalization
- Mechanical ventilation for more than 5 days
- Caregiver concern regarding speech, language, hearing, developmental delay
- Presence of syndromes associated with hearing loss (Down syndrome, Pierre Robin syndrome, Arnold-Chiari malformation, neurofibromatosis, osteopetrosis, Hunter syndrome) (Joint Committee on Infant Hearing, 2007, 2008)

Common causes of conductive hearing loss include impacted cerumen, the most frequent reason for conductive loss; outer ear infection ("swimmer's ear"); trauma; or a foreign

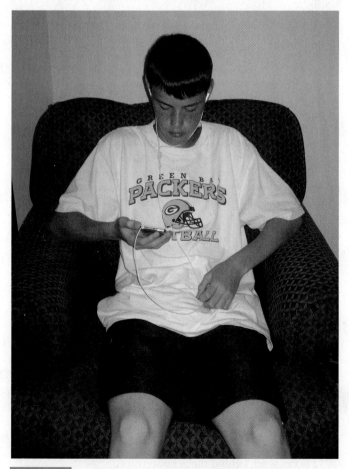

Figure 19–7 **Listening to loud music with headphones or at rock concerts is a frequent cause of hearing loss among teenagers and young adults. This adolescent needs to be informed about the possible outcomes of this activity.**

body. Conductive loss also occurs if the tympanic membrane does not fully vibrate, as in otitis media. In these cases, hearing loss may be restored after the infection clears. Chronic and untreated ear infections may lead to structural changes in the ear and permanent hearing impairment. The loss of acuity may be gradual or rapid and results in diminished hearing in all ranges.

Conditions leading to sensorineural hearing loss may be congenital (maternal rubella), genetic (Tay-Sachs disease), or acquired (such as from ototoxic drugs, bacterial meningitis, or loud noise). In sensorineural hearing loss, high-frequency sounds are most affected. Such hearing loss may be preceded by **tinnitus** or ringing in the ears. Teenagers who use earphones at high volumes or attend many rock concerts are at risk for hearing loss (Figure 19–7). Other noise hazards include firecrackers, guns, and power and farm equipment.

CLINICAL MANIFESTATIONS

Hearing is both an innate and a learned behavior. Infants and children who have hearing impairments exhibit a range of behaviors, depending on their age and the severity of the deficit. Infants who hear normally respond to sound in both obvious and subtle ways that do not occur in those who have hearing impairments (Table 19–9). As children mature, their hearing impairments affect their language skills. Hearing loss is often manifested as a cognitive deficit, a behavioral problem, or both.

TABLE 19–9 Behaviors Suggestive of Hearing Impairment

AGE	BEHAVIOR
Infant	Has a diminished or absent startle reflex to loud sound.
	Does not awaken when environment is very noisy.
	Awakens only to touch.
	Does not turn head to sound at 3–4 months.
	Does not localize sound at 6–10 months.
	Babbles little or not at all.
Toddler and preschooler	Speaks unintelligibly, in a monotone, or not at all.
	Communicates needs through gestures.
	Appears developmentally delayed.
	Appears emotionally immature, yells inappropriately.
	Does not respond to doorbell or telephone.
	Appears more interested in objects than people and prefers to play alone.
	Focuses on facial expressions rather than verbal communications.
School-age child and adolescent	Asks to have statements repeated.
	Answers questions inappropriately, except when able to view speaker's face.
	Daydreams and is inattentive.
	Performs poorly at school or is truant.
	Has speech abnormalities or speaks in a monotone.
	Sits close to or turns television or radio up loudly.
	Prefers to play alone.

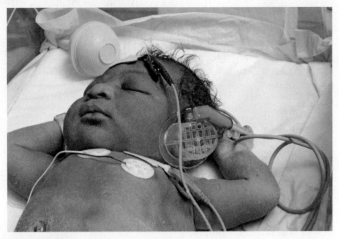

Figure 19–8 Newborn hearing screening is an effective tool in diagnosing some causes of hearing impairment very early in life.

CLINICAL THERAPY

Early identification of hearing loss is a key element in successful treatment (see *Growth and Development*). Detection of hearing loss in infants is important to ensure optimal development. Universal screening of all infants is recommended before 1 month of age, with diagnostic audiologic evaluation before 3 months, and beginning of early intervention programs by 6 months of age for those with hearing impairment. State laws now mandate screening of newborns, and national data are maintained on outcomes. Observations of response to noise in all newborns should be accompanied by more sophisticated testing such as auditory brain stem response or transient evoked otoacoustic emissions, especially in those at high risk of deficits (Figure 19–8). All children should be evaluated for communication development beginning at 2 months of age during all well-child visits (American Academy of Pediatrics Committee on Practice and Ambulatory and Bright Futures Periodicity Schedule Work Group, 2014). See Table 19–10.

Growth and Development

Children with hearing loss can easily fall behind their peers in language milestones because they cannot hear and speak in the same manner as other children. Without interventions to enable them to learn language, they can also fail to develop reading and other literacy skills, related cognitive processes, and social-emotional development (Joint Committee on Infant Hearing, 2007). Carefully evaluate hearing and all developmental milestones during each regularly scheduled healthcare visit. Refer infants and children with abnormalities for further evaluation. When hearing loss is identified as a cause of delayed development, interventions guided by healthcare providers with expertise in hearing loss are needed.

An otoscopic examination with a tympanogram can be performed on an older infant to determine conductive hearing loss. The **tympanogram** is a test that provides a graph of the ability of the middle ear to transmit sound. An airtight probe is inserted into the external ear canal and a tone is emitted. The probe measures the pressure, which is plotted on a graph. A "flat" tympanogram suggests conductive hearing loss. **Audiography** can be used with cooperative children over 3 years of age. Sounds

TABLE 19–10 Screening Tests for Newborn Hearing

TEST	MECHANISM OF ACTION
Otoacoustic emission (OAE) (either transient-evoked [TEOAE] or distortion-product [DPOAE])	A measure of low-intensity sounds from the cochlear hair cells in response to clicks from a probe placed in the ear canal
	Sensitive in frequency range above 1500 Hz
	May show false negative for loss below 1000–1500 Hz
	Detects inner ear hearing loss by evaluating cochlear and hair cell function
	Does not detect neural damage to cranial nerve VIII
	Can be sensitive to outer ear canal obstruction or middle ear effusion, leading to false positive result
Auditory brainstem response (ABR)	Electrical response to auditory stimuli from three surface scalp electrodes
	Reflects activity of cochlea, cranial nerve VIII, and auditory brainstem pathways
	Detect hearing loss from 1000–8000 Hz
	May show false-negative results for losses in the 500- to 2000-Hz levels
	Will give a positive result if there is damage to cranial nerve VIII or brainstem pathways even if cochlear loss is not present

of various frequencies and intensities are presented to the child through earphones, and the child is instructed to raise a hand when the sound is heard. Audiography cannot detect hearing loss caused by middle ear effusion but can indicate sensorineural loss.

The hearing of preschool and school-age children is tested by asking them to repeat whispered words. Hearing of school-age children and adolescents also is assessed with the Weber and Rinne tests (see Chapter 5).

If a hearing loss is uncorrectable, a collaborative care team composed of pediatrician, audiologist, otolaryngologist, speech–language pathologist, nurse, teacher, and social worker should help the child and family adapt to the disability. If the deficit is due to recurrent ear infections, tympanostomy tube insertion may improve hearing.

A hearing aid may be prescribed for a conductive loss. A sensorineural loss is more difficult to treat, but cochlear implants and bone conduction hearing aids have been used in some children. A cochlear implant is a small electronic device that helps to provide sound for those who are deaf or profoundly hard of hearing. It consists of the following:

1. A microphone to pick up sound that is located outside of the body; worn as a headpiece behind the ear

2. A speech processor that organizes sound from the microphone; worn behind the ear or on a belt

3. A transmitter that transfers the sound into electrical impulses; part of the headpiece behind the ear

4. Electrodes that send the signals to the brain; this receiver is implanted in the skin behind the ear with a wire leading to the cochlear fluid in the middle ear

TABLE 19–11 Communication Techniques for Children Who Have a Hearing Impairment

TECHNIQUE	DESCRIPTION
Cued speech	Supplement to lipreading; eight hand shapes represent groups of consonant sounds and four positions about the face represent groups of vowel sounds; based on the sounds the letters make, not the letters themselves; child can "see-hear" every spoken syllable a hearing person hears
Oral approach	Uses only spoken language for face-to-face communication; avoids use of formal signs; uses hearing aids and residual hearing
Total communication	Uses speech and sign, fingerspelling, lipreading, and residual hearing simultaneously; child selects communication technique depending on the situation

For children with uncorrectable hearing loss, several approaches are used to enhance communication (Table 19–11). Children with hearing impairments may receive speech therapy and instructions in lipreading, sign language, cuing, and fingerspelling.

Growth and Development

Infants and young children respond automatically with a blink or the startle reflex to unexpected or loud noises. As they mature, they localize the sound source, then understand speech, and then communicate verbally.

Nursing Management

For the Child With a Hearing Impairment

Nursing Assessment and Diagnosis

Nurses conduct newborn hearing tests soon after birth and make observations of the infant's responses to sound. As the child grows, assess hearing at every well-child visit. The best judges of hearing are parents; ask them if they have any concerns about their child's hearing. An infant's reaction to rattles, bells, or handclapping (about 30 cm [12 in.] from the ear) is an important observation. Evaluate language milestones when examining the older infant and child. Language development is a major area of focus in deaf children. Deaf infants begin to babble at about 5 to 6 months of age, the same age as hearing infants. However, this babbling ceases several months later in the child who has a hearing impairment.

School nurses use audiometers to evaluate hearing during screening programs in schools, and refer children who do not pass the screening test (see the *Clinical Skills Manual* SKILLS). Measures to promote speech and communication development as well as safety are implemented.

Common nursing diagnoses for the child with impaired hearing include the following (NANDA-I © 2014):

- *Communication: Verbal, Impaired,* related to abnormal sound transmission
- *Development: Delayed, Risk for,* related to communication impairment

- *Coping: Family, Readiness for Enhanced,* related to caring for a child with a hearing impairment

Planning and Implementation

Nurses can encourage prevention of hearing loss from exposure to loud noises such as loud music and power and farm equipment. Music should be turned down and ear protection worn for other activities. School nurses should be active in hearing conservation education programs in school. Several programs are available to assist the school nurse in teaching children at targeted ages about noise-induced hearing loss. The nurse should develop and deliver hearing conservation curricula to children at elementary, middle, and high school levels; inform teachers and other professionals about noise-induced hearing loss; and train volunteers to assist with school programs.

Newborn screening, developmental assessment, and childhood hearing screening facilitate identification of hearing loss in newborns, infants, and children. Newborns and infants should be tested for hearing loss by 1 month of age. In cases of loss, intervention should begin before 6 months of age (Joint Committee on Infant Hearing, 2007).

Nursing care of the child with a hearing impairment focuses on facilitating the child's ability to receive spoken language and to send information, helping parents meet the child's schooling needs, and providing emotional support to parents. Refer the parents to an early intervention program as soon as the diagnosis of hearing impairment is made, in order to foster the child's development. If a cochlear implant is planned, the child needs surgical care and follow-up to monitor results and integrate sound gradually into the child's life. Pneumococcal and meningococcal vaccines and ongoing speech therapy are needed.

FACILITATE ABILITY TO RECEIVE SPOKEN LANGUAGE

Be aware of how the child compensates for hearing loss and use these strategies in communication:

- If hearing loss is mild or temporary or if the child reads lips, first obtain the child's visual attention by lightly touching the child or saying the child's name.

- Position your face 1 to 2 m (3 to 6 ft) from the child's face and make sure that the child's eyes are focused on your face and lips. Make sure the room is well lit, with no backlighting. Speak at a normal rate and tone, and use facial expressions that show caring or concern. If the child does not understand, rephrase the information in shorter, simpler sentences. Use specific, concrete explanations, and give the child time to comprehend. Watch for subtle signs of misinterpretations and give consistent and immediate feedback since only 30% of the English language is visible on the lips.

- Be familiar with the different types of hearing aids. Hearing aids, which are microphones that amplify all sounds, can be worn in or behind the ear, in the frame of glasses, or on the body with a wire attached to the ear. Place the hearing aid in the ear with the volume off, then slowly turn up to half volume. Adjust as needed. When talking to a child with a hearing aid, speak slowly within 15 to 45 cm (6 to 18 in.) of the microphone using a normal conversational tone. Talk to the child even if the child is not looking at you. Make sure the batteries are fresh for the best reception. Since all sound is amplified, reduce background noise as much as possible. Clean the hearing aid daily with a damp cloth. Change the batteries as needed, usually about once a week. The child's growth necessitates a new fitting, usually about once annually.

Health Promotion The Child With a Hearing Impairment

Growth and Developmental Surveillance

- Ensure that the child receives all immunizations at scheduled times. All children with cochlear implants should have pneumococcal vaccine (PCV7 for under 5 years of age or PPV23 for over 5 years). The immunization should be completed 2 weeks before surgery for cochlear implant. Children should be up-to-date on all immunizations, but rubella, mumps, and measles are especially important since infections with the diseases could cause further hearing loss.

- Complete developmental assessment, including receptive and expressive verbal skills at each visit.

- Teach about safety precautions for those with hearing impairment, such as inability to hear announcements at school, fire alarms at home, or sirens when traveling. Assist the family to install visual stimuli for fire alarms and other safety needs.

Communication

- Review the type of communication used by the child and the family's satisfaction.

- Ask about relationships with other children, both those with hearing impairments and those without.

- Review discipline techniques used by the parents and consistency of limit setting.

Nutrition and Physical Activity

- Complete 24-hour diet recall and be sure the child receives adequate nutrition appropriate in energy for activities.

- Review the child's exercise patterns since some children with hearing impairment may avoid interactions with other children in sports.

- Refer the family to community activity programs as needed.

Mental Health

- Determine stressors parents may feel.

- Locate community resources for early intervention and ongoing programs.

- Assist the youth and family to plan for moves to new schools and communities, and for plans related to transition to young adulthood, including college, trade schools, or work in the community.

Disease Prevention Strategies

- Be sure signs of ear infection such as fever, irritability, disturbed sleep, rubbing ear, or ear drainage are promptly evaluated in the pediatric healthcare home.

- Teach parents to administer antibiotics for ear infections exactly as prescribed.

- Encourage breastfeeding of infants and avoiding smoking to minimize incidence of ear infections.

- Be sure the child has all recommended immunizations.

Injury Prevention Strategies

- Encourage family to preserve any hearing the child may have by avoiding exposure to loud sounds; when children are old enough to understand, be sure they safeguard against exposure to loud music, guns, and other risks.

- Teach the child and family to plan for safety when crossing streets, driving cars, escaping house fires, and other situations that normally rely on hearing.

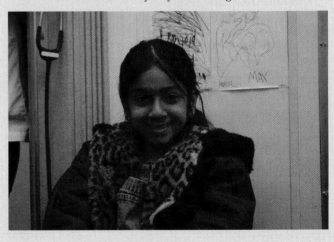

Acoustic feedback, an audible whistling sound that cannot always be heard by the child, is one of the most common problems with hearing aids. To eliminate this sound, readjust the hearing aid to make sure that it is inserted properly and that no hair or ear wax is caught between the ear mold and canal. Turning down the volume may also help. (See *Health Promotion: The Child With a Hearing Impairment*.)

A remote microphone system is another type of device designed to improve hearing. This is often used in the classroom situation because it eliminates background noise. The speaker wears a transmitter that picks up the voice and transmits it to a receiver worn by the child.

FACILITATE ABILITY TO SEND INFORMATION

Maintain the child's hearing aid in proper condition. Many children with impaired hearing communicate using speech, which is enhanced through speech therapy. In addition, they are taught to sign, fingerspell, or use cued speech (Figure 19–9). Articulation may be difficult, and understanding what the child is trying to say may be frustrating for both the nurse and the child. Taking time to listen carefully is important.

Take measures to promote speech and communication development as well as safety. Ask the parents to explain the child's communication techniques and to help interpret words. Have younger children point to pictures. Use assisted technologies such as a computer or picture board as well as drawings or gestures if necessary. This is especially helpful for communicating feelings of pain and hunger during hospitalization. If the child signs or fingerspells, make sure that you understand the signs for important functions. Give older children a pad of paper and pencil to write requests. People other than parents should be able to understand what the child is trying to communicate. Have an interpreter available if the child uses American Sign Language. Learn some common signs to communicate simple

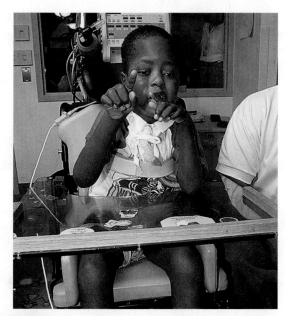

Figure 19-9 This child with a hearing impairment and tracheostomy is communicating by means of American Sign Language (ASL).

words or phrases. Orient the child carefully to new settings such as the hospital room or a new school.

HELP PARENTS MEET CHILD'S EDUCATIONAL NEEDS

Public laws apply to the education of children who have a hearing impairment (see Chapter 1). After diagnosis, the parents and healthcare professionals together agree on an individualized education plan (see discussion in Chapter 12). Day care and preschool are recommended for children with hearing problems.

- Give parents information about adjustments that may have to be made for a child with a hearing impairment who attends public school. By sitting at the front of the classroom, the child may be able to hear and see more clearly. The teacher should always face the child when speaking, and background noise should be reduced.

- Tell parents that children who have hearing impairments have the same intelligence quotient (IQ) distribution as children without a hearing impairment. However, communication and learning can be difficult, and extra support is needed.

- Children with a hearing impairment should reach their intellectual potential, although development in certain areas may take place more slowly than it does in children without a hearing impairment.

PROVIDE EMOTIONAL SUPPORT

By recognizing the effects of the diagnosis on the family, the nurse can help the family deal with their reaction to the child's hearing loss. Supporting healthy coping is an important intervention to help the parents carry on with their lives.

- Help the parents understand the child's disability and its effect on speech and language development. Provide accurate information about their concerns. Work jointly with other healthcare professionals and social service workers if necessary.

- Tell the family about the community services available for medical, nursing, psychologic, and financial assistance.

Evaluation

Expected outcomes of nursing care for a child with a hearing impairment include the following:

- The child is assisted in establishment of communication method.
- The child manifests growth and development to maximum potential.
- A successful individualized education plan is established.
- The family demonstrates positive coping and healthcare management.

Injuries of the Ear

Ear injuries of many types commonly occur in children. Lacerations, infections, and hematomas may occur in the external ear structures, especially the pinna. Children may place foreign objects in the ear, and insects may enter the ear canal. Rupture of the tympanic membrane may result from head injuries, blows to the ear, or insertion of objects into the ear canal. Caution children and parents not to place anything into the ear, including cotton swabs for cleaning.

See Table 19-12 for information on the emergency treatment of ear injuries. Any injury resulting in earache, decreased hearing, persistent bleeding, or other discharge should be seen by a healthcare provider.

Disorders of the Nose and Throat

Epistaxis

Epistaxis, or nosebleed, is common in school-age children, especially boys. The Kiesselbach plexus, an area of plentiful veins located in the anterior nares, is the most common source of bleeding. The most common cause is irritation from nosepicking, foreign bodies, or low humidity. Other causes include forceful coughing, allergies, or infections resulting in congestion of the nasal mucosa. Posterior nosebleeds have a variety of causes, some of which may indicate systemic disease (i.e., bleeding disorder) or injury. Bleeding from the posterior septum is more serious and may be life threatening. Hospitalization may be necessary.

Nursing Management

Children with nosebleeds are sometimes brought to the emergency department by a parent who has been unable to stop the flow of blood within a few minutes. Both parent and child may be frightened. Ask the parent briefly about any history of nosebleeds and other contributing factors, including medications. Take the child's pulse and blood pressure to assess for excessive blood loss. Carefully examine the nasal mucosa by asking the child to blow any clots out gently, if possible. Suctioning may be necessary.

Observing the flow may help determine whether the blood is coming from an anterior or a posterior location. A nosebleed confined to one side of the nose is almost always anterior, but posterior bleeding can flow on one or both sides. If blood cannot be seen, the child may be swallowing it and may become nauseated. Suspect posterior bleeding in children who have sustained blunt trauma to the head.

TABLE 19–12 Emergency Treatment of Ear Injuries

INJURY	TREATMENT
PINNA	
Minor cuts or abrasions	Wash thoroughly with soap and water and rinse well; leave exposed to air if possible or apply adhesive bandage; monitor for infection.
Hematomas	Needle aspiration should be performed and pressure dressing applied; undrained hematomas may become fibrotic; "cauliflower ear" deformity may develop.
Cellulitis or abscesses	Apply moist heat intermittently; make sure that prescribed antibiotic is taken; minor surgery may be performed for an abscess.
Deep lacerations	Apply pressure to stop bleeding; transport to healthcare provider's office or emergency department for suturing.
EAR CANAL	
Foreign bodies	Have child lie on back and turn head over edge of bed, with affected side down; wiggle earlobe and have child shake head; foreign object may fall out as result of gravity; if object remains in ear, call healthcare provider; do not try to remove foreign body with tweezers since this may push the object further into the ear.
Insects	Shine flashlights into ear to try to attract insect; instilling a few drops of mineral oil, olive oil, or alcohol kills insect, and irrigating ear canal gently may remove dead insect. See the *Clinical Skills Manual* SKILLS.
TYMPANIC MEMBRANE	
Ruptures	Call healthcare provider if child has persistent ear pain after blow, blast injury, or insertion of foreign object; cover external ear loosely with piece of sterile cotton or gauze; if tympanic membrane has been ruptured, systemic antibiotics are prescribed.

The child with anterior bleeding should sit upright quietly. The head should be tilted forward to prevent blood from trickling down the throat, which can lead to vomiting. The nares should be squeezed just below the nasal bone and held for 10 to 15 minutes while the child breathes through the mouth. If the bleeding does not stop, a cotton ball or swab soaked with Neo-Synephrine, epinephrine, thrombin, or lidocaine may be inserted into the affected nostril to promote topical vasoconstriction or anesthesia. Once the bleeding has stopped, the nostril may have to be cauterized with silver nitrate or electrocautery. If the bleeding cannot be stopped, absorbable packing may be used.

Posterior bleeding must also be stopped by packing, and the child must be monitored carefully. Arterial ligation is occasionally needed. Repeated or severe nosebleeds need further evaluation (Montague, Whymark, Howatson, et al., 2011).

Assess the child's hematocrit or hemoglobin if significant bleeding has occurred. Take a complete history and do a physical examination of children with frequent epistaxis to rule out systemic disease. (See *Families Want to Know: Prevention and Home Management of Epistaxis*.)

After the nosebleed has stopped, the child is more vulnerable to recurrent bleeding and should avoid bending over, stooping, strenuous exercise, hot drinks, and hot baths or showers for the next 3 to 4 days. Sleeping with the head elevated on two or three pillows and humidifying the air with a vaporizer may also prevent a recurrence. Give parents suggestions for prevention and home management of epistaxis.

Families Want to Know
Prevention and Home Management of Epistaxis

Prevention

- Humidify the child's room, especially during the winter.
- Discourage the child from picking or rubbing the nose or inserting foreign objects in the nose.
- Instruct the child to blow the nose gently and release sneezes through the mouth.

Home Management

- Keep the child calm.
- Sit the child upright with head tilted slightly forward so blood does not run down the nasopharynx.
- Press a roll of cotton under the upper lip to compress the labial artery.
- Apply steady pressure to both nostrils just below the nasal bone with the thumb and forefinger for 15 to 20 minutes. Time by the clock.
- Apply an ice pack or cold compress to the bridge of the nose or the back of the neck.
- Call healthcare provider if the bleeding does not stop.
- Avoid vigorous exercise and aspirin or other noncoagulant drugs during the first few days after an episode of epistaxis.

Source: Adapted from Melia, L., & McGarry, G. W. (2011). Epistaxis: Update on management. Current Opinion in Otolaryngology & Head and Neck Surgery, 19, 30–35.

Nasopharyngitis

Nasopharyngitis, also known as upper respiratory infection (URI) or the "common cold," causes inflammation and infection of the nose and throat and is a common illness of infancy and childhood. More than 200 viruses and numerous bacteria can cause this condition. The most common viruses include rhinovirus and coronavirus, and the most frequently occurring bacterium is group A *Streptococcus*. See Chapter 20 for a discussion of respiratory syncytial virus (RSV), a common cause of both upper and lower respiratory illness. The organisms incubate in 1 to 3 days, and the infection is communicable several hours before symptoms develop and for 1 to 2 days after they begin. Symptoms may last 4 to 10 days or longer. The pathogens spread when the infected person touches the hand of an uninfected person, who then touches the mouth or nose, resulting in self-inoculation with infected droplets.

A red nasal mucosa with clear nasal discharge and an infected throat with enlarged tonsils may be apparent in children with nasopharyngitis. Vesicles may be present on the soft palate and in the pharynx. Accompanying symptoms may vary, depending on the child's age (Table 19–13).

Between episodes of nasopharyngitis, the child should be asymptomatic. If a child continues to have upper respiratory infections, an underlying condition such as allergy, asthma, or polyps should be ruled out.

Nursing Management

For infants who cannot breathe through the mouth, normal saline nose drops can be administered every 3 to 4 hours, especially before feeding, and followed by bulb suctioning if needed

TABLE 19–13 Manifestations of Nasopharyngitis

INFANTS YOUNGER THAN 3 MONTHS OF AGE	
Lethargy	Feeding poorly
Irritability	Fever (may be absent)

INFANTS 3 MONTHS OF AGE OR OLDER	
Fever	Anorexia
Vomiting	Irritability
Diarrhea	Restlessness
Sneezing	

OLDER CHILDREN	
Dry, irritated nose and throat	Anorexia
Chills, fever	Thin nasal discharge, which may later become thick and purulent
Generalized muscle aches	
Headache	
Malaise	Sneezing

(see the *Clinical Skills Manual* SKILLS). For infants over 9 months of age, nasal stuffiness can be treated with normal saline. Children over 6 years of age can use nasal sprays.

Decongestant nose drops and sprays should not be used for more than 4 or 5 days or more often than recommended. Antihistamines may be helpful for children with allergic rhinitis or profuse nasal drainage. Long-acting nasal sprays and medications with several ingredients are not recommended. (See *Families Want to Know: Over-the-Counter Cough and Cold Medications.*)

Families Want to Know

Over-the-Counter Cough and Cold Medications

Parents may try to treat children who have upper respiratory infections with the same medications they are accustomed to taking for a cold. Work with parents during a health promotion visit and help them plan for how to handle medications for the child. Guidelines are as follows:

- Do NOT use cough and cold products in children under 2 years of age unless given specific directions to do so by a healthcare provider.

- Read the label to be sure the medication is recommended for the child's age and condition. Give only the dose recommended for the age and weight of the child. Do NOT use products packaged for adults.

- Be sure you know how to measure the medication. Tablespoon and teaspoon are not the same, and using household spoons may lead to incorrect dosing. Use only the measuring device that is provided with liquid medications to ensure accuracy. If one is not provided, purchase one at the pharmacy that is precisely labeled. Use only a measuring device with the precise marking to match the dose you need to give.

- Consult the pharmacist, nurse, or other healthcare provider if you have questions, if the child is taking other medicines, if the medication is not recommended for the age of the child, if the child's condition does not improve, or if other symptoms appear.

- Use the child-resistant cap after each opening of the bottle. Store the medication out of reach of all children, preferably in a locked location.

- Inspect containers and do not buy those that may have tears, imperfections, or tampering. Review all of the information in the "Drug Facts" box on the package label.

- If you use home remedies or other herbal products to treat colds, be sure to check on their safety with your healthcare provider first.

- If the child becomes more ill or does not improve, stop the medicine and contact the healthcare provider. If you do not understand instructions on the package contact a healthcare provider before using it.

Source: Adapted from Budnitz, D. S., Lovegrove, M. C., & Rose, K. O. (2014). Adherence to label and device recommendations for over-the-counter pediatric liquid medications. *Pediatrics, 133*, e283–e290; U.S. Food and Drug Administration. (2011). *Public Health Advisory—FDA recommends that over-the-counter (OTC) cough and cold products not be used for infants and children under 2 years of age.* Retrieved from http://www.fda.gov/drugs/drugsafety; U.S. Food and Drug Administration. (2014). *OTC cough and cold products—Not for infants and children under 2 years of age.* Retrieved from http://www.fda.gov/ForConsumers/ConsumerUpdates/ucm048682.htm

Room humidification may help prevent drying of nasal secretions. Antipyretics such as acetaminophen reduce fever and make the child more comfortable. Aspirin is not recommended because of its association with Reye syndrome (refer to Chapter 27).

Children should avoid strenuous physical activity and engage in quiet play such as reading, listening to music or stories, or watching television or videotapes. Children should not be forced to eat. Encourage the intake of favorite fluids to liquefy secretions. Tell parents that no medicine or vaccine can prevent the common cold, but eliminating contact with infected persons can reduce the spread of infection. Proper hand hygiene and disposal of tissues helps to decrease the spread of the infection. Cleaning counters, toys, door knobs, and other surfaces on a daily basis can decrease the spread of infections. Discourage sharing of food, dishes, and utensils at meals.

> ## Developing Cultural Competence Hot and Cold Disease Theory
>
> Many Hispanic and Asian cultural groups believe in the "hot and cold theory" of disease, in which health problems are viewed as the result of imbalance. For example, some Mexican Americans traditionally treat a "cold disease" such as an earache or common cold with "hot" substances. Ask families if they prefer to eat certain foods or use complementary treatments during an illness. Incorporating such preferences may help the child and increase the confidence of the family in healthcare providers.

Sinusitis

Sinusitis is an inflammation of one or more of the paranasal sinuses. These sinuses, which have respiratory epithelium and are continuous with the respiratory tract, include the maxillary, ethmoid, frontal, and sphenoid sinuses. The sinuses may become infected with bacteria following a viral upper respiratory infection or allergic inflammation, and therefore sinusitis is a common occurrence in children (Wald et al., 2013).

Sinusitis can be viral or bacterial. Signs and symptoms of sinusitis in children are sometimes nonspecific. A history of recent upper respiratory infection is common, persistent cough from postnasal drip can occur, and nasal discharge or swelling can be apparent. Malodorous breath, fever, mouth breathing, hyponasal speech, and cervical lymphadenopathy may be present. Young children may be anorexic or have difficulty feeding, and older children may complain of headache.

Diagnosis of sinusitis is usually based on history and physical examination findings. Acute bacterial sinusitis is diagnosed when a child with upper respiratory infection (URI) presents persistently (10 days or more) with nasal discharge and or daytime cough, worsening course, or severe onset with temperature 39.0°C (102.2°F) or above and purulent nasal discharge for 3 days or more (Wald et al., 2013). Percussion and illumination of sinuses, computed tomography (CT), magnetic resonance imaging (MRI), and ultrasound are not generally useful in diagnosing sinusitis in children. CT or MRI may be used when orbital or central nervous system complications are suspected. For the child with repeated sinusitis or who appears toxic, aspiration of sinus aspirate may be performed for culture by an otolaryngologist.

Antibiotics are prescribed if there is severe onset or worsening course of illness, and often when there is persistent illness (Wald et al., 2013). Amoxicillin is the first choice for therapy; amoxicillin/clavulanate, cefuroxime, cefdinir, azithromycin, and clarithromycin are also sometimes used. Children with recurrent sinusitis should be referred for further care by an otolaryngologist and allergy specialist. Efficacy of decongestants, antihistamines, and nasal irrigation has not been demonstrated (Shaikh & Wald, 2014).

Parents whose child has persistent and purulent nasal drainage should be told to see a healthcare provider, particularly if the drainage is accompanied by facial pain, headache, and fever. Nurses should teach parents to correctly administer antibiotics (e.g., to take medications for the full course) if prescribed, and to use saline nose drops if needed for comfort. Infants may need their noses cleared with nose drops and a bulb syringe prior to feedings. (Refer to the *Clinical Skills Manual* SKILLS for correct use of a bulb syringe.) Antipyretics can be given for fever and to relieve pain.

Pharyngitis

Acute pharyngitis is an infection that primarily affects the pharynx, including the tonsils. It is seen most frequently in children 4 to 7 years of age and is rare in children less than 1 year of age. Approximately 80% of these infections are caused by viruses; the rest are caused by bacteria. Bacterial pharyngitis is commonly known as "strep throat," since in many cases it is caused by group A beta-hemolytic streptococcus (GABHS) (Ebell, 2014).

The major complaint is a sore throat. Children with symptoms of strep throat who have minimal throat redness and pain, exudate, mild lymphadenopathy, and a low-grade fever, and who have been exposed to someone who has strep pharyngitis should have a throat culture. The classic signs of purulent drainage and white patches are not present in all cases of strep throat.

A child who finds swallowing difficult or extremely painful, who drools, or who exhibits signs of dehydration or respiratory distress should be seen by a healthcare professional immediately. These signs could be indicators of serious conditions such as peritonsillar or retropharyngeal abscess, epiglottitis (Chapter 20), or diphtheria (Chapter 16).

Peritonsillar abscess (a tonsil infection that spreads into surrounding tissues and causes cellulitis) or retropharyngeal abscess (an infection of the lymph nodes that drain the adenoids, nasopharynx, and paranasal sinuses) are serious conditions. These conditions may have additional symptoms such as decreased neck movement, neck edema or pain, and respiratory distress. CT scan or MRI may be helpful in diagnosis of abscess. See Table 19–14 for manifestations of viral pharyngitis, strep throat, peritonsillar abscess, and retropharyngeal abscess.

The diagnosis of strep throat is made by throat culture, using the rapid or traditional strep tests (see the *Clinical Skills Manual* SKILLS). Results of the rapid strep test may be available within minutes; those for the traditional test are available in 24 to 48 hours. A negative rapid test is followed by a traditional test in order to verify results.

Streptococcal pharyngitis is treated with oral penicillin for 10 days or with long-acting penicillin given in one injection. If the child is allergic to penicillin, erythromycin, azithromycin, or clarithromycin is given. Acute symptoms should resolve within 24 hours of therapy, at which time, the child is no longer contagious. For viral pharyngitis, symptomatic treatment alone is used.

Clinical Tip

Throat cultures must be properly performed for accurate diagnosis. Swab a sterile cotton-tip applicator across the tonsils, posterior edge of the soft palate, and uvula. Ask cooperative children to put their hands under their buttocks, open their mouth, and laugh or pant like a dog. Quickly swab the throat. You can place uncooperative and young children on their backs with their hands next to their heads and have a parent or an assistant hold them. Depress the tongue gently with a tongue blade and swab the throat and both tonsils.

TABLE 19–14 Clinical Manifestations of Viral Pharyngitis, Strep Throat (Group A Beta-Hemolytic Streptococcus [GABHS]), Peritonsillar Abscess, and Retropharyngeal Abscess

VIRAL PHARYNGITIS	STREP THROAT	PERITONSILLAR ABSCESS	RETROPHARYNGEAL ABSCESS
Nasal congestion	Abrupt onset	Fever	Fever
Mild sore throat	Tonsillar exudate	Malaise	Sore throat
Conjunctivitis	Painful cervical lymphadenopathy	Sore throat, more severe on one side	Inability to eat
Cough	Anorexia, nausea, vomiting, abdominal pain	Marked erythema and edema, especially of one side of throat, tonsil, and soft palate, sometimes with deviated uvula	Neck pain and edema
Hoarseness	Severe sore throat		Pharyngitis
Mild pharyngeal redness	Headache, malaise	Mouth odor	Respiratory distress and stridor
Minimal tonsillar exudate	Fever > 38.3°C (101.0°F)	Difficulty speaking	
Mildly tender anterior cervical lymphadenopathy	Petechial mottling of soft palate	Difficulty opening mouth wide	
Fever < 38.3°C (101.0°F)		Cervical lymphadenitis	
		Ear pain	

Note: Children 6 months to 3 years of age may have streptococcal pharyngitis with symptoms that resemble those of viral pharyngitis. Children with scarlet fever have the symptoms of strep throat plus a sandpaper-textured erythematous generalized rash and pallor around the lips.

Source: Data from Hsiao, H. J., Huang, Y. C., Hsia, S. H., Wu, C. T., & Lin, J. J. (2012). Clinical features of peritonsillar abscess in children. *Pediatric Neonatology, 53,* 366–370; Hoffman, C., Pierrot, L., Contencin, P., Morisseau-Durand, M. P., Manach, Y., & Couloigner, V. (2011). Retropharyngeal infections in children: Treatment strategies and outcomes. *International Journal of Pediatric Otorhinolaryngology, 75,* 1099–1103.

Peritonsillar abscess is treated by draining the abscess, providing antibiotics effective in treating the fluid cultured from the abscess, and hydration. Commonly administered antibiotics include ampicillin/sulbactam, penicillin G, and clindamycin. Once treatment has resolved the infection, the child is evaluated for possible tonsillectomy (Hsaio, Huang, Hsia, et al., 2012). Retropharyngeal abscess is also frequently treated by drainage of the abscess, although intravenous antibiotics alone are effective in some cases. Ampicillin/sulbactam, clindamycin, cephalosporin, and penicillin are common antibiotics. Respiratory management may be needed.

Nursing Management

Nursing care focuses on symptomatic relief. Acetaminophen reduces throat pain and generalized fever. Cool, nonacidic fluids and soft foods, ice chips, or frozen juice pops given frequently in small amounts facilitate swallowing and prevent dehydration. Humidification and gargling with warm salt water (5 g [1 teaspoon] salt to 250 mL [8 oz] water) soothe an irritated throat. Alternatively, the salt water can be placed in a spray bottle and sprayed gently toward the throat. Commercial throat sprays or throat lozenges are not generally more effective than these home remedies. Encourage the child to rest to conserve energy and promote recovery.

Teach parents the importance of completing the 10-day course of antibiotics if prescribed for bacterial pharyngitis. Reinforce to parents the importance of treating streptococcal infections because untreated infections may lead to rheumatic fever, cervical adenitis, sinusitis, glomerulonephritis, or meningitis.

Tonsillitis and Adenoiditis

Tonsillitis is an infection or inflammation (hypertrophy) of the palatine tonsils. Although most children with pharyngitis may have infected tonsils, they do not necessarily have tonsillitis. The adenoids are lymphatic tissue located on the posterior pharyngeal wall and are sometimes called the pharyngeal tonsils; they can manifest with acute or chronic infection.

ETIOLOGY AND PATHOPHYSIOLOGY
Like pharyngitis, tonsillitis and adenoiditis may be caused by a virus or bacterium. The primary site of infection is the tonsils.

CLINICAL MANIFESTATIONS
Symptoms suggestive of tonsillitis include frequent throat infections with breathing and swallowing difficulties, persistent redness of the anterior pillars, and enlargement of the cervical lymph nodes. If children breathe through their mouths continuously, the mucous membranes may become dry and irritated. Adenoiditis is characterized by nasal stuffiness, discharge, and postnasal drip, which result in coughing or excessive clearing of the throat.

CLINICAL THERAPY
Diagnosis is made on the basis of visual inspection and clinical manifestations. Tonsils appear large and inflamed. Enlarged adenoids are diagnosed by radiologic studies.

Symptomatic treatment for tonsillitis is the same as for pharyngitis. Recent guidelines provide clear recommendations for surgery involving repeated infections and sleep-disordered breathing. Watchful waiting is recommended in most cases. Tonsillectomy can be considered when there are at least seven episodes of tonsillitis in the previous year, at least five episodes per year for 2 years, or at least three episodes annually for 3 years. In these cases, tonsillitis diagnosis requires a sore throat and at least one of the following symptoms: temperature above 38.3°C (101.0°F), cervical adenopathy, tonsillar exudate, and positive group A beta-hemolytic streptococcal infection (Giordano et al., 2011). Sleep-disordered breathing that exists with tonsillar hypertrophy and a condition such as growth abnormality, poor school performance, enuresis, or behavioral problem is also appropriate reason for surgical tonsillectomy (Mitka, 2011). One intraoperative dose of intravenous dexamethasone is recommended, but routine operative antibiotics are not needed.

Nursing Management

For the Child With Tonsillitis and Adenoiditis

Nursing Assessment and Diagnosis

Assess the throat carefully during each physical examination. Observe for tonsils that are simply large (a common finding in childhood) and those that are inflamed. Look for the degree of redness and presence of any exudate. Ask if the child has pain or difficulty swallowing. Ask about the history of past tonsillar infections and the length of time of the present discomfort.

If surgery is indicated, take a complete history of the child preoperatively. Monitor vital signs and observe for respiratory distress, hemorrhage, and dehydration postoperatively.

Several nursing diagnoses may apply to the child with tonsillitis. They include the following (NANDA-I © 2014):

- *Pain, Acute,* related to inflammation of the pharynx
- *Fluid Volume: Deficient, Risk for,* related to inadequate intake
- *Breathing Pattern, Ineffective,* related to obstruction by enlarged tonsils
- *Swallowing, Impaired,* related to inflammation and pain
- *Knowledge, Readiness for Enhanced,* related to home care following discharge

Planning and Implementation

The nurse provides general supportive care and, if medication is prescribed, encourages completion of the full course of treatment. The nursing management of children with tonsillitis is similar to that of children with pharyngitis (see earlier discussion).

If surgery is indicated, help the parents prepare their child for a short-term surgical procedure with a possible overnight stay in the hospital (see Chapter 11). Children should be free of sore throat, fever, or upper respiratory infection for at least 1 week before surgery. They should not be given aspirin or ibuprofen for 2 weeks before surgery since these medications can increase postoperative bleeding. Check if any herbal medications are taken and report them to the surgeon and anesthesiologist since some may interfere with anesthetic drugs used in surgery.

DISCHARGE PLANNING AND HOME CARE TEACHING

Discharge planning includes teaching parents about pain management, fluid and nutrition intake, activity restrictions, and possible complications in the postoperative period. Most children have a sore throat for 7 to 10 days after tonsillectomy. Advise parents how to relieve the child's throat pain. (See *Families Want to Know: Care After Tonsillectomy.*)

Families Want to Know

Care After Tonsillectomy

After tonsillectomy, the parent can take the following measures to increase the child's comfort:

- Have the child drink adequate cool fluids to reduce spasms in the muscles surrounding the throat.
- Ensure that the child drinks recommended amount of fluid to avoid dehydration.
- Apply an ice collar around the child's neck.
- Give acetaminophen elixir or other analgesic as prescribed.
- Have the child gargle with a solution of 2.5 g (1/2 teaspoon) each of baking soda and salt in a glass of water.
- If ordered by the healthcare provider, have the child rinse the mouth well with viscous lidocaine or other local anesthetic.

Families Want to Know

Complications of Tonsillectomy and Adenoidectomy

Bleeding

- To prevent bleeding, aspirin or ibuprofen should not be given for pain for the first postoperative week. Use acetaminophen instead.
- Bleeding is most likely to occur within the first 24 hours or 7 to 10 days after the tonsillectomy, when the scar is forming. Report any trickle of bright red blood or increased swallowing to the healthcare provider immediately.

Infection

- The back of the throat will look white and have an odor for the first 7 to 8 days after the surgery. The child may also have a low-grade fever. These are not signs of infection.
- For temperatures over 38.3°C (101.0°F), acetaminophen may be used.
- Call the healthcare provider if the child develops a fever above 38.8°C (102.0°F).

Pain

- Administer acetaminophen as ordered.
- Offer frequent small amounts of cool liquids. Avoid citrus juice.
- Provide for rest and quiet activities for several days.

Families Want to Know

Care of a Tooth Avulsion

When a tooth is removed during an injury, prompt treatment may improve the chance that it can be reimplanted. If the child's condition is stable, try to reimplant the tooth and then transfer to an emergency dental facility.

- Handle the tooth only by the crown (its top) rather than the root to avoid further damage.
- Gently rinse the tooth with a stream of sterile saline. Do NOT place it under running water.
- Insert into the socket.
- Have the child provide gentle pressure by biting a piece of gauze or a moistened tea bag. If the child is unstable or has other injuries, enlist emergency medical transportation (call 9-1-1). In this case, the tooth is transported with the child.
- If a dental aid kit is available, it may contain a transport liquid such as ViaSpan or Hank's Balanced Salt Solution. If these are not available, alternatives include cold milk, saline, saliva, or water. Place the tooth in one of these transfer liquids to keep it moist and send it with the child to the healthcare facility.

Source: Adapted from American Association of Endodontists. (2013). *The treatment of traumatic dental injuries*. Retrieved from http://www.nxtbook.com/nxtbooks/aae/traumaguidelines/index.php#/0

Children may experience ear pain, especially when swallowing, between 4 and 8 days after tonsillectomy. Advise parents that this pain is referred from the tonsillar area and does not indicate an ear infection.

Emphasize to parents the importance of adequate fluid intake. Children should be given any liquid they prefer for the first week, except citrus juices, which may produce a burning sensation in the throat. Soft foods such as gelatin, applesauce, frozen juice pops, and mashed potatoes can be added as tolerated.

Children do not need to be confined to bed, but they should avoid vigorous exercise for the first week after surgery. Advise parents that the child may return to school approximately 10 days after tonsillectomy.

Any surgery carries the risk of postoperative complications. Teach parents the normal signs of healing in the postoperative period, as well as signs of complications. (See *Families Want to Know: Complications of Tonsillectomy and Adenoidectomy*.)

Evaluation

Expected outcomes of nursing care for the child with tonsillitis include the following:

- The child has adequate intake of food and fluids.
- Pain and fever are effectively managed.
- There is an absence of postoperative complications such as bleeding, hemorrhage, and dehydration.
- Healing occurs without impairment following tonsillectomy.

Disorders of the Mouth

The mouth is an important structure that is directly linked to both the gastrointestinal and respiratory systems. Structural problems can occur in the mouth, often in conjunction with other defects such as tracheoesophageal fistula or cleft lip and palate (see Chapter 25). A second type of mouth disorder in children is ulceration. Children sometimes have changes in the mucous membranes of the mouth, associated with illnesses, infections, or as a side effect of drug treatments. Trauma is a third cause for mouth disorders in children. Accidents can cause fractures of the jaw, dental emergencies, or other trauma.

Nursing Management

Most mouth ulcers are treated symptomatically. Since the oral mucosa is fast growing, the cells can rapidly heal. Keeping the mouth clean and administering systemic or topical analgesics can assist with comfort. Foods should be mild and nonirritating. Acyclovir may be administered for treatment of herpes infections. Antibiotics are needed for bacterial infection of oral lesions. Stevens-Johnson syndrome necessitates removing the drug that causes the reaction, and treating the child with oral antihistamines and supportive therapy.

Nurses inform parents of proper treatment for injuries and may provide emergency treatment in schools and other community settings. Injury prevention is encouraged through use of protective gear during sports. Mouth guards can be helpful to prevent dental damage. See Chapter 17 for a discussion of protective sporting gear and of body piercing that may involve the oral cavity. Because the mouth has a profuse blood supply, bleeding may be extensive for even minor injuries. It is best to use clean cloths to absorb the blood and prevent choking on it, and get the child to an emergency facility to have the lesion examined.

Dental injuries may involve fracture of a tooth, luxation (partial extrusion), or avulsion (complete removal). The periodontal ligament holds the tooth in the socket but its attachment is torn during a tooth avulsion. When avulsion has occurred, fast care improves the chance that a permanent tooth can be reimplanted and kept alive. When reimplanted within 30 minutes, the chances of survival of the tooth are best (American Association of Endodontists, 2013). The nurse or family provides immediate care and the child should be transported immediately to an emergency facility. (See *Families Want to Know: Care of a Tooth Avulsion*.)

Chapter Highlights

- Health conditions affecting the eyes and ears are common in childhood, partially because of anatomic differences in structure, and can lead to developmental and communication disorders.

- Conjunctivitis can occur in the newborn and throughout childhood.

- Children manifest a wide array of visual disorders, such as hyperopia, myopia, and astigmatism.

- Strabismus, amblyopia, cataracts, glaucoma, and retinopathy of prematurity are serious conditions that can affect vision.

- Nurses commonly screen vision of children in schools and healthcare facilities to identify those with visual impairment.

- Otitis media is a common childhood health condition, with monitoring and antibiotics as potential treatments.

- Newborns should be screened for response to sounds, and those at high risk of hearing impairment should be carefully monitored in early childhood.

- Hearing loss may be conductive, sensorineural, or mixed.

- Nursing interventions for the child with vision or auditory impairment should focus on maximizing development and communication.

- Common disorders of the nose, throat, and mouth include epistaxis, nasopharyngitis, pharyngitis, tonsillitis, and oral ulcers.

- Nurses are influential in providing preventive teaching and emergency care when trauma occurs to the eyes, ears, and mouth.

Clinical Reasoning in Action

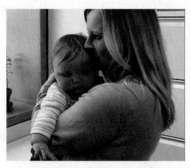

You are working at a local children's urgent care facility when a couple comes in carrying their screaming 9-month-old child, Becky. The parents are worried, as Becky has been crying steadily for the past 2 hours. You ask about recent illnesses or injuries and they tell you that she has had only two colds in her life and the most recent was about a week ago.

You assess Becky's vital signs as follows: weight 19 lb (8.6 kg), temperature 101°F, respirations 60 breaths per minute without retractions, and heart rate 120 beats per minute. She does not have any rashes or evidence of injuries, and upon examination, she appears well nourished but clearly in distress. Her heart rate is regular and rhythmic, and breath sounds are equal bilaterally and clear to auscultation. Both tympanic membranes are red and bulging. Her abdomen is soft and without organomegaly. The healthcare provider diagnoses bilateral acute otitis media and administers analgesic ear drops and ibuprofen in the office. Within 15 minutes, Becky has settled down, stopped crying, and is resting in her father's arms. The family is sent home with instructions to administer analgesics and return within 48 hours for further assessment.

1. What are the three main organisms that may have caused Becky's otitis media?

2. What are some of the guidelines you can give Becky's parents about otitis media treatment?

3. The mother says she has family members who have had tubes placed in their ears because of ear infections and wants to know if this is something that Becky will need to have done. How will you answer the mother's question?

4. What are some methods parents can use to prevent future otitis media episodes?

References

Adams A. J., Verdon W. A., & Spivey B. E. Color vision. (2012). In W. Tasman & E. A. Jaeger (Eds.), *Duane's foundations of clinical ophthalmology*. Philadelphia: Lippincott Williams & Wilkins.

American Academy of Pediatrics (AAP). (2011). *Vision screenings*. Retrieved from http://healthychildren.org

American Academy of Pediatrics (AAP) Committee on Practice and Ambulatory Medicine and Bright Futures Periodicity Schedule Work Group. (2014). Policy statement: 2014 recommendations for pediatric preventive health care. *Pediatrics, 133*(3), 568–570.

American Association for Pediatric Ophthalmology and Strabismus. (2014). *Strabismus*. Retrieved from http://www.aapos.org/terms/conditions/100

American Association of Endodontists. (2013). *The treatment of traumatic dental injuries*. Retrieved from http://www.nxtbook.com/nxtbooks/aae/traumaguidelines/index.php#/0

American Foundation for the Blind. (2011). *Children and youth with vision loss*. Retrieved from http://www.afb.org/Section/asp?SectionID=15&TopicID=411&DocumentID=4896

American Speech-Language-Hearing Association (ASLHA). (2011). *Type, degree, and configuration of hearing loss*. Retrieved from http://www.asha.org/public/hearing/disorders/types.htm

American Speech-Language-Hearing Association (ASLHA). (2014). *The prevalence and incidence of hearing loss in children*. Retrieved from http://www.asha.org/public/hearing/disorders/children.htm

Bradfield, Y. S. (2013). Identification and treatment of amblyopia. *American Family Physician, 87*, 348–352.

Budnitz, D. S., Lovegrove, M. C., & Rose, K. O. (2014). Adherence to label and device recommendations for over-the-counter pediatric liquid medications. *Pediatrics, 133*, e283–e290.

Centers for Disease Control and Prevention (CDC). (2012). *Summary of 2009 national CDC EHDI data.* Retrieved from http://www.cdc.gov/ncbddd/hearingloss/2009-data/2009_ehdi_hsfs_summary_508_ok.pdf

Chou, R., Dana, T., & Bougatsos, C. (2011). *Screening for visual impairment in children ages 1–5 years: Systematic review to update the 2004 U.S. Preventive Services Task Force recommendation* (Report No. 11-05151-EF-1). Rockville, MD: Agency for Healthcare Research and Quality.

Cohen, S. M. (2011). Orbital cellulitis as a complication of sinusitis. *Journal for Nurse Practitioners, 7*, 38–44.

Davidson, S., & Quinn, G. E. (2011). The impact of pediatric vision disorders in adulthood. *Pediatrics, 127*, 334–339.

Ebell, M. H. (2014). Diagnosis of streptococcal pharyngitis. *American Family Physician, 89*, 976–977.

Farboud, A., Skinner, R., & Pratap, R. (2011). Otitis media with effusion ("glue ear"). *British Medical Journal, 343.* doi:10.1136/bmj.d3770

Giordano, T., Litman, R. S., Li, K. K., Mannix, M. E., Schwartz, R. H., Setzen, G., . . . Patel, M. M. (2011). Clinical practice guideline: Tonsillectomy in children. *Otolaryngology—Head and Neck Surgery, 144.* doi:10.1177/0194599810389949

Gold, R. S. (2011). Treatment of bacterial conjunctivitis in children. *Pediatric Annals, 40*, 95–105.

Granet, D. B. (2011, May). Treating bacterial conjunctivitis. *Infectious Diseases in Children,* 10–15.

Granet, D. B., & Khayali, S. (2011, February). Amblyopia and strabismus. *Pediatric Annals,* 89–94.

Harmes, K. M., Blackwood, A., Burrows, H. L., Cooke, J. M., Van Harrison, R., & Passamani, P. P. (2013). Otitis media: Diagnosis and treatment. *American Family Physician, 88*, 435–440.

Hartnett, M. E., Morrison, M. A., Smith, S., Yanovitch, T. L., Young, T. L., Colaizy, T., . . . Cotton, C. M. (2014). Genetic variants associated with severe retinopathy of prematurity in extremely low birth weight infants. *Investigative Ophthalmology and Visual Science, 55*, 6194–6203.

Hoberman, A., Paradise, J. L., Rockette, H. E., Shaikh, N., Wald, E. R., Kearney, D. H., . . . Barbadora, K. A. (2011). Treatment of acute otitis media in children under 2 years of age. *New England Journal of Medicine, 364*, 105–115.

Hoffman, C., Pierrot, L., Contencin, P., Morisseau-Durand, M. P., Manach, Y., & Couloigner, V. (2011). Retropharyngeal infections in children: Treatment strategies and outcomes. *International Journal of Pediatric Otorhinolaryngology, 75*, 1099–1103.

Hou, C., Norcia, A. M., Madan, A., Tith, S., Agarwal, R., & Good, W. V. (2011). Visual cortical function in very low birth weight infants without retinal or cerebral pathology. *Investigative Ophthalmology and Visual Science, 25*, 9091–9098.

Hsiao, H. J., Huang, Y. C., Hsia, S. H., Wu, C. T., & Lin, J. J. (2012). Clinical features of peritonsillar abscess in children. *Pediatric Neonatology, 53*, 366–370.

International Committee for the Classification of Retinopathy of Prematurity. (2005). The international classification of retinopathy of prematurity revisited. *Archives of Ophthalmology, 123*, 991–999.

Joint Committee on Infant Hearing. (2007). Year 2007 position statement: Principles and guidelines for early hearing detection and intervention programs. *Pediatrics, 120*, 898–921.

Joint Committee on Infant Hearing. (2008). *Clarification for year 2007 JCIH position statement.* Retrieved from http://www.jcih.org/clarification%20year%20207%20statement.pdf

Kemper, A. R., Helfrich, A., Talbot, J., & Patel, N. (2012). Outcomes of an elementary school-based vision screening program in North Carolina. *Journal of School Nursing, 28*, 24–30.

Kliegman, R. M., Stanton, B., St. Geme, J., & Schor, N. (Eds.). (2016). *Nelson textbook of pediatrics* (20th ed.). Philadelphia, PA: Saunders.

Lieberthal, A. S., Carroll, A. E., Chonmaitree, T., Ganiats, T. G., Hoberman, A., Jackson, M. A., . . . Tunkel, D. E. (2013). The diagnosis and management of acute otitis media. *Pediatrics, 131*, e964–e999.

Liu, S., Pavan-Langston, D., & Colby, K. A. (2012). Pediatric herpes simplex of the anterior segment: Characteristics, treatment, and outcomes. *Ophthalmology, 119*, 2003–2008.

Melia, L., & McGarry, G. W. (2011). Epistaxis: Update on management. *Current Opinion in Otolaryngology & Head and Neck Surgery, 19*, 30–35.

Mitka, M. (2011). Guideline cites appropriateness criteria for performing tonsillectomy in children. *Journal of the American Medical Association, 305*, 661–662.

Montague, M. L., Whymark, A., Howatson, A., & Kubba, H. (2011). The pathology of visible blood vessels on the nasal septum in children with epistaxis. *International Journal of Otorhinolaryngology, 75*, 1032–1034.

National Association of School Nurses (NASN). (2012). *The use of volunteers in school health services.* Silver Spring, MD: Author.

National Eye Institute. (n.d.). *Sports-related eye injuries.* Retrieved from http://www.nidcd.nih.gov/health/hearing/coch.asp

National Eye Institute. (2014). *Facts about retinopathy of prematurity (ROP).* Retrieved from https://www.nei.nih.gov/health/rop/rop

National Institute of Deafness and Other Communication Disorders (NIDCD). (2014). *Quick statistics.* Retrieved from http://www.nidcd.nih.gov/health/statistics/Pages/quick.aspx

National Institutes of Health. (2013). *Retinopathy of prematurity.* Retrieved from http://www.nlm.nih.gov/medlineplus/ency/article/001618.htm

O'Brien, T. P. (2012). Comparative analysis of current antibiotics' potency, safety, and efficacy in treating bacterial conjunctivitis as well as potential impact on bacterial resistance. *Infectious Diseases in Children,* (Suppl), 9–14.

Ortiz, G. (2013, January). Va conjunctivitis. *Clinical Advisor,*

Qureishi, A., Lee, Y., Belfield, K., Birchall, M. (2014). Update on otitis media—Prevention treatment. *Infection and Drug Resistance, 7,* 15

Rudolph, C., Rudolph, A., Lister, G., First, L., & Gershon, A. (Eds.). (2011). *Rudolph's pediatrics* (22nd ed.). New York, NY: McGraw-Hill.

Rye, M. S., Blackwell, J. M., & Jamieson, S. E. (2012). Genetic susceptibility to otitis media in childhood. *Laryngoscope, 122*, 665–675.

Seltz, L. B., Smith, J., Durairaj, V. D., Enzenauer, R., & Todd, J. (2011). Microbiology and antibiotic management of orbital cellulitis. *Pediatrics, 127*, e566–e572.

Shaikh, N., & Wald, E. R. (2014). Decongestants, antihistamines and nasal irrigation for acute sinusitis in children. *Cochrane Database Systematic Review, 9,* CD007909.

Sharma, A., Congdon, N., Patel, M., & Gilbert, C. (2012). School-based approaches to the correction of refractive error in children. *Survey of Ophthalmology, 57,* 272–283.

Sides, M., & Sigmon, P. (2013). Innovative solutions for mandated vision screenings. *NASN School Nurse, 28,* 185–186.

Steele, R. W. (2012). Differentiating pediatric acute bacterial conjunctivitis from other etiologies. *Infectious Diseases in Children,* (Suppl), 3–8.

Trumler, A. A. (2011). Evaluation of pediatric cataracts and systemic disorders. *Current Opinion in Ophthalmology, 22,* 365–379.

Tschudy, M. M., & Arcara, K. M. (2012). *The Harriet Lane handbook* (19th ed.). St. Louis, MO: Elsevier Mosby.

U.S. Food and Drug Administration. (2011). *Public health advisory—FDA recommends that over-the-counter (OTC) cough and cold products not be used for infants and children under 2 years of age.* Retrieved from http://www.fda.gov/drugs/drugsafety

U.S. Food and Drug Administration. (2014). *OTC cough and cold products—Not for infants and children under 2 years of age.* Retrieved from http://www.fda.gov/ForConsumers/ConsumerUpdates/ucm048682.htm

U.S. Preventive Services Task Force. (2011). *Vision screening.* Retrieved from http://www.ahrq.gov/news/visioneng.htm

Wald, E. R., Applegate, K. E., Bordley, C., Darrow, D. H., Glode, M. P., Marcy, M., . . . Weinberg, S. T. (2013). Clinical practice guideline for the diagnosis and management of acute bacterial sinusitis in children ages 1 to 18 years. *Pediatrics, 132,* e262–e280.

Wang, J., Spencer, R., Leffler, J. N., & Birch, E. E. (2012). Characteristics of peripapillary retinal nerve fiber layer in preterm children. *American Journal of Ophthalmology, 153,* 850–855.

Williamson, I. (2011, January 12). Otitis media with effusion in children. *Clinical Evidence,* pii:0502.

Yeung, H. H., & Walton, D. S. (2012). Recognizing childhood glaucoma in the primary care setting. *Contemporary Pediatrics, 29*(5), 32–40.

Chapter 20
Alterations in Respiratory Function

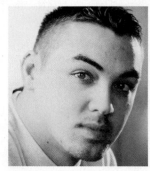

Emily gets sick so much faster than my other children. I guess the chronic lung disease and her tracheostomy make her more susceptible to infections. I really get concerned because she struggles so hard to breathe when she gets an infection. I have learned to suction and change her tracheostomy, but I'm afraid that one day her tracheostomy tube will get completely blocked. I just hope I remember all the things I've learned if that happens, and that the emergency medical personnel come quickly.

—Father of Emily, 8 months old

Ron Chapple/Getty Images

∨ Learning Outcomes

20.1 Describe unique characteristics of the pediatric respiratory system anatomy and physiology and apply that information to the care of children with respiratory conditions.

20.2 Contrast the different respiratory medical conditions that can cause respiratory distress in infants and children.

20.3 Explain the visual and auditory observations made to assess a child's respiratory effort or work of breathing.

20.4 Assess the child's respiratory status and analyze the need for oxygen supplementation.

20.5 Distinguish between conditions of the lower respiratory tract that cause illness in children.

20.6 Create a nursing care plan for a child with a common acute respiratory condition.

20.7 Develop a school-based nursing care plan for the child with asthma.

20.8 Develop a home nursing care plan for the child with cystic fibrosis.

20.9 Contrast the signs of different injuries to the respiratory system.

Respiratory conditions are the most common cause of hospitalization in children between 1 and 17 years of age when numbers for pneumonia and asthma are combined (Pfuntner, Wier, & Stocks, 2013). Some respiratory conditions are chronic and have a significant impact on the child's growth and development. However, most respiratory problems in children produce mild symptoms, last a short time, and can be managed at home.

Respiratory Distress and Respiratory Failure

Many respiratory conditions associated with breathing difficulty can progress to respiratory distress. If the condition is not managed effectively, it can progress to respiratory failure. Foreign-body aspiration is a common cause of airway obstruction and respiratory distress.

Text continues on page 478

FOCUS ON:
The Respiratory System

Anatomy and Physiology

The respiratory system is composed of both the upper and lower airways. The upper airway, containing the nasopharynx and oropharynx, serves as the pathway for gases exchanged during ventilation, the movement of oxygen into the lungs and carbon dioxide out of the lungs. The larynx divides the upper and lower airways. The lower airways (trachea, bronchi, and bronchioles) serve as the pathway of gases to and from the alveoli in the lungs. The left lung is divided into two lobes, and the right lung is divided into three lobes. Alveolar sacs surrounded by capillaries are located at the end of the airways and are the site of gas exchange, where oxygen diffuses across the alveolocapillary membrane. Surfactant secreted by alveolar cells coats the inner surface of the alveolus to allow expansion during inspiration. The lung tissue surrounding the airways keeps them from collapsing as the oxygen moves in and carbon dioxide moves out during ventilation. The lungs are positioned in the thoracic cavity, where the ribs and muscles protect the lungs from injury.

The intercostal muscles work with the diaphragm to perform the work of breathing. The diaphragm is a muscle that separates the abdominal and thoracic cavity contents. When the diaphragm contracts, it creates negative pressure that increases the thoracic volume and pulls air into the lungs. The lungs and chest wall have the ability to expand during inspiration (compliance) and then to recoil or return to the resting state with expiration. The work of breathing is tied to the muscular effort required for ventilation, which can be increased in cases of airway obstruction or disorders that increase the stiffness of the lungs.

The respiratory center in the brain controls respiration, sending impulses to the respiratory muscles to contract and relax. Breathing is usually automatic as the nervous system adjusts the ventilatory rate and volume to maintain normal gas exchange (Brashers, 2014). Chemoreceptors monitor the pH, $PaCO_2$, and PaO_2 in the arterial blood and send signals to the respiratory center to increase ventilation in cases of arterial hypoxemia. Effective gas exchange requires a near even distribution of ventilation and perfusion (oxygenated blood flow to all portions of the lungs). As oxygen diffuses across the alveolocapillary membrane, it dissolves in the plasma and the resulting increased partial pressure of oxygen (PaO_2) helps bind the oxygen to the hemoglobin molecules for transport to the cells for metabolism. Carbon dioxide produced by cellular metabolism is dissolved in the plasma (PCO_2) and/or as bicarbonate and travels back to the lungs where it diffuses across the alveolocapillary membrane (Brashers, 2014).

Pediatric Differences

The child's respiratory tract constantly grows and changes until about 12 years of age. The young child's neck is shorter than an adult's, resulting in airway structures that are closer together.

Upper Airway Differences

The child's airway is shorter and narrower than an adult's. These differences create a greater potential for obstruction (see *As Children Grow: Airway Development*). The infant's airway diameter is approximately 4 mm (0.16 in.), about the width of a drinking straw, in contrast to the adult's airway diameter of 20 mm (0.8 in.). The child's little finger is a good estimate for the child's tracheal diameter and can be used for a quick assessment of airway size. The trachea primarily increases in length rather than diameter during the first 5 years of life.

The tracheal division of the right and left bronchi is higher in a child's airway and at a different angle than the adult's (see *As Children Grow: Trachea Position*). The cartilage that supports the trachea is more flexible, and the airway may be compressed when the head and neck are flexed toward the chest. The child's narrower airway causes a greater increase in **airway resistance** (the effort or force needed to move oxygen through the trachea to the lungs) in any condition causing airway inflammation or edema (see *Pathophysiology Illustrated: Airway Diameter*).

Newborns are obligatory nose breathers. The only time newborns breathe through the mouth is when they are crying. The coordination of mouth breathing is controlled by maturing neurologic pathways, and infants up to 2 to 3 months of age do not automatically open the mouth to breathe when the nose is obstructed. It is important to keep the newborn's nose patent for breathing and eating.

Lower Airway Differences

The tracheobronchial tree is complete in the full-term newborn, but the child's lower airway is constantly growing. Beginning at 24 weeks' gestation, the lung sacs begin forming to support future gas exchange. The lung sacs begin differentiating into alveoli at 36 weeks' gestation (Rozance & Rosenberg, 2012). Alveoli continue developing and increasing in number for the first 5 to 8 years of age, followed by further development in size and complexity (Brashers & Huether, 2014). The bronchi and bronchioles are lined with smooth muscle that develops after birth.

Children under 6 years of age use the diaphragm to breathe because the intercostal muscles are immature. By 6 years of age the child uses the intercostal muscles more effectively. The ribs are primarily cartilage and very flexible. In cases of respiratory distress, the negative pressure caused by the diaphragm movement causes the chest wall to be drawn inward, causing **retractions** (see *Pathophysiology Illustrated: Retraction Sites*).

Children consume more oxygen than adults because of their higher metabolic rate. This rate of oxygen consumption increases when the child is in respiratory distress. The child also has fewer muscle glycogen reserves, leading to more rapid muscle fatigue when accessory muscles must be used for breathing (Brashers & Huether, 2014).

Use *Assessment Guide: The Child in Respiratory Distress* to perform a nursing assessment of the respiratory system. See Table 20–1 for a list of diagnostic and laboratory tests used to evaluate respiratory conditions. See Appendix D for expected laboratory values and Appendix E for information about diagnostic procedures.

As Children Grow: **Airway Development**

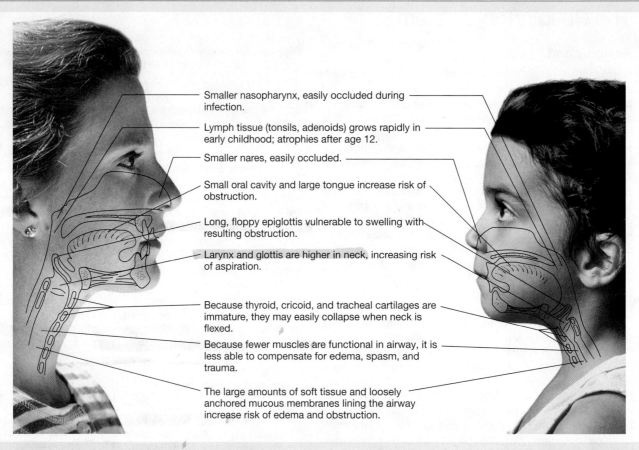

Smaller nasopharynx, easily occluded during infection.

Lymph tissue (tonsils, adenoids) grows rapidly in early childhood; atrophies after age 12.

Smaller nares, easily occluded.

Small oral cavity and large tongue increase risk of obstruction.

Long, floppy epiglottis vulnerable to swelling with resulting obstruction.

Larynx and glottis are higher in neck, increasing risk of aspiration.

Because thyroid, cricoid, and tracheal cartilages are immature, they may easily collapse when neck is flexed.

Because fewer muscles are functional in airway, it is less able to compensate for edema, spasm, and trauma.

The large amounts of soft tissue and loosely anchored mucous membranes lining the airway increase risk of edema and obstruction.

It is easy to see that a child's airway is smaller and less developed than an adult's airway, but why is this important? An upper respiratory tract infection, allergic reaction, positioning of the head and neck during sleep, and the small objects children play with can have serious consequences in the child.

As Children Grow: **Trachea Position**

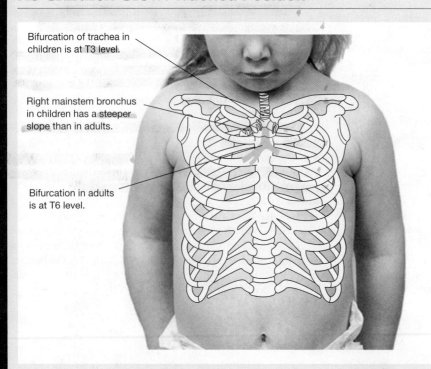

Bifurcation of trachea in children is at T3 level.

Right mainstem bronchus in children has a steeper slope than in adults.

Bifurcation in adults is at T6 level.

In children, the trachea is shorter and the angle of the right bronchus at bifurcation is more acute than in the adult. When you are resuscitating or suctioning, you must allow for these differences. Do you think that the angle of the right bronchus is significant in foreign-body aspiration? Why?

Pathophysiology Illustrated: **Airway Diameter**

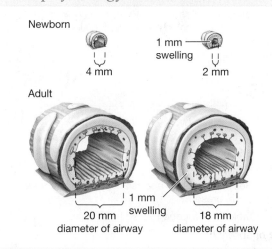

An infant's airway diameter is approximately 4 mm (0.16 in.), in contrast to the adult's 20–mm (0.8-in.) airway diameter. An inflammatory process in the airway causes swelling that narrows the airway, and airway resistance increases. Note that swelling of 1 mm (0.04 in.) reduces the infant's airway diameter to 2 mm (0.08 in.), but the adult's airway diameter is only narrowed to 18 mm (0.7 in.). Air must move more quickly in the infant's narrowed airway to get the needed amount of air into the lungs. The friction of the quickly moving air against the side of the airway increases airway resistance. The infant must use more effort to breathe and must breathe faster to get adequate oxygen.

Pathophysiology Illustrated: **Retraction Sites**

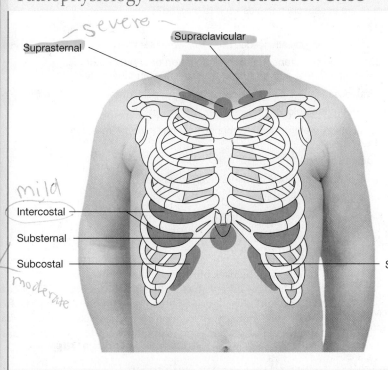

Infants and young children have immature chest muscles and ribs of cartilage, making the chest wall very flexible. The negative pressure created by the downward movement of the diaphragm is increased in cases of respiratory distress, and the chest wall is pulled inward, causing retractions. Intercostal retractions are seen in mild respiratory distress. As respiratory distress severity increases, substernal and subcostal retractions are seen. In cases of severe distress, supraclavicular and suprasternal retractions occur as the accessory muscles (sternocleidomastoid and trapezius muscles) are used.

TABLE 20–1 Diagnostic and Laboratory Procedures/Tests for the Respiratory System*

DIAGNOSTIC PROCEDURES	LABORATORY TESTS
Bronchoscopy	Arterial blood gas analysis
Chest radiograph	Cultures
Polysomnography (sleep study)	Neonatal screening for cystic fibrosis
Pulse oximetry	Protein-purified derivative (PPD), the Mantoux test
Spirometry (pulmonary function tests)	
Sweat chloride test	

* See Appendices D and E for information about these diagnostic procedures and tests.

Pediatric respiratory conditions may occur as a primary problem or as a complication of nonrespiratory conditions. Respiratory problems may result from structural problems, functional problems, or a combination of both. Structural problems involve alterations in the size and shape of parts of the respiratory tract. Functional problems involve alterations in gas exchange and threats to the process of ventilation due to irritation by large particles and chemicals or infection. Alterations in other organ systems, especially the immune and neurologic systems, may also threaten respiratory function. See Chapter 19 for upper respiratory conditions such as otitis media, sinusitis, and pharyngitis.

ASSESSMENT GUIDE | The Child in Respiratory Distress*

Assessment Focus	Assessment Guideline
Position of comfort	• Is the child comfortable lying down?
	• Does the child prefer to sit up or in the **tripod position** (sitting forward with arms on knees for support and extending the neck)?
Vital signs	• Assess the rate and depth of respirations. See Table 5–9 for age-related respiratory rates. Is **tachypnea** (abnormally rapid respiratory rate) present?
	• Assess the pulse for rate and rhythm. See Table 5–11 for age-related heart rates.
Lung auscultation	• Are breath sounds bilateral, diminished, or absent?
	• Are **adventitious sounds** (wheezes, crackles, or rhonchi) present?
Respiratory effort (work of breathing)	• Is **stridor** (audible crow-like inspiratory and expiratory breath sounds) or wheezing present? Is grunting heard on expiration?
	• Is breathing easy or labored?
	• Are retractions present or are accessory muscles used to breathe?
	• Is nasal flaring present?
	• Can the child say a full sentence or is a breath needed every few words? Is the cry strong or weak?
	• Do the chest and abdomen rise simultaneously with inspiration or is **paradoxical breathing** present in which the chest and abdomen do not rise simultaneously?
Color	• What is the color of the mucous membranes, nail beds, or skin (pink, pale, cyanotic, or mottled)?
	• Does crying improve or worsen the color?
Cough	• Is the cough dry (nonproductive), wet (productive, mucousy), brassy (noisy, musical), or croupy (barking, seal-like)?
	• Is the coughing effort forceful or weak?
Behavior change	• Is irritability, restlessness, or change in level of responsiveness present?

Refer to Chapter 5 for the assessment techniques mentioned in this table.

Foreign-Body Aspiration

Foreign-body aspiration is the inhalation of any object (solid or liquid, food or nonfood) into the respiratory tract. It is a major health threat for infants and young toddlers because of their increasing mobility and tendency to put objects into their mouths. Aspiration occurs most often during feeding and reaching activities, while crawling, or during playtime. However, aspiration may occur in children of any age. Approximately 100,000 cases occur each year, most often in children between 1 and 3 years old (Brashers & Huether, 2014). Some children die as a result of complete airway obstruction.

ETIOLOGY AND PATHOPHYSIOLOGY

In infants over 6 months of age and young children, any number of small objects that enter the child's mouth may cause aspiration. Foods such as nuts, popcorn, or small pieces of raw vegetables or hot dog and small objects such as toy parts, beads, safety pins, coins, buttons, or latex balloon pieces are frequent causes of airway obstruction. Partial and sometimes complete airway obstruction can occur.

The severity of the obstruction depends on the size and composition of the object or substance and its location within the respiratory tract. Most aspirated foreign bodies (AFBs) usually cause bronchial, not tracheal, obstruction. An object lodged high in the airway above the vocal cords is more easily removed by coughing or by back blows and chest thrusts.

The right lung is the most common site of the AFB because of the angle of its mainstem bronchus. Objects may migrate from higher to lower airway locations. An object may also move back up to the trachea, creating extreme respiratory difficulty. If the AFB is lodged in the trachea, it becomes life threatening.

CLINICAL MANIFESTATIONS

In many cases, the aspiration is unobserved. The child may have a sudden onset of choking, spasmodic coughing, shortness of breath, or **dysphonia** (muffled, hoarse, or absent voice sounds). These signs may be brief or may persist for several hours if the object drops below the trachea into a mainstem bronchus. Some children become asymptomatic after coughing for 15 to 30 minutes. The child may develop increased respiratory effort such as **dyspnea** (difficulty breathing), tachypnea, nasal flaring, and retractions. As respiratory distress progresses, the child may have a concentrated focus on breathing, an anxious expression, and an upright position with the neck extended. As **hypoxia** (lower than normal oxygen in the tissues) increases, behavior changes such as irritability and decreased responsiveness are seen.

If the AFB drops into the right bronchus and lower airway and is not removed, the child may present weeks later with a chronic cough, persistent or recurrent pneumonia, or a lung abscess.

CLINICAL THERAPY

Clinical therapy focuses on taking a careful history to determine whether aspiration could have occurred. Witnessed coughing, gagging, or choking associated with feeding or crawling on the floor may confirm the aspiration. Decreased breath sounds, stridor, and respiratory distress increase suspicion in the child without a witnessed aspiration. Many aspirated objects are organic, such as food, and cannot be seen on a radiograph. See Figure 20–1. A special radiograph, called a forced expiratory film, may show local hyperinflation (air trapping) and a mediastinal shift away from the affected side, abnormalities that an AFB may cause.

An object lodged in the trachea is life threatening. Back blows and chest thrusts or abdominal thrusts are used to remove an object from an obstructed airway. (See the *Clinical Skills Manual* SKILLS .) Fluoroscopy and fiberoptic bronchoscopy may be used to identify, locate, and extract the AFB. The child may develop pneumonia if an AFB is not recognized as a cause of respiratory distress. See the section on pneumonia later in the chapter.

Nursing Management

For the Child With Foreign-Body Aspiration

Nursing Assessment and Diagnosis

PHYSIOLOGIC ASSESSMENT

Perform the respiratory assessment following the guidelines given in *Assessment Guide: The Child in Respiratory Distress*. The child with an acute AFB will be in respiratory distress and must be constantly monitored. If the object remains lodged, observe the child for signs of increasing respiratory distress, especially vital signs, altered mental status, and audible wheezing on auscultation. Note changes in breath sounds, from noisy to decreasing to absent, on the affected side. This can indicate that the object is moving and blocking a mainstem bronchus. Document any subtle changes in the child's respiratory status and report promptly.

Attach the child to a cardiorespiratory monitor and pulse oximeter (a transcutaneous assessment method to detect the amount of hemoglobin saturated with oxygen [SpO_2]) to assess the child for subtle signs of increasing hypoxia. A pulse oximetry reading (SpO_2) of less than 95% indicates **hypoxemia** (lower than normal oxygen level in the blood).

PSYCHOSOCIAL ASSESSMENT

The unexpected and acute nature of the event creates anxiety for both parents and child. The child will be fearful because of difficulty breathing. Assess the family's level of distress and coping ability.

DEVELOPMENTAL ASSESSMENT

As the child's condition stabilizes, observe how well the child's abilities match the parents' understanding of age-appropriate behaviors. See Chapter 4.

Common nursing diagnoses for a child with an AFB include the following (NANDA-I © 2014):

- *Airway Clearance, Ineffective,* related to obstruction by a foreign body
- *Ventilation: Spontaneous, Impaired,* related to respiratory muscle fatigue
- *Anxiety (Child)* related to difficulty breathing, unfamiliar surroundings, and procedures
- *Injury, Risk for,* related to small objects in environment

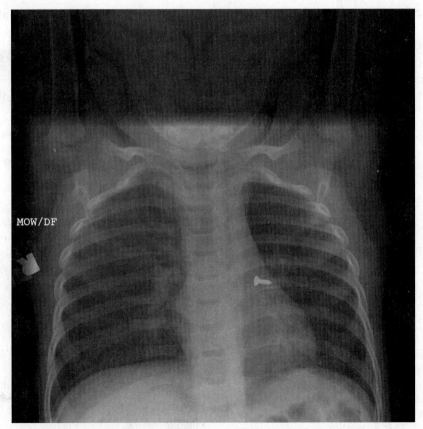

Figure 20–1 An aspirated screw is clearly visible in the child's left mainstem bronchus on this chest radiograph.

SOURCE: Courtesy of Evelyn Anthony, MD, Department of Radiology, Brenner Children's Hospital, Wake Forest University Health System.

Planning and Implementation

Be prepared to perform back blows and chest thrusts for an infant or abdominal thrusts for the child with complete obstruction. (See the *Clinical Skills Manual* SKILLS .) When the child has a partial obstruction, remain with the child and have resuscitation equipment at the bedside. Permit the child to stay in a position of comfort. Avoid performing procedures that increase the child's anxiety because sudden movements and increased respiratory efforts may cause the obstruction to move and completely obstruct the airway.

After the AFB is removed, the child is stabilized and observed for a few hours in a short-stay unit to ensure that there are no respiratory complications.

Clinical Tip

Accuracy of pulse oximetry readings (SpO$_2$) can be improved by doing the following:

- Place the sensor over clean dry skin (e.g., finger, foot, ear lobe). Select a site or extremity that will not be moved extensively and where perfusion is adequate. Make the sensor secure to prevent movement of the sensor.
- Position the sensor for a reading at the level of the heart.
- Avoid placing the sensor probe over sites covered with dark nail polish or false nails.
- Cover the sensor with a light barrier when the child is in intense internal or external light to reduce interference.
- Confirm that the child's heart rate matches that detected by the pulse oximeter.
- Shivering, vasoconstriction, poor capillary refill, hypothermia, intravenous dyes, and electromagnetic interference may result in a false low reading (Fouzas, Priftis, & Anthracopoulos, 2011). Anemia may result in a false high reading.

DISCHARGE PLANNING AND HOME CARE TEACHING

Prevention of future aspirations is a major focus for nursing care. Educate the family on the child's developmental characteristics and how to identify potential safety hazards in the home. Food should be cut in small pieces. Check toys for small or broken parts and remove from young children. Store small objects (e.g., batteries, screws, buttons, earrings, and coins) out of a child's reach. Encourage the parents to learn rescue breathing, back blows, chest thrusts, or abdominal thrusts.

Evaluation

Expected outcomes of nursing care include the following:

- The child breathes spontaneously after removal of the foreign body.
- Parents complete a home safety check to prevent future aspiration incidents.

Respiratory Failure

Respiratory failure occurs when the body can no longer maintain effective gas exchange. Poor ventilation of the alveoli initiates the process that leads to respiratory failure. Hypoventilation occurs when oxygen need exceeds oxygen intake, the airway is partially occluded, or the exchange of oxygen and carbon dioxide in the alveoli is disrupted. This disruption may occur when a malfunction of respiratory center stimulation occurs (the alveoli do not receive the message to diffuse, e.g., a narcotic overdose), muscles of ventilation are fatigued and do not work effectively (e.g., status asthmaticus), or the relationship between ventilation and blood flow to the alveoli (perfusion) is impaired. Hypoxemia and **hypercapnia** (an excess of carbon dioxide in the blood) result from hypoventilation. When the blood levels of oxygen and carbon dioxide reach abnormal levels, hypoxia occurs and respiratory failure begins.

Signs of impending respiratory failure include worsening respiratory distress with increased respiratory effort (dyspnea, tachypnea, nasal flaring, and intercostal retractions), irritability, lethargy, and cyanosis. Grunting in infants is a sign of severe disease and the potential need for mechanical ventilation (Prodhan, Sharoor-Karni, Lin, et al., 2011). *Hypoxemia that persists when supplemental oxygen is given is a sign of respiratory failure.* See Table 20–2.

CLINICAL THERAPY

Arterial blood gas values help identify hypoxemia and hypercapnia. Pulse oximetry helps determine when an arterial blood gas measurement is needed. When pulse oximetry (SpO$_2$) readings are between 76% and 90%, an arterial blood gas should be obtained as the SpO$_2$ reading may be falsely high (Ross, Newth, & Khemani, 2014). See Appendix D for expected arterial blood gas values and the *Clinical Skills Manual* SKILLS . Refer to Chapter 18 for interpretation of acidosis and alkalosis that must be considered simultaneously.

Medical management is focused on treating the cause of respiratory failure and reversing the severe hypoxemia with oxygen, mechanical ventilation, and positive end-expiratory pressure (PEEP) to increase functional residual capacity. These children are admitted to the pediatric intensive care unit (PICU).

TABLE 20–2 Clinical Manifestations of Respiratory Failure and Imminent Respiratory Arrest

PHYSIOLOGIC CAUSE	CLINICAL MANIFESTATIONS
INITIAL SIGNS OF RESPIRATORY FAILURE	
The child is trying to compensate for oxygen deficit and airway blockage. Oxygen supply is inadequate; behavior and vital signs reflect compensation and beginning hypoxia.	Restlessness Tachypnea Tachycardia Diaphoresis
EARLY DECOMPENSATION	
The child tries to use accessory muscles to assist oxygen intake; hypoxia persists and efforts now waste more oxygen than is obtained.	Nasal flaring Retractions Grunting Wheezing Anxiety, irritability Mood changes Headache Hypertension Confusion
SEVERE HYPOXIA AND IMMINENT RESPIRATORY ARREST	
The oxygen deficit is overwhelming and beyond spontaneous recovery. Cerebral oxygenation is dramatically affected; central nervous system changes are ominous.	Dyspnea Bradycardia Cyanosis Stupor and coma

The child's ability to maintain an open airway decreases as the level of responsiveness declines. Endotracheal (ET) intubation is a short-term, emergency measure to stabilize the airway by placing a tube in the trachea. The ET tube must be protected and stabilized to prevent its displacement. End-tidal CO_2 monitoring is used to ensure that the tube is correctly positioned in the trachea (see the *Clinical Skills Manual* SKILLS). A **tracheostomy**, the creation of a surgical opening into the trachea through the anterior neck at the cricoid cartilage, is performed when long-term airway management is needed.

Assisted ventilation may be needed until mechanical ventilation is provided or the child breathes spontaneously. Children are often sedated to improve ventilation. Continuous positive airway pressure is one therapy used to improve oxygenation and lung compliance. Respiratory arrest results if respiratory failure cannot be managed.

Nursing Management

Early recognition of impending respiratory failure is the most important aspect of care for a child with any signs of respiratory compromise. Assess the child using guidelines found earlier in this chapter in the *Assessment Guide*. Monitor the child for changes in vital signs, respiratory status, SpO_2, and level of responsiveness. When the child has a chronic respiratory condition, development of respiratory failure may be gradual and signs will be subtle. Be particularly alert to behavior changes in addition to respiratory signs. Serial blood gases may be needed to monitor the child.

SAFETY ALERT!
As the child tires from the prolonged effort of breathing, the respiratory rate may begin to decrease. This is an ominous sign and may progress to respiratory arrest without intervention.

Place a child who has respiratory compromise in an upright position (elevate the head of the bed). Respiratory distress, anxiety, excessive crying, and even fever can deplete metabolic reserves and increase the child's need for oxygen. Administer oxygen as ordered and keep emergency equipment at the child's bedside. Be prepared to provide assisted ventilation if the respiratory status deteriorates. (See the *Clinical Skills Manual* SKILLS .)

> **Clinical Reasoning** Oxygen Delivery Devices
> Oxygen delivery devices are selected to match the concentration of oxygen needed by the child. In respiratory failure, a higher concentration of oxygen is needed to reverse the hypoxemia. Which oxygen delivery device should be used? Are there any contraindications to oxygen use in a child who is hypoxic?

The child with an endotracheal or tracheostomy tube cannot talk or cry because vocal cord vibration is obstructed. Infants and young children often express initial frustration when they realize they cannot communicate verbally. When the child is alert, provide a bell or noisemaker as a way to gain attention. A communication board can be used with older children. Suction airway secretions as needed and provide tracheostomy care if present. (See the *Clinical Skills Manual* SKILLS .)

Many children are discharged from the hospital and cared for at home for an extended period with a tracheostomy tube in place. Parents must demonstrate competence in all aspects of tracheostomy care (how to maintain and suction the airway, clean the tracheostomy site, and change the tube), as well as emergency resuscitation skills adapted to the tracheostomy. A home healthcare nurse can provide follow-up care and support for the child and family. (See the *Clinical Skills Manual* SKILLS .)

Apnea

Infants commonly have **periodic breathing**, an irregular rhythm, and may have pauses of up to 20 seconds between breaths. This breathing pattern is not apnea. **Apnea** is the cessation of respiration lasting longer than 20 seconds, or any pause in respiration associated with cyanosis, marked pallor, hypotonia, or bradycardia. Apnea may be the first major sign of respiratory dysfunction in the newborn.

Apparent Life-Threatening Event (ALTE)

Apparent life-threatening event (ALTE) is defined as a frightening episode of apnea accompanied by a color change (e.g., cyanosis or pallor), limp muscle tone, choking, or gagging. Most affected infants are younger than 6 months of age (Chu & Hageman, 2013).

Potential causes of ALTE include gastroesophageal reflux, seizures, and lower respiratory disorders. Other causes may include ear, nose, and throat abnormalities; trauma; metabolic disorder; cardiac arrhythmias; sepsis; pertussis; and child abuse. ALTE and sudden infant death syndrome (SIDS) have different clinical and epidemiologic factors; however, some infants with ALTE are at increased risk for mortality (Chu & Hageman, 2013).

A detailed history helps identify the potential condition associated with ALTE. Diagnostic tests may include an electrocardiogram, complete blood count with differential, serum electrolytes, swallowing studies, gastrointestinal imaging, cultures, serum ammonia levels, and a chest radiograph. A medical cause is found for about 50% of ALTE cases (Chu & Hageman, 2013). Physical stimulation or emergency resuscitation may be required to revive the infant. Treatment is targeted at the underlying condition.

Nursing Management

After ALTE, many infants are admitted to the hospital for evaluation and cardiorespiratory monitoring. Assess the infant's responsiveness and behavior (e.g., irritability or unexplained sleepiness). Monitor vital signs, and assess the child's growth. The focus of the physical examination is to detect signs of injury, infection, neurologic abnormalities, or features suggestive of a genetic or metabolic syndrome.

Attach a cardiorespiratory monitor and pulse oximeter to continuously assess the heart rate, respiratory rate, and oxygenation status while the infant is awake and asleep. Because the infant who has had ALTE may be at risk for cardiopulmonary arrest, keep emergency resuscitation equipment and drugs readily accessible at all times.

Provide emotional support. Establishing rapport and open communication with the parents is essential for creating a sense of trust. To obtain further information about the episode, use open-ended questions and active listening skills. Parents are fearful and anxious about the infant's prognosis. Explanations of tests and treatment help to decrease their anxiety and increase their understanding of the situation.

Encouraging parents' participation in the infant's care helps to promote the infant's sense of security, and it promotes family bonding. Teach parents how to hold the infant without disconnecting the monitoring cables. Wrapping the cable inside the infant's blanket helps secure the wires, increasing parents' feelings of confidence in handling the infant.

Support the mother to continue breastfeeding and maintaining a supply of breast milk by pumping, if necessary. Ensure that the mother gets adequate fluids and nutrition. Provide privacy for breast pumping, and store breast milk for future feedings.

DISCHARGE PLANNING AND HOME CARE TEACHING

Address home care needs in advance of the infant's discharge. Review guidelines for safe sleep positions. Some infants may be discharged with a cardiorespiratory monitor. Teach parents how to operate the monitor, what to do when the infant has an apnea episode, and how to perform cardiopulmonary resuscitation (CPR) and choking-intervention techniques (see the *Clinical Skills Manual* SKILLS). See *Families Want to Know: Home Care Instructions for the Infant Requiring a Cardiorespiratory Monitor.*

Obstructive Sleep Apnea

Obstructive sleep apnea syndrome (OSAS) is a disorder of breathing during sleep that involves increased respiratory resistance leading to recurrent episodes of partial and complete upper airway obstruction that disrupt normal ventilation during sleep and sleep patterns (Marcus et al., 2012). This results in labored breathing and snoring when the child tries to move air past the obstruction. OSAS is believed to affect 1% to 5% of school-age children (Marcus et al., 2012).

The upper airway contains about 30 muscles that permit the pharynx to collapse, enabling the child to talk and swallow, but also maintain airway patency. When the child is awake, muscle tone is maintained and the airway remains patent even when potential obstructions are present. During sleep, the airway muscles relax, the pharynx becomes obstructed, and airway resistance increases, leading to snoring. Reduced upper airway tone and obstruction cause apnea episodes that lead to hypoxemia, hypercapnia, and an elevated blood pressure. Hypertrophy of the adenoids and tonsils is the most common

---

Families Want to Know

Home Care Instructions for the Infant Requiring a Cardiorespiratory Monitor

Apnea Equipment

- Review how the monitor operates, the lead wires, placement of skin electrodes and pulse oximetry sensor, and how to set the event recorder. Keep the battery fully charged, and keep the manual for troubleshooting handy.

Emergency Preparation

- Have an emergency plan and complete an emergency information form about the infant's health problem. Notify the telephone company, electric company, local ambulance service, and the local emergency department (to get priority service status).
- Post the emergency response phone numbers by all phones and save in cell phones, along with the phone numbers for the healthcare provider, medical equipment company, power company, neighbor, and key family members.
- Take a cardiopulmonary resuscitation (CPR) course.

Safety Precautions

- Place monitor on firm surface; keep away from other appliances (television, microwave oven) and water.
- Ensure that alarms are audible from all locations.
- Double-check that the monitor and event recorder are on before putting the infant down for a nap or at bedtime.
- Thread cable and wires through lower end of infant's clothes.
- Ensure integrity of leads, monitor cable, and power cord (replace if frayed).

Routine Care

- Explain the reasons for the apnea monitor and frequency of use. Use it whenever the infant sleeps. Review the manual for troubleshooting.
- Show how to attach and detach infant chest leads and belt. Evaluate the skin for irritation or sores under the electrodes, and move the electrode if skin is irritated. Use no oils or lotions on the chest.

Responding to an Alarm

- Observe the infant for breathing first to determine if this is a real event or a loose lead.
- Stimulate the infant if respirations are absent or infant is lethargic. Start by calling the infant's name and gently touching, proceeding to vigorous touch if needed.
- If no response, proceed with CPR and call 9-1-1.
- If a loose lead is suspected, determine if electrode patches are loose. Check the wires from the electrode or monitor cable. Check the power supply. Is the monitor malfunctioning?

cause of OSAS, followed by craniofacial abnormalities, obesity, and neuromuscular disorders (e.g., cerebral palsy, muscular dystrophy).

Children with OSAS snore and have labored breathing during sleep such as retractions and paradoxical breathing. After snoring or breathing pauses, the child may snort, gasp, choke, move, or arouse to take a breath. Sleep is restless and the child may sleep in unusual positions to hyperextend the neck and airway. Symptoms of sleep deprivation (daytime sleepiness, poor attention, aggression, acting-out behavior, and poor school performance) may be noted. The child may also have enuresis, a morning headache, obesity, hypertension, failure to thrive, and cardiac dysfunction.

Healthy People 2020

(SH-1) Increase the proportion of persons with symptoms of obstructive sleep apnea who seek medical evaluation

---

Initial diagnosis occurs with a detailed history about snoring. **Polysomnography**, a sleep study that simultaneously records the sleep state, gas exchange, breathing efforts, cardiac rhythm, and muscle activity and movement, is performed. Adenotonsillectomy (adenoidectomy and tonsillectomy) is the most common treatment for OSAS, and the condition resolves in the majority of children. Children are evaluated 6 to 8 weeks after adenotonsillectomy to determine if some degree of OSAS persists that needs other treatment. Continuous positive airway pressure (CPAP) is used for children with surgical contraindications or those with persistent OSAS (craniofacial anomalies or neuromuscular disorders) after adenotonsillectomy. Weight loss strategies may be implemented for children with obesity. Some children with mild OSAS may be treated with nasal steroids. Without treatment, complications can include failure to thrive, pulmonary hypertension, **cor pulmonale** (obstruction of pulmonary blood flow that leads to right ventricular hypertrophy and heart failure), systemic hypertension, and cognitive impairment.

Nursing Management

In the community setting, all children should be screened for snoring as part of their routine health care. Assess the child for signs of nasal obstruction, mouth breathing, and enlarged tonsils. Determine if the child has symptoms of sleep deprivation or if a condition is present that places the child at high risk for OSAS. When snoring is present, encourage the family to keep a sleep diary.

When a polysomnogram is ordered, talk with the parents about how to prepare the child for the strange setting and wires that will be attached during the sleep study. Most pediatric centers will allow the parent to stay with the child during the study.

Following adenotonsillectomy, the child with OSAS is commonly hospitalized overnight because respiratory complications may occur. The hospital nurse monitors the child for bleeding and respiratory distress, such as obstructive sleep apnea and pulmonary edema. Continuous pulse oximetry is used to detect oxygen desaturation. See Chapter 19 for care of the child having adenoidectomy and tonsillectomy.

Sleep center nurses provide education and support to families of children who need to use CPAP to treat OSAS. The nurse helps identify the best fitting mask or nasal prong system for CPAP delivery. Parents may need guidance about helping children go to sleep wearing the mask until they are accustomed to it.

Sudden Infant Death Syndrome

Sudden and unexpected infant death (SUID) is a leading cause of infant mortality. Sudden infant death syndrome (SIDS), a subset of SUID, is defined as the sudden death during sleep of an infant under 1 year of age that remains unexplained after a thorough investigation, including an autopsy, a review of the circumstances of death, and the clinical history. Some unexpected infant deaths may be classified as accidental suffocation or positional asphyxia (e.g., face against bedding or rolled from side to abdomen) depending on the circumstances. SIDS is the third leading cause of infant mortality in the United States (Heron, 2013). Most SIDS deaths occur in infants between 2 and 4 months of age, and it accounts for 50% of SUID cases (Matthews & Moore, 2013). SIDs is currently unpredictable and, in some cases, unpreventable.

SIDS is called a "syndrome" because infants are believed to have a vulnerability that increases their risk for sudden death during the first 6 months of life, a critical period of developing homeostatic control. An environmental stressor (e.g. secondhand smoke, overheating, soft bedding, prone or side-lying position) compounds the vulnerability. Abnormalities associated with the neurotransmitter serotonin in the medulla oblongata may interfere with arousal responses during sleep in a critical development period (Matthews & Moore, 2013). See Table 20–3 for factors that place infants at risk for sudden infant death.

Typically, parents find the infant unresponsive in the crib in the morning or after a nap. They usually report hearing no cries or disturbances during the night. Clinical findings include evidence of a struggle or change in position during sleep and the presence of frothy, blood-tinged secretions from the mouth and nose.

TABLE 20–3 Risk Factors for Sudden Infant Death

INFANT RISK FACTORS

- Preterm or low birth weight, small for gestational age, multiple birth
- Native American and African American infants are at higher risk; Whites, Asians, and Hispanics are at lower risk
- Males are at higher risk
- Maternal smoking, alcohol use disorder, or substance abuse
- Socioeconomic disadvantages

ENVIRONMENTAL RISK FACTORS

- Sleeping prone or side-lying position
- Bed sharing—higher risk in infants 0–3 months old
- Soft bedding, pillows, blankets, and stuffed animals that infants roll into—higher risk in infants over 3 months old
- Overheating
- Secondhand tobacco smoke exposure

Source: Data from Gelfer, P., & Tatum, M. (2014). Sudden infant death syndrome. *Journal of Pediatric Health Care, 28*(5), 470–474; Colvin, J. D., Collie-Akers, V., Schunn, C., & Moon, R. Y. (2014). Sleep environment risks for younger and older infants. *Pediatrics, 134*(2), e406–e412; Van Nguyen, J. M., & Abenhaim, H. A. (2013). Sudden infant death syndrome: Review for the obstetric care provider. *American Journal of Perinatology, 30*(09), 703–714.

Nursing Management

The sudden, unexpected nature of the infant's death is often confirmed in the emergency department. The nurse's role is to be empathetic and provide support during one of the greatest crises a family must face. The focus is on supporting the family during the communication of bad news and the shock of the infant's death. See Chapter 13.

Reassure the parents that they are not responsible for the infant's death and help them contact other family members and mobilize support. Older children may need reassurance that SIDS will not happen to them. They may also believe that bad thoughts or wishes about their baby brother or sister caused the death. Support groups can help parents, siblings, and other family members express these fears and work through their feelings about the infant's death. The First Candle organization can help families locate a support group in their area.

Nurses play an important role in SUID and SIDS prevention. Educate the parents of all newborns and infants about the recommended infant sleep position—on the back on a firm surface. The Safe to Sleep Campaign, encouraging the placement of infants in the supine position for sleeping, was initiated in 1992 and has led to a 50% decrease in SIDS deaths (Flook & Vincze, 2012). However, no further reduction in deaths due to SUID or SIDS has been noted for the last decade. Ask parents to make sure the infant is placed to sleep on the back when cared for by another family member or childcare provider. Parents should also use a firm mattress and avoid the use of loose bedding, toys, and pillows. A sleeper suit rather than a blanket should be used to keep the infant warm while sleeping. See *Evidence-Based Practice: Infant Sleep Environment and Positioning*. A pacifier is also recommended for nap and bedtime (Task Force on Sudden Infant Death Syndrome, 2011). See Chapter 27 for issues related to infant skull flattening from sleeping on the back.

EVIDENCE-BASED PRACTICE | Infant Sleep Environment and Positioning

Clinical Question

In 2010, 13.5% of all infants were reported to be placed to sleep in the prone position (Matthews & Moore, 2013). An unknown number of infants are placed to sleep in a manner that increases their risk of suffocation. What strategies might help increase safe sleep environments and positioning for young infants?

The Evidence

A study used focus groups and interviews with 83 African American mothers from diverse socioeconomic groups to learn about surfaces and soft bedding used for their infants. Findings revealed that parents had different interpretations of firm bedding, and they believed that soft bedding (pillows, blankets, and crib bumper pads) increased the infant's comfort and, in some cases, safety. For example, parents believed that the surface was firm if a pillow or blanket was placed between the mattress and the sheet and the sheet was tucked tautly around the pillow or blanket. Misconceptions about firm and soft bedding increase the risk for suffocation and SIDS as the infant sleeps (Ajao, Oden, Joyner, et al., 2011).

A bed audit in a large neonatal intensive care unit (NICU) identified that only 39% of infants were sleeping in supine position, and 45% had no soft objects in their bed. A telephone survey to parents of infants discharged from the NICU identified only 23% of infants had safe sleep practices that met all criteria. A quality improvement initiative led to nursing guidelines and nursing education on safe sleep practices. An algorithm was developed to assess when an infant could be transitioned to supine sleep position. Cue cards were placed in an infant's crib when the infant met criteria to begin supine sleep positioning. The card reminded nurses to use and to begin educating parents about safe sleep practices. Parent education about safe sleep practices included a DVD and written discharge guidelines. A crib audit revealed an increase in supine sleep position use in eligible infants from 39% before interventions to 83% 3 months after the intervention. Rates also increased for firm bedding surface and no soft items in the bed. A follow-up survey of parents after

discharge also reflected a significant increase in safe sleep practices (23% before interventions and 82% after the intervention) (Gelfer, Cameron, Masters, et al., 2013).

A study investigated factors in the sleep environment by age of infants who died of SIDS or SUID. Data collected by state child death review teams for infants less than 12 months of age who died during sleep or in the sleep environment were analyzed for the following factors: infant and caregiver characteristics, object (e.g., clothing, blanket, bumper pads, stuffed toys) in the sleep environment, and sleep place and position. Bedsharing was associated with 69.2% of study infant deaths, and the rate was significantly higher in infants less than 3 months of age (73.8%) than in older infants (58.9%). Deaths in younger infants were less likely to be associated with an object in the sleep environment or a change in sleep position for supine or side-lying to prone. Older infants were more likely to die in the prone position and to have objects in the sleep environment (Colvin, Collie-Akers, Schunn, et al., 2014).

Best Practice

While the Safe to Sleep Campaign has successfully promoted supine sleep positions for infants, additional sleep environment factors can increase the risk for an infant's death during sleep. Parent education needs to focus on more than just supine positioning. Modeling the safe sleep environment and position for parents when infants are hospitalized is an effective message. As infants develop an ability to roll over and move in the bed, parents should be reminded to keep objects out of the bed, especially soft objects that can suffocate when the infant rolls from supine to prone. Nurses also need to understand a parent's perspective on issues such as bedding and bedsharing so that education can appropriately address beliefs and concerns.

Clinical Reasoning

Identify if policies exist for infant sleep position in the maternity and pediatric sections of your hospital. Conduct an audit of cribs and bassinets to determine what proportions of infants are sleeping in the supine position and if any objects are in the bed.

Croup Syndromes

Croup is a term applied to a broad classification of upper airway illnesses that result from inflammation and swelling of the epiglottis and larynx. The swelling usually extends into the trachea and bronchi. Viral croup syndromes include acute spasmodic laryngitis (spasmodic croup) and laryngotracheobronchitis (LTB). Bacterial croup syndromes include bacterial tracheitis and epiglottitis (see *Pathophysiology Illustrated: Airway Changes With Croup*).

Acute spasmodic laryngitis, LTB, and bacterial tracheitis affect a large number of children across all age groups in both genders. Epiglottitis, previously a common serious respiratory illness, is rare in the United States because of the *Haemophilus influenzae* type B vaccine. The initial symptoms of all four conditions include inspiratory stridor (a high-pitched, musical sound that is created by narrowing of the airway), a "seal-like" barking cough, and hoarseness. Acute spasmodic croup and LTB are the most common disorders, but epiglottitis and bacterial tracheitis are more serious. See Table 20–4 for information on the etiology, clinical manifestations, and clinical therapy for these disorders.

Developing Cultural Competence Safe Sleep for Infants

While African American infants are at higher risk for SIDS, many of these families do not follow guidelines for safe sleep practices, even when stating they have heard about recommendations to avoid bed sharing and to use supine sleep positioning for the infant. Reasons parents gave for not following medical advice included perceived safety (less risk of aspiration), convenience (do not have to walk to the crib), and better infant sleep quality when prone. Cultural and familial influences were a factor in not following medical advice (Gaydos et al., 2015). Nurses, when counseling about safe sleep, should more thoroughly explain the rationale for the safe sleep recommendations and address cultural and familial beliefs.

Clinical Tip

A review of several studies evaluated the relationship between breastfeeding and SIDS. Findings revealed that breastfeeding for any period of time is protective, and greater protection occurs if breastfeeding is exclusive (Hauck, Thompson, Tenabe, et al., 2011). Place hospitalized infants to sleep in supine position rather than side-lying or prone.

SAFETY ALERT!

Throat cultures and visual inspection of the inner mouth and throat are contraindicated in children with LTB and epiglottitis. These procedures can cause **laryngospasms** (spasmodic vibrations that close the larynx) as a result of the child's anxiety or of probing this reactive and already compromised area. A complete airway obstruction may result.

Pathophysiology Illustrated: **Airway Changes With Croup**

Upper airway tissues respond to the invading virus with inflammation and edema. The epiglottis swells, occluding the airway, and the trachea swells against the cricoid cartilage, narrowing the airway. Copious secretions increase the respiratory distress and can obstruct the airway.

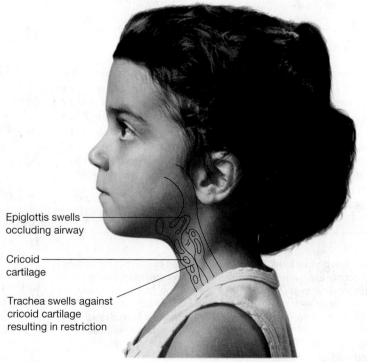

Epiglottis swells occluding airway

Cricoid cartilage

Trachea swells against cricoid cartilage resulting in restriction

TABLE 20–4 Summary of Croup Syndromes

| | VIRAL SYNDROMES | | BACTERIAL SYNDROMES | |
	ACUTE SPASMODIC LARYNGITIS (SPASMODIC CROUP)	LARYNGOTRACHEITIS/ LARYNGOTRACHEO- BRONCHITIS (LTB)	BACTERIAL TRACHEITIS	EPIGLOTTITIS (SUPRAGLOTTITIS)
Etiology	Recurrent; suspect allergies with sensitivity to viruses that cause LTB; also associated with gastroesophageal reflux	Parainfluenza, types I, II and III, RSV, influenza, enteroviruses, adenoviruses, or *Mycoplasma pneumoniae*	*Staphylococcus*, *Moraxella catarrhalis*, and nontypeable *H. influenzae*; may follow viral LTB as a secondary infection	*Haemophilus influenzae*, Group A beta-hemolytic streptococcus, staphylococcus
Severity	Least serious	Serious; progresses if untreated	Can be life threatening; requires close observation	Most life threatening (medical emergency)*
Age affected	3 months to 8 years	3 months to 3 years	1 month to 13 years*	2 years to 8 years
Onset	Abrupt nighttime onset; resolves over 24 to 48 hours; recurs*	Gradual onset as a URI, progressing to respiratory distress and potential airway obstruction over 24 to 48 hr	Progressive over 2 to 5 days, may present like LTB initially but condition worsens after LTB treatment	Progresses rapidly (hours)*; may progress to complete airway obstruction
Clinical manifestations	Afebrile; mild respiratory distress; barking-seal cough; signs of respiratory infection are not present*	*Early:* mild fever (less than 40.0°C [102.2°F]); barking-seal, brassy, croupy cough; rhinorrhea; sore throat; stridor (inspiratory); apprehension; restless or irritable May progress to retractions; increasing stridor; cyanosis	High fever (higher than 39.0°C [102.2°F]); URI appears as viral croupy cough and croup initially; stridor (tracheal); purulent secretions; child often prefers to lie flat; toxic appearance; dysphagia and drooling area rarely present	High fever (higher than 39.0°C [102.2°F]); URI; intense sore throat; dysphagia*; drooling*; increased pulse and respiratory rate; prefers upright position (tripod position with neck extended)*; cherry red epiglottis; barking cough is absent*
Clinical therapy	Oral dexamethasone; treatment for gastroesophageal reflux may reduce recurrences; other airway disorders may need to be considered such as aspirated foreign body	Oral dexamethasone; nebulized epinephrine for severe symptoms; supplemental oxygen if hypoxic; monitor for airway obstruction	May have initial treatment for LTB but condition worsens; blood cultures, endotracheal intubation to protect the airway, and intravenous antibiotics	Immediate endotracheal intubation to protect the airway, supplemental oxygen, blood cultures, culture of epiglottis, intravenous antibiotics for gram-positive organisms that are changed as needed to match culture sensitivities

* Classic signs that distinguish the condition.

Source: Data from Roosevelt, G. E. (2016). Acute inflammatory upper airway obstruction (croup, epiglottitis, laryngitis, and bacterial tracheitis). In R. M. Kliegman, B. F. Stanton, J. W. St. Geme, & N. F. Schor (Eds.), *Nelson textbook of pediatrics* (20th ed., pp. 2031–2036). Philadelphia, PA: Elsevier; Sharma, G. D., & Conrad, C. (2011). Croup, epiglottitis, and bacterial tracheitis. In American Academy of Pediatrics Section on Pediatric Pulmonology, *Pediatric pulmonology* (pp. 347–363). Elk Grove Village, IL: Author; Zoorob, R., Sidani, M., & Murray, J. (2011). Croup: An overview. *American Family Physician*, 83(9), 1067–1073.

Emergency management consists of maintaining and improving respiratory effort with medications, and, in some cases, supplemental oxygen. Children with acute spasmodic croup and LTB who respond well to oral medication are often sent home from the emergency department after an observation period. Children with moderate to severe symptoms may need additional nebulized epinephrine, and may be admitted for further treatment if the respiratory status does not improve. Most children who are admitted respond to medications and oxygen therapy and are discharged within 48 to 72 hours.

Clinical Tip

No studies of therapies for acute spasmodic croup or LTB support routine exposure of the child to cold air, decongestants, or cough medications (Zoorob, Sidani, & Murray, 2011). However, some children with mild recurrent acute spasmodic croup get relief from exposure to cold air or warm humidity in a closed bathroom with warm steam. Children who do not have relief from these complementary therapies should be seen by a healthcare provider for treatment.

Children with bacterial tracheitis and epiglottitis have a more severe airway obstruction. These children usually are intubated in the operating room because the obstruction can rapidly become life threatening. These children are then transferred to the PICU for care.

Nursing Management

For the Child With Croup Syndrome

Nursing Assessment and Diagnosis

The initial and ongoing physical assessment of the child with one of the croup syndrome disorders focuses on adequacy of respiratory functioning and severity of illness. Attach a cardiorespiratory monitor and pulse oximeter. Have the child in an area where continuous visual monitoring is possible to detect changes in severity of respiratory distress. Assess vital signs, including temperature.

Pay particular attention to any progressive changes in the child's respiratory effort that may signal the need for intubation. Regularly assess the respiratory rate, heart rate, retractions, use of accessory muscles, stridor, breath sounds, preferred position, and responsiveness (Figure 20–2). Exhaustion can diminish the intensity of retractions and stridor. As the child uses remaining energy reserves to maintain ventilation, breath sounds may actually diminish. Noisy breathing (audible airway congestion, coarse breath sounds) in this situation verifies adequate energy stores. Responsiveness decreases as hypoxemia increases.

SAFETY ALERT!

If the child is suspected of having epiglottitis or a severe airway obstruction, do not leave the child's side until intubation occurs. Observe the child continuously for inability to swallow, absence of voice sounds, increasing degree of respiratory distress, and acute onset of drooling. A change in the child's level of consciousness—from anxiety to lethargy to stupor—occurs as hypoxia increases. If any of these signs occur, get medical assistance immediately. The quieter the child, the greater the cause for concern.

The following nursing diagnoses might be appropriate for the child with a croup syndrome disorder (NANDA-I © 2014):

- *Breathing Pattern, Ineffective*, related to airway narrowing, decreased energy, and fatigue
- *Fluid Volume: Deficient, Risk for*, related to fever and swallowing difficulty
- *Fear (Child)* related to dyspnea, unfamiliar surroundings, procedures, and separation from support system

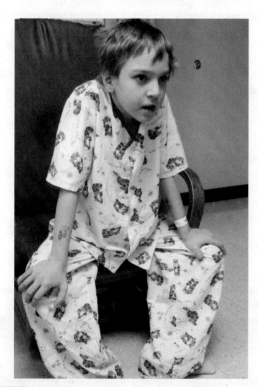

Figure 20–2 Children with severe respiratory distress and a narrowed airway often sit in a tripod position, leaning forward with arms on the legs. The head and neck are extended with the jaw thrust forward to help keep the airway open. This position may also be seen in a child with an acute asthma flare.

Planning and Implementation

MAINTAIN AIRWAY PATENCY

Allow the child to assume a comfortable position. Be immediately available to attend to the child's respiratory needs, and keep resuscitation equipment and an intubation tray at the bedside. Supplemental oxygen with humidity may be needed for hypoxemia. Ensure that a means of communication (sign language or simple word cues) is established so the older child can alert nursing staff to respiratory difficulty.

Postpone anxiety-provoking procedures such as venipuncture until the airway is considered to be secure. Anxiety associated with procedures often causes increased respiratory distress. Crying stimulates the airway, increases oxygen consumption, and in some cases, such as epiglottitis, can precipitate laryngospasm that can obstruct the airway.

When the child is intubated, care is provided in the PICU to ensure continual observation (see the *Clinical Skills Manual* SKILLS). Provide humidified air or supplemental oxygen if prescribed. The child with bacterial tracheitis needs frequent suctioning because of thick tracheal secretions that pool in the upper airway.

MEET FLUID AND NUTRITIONAL NEEDS

The illness preceding the emergency department visit may have compromised the child's fluid status, or the child may have difficulty swallowing because of inflammation. Recognize the potential fluid deficit and monitor the child's hydration and nutritional status. Fluids help thin secretions and provide calories for energy and metabolism.

When the child can drink fluids provide cool, noncarbonated, nonacidic drinks such as oral rehydration fluids or fruit-flavored drinks, gelatin, and popsicles. Encourage the parents to gain the child's cooperation in taking oral fluids. When the child's airway is compromised an intravenous infusion is needed to rehydrate the child, maintain fluid balance, or provide emergency access.

ADMINISTER MEDICATIONS

Administer medications as prescribed. Children with acute spasmodic laryngitis and LTB are treated with oral dexamethasone, and some children need nebulized epinephrine. Children with bacterial tracheitis or epiglottitis are initially treated with IV antibiotics until inflammation is reduced and the airway becomes stable without an endotracheal tube. Antibiotics are then administered orally.

PROVIDE FAMILY SUPPORT

Support parents who may be very anxious about the abrupt onset of life-threatening respiratory distress. When the child is intubated, reassure the child and family that their inability to make sounds is temporary. Explain the need for various pieces of equipment to help reduce the child's stress.

DISCHARGE PLANNING AND HOME CARE TEACHING

During the child's observation period for acute spasmodic laryngitis and LTB, educate the parents about actions to take if symptoms recur. For example, the child should return to the healthcare provider if:

- Mild symptoms do not improve after 1 hour of exposure to cool outdoor air or air conditioning.
- The child's breathing is rapid and labored with nasal flaring and retractions.
- The child does not drink adequate fluids and the urine output is reduced.

Ensure that parents of children with bacterial tracheitis or epiglottitis understand the importance of completing the full course of antibiotics.

Evaluation

Expected outcomes of nursing care include the following:

- The child responds to medications with decreased respiratory distress.
- The child's fear and anxiety is managed with family support and explanations about care.

Lower Airway Disorders

Lower airway disorders occur because a structural or functional problem interferes with the lungs' ability to complete the respiratory cycle. Disorders of the lower airway include bronchitis, bronchiolitis, pneumonia, and tuberculosis.

Bronchitis

Acute bronchitis, inflammation of the trachea and bronchi, rarely occurs in childhood as an isolated problem. The bronchi can be affected simultaneously with adjacent respiratory structures during a respiratory illness. Bronchitis occurs most commonly in the winter months.

The classic symptom of bronchitis is a dry, hacking cough that increases in severity at night. The cough may or may not be productive. The child may swallow sputum and vomit as a result. The chest and ribs may be sore because of the deep and frequent coughing. Over several days breath sounds may become coarse with fine crackles, and some scattered high-pitched wheezing may be heard. Treatment is palliative unless a secondary bacterial infection occurs that needs antibiotic therapy.

Nursing Management

Nursing management includes supporting respiratory function through rest, humidification, hydration, and symptomatic treatment. Refer to the sections in this chapter on asthma and pneumonia for detailed information on treatment measures.

Home care should emphasize the self-limiting nature of the disorder. Advise parents who smoke that quitting or not smoking in the child's presence may benefit the child.

Bronchiolitis and Respiratory Syncytial Virus

Bronchiolitis is a lower respiratory tract illness that occurs when a viral or bacterial organism causes inflammation and obstruction of the bronchioles. It is a leading cause of hospitalization during the first year of life (Weinberger, 2011). Infants who develop bronchiolitis have an increased risk for recurrent wheezing during the first year of life (Blanken et al., 2013).

ETIOLOGY AND PATHOPHYSIOLOGY

Respiratory syncytial virus (RSV) is the most common cause of bronchiolitis, but adenovirus, parainfluenza virus, and human metapneumovirus may also be responsible. RSV occurs in annual epidemics from October to March. It is transmitted through direct contact with respiratory secretions or indirectly through contaminated surfaces. The infected child sheds the virus for 3 to 8 days, and the incubation period is 2 to 8 days. Nearly all children have been infected with RSV by 2 years of age, and reinfection throughout life is common (American Academy of Pediatrics

[AAP], 2015, p. 667–668). Risk factors for severe RSV infection include immunosuppression, very low birth weight, lung disease, severe neuromuscular disease, or complicated congenital heart defects (Brashers & Huether, 2014).

Viruses, acting as parasites, are able to invade the mucosal cells that line the small bronchi and bronchioles. The invaded cells die when the virus bursts from inside the cell to invade adjacent cells. The membranes of the infected cells fuse with adjacent cells, creating large masses of cells or "syncytia." The resulting cell debris clogs and obstructs the bronchioles and irritates the airway. In response, the airway lining swells and produces excessive mucus. Despite this protective effort by the bronchioles, the actual effect is partial airway obstruction and bronchospasms.

The cycle is repeated throughout both lungs as the airway cells are invaded by the virus. The partially obstructed airways allow air in, but the mucus and airway swelling cause air trapping, and hyperinflation of the alveoli. Areas of atelectasis may occur. Normal gas exchange is affected, leading to hypoxemia. The child with severe RSV is at risk for apnea and respiratory failure as hypoxemia and hypercarbia develop.

CLINICAL MANIFESTATIONS

Some children have mild symptoms such as rhinitis, cough, low-grade fever, wheezing, tachypnea, poor feeding, vomiting, and diarrhea. Dehydration may be present if the child has been sick for several days. Parents report that the infant or child is acting more ill—appearing sicker, less playful, and less interested in eating. Infants, especially, may refuse to feed or may spit up what they eat along with thick, clear mucus.

The infant or child with a more severe infection has tachypnea greater than 70 breaths per minute, grunting, increased wheezing, crackles, retractions, nasal flaring, irritability, lethargy, poor fluid intake, and a distended abdomen from overexpanded lungs. As hypoxia develops the infant becomes cyanotic and has decreasing mental status. As the airflow continues to decrease, breath sounds diminish. Thus the noisier the lungs, the better, as this indicates that the child is still able to move air in and out of the lungs. Although RSV bronchiolitis resolves in 5 to 7 days, increased airway resistance and airway hypersensitivity may persist for weeks or even months.

CLINICAL THERAPY

The history and physical examination provide the data needed to diagnose bronchiolitis. Chest radiographs show hyperinflation, patchy atelectasis, and other signs of inflammation. Enzyme-linked immunoabsorbent assay (ELISA) or immunofluorescent assay performed on a posterior nasopharyngeal wash or swab specimen are used to identify the virus causing bronchiolitis (see the *Clinical Skills Manual* SKILLS).

Treatment is supportive. Most children have mild disease and can be managed at home. See *Families Want to Know: Home Care for the Infant With Mild Bronchiolitis*. The child is placed on respiratory and contact isolation when hospitalized to minimize the spread of the virus to other hospitalized children. Humidified oxygen is provided to infants with severe hypoxemia. Other supportive care includes hydration with oral or IV fluids and nasal suctioning before feeding. Continuous positive airway pressure (CPAP) may be used in the child with moderate to severe bronchiolitis. Chest physiotherapy is not recommended (Niergarten, 2015).

Few medications are prescribed for RSV and bronchiolitis. Bronchodilators, corticosteroids, and epinephrine are not recommended. Antipyretics may be used. Nebulized hypertonic saline (3%) may be used in hospitalized infants. Antibiotics are used only when a bacterial infection is present (Nierengarten, 2015).

Families Want to Know
Home Care for the Infant With Mild Bronchiolitis

General care instructions:

- Use the bulb syringe to suction the nares of an infant under 1 year of age.
- Give fluids to help thin secretions and provide calories for energy.
- Encourage active toddlers to rest and take naps during recovery.

Advise parents to call the physician if:

- Respiratory symptoms interfere with sleeping or eating.
- Breathing is rapid or difficult.
- Symptoms persist in a child who is less than 1 year old, has heart or lung disease, or was premature and had lung disease after birth.
- The child acts sicker—appears tired, less playful, and less interested in food (parents just "feel" the child is not improving).

Prevention of RSV is a focus for children at highest risk for severe bronchiolitis. Examples include infants born prematurely (less than 32 weeks' gestation) and those who required supplemental oxygen for several weeks after birth. Some children less than 2 years of age being treated for chronic lung disease of prematurity, congestive heart failure, or pulmonary hypertension are also at higher risk. The American Academy of Pediatrics has specific criteria for selecting children to receive passive immunity protection (AAP, 2015, pp. 673–675).

Intramuscular palivizumab (Synagis) provides passive immunity to help protect these high-risk infants. A dose of 15 mg/kg is given every 30 days for 5 months beginning in October or November at the onset of the RSV season. Palivizumab is expensive, but it is believed to offer benefits to the infants at high risk who might require hospitalization for RSV. Palivizumab does not interfere with administration of normal recommended childhood vaccines (AAP, 2015, p. 40).

Nursing Management
For the Child With Bronchiolitis and RSV

Nursing Assessment and Diagnosis

PHYSIOLOGIC ASSESSMENT

Assess airway and respiratory function carefully. Good observation skills are important to ensure timely interventions for worsening respiratory symptoms and prevention of respiratory failure (see the *Assessment Guide* and Table 20–2 earlier in this chapter). Assess the child's hydration status, weigh the child daily, and monitor the intake and output. Attach a cardiorespiratory monitor and pulse oximeter. An oxygen saturation level below 90% is the best indicator of the condition's severity.

SAFETY ALERT!

RSV bronchiolitis often increases in severity before beginning to resolve. Stay alert for signs of increasing respiratory distress and a greater need for oxygen. Signs of life-threatening illness include central cyanosis, respiratory rate greater than 70 breaths a minute, listlessness, diminished breath sounds, and apneic episodes. Inform the physician immediately of any significant changes in respiratory status.

PSYCHOSOCIAL ASSESSMENT

Observe children and their parents for signs of fear and anxiety. The unfamiliar hospital environment and procedures can increase stress. Parents' questions, as well as their nonverbal cues, help direct nursing interventions during admission and throughout hospitalization.

The accompanying *Nursing Care Plan: The Child With Bronchiolitis* lists common nursing diagnoses for the child with bronchiolitis. Others that might also be appropriate include (NANDA-I © 2014):

- *Airway Clearance, Ineffective,* related to increased airway secretions in bronchioles
- *Activity Intolerance* related to imbalance between oxygen supply and demand
- *Family Processes, Interrupted,* related to sudden acute illness of the infant

Planning and Implementation

Nursing management of the hospitalized child with bronchiolitis focuses on maintaining respiratory function, supporting overall physiologic function and hydration, reducing the child's and family's anxiety, and preparing the family for home care.

MAINTAIN RESPIRATORY FUNCTION

Close monitoring is essential to evaluate the child's improvement or to spot early signs of deterioration. Patent nares are important to promote oxygen intake. A bulb syringe and saline nose drops can be used to quickly clear the nasal passages. Elevate the head of the bed to ease the work of breathing and drain mucus from the upper airways. Supplemental oxygen with humidity may be provided via nasal cannula, mask, hood, or tent. When the child resists or is frightened by the oxygen apparatus, engage the parent to soothe the child and promote acceptance of the therapy.

SUPPORT PHYSIOLOGIC FUNCTION

Group nursing tasks to decrease stress and promote rest. Medications may be administered to control temperature and promote comfort as needed. Infants may have feeding difficulty and are at risk for aspiration. Suction the nasal passages before giving oral feedings. Feed smaller volumes more frequently to help conserve energy in infants who are formula-fed or breastfed. When the risk of aspiration is high, nasogastric tube feedings may be used to provide nutrition. An IV infusion may be ordered to rehydrate the child and maintain fluid balance until oral fluid intake is adequate.

Nursing Care Plan: The Child With Bronchiolitis

1. Nursing Diagnosis: *Breathing Pattern, Ineffective,* related to increased work of breathing (NANDA-I © 2014)

GOAL: The child will return to respiratory baseline and will not experience respiratory failure.

INTERVENTION	RATIONALE
• Assess respiratory status (see *Assessment Guide*) when child is calm and not crying at least every 2–4 hr, or more often as indicated for an increasing or decreasing respiratory rate and episodes of apnea.	• Changes in breathing pattern may occur quickly as the child's energy reserves are depleted. Baseline and subsequent assessments help detect changes in the respiratory rate and respiratory effort.
• Attach a cardiorespiratory monitor and pulse oximeter with alarms set. Record and report changes promptly to physician.	• The alarm can alert the nurse to any sudden respiratory changes and lead to more rapid interventions.

EXPECTED OUTCOME: Child will return to respiratory baseline within 48–72 hr.

GOAL: The child's oxygenation status will return to baseline.

INTERVENTION	RATIONALE
• Administer humidified oxygen via mask, nasal cannula, hood, or tent.	• Humidified oxygen loosens secretions, helps maintain oxygenation status, and eases respiratory distress.
• Assess and compare the child's SpO_2 level on room air and when on supplemental oxygen.	• Comparison of SpO_2 levels provides information about improvement status.
• Note child's response to ordered medications.	• Medications act systemically to improve oxygenation and decrease inflammation.
• Position head of bed up or place child in position of comfort on parent's lap, if crying or struggling in crib or bed.	• Position facilitates improved aeration and promotes decrease in anxiety (especially in infants) and energy expenditure.
• Assess tolerance to feeding and activities.	• Provides an assessment of condition improvement.

EXPECTED OUTCOME: Child's respiratory effort will ease. The SpO_2 level will remain above 90% during treatment. Child will tolerate therapeutic measures with no adverse effects. Child will rest quietly in position of comfort.

2. Nursing Diagnosis: *Fluid Volume: Deficient, Risk for,* related to inability to meet body requirements and increased metabolic demand (NANDA-I © 2014)

GOAL: The child's immediate fluid deficit will be corrected.

INTERVENTION	RATIONALE
• Evaluate need for intravenous fluids. Maintain IV, if ordered.	• Previous fluid loss may require immediate replacement.

EXPECTED OUTCOME: Child's hydration status will be maintained during acute phase of illness as demonstrated by appropriate urine output and moist mucous membranes.

GOAL: The child will be adequately hydrated, be able to tolerate oral fluids, and progress to normal diet.

INTERVENTION	RATIONALE
• Calculate maintenance fluid requirements and give oral fluids, IV fluids, or both.	• Assessment of fluid requirements enables the child to maintain hydration while transitioning to oral fluids.
• Offer clear fluids and incorporate parent in care. Offer fluid choice when tolerated.	• Choice of fluid offered by parent gains the child's cooperation.
• Maintain strict intake and output monitoring and evaluate specific gravity at least every 8 hours.	• Monitoring provides objective evidence of fluid loss and ongoing hydration status.
• Perform daily weight measurement on the same scale at the same time of day. Evaluate skin turgor.	• Further evidence of improvement of hydration status.
• Assess mucous membranes and presence of tears.	• Moist mucous membranes and tears are signs of adequate hydration.

EXPECTED OUTCOME: Child will take adequate oral fluids after 24–48 hr to maintain hydration. Child will accept beverage of choice from parent or nursing staff. Child's weight will stabilize after 24–48 hr; skin turgor will be supple. Child will show evidence of improved hydration.

3. Nursing Diagnosis: *Anxiety (Child and Parent)* related to acute illness, hospitalization, uncertain course of illness and treatment, and home care needs (NANDA-I © 2014)

GOAL: The child and parents will demonstrate behaviors that indicate less anxiety.

INTERVENTION	RATIONALE
• Encourage parents to express fears and ask questions; provide direct answers and discuss care, procedures, and condition changes.	• Parents have the opportunity to vent feelings and receive timely, relevant information. This helps reduce parents' anxiety and increase trust in nursing staff.
• Incorporate parents in the child's care. Encourage parents to bring familiar objects from home. Ask about and incorporate in care plan the home routines for feeding and sleeping.	• Familiar people, routines, and objects decrease the child's anxiety and increase parents' sense of control over an unexpected, uncertain situation.

EXPECTED OUTCOME: Parents and child will show less anxiety as symptoms improve and as child and parents feel more secure in hospital environment. *Parents* will freely ask questions and participate in the child's care. *Children* will cry less and allow themselves to be touched or held by staff.

GOAL: Parents will verbalize knowledge of bronchiolitis symptoms and use of home care methods before the child's discharge from the hospital.

INTERVENTION	RATIONALE
• Explain symptoms, treatment, and home care of bronchiolitis.	• Anticipating the potential for recurrence assists the family to be prepared should respiratory symptoms recur after discharge.
• Provide written instructions for follow-up care arrangements, as needed.	• Written and verbal instructions reinforce knowledge. Parents may not "hear" and remember details if only given verbally.
• Make sure parents can read the instructions provided in family's primary language.	• Many families have reading difficulties or may read a language other than English.

EXPECTED OUTCOME: Parents will accurately describe respiratory symptoms and initial home care actions.

REDUCE ANXIETY

The need for hospitalization and assistive therapies creates anxiety and fear in the child and parents. The parents may be frightened by the child's continued respiratory difficulty. Infants may respond to their parents' anxiety and be more irritable. Provide parents with thorough explanations and daily updates, and encourage their participation in the child's care. Reassure them that holding or touching the child will not dislodge wires or tubing, and that their presence will calm and support the child.

If the child has been ill for a few days before admission, the parents are likely to be tired. Acknowledging parents' physical and emotional needs creates a spirit of caring and enhances communication between staff and family. Encourage the parents to take turns at the child's bedside and to take breaks for meals and rest.

DISCHARGE PLANNING AND HOME CARE TEACHING

The child is discharged once oxygenation is stable (pulse oximetry at least 90%) on room air and full oral feedings have been possible for at least 12 hours (Weinberger, 2011). In most children, respiratory efforts and decreased mucus production decrease within 24 to 72 hours, but all symptoms like coughing may take weeks to resolve.

Teach the parents proper administration of medications. Acetaminophen or ibuprofen may be prescribed for persistent low-grade fevers and general discomfort. Advise parents that RSV infection can recur. Educate them to recognize symptoms and when to call the healthcare provider.

Evaluation

Expected outcomes of nursing care for the child with bronchiolitis are provided in the *Nursing Care Plan*.

Pneumonia

Pneumonia, an inflammation or infection of the bronchioles and alveolar spaces of the lungs, occurs most often in infants and young children. More than 150,000 children are hospitalized for pneumonia annually in the United States (Queen et al., 2014). Pneumonia can be community acquired (CAP) or hospital acquired (e.g., associated with mechanical ventilation). The focus of this discussion is CAP.

Pneumonia may be viral, mycoplasmal, or bacterial in origin. Viral-bacterial coinfection also occurs. Children under 5 years of age most often have viral pneumonia caused by RSV, human metapneumovirus, influenza virus, parainfluenza virus, or adenovirus. Bacterial pneumonia occurs in all age groups. Mycoplasmal pneumonia is more common in children 5 years and older. Common bacterial organisms include *Streptococcus pneumoniae*, *Chlamydophila pneumoniae*, and *Staphylococcus aureus*. Group B streptococcus, enteric gram-negative bacilli, and *Chlamydia trachomatis* are found in infants younger than 3 months of age. Children with cystic fibrosis or immunosuppression are susceptible to other bacterial, parasitic, or fungal infections.

Bacterial and viral invaders act differently within the lungs:

• Bacteria enter the lungs after aspiration of nasopharyngeal bacteria and colonize in the trachea and bronchi.

Prior damage by a viral infection may damage the epithelium and reduce the child's ability to clear the organisms. Inflammation leads to edema and purulent exudates. Cellular debris and mucus cause airway obstruction. Bacteria tend to be distributed evenly throughout one or more lobes of a single lung, a pattern termed *unilateral lobar pneumonia*.

- Viruses enter through the upper respiratory tract, damaging the ciliated epithelium in the distal airway. Viruses invade and kill cells causing cell debris. The alveoli become infiltrated nearest the bronchi of one or both lungs. Adjacent areas become invaded in a scattered, patchy pattern referred to as bronchopneumonia.

- Aspiration of food, emesis, gastric reflux, or hydrocarbons causes a chemical injury and inflammatory response, which sets the stage for bacterial invasion.

Community acquired pneumonia is often preceded by an upper respiratory tract infection including rhinitis and a cough. Other symptoms include fever, rhonchi, crackles, wheezes, dyspnea, tachypnea, chest pain, restlessness, and abdominal pain. Newborns and infants may have tachypnea, grunting, nasal flaring, retractions, irritability, lethargy, and a poor appetite. Diminished breath sounds may be noted.

Diagnosis is based on history and physical findings. Rapid influenza and other respiratory virus testing is recommended to help distinguish between viral and bacterial causes of CAP. Bacterial pneumonia is more often associated with a higher fever, absolute neutrophil count, and percentage of bands (Brashers & Heuther, 2014). A chest radiograph and blood cultures may be performed when the child requires hospitalization.

Clinical management for all types of pneumonia includes pain and fever control, and supportive care through airway management, fluids, and rest. Children with severe CAP are hospitalized, and may be treated with antibiotics, supplemental oxygen, and IV fluids. Current antibiotic guidelines are high-dose ampicillin or amoxicillin for 5 days in children with uncomplicated CAP (Greenberg, Givon-Lavi, Sadaka, et al., 2014). Antiviral therapy is prescribed for some children.

Nursing Management

If the child with CAP is hospitalized, assess the child, paying particular attention to respiratory rate, heart rate, and temperature, and observe color for pallor or cyanosis. Attach a pulse oximeter to monitor the SpO$_2$ level. Assess hydration status. Assess for the presence of pain with coughing.

Nursing measures used for the child with bronchiolitis are generally applicable (see earlier section in this chapter). Teach the child and parent how to splint the chest by hugging a small pillow or teddy bear to make coughing less painful. Acetaminophen or ibuprofen may be prescribed for pain management and temperature control. Administer antibiotics as prescribed. Promote hydration and nutrition by encouraging the intake of preferred clear liquids and small servings of soft foods.

For home management, teach parents about administering prescribed antibiotics, any potential side effects, and the need to give the full course. Educate parents about signs that the child's condition may be worsening (increased breathing difficulty or refusal to take fluids). Most children recover uneventfully, but some continue to have worsening reactive airway problems or abnormal results on pulmonary function tests.

Preventive measures are limited. The *Haemophilus influenzae* type B (Hib) and pneumococcal conjugate (PCV13) vaccines protect against some causes of pneumonia. The 23-valent pneumococcal vaccine is recommended for children over 2 years of age with immunosuppression or some chronic conditions (see Chapter 16).

Tuberculosis

Tuberculosis (TB) is an infection caused by *Mycobacterium tuberculosis*, which is transmitted through the air in infectious particles called *droplet nuclei*. About 1000 active TB cases occur in children each year, and rates are highest among children and adolescents with at least one foreign parent (Starke & Cruz, 2014). Children account for 7% of all cases reported in the United States each year (Winston & Menzies, 2012).

ETIOLOGY AND PATHOPHYSIOLOGY

Children usually acquire a TB infection from infected adults who cough, sneeze, speak, or sing, and send out tiny droplets containing the bacillus. When inhaled, the bacillus is small enough to travel directly to the alveoli and cause infection. When the organism reaches the alveoli, an immune response is initiated, and macrophages surround and wall off the bacillus in a small hard capsule, called a *tubercle*. The tubercle bacilli grow slowly, dividing every 25 to 32 hours. The bacilli grow for 2 to 12 weeks until they number 1000 to 10,000, at which point the cellular immune response to a TB skin test (TST) would occur if the test were administered.

In persons with intact cell-mediated immunity, activated T cells and macrophages form granulomas around the tubercles that limit multiplication. The proliferation of TB is arrested, but small numbers of viable bacilli remain in the tubercle. These individuals have latent tuberculosis infection (LTBI), a positive TST, and no clinical or radiographic signs of disease. They are not infectious and cannot transmit the disease.

Active TB can develop as the bacilli grow, divide within the tubercle, and break free. Progression to active TB generally occurs within 1 year of infection in infants and adolescents, who have the greatest risk of transitioning from LTBI to active TB (Perez-Velez & Marais, 2012). Factors further increasing that risk include immunosuppressive therapy, HIV coinfection, immunodeficiency, malnutrition, and chronic medical conditions (AAP, 2015, p. 808). Most children under age 10 years with active TB are not contagious because they have small pulmonary lesions and unproductive coughing during which few or no bacilli are expelled (AAP, 2015, pp. 827).

Disseminated, or extrapulmonary, TB occurs more commonly in infants and young children. Bacilli are released from the primary site into the bloodstream, spreading to the liver, spleen, kidney, bone marrow, or meninges (miliary TB).

CLINICAL MANIFESTATIONS

Children with LTBI are asymptomatic. Children with pulmonary TB may have a persistent cough, weight loss or failure to gain weight, fever, fatigue, wheezing, and decreased breath sounds. Adolescents may have fever, anorexia, weight loss or growth delay, productive cough, and night sweats. **Hemoptysis** (coughing up blood from the respiratory tract) is a late sign of advanced pulmonary TB. When TB spreads outside the pulmonary system, additional signs are specific to the system invaded:

- *Superficial lymphadenitis:* firm, nontender, matted lymph nodes

- *Miliary:* high fever, vomiting, lethargy, headache, seizures, nuchal rigidity, cranial nerve palsies, and irritability; also hepatosplenomegaly and generalized lymphadenopathy
- *Osteoarticular:* inflammation, pain, swelling, fever, and limited range of motion of the affected bone or joint

CLINICAL THERAPY

Screening to identify a child's risk for LTBI should occur during the first health visit, every 6 months until age 2 years, and then annually. Administer a tuberculin skin test (intradermal purified protein derivative [PPD]) or collect blood for an interferon-gamma release assay (IGRA) if one or more of these risk factors are present (AAP, 2015, p. 812; Desale, Bringardner, Fitzgerald, et al., 2013; Rose et al., 2014; Seddon, Hesseling, Godfrey-Faussett, et al., 2013):

- The child's parents or family members immigrated from a country or region where TB is an established health problem, such as Asia, India, the Middle East, Africa, or Latin America.
- The child was born in one of the countries or regions mentioned.
- The child traveled to any of the countries or regions mentioned and had close contact with residents, such as residing in the home of residents, for a week or longer.
- A family member has tested positive with a PPD or IGRA.
- The child has clinical signs or radiologic findings that could be associated with TB.
- The child infected with HIV should have annual tuberculin testing.

A positive PPD or IGRA indicates that the child has been exposed to and infected with TB, and antibodies have been produced against the bacillus.

An interferon-gamma release assay (IGRA; e.g., quantiFERON or T.Spot.TB) may help clarify PPD findings. For example, a child vaccinated with bacille Calmette-Guérin (BCG) may have a false-positive response to multiple PPDs, but IGRA does not cross-react with BCG and gives a more accurate result (Riazi et al., 2012). Like the PPD, the IGRA cannot distinguish between latent or active TB. Other diagnostic tests include acid-fast stains of blood, gastric aspirate, sputum cultures, and a chest radiograph.

Active and latent TB are treated with isoniazid, rifampicin, pyrazinamide, and ethambutol. Therapy for active TB usually involves a 6-month regimen consisting of isoniazid, rifampin, pyrazinamide, and ethambutol for the first 2 months and isoniazid and rifampin for the remaining 4 months. LTBI in children less than 12 years of age is treated with a single daily dose of isoniazid for 9 months (or rifampin for 6 months if TB is drug resistant to isoniazid). Direct-observed drug therapy administered by a healthcare provider 2 times a week for the duration of treatment is recommended for children with active TB and when daily therapy adherence is not assured for children with LTBI (AAP, 2015, p. 816). Healthy youth with LTBI, ages 12 years and older, may receive once-weekly direct-observed drug therapy with isoniazid and rifampin for 12 weeks (Jereb, Goldberg, Powell, et al., 2011). Children with a positive PPD and negative IGRA who do not receive treatment for LTBI should be followed for 1 to 2 years to monitor for transition to active disease (Amanatidou, Syridou, Mavrikou, et al., 2012).

The local public health department is notified to search for disease contacts of the child with newly diagnosed LTBI or active TB. The child is considered a sentinel case and the adult contact with active TB must be identified.

Nursing Management

Assessment focuses on identifying children at high risk of TB exposure and performing a PPD as appropriate. Infant and young children with a positive PPD are at greater risk to develop active TB, so assess them carefully for weight loss, fever, fatigue, coughing, and respiratory status. Consider the child's immunosuppression status. If active TB is suspected, implement airborne isolation precautions until the infection status is known.

SAFETY ALERT!

Airborne isolation precautions are intended to protect the nurse as well as to reduce the risk for transmission of infection to other clients. Use all recommended personal protective equipment (PPE) correctly, perform hand hygiene, and appropriately dispose of linens, PPE, and trash to protect yourself and others from infection.

Nursing care of the child with LTBI focuses on administering medications and providing supportive care. Teach parents about the disease process, medications, possible side effects, and the importance of completing long-term therapy. Emphasize the importance of taking medications as prescribed on an empty stomach. Initiate direct-observed drug therapy twice a week if poor adherence is suspected.

Encourage proper nutrition and rest to promote normal growth and development. The child can return to school or child care when effective therapy has been instituted, adherence to therapy has been documented, and clinical symptoms have diminished substantially (AAP, 2015, p. 829). Children should receive all usual immunizations. Most children treated for TB can lead essentially normal lives. See the discussion of pneumonia earlier in this chapter and of tubercular meningitis in Chapter 27 for other nursing care measures.

Chronic Lung Conditions

Bronchopulmonary Dysplasia (Chronic Lung Disease)

Bronchopulmonary dysplasia (BPD), also called chronic lung disease of prematurity, is defined as the need for supplemental oxygen for at least 28 days after premature birth. BPD more commonly develops in infants born at less than 28 weeks' gestation when lungs are immature. It is estimated to occur in 35% to 50% of newborns born at less than 28 weeks' gestation (Strueby & Thébaud, 2014).

ETIOLOGY AND PATHOPHYSIOLOGY

Preterm infants less than 28 weeks' gestation are born before alveolar development occurs. BPD results from positive-pressure ventilation and oxygen needed to treat respiratory failure and respiratory distress syndrome. The treatment injures the immature lungs leading to fewer and larger alveoli with less functional surface area and a smaller vascular bed in the lungs, which has greater tone and reactivity. These changes potentially lead to long-term chronic lung disease (Strueby & Thébaud, 2014). A patent ductus arteriosus may also contribute to BPD development. Antenatal corticosteroids and surfactant replacement therapy have reduced the incidence of BPD in more mature preterm infants.

Pathophysiology Illustrated: **Barrel Chest**

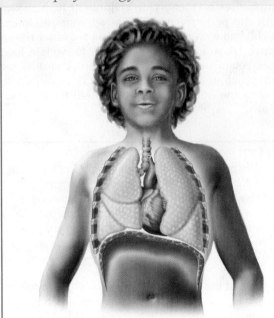

A barrel chest may result from chronic respiratory conditions such as asthma or bronchopulmonary dysplasia, in which air trapping or hyperinflation of the alveoli occurs. The chest's anterioposterior diameter increases to give a rounded chest shape.

CLINICAL MANIFESTATIONS

The infant with BPD has persistent signs of respiratory distress: tachypnea, nasal flaring, grunting, retractions, wheezing, crackles, and irritability. Normal activities like feeding create increased oxygen demands and fatigue that may lead to failure to thrive. The infant has intermittent bronchospasms, mucous plugging, and chronic air trapping, which may lead to a barrel-shaped chest (see *Pathophysiology Illustrated: Barrel Chest*). Cyanosis may be seen in severe cases.

CLINICAL THERAPY

Medical management for BPD involves therapies to support respiratory function and good nutrition, which helps to accelerate lung maturity. Medications are administered such as surfactant, corticosteroids, vitamin A, and caffeine (Strueby & Thébaud, 2014). Supplemental oxygen with humidity is used. Nasal continuous or intermittent positive pressure ventilation is often used. An endotracheal tube or tracheostomy may be needed for long-term airway management to prevent narrowing of the trachea in more severe cases. Infants with severe BPD are carefully weaned off of assisted ventilation. Increased calories are needed to support growth, but fluids are restricted to prevent pulmonary edema. Some infants need gastrostomy or nasogastric tube feeding to get adequate calories.

Severity of BPD is determined at 36 weeks' corrected gestational age by the ongoing need for supplemental oxygen or positive-pressure ventilation in an infant who required supplemental oxygen at 28 days of life. Pulmonary artery hypertension is a complication when severe lung disease exists (see Chapter 21). Surviving infants are at risk for cognitive delays, cerebral palsy, growth failure, and abnormal lung function. Infants with severe BPD often have chronic lung disease.

After discharge from the neonatal ICU (NICU), some infants require ongoing oxygen therapy and some may have a tracheostomy. Infants with severe BPD often require frequent hospitalization because of respiratory infections or pulmonary hypertension. Antibiotics are used to aggressively treat infections. An annual influenza vaccine is recommended, and palivizumab may be given monthly to prevent RSV (see the section on bronchiolitis earlier in this chapter). Infants and children with continuing airway hyperactivity may have bronchodilator therapy and asthma controller medications prescribed (see the section on asthma later in this chapter).

Nursing Management

For the Child With Bronchopulmonary Dysplasia

Nursing management focuses on assessing and managing the infant's acute episodes, ensuring adequate nutrition, and promoting growth and development.

Nursing Assessment and Diagnosis

At each healthcare visit, assess the infant's respiratory status and growth. The infant may have poor weight gain because the work of breathing requires extra calories. Assess how well the family is managing care for the child in the home and any stressors that might exist. Evaluate development regularly because the infant may have motor, language, and cognitive delays. Coordinate a periodic assessment of hearing and vision. Infants with BPD may become acutely ill at any time, so observe for signs of infection.

During hospitalization for acute infections, a cardiorespiratory monitor and pulse oximeter are used. Assess airway and respiratory function, vital signs, color, and behavior changes to identify signs of worsening respiratory symptoms even when oxygen is provided. Observe for airway obstruction when the infant has a tracheostomy and suction as needed. See the *Clinical Skills Manual* SKILLS for tracheostomy care.

Nursing diagnoses that may be appropriate include (NANDA-I © 2014):

- *Gas Exchange, Impaired,* related to ventilation-perfusion imbalance
- *Nutrition, Imbalanced: Less than Body Requirements,* related to high metabolic needs and fatigue associated with feeding
- *Caregiver Role Strain* related to 24-hour responsibility for infant with BPD
- *Development: Delayed, Risk for,* related to chronic condition and limited opportunities to practice motor skills

Planning and Implementation

Organize care for the hospitalized child to reduce unnecessary physical stimulation. Position the infant to facilitate breathing.

Administer medications as prescribed. Careful fluid management is essential to reduce the risk for pulmonary edema. Provide nutrition to meet energy needs. Support the mother who desires to breastfeed. A high-calorie formula (24 to 30 calories/oz) may be given to promote weight gain. Some children need nasogastric or enteral feedings to get adequate nutrition when cyanosis is noted with feeding.

Once home, many infants need oxygen, tracheostomy care, multiple medications, and high-calorie feedings (Figure 20–3). Make referrals for needed oxygen, respiratory supplies, medications, an early intervention program, and follow-up care well in advance of the infant's discharge. Some families need home health nursing assistance, especially during the initial transition

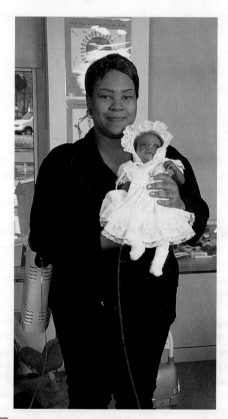

Figure 20–3 | **Many children with BPD are cared for at home, with the support of a home care program to monitor the family's ability to provide airway management, oxygen, and ventilator support. This premature infant girl, who is now 4 months old but weighs only about 5 lb, still requires supplemental oxygen.**

period. Teach parents to provide the complex care needed by the infant and to identify the signs of respiratory compromise indicating a need for rapid intervention.

All infants with BPD need more frequent health promotion visits and all immunizations. Suggest ways to provide for the infant's normal development through rest, nutrition, stimulation, and family support (see *Health Promotion: The Child With Bronchopulmonary Dysplasia*).

Clinical Reasoning Infant With BPD

Emily is an 8-month-old infant with BPD cared for at home by her parents. She has a tracheostomy and receives humidification. Emily has periodic infections and episodes of respiratory distress that require hospitalization. When she develops a fever, more secretions than usual collect in the trachea. Suctioning is needed to ease Emily's breathing. What signs indicate that Emily needs to be suctioned? How do you select the correct size of suction catheter? How do you suction Emily without causing hypoxia? When is it necessary to change Emily's tracheostomy tube?

Evaluation

Expected outcomes of nursing care may include:

- The infant receives adequate calories to sustain growth.
- The family identifies acute illness episodes rapidly and seeks appropriate care.
- The infant's acute respiratory decompensation episodes are effectively managed.

Asthma

Asthma is a common chronic disorder in children characterized by bronchial constriction, hyperresponsive airways, and airway inflammation. An estimated 10.5 million (14%) of children in the United States have received an asthma diagnosis, and 7.1 million children continue to have asthma episodes. Children report that asthma episodes result in missing 1 or more days of school and some activity limitation (Centers for Disease Control and Prevention, 2013). Asthma results in an increased number of health center and emergency department visits for treatment; sometimes hospitalization is necessary. The rate of death due to asthma in children and youth in the United States is 2.6 per million (Centers for Disease Control and Prevention, 2013). See *Developing Cultural Competence: Asthma Prevalence.*

Healthy People 2020

(RD-1) Reduce asthma deaths

(RD-2) Reduce hospitalizations for asthma

(RD-3) Reduce emergency department (ED) visits for asthma

Developing Cultural Competence Asthma Prevalence

Current asthma prevalence in children was higher among males (10%) compared to females (7.1%). Among racial and ethnic groups, Black children (14.0%) and multirace children (13.2%) have a higher prevalence than White children (7.4%) (Centers for Disease Control and Prevention, 2013).

Health Supervision

- Assess blood pressure to detect abnormal findings associated with pulmonary hypertension.

- Coordinate vision screening by an ophthalmologist every 2 to 3 months during the first year of life. Myopia and strabismus are common in children who were born prematurely.

- Coordinate pulmonary function tests annually or as needed for clinical condition.

- Perform hearing and other screening tests as recommended for age.

Growth and Developmental Surveillance

- Assess growth and plot measurements on a growth chart corrected for gestational age. Even if length and weight are lower than normal, monitor for continued growth following the growth curves.

- Perform a developmental assessment, correcting for gestational age.

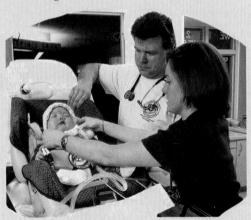

Nutrition

- Review caloric intake. Ensure that increased calories are provided to support growth. Assess feeding difficulties related to oral motor function associated with long-term enteral feeding. Refer to a nutritionist as necessary.

Physical Activity

- Organize care to provide rest periods during the day.

- Give parents ideas for promoting the infant's motor development, such as reaching for and moving toward toys and objects of interest.

Family Interactions

- Identify ways to coordinate nighttime care to reduce child and family sleep disturbances.

- Provide discipline appropriate for developmental age.

Disease Prevention Strategies

- Reduce exposure to infections. Encourage selection of a childcare provider who cares for a small number of children, if one is used. If possible, avoid the use of childcare centers during respiratory syncytial virus (RSV) season.

- Immunize the child with the routine vaccine schedule based on chronologic age.

- Administer the 23-valent pneumococcal vaccine at 2 years of age.

- Provide monthly injections of palivizumab throughout the RSV season.

Condition-Specific Guidance

- Develop an emergency care plan for times when the infant's condition rapidly worsens.

ETIOLOGY AND PATHOPHYSIOLOGY

Asthma is a chronic inflammatory disease caused by multiple factors (e.g., environmental exposures, viral illnesses, allergens, and a genetic predisposition) that occur at a crucial time in the immune system's development. Asthma is now considered to be a collection of several diseases that have similar characteristics and symptoms (Custovic, Lazic, & Simpson, 2013).

Many potential genes or regions of chromosomes are associated with asthma, such as those that are associated with increased immune and inflammatory response and airway remodeling. Approximately 70% of children have an allergic or atopic form of asthma, whereas other children have genetic factors that reduce their responsiveness to beta-adrenergic inhaled medications (Brashers & Huether, 2014; Chang, 2012). Environmental exposures also increase the risk for asthma, including passive tobacco smoke, indoor air contaminants (e.g., pet dander, cockroach feces), and outdoor air pollutants. Recurrent respiratory viral infections also increase risk. Protective factors are believed to include a large family size, later birth order, childcare attendance, and exposure to certain organisms. In theory, these factors increase exposure to infections early in life, enabling the child's immune system to develop along a nonallergic pathway (Brashers & Huether, 2014).

Persistent inflammation causes the normal protective mechanisms of the lungs (mucous formation, mucosal swelling, and airway muscle contraction) to overreact in response to a **trigger** (an inflammatory or noninflammatory stimulus that initiates an asthma episode). Triggers include exercise, infectious agents, allergens, fragrances, food additives, pollutants, weather changes, emotions, and stress. Inflammatory mechanisms enhance airway responsiveness, and triggers stimulate bronchospasms (smooth muscle contractions).

The trigger leads B cells to activate IgE and cytokines that then activate the migration and proliferation of eosinophils and the release of proinflammatory mediators. Direct tissue injury, increased bronchial hyperresponsiveness, fibroblast proliferation, and airway scarring result. An exaggerated inflammatory response leads to vasodilation, increased capillary permeability, mucosal edema, contraction of smooth bronchial muscle, and secretion of thick mucus, which narrow and obstruct the airways. Impaired expiration leads to air trapping, hyperinflation, and dyspnea, the physiologic sequence that results in an acute asthma episode (see *Pathophysiology Illustrated: Asthma*). Decreased perfusion of the alveolar capillaries results from hypoxic vasoconstriction and increased pressure due to hyperinflation of the alveoli. Hypoxemia leads to an increased respiratory rate, but because of airway resistance, less air is inspired per minute, worsening hypoxemia.

Pathophysiology Illustrated: **Asthma**

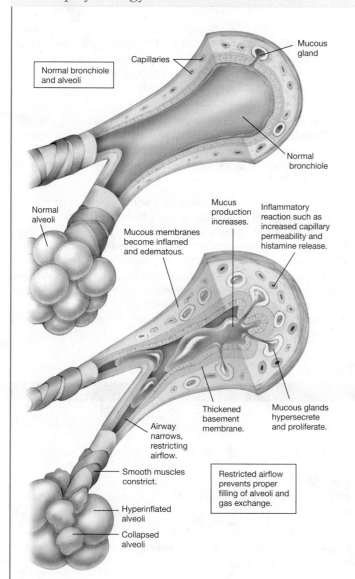

Normal bronchiole and alveoli

Capillaries

Mucous gland

Normal bronchiole

Normal alveoli

Mucous membranes become inflamed and edematous.

Mucus production increases.

Inflammatory reaction such as increased capillary permeability and histamine release.

Thickened basement membrane.

Mucous glands hypersecrete and proliferate.

Airway narrows, restricting airflow.

Smooth muscles constrict.

Restricted airflow prevents proper filling of alveoli and gas exchange.

Hyperinflated alveoli

Collapsed alveoli

Some asthma triggers are exercise, infection, and allergies. Airflow is obstructed through constriction and narrowing of the airway, along with increased production of mucus. Alveoli may become hyperinflated or collapse because of obstruction, leading to impaired gas exchange.

CLINICAL MANIFESTATIONS

The sudden onset of breathing difficulty (cough, wheeze, or short-ness of breath) is an acute asthma episode or asthma attack. The infant or child who has had frequent episodes of coughing or respiratory infections should be evaluated for asthma. Frequent coughing, especially at night, is a signal that the child's airway is very sensitive to stimuli, and this could be a sign of "silent" asthma.

During an acute episode, respirations are rapid and labored and the child often appears tired because of the ongoing effort to breathe. Nasal flaring and intercostal retractions may be visible. The child exhibits a productive cough and expiratory wheezing, a prolonged expiratory phase, decreased air movement, accessory muscle use, and respiratory fatigue. The child may complain of chest tightness. Anxiety increases as the acute episode worsens, and the increasing anxiety intensifies the child's physical responses.

In a severe acute episode, wheezing may not be heard because of low airflow. Head bobbing may be seen in young children using the accessory muscles to breathe. Hypoxia and the cumulative effect of administered medications may cause behaviors ranging from wide-eyed agitation to lethargic irritability. In children who have repeated acute episodes, a barrel chest and accessory muscle use are common findings.

CLINICAL THERAPY

Diagnosis is made by history, physical examination and pulmonary function testing (spirometry) that shows evidence of episodic airflow obstruction (that is at least partially reversible), and airway hyperresponsiveness. Spirometry readings are most commonly measured as forced expiratory volume in 1 second (FEV_1) and expressed as a percentage of predicted FEV_1 for the child's height, age, gender, and race. A chest radiograph may help determine if a foreign body could account for symptoms. Skin testing may be used to identify allergens (asthma triggers).

Spirometry testing is performed when the child is able to cooperate, usually by 5 to 6 years of age. Coughing interferes with a good result, so perform testing when asthma is well controlled. Coach the child to give the best effort each time. Allow children to practice using the mouthpiece and nose clip. To perform the test, have the child exhale forcefully. With the mouth forming a tight seal around the mouthpiece, ask the child to take a rapid deep breath without breathing through the nose. Have the child to keep a tight seal around the mouthpiece and to exhale forcibly for at least 6 seconds. Three acceptable readings are obtained, but limit the child to eight efforts (Banasiak, 2014). Be sure to record the child's age, height, weight, gender, race, and time and dose of the last medications, which are used for interpretation of the test.

Several clinical patterns (phenotypes) of asthma have been noted and can sometimes be identified from the history. Asthma management that specifically addresses a child's clinical pattern is being investigated. Examples of clinical patterns include the following (Howrylak et al., 2014):

- Intermittent asthma is triggered only by a viral respiratory infection. No allergic component exists, and lung function is not impaired. Symptoms are seasonal, matching the timing of increased viral infections. The most effective asthma maintenance treatments do not prevent the viral infection trigger.

- Persistent or chronic asthma presents daily and has year-round symptoms. Most have an allergic component to their disease, such as atopic dermatitis. Viral infections may also trigger symptoms. Airway hyperresponsiveness is present and lung function is affected. Symptom-free days occur only with effective maintenance treatment.

- Seasonal allergic asthma is triggered by inhalant allergens (mold, grasses, other pollens) and cause daily symptoms during that allergy season. Seasonal asthma treatment versus continuous asthma treatment may be an effective strategy.

Asthma may go into remission or increase in severity over time. Asthma severity is categorized by how often the child has symptoms and nighttime awakening, how many days a week a short-acting beta$_2$-agonist (SABA) medication is needed, and how many times a year a child needs oral corticosteroid therapy. Spirometry measurement of lung function is an additional method used to determine asthma severity in children 5 years and older. See Table 20–5 for classification of asthma severity in children. See accompanying *Medications Used to Treat: Asthma*.

TABLE 20–5 Classification of Asthma Severity in Children

ASTHMA SEVERITY	CHARACTERISTICS
Intermittent	Symptoms 2 or fewer days a week
	No nighttime awakenings
	SABA use for symptom control 2 or fewer days a week
	No interference with activity
	Oral corticosteroid use no more than once a year
	Normal FEV$_1$ between exacerbations, FEV$_1$ greater than 80% predicted, FEV$_1$/FVC greater than 85% (5–11 years) or normal (12 years and older)
Mild persistent	Symptoms greater than 2 days a week, but not daily
	Nighttime awakenings 1 to 2 times a month (age under 5 years) or 3 to 4 times a month (5 years and older)
	SABA use for symptom control 2 or more days a week, but not daily
	Minor activity limitation
	Oral corticosteroid use 2 or more times a year
	FEV$_1$ greater than 80% predicted, FEV$_1$/FVC greater than 80% (5–11 years) or normal (12 years and older)
Moderate persistent	Daily symptoms
	Nighttime awakenings 3 to 4 times a month (age under 5 years) or more than once a week but not nightly (5 years and older)
	SABA use for symptom control daily
	Some activity limitation
	Oral corticosteroid use 2 or more times a year
	FEV$_1$ equals 60%–80% predicted, FEV$_1$/FVC equals 70%–80% (5–11 years) or FEV$_1$/FVC reduced more than 5% (12 years and older)
Severe persistent	Symptoms throughout the day
	Nighttime awakening greater than 1 time a week (age under 5 years) or every night (5 years and older)
	SABA use several times a day
	Extremely limited activity
	Oral corticosteroid use 2 or more times a year
	FEV$_1$ less than 60% predicted, FEV$_1$/FVC less than 75% (5–11 years) or FEV$_1$/FVC reduced more than 5% (12 years and older)

Note: SABA = short-acting beta$_2$-agonist; FEV$_1$ = forced expiratory volume in 1 second; FVC = forced vital capacity.

Source: Adapted from National Asthma Education and Prevention Program (NAEPP). (2007). *Expert panel report 3: Guidelines for the diagnosis and management of asthma* (pp. 307–309). Bethesda, MD: National Heart Lung and Blood Institute, National Institutes of Health. Retrieved from http://www.nhlbi.nih.gov/guidelines/asthma

Medications Used to Treat: Asthma

QUICK RELIEF MEDICATIONS, ROUTE, AND ACTION	NURSING MANAGEMENT
Short-acting beta$_2$–agonists (SABA) Albuterol, levalbuterol, pirbuterol *Metered-dose inhaler or nebulizer* Relaxes smooth muscle in airway leading to rapid bronchodilation (within 5–10 min) and mucus clearing. Drug of choice for acute therapy and prevention of exercise-induced bronchospasm.	• Use before inhaled steroid, wait 1–2 min between puffs, wait 15 min to give inhaled steroid. Child should hold breath 10 sec after inspiring. Then rinse mouth and avoid swallowing medication. Use a spacer. • Differences in potency exist, but all products are comparable on a per puff basis. • Dose-related side effects include tachycardia, nervousness, nausea and vomiting, headaches. • Regular use more than 2 days a week for symptom control indicates a loss of control and need for additional therapy.
Corticosteroids Methylprednisolone, prednisone, prednisolone *Oral* Diminishes airway inflammation, secretions, and obstruction; enhances bronchodilating effect of beta$_2$–agonists. Used for acute episodes not fully responsive to beta$_2$–agonists; reduces hospitalization rates.	• Short-term therapy should continue until child achieves 80% peak expiratory flow personal best, or until symptoms resolve. • Give with food to reduce gastric irritation. • Give oral dose in early morning to mimic normal peak corticosteroid blood level. • Assess for potential adverse effects of long-term therapy, such as decreased growth, unstable blood sugar, immunosuppression.
Anticholinergic Ipratropium *Metered-dose inhaler or nebulizer* Inhibits bronchoconstriction and decreases mucus production.	• Not for primary emergency treatment because of 30- to 90-min time of onset. • Rinse mouth afterward to get rid of bitter taste. • Side effects include increased wheezing, cough, nervousness, dry mouth, tachycardia, dizziness, headache, palpitations. • Prevent medication contact with eyes.

DAILY CONTROL MEDICATIONS, ROUTE, AND ACTION	NURSING MANAGEMENT
Long-acting beta$_2$–agonists (LABA) Salmeterol, formoterol *Dry powder inhaler* Relaxes smooth muscle in airway; increases ciliary motility. Used for nocturnal symptoms and prevention of exercise-induced bronchospasm. Used as an add-on therapy.	• Do not use for acute asthma episode. • Take preexercise dose 30–60 min before activity. Do not use additional dose before exercise if already using twice daily doses, which should be 12 hr apart. • Caution against overdosage because side effects such as tachycardia, tremor, irritability, insomnia will last 8–12 hr. • Report failure to respond to usual dose because this may indicate need for stepped-up therapy.
Inhaled corticosteroids (ICS) Beclomethasone, budesonide, flunisolide, fluticasone, mometasone, triamcinolone *Metered-dose inhaler or nebulizer* Anti-inflammatory, controls seasonal, allergic, and exercise-induced asthma; effectively reduces mucosal edema in airways.	• Administer with spacer or holding chamber. • Separate parts and clean inhaler daily. • Rinse mouth and gargle following treatment to remove drug from oropharynx to reduce chance of cough, thrush, and dysphonia. • Prevent eye exposure through proper metered-dose inhaler, nebulizer, or dry powder inhaler (DPI) administration. • Monitor for headache, gastrointestinal upset, dizziness, infection. • Use exactly as prescribed.

Medications Used to Treat: Asthma (*continued*)

Methylxanthines Theophylline *Oral* Relaxes muscle bundles that constrict airways; dilates airway; provides continuous airway relaxation. Used for long-term control; may help reduce need for increased corticosteroid dosages. Less commonly used than inhaled medications because of side effects.	• Do not crush or chew tablet. Give at same time each day. • Maintain therapeutic serum level of 10–20 mcg/L; requires serum level checks and dose adjustment. • Limit caffeine intake. • Side effects include tachycardia, dysrhythmias, restlessness, tremors, seizures, insomnia, hypotension, severe headaches, vomiting, and diarrhea.
Mast cell inhibitors Cromolyn sodium, nedocromil *Metered-dose inhaler or nebulizer* Anti-inflammatory, inhibits activation and release of inflammatory mediators for early and late phase asthma response to allergens and exercise-induced bronchospasm. May be used for unavoidable allergen exposure.	• Do not use at time of symptom development or acute episode. • Must be used up to 4 times a day to be effective. • Therapeutic response seen in 2 weeks, maximum benefit may not be seen for 4–6 weeks. • Adverse reactions include wheezing, bronchospasm, throat irritation, nasal congestion, and anaphylaxis. Immediately report these symptoms to physician.
Leukotriene receptor antagonist (LTRA) Montelukast, zafirlukast *Oral* Reduces inflammation cascade responsible for airway inflammation; improves lung function and diminishes symptoms and need for quick-relief medications.	• Available in granules for infants and chewable tablets for young children. • Administer montelukast in the evening; may be given with food or without. • Make sure child chews montelukast chewable tablet rather than swallowing whole. Granules may be mixed in applesauce or ice cream; do not mix in liquid. • Administer zafirlukast 1 hour before or 2 hr after meal. • Report fever, acute asthma episodes, flulike symptoms, severe headaches or lethargy. • Take as prescribed; do not withdraw abruptly.
Immunotherapy Omalizumab *Subcutaneous* A therapeutic antibody that blocks IgE from causing reactions leading to asthma symptoms.	• Approved for children 12 years and older with moderate or severe persistent asthma. • Injections required every 2–4 weeks based on serum IgE levels. • Be alert for anaphylaxis; it should be administered in a health center prepared to treat anaphylaxis.
Other Hyposensitization (allergy shots) *Subcutaneous* Series of injections with gradual dose increase that can increase the child's tolerance of unavoidable allergens (e.g., mold, pollen).	• May be of value for child with persistent asthma having allergies that can be addressed by immune therapy.

Source: Data from Wilson, B. A., Shannon, M. T., & Shields, K. M. (2016). *Nurse's drug guide 2016.* Hoboken, NJ: Pearson; Taketomo, C. K., Hodding, J. H., & Kraus, D. M. (2014). *Pediatric and neonatal dosage handbook* (21st ed.). Hudson, OH: Lexicomp; Chang, C. (2012). Asthma in children and adolescents: A comprehensive approach to diagnosis and management. *Clinical Reviews in Allergy and Immunology, 43*(1–2), 98–137.

Recommended therapy is tied to asthma severity classification. Clinical therapy includes medications, hydration, education, and support of parents and child. Pharmacologic treatment is matched to the severity of asthma for daily control and for management of acute episodes. The goal is to maintain asthma control long term, using the least amount of medication and reducing the risk for adverse effects.

Clinical Tip

Signs of good control in children during a week include few or no episodes of dyspnea or wheezing during the day or waking the child at night, no interference with normal activity, school, or exercise, and few uses of a short-acting beta$_2$-agonist for symptom control (Nguyen et al., 2014). Various questionnaires to measure asthma control in children have been proposed and studies to validate them are in process.

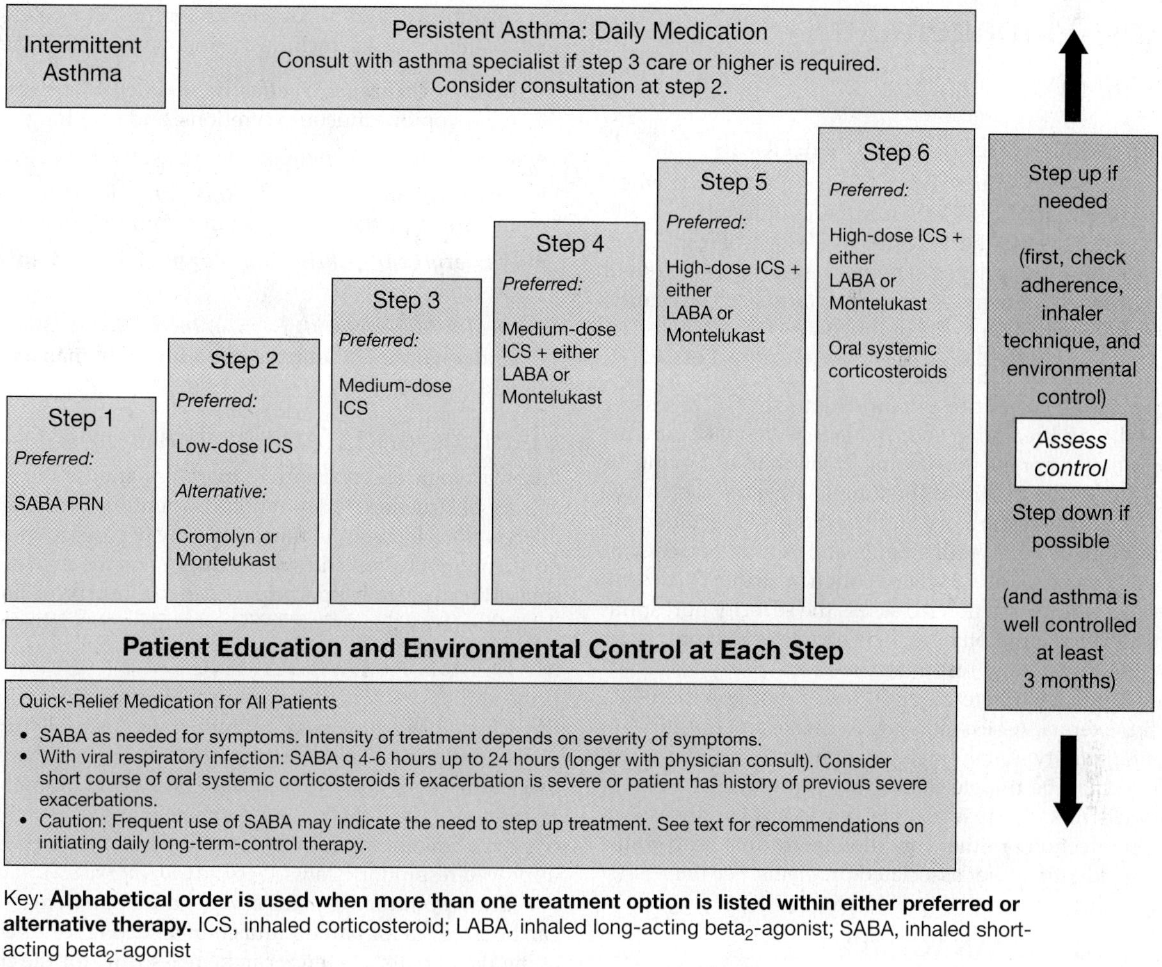

Intermittent Asthma	Persistent Asthma: Daily Medication
	Consult with asthma specialist if step 3 care or higher is required. Consider consultation at step 2.

Step 1

Preferred:

SABA PRN

Step 2

Preferred:

Low-dose ICS

Alternative:

Cromolyn or Montelukast

Step 3

Preferred:

Medium-dose ICS

Step 4

Preferred:

Medium-dose ICS + either LABA or Montelukast

Step 5

Preferred:

High-dose ICS + either LABA or Montelukast

Step 6

Preferred:

High-dose ICS + either LABA or Montelukast

Oral systemic corticosteroids

Step up if needed

(first, check adherence, inhaler technique, and environmental control)

Assess control

Step down if possible

(and asthma is well controlled at least 3 months)

Patient Education and Environmental Control at Each Step

Quick-Relief Medication for All Patients

- SABA as needed for symptoms. Intensity of treatment depends on severity of symptoms.
- With viral respiratory infection: SABA q 4-6 hours up to 24 hours (longer with physician consult). Consider short course of oral systemic corticosteroids if exacerbation is severe or patient has history of previous severe exacerbations.
- Caution: Frequent use of SABA may indicate the need to step up treatment. See text for recommendations on initiating daily long-term-control therapy.

Key: **Alphabetical order is used when more than one treatment option is listed within either preferred or alternative therapy.** ICS, inhaled corticosteroid; LABA, inhaled long-acting beta$_2$-agonist; SABA, inhaled short-acting beta$_2$-agonist

Figure 20–4 Stepwise approach to managing asthma in children 0 to 4 years of age.

SOURCE: From National Asthma Education and Prevention Program. (2007). *Expert panel report 3: Guidelines for the diagnosis and management of asthma* (p. 305). Bethesda, MD: National Institutes of Health, National Heart Lung and Blood Institute. Retrieved from http://www.nhlbi.nih.gov/guidelines/asthma

The main goal of asthma therapy is to manage symptoms and the disorder. Medication therapy and other therapies are divided into six progressive steps intended to match the child's asthma severity. Specific step guidelines are established for different age groups: 0 to 4 years, 5 to 11 years, and 12 years and older. The child's response to therapy is reviewed periodically to determine if medications should be stepped up or down to correspond to the child's symptoms. See Figure 20–4 for the nationally recommended stepwise approach for children aged 0 to 4 years. An asthma action plan is recommended to guide home management of asthma symptoms.

Recommendations for children with persistent asthma include the use of daily inhaled corticosteroids and additional long-term control medications as severity increases. A peak flow meter is often recommended in addition to an asthma management plan to guide the parents and child in treating asthma episodes. Children with intermittent asthma may only need short-acting beta$_2$-agonist. When asthma control is difficult to achieve, the child is referred to an asthma specialist.

Acute Asthma Episodes. Most children with acute exacerbations respond to aggressive management in the emergency department with continuous albuterol by nebulizer, oral systemic corticosteroids, and inhaled ipratropium. Children who do not respond or who are already being managed at home on corticosteroids have a greater chance of hospital admission.

Exercise-Induced Asthma. Up to 70% of children and youth report shortness of breath, wheezing, coughing, difficulty taking a deep breath, noisy breathing, or chest tightness to occur during and after exercise. Pretreatment with a short-acting beta$_2$-agonist 5 to 20 minutes before exercise often prevents exercise-induced asthma and provides relief for 2 to 4 hours (Parsons et al., 2013).

Severe Asthma Episodes. Some asthma episodes do not respond to repeated doses of albuterol and corticosteroids, and progress to potentially life-threatening episodes. The child has increased hypoxemia, decreased expiration due to air trapping, and ineffective ventilation. Respiratory acidosis develops. Children often require treatment in the intensive care unit. Intravenous magnesium sulfate may be added to other medications, such as theophylline and intravenous beta$_2$ agonists, for the acute episode. Heliox (70% helium:30% oxygen or 80% helium:20% oxygen) gas is less dense than supplemental oxygen and causes less airflow resistance in narrowed airways. Ketamine and inhaled anesthetics are used in some critical cases along with assisted ventilation (Wong, Lee, Turner, et al., 2014). A few children progress to respiratory failure and die.

Nursing Management

For the Child With Asthma

Nursing Assessment and Diagnosis

The nurse usually encounters the child and family in the emergency department, health center, or nursing unit. Often, acute care has become necessary because the child's level of respiratory compromise cannot be managed at home. In some cases, the child and family are seen following acute episodes to have education for asthma management at home or in school.

PHYSIOLOGIC ASSESSMENT

Identify the child's current respiratory status first by assessing the ABCs—airway, breathing, and circulation—to make sure the child's condition is not life threatening. If the child is moving air or talking, assess the quality of breathing. Observe the child's color, and assess the respiratory and heart rates. Auscultate the lungs for the quality of breath sounds and for the presence or absence of wheezing. Note whether a cough or stridor is present. Inspect the chest for retractions to assess the severity of respiratory distress. Move on to other aspects of assessment only after finding no life-threatening respiratory distress.

Attach a pulse oximeter; a SpO_2 reading of less than 92% indicates hypoxemia. Assess skin turgor, intake and output, and urine specific gravity. A spirometry reading may be attempted, but the child may be unable to use the spirometer because of respiratory distress. Because asthma symptoms can be associated with an infection or other condition, perform a head-to-toe assessment to identify other associated problems. See the *Assessment Guide* at the beginning of this chapter.

ASSESS ASTHMA MANAGEMENT

Key questions to consider asking parents and older children or adolescents include the following:

- How often in the past month has the child had shortness of breath, coughing, chest tightness, or chest pain during the day? During the night?
- How many times a week does the child need to use rescue medications?
- Have asthma symptoms limited the child's work or play at school or home?
- Which medicines is the child currently taking? How often?
- Have any medication dosages been missed in the last week? How many?
- What are your concerns about the medicines prescribed (e.g., not really needed, side effects, worried about "steroids")?
- Is there any issue with the cost or ability to obtain the medicines?
- Have you tried any other treatments for asthma (e.g., complementary therapies recommended by a healer)?
- Show me how you use your inhaler.

Additionally, several questionnaires have been developed to help health professionals assess an adolescent's asthma control, such as the Asthma Control Test.

PSYCHOSOCIAL ASSESSMENT

Assess the child's anxiety or fear related to the asthma episode or hospitalization. How are parents responding to the current acute episode? Are they anxious, concerned, or frustrated? Do they potentially have concerns about finances, missing work, or other family members at home? Assess whether the child thinks this episode could have been avoided if medications had been used.

Examples of nursing diagnoses for the child experiencing an acute asthma episode include the following (NANDA-I © 2014):

- *Airway Clearance, Ineffective,* related to airway compromise, copious mucous secretions, and coughing
- *Gas Exchange, Impaired,* related to airway obstruction
- *Fluid Volume: Deficient, Risk for,* related to inability to drink adequate fluids when in respiratory distress
- *Anxiety/Fear (Child and Parents)* related to difficulty breathing
- *Health Management, Family, Ineffective,* related to lack of understanding about the need for daily management of a chronic disease

Planning and Implementation

Pharmacologic and supportive therapies are used to reverse the airway obstruction and promote respiratory function. Nursing interventions focus on maintaining airway patency, meeting fluid needs, promoting rest and stress reduction for the child and parents, supporting the family's participation in care, and providing the family with information to enable them to manage the child's disease.

MAINTAIN AIRWAY PATENCY

If the child is exhibiting breathing difficulty, give supplemental humidified oxygen by nasal cannula or face mask. Humidity prevents drying and thickening of mucous secretions. Place the child in a sitting (semi-Fowler) or upright position to promote and ease respiratory effort. Evaluate the effectiveness of positioning and oxygen administration by pulse oximeter and by observing for improved respiratory status. (See the *Clinical Skills Manual* SKILLS.)

The respiratory distress and need for supplemental oxygen can be stressful for parents and child alike (Figure 20–5). Encouraging the parents' presence can be reassuring for the child. Keep the parents informed of procedures and results, and get their input when developing the treatment plan.

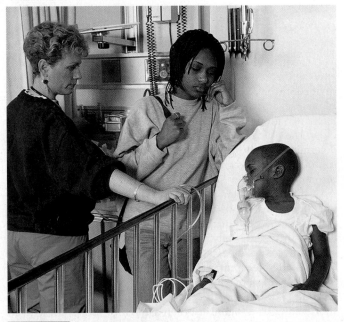

Figure 20–5 An acute asthma episode requires management in the emergency department. The child is placed in a semi-Fowler position to facilitate respiratory effort. Support both the child and parent during these acute episodes. This mother looks exhausted after a sleepless night of caring for her son.

Growth and Development

Metered-dose inhalers (MDIs), nebulizers, and dry powder inhalers (DPIs) are devices used for inhalation therapy. These devices cause special challenges for infants and young children because many devices require cooperation and coordination. The appropriate technique must be taught and reinforced frequently.

- Children over 5 years usually have the ability to use an MDI. Using the closed mouth technique, have the child insert the mouthpiece in the mouth between the teeth and seal the lips. Look straight ahead, and keep the tongue away from the mouthpiece opening. Just as the child starts to breathe, press down on the canister to release the medication. Continue to breathe in slowly through the mouth for at least 5 seconds, and then hold the breath for another 10 seconds. No mist should be seen coming from the mouth after the breath or from the top of the inhaler after actuation, both of which are signs the technique was not good. Teach the child to use an MDI without a spacer, by breathing slowly through a straw.

- Younger children need a spacer with a mask attachment, while other children prefer to use a spacer with the MDI. Select a spacer with a mask for infants and young children that fits from the top of the nose to just under the mouth. The seal should be flexible to prevent an air leak. Crying leads to prolonged exhalation and short inspiration, reducing lung deposition. Use play and distraction to improve cooperation for medication delivery. When use of a spacer or holding chamber is preferred, put the mask on firmly over the nose and mouth or the mouthpiece in the mouth with mouth closed around it. Release a puff of medication and have the child take 4 to 6 quiet deep breaths over 10 seconds. Move the spacer away from the face or mouth, and have the child hold a breath for 10 seconds. Follow this with the second puff. Wash the child's face after using a spacer with a mask. Wash the plastic spacer with household detergent and air dry it to reduce the static charge that can attract medication particles.

- A nebulizer changes liquid medication into aerosol particles. No coordination of breathing is required, making nebulizers easier for young children to use. Nebulizers are not more efficient than MDIs with a spacer, but the outcome may be better since the child can breathe normally. Make sure the nebulizer mouthpiece is sealed by the lips, and mouth breathing is used. If the child cannot coordinate mouth breathing, use a face mask. Nebulizers take 8 to 10 minutes per treatment, so distraction may be needed to improve the cooperation of infants and young children for that duration.

- Dry powder inhalers are activated when the child takes a breath, so puffs do not need to be coordinated with inhalation. No spacer or propellant is used. Children starting at age 5 years may be able to take the rapid, deep, and sustained breath needed to effectively use the device. Children less than 6 years of age who are wheezing may not be able to inspire at a rate fast enough to obtain the optimal amount of medication. Steps for using DPI include the following: Remove the lid, load the dose (puncturing the blister or capsule), fully breathe out away from the device, put the mouthpiece between the lips and teeth, and breathe in deeply and forcefully. Hold the breath for 10 seconds and remove the mouthpiece from the mouth.

- Some MDIs or DPIs have a whistle. It may warn that the inhaled breath is too fast or too shallow, but in other devices, it indicates the breath was adequate. Be sure to inform the child and family about what the whistle on the child's inhaler indicates.

Source: Data from Dinakar, C., & Welch, M. J. (2014). Device how-tos. *Contemporary Pediatrics, 31*(May). Retrieved from http://contemporarypediatrics. modernmedicine.com/contemporary-pediatrics/content/tags/asthma/device-how-tos; Sleath, B., Ayala, G. X., Gillette, C., Williams, D., Davis, S., Tudor, G., . . . Washington, D. (2011). Provider demonstration and assessment of child device technique during pediatric asthma visits. *Pediatrics, 127*(4), 642–648; Asthma Initiative of Michigan for Healthy Lungs. (2011). *How to use a metered-dose inhaler the right way.* Retrieved from http://www.getasthmahelp.org/inhalers_main.asp

Most medications are given by inhalation (Figure 20–6). (See the *Clinical Skills Manual* SKILLS.) The aerosol droplets provide the added benefit of moisture. Continuous nebulizer treatments may be used for some children with severe acute episodes. See *Growth and Development* for considerations in administering medications with inhalation devices. Monitor the child for medication side effects. The frequency of vital sign assessment is determined by the severity of symptoms.

MEET FLUID NEEDS

Fluid therapy is often necessary to restore and maintain adequate fluid balance. Adequate hydration is essential to thin and break up trapped mucous plugs in the narrowed airways. An intravenous infusion may be needed if the child cannot meet fluid needs by mouth, and for administering certain medications and glucose. Monitor the child's intake, output, and specific gravity to avoid overhydration that could lead to pulmonary edema in severe asthma episodes.

As respiratory difficulty diminishes, offer oral fluids slowly. The child's fluid preferences should be determined and choices given where possible. Involve parents to help gain the child's cooperation in taking oral fluids.

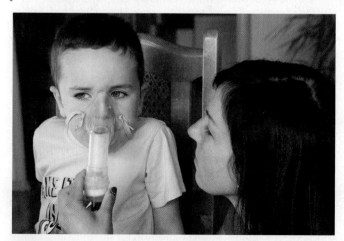

Figure 20–6 **Medications given by inhalation therapy reach the bloodstream rapidly while minimizing the systemic effects. A nebulizer works well for young children because it does not require coordination of breathing with medication inhalation.**

SOURCE: greenland/Shutterstock

Clinical Tip

Iced beverages precipitate bronchospasms in some children with asthma. Offer room-temperature or slightly cooled fluids instead.

PROMOTE REST AND STRESS REDUCTION

The child having an acute asthma episode is usually very tired from prolonged labored breathing when admitted to the nursing unit. Put the child in a quiet room that is accessible for frequent monitoring to promote relaxation and rest. Group tasks to avoid repeatedly disturbing the child.

SUPPORT FAMILY PARTICIPATION

Recognize that parents may be exhausted after spending hours with their child in respiratory distress. Give parents the *option* of assisting with the child's treatments, rather than *expecting* them to help, in addition to comforting the child. Provide frequent updates about the child's condition and encourage the parents to take breaks as needed.

Length of hospitalization depends on the child's response to therapy. Any underlying or accompanying health problem, such as preexisting lung disease or pneumonia, can complicate and extend the child's hospital stay. Communicate with the family of the hospitalized child frequently about the child's condition.

DISCHARGE PLANNING AND HOME CARE TEACHING

Parents need a thorough understanding of asthma—how to prevent asthma episodes and how to follow the child's asthma action plan to manage symptoms. Support of parents and the child should focus on helping them to understand and cope with the diagnosis and the need for daily management to promote near-normal respiratory function while the child continues to grow and develop normally.

Discharge planning for the child with asthma focuses on increasing the family's knowledge about the disease, medication therapy, and the need for follow-up care. Make sure the child receives an appointment with an allergist or asthma specialist if moderate to severe persistent asthma exists. Refer the child and parents to a healthcare provider for more comprehensive education that considers cultural factors for asthma management. See *Developing Cultural Competence: Asthma Disparity Factors.*

COMMUNITY-BASED NURSING CARE

Nurses provide care to children with asthma in pediatricians' offices, specialty asthma clinics, schools, and summer camps. The child's asthma control and management should be assessed at each visit.

Promoting Asthma Management Skills

Review the family's daily plan for monitoring the child's respiratory status. Encourage the school-age child or the parents of younger children to keep a symptom diary that includes peak exploratory flow rate (PEFR) for 2 weeks prior to a health visit as well as all daytime and nighttime symptoms. The Asthma Tracker is one tool a family can use to monitor the young child's asthma symptoms (Nkoy et al., 2013). Evaluate the child's use of the MDI or DPI, and correct the child's technique as needed. Teach the family or review the child's technique about how to measure and interpret peak expiratory flow readings (see *Families Want to Know: Using a Peak Expiratory Flow Meter*).

Clinical Tip

A study revealed that using a peak expiratory flow meter provided parents with an objective measure of the child's asthma symptoms and empowered them to initiate treatment earlier than without the meter. Communication with the child's healthcare provider was more effective when a peak expiratory flow meter was used (Burkhart, Rayens, & Oakley, 2012).

Assess the parent's ability to identify the timing and type of stepped-up care needed to manage worsening symptoms identified on the child's asthma action plan. The asthma action plan

Developing Cultural Competence Asthma Disparity Factors

African American and Hispanic children have a higher prevalence rate for asthma. A major factor may be lower access to high-quality ambulatory care that does not provide education within the cultural beliefs of the family. Other factors associated with the high prevalence rate may include (Kueny, Berg, Chowdhury, et al., 2013):

- Environmental housing conditions (indoor allergen exposure to rodents, molds, and cockroaches)
- Employment options that increase potential introduction of allergens into the home
- Air pollution in urban areas such as nitrogen dioxide from engine exhaust fumes
- Medication beliefs associated with concerns over safety of inhaled corticosteroids and development of tolerance with daily use, or following the advice of healers
- Emotional stress within the home

Identify potential factors contributing to the child's asthma to provide effective education and support to the child and family.

should include the daily control medications, quick-relief medications to take once symptoms of an asthma episode are identified, and when to call the healthcare provider. Identify routines that may improve adherence to daily medication use, such as keeping medications where they will be seen at mealtime. The goal is to bring asthma episodes under control with stepped-up care before emergency care is needed. Reassure the family that most children with asthma can lead a normal life with some modifications.

Healthy People 2020

(RD-6) Increase the proportion of persons with current asthma who receive formal patient education

(RD-7.1) Increase the proportion of persons with current asthma who receive written asthma management plans from their healthcare provider according to National Asthma Education and Prevention Program (NAEPP) guidelines

Refer parents to a local support group to gain additional knowledge and confidence in asthma management. Many hospitals have family resource centers that can assist parents to find helpful information on the Internet.

Child-Focused Education

Engage the child in learning about how the lungs work and what happens when an acute asthma episode occurs. Teach the child how to begin steps toward self-management as appropriate. Encourage the child to ask questions. Provide an activity or coloring book for the child and printed educational materials for the parents. See *Families Want to Know: Home Care for the Child With Asthma* to guide asthma education for the child and family.

Encourage school-age children to assume more responsibility for care, including avoidance of known triggers, early symptom recognition, relaxation breathing, and the proper use of inhaled medication. Help the child learn the early signs of an asthma episode (coughing, breathlessness, or peak expiratory flow meter reading) and to take quick-relief medication before signs become more serious.

Families Want to Know

Using a Peak Expiratory Flow Meter

A peak expiratory flow meter is a useful tool for asthma self-management. It measures the child's ability to push air forcefully out of the lungs. Changes in the peak expiratory flow rate (PEFR) signal worsening lung function and the beginning of an asthma episode. To use a peak expiratory flow meter:

- Set the device at zero or the base level.

- Stand up and take as deep a breath as possible.

- Put the mouthpiece of the meter in the mouth and firmly close the lips around it. Do not cough or let your tongue block the mouthpiece. Blow out as hard and fast as possible over 1 to 2 seconds. To help toddlers learn how to use a peak flow meter, have them practice by blowing into a noisemaker or party favor.

- Write down the reading.

- Repeat the process 2 times and record the highest of the 3 numbers on the chart.

- Measure and record the best PEFR reading twice a day for 2 weeks so the healthcare provider can determine the child's personal best reading. (Make sure the child is optimally treated with medications during the day to obtain the best reading.)

- The physician will use the child's personal best average readings to set the green, yellow, and red color zones to guide treatment in the child's asthma action plan. The child's personal best changes as the child grows taller, so the child's personal best should be measured every year.

- The physician provides guidelines for the child and family to use when monitoring the PEFR. If the child or parent suspects the child might have the onset of breathing difficulty, the peak flow meter can be used. Some children have problems identifying early symptoms of an acute asthma episode onset (increased cough, wheezing, or shortness of breath). The peak flow meter measures the change in how hard the child can blow out air. Using the zones established by the healthcare provider, the child and family can determine what action to take.

- **Green zone**: The PEFR reading is between 80% and 100% of the child's personal best. Air is moving well in the child's lungs. In this case, the child has good asthma control and can continue daily activities. No modification of the treatment plan is needed.

- **Yellow zone**: The PEFR reading is between 50% and 80% of the child's personal best. In this case, the child is developing breathing problems. The parents should follow directions in the child's asthma action plan, which usually involves quick-relief medications. The child should feel better and the PEFR should improve over the next hour. If symptoms and the PEFR do not improve, contact the child's healthcare provider for additional treatment guidance.

- **Red zone**: The PEFR is less than 50% of the child's personal best. In this case, the child has a severe asthma episode and needs urgent treatment with quick-relief medication. Call the child's healthcare provider for additional care guidelines or take the child to the emergency department.

Source: Data from American Academy of Allergy, Asthma, and Immunology (AAAAI). (2014). *Peak flow meter*. Retrieved from http://www.aaaai.org/conditions-and-treatments/library/at-a-glance/peak-flow-meter.aspx; Johns Hopkins Medicine. (2012). *Peak flow measurement*. Retrieved from http://www.hopkinsmedicine.org/healthlibrary/test_procedures/pulmonary/peak_flow_measurement_92,P07755; WebMD. (2012). *Asthma and the peak flow meter*. Retrieved from http://www.webmd.com/asthma/guide/peak-flow-meter

Health Maintenance

Provide routine health promotion and maintenance care, including immunizations. Live virus vaccines may need to be postponed if the child has used oral corticosteroids recently. Carefully monitor the child's growth, especially when the child uses inhaled corticosteroids and episodic oral corticosteroids, which can slow growth and result in reduced adult height by an average of 1.2 cm (0.47 in.) (Kelly et al., 2012).

Assess the child's activity and exercise level, and any symptoms experienced such as chest tightening, wheezing, or shortness of breath. Exercise-induced bronchospasm typically occurs 5 to 10 minutes after stopping the activity and resolves 20 to 30 minutes later. First, make sure the child gets some exercise to improve fitness, and then assess how frequently the child has exercise-induced symptoms. Compare that information to the classification of asthma severity in Table 20–4. Teach the child about the timing of rescue medications before exercise to prevent exercise-induced bronchospasm. Make sure the child uses the daily control and quick-relief medication asthma action plan.

Environmental Control

Reducing allergens in the environment is an important part of asthma management. Focus efforts on reducing molds in the home with lowered humidity and removal of houseplants. When possible, remove pets from the home (especially from the child's bedroom). Dust mites live in the carpets, mattresses, upholstered

Professionalism in Practice Asthma Management by School Nurses

The National School Nurses Association joined eight organizations in a position statement to improve asthma management in school settings. School nurses are encouraged to implement a comprehensive asthma plan for the management of students with asthma in the school setting that includes identifying and monitoring all students with asthma and obtaining their asthma action plans. School nurses are additionally encouraged to collaborate with school officials to adopt and implement an environmental assessment and management plan that addresses environmental asthma triggers (American Lung Association, 2013). See Chapter 10 for more information on nursing care in the school setting.

furniture, bedcovers, soft toys, and clothes. Vacuum carpets and upholstered furniture frequently using a high-efficiency vacuum filter. Buy soft toys that can be washed. Controlling dust mites in the child's bed and bedroom is a high priority. Encase the child's mattress and pillow in plastic covers. Bathe pets frequently to reduce pet dander. Initiate cockroach eradication. Smoke from cigarettes, wood stoves, and fireplaces should be eliminated when possible. See Chapter 22 for *Families Want to Know: Removing Common Allergens From the Home*.

Families Want to Know

Home Care for the Child With Asthma

Identify current knowledge about the condition and its impact on the child:

- What happens in the lungs during an asthma episode?
- What are the child's early warning signs of an asthma episode?
- What are the child's symptoms (wake up at night, cough a lot)? How does the child respond to them?
- Is the child involved in any exercise activity? If no, why not? Do asthma symptoms occur when the child is exercising?
- Does asthma interfere with social activities or activities with friends?
- What are the child's personal asthma triggers? (Suggest keeping a log of symptoms that occur during the day and night, including when and where, that will help identify triggers [e.g., home, school, outdoors, with exercise].) The symptom diary is very helpful in determining the need for more education or for stepped-up or stepped-down medications.

Set up a schedule for parents to learn asthma management:

- Make sure the parents and child know that asthma is a chronic condition that needs daily management and environmental control to reduce or prevent acute asthma episodes.
- Review the asthma action plan for daily management, quick relief, and when to call the physician or to seek emergency care.
- Assess the child's technique with a peak expiratory flow meter, and correct technique as needed. Discuss when to use the meter and how to interpret and use the results for asthma control. Keep a record of peak flow readings for 2 weeks prior to each health visit.

Review parents' understanding of medication therapy:

- Provide information about medications: name, type of drug, dose, method of administration, expected effect, possible side effects. Make sure families understand that daily control medications help prevent acute asthma episodes; the child will not feel them work like the quick-relief medications. Discuss any concerns the family has about the use of "steroid" medication, and describe how they differ from the anabolic steroids abused by athletes.
- Assess the child's MDI or DPI technique and correct as needed.
- When a nebulizer is used to treat an infant or young child, suggest diversions to promote cooperation during the 8- to 10-minute treatment.

Address associated issues:

- What are the financial considerations of medication cost and lifestyle changes?
- Have arrangements been made for the child to use medications at child care or school?
- Does the child have a medical identification bracelet or tag?
- Would a self-help group or camp experience be helpful for the child?

School Management

Provide a healthcare provider order so the child's asthma symptoms can be treated at school or at child care. The parents should work with school administrators to have an individualized health plan (that includes an asthma action plan) developed so the child can carry a rescue inhaler and medications can be administered, including pretreatment for exercise. Provide a supply of medications to the school or childcare organization. Make sure teachers of young children can help recognize signs of an acute asthma episode and reduce a child's anxiety about going to the nurse for quick-relief medications. Many schools are attempting to improve the environment and reduce asthma triggers.

Clinical Tip

All 50 states and the District of Columbia have legislation that entitles a child with asthma to carry and self-administer asthma medications at school (Allergy and Asthma Network, 2014). Families of children old enough to recognize worsening asthma symptoms and to self-administer rescue medications should make sure the school knows about the state law.

Evaluation

Expected outcomes of nursing care include the following:

- The child recognizes early asthma symptoms and promptly uses quick-relief medications, fluids, and relaxation breathing before severe respiratory distress occurs.

- The child learns to identify and avoid asthma triggers.
- The child and family implement the prescribed daily treatment plan and asthma action plan to reduce the number of asthma episodes the child has.
- The child with a serious asthma episode responds to oxygen, fluids, and medication therapy, avoiding hospital admission.

Cystic Fibrosis

Cystic fibrosis (CF) is a common inherited autosomal recessive disorder of the exocrine glands, leading to physiologic alterations in the respiratory, gastrointestinal, and reproductive systems. The incidence of CF varies by race—1:2500–3500 in non-Hispanic Whites, 1:4000–10,000 in Hispanics, 1:15,000–20,000 in non-Hispanic Blacks, 1:32,000 in Asian Americans, and 1:1500–3970 in Native Americans (Nakano & Tluczek, 2014). Gender is not a factor in disease incidence. Approximately 30,000 children and adults have CF in the United States, and approximately 50% are older than age 18 years. The median life span for individuals with CF is mid-40s (Cystic Fibrosis Foundation [CFF], 2014) (Figure 20–7).

ETIOLOGY AND PATHOPHYSIOLOGY

A gene isolated on the long arm of chromosome 7 directs the function of the transmembrane conductance regulator (*CFTR*), which regulates the hydration of epithelial cells of many body organs. More than 1900 mutations of the *CFTR* gene have been identified, but only 127 of these mutations produce CF symptoms (Nakano & Tluczek, 2014). An estimated 10 million persons in the United States are carriers of a defective *CFTR* gene, and have

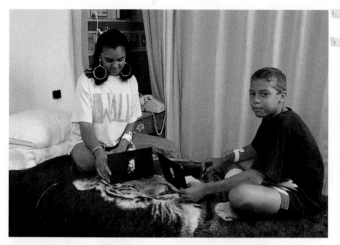

Figure 20–7 Cystic fibrosis is an inherited autosomal recessive disorder of the exocrine glands, so it is not uncommon to see siblings with it such as this brother and sister.

no symptoms (Brashers & Huether, 2014). Disease severity varies by number of symptom-causing *CFTR* mutations. Children with more severe CF have 2 symptom-causing *CFTR* mutations (Nakano & Tluczek, 2014).

With a defective CFTR protein, chloride-ion transport across the exocrine and epithelial cells is impaired and increased sodium absorption reduces water movement across cell membranes. Secretions become thickened in the sweat ducts, the airways, pancreas, intestine, bile ducts, and vas deferens. The small airways in the lungs become clogged with thickened mucus that can harbor bacteria. The lubricating layer between the airway epithelium and mucus inhibits normal ciliary action and cough clearance.

Air becomes trapped in the small airways, leading to hyperinflation, atelectasis, and secondary respiratory infections. Even with antibiotics and a good response, over time the airways develop chronic bacterial and fungal colonization and **bronchiectasis** (a persistent abnormal dilation of the bronchi), followed by respiratory failure. Pneumothorax and hemothorax may occur in older children. The rate of disease progression is related to disease severity.

Obstructions in the pancreatic ducts impede the natural enzyme flow that enables the body to digest fats, fat-soluble vitamins, and proteins. Nutritional deficits may cause failure to thrive. As the child ages, the pancreas may stop producing sufficient insulin, leading to glucose intolerance and the development of cystic fibrosis–related diabetes mellitus.

Failure to secrete enough chloride and fluid into intestines causes meconium ileus (a small bowel obstruction in newborns), affecting 15% of newborns with CF (Henderson et al., 2012). Older children may have intermittent and recurrent episodes of partial small bowel obstruction that can progress to total obstruction, abdominal distention, and vomiting. Chronic inflammation may occur in the intestines, leading to the development of Crohn disease. In rare cases, children with CF develop liver disease.

TABLE 20–6 Clinical Manifestations of Cystic Fibrosis

PATHOPHYSIOLOGY	CLINICAL MANIFESTATIONS
UPPER RESPIRATORY	
Clogged sinuses	Nasal polyps
	Chronic sinusitis, frontal headaches, purulent nasal discharge, postnasal discharge
LOWER RESPIRATORY	
Reduced ciliary clearance; obstructed airways; air trapping and hyperinflation; bacterial colonization	Chronic moist, productive cough; wheezing; coarse crackles
Chronic fibrotic lung changes	Frequent infections
	Shortness of breath, decreased exercise tolerance
	Barrel chest
	Clubbing of fingers and toes (Figure 20–8)
PANCREAS	
Damaged pancreatic ducts obstruct enzymes needed for digestion	Poorly digested food
Produced enzymes damage the pancreas, leading to inadequate insulin secretion	Vitamin A, D, E, and K deficiencies
	Poor weight gain or failure to thrive; delayed onset of puberty
	CF-related diabetes mellitus
GASTROINTESTINAL	
Thickened intestinal secretions and decreased gut mobility	Meconium ileus at birth
Obstructed bile ducts	Abdominal distention
	Greasy, bulky stools (steatorrhea) that are frothy, foul smelling, and floating
	Constipation or intestinal obstruction
	Rectal prolapse
	Liver cirrhosis
REPRODUCTIVE	
Males—absence of vas deferens, low sperm count	Males—infertility
Females—thick vaginal discharge and decreased cervical secretions	Females—may have difficulty conceiving
SWEAT GLANDS	
Excess chloride and sodium electrolyte loss in the sweat	Salty sweat
	Salt depletion, hyponatremia

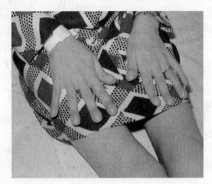

Figure 20–8 Digital clubbing, enlargement of the distal phalanges, occurs in children with cystic fibrosis because of chronic fibrotic changes within the lungs.

The imbalances created by excessive electrolyte loss through perspiration, saliva, and mucous secretion alter metabolic function. These children are at risk for hyponatremic dehydration secondary to electrolyte imbalance.

CLINICAL MANIFESTATIONS
One of the first signs of CF is that newborns fail to pass meconium in the first few days of life. Parents may notice a salty taste to the skin of their infant. Other primary symptoms are associated with thick, sticky mucus. See Table 20–6.

CLINICAL THERAPY
Cystic fibrosis is usually diagnosed in infancy. Newborn screening is performed (in all 50 states and the District of Columbia) on dried blood samples to measure pancreatic enzyme immunoreactive trypsinogen (IRT) concentrations, which are high in newborns with CF. If the reading is high, a second IRT concentration test is performed in 2 to 3 weeks. Some states perform a DNA analysis for the most common *CFTR* mutations on the same blood sample if the second IRT concentration is high. Newborn screening is positive if the IRT is elevated and DNA analysis identifies one or more *CFTR* mutations (Nakano, & Tluczek, 2014).

A sweat chloride test by pilocarpine iontophoresis, the gold standard for diagnosis of CF, is performed if the newborn screening is positive or if a *CFTR* mutation is found (Figure 20–9). A chloride concentration of 60 mEq/L or higher is diagnostic for all age groups. A sweat chloride concentration of 30 to 59 mEq/L in infants less than 6 months old or a concentration between 40 to 59 mEq/L for children and adults is suspicious. If suspicious, a repeat sweat chloride test or DNA analysis for additional *CFTR* mutations maybe performed. Genetic testing is also available for adults with a positive family history, partners of individuals with CF, and couples seeking prenatal testing to identify carriers of CF gene mutations.

A spirometer is used to monitor pulmonary function in children 6 years and older (see *Clinical Tip* on spirometry testing in the section on asthma). Forced vital capacity (FVC) and forced expiratory volume in 1 second (FEV$_1$) readings are taken. Sputum cultures are obtained to identify infectious organisms and antibiotic sensitivities.

Clinical therapy focuses on maintaining respiratory function, managing infections, promoting optimal nutrition and exercise, and preventing gastrointestinal blockage (Table 20–7). Newly diagnosed children without symptomatic lung disease are aggressively treated to slow the development of inflammation, chronic respiratory infections, reduction in pulmonary function, and to improve nutrition and support growth.

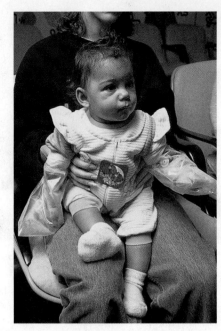

Figure 20–9 This 6-month-old girl is being evaluated for cystic fibrosis using the sweat chloride test.

Treatment is focused on controlling inflammation of the airways, treating infection, and on reducing mucus accumulation. Various devices and airway clearance techniques are used regularly to reduce the accumulation of mucus in the lungs, such as chest physiotherapy, forced expiratory technique (huffing), oscillating positive expiratory pressure, and high-frequency chest wall oscillation. Chest physiotherapy is often performed on infants and young children, but older children can learn to use other airway techniques independently.

Frequent prolonged courses of antibiotics for infections may be prescribed to improve pulmonary function, exercise tolerance, and quality of life. Sputum culture results and sensitivities help guide the selection of the specific antibiotics. Children with *Pseudomonas aeruginosa* or *Burkholderia cepacia* infections have a poorer outcome. Medications are used to reduce sputum viscosity and to dilate the airways. Anti-inflammatory treatment is sometimes prescribed. Vitamins and pancreatic enzymes are also provided to improve the child's nutritional status. A new medication, ivacaftor (Kalydeco), has been approved only for children 6 years and older who have the G551D *CFTR* mutation. See the following *Medications Used to Treat: Cystic Fibrosis.*

Collaborative care by healthcare providers including physicians, nurses, respiratory therapists, and nutritionists has resulted in improved medical management and nutrition that prolongs the lives of children and adults with CF. However, new complications such as CF-related diabetes (often with insulin insufficiency and insulin resistance) that develops in 20% of adolescents must be carefully managed along with the progression of the disease (see Chapter 30) (Delaney & Windemuth, 2014). CF-related diabetes is difficult to manage because the child needs a large caloric intake that must be balanced by insulin dosage.

End-stage lung disease from cystic fibrosis is the third most common reason for a lung transplant in the United States. About 67.8% of cases survive 1 year, 60% survive 5 years, and 43% survive 10 years (Dorgan & Hadjiliadis, 2014). Persons infected with *Burkholderia cepacia* have a lower rate of survival, making them ineligible for transplant at many centers. Respiratory failure from end-stage lung disease is the cause of death in most patients with cystic fibrosis.

Medications Used to Treat: Cystic Fibrosis

MEDICATIONS AND ACTIONS	NURSING MANAGEMENT
Beta$_2$–adrenergic receptor agonist bronchodilators *Aerosol* Used for airway hyperresponsiveness; may help prevent bronchospasm associated with inhaled therapies.	• Use before airway clearance procedure. Have the child hold the breath 10 sec after inhalation. • Avoid swallowing the medicine, and rinse the mouth afterward.
Dornase alpha (DNAse or Pulmozyme) [*a lfa-recombinant DNA*] *Aerosol* Loosens, liquefies, and thins pulmonary secretions to reduce exacerbations.	• Keep refrigerated until placed in the nebulizer. • Monitor for improvement in dyspnea and mucus clearance.
Hypertonic saline (7%) *Aerosol* Hydrates the airway mucus and stimulates coughing to improve lung function and reduce exacerbations.	• Use following a bronchodilator.
Ivacaftor (Kalydeco) *Oral* Promotes chloride ion transport and improves regulation of salt and water absorption and secretion in the tissues (Taketomo, Hodding, & Kraus, 2014). Only for children with G551D *CFTR* mutation.	• Monitor child's hepatic enzyme levels; hold medication if levels are significantly elevated. • Administer with high-fat foods. • Do not eat grapefruit or Seville oranges while taking medication.
Ibuprofen *Oral* Can slow the progression of lung pulmonary function decline (Mogayzel et al., 2013).	• Educate the child and parents to monitor for signs of gastrointestinal bleeding. • Ensure that the child does not take aspirin or other NSAIDs unless approved by healthcare provider.
Antibiotics (e.g., tobramycin, azithromycin, aztreonam, and others identified by culture sensitivity) *Aerosol, oral, or IV* Used to treat and suppress infections.	• Higher doses than normal and prolonged courses may be prescribed. • Teach the child and family to develop a schedule to give the correct dose at appropriate intervals.
Pancreatic enzyme supplements (Cotazym-S, Pancrease, Viokase) *Oral* Assists in digestion of nutrients decreasing fat and bulk.	• Given prior to food ingestion. • Ensure that enzymes are taken with meals and snacks.
Vitamins (A, D, E, and K) and antioxidants (selenium, zinc, and ascorbate) *Oral* Supplements vitamins not produced.	• Ensure that vitamins are prescribed in non–fat-soluble form to promote absorption. • Give twice a day.

Nursing Management

For the Child With Cystic Fibrosis

Care of the child with previously diagnosed CF is the focus of the following discussion.

Nursing Assessment and Diagnosis

PHYSIOLOGIC ASSESSMENT

Physical assessment of the child focuses on respiratory function. Inquire about the frequency and characteristics of the child's cough and sputum. Compare this information with the child's baseline. Changes in the cough may be more important than its presence or absence related to the development of a new infection. Auscultate the chest for breath sounds, crackles, and wheezes. Note any cyanosis or clubbing of the extremities. Obtain SpO$_2$ and spirometry readings if changes in respiratory status are suspected.

Determine if the child is maintaining an appropriate growth pattern by plotting the weight, height, and body mass index on a growth curve. Children with significantly lower percentiles for height and weight should be considered malnourished. Inquire about the child's appetite and dietary intake. Ask how nutritional supplements, pancreatic enzymes, and

TABLE 20–7 Clinical Therapy for Cystic Fibrosis

CLINICAL THERAPY	RATIONALE
RESPIRATORY THERAPY	
Exercise and physical fitness	Promotes maintenance of lung function.
Airway clearance techniques—chest physiotherapy twice a day for all lung segments (percussion or vibration with the child positioned to promote sputum drainage), oscillating chest vests, or other expiratory techniques	Helps secretions move to bronchi from smaller airways. Coughing and breathing airway clearance techniques help expel secretions.
Immunizations	Prevents viral and some bacterial infections.
Chest tube drainage of air leaks	Resolves pneumothorax.
Thoracoscopy to sew over ruptured alveoli	Repairs area of recurrent pneumothorax and prevents future episode in same location.
Lung transplantation	Reverses respiratory failure.
GASTROINTESTINAL TRACT THERAPY	
Acid suppression therapy	Gastroesophageal reflux worsens lung function; enteric coating of enzyme supplements is affected by high acid content in duodenum.
Hyperosmolar enemas, isotonic fluid lavage of the intestines (oral or by nasogastric tube)	Enema relieves meconium ileus in most infants; fluid lavage reduces distal intestinal obstruction.
NUTRITION	
Well-balanced, high-calorie, high-fat diet	Promotes essential nutrient balance for health, growth, weight maintenance, and increased lung capacity and survival.
Pancreatic enzyme supplements	Promotes digestion of fats and proteins.

vitamins are used. Observe the adolescent for the appearance of secondary sex characteristics, which are often delayed because of nutritional status.

Assess the child's stooling pattern. Identify whether the child has problems with abdominal pain or bloating, and whether these problems can be related to eating, stooling, or other activities. Palpate the abdomen for liver size, fecal masses, and evidence of pain.

PSYCHOSOCIAL ASSESSMENT

The emotional stress of this chronic disease may not be readily apparent, particularly if the child's symptoms are mild and not imminently life threatening. Ongoing observation of child and parent behaviors helps direct nursing interventions. Parents may feel guilt as carriers of the disease. Siblings may also show signs of difficulty in dealing with the illness, particularly if not affected by the disease. Siblings with CF may be affected if the child is showing signs of significant deterioration, being forced to acknowledge their own future course with the disease.

Ask parents how the child's illness has affected day-to-day functioning, potential conflicts with family activities, and how they have adapted to the child's plan of care. Investigate the need for respite care. Ask what the parents have told the child and siblings about the disease. What questions have the child and siblings asked about CF, and how have parents answered them? Has the child ever asked about the life expectancy of someone with CF? If not, what would parents say if asked?

Common nursing diagnoses for the child with CF include the following (NANDA-I © 2014):

- *Airway Clearance, Ineffective,* related to thick mucus in lungs
- *Nutrition, Imbalanced: Less than Body Requirements,* related to need for increased calories to meet growth and metabolic needs

- *Infection, Risk for,* related to the presence of mucous secretions conducive to bacterial growth
- *Role Conflict, Parental,* related to interruptions in family life due to the home care regimen and child's frequent exacerbations

Planning and Implementation

Nursing management involves supporting the child and family initially, when the diagnosis is made, during subsequent hospitalizations, and during visits to specialty and primary healthcare providers. The nurse's role begins with implementing specific medical therapies and providing nursing care to meet the child's physiologic and psychosocial needs. Airway clearance techniques, medications, and nutrition must be coordinated to promote optimal body function. Psychosocial support and reinforcement of the child's daily care needs are important in preparation for home care.

Children with CF require periodic hospitalization when a severe infection occurs or for a pulmonary and nutritional assessment. The child is often placed in a private room with standard precautions to reduce the spread of infectious organisms. Children with CF are not roomed together to reduce the risk for transmission of *Pseudomonas aeruginosa* and *Burkholderia cepacia* between them.

Respect the parents' experiences as the child's primary care provider and include them in the child's routine care as much as possible. However, parents may view the hospital stay as a break from the rigorous daily pulmonary routine at home and need support to take advantage of the respite. While the family is often proficient at providing physical care to the child, the nurse should take the opportunity to review basic and new information about airway clearance techniques, medications, and nutrition. This is especially important as the child matures and begins to assume some self-care responsibilities.

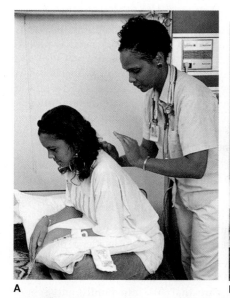
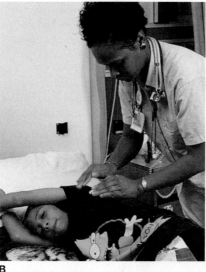
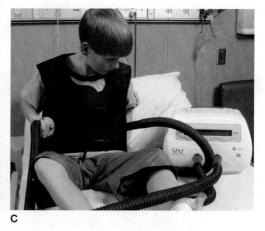

A **B** **C**

Figure 20–10 Chest physiotherapy with postural drainage can be achieved by clapping with a cupped hand on the chest wall over the segment to be drained to create vibrations that are transmitted to the bronchi to dislodge secretions. *A*, If the obstruction is in the posterior apical segment of the lung, the nurse can do this with the child sitting up. *B*, If the obstruction is in the left posterior segment, the child should be lying on the right side. Several other positions can be used depending on the location of the obstruction. *C*, A high-frequency chest wall oscillation vest is another option for airway clearance that the child can independently manage.

PROVIDE RESPIRATORY THERAPY

Chest physiotherapy or an alternate airway clearance technique is usually performed 1 to 3 times per day to facilitate the removal of secretions from the lungs. (See the *Clinical Skills Manual* SKILLS .) Perform this before meals because coughing may stimulate vomiting. Aerosol treatments with a bronchodilator, as well as DNAse and hypertonic saline to help thin respiratory secretions, may precede the airway clearance procedure. Respiratory therapists and nurses often collaborate in teaching parents and other family members the skills for these necessary treatments. Some children use an oscillating vest for 30 minutes twice a day rather than chest physiotherapy (Figure 20–10).

ADMINISTER MEDICATIONS AND MEET NUTRITIONAL NEEDS

Antibiotics for acute exacerbation are provided by oral, inhalation, and intravenous routes. Because children with CF have an increased clearance of most antibiotics, they need higher doses and longer treatment courses, often for at least 14 days until the child achieves the best possible lung function. Serum antibiotic drug levels may be ordered to ensure therapeutic dosing; however, monitor renal function tests to detect problems related to higher antibiotic dosages. In some cases, a portacath or peripherally inserted central catheter (PICC) line is placed so that IV antibiotics can be given at home.

Digestive problems can be eased with pancreatic enzymes and dietary modification. Pancreatic enzyme supplements come in powder sprinkles and capsule form and are taken orally with all meals and large snacks. The amount needed is individualized based on the child's nutritional needs and digestive response to these supplements. Help families identify any foods that contribute to a child's gastrointestinal problems. The goal is to achieve near-normal, well-formed stools and adequate weight gain.

Fat-soluble vitamins (A, D, E, and K) are not completely absorbed from food; therefore, they must be taken in water-soluble form. Multivitamins taken twice daily usually are sufficient to prevent deficiency.

Respiratory complications and a higher metabolic rate make additional calories essential. Some children and youth need supplemental nasogastric or gastrostomy feedings to gain and maintain weight. The diet should be well balanced, with an emphasis on high caloric value and high-fat content. Salt is also needed in the diet.

PROVIDE PSYCHOSOCIAL SUPPORT

Help the parents and child learn what they must do to maintain health after discharge. Emotional support is essential because the diagnosis of CF creates anxiety and fear in both the parents and the child. They need assistance with emotional and psychosocial issues relating to discipline, body image (stooling odor, barrel chest), frequent rehospitalization, the potential terminal nature of the illness, the child's feeling of being different from friends, and overall financial, social, and family concerns. Because CF is inherited, families may have more than one child with CF. Refer families to genetic counseling and support groups.

DISCHARGE PLANNING AND HOME CARE TEACHING

The financial burden of medications, supplies, and medical follow-up may not be recognized immediately by a family overwhelmed by the diagnosis. Initially, parents need assistance in obtaining necessary equipment. If the parents require financial assistance, refer them to social services and the Cystic Fibrosis Foundation. Home care of the child with CF is expensive and can impact the family's finances.

COMMUNITY-BASED NURSING CARE

Nurses may encounter the child with CF in specialty clinics, health centers, and schools. Use the assessment guidelines found earlier in this chapter to assess the child. Observe the child's physical appearance, noting overall body proportions and any changes characteristic of CF. Respiratory function tests are usually performed every 6 months during CF visits. Assess hearing acuity on a regular basis, especially if the antibiotic tobramycin is used.

A psychosocial assessment is especially important when the child is going through major developmental stages. School-age children and adolescents are often embarrassed at being viewed as different from peers. Ask how the child or adolescent feels about the need to consume such a large amount of food, to take medications, and to follow the daily respiratory care routine.

Review the child's airway clearance technique. If additional short-term therapies are prescribed to help improve pulmonary status, educate the child and family about the techniques to use and help them identify the best time to fit the additional treatment into the daily schedule. Having to do the chest physiotherapy regimen 3 or 4 times a day has a significant impact on family time. Alternate airway clearance therapy techniques, such as a vest, huffing, or oscillating positive expiratory pressures, may be more easily accepted by the family, especially since the parent does not have to physically perform the percussion and vibration. Daily aerobic exercise is recommended to promote airway clearance and overall health.

Managing the child's nutrition is important and takes time and energy. Refer the parents to a nutritionist to customize a meal plan for the child's caloric needs. Despite the child's voracious appetite, parents may have difficulty getting the child with CF to eat enough calories for optimal nutrition and growth. Parents need suggestions for preparing calorie-dense meals and snacks. A gastrostomy tube for nighttime feeding may be needed when the child's weight is 85% to 90% of ideal for height. Children with adequate nutrition have a longer life expectancy.

Clinical Tip

Use of cream or half and half added to soups, casseroles, and puddings; cream cheese spread on breads, muffins, and crackers; sour cream added to casseroles; and powdered milk added to regular milk, meatloaf, and custards are all ways to increase the calories in food eaten. Adolescents should have high-calorie snacks they can store in their school locker to eat before after-school activities.

Children with CF lose more than normal amounts of salt in their sweat, especially during hot weather, strenuous exercise, and fever. During periods of exercise and increased sweating, encourage the child to drink more fluids and increase salt intake. Allow the child to add extra salt to food and permit some salty snacks (pretzels with salt, pickles, carbonated soda). Teach parents to recognize early symptoms of salt depletion, including fatigue, weakness, abdominal pain, and vomiting, and to contact the child's healthcare provider if these symptoms occur.

Gradual assumption of responsibility for daily disease management is necessary and may be challenging if the child rebels or is defiant regarding therapy. Individualize the child's daily care regimen to facilitate time for interaction with peers and participation in school activities. Link adolescents to vocational service planning programs to help plan for their future. Initiate palliative care planning when the child's disease progresses toward respiratory failure.

Adolescents with CF need special assistance in coping with their disorder, especially since the median survival is now more than 40 years. Help them identify normal adolescent changes versus those related to CF. Discuss ways to cope with the difference they know exists between themselves and peers. They need to develop normal relationships and establish intimacy with a partner. Information about potential infertility must be provided along with the guidelines for safe sexual practices to reduce the risk for sexually transmitted infections. Females with CF may be able to conceive and should be offered contraception.

Evaluation

Expected outcomes of nursing care include the following:

- The child and family develop proficiency in providing the daily pulmonary care and reducing the incidence of respiratory infections.
- The child and family develop a schedule and routine for daily pulmonary care that fits into family and school activities.
- The child consumes adequate calories and pancreatic enzymes to support growth and to stay within desirable weight ranges.
- The child and family cope effectively with the child's disease.

Injuries of the Respiratory System

Airway compromise after an injury to the respiratory system can cause death if not managed quickly and effectively. Children are vulnerable to changes in respiratory function after injury because their airway is small and can become easily obstructed. Airway obstruction can be caused by the tongue, small amounts of blood, mucus, or foreign debris, and swelling in the respiratory tract or adjacent neck tissue, leading to hypoxia. If the child's neck is flexed or hyperextended, the soft laryngeal cartilage may also compress and obstruct the airway.

Smoke-Inhalation Injury

Exposure of the child's face and airway to smoke or extreme heat leads to dramatic responses in the child's respiratory tract. Smoke and heat increase the child's risk for airway obstruction, carbon monoxide poisoning, acute respiratory distress syndrome, late complications such as pneumonia, and death. The child's higher respiratory rate also increases exposure to noxious chemicals.

The severity of the smoke-inhalation injury is influenced by the type of material burned and is more severe if the child was found in a closed space. Smoke, a product of the burning process that is composed of gases and particles, such as cyanide from synthetic materials, is generated in varying volumes and density. The type and concentration of toxic gases, which are usually invisible, affect the severity of pulmonary damage. The duration of exposure to the smoke and toxic gases contributes significantly to the child's prognosis.

Exposure to extreme heat, common in house fires, leads to surface injury and upper airway damage. The upper airway normally removes heat from inhaled gases, sparing the lower airway from thermal damage. Airway edema develops rapidly over a few hours and potentially leads to acute respiratory distress syndrome.

Carbon monoxide (CO) is a clear, colorless, odorless, and tasteless gas that develops as a fire consumes oxygen or from poorly ventilated heating systems. The CO molecule binds more firmly to hemoglobin than does oxygen. As a result, reduced amounts of oxygen in the blood rapidly produce tissue hypoxia in the child. The brain receives inadequate oxygen, resulting in confusion and progressing to loss of consciousness. This is one reason fire victims have difficulty escaping. The process can be rapidly reversed by the timely administration of 100% oxygen, if provided before hypoxia becomes too severe (Hampson, Piantadosi, Thom, et al., 2012).

Damage to the lower airway often results from chemical or toxic gas inhalation. Soot carried deeply into the lungs combines with water to deposit acid-producing chemicals on the lung tissue. These acids burn the tissue and destroy the cilia and surfactant. Tissue destruction, pulmonary edema, and disrupted gas exchange are the initial insult to the lungs. Days later, the damaged tissue sloughs off, obstructing the airways. The lungs become a breeding ground for microorganisms, leading to pneumonia. Healing leaves scars in the damaged alveoli that can reduce future lung function.

Clinical manifestations of inhalation injury associated with fire include burns of the face and neck, singed nasal hairs, soot around the mouth or nose, and hoarseness with stridor or voice change, even when the child initially has no respiratory distress. Edema develops rapidly over a few hours and may lead to airway obstruction with signs such as tachypnea, stridor, coughing, and wheezing. Respiratory distress develops and can lead to respiratory failure. If carbon monoxide poisoning is present, the child may have headache, dizziness, confusion, shortness of breath, and loss of consciousness.

Diagnosis is based on history of smoke exposure in a closed area, and physical signs of soot around the nose and mouth. Arterial blood gases and a carboxyhemoglobin level are obtained. The child with minimal signs and symptoms when seen in the emergency department may be admitted to monitor for progression of respiratory distress. Initial treatment is 100% humidified oxygen. If respiratory distress develops, aggressive airway management with endotracheal tube insertion and monitoring are provided in the PICU. Mechanical ventilation and high concentration oxygen may be necessary. Chest physiotherapy and suctioning may be provided in an effort to keep the airway clear. All other injuries sustained in the fire are treated.

Nursing Management

Assess the child for the development of respiratory distress. Check vital signs frequently, and monitor the SpO_2. Auscultate the lungs for crackles, wheezes, and decreased breath sounds. Assess for level of consciousness and behavior changes that could indicate increasing hypoxia.

Provide oxygen as ordered. Position the child to promote respiratory function. If the child's condition deteriorates, assist with procedures to secure the child's airway and prepare the child for transfer to the ICU. Assess the family's response to the life-threatening crisis and offer support with information about the child's condition (see Chapter 13).

Blunt Chest Trauma

Blunt chest trauma in infants and toddlers is most often due to motor vehicle crashes and abuse. Bicycles, scooters, skateboards, and skates are more commonly associated with blunt chest trauma in school-age children. Injuries from high-energy motor vehicle crashes more commonly occur in adolescents. Chest injuries may not be obvious and can be extremely difficult to evaluate.

Most children who die after sustaining severe blunt chest trauma were hypoxic because of poor airway and ventilatory control. A child's elastic, pliable chest wall and thin abdominal muscles provide minimal protection to underlying organs. This elasticity of the ribs often prevents rib fractures in children less than 12 years of age, but the energy from blunt trauma is transferred directly to the internal organs. A pulmonary contusion or pneumothorax may result.

Pulmonary Contusion

A pulmonary contusion is defined as bruising damage to the tissues of the lung that often results from the transfer of energy from a strong blow to the chest. It often occurs without rib fracture. The lung tissue is indirectly injured, causing capillaries to bleed into the alveoli. Edema develops in the lower airways. The blood and fluid from damaged tissues accumulate over a couple of days and may interfere with gas exchange. Acute respiratory distress syndrome and long-term respiratory dysfunction may result.

The child may initially appear asymptomatic if it is an isolated injury. With a large pulmonary contusion the child may develop respiratory distress, along with fever, wheezing, hemoptysis, and crackles over several hours. Careful observation is required during the first 12 hours after the injury to detect decreased perfusion related to ventilatory impairment.

Chest radiographs or computed tomography may be diagnostic for a pulmonary contusion several hours after the injury. Therapy includes supplemental oxygen, pain control, incentive spirometry, and avoiding prolonged immobilization. Children with severe injury to the lungs will require mechanical ventilation with low airway pressures. Pneumonia is a potential complication.

Nursing Management

Nursing care centers on providing necessary physiologic support, such as oxygen therapy, positioning, incentive spirometry, fluid management, and comfort measures. Observe for hemoptysis, dyspnea, decreased breath sounds, wheezes, crackles, and a transient temperature elevation. Agitation and lethargy can signal increasing hypoxia. Inspect the thorax for symmetric chest wall movement, and auscultate for breath sounds in both lungs. The child may initially appear well but requires careful monitoring to detect signs of deterioration. Children with significant injuries are cared for in the ICU. Some children require ventilator support as the pulmonary tissues heal.

Pneumothorax

A pneumothorax occurs when air enters the pleural space because of a penetrating chest injury or tears in the tracheobronchial tree, the esophagus, or the chest wall. If blood collects in the pleural space, it is called a *hemothorax*, and if blood and air collect, it is called a *pneumohemothorax*. A pneumothorax is one of the more common thoracic injuries in pediatric trauma patients. The three types of pneumothorax are open, closed, and tension.

An *open pneumothorax* results from any penetrating injury that exposes the pleural space to atmospheric pressure, thereby collapsing the lung. A sucking sound may be heard as the air moves through the opening on the chest wall. The child may show signs of restlessness, cyanosis, and subcutaneous emphysema (air leakage in the tissue). Emergency treatment involves placing a water-tight bandage sealed on three sides over the opening to prevent more air from entering the chest during inspiration. The fourth side is left open so accumulated air can escape on expiration. A thoracostomy is performed, and a chest tube is inserted (see the *Clinical Skills Manual* SKILLS). A closed drainage

Pathophysiology Illustrated: **Pneumothorax**

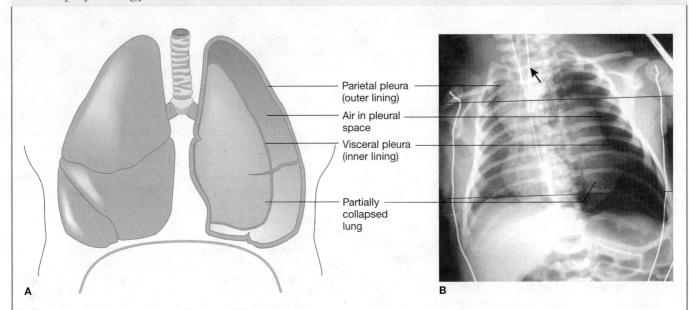

Parietal pleura (outer lining)

Air in pleural space

Visceral pleura (inner lining)

Partially collapsed lung

A

B

A, A pneumothorax is air in the pleural space that causes a lung to collapse. Whether the air results from an open injury or from bursting of alveoli due to a blunt injury, it is important to focus on airway management and maintain lung inflation. *B,* Tension pneumothorax. Note the collapsed lung on the child's left side and the deviation of the child's heart and trachea to the right side of the chest (see arrow).

SOURCE: Courtesy of Dorothy Bulas, MD, Professor of Radiology and Pediatrics, Children's National Medical Center, Washington, DC.

system is attached to remove the air and reinflate the lung by reestablishing negative pressure.

A *closed pneumothorax* is sometimes caused by blunt chest trauma with no evidence of rib fracture (see *Pathophysiology Illustrated: Pneumothorax*). The chest may be compressed against a closed glottis (such as with breath holding), causing a sudden increase in pressure within the thoracic cavity. The pressure increase is transferred to the alveoli, causing them to burst. A single burst alveolus may be able to seal itself off, but the lung collapses when many alveoli are damaged. Breath sounds are decreased or absent on the injured side, and the child is in respiratory distress. A thoracostomy is performed and a chest tube inserted and attached to a closed drainage system.

A *tension pneumothorax* is a life-threatening emergency that results when the air leaks into the chest during inspiration but cannot escape during expiration. Internal pressure continues to build, compressing the chest contents and collapsing the lung. Venous return to the heart is impaired as the mediastinum shifts and the trachea, heart, vena cava, and esophagus are compressed

toward the unaffected lung, leading to decreased cardiac output. Signs of tension pneumothorax include increasing respiratory distress, decreased breath sounds, and paradoxical breathing. Immediate care for a tension pneumothorax is a needle thoracentesis to allow air to escape and relieve the tension. A chest tube is then inserted and attached to a closed drainage system.

Nursing Management

Nursing management focuses on airway management and maintaining lung inflation. The child arrives on the nursing unit with a chest tube and drainage system in place. Continued close observation for respiratory distress is essential. Carefully monitor vital signs. When the chest tube is removed, the site is covered with an occlusive dressing and the child's respiratory status is monitored for signs of respiratory distress. Complications include hemothorax (if the thoracostomy and chest tube are improperly placed), lung tissue injury, and scarring from poor tube placement (especially if the tube is placed too near the breast in girls).

Chapter Highlights

- Respiratory conditions are a leading cause of hospitalization for all children between 1 and 19 years of age.

- The child's airway is shorter and narrower than an adult's, increasing the risk for obstruction. The lungs have no muscles; the diaphragm and intercostal muscles power ventilation.

- Foreign-body aspiration is a major health problem for infants and toddlers, often related to their increasing mobility and tendency to put small objects such as food and small toy parts in their mouths.

- Signs of impending respiratory failure in infants and children include worsening respiratory distress, irritability, lethargy, mottled color or cyanosis, diaphoresis, and increased respiratory effort such as dyspnea, tachypnea, nasal flaring, grunting, and retractions.

- An apparent life-threatening event (ALTE) is an episode of apnea accompanied by a color change (e.g., cyanosis or pallor), limp muscle tone, choking, or gagging in an infant less than 12 months of age.

- Obstructive sleep apnea syndrome (OSAS) in children is commonly caused by enlarged tonsils and adenoids. Children snore loudly and have labored breathing during sleep.

- Sudden infant death syndrome (SIDS) is a leading cause of death in infants. Onset of the fatal episode occurs during sleep and remains unexplained after a thorough investigation, including an autopsy, a review of the circumstances of death, and the clinical history.

- Laryngotracheobronchitis (LTB) is a viral croup syndrome with signs of an upper respiratory illness, hoarseness, tachypnea, inspiratory stridor, and a seal-like barking cough. Fever may or may not be present.

- Epiglottitis is a bacterial infection that can cause a life-threatening airway obstruction. It is commonly prevented by the pneumococcal vaccine. Classic signs include dysphonia, dysphagia, drooling, and distressed respiratory effort.

- Respiratory syncytial virus (RSV) is the most common cause of bronchiolitis, a lower respiratory tract infection that causes inflammation and obstruction of the bronchioles.

- Symptoms of pneumonia in infants and children include elevated temperature, rales, crackles, wheezes, cough, dyspnea, tachypnea, restlessness, and decreased breath sounds if consolidation occurs.

- Children under 2 years are at increased risk for developing active tuberculosis, including tubercular meningitis and disseminated TB.

- Chronic lung disease or bronchopulmonary dysplasia (BPD) usually develops in neonates with a birth weight of 1000 g (2.2 lb) or less. Treatment with oxygen and positive-pressure ventilation causes inflammation and damages the bronchioles, resulting in fibrosis, edema of the bronchioles, and smooth muscle hypertrophy.

- An asthma episode results from inflammation and a stimulus causing excessive mucus formation, mucosal swelling, and airway muscle contraction, leading to airway obstruction.

- In cystic fibrosis, defective chloride-ion transport across the exocrine and epithelial cell walls results in an abnormal accumulation of viscous, dehydrated mucus that affects the respiratory, gastrointestinal, and reproductive systems.

- Signs of smoke-inhalation injury in children include burns of the face and neck, singed nasal hairs, soot around the mouth or nose, and hoarseness with stridor or voice change.

- A pneumothorax may become life threatening when air leaking into the chest cavity during inspiration cannot escape during expiration, increasing compression. Venous blood return to the heart is impaired as the mediastinum shifts toward the unaffected lung.

Clinical Reasoning in Action

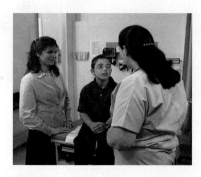

Adam and his mother have come to the health center to follow up on his hospitalization to get an asthma action plan and to discuss how to reduce his asthma episodes. Adam, who is 7 years old, has a history of episodic wheezing and nebulizer treatments, but he had never been hospitalized for asthma until last week. During his 2-day hospitalization, his parents were given initial education about how to manage his moderate persistent asthma.

His mother has brought along Adam's medications (inhaled corticosteroid and salmeterol MDI for daily control, and an albuterol MDI for quick relief), his peak flow meter, spacer, and his asthma action plan. She tells you that he is also completing a dose of oral corticosteroids. You discuss the peak flow meter, the guidelines, and what type of action to take as needed. Based on his height of 48 in., his peak flow meter green zone is 160–128, his yellow zone is 128–80, and his red zone is 80 or below. Adam is to use his daily control medications twice a day. If he has symptoms, he is to take his albuterol MDI with spacer, two puffs every 4–6 hours as needed.

1. What are some of the side effects associated with Adam's albuterol MDI?
2. What is the benefit to using a spacer on Adam's albuterol and inhaled corticosteroid MDI?
3. Address the concerns of Adam's mother about the daily use of inhaled corticosteroids.
4. What are the signs of respiratory distress to observe for with Adam?
5. What information should be shared with the school nurse for Adam's symptom management while at school?

References

Ajao, T. I., Oden, R. P., Joyner, B. I., & Moon, R. Y. (2011). Decisions of black parents about infant bedding and sleep surfaces. A qualitative study. *Pediatrics, 128*(3), 494–502.

Allergy and Asthma Network. (2014). *Medications at school*. Retrieved from http://www.aanma.org/advocacy/meds-at-school/

Amanatidou, V., Syridou, G., Mavrikou, M., & Tsolia, M. N. (2012). Latent tuberculosis infection in children: Diagnostic approaches. *European Journal of Clinical Microbiologic Infectious Disease, 31*, 1285–1294.

American Academy of Allergy, Asthma, and Immunology (AAAAI). (2014). *Peak flow meter*. Retrieved from http://www.aaaai.org/conditions-and-treatments/library/at-a-glance/peak-flow-meter.aspx

American Academy of Pediatrics (AAP). (2015). *Red book: 2015 report of the Committee on Infectious Diseases* (30th ed.). Elk Grove Village, IL: Author.

American Lung Association. (2013). *Joint statement on improving asthma management in schools*. Retrieved from http://www.lung.org/lung-disease/asthma/becoming-an-advocate/national-asthma-public-policy-agenda/joint-statement-improve-asthma-mgmt-schools.pdf

Asthma Initiative of Michigan for Healthy Lungs. (2011). *How to use a metered-dose inhaler the right way*. Retrieved from http://www.getasthmahelp.org/inhalers_main.asp

Banasiak, N. C. (2014). Spirometry in primary care for children with asthma. *Pediatric Nursing, 40*(4), 195–198.

Blanken, M. O., Rovers, M. M., Molenaar, J. M., Winkler-Seinstra, P. L., Meijer, A., Jan, L. L., . . . Bont, L. (2013). Respiratory syncytial virus and recurrent wheeze in healthy preterm infants. *New England Journal of Medicine, 368*(19), 1791–1799.

Brashers, V. L. (2014). Structure and function of the pulmonary system. In K. L. McCance, S. E. Huether, V. L. Brashers, & N. S. Rote (Eds.), *Pathophysiology: The biologic basis for disease in adults and children* (7th ed., pp. 1225–1247). St. Louis, MO: Elsevier Mosby.

Brashers, V. L., & Huether, S. E. (2014). Alterations in pulmonary function in children. In K. L. McCance, S. E. Huether, V. L. Brashers, & N. S. Rote (Eds.), *Pathophysiology: The biologic basis for disease in adults and children* (7th ed., pp. 1290–1318). St. Louis, MO: Elsevier Mosby.

Burkhart, P. V., Rayens, M. K., & Oakley, M. G. (2012). Effect of peak flow monitoring on child asthma quality of life. *Journal of Pediatric Nursing, 27*, 18–25.

Centers for Disease Control and Prevention. (2013). *Asthma facts—CDC's national asthma control program grantees*. Retrieved from http://www.cdc.gov/asthma/pdfs/asthma_facts_program_grantees.pdf

Chang, C. (2012). Asthma in children and adolescents: A comprehensive approach to diagnosis and management. *Clinical Reviews in Allergy and Immunology, 43*(1–2), 98–137.

Chu, A., & Hageman, J. R. (2013). Apparent life-threatening events in infancy. *Pediatric Annals, 42*(2), 78–83.

Colvin, J. D., Collie-Akers, V., Schunn, C., & Moon, R. Y. (2014). Sleep environment risks for younger and older infants. *Pediatrics, 134*(2), e406–e412.

Custovic, A., Lazic, N., & Simpson, A. (2013). Pediatric asthma and development of atopy. *Current Opinion in Allergy and Clinical Immunology, 13*(2), 173–180.

Cystic Fibrosis Foundation (CFF). (2014). *About cystic fibrosis: What is cystic fibrosis?* Retrieved from http://www.cff.org/AboutCF/

Delaney, R. A., & Windemuth, B. (2014). The unique management of cystic fibrosis-related diabetes and the importance of glycemic control. *The Journal for Nurse Practitioners, 10*(9), 682–686.

Desale, M., Bringardner, P., Fitzgerald , S., Page, K., & Shah, M. (2013). Intensified case-finding for latent tuberculosis infection among the Baltimore City Hispanic population. *Journal of Immigrant Minority Health, 15*, 680–685.

Dinakar, C., & Welch, M. J. (2014). Device how-tos. *Contemporary Pediatrics, 31*(May). Retrieved from http://contemporarypediatrics.modernmedicine.com/contemporary-pediatrics/content/tags/asthma/device-how-tos

Dorgan, D. J., & Hadjiliadis, D. (2014). Lung transplantation in patients with cystic fibrosis: Special focus to infection and comorbidities. *Expert Reviews in Respiratory Medicine, 8*(3), 315–326.

Flook, D. M., & Vincze, D. L. (2012). Infant safe sleep: Efforts to improve education and awareness. *Journal of Pediatric Nursing, 27*(2), 186–188.

Fouzas, S., Priftis, K. N., & Anthracopoulos, M. B. (2011). Pulse oximetry in pediatric practice. *Pediatrics, 128*(4), 740–751.

Gaydos, L. M., Blake, S. C., Gazmararian, J. A., Woodruff, W., Thompson, W. W., & Dalmida, S. G. (2015). Revisiting safe sleep recommendations for African-American infants: Why current counseling is insufficient. *Maternal Child Health Journal, 19*, 496–503.

Gelfer, P., Cameron, R., Masters, K., Six Sigma Black Belt, & Kennedy, K. (2013). Integrating "Back to Sleep" recommendations into neonatal ICU practice. *Pediatrics, 131*(4), e1264–e1270.

Gelfer, P., & Tatum, M. (2014). Sudden infant death syndrome. *Journal of Pediatric Health Care, 28*(5), 470–474.

Greenberg, D., Givon-Lavi, N., Sadaka, Y., Ben-Shimol, S., Bar-Ziv, J., & Dagan, R. (2014). Short-course antibiotic treatment for community-acquired alveolar pneumonia in ambulatory children: A double-blind, randomized, placebo-controlled trial. *Pediatric Infectious Disease Journal, 33*(2), 136–142.

Hampson, N. B., Piantadosi, C. A., Thom, S. R., & Weaver, L. K. (2012). Practice recommendations in the diagnosis, management, and prevention of carbon monoxide poisoning. *American Journal of Respiratory Critical Care Medicine, 186*(11), 1095–1101.

Hauck, F. R., Thompson, J. M. D., Tenabe, K. O., Moon, R. Y., & Vennemann, M. M. (2011). Breastfeeding and reduced risk of sudden infant death syndrome: A meta-analysis. *Pediatrics, 128*(1), 103–110.

Henderson, L. B., Doshi, V. K., Blackman, S. M., Naughton, K. M., Pace, R. G., Moskovitz, J., . . . Cutting, G. R. (2012). Variation in MSRA modifies risk of neonatal intestinal obstruction in cystic fibrosis. *PLoS Genetics, 8*(3), e1002580.

Heron, M. (2013). Deaths: Leading causes for 2010. *National Vital Statistics Reports, 62*(2), 1–96.

Howrylak, J. A., Fuhlbrigge, A. L., Strunk, R. C., Zeiger, R. S., Weiss, S. T., & Raby, B. A. (2014). Classification of childhood asthma phenotypes and long-term clinical responses to inhaled anti-inflammatory medications. *Journal of Allergy and Clinical Immunology, 133*(5), 1289–1300.

Jereb, J. A., Goldberg, S. V., Powell, K., Villarino, M. E., & LoBue, P. (2011). Recommendations for use of an isoniazid-rifapentine regimen with direct observation to treat latent *Mycobacterium tuberculosis* infection. *Morbidity and Mortality Weekly Report, 60*(48), 1650–1653.

Johns Hopkins Medicine. (2012). *Peak flow measurement*. Retrieved from http://www.hopkinsmedicine.org/healthlibrary/test_procedures/pulmonary/peak_flow_measurement_92,P07755

Kelly, H. W., Sternberg, A. L., Lescher, R., Fuhlbrigge, A. L., Williams, P., Zeiger, R. S., . . . Strunk, R. C. (2012). Effect of inhaled glucocorticoids in childhood on adult height. *New England Journal of Medicine, 367*(10), 904–912.

Kueny, A., Berg, J., Chowdhury, Y., & Anderson, N. (2013). Poquito a poquito: How Latino families with children who have asthma make changes in their home. *Journal of Pediatric Health Care, 27*(1), e1–e11.

Marcus, C. L., Brooks, L. J., Draper, K. A., Gozal, D., Halbower, A. C., Jones, J., . . . Shiffman, R. N. (2012). Clinical practice guideline: Diagnosis and management of childhood obstructive sleep apnea syndrome. *Pediatrics, 130*(3), 576–584.

Matthews, R., & Moore, A. (2013). Babies are still dying of SIDS. *American Journal of Nursing, 113*(2), 59–64.

Mogayzel, P. J., Naureckas, E. T., Robinson, K. A., Mueller, G., Hadjiliadis, D., Hoag, J. B., . . . Pulmonary Clinical Practice Guidelines Committee. (2013). Cystic fibrosis pulmonary guidelines: Chronic medications for maintenance of lung health. *American Journal of Respiratory Critical Care Medicine, 187*(7), 680–689.

Nakano, S. J., & Tluczek, A. (2014). Genomic breakthroughs in the diagnosis and treatment of cystic fibrosis. *American Journal of Nursing, 114*(6), 36–43.

National Asthma Education and Prevention Program (NAEPP). (2007). *Expert panel report 3: Guidelines for the diagnosis and management of asthma*. Bethesda, MD: National Institutes of Health, National Heart Lung and Blood Institute. Retrieved from http://www.nhlbi.nih.gov/guidelines/asthma

Nguyen, J. M., Holbrook, J. A., Wei, C. Y., Gerald, L. B., Teague, W. G., & Wise, R. A. (2014). Validation and psychometric properties of the Asthma Control Questionnaire among children. *Journal of Allergy and Clinical Immunology, 133*, 91–97.

Nierengarten, M. B. (2015). Bronchiolitis guidelines: Diagnosis, management, and prevention. *Contemporary Pediatrics, 32*(1), 20–22.

Nkoy, F. L., Stone, B. L., Fassl, B. A., Uchida, D. A., Koopmeiners, K., Sarah Halbern, S., . . . Maloney, C. G. (2013). Longitudinal validation of a tool for asthma self-monitoring. *Pediatrics, 132*(6), e1554–e1561.

Parsons, J. P., Hallstrand, T. S., Mastronarde, J. G., Kaminsky, D. A., Rundell, K. W., Hull, J. H., . . . Anderson, S. D. (2013). An official American Thoracic Society clinical practice guideline: Exercise-induced bronchoconstriction. *American Journal of Respiratory Critical Care Medicine, 187*(9), 1016–1027.

Perez-Velez, C. M., & Marais, B. J. (2012). Tuberculosis in children. *New England Journal of Medicine, 367*(4), 348–361.

Pfuntner, A., Wier, L. M., & Stocks, C. (2013). Most Frequent Conditions in U.S. Hospitals, 2011, *H-CUP Statistical Brief #162*. Retrieved from http://www.hcup-us.ahrq.gov/reports/statbriefs/sb162.pdf

Prodhan, P., Sharoor-Karni, S., Lin, J., & Noviski, N. (2011). Predictors of respiratory failure among previously healthy children with respiratory syncytial virus infection. *American Journal of Emergency Medicine, 29*, 168–173.

Queen, M. A., Myers, A. L., Hall, M., Shah, S. S., Williams, D. J., Auger, K. A., . . . Tieder, J. S. (2014). Comparative effectiveness of empiric antibiotics for community-acquired pneumonia. *Pediatrics, 133*(1), e23–e29.

Riazi, S., Zeligs, B., Yeager, H., Peters, S. M., Benavides, G. A., Mita, O. D., & Bellanti, J. A. (2012). Rapid diagnosis of *Mycobacterium tuberculosis* infection in children using interferon-gamma release assays (IGRAs). *Allergy and Asthma Proceedings, 33*(3), 217–226.

Roosevelt, G. E. (2016). Acute inflammatory upper airway obstruction (croup, epiglottitis, laryngitis, and bacterial tracheitis). In R. M. Kliegman, B. F. Stanton, J. W. St. Geme, & N. F. Schor (Eds.), *Nelson textbook of pediatrics* (20th ed., pp. 2031–2036). Philadelphia, PA: Elsevier Saunders.

Rose, W., Kitai, I., Kakkar, F., Read, S. E., Behr, M. A., & Bitnun, A. (2014). Quantiferon gold-in-tube assay for TB screening in HIV infected children: Influence of quantitative values. *BMC Infectious Diseases, 14*, 516–521.

Ross, P. A., Newth, C. J. L., & Khemani, R. G. (2014). Accuracy of pulse oximetry in children. *Pediatrics, 133*(1), 22–29.

Rozance, P. J., & Rosenberg, A. A. (2012). The neonate. In S. G. Gabbe, J. R. Niebyl, H. L. Galen, E. Jauniaux, M. B. Landon, J. L. Simpson, . . . D. A. Driscoll (Eds.), *Obstetrics: Normal and problem pregnancies* (6th ed., pp. 481–516). Philadelphia, PA: Elsevier Saunders.

Seddon, J. A., Hesseling, A. C., Godfrey-Faussett, P., Fielding, K., & Schaaf, H. S. (2013). Risk factors for infection and disease in child contacts of multidrug-resistant tuberculosis: A cross-sectional study. *BMC Infectious Diseases, 13*, 392–401.

Sharma, G. D., & Conrad, C. (2011). Croup, epiglottitis, and bacterial tracheitis. In American Academy of Pediatrics Section on Pediatric Pulmonology, *Pediatric Pulmonology* (pp. 347–363). Elk Grove Village, IL: Author.

Sleath, B., Ayala, G. X., Gillette, C., Williams, D., Davis, S., Tudor, G., . . . Washington, D. (2011). Provider demonstration and assessment of child device technique during pediatric asthma visits. *Pediatrics, 127*(4), 642–648.

Starke, J. R., & Cruz, A. T. (2014). The of childhood tuberculosis. *Pediatrics,* e725–e727.

Strueby, L., & Thébaud, B. (2014). Advances in bro chopulmonary dysplasia. *Expert Reviews in Respira tory Medicine, 8*(3), 327–338.

Taketomo, C. K., Hodding, J. H., & Kraus, D. M. (2014). *Pediatric and neonatal dosage handbook* (21st ed.). Hudson, OH: Lexicomp.

Task Force on Sudden Infant Death Syndrome. (2011). SIDS and other sleep-related infant deaths: Expansion of recommendations for a safe infant sleeping environment. *Pediatrics, 128*(5), 1030–1039.

Van Nguyen J. M., & Abenhaim H. A. (2013). Sudden infant death syndrome: Review for the obstetric care provider. *American Journal of Perinatology, 30*(09), 703–714.

WebMD. (2012). *Asthma and the peak flow meter*. Retrieved from http://www.webmd.com/asthma/guide/peak-flow-meter

Weinberger, M. M. (2011). Bronchiolitis. In American Academy of Pediatrics Section on Pediatric Pulmonology, *Pediatric pulmonology* (pp. 377–390). Elk Grove Village, IL: Author.

Wilson, B. A., Shannon, M. T., & Shields, K. M. (2016). *Nurse's drug guide 2016*. Hoboken, NJ: Pearson.

Winston, C. A., & Menzies, H. J. (2012). Pediatric and adolescent tuberculosis in the United States, 2008–2010. *Pediatrics, 130*(6), e1425–e1432.

Wong, J. J. M., Lee, J. H., Turner, D. A., & Rehder, K. J. (2014). A review of the use of adjunctive therapies in severe acute asthma exacerbation in critically ill children. *Expert Reviews in Respiratory Medicine, 8*(4), 423–441.

Zoorob, R., Sidani, M., & Murray, J. (2011). Croup: An overview. *American Family Physician, 83*(9), 1067–1073.

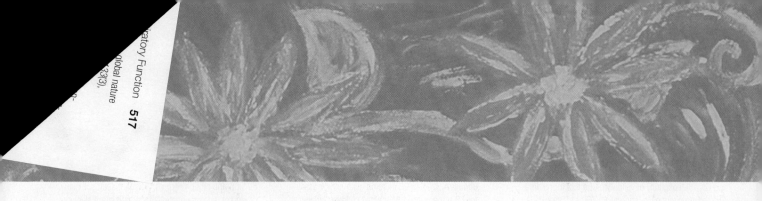

Chapter 21
Alterations in Cardiovascular Function

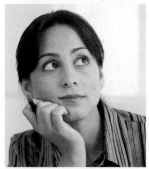

Brandy got sick so fast. Look how fast she is breathing. She gets tired before she can finish her formula. We didn't expect her to need heart surgery when she was still so small. We were told her chances for successful surgery would improve if she grew some more. I just want her to get stronger and have the chance to grow up to be like other kids.

—Mother of Brandy, 1 month old

Blend Images/Shutterstock

∨ Learning Outcomes

21.1 Describe the anatomy and physiology of the cardiovascular system, focusing on the flow of blood and the action of heart valves.

21.2 Describe the pathophysiology associated with congenital heart defects with increased pulmonary circulation, decreased pulmonary circulation, mixed defects, and obstructed systemic blood flow.

21.3 Develop a nursing care plan for the infant with a congenital heart defect cared for at home prior to corrective surgery.

21.4 Create a nursing care plan for the child undergoing open heart surgery.

21.5 Recognize the signs and symptoms of congestive heart failure in an infant and child.

21.6 Develop a nursing care plan for a child with congestive heart failure.

21.7 Differentiate among the heart diseases that are acquired or begin development during childhood.

21.8 Develop a nursing care plan for a child with Kawasaki syndrome.

21.9 List strategies to reduce a child's risk of adult-onset cardiovascular disease.

21.10 Plan the nursing management of hypovolemic shock.

Alterations in cardiovascular function may result from a congenital defect, acquired infection, or injury. Congenital heart defects are one of the most common birth defects, occurring in approximately 1% of all live births (Peterson et al., 2014). More than 35 types of heart defects have been documented. Examples of acquired cardiovascular conditions include rheumatic fever, Kawasaki disease, and hypertension.

Text continues on page 522

FOCUS ON:
The Cardiovascular System

Anatomy and Physiology

The heart is divided into four chambers: two atria and two ventricles. Atrioventricular valves (tricuspid and mitral) separate the atria from the ventricles. They open and close to control the flow of blood to the ventricles. The semilunar valves (pulmonary and aortic) open when the ventricles pump blood and close to prevent the backflow of blood to the ventricles. The great arteries (aorta and pulmonary artery) carry blood away from the heart to either the body or the lungs. Pulmonary veins and the superior and inferior venae cavae return blood to the heart. See Figure 21–1 for the anatomy of the heart and pressures generated by the blood.

The heart is the pump that circulates the blood through the systemic and pulmonary systems. Blood flows to the lungs for oxygen and carbon dioxide exchange. The oxygenated blood returns to the heart for distribution to the systemic circulation, organs, and tissues. See Table 21–1 for **hemodynamics** (passage of blood through the heart and pulmonary system and action of the valves) of the normal heart. The heart's electrical conduction system controls the rhythmic pumping (Figure 21–2).

TABLE 21–1 Hemodynamics of the Normal Heart

ACTION	RIGHT SIDE OF HEART	LEFT SIDE OF HEART
Blood return to heart	From the systemic circulation by way of the superior and inferior venae cavae.	From the lungs by way of the left and right pulmonary veins.
Diastolic phase	Pulmonary valve closes and tricuspid valve opens.	Aortic valve closes and mitral valve opens.
	Blood flows from the venae cavae through the right atrium and tricuspid valve into the right ventricle.	Blood flows from the pulmonary veins through the left atrium and mitral valve into the left ventricle.
Systolic phase	Tricuspid valve closes and pulmonary valve opens.	Mitral valve closes and aortic valve opens.
	Blood is pumped into the pulmonary artery and passes into the right and left pulmonary arteries and lungs.	Blood is pumped into the aorta where it enters the systemic circulation.

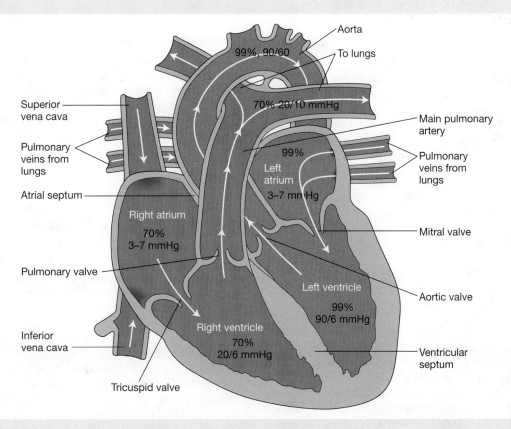

Figure 21–1 Anatomy of the heart, direction of blood flow, and the normal pressure gradients and oxygen saturation levels in the heart chambers and great arteries. The right ventricle has a lower pressure during systole than the left ventricle because less pressure is needed to pump blood to the lungs than to the rest of the body.

(continued)

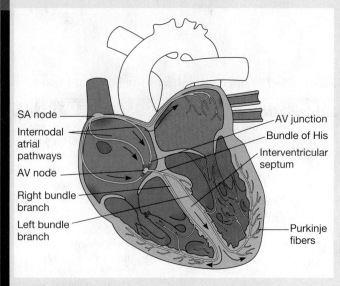

SA node
Internodal atrial pathways
AV node
Right bundle branch
Left bundle branch

AV junction
Bundle of His
Interventricular septum

Purkinje fibers

Figure 21–2 Electrical conduction system of the heart. Depolarization normally follows a sequence that begins in the sinoatrial (SA) node and travels through the atrial muscle to the atrioventricular (AV) junction, and then through the AV node to the ventricular muscles. The pathway in the ventricles begins in the bundle of His and divides into the right and left bundle branches. The pathway terminates in the Purkinje system so that the impulse spreads across the myocardium.

Transition From Fetal to Pulmonary Circulation

The transition from fetal to pulmonary circulation occurs within a few hours of birth (see *As Children Grow: Transition of Fetal Circulation to Pulmonary Circulation*). Permanent closure of the ductus arteriosus occurs by 10 to 21 days after birth, unless oxygen saturation remains low. Fetal tissues are accustomed to low oxygen saturation. This may explain why newborns with heart conditions with decreased pulmonary blood flow (cyanotic defects) appear relatively comfortable even when their arterial partial pressure of oxygen (PaO$_2$) is very low.

Pediatric Differences

Cardiac Functioning

Infants have a greater risk of heart failure than older children because the immature heart is more sensitive to volume or pressure overload. During infancy the heart's muscle fibers are less developed and less organized, resulting in limited functional capacity. Less **compliance** (amount of expansion the ventricles can achieve to increase stroke volume) of the heart muscle means that the **stroke volume** (the amount of blood ejected with each contraction) cannot increase substantially. The heart muscle fibers develop during early childhood, and by 9 years of age, the weight of the heart has increased by six times (McDaniel, 2014). As the child's heart grows and develops, the systolic blood pressure rises, reaching adult levels by puberty.

The infant maintains a high heart rate and high **cardiac output** (volume of blood ejected from the left ventricle each minute) to

meet high metabolic rate and oxygen requirements. Infants and children with a fever, exercise, stress, or respiratory distress respond with tachycardia rather than increased stroke volume to increase their cardiac output. The newborn has little cardiac output reserve capacity until oxygen requirements begin to decrease at about 2 months of age (McDaniel, 2014).

Oxygenation

Oxygen bound to hemoglobin is transported to the tissues by the systemic circulation. Hematocrit and hemoglobin concentrations appropriate for the child's age are necessary for adequate oxygen transport (see Chapter 23). The arterial oxygen saturation is the amount of oxygen that can potentially be delivered to the tissues. **Desaturated blood** results when oxygenated and unoxygenated blood mix because of a congenital heart defect. Cyanosis, which indicates **hypoxemia** (lower than normal amounts of oxygen in the blood), results when a concentration of 5 g/dL of deoxygenated hemoglobin is present in the blood or from arterial oxygen saturation less than 85% (McDaniel, 2014).

The child's bone marrow responds to chronic hypoxemia by producing more red blood cells to increase the amount of hemoglobin to be oxygenated. This increase is known as **polycythemia**. A hematocrit value of 50% or higher is common in children with heart defects with decreased pulmonary blood flow.

Children respond to severe hypoxemia with bradycardia. Cardiac arrest in children generally results from prolonged hypoxemia related to respiratory failure or shock rather than from a primary cardiac insult as in adults. Bradycardia is therefore a significant warning sign of cardiac arrest. Appropriate management of hypoxemia often reverses bradycardia and prevents cardiac arrest.

Cardiac Assessment

Performing a nursing assessment of the child with a potential or actual cardiac condition involves a careful review of the signs and symptoms in many body systems and analysis of their relationship to cardiac functioning. Use *Assessment Guide: The Child With a Cardiac Condition* to perform a comprehensive nursing assessment of the cardiovascular system. Numerous diagnostic procedures and laboratory tests are used for the diagnosis of cardiac conditions. See Table 21–2.

TABLE 21–2 Diagnostic Procedures and Laboratory Tests Used to Evaluate Cardiac Conditions*

DIAGNOSTIC PROCEDURES	LABORATORY TESTS
Cardiac catheterization	Complete blood count
Chest radiograph	Arterial blood gases
Echocardiogram (transthoracic and transesophageal)	Antistreptolysin-O antibody titer
Electrocardiography (ECG) and ambulatory ECG (Holter monitor)	Erythrocyte sedimentation rate
Exercise testing	C-reactive protein
Hyperoxitest	Serum lipid panel
Computed tomography	Serum drug tests (e.g., digoxin)
Magnetic resonance imaging	

*See Appendices D and E for information about these diagnostic procedures and expected laboratory values.

As Children Grow: **Transition of Fetal Circulation to Pulmonary Circulation**

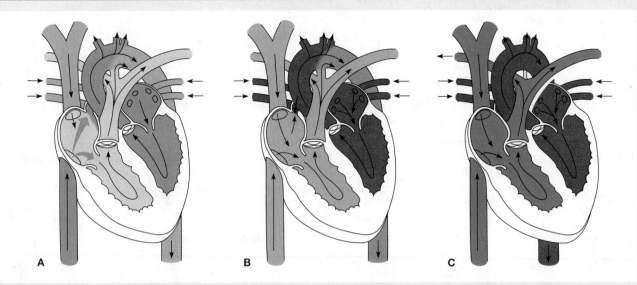

A, During pregnancy blood flows to the fetus through the umbilical vein to the ductus venosus (the fetal vascular channel between the umbilical vein and the inferior vena cava) and into the heart's RA. The foramen ovale, an opening between the atria of the fetal heart, allows blood to flow from the RA to the LA and then into the LV. Blood then flows into the aorta and systemic circulation. Some blood returns from the head and upper extremities to the superior vena cava and RA. Some blood travels to the RV where it is pumped into the pulmonary artery, through the ductus arteriosus (the vascular channel between the pulmonary artery and the aorta), and into the systemic circulation. A small amount of the blood from the pulmonary artery goes to the fetal lungs. Blood eventually returns to the placenta by way of the umbilical arteries. After the umbilical cord has been cut, the newborn must quickly adapt to receiving oxygen from the lungs.

B, The first breath expands the lungs, and blood that previously flowed through the ductus arteriosus to the aorta begins flowing to the lungs. Pulmonary blood flow increases and pulmonary vascular resistance decreases. Pressure in the LA increases as increased blood flow is returned from the lungs through the pulmonary veins. Systemic vascular resistance (the force or resistance of the blood in the body's blood vessels that helps return blood to the heart) increases and pressure in the RA falls. Increased pressure in the left atrium stimulates closure of the foramen ovale unless there is excess pressure on the right side of the heart.

C, The ductus arteriosus, responding to higher oxygen saturation, normally constricts and closes within 10 to 15 hours after birth.

KEY: LA, left atrium; LV, left ventricle; RA, right atrium; RV, right ventricle.

ASSESSMENT GUIDE | The Child With a Cardiac Condition*

Assessment Focus	Assessment Guidelines
Respirations	• What is the respiratory rate and depth?
	• Are signs of increased respiratory effort present (e.g., tachypnea, dyspnea, retractions, nasal flaring, expiratory grunting)?
	• Is a cough present?
	• Auscultate breath sounds. Are any adventitious sounds present (e.g., wheezes, crackles)?
Pulse characteristics	• Assess the pulse rate, rhythm, and quality.
	• Compare pulse sites for strength and rate (apical to brachial, radial, femoral, pedal).
Blood pressure	• Compare the blood pressure to expected value for age, gender, and height percentile. (See Appendix B.)
	• Compare blood pressure values between upper and lower extremities.

(continued)

Assessment Focus	Assessment Guidelines
Color	• Observe overall color. Note pallor, dusky color, or cyanosis. • Compare the color in peripheral and central locations (e.g., nail beds to mucous membranes). Does crying improve or worsen the color? • Assess pulse oximetry.
Chest	• Inspect the anterior chest for bulging or **heaving** (lifting of the chest wall during contraction). • Palpate the chest wall over the heart for pulsations, heaves, or vibrations. • Locate the point of maximum intensity.
Heart auscultation	• Auscultate the heart for the heart sounds and their quality (loud versus weak, distinct versus muffled). • Are any extra heart sounds or murmurs present? Describe murmurs by their intensity, location, radiation, timing, and quality. • Auscultate the heart with the child sitting and reclining to detect differences in heart sounds.
Fluid status	• Observe for signs of periorbital, facial, or peripheral edema, or for dehydration. • Observe for abdominal distention. • Palpate the liver to detect hepatomegaly. • Assess capillary refill.
Activity and behavior	• Is exercise tolerance present? Does the child tire with feeding? • Note presence of diaphoresis and when it occurs. • Identify changes in activity level or behavior (lethargy, restlessness, irritability, and decreased responsiveness).
General	• Assess pattern of growth.

*See Chapter 5 for assessment techniques.

Congenital Heart Disease

Congenital heart disease refers either to a defect in the heart or great vessels or to persistence of a fetal structure (e.g., patent foramen ovale or patent ductus arteriosus) after birth. The incidence is about 8 to 12 per 1000 live births (Park, 2014, p. 7). A critical congenital heart defect is life threatening and requires emergency care, surgery, or catheter intervention within the first days or weeks of life. These defects account for 25% of infant deaths related to a birth defect during the first year of life (Peterson et al., 2014).

Etiology and Pathophysiology

Most congenital heart defects develop during the first 8 weeks of gestation. They can develop as the result of a combined or interactive effect of genetic and environmental factors, such as:

- Fetal exposure to drugs (e.g., phenytoin, angiotensin-converting enzyme [ACE] inhibitors, lithium, warfarin, valproic acid, retinoic acid) and alcohol
- Maternal viral infections such as rubella or coxsackievirus B5
- Maternal metabolic disorders such as phenylketonuria, diabetes mellitus, and hypercalcemia
- Increased maternal age
- Multifactorial genetic patterns
- Chromosomal abnormalities (e.g., Turner, Noonan, Marfan, DiGeorge, and trisomy [13, 18, 21] syndromes)

Because of the genetic component, the incidence of congenital heart defects (CHDs) is expected to slowly rise; for example, a mother with a CHD has an increased risk of having an affected child.

Congenital heart defects are categorized by pathophysiology and hemodynamics rather than by the presence of cyanosis. These categories are described in more detail later in this chapter and include the following:

- Increased pulmonary blood flow
- Decreased pulmonary blood flow
- Obstructed systemic blood flow

Mixed defects fall into one of these three classifications, but the infant's survival depends on mixing systemic and pulmonary blood. Children with mixed defects and decreased pulmonary blood flow have similar clinical therapy and nursing management, so these categories will be discussed together.

Clinical Manifestations

The presence of a heart murmur is often the first indication of a congenital heart defect. A murmur indicates blood is flowing with higher pressure than normal to get through a narrowed valve or vessel or through a **shunt** (an abnormal anatomic opening in the septum between the systemic and pulmonary circulation). Other clinical manifestations and the timing of their appearance vary by the pathophysiology and severity of the defect. See Table 21–3. Newborns may become symptomatic as soon as the umbilical cord is cut or within the first few days of life. Some children may be asymptomatic except for a heart murmur. Signs and symptoms in older children may include exercise intolerance, chest pain, arrhythmias, syncope, and sudden death.

TABLE 21–3 Clinical Manifestations of Heart Defects by Pathophysiology

PATHOPHYSIOLOGY AND TYPE OF DEFECT	CLINICAL MANIFESTATIONS
Increased pulmonary blood flow (PDA, ASD, VSD, AV canal)	Tachypnea, tachycardia, murmur, congestive heart failure (CHF), poor weight gain, diaphoresis, periorbital edema, frequent respiratory infections
Decreased pulmonary blood flow (PS, TOF, pulmonary or tricuspid atresia, TGA)	Cyanosis, hypoxic spells, poor weight gain, polycythemia
Obstruction to systemic blood flow (COA, AS, HLHS, MS, interrupted aortic arch)	Diminished pulses, poor color, delayed capillary refill time, decreased urine output, CHF with pulmonary edema
Mixed defects—postnatal survival is dependent on mixing of systemic and pulmonary blood (TGA, TAPVR, truncus arteriosus, double outlet right ventricle)	Cyanosis, poor weight gain, pulmonary congestion, CHF may occur with increased shunting

Key: AS, aortic stenosis; ASD, atrial septal defect; AV, atrioventricular; COA, coarctation of aorta; HLHS, hypoplastic left heart syndrome; MS, mitral stenosis; PDA, patent ductus arteriosus; PS, pulmonic stenosis; TAPVR, total anomalous pulmonary venous return; TOF, tetralogy of Fallot; TGA, transposition of great arteries; VSD, ventricular septal defect

Clinical Therapy

Multiple tests are used to diagnose cardiac defects (Table 21–2). Blood tests such as a hematocrit and hemoglobin are taken to assess for anemia or polycythemia. Arterial blood gases may be obtained, especially when cyanosis or a complex heart defect is suspected. Newborn screening with pulse oximetry is used to identify critical congenital heart disease (Association of Maternal and Child Health Programs, 2013).

Treatment for congenital heart defects depends on the severity of symptoms and whether the condition is imminently life threatening. Interventional cardiac catheterization or surgical correction with restoration of normal hemodynamics and physiology is the treatment of choice for many defects. A **palliative procedure** (a surgical procedure that does not create normal anatomic or hemodynamic results) may be performed in children with a potentially fatal or lethal condition. It may also be performed as an initial procedure, allowing an infant to grow before definitive corrective surgery. Table 21–4 lists the types of interventions during cardiac catheterization and surgical procedures performed on children with congenital heart defects.

TABLE 21–4 Clinical Interventions for Congenital Heart Defects

CARDIAC CATHETERIZATION INTERVENTIONS AND THERAPEUTIC USE	PURPOSE
Balloon atrial septostomy—Rashkind, or with transatrial needle puncture and balloon dilation Palliative for TGA	Creates a larger defect (at the foramen ovale) between atria to increase blood mixing.
Balloon dilation procedure Corrective for PS and MS; palliative for AS, COA	A deflated balloon is inserted and inflated to open a narrowed valve or blood vessel. A stent may be inserted to keep the vessel (e.g., ductus arteriosus) open.
Device closure Corrective for PDA, ASD, VSD	Closure of ductus arteriosus by an umbrella or coil device, and closure of a septal defect by a septal occluder.
SURGICAL PROCEDURES AND THERAPEUTIC USE	**PURPOSE**
Aorta end-to-end anastomosis Corrective for COA	Resection of the narrowed section of the aorta and connection of the proximal and distal sections.
Blalock-Taussig shunt, modified Palliative for TOF, single ventricle lesions with pulmonary outflow obstruction	Creation of aortopulmonary conduit (from the brachiocephalic artery to pulmonary artery) to increase pulmonary blood flow.
Brock Corrective for PS	Blind incision of pulmonary valve.
Damus-Kaye-Stansel—pulmonary artery-to-aortic anastomosis Corrective for TGA, complex single ventricle defects	Pulmonary artery is cut in two with the proximal section attached to the ascending aorta; the distal section is sewn over, and a shunt is created between the systemic circulation and the pulmonary artery to send blood to the lungs.
Fontan Palliative for HLHS, single ventricle defects	Creation of a conduit between inferior vena cava and pulmonary artery to increase pulmonary blood flow—total right heart bypass. The single ventricle assumes responsibility for the systemic circulation and ejects blood into the aorta.

(continued)

TABLE 21–4 Clinical Interventions for Congenital Heart Defects (*continued*)

SURGICAL PROCEDURES AND THERAPEUTIC USE	PURPOSE
Glenn or Bidirectional Glenn Palliative for HLHS, single ventricle defects	Superior vena cava connected to right pulmonary artery along with closure of aortopulmonary shunt. Systemic venous blood from the head is sent to the lungs directly without ventricular pumping.
Jatene—arterial switch Corrective for TGA	Aorta and pulmonary arteries are transected and reattached to the opposite stumps; coronary arteries are moved to new aorta area.
Nikaidoh Corrective for TGA when a VSD and severe PS are present	The aortic root is translocated from the right ventricle, with attached coronary vessels, to the left ventricle after reconstructing the left and right outflow tracts and patching the VSD.
Norwood Palliative for aortic hypoplasia, single ventricle defects (e.g., HLHS)	Atrial septectomy, anastomosis of the main pulmonary artery to the aorta, and an arterial-pulmonary shunt (e.g., modified Blalock-Taussig shunt).
Norwood with Sano modification Palliative for HLHS	Creation of a right ventricle to pulmonary artery conduit so that both the direct pulmonary and aorta blood flow originate in the right ventricle.
Patch aortoplasty Corrective for COA	Insertion of a Dacron patch or opened left subclavian vein to expand the lumen of the aorta.
Pulmonary artery banding Palliative for VSD, AV canal, single ventricle defects	Placement of constricting band around pulmonary artery to reduce pulmonary blood flow and pressure.
Rastelli Corrective for TGA with pulmonic stenosis, TOF, tricuspid atresia, truncus arteriosus, and some cases of double outlet right ventricle	Creation of a conduit between the right ventricle to pulmonary artery with closure of the ventricular septal defect. In the case of truncus arteriosus, the pulmonary arteries are removed from the truncus.
Ross Corrective for AS	The diseased aortic valve is replaced with the patient's pulmonic valve (pulmonary autograft), and a homograft (valve from a human donor) replaces the pulmonic valve.
Subclavian flap aortoplasty Corrective for COA	Division of the distal subclavian artery and insertion of a flap into the aorta through the coarcted segment.
Transplant Corrective for HLHS, complex defects, cardiomyopathies	Replacement of diseased heart with donor heart.

Key: AS, aortic stenosis; ASD, atrial septal defect; AV, atrioventricular; COA, coarctation of aorta; HLHS, hypoplastic left heart syndrome; MS, mitral stenosis; PDA, patent ductus arteriosus; PS, pulmonic stenosis; TOF, tetralogy of Fallot; TGA, transposition of great arteries; VSD, ventricular septal defect.

Nursing Management

For the Child Having Cardiac Catheterization

Cardiac catheterization performed for examination or for therapeutic intervention is often an outpatient procedure. The child is NPO for several hours, except for medications, and arrives at the catheterization laboratory 1 to 2 hours before the procedure. In preparation for the procedure, the child is asked to void and is given an oral sedative. Infants and young children often need sedation to keep them still during the procedure.

Nursing Assessment and Diagnosis

Before the procedure, assess the child using the assessment guidelines found earlier in this chapter, *Assessment Guide: The Child With a Cardiac Condition.* Collect baseline data on skin temperature, color, strength of pedal and popliteal pulses, and hematocrit and hemoglobin levels for comparison with postcatheterization assessments.

After the procedure, monitor the child for potential complications such as arrhythmia, bleeding, hematoma development,

thrombus formation, and infection for several hours. No bleeding should occur at the catheterization site. Assess vital signs and perfusion of the lower extremities (pulses, temperature, color, capillary refill, and sensation) and compare to precatheterization status. The child's temperature and vital signs should remain stable. Monitor intake and output because the contrast medium may cause diuresis.

Clinical Tip

A pulse oximeter provides a noninvasive measurement of the percutaneous arterial oxygen saturation level (SpO_2) and may provide an early clue that hypoxemia is developing before cyanosis is visualized. A reading of 95% to 98% is normal in children. See Chapter 20 for a review of pulse oximetry use.

The following nursing diagnoses may apply to the child who undergoes cardiac catheterization (NANDA-I © 2014):

- *Fear* related to separation from support system in a stressful situation

- *Fluid Volume: Imbalanced, Risk for,* related to inadequate fluid intake due to NPO status and diuretic effect of contrast medium
- *Tissue Perfusion: Peripheral, Risk for Ineffective,* related to mechanical reduction of arterial and venous blood flow to lower extremity

Planning and Implementation

Prepare the child for cardiac catheterization with age-appropriate information. Because the child will be sedated but arousable for the procedure, explain the sensations that will be experienced (e.g., restraints on arms, equipment noises, cold liquid cleanser for catheter site, and warm feeling of contrast injection).

Nursing care during a cardiac catheterization focuses on monitoring the child's vital signs, reassuring the child, and providing emergency care if necessary. After the catheters and guidewires are removed at the end of the procedure, direct pressure must be applied for 15 minutes. A pressure dressing is then placed over the site for several hours.

SAFETY ALERT!

Assess the pressure dressing over the catheterization site every 5 minutes for 15 minutes, every 15 minutes for 1 hour, and hourly, or as directed by the healthcare provider or facility guidelines. Do not remove or loosen the dressing to observe the site until the ordered time for the pressure dressing has elapsed. Check under the buttocks to make sure blood does not ooze out and run under the child. Seek immediate medical intervention if the leg has reduced warmth and decreased perfusion, or bleeding is noted.

The child is kept on bed rest for 4 to 6 hours with an effort to keep the leg straight for several hours. Avoid elevating the head of the bed as flexion of the hips is not permitted during this period. Activity is limited for 24 hours, and in some cases, the child is hospitalized. Provide quiet diversional activities.

Encourage the child to drink small amounts of clear liquids initially, and then progress to other fluids and food as the child tolerates them. Provide adequate fluids to maintain hydration status, especially if the child takes diuretics. The child's intake and output should be balanced.

DISCHARGE PLANNING AND HOME CARE TEACHING

Children are routinely discharged several hours after the cardiac catheterization. Teach the parents to watch the child for signs of complications and make sure they know when to notify the healthcare provider. See *Families Want to Know: Home Care After Cardiac Catheterization.*

Evaluation

Expected outcomes of nursing care include the following:

- Any potential complications (thrombosis or hemorrhage) following cardiac catheterization are rapidly identified and cared for.
- The child maintains fluid balance.

Congenital Heart Defects That Increase Pulmonary Blood Flow

The most common congenital heart defects result from a connection between the left and right side of the heart (septal defect) or between the great arteries (patent ductus arteriosus) that allows blood to flow between the left and right side of the heart.

Etiology and Pathophysiology

The pressures on the left side of the heart are higher. When a connection occurs between the left and right side of the heart, blood shunts from the left to the right side of the heart and increases the amount of blood pumped to the lungs. The size of the connection and how much blood passes through it determine how quickly the child develops signs of congestive heart failure (CHF) (see the section on CHF later in this chapter). The increased blood flow to the lungs causes increased pulmonary vascular resistance (constriction of the pulmonary vascular bed) in an effort to reduce the blood flow, and pulmonary artery hypertension (see the section later in this chapter). Right ventricular hypertrophy (RVH) develops to overcome the increasing pulmonary vascular resistance and to deliver the blood to the lungs.

Clinical Manifestations

The infant's heart rate, respiratory rate, and metabolic rate are increased because of the high pulmonary blood flow. Sucking to feed takes energy and diaphoresis often occurs. If the infant is unable to take in enough calories to support the metabolic rate and growth, poor weight gain is noted. If CHF develops, signs include dyspnea, tachypnea, intercostal retractions, and periorbital edema. Frequent respiratory infections occur as the wet environment in the lungs caused by CHF supports bacterial growth. See Table 21–5 for the pathophysiology, clinical manifestations, diagnostic tests, clinical therapy, and prognosis for the specific congenital heart defects that increase pulmonary blood flow.

Families Want to Know
Home Care After Cardiac Catheterization

- Check for signs of complications several times in the first 24 hours after catheterization and notify the healthcare provider immediately if any of these signs are noted:
  - Bleeding or a bruise increasing in size at the catheterization site
  - Foot on side of catheterization site is cooler than other foot
  - Loss of feeling in foot on side of catheterization
  - Fever
- If the child is treated with diuretics, observe for signs of dehydration (dry mucous membranes, absence of tears, and strong urine).
- Encourage fluids to help flush the dye out of the body and to prevent dehydration.
- Permit quiet play such as computer games, puzzles, and videos for the first 24 hours after the procedure.

TABLE 21–5 Pathophysiology, Clinical Manifestations, Diagnostic Tests, Clinical Therapy, and Prognosis for Defects That Increase Pulmonary Blood Flow

ANATOMY

PATENT DUCTUS ARTERIOSUS (PDA)

handwritten: ductus arteriosus doesn't close

Pathophysiology

A common congenital defect caused by persistent fetal circulation that accounts for 5% to 10% of all infants with congenital heart disease (Park, 2014). When pulmonary circulation is established and systemic vascular resistance increases at birth, pressures in the aorta become greater than in the pulmonary arteries. Blood is then shunted from the aorta to the pulmonary arteries, increasing circulation to the pulmonary system. It is a common problem of preterm infants who have respiratory distress syndrome or hypoxemia that work to keep the ductus arteriosus open (Park, 2014).

Clinical Manifestations

Dyspnea; tachypnea; tachycardia; full, bounding pulses; widened pulse pressure; hypotension may be noted when cardiac output is low. May be asymptomatic.

CHF, intercostal retractions, hepatomegaly, and poor growth when a large PDA exists.

A continuous "machinery" murmur during systole and diastole, and a thrill in the pulmonic area.

High risk for frequent respiratory infections and pneumonia.

Diagnostic Tests

The chest radiograph and ECG show left ventricular hypertrophy.

The PDA can be visualized, and PDA blood flow can be measured on echocardiogram.

Clinical Therapy

Transcatheter closure by obstructive device is the standard therapy in most centers. Video-assisted thoracoscopic surgery with clip ligation of the PDA may be performed.

Intravenous ibuprofen or indomethacin often stimulates closure of the ductus arteriosus in preterm infants, but cannot be used if CHF is present; it is not used in term infants.

Prognosis

No long-term sequelae occur if treated before pulmonary vascular disease (pulmonary hypertension or pulmonary vascular obstructive disease) develops.

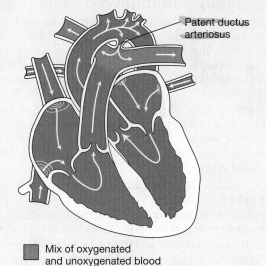

Patent ductus arteriosus

Mix of oxygenated and unoxygenated blood

ATRIAL SEPTAL DEFECT (ASD)

Pathophysiology

The opening in the atrial septum permits left-to-right shunting of blood. The opening may be small, as when the foramen ovale fails to close, or large (the septum may be completely absent). Of children with congenital heart disease, 30% to 50% have an ASD in combination with other defects, but it may occur as an isolated defect in 5% to 10% of children (Park, 2014).

Clinical Manifestations

Infants and young children with small or moderate-size ASDs usually have no symptoms. Large ASDs may cause CHF, easy tiring, and poor growth.

A soft systolic ejection murmur occurs in the pulmonic area with fixed, wide splitting of S_2 through all phases of respiration.

Diagnostic Tests

Echocardiogram identifies a dilated right ventricle due to blood overload and the shunt size.

The chest radiograph and ECG reveal little information unless the ASD is large, has excessive shunting, and right ventricular hypertrophy is present.

Clinical Therapy

Spontaneous closure of some small ASDs occurs within the first 4 years of life. No activity limitations are needed.

Secundum ASDs are usually closed by a septal occluder during cardiac catheterization. Aspirin at 81 mg per day is prescribed for 6 months after the procedure.

Surgery to close or patch the ASD is performed when significant increased pulmonary blood flow causes CHF. Arrhythmias may develop in postoperative period.

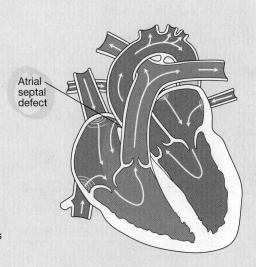

Atrial septal defect

Prognosis

Middle-aged adults with uncorrected small- and moderate-size ASDs may have no symptoms but are at risk for a stroke. Small clots that commonly develop in the right atrium can pass through the ASD into the left atrium and systemic circulation. CHF, atrial arrhythmias, and pulmonary artery hypertension may develop in untreated adults.

VENTRICULAR SEPTAL DEFECT (VSD)

Pathophysiology

An opening in the ventricular septum results in increased pulmonary blood flow. Blood is shunted from the left ventricle directly across the open septum into the pulmonary artery. This is the most common congenital heart defect. It occurs as a single defect in about 15% to 20% of cases but also is found in combination with other defects (Park, 2014).

Clinical Manifestations

Infants and children with small VSDs may have no symptoms. Moderate or large VSDs may be associated with CHF, poor growth, decreased exercise tolerance, an increased number of pulmonary infections, and pulmonary hypertension.

A systolic murmur is auscultated at the third or fourth left intercostal space at the sternal border. A thrill may be present.

Diagnostic Tests

A chest radiograph and ECG reveal little when VSDs are small. An enlarged heart and pulmonary vascular markings on chest radiograph occur in cases of large VSDs with shunting. Right and left ventricular hypertrophy may be seen on ECG. Echocardiogram identifies the size and location of the defect.

Clinical Therapy

Most small VSDs close spontaneously within the first 6 months of life. Treatment is conservative when no signs of CHF or pulmonary artery hypertension are present.

See the section on treatment of the child with CHF later in this chapter. VSD surgical closure is performed after 1 year of age unless CHF cannot be managed medically. Surgery for these infants is performed within the first 6 months of life.

Device closure of VSD during cardiac catheterization may be attempted for some VSDs that are not too close to the heart valves.

Prognosis

Highest risk associated with surgical repair is in the first 2 months of life. Children respond well to surgery and experience substantial catch-up growth. Arrhythmias, right bundle branch block, and complete heart block are possible complications. Some children need a pacemaker.

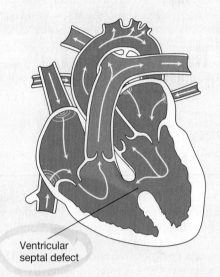

Ventricular septal defect

ATRIOVENTRICULAR CANAL (ENDOCARDIAL CUSHION) DEFECT (AV CANAL)

Pathophysiology

Endocardial cushions are fetal growth centers for the mitral and tricuspid valves and atrioventricular (AV) septum. The most complex AV canal defect results in one AV valve and large septal defects between both atria and ventricles. An AV canal defect occurs in about 2% of congenital heart defect cases, and 70% of these children have Down syndrome (Park, 2014).

Clinical Manifestations

Infants often develop CHF, tachypnea, tachycardia, avoidant/restrictive food intake disorder (failure to thrive), recurrent respiratory infections, and repeated respiratory failure.

S_1 is accentuated and S_2 is split. A holosystolic murmur is loudest at the left lower sternal border, and a thrill may be palpated. The murmur may be transmitted to the left axilla when mitral regurgitation is present (see Chapter 5 for a description of heart sounds).

Diagnostic Tests

On chest radiograph, cardiomegaly and pulmonary vascular markings are present. On ECG, a prolonged PR interval and enlarged ventricles are noted.

Echocardiogram reveals dilation of the ventricles, septal defects, and details of valve malformation.

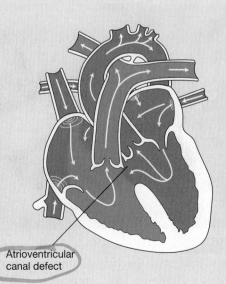

Atrioventricular canal defect

(continued)

TABLE 21–5 Pathophysiology, Clinical Manifestations, Diagnostic Tests, Clinical Therapy, and Prognosis for Defects That Increase Pulmonary Blood Flow (*continued*)

ANATOMY

Clinical Therapy

CHF is treated as described later in this chapter.

Surgery is performed between 2 and 4 months of age to prevent pulmonary vascular disease. Patches are placed over septal defects, and valve tissue is used to form functioning valves. The mitral valve may be replaced.

Infective endocarditis prophylaxis is required until 6 months after corrective surgery.

Prognosis

Arrhythmias and mitral valve regurgitation, a residual septal defect, and subaortic stenosis may occur postoperatively. Short-term survival rates among infants with and without Down syndrome are similar.

Clinical Therapy

See Table 21–2 for tests used to diagnose the heart condition. In addition to a chest radiograph, complete blood count, and urinalysis, coagulation studies, platelet counts, and serum electrolytes are often obtained for children having open heart surgery.

Surgery is often performed early in infancy to prevent irreversible pulmonary vascular disease. See Figure 21–3. Unless complications develop before surgery, infants and children usually make a complete recovery without limitations. The major complication of these defects is pulmonary artery hypertension, which is described later in this chapter.

Conservative treatment, such as waiting until the child is symptomatic or older, may be selected for some children with these defects. For example, a small ventricular septal defect may close spontaneously, or closure of an atrial septal defect may be postponed until preschool or early school-age years. Ibuprofen or indomethacin may be given to preterm infants with a patent ductus arteriosus when immediate closure of the ductus is needed. Interventional cardiac catheterization with a septal closing device is performed in an increasing number of cases.

Postpericardiotomy syndrome occurs as a complication in 25% to 30% of children when surgery involves an incision through the pericardium, leading to pericardial and pleural inflammation (Park, 2014, p. 364). It may result from an autoimmune response

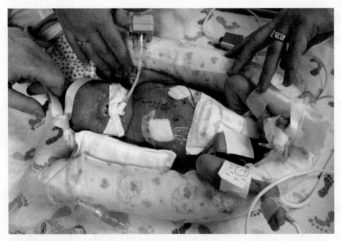

Figure 21–3 **A newborn with a ventricular septal defect repair. Surgery is performed on this type of defect to prevent pulmonary vascular disease and pulmonary artery hypertension.**

SOURCE: Barbara Davidson/Dallas Morning News/KRT/Newscom.

to damaged myocardium or pericardium or blood in the pericardial sac. The syndrome generally develops within a few weeks to a few months after surgery, more often in children over 2 years of age. It is characterized by a high fever up to 40°C (104°F) and sometimes severe chest pain that worsens with deep inspiration. The median duration of the condition is 2 to 3 weeks. Mild cases are treated with bed rest and NSAIDs or indomethacin. Severe cases may need corticosteroids, diuretics, or emergency pericardiocentesis.

Nursing Management
For the Child Prior to Surgery

Nursing Assessment and Diagnosis

PHYSIOLOGIC ASSESSMENT

Prior to surgery, the infant or child is seen regularly to assess growth and for signs of worsening CHF. See *Assessment Guide: The Child With a Cardiac Condition* (earlier in the chapter) for assessment guidelines. Failure to gain weight is an indication of an increased metabolic rate and inability to consume adequate calories for both metabolic function and growth. Assessment of length and head circumference helps to determine the full impact of the condition on growth.

PSYCHOSOCIAL ASSESSMENT

Assess the ability of the parents to cope with the infant's diagnosis. Parents may initially feel shock, guilt, or anxiety. They need an opportunity to express their feelings and to begin learning to manage the child's illness. The diagnosis, hospitalization, and early care of the infant at home are very stressful. Parents need special support if their infant has a life-threatening heart defect.

Examples of nursing diagnoses associated with heart defects having increased pulmonary blood flow and their complications include the following (NANDA-I © 2014):

- *Fluid Volume: Excess* related to heart failure and pulmonary vasculature overload
- *Infant Feeding Pattern, Ineffective,* related to shortness of breath and fatigue
- *Infection, Risk for,* related to pulmonary vascular congestion and chronic illness
- *Family Processes, Interrupted,* related to crisis of child's serious illness

Planning and Implementation

When the child has a large defect, CHF may be present. See the section on CHF later in this chapter for care guidelines.

FAMILY EDUCATION

Participate with members of the cardiology team to provide information and educate the family about the child's condition. Information may include the following:

- General information about the congenital heart disease, including a description of the heart's anatomy and physiology and the defect
- Information about genetic and environmental influences associated with congenital heart disease
- Signs of CHF and treatment if it develops
- Overview of the child's prognosis and timing of medical and surgical interventions, including some sample cases with good and poor outcomes

---

Clinical Tip

Some valuable resources for parents of a child with a congenital heart defect are as follows:

- *It's My Heart* by the Children's Heart Foundation
- *Hope for Families of Children with Congenital Heart Defects* by Lynda T. Young
- *The Heart of a Child: What Families Need to Know About Heart Disorders in Children* by C. A. Neill, E. A. Clark, and C. Clark, Johns Hopkins Press
- *Heart Warriors: A Family Faces Congenital Heart Disease* by Amanda Rose Adams, Behler Publications

---

PSYCHOSOCIAL SUPPORT

Parents are often anxious about an uncertain surgical outcome. Determine if parents have a support system as they learn about the infant's diagnosis and make difficult decisions about the child's surgery. Some parents may be concerned that signing consent for surgery places the child in even more danger of illness or even death. Identify some resources for support, such as social services, pastoral services, or a parent of a child with a similar heart defect.

Parents should be offered genetic counseling if planning a future pregnancy.

HOME CARE

Children are managed at home until surgery. Parents should encourage feeding to promote growth, but allow the infant to feed only for 30 minutes or as directed by healthcare providers for infants with complex heart defects or CHF. Breastfeeding or breast milk is encouraged because of its beneficial effects for the infant. Infants should be held at a 45-degree angle to reduce tachypnea. If the infant has difficulty gaining weight, formula or breast milk can be pumped and fortified with products that increase calorie density. Transpyloric, nasogastric, or gastrostomy tube feedings may also be given at night or 24 hours a day to ensure that adequate calories are ingested. See Figure 21–4. Salt intake is rarely limited in infants. When tube feedings are used, encourage the infant to take some formula orally to provide positive oral stimulation. See feeding suggestions for the infant with CHF later in this chapter.

Reduce the infant's exposure to infectious diseases, and encourage frequent hand hygiene. Respiratory infections increase hypoxemia in children with cyanosis. Fever increases

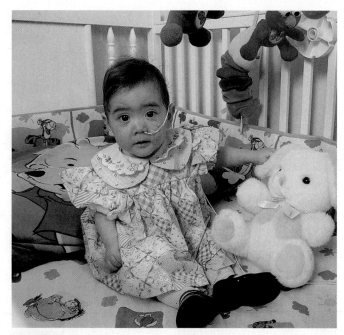

Figure 21–4 Infants with cardiac conditions often require supplemental feedings to provide sufficient nutrients for growth and development. The parents of this infant girl have been taught how to give her nasogastric feedings at home.

the metabolic rates and oxygen demands. Vomiting and diarrhea may cause an electrolyte disturbance. Notify the healthcare provider about fever, poor feeding, vomiting, and diarrhea.

Health promotion visits are important and all immunizations are provided according to the recommended schedule. Provide monthly prophylaxis for respiratory syncytial virus (RSV) with palivizumab to infants who have complex heart defects during the peak season. See Chapter 20.

PREPARATION FOR SURGERY

When the child is preschool age or older, prepare the child for the settings, equipment, and experiences to expect before and after surgery. Follow guidelines for preoperative treatment described in Chapter 11. If an infant or toddler is having surgery, inform the parents about how the child will look, equipment that will be used, and what care will be provided in the immediate postoperative period.

Evaluation

- Nutritional intake is adequate with oral and supplemental tube feeding as necessary.
- The child maintains a growth pattern that follows the established growth curve percentile.
- The child receives all immunizations and RSV prophylaxis to reduce the potential for acute illnesses.

Nursing Management

For the Child Having Surgery for Increased Pulmonary Blood Flow

The goal of nursing management is to perform assessments, provide supportive care to the family, and meet the child's nursing care needs before and after surgery.

Nursing Assessment and Diagnosis

At the time of surgery, the child needs a careful history and physical examination to detect any acute illnesses as well as the child's physiologic status. Assess the child's behavioral patterns, cardiac function, respiratory function, weight, and fluid status. See the *Assessment Guide* earlier in this chapter.

In the immediate postoperative period, the child will be cared for in the intensive care unit. When the child returns to the general nursing unit, assessment focuses on signs of surgical complications such as infection, arrhythmias, and impaired tissue perfusion. Monitor the child's temperature and inspect the surgical incision site. Fever, excessive incisional pain, spreading erythema around the incision, and wound drainage beginning 3 to 4 days postoperatively may be early signs of infection. Assess the chest and lungs for breath sounds, respiratory effort, and signs of distress that may indicate pneumonia or fluid in the pleural space.

Monitor the vital signs, including blood pressure and SpO_2. Auscultate the apical pulse to detect an irregular heart rate or bradycardia because either finding is a sign of reduced cardiac output that requires immediate intervention. Check capillary refill, extremity warmth, pedal pulses, level of consciousness, and urine output to assess tissue perfusion. Reduced urine output is a sign of decreased cardiac output. Continue to assess the child's pain.

Examples of nursing diagnoses following cardiac surgery include the following (NANDA-I © 2014):

- *Breathing Pattern, Ineffective,* related to respiratory muscle fatigue
- *Pain, Acute,* related to surgical incision and expansion of chest with coughing and deep breathing exercises
- *Fluid Volume: Imbalanced, Risk for,* related to impact of surgery on heart's pumping action
- *Infection, Risk for,* related to surgery and chronic disease status

Planning and Implementation

PAIN MANAGEMENT

Pain management with 24-hour intravenous opioids is provided for 1 to 2 days postoperatively or until the child is taking fluids. Then give oral analgesics around the clock. Follow the guidelines for pain management provided in Chapter 15. Teach parents and caregivers to move the child without lifting under the arms to reduce stress on the incision and pain.

PROMOTE RESPIRATORY FUNCTION

Encourage the child to take deep breaths and cough or to perform spirometry exercises regularly to promote full lung expansion (see the *Clinical Skills Manual* SKILLS). Bubbles or pinwheels may help young children to take deep breaths. Splint the chest with a pillow or stuffed animal to reduce pain from coughing and deep breathing. Chest physiotherapy may be performed in children under 3 years of age.

NUTRITION AND GENERAL CARE

Encourage the infant or child to begin oral fluids and nutrition when permitted. Oral fluids are rarely limited following surgery for defects with increased pulmonary blood flow, but assess intake and output carefully. Allow parents to bring in the child's favorite foods to encourage eating when they can be tolerated. Promote bowel elimination following surgery and when opioids are used.

Administer antibiotics as prescribed. If intravenous antibiotics are continued after the child's oral intake is established, the IV line can be converted to a heparin or saline lock.

Encourage the child to increase activity gradually with longer periods out of bed every day, but ensure adequate rest periods to promote healing. Provide diversional activities and opportunities for therapeutic play so the child can better manage the stresses associated with pain and frightening procedures.

DISCHARGE PLANNING AND HOME CARE TEACHING

Infants and children may be discharged from the hospital within a few days of surgery. Parents need information spread over several days to prepare for care of the child at home. See *Families Want to Know: Care of the Child After Cardiac Surgery.*

Prepare parents for potential behavior problems of young children that may result from the stress of hospitalization, such as nightmares, separation anxiety, and overdependence on parents. Encourage parents to reassure children about their security, and to promote play and other means to deal with their feelings. If the child's behavioral symptoms continue for several weeks, referral for psychologic assessment and support may be needed for posttraumatic stress disorder. See Chapter 28.

Reassure parents of children with a complete correction of the cardiac defect that no further cardiovascular problems should occur. Provide parents with full information about the child's defect and the surgery performed to share with the child's healthcare providers. Encourage parents to allow the child to live a normal and active life.

Evaluation

Examples of expected outcomes of nursing care include the following:

- Full lung expansion is achieved with spirometry exercises or chest physiotherapy.
- The child's pain is effectively managed.
- The child's incision heals without infection.
- Catch-up growth occurs over the next few months to years.

Defects Causing Decreased Pulmonary Blood Flow and Mixed Defects

Information about these defect categories is combined in this section because the clinical therapy and nursing interventions are similar.

Etiology and Pathophysiology

DEFECTS CAUSING DECREASED PULMONARY BLOOD FLOW

Defects that obstruct the flow of blood from the right side of the heart to the lungs decrease the amount of blood that gets oxygenated by the lungs. If an atrial or ventricular septal opening exists, the obstructed pulmonary blood raises pressures on the heart's right side higher than the left, leading to right-to-left shunting. Hypoxemia and cyanosis result because of the increased amount of unoxygenated blood in the systemic circulation.

Families Want to Know

Care of the Child After Cardiac Surgery

- Place infants and children in car safety seats for travel home from the hospital. Place a small blanket over the incision to prevent the straps from rubbing.

- Sponge bathe the infant or use a tub bath with a low water level. Avoid soaking the incision until sutures are out, the Steri-Strips fall off, or the Dermabond has flaked off and the incision is healed. Clean the incision daily as directed by the health-care provider. Do not use oils, creams, lotions, or ointments on the incision. Cover the incision with a clean shirt or bib to keep it clean and dry.

- Pick up infants and young children by placing one hand under the head and the other hand under the hips. Do not lift the child by grasping under the arms to decrease stress on the incision and sternum.

- Encourage a nutritious diet and snacks to promote healing and catch-up growth.

- Allow the child to increase activity gradually as tolerated. Report increased fatigue or decreased activity tolerance to the healthcare provider. Do not permit rough play, bike riding, and climbing for 6 weeks until the sternum incision has healed completely. The child can return to school in about 3 weeks, but no backpack should be used for several weeks.

- Report any signs of wound infection, fever over 40.3°C (101.0°F), flulike symptoms, chest pain, increased respiratory rate or respiratory distress, appetite change, or irritability to the healthcare provider.

- Give acetaminophen or ibuprofen for pain control. Use the recommended dose for the child's weight.

- When a prosthetic heart valve or material is used, give antibiotic prophylaxis for infective endocarditis for dental and invasive respiratory procedures as directed for 6 months after corrective surgery. See *Medications Used for Infective Endocarditis: Prophylaxis for Dental and Invasive Respiratory Procedures* later in this chapter. Report any unexplained fever or illness during the first 2 months following surgery.

- When blood products have been used during cardiac surgery, live virus vaccination should be delayed to ensure a full immunologic response. Check other references for the specific interval as it varies by type of blood product administered.

The bone marrow is stimulated to produce more red blood cells so more hemoglobin is available to carry oxygen. Polycythemia, an above-normal increase in the number of red blood cells, may result and place the child at risk for thromboembolism. Over time, platelet survival is reduced and clotting factors are impaired, increasing the infant's risk of bleeding with surgery. Bacteria in the unoxygenated blood (which is usually filtered out by the lung's capillaries) may cross into the systemic circulation through the septal defect, leading to a brain abscess (Park, 2014, p. 141).

When infants and children with cyanosis rise in the morning, they may experience an abrupt decrease in systemic vascular resistance. This increases the blood shunted from right to left across the VSD, and less blood flows to the lungs, leading to increased hypoxemia. Crying, feeding, increased activity, a warm bath, and straining with defecation are all events that can suddenly lower the systemic vascular resistance and trigger a hypoxic episode or spell. Hypovolemia may also trigger a hypoxic episode. The partial pressure of oxygen (Po_2) is lowered, and the partial pressure of carbon dioxide (Pco_2) rises. Hypoxemia becomes progressively worse as the respiratory center in the brain overreacts, increasing the respiratory effort. The extra respiratory effort further worsens the hypoxic episode that can become life-threatening unless rapid intervention is successful.

MIXED DEFECTS

Many complex congenital heart defects involve a combination of defects that increase and decrease pulmonary blood flow, making the newborn dependent on mixing of the pulmonary and systemic circulations for survival during the postnatal period. The mixed oxygen-saturated and oxygen-desaturated blood results in a general desaturated systemic blood flow and cyanosis. Pulmonary congestion occurs because of increased pulmonary blood flow and obstruction of systemic flow.

Clinical Manifestations

DEFECTS CAUSING DECREASED PULMONARY BLOOD FLOW

Clinical manifestations in infants initially include cyanosis shortly after birth, dyspnea, and a loud murmur. The skin may initially be ruddy or mottled before cyanosis is observed. Cyanosis that does not respond as expected to supplemental oxygen is a classic sign of decreased pulmonary blood flow. Signs and symptoms of chronic hypoxemia include fatigue, clubbing of the fingers and toes, exertional dyspnea, and delayed developmental milestones (Figure 21–5). Infants may need to stop sucking periodically during feedings to breathe, and diaphoresis may be seen with the increased work of feeding. These infants have a higher metabolic rate, and inadequate calories may be consumed, resulting in poor weight gain. See Table 21–6 for the pathophysiology, clinical manifestations, diagnostics tests, clinical therapy, and prognosis for these defects.

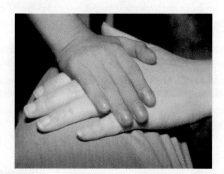

Figure 21-5 Clubbing of the fingers in an older child is one manifestation of a heart defect that reduces pulmonary blood flow.

TABLE 21–6 Pathophysiology, Clinical Manifestations, Diagnostic Tests, Clinical Therapy, and Prognosis for Defects That Decrease Pulmonary Blood Flow

ANATOMY

PULMONIC STENOSIS (PS)

Pathophysiology

Stenosis (narrowing of a valve or valve area) can be above, below, or at a valve. Stenosis obstructs blood flow into the pulmonary artery, increases preload, and results in right ventricular hypertrophy. PS as a single defect accounts for 8% to 12% of all congenital heart defects, but it also occurs with other defects (Park, 2014). Stenosis in the subvalvular area may develop as the heart muscle grows.

Clinical Manifestations

Children with mild stenosis may have no symptoms and grow normally.

In moderate to severe stenosis, dyspnea and fatigue occur on exertion. Signs of CHF, heart failure, and chest pain on exertion occur in severe cases.

A loud systolic ejection murmur with a widely split S_2 and thrill may be found in the pulmonic listening area. A murmur heard louder and longer indicates increased severity.

Diagnostic Tests

The chest radiograph may show an enlarged pulmonary artery with normal heart size and normal pulmonary vascularity.

The ECG may show right atrial enlargement and right ventricular hypertrophy.

An echocardiogram provides information about the thickness of the valve, the pressure gradient across the valve, and size of the valve ring.

Cardiac catheterization findings include increased right ventricular pressure and a normal or slightly lowered pulmonary artery pressure.

Clinical Therapy

Balloon dilation of the valve, performed during cardiac catheterization, is the preferred treatment. Pulmonary regurgitation may result but is not a significant problem.

Surgical valvotomy is performed when balloon dilation is not indicated or unsuccessful. On occasion the pulmonary valve is replaced.

Prognosis

Newborns with critical PS have a mortality rate of 10%. PS does not typically increase in severity. Lifelong infective endocarditis prophylaxis may be needed.

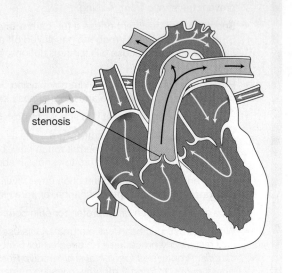

Pulmonic stenosis

☐ Decreased unoxygenated blood flow

TETRALOGY OF FALLOT (TOF)

Pathophysiology

Four defects are involved: stenosis of the pulmonary outflow tract or valve, right ventricular hypertrophy, ventricular septal defect (VSD), and overriding of aorta. The overriding aorta and VSD allow unoxygenated blood to pass into the systemic circulation. TOF accounts for about 5% to 10% of all cases of congenital heart disease (Park, 2014).

Clinical Manifestations

The newborn becomes hypoxic and cyanotic as the ductus arteriosus closes. The degree of pulmonary stenosis determines severity of symptoms. Older infants and children have tachypnea and cyanosis.

Polycythemia, hypoxic spells, metabolic acidosis, poor growth, clubbing, and exercise intolerance may develop.

Toddlers with uncorrected defects instinctively squat (assume a knee–chest position) to decrease the return of systemic venous blood to the heart.

A systolic murmur is heard in the pulmonic area and transmitted to the suprasternal notch. A thrill may be palpated in the pulmonic area.

Diagnostic Tests

A chest radiograph shows the boot-shaped heart due to the large right ventricle, decreased pulmonary vascular markings, and a prominent aorta.

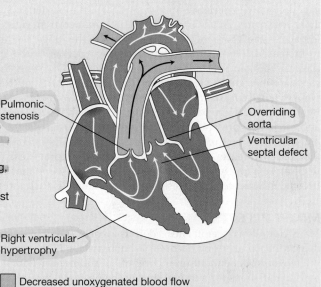

Pulmonic stenosis

Overriding aorta

Ventricular septal defect

Right ventricular hypertrophy

☐ Decreased unoxygenated blood flow

☐ Mixed oxygenated and unoxygenated blood

Diagnostic Tests (continued)

The ECG shows right ventricular hypertrophy.

The echocardiogram shows the VSD, obstruction of pulmonary outflow, an overriding aorta, and the size of the pulmonary arteries. The condition may be detected by fetal echocardiography.

Blood tests reveal an elevated hematocrit and hemoglobin and an increased clotting time. Iron deficiency may be detected.

Clinical Therapy

See the section on hypercyanotic episode management later in this chapter. Monitoring the child for metabolic acidosis or prolonged unconsciousness is critical.

Most infants have corrective surgery by 1 to 2 years of age unless a hypercyanotic spell occurs earlier. Symptomatic children have corrective surgery any time after 3 to 4 months of age. Some children need palliative surgery (modified Blalock-Taussig shunt) to delay total corrective surgery. A right bundle branch rhythm pattern may result from surgery.

If prosthetic material is used for the corrective surgery, infective endocarditis prophylaxis is required until 6 months after corrective surgery.

Prognosis

Not all children are cured by surgery, but most have improved quality of life and improved longevity. Pulmonary regurgitation may become severe and require a valve replacement 10 to 20 years after corrective surgery. Ventricular arrhythmias may occur many years after surgery and may cause sudden death (Park, 2014, p. 231).

PULMONARY OR TRICUSPID ATRESIA

In pulmonary atresia (a severe form of PS), no valve or opening exists to allow blood to flow between the right atrium and right ventricle. In tricuspid atresia, no valve or opening exists to allow blood to flow between the right atrium and ventricle. The right ventricle is **hypoplastic** (small and nonfunctional). Blood flows to the left side of the heart through the foramen ovale. The ductus arteriosus provides the only flow of blood to the pulmonary arteries and lungs. Tricuspid atresia accounts for 1% to 3% of congenital heart defects, while pulmonary atresia accounts for less than 1% (Park, 2014).

Clinical Manifestations

Cyanosis is present and severe at birth.

Tachypnea, poor feeding, CHF, pulmonary edema, hepatomegaly, acidosis, hypoxic spells, clubbing, polycythemia, and growth delays occur.

A continuous murmur from the PDA is heard in the pulmonic area. A single S_2 is heard in the aortic area, and a harsh systolic murmur may be heard at the lower left sternal border.

Diagnostic Tests

The chest radiograph may reveal a normal size or slightly enlarged right atrium and left ventricle.

The ECG may reveal left ventricular hypertrophy.

The echocardiogram shows a small hypoplastic right ventricular cavity and tricuspid valve, an absent right ventricular outflow tract, a dilated right atrium, and right-to-left shunting across the atrial septum.

Clinical Therapy

Prostaglandin E_1 is given immediately to maintain a patent ductus arteriosus. Treatment for CHF may be needed.

A balloon atrial septostomy is performed to increase the atrial opening size. Other palliative procedures may be performed, such as a Blalock-Taussig shunt or pulmonary artery banding, before a staged Fontan procedure for the single ventricle defect.

Prophylaxis for thromboembolism and infective endocarditis is recommended. Digoxin and diuretic medications may be needed long term.

Prognosis

The child has an increased risk for arrhythmia and right ventricular dysfunction. Survival after a successful Fontan procedure is greater than 95% (Park, 2014).

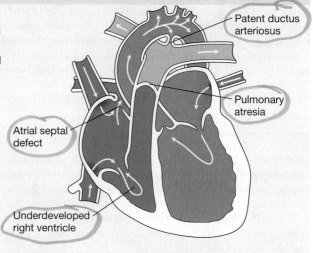

Patent ductus arteriosus

Pulmonary atresia

Atrial septal defect

Underdeveloped right ventricle

☐ Decreased unoxygenated blood flow

☐ Mixed oxygenated and unoxygenated blood

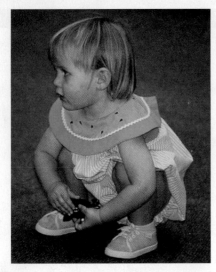

Figure 21–6 Children compensate for inadequate blood flow. A young child with an uncorrected or partially corrected defect that reduces pulmonary blood flow may squat (assume a knee–chest position) to reduce systemic blood flow return to the heart.

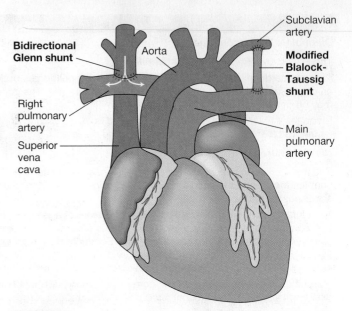

Figure 21–7 Anatomic location of the modified Blalock-Taussig and Glenn shunts for palliative procedures.

Toddlers with uncorrected cyanotic heart disease often squat in the knee–chest position to relieve dyspnea (Figure 21–6). This position reduces the cardiac output by decreasing the blood return from the lower extremities and by increasing the systemic vascular resistance. Blood flow to the lungs is increased. Hypoxic episodes can occur suddenly between 2 months and 2 years of age. Signs include increased cyanosis, increased rate and depth of respirations, tachycardia, poor tissue perfusion, diaphoresis, and seizures and loss of consciousness.

SAFETY ALERT!

Infants and young children respond to severe hypoxemia with bradycardia. Cardiac arrest in children often results from prolonged hypoxemia related to respiratory failure or shock rather than from a primary cardiac arrhythmia as in adults (Perkin, deCaen, Berg, et al., 2013). Bradycardia is a significant warning sign that cardiac arrest is imminent. Treating hypoxemia often reverses bradycardia and prevents cardiac arrest.

Older children may have additional symptoms such as exercise-induced dizziness and **syncope** (transient loss of consciousness and muscle tone), which are both serious signs indicating a need for medical evaluation.

MIXED DEFECTS

These complex congenital heart defects cause varying degrees of cyanosis and CHF. See Table 21–7 for the pathophysiology, clinical manifestations, diagnostic tests, clinical therapy, and prognosis for these complex mixed defects.

Clinical Therapy

Early management of these defects is important to prevent secondary damage to the heart, lungs, and brain, including the adverse effects of hypoxemia on the child's cognitive and psychomotor development. Corrective surgery is usually performed on newborns and young infants. A palliative procedure may be performed first for some potentially lethal conditions. See Figure 21–7 for various palliative shunts (surgically created channels for blood flow) that may be performed. In other

cases, corrective surgery is preferred to give the newborn a better outcome. CHF is treated aggressively as described later in this chapter. See Tables 21–7 and 21–8 for clinical therapy for specific congenital heart defects.

If closure of the ductus arteriosus causes life-threatening cyanosis in newborns, prostaglandin E_1 (PGE_1) is given to reopen the ductus arteriosus and improve pulmonary or systemic blood flow. Treatment with PGE_1 provides time to transfer the newborn to a cardiac center for diagnostic evaluation and surgical intervention. Adverse effects include respiratory depression and apnea, so the infant must be closely monitored and sometimes ventilation must be assisted.

The child's hemoglobin and hematocrit values are monitored for polycythemia or anemia. If the blood viscosity becomes too high, red cell apheresis may be performed. Anemia is not well tolerated because the infant has less oxygen-carrying hemoglobin.

HYPOXIC EPISODES

Hypoxic or hypercyanotic episodes are treated aggressively. Place the infant in the knee–chest position to reduce blood return to the legs, increasing systemic vascular resistance. Reduce any irritating or painful stimuli, and try to calm the infant. Provide supplemental oxygen. If these measures do not relieve the hypoxic spell, more aggressive treatment may include IV morphine, sedation (ketamine), sodium bicarbonate to treat acidosis, or a vasoconstrictor medication such as phenylephrine. Metabolic acidosis is treated if present. Postpone all unpleasant procedures. Immediate palliative or corrective surgery is often scheduled. Propanolol may be prescribed to prevent hypoxic episodes.

INFECTIVE ENDOCARDITIS

Prophylactic antibiotics for infective endocarditis are required for most children with complex cardiac defects prior to surgery and for 6 months after surgery. See *Medications Used for Infective Endocarditis: Prophylaxis for Dental and Invasive Respiratory Procedures* later in this chapter. Children whose surgery involved prosthetic valves or patches and those who have unrepaired cyanotic congenital heart disease, including palliative shunts and conduits, need lifelong infective endocarditis prophylaxis (Kharouf & Torchen, 2011).

TABLE 21–7 Pathophysiology, Clinical Manifestations, Diagnostic Tests, Clinical Therapy, and Prognosis for Mixed Defects

ANATOMY

TRANSPOSITION OF THE GREAT ARTERIES (TGA)

The pulmonary artery is the outflow tract for the left ventricle, and the aorta is the outflow tract for the right ventricle, creating parallel circulations. The condition is life threatening at birth, and survival initially depends on an open ductus arteriosus and foramen ovale. This common defect accounts for 5% to 7% of all congenital heart defects and is more common in males (Park, 2014). An ASD or VSD may also be present with TGA.

Clinical Manifestations

Cyanosis, apparent soon after birth, progresses to hypoxemia and acidosis. Cyanosis does not improve with oxygen administration. Cyanosis may be less apparent when a large VSD is present.

Infants take a long time to feed and need frequent rest periods because of rapid respiratory rate and fatigue. Growth failure may be evident as early as 2 weeks of age if corrective surgery is not performed.

CHF may develop immediately or over days or weeks. Tachypnea (60 breaths/min) is often present without retractions or dyspnea unless CHF is present.

A systolic murmur is present if a VSD is present; no other murmur is generally heard. S_2 is loud and heard as a single sound.

Diagnostic Tests

A chest radiograph may reveal a classic egg-shaped heart on a string with enlarged ventricles and increased pulmonary vascular markings.
The ECG reveals right ventricular hypertrophy.
The echocardiogram often shows the abnormal position of the great arteries rising from the ventricles and any associated defects.
Blood tests reveal an increased hematocrit and hemoglobin or polycythemia and acidosis.

Clinical Therapy

Prostaglandin E_1 is ordered to maintain a patent ductus arteriosus until a palliative procedure (balloon atrial septostomy) is performed during cardiac catheterization to permit oxygenated and unoxygenated blood to mix.
CHF is treated with diuretics and digoxin.
Corrective surgery (arterial switch) is usually performed in the neonatal period.

Prognosis

Survival without surgery is impossible. Complications may occur such as stenosis of the pulmonary artery or aorta in the vessels beyond the valves or coronary artery obstruction. Arrhythmias (sick sinus syndrome, atrial flutter, and atrial fibrillation), tricuspid valve insufficiency, right ventricular dysfunction or failure, and sudden death may be long-term complications associated with formerly used surgical procedures (e.g., Mustard and Senning) (Park, 2014, p. 213).

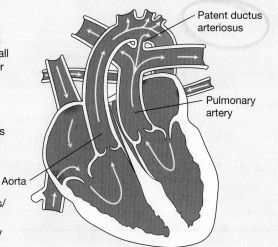

Patent ductus arteriosus
Pulmonary artery
Aorta

TRUNCUS ARTERIOSUS

A single large vessel empties both ventricles and provides circulation for the pulmonary, systemic, and coronary circulations. A VSD is usually present. This occurs in about 1% of congenital heart defects (Park, 2014).

Clinical Manifestations

Cyanosis develops soon after birth; however, this is also a condition of increased pulmonary blood flow. CHF develops within 2 weeks after birth with tachypnea, dyspnea, retractions, poor feeding, poor growth, clubbing, increased pulse pressure, bounding peripheral pulses, a widened pulse pressure, and frequent respiratory infections.

A systolic click may be heard in the apex and pulmonic area. The VSD produces a harsh systolic murmur in the lower sternal border.

Diagnostic Tests

The chest radiograph shows cardiomegaly, increased pulmonary vascular markings, and sometimes a right aortic arch.
The ECG reveals bilateral ventricular hypertrophy.
The echocardiogram shows a VSD, a large single great artery, and one semilunar valve.

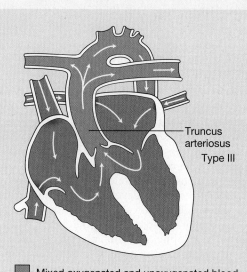

Truncus arteriosus
Type III

Mixed oxygenated and unoxygenated blood

(continued)

TABLE 21–7 Pathophysiology, Clinical Manifestations, Diagnostic Tests, Clinical Therapy, and Prognosis for Mixed Defects (*continued*)

ANATOMY

Clinical Therapy

CHF is treated with diuretics and digoxin.

A Rastelli procedure is performed within a week of birth to close the VSD, enabling the left ventricle to empty into the single large great artery. A conduit is created to the pulmonary arteries. Repeated surgery is necessary to enlarge the pulmonary artery conduit or to repair the truncal valve.

Prophylaxis for infective endocarditis is needed for life.

Prognosis

Surgical mortality varies from 10% to 30% (Park, 2014). Ventricular arrhythmias may develop. The child should not participate in competitive or strenuous sports.

TOTAL ANOMALOUS PULMONARY VENOUS RETURN

The pulmonary veins empty into the right atrium or veins leading to the right atrium rather than into the left atrium. Mixed blood must pass through the foramen ovale or an ASD to provide the systemic circulation. Any obstruction of the pulmonary veins increases the condition's severity. This accounts for 1% of congenital heart defects (Park, 2014).

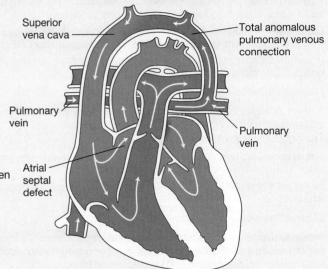

Clinical Manifestations

The newborn may have mild cyanosis and tachypnea. Signs of CHF (tachypnea, dyspnea, tachycardia, and enlarged liver) and pulmonary edema develop along with poor growth and frequent respiratory infections.

A precordial bulge may be palpated. The S_2 has a wide, fixed split when there is no pulmonary vein obstruction. A systolic murmur is heard in the pulmonic area.

Diagnostic Tests

The chest radiograph shows enlargement of the right atrium and ventricle and increased pulmonary blood flow.

The ECG reveals right ventricular hypertrophy.

The echocardiogram shows a dilated right atrium and ventricle, smaller left-sided chambers, dilated pulmonary arteries, and a patent foramen ovale. It can determine the type of pulmonary drainage and if the pulmonary venous return is obstructed.

Clinical Therapy

Prostaglandin E_1 is given to maintain the patent ductus arteriosus for some newborns.

Diuretics are given to treat CHF.

Surgery is performed to move or create a conduit to connect the pulmonary veins to the left atrium.

Prognosis

Surgery is required for survival. Postoperative mortality ranges from 5% to 10% (Park, 2014). Children may develop pulmonary hypertension, pulmonary vein obstruction, or atrial arrhythmias.

OUTCOMES AND PROGNOSIS

Most children with congenital heart disease have normal IQ scores, and children with corrected simple defects can lead normal lives; however, neurologic insults can occur for many reasons. Conditions such as congestive heart failure and cyanosis can affect gross motor development. Infants with complex congenital heart defects are at risk for preoperative neurologic insult. Inadequate nutrition during the first year of life, when rapid brain development occurs, places the infant at greater risk. Some infants have structural brain abnormalities, abnormal cerebral blood flow, chromosomal abnormalities, cerebral ischemia, and other chromosomal disorders documented prior to surgery. Infants with cyanosis who also have iron deficiency anemia may develop a stroke. See *Evidence-Based Practice: Neurodevelopmental Outcomes in Children With Complex Congenital Heart Disease*.

Children with complex congenital heart defects need multiple stages of surgery, revisions of previous surgeries, valve replacements, or interventional catheterization to reopen valves or vessels that have become obstructed. However, rates of survival to adulthood have been improving for children with complex CHD. A pacemaker may be needed for children with potential life-threatening AV block or ventricular dysfunction (Park, 2014, p. 442).

| Neurodevelopmental Outcomes in Children With Complex Congenital Heart Disease

Clinical Question

What information do parents and school officials need to plan for educational supports for children who have had surgery for complex congenital heart defects?

The Evidence

Fifty infants who had cardiac surgery at less than 8 weeks of age were assessed for gross motor performance at 4, 8, 12, and 16 months of age using the Alberta Infant Motor Scale. Infants with chromosomal abnormalities were excluded. Gross motor skill development was delayed at all ages. More than 50% of study infants had persistent delay in gross motor skills across all ages, while some showed improvement over time (Long, Harris, Elderidge, et al., 2012).

Gross motor skills were evaluated in 55 children, ages 6 to 11 years, who previously had a Fontan procedure. None had a physical activity contraindication. Each child was asked to perform locomotor skills (run, gallop, hop on one foot, standing jump, running leap, sideways slide) and object control skills (overhand throw, batting, kicking, dribbling, catching, and rolling a ball). Girls were found to have age-appropriate scores for all gross motor skills. Boys had age-appropriate locomotor skills but lower than expected object control skills. Skill mastery for running and catching were delayed at all ages. Jumping, sliding, and throwing skills were age-appropriate at younger ages but declined in older children. Lower scores were found in boys and children with more complicated medical history or who were sedentary. Children who participated on team sports or perceived family or peer expectations of activity performed better than expected for age (Longmuir, Banks, & McCrindle, 2012).

Forty children who had had corrective or palliative surgery for a significant congenital heart defect (CHD) were evaluated for behavior and competencies at school age. Children with diagnosed chromosomal abnormalities were excluded from the study. Healthy siblings closest in age to study children served as a comparison group. Parents completed the Child Behavior Checklist, while teachers completed the teacher version of the same test. Results indicated that in comparison with siblings, parents perceived that children with CHD had more behavior problems. Both teachers and parents identified reduced school competencies. Children with CHD missed more days of school, participated less in physical education, needed more remedial help, and had lower attainment than siblings (McCusker, Armstrong, Mullen, et al., 2013).

Best Practice

Children with complex CHDs and subsequent surgery often have motor and cognitive problems, such as difficulties with executive functioning skills, problem solving, and memory. These cognitive deficits may lead to learning disabilities, and poorly developed motor skills may interfere with social interactions with peers. Regular developmental screening is needed to identify the specific neurodevelopmental problems that a child could have prior to school entry. Educating families to encourage the child's participation in physical activities may help improve motor skills. Children with complex CHD may need an individualized education plan when disabilities affect learning.

Clinical Reasoning

Develop an outline of important information for a parent of a child with a complex congenital heart defect to discuss with the child's teacher and school officials when the child enters school, including physical and education issues.

Nursing Management

For the Child With Decreased Pulmonary Blood Flow

Nursing management of the hospitalized child focuses on monitoring PGE_1 therapy for newborns, treating hypercyanotic episodes, supporting families to care for the child at home, and providing postsurgical care.

Nursing Assessment and Diagnosis

PHYSIOLOGIC ASSESSMENT BEFORE SURGERY

Infants receiving PGE_1 therapy are cared for in an intensive care nursery where their cardiovascular status can be closely monitored until palliative procedures or corrective surgery is performed.

Prior to or between stages of surgery, the infant or child is seen regularly to assess growth and monitor for signs of CHF (tachycardia, tachypnea, crackles, frothy secretions, low urine output, and pulmonary edema) or worsening condition. The child's poor growth may affect weight, height, and head circumference, so plot serial measurements on the same growth curve to monitor the significance of the growth problems. Monitor physiologic status using the guidelines given in the *Assessment Guide* at the beginning of this chapter.

The child needs careful observation for signs of increased cyanosis in the morning or at other high-risk times. Observe for neurologic signs of thromboembolism due to polycythemia such as headache, dizziness, excessive irritability, and paralysis. Older children with cyanotic defects may have clubbing of the fingers and toes.

ASSESSMENT FOLLOWING SURGERY

Children are admitted to the ICU following surgery. Children undergoing video-assisted thoracostomy surgery may go to the postanesthesia unit and a short-stay unit for discharge the same day. See the nursing care guidelines in the section on nursing assessment of the child following cardiac surgery for increased pulmonary blood flow earlier in this chapter. When the child returns to the general nursing unit, monitor the child's heart functioning. Assess vital signs, pulse oximetry, skin color, and perfusion of the skin by capillary refill and distal pulses. Monitor fluid intake and output. A sudden sustained increase in pulse and respirations and a decrease in peripheral perfusion may be early signs of hemorrhage. Signs of respiratory distress may indicate the development of a pneumothorax or CHF.

PSYCHOSOCIAL ASSESSMENT

Assess the parents' need for information and emotional support. In some cases, the infant's condition is first identified at birth; however, defects are often identified by fetal sonography.

The parents will be grieving the loss of a perfect newborn and be extremely anxious about the infant's condition and prognosis.

Examples of nursing diagnoses that may apply to a child with decreased pulmonary blood flow include the following (NANDA-I © 2014):

- *Cardiac Output, Decreased,* related to ventricular restriction and an obstructed outflow tract

- *Infection, Risk for,* related to unfiltered bacteria in the blood and sites of blood shunting that promote bacterial growth

- *Health Management, Family, Ineffective,* related to complexity of therapeutic regimen: assessment and management of hypoxic spells, which are unpredictable events

- *Activity Intolerance* related to cyanosis and dyspnea on exertion

- *Development: Delayed, Risk for,* related to profound hypoxemia

Planning and Implementation

HOME CARE OF THE CHILD BEFORE SURGERY

Many infants with tetralogy of Fallot and other serious defects are managed at home to grow and potentially improve surgical outcome. Parents are usually anxious during the wait for surgery. They may fear that the infant will not survive until surgery or that they will be unable to manage any problems the infant may have. Provide information and teach parents how to care for the infant at home. Arrange for home health nursing and other community services if required. Many of these children require supplemental nutrition and oxygen for emergencies. Because unoxygenated and oxygenated blood mix, supplemental oxygen does not improve the child's usual oxygen saturation (SpO_2) level.

Cyanosis with or without CHF often results in delayed gross motor skills. Make referrals to community-based early intervention programs to help parents learn about realistic developmental goals and to promote the infant's development. Encourage parents to treat the infant as normally as possible.

SAFETY ALERT!

The infant with moderate to severe disease should be able to tolerate crying for a few minutes. Do not permit prolonged crying because it worsens cyanosis and causes more hypoxemia.

Hypoxic episodes become life threatening if not treated immediately. The child becomes progressively more hypoxic and limp, loses consciousness, is likely to have a seizure or stroke, and may die. Teach parents to observe for signs of worsening cyanosis, particularly in the morning, that could signal the beginning of a hypercyanotic episode. Some families use a pulse oximeter daily to monitor the infant's SpO_2 and identify a change that may indicate an emergency.

Provide guidelines for the initial care of a hypoxic episode. The parents should call for an ambulance and try to calm and reassure the infant. The infant should be placed in a knee–chest position by holding the infant facing the parent's chest, placing one arm under the knees, and folding the legs upward toward the infant's chest. Use the other arm to support the infant's head and back. Alternatively, the infant can be placed supine with knees bent up to the chest. If oxygen is available, provide it in a manner that does not further upset the infant. If none is available in the home, it will be administered in the ambulance during transport to the emergency department.

Teach parents to report signs of illness to the healthcare provider. Vomiting and diarrhea may cause dehydration, a particular risk in children with polycythemia (the blood becomes more viscous and may form thrombi). Fever increases the metabolic rate and further stresses the heart. Aggressive management with antipyretic medication and fluid volume replacement is necessary.

Signs of infective endocarditis (low-grade fever, fatigue, and malaise) occurring within 2 months of surgery or a high-risk procedure should be reported. Teach parents to request antibiotic prophylaxis for the child when appropriate.

Although parents may travel with cyanotic children, they should talk with the healthcare provider before taking them to areas of high altitude or on an airplane. Supplemental oxygen when traveling may be necessary.

Clinical Tip

Develop an emergency plan for the infant in anticipation of acute problems such as a hypoxic episode or respiratory distress. The parents should learn cardiopulmonary resuscitation. Provide the parents with a card or form that has information about the child's condition, medications, necessary emergency care, and the healthcare provider's name so emergency care providers have vital information for initial medical care.

HOSPITAL-BASED CARE OF THE INFANT AND CHILD

The newborn receiving continuous infusion of PGE_1 is cared for in the NICU. Side effects of prostaglandin E_1 treatment such as cutaneous vasodilation, bradycardia, tachycardia, hypotension, seizure activity, fever, and apnea are monitored and managed.

Avoid any unpleasant or anxiety-provoking procedures in an effort to prevent a hypoxic episode. If a hypoxic episode occurs, follow guidelines for treatment.

Following surgery, the child is initially cared for in the ICU until heart function has stabilized. Once the child returns to the general nursing unit, nursing care is the same as described for the child having surgery for increased pulmonary blood flow earlier in this chapter.

COMMUNITY-BASED NURSING CARE AFTER SURGERY

Support adolescents to transition to self-care, especially those with a complex congenital heart defect. Coordination between a primary healthcare provider and cardiologist with expertise in adults with CHD is recommended when adolescents transition to adult healthcare providers. See *Health Promotion: The Adolescent With Congenital Heart Disease.*

Evaluation

Examples of expected nursing care outcomes include the following:

- The parents recognize a hypoxic episode and initiate appropriate emergency treatment.

- The parents manage fever and medical illnesses to prevent dehydration and thromboembolism.

- The family copes with the stress of the child's condition and other family demands.

- The child demonstrates progressive development in gross motor, fine motor, and language skills following surgical repair.

Health Promotion The Adolescent With Congenital Heart Disease

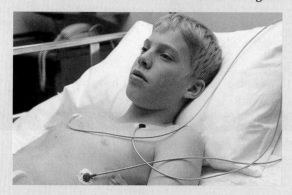

Preventive Care

- Ensure that the adolescent has a healthcare home for general health and illness care. Perform health screening according to recommended schedules (see Chapter 9). Give all recommended immunizations, including the influenza vaccine.
- Encourage routine dental visits twice a year. Make sure the adolescent knows that regular dental care can help reduce endocarditis risk and to seek antibiotic prophylaxis if needed.
- Encourage female adolescents to initiate gynecologic care to ensure that appropriate care is provided for sexual health and contraception. For example, contraceptives containing estrogen are not recommended for individuals with cyanosis, mechanical prosthetic heart valves, or Fontan circulation because of the risk of venous thrombosis (Warnes, 2014). Educate the adolescent about the potential need for special care during pregnancy.
- Provide counseling about health risks associated with tobacco use, alcohol and drug use, and unprotected sex.

Physical Activity

- Ensure that the adolescent with complex CHD has graded exercise testing on a treadmill or bicycle to determine the sports, exercises, and physical activity recommended.
- Clearly explain the importance of physical activity for long-term health. Inquire about the adolescent's beliefs about allowable exercise and activity level, and provide education if differences in recommended and perceived activity levels are found. Explain any activity limitations, such as avoidance of body blocking if a pacemaker is used.

Nutrition

- Encourage the adolescent to eat nutritious meals and snacks, and to avoid excess weight gain that could stress the heart function.
- Educate adolescents with polycythemia to maintain hydration.

Mental and Spiritual Health

- Talk with adolescents about their self-identify, as they have scars, may be smaller than their peers, may be less physically active, and have more frequent healthcare visits.
- Discuss the adolescent's concerns for the future because there may be significant uncertainty about the disease course and outcome.
- Identify and refer adolescents as needed for counseling or to a support group of adolescents of similar age with congenital heart disease.

Education for Self-Care

- Begin the process of transitioning the adolescent to adult health care. Provide education about the congenital heart defect, surgeries that have been performed, and the types of symptoms resulting. Provide information about specific signs that require healthcare provider notification. Remember that previous education has been targeted to the parents. Correct any misperceptions that prior surgery resulted in a normal heart if that is not the case.
- Provide a written succinct summary of the adolescent's condition and medical management that can be shared with other healthcare providers.
- Provide education about infective endocarditis prophylaxis if needed. Describe situations that may increase risk, such as tattooing, acupuncture, dental care, electrolysis, and various diagnostic and surgical procedures.
- Discuss the medications needed and why. Develop plans for the adolescent to assume responsibility for self-administration. Educate the adolescent to seek guidance before using over-the-counter medications and herbal medications because of the potential for medication interaction.
- Discuss the genetic aspects of the condition and provide resources for genetic counseling if desired.
- Discuss the danger signs of the condition (such as arrhythmias, or the potential of dehydration in an adolescent with cyanosis) and how to seek urgent or emergency care.

Vocational Education

- Reassure adolescents who have had complete repairs of the congenital heart defect and have no disabilities that they have no limitations in their career or vocational selection.
- Provide career and vocational counseling to adolescents with cardiac disabilities that matches their interests, academic abilities, and clinical limitations. Encourage preparation for employment that can be maintained throughout the working career. Inform adolescents about their rights under the Americans with Disabilities Act of 1990.
- Encourage families and adolescents to identify health insurance options and policies that are a better match for the level of healthcare interventions needed.

Defects Obstructing Systemic Blood Flow

Etiology and Pathophysiology

An anatomic stenosis (narrowing of a valve, of the area around a valve, or in the great artery above a valve) causes obstruction to blood flow and results in a pressure load on the left ventricle and decreased cardiac output. The greater the narrowing, the more obstructed the blood flow is to the circulation. This results in higher pressure in the ventricle and decreased cardiac output. Newborns with severe left outflow obstruction or left ventricular dysfunction may develop decreased cardiac output and shock.

Clinical Manifestations

Low cardiac output is responsible for the following clinical manifestations: diminished pulses, poor color, delayed capillary refill time, and decreased urinary output. The blood cannot move past the obstruction, so it backs up into the left atrium and then the lungs, causing CHF and pulmonary edema. The child with mild obstructions may have leg cramps, cooler feet than hands, and stronger pulses in the arms than the legs. Decreased blood supply to the gastrointestinal tract may lead to necrotizing enterocolitis. See Chapter 25. See Table 21–8 for the pathophysiology, clinical manifestations, diagnostic tests, clinical therapy, and prognosis for congenital heart defects that obstruct systemic blood flow.

TABLE 21–8 Pathophysiology, Clinical Manifestations, Diagnostic Tests, Clinical Therapy, and Prognosis for Defects That Obstruct the Systemic Blood Flow

ANATOMY

AORTIC STENOSIS (AS)

Narrowing of the aortic valve obstructs blood flow to the systemic circulation. The valve often has two valve leaflets (bicuspid), rather than three, that may be partially fused. The left ventricle must work harder to force blood past the narrowed valve opening. Aortic stenosis accounts for up to 10% of congenital heart defects (Park, 2014, p. 188).

Clinical Manifestations

Most infants and children with mild AS are asymptomatic. Life-threatening AS occurs in some newborns. CHF develops in infants with significant stenosis. Peripheral pulses may be weak and thready. The child may complain of chest pain after exercise, and exercise intolerance may be noted. Fainting and dizziness (syncope) are serious signs that require intervention.

The systolic blood pressure may be higher in the right arm than the left.

A systolic heart murmur and thrill may be detected in the aortic area with transmission to the neck. An ejection click may be heard. Splitting of the S_2 may be noted. Interventions may result in aortic insufficiency causing a high-pitched diastolic decrescendo murmur along the left sternal border near the mitral area.

Diagnostic Tests

The chest radiograph may reveal a normal-sized heart, but a dilated ascending aorta may be seen.

The ECG may show mild left ventricular hypertrophy in severe AS.

An echocardiogram reveals the number of valve leaflets, pressure gradient across the valve, and size of the aorta.

Exercise testing may be used in asymptomatic children to determine the amount of obstruction present.

Clinical Therapy

Newborns with life-threatening AS need PGE_1 to maintain a patent ductus arteriosus as well as dopamine and diuretics to treat CHF until the aortic valve can be dilated.

Treatment involves balloon dilation during cardiac catheterization or surgical valvotomy. Surgical treatment is palliative rather than curative.

Aortic valve replacement is performed when stenosis is severe or if significant regurgitation results from other interventions.

Prognosis

Chest pain, syncope, and sudden death can occur in symptomatic children, particularly during vigorous exercise. Untreated mild AS may progress after several decades as the valve calcifies. Stenosis may also recur after intervention. Valve replacement may become necessary, requiring lifelong anticoagulant therapy.

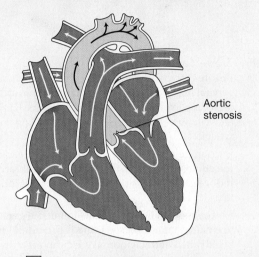

Aortic stenosis

☐ Decreased oxygenated blood flow

COARCTATION OF THE AORTA (COA)

Narrowing or constriction in the descending aorta, often near the ductus arteriosus or left subclavian artery, obstructs the systemic blood outflow. This defect occurs in 8% to 10% of congenital heart defects and is found in 30% of children with Turner syndrome (Park, 2014, p. 195).

Clinical Manifestations

Many children are asymptomatic and grow normally. Reduced blood flow through the descending aorta causes lower blood pressure in legs and higher blood pressure in arms, neck, and head. Brachial and radial pulses are typically bounding, but femoral and leg pulses are weak or absent. Older children may complain of weakness and pain in the legs after exercise.

Clinical Manifestations

Infants with moderate constriction are pale; may have poor feeding, avoidant/restrictive food intake disorder (failure to thrive), and increased respiratory effort. They may develop CHF. Newborns with severe constriction may have cyanosis in the lower extremities, heart failure, and shock as the ductus arteriosus closes. Renal failure and necrotizing enterocolitis may develop.

On auscultation, S_2 is heard as a loud single sound. A systolic ejection murmur may be heard at the upper right and middle or lower left sternal border. A thrill may be palpated in the suprasternal notch.

Diagnostic Tests

The chest radiograph may reveal cardiomegaly, pulmonary venous congestion, and indentation of the descending aorta. Dilation of the ascending aorta may be seen. Rib notching is rarely seen before 5 years of age. MRI is preferred for imaging to see the aortic arch, site of coarctation, and collateral circulation.

ECG may be normal or show left ventricular hypertrophy.

Echocardiogram shows the size of the aorta and functioning of the aortic valve and left ventricle.

Clinical Therapy

In symptomatic newborns, PGE_1 is given to reopen the ductus arteriosus and promote blood flow to the kidneys and lower extremities. Treatment to prevent CHF may be initiated with inotropic medications, diuretics, and oxygen (Park, 2014, p. 198).

Surgical resection is often preferred to balloon dilation during cardiac catheterization to reduce the risk for recoarctation. Balloon dilation with stent placement may be performed for sick newborns who will eventually need surgical repair and stent removal (Park, 2014, p. 199). Balloon angioplasty may be performed if coarctation recurs.

Prognosis

Balloon dilation and surgical resection are palliative because coarctation may recur with either procedure. Lifelong follow-up is necessary. Persistent hypertension occurs in some children.

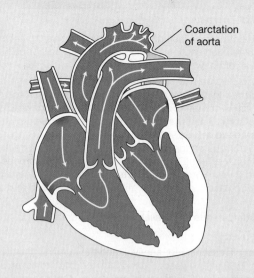

Coarctation of aorta

HYPOPLASTIC LEFT HEART SYNDROME (HLHS)

The mitral and aortic valves are absent or stenosed along with an abnormally small left ventricle and small aorta. HLHS accounts for about 1.5% of congenital heart defects (Awad & Busse, 2011). About 10% of cases are associated with Turner syndrome, trisomy 18, and other genetic disorders (Park, 2014, p. 258).

Clinical Manifestations

Within hours after birth, the newborn has progressive cyanosis and signs of CHF (tachycardia, tachypnea, dyspnea, retractions, and decreased peripheral pulses) as the ductus arteriosus closes.

Poor peripheral perfusion, pulmonary edema, and CHF lead to shock, acidosis, and death, without intervention.

On auscultation, S_2 is single and loud. No heart murmur is present.

Diagnostic Procedures

The chest radiograph shows cardiomegaly and increased pulmonary venous congestion.

The ECG shows right ventricular hypertrophy.

The echocardiogram shows the small left ventricle and enlarged right ventricle. This condition is often diagnosed prenatally.

Clinical Therapy

Prostaglandin E_1 is given immediately to maintain a patent ductus arteriosus.

Intubation and ventilation are performed, and supplemental oxygen is provided. Metabolic acidosis is treated.

Genetic, ophthalmologic, and neurologic evaluations are often performed before surgery.

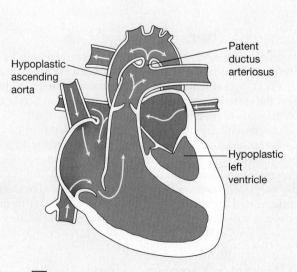

Hypoplastic ascending aorta

Patent ductus arteriosus

Hypoplastic left ventricle

■ Mixed oxygenated and unoxygenated blood

(continued)

TABLE 21–8 Pathophysiology, Clinical Manifestations, Diagnostic Tests, Clinical Therapy, and Prognosis for Defects That Obstruct the Systemic Blood Flow *(continued)*

ANATOMY

Clinical Therapy

Treatment options include surgery or a heart transplant (see the heart transplantation section later in chapter). Comfort or palliative care is chosen less often with advances in surgery.

Norwood surgery is performed in three stages. Stage 1 procedure is performed by 1 week of age. The aorta is reconstructed and the right ventricle is committed to pumping blood through the pulmonary valve to the aorta. The atrial septum is removed so blood can mix. A shunt is created to send adequate blood to the lungs. Stage 2, performed at 3 to 6 months of age, connects the superior vena cava directly to the pulmonary artery (Glenn shunt). Stage 3 Fontan procedure, performed at 1 to 2 years of age, connects the inferior vena cava to the pulmonary circulation, ending the mixing of oxygenated and unoxygenated blood.

Few infant hearts are available for transplantation.

Prognosis

Surgery is essential for survival, and the survival rate after stage 3 Fontan is 95% after 4 years (Park, 2014, p. 261). However, some infants die during intervals between surgical stages. Heart failure, arrhythmias, and sudden cardiac death may occur in children and adolescents several years after stage 3 Fontan surgery. The child will have physical activity limitations because of a single ventricle. Approximately 50% of surviving children have significant cognitive and neurologic impairment (Paris, Moore, & Schreiber, 2012) (see *Evidence-Based Practice* earlier in this chapter).

Clinical Tip

The systolic blood pressure is usually 10 to 15 mmHg higher in the legs than the arms in healthy children. In children with coarctation of the aorta, the systolic blood pressure in the legs may be equal to or lower than in the arms, as the defect obstructs systemic blood flow to the abdomen and lower extremities.

Clinical Therapy

Neonates with severe systemic outflow obstruction or left ventricular dysfunction may develop decreased cardiac output and shock. PGE_1 and inotrope medications may be required to support the systemic circulation until the obstruction is relieved or ventricular function improves.

Some children (e.g., after Fontan procedure or aortic valve replacement) need long-term treatment with aspirin or warfarin to prevent the development of thrombi. Caution parents of children who take warfarin (Coumadin) to avoid using herbal products because of interactions. For example, children will have an increased warfarin effect with ginkgo biloba or a decreased effect with St. John's wort (Yu, Bostwick, & Hallman, 2011).

Nursing Management

See the sections on *Congenital Heart Defects That Increase Pulmonary Blood Flow* for nursing care management of children with aortic stenosis and coarctation of the aorta earlier in this chapter and on *Defects Causing Decreased Pulmonary Blood Flow and Mixed Defects* for nursing care management of infants with hypoplastic left heart syndrome (HLHS) earlier in this chapter.

Parents of children with life-threatening defects such as HLHS are under intense pressure to make a decision about the best treatment for their newborns (palliative care, Norwood procedure, or heart transplant). Nurses have an important role in providing parent support during the decision making process as they may get conflicting recommendations by neonatologists and surgeons (Toebbe, Yehle, Kirkpatrick, et al., 2013). Share information with the parents so they are fully informed about treatment options and their associated mortality, the intense care needed by the surviving child, the potential for disabilities, and the unknown long-term survival. Identify family members, clergy, or social workers who can support the parents through this period. If parents choose comfort or palliative care, interventions such as PGE_1 are discontinued, and the infant is given appropriate pain medication and comfort (see Chapter 13). Reassure parents that they are good parents, no matter what decision they make.

Congestive Heart Failure

Congestive heart failure (CHF) occurs when heart function is impaired and cardiac output is inadequate to support the body's circulatory and metabolic needs. It may result from a congenital heart defect that either increases pulmonary blood flow or obstructs the systemic blood outflow tract. Other causes include arrhythmias, pathologic conditions that require high cardiac output (e.g., severe anemia, acidosis, or bronchopulmonary dysplasia), and acquired heart disease (e.g., cardiomyopathy or Kawasaki disease).

Etiology and Pathophysiology

Pulmonary blood volume overload associated with congenital heart defects is a common cause of CHF in infants. Many infants with this pathophysiology develop CHF within the first 6 months of life (McDaniel, 2014). Defects that allow blood to shunt from the left side of the heart to the right increase the amount of blood pumped to the lungs. The pulmonary system is overloaded, and if prolonged can lead to pulmonary artery hypertension (see the section later in this chapter). Obstructive congenital defects restrict the flow of blood, so the heart muscle hypertrophies to work harder to force blood through these structures. Eventually the heart muscle cannot keep up with the demand.

When cardiac output remains insufficient, blood pressure is decreased and hypoxia occurs in the organs and tissues. The sympathetic nervous system is activated and catecholamines are released, leading to tachycardia, improved heart muscle contraction, and improved smooth muscle tone that returns blood to the heart. The sympathetic nervous system also reduces blood flow to the kidneys, which in turn stimulates the release of rennin, angiotensin, and aldosterone. Sodium and fluid are retained to increase circulatory volume. The myocardium stretches temporarily to manage the increased blood flow and force of contraction. These physiologic responses are unable to maintain the cardiac output and maintain blood pressure as CHF progresses and the maximum myocardial stretch is reached. Progressive systemic edema and pulmonary congestion leads to right- or left-sided heart failure that may become bilateral.

Clinical Manifestations

Initial signs of CHF may be subtle and not immediately recognized. The infant tires easily, especially during feeding. Weight loss or lack of normal weight gain, diaphoresis, irritability, and frequent respiratory infections may be evident. Pallor or mottling of the skin may be present. Older children may have exercise intolerance, dyspnea, abdominal pain or distention, and peripheral edema.

As the disease progresses, tachypnea, tachycardia, pallor or cyanosis, nasal flaring, grunting, retractions, cough, or crackles may develop. A third heart sound may be auscultated. Generalized fluid volume overload is seen more commonly in toddlers and older children. Periorbital and facial edema and hepatomegaly are signs of fluid volume excess. Peripheral edema is less common in infants and young children. Jugular vein distention is seen in older children. See Table 21–9 for more detailed clinical manifestations.

Cardiomegaly, enlargement (hypertrophy) of the heart muscle, occurs in an effort to maintain cardiac output. Cyanosis, weak peripheral pulses, cool extremities, hypotension, and heart murmur are precursors of cardiogenic shock, which can occur if CHF is not adequately treated (see the section on cardiogenic shock later in this chapter).

Clinical Therapy

Diagnosis is based primarily on physical findings. A chest radiograph reveals cardiac enlargement and venous congestion or signs of pulmonary edema. Echocardiography confirms the diagnosis and severity of CHF. An electrocardiogram may identify an arrhythmia cause of CHF. Electrolytes, lactic acid, arterial blood gases, and a complete blood count are obtained. Renal function is evaluated with creatinine and blood urea nitrogen (BUN) levels. Liver function tests may be elevated.

TABLE 21–9 Clinical Manifestations of Congestive Heart Failure

PATHOPHYSIOLOGY	CLINICAL MANIFESTATIONS
Pulmonary venous congestion	Mild resting tachypnea, wheezing, crackles, retractions, cough, grunting, nasal flaring, recent onset of poor feeding, increased tachypnea and diaphoresis with feeding
	Tiring with play and orthopnea may be seen in older children
Systemic venous congestion	Hepatomegaly, ascites, periorbital edema, fluid retention weight gain
	Jugular venous distention and dependent edema in older children
Impaired cardiac output	Tachycardia, weak pulses, hypotension, capillary refill time greater than 2 sec, pallor, cool extremities, oliguria, restlessness, irritability
High metabolic rate	Avoidant/restrictive food intake disorder (failure to thrive) or slow weight gain, diaphoresis

The initial goal is to identify and treat the cause of CHF, such as an arrhythmia or surgical correction of a heart defect. Then efforts are made to decrease the work of the heart and improve systemic circulation. Diuretics, such as furosemide, thiazides, and spironolactone, are given to promote fluid excretion. Afterload-reducing agents (angiotensin-converting enzyme [ACE] inhibitors) are often prescribed to lessen the workload on the heart. Digoxin is less commonly prescribed with availability of ACE inhibitors. Inotropic medicines such as dopamine, dobutamine, isoproterenol, and epinephrine are used for critical care management. See *Medications Used to Treat: Congestive Heart Failure*.

Surgery or interventional cardiac catheterization for a congenital heart defect may become the treatment of choice. Cardiac transplantation may be performed for children with end-stage cardiomyopathy or complex congenital heart defects such as hypoplastic left heart syndrome.

Supportive medical therapies (supplemental oxygen, positioning to reduce respiratory distress, rest, and fluid and nutrition management) are part of the treatment plan. Most children improve rapidly after medication is administered.

Nursing Management

For the Child With Congestive Heart Failure

Nursing Assessment and Diagnosis

PHYSIOLOGIC ASSESSMENT

The diagnosis of CHF depends primarily on physical symptoms. Assess the child's vital signs, behavioral patterns, cardiac function, respiratory function, and fluid status using guidelines in the *Assessment Guide* earlier in this chapter. Use the age-specific heart and respiratory rates in Chapter 5 to identify tachycardia and tachypnea. Obtain a detailed history of the onset of symptoms from the parents because CHF often develops slowly.

Medications Used to Treat: Congestive Heart Failure

MEDICATIONS AND ACTIONS	NURSING MANAGEMENT
Digoxin (Lanoxin) Slows the heart rate, increases cardiac filling time, and increases cardiac output; used with increased pulmonary blood flow.	• Assess the heart rate for bradycardia for 1 min prior to giving a dose or for changes in heart rhythm or quality. • Monitor the child for digoxin toxicity. • See the CHF nursing management section for more information.
Furosemide (Lasix) Rapid diuresis; blocks reabsorption of sodium and water in renal tubules.	• Monitor patients during rapid diuresis for vital signs, intake and output, and fluid and electrolyte imbalances (e.g., hypokalemia and hypochloremia). • Assess for digoxin toxicity if hypokalemia is present.
Thiazides (Diuril) Chlorothiazide (suspension); hydrochlorothiazide (tablets). Maintains diuresis, decreases absorption of sodium, water, potassium, chloride, and bicarbonate in renal tubules.	• Monitor blood pressure and intake and output rates and patterns. • Monitor lab values for hypokalemia. Assess for digoxin toxicity if present.
Spironolactone (Aldactone) Maintains diuresis (potassium sparing).	• Assess for signs of fluid and electrolyte imbalance and digitoxicity.
ACEi (angiotensin-converting enzyme inhibitor) (e.g., Captopril, Enalapril) Promotes vascular relaxation and reduced peripheral vascular resistance, reduces afterload.	• Monitor for hypotension with initiation of therapy and dosage changes. • Assess for common side effects such as cough, hyperkalemia, and worsening renal function.
Carvedilol (Coreg) Improves left ventricular function, promotes vasodilation of systemic circulation; used for chronic heart failure and dilated cardiomyopathy.	• Give with food. • Assess the heart rate for bradycardia when the dose is increased. • Assess cardiac output by monitoring tissue perfusion, peripheral pulses, blood pressure, and urine output. • Monitor for dizziness and hypotension. • Monitor digoxin levels because drug may increase plasma digoxin concentration. • Monitor liver function periodically.

Source: Data from Wilson, B. A., Shannon, M. T., & Shields, K. M. (2016). *Pearson nurses' drug guide 2016*. Hoboken, NJ: Pearson Education; Park, M. K. (2014). *Pediatric cardiology for practitioners* (6th ed., pp. 457–464). Philadelphia: Elsevier Saunders; Satou, G. M., & Halnon, N. J. (2013). *Pediatric congestive heart failure*. Retrieved from http://emedicine.medscape.com/article/2069746-medication#1

Measure intake and output carefully. Weigh the infant's diapers before use and after changing (each 1-g difference in weight equals 1 mL of urine). Weigh the child at the same time each day. Observe for periorbital or peripheral edema and circulatory changes. If ascites is present, take serial abdominal measurements to monitor changes. (See the *Clinical Skills Manual* SKILLS for guidelines.) Turn the child frequently and assess the skin for redness and breakdown.

FAMILY ASSESSMENT

Review the child's previous hospitalizations and assess the family's knowledge about the child's condition. Families of children with CHF are anxious about the potential deterioration of the child's condition and their ability to provide ongoing care.

Assess the family's anxiety level and coping strategies. Evaluate the family's economic status. Medication is crucial to treatment, and a family's inability to obtain the necessary medications jeopardizes the child's outcome. Identify the parent's ability to recognize changes in the child's condition and to provide needed care. Determine if another family member is available who could assist young parents or provide respite care.

DEVELOPMENTAL ASSESSMENT

Because fatigue limits the activities of the infant and young child with CHF, the opportunity to practice the skills needed to attain normal developmental milestones is more limited. Use a developmental assessment tool to document current status (see Chapter 6). Ask parents when the child attained expected developmental milestones such as sitting, manipulating objects, standing, or walking; also ask about contact and play with other children and a typical day's activity schedule. Parents may limit the child's contact with other children because of frequent infections and exercise intolerance. When CHF is well controlled, the child's energy level increases and developmental skills often improve. Repeating assessments every 2 to 3 months in infants and toddlers provides useful information about development and disease management.

Several nursing diagnoses that may apply to the child with CHF can be found in the accompanying *Nursing Care Plans*. The primary nursing diagnosis is **Cardiac Output, Decreased,** related to cardiac anomaly (NANDA-I © 2014).

Planning and Implementation

Nursing care for the child with CHF focuses on administering and monitoring effects of medications, maintaining adequate oxygenation and myocardial function, promoting rest, fostering development, providing adequate nutrition, and providing emotional support to the child and family (Figure 21–8). (See *Nursing Care Plan: The Child Hospitalized With Congestive Heart Failure*.)

ADMINISTER AND MONITOR PRESCRIBED MEDICATIONS

Children with CHF usually receive furosemide and an ACE inhibitor, and they may receive intravenous inotropic medications while in the PICU. In some cases, digoxin is prescribed. These medications are potent and must be administered correctly.

SAFETY ALERT!

Before giving the digitalizing dose of digoxin (a higher dose to establish a blood level more rapidly), assess baseline vital signs, the quality of peripheral pulses, and clinical symptoms, and also obtain an electrocardiogram (ECG). Check the levels of serum electrolytes, and check hepatic and renal functions. Assess hydration status, and hydrate if hypovolemic. The risk for digoxin toxicity is increased when hypokalemia is present. Repeated ECGs are used for early detection of toxicity for several days after digitalization (Park, 2014, p. 461).

Before giving any dose of digoxin, take the apical pulse for 1 minute. Call for a healthcare provider's advice before administering the digoxin in the following conditions:

- The heart rate is less than 60 to 100 beats/min, depending on the age, or is higher or lower than the guideline noted in the healthcare provider's order.
- Changes in heart rhythm or quality are noted.

MAINTAIN OXYGENATION AND MYOCARDIAL FUNCTION

Oxygen therapy may be ordered. Make sure that tubing is patent, the oxygen flow rate is correct, the oxygen delivery device is working properly, and humidification is provided. Keep the child calm and quiet. Position the child in semi-Fowler or a 45-degree angle position to promote maximum oxygenation. An infant car safety seat is an option.

PROMOTE REST

Group assessments and interventions together to ensure that the child has some uninterrupted rest each hour. Rocking is restful for infants. Encourage older children to engage in quiet activities such as computer games and videos.

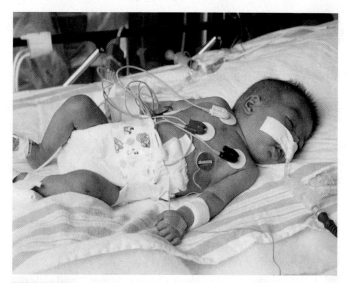

Figure 21–8 Jooti is receiving intravenous fluids and oxygen. Her condition is being continuously monitored for congestive heart failure.

FOSTER DEVELOPMENT

Encourage parents to play with the child, using toys to stimulate eye–hand coordination and fine motor movements. Such toys include rattles, blocks, and stuffed animals for infants and books, paper and crayons, and dolls for older children. Encourage sitting, standing, or walking for short periods with adequate rest afterward to promote the development of large muscles. Singing, talking, and playing music facilitate cognitive and language skills.

PROVIDE ADEQUATE NUTRITION

Teach parents about feeding techniques. Encourage the mother who chooses to breastfeed the infant. The antibodies in breast milk reduce infections, and the milk is naturally low in sodium. However, the sucking involved in breastfeeding or bottle feeding may cause dyspnea that forces the infant to rest frequently during feeding. Feedings should last no more than 30 to 40 minutes, but some infants should feed no longer than 20 minutes. Frequent small feedings generally work best, with burping after every half ounce of intake to minimize vomiting. Holding the infant at a 45-degree angle or positioned in an infant seat decreases venous return to the heart and decreases its metabolic demand. Make sure parents understand that changes in feeding habits (decreased intake, vomiting, sleeping through feedings, and increased perspiration with feedings) may indicate deteriorating cardiac status.

Infants with CHF need adequate nutrition to support growth because their metabolic rate is elevated. Some infants need a higher caloric formula (24 to 30 calories per ounce) to obtain adequate nutrition. For example, regular powdered formula can be prepared with less water or a human milk fortifier can be added to breast milk. In some cases, low-osmolarity glucose polymers or medium-chain triglyceride (MCT) oil is recommended for addition to standard formula (Park, 2014, p. 457). Nutritional supplementation by nasogastric, transpyloric, or gastrostomy tube may be prescribed. Parents are often advised to have the infant feed normally for a specific period to promote oral stimulation and bonding. The remainder of the formula is then given by tube feeding. (See the *Clinical Skills Manual* SKILLS.)

Nursing Care Plan: The Child Hospitalized With Congestive Heart Failure

1. Nursing Diagnosis: *Cardiac Output, Decreased,* **related to cardiac anomaly (VSD) (NANDA-I © 2014)**

GOAL: The child's cardiac output will be sufficient to meet the body's metabolic demands.

INTERVENTION	RATIONALE
• Administer digoxin as ordered.	• Digoxin increases contractility of the heart and force of contraction.
• Regularly count the apical pulse and listen to heart sounds, especially before each dose of digoxin. Record the apical pulse rate with each dose of digoxin.	• Digoxin may cause bradycardia. Pulse and heart sounds provide information about heart functioning.
• Use cardiac monitor if prescribed.	• Monitor notes bradycardia and arrhythmias.
• Monitor serum potassium level and for digitoxicity.	• Hypokalemia increases risk of digoxin toxicity.
• Provide for rest periods each hour.	• Rest decreases need for high cardiac output.

EXPECTED OUTCOME: Child's cardiac output will be sufficient as indicated by increased energy, adequate feeding intake, and decreased edema. Child will maintain normal serum potassium levels and therapeutic levels of digoxin. Child will rest hourly and have adequate energy to eat and play.

GOAL: The child will manifest adequate oxygenation.

INTERVENTION	RATIONALE
• Evaluate respiratory rate and breath sounds. Observe for diaphoresis, a sign of increased respiratory effort. Use pulse oximetry to determine oxygen saturation readings.	• Provides information about oxygenation and ease of respiration.
• Provide oxygen and humidification if prescribed.	• Supplemental oxygen decreases tachypnea, and humidification moistens secretions to keep airway clear.
• Place child in semi-Fowler position.	• This position facilitates lung expansion.

EXPECTED OUTCOME: Child will maintain a normal SpO$_2$ level and respiratory rate for age without evidence of adventitious sounds or diaphoresis.

2. Nursing Diagnosis: *Fluid Volume: Excess* **related to heart failure (NANDA-I © 2014)**

GOAL: Intake and output will be balanced once excess fluid is excreted.

INTERVENTION	RATIONALE
• Administer diuretics as ordered.	• Diuretics mobilize fluids and facilitate excretion.
• Measure intake and output carefully. Weigh diapers to assess output of infants. Weigh daily. Measure abdominal girth daily. Observe for peripheral edema.	• Adequate output is a good indicator of renal perfusion. Assessments demonstrate effectiveness of treatment.
• Monitor electrolytes.	• Electrolyte imbalance is common when diuretics are given.
• Maintain fluid restrictions if prescribed.	• Fluid restriction may help decrease the cardiac load.

EXPECTED OUTCOME: Child's intake and output will be proportional, and electrolyte levels will remain within normal ranges.

3. Nursing Diagnosis: *Skin Integrity, Risk for Impaired,* **related to altered fluid status (NANDA-I © 2014)**

GOAL: The child's peripheral and central edema will decrease.

INTERVENTION	RATIONALE
• Change child's position frequently.	• Position changes promote circulation to skin over pressure points.
• Inspect skin frequently for redness and skin breakdown over pressure points.	• Inspection identifies earliest stages of skin breakdown.

EXPECTED OUTCOME: Child will have no skin breakdown after edema resolves.

4. Nursing Diagnosis: *Nutrition, Imbalanced: Less than Body Requirements*, **related to high metabolic needs and rapid tiring while feeding (NANDA-I © 2014)**

GOAL: The child will receive adequate nutrition to meet metabolic needs.

INTERVENTION	RATIONALE
• Hold infant at 45-degree angle for feeding.	• Position facilitates breathing while eating.
• Record intake carefully.	• Evaluation of intake indicates whether caloric and other nutritional needs are met.
• Weigh child daily.	• Weight gain indicates growth (in absence of fluid retention).
• Give frequent small meals with rest periods in between.	• Digesting small meals requires less energy.
• Use high-calorie formula or give high-calorie snacks.	• High-calorie formulas and snacks provide calories efficiently.
• Use soothing approaches such as holding infants for feeding and having parents eat with older child.	• Restful approach facilitates intake with minimum cardiac work.
• Transition to supplemental tube feedings if the infant is not able to gain weight.	• Tube feedings provide added calories without taxing the infant's energy.

EXPECTED OUTCOME: Infant or child will gain recommended weight according to growth grids. All dietary requirements will be met, and mealtimes will be pleasant.

PROVIDE EMOTIONAL SUPPORT

The family is often anxious about the condition of the child hospitalized with CHF. Give parents a chance to express concerns about their child's condition. Explain the child's treatment regimen, and make sure family members understand the child's need for nutrition and rest. Refer parents to the appropriate support groups; talking with parents of children with cardiac conditions may be a source of emotional support.

DISCHARGE PLANNING AND HOME CARE TEACHING

Identify and address home care needs well in advance of discharge. Show parents how to prepare formula or supplement breast milk, and then offer guidance to help maximize the child's nutritional intake. While the child is hospitalized, teach the family about medication administration and signs of a worsening condition (e.g., increased feeding difficulty, irritability, lethargy, breathing difficulty, and puffiness around the eyes or extremities). Arrange for home care nursing visits to reinforce the education provided, to monitor the child's condition, and to assess the family's ability to manage the child's care. Ensure that the family has a phone contact for questions and emergency assistance. (See *Nursing Care Plan: The Child With Congestive Heart Failure Being Cared for at Home.*)

Demonstrate administration of drugs, and then supervise while the parents measure and administer medications. If digoxin is prescribed, teach parents about the signs of digoxin's toxic effects. Parents are frequently taught to take the child's pulse and to report any significant change to the healthcare provider and any signs of medication side effects. Teach parents about the potential interaction between digoxin and macrolide antibiotics so they can remind the primary care provider to prescribe safe antibiotics when they are needed.

Teach parents to take special care with an acute illness that involves a fever and diarrhea or vomiting. An acute illness could lead to dehydration more quickly when the child takes diuretics, and urgent care will be needed.

These children are evaluated frequently by healthcare providers for progression in signs and symptoms, appropriate weight gain, and developmental progress. Families are evaluated for their ongoing ability to manage the child's condition and cope with the stress of caring for a sick child.

Evaluation

Expected outcomes of nursing care can be found in the *Nursing Care Plans*.

Clinical Reasoning **The Infant With Ventricular Septal Defect**

Brandy, who is 1 month old, was diagnosed with a ventricular septal defect (VSD) at birth and started developing signs of respiratory distress and difficulty with feeding.

Brandy's mother had been alerted to watch for these signs as a possible indication of congestive heart failure. Brandy was quickly hospitalized so her CHF could be treated with intravenous furosemide, dopamine, and potassium. Over the next 2 days, she lost the weight she had gained as a result of fluid retention.

Corrective surgery was performed to place a patch over the septal opening. Brandy was cared for in the intensive care unit before being transferred to another unit.

- Why did Brandy develop CHF? Why was corrective surgery performed when she is so young?
- What teaching and support do Brandy's parents need to care for her at home after the heart surgery?

Acquired Heart Diseases
Cardiomyopathy

Cardiomyopathy is a serious disorder of the heart's muscle that affects chamber size, wall thickness, or contraction and leads to problems with ventricular systolic or diastolic function.

Nursing Care Plan: The Child With Congestive Heart Failure Being Cared for at Home

1. Nursing Diagnosis: *Development: Delayed, Risk for,* related to effects of physical disability (NANDA-I © 2014)

GOAL: The child will meet developmental milestones for age group.

INTERVENTION	RATIONALE
• Perform baseline developmental assessment.	• Assessment provides comparison for later assessments and basis for planning specific games, toys, and activities.
• Plan for short play periods after rest.	• Short play periods maintain energy and facilitate play.
• Introduce age-appropriate toys and activities such as rattles and blocks for infants and art projects for older children.	• Play activities facilitate learning and mastery of developmental tasks.
• Plan for interactions with healthy children.	• Social skills are learned through contact with others.

EXPECTED OUTCOME: Child will display normal language, fine motor, and gross motor activity.

2. Nursing Diagnosis: *Health Management, Family, Ineffective,* related to complexity of therapeutic regimen (NANDA-I © 2014)

GOAL: Parents will demonstrate correct administration of medications.

INTERVENTION	RATIONALE
• Have parents prepare the medication dosages and administer the digoxin, diuretics, and other medications to the child while observed by the nurse.	• Demonstrating techniques used to administer medications provides opportunities to identify dosage errors and to suggest methods to help ensure the child gets all needed medications.

EXPECTED OUTCOME: Parents will demonstrate ability to prepare correct medication dosage and administer it to the child.

GOAL: Parents will state side effects of medications and symptoms of congestive heart failure.

INTERVENTION	RATIONALE
• Describe side effects of medications. Give parents handouts with telephone number to call to ask questions or report side effects.	• If side effects are understood, serious complications can be avoided.
• Describe subtle onset of CHF symptoms (increasing weakness, exhaustion, irritability, difficulty feeding, cough or difficult respirations, edema).	• Parents can evaluate child regularly and note subtle changes requiring medical management.

EXPECTED OUTCOME: Parents will report that child continues to demonstrate improvement and adequate cardiac output without signs of congestive heart failure.

3. Nursing Diagnosis: *Nutrition, Imbalanced: Less than Body Requirements,* related to chronic illness and tiring while feeding (NANDA-I © 2014)

GOAL: The infant or child will demonstrate normal weight gain for age.

INTERVENTION	RATIONALE
• Teach parents methods to promote food intake related to positioning, size of feedings, and food choices.	• Positioning, frequency of feedings, size of feedings, and use of high-caloric foods can enhance nutritional intake.
• Observe feeding during home visit.	• Feedback can assist parents in integrating positive feeding techniques.

EXPECTED OUTCOME: Infant or child will show normal weight gain. Parents will report and demonstrate successful feedings of child.

4. Nursing Diagnosis: *Activity Intolerance* related to poor cardiac output (NANDA-I © 2014)

GOAL: The child will perform all necessary activities of daily living without undue tiring.

INTERVENTION	RATIONALE
• Suggest activities parents can alternate with rest throughout the child's day.	• Activities to promote development must be alternated with rest because of decreased cardiac output.
• Have parents limit child's exposure to persons with contagious disease.	• When the child is ill and tired, the immune system can be compromised.

- Help family plan quiet surroundings to provide for child's rest.
- Home setting may need to be altered to promote rest.

EXPECTED OUTCOME: Child will perform necessary activities and rest frequently each day.

5. Nursing Diagnosis: *Caregiver Role Strain* related to 24-hour responsibility for child's care (NANDA-I © 2014)

GOAL: Parents will express ability to meet own needs.

INTERVENTION	RATIONALE
• Assess family and community supports. Provide information related to respite care.	• Variable family and community supports are available.
• Encourage parents to seek activities to meet personal needs.	• Parents need time for own personal needs to successfully care for child.

EXPECTED OUTCOME: Parents will report some time away from the child and report renewal in caring for the child.

Dilated cardiomyopathy is the most common form, in which the four chambers dilate and systolic contraction is weakened. Clots may form as blood pools in the heart, increasing the child's risk for pulmonary or brain embolism. An estimated 20% to 35% have an inherited form with autosomal dominant, autosomal recessive, X-linked, or mitochondrial inheritance pattern (Park, 2014, p. 330). Other common causes are myocarditis, neuromuscular disease, such as muscular dystrophy, or other infections. The child usually presents with fatigue, weakness, and exertional dyspnea. Arrhythmias may develop that can cause cardiac arrest. The child is treated for CHF (diuretics, digoxin, and ACE inhibitors), including aspirin to reduce throboembolisms, antiarrhythmic medications, and beta-adrenergic medications (e.g., carvedilol). Ultimately a heart transplant may be considered. Activity is restricted.

In hypertrophic cardiomyopathy, enlargement or hypertrophy of the left ventricle and the ventricular septum occurs, making the ventricular walls rigid. About 50% of hypertrophic cardiomyopathy cases are genetically transmitted as an autosomal dominant trait involving mutations on 1 of 10 genes (Park, 2014, p. 321). Myocardial cells become enlarged with some scarring, and coronary arteries may be affected. The outflow tract may become obstructed. Because the left ventricle is stiff, diastolic filling is affected, potentially causing enlargement of the left atrium and pulmonary venous congestion. Symptoms include exertional dyspnea, fatigue, dizziness, fainting, and angina-like chest pain. Palpitations may occur because of atrial or ventricular arrhythmia. It is the most common cause of sudden unexpected cardiac death in adolescents and young adult athletes (Park, 2014, p. 321). Treatment involves beta-adrenergic blockers (e.g., propranolol or metoprolol) or calcium channel blockers (e.g., verapamil). An implantable cardioverter/defibrillator or surgical myomectomy to relieve the obstruction may be considered. Strenuous exercise and competitive sports are prohibited.

Nursing Management

Nursing management for dilated cardiomyopathy is similar to that for children with CHF unless or until a heart transplant is performed. Nursing management for cardiomyopathy involves frequent visits to assess the child's condition and to review treatments.

Heart Transplantation

Approximately 450 heart transplants are performed on children and adolescents each year in the United States (Meaux et al., 2014). The number of donor hearts available for transplantation in children is limited. Ventricular assist devices are used in some pediatric centers to maintain function in other vital organs until

a heart is available for transplant. In 2010, the median survival of infants receiving heart transplants was 18.3 years and for adolescents 11.3 years (Meaux et al., 2014). The primary reasons for heart transplantation in infants and children are cardiomyopathy and congenital heart disease. The number of adults with complex congenital heart defects who seek heart transplantation is increasing as survival through childhood has increased.

Acute rejection is a leading cause of early mortality after transplantation. Signs in infants and children are often nonspecific, including low-grade fever, increasing resting heart rate, fatigue, abdominal pain, nausea, vomiting, decreasing exercise tolerance, and irregular rhythm. Endomyocardial biopsy performed during cardiac catheterization is used to diagnose rejection and may be performed frequently. Research continues for identify biomarkers that can be used to diagnose and monitor rejection in children. The immunosuppression regimen usually includes calcineurin inhibitors (cyclosporin or tacrolimus), azathioprine or mycophenolate mofetil, and corticosteroids. Selecting the correct dosage for children is essential as too much increases the risks for infection, malignancy, and toxic effects, while too little increases the risk for rejection (Andrikopoulou & Mather, 2014).

Early deaths are due to graft failure or infection. Hyperlipidemia and blood vessel thickening in the transplanted heart are leading causes of death for long-term survivors. Statin medications are prescribed to control hyperlipidemia, and hypertension is treated with calcium channel blockers.

While bacterial, fungal, and viral (i.e., cytomegalovirus) infections are a cause of mortality, more common childhood illnesses (acute otitis, colds) may be well tolerated. Antibiotics and other new medications prescribed must be carefully considered because of potential interactions with immunosuppression medications.

Nursing Management

Depending on the age at time of transplant, the child may not have had all immunizations (see Chapter 16). Live virus vaccines should be given at least 1 month prior to the heart transplant, and are usually contraindicated following the transplant (AAP, 2015, pp. 84–86). Help parents arrange for schools and childcare centers to provide early notification of cases of measles, mumps, rubella, and chickenpox. Provide preventive treatment for the child as needed. Encourage good hand hygiene to reduce the spread of infection at home and at school.

After recovery from surgery, children may have near-normal exercise capabilities, normal heart function, and be able to return to school and other activities. Immunosuppressive medications will be continued long term and can cause a variety of physical side effects such as hirsutism, gum hyperplasia, weight gain, moon face, acne, rashes, and osteoporosis. Children and adolescents may need support to develop positive self-esteem.

Organ rejection is a major concern of families. Provide education for the parents and child about the need to adhere to the immunosuppression protocol and to keep appointments for evaluation. Adolescents need special attention to promote adherence to the immunosuppression protocol.

Pulmonary Artery Hypertension

Pulmonary artery hypertension (PAH) is a sustained increased pressure in the pulmonary artery. It is a complication of congenital heart defects that increases pulmonary blood flow in about 43% of cases (Maxwell, Nies Ajuba-Iwuji, et al., 2015). Other potential causes include pulmonary conditions (e.g., meconium aspiration, acute respiratory distress syndrome in the newborn, and prematurity-related chronic lung disease) and congenital diaphragmatic hernia.

Local mediators help the pulmonary vascular smooth muscles stay relaxed to allow blood to flow easily to the lungs. Excessive pulmonary blood flow, such as from a patent ductus arteriosus or ventricular septal defect, causes blood to back up in the lungs and pulmonary vascular constriction to decrease blood flow to the lungs. If excess pulmonary blood flow is not controlled, pulmonary vasoconstriction is maintained. Right ventricular hypertrophy develops to increase the pulmonary artery pressure and push blood across the constricted pulmonary vascular bed. Inflammation, hypertrophy of small pulmonary arteries, and fibrosis develop. The increased pressure leads to a right-to-left shunt, and right heart failure may occur. PAH may become progressive and irreversible.

The child has dyspnea with activity, retractions, fatigue, tachypnea, cyanosis with or without clubbing, diaphoresis, feeding difficulty, and avoidant/restrictive food intake disorder (failure to thrive). Cough with wheezing may occur. As right-sided heart failure occurs, signs of CHF develop. Older children also have distended neck veins, palpitations, chest pain, and syncope.

Cardiac catheterization is used to diagnose the severity of the condition. Therapy for pulmonary hypertension involves supplemental oxygen as needed. Surgery is used to treat the condition in cases of CHD that increases pulmonary blood flow. Treatments for other pulmonary conditions causing PAH, such as meconium aspiration and acute respiratory distress disorder,

are initiated. Medications used to treat chronic PAH include calcium channel blockers, diuretics, and anticoagulants. Other medications used but still being tested for use in children include bosentan, ambrisentan, and sildenafil (Buck, 2013). No cure is available, but life can be prolonged with these measures.

Nursing Management

Nursing care in the community focuses on promoting rest for oxygen conservation, monitoring fluid intake and output carefully, and administering medications and oxygen. Airplane travel may be possible with supplemental oxygen. Exercise should be tailored to avoid dyspnea. Give parents needed support and information about their child.

Infective Endocarditis

Infective endocarditis is a potentially life-threatening but uncommon infection in an individual with endocardial cell damage. While it is a rare condition in children, it may be associated with a congenital heart defect (CHD), rheumatic heart disease, a central venous catheter, heart surgery, or intravenous drug abuse. Among children with a CHD, those with a bicuspid aortic valve, cyanotic lesion, or cardiac surgery within the prior 6 months are at greater risk for endocarditis (Leggiadro, 2014; Park, 2014, p. 343). The rate of endocarditis has increased, potentially because of the use of medical devices and hospital-acquired infections (Bor, Woolhandler, Nardin, et al., 2013).

The endocardium may be injured by a high-velocity or turbulent blood flow due to a heart defect or an indwelling catheter in the right side of the heart. Implanted vascular grafts, patches, prosthetic valves used during cardiac surgery, or implanted devices (e.g., for dialysis) may be a site of infection. Staphylococcal and streptococcal organisms are the most commonly reported bacteria causing endocarditis (Williams & Fagan, 2014). Infectious organisms introduced into the bloodstream by dental or medical procedures adhere to the injury site and colonize (see *Pathophysiology Illustrated: Infective Endocarditis*).

The onset is often slow with symptoms such as recurrent low-grade fever, fatigue, weakness, joint and muscle aches, loss of appetite, weight loss, and diaphoresis. Other signs may include a new heart murmur, or a change in intensity of an existing murmur, and splenomegaly. Petechiae, splinter hemorrhages under

Pathophysiology Illustrated: **Infective Endocarditis**

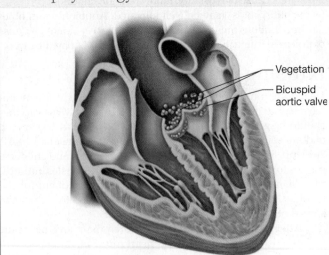

Vegetation

Bicuspid aortic valve

The endocardium is injured by high velocity blood flow through a stenotic valve, by turbulent blood flow across a septal defect, or by the positioning of a central venous catheter. Fibrin and platelets migrate to the site of the endothelial damage, becoming the foundation for nonbacterial thrombotic emboli where the infective organisms settle. In some cases, a vegetation forms near the site of the injury, as in this illustration around the aortic valve.

Medications Used for Infective Endocarditis: Prophylaxis for Dental and Invasive Respiratory Procedures

ANTIBIOTIC RECOMMENDATIONS

Amoxicillin for oral use

Ampicillin for IM or IV use

If allergic to penicillin:

    Cephalexin

    Clindamycin

    Azithromycin

    Clarithromycin

NURSING MANAGEMENT

- Give 1 large dose 30–60 min before procedures, or up to 2 hr after the procedure if preprocedure dose is missed.
- Teach parents and the child to keep at least 1 dose in the home for dental visits or emergencies.
- Have parents inform each healthcare provider of the child's need for prophylaxis.

Source: Data from American Academy of Pediatrics (AAP). (2015). *Red book: 2015 report of the Committee on Infectious Diseases* (30th ed., p. 971). Elk Grove Village, IL: Author; Sabe, M. A., Shrestha, N. K., & Menon, V. (2013). Contemporary drug treatment of infective endocarditis. *American Journal of Cardiovascular Drugs, 13*, 251–258; Park, M. K. (2014). *Pediatric cardiology for practitioners* (6th ed., p. 349). Philadelphia: Elsevier Saunders.

nails, Roth spots (exudative lesions of the retina), Osler nodes (red, painful nonhemorrhagic nodules on the pads of the fingers and toes), and Janeway lesions (nontender, blanching macular lesions on the palms and soles) may be seen in adolescents (Park, 2014, pp. 343–344). Signs of CHF may be seen in some children. Those with indwelling catheters may initially have pulmonary signs related to septic pulmonary embolism.

The Duke criteria, a positive blood culture, echocardiographic findings, and clinical signs provide guidelines for diagnosis and management of infective endocarditis. The condition is most often diagnosed by transthoracic and transesophageal echocardiography, which reveals the site of infection, valve damage, and heart function. Blood culture identifies the infective organism.

Clinical therapy consists of intravenous antibiotics such as nafcillin, oxacillin, or methacillin and gentamycin initially until blood cultures reveal the specific organism. Vancomycin is used in some cases. Once the organism is identified, the antibiotics are changed and administered for a minimum of 4 to 6 weeks depending on the infective organism. Surgery to replace an affected valve is performed in some children. The majority of children recover.

Prevention of infective endocarditis is preferred. Antibiotic prophylaxis is recommended for dental procedures and invasive respiratory procedures for selected individuals at highest risk for adverse outcomes from infective endocarditis (see the section on defects causing decreased pulmonary blood flow earlier in this chapter). See the accompanying *Medications Used for Infective Endocarditis: Prophylaxis for Dental and Invasive Respiratory Procedures.*

Nursing Management

Nursing care focuses on assessing the child's respiratory and cardiovascular status, administering medications, and teaching the parents about the child's care. Assess the child's vital signs, SpO$_2$, and level of consciousness because CHF and embolism may occur. The parents will be anxious about the child's condition, especially if this occurs following surgery for a congenital heart defect or in a critically ill child or newborn. Monitor the parents' coping skills and need for information.

Administer medications as prescribed and monitor serum antibiotic levels. Monitor for side effects of antibiotics and for infiltration at the infusion site. Keep invasive procedures to a minimum. Use careful aseptic technique when managing central lines and venous access devices.

The child is often lethargic and on bed rest. Encourage parents to participate in the child's care and plan quiet age-appropriate activities. Home infusion therapy is often ordered so care can continue on an outpatient basis. Instruct parents about care procedures and reinforce the importance of follow-up visits. Home schooling may be needed during the recovery period.

Nursing care also focuses on prevention of endocarditis. Good oral hygiene and regular dental care are important preventive measures. Stress the importance of telling future healthcare providers, including dentists and surgeons, about the child's infective endocarditis history so prophylactic antibiotics can be given for invasive dental and respiratory procedures.

Acute Rheumatic Fever

Acute rheumatic fever (ARF) is an inflammatory disorder of connective tissue that results from an autoimmune response to some strains of group A beta-hemolytic streptococci (GAS). This disorder may cause long-term damage to heart valves, and affects the joints, brain, and skin tissues. While ARF is a significant health problem in developing countries, the incidence is very low in the United States and developed countries because GAS infections are treated earlier.

Only a small number of individuals infected with a strain of GAS that causes pharyngitis develop ARF, but specific serotypes have not been identified (AAP, 2015, p. 733). It occurs most commonly in children between 5 and 15 years old. A genetic susceptibility to the disease may exist, such as in Pacific Islanders, predisposing children to the disorder. An estimated 60% of patients with ARF develop rheumatic heart disease (Chang, 2012).

One to 3 weeks after an untreated streptococcal infection, the major or hallmark signs of ARF may occur. Carditis involving the mitral or aortic valve may be detected by the development of a new murmur. Chest pain may be caused by pericardial inflammation. Two or more large joints become inflamed with pain, swelling, tenderness, erythema, and heat. The signs may migrate from joint to joint (migratory polyarthritis). Subcutaneous nodules may be palpated over bony prominences and along extensor tendons. A nonpruritic skin rash (erythema marginatum) with pink macules and blanching in the middle of the lesions appears on the trunk, but never on the face and hands. If the central nervous system is affected, Sydenham chorea (St. Vitus dance), characterized by aimless movements of the extremities and facial grimacing, is present.

Diagnosis is based on the Jones criteria, the presence of two or more of the major signs noted above and evidence of a recent streptococcal infection (e.g., a positive throat culture or an elevated or rising antistreptolysin-O titer of 333 Todd units). ARF is suspected when one major sign, evidence of a recent streptococcal infection and one or more minor signs (arthralgia, fever, elevated erythrocyte sedimentation rate or C-reactive protein, or a prolonged PR interval on electrocardiogram) are present (Park, 2014, p. 368). Echocardiography is used to diagnose subclinical signs of carditis that are not evident by auscultation (Gerwitz, Baltimore, Tani, et al., 2015).

Clinical therapy includes antibiotics (penicillin or erythromycin) to eradicate the streptococcal infection. Aspirin is used for fever, arthritis, and arthralgias. Corticosteroids are recommended in cases of severe carditis. Most children recover fully, but they are at risk for subsequent episodes of rheumatic fever. Children should be monitored carefully by echocardiogram for potential cardiac complications. Antibiotic prophylaxis (oral penicillin V or amoxicillin, or intramuscular benzathine penicillin G) is prescribed to children with ARF to reduce the risk for recurrent episodes until at least 21 years of age or 10 years after ARF (Park, 2014, p. 373). Persons allergic to penicillin are often prescribed azithromycin or clindamycin (Chang, 2012).

Nursing Management

An important role of the nurse is prevention of ARF. Nurses in clinics, offices, and schools need to ensure that all children with possible streptococcal infections obtain a rapid strep test or throat culture. Even if the sore throat is mild, testing is needed if family members or other contacts have had a streptococcal infection. Emphasize to the family the importance of giving all doses of the antibiotic prescribed when the test result is positive.

The child with ARF is hospitalized for a period of time. During the acute inflammatory phase, monitor temperature and vital signs at least every 4 hours. Auscultate the child's heart and note any unusual sounds. Observe the child for changes in skin, joints, or behavior. The child is on bed rest for several weeks if carditis is present, or only a week if arthritis is the major manifestation. Be sure family members obtain throat cultures to identify possible asymptomatic streptococcal carriers.

Administer antibiotics and aspirin as prescribed. The child is usually lethargic and often has joint pain. Aspirin often relieves pain dramatically after a few doses. Position and handle the child's joints carefully. Provide quiet activities, and encourage visits or telephone calls from family members and friends. Provide emotional support for the child with chorea; the purposeless involuntary movements are disturbing and can last for 5 to 15 weeks.

The child is generally cared for at home during the recovery phase. Activities may be limited, especially if heart damage is suspected. Help parents plan quiet activities, such as playing board games or computer games, watching videos, or reading. Arrange rest periods after the child returns to school. Reassure the child and parents that the effects of chorea will eventually subside.

After discharge, long-term antibiotic prophylaxis is initiated. Make sure the child and parents understand the importance of taking prescribed medication until adulthood to prevent recurrent rheumatic fever. Make sure the parents understand that the child's future sore throats may be streptococcal and a rapid strep test or throat culture should be obtained even when the child is taking daily antibiotics. The child may need a different antibiotic for the infection. Emphasize the importance of follow-up care to prevent new infections and to monitor heart function.

Kawasaki Disease

Kawasaki disease is an acute febrile, systemic vascular inflammatory disorder that affects small and midsize arteries, including the coronary arteries. It is the leading cause of acquired heart disease in children in the United States and leads to more than 5000 hospitalizations per year (O'Connell & Sloand, 2013). Children under 5 years of age account for 80% of cases, and 50% of cases occur in children under 2 years (AAP, 2015, p. 497). In the United States, Kawasaki disease has a higher incidence in children of Asian and Pacific Island origin (Park, 2014, p. 354).

ETIOLOGY AND PATHOPHYSIOLOGY

The etiology of Kawasaki disease is unknown. It is thought to be caused by or related to an infectious agent that has not yet been identified. The disorder appears to result in an exaggerated immune response to the infection in a genetically susceptible child. The inflammatory disease involves the small and midsize arteries and sometimes causes coronary artery aneurysms. Coronary artery abnormalities may occur within a week of fever onset (Rowley, 2012). Without treatment, up to 25% of children develop coronary artery aneurysms that can lead to a myocardial infarction (Park, 2014, p. 360).

CLINICAL MANIFESTATIONS

The three stages of the disease are acute, subacute, and convalescent:

- The acute stage of Kawasaki disease, lasting 1 to 2 weeks, is characterized by irritability, high fever that persists for more than 5 days, hyperemic conjunctivae, red throat, swollen hands and feet, maculopapular or erythema multiforme-like rash on the trunk and perineal area, unilateral enlargement of the cervical lymph nodes, diarrhea, and hepatic dysfunction.

- The subacute stage, lasting 2 or more weeks, is characterized by no fever, cracking lips and fissures, desquamation of the skin on the tips of the fingers and toes, joint pain, cardiac disease, and thrombocytosis (Figure 21–9).

- In the convalescent stage, 6 to 8 weeks after disease onset, the child appears normal but lingering signs of inflammation may be present. Deep transverse grooves (Beau lines) may appear across nails on the hands and feet.

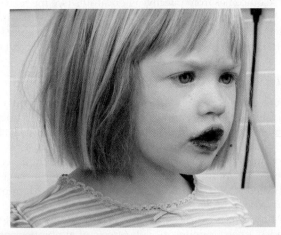

Figure 21–9 This child shows many of the signs of the subacute stage of Kawasaki disease: strawberry tongue, dry cracking lips, and buccal mucosa erythema.

TABLE 21–10 Diagnostic Criteria for Kawasaki Disease

Kawasaki disease is diagnosed when a high spiking fever over 39.0°C (102.2°F) for 5 days or longer is accompanied by four of the five principal features not explained by another disease process. When fewer than four criteria are present, but echocardiography or angiography reveals coronary artery abnormalities, Kawasaki disease is also diagnosed.

BODY PART AFFECTED	PRINCIPAL FEATURES
Eyes	Bilateral bulbar conjunctivitis without exudate
Skin	Intense erythema of the buccal and pharyngeal surfaces with dry, swollen, cracked, and fissuring lips and a strawberry tongue
	Erythema of the palms and soles, edema of the hands and feet, and then desquamation after 2 or more weeks of symptoms
	Dermatitis of the trunk with an erythematous maculopapular rash
Lymph nodes	Cervical lymphadenopathy, frequently unilateral, with a lymph node over 1.5 cm (0.60 in.) in diameter found early in the disease

Source: Data from McLellan, M. C., & Baker, A. L. (2011). At the heart of the fever: Kawasaki disease. *American Journal of Nursing, 111*(6), 57–63; Rowley, A. H. (2012). Kawasaki disease genetics, pathology, and need for earlier diagnosis and treatment. *Contemporary Pediatrics, 29*(12), 18–24; Park, M. K. (2014). *Pediatric cardiology for practitioners* (6th ed., pp. 355–357). Philadelphia: Elsevier Saunders.

Other clinical manifestations may occur during the acute phase, such as arthralgias, abdominal pain with diarrhea, liver dysfunction, gallbladder hydrops, and aseptic meningitis. During the acute phase of Kawasaki disease, its signs and symptoms are commonly confused with other diseases.

CLINICAL THERAPY

Diagnosis is based on clinical signs using the criteria given in Table 21–10 because there is no specific diagnostic laboratory test. Blood studies may reveal elevations of the erythrocyte sedimentation rate, white blood cell count, C-reactive protein, platelet counts, bilirubin, alanine aminotransferase levels, and lipid levels (Park, 2014, pp. 356). Initial and repeat echocardiography is used to identify specific vascular changes in the heart and coronary arteries.

Kawasaki disease is treated with a single high dose (2 g/kg) IV infusion of immune globulin (IVIG) over 10 to 12 hours. Administering IVIG within 7 to 10 days of onset reduces the risk for coronary artery aneurysm. Some children receive IV diphenhydramine before IVIG to reduce the risk of allergic response. High doses of aspirin (80 to 100 mg/kg/day in 4 divided doses) are given for the high fever and to promote comfort. A lower aspirin dose (2 to 5 mg/kg once daily) is given once the child is afebrile for 2 to 3 days. Low-dose aspirin is continued to reduce clot formation until the platelet count is normal or longer term if coronary artery abnormalities occur. When the fever persists or returns within 36 hours after the first IVIG dose, a second IVIG infusion of 2 g/kg is given. If the second IVIG dose is not effective, corticosteroid therapy may be used. Infliximab, a monoclonal antibody, has been used in some U.S. children, but studies of its effectiveness have not yet been completed (Park, 2014, p. 360).

The duration of hospitalization depends on the presence of cardiac lesions and how long the fever persists. Most children recover fully, but they are monitored for cardiac disease for several months. Coronary aneurysms develop in 5% and giant aneurysms occur in 1% of children treated with IVIG, but about 50% to 67% of coronary artery aneurysms resolve within 2 years (Park, 2014, pp. 360–361). Some children with coronary artery involvement have a myocardial infarction, often within the first year after disease onset.

Nursing Management

Nursing care focuses on promoting comfort, monitoring for early signs of complications or disease progression, and supporting the family.

When the child is hospitalized, take the temperature every 4 hours and before each aspirin dose. Assess the extremities for edema, redness, and desquamation every 8 hours. Examine the eyes and the mucous membranes for inflammation. Monitor the child's dietary and fluid intake, and weigh the child daily. Carefully assess heart sounds and rhythm.

Administer aspirin and monitor for side effects such as bleeding and gastrointestinal upset. Administer IVIG as a blood product. Start the infusion rate at a rate of 0.5 mL/kg/hr for 30 minutes and gradually increase the rate to 2 mL/kg/hr. Carefully monitor the child and stop the infusion immediately if a reaction occurs (see Chapter 22).

Promote the child's comfort. Assess pain and provide analgesics and complementary therapies to manage pain. Keep the child's skin clean and dry, and lubricate the lips. Use cool compresses and tepid sponges to make the feverish child more comfortable. Change the child's clothes and bed linens frequently. Give the child frequent small feedings of soft foods and liquids that are neither too hot nor too cold.

Use passive range-of-motion exercises to facilitate joint movement. Because the child with Kawasaki disease is often lethargic and irritable, plan rest periods and quiet age-appropriate activities. Encourage the parents to participate in their child's care to promote comfort and reassure the child. Give the parents information about the disease and the child's treatment.

Before the child is discharged, teach the parents to administer aspirin as ordered and to watch for side effects. Have them measure the child's temperature daily for the first 2 weeks and record it on a log. Any fever above 38.3°C (101.0°F) should be reported to the healthcare provider. Advise the parents that the child needs to avoid contact sports or other activities that could cause bleeding when aspirin or warfarin is prescribed long term. The child who recovers without cardiovascular complications is encouraged to live an active lifestyle without exercise limitations. Limitation of strenuous activity is recommended for all children with coronary aneurysms or stenoses.

Emphasize the need for follow-up care to monitor for cardiac complications, hypertension, and hyperlipidemia. Postpone needed live virus vaccines (measles and varicella) for 11 months after IVIG administration, but other immunizations may be given on schedule.

Cardiac Arrhythmias

Cardiac **arrhythmias** (abnormal heart rhythms or dysrhythmias) occur frequently in children, but less often than in adults. Three categories of arrhythmias are tachyarrhythmias (sinus tachycardia), bradyarrhythmias (sinus bradycardia), and no pulse (ventricular tachycardia, ventricular fibrillation, pulseless electrical activity, or asystole). Less common arrhythmias are often associated with postoperative complications of congenital heart disease, Kawasaki disease with coronary artery involvement, rheumatic heart disease, cardiomyopathy, and electrolyte abnormalities. Arrhythmias may cause decreased cardiac output and CHF. More serious arrhythmias may result in syncope or sudden death.

BRADYCARDIA

Bradycardia is a heart rate less than the lower limit of normal for the child's age (usually a heart rate less than 80 in infants and less than 60 in children and adolescents). Some athletes may normally have a heart rate of 60. It is associated with beta-adrenergic medications and conditions such as hypothermia, hypoxia, hyperkalemia, and increased intracranial pressure. See Chapter 5 for normal heart rate ranges by age.

General symptoms of bradycardia include fatigue, exercise intolerance, dizziness, and syncope. The underlying cause is treated. Other treatment may include supplemental oxygen and medications (epinephrine, atropine, isoproterenol, glucagon). Chronic bradycardia may require a pacemaker.

SUPRAVENTRICULAR TACHYCARDIA

Supraventricular tachycardia (SVT), the most common pathologic tachycardia, is the abrupt onset of a rapid, regular heart rate, often too fast to count. The presenting heart rate with SVT will be greater than 220 beats/min in infants and greater than 180 beats/min in children. Potential causes include Wolff–Parkinson–White syndrome, congenital heart defects (e.g., single ventricle and corrected transposition of the great arteries), and postoperative cardiac surgery. Often no heart disease is present. Cardiac output is affected because diastolic filling cannot occur with such a rapid heart rate. Prolonged episodes of continuous SVT (more than 6 to 12 hours) can progress to CHF or cardiogenic shock if untreated.

Early signs in infants include poor feeding, irritability, and pallor. Older children may have palpitations, chest pain, dizziness, shortness of breath, decreased exercise tolerance, and syncope. Palpitations felt in the neck may be present. Recurrent attacks are common.

Treatments focus on reducing the heart rate. Initial steps involve vagal stimulation (applying ice-water bag to the face for 10 seconds or rectal stimulation with a thermometer) or having the child perform a Valsalva maneuver (e.g., holding the breath and straining, or blowing forcefully on the thumb to increase intrathoracic and venous pressures). Amiodarone by IV bolus is the preferred medication to lower the heart rate. Synchronized cardioversion is used for life-threatening episodes unresponsive to medications. Recurrent episodes of SVT are common, and propranolol, verapamil, or atenolol may be prescribed long term to reduce the frequency of episodes. **Radio-frequency ablation**, the use of radio energy (heat) to destroy a very small section of the myocardium through which an accessory conduction pathway passes, may be performed during cardiac catheterization.

LONG QT SYNDROME

Long QT syndrome (LQTS) is an inherited rhythm disturbance of ventricular tachycardia with a prolonged QT interval and abnormal T waves that puts children at risk for ventricular fibrillation and sudden death. Electrolyte disorders and certain drugs may trigger long QT arrhythmia in some children genetically predisposed to the disorder. In some children, arrhythmia is triggered by demanding physical exercise (e.g., swimming), a strong emotional reaction, or an abrupt loud noise (e.g., doorbell or alarm clock). In some genetic forms, the arrhythmia

more often occurs during rest or sleep. Arrhythmia may occur without warning and result in sudden death. Presenting signs include episodic dizziness, palpitations, syncope, seizure, or cardiac arrest.

Professionalism in Practice Sports Preparticipation Screening

The American Academy of Pediatrics recommends sports preparticipation screening to identify children and youth at risk for sudden cardiac death (American Academy of Pediatrics Section on Cardiology and Cardiac Surgery, 2012). Nurses can play an important role in identifying children and youth at risk by asking questions during the history for any child symptomatic of an arrhythmia or presenting for a physical assessment to play sports. Important questions include the following:

- Has the child passed out or had a seizure suddenly and without warning, either during exercise or in response to a loud noise (e.g., doorbell, alarm clock)?
- Has the child ever experienced chest pain or shortness of breath when exercising?
- Has any family member died suddenly and unexpectedly before age 50 years?
- Has any family member been diagnosed with an enlarged heart (cardiomyopathy) or rhythm disorder like long QT syndrome?

If the child is resuscitated or evaluated because of presenting signs or family history, the arrhythmia is commonly detected by electrocardiogram. The disorder is treated by beta-blockers (e.g., propranolol). A cardioverter/defibrillator (ICD) may be implanted in children and adolescents considered at high risk for sudden death. Do not permit the child to participate in competitive sports and supervise the child when swimming. Other triggers and medications that prolong the QT interval are avoided.

Nursing Management

Children with severe arrhythmias are treated in the emergency department or intensive care unit. The child is placed on a cardiac monitor and pulse oximeter. Frequently assess the vital signs and keep the healthcare provider informed about continuing abnormal rates or rhythms. Observe and record changes in level of consciousness, color, weakness, irritability, and feeding patterns. Administer medications as ordered. Have emergency drugs and resuscitation equipment available at the bedside. When sedation is ordered for invasive procedures such as synchronized cardioversion, follow the institution's guidelines for frequent assessment and intervention.

Episodes of arrhythmia and the potential for future episodes are frightening for both the child and parents. Provide written information about the danger signs indicating an arrhythmic episode and how to obtain emergency care. Educate the child and parents about the home treatment plan, including the importance of medication adherence that may prevent or reduce the frequency of episodes. Encourage parents to obtain cardiopulmonary resuscitation training. Help the child and family to avoid medications that can trigger another episode: for SVT, cardiac stimulant drugs such as decongestants; and for

LQTS, medications that prolong the QT interval (e.g., antihistamines, antidepressants, and macrolide antibiotics). An updated list of these medications can be found online. If the child has an ICD, parents need education about signs of defibrillation discharges (crying, grabbing chest, chest pain) and when to notify the healthcare provider.

Dyslipidemia

Dyslipidemia is an abnormal concentration of one or more lipids (total cholesterol, low-density lipoproteins [LDL], triglycerides, high-density lipoproteins [HDL]) in the blood. Children who have a genetic history or lifestyle that makes them more susceptible to future coronary heart disease (atherosclerosis) should be identified so preventive health measures can be implemented. A high LDL level, reduced HDL level, elevated blood pressure, type 1 or 2 diabetes mellitus, cigarette smoking, and obesity are major risk factors (National Heart Lung and Blood Institute [NHLBI], 2012).

Abnormalities in the lipid levels may be the result of excessive production, lack of clearance of the lipoprotein particles, a genetic defect in lipid metabolism, or other defects such as enzyme deficiencies. Some children have dyslipidemia due to genetic factors that cause abnormalities in lipid-metabolizing enzymes or abnormal cellular lipid receptors. Obesity is another leading cause of dyslipidemia. Examples of other causes include hypothyroidism, diabetes, nephritic syndrome, and certain drugs such as corticosteroids, beta-blockers, and isotretinoin (Brashers, 2014). More commonly, children have mild lipid abnormalities due to a combination of heredity and lifestyle factors. The child with dyslipidemia has no clinical manifestations of the condition.

A blood test for total cholesterol, HDL, and triglycerides identifies the condition. The LDL level is calculated from the triglyceride, HDL, and total cholesterol levels. See Table 21–11. Children between 2 and 8 years of age with the following risk factors should be screened for hyperlipidemia with a fasting lipid panel: a positive family history of dyslipidemia or cardiovascular disease (e.g., myocardial infarction, angina, stroke, coronary bypass surgery, or angioplasty) before 55 years in men or 65 years in women, parent with total cholesterol of 240 mg/dL or higher, or the child has cardiovascular risk factors (body mass index greater than 95th percentile, hypertension, cigarette smoking, diabetes mellitus, or a condition that causes secondary dyslipidemia). All children should have lipid screening once between 9 and 11 years of age and again between 17 and 21 years of age (NHLBI, 2012).

The primary management of dyslipidemia in most children includes dietary modifications, exercise, and other changes in lifestyle. The child's diet is carefully analyzed and changes are made to satisfy the dietary guidelines so that saturated fats are less than 7% and monosaturated fats are 20% of total caloric intake, cholesterol intake is less than 200 mg/day for treatment of elevated LDL levels, and trans fats are avoided (NHLBI, 2012). A healthy total fat intake is 20% to 35% of daily calories. High dietary fiber is encouraged. If the child is obese, weight loss is encouraged.

If a child age 10 years or older continues to have high serum lipid levels after dietary changes and increased physical activity, medications may be prescribed. Cholestyramine or colestipol, which bind bile acid in the intestine, niacin, statins, and fish oil may be prescribed. The goal is to lower LDL concentration to less than 130 mg/dL or a 50% level reduction (Giddings, 2012). Children and adolescents taking statins should have periodic creatine kinase and liver transaminase monitoring.

TABLE 21–11 Laboratory Values for Assessment of Dyslipidemia in Children Between 2 and 19 Years Old

TEST	RECOMMENDED LEVEL	LEVELS OF HIGHER RISK
Total cholesterol	Under 170 mg/dL	Borderline: 170–199 mg/dL Abnormal: 200 mg/dL or higher
LDL-C	Under 110 mg/dL	Borderline: 110–129 mg/dL Abnormal: 130 mg/dL or higher
Triglyceride 0–9 years	Under 75 mg/dL	Borderline: 75–99 mg/dL Abnormal: 100 mg/dL or higher
10–19 years	Under 90 mg/dL	Borderline: 90–129 mg/dL Abnormal: 130 mg/dL or higher
HDL-C	45 mg/dL or higher	Borderline: 40–45 mg/dL Abnormal: Under 40 mg/dL

Source: Adapted from National Heart Lung and Blood Institute (NHLBI). (2012). *Expert panel on integrated guidelines for cardiovascular health and risk reduction in children and adolescents*. Retrieved from http://www.nhlbi.nih.gov/guidelines/cvd_ped/index.htm

Nursing Management

Nursing care focuses on identifying children at risk for dyslipidemia, providing education about diet and exercise, and monitoring eating patterns. Identification and management of dyslipidemia takes place in many community settings. Office and clinic nurses identify children who need to have serum lipid measured. Nurses in schools provide education on ways to reduce risk factors. The child's history of exercise patterns, weight percentile, and dietary intake provides important information. Obtain information on familial heart disease, hypertension, diabetes, and smoking to determine risk factors.

Work with nutritionists to provide dietary teaching and monitor family eating patterns. The food plan for the child and entire family should consist primarily of fruit, vegetables, whole grain breads and cereals, low-fat and nonfat dairy products, lean meat and fish, legumes, and nuts. Processed foods, juices, sugar-sweetened drinks, and simple carbohydrates (foods with sugar and white flour) should be limited. Help parents understand that modeling food choices helps children learn to select and eat better food choices and reduce lipid levels. For children with familial hypercholesterolemia, lifelong dietary management is essential.

Healthy People 2020

(NWS-18) Reduce consumption of saturated fat in the population aged 2 years and older

Help the child select an enjoyable moderate to intense activity for daily participation, and then perform 30 minutes of aerobic exercise (e.g., jogging, swimming, biking, roller blading, soccer) at least 3 to 4 times a week to promote cardiovascular fitness. Discourage smoking by the child or the parents to reduce the risk for cardiovascular disease.

Educate children and adolescents taking statin medications to report any adverse effects to their healthcare provider: myalgia, muscle soreness, weakness, tenderness, or dark-colored urine. Include the entire family in the treatment plan; it is difficult for a single family member to change eating and exercise patterns.

Hypertension

Hypertension in children and adolescents is defined as a systolic or diastolic blood pressure reading that is equal to or greater than 95th percentile for age, gender, and height percentile. Normal blood pressure is defined as a systolic or diastolic reading that falls below the 90th percentile for age, gender, and height percentile. An estimated 3% to 5% of children and adolescents have hypertension (Hylick, Grubbs, Johnson, et al., 2014). Detection during childhood is important as it is a major risk factor for heart disease and stroke during adulthood.

Healthy People 2020

(HDS-5) Reduce the proportion of persons in the population with hypertension

---

Primary hypertension occurs in about 5% of the pediatric population and is related to the increasing rate of obesity in children (Dennison, 2012). The most common causes of secondary hypertension in children include coarctation of the aorta, renal disorders, neurofibromatosis, obstructive sleep apnea, and endocrine disorders (Daniels, 2012).

Because children rarely have symptoms of hypertension, the condition is detected during a health examination. Symptoms of severe hypertension may include headaches, epistaxis, dizziness, and visual changes.

CLINICAL THERAPY

Hypertension is diagnosed after three or more separate blood pressure readings a week apart or when ambulatory blood pressure monitoring shows systolic or diastolic readings at the 95th percentile or higher for gender, age, and height. Initial evaluation includes a urinalysis, serum creatinine, electrolyte levels, blood urea nitrogen, and a complete blood count. A urine culture and renal ultrasound are performed if an initial test is positive. Serum lipid studies, fasting glucose, and serum insulin are obtained to identify dyslipidemia or diabetes. Other potential testing may include thyroid and adrenal hormone levels to identify hyperthyroidism and an echocardiogram to assess for coarctation of the aorta or left ventricular hypertrophy. Polysomnography may be performed to identify a sleep disorder.

Developing Cultural Competence Blood Pressure

A recent study investigated the blood pressure readings of 199,513 children between 3 and 17 years of age along with height, weight, and body mass index (BMI). The sample was well represented by the following racial and ethnic groups: White, Black, Asian, and Hispanic. The rate of prehypertension (90th to less than 95th percentile) was 12.7%, whereas 5.4% were in the hypertension range (95th percentile or greater). The highest prevalence of hypertension was found among the Black and Asian children in the study (Lo et al., 2013).

Nonpharmacologic measures for reduction of blood pressure include weight reduction and increased exercise (30 to 60 minutes a day). The Dietary Approaches to Stop Hypertension (DASH) diet is recommended for children and adolescents with elevated blood pressure. It is low in sodium and encourages fruits, vegetables, low-fat or fat-free dairy products, whole grains, fish, poultry, beans, seeds, and nuts (NHLBI, 2012). Discourage the child from smoking and the use of alcohol or drugs.

Medications are used for children with persistent, severe hypertension that is not resolved with dietary changes and exercise. Medications prescribed may include diuretics, beta-blocking agents, angiotensin-converting enzyme (ACE) inhibitors, angiotensin receptor blockers (ARB), and calcium channel blockers (Daniels, 2012).

Nursing Management

Children should have their blood pressure measured annually beginning at 3 years of age. Take a complete history for the child with persistent high blood pressure to identify potential risk factors such as family history for hypertension, smoking, or a systemic disease. Is the child obese? Assess the diet for salt intake and servings of fruits and dairy products eaten daily. What are the child's daily exercise routines? Review any medications or other potential agents used by the child or adolescent.

Assess the child's blood pressure and consistently use the right arm and an appropriately sized cuff (see the *Clinical Skills Manual* SKILLS). Compare the leg blood pressure to that in the arm. Compare readings to the blood pressure values for gender, age, and height percentile (see Appendix B). Monitor the child with borderline hypertension every 3 to 6 months. Take at least two readings during the visit and average them if they differ.

Teach both the child and the parents how to improve the diet and develop exercise routines. Provide suggestions about seasoning substitutes for salt and a list of salty foods to avoid. Increasing intake of low-fat dairy products and fruits can contribute to blood pressure control.

Discuss ways to increase activity and reduce time watching television or playing computer games. Provide suggestions for the management of stress and stressful situations. Emphasize the need to avoiding smoking, alcohol, and drugs. Teaching that involves the entire family is usually the most effective. Instruct the family on correct administration of prescribed medications when used.

Injuries of the Cardiovascular System

Shock

Shock is an acute, complex state of circulatory dysfunction resulting in failure to deliver sufficient oxygen and other nutrients to cells and tissues. It can be caused by a variety of conditions such as hemorrhage, dehydration, sepsis, obstruction of blood flow, and cardiac pump failure.

Hypovolemic Shock

Hypovolemic shock is a clinical state of inadequate tissue and organ perfusion resulting from inadequate blood or plasma volume in the vascular space (see *Pathophysiology Illustrated: Hypovolemic Shock*). The blood or plasma in the vascular space may be decreased because of hemorrhage or fluid movement into the interstitial spaces.

Pathophysiology Illustrated: **Hypovolemic Shock**

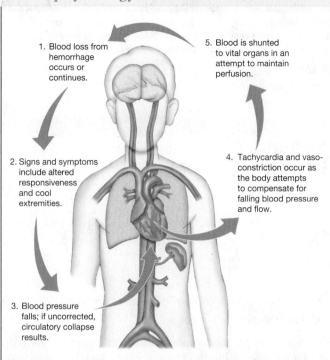

1. Blood loss from hemorrhage occurs or continues.

2. Signs and symptoms include altered responsiveness and cool extremities.

3. Blood pressure falls; if uncorrected, circulatory collapse results.

4. Tachycardia and vaso-constriction occur as the body attempts to compensate for falling blood pressure and flow.

5. Blood is shunted to vital organs in an attempt to maintain perfusion.

If hemorrhage reduces the circulating blood volume, the body compensates by increasing the heart rate and constricting the peripheral blood vessels. This allows the remaining blood to be circulated to the vital organs. When blood loss exceeds 20% to 25%, the child's body can no longer compensate; blood pressure falls, and circulatory collapse is imminent.

ETIOLOGY AND PATHOPHYSIOLOGY

Major causes of decreased intravascular blood volume include the following:

- Hemorrhage from significant injury
- Plasma loss from burns, nephrotic syndrome, and sepsis
- Fluid and electrolyte loss associated with dehydration, diabetic ketoacidosis, and diabetes insipidus

Decreased blood volume results in inadequate delivery of oxygen and nutrients to cells and accumulation of toxic wastes in the capillaries. Less blood returns to the heart to fill the ventricles, resulting in a lower stroke volume. Decreased cardiac output and mean arterial pressure then occur. The kidneys receive less blood, leading to decreased ability to filter toxins. Cellular hypoxia (reduced oxygenation of the tissues) and acidosis develop simultaneously. The accumulation of toxins and inadequate tissue oxygenation cause cellular damage.

When the child's brain senses inadequate oxygen, adrenergic and renal mechanisms help compensate:

- Catecholamine and cortisol levels rise to increase the heart rate, blood pressure, and heart muscle contractions to improve cardiac output.
- The renin–angiotensin–aldosterone system works to retain sodium and fluid in the vascular space when kidney perfusion is decreased.
- Antidiuretic hormone is secreted when the atria have reduced blood volume leading to water retention.
- Glucagon is released to provide energy for life-preserving functions.
- An increased respiratory rate improves oxygenation and decreases waste accumulation in the cells.
- The hydrostatic pressure falls, permitting fluid to shift into the vascular space and increase circulating blood volume.

- Peripheral vessels constrict to maintain systemic vascular resistance and increase perfusion to vital organs as long as possible.

When the child can no longer compensate (20% to 25% of volume loss), hypotension results. Life-threatening end-organ failure occurs without immediate therapy.

CLINICAL MANIFESTATIONS

Signs of early hypovolemic shock in children are nonspecific as the child is compensating for decreased blood volume. The blood pressure may be normal for age. The child has sustained tachycardia (usually higher than 130 beats per minute), increased respiratory effort, delayed capillary refill (greater than 2 seconds), weak peripheral pulses, pallor, and cold extremities (signs of decreased perfusion). Urine output decreases (to less than 0.5 to 1 mL/kg/hr in infants and young children) when renal blood flow drops. In cases of dehydration, dry mucous membranes and poor skin turgor are also present. See Table 21–12.

CLINICAL THERAPY

Clinical signs are used to diagnose the condition as no laboratory tests detect the blood volume deficit quickly enough. After hypovolemic shock is diagnosed or suspected, treatment is initiated. The hematocrit and hemoglobin, arterial blood gases, serum electrolytes, glucose, osmolality, blood urea nitrogen, and urinalysis are obtained during initial care.

Emergency care focuses on improving tissue perfusion. An open airway is established, oxygen is administered, and ventilation is assisted if necessary. Bleeding is controlled, and an IV or intraosseous line is inserted to provide large volumes of crystalloid fluids (normal saline or lactated Ringer). A fluid bolus of 20 mL/kg is administered rapidly over 5 minutes. The same amount of fluid is given in 5 minutes if the child's physiologic condition does not improve after the first fluid bolus. When the child is injured and no improvement is seen after the second fluid

TABLE 21–12 Clinical Manifestations of Hypovolemic Shock

SYSTEM	EARLY COMPENSATED SHOCK	MODERATE UNCOMPENSATED SHOCK	SEVERE UNCOMPENSATED SHOCK
Cardiac	Mild tachycardia, weak distal pulses, strong central pulses, normal blood pressure	Moderate tachycardia, thready distal pulses, weak central pulses, decreasing systolic blood pressure	Extreme tachycardia, hypotension, narrow pulse pressure, absent distal pulses, thready central pulses
Respiratory	Mild tachypnea	Moderate tachypnea	Severe tachypnea
Neurologic	Normal, anxious, irritable, or combative behavior	Confusion, agitation, combativeness, lethargy, decreased pain response	Comatose state
Skin	Mottled appearance; capillary refill time greater than 2 sec; cool, clammy extremities	Pallor; capillary refill time greater than 3 sec; cold, dry extremities; sunken eyes	Pale, cold skin; cyanosis; capillary refill greater than 5 sec
Renal	Decreased urine output; increased specific gravity in older infants and children (newborns cannot concentrate urine)	Oliguria; increased specific gravity	No urine output

Source: Data from Chamiedes, L., Samson, R. A., Schexnadyer, S. M., & Hazinski, M. F. (Eds.). (2011). *Pediatric advanced life support* (p. 97). Dallas, TX: American Heart Association; Hazinski, M. F., Mondozzi, M. A., & Baker, R. A. U. (2014). Shock, multiple organ dysfunction syndrome, and burns in children. In K. L. McCance, S. E. Huether, V. L. Brashers, & N. R. Rote (Eds.), *Pathophysiology: The biologic basis for disease in adults and children* (7th ed., pp. 1699–1727). St. Louis, MO: Mosby Elsevier; Steffen, K. M. (2011). Trauma, burns, and common critical care emergencies. In M. M. Tschudy & K. M. Arcara (Eds.), *The Harriet Lane handbook* (19th ed., p. 109), Philadelphia, PA: Elsevier Mosby.

bolus, blood is often administered. Once the child's physiologic condition is stabilized, the cause of the hypovolemic shock becomes the focus of examination and treatment.

Nursing Management

For the Child With Hypovolemic Shock

Nursing Assessment and Diagnosis

Ask the parent (or child, if appropriate) about possible injuries or the duration and severity of acute illnesses. If no external bleeding is evident, determine whether an injury may be causing internal bleeding. For example, the liver and spleen are highly vascular organs and if injured could bleed enough to cause hypovolemic shock without evidence of bleeding. An acute illness such as gastroenteritis with prolonged vomiting and diarrhea can also result in dehydration and hypovolemic shock.

If external bleeding is apparent, determine the amount of blood lost. Although children lose the same amount of blood from a laceration as adults, the total volume of blood lost is proportional to their weight.

Growth and Development

The child's total blood volume varies by weight. The child has approximately 80 mL of blood for every kilogram of body weight.

- Newborn: 3 kg × 80 mL = 240 mL (1 cup)
- 5-year-old child: 25 kg × 80 mL = 2000 mL (2 quarts)
- 13-year-old child: 50 kg × 80 mL = 4000 mL (1 gallon)

Frequently assess the child's heart rate, respiratory rate, blood pressure, capillary refill time, level of consciousness with the Glasgow Coma Scale (see Chapter 27), color, and skin temperature to identify any changes that indicate improvement or deterioration in the child's condition. Monitor urine output and specific gravity hourly. Signs of the child's improved status include:

- A decrease in heart rate, respiratory rate, and capillary refill time
- An increase in systolic blood pressure and urine output

- Improved color, level of consciousness, and skin temperature
- Regaining of lost weight

Assess the parents' response and coping mechanisms to the child's potentially life-threatening injury. Families are unprepared for the abrupt change in the child's condition because of the unpredictability of the injury. See Chapter 13.

Examples of nursing diagnoses that may apply to the child with hypovolemic shock include (NANDA-I © 2014):

- ***Cardiac Output, Decreased,*** related to hypovolemia
- ***Fluid Volume: Deficient*** related to active fluid volume loss
- ***Tissue Perfusion: Peripheral, Ineffective,*** related to impaired transport of oxygen across alveolar and capillary membrane
- ***Coping: Family, Compromised,*** related to life-threatening condition of the child

Planning and Implementation

Nurses in the emergency department, operating room, and intensive care unit more commonly participate in the resuscitation of the child in hypovolemic shock, often using guidelines or protocols for nursing actions. Assist with the child's assessment and establish IV access. Calculate and prepare the amount of IV fluid needed for the child's weight (20 mL/kg). The IV fluid is often warmed because hypothermia interferes with the child's response to treatment. Ensure rapid fluid administration by IV push or pressure bag. Monitor the child's physiologic response to the fluid bolus within 5 minutes. Prepare a second and third fluid bolus. Keep the child covered or use heat lamps to reduce body-heat loss.

When packed red blood cells are administered, verify that the correct blood has been obtained for the child. Ensure that the IV fluid is normal saline to prevent clotting during blood administration (see the *Clinical Skills Manual* SKILLS). Assess the child carefully for a transfusion reaction (see Chapter 23). Monitor the child's physiologic circulatory responses for improvement or deterioration in status. Notify the healthcare provider of any deterioration.

Parents and children with hypovolemic shock resulting from injury are usually apprehensive. The child may be fearful because of the sudden hospitalization or agitated because of an

Pathophysiology Illustrated: **Obstructive Shock Due to Mediastinal Shift**

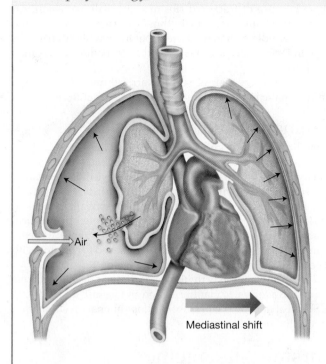

Air

Mediastinal shift

Obstructive shock can occur when a tension pneumothorax obstructs blood flow to and from the heart (see Chapter 20). Here, the great vessels are compressed during the mediastinal shift, obstructing blood return to the heart.

altered level of consciousness. Because parents often fear for the child's life in cases of severe injury, update them about the child's condition frequently. Provide support and explain the care being provided and how it helps the child. Listen to their concerns and correct any misconceptions.

Evaluation

Examples of expected nursing care outcomes include the following:

- The child receives adequate fluid resuscitation or blood to prevent progression to severe uncompensated shock.
- The family copes with the stress of the child's injury.

Distributive Shock

Distributive shock is an abnormal distribution of blood volume, usually resulting from a decrease in systemic vascular resistance. The blood accumulates in the extremities because of vasodilation and capillary permeability. Less blood is returned to the heart, so **preload** (amount of blood in the ventricle at the end of diastole that stretches the heart muscle before contraction) drops and cardiac output falls. Blood flow is inadequate to all tissue beds. Causes of distributive shock include anaphylaxis, sepsis, and spinal cord injury. See Chapter 16 for a discussion of sepsis and septic shock.

Nursing Management

The child with distributive shock is cared for in the intensive care unit. Nursing care focuses on detecting and managing subtle changes in the child's physiologic status to improve the child's condition. Parents are supported as described in Chapter 13.

Obstructive Shock

Obstructive shock occurs from a mechanical blockage of blood flow into and through the heart and great vessels (see *Pathophysiology Illustrated: Obstructive Shock Due to Mediastinal Shift*). Causes in children include compression of the vena cava, pericardial tamponade, pulmonary embolism, tension pneumothorax, pleural effusion, and congenital heart defects with outflow obstruction (e.g., severe aortic stenosis, coarctation of the aorta). Management is focused on treatment of the underlying condition to relieve the obstruction.

Nursing Management

The child is usually cared for in the intensive care unit with nursing care focused on supporting the child's respiratory and cardiovascular functioning. See Chapter 20 for care of the child with a tension pneumothorax.

Cardiogenic Shock

Cardiogenic shock is an impairment of myocardial function that causes low cardiac output and poor tissue perfusion even though blood volume is adequate. Causes of cardiogenic shock in children may include pump failure, severe obstructive congenital heart disease such as hypoplastic left heart syndrome, cardiomyopathy, myocarditis, severe electrolyte or acid–base imbalance, a complication of shock, and early septic shock (Hazinski, Mondozzi, & Baker, 2014).

Compensatory responses divert blood to the heart and brain; however, reduced blood flow to the kidneys, liver, and intestines can lead to ischemia and end-organ failure. Increased systemic vascular resistance puts more stress on the failing heart. Each contraction causes more blood to accumulate in the heart and pulmonary vessels, eventually leading to CHF, metabolic acidosis, and circulatory collapse.

Clinically, cardiogenic shock resembles hypovolemic shock with low cardiac output. Tachycardia, tachypnea, decreased oxygen saturation, hypotension, diminished peripheral pulses, and cool, mottled extremities are common signs. Disorientation and restlessness occur as the compensatory mechanisms fail. Signs of respiratory distress associated with CHF and pulmonary edema are often present.

An enlarged heart and pulmonary congestion may be seen on a chest radiograph. The goals of medical treatment are rapid restoration of myocardial function. Diuretics and vasodilators are given along with adequate ventilatory support, sedatives, analgesics, and antipyretics. Inotropic agents may be used in some cases.

Nursing Management

The child will be cared for in the intensive care unit. Nursing care focuses on monitoring and supporting the respiratory and cardiovascular status, fluid management, and medication administration. See Chapter 13 for care of the child with a life-threatening condition.

Myocardial Contusion

Myocardial contusion, a rare injury in children, results from a strong, blunt force against the chest wall that injures the heart muscle in the right ventricle. Blood flow to areas of the heart muscle is disrupted, or myocardial cells are directly destroyed. This potentially life-threatening condition most often occurs with striking the steering wheel of a motor vehicle during a crash, a crush injury, or a fall.

A myocardial contusion should be suspected in cases of injury to the anterior chest. The child has chest wall tenderness or pain because of fractured ribs or chest wall contusion. An electrocardiogram reveals arrhythmias or signs of myocardial infarct. A two-dimensional echocardiogram may show an abnormality in heart wall movement. Cardiac troponin I levels may be elevated.

Because of the risk of sudden arrhythmias, the child is admitted to the intensive care unit for cardiac monitoring.

Commotio Cordis

Commotio cordis, also known as a cardiac concussion, is a blunt, nonpenetrating blow to the precordium that causes ventricular fibrillation and sudden death. The majority of victims are healthy children and youth without an underlying cardiovascular disease participating in sports such as baseball, softball, ice hockey, and lacrosse. In some cases, the event is triggered by physical contact with another person, such as a fist, elbow, knee, or head. The impact timing on the precordium is believed to coincide with the period of vulnerable cardiac repolarization.

The most common arrhythmias recorded after the victim's collapse include ventricular fibrillation and ventricular tachycardia. Survival improves if prompt cardiopulmonary resuscitation or defibrillation is provided.

Nursing Management

The role of the nurse is to implement rapid cardiopulmonary resuscitation and to facilitate defibrillation. Nursing care is then focused on monitoring for cardiac arrhythmias, often in the intensive care unit.

Chapter Highlights

- Congenital heart defects occur in approximately 1% of all live births, making them the most common birth defect.

- Infants and children under 5 years of age increase their cardiac output by increasing the heart rate. After that age, the muscle fibers in the myocardium are developed enough to stretch and increase stroke volume.

- Most congenital heart defects develop during the first 8 weeks of gestation, often the result of genetic and environmental factors.

- Congenital heart defects are categorized by pathophysiology and hemodynamics:

  - Defects that increase pulmonary blood flow include the following: patent ductus arteriosus, atrial septal defect, ventricular septal defect, and atrioventricular canal.

  - Defects that decrease pulmonary blood flow include the following: pulmonic stenosis, tetralogy of Fallot, pulmonary atresia, and tricuspid atresia.

  - Defects that decrease systemic blood flow include the following: aortic stenosis, coarctation of the aorta, and hypoplastic left heart syndrome.

- Transposition of the great arteries and truncus arteriosus are examples of mixed defects that require mixing of the pulmonary and systemic circulations for survival during the neonatal period.

- Cardiac catheterization is more commonly used in children to intervene or repair some heart defects rather than to evaluate the hemodynamics and pressure gradients within the heart.

- Infants with congenital heart defects that increase pulmonary blood flow are at high risk for development of congestive heart failure.

- The child with a congenital heart defect that decreases pulmonary blood flow may have life-threatening hypoxic episodes requiring emergency treatment.

- Congenital heart defects that obstruct systemic blood flow cause signs and symptoms associated with low cardiac output: diminished pulses, poor color, prolonged capillary refill time, and decreased urinary output.

- Infants are at risk of heart failure as they are more sensitive to volume or pressure overload.

- Signs of congestive heart failure may include tachypnea, tachycardia, pallor or cyanosis, nasal flaring, grunting, retractions, cough, crackles, periorbital and facial edema, jugular vein distention, and hepatomegaly.

- Cardiomyopathy during childhood occurs most often in infancy and adolescence.

- Heart transplantation is performed in infants and children for complex heart defects or cardiomyopathy. Rejection and infection are the major causes of mortality and morbidity during the first year following the transplant.

- Pulmonary artery hypertension is a life-threatening complication of congenital heart disease with excessive pulmonary blood flow. Irreversible pulmonary vascular changes include inflammation, hypertrophy of pulmonary vessels, and fibrosis.

- Infective endocarditis is a risk for children who have some congenital heart defects, following heart surgery with patching or artificial valves, rheumatic heart disease, or a central venous catheter. Not all cases of infective endocarditis are preventable.

- Rheumatic fever is an inflammatory connective tissue disease following a streptococcal infection that may affect the heart, joints, skin, or central nervous system.

- Kawasaki disease is an acute febrile, systemic inflammatory illness with an unknown etiology. Coronary artery inflammation or aneurysms may be a significant complication.

- Two potentially life-threatening cardiac arrhythmias are supraventricular tachycardia and long QT syndrome.

- Some children have familial or lifestyle-related dyslipidemia that causes undesirable levels of cholesterol or triglycerides. These children need dietary intervention and exercise regimens as initial therapies.

- All children with systolic or diastolic blood pressure at the 95th percentile for age, gender, and height percentile have hypertension.

- Hypovolemic shock is an acute, complex state of circulatory dysfunction resulting in failure to deliver sufficient oxygen and other nutrients to meet cell and tissue demands.

- Signs that a child is in compensated hypovolemic shock include tachycardia, increased respiratory effort, prolonged capillary refill time, weak peripheral pulses, pallor, and cold extremities.

- Distributive shock is an abnormal distribution of the blood volume that results from a decrease in vascular resistance. It may be caused by anaphylaxis, sepsis, or spinal cord injury.

- Obstructive shock occurs when circulation is impeded by conditions such as compression on the vena cava due to tension pneumothorax, aortic stenosis, or coarctation of the aorta.

- Myocardial contusion results from a strong, blunt force against the chest wall that injures the heart muscle and causes an arrhythmia.

Clinical Reasoning in Action

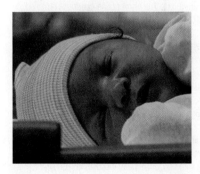

You are working in the hospital when Samantha, a 2-day-old newborn, is diagnosed with a continuous, systolic, grade 3 heart murmur in the pulmonic area of the chest. This is the parents' first child and they are extremely worried about their 6-week-premature baby. Samantha has full, bounding pulses and weighed 5 lb 6 oz at birth, but has lost 3 oz in the past 2 days. The mother's pregnancy was healthy until her water broke suddenly. The day after Samantha was born, the parents were told about the heart murmur. After an echocardiogram and chest radiograph are performed, Samantha is diagnosed with a patent ductus arteriosus (PDA). The healthcare provider prescribes 3 doses of a medication to aid in the closure of the duct. You explain that her vital signs and urine output will need to be monitored closely for decreases while she is on this medicine.

Several days later, the heart murmur is still heard; the medicine did not work. The parents want to avoid surgery if possible and the doctor explains that if the ductus closes by the time she is 9 to 12 months old, and she is without symptoms, surgery could be avoided. If the PDA is not corrected, her life span will be shortened. She is discharged from the hospital, thriving and breastfeeding well. The parents are educated to observe for poor weight gain, swelling, intercostal retractions, and breathing more than 60 times per minute. A follow-up appointment is made for 1 week later.

1. How would you explain a PDA to the parents?
2. What was the most likely cause of Samantha's initial weight loss? Is it the PDA that caused the weight loss?
3. What is the physiologic reason Samantha's life span would be shortened if the PDA does not close or get surgical correction?
4. How would you describe congestive heart failure to the parents?

References

American Academy of Pediatrics (AAP). (2015). *Red book: 2015 report of the Committee on Infectious Disease* (30th ed.). Elk Grove Village, IL: Author.

American Academy of Pediatrics Section on Cardiology and Cardiac Surgery. (2012). Pediatric sudden cardiac arrest. *Pediatrics, 129*(4), e1094–e1102.

Andrikopoulou, E., & Mather, P. J. (2014). Current insights: use of Immuknow in heart transplant recipients. *Progress in Transplantation, 24*(1), 44–50.

Association of Maternal and Child Health Programs. (2013). *Issue brief: State newborn screening and birth defects program role in screening for critical congenital heart defects (CCHD).* Retrieved from http://www.amchp.org/programsandtopics/CHILD-HEALTH/projects/newborn-screening/Documents/AMCHP_Screening_for_CCHD_Issue_Brief_FINAL-Oct2013.pdf

Awad, S. M. M., & Busse, J. (2011). Hypoplastic left heart syndrome. In R. Abdulla (Ed.), *Heart disease in children* (pp. 273–282). New York, NY: Springer.

Bor, D. H., Woolhandler, S., Nardin, R., Brusch, J., & Himmelstein, D. U. (2013). Infective endocarditis in the U.S., 1998–2009: A nationwide study. *PLOS One, 8*(3), e60033.

Brashers, V. L. (2014). Alterations in cardiovascular function. In K. L. McCance, S. E. Huether, V. L. Brashers, & N. R. Rote (Eds.), *Pathophysiology: The biologic basis for disease in adults and children* (7th ed., pp. 1129–1193). St. Louis, MO: Elsevier Mosby.

Buck, M. (2013). Update on therapies for pulmonary arterial hypertension in children. *Pediatric Pharmacotherapy, 19*(6), 1–4.

Chamiedes, L., Samson, R. A., Schexnayder, S. M., & Hazinski, M. F. (Eds.). (2011). *Pediatric advanced life support* (p. 97). Dallas, TX: American Heart Association.

Chang, C. (2012). Cutting edge issues in rheumatic fever. *Clinical Reviews in Allergy and Immunology, 42*(2), 213–237.

Daniels, S. R. (2012). Diagnosis and management of hypertension in children and adolescents. *Pediatric Annals, 41*(7), e144–e153.

Dennison, B. A. (2012). Bright futures and NHLBI integrated pediatric cardiovascular health guidelines. *Pediatric Annals, 41*(1), 31–35.

Gerwitz, M. H., Baltimore, J. S., Tani, L. Y., Sable, C. A., Shulman, S. T., Carapetis, J., . . . Kaplan, E. L. (2015). Revision of the Jones Criteria for the diagnosis of acute rheumatic fever in the era of Doppler echocardiography: A scientific statement from the American Heart Association. *Circulation, 131*, 1806–1818.

Giddings, S. S. (2012). An emerging dyslipidemia: New NHLBI and NLA treatment guidelines. *Contemporary Pediatrics, 29*(7), 24–33.

Hazinski, M. F., Mondozzi, M. A., & Baker, R. A. U. (2014). Shock, multiple organ dysfunction syndrome, and burns in children. In K. L. McCance, S. E. Huether, V. L. Brashers, & N. R. Rote (Eds.), *Pathophysiology: The biologic basis for disease in adults and children* (7th ed., pp. 1699–1727). St. Louis, MO: Mosby Elsevier.

Hylick, E. V., Grubbs, C. R., Johnson, J., & Oliver, B. (2014). Pediatric hypertension. *US Pharmacist. 39*(2), 57–60.

Kharouf, R., & Torchen, L. (2011). Infective endocarditis. In R. Abdulla (Ed.), *Heart disease in children* (pp. 333–342). New York, NY: Springer.

Leggiadro, R. J. (2014). Infective endocarditis in children with congenital heart disease. *Pediatric Infectious Disease Journal, 33*(2), 173.

Lo, J. C., Sinaiko, A., Chandra, M., Daley, M. F., Greenspan, L. C., Parker, E. D., . . . O'Connor, P. J. (2013). Prehypertension and hypertension in community-based pediatric practice. *Pediatrics, 131*(2), e415–e424.

Long, S. H., Harris, S. R., Eldridge, B. J., & Galea, M. P. (2012). Gross motor development is delayed following early cardiac surgery. *Cardiology in the Young, 22*, 574–582.

Longmuir, P. E., Banks, L., & McCrindle, B. W. (2012). Cross-sectional study of motor development among children after the Fontan procedure. *Cardiology in the Young, 22*, 443–450.

Maxwell, B. G., Nies M. K., Ajuba-Iwuji, C. C., Coulson, J. D., Lewis, H., & Romer, L. H. (2015). Trends in hospitalization for pediatric pulmonary hypertension. *Pediatrics, 136*(2), 241–250.

McCusker, C. G., Armstrong, M. P., Mullen, M., Doherty, N. N., & Casey, F. A. (2013). A sibling-controlled, prospective study of outcomes at home and school in children with severe congenital heart disease. *Cardiology in the Young, 23*, 507–516.

McDaniel, N. L. (2014). Alterations in cardiovascular function in children. In K. L. McCance, S. E. Huether, V. L. Brashers, & N. R. Rote (Eds.), *Pathophysiology: The biologic basis for disease in adults and children* (7th ed., pp. 1194–1224). St. Louis, MO: Elsevier Mosby.

McLellan, M. C., & Baker, A. L. (2011). At the heart of the fever: Kawasaki disease. *American Journal of Nursing, 111*(6), 57–63.

Meaux, J. B., Green, A., Nelson, M. K., Huett, A., Boateng, B., Pye, S., . . . Riley, L. (2014). Transition to self-management after pediatric heart transplant. *Progress in Transplantation, 24*, 226–233.

National Heart Lung and Blood Institute (NHLBI). (2012). *Expert panel on integrated guidelines for cardiovascular health and risk reduction in children and adolescents.* Retrieved from http://www.nhlbi.nih.gov/guidelines/cvd_ped/index.htm

O'Connell, J., & Sloand, E. (2013). Kawasaki syndrome and streptococcal scarlet fever: A clinical review. *The Journal for Nurse Practitioners, 9*(5), 259–264.

Ofori-Amanfo, G., & Cheifetz, I. M. (2013). Pediatric postoperative cardiac care. *Critical Care Clinics of North America, 29*, 185–202.

Paris, J. J., Moore, M. P., & Schreiber, M. D. (2012). Physician counseling, informed consent and parental decision making for infants with hypoplastic left-heart syndrome. *Journal of Perinatology, 32*, 748–751.

Park, M. K. (2014). *Pediatric cardiology for practitioners* (6th ed.). Philadelphia: Elsevier Saunders.

Perkin, R. M., deCaen, A. R., Berg, M. D., Schexnayder, S. M., & Hazinski, M. F. (2013). Shock, cardiac arrest, and resuscitation. In M. F. Hazinski (Ed.), *Nursing care of the critically ill child* (3rd ed., pp. 101–154). St. Louis, MO: Elsevier.

Peterson, C., Ailes, E., Riehle-Colarusso, T., Oster, M. E., Olney, R. S., Cassell, C. H., . . . Gilboa, S. M. (2014). Late detection of critical congenital heart disease among US infants: Estimation of the potential impact of proposed universal screening using pulse oximetry. *JAMA Pediatrics.* doi:10.1001/jamapediatrics.2013.4779

Rowley, A. H. (2012). Kawasaki disease genetics, pathology, and need for earlier diagnosis and treatment. *Contemporary Pediatrics, 29*(12), 18–24.

Sabe, M. A., Shrestha, N. K., & Menon, V. (2013). Contemporary drug treatment of infective endocarditis. *American Journal of Cardiovascular Drugs, 13*, 251–258.

Satou, G. M., & Halnon, N. J. (2013). *Pediatric congestive heart failure.* Retrieved from http://emedicine.medscape.com/article/2069746-medication#1

Steffen, K. M. (2011). Trauma, burns, and common critical care emergencies. In M. M. Tschudy, & K. M. Arcara (Eds.), *The Harriet Lane handbook* (19th ed., p. 109). Philadelphia, PA: Elsevier Mosby.

Toebbe, S., Yehle, K., Kirkpatrick, J., & Coddington, J. (2013). Hypoplastic left heart syndrome: Parent support for early decision making. *Journal of Pediatric Nursing, 28*, 383–392.

Warnes, C. A. (2014). Pregnancy and heart disease. In D. L. Mann, D. P. Zipes, P. Libby, R. O. Bonow, & E. Braunwald (Eds.), *Braunwald's heart disease: A textbook of cardiovascular medicine* (10th ed., pp. 1755–1770). Philadelphia, PA: Elsevier Saunders.

Williams, J. T. B., & Fagan, H. A. (2014). A 15-year-old boy with congenital heart disease, fevers, and acute onset of dysarthria. *Pediatric Annals, 43*(2), 64–67.

Wilson, B. A., Shannon, M. T., & Shields, K. M. (2016). *Pearson nurses' drug guide 2016.* Hoboken, NJ: Pearson Education.

Yu, M. A., Bostwick, J. R., & Hallman, I. S. (2011). Warfarin drug interactions: Strategies to minimize adverse drug events. *Journal for Nurse Practitioners, 7*(6), 506–512.

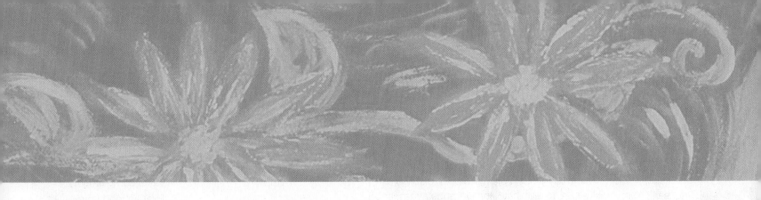

Chapter 22
Alterations in Immune Function

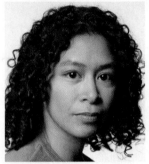

Barbara Penoyar/Getty Images

We knew that Raymond might have AIDS—my sister was HIV positive. But we have taken him in as our own child and cared for him. Somehow we thought he would be fine. Now, to find out that he does have AIDS is devastating, especially since my sister is also very ill. We need to learn a lot about how to help him. Can we send him to a preschool next year as we had planned? How will we get money to pay for his medicines? What do we tell other people? How do we get him to eat better? We just don't know where to turn right now.

—Aunt of Raymond, 2 years old

∨ Learning Outcomes

22.1 Describe the structure and function of the immune system and apply that knowledge to the care of children with immunologic disorders.

22.2 Summarize infection control measures needed for children with an immunodeficiency.

22.3 Develop a nursing care plan in partnership with the family for a child with human immunodeficiency virus (HIV infection).

22.4 Plan nursing care for the child with an autoimmune condition such as systemic lupus erythematosus or juvenile arthritis.

22.5 Identify exposure prevention measures for the child with latex allergy.

22.6 Determine nursing interventions and prevention measures for the child experiencing hypersensitivity reactions.

Signs and symptoms of immunologic disorders in children are often nonspecific. The immune system is one of the few body systems that regulate, either directly or indirectly, all other body functions. Thus a problem with the immune system can result in multisystem consequences and may be life threatening. The child with recurring infections may have an undiagnosed immunologic disorder. Congenital abnormalities sometimes signal a defect in cellular immunity. This chapter will examine some of the more common disorders of immune function and discuss nursing care of children and families who have these diseases.

Immunodeficiency Disorders

Immunodeficiency, a state of decreased responsiveness of the immune system, can occur to varying degrees in response to any number of events. Children with congenital immune deficiency, or **primary immune deficiency**, are born with a failure of humoral antibody formation (B-cell disorder), a deficient cellular immune system (T-cell disorder), or a combination of both defects. In congenital disorders, the immune deficiency is not caused by another condition. However, immunodeficiency may also be acquired, as in human immunodeficiency virus (HIV) infection. Acquired immune deficiency is also called **secondary immune deficiency**.

Text continues on page 566

FOCUS ON:
The Immune System

Anatomy and Physiology

The function of the immune system is to recognize any foreign substances within the body—in simple terms, to distinguish "nonself" from "self"—and to eliminate foreign substances as efficiently as possible. When the body recognizes the presence of a substance that it cannot identify as part of itself, the body protects itself through the immune response. Normally, the immune system responds to an invasion of foreign substances, or antigens, in numerous ways. It produces **antibodies**, or proteins that work against **antigens**, the foreign substances that trigger the immune response. There are many types of antibodies, which are described later in this section. The immune system also produces other types of cells, such as T lymphocytes and natural killer (NK) cells.

Immunity is either natural or acquired. **Natural immunity** comprises the defenses present at birth, such as intact skin, body pH, natural antibodies from the mother, and inflammatory and phagocytic properties. **Acquired immunity** consists of humoral (antibody-mediated) and cell-mediated immunity and is not fully developed until a child is about 6 years of age.

Humoral immunity is responsible for destroying bacterial antigens. B lymphocytes, produced in the bone marrow, gut, and other lymphoid tissue, are the central factor in humoral immunity and develop into plasma cells that produce antibodies. Antibodies are a type of protein called **immunoglobulins**, of which there are five types: IgM, IgG, IgA, IgD, and IgE (Table 22–1). IgM, IgG, and IgA act to control a number of body infections, whereas IgE is useful in combating parasitic infections and is part of the allergic response. The role of IgD is unknown (Orduño, Grimaldi, & Diamond, 2013).

Antibodies are found in serum, body fluids, and certain tissues. When a child is first exposed to an antigen, the B-lymphocyte system begins to produce antibodies that react specifically to that antigen (see *Pathophysiology Illustrated: Primary Immune Response*). It takes approximately 3 days for this process, known as a **primary immune response**, to occur. Subsequent encounters with the antigen trigger memory cells, resulting in a **secondary immune response** within 24 hours.

Cellular immunity or *cell-mediated immunity* uses T lymphocytes, produced mainly in the thymus, to provide cellular

TABLE 22–1 Classes of Immunoglobulins

IMMUNO-GLOBULIN	LOCATION	ACTION
IgM	Present in intravascular spaces (blood and lymph)	Mediates cytotoxic response and activates complement First antibody produced with primary immune response
IgG	Present in all body fluids	Active against bacteria, bacterial toxins, and viruses Activates complement Only immunoglobulin to cross the placenta
IgA	Present in secretions of gastrointestinal, respiratory, and genitourinary tracts	Prevents binding of viruses to cells of the respiratory and gastrointestinal tracts
IgD	Present in blood, lymph, and surfaces of B cells	Function not fully understood
IgE	Present in internal and external body fluids	Releases chemical mediators responsible for immediate hypersensitivity response

Pathophysiology Illustrated: **Primary Immune Response**

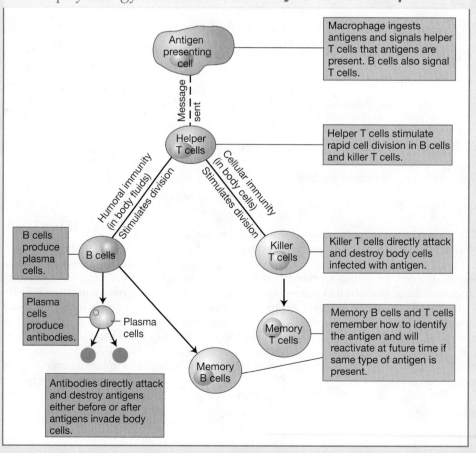

immunity and protect against most viruses, fungi, slowly developing bacterial infections such as tuberculosis, and tumors. In addition, they control the timing of the response in delayed hypersensitivity reactions, such as the purified protein derivative (PPD) test, and they are responsible for the rejection of foreign grafts, such as transplants. Specialized types of T lymphocytes include killer T cells, suppressor T cells, and helper T cells. Suppressor T cells inhibit B lymphocytes from differentiating into plasma cells. Helper T cells aid in the proliferation and immunologic function of other cells. T lymphocytes have proteins on their surfaces that attract and trap receptors; these proteins can be used to measure the immune activity of these cells. For example, some of the common proteins are CD2, CD3, CD4, CD5, CD7, and CD8. Natural killer (NK) cells (also known as non-B/non-T lymphocytes) originate in the bone marrow and thymus and migrate to the blood and spleen. They play a role in control of viral infection, tumors, and autoimmune diseases.

Complement is a component of blood serum consisting of 11 protein compounds. It is an inactive enzyme that activates in response to antigen–antibody functions, resulting in a generalized inflammatory reaction that kills foreign cells. It also plays a role in causing some autoimmune diseases.

Immune cells also secrete proteins called cytokines that carry messages for immune system function. Lymphocytes, monocytes, and macrophages all secrete cytokines that have a variety of effects on the target cells. Effects may include stimulation of growth through proliferation of cells, differentiation of cellular actions, production of inflammation, sensitization to pain, and other actions. Interleukins, a type of cytokine, were first identified in white blood cells but now are known to be present in many cells. Many types of interleukins have been identified, and some are known to influence the function of the immune system.

Pediatric Differences

Immune system development is a complex and multifactorial process. Early in-utero experiences, environmental exposures after birth, and other factors influence this important feedback system. It protects children from harmful diseases but also leads to conditions such as asthma (Chapter 20), food allergy (Chapter 14), or skin atopy (Chapter 31).

Infants and children have differing amounts of some immunoglobulins. IgG is the only immunoglobulin that crosses the placenta; as a result, a newborn's levels are similar to those of the mother (Buckley, 2016a). This maternal IgG disappears by 6 to 8 months of age. The infant's IgG then increases gradually until mature levels are reached at 7 to 8 years. IgM levels are low at birth, rise markedly at 1 week of age, and continue to increase until adult levels are reached at about 1 year. IgA and IgE are not present at birth. Manufacture of these immunoglobulins begins by 2 weeks of age; however, normal values are not achieved until 6 to 7 years. Thus it is easy to see why children under 6 years of age become ill so often—they do not have a full complement of immunoglobulins.

In contrast, cell-mediated immunity achieves full function early in life. Early in fetal life, the thymus begins producing T cells. By birth, many of these cells are present. The thymus is large at birth, grows during childhood, reaches peak size just before puberty, and then decreases in size (Buckley, 2016a). Other lymphoid tissues, such as the spleen and tonsils, are also comparatively large in young children. Because of the well-developed cellular immunity, any blood infused into newborns is generally irradiated to prevent **graft-versus-host disease** (a series of immunologic reactions in response to transplanted cells) from transfused

As Children Grow: **Immunoglobulins Throughout Childhood**

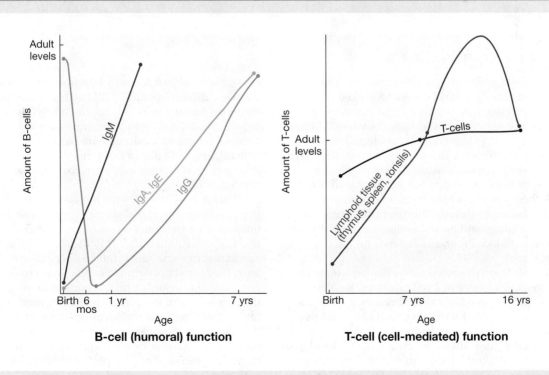

B-cell (humoral) function

T-cell (cell-mediated) function

(continued)

lymphocytes (see *As Children Grow: Immunoglobulins Throughout Childhood*).

Newborns have somewhat lower numbers of NK cells than older children and adults, decreasing their ability to respond to certain antigens. The levels of some complement proteins are lower in newborns than in older children and adults, thus delaying and hampering response to certain infections.

Growth and Development

Newborns are most prone to development of infection, particularly when born prematurely, because they have lower levels of their own immune protections. Human milk contains immunologic components that can influence the immune response in the infant and protect against infection (Hassiotou et al., 2013).

Table 22–2 provides examples of diagnostic and laboratory tests used to evaluate immune system function. Use *Assessment Guide: The Child With an Immune System Alteration* to perform a nursing assessment of the immune system.

TABLE 22–2 Diagnostic Tests and Laboratory Procedures for the Immune System*

DIAGNOSTIC TEST	LABORATORY TEST
Intradermal skin testing	Complete blood count
	Complement
	Immunoglobulins
	HIV tests—see information later in the chapter

*See Appendices D and E for information about these diagnostic procedures and tests.

ASSESSMENT GUIDE | The Child With an Immune System Alteration

Assessment Focus	Assessment Guidelines
Family history	• Does a family member have a history of allergy?
	• Does the mother or other family member have a history of HIV or other immune system disorder?
	• Has the child been treated prophylactically for HIV due to the mother's positive status?
Growth and development	• Is growth regular? Is the child meeting developmental milestones?
	• What is the child's food intake and appetite?
Skin and mucous membranes	• Is the skin intact? Are there lesions of the mucous membranes?
	• Do lesions heal quickly without additional infection?
Evidence of disease	• Does the child have a history of recurring or unusual infections?

B-Cell and T-Cell Disorders

In B-cell disorders, immunoglobulins may be present in inadequate numbers or nearly absent. X-linked agammaglobulinemia, selective IgA deficiency, and common variable immunodeficiency are examples of such disorders (Michaels & Green, 2016). Because newborns are protected from infection by maternal antibodies in the first months after birth, symptoms of B-cell disorders usually become apparent after 3 months of age once the infant loses maternal antibodies. Infants with these disorders have frequent recurrent bacterial infections and failure to thrive. With treatment, consisting of intravenous immunoglobulins and antibiotics, most children survive into adulthood. Prognosis depends on the degree of antibody deficiency.

T-cell disorders are characterized by inadequate numbers of T lymphocytes or absence of T-cell functions. Isolated T-cell disorders are rare, are usually accompanied by a B-cell disorder, and may be associated with congenital abnormalities (as in DiGeorge syndrome) or of unknown cause. DiGeorge syndrome, a T-cell disorder caused by chromosome deletion at 22q11.2, is usually diagnosed soon after birth. The syndrome is characterized by the absence (complete DiGeorge) or hypoplasia (partial DiGeorge) of the parathyroid glands or thymus gland, hypocalcemia with tetany within 24 to 48 hours after birth, cardiac defects, low-set ears, hypertelorism (widely set eyes), and viral and bacterial infections in the neonatal period (Buckley, 2016b; Fernandez, 2013). There is generally a mild to moderate decrease in T-lymphocyte counts (McDonald-McGinn & Sullivan, 2011). Prophylactic antibiotics are used to prevent bacterial infections. Children with partial DiGeorge are treated with calcium and vitamin D supplements. Those with complete DiGeorge need thymus transplantation in order to survive (Fernandez, 2013).

Immunodeficiency with hyper-IgM is a T-cell disorder that primarily affects males and causes decreased T-cell function, variable abnormal levels of immunoglobulins, and high titers of some antibodies. It is usually X linked but may be autosomal in some cases. Infections caused by viruses, bacteria, fungi, and opportunistic infections are common in children with this disorder. Intravenous immune globulin (IVIG) therapy is helpful in decreasing the frequency of lower respiratory tract infections and severe infections but does not affect the frequency of upper respiratory infections or other infections. Bone marrow or stem cell transplantation with cord blood has been used as an aspect of treatment in some patients with varying outcomes (Park, 2012). Table 22–3, shown later, compares laboratory values for selected congenital immunodeficiency disorders.

Severe Combined Immunodeficiency Disease

Severe combined immunodeficiency disease (SCID) is a congenital condition characterized by the absence of both humoral and cellular immunity that is manifested by lack of appropriately functioning T cells and B cells (Schwartz & Sinha, 2013). SCID occurs in X-linked recessive and autosomal recessive forms. In some cases, SCID may be the result of chromosomal abnormalities. The disorder is estimated to occur in 1 per 50,000–100,000 live births (Pai & Notarangelo, 2013). Without appropriate treatment, children born with SCID usually do not survive more than 1 year (Buckley, 2016c)

ETIOLOGY AND PATHOPHYSIOLOGY

Severe combined immunodeficiency disease is caused by genetic mutations that lead to absence of immune function and, in some cases, absence of natural killer (NK) cells (Buckley, 2016c). The B lymphocytes are also generally defective, but even if they are normal, their function is compromised because of the severe T-cell deficiency (Kwan et al., 2014).

CLINICAL MANIFESTATIONS

Symptoms of SCID develop early in life. The infant often demonstrates a susceptibility to infection, presenting during the first few months of life with persistent respiratory infections and diarrhea (Buckley, 2016c). Recurrent oral candidiasis, failure to thrive, and skin infections are also frequently seen in affected children. Additionally, failure to recover completely from infection, frequent reinfection, and infection with viruses such as cytomegalovirus and the bacterium *Pneumocystis jiroveci* (formerly called *P. carinii*) are common in the child with SCID (Buckley, 2016c). Children are also highly susceptible to serious infections such as meningitis, skin or organ infection, osteomyelitis, or sepsis.

CLINICAL THERAPY

Refer to Table 22–3 for laboratory findings in SCID. Diagnosis is usually made only after extensive laboratory testing. In addition to a complete blood count, erythrocyte sedimentation rate, and B- and T-cell lymphocyte counts, other studies including IgA, IgG, and IgM antibody titers to immunizations received, and neutrophil count, may be performed (Table 22–4). A chest radiograph is conducted to assess thymus size.

TABLE 22–3 Laboratory Findings for Selected Congenital Immunodeficiency Disorders

DISORDERS	LABORATORY FINDINGS
B CELL	
X-linked hypogammaglobulinemia	Reduced IgA, IgM, IgE, IgG (<100 mg/dL), absence of B cells in peripheral blood, normal T cells
Selective IgA deficiency	IgA less than 10 mg/dL
Common variable immunodeficiency	Reduced IgG, IgA, and IgM
T CELL	
DiGeorge syndrome	Lymphopenia; absent T-cell functions, decreased T cells, normal B cells
X-linked immunodeficiency with hyper-IgM	Reduced IgG, IgA; elevated IgM; mutations in T-cell surface proteins
COMBINED	
Severe combined immunodeficiency syndrome (SCID)	Complete absence of T- and B-cell and NK immunity
Wiskott-Aldrich syndrome	Thrombocytopenia, low platelet volume, nonfunctional B-cells, normal IgG, decreased IgM, increased IgA, increased IgE; inability to respond to polysaccharide antigens

The standard therapy for severe combined immunodeficiency disease is the administration of intravenous immune globulin (IVIG), which is administered to provide protection until humoral immunity is established. Hematopoietic stem cell transplantation (see Chapter 23) offers the best hope for children with SCID. T-cell function is restored with the transplantation, and new cells appear 3 to 4 months after infusion of the donor stem cell. Gene therapy may also be used to treat SCID. Prognosis for the child is poor without aggressive therapy and transplant.

Prevention and prompt treatment of infection are essential. Antibiotic therapy is targeted at infectious agents. Antibiotic

TABLE 22–4 Cells Evaluated in Laboratory Studies for Immune Conditions

TEST AND TYPE OF CELL EVALUATED	ACTION	IMPLICATION OF INCREASED OR DECREASED LEVELS
WHITE BLOOD CELL (WBC) COUNT		
Neutrophil (54%–62%)	Phagocytic cell that defends against bacteria	Increased in bacterial infection, inflammatory processes, and some malignancies
Eosinophil (1%–3%)	Associated with antigen–antibody reaction	Increased in allergic reaction; decreased in children receiving corticosteroids
Basophils (0%–3%)	Phagocytic cell; involved in immediate hypersensitivity reaction; stores histamine and has receptor sites for IgE	Increased in leukemia; decreased in allergy, acute infection, collagen, and chronic diseases
Monocytes (4%–9%)	Phagocytic cell active in chronic infection	Increased in tuberculosis, protozoan infection, monocytic leukemia
Lymphocytes (T, B, non-B/non-T [NK]) (25%–33%)	Major components of immune system	Increased in many infections; decreased in children with immune deficiency
IMMUNOGLOBULINS		
(IgM, IgG, IgA, IgD, IgE) (See Appendix D for age-specific values.)	Many roles in a number of immunologic reactions	Increased in presence of infection or allergic response; decreased in children with immune deficiency

prophylaxis and special immunization recommendations are needed. Children with T-cell deficiencies should receive lymphocyte-depleted and irradiated blood products because of the risk of infection and graft-versus-host disease from lymphocytes in the donor blood (Schwartz & Sinha, 2013).

Nursing Management

For the Child With SCID

Nursing Assessment and Diagnosis

Obtain a thorough history of infections, including age of onset, type of causal organism, frequency, and severity. Assess family history, and determine if the child has had any unusual reactions to vaccines, medications, or foods. Measure the child's height and weight and plot on a growth chart to identify failure to thrive. Assess the child's nutritional intake and fluid and electrolyte balance. Assess for evidence of infections involving the skin, subcutaneous tissues, respiratory system, and mucous membranes. Palpate the abdomen for hepatomegaly and the lymph nodes for lymphadenopathy. Perform a developmental assessment and assess for delays in achievement of developmental milestones. Assess family support systems and coping mechanisms when a child is diagnosed with the disorder.

The primary nursing diagnosis for a child with SCID is *Infection, Risk for,* related to immunodeficiency. Other nursing diagnoses may include the following (NANDA-I © 2014):

- *Nutrition, Imbalanced: Less than Body Requirements,* related to illness
- *Skin Integrity, Risk for Impaired,* related to immunologic deficit
- *Caregiver Role Strain, Risk for,* related to a child with a chronic, life-threatening illness
- *Development: Delayed, Risk for,* related to physical disability and chronic illness

Planning and Implementation

Nursing care of the immunodeficient child focuses on preventing infection (see *Families Want to Know: Reducing Risk of Infection in the Child With Immunodeficiency Disease*). However, even with the use of environmental controls, such as keeping children inside special units (positive-pressure rooms) to maintain a sterile environment, these children are prone to **opportunistic infections** (those caused by normally nonpathogenic organisms in persons who lack normal immunity).

PREVENT SYSTEMIC INFECTION

Frequent and thorough handwashing is important. Standard precautions are always used and transmission-based precautions are established when indicated. Implement sterile aseptic technique when caring for all sites where needles, catheters, central lines, endotracheal tubes, pressure-monitoring lines, and peripheral intravenous lines, or other invasive equipment enter the child's body (see the *Clinical Skills Manual* SKILLS). The child should be placed in a positive-pressure isolation room, and contact with infectious individuals should be avoided. Inform parents that because of the risk of infection to the child, live vaccines are avoided for the child as well as siblings, parents, and other household members. Refer to the current recommendations for immunizations for the immunocompromised child. (See Chapter 16.)

PROMOTE SKIN INTEGRITY

The skin is the only intact defense that many immunodeficient children have. Provide thorough and frequent skin care, and observe all possible pressure areas closely for signs of breakdown or infection. Reposition the child frequently and encourage range-of-motion exercises.

PROMOTE NUTRITIONAL BALANCE

Encourage adequate fluid and nutritional intake. Provide foods that the child prefers and those with high nutritional value. Offer small frequent feedings of high-calorie, protein-rich foods. Refer to a dietitian as needed to plan with parents for the best individualized diet for the child.

MANAGE MEDICATION THERAPY

Many medications used long term in the treatment of children with SCID have numerous side effects. Monitor closely for side effects of antibiotics, such as overgrowth of resistant organisms (e.g., thrush infections in the mouth, *Clostridium difficile* infections of the gastrointestinal tract) and administer IVIG safely.

PROVIDE EMOTIONAL SUPPORT AND REFERRALS

SCID is a life-threatening and devastating disease. Even with aggressive therapy, the prognosis is poor for children who do not receive a hematopoietic stem cell transplant. Evaluate the family's knowledge about the disease and provide education about infection control measures and signs of infection. The parents may experience guilt because of the genetic nature of the disease and the difficulties of treatment. Listen closely to their concerns and encourage them to discuss their fears. Refer them to an appropriate support group or counselor if needed. Encourage genetic counseling if the parents plan to have more children. Evaluate the family's ability to care for the child at home. Offer financial resource information and other referrals as needed.

Families Want to Know

Reducing Risk of Infection in the Child With Immunodeficiency Disease

Teach family members the following practices to reduce the risk of transmission of infection:

- Wash all bottles, nipples, and pacifiers with hot water and soap, or in the dishwasher.
- Do not allow child to share utensils, cups, bottles, or pacifiers.
- Use safe food preparation practices such as peeling fruit and vegetables and using different surfaces and utensils for preparing meats versus other foods.
- Change diapers frequently and cleanse skin with mild soap and dry thoroughly.
- Wash hands before handling child, after changing diapers, and before feeding child.
- Maintain clean pets and keep the pet's environment clean.
- Avoid exposing the child to other family members' illnesses, such as colds.

The family of a child who undergoes hematopoietic stem cell transplantation requires additional support and referrals. The transplantation procedure involves surgery for both the ill child and the donor, often another child in the family. After the transplant the ill child will be hospitalized for several months until T-lymphocyte levels are sufficient to provide resistance to infection. During this period, parents may need to rely on social services to help manage the family situation, particularly if the child is hospitalized at a medical center far from the family's home. Assess the family's situation and make appropriate referrals to social services and support groups. Introduce parents to other families undergoing hematopoietic stem cell transplantation. (See Chapter 23 for discussion of hematopoietic stem cell transplantation.)

Evaluation

The success of nursing care for the child with SCID is measured by outcomes such as the following:

- The child is free of infection.
- The child has adequate nutritional status as determined by normal growth patterns.
- The child's skin remains intact.
- The family adapts to and copes with the demands of a chronic illness.
- The child performs developmentally within normal level for age.

Wiskott-Aldrich Syndrome

A combined congenital immunodeficiency syndrome, Wiskott-Aldrich syndrome (WAS) is an X-linked disorder that causes mutation in the *WAS* gene and changes in the WAS protein. The gene resides on Xp11.22–11.23 (Buckley, 2016c). The incidence is 1 in 250,000 live male births (Schwartz & Siperstein, 2013). The IgM levels are low, IgG levels are normal or slightly low, and IgA and IgE levels are elevated (Buckley, 2016c).

The diagnosis is made in the early neonatal period on the basis of the thrombocytopenia, which leads to bleeding as evidenced by petechiae, hematuria, bloody diarrhea, and hematemesis. In addition to thrombocytopenia and related symptoms, Wiskott-Aldrich syndrome is characterized by eczema and recurrent infections in infancy and childhood. Infections including otitis media, bacterial pneumonia, and skin infections are common (Albert, Notarangelo, & Ochs, 2011; Schwartz & Siperstein, 2013).

Treatment is supportive and includes antibiotic prophylaxis, platelet transfusions, and intravenous gamma globulin (IVIG). Splenectomy may reduce the risk of bleeding; however, this is done sparingly because of the risk of life-threatening infection following the procedure. The treatment of choice and the only cure for Wiskott-Aldrich syndrome is hematopoietic stem cell transplantation (HSCT). Following HSCT, the child is at risk for both rejection and graft-versus- host disease (Albert et al., 2011; Schwartz & Siperstein, 2013).

Nursing Management

Nursing care is similar to that for the child with SCID. Refer the parents for genetic counseling to help them understand the disease transmission and the probability of having another child with the same disorder. Arrange for psychologic support for parents overwhelmed with guilt from learning that the illness is inherited.

Help the parents and family cope with the knowledge that the child has a chronic and potentially fatal illness (see Chapters 12 and 13). Referral to family counseling may be appropriate. Expected outcomes are the child's return to normal immunologic function, absence of hemorrhage, and successful coping with a life-threatening illness.

Human Immunodeficiency Virus and Acquired Immune Deficiency Syndrome

Acquired immune deficiency syndrome (AIDS) is caused by the human immunodeficiency virus (HIV-1 primarily; HIV-2 less commonly) (American Academy of Pediatrics [AAP], 2015, p. 453). Because HIV destroys the body's ability to fight infection, opportunistic infections that would normally not affect healthy people destroy the immune system. AIDS is the advanced stages of HIV infection.

Most cases of HIV in children are the result of perinatal transmission. The Centers for Disease Control and Prevention (CDC) (2014a) estimates that 162 infants were born with HIV infection in the United States in 2010. The incidence of perinatally acquired HIV infection in the United States has declined by an estimated 90% since the early 1990s. This improvement is primarily due to more effective identification and treatment of mothers who are infected with HIV (CDC, 2014a). The leading cause of newly acquired HIV infection in teens is unprotected sexual intercourse, while intravenous substance use is responsible for most other cases. In many cases, both of these factors are involved.

ETIOLOGY AND PATHOPHYSIOLOGY

Children can acquire HIV in a form of **vertical transmission** from their mothers transplacentally or during delivery. Transmission can occur during birth from blood, amniotic fluid, and exposure to genital tract secretions, and after birth through breast milk from HIV-infected mothers. However, risk for perinatal transmission has been significantly reduced since mothers identified as being infected receive antiretroviral therapy (ART) during pregnancy, undergo a cesarean section, and are advised not to breastfeed (CDC, 2014a). If the mother is not treated during pregnancy, labor, or delivery, there is a 25% chance that the newborn will be infected (U.S. Department of Health and Human Services [USDHHS], 2012). Prenatal testing is essential for identifying mothers who are HIV positive so that treatment can be started and decrease the infant's chances of acquiring the infection to less than 1% (CDC, 2014a).

The virus affects multiple systems and eventually destroys the ability of the child's immune system to respond to infection. An understanding of the natural history of HIV disease is still evolving, and there are several important differences in the disease progression and clinical manifestations of pediatric and adult HIV infections.

The virus selectively targets and destroys T cells, thereby decreasing and eventually eliminating cellular immunity. HIV destroys CD4 T cells (helper cells), which are crucial to normal function of the immune system. HIV selectively targets T cells, decreasing cellular immunity, and affecting humoral immunity as well. Thus the untreated child is left unprotected against a myriad of bacterial, viral, fungal, and opportunistic infections, which are ultimately fatal. Every organ system can be affected. (See *Pathophysiology Illustrated: Human Immunodeficiency Virus.*)

CLINICAL MANIFESTATIONS

The neonate is asymptomatic at birth. The time period for the development of opportunistic infections varies; however, the interval from HIV infection to the onset of overt AIDS is shorter in children than in adults. See Table 22–5.

Early clinical signs for children with HIV infection are nonspecific findings, including lymphadenopathy, hepatosplenomegaly, oral candidiasis, failure to thrive and weight loss, delayed development, swelling of the parotid gland, and chronic diarrhea (AAP, 2015, p. 457; Kronman & Smith, 2015). Recurrent bacterial infections, lymphoid interstitial pneumonitis (LIP), and progressive neurologic deterioration are more common in children than adults. *Pneumocystis jiroveci* (formerly known as *P. carinii*) pneumonia is also common and may present early in infancy (Kronman & Smith, 2015).

CLINICAL THERAPY

There is no cure for HIV or AIDS. Care focuses on the prevention of HIV transmission, the detection of the presence of HIV, aggressive therapy to reduce progression to AIDS, and promotion of the infant's or child's growth and development and survival.

Most children with HIV infection are diagnosed early in life. Virologic tests for detection of the virus are monitored in infants born to mothers infected with HIV. Testing is recommended at 14 to 21 days, 1 to 2 months, and 4 to 6 months. The preferred tests are the HIV DNA polymerase chain reaction (PCR) or the HIV RNA assay (viral load). Any positive result is confirmed by retesting. In addition, CD4 cell counts and percentages should be performed at least every 3 to 4 months to evaluate the child's immune status. This monitoring may change to every 6 to 12 months in children and adolescents who are compliant with therapy and have stable CD4 values and clinical status for over

Pathophysiology Illustrated: **Human Immunodeficiency Virus**

① HIV uses the CD4 antigen to bind to the surface of the target cell

Helper T cell (target cell)

Nucleus with DNA

CD4 antigen

HIV

② Virus sheds protein coat

③ Viral RNA is converted with reverse transcriptase into viral DNA

④ Viral DNA integrates with host cell DNA

Virus remains latent

Virus infects daughter cells during host replication

Viral proliferation results in the lysis of the infected cell

⑤ The net result of an HIV infection is decreased cellular immunity

TABLE 22–5 Clinical Manifestations of Human Immunodeficiency Virus in Children

ETIOLOGY	CLINICAL MANIFESTATIONS	CLINICAL THERAPY
Frequent, chronic, or unusual infections due to poor immune response	Chronic bilateral otitis media Oral candidiasis *Pneumocystis jiroveci* pneumonia Skin disorders Fever Parotitis	Antimicrobial therapy for treatment of infections Recommended immunizations Limit exposure to groups of people or to individuals with known infections of any kind
Poor nutritional intake due to lack of appetite caused by disease and medications	Failure to thrive (eating disorder of childhood) Weight and body mass index below 10th percentile Chronic diarrhea Skin irritation	Monitor growth Supplemental intake such as enteral feedings at night, and total parenteral nutrition (TPN) if needed Meticulous skin care to prevent breakdown
Immune system overgrowth to compensate for lack of proper immune response	Hepatosplenomegaly and lymphadenopathy	Assess abdomen frequently Teach about safe transport to avoid injury to liver and spleen

Note: Be alert for the possibility of HIV infection in infants with combinations of listed clinical manifestations, especially in infants known to be at risk.

Source: Data from American Academy of Pediatrics (AAP). (2015). *Red book: 2015 report of the Committee on Infectious Diseases* (30th ed.). Elk Grove Village, IL: Author; Kronman, M. P., & Smith, S. (2015). Infectious diseases. In K. J. Marcdante & R. M. Kliegman, *Nelson essentials of pediatrics* (7th ed., pp. 315–416). Philadelphia, PA: Elsevier Saunders.

2 to 3 years (Panel on Antiretroviral Therapy and Medical Management of HIV-Infected Children, 2014).

Antibody tests are performed in children with no clinical signs or virologic evidence of HIV infection to see if the maternal HIV antibodies have disappeared. A diagnosis of HIV infection is definitively excluded in children with two negative antibody tests at age 6 months or older. Repeat testing is recommended between 12 and 18 months of age in children who have not yet had two negative antibody tests (Panel on Antiretroviral Therapy and Medical Management of HIV-Infected Children, 2014). See Table 22–6.

Medical management begins with prevention of the spread of HIV from mother to newborn. Because of the rapidity of disease progression in perinatally transmitted HIV infection, early identification of infected infants is important to ensure the most effective treatment. Mothers infected with HIV should be identified during pregnancy, and their infants should undergo periodic laboratory testing, as described earlier. All infected mothers should receive zidovudine antiretroviral therapy after the 14th week of pregnancy (AAP, 2015, p. 472). Early identification of mothers infected with HIV and implementation of antiretroviral therapy will lead to a decrease in the numbers of infants and children with HIV infection.

Clinical Tip

Many people who are at risk of HIV infection may not have HIV testing readily available. To reduce barriers to early detection of the virus, rapid HIV tests have been made available. Specimens are obtained from saliva or fingerstick for blood sample. Oral fluids are obtained by gently swabbing both the upper and lower outer gums of the mouth. Results are available in 20 minutes. Follow-up testing is performed to confirm positive rapid HIV tests (CDC, 2014b). Health professionals must be prepared to offer counseling during the same visit as when the test is administered.

All infants of infected mothers with indeterminate HIV infection status should start prophylaxis against *P. jiroveci* pneumonia by the age of 4 to 6 weeks and continue to 1 year of age unless the diagnosis of HIV infection is excluded. Prompt therapy with anti-infectives is used for bacterial and viral

opportunistic infections. The need for prophylaxis after 1 year of age is dependent on the child's degree of immunosuppression (AAP, 2015, p. 641).

Treatment for the child diagnosed with HIV involves combination antiretroviral therapy (cART). Initial medication therapy should include a combination of several antiretroviral (AVR) drugs. At least three drugs from a minimum of two different categories should be used. See *Medications Used to Treat: Human Immunodeficiency Virus in Children* for information related to antiretroviral drugs that may be used in children. Families should be advised that these drugs neither cure HIV nor prevent transfer from the person infected to others.

Children on antiretroviral therapy should be monitored closely for side effects and toxicity related to the medications. A complete blood count and blood chemistry along with a clinical history should be evaluated prior to beginning treatment, 4 to 8 weeks later, and then every 3 to 4 months. In addition, CD4 cell counts and HIV RNA levels are recommended at the same time intervals to evaluate compliance with the medication regimen and effectiveness of the treatment. A lipid panel is also recommended prior to initiating treatment and every 6 to 12 months to monitor for signs of elevated cholesterol and triglyceride levels. Additional testing may be recommended depending on the particular drug regimen (Panel on Antiretroviral Therapy and Medical Management of HIV-Infected Children, 2014). With rapid advances in the treatment of HIV infection, HIV is thought of more as a chronic illness as opposed to a terminal disease (Mawn, 2012).

TABLE 22–6 HIV Pediatric Classification System: Clinical Categories

WHEN INFECTED, THE CHILD WITH HIV IS CLASSIFIED AS:

- Category N (not symptomatic)
- Category A (mildly symptomatic)
- Category B (moderately symptomatic)
- Category C (severely symptomatic; multiple, recurrent serious bacterial infections)

Source: Adapted from Panel on Antiretroviral Therapy and Medical Management of HIV-Infected Children. (2014). *Guidelines for the use of antiretroviral agents in pediatric HIV infection.* Retrieved from http://aidsinfo.nih.gov/contentfiles/lvguidelines/pediatricguidelines.pdf

Medications Used to Treat: Human Immunodeficiency Virus in Children

MEDICATION AND ACTION/INDICATION	NURSING IMPLICATIONS
Nucleoside and nucleotide analog reverse transcriptase inhibitors	
Inhibits action of viral reverse transcriptase, an enzyme in the conversion of RNA to DNA. Abacavir Didanosine Emtricitabine Lamivudine Stavudine Tenofovir Zidovudine (AZT)	Common side effects include fever, headache, insomnia, myalgia, nausea, vomiting, diarrhea, anorexia, bone marrow suppression with resulting granulocytopenia and anemia, dyspnea, cough, skin rash. Teach signs and symptoms of infection.
Protease inhibitors	
Blocks the function of the enzyme protease needed for viral formation and growth. Atazanavir Darunavir Fosamprenavir Lopinavir/Ritonavir Nelfinavir Ritonavir Tipranavir	Side effects include CNS, CV changes, life-threatening hematologic changes, respiratory distress, and allergy; monitor for specific side effects of the particular drug administered. Take oral forms within 2 hr of a full meal.
Nonnucleoside reverse transcriptase inhibitors (NNRTIS)	
Binds to viral reverse transcriptase and disrupts the conversion of RNA to DNA. Efavirenz Etravirine Nevirapine	Side effects include fever, headache, nausea, diarrhea, hepatitis, altered liver function, anemia, neutropenia, drowsiness and fatigue, altered mental status, rash, Stevens–Johnson syndrome. Teach the family to notify healthcare provider immediately if rash appears.
Fusion inhibitors	
Prevents viral entry. Enfuvirtide	Requires subcutaneous injection twice a day. There is a high incidence of local reaction at the injection site, limiting the use of this medication in children.
Integrase inhibitors	
Blocks the action of the viral enzyme integrase. Raltegravir	Side effects include rash, nausea, diarrhea, headache, insomnia, fever, and muscle weakness. Give orally without regard to food intake.

Source: Data from Panel on Antiretroviral Therapy and Medical Management of HIV-Infected Children. (2014). *Guidelines for the use of antiretroviral agents in pediatric HIV infection*. Retrieved from http://aidsinfo.nih.gov/contentfiles/lvguidelines/pediatricguidelines.pdf; Rivera, D. M., & Frye, R. E. (2014). *Pediatric HIV infection treatment & management*. Retrieved from http://emedicine.medscape.com/article/965086-treatment\#aw2aab6b6b2

Nursing Management

For the Child With HIV Infection

Nursing Assessment and Diagnosis

For infants at risk of HIV infection, obtain the HIV test results of the mother if available. When the mother's results are positive, the infant will need to be screened for HIV infection according to CDC guidelines as described in the previous section. Facilitate the screening and explain its necessity to the family.

PHYSIOLOGIC ASSESSMENT

Assessment centers on observation and evaluation of potential sites of infection. Assess breath sounds, respiratory status, arterial blood gases, level of consciousness, and mental status, and report any abnormal findings. Assess the child's height and weight frequently. Observe for signs of failure to thrive and assess for anemia. Assess for *Candida* infections in the mouth and the diaper area. Note any developmental delays in motor skills or intellectual functioning, which could result from encephalopathy and poor nutrition, and can signal an increasing severity in symptom level. These findings should be reported immediately so that further medical evaluation can be implemented.

PSYCHOSOCIAL ASSESSMENT

Assess family support systems and coping mechanisms because the stress of caring for a child with HIV infection may overwhelm the parents. Assess the family's ability to care for the child. Inquire about the extended family's ability to provide daily care as well as emotional support. Support the family when they decide to inform a school-age child or adolescent of the diagnosis. When assessing an adolescent with HIV infection, evaluate the teen's understanding of how HIV is transmitted and the response to the diagnosis.

The accompanying *Nursing Care Plan* includes common nursing diagnoses that may apply to a child hospitalized with HIV infection. Other nursing diagnoses may include the following (NANDA-I © 2014):

- *Diarrhea* related to gastrointestinal infection, malignancy, or drug reactions
- *Mucous Membrane: Oral, Impaired,* related to infection
- *Development: Delayed, Risk for,* related to chronic infection and poor nutrition
- *Coping: Family, Compromised,* related to life-threatening illness
- *Caregiver Role Strain* related to anxiety about child's condition and demands of providing care

Planning and Implementation

The first step in managing HIV infection is prevention. Nurses must be active in instituting measures to prevent vertical transmission of HIV to the infants of infected mothers. Measures advised include adequate testing, prophylaxis for HIV-exposed infants and opportunistic infections, and follow-up visits for evaluation of general health and development for all infants at risk of the disease.

Education related to HIV infection, transmission of the disease, and testing should be a routine part of anticipatory guidance provided to adolescents. Adolescents who are sexually active should be offered HIV testing. Nurses can be instrumental in developing educational programs related to HIV prevention in school settings.

If the child is diagnosed with HIV, close health supervision is needed to ensure that medications are taken and examinations are carried out. When HIV progresses to clinical AIDS, nursing care is similar to that of a child with any serious, chronic, life-threatening disease. Nursing care focuses on preventing infection, managing pain, promoting respiratory and other organ function, promoting adequate nutritional intake, and providing emotional support to the parents and child, while promoting the child's growth and development. The accompanying *Nursing Care Plan* summarizes nursing care for the child hospitalized with AIDS.

PREVENT INFECTION

Immunosuppressed children become infected with bacteria as well as other organisms that are common in the environment. Protect the neonate from HIV-infected maternal secretions. Bathe the newborn as soon as possible after delivery and wash the eyes and face before administering prophylactic eye drops or ointment. Avoid invasive procedures in the newborn and encourage the mother to formula-feed the baby rather than breastfeed.

Proper disposal of needles and contaminated materials or equipment is essential to reduce the transmission of HIV (Figure 22–1). Standard precautions (see the *Clinical Skills Manual* SKILLS) are implemented to prevent exposure to HIV.

Frequent hand hygiene and limiting exposure of the child to individuals with upper respiratory or other infections are the best interventions to protect the child with HIV from acquiring other infections. Vaccines are administered to children with HIV infection

following guidelines that have been established (see Chapter 16). Benefits and risks of vaccines are weighed and the child should receive the immunization if appropriate. The live measles-mumps-rubella and the varicella vaccines can be administered to children and adolescents with HIV infection who are asymptomatic and have adequate T-lymphocyte and CD4 values (AAP, 2015, p. 469). See Chapter 16 for further immunization recommendations for the child who is immunocompromised. Educate sexually active adolescents on the importance of practicing safe sex and the ramifications of high-risk sexual behaviors and intravenous drug abuse.

Clinical Tip

Older school-age children and adolescents with HIV should be informed of their diagnosis and counseled appropriately regarding sexual transmission. Telling the child is difficult for parents and they often avoid doing so. Because parents usually want to be the ones to tell the child, they need help to plan how to discuss the issue and ongoing support in the process of communication. Nurses can assist in the following ways:

- Help parents understand the need to discuss the diagnosis with the child.
- Provide information about how to tell the child. Role-play with the parents how to tell the child and use information at the child's developmental understanding to assist parents to be honest.
- Provide sources of hope—the success of treatment, children living with HIV, and maintaining an active life.
- Assist the family to join support groups or web-based groups.
- Help the family plan for respite care as needed.
- Provide emotional support for this difficult task and allow for ongoing opportunities to express concerns, fears, and anxieties.

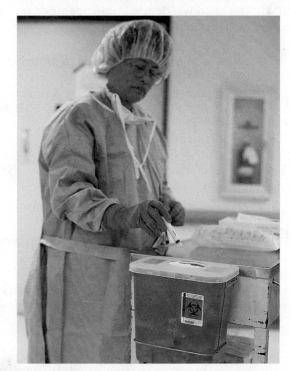

Figure 22–1 Biohazard disposal. This nurse is disposing of a needle and syringe in a biohazard container, a necessary practice to avoid the transmission of HIV through needlesticks with contaminated needles. Standard precautions provide protection even when the immune status of the patient is not known.

Nursing Care Plan: The Child With Acquired Immunodeficiency Syndrome

1. Nursing Diagnosis: *Infection, Risk for,* **related to immunosuppression (NANDA-I © 2014)**

GOAL: Risk factors for infection will be reduced as evidenced by absence of signs of infection.

INTERVENTION	RATIONALE
• Assess the child every 2–4 hr for fever; lesions in the mouth; and redness, inflammation, soreness, and lesions on the skin or around intravenous lines.	• Fever is one of the few signs of infection in the immunosuppressed child who does not have a sufficient number of white blood cells.
• Auscultate for changes in breath sounds every 2 hr. Perform pulmonary toilet (coughing, deep breathing, incentive spirometry) every 2–4 hr.	• Pneumonia is a likely infection in the child HIV infection.
• Enforce good hand hygiene. Allow no fresh flowers, fruits, or vegetables in child's room. Screen visitors for colds or recent exposure to varicella. Use blood and body fluid precautions (refer to the *Clinical Skills Manual* SKILLS). Practice strict asepsis for dressing changes and suctioning.	• Control of environmental factors helps prevent infection.
• Coordinate patient care assignments to avoid exposing the child to individuals with recent infections or immunizations.	• Planning minimizes chances for infection.
• Organize patient care activities to allow for adequate periods of rest.	• Rest periods allow the child to regain energy.
• Follow recommendations of CDC and AAP for immunizing immunosuppressed children. Avoid varicella vaccine. Perform annual TB testing.	• Special recommendations consider the child's decreased immune response and the danger of acquiring disease from certain live virus vaccines.

EXPECTED OUTCOME: Child will have no fever and show no other signs of infection.

2. Nursing Diagnosis: *Nutrition, Imbalanced: Less than Body Requirements,* **related to loss of appetite and decreased absorption of nutrients (NANDA-I © 2014)**

GOAL: The child will demonstrate adequate nutritional status to meet metabolic needs as evidenced by adequate weight gain for age.

INTERVENTION	RATIONALE
• Encourage frequent small meals to promote nutritional and fluid intake.	• Additional nutrition is required to rebuild the immune system.
• Maintain nasogastric tube feeding, if ordered. Total parenteral nutrition may be necessary to ensure adequate nutrition.	• Supplementation may be needed to ensure adequate calories.
• Eliminate unpleasant stimuli and odors from the environment during meals.	• Unpleasant stimuli decrease the desire for food.
• Monitor skin turgor every shift.	• Skin turgor reflects hydration status.
• Weigh daily.	• It is important to monitor weight status.
• Involve a nutritionist in planning a diet for the child that includes favorite foods.	• Including favorite food encourages intake.

EXPECTED OUTCOME: Child will eat frequent meals of adequate nutritional content. Child's weight will stay within normal limits.

3. Nursing Diagnosis: *Skin Integrity, Risk for Impaired,* **related to skin infection, immobility, or diarrhea (NANDA-I © 2014)**

GOAL: The child will have intact skin.

INTERVENTION	RATIONALE
• Observe all pressure areas closely for signs of infection or breakdown.	• Skin care is important in the immunocompromised child. The skin may be the only intact defense the child has.
• Keep skin clean and dry. Provide perineal care to minimize irritation from diarrhea.	• Prevents breaking or cracking of skin.

EXPECTED OUTCOME: Child will be free of preventable skin breakdown.

4. Nursing Diagnosis: *Knowledge, Deficient (Parent)*, related to home care of child with AIDS (NANDA-I © 2014)

GOAL: The parent(s) will demonstrate knowledge about home care including medication regimen, measures to prevent infection, and signs and symptoms to report to healthcare providers.

INTERVENTION	RATIONALE
• Explain the importance of optimizing the child's health status and reducing risk of complications through diet, rest, and meticulous personal hygiene. Be sure that parents and other family members understand how HIV infection is spread and take appropriate precautions.	• Knowledge about the disorder and preventive measures is necessary to provide safe and effective home care for the child.
• Be sure that parents understand the need for adherence to the medication regimen and understand how to administer medications.	• Knowledge of rationale increases compliance.
• Inform the family about signs and symptoms of infection that should be reported promptly to the healthcare provider or nurse (fever, chills, cough, mild erythema).	• Prompt treatment increases outcome.

EXPECTED OUTCOME: Parent will describe appropriate home care and preventive measures for a child with AIDS.

Clinical Tip

Work with the family of the child with HIV infection to establish a plan for medication administration. Assist them to establish a time schedule that limits the administration of several large amounts of medication at the same time. Stress the importance of disguising the taste of bitter medications to increase the child's willingness to take the medication.

PROMOTE MEDICATION REGIMEN ADHERENCE

The treatment regimen with the use of antiretroviral therapies for the child with HIV infection may be complex, time consuming, and costly, presenting an overwhelming challenge to the child and the family. Adherence to the prescribed antiretroviral regimen is imperative as nonadherence will likely result in disease progression (Buchanan et al., 2012). Some common reasons for nonadherence include frequent dosing, restrictions on daily schedules, pill taste, side effects, and dietary restrictions (Malee et al., 2011). Strategies for achieving optimal management of the treatment regimen include educating the parent or childcare provider, and the affected child when doing so is developmentally appropriate, about the purpose of the medication, the benefits of adhering to the regimen, and the potential consequences of failure to adhere to the regimen. Behavior modification techniques, using positive reinforcement, can be very effective in promoting the child's adherence. Provide support to the family, and tailor the medication regimen to the family's routine when possible. Offer praise to the child and parent for adhering to the regimen. If problems exist in managing the treatment regimen, carefully listen to the family to help determine the cause. Collaborate with the family in establishing goals to help meet the prescribed treatment regimen. If further intervention is required, options include direct observational therapy or home visits. Consider the effect of cultural beliefs on medication adherence (see *Developing Cultural Competence: HIV/AIDS and African Americans* and *Evidence-Based Practice: Adolescents With HIV Infection and Medication Regimen Adherence*).

Developing Cultural Competence   HIV/AIDS and African Americans

HIV affects African Americans more than any other racial/ethnic group. The incidence of HIV in African Americans is 8 times greater than that of Whites. According to 2010 data, African Americans accounted for approximately 44% of new HIV infections in adults and children over 13 years of age. The CDC has implemented programs focusing on maximizing the effectiveness of HIV prevention methods (CDC, 2015). It is essential that efforts are focused on high-risk populations so that they receive education regarding prevention, testing, and resources.

PROMOTE RESPIRATORY FUNCTION

Because many children with HIV infection develop pneumonia, encourage the child to cough and deep breathe every 2 to 4 hours. In the community, regular physical activity encourages lung aeration. When in the hospital, blowing cotton balls with a straw, blowing bubbles, or other games may engage the interest of a younger child. Reposition infants frequently so all areas of the lungs can aerate. The plan of care should include rest periods to conserve energy and lower the body's demand for oxygen.

PROMOTE ADEQUATE NUTRITIONAL INTAKE

Because many children with HIV infection fail to thrive, nutrition is an important part of their care. (See Chapter 14 for information to include in a detailed nutritional assessment.) A nutritionist should be involved in planning an appropriate diet for the child that provides necessary calories, protein, and other nutrients. Vitamins may be especially lacking in the diets of infected children. Antioxidants (vitamin A, vitamin E, zinc, and selenium) are known to enhance general immune system function; children should consume these nutrients at recommended levels. It is important, however, to verify that there are no interactions between specific vitamins and the child's prescribed antiretroviral medications. Periodic dietary analysis and teaching are needed. Adequate nutrition is sometimes provided through total parenteral nutrition or through nasogastric or gavage feeding.

Diarrhea resulting from gastrointestinal infection and lactose intolerance is a common finding in children with HIV infection, and it complicates other nutritional disturbances. Alternative formulas may be recommended. Although antidiarrheal medications are not generally used in infants, they may be prescribed for older children. Carefully monitor hydration status, skin turgor, and urine output. Provide careful perineal skin care to prevent infection.

The frequency of *Candida* infections leads to blisters, cracking, and discharge involving the oral mucous membranes. To keep the child's lips and mouth moist, mouth care should be performed every 2 to 4 hours with a non–alcohol-based solution such as normal saline. The child may need a prescription mouthwash.

PROVIDE EMOTIONAL SUPPORT
The family of the child with HIV infection is under emotional stress, and this is compounded if others in the family are infected. The infected teen may see progression of disease in the parent and lose hope. Integrate social services and support groups into the care of the child as soon as the diagnosis is made. Spend time talking with the family to provide them with an opportunity to discuss their fears and feelings. In many parts of the United States, HIV infection still carries a tremendous stigma, and the family may not be able to discuss their feelings outside the healthcare environment. Safeguard the family's wishes about the privacy of the diagnosis.

Clarify any misconceptions the older child with HIV infection may have about transmission of the disease. Routes of transmission and the need for safe sexual practices must be discussed openly and clearly with adolescents. Providing support for adolescents is particularly important because the dependence on family or other caregivers that this chronic and terminal disease brings can make it difficult to meet the

---

EVIDENCE-BASED PRACTICE | Adolescents With HIV Infection and Medication Regimen Adherence

Clinical Question
What factors are associated with medication adherence in the adolescent with HIV infection?

The Evidence
MacDonell, Naar-King, Huszti, et al. (2013) utilized a cross-sectional multisite sample to examine barriers to antiretroviral medication adherence in behaviorally and perinatally HIV-infected youth. The subjects for the study were 484 youth, ages 12 to 24, who were prescribed medication for HIV. The most common barriers reported were forgetting to take the medication, not feeling like taking the medication, and not wanting to be reminded of their disease. While the top barriers were similar for behaviorally and perinatally infected participants, those infected perinatally reported significantly more barriers. There was a significant correlation in those with perinatally acquired infection between the number of barriers and percentage of doses missed, psychologic distress, and viral load. For those with behaviorally acquired infection, there was a significant correlation between number of barriers and number of doses missed, psychologic distress, and substance use. Forgetting to take the medication was the top barrier listed for the full study sample. Other top barriers included not feeling like it/needing a break, medicine reminded them of the disease, medication made them sick to their stomach/tasted bad, and running out of the prescription.

A qualitative study by Udomkhamsuk, Fongkaew, Grimes, et al. (2014) examined the concerns and needs related to adherence to treatment for HIV infection. Data were collected using participatory activities and interviews with 25 youth ages 14 to 21. Five themes emerged from the interviews: Lack of drug knowledge; boredom, discouragement, and denial; fear of disclosure; not managing medication; and risk taking. Some of the subthemes included not knowing about side effects of antiretroviral therapy (ART), being bored with repeatedly taking medications, feeling discouraged by having an incurable disease, denial, fear of losing friendships, disclosure of their infection, forgetting to carry the medicine with them, not taking medicine on time, lack of negotiation skills, curiosity, and poor safe sex planning skills. The study concluded that lack of full adherence to the ART regimen was related to cognitive and psychosocial factors and that youth with HIV infection lack knowledge related to ART.

Navarra, Neu, Toussi, and colleagues (2014) used a cross-sectional descriptive survey design to evaluate the relationship between functional literacy (the ability to read and write), health literacy (the skill to access and understand health information), beliefs about antiretroviral therapy (ART), media use, and adherence to ART. Fifty youth ages 13 to 24 participated in the study. The instruments used in the study included The Test of Functional Health Literacy in Adults (TOFHLA), the Rapid Estimate of Adult Literacy in Medicine-teen (REALM-teen), the Media Use Questionnaire, and the Beliefs About Medication Scale (BAMS). The BAMS assessed intent regarding oral medication adherence, perceived threat of illness, negative outcome expectancy, and positive outcome expectancy. Data from these instruments were collected during a clinic visit using face-to-face interviews after the investigator asked the youth to recall how many doses of their antiretroviral medication had been missed in the past 3 days. While health literacy was not a predictor of adherence in these subjects, higher positive outcome expectancy scores were associated with increased adherence. Subjects with below-grade level reading were associated with a lower level of adherence. This study indicated the importance of a comprehensive care model that includes assessing both health beliefs and reading skills in HIV-infected youth.

Best Practice
Adherence to antiretroviral therapy is a concern in the adolescent population. Concerns and knowledge related to the disease and the treatment plan should be assessed. It is essential that adolescents have adequate medical care and receive comprehensive education related to the importance of adherence to their medication regimen and the positive effects of adhering to antiretroviral therapy. Regimens that are simple, palatable, and with the fewest side effects possible are important in order to increase adherence (MacDonnell et al., 2013). Measures that increase adolescents' confidence in their ability to comply with the treatment plan should be implemented. Discuss strategies with adolescents that will assist them in remembering to take their medication.

Clinical Reasoning
What barriers does your health center address in its care of children with HIV that may lead to medication nonadherence in the HIV-infected adolescent? What support does the adolescent need to improve medication adherence? What measures can the nurse take to improve medication adherence in the adolescent?

developmental task of independence. Adolescents may benefit from contact with other infected peers.

DISCHARGE PLANNING

The diagnosis of HIV infection is surrounded by strong emotions and fears. Be honest and direct. Education is essential. Explain that there is no evidence that casual contact among family members can spread the infection. For the child who has been hospitalized, home care needs should be identified in advance of discharge.

Discuss the family's finances as well as health insurance coverage for the child's care. Assess the family's ability to provide nutritious food, pay for required medications, and to provide a supportive environment. Refer to services as needed to ensure provision of quality care after discharge.

Support groups, home healthcare nursing services, financial assistance, and psychologic counseling are usually needed at some point during the child's illness, and the family should be aware that such services are available. Assist the family with coping mechanisms to deal with feelings of guilt and/or fear about the child's condition.

Clinical Reasoning **The Toddler With HIV Infection**

Raymond, a 2-year-old child, has had recurrent infections since he was born. After a recent illness with fever, vomiting, and diarrhea, blood tests were done to evaluate his immune function. He was diagnosed with HIV infection and admitted to the hospital for children.

- What physical needs does Raymond have at this time?
- What information does Raymond's family need?
- What can you do to provide emotional support to Raymond's family?

COMMUNITY-BASED NURSING CARE

Much of the care of the child with HIV infection takes place in the community. With the continued success of aggressive therapy, the majority of children infected with HIV can be expected to attend child care and school. Additionally, a substantial number of these children will reach adolescence, and some will reach adulthood. Assess the family and community support systems and provide resources and referrals as needed to help parents provide adequate care for their child and to assist adolescents as they transition to adulthood. Many children with HIV infection are placed in foster homes, and these families need careful instruction to manage this multifaceted illness.

School attendance guidelines recommend unrestricted school attendance and/or childcare center attendance for children with HIV infection. In addition, children should be allowed to participate in all activities to the extent that their health and other recommendations for management of infectious diseases permit (AAP, 2015, pp. 158–159). Contraindications to school attendance include lack of control of body secretions, biting, and open wounds that cannot be covered. CDC guidelines for standard precautions should always be followed in the school, child care, and home settings. The nurse or assigned school personnel may be responsible for providing medicines or other care at school for children infected with HIV.

Assist the family in altering the home environment to provide standard precautions during care. To reduce the likelihood of transmission of HIV, make sure the child and family understand that the virus is transmitted through blood, urine, stool, and other body fluids. Instruct parents to use recommended precautions when handling body fluids. Explain that they should wear gloves when changing diapers; disposing of urine, stool, and emesis; or treating the child's cuts and scrapes. In addition, teach them to wash their hands immediately after contact with blood or other body fluids. To reduce the risk of spread of infectious organisms to the child with HIV, educate family members about the importance of proper hand hygiene. Instruct parents to use a bleach solution for disinfection of objects when necessary and to avoid contact with people with infectious illnesses.

Precautions to guard against foodborne illness are particularly important for the child with HIV infection. Parents also need instruction on correct administration and side effects of any medications the child is taking. Giving a child a complicated combination of drugs can be challenging for all families; therefore, teaching should be tailored to the particular family and should be followed by repeated evaluation of the family's success with medication administration.

SAFETY ALERT!

When a child has been diagnosed with HIV, even common childhood infections are a cause for concern. Conditions such as respiratory infection, fever, chickenpox, or gastrointestinal illness can progress rapidly to a life-threatening stage. Teach families to seek prompt treatment at the first sign of illness.

The parent's close observation and feeling that something is not right should be cause for concern and medical evaluation.

Emphasize the importance of promoting the child's development. Perform frequent developmental screenings. Teach the parents how to support the child in achieving developmental milestones. Encourage contact with other children and adults, provide for appropriate toys, teach parents how to encourage the child's communication, and praise the family for what the child has already accomplished. Children who manifest decreasing achievement of developmental milestones or other neurologic symptoms should be assessed by the primary healthcare provider for HIV-induced encephalopathy. The nurse's record of development will be of great importance in this situation. The child needs regular health maintenance care, such as child health supervision visits, immunizations, and care for any other health conditions.

Evaluation

There are many desired outcomes of care for the child with HIV infection or AIDS. Expected outcomes of nursing care include the following:

- The numbers of cases of pediatric HIV due to vertical transmission from known infected mothers decrease.
- Infectious diseases in children with HIV infection are prevented.
- The child has adequate respiratory function and perfusion.
- The child has adequate nutritional intake to support normal growth patterns and prevent malnutrition.

- The family adequately copes with the stress of a chronic disease.
- The child attends school and is supported in the educational process.

Autoimmune Disorders

In an immune system damaged by pathologic changes, an immune response may occur to some of the body's own proteins, resulting in the production of autoantibodies. These pathologic conditions in which the body directs the immune response against itself—identifying "self" as "nonself"—are called *autoimmune disorders*.

The primary feature of autoimmune disorders is tissue injury caused by a probable immunologic reaction of the host with its own tissues. Structural or functional changes occur as immune cells attack other cells in the body. Autoimmune disorders are grouped into systemic and organ-specific diseases. Systemic diseases, which generally involve more than one organ, include systemic lupus erythematosus and juvenile arthritis, which are discussed in this chapter. Organ-specific diseases, which primarily affect a single organ, include type 1 diabetes (see Chapter 30) and thyroiditis. Immune thrombocytic purpura is an immune disease affecting blood platelets and clotting and is discussed in Chapter 23. Psoriasis is a T-cell–mediated autoimmune disease of the skin and is discussed in Chapter 31.

Systemic Lupus Erythematosus

Systemic lupus erythematosus (SLE) is a chronic inflammatory, autoimmune disease of unknown origin that involves many organ systems (Silverman & Eddy, 2011). Although it is primarily diagnosed in adulthood, approximately 15% to 20% of cases are diagnosed in childhood (Fortuna & Brennan, 2013). SLE affects 1.5 million people in the United States. It is more common among African Americans, Native Americans, Hispanics, and Asians than Whites. More severe disease and higher morbidity and mortality are seen in African Americans with SLE (Mattingly, 2011). SLE is 9 times more common in females than males (Ferenkeh-Koroma, 2012).

ETIOLOGY AND PATHOPHYSIOLOGY

The exact etiology of SLE is unknown. A genetic component is suspected because the disease is often more prevalent in members of the same family. It is believed that in those genetically predisposed, an outside environmental agent causes the body to initiate an abnormal immune system response to its own tissues (Lupus Foundation of America, 2014; Silverman & Eddy, 2011). The body produces autoantibodies and combines with antigens to form immune complexes. These antigen–antibody complexes are deposited in the connective tissue, triggering an inflammatory response. The chronic inflammation then destroys connective tissue. The tissue damage varies according to the organ involvement, although the tissues most likely to be affected are the small blood vessels, glomeruli, joints, spleen, and heart valves. Because many systems can be affected simultaneously, organ damage with subsequent multisystem failure may occur.

CLINICAL MANIFESTATIONS

Manifestations of SLE may be acute, with onset of nephritis, arthritis, or vasculitis, or may be noted as a gradual onset with nonspecific symptoms. Symptoms depend on the organ involved and the amount of tissue damage that has occurred and include fever, fatigue, malaise, and weight loss. Other clinical manifestations include rash, arthritis, and nephritis (Defendi, 2011; Mattingly, 2011). A butterfly rash on the face, consisting of a pink or red rash over the bridge of the nose extending to the cheeks, is a characteristic finding (Ferenkeh-Koroma, 2012) (Figure 22–2). Children with SLE may have anemia, leukopenia, and thrombocytopenia (Mattingly, 2011). Renal disease, the leading cause of morbidity and mortality in children with SLE, is evident at diagnosis in 50% of these children and in 80% to 90% within the

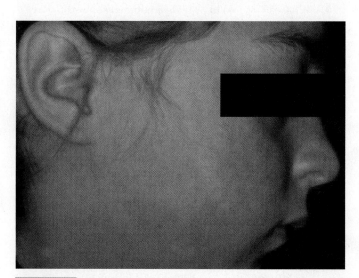

Figure 22–2 This child displays a "butterfly" rash across the cheeks and bridge of the nose. It is often seen in the child with SLE.

SOURCE: BSIP/Science Source.

first year of diagnosis. Central nervous system disorders may occur in children with SLE and include headaches, mood disorders, seizure disorders, and cerebrovascular disease (Silverman & Eddy, 2011). See Table 22–7.

Systemic lupus erythematosus is characterized by periods of remission and exacerbation (flares). Flares are triggered by a variety of causes, including sun exposure, an upper respiratory infection or other infection, and stress. The child or family may be able to identify other triggers to flares, such as particular events, activities, or situations.

CLINICAL THERAPY

Blood tests reveal anemia, an elevated blood urea nitrogen (BUN), abnormal plasma proteins, abnormal erythrocyte sedimentation rate (ESR), presence of antinuclear antibodies, and a positive LE (lupus erythematosus) cell reaction, which indicates nonspecific inflammation. The Coombs test is positive. Radiologic examinations include chest radiographs and computed tomography (CT) scans, as well as magnetic resonance imaging (MRI) of affected joints. A 24-hour urine collection and imaging studies, as well as renal biopsies, may be performed to evaluate lupus nephritis. Urinalysis may reveal proteinuria.

The goals of medical management are to create a remission of symptoms and to prevent complications. Corticosteroids, such as prednisone or methylprednisolone, are prescribed to control inflammation. Antimalarial preparations, such as hydroxychloroquine, are used to treat symptoms associated with skin lesions and renal and arthritic problems. Although the exact action of these drugs on SLE is not known, they often permit continued remission with a lowered dose of steroids. Nonsteroidal anti-inflammatory drugs (ibuprofen, naproxen) are used to relieve muscle and joint pain. Immunosuppressant drugs, such as cyclophosphamide, azathioprine, mycophenolate mofetil, cyclosporine, and methotrexate, have been used to help control SLE (Klein-Gitelman, 2013; Mattingly, 2011; Silverman & Eddy, 2011). Patients with SLE who are on corticosteroids or those who have arthritis are at increased risk for osteopenia. Vitamin D_3 and calcium carbonate improve bone health in these patients (Klein-Gitelman, 2013). Diet may be restricted if the child has excessive weight gain or fluid retention from steroids and renal damage. Prognosis depends on the severity of the internal organ involvement. Whereas SLE was once considered a fatal disease, 5-year survival rates for SLE are 92% or as high as 100%, and 10-year survival rates of 85% have been cited (Defendi, 2011). Survival rates decrease to 80% at 15 years after diagnosis (Mattingly, 2011). Kidney failure is managed by hemodialysis or peritoneal dialysis. Renal transplantation has been very successful for treatment of renal failure secondary to lupus nephritis.

Growth and Development

The side effects of the corticosteroids, immunosuppressants, and antimalarial drugs used in the treatment of children with SLE include hair loss, susceptibility to infection, "moon face," retinal damage, and bone loss. These are significant side effects for the adolescent, who is commonly concerned about appearance. Teens with SLE may need special teaching, guidance, and support. Support groups or Internet chat rooms may be helpful.

Nursing Management

For the Child With SLE

Nursing Assessment and Diagnosis

PHYSIOLOGIC ASSESSMENT

Assess the child's nutritional status, including comparison of prior and current weight for evidence of recent weight loss or weight gain. Assess the skin for rashes, ulcers, photosensitivity, ecchymosis, petechiae, cyanosis, and hair loss. Respiratory assessment includes breath sounds, respiratory rate, and assessing for extra sounds associated with pleural effusion or pleuritis. Cardiovascular assessment includes vital signs as well as assessing heart sounds and for signs of pericarditis or friction rub. Musculoskeletal assessment includes joint pain, joint swelling, joint deformity, pain, weakness, and ability to perform activities of daily living. Assess the neurologic system for changes in affect or cognitive abilities and seizure activity. Palpate the spleen to detect splenomegaly.

TABLE 22–7 Clinical Manifestations of Systemic Lupus Erythematosus

SYSTEM	CLINICAL MANIFESTATIONS
Integumentary	A butterfly rash on the face, consisting of a pink or red rash over the bridge of the nose extending to the cheeks, is a characteristic finding Photosensitivity Alopecia Mouth or nose ulcers
Hematologic	Fatigue Fever Easy bruising Nosebleeds
Musculoskeletal	Joint pain Swollen inflamed joints Myalgias Muscle weakness
Neurologic	Headache Peripheral neuropathy Psychosis Seizures Mood disorder Cognitive disorder Stroke
Pulmonary	Chest Pain Dyspnea Pulmonary hypertension Pulmonary embolism
Cardiac	Arrhythmias Chest pain Friction rub Raynaud phenomenon (fingers turning white and/or blue in the cold)
Renal	Hematuria Hypertension Proteinuria Edema
Gastrointestinal	Abdominal pain (may radiate to the shoulder) Diarrhea

Source: Adapted from Mattingly, E. (2011). Lupus in adolescents. *Advance for NPs & PAs, 2*(4), 27–32; Klein-Gitelman, M. S. (2013). *Pediatric systemic lupus erythematosus*. Retrieved from http://emedicine.medscape.com/article/1008066-overview; Silverman, E., & Eddy, A. (2011). Systemic lupus erythematosus. In J. T. Cassidy, R. E. Petty, R. M. Laxer, & C. B. Lindsley (Eds.), *Textbook of pediatric rheumatology* (6th ed., pp. 315–343). Philadelphia, PA: Elsevier Saunders.

PSYCHOSOCIAL ASSESSMENT

Because SLE is a chronic disease that primarily affects adolescents, psychosocial assessment is indicated. Assess family interactions, exploring stressful situations such as divorce or trauma. Treatment-related restrictions associated with medications and changes in appearance such as weight gain, cushingoid appearance, and skin rashes can lead to withdrawal, depression, and risk for suicide. Perform psychosocial assessments periodically as the child grows and adapts to the disorder or faces new developmental challenges with a chronic disease.

Several nursing diagnoses may apply to the child with SLE. These include the following (NANDA-I © 2014):

- *Skin Integrity, Risk for Impaired,* related to photosensitivity
- *Activity Intolerance, Risk for,* related to joint pain and fatigue
- *Body Image, Disturbed,* related to side effects of medications and skin alterations
- *Infection, Risk for,* related to immunosuppressive medications
- *Pain, Acute,* related to joint inflammation and injury
- *Health Management, Family, Ineffective,* related to complexity of therapeutic regimen

Planning and Implementation

The goals of nursing care are to assist the child to manage and cope with a chronic disease, prevent infection, maintain fluid balance, promote adequate nutrition, promote skin integrity, promote rest and comfort, manage side effects of medication, avoid triggers for disease flares, and provide emotional support.

PREVENT INFECTION

Infections are a leading cause of death for those with SLE. Prophylactic antibiotics may be required for dental work and surgical procedures. Instruct the patient and family to inform all healthcare providers of the disease to plan for prophylactic measures. Emphasize the importance of receiving recommended immunizations including pneumococcal, meningococcal, and influenza. Instruct the family on hand hygiene and infection control measures in the home. Warn adolescents about the dangers of tattooing and body piercing because of the risk of infection.

MAINTAIN FLUID BALANCE

Because most children with SLE have renal involvement, nursing care includes maintaining accurate intake and output measurements and frequent evaluation of the child's fluid and electrolyte status and weight.

PROMOTE ADEQUATE NUTRITION

Currently, there are no specific dietary plans for the child with SLE; however, the diet may be restricted according to renal involvement, weight gain, weight loss, or other complications. The child is at risk for weight gain associated with treatment with steroids and a decreased activity level during exacerbations of this disease. A well-balanced, nutritious diet with calcium and vitamin D supplements to support bone density as well as appropriate fluid intake for age should be encouraged.

PROMOTE SKIN INTEGRITY

The presence of ulcers on mucous membranes can cause weakening of the tissues, placing the child at increased risk for infection. Provide instructions on oral care to maintain intact oral mucosa. Encourage the use of good hygienic measures and a mild soap for the skin. Recommend that adolescents limit their use of cosmetics, especially oil-based ones. Reinforce the importance of avoiding sunlight as much as possible and the use of sun protection factor (SPF) of 30 or higher at all times when in the sun. Encourage the child to wear protective clothing to limit exposure to sunlight (see Chapter 31 for discussion of sun exposure). Additionally, avoidance of unprotected fluorescent lighting is recommended since exacerbations of systemic lupus erythematosus have been reported following this type of exposure. Advise adolescents with lupus to avoid the use of tanning beds since these devices produce ultraviolet light and can cause or worsen lupus skin lesions (Lupus Foundation of America, 2014). Provide instructions on oral care to maintain intact oral mucosa. Provide instructions on the care of the head if alopecia occurs.

PROMOTE REST AND COMFORT

The child with SLE experiences fatigue and joint pain, leaving little energy reserve during acute episodes of the disease. Encourage frequent rest periods and a nutritious diet to maximize energy stores. A physical therapist can plan a program to encourage mobility and increase muscle strength. Implement measures such as application of heat to painful areas.

MANAGE SIDE EFFECTS OF MEDICATIONS

Observe for side effects of medications used for treatment, and teach the child and family about these effects. For example, immunosuppressant drugs can reduce the body's resistance to infection, and nonsteroidal anti-inflammatory drugs commonly cause gastric distress and bleeding of the gastrointestinal tract. The antimalarial drug hydroxychloroquine increases the risk of retinopathy and blindness; therefore, eye examinations should be performed every 6 months (Ilowite & Laxer, 2011). Corticosteroid side effects include cushingoid effects, weight gain, and hypertension. Sulfa drugs should be avoided because they increase photosensitivity.

AVOID TRIGGERS FOR DISEASE FLARES

Many children and their parents can recognize the signs of an impending flare and the triggers that precede them. Some of the triggers that might cause a flare include sunlight, stress, illness, and medications. Partner with the parents and child to implement measures to avoid these triggers. Discuss preventive behaviors such as avoiding sun exposure and avoiding stressors. Stress-reducing techniques such as guided imagery, reading, yoga, and quiet games can benefit the child or adolescent and reduce exacerbations of SLE. It may be necessary to discontinue a sport, music lesson, or other activity temporarily to provide a chance for the child to relax each day. Adolescents should be warned that alcohol, smoking, and drugs also pose an increased risk due to the potential to stimulate flares. Female adolescents who are sexually active should avoid birth control pills that contain the hormone estrogen, since the extra estrogen may exacerbate symptoms. Alternative birth control methods should be discussed with the adolescent.

PROVIDE EMOTIONAL SUPPORT

Adolescents may have an altered body image as a result of rash, alopecia, arthritic changes in the joints, and chronic disease. Referral to a lupus support group, social services, or counseling may be helpful. The Lupus Foundation of America can provide information to help parents and children adjust to the disease. Internet support groups are also available for those with SLE.

Evaluation

Successful outcomes of nursing care involve management of this chronic disease. Expected outcomes of nursing care include the following:

- The child has absence of pain.
- The child has absence of infection.
- The child has adequate intake and output levels, with demonstrated fluid and electrolyte balance and renal function.
- The child maintains intact skin.
- The child has a positive body image.

Juvenile Idiopathic Arthritis

Arthritis in children has long been referred to as *juvenile rheumatoid arthritis (JRA)* in the United States. The International League of Associations for Rheumatology now uses the term *juvenile idiopathic arthritis (JIA)* to describe arthritis with an unknown cause in children (Wedderburn & Nistala, 2013).

Juvenile idiopathic arthritis refers to inflammation involving one or more joints, lasting more than 6 weeks, and diagnosed prior to 16 years of age (Wedderburn & Nistala, 2013). This disease results in decreased mobility, swelling, and pain. The peak age of onset for JIA is between 1 and 3 years of age, with the illness occurring twice as often in females as in males (Petty & Cassidy, 2011). Approximately 1 of every 1000 children in the United States has JIA (Stanley & Ward-Smith, 2011).

Juvenile arthritis affects joints and surrounding tissues in addition to potential effects on other organs such as the heart, lungs, liver, and eyes. During the disease's course, the child may experience pain, impaired mobility, and interference with normal growth and development. Children may enter remission or manifest continued symptoms of a chronic disease. Remission may last for months, years, or a lifetime. Rarely, the disease is unresponsive to treatment or the child may suffer lasting impairment such as bone and joint changes. Children with early onset have a better prognosis for complete recovery.

ETIOLOGY AND PATHOPHYSIOLOGY

The cause of JIA is unknown, but it is thought to have an autoimmune basis. Inflammation begins in the joint and leads to pain and swelling (Figure 22–3). Scar tissue eventually develops,

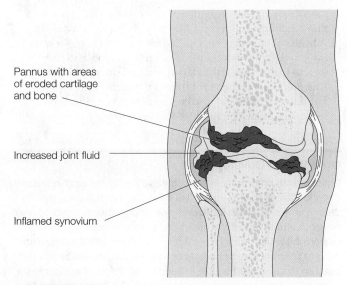

Pannus with areas of eroded cartilage and bone

Increased joint fluid

Inflamed synovium

Figure 22–3 **Joint inflammation and destruction in juvenile arthritis.**

resulting in limited range of motion. Altered growth related to early closure of epiphyseal plates, small joint contractures, and synovitis may occur. Although terminology varies among the different classifications, the three major types of juvenile arthritis under the most current classification of JIA are oligoarthritis, polyarthritis, and systemic arthritis (Petty & Cassidy, 2011):

- *Oligoarthritis* involves one to four joints and is the most common type of JIA. Approximately 30% to 60% of children with JIA have oligoarthritis. **Uveitis** (inflammation of the middle layer of the eye) occurs in approximately 17% to 26% of children with oligoarthritis (Hsu, Lee, & Sandborg, 2013).
- *Polyarthritis* involves five or more joints. Rheumatoid factor–negative polyarthritis affects 10% to 30% of children with JIA, while rheumatoid factor–positive polyarthritis affects 5% to 10% of children with JIA. Uveitis occurs in approximately 4% to 25% of children with rheumatoid factor–negative JIA and 0% to 2% of those with rheumatoid factor–positive JIA (Hsu et al., 2013).
- *Systemic arthritis* is characterized by high fever; swollen, painful joints; and rash. Systemic arthritis affects internal organs and joints. Approximately 10% of children with JIA have systemic arthritis (Hsu et al., 2013; Nierengarten & Oski, 2014).

CLINICAL MANIFESTATIONS

Juvenile idiopathic arthritis may be restricted to a few joints or be systemic with involvement of multiple joints. Symptoms can include fever, rash, lymphadenopathy, splenomegaly, and hepatomegaly. The child with JIA may develop a limp or obviously favor one extremity over the other. A slow rate of growth or uneven growth of extremities may also be noted. Pain, stiffness, loss of motion, and swelling occur in the large joints such as the knees. Older children may develop symmetric involvement of the small joints of the hand. The disease is frequently chronic, extending over several years after an initial manifestation with pain and other symptoms. Remissions and exacerbations are characteristic.

CLINICAL THERAPY

No specific laboratory tests confirm the diagnosis; however, there are some tests to help support the diagnosis. The child may present with anemia and leukocytosis. Erythrocyte sedimentation rate (ESR) and C-reactive protein (CRP) tests may be helpful in determining the amount of inflammation. Rheumatoid factor and antinuclear antibody (ANA) tests may be positive (Petty & Cassidy, 2011). Radiographs are generally performed to exclude other causes, such as fractures, rather than as a definitive diagnosis, although radiographs are useful in monitoring for joint damage and bone development.

The goals of treatment are to relieve pain, control inflammation, preserve joint function, prevent deformities, achieve remission of the disease, minimize side effects of the disease and treatment, and promote normal growth and development (Petty & Cassidy, 2011). Nonsteroidal anti-inflammatory drugs (NSAIDs) such as ibuprofen, naproxen, indomethacin, diclofenac, and meloxicam are used to reduce inflammation and pain. Children who do not respond to NSAIDs may be treated with disease-modifying antirheumatic drugs such as methotrexate. Steroids such as prednisone and methylprednisolone may be used with children with more severe forms of juvenile arthritis. Biologic response modifiers such as etanercept, infliximab, and adalimumab have also been used to treat JIA (Petty & Cassidy, 2011; Stanley & Ward-Smith, 2011).

Complications such as chronic uveitis, which results from chronic inflammation, may occur in children with juvenile arthritis. Children with oligoarthritis and polyarthritis will need eye examinations either every 3 to 4 months or 4 to 6 months depending on their age and the presence or absence of ANA. Because uveitis is rare in children with systemic arthritis, the recommended frequency for eye examinations is every 12 months (Petty & Rosenbaum, 2011).

Growth interference for the child with JIA is a potential complication. The specific disorder may result in bone growth disturbance such as contractures or effusions. The administration of corticosteroids can also inhibit growth.

Nursing Management

For the Child With JIA

Nursing Assessment and Diagnosis

A careful history is important, as it is sometimes the primary mode of diagnosis. Assess for joint swelling and deformities, pain, decreased mobility, morning stiffness, fever, nodules under the skin, growth delays, and enlarged lymph nodes. The following nursing diagnoses may apply to the child with juvenile arthritis (NANDA-I © 2014):

- *Activity Intolerance* related to chronic pain
- *Mobility: Physical, Impaired,* related to joint stiffness and inflammation
- *Pain, Chronic,* related to joint inflammation
- *Body Image, Disturbed,* related to condition and physical appearance

Planning and Implementation

Nursing care focuses on promoting mobility, encouraging adequate nutrition, and teaching the parents and child about the disease and its management. Most care will occur in the community, including physical therapy, with only occasional hospitalizations at the time of an exacerbation of the disease.

PROMOTE IMPROVED MOBILITY

The goals of physical therapy are to maintain joint function, strengthen muscles, increase tone, maintain body alignment, and prevent permanent deformities such as contractures. Range-of-motion exercises, stretching, hydrotherapy, and swimming exercises help to prevent deformities (Figure 22–4). Encourage the child to perform activities of daily living. Exercise may be painful or even difficult for the child, but it is important because it strengthens and stretches the muscles and prevents potential contractures. Emphasize the importance of establishing a regular exercise and activity routine. Encourage periods of rest during exacerbations, as the child fatigues more easily. Medications may be given to reduce joint swelling and inflammation. In addition, warm compresses to the involved joints are soothing.

PROMOTE ADEQUATE NUTRITION

Promote general health by encouraging a well-balanced diet. Children with decreased mobility may have reduced metabolic needs, and excess weight causes additional muscle strain. Periodically perform diet recalls and nutritional assessments. Plot growth carefully and watch for changes in growth percentiles. (See Chapter 14 for additional information regarding nutrition assessment.)

COMMUNITY-BASED NURSING CARE

The child with JIA may never, or rarely, be hospitalized. Most care takes place during visits to healthcare offices, clinics, and physical therapy. Educate parents on the child's condition and prognosis, and answer their questions about the child's treatment. The child may need support to adjust to the diagnosis of a chronic illness. Allow the child to express anger and frustration about the diagnosis of arthritis. Allow the opportunity for the child and parents to express feelings regarding the crippling effects of the disease. Social services, a child-life specialist, or a psychologist may be consulted as needed.

Encourage the child to maintain contact with peers and to attend school whenever possible. Explain to the child and parents that overexertion may exacerbate the disease. Inform parents about possible complications of JIA, such as altered growth related to early closure of epiphyseal plates, small joint contractures, and synovitis. Partner with the family and school officials to meet the child's needs.

> **Professionalism in Practice** Accommodations for Children With JIA
>
> Section 504 of the Rehabilitation Act of 1973 and the Individuals with Disabilities Education Act (IDEA) protect children with disabilities from discrimination. A formal plan such as an individualized education plan (IEP) should be developed for the child with arthritis that outlines accommodations and modifications that are needed at school (Solomon, 2014). The school nurse can work with the family and school administration to determine the plan. Accommodations at school may include providing a set of books for the home so that the child is not required to carry the books home daily. Additional time may be required for the child to move from class to class. The school nurse can refer parents and children to the Arthritis Foundation and the American Juvenile Arthritis Organization for further information and support. The adolescent should also be referred for vocational counseling and offered support for transition to adult services.

Growth and Development

Children with chronic illnesses such as JIA may develop increased dependence on their parents. It is essential that school-age children maintain as much independence as possible to promote their development of industry. These children should also have some responsibility for their treatment plan. Children with JIA may also need to miss school for periods of time. A plan should be developed so that the child is able to keep up with school assignments. In addition, ongoing contact with peers should be maintained to promote the child's social development.

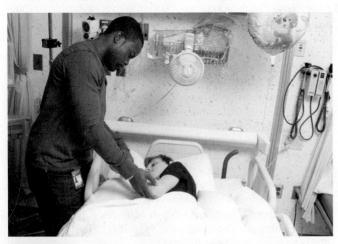

Figure 22–4 Passive range-of-motion exercises are an important aspect of physical therapy for a child or adolescent with juvenile idiopathic arthritis.

TABLE 22–8 Characteristic Findings in Children With Allergies

SYSTEM/ORGAN	FINDINGS
Respiratory system	Wheezing, rhinitis (seasonal and perennial), cough, adventitious breath sounds, inspiratory stridor, edema of glottis, nasal congestion or discharge
Gastrointestinal system	Abdominal pain and colic, mouth sores, constipation, diarrhea, bloody stools, geographic tongue, vomiting
Skin	Angioedema, urticaria, eczema, atopic dermatitis, erythema multiforme, purpura, drug and food rashes, contact dermatitis
Nervous system	Headache, tension, fatigue, seizures, tremors, irritability, sleep disorders, decreased concentration
Eye	Conjunctivitis, ciliary spasm, iritis, itching of eyes, tearing
Blood	Thrombocytopenic purpura, hemolytic anemia, leukopenia, agranulocytosis
Musculoskeletal system	Arthralgia, myalgia, torticollis
Genitourinary system	Dysuria, vulvovaginitis, enuresis
Miscellaneous	Anaphylactic shock, serum sickness

Evaluation

Expected outcomes of nursing care for the child with juvenile arthritis include the following:

- The child maintains joint mobility and has absence of joint deformity.
- The child has absence of pain.
- The child has a positive body image.
- The child has absence of infection.
- The parents understand and support the therapeutic process.

Allergic Reactions

For unclear reasons, an increasing number of children are diagnosed with some types of allergy, such as allergic rhinitis and asthma. Why are some children allergic to cats, for instance, while no one else in the family has allergies? To answer this question, the nurse needs a basic understanding of the mechanisms of allergy.

An **allergy** is an abnormal or altered reaction to an antigen. Antigens responsible for clinical manifestations of allergy are called **allergens**. Allergens can be ingested in food or drugs, injected or absorbed through contact with unbroken skin, and inhaled. Food allergies are discussed in Chapter 14. Common allergens in children include:

- Medications (such as penicillin)
- Animal dander
- Dust, mites, and mold
- Plant pollens
- Foods (such as nuts, seafood, or egg white)

An allergic reaction is an antigen–antibody reaction and can manifest itself as anaphylaxis, atopic disease, serum sickness, or contact dermatitis. Therefore, the symptoms can be mild to severe or life threatening, and they can be localized or systemic. Characteristic findings in children with allergies are summarized in Table 22–8.

The **hypersensitivity response**, an overreaction of the immune system, is responsible for allergic reactions. Hypersensitivity reactions have been classified into four types (Table 22–9). Type I hypersensitivity reactions, the most common allergic reactions, occur within seconds or minutes of exposure to the antigen and may progress to anaphylaxis. The release of chemical substances such as histamine is responsible for the signs and symptoms exhibited. The first time a child is exposed to the allergen,

TABLE 22–9 Clinical Manifestations of Types of Hypersensitivity Reactions

TYPE	ETIOLOGY	CLINICAL MANIFESTATIONS	EXAMPLES
Type I: localized or systemic reactions (anaphylaxis)	Antibodies bind to certain cells, causing release of chemical substances such as histamine that produce an inflammatory reaction.	Hypotension, wheezing, spasm of smooth muscle; stridor, wheal, urticaria edema, vomiting, diarrhea	Anaphylaxis Extrinsic asthma
Type II: tissue-specific reactions	Antibodies cause activation of complement system, which leads to tissue damage.	Variable; may include dyspnea or fever	Transfusion reaction ABO incompatibility Hemolytic anemia
Type III: immune-complex reactions	Immune complexes are deposited in tissues, where they activate complement, which results in a generalized inflammatory reaction.	Urticaria, fever, joint pain	Acute glomerulonephritis Serum sickness
Type IV: delayed reactions	Antigens stimulate T cells that release lymphokines, which cause inflammation and tissue damage.	Variable; may include fever, erythema, pruritus, contact dermatitis, blistering	Contact dermatitis Tuberculin skin test Graft-versus-host disease Stevens–Johnson syndrome Allograft rejection

there is no reaction. With every exposure thereafter, however, the allergic child may have a reaction to the allergen.

Type II sensitivity reactions occur within 15 to 30 minutes after exposure to the antigen. Type III hypersensitivity reactions may be difficult to distinguish from type II reactions. Hypersensitivity reactions generally peak within 6 hours.

Type IV reactions are delayed responses that do not appear until several hours after exposure and require 24 to 72 hours to fully develop. A type IV reaction, which is not confined to any specific tissue, is elicited by relatively complex antigens such as those of bacteria and viruses and by simple antigens such as drugs and metals.

Assessment of the child with an allergy includes a complete physical examination; laboratory, radiography, and pulmonary function studies; tests of nasal function; and serum and/or skin testing. Treatment generally involves avoidance of the allergen, such as substitution of a different drug when the child has a drug allergy. Desensitization may sometimes be used with increasing doses of the allergen administered subcutaneously in an office where resuscitation is readily available. This treatment is useful for allergy to bees or some pollens. For skin allergies, the allergen is avoided, skin is kept well lubricated, and topical steroids may be used. Oral antihistamines are sometimes used to treat allergy. Emergency medical care may be required to treat anaphylaxis.

Nursing Management

The child with allergies requires a thorough assessment, including a complete past medical history, family history, personal and social history, and review of symptoms. The history focuses on the following areas:

- What symptoms does the child experience? Children should be encouraged to describe the difficulty in their own words.
- Are the symptoms continuous or intermittent? What are the frequency and duration of episodes?
- When did the child first begin to experience symptoms? Did the child have eczema/atopic dermatitis or a feeding problem in infancy or childhood? Did the infant have frequent bouts of colic or skin problems when new foods were introduced? Was there a change in symptoms at puberty? Are the symptoms becoming worse or spontaneously improving?
- What known agents in the environment cause difficulties?
- Are there seasonal variations in symptoms? At what time of the day or night do symptoms usually occur?

The nurse may be responsible for performing intradermal skin tests for allergies (Figure 22–5). Nursing care focuses on treating the symptoms, alleviating the anxiety of the child and parents, and identifying the allergens. Educating the child and family on methods to minimize or avoid exposure to allergens is important.

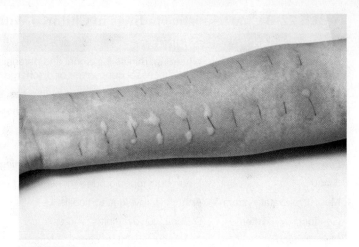

Figure 22–5 **Results of intradermal skin testing on the forearm. Injections are given on each side of the markings. Note the positive results marked by induration and erythema in response to certain antigens.**

SOURCE: Southern Illinois University/Science Source.

Teach parents of children who have had severe reactions to bee or wasp stings how to take precautions and how to provide emergency treatment if the child is stung. An EpiPen may be prescribed, and the parents and child will require instructions on its proper use.

Families may need instructions on allergy-proofing the home. Pets, dust, carpets, fabrics, feather pillows and bedding, and cigarette smoke can all cause allergic reactions. If families are reluctant to give up pets, frequent baths can reduce dander, which is the usual allergen. Instruct the family on proper use of epinephrine.

When the child has type I reactions to an environmental substance, avoidance of the allergen is most critical. In addition, childcare providers, families, and school personnel must be able to treat anaphylaxis if exposure to the allergen occurs. When the child is hospitalized, be sure to label the child's chart and bed and apply a red armband to alert others to allergies. School nurses keep records about children's allergies and inform school personnel about the allergies and cautions that need to be followed. See Chapter 14 for more information about serious reactions to food, such as peanut allergy. Nurses must be aware of the resuscitation procedures and equipment in all facilities such as hospital units, offices, childcare centers, and schools. See Chapter 19 for airway maintenance.

Latex Allergy

Latex is a sap from the rubber tree. It is prevalent in the environment and is a component of many commercial products (Asthma and Allergy Foundation of America, 2014). Latex allergy is caused by an IgE-mediated response that develops after repeated exposure to latex. A reaction to latex products can be manifested as an irritant reaction of the skin; as a type IV delayed hypersensitivity reaction with contact dermatitis; or as a type I hypersensitivity, which is immediate and often has systemic manifestations (itchy eyes, asthma, or anaphylaxis) (Katrancha & Harshberger, 2012; Wade, 2012).

Latex allergy is present in approximately 1% of the general population (Katrancha & Harshberger, 2012). It is more common among certain occupations, including healthcare workers, and in specific types of clients. An estimated 8% to 17% of healthcare workers and up to 68% of children with spina bifida are allergic to latex (American Latex Allergy Association, 2014). In addition, children who have frequent medical procedures or multiple surgeries involving latex are at increased risk of developing allergy to latex (Asthma and Allergy Foundation of America, 2014).

Clinical Tip

In 1998, the U.S. Food and Drug Administration ordered that warning labels be placed on any medical products that contain latex, advising that use of the product might cause an allergic reaction (U.S. Food and Drug Administration, 2014). Check product labels in your healthcare facility for this warning. What products should have a label?

Children and adolescents at high risk should receive allergy testing for latex. When a positive skin test has occurred or when the person has had a reaction to latex, all latex products must be removed from the allergic individual's environment. Alternative products, such as nonlatex gloves and catheters, must be used when providing health care. People allergic to latex should also wear a medical identification bracelet at all times and should have an epinephrine kit readily available at home and school. Nurses should be alert for any signs of hypersensitivity when the child is receiving health care, and be prepared with drugs and equipment to treat anaphylaxis. This is especially important in operative settings when acute anaphylaxis is often life threatening. Nurses should emphasize to parents and children that many everyday products contain latex, including latex balloons and condoms (Table 22–10).

TABLE 22–10   Latex Sources in the Home and Community

• Art supplies	• Diapers
• Balloons	• Feeding nipples
• Koosh balls	• Handles on racquets, tools, and bikes
• Tennis balls	• Kitchen cleaning gloves
• Gym mats	• Pacifiers
• Chewing gum	• Paints and sealants
• Sneakers	• Condoms
• Sandals	• Rubber bands
• Toothbrushes	• Water toys and equipment

Source: Data from Spina Bifida Association. (2012). *Latex in the home and community.* Retrieved from http://www.spinabifidaassociation.org/atf/cf/%7B85f88192-26e1-421e-9e30-4c0ea744a7f0%7D/SBA-LATEXLIST-2012-ENGLISH.PDF

Clinical Tip

Healthcare personnel are at high risk of developing latex allergy because of intense exposure to products containing latex. Nurses can protect themselves by using the following measures:

- Decrease exposure by using alternative products whenever available (use synthetic rubbers, polyethylene, nitrile, neoprene, vinyl gloves).
- Use powder-free gloves if using latex gloves (the powder has high amounts of latex, which are inhaled).
- Avoid oil-based hand creams and lotions before putting on latex gloves, as these preparations break down the latex.
- When symptoms of sensitivity to latex occur on exposure (rash, hives, nasal congestion, conjunctivitis, cough, or wheeze), contact the employee health department of your facility.
- If diagnosed as latex allergic, avoid all contact and wear a medical identification bracelet.

Graft-Versus-Host Disease

Graft-versus-host disease can occur when organs are transplanted or when bone marrow or stem cells are transfused into a recipient, typically as treatment for leukemia or severe combined immunodeficiency disease. The donated cells attach to the recipient child's bone marrow and begin production. The child's

Families Want to Know

Removing Common Allergens From the Home

Preventing exposure to the known allergens in the home setting is important. Families can take several measures to minimize contact with allergens. These include:

- Keep pets out of the child's bedroom.
- Clean frequently with moist cloths and mops to remove dust.
- Use plastic covers on mattresses and pillows.
- Avoid using carpeting whenever possible; hard-surface floors are preferable.
- Avoid toys that collect dust (plastic and wood toys are better alternatives than stuffed fabric toys).
- Use high-efficiency air filters.
- Repair homes to prevent entry of water and subsequent molds.
- Consider dehumidification in moist climates, especially in the child's bedroom.

lymphocyte production increases and an immune response develops. However, despite blood and tissue typing, sometimes the donor cells are incompatible with the recipient cells and the new cells begin to mount an immunologic response in the child who has received the transplant. The incidence of the disease is lower in matched siblings than in matched nonsibling transplants (Velardi & Locatelli, 2016).

Graft-versus-host disease may be either acute or chronic. Acute disease has generally been thought of as occurring during the first 100 days after transplant, while chronic disease has been labeled as occurring 100 days posttransplant. In acute disease, the skin, liver, and upper and lower gastrointestinal tract are affected. Symptoms include a pruritic or painful rash, diarrhea, and abdominal pain. The diarrhea may be voluminous and lead to fluid and electrolyte imbalance. Liver enzymes and bilirubin are also elevated (Mandanas, 2014).

Chronic graft-versus-host disease is similar to an autoimmune reaction in the recipient's body and affects multiple systems, including skin, oral cavity, eyes, gastrointestinal tract, liver, lungs, and joints. Specific symptoms may include but are not limited to a rash, mouth sores, diarrhea, anorexia, nausea, vomiting, shortness of breath, chronic cough, itching, muscle weakness, and photophobia (Liu & Hockenberry, 2011).

Careful physical examination and laboratory tests assist in determining the presence of the disease and stage of reaction. Early identification is key to beginning therapy and stopping progression of this life-threatening condition. Several drugs have been used in treatment of graft-versus-host disease and include cyclosporine, tacrolimus, and prednisone or methylprednisolone. Topical corticosteroids such as triamcinolone 0.1% may be used for skin involvement (Mandanas, 2014).

Nursing care focuses on careful physical assessment of all children who have received transplants to assist in early identification of the disease process. All body systems can be involved, especially in chronic disease, so frequent and thorough assessments are needed. Place particular emphasis on skin examination and report rashes that occur. Monitor gastrointestinal functioning by asking about nausea, vomiting, diarrhea, abdominal pain, bloody stools, and dietary intake. Weigh and measure the child and compare to earlier findings. Auscultate the lungs and be alert for signs of infection. Inquire about pain in joints or other body parts. Perform regular eye examinations and ask about burning or itching of eyes. Perform prescribed blood tests to monitor for liver and bone marrow function.

Nursing care for the child who has had a bone marrow or stem cell transplant is complex. Emphasize the need for regular examinations to identify any signs of disease. Children and their families need information and support about this immune system complication of transplantation of bone marrow or stem cells.

Chapter Highlights

- The immune system recognizes any foreign substances within the body and eliminates them as efficiently as possible.

- The immune system is composed of antibodies, leukocytes (white blood cells), and lymphoid tissue.

- The infant is born with natural immunity from the mother and develops acquired immunity gradually in the first 6 years of life.

- Acquired immunity is humoral (antibody mediated) and cell mediated.

- B cells, T cells, natural killer (NK) cells, and complement proteins are the major components of a healthy immune system.

- Disorders of the immune system can have genetic causes (primary immunodeficiency) or they can be acquired (secondary immunodeficiency).

- Severe combined immunodeficiency disease (SCID) is life threatening and requires careful medical and nursing management.

- Human immunodeficiency virus (HIV) can lead to acquired immune deficiency syndrome (AIDS); care focuses on prevention of this viral infection.

- When the child is infected with HIV/AIDS, nursing care centers on preventing infection, promoting adherence to the medication regimen, managing pain, promoting respiratory and other organ function, promoting adequate nutritional intake, and providing emotional support to the parents and child while promoting the child's growth and development.

- Autoimmune disorders such as juvenile idiopathic arthritis and systemic lupus erythematosus occur when the body perceives its own tissue as being foreign and mounts a defense against it.

- Systemic lupus erythematosus (SLE), a generalized disorder mainly occurring in females, is a chronic inflammatory, autoimmune disease of unknown origin that involves many organ systems.

- Juvenile idiopathic arthritis (JIA) is a chronic autoimmune inflammatory disease characterized by joint inflammation resulting in decreased mobility, swelling, and pain. JIA occurs twice as often in females as in males.

- There continues to be a rise in the number of children diagnosed with some types of allergy. A thorough assessment and careful teaching can help the child with allergies to successfully manage reactions.

- Allergy to latex products is commonly seen in children, healthcare workers, and the general population. Children most at risk for latex allergy include those with spina bifida and those undergoing frequent medical procedures or multiple surgeries involving latex.

- Graft-versus-host disease can occur when organs are transplanted or when bone marrow or stem cells are transfused into a recipient.

Clinical Reasoning in Action

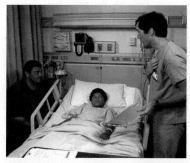

You are working at a pediatrician's office when 11-year-old Nirah and his parents come in. The husband, wife, and Nirah have all been infected with the human immunodeficiency virus (HIV). Nirah does not know he is HIV infected, but he has been very compliant with taking his antiretroviral medications. However, he has recently developed a cough and his parents decided to visit the pediatrician's office.

The pediatrician finds that Nirah has a fever of 102.0°F (38.8°C), respiratory rate of 60 breaths per minute, no visible retractions during respiration, and a pulse of 120 beats per minute. The healthcare provider decides to admit him to the hospital.

After the laboratory tests and radiographs are completed in the hospital, the healthcare provider tells the family that Nirah has pneumonia and strep throat. Nirah is started on IV antibiotics and shows improvement after 3 days of treatment. You monitor Nirah frequently and have him deep breathe. You also teach the parents how to encourage deep-breathing exercises.

1. How does HIV interfere with normal function of the child's immune system?
2. What are some of the measures of infection control for Nirah while he is hospitalized with HIV?
3. How can you promote Nirah's respiratory function?
4. When children, especially those with an immune system problem, are on antibiotics, they can develop thrush (*Candida* in the mouth). What is the treatment to prevent this side effect?

References

Albert, M. H., Notarangelo, L. D., & Ochs, H. D. (2011). Clinical spectrum, pathophysiology, and treatment of the Wiskott-Aldrich syndrome. *Current Opinion in Hematology, 18*, 42–48.

American Academy of Pediatrics (AAP). (2015). *Red book: 2015 report of the Committee on Infectious Diseases* (30th ed.). Elk Grove Village, IL: Author.

American Latex Allergy Association. (2014). *About latex allergy.* Retrieved from http://latexallergyresources.org/about-latex-allergy

Asthma and Allergy Foundation of America. (2014). *Latex allergy.* Retrieved from http://www.aafa.org/display.cfm?id=9&sub=21&cont=383

Buchanan, A. L., Montepiedra, G., Sirois, P. A., Kammerer, B., Garvie, P. A., Storm, D. S., & Nichols, S. L. (2012). Barriers to medication adherence in HIV-infected children and youth based on self- and caregiver report. *Pediatrics, 129*(5), e1244–1251.

Buckley, R. H. (2016a). T lymphocytes, B lymphocytes, and natural killer cells. In R. M. Kliegman, B. F. Stanton, J. W. St. Geme, & N. F. Schor (Eds.), *Nelson textbook of pediatrics* (20th ed., pp. 1006–1012). Philadelphia, PA: Elsevier.

Buckley, R. H. (2016b). Primary defects of cellular immunity. In R. M. Kliegman, B. F. Stanton, J. W. St. Geme, & N. F. Schor (Eds.), *Nelson textbook of pediatrics* (20th ed., pp.1019–1022). Philadelphia, PA: Elsevier.

Buckley, R. H. (2016c). Primary combined antibody and cellular immunodeficiencies. In R. M. Kliegman, B. F. Stanton, J. W. St. Geme, & N. F. Schor (Eds.), *Nelson textbook of pediatrics* (20th ed., pp. 1022–1032). Philadelphia, PA: Elsevier.

Centers for Disease Control and Prevention (CDC). (2014a). *HIV among pregnant women, infants, and children.* Retrieved from http://www.cdc.gov/hiv/risk/gender/pregnantwomen/facts/

Centers for Disease Control and Prevention (CDC). (2014b). *HIV/AIDS.* Retrieved from http://www.cdc.gov/hiv/default.html

Centers for Disease Control and Prevention (CDC). (2015). *HIV among African Americans.* Retrieved from http://www.cdc.gov/hiv/risk/racialethnic/aa/facts/index.html

Defendi, G. L. (2011). Systemic lupus erythematosus. *Consultant for Pediatricians, 10*(1), 26–27.

Ferenkeh-Koroma, A. (2012). Systemic lupus erythematosus: nurse and patient education. *Nursing Standard, 26*(39), 49–57.

Fernandez, J. (2013). DiGeorge. *Merck Manual Online.* Whitehouse Station, NJ: Merck Research Laboratories. Retrieved from http://www.merckmanuals.com/professional/immunology_allergic_disorders/immunodeficiency_disorders/digeorge_syndrome.html

Fortuna, G., & Brennan, M. T. (2013). Systemic lupus erythematosus: Epidemiology, pathophysiology, manifestations, and management. *Dental Clinics of North America, 57*(4), 631–655.

Hassiotou, F., Hepworth, A. R., Metzger, P., Lai, C. T., Trengove, N., Hartmann, P. E., & Filgueira, L. (2013). Maternal and infant infections stimulate a rapid leukocyte response in breastmilk. *Clinical and Translational Immunology, 2*(e3), 1–10.

Hsu, J. J., Lee, T. C., & Sandborg, C. I. (2013). Treatment of juvenile idiopathic arthritis. In G. S. Firestein, R. C. Budd, R. C. Gabriel, I. B. McInnes, & J. R. O'Dell (Eds.), *Kelley's textbook of rheumatology* (9th ed., pp. 1752–1770). Philadelphia, PA: Elsevier Saunders.

Ilowite, N., & Laxer, R. M. (2011). Pharmacology and drug therapy. In J. T. Cassidy, R. E. Petty, R. M. Laxer, & C. B. Lindsley (Eds.), *Textbook of pediatric rheumatology* (6th ed., pp. 71–126). Philadelphia, PA: Elsevier Saunders.

Katrancha, E. D., & Harshberger, L. A. (2012). Nursing students with latex allergy. *Nurse Education in Practice, 12*, 328–332.

Klein-Gitelman, M. S. (2013). *Pediatric systemic lupus erythematosus.* Retrieved from http://emedicine.medscape.com/article/1008066-overview

Kronman, M. P., & Smith, S. (2015). Infectious diseases. In K. J. Marcdante & R. M. Kliegman (Eds.), *Nelson essentials of pediatrics* (7th ed., pp. 315–416). Philadelphia, PA: Elsevier Saunders.

Kwan, A., Abraham, R. S., Currier, R., Brower, A., Andruszewski, K., Abbott, J. K., . . . Puck, J. M. (2014). Newborn screening for severe combined immunodeficiency in 11 screening programs in the United States. *JAMA, 312*(7), 729–738.

Liu, Y-M., & Hockenberry, M. (2011). Review of chronic graft-versus-host disease in children after allogeneic stem cell transplantation: Nursing perspective. *Journal of Pediatric Oncology Nursing, 28*(1), 6–15.

Lupus Foundation of America. (2014). *Living well with lupus.* Retrieved from http://www.lupus.org/answers/topic/living-well-with-lupus

MacDonell, K., Naar-King, S., Huszti, H., & Belzer, M. (2013). Barriers to medication adherence in behaviorally and perinatally infected youth living with HIV. *AIDS and Behavior, 17*(1), 86–93.

Malee, K., Williams, P., Montepiedra, G., McCabe, M., Nichols, S., Sirois, P. A., . . . Kammerer, B. (2011). Medication adherence in children and adolescents with HIV infection: Associations with behavioral impairment. *AIDS Patient Care and STDs, 25*(3), 191–200.

Mandanas, R. A. (2014). *Graft versus host disease.* Retrieved from http://emedicine.medscape.com/article/429037-overview

Mattingly, E. (2011). Lupus in adolescents. *Advance for NPs & PAs, 2*(4), 27–32.

Mawn, B. E. (2012). The changing horizons of U.S. families living with pediatric HIV. *Western Journal of Nursing Research, 34*(2), 213–229.

McDonald-McGinn, D. M., & Sullivan K. E., (2011). Chromosome 22q11.2 deletion syndrome (DiGeorge syndrome/velocardiofacial syndrome). *Medicine, 90*(1), 1–18.

Michaels, M. G., & Green, M. (2016). Infections in immunocompromised persons. In R. M. Kliegman, B. F. Stanton, J. W. St. Geme, & N. F. Schor (Eds.), *Nelson textbook of pediatrics* (20th ed., pp. 1287–1295). Philadelphia, PA: Elsevier.

Navarra, A-M, Neu, N., Toussi, S., Nelson, J., & Larson, E. L. (2014). Health literacy and adherence to antiretroviral therapy among HIV-infected youth. *Journal of the Association of Nurses in AIDS Care, 25*(3), 203–213.

Nierengarten, M. B., & Oski, J. A. (2014). Juvenile idiopathic arthritis: Rethinking remission. *Contemporary Pediatrics, 31*(7), 14–19.

Orduño, N. M., Grimaldi, C., & Diamond, B. (2013). B cells. In G. S. Firestein, R. C. Budd, R. C. Gabriel, I. B. McInnes, & J. R. O'Dell (Eds.), *Kelley's textbook of rheumatology* (9th ed., pp. 191–214). Philadelphia, PA: Elsevier Saunders.

Pai, S-Y, & Notarangelo, L. D. (2013). Congenital disorders of lymphocyte function. In R. Hoffman, E. J. Benz, L. E. Silberstein, H. Heslop, J. I. Weitz, & Anastasi, J. (Eds.), *Hematology: Basic principles and practice* (6th ed., pp. 674–685). Philadelphia, PA: Elsevier Saunders.

Panel on Antiretroviral Therapy and Medical Management of HIV-Infected Children. (2014). *Guidelines for the use of antiretroviral agents in pediatric HIV infection.* Retrieved from http://aidsinfo.nih.gov/contentfiles/lvguidelines/pediatricguidelines.pdf

Park, C. L. (2012). *X-linked immunodeficiency with hyper IgM.* Retrieved from http://emedicine.medscape.com/article/889104-overview

Petty, R. E., & Cassidy, J. T. (2011). Chronic arthritis in childhood. In J. T. Cassidy, R. E. Petty, R. M. Laxer, & C. B. Lindsley (Eds.), *Textbook of pediatric rheumatology* (6th ed., pp. 211–235). Philadelphia: Elsevier Saunders.

Petty, R. E., & Rosenbaum, J. T. (2011). Uveitis in juvenile idiopathic arthritis. In J. T. Cassidy, R. E. Petty, R. M. Laxer, & C. B. Lindsley (Eds.), *Textbook of pediatric rheumatology* (6th ed., pp. 305–314). Philadelphia: Elsevier Saunders.

Rivera, D. M., & Frye, R. E. (2014). *Pediatric HIV infection treatment & management.* Retrieved from http://emedicine.medscape.com/article/965086-treatment\#aw2aab6b6b2

Sampson, H. A., Wang, J., & Sicherer, S. H. (2016). Anaphylaxis. In R. M. Kliegman, B. F. Stanton, J. W. St. Geme, & N. F. Schor (Eds.), *Nelson textbook of pediatrics* (20th ed., pp. 1131–1136). Philadelphia, PA: Elsevier.

Schwartz, R. A., & Sinha, S. (2013). *Pediatric severe combined immunodeficiency.* Retrieved from http://emedicine.medscape.com/article/888072-overview

Schwartz, R. A., & Siperstein, R. (2013). *Pediatric Wiskott-Aldrich syndrome.* Retrieved from http://emedicine.medscape.com/article/888939-overview

Silverman, E., & Eddy, A. (2011). Systemic lupus erythematosus. In J. T. Cassidy, R. E. Petty, R. M. Laxer, & C. B. Lindsley (Eds.), *Textbook of pediatric rheumatology* (6th ed., pp. 315–343). Philadelphia, PA: Elsevier Saunders.

Solomon, L. (2014). *Educational rights for your child with juvenile arthritis: Understanding the educational rights of your child with arthritis is the key to school success.* Retrieved from http://www.arthritistoday.org/about-arthritis/types-of-arthritis/juvenile-arthritis/daily-life/educational-rights-and-resources/individual-education-plan.php

Spina Bifida Association. (2012). *Latex in the home and community.* Retrieved from http://www.spinabifidaassociation.org/atf/cf/%7B85f88192-26e1-421e-9e30-4c0ea744a7f0%7D/SBA-LATEX-LIST-2012-ENGLISH.PDF

Stanley, L. C., & Ward-Smith, P. (2011). The diagnosis and management of juvenile idiopathic arthritis. *Journal of Pediatric Health Care, 25*(3), 191–194.

Udomkhamsuk, W., Fongkaew, W., Grimes, D. E., Viseskul, N., & Kasatpibal, N. (2014). Barriers to HIV treatment adherence among Thai youth living with HIV/AIDS: A qualitative study. *Pacific Rim International Journal of Nursing Research, 18*(3), 203–215.

U.S. Department of Health and Human Services (USDHHS). (2012). *Can I transmit HIV to my baby?* Retrieved from http://aids.gov/hiv-aids-basics/prevention/reduce-your-risk/pregnancy-and-childbirth/

U.S. Food and Drug Administration. (2014). *New type of latex glove cleared.* Retrieved from http://www.fda.gov/forconsumers/consumerupdates/ucm048052.htm

Velardi, A., & Locatelli, F. (2016). Graft versus host disease, rejection, and venoocclusive disease. In R. M. Kliegman, B. F. Stanton, J. W. St. Geme, & N. F. Schor (Eds.), *Nelson textbook of pediatrics* (20th ed., pp. 1069–1071). Philadelphia, PA: Elsevier.

Wade, J. (2012). Care of the type 1 latex allergy patient. *Australian Nursing Journal, 12*(19), 30–33.

Wedderburn, L. R., & Nistala, K. (2013). Etiology and pathogenesis of juvenile idiopathic arthritis. In G. S. Firestein, R. C. Budd, R. C. Gabriel, I. B. McInnes, & J. R. O'Dell (Eds.), *Kelley's textbook of rheumatology* (9th ed., pp. 1741–1751). Philadelphia, PA: Elsevier Saunders.

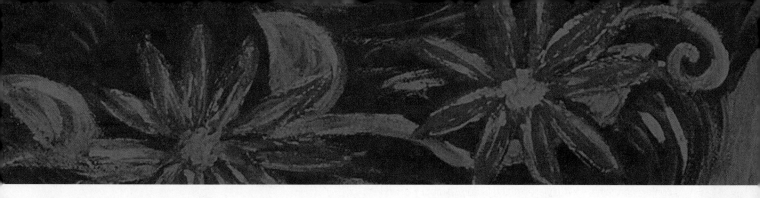

Chapter 23
Alterations in Hematologic Function

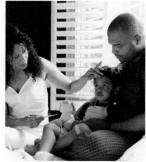

Having a child with sickle cell disease is very difficult for us. We know this is a genetic disease, and we feel responsible for Michael's pain. We also never seem to expect the bad times when they come. He'll be doing well and we almost forget . . . then he gets sick or doesn't drink enough and we're in the hospital again. His older sister has started talking about how she worries that sometime she'll have a child with sickle cell disease and we don't know what to tell her.

—Father of Michael, 3 years old

Blend Images/Alamy

Learning Outcomes

23.1 Describe the function of red blood cells, white blood cells, and platelets.

23.2 Discuss the pathophysiology and clinical manifestations of the major disorders of red blood cells affecting the pediatric population.

23.3 Discuss the pathophysiology and clinical manifestations of the selected disorders of white blood cells affecting the pediatric population.

23.4 Discuss the pathophysiology and clinical manifestations of the major bleeding disorders affecting the pediatric population.

23.5 Plan the nursing management and collaborative care of a child with a hematologic disorder.

23.6 Prioritize nursing interventions for a child receiving hematopoietic stem cell transplantation (HSCT).

The hematologic system is one of a few body systems that regulate, directly or indirectly, all other body functions. Because blood is involved in the function of all tissues and organs, changes in the blood may result in altered functioning of many body organs and structures. This chapter discusses the most common disorders of the blood and blood-forming organs in children. (See Chapter 24 for a discussion of leukemia.)

Anemias

Anemia is defined as a reduction in the number of red blood cells (RBCs), the quantity of hemoglobin, and the volume of packed red cells to below-normal levels. This condition can be caused by loss or destruction of existing RBCs or by an impaired or decreased rate of red cell production. Anemia also can be a clinical manifestation of an underlying disorder, such as lead poisoning or **hypersplenism** (a syndrome characterized by splenomegaly and blood cell deficiencies). Common childhood anemias are discussed in this section.

Iron Deficiency Anemia

Iron deficiency anemia is the most common type of anemia and the most common nutritional deficiency in children. Iron deficiency anemia can occur secondary to blood loss, malabsorption, or poor nutritional intake. See Chapter 14 for a discussion of iron deficiency anemia due to deficits in nutritional intake. Increased physiologic demands (such as rapid growth periods) for blood production can also lead to anemia.

Rapidly growing adolescents whose diets are high in fat and low in vitamins and minerals are particularly susceptible to iron deficiency anemia. Infants who do not consume adequate solid foods after 6 months of age and are fed only breast milk

Text continues on page 592

FOCUS ON:
The Hematologic System

Anatomy and Physiology

Blood has two components: a fluid portion called *plasma* and a cellular portion known as the *formed elements* of the blood. Plasma contains proteins, electrolytes, clotting factors, antibodies, and anticoagulants. The cellular elements are red blood cells or RBCs (erythrocytes), white blood cells or WBCs (leukocytes), and platelets (thrombocytes) (Figure 23–1). Table 23–1 gives normal values for these blood components in children.

Red Blood Cells

Red blood cells, or erythrocytes, are the most abundant of the cellular elements of blood. They are formed through a process called **erythropoiesis**. The primary function of red blood cells is to transport oxygen from the lungs to the tissues. These cells also help carry carbon dioxide from the tissues back to the lungs. Hemoglobin, a red pigment composed of protein and iron, is essential to this function.

Polycythemia is an above-average increase in the number of red cells in the blood. **Anemia** is a reduction in the number of red blood cells; the various types of anemia are discussed in the following main section.

White Blood Cells

White blood cells, or leukocytes, are the mobile units of the body's protective system. They are formed in bone marrow and lymphoid tissue. There are five types of white blood cells, each with a distinct function (Table 23–2).

A differential blood count indicates the percentages of the different types of white cells in the blood and is sometimes useful in identifying the cause of an illness. For example, infections cause an increase in neutrophils, and allergies are related to an increase in eosinophils. The role of lymphocytes is discussed with acquired immunodeficiency syndrome in Chapter 22. A decrease in the number of white blood cells is called **leukopenia**, and can be caused by immune or bone marrow disorders.

Platelets

Platelets, or thrombocytes, are cell fragments that can form hemostatic plugs to stop bleeding. They are synthesized from components in the red bone marrow and are stored in the spleen. A deficiency of platelets can lead to bleeding disorders and is termed **thrombocytopenia**.

Pediatric Differences

Production of red blood cells begins in the embryo by the second week of gestation. White blood cell and platelet production begins at 8 weeks. Most of this early production occurs first in the embryonic yolk sac and then in the liver; however, by 20 to 24 weeks' gestation, liver production decreases as bone marrow production begins to dominate (Christensen & Ohls, 2016). At birth, **hematopoiesis**, or blood cell production, occurs in the marrow of almost every bone. The flat bones, such as the sternum, ribs, pelvic and shoulder girdles, vertebrae, and hips, retain most of their hematopoietic activity throughout life.

At birth, the newborn has a naturally occurring elevation in RBCs due to a high level of erythropoietin, which stimulates red cell production. Once the newborn begins breathing air and the oxygen level in the blood increases, this production slows. Levels of RBCs fall until about 2 to 3 months of age (to about 9 to 11 g/dL) and then begin increasing. Adult levels are reached during adolescence. Male adolescents have RBC levels slightly higher than those of female adolescents (see Appendix D).

The white blood cell count is highest at birth, although levels vary greatly among newborns. Values begin to decline after 12 hours of life and continue to do so during the first week. By 1 week of age, white blood cell values stabilize and remain stable until 1 year of age. After that, the white blood cell count slowly decreases until the adult value is reached in adolescence (Walovich & Newberger, 2016).

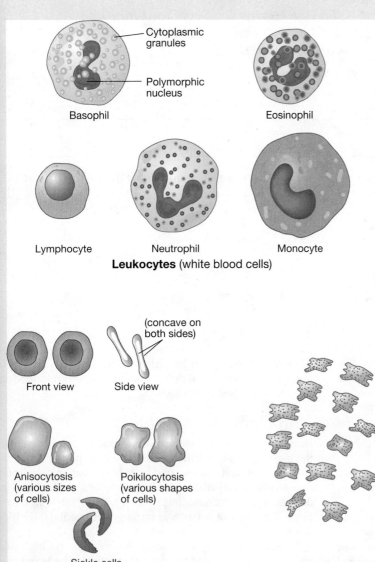

Cytoplasmic granules

Polymorphic nucleus

Basophil

Eosinophil

Lymphocyte   Neutrophil   Monocyte

Leukocytes (white blood cells)

(concave on both sides)

Front view   Side view

Anisocytosis (various sizes of cells)

Poikilocytosis (various shapes of cells)

Sickle cells

Erythrocytes (red blood cells)   **Thrombocytes** (platelets)

Figure 23–1   **Types of blood cells.**

TABLE 23–1 Mean Values for Common Hematology Tests in Children

TEST*	MEAN VALUE
Red blood cell (RBC)	$3.8–5.03 \times 10^{12}/L$
Hemoglobin (Hb)	10.2–13.4 g/dL
Hematocrit (Hct)	31.7%–39.8%
White blood cell (WBC)	$4.86–11.4 \times 10^9/L$
Platelets	$203–367 \times 10^9/L$

*See additional blood values in Appendix D.

Source: Adapted from Soldin, S. J., Wong, E. C., Brugnara, C., & Soldin, O. P. (2011). *Pediatric reference ranges* (7th ed.). Washington, DC: AACC Press; data from Lo, S. F. (2016). Reference intervals for laboratory tests and procedures. In R. M. Kleigman, B. F. Stanton, J. W. St. Geme, & N. F. Schor (Eds.), *Nelson textbook of pediatrics* (20th ed., pp. 3464–3473). Philadelphia, PA: Elsevier.

TABLE 23–2 White Blood Cells and Their Functions

TYPE	FUNCTION
Neutrophils	Phagocytosis
Eosinophils	Allergic reactions
Basophils	Inflammatory reactions
Monocytes (macrophages)	Phagocytosis, antigen processing
Lymphocytes	Humoral immunity (B cell), cellular immunity (T cell)

TABLE 23–3 Laboratory Tests for the Hematologic System*

- Complete blood count
- Clotting indices (prothrombin time, thrombin time, platelets, reticulocyte count)
- Fetal hemoglobin level
- Hemoglobin electrophoresis
- Iron indices (ferritin, iron, iron-binding capacity)
- Red blood cell indices (mean corpuscular volume [MCV], mean corpuscular hemoglobin [MCH], mean corpuscular hemoglobin concentration [MCHC])
- White blood cell differential

*See Appendix D for information about these laboratory tests.

Platelet levels in newborns are lower than in older children and adults. Levels of many clotting factors are also lower in newborns (Scott & Raffini, 2016). Vitamin K is required for the synthesis of clotting factors II, VII, IX, and X. For this reason, all newborns receive a prophylactic injection of vitamin K at birth (Greenbaum, 2016).

Table 23–3 provides examples of diagnostic and laboratory tests used to evaluate the hematologic system; see Appendices D and E for more detailed descriptions. Use *Assessment Guide: The Child With a Hematologic Condition* to perform a nursing assessment of this system.

ASSESSMENT GUIDE | The Child With a Hematologic Condition

Assessment Focus	Assessment Guidelines
Family history	<ul><li>Does a family member have sickle cell disease/trait or other blood disorder?</li><li>Does a family member have hemophilia or other inherited clotting alteration?</li></ul>
Growth and development	<ul><li>Measure height and weight on a regular basis and plot on standardized growth charts.</li><li>Perform nutritional assessment to see if child is getting enough calories.</li><li>Assess child for attainment of developmental milestones.</li></ul>
Skin	<ul><li>Assess for pallor, flushing, rashes, and ecchymosis.</li><li>Observe for prolonged bleeding/clotting time and easy bruising.</li></ul>
Joints	<ul><li>Observe for edema, pain, inflammation, and range of motion.</li></ul>
Additional assessments	<ul><li>Assess pain in various body parts.</li><li>Identify frequency of infections.</li><li>Assess for history of fatigue and lethargy.</li></ul>

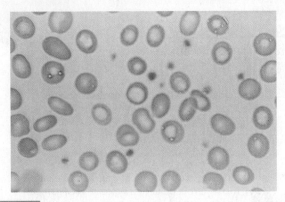

Figure 23–2 In iron deficiency anemia, red blood cells appear hypochromic as a result of decreased hemoglobin synthesis.

SOURCE: Biophoto Associates/Science Source.

or formula that is not fortified with iron are also at risk for iron deficiency because neonatal iron stores have been depleted by this time and their iron needs are not being met. In addition, if the mother's nutritional status during pregnancy was inadequate, or the infant was born prematurely or as part of a multiple birth, insufficient iron may have been stored in the latter part of pregnancy, placing the infant at higher risk for anemia in the first months of life.

Chronic blood loss is always a potential cause of iron deficiency anemia. Those at risk of anemia include the infant who has had bleeding in the neonatal period; the child who loses blood as a result of conditions such as Crohn disease, celiac disease, or parasitic gastrointestinal illness; and the female adolescent who has **menorrhagia** (heavy menstrual bleeding).

Clinical manifestations and severity of symptoms are directly related to the amount of iron deficiency or degree of iron deficiency anemia. Infants with mild to moderate anemia may be asymptomatic, while those with severe anemia may present with pallor, fatigue, irritability, poor feeding, tachypnea, and cardiomegaly (Mahoney, 2014). *Pica*, or consumption of nonfood items, is also a symptom of iron deficiency anemia (Harper & Conrad, 2014).

Diagnosis is made on the basis of clinical presentation and laboratory studies. The hemoglobin, hematocrit, mean corpuscular volume, mean corpuscular hemoglobin, red blood cell count, and reticulocyte count are evaluated to confirm the diagnosis (Harper & Conrad, 2014). A hemoglobin value less than 11 g/dL is indicative of anemia. For children with severe anemia, additional recommended testing includes serum iron, serum ferritin, total iron-binding capacity, transferrin saturation levels, and stool testing for occult blood. Microscopic analysis reveals RBCs to be microcytic (small) in size and hypochromic (pale) in appearance (Mahoney, 2014). (See Figure 23–2.) A diet history and analysis can provide information about food intake; see Chapter 14 for guidelines about diet history.

Treatment involves correction of the iron deficiency with oral elemental iron preparations. Ferrous sulfate at a dose of 3 to 6 mg/kg/day is a common treatment, followed by evaluation for its effectiveness (Mahoney, 2014; Powers & Buchanan, 2014). Oral iron preparations cause several side effects such as constipation and gastrointestinal discomfort; therefore, the child may receive iron medications (to restore blood levels of iron) while the iron content of the diet is increased above the recommended dietary allowances (RDAs). Oral iron medications can then be tapered off once the child's food intake can supply the needed iron; the child is evaluated in about 6 months for recurring anemia.

Nursing Management

Children with iron deficiency anemia are usually identified and treated in the community unless they have another serious illness. Nursing care focuses on screening for the disorder and educating the parents and child about the causes of iron deficiency anemia, dietary management, and the importance of complying with the medication regimen.

Screening for iron deficiency is recommended for all children at approximately 12 months of age (Mahoney, 2014; Powers & Buchanan, 2014). Rescreening is needed in children if risk factors are identified (Mahoney, 2014). Frequency of screening for anemia during adolescence should be determined on an individual basis. Male teens should be screened at least once during peak growth spurts. Female teens should be screened at least every 5 years beginning at 13 years of age. Risk assessment for anemia should be performed annually in adolescents. If risk factors are identified, the adolescent is screened more frequently (Abrams, 2014) (see Chapters 6 and 9). A hematocrit or hemoglobin level is obtained for screening. More detailed tests are performed if the blood test is abnormal. Children at high risk for nutritional deficiencies, such as those in low-income groups and WIC programs (Special Supplemental Nutrition Program for Women, Infants, and Children), may require tests earlier. Most children in Head Start are screened annually by nurses. In addition, children showing signs of anemia such as low energy and pallor should be screened. Height and weight measurements are obtained at each healthcare visit, plotted on growth charts, and compared with percentiles obtained at previous visits. Slow downward trends in percentiles are of concern and require further nutritional analysis (see Chapter 14). Perform developmental screening tests to assess for developmental delays (see Chapter 4).

Dietary management is the preferred long-term treatment for iron deficiency anemia. Teach the child and family to plan for foods that are rich in iron. Include teaching about foods with vitamin C since this vitamin may increase the absorption of iron (Powers & Buchanan, 2014). The infant over 6 months of age should have a diet that includes breast milk or iron-fortified formula and baby cereals with iron fortification. Avoid cow's milk in the first year of life because it can cause bleeding from the gastrointestinal tract, contributing to anemia. If the older infant or toddler consumes large quantities of milk and refuses to eat solid food, restrictions on milk intake may be required. Older infants and toddlers can eat finger foods such as thinly sliced meats. Adolescents can be encouraged to eat foods with high iron content and vitamin C such as hamburgers with a slice of tomato.

Oral iron preparations are given to correct anemia. Instruct the family about side effects such as black stools, constipation, and a foul aftertaste. Emphasize the importance of drinking fluids and eating foods high in dietary fiber to minimize constipation. The medicine should be stored safely to avoid accidental poisoning. Expected outcomes of care are intake of recommended levels of iron and return to normal hematocrit level.

Normocytic Anemia

In normocytic anemia, there is an increase in the destruction of red blood cells or decreased production of red blood cells. This type of anemia may be related to parvovirus B19, Epstein-Barr virus or other infections; bone marrow disorders such as leukemia; renal disease, G6PD (glucose-6-phosphate dehydrogenase) deficiency; inflammatory disorders or several other conditions (Lerner, 2016; Panepinto, Punzalan, & Scott, 2015). Clinical manifestations of normocytic anemia are similar to those seen in iron deficiency anemia, with the possible occurrence of hepatomegaly and splenomegaly as well.

Treatment of normocytic anemia depends on the underlying cause. When the anemia is associated with inflammation or infection, the underlying condition is treated. When hemorrhage is the underlying cause, the source of the bleeding is identified and treated. In acute emergencies, blood products are infused to make up for some of the losses.

Nursing Management

Nursing management of normocytic anemia depends on the cause of the decreased RBCs. Children with inflammatory or infectious diseases require careful assessment and management of medication and other treatment regimens. Administer blood products and other intravenous fluids as ordered to restore blood volume. Use follow-up or home visits to assess hematocrit, hemoglobin, and dietary intake. (Refer to the discussion later in this chapter for management of disseminated intravascular coagulation, to Chapter 25 for management of intestinal infections, and to Chapter 26 for management of hemolytic uremic syndrome.)

Sickle Cell Disease

Sickle cell disease (SCD) is a hereditary **hemoglobinopathy** characterized by the partial or complete replacement of normal hemoglobin with abnormal hemoglobin S (Hgb S) in red blood cells (Table 23–4). This causes occlusion of small blood vessels, ischemia, and damage to affected organs. Sickle cell trait (carrying one gene for the disease) affects approximately 2 million Americans. Approximately 1 in 12 African Americans are carriers of the disease (Maakaron & Taher, 2014). Individuals with sickle cell trait have one sickle cell hemoglobin gene and one normal hemoglobin gene. They are carriers of the disease and generally do not have symptoms, although symptoms have been known to occur when the body is under extreme conditions (Centers for Disease Control and Prevention, 2014).

ETIOLOGY AND PATHOPHYSIOLOGY

Sickle cell disease is an autosomal recessive disorder. If both parents have the trait, with each pregnancy the risk of having a child with the disease is 25%. (See Chapter 3 for a discussion of recessive gene transmission.)

In the most common type of sickle cell disease (HbSS, also referred to as sickle cell anemia), the hemoglobin in the RBC acquires an elongated crescent or sickle shape (Figure 23–3). The sickled cells are rigid and obstruct capillary blood flow. Microscopic obstructions lead to engorgement and tissue ischemia. This local tissue hypoxia causes further sickling and ultimately large infarctions. Organ tissues become damaged by infarctions, leading to scarring and impaired function by 2 to 3 months of age. Levels of fetal hemoglobin decline, leading to splenic impairment (Yawn et al., 2014). Most children with HbSS disease will have functional asplenia by 5 years of age (DeBaun, Frei-Jones, & Vichinsky, 2016). Children with sickle cell disease may suffer from splenic sequestration when blood is trapped in the spleen, a life-threatening complication. Many children must undergo splenectomy in early childhood, leading to severely compromised immunity. Infection rate is high because of impaired immunity. Bacterial infections are the leading cause of death in young children with sickle cell disease.

A stroke occurs in some children with sickle cell disease. Eleven percent of children experience this complication by 20 years of age (Lovett, Sule, & Lopez, 2014). Other complications of sickle cell disease may include acute chest syndrome with pulmonary infiltrate and infection, priapism (sustained and painful penile erection), retinopathy, kidney damage, and gallstone formation (de Montalembert, Ferster, Colombatti, et al., 2011; Meier & Miller, 2012; Tanabe, Dias, & Gorman, 2013).

Sickling may be triggered by fever, hypoxia, emotional stress, or physical stress. Precipitating factors for sickle cell crisis include increased blood viscosity (such as from a low fluid intake or fever) and hypoxia or low oxygen tension. Potential causes of hypoxia or low oxygen tension include high altitudes, poorly pressurized airplanes, hypoventilation, vasoconstriction when cold, or an emotionally stressful event. Any condition that increases the body's need for oxygen or alters the transport of oxygen (such as infection, trauma, or dehydration) may result in sickle cell crisis.

TABLE 23–4 Types of Sickle Cell Disease

DISORDER	CHARACTERISTICS
Sickle cell anemia (HbSS)	Most common type of sickle cell disease
	RBCs are crescent shaped
	Homozygous condition (child has two sickle hemoglobin genes)
	Child is subject to sickle cell crises
	Average life span is 45 years of age
Sickle C disease (HbSC)	Child inherits one HbS gene and one HbC gene
	RBCs are C shaped
	Anemia is generally milder than in HbSS disease
	Painful crises occur about 50% as often as in HbSS disease
	Average life span is 64 years of age
Sickle beta + thalassemia disease (Hb + Sβ) and sickle beta 0 thalassemia disease (Hb0 Sβ)	Combination of sickle cell trait and thalassemia trait. In sickle cell beta+, there is a reduced amount of hemoglobin A, and the life span is near normal. In sickle cell beta 0, there is no hemoglobin A and the life span is mid-50s.

Source: Data from DeBaun, M. R., Frei-Jones, M., & Vichinsky, E. (2016). Hemoglobinopathies. In R. M. Kliegman, B. F. Stanton, J. W. St. Geme III, & N. F. Schor (Eds.), *Nelson textbook of pediatrics* (20th ed., pp. 2336–2353). Philadelphia, PA: Elsevier Saunders; Saunthararajah, Y., & Vichinsky, E. P. (2013). Sickle cell disease: Clinical features and management. In R. Hoffman, E. J. Benz, L. E. Silberstein, H. Heslop, J. I. Weitz, & J. Anastasi (Eds.), *Hematology: Basic principles and practice* (6th ed., pp. 548–572). Philadelphia, PA: Elsevier Saunders; Vichinsky, E. P. (2014). *Variant sickle cell syndromes*. Retrieved from uptodate.com

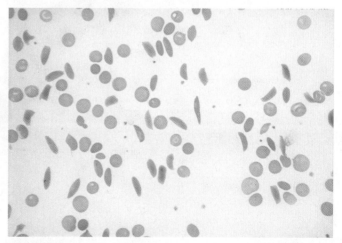

Figure 23–3 **Many of these red blood cells show the elongated crescent shape characteristic of sickle cell disease.**

SOURCE: Bruce Coleman Inc./Alamy.

Pathophysiology Illustrated: **Sickle Cell Disease**

The clinical manifestations of sickle cell disease result from pathologic changes to structures and systems throughout the body.

Hemoglobin S and Red Blood Cell Sickling

Sickle cell anemia is caused by an inherited autosomal recessive defect in Hb synthesis. Sickle cell hemoglobin (HbS) differs from normal hemoglobin only in the substitution of the amino acid valine for glutamine in both beta chains of the hemoglobin molecule.

When HbS is oxygenated, it has the same globular shape as normal hemoglobin. However, when HbS loses its oxygen, it becomes insoluble in intracellular fluid and crystallizes into rodlike structures. Clusters of rods form polymers (long chains) that bend the erythrocyte into the characteristic crescent shape of the sickle cell.

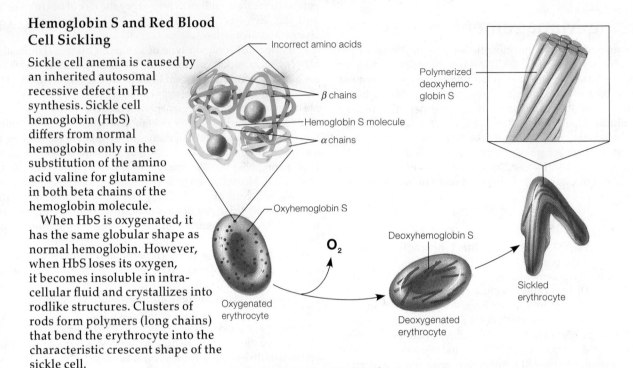

The Sickle Cell Disease Process

Sickle cell disease is characterized by episodes of acute painful crises. Sickling crises are triggered by conditions causing high tissue oxygen demands or that affect cellular pH. As the crisis begins, sickled erythrocytes adhere to capillary walls and to each other, obstructing blood flow and causing cellular hypoxia. The crisis accelerates as tissue hypoxia and acidic metabolic waste products cause further sickling and cell damage.

Sickle cell crises cause microinfarcts in joints and organs, and repeated crises slowly destroy organs and tissues. The spleen and kidneys are especially prone to sickling damage.

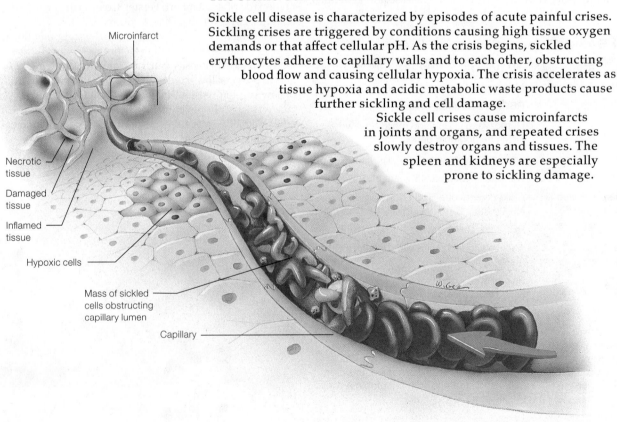

Sickled cells can resume a normal shape when rehydrated and reoxygenated. However, the membranes of these cells become more fragile, and cell life is shortened to about 10 to 20 days rather than the usual 120 days. Chronic hemolytic anemia develops because of the continued destruction of RBCs (Maakaron & Taher, 2014; Myers & Eckes, 2012). (See *Pathophysiology Illustrated: Sickle Cell Disease.*)

CLINICAL MANIFESTATIONS

Affected children are usually asymptomatic until 4 to 6 months of age because sickling is inhibited by high levels of fetal hemoglobin. Clinical manifestations are directly related to the shortened life span of blood cells (hemolytic anemia) and tissue destruction resulting from **vaso-occlusion** (blockage of a blood vessel). Illness results from recurrent vaso-occlusive events that involve painful crises and chronic organ damage. Pathologic changes happen in most body systems, resulting in multiple signs and symptoms. Examples of common organs affected include the following:

- Brain—stroke, often manifested by headache, aphasia, convulsions, visual changes
- Eyes—retinopathy, retinal detachment, diminished vision
- Bones—chronic ischemia of bones with susceptibility to infection and bone degeneration, manifested by osteoporosis, osteomyelitis, spinal deformities, or aseptic necrosis of the femoral head
- Liver—impaired blood flow from capillary obstruction leads to enlargement and scarring of the liver, manifested by hepatomegaly or cirrhosis
- Spleen—splenic infarct leads to fibrosis and increased rates of infection
- Kidneys—ischemia of kidneys causes enuresis, hematuria, inability to concentrate urine
- Penis—microcirculatory obstruction and engorgement (priapism)
- Extremities—vaso-occlusion and chronic ischemia manifests as peripheral neuropathy, weakness, or arthralgia
- Skin—decreased peripheral circulation causes ulcerations

Sickle cell crises are acute exacerbations of the disease that vary markedly in severity and frequency. Table 23–5 outlines the most common types of crises affecting children with sickle cell disease. The most common reason for a visit to the emergency department for the child with sickle cell disease is acute pain crisis (Shihabuddin & Scarfi, 2014). Additionally, 60% to 80% of hospitalizations for children with SCD are related to pain (Meier & Miller, 2012). The sickled RBCs cannot move through the blood vessels and capillaries. Blood vessel occlusion occurs, leading to restricted blood flow and subsequent tissue ischemia. This is referred to as vaso-occlusive crisis (Myers & Eckes, 2012). Pain results from tissue ischemia. Pain is typically experienced in the back or extremities but can occur in other areas (Lovett et al., 2014). Children with sickle cell disease can also develop acute chest syndrome (ACS), a life-threatening complication of sickle cell disease in which a new pulmonary infiltrate is present on chest radiograph. Symptoms of ACS include fever, chest pain, tachypnea, coughing, and wheezing (Meier & Miller, 2012).

CLINICAL THERAPY

Newborns are screened for sickle cell disease. If the test is positive, hemoglobin electrophoresis should be repeated to confirm the diagnosis (Maakaron & Taher, 2014). (See *Developing Cultural Competence: Sickle Cell Disease.*)

Developing Cultural Competence Sickle Cell Disease

Historically, sickle cell disease has been thought of as occurring only in the African American population. In recent years, the disease has been diagnosed in those of Mediterranean, South American, Arabian, and East Indian descent. All newborns in the United States are screened for sickle cell disease as part of the newborn screening panel (March of Dimes, 2014). While African American families may be familiar with the need for screening, parents of children from other cultures may question this practice. Explain the importance of early diagnosis of sickle cell disease and reinforce the fact that heritage cannot be predicted from appearance or name alone.

TABLE 23–5 Types of Sickle Cell Crises

TYPE	CAUSE/PRECIPITATING EVENTS	CLINICAL MANIFESTATIONS	SEVERITY
Vaso-occlusive crisis (pain crisis); most common type of crisis.	Stasis of blood with clumping of cells in the microcirculation, ischemia, and infarction Precipitated by: • Dehydration • Temperature extremes • Infection • Localized hypoxemia • Physical or emotional stress	Extremely painful Symptoms include: • Fever • Tissue engorgement • Painful swelling of joints in hands and feet • Priapism • Severe abdominal pain	Thrombosis and infarction of local tissue may occur if the crisis is not reversed. Cerebral occlusion can result in stroke, manifested by paralysis and/or other central nervous system complications.
Splenic sequestration	Pooling of blood in the spleen	Profound anemia, hypovolemia, and shock	Life-threatening crisis—death can occur within hours.
Aplastic crisis	Triggered by infection with parvovirus B19 or depletion of folic acid	Diminished production and increased destruction of red blood cells Signs include profound anemia, pallor	Is life threatening.

Source: Data from Lovett, P. B., Sule, H. P., & Lopez, B. L. (2014). Sickle cell disease in the emergency department. *Emergency Medicine Clinics of North America, 32*(3), 629–647; Maakaron. J. E., & Taher, A. T. (2014). *Sickle cell anemia.* Retrieved from http://emedicine.medscape.com/article/205926-overview; Meier, E. R., & Miller, J. L. (2012). Sickle cell disease in children. *Drugs, 72*(7), 895–906; Myers, M., & Eckes, E. J. (2012). A novel approach to pain management in persons with sickle cell disease. *MEDSURG Nursing, 21*(5), 293–298.

Management focuses on pain control, hydration, oxygenation, prevention of infection, and prevention of associated complications. Treatment of crises involves aggressive hydration, oxygen administration, pain management, and bed rest to reduce energy expenditure. Parenteral analgesics, such as morphine and hydromorphone (Dilaudid), are generally administered around the clock or via patient-controlled analgesia. In addition to parenteral narcotics, the child may also receive intravenous ketorolac (Toradol) or oral ibuprofen (Motrin) every 6 hours around the clock as adjunctive therapy. Oral and intravenous fluid replacement also promotes pain relief since dehydration is often a cause of crisis. Fluids also reduce the viscosity of the blood, so adequate hydration is essential. Oxygen is usually administered to provide comfort and decrease the incidence of pulmonary complications.

Infection in a child with sickle cell disease is a serious condition requiring immediate attention. When an infection is suspected, cultures (blood, urine, and throat) are obtained to identify the source of infection and the offending organism. Aggressive antibiotic therapy is implemented immediately.

Penicillin prophylaxis should be started in the newborn period or as soon as the child is diagnosed and continued until 5 years of age to prevent a potentially life-threatening bacterial infection with the *Streptococcus pneumoniae*. Newborn screening has led to earlier diagnosis and, therefore, earlier initiation of prophylaxis (Yawn et al., 2014). The medication may be continued past 5 years of age if the child has a history of severe pneumococcal sepsis, or if the healthcare provider feels the child is still at high risk for infection caused by *S. pneumoniae* (Saunthararajah & Vichinsky, 2013).

To prevent life-threatening infection in the child with sickle cell disease, it is essential for the child to receive recommended immunizations including the pneumococcal conjugate vaccine, HIB vaccine, hepatitis B vaccine, and influenza vaccine (see Chapter 16). In addition, children with SCD should receive the 23-valent pneumococcal vaccine (Pneumovax) at age 2 and age 5 and every 5 years as an adult (Saunthararajah & Vichinsky, 2013). Children with anatomic or functional asplenia should also receive the meningococcal vaccine beginning at 2 months of age. Specific guidelines are provided by the CDC (Centers for Disease Control and Prevention, 2015). Blood transfusions improve tissue oxygenation, reduce sickling, correct anemia, and temporarily reduce the percentage of HbS (Inati, Khoriaty, & Musallam, 2011).

Annual transcranial Doppler testing is recommended for children with SCD between the ages of 2 and 16 (Maakaron & Taher, 2014). Prophylactic transfusions are recommended for children with abnormal transcranial Doppler testing to prevent or decrease the risk of stroke (Lovett et al., 2014; Maakaron & Taher, 2014). However, frequent transfusions may result in an overload of iron in the body. The iron is stored in tissues and organs (**hemosiderosis**) because the body has no way of excreting it (Lovett et al., 2014). An iron-chelating drug such as deferoxamine (Desferal), which binds excess iron so it can be excreted by the kidneys, is administered. An oral chelator, deferasirox (Exjade), has been used in some patients since approval by the U.S. Food and Drug Administration (FDA) in 2005 and has demonstrated similar efficacy to deferoxamine infusion (Meier & Miller, 2012). Deferasirox could potentially simplify treatment and improve compliance by use of oral administration for patients requiring chelation therapy.

Treatment with hydroxyurea has been helpful in adults, and is being used frequently in children. This medication improves fetal hemoglobin levels and increases total hemoglobin concentration (Strouse & Heeney, 2012). The presence of fetal hemoglobin reduces sickling and subsequently the frequency of painful crisis secondary to vaso-occlusion. Although studies have demonstrated the effectiveness of hydroxyurea in children, the FDA labeling related to indications for the use of this drug refers only to adults, necessitating off-label usage in the pediatric population (Strouse & Heeney, 2012).

Hematopoietic stem cell transplantation (HSCT) is the only known cure for sickle cell disease and has been used in children with severe complications related to SCD. Only a few hundred people with sickle cell disease worldwide have received a stem cell transplant as a cure for sickle cell disease because its use is limited to those children who have a human leukocyte antigen (HLA)–compatible sibling. It is estimated that less than 20% of children with SCD have a sibling who is a match. The survival rate for children with sickle cell disease who have been able to receive a stem cell transplant is 93% to 97% (Meier & Miller, 2012). (See discussion regarding HSCT later in this chapter.)

SAFETY ALERT!
It is important for all health facilities to have current guidelines for transfusion protocols. Become familiar with the policies and procedures where you work. For example, the child's blood type and patient identification need to be checked by two registered nurses before starting the infusion. See the *Clinical Skills Manual* SKILLS for further information on blood transfusions.

Prognosis depends on the severity of the child's disease; children with more frequent exacerbations and hospitalizations have poorer prognosis. Newborn screening has led to early intervention in babies who have SCD (Maakaron & Taher, 2014). Early diagnosis, prophylactic antibiotics, and monthly transfusions for those at risk for stroke have extended life spans in individuals with sickle cell disease, with a median life span of 42 years of age for males and 48 for females (Tanabe et al., 2013). The life span of individuals with sickle cell trait is normal (Sickle Cell Information Center, 2012).

Nursing Management
For the Child With Sickle Cell Disease

Nursing Assessment and Diagnosis

The nurse may be involved in sickle cell gene testing to identify carriers and children who have the disease. Once a child is diagnosed with the disease, a comprehensive physical assessment is essential because sickle cell disease can affect any body system.

Professionalism in Practice Newborn Screening for SCD

Newborn screening for sickle cell disease is mandatory in all 50 states (National Newborn Screening and Genetics Resource Center, 2014). Nurses play an important role in educating parents about the importance of newborn screening and about the diagnosis and treatment plan once a diagnosis of sickle cell disease is made.

PHYSIOLOGIC ASSESSMENT

In children who are known to have sickle cell disease, obtain a detailed history from the parents or child about past crises, precipitating events, medical treatment, and home management. Measure the child's height and weight accurately and compare to past measurements since failure to thrive is common. Ask about chronic or acute pain that the child is experiencing. Pain may occur in nearly any body part, but most commonly manifests as headache, extremity pain, or abdominal discomfort. The ill child with sickle cell disease should receive a careful multisystem assessment. Fever, neurologic changes such as decreased alertness or behavioral changes, and respiratory symptoms are emergency conditions that necessitate prompt treatment. When the child is in crisis, assess pain and note the presence of any signs of inflammation or infection. Carefully monitor the child for signs of shock (see Chapter 21).

Clinical Reasoning Sickle Cell Disease

Michael is a 3-year-old African American child with sickle cell disease who is admitted to the hospital with severe abdominal pain. What are the most important nursing assessments and interventions to integrate within Michael's care?

PSYCHOSOCIAL ASSESSMENT

The family of a child with sickle cell disease requires a thorough psychosocial assessment. Ask if other family members have the diagnosis. If the child is newly diagnosed with the disorder, the family needs assistance to deal with feelings related to the serious, life-threatening nature of the disease. Assess parents' understanding of the disease transmission and ask whether genetic counseling has been obtained. Determine whether the family has adequate healthcare coverage to pay for the child's medical expenses and whether the child qualifies for assistance because of the disability associated with the disease. Ask older children about their knowledge of the disease, and explore their feelings related to the management of a chronic condition. When siblings or other family members are carriers, periodic counseling is needed so they can understand implications for dating, marriage, and having children.

Several nursing diagnoses that might apply to the child with sickle cell disease are presented in the accompanying *Nursing Care Plan*. Other nursing diagnoses might include the following (NANDA-I © 2014):

- *Caregiver Role Strain* related to illness chronicity
- *Parenting, Risk for Impaired*, related to having a child with a physical illness
- *Development: Delayed, Risk for*, related to effects of physical disability
- *Mobility: Physical, Impaired*, related to pain
- *Knowledge, Deficient (Child or Parents)*, related to lack of exposure about cause and treatment of sickle cell disease

Planning and Implementation

The accompanying *Nursing Care Plan* summarizes nursing care for the child with sickle cell disease. Nursing management for the child in crisis focuses on increasing tissue perfusion, promoting hydration, controlling pain, preventing infection, ensuring adequate nutrition, preventing complications, and providing emotional support to the child and family.

INCREASE TISSUE PERFUSION

Administer blood transfusions and oxygen as ordered. To prevent hemolysis, the intravenous fluid used before and after a blood transfusion must be saline rather than D_5W. Monitor for transfusion reactions (Table 23–6). Encourage the child to rest. Work with the child and family to avoid emotional stress. Any activities that increase cellular metabolism also result in tissue hypoxia. Schedule caregiving activities and play to allow for optimal rest.

PROMOTE HYDRATION

The child with sickle cell disease is adversely affected by dehydration. Calculate the child's fluid maintenance requirements (minimum daily fluid intake) (see Chapter 18) and monitor the child's oral fluid intake. Administer intravenous fluids as ordered. Adjust oral intake as necessary to keep the child well hydrated.

CONTROL PAIN

Administer prescribed analgesics around the clock during crises. If patient-controlled analgesia is used, be sure that the constant infusions run as ordered and that the parent or child understands the use of the button for dosing when needed (see Chapter 15). Help the child assume a comfortable position. Avoid putting stress on painful joints. See *Evidence-Based Practice: Sickle Cell Disease and Pain Management*.

SAFETY ALERT!

Blood reactions can occur as soon as a blood transfusion begins. Administer the first 20 mL of blood slowly and observe the child carefully for a reaction. Assess the child according to agency policy and promptly report changes in condition. If a reaction occurs, stop the transfusion immediately, call the healthcare provider, monitor vital signs, keep the intravenous line open with normal saline, check for hematuria, and administer medications as ordered.

PREVENT INFECTION

Infection makes the child more susceptible to a crisis, and the crisis, in turn, increases susceptibility to infection. Teach the parents how to administer antibiotics for prophylaxis or treatment of infection. Because infections are particularly virulent in these children, tell parents to get immediate care when the child is ill. Emphasize the importance of immunizations. See the discussion earlier in this chapter and Chapter 16 for further information about recommended and supplemental immunizations.

TABLE 23–6 Clinical Manifestations of Blood Transfusion Reactions

TYPE OF REACTION AND ETIOLOGY	CLINICAL MANIFESTATIONS
Allergic reaction related to immune response to protein in the blood	Urticaria, itching, respiratory distress
Hemolytic reaction related to mismatched blood, history of multiple transfusions, or infusion with a solution containing dextrose or other additives	Fever, chills, hematuria, headache, chest pain; can progress to shock
Febrile or septic related to contamination of blood; may also be caused by idiopathic conditions	Chills, fever, headache, decreased blood pressure, nausea or vomiting, and leg and back pain
Circulatory overload related to infusions of excessive amounts of fluid or too rapid administration	Labored breathing, chest or low back pain, productive cough, rales upon auscultation, distended neck veins, increased central venous pressure

Nursing Care Plan: The Child With Sickle Cell Disease

1. Nursing Diagnosis: *Tissue Perfusion: Peripheral, Ineffective,* related to affinity of hemoglobin for oxygen (NANDA-I © 2014)

GOAL: The child will show few signs and symptoms of tissue hypoxia.

INTERVENTION	RATIONALE
• Instruct child to avoid physical exertion, emotional stress, low-oxygen environments (e.g., airplanes, high altitudes), and known sources of infection.	• Decreased activity and exposure reduce the body's need for oxygen.

EXPECTED OUTCOME: Child will have no shortness of breath and shows no signs of hypoxia.

GOAL: Repeated stroke will be avoided.

INTERVENTION	RATIONALE
• Administer blood transfusions as ordered.	• Packed cells increase number of red blood cells available to carry oxygen to tissue cells. Transfusions promote circulation.
• Perform several caregiving activities together whenever possible.	• Grouping activities allows for optimum rest.
• Give oxygen as ordered.	• A high concentration of oxygen in alveoli increases diffusion of gas across membranes.
• Administer and teach the family about prophylactic transfusions for the child who has had a stroke.	• Lowers potential for a future stroke.

EXPECTED OUTCOME: Child does not suffer a stroke.

2. Nursing Diagnosis: *Fluid Volume: Deficient, Risk for,* related to inadequate fluid intake and dehydration (NANDA-I © 2014)

GOAL: The child will maintain or be restored to adequate hydration.

INTERVENTION	RATIONALE
• Calculate the child's daily fluid requirements. Monitor the child's usual fluid consumption and make necessary adjustments. Encourage the child to take fluids. Observe for signs of dehydration.	• Optimizing fluid intake ensures that the child gets needed fluid. Dehydration exacerbates crises.
• Record intake and output.	• Early intervention can be effective in minimizing complications from dehydration. Child may need oral or intravenous rehydration therapy.

EXPECTED OUTCOME: Child will show signs of adequate hydration.

3. Nursing Diagnosis: *Pain, Chronic,* related to physical disability and clustering of sickled cells (NANDA-I © 2014)

GOAL: The child will verbalize that pain is controlled.

INTERVENTION	RATIONALE
• Administer analgesics, such as morphine or hydromorphone (Dilaudid), as ordered. Continuous intravenous infusion is used for the duration of a painful crisis.	• Pain of sickle cell crises is excruciating.
• Position carefully.	• Joints and extremities can be extremely painful.

EXPECTED OUTCOME: Child will be pain free or pain control will be significantly improved.

4. Nursing Diagnosis: *Infection, Risk for,* **related to chronic disease and splenic malfunction (NANDA-I © 2014)**

GOAL: The child will not develop infection.

INTERVENTION	RATIONALE
• Ensure adequate nutrition by providing high-calorie, high-protein diet. Ensure that the child's immunizations are up-to-date and that children less than age 5 years are receiving prophylactic antibiotics. Make sure that parents have a thermometer in the home and know how to use it. Report any signs of infection to a healthcare provider immediately.	• Children with a chronic illness are at greater risk of infection.
• Isolate the child from possible sources of infection. Instruct parents about signs of infection and encourage them to seek prompt health care.	• Restriction of persons with infection decreases the child's contact with infectious agents. Prompt care for infection reduces the chance of sickle cell crisis.

EXPECTED OUTCOME: Child will be free of infection.

EVIDENCE-BASED PRACTICE | Sickle Cell Disease and Pain Management

Clinical Question

What are effective pain management strategies for children with sickle cell disease? How well is pain assessed and managed in children with sickle cell disease?

The Evidence

Severe episodes of sickle cell crisis require visits to the emergency department (ED) and/or hospitalization for pain management. Relief of pain is the primary goal for healthcare providers and is most significant to the child experiencing pain.

Zempsky, Corsi, and McKay (2011) performed a retrospective chart review of 77 patients with sickle cell disease (SCD), ages 3 to 21 years, to evaluate the relationship between pain scores and time to administration of pain medication. Triage pain scores using the visual analog scale (VAS) in the ED for patients with sickle cell disease averaged 7.7, whereas those for patients with long bone fractures averaged 6.7. For every point increase on the VAS for patients with fractures, the time to administration of pain medication decreased by 5.6 minutes. There was no relationship between the pain score for patients with SCD and time to administration of pain medication. This suggests that pain scores are not used initially when making decisions in the ED regarding pain management for individuals with sickle cell disease but are used for patients with other painful conditions.

Ender et al. (2014) evaluated the use of a clinical pathway in the acute management of pain in children with sickle cell disease. Data were collected from 35 patients before the pathway was introduced and from 33 patients after the pathway was introduced. All patients with sickle cell disease older than 6 months of age who presented to the pediatric ED with sickle cell pain were eligible to be included in the study. Patients with SCD with pain from another cause or those in whom a stroke was suspected were excluded from the study. Data collected at triage included time of patient registration and first set of vital signs, patient weight, time of first pain medication administration, type of medication and dosage administered, pain score, and whether or not the child was admitted to the hospital. The

pathway included a checklist that provided instructions for triage, monitoring, timing of assessments and interventions, and medication administration. Results of the study showed that after the clinical pathway was introduced, the mean time interval for administration of the first analgesic was reduced from 74 minutes to 42 minutes. The mean time interval for administration of the first opioid was reduced from 94 minutes to 46 minutes. This represented significant improvement in administration of the first analgesic and first opiod and was statistically significant. The mean time interval for pain reassessment showed improvement, with the time reduced from 110 minutes to 72 minutes, but was not statistically significant. The study concluded that use of a clinical pathway can lead to improvement in pain management of patients with SCD.

Dobson and Byrne (2014) evaluated the effects of guided imagery training on school-age children ages 6 to 11 years with a diagnosis of sickle cell disease. Changes in pain perception, use of analgesia, self-efficacy, and imaging ability were described. Twenty children who had been treated in the clinic for at least a year served as the sample for the study. The children completed pain diaries every day for 2 months. Baseline and end-of-treatment imaging ability and self-efficacy were measured. The results of the study showed that training in the use of guided imagery led to reductions in pain intensity, decreased use of analgesics, and a significant increase in self-efficacy. The study concluded that guided imagery is effective in the management of pain related to sickle cell disease.

Best Practice

Children and adolescents with sickle cell disease who present to the ED with a painful episode have high levels of pain. These patients may have been in pain for several days prior to coming to the hospital. They may wait for a period of time before receiving opioid pain medication.

Protocols or clinical pathways should be established to ensure that children and adolescents who present to the ED with a painful episode receive pain medication in a timely

(continued)

manner. While in the ED and if hospitalized, pain intensity should be evaluated on a regular basis using an appropriate pain scale and the pain regimen adjusted as needed.

Clinical Reasoning
How will you determine which pain assessment tool is most appropriate to assess pain in children of different ages? How will you determine if the child in sickle cell crisis is obtaining adequate pain relief? (Consult Chapter 15 for ideas.) In addition to analgesics, what are appropriate nonpharmacologic methods that you can use to decrease pain in children with SCD?

ENSURE ADEQUATE NUTRITION

Emphasize the importance of adequate nutrition to promote growth. Encourage the child to eat a high-protein, high-calorie diet. Stress the importance of folic acid and vitamin C as supplements as prescribed. Perform regular growth measurements, and if slow growth is apparent, perform 24-hour recalls and other nutritional assessments.

Growth and Development

To encourage fluid intake in a small child:

- Use a favorite cup or glass.
- Use straws.
- Take advantage of times the child is thirsty, such as on awakening or after play.
- Leave a cup within easy reach of the child.
- Offer frozen juice pops and crushed ice drinks.

PREVENT COMPLICATIONS OF CRISES

Observe the child for signs of increasing anemia, infection, shock, and acute chest syndrome. Assess vital signs frequently and note changes that might be indicative of complications. Maintain ongoing monitoring of the child's neurologic status for evidence of altered cerebral function. Monitor the child's respiratory status for signs of acute chest syndrome. Assess for an enlarged spleen by gentle palpation. Administer blood transfusions and observe the child for any adverse reaction. Assess growth and developmental milestones.

PROVIDE EMOTIONAL SUPPORT

Sickle cell disease is a chronic disease accompanied by life-threatening episodic crises. Family members often need help to deal with their feelings about the diagnosis and its implications. Explore resources in the home and community to see if parents will be able to administer medications and fluids and to provide adequate nutrition. Assess parents' knowledge of signs of infection and of sickle cell crisis and when to seek medical care for the child. Refer the parents for genetic counseling, particularly if they plan to have more children. Encourage adolescents and young adults in the family to receive genetic counseling and testing as well. Referrals to support groups and contact with others with the disease can be helpful.

DISCHARGE PLANNING AND HOME CARE TEACHING

Identify and address home care needs well in advance of discharge. Give parents information about sickle cell disease and the child's treatment. Even parents of a child previously diagnosed with the disorder may benefit from information about the disease process and its management. Explain the basic effect of tissue hypoxia and the effects of sickling on circulation. Assist the family to explore resources in the home and community and determine if parents will be able to administer medications and fluids and to provide adequate nutrition.

Teach parents to look for signs of dehydration, such as dry mucous membranes, weight loss, and a sunken fontanelle in infants. Give specific instructions about how many ounces of liquid the child needs to drink each day. Emphasize that increased fluid intake is needed to replace the fluids lost from overheating or exposure to hot weather. Make sure both the child and family understand the triggers and precipitating factors for sickle cell crises. Encourage them to avoid situations that cause crises. Instruct the child and parents about signs and symptoms of crises that should be reported to their healthcare provider.

When regular blood infusions are used, the resulting iron overload is damaging to body organs. Provide the family with instructions about the treatment for iron overload.

Tell parents that it is important to inform all treating healthcare providers and dentists of the child's medical condition. The child should also wear medical identification (e.g., a medical identification bracelet). Special precautions are necessary when the child undergoes surgery of any kind because hypoxia resulting from anesthesia is a major surgical risk.

Family members need ongoing support to deal with the stress of having a child with a chronic condition. Provide resources, respite care for parents, and information as needed for siblings.

Encourage older children with sickle cell disease to participate in activities with other children between crises but to avoid strenuous physical exertion and contact sports. Play and social interactions that promote learning and development are important.

Evaluation

Expected outcomes of nursing care for the child with sickle cell disease include the following:

- Pain is managed to facilitate comfort level.
- The child maintains an adequate hydration state to prevent cell sickling.
- Side effects of the disease are absent in the respiratory system, central nervous system, and body organs.
- The child maintains a normal immune status and prevents infection.
- The family or child promptly recognizes and treats the complications of the disease.
- The child maintains normal growth and development.
- The nurse provides necessary services and resources for the parents and other family members.
- The family has knowledge of disease and its treatment.

Families Want to Know

Home Care Considerations for the Child With Sickle Cell Disease

- Follow recommended schedules for health promotion visits.
- Keep scheduled appointments with the child's hematologist.
- Be sure the child's immunizations are up-to-date.
- Special testing, such as heart and eye examinations, may be needed periodically to check for sequelae of the disease.
- Follow instructions for antibiotic administration.
- Assess the child's pain and give pain medication as prescribed for acute and chronic pain.
- Ensure that the child gets extra fluids in hot weather, when ill, during physical activity, and during travel. Dehydration can lead to crisis.
- As the child develops, provide information about the disease and encourage self-care.
- Be sure the school personnel understand the child's diagnosis and any care required during school hours.
- Contact your healthcare provider if the child has a high fever, a common illness that lasts more than 1 day, seizures, change in behavior, severe pain, abnormal skin color or breathing pattern, or any other symptoms that concern you.
- Inform all care providers of the child's condition and need for special planning prior to surgery.

Thalassemias

The thalassemias are a group of inherited blood disorders of hemoglobin synthesis characterized by anemia that can be mild or severe. There are three types of beta-thalassemias (β-thalassemias): thalassemia minor, or thalassemia trait (produces mild anemia); thalassemia intermedia (produces moderate anemia and may require transfusions); and thalassemia major, also known as Cooley's anemia (produces anemia requiring transfusion). Clinical manifestations of β-thalassemia are caused by the defective synthesis of hemoglobin, structurally impaired RBCs, and the shortened life span of the RBCs. Symptoms of thalassemia major generally develop during the second 6 months of age and include pallor, jaundice, growth retardation, irritability, hepatomegaly, and splenomegaly (Giardina & Rivella, 2013). In alpha-thalassemia (α-thalassemia), the child may have a one-gene defect (α-thalassemia silent carrier) and generally be symptom free; have a two-gene defect (α-thalassemia trait) and have mild anemia; or have α-thalassemia major, which results in hydrops fetalis. Intrauterine transfusion can increase the survival rate in the fetus with α-thalassemia major. Those who survive will be transfusion dependent. Hematopoietic stem cell transplant is the only cure (DeBaun et al., 2016).

Diagnosis is made by hemoglobin electrophoresis, which reveals a decreased production of one of the globin chains in hemoglobin and an elevated F and A hemoglobin. A complete blood count shows a decreased hemoglobin, hematocrit, and reticulocyte count (DeBaun et al., 2016). Prenatal testing using chorionic villi sampling or amniocentesis can detect the disease in the fetus. Treatment is supportive. The goal of medical management is to maintain normal hemoglobin levels. A chronic transfusion program, in which blood transfusions are administered every 2 to 4 weeks, is the conventional therapy used to treat children with severe disease. Since iron overload is a side effect of this treatment, children may need to receive an iron-chelating drug such as deferoxamine or deferasirox (Exjade). (See previous discussion.) A splenectomy may be required for the child with splenomegaly. Hematopoietic stem cell transplantation (HSCT) may be offered as an alternative therapy for children newly diagnosed with the disorder.

Nursing Management

Nursing care focuses on observing for complications of transfusion therapy, supporting the child and family in dealing with a chronic life-threatening illness, and referring the family for genetic counseling. Encourage parents to take an active role in the child's treatment regimen. Teach parents the technique for subcutaneous infusion of deferoxamine if that route is to be used for therapy at home.

Compliance with transfusion therapy often becomes an issue as children reach adolescence. Offering the adolescent treatment options, such as when to undergo transfusion, can help improve compliance. Adolescents with β-thalassemia and parents of newly diagnosed children can be referred to the Thalassemia Action Group, a national organization for those with this disease, or to the Cooley's Anemia Foundation. Expected outcomes of nursing care include maintenance of normal hemoglobin and hematocrit, safe transfusion of blood products, maintenance of recommended body iron levels, and family understanding about the genetic transmission of the disease.

Hereditary Spherocytosis

Hereditary spherocytosis (HS) is a hemolytic disorder occurring in 1 in 5000 people of Northern European descent. The inheritance pattern of hereditary spherocytosis is most commonly autosomal dominant, but in some cases is autosomal recessive. Additionally, up to 25% of cases have no family history (Segel & Casey, 2016). Erthrocytes assume a spherical shape due to an intrinsic membrane defect. Spectrin deficiency is most common (Gonzalez & Eichner, 2014). The erythrocytes are retained and removed by the spleen, leading to splenomegaly in the child (Hsiao et al., 2013).

Clinical manifestations appear in the neonatal period or during early infancy. Severity of the anemia varies, but mild jaundice is usually evident. Aplastic crisis (discussed in Table 23–5) is the most serious complication the child experiences. Gallstones are a complication associated with hereditary spherocytosis. Complete blood count reveals anemia, and microscopic examination reveals the abnormally shaped cells (Gonzalez & Eichner, 2014).

Treatment of children with hereditary spherocytosis includes daily folic acid and red blood cell transfusions when indicated. Children with mild, uncomplicated disease may be managed without surgery (Gonzalez & Eichner, 2014). Splenectomy is indicated in children with severe disease and in those with moderate disease who show signs of growth failure or significant signs and symptoms of anemia. Removal of the spleen increases the risk of infection and sepsis (Das et al., 2014; Gonzalez & Eichner, 2014). Infants and young children are especially at risk. Delaying the surgery until after age 6 reduces the risk of bacterial infection and sepsis (Gonzalez & Eichner, 2014). Nursing care for the child with hereditary spherocytosis is the same as care for the child with anemia.

Aplastic Anemia

Aplastic anemia is a deficiency in the number of blood cells that results from failure of the bone marrow to produce adequate numbers of all types of circulating blood cells. The condition may be congenital or acquired. Eighty percent of cases of aplastic anemia are acquired, and it is thought to be an autoimmune disease (Bakhshi, 2014).

Acquired aplastic anemia in children can develop after treatment with radiation or after ingestion of drugs such as chloramphenicol, NSAIDS, or anticonvulsants. This type of anemia can also be a result of an infectious process such as viral hepatitis, mononucleosis, or cytomegalovirus; related to nutritional deficiencies in vitamin B_{12} or folic acid; or related to exposure to chemicals such as insecticides and pesticides (Hartung, Olson, & Bessler, 2013).

Symptoms are related to the degree of bone marrow failure and include **petechiae** (small pinpoint red or purple spots on the mucous membranes or skin), **purpura** (irregular bluish purple areas of bleeding into the tissues), menorrhagia in postmenarchal girls, and epistaxis. Symptoms associated with anemia include pallor, fatigue, and exercise intolerance. Symptoms related to neutropenia include fever and bacterial infections (Hartung et al., 2013). Death can result from complications associated with hemorrhage and sepsis.

Diagnosis is made by complete blood count studies, which reveal leukopenia with marked neutropenia, thrombocytopenia, and **pancytopenia** (decreased number of blood cell components), and by bone marrow aspiration, which reveals yellow, fatty bone marrow instead of red bone marrow.

Supportive treatment includes transfusions of packed cells, platelets, or both. Immunosuppressive drug therapy is effective for many children because it is believed the child's immune system is attacking the bone marrow. Immunosuppressive agents generally include antithymocyte globulin (ATG) and cyclosporine. The treatment of choice for children with severe aplastic anemia is hematopoietic stem cell transplantation (HSCT) from an HLA-matched sibling donor (Bakhshi, 2014).

Nursing Management

Nursing interventions focus on preventing bleeding, administering and monitoring blood transfusions, preventing infection, encouraging mobility as tolerated, educating the parents and child about the disorder, and providing emotional support. Families need support in dealing with a child who has a life-threatening disease. Refer them to support groups for counseling, if indicated, and to social services. Expected outcomes of nursing care include absence of infection, no bleeding, and parental education related to the disease and treatment.

Bleeding Disorders
Hemophilia

Hemophilia refers to a group of hereditary bleeding disorders that result from a deficiency in specific clotting factors. Hemophilia A, or classic hemophilia, is caused by a deficiency of factor VIII in the blood and occurs in 1 in 5000 male births (Ozgonenel et al., 2013). Hemophilia B, also known as Christmas disease, is caused by a deficiency of factor IX and occurs in 1 in 25,000–30,000 male births (Zaiden, 2014). Hemophilia A accounts for 85% of persons with hemophilia, and 10% to 15% have hemophilia B (Scott, 2016).

ETIOLOGY AND PATHOPHYSIOLOGY

Hemophilias A and B are X-linked recessive disorders, which manifest almost exclusively as affected males and carrier females. Genes for clotting factors VIII and IX are located near the terminal long arm of the X chromosome (Scott, 2016). A daughter will inherit the gene from her father with hemophilia and may transmit it to her sons. (See Chapter 3 for a description of genetic transmission.) Some children affected by hemophilia do not have a family member with a history of a clotting disorder. In these cases, the disorder is caused by a new mutation. (Scott, 2016). The degree of bleeding is related to the amount of clotting factor and the severity of the injury.

CLINICAL MANIFESTATIONS

Hemophilia is manifested in different children by bleeding tendencies that range from mild to moderate or severe. Children with hemophilia often do not demonstrate symptoms until after 6 months of age as they become more mobile and incur injuries and bleeding from falls.

Spontaneous bleeding, **hemarthrosis** (bleeding into a joint space), and deep tissue hemorrhage occur. Affected children frequently experience bleeding into the joint spaces of the knees, ankles, and elbows. Bleeding into joint spaces causes the child to have limited motion because of pain and swelling. Bone changes and flexion deformities can result from the effects of blood in the joint structures (Rodriguez-Merchan, 2012).

Males may have bleeding after circumcision. Other symptoms include easy bruising (**ecchymosis**), hematuria, and bleeding after tooth extraction, minor trauma, or minor surgical procedures. Subcutaneous, intramuscular hemorrhages and gastrointestinal bleeding can occur. Intracranial bleeding occurs in 10% of patients with severe hemophilia and has a mortality rate of 30%. Females who carry the trait for hemophilia do not usually manifest symptoms of the disease (Zaiden, Furlong, Crouch, et al., 2014).

CLINICAL THERAPY

Diagnosis of affected children and carriers can be done before birth through chorionic villus sampling or amniocentesis. Genetic testing of family members is increasingly being used to identify carriers. Diagnosis can also be made on the basis of the history, physical examination, and laboratory data. Laboratory tests show low levels of factor VIII or IX, and prolonged activated partial thromboplastin time (aPPT). Prothrombin time (PT), thrombin time (TT), fibrinogen, and platelet count are normal.

The goal of medical management is to control bleeding by replacing the missing clotting factor. Desmopressin (DDAVP), an analog of vasopressin, stimulates the release of factor VIII stored in the blood vessels, thereby increasing the percentage of available factor by approximately threefold. DDAVP is effective in some patients with mild and moderate hemophilia A (Roman, Larson, & Manno, 2013).

Many recombinant factor VIII concentrates are available as replacement therapy for hemophilia A (Zaiden et al., 2014). Factor IX concentrates are also available to treat hemophilia B (Zaiden, 2014). The child with severe hemophilia may be on a prophylactic regimen of replacement therapy, whereas the child with mild to moderate hemophilia may only receive episodic therapy. Prophylaxis decreases bleeding episodes and joint damage that may result from repeated episodes of hemarthrosis (Koerper, 2012). Prompt and adequate treatment is needed to prevent serious bleeding episodes and their sequelae. Gene therapy is being explored for treatment of hemophilia in hopes that an eventual cure will be found (Chuah, Evens, & Vandendriessche, 2013).

Nursing Management

For the Child With Hemophilia

Nursing Assessment and Diagnosis

PHYSIOLOGIC ASSESSMENT

Obtain a complete medical history from the parents or child. In particular, ask about previous episodes of bleeding and the occurrence of hemophilia or any other bleeding disorders in family members. The history of bleeding will vary, depending on the severity of the disease.

Assess the child for any joint pain, swelling, or permanent deformity, particularly around the knees, elbows, ankles, and shoulders. Observe for prolonged bleeding or oozing of blood. Note the presence of hematuria and mild flank pain. Conduct a neurologic assessment because the risk for intracranial hemorrhage and bleeding can lead to peripheral neuropathies.

PSYCHOSOCIAL ASSESSMENT

It is difficult for families to manage care of the child with hemophilia, especially if the disease is severe. Assess the family's coping mechanisms and support systems. Determine the family's ability to manage procedures and treatments; the factor concentrates and infusion equipment are costly. Assess older children's understanding of the disease, limitations, and their adaptation to the disease.

DEVELOPMENTAL ASSESSMENT

Because the child with hemophilia may have physical activity restrictions, physical skills may be delayed. Perform frequent developmental assessments, being particularly attentive to fine and gross motor skills.

The most important nursing diagnosis for the child with hemophilia is *Injury, Risk for,* related to bleeding disorder. Some of the other nursing diagnoses that might apply include the following (NANDA-I © 2014):

- *Pain* related to bleeding episodes
- *Mobility: Physical, Impaired,* related to joint stiffness or contractures
- *Home Maintenance, Impaired,* related to challenges of hemophilia
- *Family Processes, Interrupted,* related to family role shift required to care for a child with a chronic illness
- *Development: Delayed, Risk for,* related to effects of physical disability

Planning and Implementation

Nursing care focuses on preventing and controlling bleeding episodes, limiting joint involvement and managing pain, and providing emotional support. Both short-term interventions and long-term management are necessary.

PREVENT AND CONTROL BLEEDING EPISODES

Bleeding problems are rare in infants with hemophilia. However, as children learn to walk and develop other motor skills they often fall and suffer cuts and bruises. The risk of injury can be reduced by emphasizing to parents the need for close supervision and a safe environment. Parents should encourage children to play with safe, age-appropriate toys.

When the child is hospitalized, use nursing approaches to minimize the possibility of bleeding. Ensure that the hospital environment is safe by orienting the child to the room and keeping the floor and room clear of hazards as much as possible. If significant bleeding does occur, offer supportive measures and assist with factor replacement therapy. Carefully monitor the child's condition for any side effects when factor replacement therapy is administered. Control any superficial bleeding by applying pressure to the area for at least 15 minutes. Immobilize and elevate the affected area, and apply ice packs to promote vasoconstriction.

LIMIT JOINT INVOLVEMENT AND MANAGE PAIN

During bleeding episodes, hemarthrosis is managed by the administration of factor replacement as quickly as possible, elevating and immobilizing the joint and applying ice packs, and administering analgesics for pain. Once bleeding has been controlled, range-of-motion exercises strengthen muscles and joints and prevent flexion contractures. Physical therapy may be needed. Because excessive weight can place added stress on joints, encourage the child to maintain an appropriate weight.

PROVIDE EMOTIONAL SUPPORT

The needs of families with children who have hemophilia are best met through a comprehensive team approach. Refer the parents for genetic counseling as soon as possible after diagnosis. It is important to identify family members who carry the trait because they may suffer excessive bleeding during surgery.

Encourage the parents to verbalize their feelings. Be understanding and sensitive to their needs. Teach the parents about hemophilia and explain how the disorder affects both the child and other family members. Refer the parents and child to organizations such as the National Hemophilia Foundation for further information.

DISCHARGE PLANNING AND HOME CARE TEACHING

The child may be hospitalized briefly during the first manifestation of bleeding for diagnosis and management. Most care will subsequently take place in the home. Home care needs should be identified and addressed well in advance of discharge. Advise parents to have the child wear a medical identification bracelet. Dentists and all other healthcare providers should be aware of the diagnosis.

Explain the cause of bleeding so both the child and parents understand the disease process. Teach the child and family how to identify internal bleeding. Signs and symptoms such as joint pain, abdominal pain, and obvious bleeding are indicators for immediate factor infusion. Make sure the child and parents know what situations could cause bleeding to occur. Teach parents to give acetaminophen instead of aspirin and aspirin-containing products.

Instruct the parents and the child, when appropriate, to prepare and administer factor concentrate. If infusion of the missing factor is scheduled regularly, bleeding episodes can be controlled or avoided. Have the parents demonstrate the procedure and make sure they can administer the product correctly. Ensure that parents know where they can get the factor concentrate.

The child will need an individualized school health plan (see Chapter 12). Members of the school staff should be instructed in management of emergencies. The nurse can identify key staff members in the school and teach them the actions that need to be taken.

Help the family and school in planning an appropriate schedule of activities for the child. Explain how the parents can coordinate their child's care with a number of healthcare professionals. Provide ongoing case management, assisting the family to take on this task if able.

Hemophilia is a debilitating disorder for the child, and it also can be financially draining for the family. Frequent outpatient visits, emergency department visits, hospital admissions, and the cost of factor replacement can exhaust a family's resources. If indicated, refer families to appropriate social services (e.g., the state's maternal and child health program for children with special healthcare needs) and organizations such as the National Hemophilia Foundation. Sharing experiences with other families of children with hemophilia can provide support.

Evaluation

Expected outcomes of nursing care include the following:

- Injury to the child is prevented.
- Pain is managed to promote comfort level.
- The nurse and family promote normal growth and development for the child.
- The child and family have adequate knowledge of disease management, including recognition of bleeding and prompt initiation of infusions.

Clinical Tip

Use the acronym RICE (**r**est, **i**ce, **c**ompression, **e**levation) to help you remember important measures to control a bleeding episode.

Clinical Tip

Take the following precautions when caring for children with bleeding disorders:

- Avoid taking temperatures rectally or giving suppositories.
- Avoid intramuscular injections unless absolutely necessary and only after factor replacement has been given. Children should receive recommended immunizations subcutaneously with firm pressure to the injection site for 5 minutes following the injection.
- Apply firm, continuous pressure to venipuncture sites 5 minutes after any venipuncture procedure.
- Do not give aspirin or aspirin-containing products.

Von Willebrand Disease

Von Willebrand disease is the most common hereditary bleeding disorder. The various subtypes of this disorder are classified based on the amount and functionality of the von Willebrand factor (vWF), a plasma protein and the carrier for clotting factor VIII.

The most common form of the disorder is transmitted as an autosomal dominant trait, and can occur in both males and females (Acharya, 2014).

The characteristic manifestations are prolonged and excessive mucocutaneous bleeding. In children, this is generally exhibited through easy bruising and recurrent epistaxis. Increased bleeding also occurs during surgery and dental extractions. Affected female teenagers may have menorrhagia (increased menstrual bleeding) (Acharya, 2014; Weickert, Miesbach, Alesci, et al., 2014).

Growth and Development

Encourage children with hemophilia to participate in leisure activities such as computer games, reading clubs, and crafts as well as social clubs such as Boy Scouts. Swimming, bicycle riding, hiking, and other noncontact sports are excellent options for the child. Protective equipment appropriate to the sport or recreational activity the child is participating in should be worn. Activities important to development can be encouraged when coaches, teachers, and others know how to treat bleeding episodes.

Diagnosis of von Willebrand disease is made after laboratory studies reveal decreased von Willebrand factor levels, von Willebrand factor antigen levels, and factor VIII activity; reduced platelet agglutination; and prolonged or normal activated partial thromboplastin time (aPPT).

Treatment is similar to that for the child with hemophilia and involves infusion of von Willebrand protein concentrate. Desmopressin (DDAVP) is administered to promote release of stored vWF and to prevent bleeding associated with dental or surgical procedures (Thiagarajan, 2014).

Nursing Management

Teach parents about the disorder and instruct them not to give the child any aspirin or other drugs that can cause bleeding or inhibit platelet function. Teach management of bleeding episodes and intravenous infusion techniques, as for hemophilia. The prognosis is good, and children with von Willebrand disease usually have a normal life expectancy. Expected outcomes of nursing care include prompt management of bleeding and prevention of disease complications.

Disseminated Intravascular Coagulation

Disseminated intravascular coagulation (DIC) is a life-threatening, acquired pathologic process in which the clotting system is abnormally activated, resulting in widespread clot formation in the small vessels throughout the body. Excess thrombin is generated, followed by deposition of fibrin strands in body tissues. The circulating fibrin fragments later begin to interfere with platelet aggregation and other aspects of the clotting mechanism, resulting in bleeding or hemorrhage (LeMone, Burke, Bauldoff, et al., 2015).

The most common cause of DIC is sepsis. Infections caused by gram-negative and gram-positive bacteria, fungi, viruses, and protozoa may lead to DIC (LeMone et al., 2015). Symptoms can include gingival bleeding, mucosal bleeding, hemoptysis, petechiae, purpura, bruising, oozing of blood after an injection, hematuria, frank bleeding from incisions, tachycardia, and hypotension (LeMone et al., 2015; Levi & Schmaier, 2014).

Medical management includes platelet and factor replacement so that platelets and clotting factors are restored. Although controversial, heparin may be administered to treat uncontrolled thrombosis (LeMone et al., 2015; Levi & Schmaier, 2014).

Nursing Management

Disseminated intravascular coagulation is a complex disorder managed by a critical care team. Nursing care focuses on assessing the bleeding, preventing further injury, and administering prescribed therapies. Observe for petechiae, ecchymoses, and all body orifices and skin breaks for oozing every 1 to 2 hours. Careful monitoring of dependent areas is essential because blood will pool in these locations. Intravenous sites are particularly prone to oozing and should be assessed every 15 minutes. Examine stool for the presence of blood, and measure blood loss as accurately as possible. Measure intake and output.

Because all body systems can be involved, careful, continuous assessment of all systems is needed. Institute bleeding control precautions, monitor prescribed therapy (transfusion, anticoagulant therapy), and report any signs of complications. Desired outcomes of nursing care are management of bleeding and adequate function of all body systems. Adequate family support in this life-threatening situation is a focus of nursing care.

Immune Thrombocytopenic Purpura

Immune thrombocytopenic purpura (ITP), also known as *idiopathic thrombocytopenic purpura,* is a bleeding disorder characterized by increased destruction of platelets in the spleen. Platelets are destroyed as a result of the binding of autoantibodies to platelet antigens (Kessler & Sandler, 2014). When the rate of platelet destruction exceeds the rate of platelet production, the number of circulating platelets decreases and blood clotting slows. The cause of ITP is unknown, but it usually follows an infectious illness.

Symptoms include multiple ecchymoses and petechiae and mucosal bleeding in the mouth or nose. Diagnosis is made by history and through physical and laboratory findings, which show a decreased platelet count (generally less than 20,000 mm^3/dL) (Kessler & Sandler, 2014; Warrier & Chauhan, 2012). The child has normal hemoglobin and white blood cell counts. A bone marrow aspiration may be performed to rule out other diagnoses (Warrier & Chauhan, 2012).

Patients with a platelet count greater than 10,000 and little bleeding may be carefully observed without the need for additional treatment. Modalities of treatment vary among healthcare providers and may include corticosteroids, intravenous immune globulin (IVIG), and intravenous anti-D immunoglobulin. Platelet administration is not generally an aspect of treatment, except in cases of severe hemorrhage (Heiner & Morgan, 2014). With ITP, platelet administration will control bleeding temporarily since the administered platelets will be destroyed.

It is estimated that 20% of children with ITP will develop chronic disease (Warrier & Chauhan, 2012). Children who fail to respond to treatment for acute ITP and persist with thrombocytopenia for longer than 12 months are considered to have chronic ITP (Generali & Cada, 2013). Splenectomy may be an option for children with persistent or chronic disease, significant bleeding, lack of response to drug therapy, or altered quality of life (Neunert, 2011).

Nursing Management

Nursing care focuses on controlling and reducing the number of bleeding episodes. Preventive measures are similar to those for the child with hemophilia. Teach parents to use acetaminophen, rather than aspirin, to control pain. Provide emotional support to the family. Have the child avoid contact sports. Perform careful assessments of bleeding and take vital signs. Expected outcomes of care are prevention of bleeding and restoration of normal coagulation patterns.

Hematopoietic Stem Cell Transplantation

Hematopoietic stem cell transplantation (HSCT) is a treatment used for diseases such as severe combined immunodeficiency disease, severe and unresponsive aplastic anemia, and leukemia (refer to Chapters 22 and 24). Hematopoietic stem cells exist primarily in the bone marrow but also circulate in the peripheral blood. These cells can grow into new body cells, and have become useful in treatment of immune and hematologic diseases when restoration of normal cells is needed. Stem cells can be obtained from bone marrow, cord blood, or peripheral blood (Kolins, Zbylut, McCollom, et al., 2011; Moore & Ikeda, 2014).

Hematopoietic stem cell transplants are either autologous or allogeneic. In **autologous transplantation**, the child's own marrow is taken, treated, stored, and reinfused after the child has received chemotherapy. **Allogeneic transplantation** may be syngeneic (from an identical twin), related, or unrelated. In allogeneic transplantation, the donor, often a sibling (related), has a compatible human leukocyte antigen (HLA). HLAs are proteins found on the surface of nearly all nucleated cells within the body, and they are responsible for regulating the immune response. When no relative is found to match the child, a histocompatible donor (unrelated) may be sought from the National Marrow Donor Program or a cord blood bank (Kolins et al., 2011; Moore & Ikeda, 2014). With the development of this registry, bone marrow transplantation from HLA-matched unrelated donors has become possible for some children.

The transplantation procedure begins with chemotherapy and, sometimes, total body irradiation directed at destroying circulating blood cells and the diseased bone marrow in the ill child. The chemotherapy program for destruction of bone marrow ranges from 7 to 10 days (Moore & Ikeda, 2014). During this time, the child is cared for in strict isolation in a special unit that provides a germ-free environment (Figure 23–4). Following

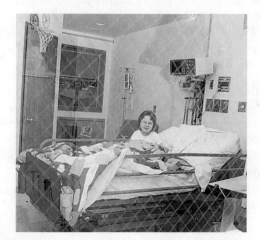

Figure 23–4 The child undergoing bone marrow transplantation is hospitalized in a special sterile unit while receiving chemotherapy before the transfusion. The child remains in the unit for several weeks afterward until the new marrow produces enough cells to maintain health.

the immunosuppression procedure, the child receives an intravenous transfusion with the donor stem cells. This procedure is similar to administration of a blood product. The healthy stem cells migrate to the bone marrow. Healthy bone marrow, capable of making blood cells, is the anticipated result. If the transplantation is successful, the cells implant in the child's marrow and begin to produce blood cells within approximately 2 to 4 weeks.

Pancytopenia (marked decrease in RBCs, WBCs, and platelets) lasts for several weeks following the transplant. Major risks during this period are anemia, infections, and bleeding. Once the bone marrow begins to produce new cells, graft-versus-host disease (rejection) is the major threat. Refer to Chapter 22 for a discussion of graft-versus-host disease.

Monitor the child undergoing HSCT by assessing the skin, mucous membranes, gastrointestinal function, respiratory function, cardiac function, and hydration status. Because graft-versus-host disease may occur at any time, even after the child returns home, frequent thorough assessments are necessary after discharge.

Supportive care after the transplantation procedure focuses on preventing infection, controlling bleeding, maintaining a nutritious diet and hydration, monitoring for signs of rejection, and providing psychosocial support. The treatment is lengthy, the child is often critically ill, and parents may have traveled to a medical center many miles from home for the procedure. Ask parents about other family members and how they are managing. Provide information about inexpensive housing available near the medical center. Encourage parents to discuss their feelings with other parents of children receiving bone marrow transplantation. Organizations such as the Bone Marrow Transplant Family Support Network can serve as resources for families.

When the child is ready for discharge, be sure the family is prepared to administer medications, recognize signs of graft-versus-host disease, provide adequate nutrition for the child, and perform other necessary care. Arrange for follow-up visits and provide the names of local healthcare contact people who can offer support and provide information. The child may need tutors or other educational assistance to promote integration back into the school setting. The major expected outcome of nursing care is the proper activity of bone marrow in the child with resulting normal levels and function of blood cells. Other outcomes are provision of family support, ongoing care and education for the child, adequate nutrition, and prevention of infection. See *Health Promotion: The Child With Hematopoietic Stem Cell Transplantation (HSCT)*.

Health Promotion The Child With Hematopoietic Stem Cell Transplantation (HSCT)

Growth and Development

- Measure and plot height and weight at each visit using standard growth curve charts.
- Measure onset and progression of puberty using Tanner staging.
- An individualized education plan (IEP) should be performed yearly to identify learning problems.
- Routine hearing screening is advised since hearing loss may occur as a result of ototoxic drug therapy.
- Vision should be screened at each primary care visit since corticosteroid use can cause cataracts, graft-versus-host disease (GVHD) can result in keratoconjunctivitis, and cytomegalovirus (CMV) can cause retinitis.
- Blood pressure should be monitored at each visit because children are commonly placed on medication for hypertension after HSCT because of nephrotoxic medications.
- Instruct parents to measure and record blood pressure at home if necessary.

Nutrition

- Teach family to avoid foods with potential vectors for infection, such as unpasteurized products and undercooked meats.
- A low-sodium diet may be required if the child has hypertension.
- Calcium supplements may be administered to reduce the risk of osteopenia.

Physical Activity

- If the child has thrombocytopenia, physical activity may be restricted.
- The child may experience fatigue. Ask about activity tolerance.

Oral Health

- Dental screening and any required restorative care should be done before transplant to reduce potential sources of infection.
- Routine dental care is resumed once the child's immune system is restored. Ask the family about the child's routine dental care.

Mental and Spiritual Health

- Apply developmental approaches to assess the child's feelings after a HSCT.
- Ask the child about coping with being in the hospital and at home rather than attending school.
- Many physical changes occur with treatment that may interfere with body image. Assess the child's or adolescent's body image in a manner appropriate to age.

Relationships

- In-hospital or in-home schooling is required after HSCT for 6 to 12 months until immune function has been obtained to reduce the risk of infection.
- Encourage peer contact, telephone calls, e-mail, and letters to reduce the child's feelings of isolation.
- On returning to school, the child is encouraged to participate fully in school activities.
- For the adolescent, sex education is important, especially to avoid sexually transmitted infections.

Disease Prevention Strategies

- Teach the family that hand hygiene is essential to prevent the spread of infection.
- Dishes should be washed in a dishwasher. Teach safe food preparation techniques.

- In-home child care is recommended because of the risk of infection in other childcare settings.
- Teach the family that the child should have minimal direct contact with animals to avoid infections.

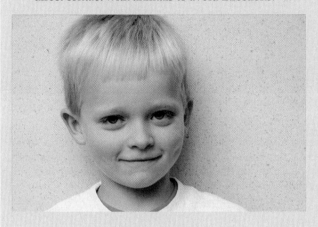

- Determine the child's need for an altered immunization schedule after HSTC.
- Instruct parents to monitor the child for infection and report any temperature elevation to the healthcare provider.
- Encourage the family to obtain an influenza vaccine annually for the child and all household or close contacts.
- Teach signs and symptoms of infection and stress the importance of prompt reporting.

Injury Prevention Strategies
- Review safe medication storage with the family.
- Help the family develop a plan for the safe disposal of used needles and syringes.

Chapter Highlights

- Erythrocytes (red blood cells) are a major component of the blood and transport oxygen from the lungs to body tissues.
- Polycythemia is an increase in the number of red blood cells. Anemia is characterized by a decrease in red blood cell number.
- Leukocytes (white blood cells) are important in the cell's defenses against disease.
- Thrombocytes (platelets) are necessary for normal clotting of blood.
- The major anemias of childhood include iron deficiency anemia, normocytic anemia, sickle cell disease, thalassemia, hereditary spherocytosis, and aplastic anemia.
- Sickle cell disease is a genetic disease in which an abnormal shape, or sickling, of red blood cells prevents the normal flow of blood.
- Children with sickle cell disease are at risk for vaso-occlusive (pain) crisis, splenic sequestration, and aplastic crisis.
- Complications of sickle cell disease include stroke, acute chest syndrome with pulmonary infiltrate and infection, priapism, retinopathy, kidney damage, and gallstone formation.
- Nurses assist families in dealing with chronic diseases such as sickle cell disease by providing information about the disorder and resources that can provide assistance, monitoring child growth and development, instituting preventive care, and managing exacerbations of the disease.
- The thalassemias are a group of genetic diseases of red blood cells, which cause defective synthesis of hemoglobin.

- Children who receive chronic blood transfusions for sickle cell disease or thalassemia are at risk to develop iron overload and may need to receive an iron-chelating drug such as deferoxamine or deferasirox (Exjade).
- Hereditary spherocytosis (HS) is a hemolytic disorder in which the erythrocytes assume a spherical shape due to an intrinsic membrane defect. The erythrocytes are retained and removed by the spleen, leading to splenomegaly in the child.
- Aplastic anemia is a deficiency of all blood cells related to poor bone marrow function; it can be congenital or acquired after exposure to certain drugs or harmful environmental toxins.
- Hemophilia is a bleeding disorder transmitted by genes; hemophilia A is most common and results in a decrease in clotting factor VIII.
- The goal of treatment for hemophilia is to control bleeding by preventive care and replacement of the missing factor.
- Major nursing concerns for the child with hemophilia include managing bleeding episodes, controlling pain during bleeds, minimizing physical immobility, supporting the family in learning management of this chronic disease, and explaining genetic implications of the disease.
- Von Willebrand disease is a hereditary bleeding disorder characterized by a deficiency of von Willebrand factor, a plasma protein that is a carrier for clotting factor VIII.
- Disseminated intravascular coagulation is a serious condition in which clotting mechanisms are disturbed, leading to extensive clotting and tissue damage.

- Immune thrombocytopenic purpura causes destruction of platelets and most frequently follows a childhood viral disease.

- Management of immune thrombocytopenic purpura includes corticosteroids, intravenous immune globulin (IVIG), and intravenous anti-D immunoglobulin. The disease is considered to be autoimmune in nature.

- Hematopoietic stem cell transplant (HSCT) is a useful treatment in some diseases of the hematologic system and some cancers; it involves infusion of bone marrow, peripheral stem cells, or neonatal stem cells from a donor into the blood of the recipient where it circulates, implants into the bone marrow, and begins making new blood cells.

- Nursing care before and after HSCT includes infection prevention, careful physical assessment, administration of medications, and support for the family.

Clinical Reasoning in Action

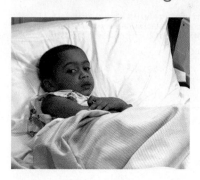

Frederick is admitted to the hospital with severe abdominal pain. He has been hospitalized for his sickle cell disease several times in the past and now, as an 8-year-old, he and his mother are very familiar with the routine. The disease is stable most of the time, but about twice annually he is admitted to the hospital for complications of the disorder. His mother expresses how upsetting it is to watch her son suffer pain from this disease.

In the hospital, a priority nursing intervention is to control Frederick's pain. The doctor diagnoses that the abdominal pain is caused by sickled cells in his spleen. Frederick's hemoglobin is 6 g/dL, and a blood transfusion is ordered. Fluids and oxygen are also administered. Frequent vital signs and other monitoring are performed to identify any infections.

1. Besides correcting the anemia, what is another reason Frederick would be given a transfusion?

2. What is happening to Frederick's spleen such that it is causing his abdominal pain?

3. In what way does sickle cell disease affect the various systems of the body?

4. When giving a blood transfusion to Frederick, should warm or cold blood be given? What is the reason for your answer?

References

Abrams, S. A. (2014). *Iron requirements and iron deficiency in adolescents*. Retrieved from www.uptodate.com

Acharya, S. S. (2014). *Pediatric Von Willebrand disease*. Retrieved from http://emedicine.medscape.com/article/959825-overview

Bakhshi, S. (2014). *Aplastic anemia*. Retrieved from http://emedicine.medscape.com/article/198759-overview

Centers for Disease Control and Prevention. (2014). *What you should know about sickle cell trait*. Retrieved from http://www.cdc.gov/ncbddd/sicklecell/documents/SCD%20factsheetSickle%20Cell%20Trait.pdf

Centers for Disease Control and Prevention. (2015). *Summary of recommendations for child/teen immunization*. Retrieved from http://www.immunize.org/catg.d/p2010.pdf

Christensen, R. D., & Ohls, R. K. (2016). Development of the hematopoietic system. In R. M. Kliegman, B. F. Stanton, J. W. St. Geme III, & N. F. Schor (Eds.), *Nelson textbook of pediatrics* (20th ed., p. 2304–2309). Philadelphia, PA: Elsevier Saunders.

Chuah, M. K., Evens, H., & Vandendriessche, T. (2013). Gene therapy for hemophilia. *Journal of Thrombosis and Haemostasis, 11*(Suppl 1), 99–110.

Das, A., Bansal, D., Ahluwalia, J., Das, R., Rohit, M. K., Attri, S. V., . . . Marwaha, R. K. (2014). Risk factors for thromboembolism and pulmonary artery hypertension following splenectomy in children with hereditary spherocytosis. *Pediatric Blood and Cancer, 61*(1), 29–33.

DeBaun, M. R., Frei-Jones, M., & Vichinsky, E. (2016). Hemoglobinopathies. In R. M. Kliegman, B. F.

Stanton, J. W. St. Geme III, & N. F. Schor (Eds.), *Nelson textbook of pediatrics* (20th ed., pp. 2336–2353). Philadelphia, PA: Elsevier Saunders.

de Montalembert, M., Ferster, A., Colombatti, R., Rees, D. C., & Gulbis, B. (2011). ENERCA clinical recommendations for disease management and prevention of complications of sickle cell disease in children. *American Journal of Hematology, 86*(1), 72–75.

Dobson, C. E., & Byrne, M. W. (2014). Using guided imagery to manage pain in young children with sickle cell disease. *American Journal of Nursing, 114*(4), 26–36.

Ender, K. L., Krajewski, J. A., Babineau, J., Tresgallo, M., Schechter, W., Saroyan, J. M., & Kharbanda, A. (2014). Use of a clinical pathway to improve the acute management of vaso-occlusive crisis pain in pediatric sickle cell disease. *Pediatric Blood & Cancer, 61*(4), 693–696.

Generali, J. A., & Cada, D. J. (2013). Dexamethasone: Idiopathic thrombocytopenic purpura in children and adolescents. *Hospital Pharmacy, 48*(2), 108–110.

Giardina, P. J., & Rivella, S. (2013). Thalassemia syndromes. In R. Hoffman, E. J. Benz, L. E. Silberstein, H. Heslop, J. I. Weitz, & J. Anastasi (Eds.), *Hematology: Basic principles and practice* (6th ed., pp. 505–535). Philadelphia, PA: Elsevier Saunders.

Gonzalez, G., & Eichner, E. R. (2014). *Hereditary spherocytosis*. Retrieved from http://emedicine.medscape.com/article/206107-overview

Greenbaum, L. A. (2016). Vitamin K deficiency. In R. M. Kliegman, B. F. Stanton, J. W. St. Geme III, & N. F.

Schor (Eds.), *Nelson textbook of pediatrics* (20th ed., pp. 342–343). Philadelphia, PA: Elsevier Saunders.

Harper, J. L., & Conrad, M. E. (2014). *Iron deficiency anemia*. Retrieved from http://emedicine.medscape.com/article/202333-overview

Hartung, H. D., Olson, T. S., & Bessler, M. (2013). Acquired aplastic anemia in children. *Pediatric Clinics of North America, 60*(6), 1311–1336.

Heiner, J. D., & Morgan, T. L. (2014). Progressive bruising in an otherwise healthy child: Immune thrombocytopenia purpura. *Canadian Journal of Emergency Medicine, 16*(2), 158–159.

Hsiao, M., Sathya, C., Nathens, A. B., de Mestral, C., Hill, A. D., & Langer, J. C. (2013). Is activity restriction appropriate for patients with hereditary spherocytosis? A population-based analysis. *Annals of Hematology, 92*(4), 523–525.

Inati, A., Khoriaty, E., & Musallam, K. M. (2011). Iron in sickle-cell disease: What have we learned over the years? *Pediatric Blood and Cancer, 56*, 182–190.

Kessler, C. M., & Sandler, S. G. (2014). *Immune thrombocytopenic purpura*. Retrieved from http://emedicine.medscape.com/article/202158-overview

Koerper, M. (2011). *Keeping up to date on prophylaxis and treatment strategies in patients with hemophilia*. Retrieved from http://www.medscape.org/viewarticle/750012

Kolins, J. A., Zbylut, C., McCollom, S., & Aquino, V. M. (2011). Hematopoietic stem cell transplantation in children. *Critical Care Nursing Clinics of North America, 23,* 349–376.

LeMone, P., Burke, K. M., Bauldoff, G., & Gubrud, P. (2015). Nursing care of patients with hematologic disorders. In P. LeMone, K. M. Burke, G. Bauldoff, & P. Gubrud (Eds.), *Medical surgical nursing: Clinical Reasoning in Patient Care* (6th ed., pp. 1014–1061). Hoboken, NJ: Pearson.

Lerner, N. B. (2016). The anemias. In R. M. Kliegman, B. F. Stanton, J. W. St. Geme III, & N. F. Schor (Eds.), *Nelson textbook of pediatrics* (20th ed., pp. 2309–2312). Philadelphia, PA: Elsevier Saunders.

Levi, M. M., & Schmaier, A. H. (2014). *Disseminated intravascular coagulation*. Retrieved from http://emedicine.medscape.com/article/199627-overview

Lo, S. F. (2016). Reference intervals for laboratory tests and procedures. In R. M. Kliegman, B. F. Stanton, J. W. St. Geme, & N. F. Schor (Eds.), *Nelson textbook of pediatrics* (20th ed., pp. 3464–3473). Philadelphia, PA: Elsevier.

Lovett, P. B., Sule, H. P., & Lopez, B. L. (2014). Sickle cell disease in the emergency department. *Emergency Medicine Clinics of North America, 32*(3), 629–647.

Maakaron, J. E., & Taher, A. T. (2014). *Sickle cell anemia*. Retrieved from http://emedicine.medscape.com/article/205926-overview

Mahoney, D. H. (2014). *Iron deficiency in infants and young children: Screening, prevention, clinical manifestations, and diagnosis*. Retrieved from www.uptodate.com

March of Dimes. (2014). *Sickle cell disease and your baby*. Retrieved from http://www.marchofdimes.org/baby/sickle-cell-disease-and-your-baby.aspx

Meier, E. R., & Miller, J. L. (2012). Sickle cell disease in children. *Drugs, 72*(7), 895–906.

Moore, T., & Ikeda, A. K. (2014). *Bone marrow transplantation*. Retrieved from http://emedicine.medscape.com/article/1014514-overview

Myers, M., & Eckes, E. J. (2012). A novel approach to pain management in persons with sickle cell disease. *MEDSURG Nursing, 21*(5), 293–298.

National Newborn Screening and Genetics Resource Center. (2014). *National Newborn Screening Status Report*. Retrieved from http://genes-r-us.uthscsa.edu/sites/genes-r-us/files/nbsdisorders.pdf

Neunert, C. (2011). Idiopathic thrombocytopenic purpura: Advances in management. *Clinical Advances in Hematology & Oncology, 9*(5), 404–406.

Ozgonenel, B., Zia, A., Callaghan, M. U., Chitlur, M., Rajpurkar, M., & Lusher, J. M. (2013). Emergency department visits in children with hemophilia. *Pediatric Blood and Cancer, 60*(7), 1188–1191.

Panepinto, J. A., Punzalan, R. C., & Scott, J. P. (2015). Hematology. In K. J. Marcdante & R. M. Kliegman (Eds.), *Nelson essentials of pediatrics* (7th ed., pp. 506–533). Philadelphia, PA: Elsevier Saunders.

Powers, J. M., & Buchanan, G. R. (2014). Iron deficiency anemia in toddlers to teens: How to manage when prevention fails. *Contemporary Pediatrics, 31*(5), 12–17.

Rodriguez-Merchan, E. C. (2012). Prevention of the musculoskeletal complications of hemophilia. *Advances in Preventive Medicine, 2012,* 1–8.

Roman, E., Larson, P. J., & Manno, C. S. (2013). Transfusion therapy for coagulation factor deficiencies. In R. Hoffman, E. J. Benz, L. E. Silberstein, H. Heslop, J. I. Weitz, & J. Anastasi (Eds.), *Hematology: Basic principles and practice* (6th ed., pp. 1705–1715). Philadelphia, PA: Elsevier Saunders.

Saunthararajah, Y., & Vichinsky, E. P. (2013). Sickle cell disease: Clinical features and management. In R. Hoffman, E. J. Benz, L. E. Silberstein, H. Heslop, J. I. Weitz, & J. Anastasi (Eds.), *Hematology: Basic principles and practice* (6th ed., pp. 548–572). Philadelphia, PA: Elsevier Saunders.

Scott, J. P. (2016). Factor VIII or factor IX deficiency (hemophilia A or B). In R. M. Kliegman, B. F. Stanton, J. W. St. Geme III, & N. F. Schor (Eds.), *Nelson textbook of pediatrics* (20th ed., pp. 2384–2388). Philadelphia, PA: Elsevier Saunders.

Scott, J. P., & Raffini, L. J. (2016). Hemostasis. In R. M. Kliegman, B. F. Stanton, J. W. St. Geme III, & N. F. Schor (Eds.), *Nelson textbook of pediatrics* (20th ed., pp. 2379–2381). Philadelphia, PA: Elsevier Saunders.

Segel, G. B., & Casey, D. (2016). Hereditary spherocytosis. In R. M. Kliegman, B. F. Stanton, J. W. St. Geme III, & N. F. Schor (Eds.), *Nelson textbook of pediatrics* (20th ed., pp 2330–2333). Philadelphia, PA: Elsevier Saunders.

Shihabuddin, B. S., & Scarfi, C. A. (2014). Fever in children with sickle cell disease: Are all fevers equal? *The Journal of Emergency Medicine, 47*(4), 395–400.

Sickle Cell Information Center. (2012). *FAQ: Sickle cell disease*. Retrieved from https://scinfo.org/faq/faq-sickle-cell-disease

Soldin, S. J., Wong, E. C., Brugnara, C., & Soldin, O. P. (2011). *Pediatric reference ranges* (7th ed.). Washington, DC: AACC Press.

Strouse, J. J., & Heeney, M. M. (2012). Hydroxyurea for the treatment of sickle cell disease: Efficacy, barriers, toxicity, and management in children. *Pediatric Blood & Cancer, 59,* 365–371.

Tanabe, P., Dias, N., & Gorman, L. (2013). Care of children with sickle cell disease in the emergency department: Parent and provider perspectives inform quality improvement efforts. *Journal of Pediatric Oncology Nursing, 30*(4), 205–217.

Thiagarajan, P. (2014). *Platelet disorders*. Retrieved from http://emedicine.medscape.com/article/201722-overview\#aw2aab6c21

Vichinsky, E. P. (2014). *Variant sickle cell syndromes*. Retrieved from uptodate.com

Walovich, K. J., & Newberger, P. E. (2016). Leukopenia. In R. M. Kliegman, B. F. Stanton, J. W. St. Geme III, & N. F. Schor (Eds.), *Nelson textbook of pediatrics* (20th ed., pp. 1047–1053). Philadelphia, PA: Elsevier Saunders.

Warrier, R., & Chauhan, A. (2012). Management of immune thrombocytopenic purpura. *The Ochsner Journal, 12*(3), 221–227.

Weickert, L., Miesbach, W., Alesci, S. J., Eickholz, P., & Nickles, K. (2014). Is gingival bleeding a symptom of type 1 von Willebrand disease? A case-control study. *Journal of Clinical Peridontology, 41,* 766–771.

Yawn, B. P., Buchanan, G. R., Afenyi-Annan, A. N., Ballas, S. K., Hassell, K. L., James, A. H., . . . John-Sowah, J. (2014). Management of sickle cell disease: Summary of the 2014 evidence-based report by expert panel members. *JAMA, 312*(10), 1033–1048.

Zaiden, R. A. (2014). *Hemophilia B*. Retrieved from http://emedicine.medscape.com/article/779434-overview

Zaiden, R. A., Furlong, M. A., Crouch, G. D., & Besa, E. C. (2014). *Hemophilia A*. Retrieved from http://emedicine.medscape.com/article/779322-overview

Zempsky, W. T., Corsi, J. M., & McKay, K. (2011). Pain scores: Are they used in sickle cell pain? *Pediatric Emergency Care, 27*(1), 27–28

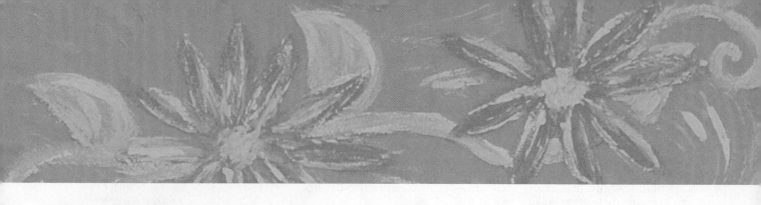

Chapter 24
The Child With Cancer

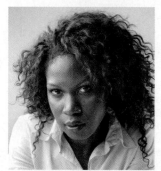

Rasheed was just diagnosed with leukemia seven months ago, but already he has been in the hospital five times. This time he had enterocolitis, an infection of the intestines. But he has now improved and is determined to fight the disease. It's his will and strength that help us all to be strong and to know that he will do well after his treatment is finished.

—Mother of Rasheed, 12 years old

Ollyy/Shutterstock

⌄ Learning Outcomes

24.1 Describe the incidence, known etiologies, and common clinical manifestations of cancer.

24.2 Synthesize information about diagnostic tests and clinical therapy for cancer to plan comprehensive care for children undergoing these procedures.

24.3 Integrate information about oncologic emergencies into plans for monitoring all children with cancer.

24.4 Recognize the most common solid tumors in children, describe their treatment, and plan comprehensive nursing care.

24.5 Plan care for children and adolescents of all ages who have a diagnosis of leukemia.

24.6 Prioritize elements of comprehensive care planning for children with soft-tissue tumors.

24.7 Analyze the impact of cancer survival on children and use this information to plan for ongoing physiologic and psychosocial care in the children's futures.

Cancer is a daunting diagnosis at any age, but in children, it seems even more profound. The diagnosis and treatment are met with shock and disbelief, they require a change in the roles of everyone in the family, and challenge all children and families involved in many ways. Nurses who work in pediatric oncology have unique opportunities to assist children and families in mobilizing resources and learning about maximizing physical, emotional, and developmental health while dealing with the challenges of the illness and treatment.

Why do children develop different types of cancers than adults? Cancer in adults is often the result of dietary practices or habits such as smoking. Some adult-onset cancers are the result of oncogenic responses to stimuli—that is, responses that stimulate cancerous changes in cells. Other cancers that occur in adults result from prolonged exposure to toxins such as coal dust and asbestos. Some cancers are known to be related to genetic causes. In adults, prevention through general lifestyle changes is a major focus of interventions. However, in children, cancer is usually embryonic (occurring during development of the fetus) or oncogenic in origin. Thus, lifestyle changes that begin in childhood have little effect on the incidence of childhood cancer, although they may help reduce the incidence of later cancer or other diseases. Occasionally, an environmental exposure is linked to the incidence of cancer in children.

Text continues on page 613

FOCUS ON:
Cellular Growth

Anatomy and Physiology

Abnormal cellular growth can occur in any area of the body. Why are some growths called cancer and others are not? Changes in cellular growth within the body are called neoplasms (meaning new growth). A neoplasm is further classified as benign or malignant. **Benign** means that a growth does not endanger life or health; it tends not to recur after treatment. **Malignant** means that progressive growth of the tumor will, if not checked by treatment, spread to other sites in the body (**metastasis**), resulting in death. The common term for this type of cellular growth is *cancer*.

Pediatric Differences

Cancers in children often have different etiology than those in adults. Most adult cancers are epithelial in origin, whereas in children the nonepithelial or embryonal cell types predominate. While many adult cancers are slow-growing and result from exposure to carcinogens over time, most childhood cancers are fast-growing, so that a child who appears healthy becomes ill over a period of days or weeks. Different types of cancers predominate at various ages in childhood, demonstrating the multiple causes and their relationship to age and development (Figure 24–1).

Although not common, some neonates have cancer that is diagnosed soon after birth. The types of cancers most common in this age group include brain tumors, neuroblastoma, leukemia, retinoblastoma, and teratomas (arising from primary germ layers). While treatments are usually as effective in neonates as in older children, rapid growth at this age makes side effects of therapy more serious.

A major physiologic difference between adults and children that affects cellular growth involves the immune system, which plays a part in preventing some cancers but functions immaturely in the young child (see the following text for further description of immune immaturity). The rate of cell growth in children can also play a role in the rapidity with which some childhood cancers progress. The continuing presence of fetal cells in small children is related to some cancers. These immature cells decrease and finally disappear as children grow but can be related to cancers such as neuroblastoma in very young children.

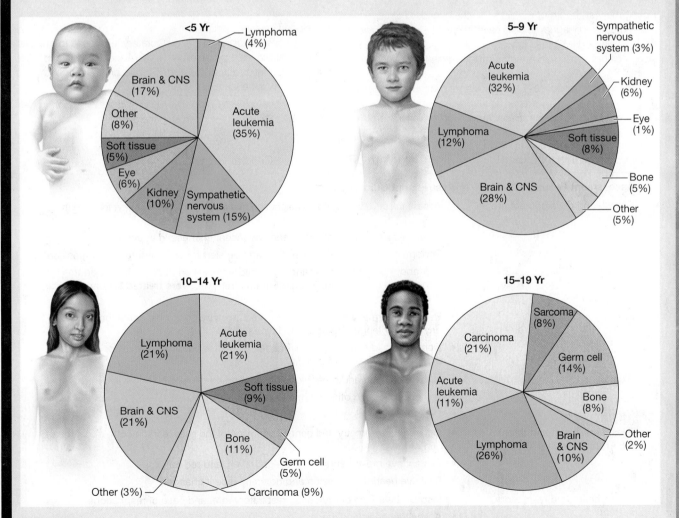

Figure 24–1 **Percentage of primary tumors by site of origin for different age groups.**

SOURCE: Data from Asselin, B. (2011). Epidemiology of childhood and adolescent cancer. In R. M. Kliegman, B. F. Stanton, J. W. St. Geme, N. F. Schor, & R. E. Behrman (Eds.), *Nelson textbook of pediatrics* (19th ed., pp. 1725–1727). Philadelphia, PA: Elsevier Saunders.

(continued)

TABLE 24–1 Diagnostic Procedures and Laboratory Tests for Cancer

DIAGNOSTIC PROCEDURES	LABORATORY TESTS
Biopsy	Complete blood count (CBC) with differential
Bone marrow aspiration and biopsy	Red and white blood cell indices
Computed tomography (CT) and computerized axial tomography (CAT)	Serum chemistry panel
Lumbar puncture	Tumor markers
Magnetic resonance imaging (MRI)	Urinalysis
Positron emission tomography (PET) scan and single-photon emission computed tomography (SPECT)	
Radiograph (x-ray)	
Nuclear medicine scans	
Ultrasound	

The immune system defends the body against foreign organisms and substances through two responses: nonspecific and specific. In a *nonspecific response,* the components of the immune system attack a variety of targets. Nonspecific components include phagocytic (cell destroying) cells such as mononuclear leukocytes, polymorphonuclear (PMN) leukocytes, natural killer (NK) cells, and complements (noncellular proteins) that work together to destroy invading cells and substances. During the first month of a child's life, the nonspecific response is immature, so phagocytic cells have little ability to move toward cancer cells and fulfill their function. The nonspecific response is also impaired in premature and small-for-gestational-age (SGA) infants.

In a *specific response,* T lymphocytes and immunoglobulin (Ig) attack only one type of invader. The specific response capability also is immature in infants. B-cell production of various proteins called immunoglobulins (IgM, IgG, and IgA) is below adult levels, so that the infant is vulnerable to bacterial and viral infections. (For a discussion of immune function, see Chapter 22.)

In children, many cells are growing quickly; this fast growth can lead to the proliferation of both cancerous and normal cells. Cell division that is out of control may normally trigger a mechanism called **apoptosis**, whereby the cell "realizes" something is wrong and destroys itself. The process of apoptosis or physiologic cell death limits the growth of cancerous cells but may not be well developed in young children.

Examples of diagnostic and laboratory tests used to evaluate cancer are provided in Table 24–1; see Appendices D and E for further information about these diagnostic procedures and tests common in cancer care.

Use *Assessment Guide: The Child With an Alteration in Cellular Growth* to identify and monitor alterations in cellular growth.

ASSESSMENT GUIDE | The Child With an Alteration in Cellular Growth

Assessment Focus	Assessment Guidelines
Growth and development parameters	• Assess the child's weight and height and plot on growth grids; be alert for weight loss.
	• Inquire about nutritional intake and any recent changes in appetite.
	• Perform developmental assessment and be alert for slow progress or regression.
	• Ask about school performance for children enrolled in school; include this information in every assessment of children who were treated for cancer in the past.
Pain	• Pain is abnormal if there is no known acute injury or chronic condition; assess any pain for length, duration, and type.
	• Does the child exhibit limping, headache, decreased activity level, or other symptoms indicative of pain?
Skin	• Is there bruising and other signs of bleeding on the skin?
	• Is there pallor and other signs of anemia?
	• Describe skin lesions.
Eyes, ears, nose, and throat (EENT) and sensory	• Inspect the symmetry and general condition of the eyes, ears, mouth, throat, head, and neck.
	• Inspect eye movements, corneal light reflex, and red reflex.
	• Evaluate hearing and vision and note any recent changes.
Chest, heart, and respiratory system	• Inspect the shape of the chest, respiratory rate, and ease of respirations.
	• Auscultate heart and lungs.
	• Ask about endurance and activity levels.

Assessment Focus	Assessment Guidelines
Abdomen	• Be alert for abdominal masses. Stop palpation immediately if any are noted and inform the physician. • Is there repeated vomiting, anorexia, or weight loss?
Urinary and gastrointestinal systems	• Evaluate frequency of urination and feces. • Assess for intake and evidence of vomiting or food intolerance. • Ask about blood or other discoloration in urine or stool. • Be alert for urinary tract infections.
Musculoskeletal system	• Observe for expected developmental tasks. • Is there asymmetry of bone or muscle? • Does the child limp or have other abnormalities of gait?

Childhood Cancer

The care of children who have cancer is a challenging specialty in pediatric nursing. In some cases, the child undergoes treatments that may continue for years and result in a variety of side effects. Today, treatments for cancer have improved prognoses in many cases, but in some, the prognosis still requires that the family deal with a life-threatening illness (see Chapter 13). The child is often cared for at home with outpatient visits for treatment and occasional hospitalization when needed. The periods of hospitalization are times of intense physical vulnerability for the child and intense emotional vulnerability for both the child and the family. To monitor the child closely, nurses need a sound knowledge of physiologic and psychologic responses, medical interventions, and nursing care. Integration of developmental knowledge into assessment and intervention is essential. Effective communication skills are necessary to support the child and family and promote realistic hope. See the *Nursing Management* sections and the *Nursing Care Plans* later in this chapter for specific interventions required.

Incidence

In the United States, cancer is diagnosed annually in approximately 11,000 children under 15 years of age, and about 1500 die from cancer annually (American Cancer Society [ACS], 2011). In children under 15 years of age, cancer is the leading cause of disease-related death, and it is the second leading cause of overall death after unintentional injury (ACS, 2011). However, mortality rates have declined by about 47% since 1975. The overall survival rate is 80% for childhood cancer. Survival rates vary related to the stage of disease at time of diagnosis and differ for specific types of cancer, ranging from 66% for neuroblastoma to 95% for Hodgkin disease (ACS, 2011; Arndt, 2011a). Figure 24–1 shows the most common forms of childhood cancers among children in different age groups.

Etiology and Pathophysiology

Alterations in cellular growth occur in response to external and internal stimuli. **Neoplasms** are caused by one or any combination of three factors: (1) external stimuli that cause genetic mutations, (2) immune system and gene abnormalities, and (3) chromosomal abnormalities.

EXTERNAL STIMULI

External stimuli may affect the child's general health and cause mutations in body cells. **Carcinogens** are chemicals or industrial processes that, when combined with genetic traits and in interaction with one another, result in cancer. Several carcinogens cause cancers that are diagnosed during childhood. Others cause cancers that begin in childhood but are not identified until adulthood. Some chemicals suspected of causing childhood cancer include diethylstilbestrol (maternal use of therapeutic estrogen hormones), anabolic androgenic steroids, alkylating chemotherapeutic agents, and immunosuppressants used for organ transplantation. Radiation exposure has been known to cause cancers such as leukemia and thyroid tumors in children exposed to nuclear fallout from atomic bombs, other nuclear accidents, and other excessive radiation sources.

External stimuli may also lead to secondary cancers in children, or those occurring after treatment for a primary cancer and of a different cellular type than the primary cancer. Secondary cancers can result when the child is treated for a primary cancer with high doses of radiation. Excessive exposure to ultraviolet radiation from the sun predisposes children to development of skin cancer in adolescence and adulthood (see Chapter 31).

IMMUNE SYSTEM AND GENE ABNORMALITIES

One critical function of a normal immune system is immune surveillance, in which phagocytic cells circulate throughout the body, detecting and destroying abnormal and cancerous cells. Children with congenital immune deficiencies, such as Wiskott-Aldrich syndrome, in which immune surveillance may fail, are at high risk for cancer. A form of non-Hodgkin lymphoma develops in some children treated with immune system–suppressing drugs. Children with acquired immunodeficiency syndrome (AIDS) may also be at higher risk of certain types of cancer, such as Hodgkin disease, non-Hodgkin lymphoma, Kaposi sarcoma, and leiomyosarcoma (Sigel et al., 2011).

Viruses and other substances may alter the immune system, thereby allowing cancer to occur (see *Pathophysiology Illustrated: Proto-Oncogene Alteration*). Their action is based on changing certain genes that normally regulate cellular growth and development (called **proto-oncogenes**) into related genes that allow unregulated cell division and cancerous growth (called **oncogenes**). Among the cancers thought to be linked to viral action and the change of proto-oncogenes to oncogenes are certain leukemias, rhabdomyosarcoma, Burkitt lymphoma, and some forms of Hodgkin disease.

Genetic changes can include autosomal dominant, autosomal recessive, and X-linked transfer. In these cases, the resulting cancers often occur relatively early in life. Cancers of these types are typically aggressive since the child has inherited the abnormal gene and it is within each cell, rather than a single mutation of one gene in a specific cell. Because of the progress made in the Human Genome Project, there is increasing ability to perform genetic testing for certain familial cancers. Examples of cancers that are sometimes caused by genetic abnormalities within families include retinoblastoma and Wilms tumor (described later in this chapter), multiple endocrine neoplasia, type 2 (thyroid cancer), and familial adenomatous polyposis (invasive colon cancer). Not all cases of these cancers are familial, but their incidence suggests the need for careful history taking to identify any other cases in the family.

Pathophysiology Illustrated:
Proto-Oncogene Alteration

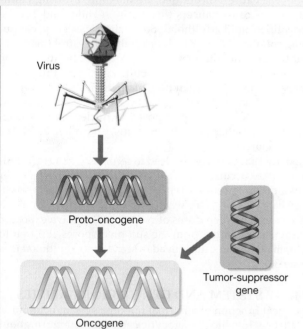

A proto-oncogene normally regulates cellular growth and development. When altered by a virus or other external cause, it can change to an oncogene, which allows unregulated genetic activity and tumor growth. Tumor suppressor genes regulate the effects of oncogenes to decrease wildly proliferating cellular growth.

Providing recommendations for referral to genetic counseling services and following up with further education and psychologic support are important nursing roles.

Tumor suppressor genes counteract the effect of oncogenes, keeping cellular growth within normal limits. When tumor suppressor genes are missing, unstemmed cellular growth can occur. These genes are commonly missing in children with retinoblastoma and Wilms tumor.

CHROMOSOMAL ABNORMALITIES

Normal chromosomes undergo change as a part of the genetic process. Most changes are not harmful. However, some result in chromosomal abnormalities such as hyperploidy (more than the normal number of chromosomes), deletion, translocation, and breakage.

Some chromosomal abnormalities have been linked to an increased incidence of cancer. Children with Down syndrome have a much higher incidence of leukemia than nonaffected children; the risk varies greatly according to the type of leukemia (Roberts & Izraieli, 2014). Children missing a band of genetic material on chromosome 13 often have retinoblastoma. Similarly, a Wilms tumor often develops in children missing part of the genetic material from chromosome 11.

Regardless of the location and cause of abnormal cellular growth, the pathophysiologic process of cancer is similar. The altered cell begins to multiply as directed by the altered genetic structure of its DNA and the absence or inactivation of tumor suppressor genes. Each new cell transmits the new or altered pattern to the next generation. As the abnormal cells replicate, they form a growing neoplastic mass. Normal cells usually die as the increased metabolic rate of the neoplastic cells depletes available nutrition. The altered DNA in the tumor cells may also cause the abnormal cells to invade adjoining tissue. Through continued growth the mass expands until it enters and disrupts a major vessel or a vital organ.

Families Want to Know

Ways to Decrease the Incidence of Cancer in Children

Many parents ask what they can do to decrease the incidence of cancer in children as they grow into adulthood. Three major teaching areas should be addressed:

1. Have children increase intake of fruits and vegetables. Most children do not eat enough of these foods, and increased intake is associated with lower rates of many cancers. Aim for a minimum of five servings daily.

2. Protect skin with sunscreen. Early excessive exposure to sun, and having had one or repeated severe sunburns during childhood, increases chances of skin cancers developing in adulthood. Tanning bed exposure is a prime risk factor for skin cancer; all children and adolescents, and particularly those with cancer, should strictly avoid tanning beds (Greinert & Boniol, 2011).

3. Discourage smoking among children and be sure children are not exposed to environmental tobacco smoke. This will decrease the future chance of developing lung cancer.

When there is a history of cancer in the family, particularly of a type associated with familial incidence such as some breast or ovarian cancers, encourage the family to learn more about the cancer and teach their children to receive regular surveillance as they enter young adulthood.

Inform youth in all families about screening, such as the Papanicolaou test, breast self-examination, and testicular examination that can lead to early detection. Encourage youth to receive the human papillomavirus quadrivalent vaccine recombinant (Gardasil) to prevent cervical cancers and other health problems caused by human papillomavirus (HPV). (See Chapter 16 for further information.)

Clinical Manifestations

Each type of childhood cancer signals its presence differently. Because many of the presenting signs and symptoms of cancer are typical of common childhood illnesses, diagnosis may be delayed. In some cases, no symptoms are noted until the cancer is advanced. Some of the common presenting symptoms of cancer follow:

- *Pain* may be the result of a neoplasm either directly or indirectly affecting nerve receptors through obstruction, inflammation, tissue damage, stretching of visceral tissue, or invasion of susceptible tissue.

- *Cachexia* is a syndrome characterized by anorexia, weight loss, anemia, asthenia (weakness), and early satiety (feeling of being full).

- *Anemia* may be experienced during times of chronic bleeding or iron deficiency. In chronic illness, the body uses iron poorly. Anemia is also present in cancers of the bone marrow when the number of red blood cells (RBCs) is reduced, in part because of the presence of large numbers of other bone marrow products. Treatment of cancer often promotes further anemia.

- *Infection* is usually a result of an altered or immature immune system. In addition, infection occurs when bone marrow cancers inhibit maturation of normal immune system cells. Infection may also occur in children treated with corticosteroids. Because their immune response is altered, the normal signs of infection may not appear.

- *Bruising* and *petechiae* can occur if the bone marrow cannot produce enough platelets; bleeding after even minor trauma can lead to ecchymosis.

- *Neurologic symptoms* may result from impingement on the brain or nervous system. Signs of increased intracranial pressure, decreased or altered consciousness, eye abnormalities, or other neurologic or behavioral changes may be evident.

- *Palpable mass* may be present for certain cancers. This is most commonly abdominal but may be mediastinal, in the neck, or at other sites.

A variety of other symptoms can occur depending on the location of the cancer. Subcutaneous nodules may appear if leukocytosis is present. Superior vena cava syndrome or respiratory difficulty can occur with mediastinal tumors (such as neuroblastoma), and enlarged lymph nodes are common with lymphomas.

Diagnostic Tests

The most common diagnostic tests performed on children with cancer are a complete blood count (CBC) with differential, bone marrow aspiration (BMA), bone marrow biopsy (BMBX), lumbar puncture (LP), peripheral blood studies, radiographic examination, magnetic resonance imaging (MRI), computed tomography (CT; Figure 24–2), ultrasound, and biopsy of tumor. See Table 24–2.

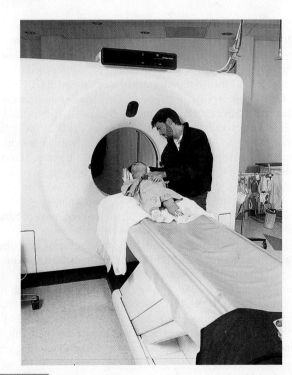

Figure 24–2 Computed tomography can be a frightening procedure for children. This 2-year-old boy is comforted by his father before the procedure.

TABLE 24–2 Selected Diagnostic Tests for Childhood Cancer

TEST	PURPOSE	NORMAL LABORATORY VALUES	DIAGNOSTIC VALUES
Bone marrow aspiration	Examines bone marrow.	Less than 5% blast cells (immature)	Greater than 25% blast cells in acute lymphoblastic leukemia, most with hypercellular marrow
Lumbar puncture	Examines cerebrospinal fluid.	Cell count (microliters) Polymorphonuclear leukocytes 0 Monocytes 0–5 RBCs 0–5	Presence of malignant cells indicates central nervous system involvement
Complete blood count and differential	Examines cellular components of blood.	WBC less than 10,000/mcL Platelets 150,000–400,000/mcL Hemoglobin 12–16 g/dL	WBC greater than 10,000/mcL OR depressed levels of WBCs Platelets 20,000–100,000/mL Hemoglobin 7–10 g/dL
Absolute neutrophil count (ANC)	Examines blood component ratio: (% of segmental neutrophils plus % of bands [immature neutrophils]) times WBC count; this number is then divided by 100.	ANC greater than 1000	ANC less than 1000 = risk of infection

---

SAFETY ALERT!

Remove all jewelry and clothes with metal snaps from the child before an MRI scan. Ask about and remove body piercings; they may not always be visible. Some metallic objects implanted in the body are compatible with MRI but others contraindicate the use of MRI. Metallic objects include orthodontic braces, metal dental bridgework, cochlear implants, surgical clips or plates, and orthopedic rods. When there are metal objects in the body or tattoos, be certain to report them to the managing healthcare provider and radiology technician so they can determine if it is safe to perform MRI.

Additional studies helpful for certain cancers are nuclear medicine scans with radioactive isotopes such as gallium or iodine, bone scan with technetium 99m, or positron emission tomography (PET) and single-photon emission computed tomography (SPECT), which combine nuclear medicine with CT. Specific tests such as pulmonary function tests and echocardiograms may be used in certain situations. Urine analysis is also performed.

The blood work is very detailed and includes RBC, WBC, platelets, hematocrit and hemoglobin, serum electrolytes, liver studies, and markers that are elevated in specific types of tumors. Absolute neutrophil count (ANC) is important; it uses both the segmented (mature) and bands (immature neutrophils) as a measure of the body's infection-fighting capability. ANC is calculated by adding the percentage of segmented neutrophils to the percentage of bands, and then multiplying this percentage by the WBC count.

The tests are aimed at identifying the source of the cancer and any metastases to additional sites. This enables the oncology specialist to stage the cancer. *Staging* refers to the process of labeling the type of cancer cells, severity, and spread, which will determine the recommended treatment and assist in teaching the family about treatment and prognosis. Stage 1 indicates less severe cancer without spread to other parts of the body; higher numbers indicate both greater severity and spread to other sites.

Clinical Therapy

Clinical therapy for cancer is extremely complex and is managed by a specialist in pediatric oncology. The cancer itself is treated, its effects on the body are addressed, and the side effects of treatment are managed. Examples of the effects of cancer on the body include altered nutritional status from anorexia due to the cancer diverting nutrients to itself, decreased immune response from impaired manufacture of white blood cells and other immune components, and a variety of symptoms as a tumor presses on vital organs. In addition, cancer treatment itself has many potential side effects that require constant monitoring and adjustments in treatment.

Cancer is treated with one or a combination of therapies: surgery, chemotherapy, radiation, **biotherapy** (treatment that uses and/or enhances the body's abilities to fight disease, particularly by using biologic agents to promote immune response), and bone marrow transplantation. The choice of treatment is determined by the type of cancer, its location, and staging. Treatments all have side effects and these will also require clinical management. Many families also choose to use some type of complementary therapy in addition to traditional medical approaches.

The goal of treatment may be curative, supportive, or provision of end-of-life care. Curative treatment rids the child's body of the cancer. Supportive treatment includes transfusions, pain management, antibiotics, and other interventions to assist the body's defenses and increase the child's comfort. End-of-life treatment is designed to make the child as comfortable as possible when no curative treatment is possible. (See Chapter 13 for a detailed discussion of end-of-life care for children.) Whatever combination of treatment is used, families have many questions and need resources for information.

SURGERY

Surgery is used to remove or debulk (reduce the size of) a solid tumor. An example of a cancer that is commonly treated with surgery is a Wilms tumor. Surgery may also determine the stage and type of cancer.

CHEMOTHERAPY

Chemotherapy is the administration of specific drugs that kill both normal and cancerous cells. The administration of various chemotherapeutic drugs is timed to achieve the greatest cellular destruction. The cell's cycle of replication determines

Protocol = Map or plan of action

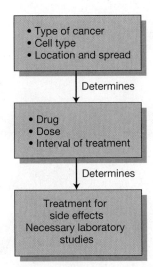

Figure 24–3 Chemotherapy protocol. **A protocol is a map or plan of action that directs therapy by identifying the drug and its accompanying treatment.**

the schedule (see *Pathophysiology Illustrated: Chemotherapeutic Drug Action*). Several chemotherapeutic drugs are administered simultaneously to maximize their lethal impact on cells at all stages of activity (see *Medications Used for: Cancer Chemotherapy*). Medications are most commonly oral, intravenous, or **intrathecal** (into spinal canal). Whereas DNA in a normal cell can repair itself after chemotherapy, the DNA in a neoplastic cell cannot. The particular chemotherapeutic treatment protocol used is based on research into different types of cancer cells. A **protocol** is a plan of action for chemotherapy based on the type of cancer, its stage, and the particular cell type (Figure 24–3).

Other drugs used in the treatment of children with cancer include colony-stimulating factors, antiemetics, and nutritional supplements. Colony-stimulating factors are hormone-like glycoproteins that enhance blood cell production and counteract the myelosuppressive effects of chemotherapeutic drugs. For example, erythropoietin is produced in the kidney, and a recombinant form (epoetin) is available that can be used to treat anemia of cancer, thereby decreasing the number of transfusions needed. Filgrastim (Neupogen) increases production of neutrophils by the bone marrow (see *Medications Used During Cancer Treatment: Colony-Stimulating Factors*). Antiemetics, such as ondansetron (Zofran), can be used to treat the nausea and vomiting that are common side effects of therapy. Nutritional supplements help maintain nutritional status.

RADIATION

Radiation therapy involves unstable isotopes that release varying levels of energy to cause breaks in the DNA molecule and thereby destroy cells. Radiation has been used as a treatment method since the early 1900s, shortly after its discovery. It is often used for the local and regional control of cancer, and in combination with surgery and chemotherapy; it may be curative or palliative.

The area to be irradiated (treatment field) includes the tumor site and sometimes other involved areas, such as lymph glands. The goal is to irradiate the tumor but not healthy adjacent tissue. The total dose of radiation is divided (or fractionated) and given over several weeks. A common course of

Families Want to Know

Cancer Therapy

Most parents are not aware of the effects of cancer treatment and how they can help children through this experience. Depending on the stage and type of treatment, there are several ways to help:

- Children in radiation therapy and chemotherapy become fatigued because of cancer and treatment effects. Provide extra rest periods with shorter activity periods between them.
- Have a suitcase ready in case the child develops a complication and needs to be taken to stay in the hospital for a few days. Several hospital stays of a few days are normal during treatment.
- Parents are often key in identifying problems early. They should be encouraged to share their observations and concerns about symptoms the child is experiencing.
- Parents are usually concerned about providing central line care but feel more comfortable after a few days of caring for the line.
- Children may not feel hungry because of anorexia from the disease and as a side effect of treatment. When they are ready to eat, intake should be nutritious.
- Remember that children with cancer are still at their normal developmental age. Treat them appropriately for their age, not as if they are older or younger. Utilize the child-life specialist in the hospital to assist with planning activities appropriate to the child's developmental age.
- Try to maintain contact with the child's peer group and family members. When school attendance or direct contact is not possible because of immune suppression, arrange for phone calls, videocam exchanges, and other methods of communication.
- Seek information from other parents, the Internet, and other resources on cancer care.
- Many families use complementary approaches to deal with the child's cancer. Most of these approaches are not contraindicated. However, be sure to tell the oncologist about what treatments you are choosing to use to be sure none of them will injure your child.
- Take time to get away and relax so that you have enough energy and are better able to deal with your child's therapy.

Pathophysiology Illustrated: **Chemotherapeutic Drug Action**

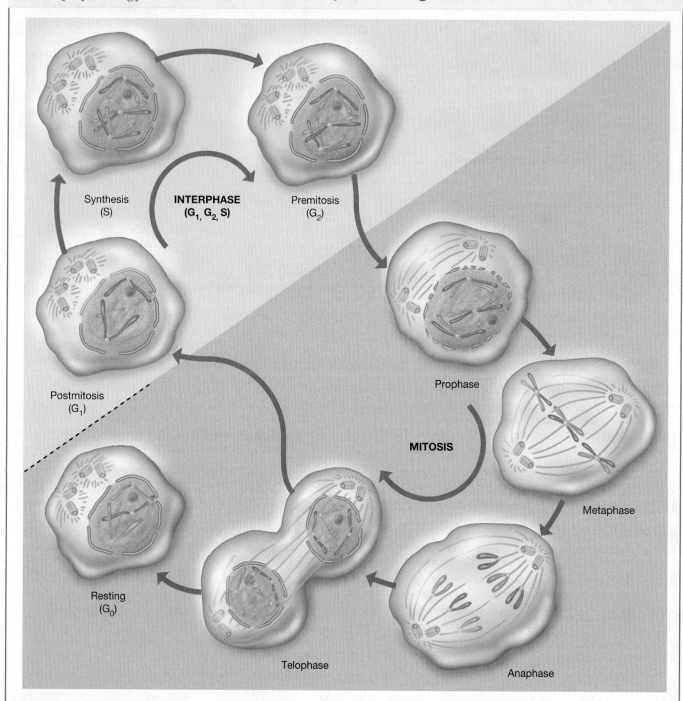

Synthesis (S)

INTERPHASE (G₁, G₂, S)

Premitosis (G₂)

Postmitosis (G₁)

Prophase

MITOSIS

Metaphase

Resting (G₀)

Telophase

Anaphase

Chemotherapeutic drugs either act at specific parts of the cell cycle or are nonspecific for action (act throughout all cell phases). See *Medications Used for: Cancer Chemotherapy* for further information about specific drugs and their site of action in the cell cycle.

radiation treatment might be once daily 4 or 5 days per week for a period of 2 to 7 weeks.

Examples of cancers treated with radiation include Hodgkin disease, Wilms tumor, retinoblastoma, rhabdomyosarcoma, and central nervous system disease in leukemia. Tumors that have a low sensitivity to radiation, such as osteosarcoma and soft-tissue sarcomas, require higher doses of radiation, or other treatments may be preferred.

Medications Used for: Cancer Chemotherapy

MEDICATION AND ACTION/INDICATION	NURSING IMPLICATIONS
Cell Cycle–Specific Agents	
Antimetabolites • 5-Azacytidine • 5-Fluorouracil • 6-Mercaptopurine • 6-Thioguanine • Cytosine arabinoside (cytarabine) • Hydroxyurea • Methotrexate The antimetabolites work at the synthesis phase of cell division; interfere with function of nucleic acid; inhibit DNA or RNA synthesis.	Various routes are used for individual agents, such as oral, intravenous, and intrathecal. Most common side effects are nausea and vomiting, myelosuppression, stomatitis. Specific agents such as methotrexate and cytarabine can cause neurologic toxicity with high doses. Consult drug books and package inserts for a detailed list of side effects. Obtain baseline CBC, liver function, renal function. Monitor intake and output and body weight. Ensure hydration and output levels ordered by oncologist. Monitor vital signs and cardiovascular and respiratory function. Watch for bleeding and signs of infection. Monitor carefully during administration for signs of anaphylaxis.
Vinca alkaloids • Etoposide • Teniposide • Irinotecan • Paclitaxel • Vinblastine • Vincristine Act during mitosis; bind with cell proteins to inhibit nucleic acid and protein synthesis.	Most are given intravenously with some drugs also available for oral route. Common side effects include nausea and vomiting, abdominal cramping and diarrhea, constipation, paralytic ileus, hair loss, hypotension or hypertension, peripheral neuropathy and neurologic toxicity (latter especially with vinblastine and vincristine). Obtain baseline blood work. Consult specific drug information for period of maximum myelosuppressive effect. Be alert for bruising, infection, and other signs of myelosuppression. Monitor carefully during administration for signs of anaphylaxis, particularly with etoposide and paclitaxel.
Miscellaneous—G_1 phase activity • L-asparaginase Causes depletion of asparagine, needed by cancer cells; makes cell in G_1 phase vulnerable to other agents; interferes with synthesis. Used in combination with other agents in leukemia and other cancers.	Administered intravenously or intramuscularly. Major side effects are severe nausea and vomiting, hypersensitivity, renal failure, myelosuppression, acid–base imbalance. Because of the risk of life-threatening hypersensitivity reactions, emergency medications and care must be immediately available. Perform CBC, serum amylase, glucose, coagulation factors, bone marrow function, liver function tests before therapy and twice weekly. Monitor intake and output, neurologic status, gastrointestinal symptoms, abdominal pain.
Miscellaneous—G_2 phase activity • Etoposide Works at G_2 phase; binds cellular proteins to cause metaphase arrest; also acts on S phase of DNA synthesis. Used with other agents, particularly in recurrent disease.	Administered orally and intravenously. Common side effects are nausea and vomiting, myelosuppression, hair loss, diarrhea. Can cause anaphylaxis; hypotension and IV site pain with rapid infusion. Perform baseline CBC, liver, and renal function tests. Check IV site frequently since extravasation can cause necrosis. Monitor vital signs during infusion and stop drug if hypotension occurs. Keep emergency drugs and equipment readily available.

(continued)

Medications Used for: Cancer Chemotherapy (*continued*)

Cell Cycle–Nonspecific Agents

Alkylating agents

- Cyclophosphamide
- Carboplatin
- Cisplatin
- Busulfan
- Chlorambucil
- Ifosfamide
- Thiotepa
- Mechlorethamine
- Melphalan
- Procarbazine
- Dacarbazine

Substitute an alkyl group for a hydrogen atom, leading to blockage of DNA replication. Used for treatment of many cancers, either alone or in conjunction with other agents.

Most are administered orally and/or intravenously. Array of side effects depending on specific drug. Some common side effects are nausea and vomiting, diarrhea, myelosuppression, hair loss, neuropathies, pulmonary toxicity, renal damage; secondary tumors later in life associated with some agents.

Obtain CBC and full blood work before and during treatment. Mesna may be administered with some alkylating agents to lower the risk of hemorrhagic cystitis. Monitor for side effects of the specific agents administered.

Ensure generous hydration and monitor intake and output.

Teach family the importance of long-term monitoring for secondary tumors.

Antibiotics

- Doxorubicin
- Mitomycin-C
- Dactinomycin
- Bleomycin
- Daunorubicin
- Idarubicin
- Mitoxantrone

Interfere with nucleic acid, inhibiting DNA or RNA synthesis. Used in combination with other agents to treat leukemia and other childhood cancers.

Most are administered intravenously.

Common side effects include nausea and vomiting, myelosuppression, oral ulcers, skin and pulmonary toxicity. Several have cumulative dose toxicity, such as cardiac abnormalities (doxorubicin) and skin/pulmonary (bleomycin); total dose the child has received must be monitored.

Obtain baseline CBC and other blood studies and monitor throughout therapy.

Monitor vital signs, lung function, cardiac function, and neurologic status throughout and following therapy. Be alert for signs of myelosuppression and mucosal ulcers.

Nitrosoureas

- Carmustine
- Lomustine

Cross-breakage in DNA strands so that DNA and RNA replication cannot occur. Used in lymphomas and other childhood cancers. Can cross blood–brain barrier.

Administered orally (lomustine) or intravenously (carmustine). Major side effect is myelosuppression.

Others include pulmonary fibrosis, eye infarction, skin changes, hair loss, nausea, and vomiting.

Obtain baseline and periodic CBC and other studies.

Monitor pulmonary function, skin, and signs of infection or bleeding such as ecchymosis or petechiae.

Hormones

- Prednisone
- Prednisolone
- Dexamethasone

Analog of hydrocortisone; anti-inflammatory; delayed and depressed immune response. Used in conjunction with other agents for many types of childhood cancer.

Often administered orally.

Numerous side effects including edema, moon face, mood lability, increased appetite, disturbed sleep, immunosuppression, disturbed glucose control, osteoporosis.

Teach child and family the effects of the drug. Minimize exposure to persons with infection. Monitor for infections in all systems.

Monitor weight regularly. Take vital signs. Teach to take as directed. Drug must be tapered slowly at end of therapy.

Topoisomerase I inhibitor

- Irinotecan
- Mitoxantrone
- Topotecan

Inhibit the enzyme topoisomerase I in the cell nucleus, relaxing DNA and preventing its duplication.

Used in conjunction with other agents to treat acute lymphocytic leukemia and other childhood cancers.

Administered intravenously: topotecan can be given intrathecally. Common side effects include nausea and vomiting, diarrhea, fever, dehydration, myelosuppression. Can alter liver function and cause skin changes.

Obtain baseline and periodic CBC and other studies, including liver function.

Monitor for signs of myelosuppression, gastrointestinal distress, change in liver function.

BIOTHERAPY

Biotherapy is the use of biologic retooling and molecular intervention to produce targeted cancer therapy. Biologic retooling uses parts of the human body that are programmed to destroy cells, and applies them to the cancer cells. An example of this technique includes development of antibodies that are tumor specific to certain cancers, and produced by the body in response to antigens of cancer cells (Smith & Reaman, 2015). These antibodies promote apoptosis or death of the cancerous cells. Another example is the group of drugs that stimulate the body's own immune response. Cancer vaccines are under development that may work to help the body fight cancers; already developed is human papillomavirus vaccine (see Chapter 16). The actions of many of these agents are not completely understood and may have different effects in children versus adults, and some agents have more than one effect. For example, interferon has both antiviral and antiproliferative effects on some malignant cells. Interferon and tumor necrosis factor (TNF) are undergoing clinical trials to study their effectiveness and to develop protocols for their safe use against selected cancers.

Molecular targeting involves interference with metabolic pathways (e.g., through enzyme disruption) in the tumor cells. It may therefore disturb the cell's growth and development and thereby depress proliferation.

Medications Used During Cancer Treatment: Colony-Stimulating Factors

MEDICATION AND ACTION/INDICATION	NURSING IMPLICATIONS
Epoetin alfa (human recombinant erythropoietin) This glycoprotein stimulates the bone marrow in RBC formation; useful when numbers of RBCs are low because of chemotherapeutic effects.	Give subcutaneously or intravenously. Do not shake and do not use if discolored or particles are present. Single-dose vials only, so discard any solution that is not used. Obtain red blood cell tests before therapy and periodically after; improvement in hematocrit should be seen in 7–14 days. Monitor blood pressure before and during therapy because hypertension can result. Monitor for change in neurologic response and headache; both seizures and strokes are possible side effects.
Filgrastim (Neupogen) and pegfilgrastim (Neulasta) These human granulocyte colony-stimulating factor preparations (G-CSF) increase the bone marrow's production of neutrophils.	Administered subcutaneously and intravenously; prepare as directed for IV infusion to prevent its absorption by IV tubing. Single-dose vials only so discard any solution that is not used. Incompatible with many medications; check package insert; do not give within 24 hr before or after chemotherapeutic drugs or their effect may be decreased. Obtain baseline and twice weekly CBC. Monitor for side effects such as bone pain and heart arrhythmias; report fevers and be alert for other signs of infection when neutrophil count is low.
Oprelvekin (Neumega) A hematopoietic growth factor, interleukin-11, that increases platelet count; useful in low platelet count due to chemotherapeutic effects on bone marrow.	Administered subcutaneously. Single-dose vials only, so discard any solution that is not used. Obtain baseline CBC and platelet count; monitor platelets throughout treatment. Monitor for side effects such as edema, fever, CNS changes, tachycardia, respiratory problems, and skin rash. Take daily weights and monitor for fluid retention.

An additional type of biologic therapy is gene therapy, or attempting to replace a faulty gene with one that is normal. Genetic technology is growing rapidly and shows promise for future treatment of cancer and other childhood diseases. This complex field includes research to identify genes that lead to disease, recombinant techniques to enable genetic engineering, and studies of enzymes active in DNA and RNA formation. Nurses need to have enhanced knowledge of this important work as technologies are increasingly applied in cancer treatment (Calzone et al., 2014; Greco et al., 2011).

BONE MARROW AND HEMATOPOIETIC STEM CELL TRANSPLANTATION

Bone marrow and hematopoietic stem cell transplantation (HSCT) are used to treat leukemia, neuroblastoma, and some noncancerous conditions such as aplastic anemia. The goal of therapy is to administer a lethal dose of chemotherapy and radiation that will kill the cancer, and then to resupply the body with stem cells either from the child's own bone marrow that was previously removed (autologous transplant) and stored or from a compatible donor (allogeneic transplant). Umbilical cord blood is a potential source of stem cells used for transplant, as are peripheral blood stem cells (obtained from the donor's circulating blood rather than from bone marrow). The donor, whether autologous or allogeneic, can be given growth factors prior to donation to stimulate production of stem cells. An advantage of peripheral stem cells is that they can be easily collected somewhat less painfully and invasively than by the procedure of a bone marrow aspiration.

Transplantation has become the treatment of choice for some cancers when a relapse occurs while the child is receiving another form of cancer therapy and for primary treatment of certain cancers. First, a histocompatible donor must be located. The child then receives intensive chemotherapy, often followed by total body irradiation. Beginning 7 to 10 days before the transplant, this treatment kills all circulating blood cells and bone marrow contents. Following this treatment, the child is intravenously transfused with the donor bone marrow or other source of stem cells. New blood cells usually form within 2 to 8 weeks. (See Chapter 23 for a description of care for the child undergoing transplantation.)

Stem cells that become established in the host child's bone marrow can also be obtained from newborn umbilical cord blood. For some children this has become a better option than waiting for a matching bone marrow donor. Cord blood can be easily collected at birth from a sibling of the ill child because histocompatible matches often occur in siblings, or cord blood banks may offer a match. The umbilical cord blood is then infused into the child undergoing treatment, and the same mechanism occurs as in transplantation of bone marrow—implantation of the stem cells into the child's bone marrow and production of normal blood cells over about 2 to 6 weeks. Advantages of umbilical cord blood are that, unlike bone marrow collection, it is not painful for the donor and does not require anesthesia, there is an opportunity to easily collect samples from many ethnic groups that are underrepresented in bone marrow donor registries, graft-versus-host disease after treatment is less prevalent, and storage of umbilical cord blood for use later in life is possible. A variety of federally funded and private blood banks are available to store and provide umbilical blood.

COMPLEMENTARY THERAPIES

Many families use **complementary therapies** in treatment of a child's cancer. These approaches to care are also referred to as alternative or unconventional, and may involve nutritional supplements, oral herbal supplements, touch therapy, and mind/body interventions. Little research has been done on complementary therapies, although up to 80% of children with cancer have used at least one such therapeutic approach (Paisley, Kang, Insogna, et al., 2011). Healthcare providers should be aware of these practices, inquire in a nonjudgmental manner about the therapies, and attempt to learn about specific therapies and practices. Although some herbs and nutritional products such as St. John's wort may decrease serum concentration of chemotherapeutic agents, or some may act as hormones in the body, most are not known to negatively affect contemporary medical treatment. The families should be assisted in seeking information and supported in use of their chosen therapies. Eating fruits and vegetables is associated with lower cancer incidence in adults, and some foods such as garlic and oranges may slow cancer growth or enhance medical chemotherapy. Some individuals use herbal supplements to treat cancer; these include cat's claw (bark of a tree root), mistletoe, and shark cartilage. The U.S. Food and Drug Administration has allowed testing of the efficacy of some herbal treatments for cancer. Some herbs can decrease nausea and vomiting, and others can boost the immune system's function. Several cancer drugs such as vincristine and paclitaxel are obtained from plant products.

END-OF-LIFE CARE

In spite of modern medical practices and complementary therapies, some children do not survive childhood cancer. In these cases, the focus of health care is to provide comfort and emotional support for the child and family. Too often, healthcare providers feel uncomfortable when a child is expected to die and may withdraw from close contact with the child or family, fail to provide adequate comfort measures, and leave the family without access to needed resources. When recognition of prognosis is delayed, children suffer more and end-of-life care is less integrated. Some symptoms for which children are commonly undertreated include pain, dyspnea, nutrition, elimination, and fatigue. Additionally, care may be required from a wide array of specialists, which can lead to fragmentation of care and lack of integrated palliative approaches.

Care for the dying child can be enhanced by an end-of-life or palliative care team; an integrated plan of care; collaboration among families and healthcare providers; and a focus on the child's developmental level and family needs. Parents state that an advanced care directive that outlines the medical care plans for the child is helpful in preserving the child's quality of life and increases the child's comfort. See Chapter 13 for a detailed description of terminal care for children with terminal disease.

Special Issues in Childhood Cancer

ONCOLOGIC EMERGENCIES

Oncologic emergencies can be organized into three groups: metabolic, hematologic, and those involving space-occupying lesions. The most common metabolic emergencies include tumor lysis syndrome and septic shock, while common hematologic emergencies include bone marrow suppression, gastrointestinal and central nervous system bleeding, and disseminated intravascular coagulation. The most common emergencies involving space-occupying lesions include brain herniation, spinal cord compression, and superior vena cava compression from a superior mediastinal mass. The next sections describe these and other oncologic emergencies in more detail.

Metabolic Emergencies. Metabolic emergencies result from the lysis (dissolving or decomposing) of tumor cells, a process called *tumor lysis syndrome*. This cell destruction results in hypocalcemia, hyperkalemia, hyperphosphatemia, and hyperuricemia. It is seen most commonly in children with non-Hodgkin

TABLE 24-3 Clinical Manifestations and Management of Tumor Lysis Syndrome

ETIOLOGY	CLINICAL MANIFESTATIONS	CLINICAL THERAPY	NURSING IMPLICATIONS
Breakdown of malignant cells releases intracellular components into blood.	Hyperuricemia Hyperkalemia Hyperphosphatemia Hypocalcemia	• Vigorous hydration with 2–4 times maintenance fluid • Correction of electrolyte imbalances • Administration of allopurinol or urate oxidase (Rasburicase) to reduce conversion of metabolic by-products to uric acid	• Administer fluids, beginning before therapy. • Carefully measure intake and output. • Record daily weight. • Monitor urine specific gravity; it should remain less than 1.010. • Monitor for desired and side effects of drug therapy.
Electrolyte imbalance causes metabolic acidosis and serious abnormalities.	Cardiac arrhythmias Impaired renal function Tetany, neurologic and mental status changes	• ECG monitoring • Medications such as furosemide to facilitate potassium excretion • Dialysis may be needed	• Administer electrolytes and medications. • Urine pH should remain 7.0–7.5. • Perform Trousseau and Chvostek signs for tetany monitoring and assess neurologic function. • Perform mental status examination. • Obtain laboratory specimens as needed.

lymphoma (especially the subtype Burkitt lymphoma), acute lymphocytic leukemia, and acute myeloid leukemia (Burns, Topoz, & Reynolds, 2014; Kishimoto et al., 2014). (See Table 24–3.) The nurse collects laboratory studies, including CBC, absolute neutrophil count (ANF), serum electrolytes, bicarbonate, uric acid, blood urea nitrogen (BUN) and creatinine, and urinalysis. The emergency can be life threatening, and the family will need ongoing support and explanations about care.

A second type of metabolic emergency is septic shock. During periods of immune suppression, the child is vulnerable to overwhelming infection, resulting in circulatory failure, inadequate tissue perfusion, and hypotension. Septic shock can be fatal (see Chapter 21 for a description of septic shock), so early and aggressive treatment improves outcome. Factors contributing to massive infection include inadequate neutrophil production, abnormal granulocytes (not able to be actively phagocytic), erosions through normal barriers such as blood vessels and mucous membranes, and altered bone marrow production caused by chemotherapy and some forms of radiation. Such infections may manifest with hyperthermia or hypothermia, tachycardia, tachypnea, hypotension, mental changes, and peripheral cyanosis and coolness, and must be vigorously treated with antimicrobial therapy and hydration management.

A third type of metabolic emergency occurs when treatment destroys large amounts of bone, resulting in hypercalcemia (elevated calcium in the serum). Hypercalcemia is most common in children with acute lymphocytic leukemia and rhabdomyosarcoma. Treatment includes hydration and adequate oral phosphate supplement (Demirkaya, Sevinir, Yalcinkaya, et al., 2012; Kolyva, Efthymiadou, Gkentizi, et al., 2014).

Some children develop syndrome of inappropriate antidiuretic hormone (SIADH) and have excessive release of ADH. The resulting decreased urinary output leads to water intoxication. See Chapter 30 for a detailed description of SIADH.

Hematologic Emergencies. Hematologic emergencies result from bone marrow suppression or infiltration of brain and respiratory tissue with high numbers of leukemic blast cells (hyperleukocytosis). Bone marrow suppression results in anemia

and thrombocytopenia with resultant hemorrhage. Gastrointestinal and central nervous system bleeding (strokes) are common. Disseminated intravascular coagulation (DIC) occurs in some children and is a life-threatening complication. See Chapter 23 for a thorough description of this condition. Disruption of normal WBC production and resulting hyperleukocytosis can lead to obstruction of small blood vessels throughout the body.

Treatment involves infusion of packed red blood cells for anemia; and platelet transfusion, vitamin K, and fresh frozen plasma for thrombocytopenia and hemorrhage. Hyperviscosity is treated by plasmapheresis, hydroxyurea, and close management of chemotherapy. Respiratory and other vital support is needed (Henry & Sung, 2015; Lewis, Hendrickson, & Moynihan, 2011).

Space-Occupying Lesion. Extensive tumor growth may result in spinal cord compression, increased intracranial pressure, brain herniation, seizures, massive hepatomegaly, and superior vena cava syndrome (obstruction of the superior vena cava by tumor). These emergencies are often caused by neuroblastoma, medulloblastoma, astrocytoma, Hodgkin disease, or lymphoma. After biopsy of the mass, treatment involves radiation therapy, chemotherapy, and corticosteroids.

PSYCHOSOCIAL NEEDS

The diagnosis of cancer is devastating for families. They cannot believe that their vibrant, young child or adolescent has a potentially life-threatening disease. Families are in a state of crisis when the diagnosis is made, with the first response being one of shock. At the same time that they are in a state of shock about the diagnosis, parents must gather resources to support the child, make treatment decisions, and adjust family life to integrate the needs of the child with cancer. Some families need to travel a great distance for the child's treatments, and others may have financial constraints that make healthcare costs a major concern. For nearly everyone, parental work schedules as well as arrangements for other children must be adjusted. Most cancer treatment will last for a minimum of several months up to several years, necessitating nearly constant adaptation. Parents, siblings, and extended families should all be included in plans of care.

The child reacts to the diagnosis based on age. Infants and toddlers are unaware of the severity of the disease, but react to a change in routine and to the anxiety of the care providers. Preschoolers are beginning to understand illness; however, they may think they caused their illness and are confused about why the parent cannot make the illness go away. School-age children can understand a diagnosis of cancer and benefit from opportunities to talk about the experience. Adolescents find contact with others who have gone through their experience reassuring and supportive. Nearly all children are hospitalized after diagnosis, and care should include proximity to parents, involvement in self-care appropriate for age, positive relationships with staff, and emotional care. Programs such as group therapy sessions, computer programs about cancer and treatment, and school reintegration all show potential for assisting youth who are adjusting to cancer. Children with cancer are commonly anxious about the treatments and disturbed schedules and routines (National Cancer Institute, 2011d).

Nursing Management

For the Child With Cancer

Nursing Assessment and Diagnosis

HISTORY
During health promotion visits of all children, nurses take into account the importance of a history of cancer in the family. Particularly when more than one person has had cancer, and when young children in the extended family have been affected, complete a family history, or genogram, to isolate cases in the family (see Chapter 3 for examples of genograms). A history of exposure to known carcinogens is also important. Does a parent work in an industry with substances like chemicals or asbestos that might remain on clothing worn home? Was the child treated with radiation or chemotherapy for a previous cancer? Does the child have an identified condition with a high incidence of some type of cancer, such as Down syndrome? Does the child have any recognized congenital anomalies? A number of conditions are more commonly associated with certain types of cancer.

PHYSIOLOGIC ASSESSMENT
When performing any physiologic assessment on children, consider the possible signs and symptoms of cancer. These include anemia, frequent infections, bleeding disorders, loss of weight, fatigue, pain, and changes in mental health and neurologic status. Assessment of children with the most significant types of childhood cancers is presented later in the chapter.

Once cancer has been diagnosed, a thorough physical assessment of all systems is needed to help identify the presence and extent of cancer (see Chapter 5). Systems needing particularly thorough assessments are neurologic, respiratory, cardiac, and gastrointestinal. Assess hydration status and the tumor site if it is visible. Carefully measure height and weight, and compare with prior findings for the child. Observe gait and coordination, as well as any changes in mental status. Evaluate immunization status, pain, nutritional intake, fatigue, infections, bruising, shortness of breath, and elimination problems. Periodic laboratory studies will be performed. Tailor assessments to the side effects of particular treatments. For example, the child on chemotherapy is likely to experience a **nadir** (lowest point) of WBC count about 10 days after drug administration so blood counts are needed then.

PSYCHOSOCIAL ASSESSMENT
Assessment of body image, stress and coping abilities, knowledge of the condition and cognitive level, support systems,

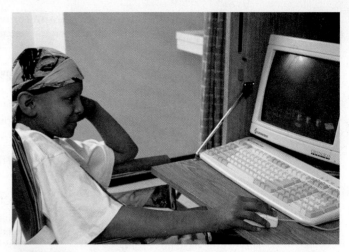

Figure 24–4 **One of the most common threats to a child's body image at any age is hair loss induced by chemotherapy. Use of hats can improve self-concept.**

and developmental level provides data that help determine the appropriate nursing interventions for the child with cancer and the family.

Body Image
Hair loss, surgical scars, and cushingoid changes are three common treatment-induced threats to body image. Most children being treated for cancer experience hair loss (Figure 24–4). Children who have cranial surgery lose hair as part of the surgical preparation. Chemotherapy frequently results in some degree of hair loss. The speed of hair loss is unique to the child and can be as rapid as overnight or slower, with hair left on the pillow and in the hairbrush.

A second challenge to the child's body image is surgery. The scars of cranial and neck surgery are obvious, as are amputation and limb salvaging. Abdominal surgery for lymphoma is more easily concealed but is still a threat to the child's body image.

A third source of altered body image is the cushingoid features, such as round and flushed face, prominent cheeks, double chin, and generalized obesity (Figure 24–5), that result from the

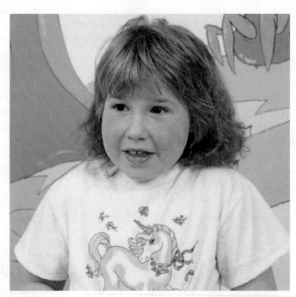

Figure 24–5 **The child with cushingoid changes frequently has a rounded face and prominent cheeks.**

As Children Grow: **Children Need Help in Coping With the Physical Effects of Cancer Treatment**

Children of different ages experience differing threats to body image as a result of cancer treatment. A preschool girl may be most upset at hair loss because she now looks like a boy. For many parents, especially of daughters, the loss of the child's hair can be devastating. Ask the parents and the child what the loss is like for them. Prepare them for the fact that hair loss can be rapid or slow. Find out how they will plan to cope. Some children want the hair cut very short so its loss will not be as traumatic. Offer resources for wigs, hats, or other ideas. Put them in touch with children who have lost hair and with those who have now regrown it.

A school-age child has the most difficult time with changes that interfere with the developmental task of industry. Amputation, which decreases the child's ability to participate in activities such as sports, dancing, and schoolwork, can be a major challenge during the school-age years. Assist children to adapt to new sports when they are able to do so. Partner with schools, coaches, and families to facilitate children's participation in activities they choose.

Teenagers are often most worried about changes like hair loss and cushingoid features, which cause them to look different from peers. Introducing adolescents to others of their own age who are coping with similar conditions can assist them in their developmental tasks.

use of corticosteroids. As the child's weight increases, stretch marks similar to those of pregnancy may occur. These stretch marks often remain after the corticosteroids are decreased.

Body image disturbances occur when a child cannot integrate changes and continues to cling to old images despite their inconsistency with reality. Common means for assessing body image are drawings, colored pictures cut out by the child to form a collage, discussion, and observation. See Chapter 11 for further discussion of these and other assessment techniques that can be used with children.

Stress and Coping

The diagnosis of cancer is a major stressor for both the child and the family. Although each child's prognosis and each family's coping mechanisms are unique, most families deal with the diagnosis in a manner similar to that of other families who have a child with a life-threatening illness (see Chapter 13). Assess the family (and child if old enough) for their understanding and acceptance of the diagnosis. Find out if the family has told the child and siblings about the diagnosis and if they need assistance in deciding how to do this. Assess the level of anxiety during healthcare visits and scheduled treatments (Figure 24–6). Evaluate the family's methods of coping, such as the ability to integrate relaxing and meaningful activities into family life, the use of

support systems in the extended family and community, and the ability to alter expectations to take into account the child's health status. Some families demonstrate resilience and the ability to assist the child and all of their members. Other families, however, may be experiencing multiple stresses, making adaptation to the new diagnosis particularly difficult. Concurrent stressors increase the difficulty of coping with childhood cancer. Evaluate the family for stressors such as illness or death of another family member, occupational changes, financial problems, relocation, and change in vacation plans. Evaluate the family's knowledge of the U.S. Family and Medical Leave Act benefits, which enable parents to use sick time, vacation, and leave without pay to care for an ill family member while safeguarding employment.

Knowledge

Anxious people tend to narrow their scope of attention and may read unintended messages into the behaviors of healthcare personnel. Anxiety also limits a person's ability to retain information.

Assess the child's knowledge of cancer and its treatment throughout the treatment period. As the child matures cognitively, reevaluate knowledge. Cancer and its treatment are complex topics. Parents are exposed to information in various forms, including written material, news reports, and Internet websites and resources. Evaluate their knowledge and information sources and provide them with opportunities to ask questions. Evaluate the learning style of the child and family in order to adapt approaches to meet their needs.

Support Systems

Cancer treatment generally occurs over a long time. The extended family is crucial in providing necessary support to the child, parents, and siblings. Identify key people in the family. They may be the parents, grandparents, or aunts and uncles. Support groups for children or other family members often help individuals and the family meet the challenges of the disease. Thoroughly assess the coping strategies the family uses to meet the various challenges posed by the child's illness. This information helps predict the success of interventions, such as home care with intravenous medications, and assists in deciding when referrals for other supportive therapies are needed.

The return to school may pose difficulties for the child with cancer or it may be a source of support to be connected again to peers. The child is encouraged to go to school, even if only for half a day per week, to stay connected to peers. Evaluate the school's ability to accept a child who is medically vulnerable into

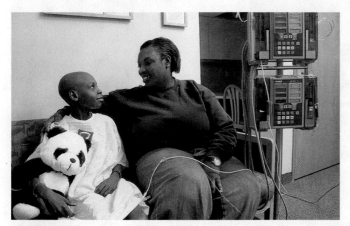

Figure 24–6 The child with cancer depends on parents and family members to provide support. Nurses can assist families and draw on their strengths to help the child.

the classroom. Assess whether the other children and teachers have been prepared for the appearance and needs of the child with cancer. Nurses who work in the oncology department of the hospital or clinic can ask if the family would give consent to visit the school, meet with the school nurse, and plan together to meet the child's educational needs. Help the teacher devise a plan to prepare the children, and offer to visit the classroom to explain what the child with cancer is experiencing. Arrangements can be made for tutors to help children keep up with schoolwork if they cannot attend school. An individualized education plan is needed. Parents need information about the legal right to home schooling and a specialized plan since the child is newly ill and they will likely not have been exposed to this in the past.

Assess family resources to identify support systems available to help the family during crises and if a child is expected to die. Extended supports include friends, jobs, insurance coverage, religious affiliations, cultural support systems, and the school system. Parents commonly lose contact with close friends after the diagnosis of cancer in a child. This is an additional stressor for the family. Jobs are often a source of support because coworkers may have gone through the same experience. It may also be comforting for parents to return to their jobs where they can feel a sense of security in tangible accomplishments. However, jobs can also be a source of stress if employers are unsympathetic to the demands of the child's hospitalization and clinic or office visits.

The nurse caring for a child and family in the end-of-life care phase can best support family members by helping them view the child's unique characteristics, conveying care and concern for the family, and continuing to have close contact with the dying child. Faith-based affiliations can be an important source of support. Evaluate whether such affiliations are meaningful for the family and, if so, plan for visits from the appropriate clergy. In some cultures, spiritual leaders are an important part of the family's support system. Enable a healer to visit the child and conduct a healing ceremony if that will be supportive to the family and child.

DEVELOPMENTAL ASSESSMENT

Developmental assessment of children should be performed regularly during treatment for cancer at times when the child is feeling well so that results are accurate. Assessment of the child's physical and neurologic development helps determine the progress made during treatment and provides a baseline for evaluating the long-term effects of treatment. Children under 6 years of age who have cancer should receive regular developmental assessment with a standardized screening tool (see Chapter 6). A home healthcare nurse can perform such testing, or it can be done by a nurse in the pediatric healthcare home (medical home) who sees the child for a general health supervision visit. Recommend referral to a neuropsychologist for testing early in treatment and if changes in developmental performance are noted. Children who have received cranial radiation and intrathecal chemotherapy need regular scholastic evaluations. Impaired neurocognitive performance may be a long-term effect of treatment. Observe developmental milestones at each contact with the child and refer for further assessment if regression has occurred. Performance in school and engagement in social activities with friends provide important information about expected developmental milestones in older children. If the parents have signed up for a clinical trial (research) treatment for the child, children should also give verbal or written assent when they have the cognitive maturity to do so.

ASSESSMENT FOR IMPACT OF CANCER SURVIVAL

Children with cancer have a variety of common psychologic and physiologic problems regardless of their specific type of

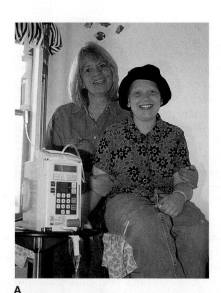
A

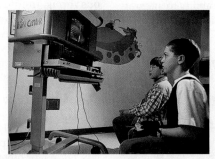
B

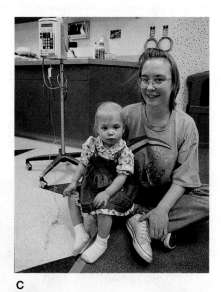
C

Figure 24–7 Survivors of childhood cancer. *A*, Nicole, 11 years old, is undergoing chemotherapy for Ewing sarcoma. Her mother emphasizes, "It's our faith that has gotten us through this. The hardest part is how busy you are coming to treatments all the time. Nicole's younger brother sometimes feels neglected." *B*, According to Jesse, who is 10 years old and waiting for a bone marrow transplant, "The thing that has helped me the most [in dealing with acute lymphoblastic leukemia] is all the mail I got from my friends." His mother adds, "We're just really positive and think that everything will turn out all right." *C*, Cassie, 19 months old, has been diagnosed with neuroblastoma. At this age, it is hard for her to understand what is happening to her. Her mother has stayed with her each time she has come to the hospital, which has helped Cassie adjust to therapy. Her caregivers are confident that she will respond well to her treatment.

cancer. They and their families are dealing with a complex illness that will influence their lives for years. The impact of this experience extends into all areas of function. During the past 20 to 30 years, treatment for childhood cancers has been increasingly successful, and 80% of children with cancer are now expected to have long-term survival. However, the success of new modalities and treatment combinations has created special healthcare needs for many survivors (Landier, Armenian, & Bhatia, 2015; Rueegg et al., 2013) (Figure 24–7).

Surgery can have many results. Body organs may be removed and manipulated, leading to adhesions, intestinal obstruction, visual impairment, neurologic disruption, and sterility. Removal of the spleen can lead to serious infections. Amputation necessitates the need for prosthetic devices and physical rehabilitation.

Radiation has several long-term effects. It can impair the growth of bones and teeth, leading to conditions such as scoliosis, leg length discrepancy, or poor dental health. Chronic pain can result from skeletal toxicity. Hypothyroidism can be observed in those who have had head and neck radiation. Cardiotoxicity and pulmonary toxicity can result from mediastinal radiation. Delayed puberty and sterility can result from radiation effects to the cranium and spinal regions. Impaired neurocognitive performance may occur as long-term effects of treatment, especially with higher doses of radiation.

Secondary cancers, most commonly solid tumors, occur in some survivors. **Secondary cancers** are also called *second malignant neoplasms (SMNs).* They occur subsequent to the primary cancer and treatment but are of a different histologic type. Cancers of the central nervous system, skin, breast, bone, and thyroid are examples of secondary neoplasms (Reulen et al., 2011). Most of these cancers can be effectively treated, emphasizing the need for thorough and frequent monitoring of the treated patient with cancer. Other chronic conditions, such as heart failure, congestive heart failure, cognitive dysfunction, and reproductive problems are more common in cancer survivors who are adults than in the general population, whereas cardiovascular risk and insulin resistance may even be more prevalent in child cancer survivors (Steinberger et al., 2012).

TABLE 24–4 Common Side Effects of Chemotherapy

SIDE EFFECT	CLINICAL MANIFESTATIONS	CLINICAL THERAPY
Bone marrow suppression	Evidence of suppression usually appears 7–10 days after administration of chemotherapy; recovery is usually complete within 3–4 weeks.	Blood transfusions are administered when anemia is severe (Hgb less than 7–8 g/dL) or platelets are very low and clinical examination reveals signs and symptoms of anemia or bleeding.
		Some institutions use a low-microbial diet to decrease the possibility that infectious organisms will colonize the intestine.
		Septra is used for *Pneumocystis jiroveci* pneumonia (formerly known as *P. carinii*) prophylaxis; additional drugs for antifungal and antibacterial prophylaxis are under investigation.
		Instruct the family and child about the importance of protecting the body from bruising during periods of mild to moderate thrombocytopenia (platelet count: 5000–20,000/mm^3).
		Careful hand hygiene is essential.
		Encourage use of masks if family or staff has nasopharyngeal infections.
Nausea and vomiting	Symptoms may occur immediately or 5–6 hr after administration of chemotherapy and may last 48 hr.	Antiemetics, such as ondansetron (Zofran), granisetron (Kytril), metoclopramide (Reglan), and diphenhydramine (Benadryl), are used to treat this side effect.
		Teach relaxation techniques, hypnosis, and systematic desensitization (a hypnotic process that progressively reduces reactions to objects that cause strong emotional or physical responses) to help decrease the child's symptoms.
		Encourage mild exercise and change of diet (eating only easily digestible foods) 12 hr before chemotherapy.
Anorexia and weight loss	May occur at any time.	Hyperalimentation is necessary if dietary changes are unsuccessful in halting the child's weight loss.
		Pay careful attention to changes in taste that affect food preferences.
		Referral to a dietitian may be helpful to achieve successful modification of the child's diet.
Oral ulcers	The oral mucositis resulting from chemotherapy usually occurs within 3–4 days and is often a contributing factor in anorexia.	Antifungal agents, such as nystatin or clotrimazole, lessen the possibility of candidal infection.
		Promote good oral hygiene, use soft foam wand or water irrigation to clean teeth; commercial mouthwashes are not recommended because they contain alcohol and increase drying of the oral cavity; specially formulated pharmacologic mouthwash may promote comfort.

(continued)

TABLE 24–4 Common Side Effects of Chemotherapy (*continued*)

SIDE EFFECT	CLINICAL MANIFESTATIONS	CLINICAL THERAPY
Constipation	Can occur at any time in treatment but becomes more common as therapy progresses and dietary intake and physical activity decrease.	Stool softeners and laxatives are used to treat this side effect (e.g., MiraLAX). Advise parents to increase fluids and fibrous foods in the child's diet.
Pain	Pain can occur at any time and is best understood by subjective explanations of the child.	Acetaminophen, morphine, steroids, and antidepressants may be used to manage pain; nonsteroidal anti-inflammatory drugs are often avoided because of their promotion of bleeding. Careful pain assessment is important; the location of the pain may provide a clue to its cause, for example, metastasis to the skull, infiltration of joints, or damage to soft tissue; pain associated with chemotherapy may also be related to oral mucositis, myalgia, or tumor embolization; painful polyneuropathy can follow treatment with vincristine or cisplatin. Acetaminophen for pain can mask the presence of fever, which signals infection; careful and complete physical assessment is needed to identify infection. Pharmacologic, nonhypnotic (deep breathing, self-control), and hypnotic methods of pain control may be used; the nonpharmacologic methods often prove helpful to children with pain from multiple etiologies.

Chemotherapy can cause a wide variety of effects, both during its administration and for years afterward (Table 24–4). Cardiomyopathy can occur with some drugs, especially the anthracyclines. Temporary or permanent pulmonary toxicity and renal complications can develop. Neurologic effects of some drugs can lead to hearing loss (e.g., cisplatin and ifosfamide), cataracts, and paraplegia (e.g., intrathecal methotrexate for leukemia). Learning disabilities or change in intelligence quotient (IQ) occurs in some children; infertility may result (Kirchhoff et al., 2011).

The diagnosis and stress of treatment, along with the risk of recurrence, are significant stressors for the child with cancer. Families may find it difficult to obtain full insurance coverage for the child who has had a prior cancer. Employment can be a potential problem for cancer survivors if employers have concerns about the earlier cancer diagnosis. Most people with cancer report fear of recurrence of the disease, which is a stressor. Some children report decreased quality of life (QOL) and emotional distress (Rueegg et al., 2013; Winick, 2011). Conversely, hopefulness and the sense of having an added purpose in life can be positive outcomes for many cancer survivors. Some meet with others who have a recent diagnosis, or work on fund-raising events that financially support cancer research. Survivorship services and care plans promote positive health outcomes (Eshelman-Kent et al., 2011).

Nurses are involved with families when a diagnosis of cancer is made, during the therapy process, and in the years that follow. For a child who survives cancer, ongoing care is essential. Evaluate the child regularly with thorough physical, psychosocial, developmental, and cognitive assessments. Carefully monitor all body systems (e.g., cardiovascular; respiratory; musculoskeletal; eye, ear, nose, and throat; genitourinary). Record height and weight, growth patterns, and nutritional patterns. Ask about the child's interactions with peers and performance at school. Children who have received cranial radiation and intrathecal chemotherapy need regular scholastic evaluations. Be alert for signs and symptoms that could indicate a secondary tumor.

Periodic laboratory studies will be performed. Ask the parents about insurance coverage and other financial difficulties during ongoing care.

Plan care to assist the family to manage any long-term effects of cancer treatment. This may involve physical rehabilitation, support related to visual impairment, or treatment for cardiac or musculoskeletal abnormalities. Provide resources for information and support. Facilitate periodic evaluations in a healthcare agency so that serious outcomes of treatment can be identified early.

The accompanying *Nursing Care Plans* include several diagnoses that may be appropriate for the child with cancer who is receiving care in the hospital or at home. Among the many other diagnoses that may be appropriate for a child with cancer are the following (NANDA-I © 2014):

- *Diarrhea* related to radiation therapy and toxins
- *Urinary Elimination, Impaired,* related to chemotherapy
- *Tissue Integrity, Impaired,* related to the effects of chemotherapy and radiation therapy on oral mucosa
- *Skin Integrity, Impaired,* related to altered nutritional state, effects of medication, radiation, and immobilization
- *Coping, Ineffective,* related to situational crisis of chronic and acute illness
- *Caregiver Role Strain* related to anxiety and disruption in family roles and patterns
- *Sleep Pattern, Disturbed,* related to biochemical agents, anxiety, and unfamiliar surroundings
- *Body Image, Disturbed,* related to chronic illness and treatments
- *Knowledge, Deficient (Child or Parents),* related to lack of exposure to disease or treatments
- *Grieving* related to actual or potential loss

Nursing Care Plan: Hospital Care of the Child With Cancer

1. Nursing Diagnosis: *Pain, Acute,* related to tissue injury (NANDA-I © 2014)

GOAL: The child will report reduced pain that is manageable.

INTERVENTION	RATIONALE
• Give analgesics as ordered.	• Adequate medications can reduce pain.
• Teach relaxation techniques, deep breathing, and distraction.	• Nonpharmacologic methods work with the medication to reduce pain.
• Insert pain management techniques appropriate for developmental age (see Chapter 15).	• Developmental level determines the pain assessment method that should be used, as well as the most appropriate intervention methods, from rocking, to distraction, to providing information.

EXPECTED OUTCOME: Child will experience pain reduced to the level that allows the child to interact appropriately and gain rest.

2. Nursing Diagnosis: *Nutrition, Imbalanced: Less than Body Requirements,* related to inability to ingest or digest food or absorb nutrients (NANDA-I © 2014)

GOAL: The child will maintain adequate nutritional intake. The child will experience reduced effects of chemotherapy (i.e., nausea and vomiting).

INTERVENTION	RATIONALE
• Offer small feedings. Encourage favorite foods. Refer to dietitian for special meals. Weigh daily.	• Measures can increase caloric intake. Taste changes and mouth sores alter desire for food.
• Teach the child distraction and relaxation techniques. Give antiemetics according to orders.	• Pharmacologic and nonpharmacologic methods are effective in helping to reduce nausea.

EXPECTED OUTCOME: Child will maintain admission weight or preillness weight. The child will have minimal side effects of nausea and vomiting.

3. Nursing Diagnosis: *Fluid Volume: Excess or Deficient* related to medications (NANDA-I © 2014)

GOAL: The child will be adequately hydrated.

INTERVENTION	RATIONALE
• Record all intake and output. Monitor intravenous rate and solution as appropriate. Monitor output from urine and other output routes such as vomiting or diarrhea.	• Some drugs (e.g., cyclophosphamide) necessitate a high level of fluid intake to prevent complications. Careful balance of intake and monitoring of output are required.
• Test specific gravity of urine daily.	• Renal function may be affected by chemotherapy.

EXPECTED OUTCOME: Child will demonstrate adequate hydration. Mucous membranes will be hydrated. Specific gravity will remain within normal range.

4. Nursing Diagnosis: *Infection, Risk for,* related to immunosuppression, invasive procedures, malnutrition, or pharmaceutical agents (NANDA-I © 2014)

GOAL: The child will remain free of infection.

INTERVENTION	RATIONALE
• Wash hands often. Maintain in isolation if needed.	• Hand hygiene is effective to reduce organisms. Transmission-based precautions may be needed to safeguard child.
• Monitor temperature. Use a noninvasive method such as tympanic; report method used when recording temperature. Report elevation to healthcare provider.	• Elevated temperature is a sign of infection. Children with oral or intestinal mucositis should not have temperature taken in these mucous cavities since it may cause increased irritation.

EXPECTED OUTCOME: Child will remain infection-free.

(continued)

Nursing Care Plan: Hospital Care of the Child With Cancer (continued)

GOAL: The child will return to normal, uninfected state.

INTERVENTION	RATIONALE
• Administer intravenous antibiotics as ordered. Monitor temperature. Use cooling mattress as ordered. Report elevations over 38°C (101°F) to healthcare provider.	• Multiple antibiotics are needed to deal with bacterial and fungal infections during neutropenia. Blood cultures may be taken to identify organism.

EXPECTED OUTCOME: The child with an infection will be effectively treated.

5. Nursing Diagnosis: *Coping, Ineffective,* **related to situational crisis (NANDA-I © 2014)**

GOAL: The child will demonstrate normal adaptive coping methods.

INTERVENTION	RATIONALE
• Encourage drawings and other therapeutic play for expression of feelings. Allow for expression of angry feelings, such as hitting dolls and throwing sponge balls. Discuss how to behave during treatments.	• Expression of feelings helps identify avoidance coping for further intervention. Play is a normal way for the child to express self and ideas. Misinterpretations can be corrected. Knowledge of appropriate and helpful behaviors supports self-esteem.

EXPECTED OUTCOME: Child will continue to use usual coping strategies expected for developmental stage.

Planning and Implementation

Nurses have many resources to assist in planning and implementing nursing care for the child with cancer. Oncology Nursing Society and the Association of Pediatric Hematology and Oncology Nurses are examples of organizations helpful to nurses. The nursing care of children newly diagnosed with cancer and their families includes immediate physiologic and psychologic support, along with anticipatory guidance about imminent and future medical interventions. Assist and support the family as they make decisions about types of treatment that are appropriate for the child.

Nursing care of the hospitalized child with cancer and the child receiving ongoing therapy at home is summarized in the accompanying *Nursing Care Plans*. These care plans are designed for the child who has progressed beyond cancer diagnosis and is receiving chemotherapy.

Physiologic care of the hospitalized child focuses on providing support during treatment. This includes ensuring optimal nutritional intake, administering medications, managing the multiple side effects of chemotherapy and radiation, ensuring adequate hydration, preventing infection, and managing pain during diagnostic procedures and treatment.

Nursing Care Plan: Home Care of the Child With Cancer

1. Nursing Diagnosis: *Health Management, Family, Ineffective,* **related to complex chemotherapeutic therapy (NANDA-I © 2014)**

GOAL: The family and child will comply with the child's medication regimen.

INTERVENTION	RATIONALE
• Educate parents and child about the importance of taking medication as prescribed.	• Understanding can assist parents and child in placing importance on medication intake.
• Set up calendar with dates, times, and medications clearly labeled.	• Visual reminders can help them recall instructions.
• Reward the child for taking medications.	• Reinforcing desired behaviors through rewards is effective with children.

EXPECTED OUTCOME: Child will take all medications according to prescription.

2. Nursing Diagnosis: *Development: Delayed, Risk for,* related to serious illness (NANDA-I © 2014)

GOAL: The child will demonstrate normal physical, emotional, and cognitive development.

INTERVENTION	RATIONALE
• Encourage play appropriate to age.	• Normal activities support self-esteem and self-knowledge.
• Encourage the child to attend school when able to do so. Arrange for tutors at home when unable to attend.	• School is the work of the child and promotes cognitive and social growth.
• Encourage seeing peers when unable to attend school.	• Peer contacts help the child in normal developmental tasks.
• Work with teachers to support reentry to school. Use puppets, videotape, and discussion with classmates.	• Classmates need to understand what has happened to their friend without asking the child directly.

EXPECTED OUTCOME: Child will continue to develop physically, emotionally, and cognitively at a normal pace.

3. Nursing Diagnosis: *Fatigue* related to disease state (NANDA-I © 2014)

GOAL: The child will maintain energy levels necessary for normal activities.

INTERVENTION	RATIONALE
• Problem solve ways to save energy for play and school.	• The child and parents are assisted to see school and play as important.
• Plan with child for quiet activities during low-energy times.	• The child is empowered to select and plan own activities.

EXPECTED OUTCOME: Child will plan use of time effectively to maintain energy for school and play. The child conserves energy during times of increased fatigue.

ENSURE OPTIMAL NUTRITIONAL INTAKE

The high metabolic rate of cancer growth depletes the child's nutritional stores. In addition, the catabolic effect of chemotherapy and radiation on normal cells necessitates additional cellular replacement. The child needs increased nutritional intake at a time when nausea and vomiting are occurring as drug side effects, and when decreased activity, treatment protocols, and general health status result in diminished appetite. This often leads to extreme concern on the part of parents, and they may focus excessive attention on the child's intake.

Administer antiemetic drugs to lessen nausea from chemotherapy. Integrate feeding methods and foods that the family and the child find most helpful for ensuring adequate intake. Allow the family to bring the child's favorite foods to the hospital. Ask the family what treatments they use to decrease the child's nausea and vomiting. Perform 24-hour dietary recalls to assess the child's intake, and evaluate height and weight regularly. Special nutritional products may be given orally, nasogastric or nasoduodenal tube feedings may be given, or total parenteral nutrition may be necessary.

ADMINISTER MEDICATIONS

An important intervention of the oncology nurse is administering medications safely. Most chemotherapeutic drugs are prescribed and calculated as dose per meter squared (dose/m²), with m² being calculated from the child's height and weight. (See the *Clinical Skills Manual* SKILLS .)

A number of chemotherapeutic drugs are commonly used in combinations. These drugs are prepared with special techniques under laminar flow devices to minimize potential toxic effects on healthcare providers. Gloves and other hazardous drug protocols are used. The Occupational Safety and Health Administration (OSHA) publishes an instruction manual entitled *Controlling Occupational Exposure to Hazardous Drugs* that outlines general guidelines, protective equipment, and procedures. Care must be taken to protect the patient as well; the nurse should avoid **extravasation** of intravenous drugs (leakage into the soft tissue around the infusion site) because permanent tissue damage can result.

In addition to chemotherapeutic drugs, the nurse administers other medications, such as antiemetics to control nausea, vitamin supplements, and antibiotics. Antiemetics such as ondansetron are given prophylactically when a cancer agent is administered that has known emetic effects. Ask parents about complementary therapy and medications they are obtaining from other sources and using at home. All medications must be safely administered and the child should be monitored for side effects. **Polypharmacy** (the use of several drugs at one time to treat multiple health conditions) can lead to multiple side effects and can challenge the body's ability to metabolize and excrete drugs.

Some children receive fluids and medications at home via central lines or by intramuscular or subcutaneous injection. Consider referral to home healthcare infusion agencies for monitoring of these treatments and provision of supplies for home use.

Families Want to Know

Nutrition and the Child With Cancer

Because of the effects of cancer and chemotherapy or other treatment, the child often has a poor appetite. Mucosal sores lead to difficulty chewing and swallowing. Parents can enhance the nutritional intake of the child in a variety of ways:

- Provide frequent small feedings rather than three meals daily.
- Integrate the child's favorite foods and the cultural foods common to the family into daily menus.
- Have nutritious snacks available for times when the child feels like eating.
- Sprinkle dried milk on top of cereals and other foods.
- Smooth, soft foods are usually preferred. Avoid acidic or spicy foods. Milkshakes with added peanut butter, puddings, and soft casseroles may be well tolerated. Try a variety of liquid protein-calorie supplements to find those the child likes.
- Avoid making food an area for disagreement. Do not force foods but rather make them readily available.
- If therapy is causing the child to vomit, do not encourage food at that time. The child may develop food aversions to foods that are vomited.
- Administer antiemetics as ordered during therapy since they can prevent nausea and vomiting.
- Report weight loss and increased fatigue.
- Bring the child in for scheduled health visits so growth, development, and effects of therapy can be monitored.
- Some children need a temporary feeding tube to ensure adequate nutrition. Feedings at night can often increase intake and promote health. Occasionally, a central line is inserted to provide total parenteral nutrition.
- Supplements and tube feedings will usually be covered by insurance if the healthcare provider writes an order for them.

MANAGE TREATMENT OF SIDE EFFECTS

All cancer treatments affect some normal body cells as well as cancer cells, causing a wide variety of side effects. Know all side effects of specific drugs administered and monitor for them. A frequent occurrence is **myelosuppression**, or suppression of blood cell production in the bone marrow. Be alert for signs of a decreased white blood cell count, such as infections. **Neutropenia** is present when the absolute neutrophil count is less than 500 cells/mm³ or if between 500 and 1000 cells/mm³ when chemotherapy is being given and falling levels are anticipated. At these levels, children will be given a broad-spectrum antibiotic; granulocyte colony-stimulating factor (G-CSF) may be given (refer to *Medications Used During Cancer Treatment: Colony-Stimulating Factors* earlier in the chapter). Take the child's temperature, isolate the child from others with infections, and perform serum laboratory studies as ordered. Although an elevated temperature generally indicates infection, in a child with immunosuppression, the temperature may be low even in overwhelming infection. A colony-stimulating factor for white cell production may be administered if necessary. A treatment known as *leucovorin rescue* is used in conjunction with high-dose methotrexate chemotherapy. Leucovorin (citrovorum factor) is a form of folic acid that helps protect normal cells from the destructive action of methotrexate. It is started within 36 hours of methotrexate administration and is given along with hydration therapy (Cohen & Wolff, 2013).

Protect the child from bruises and be alert for hemorrhage or signs of bleeding such as petechiae or the presence of blood in vomit and urine. These are all effects of **thrombocytopenia**, or decreased platelets. When thrombocytopenia occurs, minimize needlesticks and other intrusive procedures. Be ready to deal with nosebleeds and watch for bleeding gums. Report any bleeding episodes to the oncology specialist. Be sure parents know that the child should avoid contact sports or other rough activities and that any healthcare provider, such as a dentist, should be informed of the child's treatment and condition. Infusions to increase platelets are sometimes administered.

Inadequate red blood cell production can result in anemia. Encourage the child to eat iron-rich foods, and administer nutritional supplements as needed. Blood transfusions are sometimes needed to treat severe anemia.

Chemotherapy affects all rapidly growing cells in the body, but especially those of the mucous membranes. Provide good oral hygiene with a soft toothbrush, foam wand, or water irrigation device. Report oral breakdown promptly. See *Families Want to Know: Oral Care* for common techniques to manage oral hygiene. Be alert for blood in vomit and stool or dark-colored stools, all of which can indicate bleeding in the gastrointestinal tract. Blood in the urine may also occur. Know all side effects of specific drugs administered and monitor for them. Some side effects are late and may be seen after therapy is completed. Emphasize importance of all follow-up visits scheduled in the future for monitoring of late effects.

Radiation can cause burns to the skin. Examine the skin daily during hospitalization or weekly when making home visits. Leave the marks on the skin that outline the radiation target area. Avoid use of lotions, powders, and soaps on the target skin area. Some children may need to be anesthetized to ensure correct positioning for radiation; postanesthesia care will then be needed.

ENSURE ADEQUATE HYDRATION

Hydration management can be a challenge because the child may not be thirsty but is excreting large numbers of cell fragments and other substances as a result of treatment. Offer frequent small amounts of fluid. Include frozen ice pops or other fluid-containing foods such as Jell-O. Measure intake and output. To ensure adequate excretion, a number of chemotherapeutic drugs are given with intravenous fluids. It is important to administer fluids as ordered and ensure that the recommended urinary output excretion rate is maintained after drug administration.

Families Want to Know

Oral Care

Since cancer treatment and poor nutritional status can adversely affect the oral status of children, families need help to plan and carry out prophylactic and treatment measures. Children continue to lose teeth, have new teeth erupt, and require nutrients to help in building teeth not yet erupted even during cancer treatment. Some suggestions are:

- Provide a visit to the dentist early in treatment for assessment, treatment of dental disease, and establishment of a prevention plan.
- Brush teeth twice daily with a soft bristle brush and rinse with water.
- When granulocyte counts fall below 500/mm^3 or platelets fall below 40,000/mm^3, toothettes or gauze can be used to clean the teeth. Avoiding brushes will help to prevent bleeding and infection.
- Toothpaste can be used unless it causes discomfort.
- Medications may be used to prevent infection. They may include antibacterial mouthwash, nystatin, or fluconazole. Continue oral fluoride if it is not present in the drinking water.
- If bleeding, infection, or other oral care needs emerge, consult with the dentist and pediatric oncologist to develop a treatment plan.

PREVENT AND TREAT INFECTION

Children with cancer have an altered immune system, both from the disease and from the effects of immunosuppressant drugs, and must be kept away from persons with known infections. Teach parents to avoid taking the child to places that attract large gatherings of people, such as department stores, once the child returns home. Teach administration of any drugs being used to prevent infection such as pentamidine or sulfa preparations for *Pneumocystis* pneumonia prophylaxis. Emphasize the need to report any exposure to contagious diseases, especially chickenpox. Some drugs may mask signs of infection, so be alert for any signs of mild infection. Fever, malaise, and mild respiratory infection must all be reported promptly (see *Families Want to Know: Reportable Events for Children Receiving Chemotherapy*). Keep the child's immunization record so immunizations that have not been given yet can be administered in regular clinic visits after therapy is complete, using Centers for Disease Control and Prevention (CDC) recommendations for timing after treatment. Follow recommendations for the immunization of children with cancer as published by the CDC and the American Academy of Pediatrics (AAP). Usually, no immunizations are given to the child until 6 months after completing chemotherapy.

Management of infections is critical. Children are often hospitalized and central lines are used for antibiotic administration. Blood cultures and cultures of infected body parts help to establish the causative organisms. Because of lowered immune status, unusual agents are sometimes identified. Administer medication treatment on time and as ordered. Ensure standard precautions and transmission-based precautions are followed. Temperature and vital signs are taken and all body systems are assessed at admission and at least every 4 hours.

MANAGE PAIN

The child with cancer may experience pain from the disease itself and from the medical interventions, such as lumbar puncture, bone marrow aspiration, and frequent intravenous infusions and blood draws. Use all possible pain management techniques

Families Want to Know

Reportable Events for Children Receiving Chemotherapy

Parents require verbal and written instructions about signs and symptoms to report to the child's oncologist while the child is receiving chemotherapy. Have parents report the following events to the child's oncologist if they occur while the child is receiving chemotherapy:

- Temperature above 38°C (101°F)
- Any bleeding, such as nosebleeds, blood in stool or urine, petechiae, bruising
- Pain or discomfort with urination or defecation
- Sores in the mouth
- Vomiting or diarrhea
- Persistent pain anywhere, including headache
- Signs of infection, such as cough, fever, runny nose, tugging at ears
- Signs of infection in central lines, such as redness, drainage, or tenderness
- Exposure to communicable diseases, especially varicella (chickenpox)

Parents should also inform dentists and other healthcare providers that the child is receiving chemotherapy prior to procedures. Prophylactic antibiotics should be given before and after dental care.

Source: Adapted from Bindler, R. M., & Howry, L. B. (2005). *Pediatric drug guide*. Upper Saddle River, NJ: Prentice Hall.

to keep the child comfortable because this encourages cooperation throughout the long treatment period. Whenever possible, include the parents in comforting the child after painful procedures. (See Chapter 15 for suggestions on methods of pain management.) Nurses must examine research on effective pain management for children and integrate findings into practice (Fielding, Sanford, & Davis, 2013).

Sedation for diagnostic and therapeutic procedures (see Chapter 15) may be used for pain management. Administer sedation as ordered for young children who are undergoing lumbar punctures, radiation, and other procedures, and monitor them after the procedure. Coordinate other painful or intrusive tests so they can be done while the child is sedated for radiation.

Topical anesthetics such as eutectic mixture of local anesthetic (EMLA) cream may be used to numb the skin before an intravenous start, lumbar puncture, or bone marrow aspiration. Do not use EMLA on infants who are a gestational age of less than 37 weeks. Doses are individualized for infants and young children; follow guidelines for drug administration. For all infants, be certain that parents realize the importance of limiting the area and duration as ordered and to keep the cream in a safe place to avoid ingestion by any children. Other pain-prevention measures include fast-acting sprays, intradermal injection of anesthesia with lidocaine, iontophoresis (local anesthetic and electrical current), and sedation. Follow sedation monitoring protocols. (See the *Clinical Skills Manual* SKILLS .) Additional pain management techniques such as relaxation training and hypnosis may be beneficial. Having parents or other support persons present is helpful to most children.

PROVIDE PSYCHOSOCIAL SUPPORT

A diagnosis of cancer brings with it many emotions for the family. Initially, parents experience shock and anger. They need basic information about the disease and the purpose of the tests that will be performed. Instructions often need to be repeated as parents may not process information the first time it is presented because of their increased stress levels. Help the parents plan how and when to tell the child the diagnosis. What the child needs to know is based on the child's developmental level and understanding.

When family members have progressed from their initial state of shock about the diagnosis, they need to learn more about the disease. They may be interested in the pathophysiology, treatment, and expected outcome or the prognosis. Clarify their understanding of these areas and ask what questions they have. Provide verbal explanations and written material. Parents may talk with friends, purchase books, or search the Internet for information. Find out where they are getting information and provide additional resources when appropriate. Correct misconceptions and misinformation.

The family needs many strategies to deal with the challenge of long-term treatment for cancer. As the child experiences remissions and exacerbations or complications, the family feels alternately hopeful and discouraged. Identify the family's support systems and intervene as needed to enhance these systems. Facilitate contact with extended family members who might be of help, religious or spiritual connections, social service agencies, and other resources such as Internet and parent support groups. For parents who are concerned about job obligations and financial concerns, help them identify sources of financial assistance, respite from child care, and ways to take time for themselves.

Children undergoing treatment for cancer need support appropriate to their developmental stage and cognitive level. (See Chapters 4 and 11 for developmental levels and effective support strategies for children of different ages.) Younger children primarily need support during painful procedures and separation from parents. Older children need intervention strategies to help work

---

EVIDENCE-BASED PRACTICE | Cancer, Sleep, and Fatigue

Clinical Question

Inadequate amounts and quality of sleep are common problems among youth. Busy schedules and use of screen technologies contribute to poor sleep habits. Daytime sleepiness and other outcomes can result (Bartel, Gradisar, & Williamson, 2014). The child or adolescent with cancer is even more likely to have disturbed sleep, due to the cancer itself, the treatment protocols, and associated symptoms. What assessments and interventions should the nurse implement to understand sleep needs in the child with cancer?

The Evidence

A systematic review by nurses examined the measurement of sleep in adolescents with cancer by measures such as questionnaires, sleep diaries, and actigraphy (a watchlike device that measures movement and accurately displays sleep time). Primary reasons for disturbed sleep in cancer treatment included pain, frequent awakenings or fragmented sleep, and symptoms such as nausea (Erickson et al., 2011). Both mothers and children with acute lymphoblastic leukemia had disturbed sleep patterns, difficulty falling asleep, and fatigue (Matthews, Neu, Cook, et al., 2014).

Sleep disturbance may even continue after cancer treatment is completed because of brain changes that resulted from a tumor, or from treatment such as radiation or chemotherapy. In over 1400 survivors of childhood cancer, fatigue and poor sleep quality were identified (Clanton et al., 2011).

Best Practice

Cancer interfaces with normal developmental progression in several ways, one of which is sleep. Question sleep patterns at each oncology visit, provide suggestions for sleep hygiene, and refer the child and parents for sleep intervention as needed. Inquire about daytime sleepiness and fatigue. Have the family remove televisions and cell phones from the youth's bedroom, arrange for rest periods each day, and maintain routines that enable sleep.

Clinical Reasoning

Plan a series of questions to ask children and teens with cancer about the amount of sleep obtained on weekdays and weekends, patterns of sleep, and any changes in sleep since the cancer was diagnosed. Inquire about how the disease and its treatment have influenced sleep in the parents. What sleep hygiene measures can assist in acquiring needed sleep time and quality?

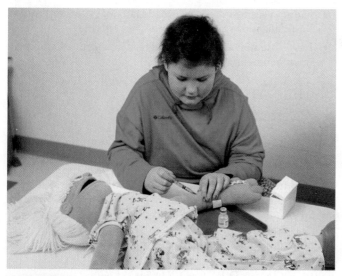

Figure 24–8 A child in a pediatric oncology clinic giving injections to a doll. This type of play therapy helps the child deal with fear, thus lowering her stress level.

through feelings about treatments (Figure 24–8). A major developmental task of adolescence is to attain independence and control, but cancer often interferes with adolescents' ability to achieve this task. Therefore, plan nursing strategies that empower adolescents as much as possible. Introduce them to other teens with similar diagnoses and allow them to make decisions and choices independent of parents when possible. An adolescent can decide which type of medication port would be best (e.g., an implantable port under the skin or a venous access device with tubing outside the body). Making this choice enables the teen to feel more in control of the disease and treatment. (See *Evidence-Based Practice: Cancer, Sleep, and Fatigue.*)

Talk with the child's teachers before the return to school after treatment to explain the child's condition. Ask them to notify the family immediately of diseases or infections in other children so the child with cancer treatment who is immunocompromised can be kept home. Arrange for tutors if necessary to assist the child with schoolwork during hospitalization and home care. Explore the option of summer camp for children with cancer. The Make-A-Wish Foundation strives to make dreams come true for ill children by sponsoring them for a desired activity or outing. Refer the child to this foundation if appropriate.

The siblings of a child who has cancer may grieve over the ill brother or sister and may feel sad and depressed. Inquire about what they know about the child's condition and their reactions or behavior changes. Consider the impact on siblings when a child is being treated for cancer. They may alternately resent and feel guilty for the sibling's illness. They may not understand the treatments or disease. School progress may be slowed and teachers may not be aware of the sibling's stress. Ask the parents if the siblings are demonstrating symptoms such as depression, behavioral changes, or decrease in school performance and suggest interventions as appropriate. Find out who is caring for siblings and whether their teachers have been informed about the family situation. Invite them to play therapy sessions and recreational activities with the ill child. They may benefit from speaking with a school counselor or can be referred to a support group for siblings of children with cancer. Some cancer summer camps welcome siblings as well as children with cancer.

Chapter 13 offers strategies to help the family of a child with cancer cope with the stressor of a life-threatening illness.

For some types of cancer, the child may experience a remission with treatment, but a recurrence of disease later as cancer cells grow again. The family may become angry or depressed about the relapse. Repeated treatments challenge the family's support systems. Waiting for the outcome of diagnostic tests can be an especially challenging time. Provide information as soon as possible. If the child's illness progresses, refer the family to hospice to help them care for the terminally ill child and work through the grieving process. Explore cancer support groups and share this information with families.

DISCHARGE PLANNING AND HOME CARE TEACHING

Preparation for home care centers on creating a normal environment while supporting the child's physiologic and psychosocial responses to the cancer and treatments. Education is the primary focus of discharge planning. Teach the parents how to ensure adequate nutritional intake, to be alert for signs of infection, to protect the child from exposure to communicable diseases during times of neutropenia, to administer medications at home, and to handle vomiting and pain. Help the parents and child deal with any obstacles to normal development and functioning. Teach the parents and family about symptoms that need to be treated immediately.

Home management of a vascular access device or central line, such as a Broviac catheter, initially challenges parents (Figure 24–9). An implanted port, which allows the child freedom to swim and engage in other activities, may be used. Parents will need information about whatever device the child has received. Demonstrate details about cleaning the site, instilling heparin in the line or reservoir, and other needed care. After teaching the parents, observe them performing the procedure before the child is discharged.

Emphasize the need for the child and family to have fun and be as normal as possible. Play distracts the child and is essential in reducing fears. Children, parents, and siblings often benefit from

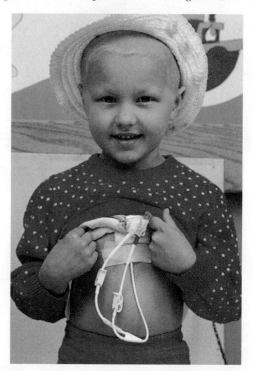

Figure 24–9 Comfort and convenience. A vascular access device allows chemotherapeutic agents to be administered without the need for repeated "sticks" to the child.

participation in cancer support groups and cancer summer camps. These activities create additional support systems, build the child's self-esteem, and enhance coping skills through role modeling. (See *Families Want to Know: Cancer Therapy* earlier in this chapter.)

Make home visits to evaluate the family's strengths and needs in the home setting. Be sure that the family has adequate support from hospice and other end-of-life services when a child's condition is terminal.

Most children are treated for cancer over a period of 2 to 3 years. Since normal developmental stages progress during this time, health promotion and health maintenance visits should still occur. Some usual care may have to be altered, but many of the same developmental concerns of all children should be addressed. Help parents to view the child as a "normal" child who is ill for a period of time, but still needs to have limits set on behavior, to develop healthy lifestyles, and to have environmental stimulation to learn to talk, read, or perform motor and cognitive tasks.

Evaluation

Expected outcomes of nursing care for the child with cancer relate to the specific disease, treatments, and responses. Some examples of outcomes include the following:

- The child demonstrates adequate intake to promote normal growth.
- Hydration is adequate to support body processes and ensure drug and cancer cell product elimination.
- Treatment side effects are promptly identified.
- Pain is managed to a level of comfort satisfactory to child and family.

- Family uses resources to provide necessary support during hospitalizations and treatments.
- Family demonstrates knowledge of management and treatment regimens.

Solid Tumors

Brain Tumors

Central nervous system (CNS) or brain tumors are the most commonly occurring solid tumors in children and the second most common malignancy, after leukemia. Each year approximately 1300 children under 5 years of age and 2200 youth up to 20 years of age are diagnosed with tumors of the brain and CNS, accounting for one in five childhood cancers; the overall survival rate is 70% ("Brain Tumor Incidence," 2011; Kuttesch, Rush, & Ater, 2011; McLendon, Adekunle, Rajaram, et al., 2011).

ETIOLOGY AND PATHOPHYSIOLOGY

The cause of most brain tumors is unknown. About 5% to 10% of brain tumors are genetic in origin. Exposure to radiation is a known risk factor, such as CNS radiation used for treatment of some other cancers. There is a higher incidence in children than adults with certain other cancers or diseases such as retinoblastoma, renal tumors, neurofibromatosis, tuberous sclerosis, or endocrine syndromes (Faria, Rutka, Smith, et al., 2011; Pollack & Jakacki, 2011).

Brain tumors in children usually occur below the roof of the cerebellum and involve the cerebellum, midbrain, and brainstem (see *Pathophysiology Illustrated: Brain Tumors*). In contrast, brain tumors in adults are usually located above the areas between the cerebrum and cerebellum.

Pathophysiology Illustrated: **Brain Tumors**

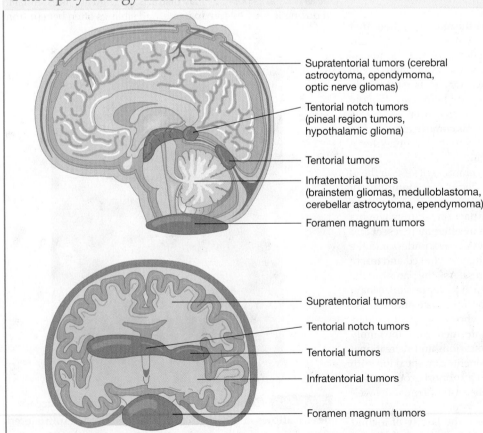

Supratentorial tumors (cerebral astrocytoma, ependymoma, optic nerve gliomas)

Tentorial notch tumors (pineal region tumors, hypothalamic glioma)

Tentorial tumors

Infratentorial tumors (brainstem gliomas, medulloblastoma, cerebellar astrocytoma, ependymoma)

Foramen magnum tumors

Supratentorial tumors

Tentorial notch tumors

Tentorial tumors

Infratentorial tumors

Foramen magnum tumors

Approximately 1700 children under the age of 14 years are diagnosed annually as having tumors of the brain and CNS. The four most common brain tumors in children are medulloblastoma, cerebral astrocytoma, ependymoma, and brainstem glioma ("Brain Tumor Incidence," 2011; Kuttesch et al., 2011; McLendon et al., 2011).

Health Promotion The Child Receiving Cancer Treatment

Cancer treatment often extends for several years, so the child needs to continue health promotion and health maintenance visits.

Growth and Development Surveillance

- The child is assessed for height, weight, and body mass index. This provides information about growth patterns, which may be altered by cancer treatment. If indicated, 24-hour diet recalls and other nutritional assessments are performed.

- Teaching is provided about age-appropriate foods. Since appetite may be impaired during periods of treatment, the child may be lacking fruits, vegetables, or other foods, as well as the nutrients they include. Encourage parents to be sure the child has a well-balanced diet during periods of remission.

- Perform developmental screening of young children. Provide suggestions for parents about the stimulation that is appropriate for the child's age. Include quiet activities that can be used when the child is fatigued or receiving therapy. These might include reading books, listening to tapes and music, and working on a computer. Have the parent plan for these activities on days that the child goes for chemotherapy or other treatment.

- Ask about the school-age child's progress in school. Performance may be altered because of neurologic effects of treatment as well as missing school. Plan for the family to partner with the school personnel for provision of tutors, computer programs, or other needed assistance.

- Encourage continued social contact with peers when blood counts are adequate to prevent infection.

Physical Assessment and Screening

- Careful physical assessments are performed to identify any abnormalities that may result from cancer or its treatment. Cardiopulmonary and neuromuscular assessments are particularly important. Vision and hearing should be assessed prior to treatment and periodically throughout. Include measurements of fine and gross motor activity.

Elimination

- Toddlers may have an interruption in toilet training during periods when they do not feel well. Help parents understand this regression and encourage them to start again when the child is feeling better.

- Some medications cause diarrhea or constipation, so evaluate bowel patterns and provide guidance as needed. Skin care instruction may be needed if the child has diarrhea and is relatively immobile. Increasing fluids and fiber foods may be needed for constipation.

- Evaluate urinary output since many medications have effects on kidney function. Encourage adequate fluids for age to ensure elimination of medications.

Sleep and Fatigue

- Children undergoing treatment often have disturbed sleep patterns. Parents of young children may become exhausted working all day, getting the child to treatments, and having disturbed sleep at night. Assess both the child's sleep patterns and the family's experiences. Encourage plans for respite care to enable rest periods.

- Provide cots, rocking chairs, and other comfortable settings for child and family members during treatments.

- Both child and parents may not expect or understand the profound fatigue that occurs during cancer treatment. They can be helped to plan for providing quiet times, and replenishing energy through naps, massage, relaxing baths, and spending time with family.

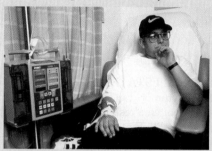

Physical Activity

- Because the child has periods of fatigue, patterns of physical activity may decrease. Emphasize the importance of integrating physical activity when the child feels well, since it is needed for learning gross motor skills, facilitating blood flow, improving mental status, and setting patterns for the future.

Disease and Injury Prevention Strategies

- The child with cancer has the same safety hazards as other children of the same age, and such topics as car safety seats, fire prevention, water safety, and violence prevention should be addressed.

- An important hazard for children with cancer is infection due to decreased immune response. Keep records of immunization status. Follow the recommendations of the CDC and AAP for other immunizations. Teach about the hazards of large groups when the child's immune system is compromised. Discuss the care of central lines and other potential sources of infection. Have families report signs of infection and exposure to known illnesses promptly.

Mental and Spiritual Health

- Evaluate the child and family for signs of anxiety and depression. Ask how they are managing the cancer treatment and what poses the greatest challenges. Refer to other families with similar circumstances for support.

- Ensure that the child has contact with friends through child care, school, or via phone, letters, and a computer.

- Find out the impact of the child's cancer on the parent's jobs. Ask how the siblings have been coping, what changes there are in school performance, and whether teachers and others are aware of the stress the sibling may be experiencing.

Transitional Care

- As the child's treatment ends, instruct the child's parents about needed periodic follow-up with the oncologist. Continue to perform neurologic examinations and ascertain school performance. Be alert for signs of secondary tumors.

- Ask about worries regarding the future. As teens grow older, have them take over more responsibility for informing healthcare providers of their cancer history and assist them to transition to adult healthcare providers.

TABLE 24–5 Clinical Manifestations of Brain Tumors

TUMOR	ETIOLOGY	CLINICAL MANIFESTATIONS	CLINICAL THERAPY
Medulloblastoma	External layer of cerebellum	Headache, vomiting, ataxia	Surgery; chemotherapy with lomustine, vincristine, cisplatin; radiation
Astrocytomas	Glial cells, supratentorial or infratentorial	Seizures, visual disturbances, increased intracranial pressure, vomiting	Surgery; chemotherapy with vincristine, dactinomycin; radiation
Ependymoma	Fourth ventricle, posterior fossa	Hydrocephalus	Surgery, radiation
Brainstem gliomas	Pons	Cranial nerve (VI + VII) tract signs, nystagmus, ataxia, motor symptoms	Surgery, radiation

CLINICAL MANIFESTATIONS

Children with brain tumors can manifest behavioral and nervous changes. These are often a result of increased intracranial pressure and may occur either rapidly or slowly and subtly. Some common symptoms include headache, nausea, vomiting, abnormal gait, dizziness, change in vision or hearing, fatigue, and mental status changes such as educational or behavioral problems.

Brainstem tumors can present with weight deficits and may be mistakenly diagnosed as an eating disorder of infancy and childhood (failure to thrive). This may delay proper treatment. See Table 24–5 for common manifestations of certain types of brain tumors.

Medulloblastomas are brain tumors in the external layer of the cerebellum. They account for 35% to 40% of childhood brain tumors, and commonly occur in children 5 to 6 years of age. *Astrocytomas* arise from glial cells and can be either above or below the area between the cerebrum and cerebellum. They account for 35% to 40% of childhood brain tumors. The presenting symptoms vary depending on the location of the tumor. Endocrine, vision, and behavioral changes are all possible, as well as increased intracranial pressure and seizures. *Ependymomas* commonly occur in the fourth ventricle of the posterior fossa and comprise 10% to 15% of childhood brain tumors. Impaired growth, hydrocephalus, seizures, and cranial nerve impairments are the most common manifestations. *Brainstem gliomas* are located in the pons and typically spread into the surrounding tissue. They account for 10% to 15% of childhood brain tumors (Kuttesch et al., 2011).

CLINICAL THERAPY

Brain tumors are diagnosed with computed tomography (CT), magnetic resonance imaging (MRI), positron emission tomography (PET), single-photon emission computed tomography (SPECT), myelography, and angiography. New technologies combine imaging with angiography to more specifically image the lesion. Examples include magnetic resonance angiography (MRA), magnetic resonance spectroscopy (MRS), perfusion and diffusion imaging, digital subtraction angiography (DSA), and CT angiography (CTA) (Paldino, Faerber, & Poussaint, 2011). Neurophysiologic tests (electroencephalography and brainstem evoked potentials) are used to assess sensory pathway integrity and disease-related or drug-related sensory dysfunction. Other tests that may be performed are tumor markers and cerebrospinal fluid cytology. Lumbar puncture identifies abnormal cells in the cerebrospinal fluid. Bone marrow aspiration and bone scans identify extracranial primary neoplastic growth since cancers in other sites can metastasize to the brain.

Treatment depends on the type of brain tumor. Surgery is common. It may be performed to obtain a biopsy specimen, to debulk (reduce the tumor by partial removal) or excise the tumor, or to treat any hydrocephalus that may be present. During surgery, radiologic images allow the neurosurgeon to see computerized images of the brain while stimulating nerves to determine their functioning. These techniques provide rapid feedback to the neurosurgeon. Laser surgery, which has delicate precise control and accuracy, is used when tumors are close to sensitive neural or vascular structures.

Use of radiation after surgery and chemotherapy has improved the survival of children with medulloblastoma and ependymoma. High-dose chemotherapy is often used, and this modality has improved the survival of children with CNS tumors. Low-dose chemotherapy can shrink and help manage some tumors. Intrathecal administration of chemotherapy is useful in some cases. An Ommaya reservoir, a dome-shaped device with a catheter, may be surgically placed under the scalp to administer chemotherapy directly to the central nervous system.

However, the blood–brain barrier reduces the effectiveness of chemotherapy for children with brain tumors. For example, when methotrexate is administered intrathecally (in the spinal canal), only a small amount crosses normal brain capillaries. Radiation is not used in children under 3 years old because of resultant damage to brain cells. Hematopoietic stem cell transplantation is increasingly used. Numerous new approaches are being investigated and will be used increasingly in the years ahead. New combinations of chemotherapeutic agents, precision-guided delivery of medications and radiotherapy, gene therapy, cytokine-producing therapy to activate the immune system, molecular analysis and epigenetic markers to guide treatment, and blood–brain barrier disruption are examples of emerging treatments (Faria et al., 2011; Pollack, 2011).

Clinical Tip

The following are examples of drugs that may be used to treat brain tumors (Kuttesch et al., 2011):

- Cyclophosphamide
- Ifosfamide
- Lomustine
- Methotrexate
- Vincristine
- VP-16
- Cisplatin
- Carboplatin
- Nitrosourea
- Temozolomide

Complications of treatment for children with brain tumors are significant. They include severe infections (associated with high-dose chemotherapy), seizure activity, sensorimotor defects, hydrocephalus, and growth problems. Care is taken to treat infections early and aggressively. If a cerebrospinal shunt is used, infection or blockage can occur. (See Chapter 27 for further discussion of cerebrospinal shunts in children.) Anticonvulsants are commonly given prophylactically after surgery. Endocrine problems, such as growth hormone changes, hypothyroidism, and panhypopituitarism, may occur when the tumor is in the hypothalamic–pituitary area. Treatment may also lead to impaired cognitive function and emotional or behavioral problems in some children. Memory deficits and selective attention deficits are the most common problems.

Diabetes insipidus is a special consideration in children with midline brain tumors, such as those that compress the hypothalamus, pituitary stalk, or posterior pituitary gland. Manifestations of diabetes insipidus include voiding of large amounts of dilute urine with a specific gravity of less than 1.005 to 1.010 (see Chapter 30).

Nursing Management

For the Child With a Brain Tumor

Nursing Assessment and Diagnosis

The focus of physiologic assessment of the child with a brain tumor is determined by its presentation (Table 24–6). Presenting signs can be categorized as follows:

- Nonspecific signs related to increasing intracranial pressure
- Secondary signs related to displacement of intracranial structures
- Focal signs suggesting direct involvement of the brain and cranial nerves

Thorough neurologic examination before surgery is essential to provide a record of baseline functioning. The neurologic examination also allows the evaluation of the child's changing physiologic status before surgery. Ask if the child has manifested slow changes over time or has had quickly developing symptoms. Measurement of head circumference and assessment of the anterior fontanelle are necessary in children under the age of 18 months.

Perform developmental screening on young children using the Denver II or other developmental test (see Chapter 6). Ask about the child's social interactions, school performance, and any behavior changes that have occurred.

Several nursing diagnoses can be identified for the child with a brain tumor depending on the type and location of the tumor. Some common examples follow (NANDA-I © 2014):

- *Nutrition, Imbalanced: Less than Body Requirements,* related to loss of appetite

TABLE 24–6 Physiologic Assessment of Brain Tumors

CLINICAL MANIFESTATIONS	ASSESSMENT
Nonspecific signs: headache, morning vomiting, somnolence, irritability	Level of consciousness, pupil response, pupil shape and size
Secondary signs: disturbances of cranial nerves; other signs depend on site of tumor	All cranial nerves
Focal signs: truncal ataxia (midline brain tumors), general nystagmus, head tilting	Motor ability, head positions when watching television or looking at people (double vision, sixth cranial nerve involvement)

- *Mobility: Physical, Impaired,* related to tumor pressure on coordination centers
- *Development: Delayed, Risk for,* related to effects of disability
- *Memory, Impaired,* related to neurologic disturbance
- *Pain, Acute,* related to compression of brain tissue

Planning and Implementation

The child with a brain tumor requires multidisciplinary care by, among others, a neurologist, neurosurgeon, pediatrician, dietitian, and social worker. Other specialists are also often needed. The nurse can act as a case manager to coordinate the complex care needed by the child.

For the nursing care of children immediately following surgery, refer to Chapter 11. In addition, close monitoring of neurologic status is needed postoperatively (refer to Chapter 27). Be especially alert for signs of increased intracranial pressure and infection. Observe for seizure activity. Administer drugs such as antibiotics and anticonvulsants as ordered.

Signs and symptoms of diabetes insipidus may occur following brain surgery (see Chapter 30 for a description of diabetes insipidus). Nursing care includes hourly measurement of intake and output, measurement of serum sodium levels every 4 to 6 hours, accurate fluid replacement, and frequent assessment of neurologic status. An indwelling urinary catheter is useful for accurate measurement of urinary output.

DISCHARGE PLANNING AND HOME CARE TEACHING

Teach the parents to watch for an increase in the child's voiding of dilute urine. Be sure they can recognize the signs of infection and changes in the child's neurologic status. Once the child is ready for discharge, chemotherapy or radiation may begin; tell parents the reason and potential side effects of these treatments. Help the family get any special equipment they may need to care for the child at home, such as a wheelchair, bed rails, or dressings. The American Cancer Society is a potential resource for assistance with these needs.

Children with brain tumors, especially those who have received radiation, often have some permanent sequelae. They may have slowed development, incoordination, learning disabilities, or other effects. These sequelae are most common in children who are 3 years of age or younger at the time of radiation therapy. Perform accurate height and weight measures at each healthcare visit. Assess developmental milestones. Ask about progress in school and any special services that might be needed. Perform thorough neurologic assessments. Support the family as they learn to deal with unknown or changed expectations for the child's performance.

Evaluation

Expected outcomes of nursing care for the child with a brain tumor depend on the site of tumor, clinical therapy, and medical outcome. Some outcomes might include the following:

- Nutritional intake is adequate to support growth and prevent malnutrition.
- A safe environment is maintained for the child.
- Physical mobility is maintained to the limits of developmental level and alterations of disease.
- An environment that supports normal developmental milestones within the capability of the child is maintained.
- Pain is managed to a level of comfort.
- Parents understand the diagnosis and treatment plan.

Neuroblastoma

Neuroblastoma is the solid tumor most commonly occurring outside the cranium of children. It is responsible for 8% to 10% of childhood cancers and 15% of cancer deaths in children. The average age at diagnosis is 17 to 22 months; it is the most common tumor in infants during the first year of life. Nearly all cases (90%) are diagnosed before 5 years of age (Zage & Ater, 2011). Prognosis varies, depending on the staging of the tumor (Table 24–7) and the age of the child, with more favorable outcomes in infants under 1 year of age and in presenting sites in the pelvis or thorax. Less favorable outcomes are associated with the presence of N-*myc* oncogen amplification. Survival rates are 90% for stages 1 and 2, but drop to 25% to 35% for stage 4 (Zage & Ater, 2011). As compared to White, Hispanic, and Asian children, more Black and Native American children have advanced disease upon diagnosis and therefore lower survival rates (Henderson et al., 2011). It is unknown if genetic differences or lack of consistent primary care contributes to this disparity.

Neuroblastoma is commonly a smooth, hard, nontender mass that can occur anywhere along the sympathetic nervous system chain. A frequent location is the abdomen, although other sites are the adrenal, thoracic, and cervical areas.

ETIOLOGY AND PATHOPHYSIOLOGY

Neuroblastoma originates in primitive neurocrest cells that form the adrenal medulla, paraganglia, and sympathetic nervous system of the cervical sympathetic chain and the thoracic chain. Approximately 50% of neuroblastomas develop in the adrenal medulla; 30% develop in the cervical, thoracic, or pelvic ganglia; and the remaining are elsewhere along the sympathetic chain (Zage & Ater, 2011). Lymph node metastasis is common because of the proximity of the tumor origin to the lymph system drainage.

TABLE 24–7 International Neuroblastoma Staging System

STAGE	DESCRIPTION
1	Localized tumor confined to the area of origin; complete gross excision, with or without microscopic residual disease; identifiable ipsilateral and contralateral lymph nodes negative microscopically
2A	Unilateral tumor with incomplete gross excision; identifiable ipsilateral and contralateral lymph nodes negative microscopically
2B	Unilateral tumor with complete or incomplete gross excision; with positive ipsilateral regional lymph nodes; identifiable contralateral lymph nodes negative microscopically
3	Tumor infiltrating across the midline with or without regional lymph node involvement; or unilateral tumor with contralateral regional lymph node involvement; or midline tumor with bilateral regional lymph node involvement
4	Dissemination of tumor to distant lymph nodes, bone, bone marrow, liver, and/or other organs (except as defined in stage 4S)
4S	Localized primary tumor as defined for stage 1 or 2 with dissemination limited to liver, skin, and/or bone marrow; bone marrow involvement should be minimal (less than 10% of cells; if greater it is stage 4 disease

Source: Data from National Cancer Institute. (2011e). *Stages of neuroblastoma*. Retrieved from http://www.cancer.gov/cancertopics/pdq/treatment/neuroblastoma/HealthProfessional/page2

The cause of neuroblastoma is unknown. A genetic defect found in many cases of neuroblastoma is a deletion of the short arm of chromosome 1 (1p del); other abnormalities include 11q, 14q, and 17q. Amplification of the proto-oncogene N-*myc* or mutation of *Phox2B* and *ALK* genes may be seen (Shuangshoti et al., 2011; Zage & Ater, 2011).

CLINICAL MANIFESTATIONS

The location of the mass determines the symptoms. A retroperitoneal mass causes altered bowel and bladder function; characteristic signs are weight loss, abdominal distention, enlarged liver, irritability, fatigue, and fever. Dyspnea or infection may occur when the tumor is mediastinal. Neck and facial edema may result from vena cava syndrome if the tumor is mediastinal and large. Intracranial lesions may be present with periorbital ecchymosis. Malaise, fever, and a limp can occur if there has been metastasis to the bone. Bone marrow disease can manifest as **pancytopenia** (abnormal depression of all cellular blood components) with neutropenia (causing infections) and anemia (causing fatigue). Metastatic spread can result in an array of symptoms affecting multiple organs.

CLINICAL THERAPY

The International Neuroblastoma Staging System (INSS) recommends different diagnostic and laboratory evaluations for diagnosis of the primary disease and of metastases (see Table 24–7). Biopsy of the tumor is used for initial diagnosis, and metastases are diagnosed by bone marrow biopsy, radiolabeled scanning, x-ray, CT, and MRI. Tumor markers include vanillylmandelic acid (VMA), homovanillic acid (HVA), dopamine, ferritin, NSE (an enzyme in neural tissue), lactic dehydrogenase (LDH), and a ganglioside GD2 (a sugar and lipid molecule on the surface of neural cells). VMA and HVA are by-products of adrenal hormones, and their levels are usually elevated in the urine and blood (see Appendix D for normal values). Areas of necrosis and calcification are readily identifiable with radiologic tests. These tests also help in the staging of the disease by identifying metastases. Urinary catecholamines are often increased.

Routine blood cell counts are needed, including CBC with differential. The test may reveal anemia and thrombocytopenia. There is no classic WBC response, although thrombocytopenia may occur in association with disseminated intravascular coagulation. **Leukocytosis** (higher than normal leukocyte count) and **leukopenia** (lower than normal leukocyte count) have been observed with bone marrow involvement. Serum electrolytes, liver function studies, LDH, coagulation studies, and urinalysis are performed. Elevations in dopamine, ferritin, NSE , LDH, and GD2 are seen. All of these laboratory findings are used initially to diagnose the disease and later to follow its progress. A biopsy or surgical removal of the tumor will be followed by analysis of its type and genetic abnormalities. Areas of necrosis and calcification in major organs are readily identifiable with radiologic tests and MRIs. These tests also help in the staging of the disease by identifying metastases.

The stage of the tumor determines the treatment protocol. Surgical excision of the mass is performed and may be the only treatment in low-risk stages. With higher risk, surgery is followed by chemotherapy with a combination of drugs. Radiation is often used, especially in disseminated disease or when tumors are not receptive to chemotherapy. Autologous stem cell transplantation may be performed for advanced disease, sometimes followed by the biologic modifier *cis*-retinoic acid and fenretinide (to promote apoptosis) (Zage & Ater, 2011).

Clinical Tip

The following are examples of drugs that may be used to treat neuroblastoma:

- Cyclophosphamide
- Cisplatin
- Ifosfamide
- Teniposide
- Etoposide
- Carboplatin

Nursing Management

For the Child With Neuroblastoma

Nursing Assessment and Diagnosis

Assess the presenting site of the tumor, such as the neck or abdomen, by observation and inspection. Palpation is contraindicated to avoid seeding tumor cells. Carefully document related functioning, such as bowel and bladder function. Take vital signs to watch for elevated temperature and vital sign changes caused by a thoracic mass. Observe gait and coordination. Take weight and height and compare to earlier percentiles for the child. Specific assessments during treatment will depend on the treatment methods used (refer to the earlier discussions of chemotherapy and radiation treatment). Psychosocial assessment and emotional assessment of the family are needed.

A variety of nursing diagnoses may be appropriate for the child with neuroblastoma, depending on the location and extent of the presenting disease. Some common diagnoses might include the following (NANDA-I © 2014):

- *Gas Exchange, Impaired,* related to ventilation-perfusion imbalance
- *Mobility: Physical, Impaired,* related to neuromuscular impairment
- *Pain, Acute or Chronic,* related to tumor pressure and injury
- *Grieving (Family)* related to potential loss of significant person

Planning and Implementation

The nursing management of the child with neuroblastoma can encompass the three phases of medical treatment: chemotherapy, surgery, and radiation. Specific postsurgical care depends on the size and site of the tumor. Normal postoperative care includes providing fluid support and respiratory care and preventing infection.

Nursing care during the chemotherapy phase includes minimizing side effects, preventing infection, teaching parents about the medications their child is receiving, and monitoring physical and emotional growth and development of the young child. When radiation is part of the treatment, use common nursing measures described earlier in the chapter.

Topics for parent and family teaching and discharge planning are presented in *Families Want to Know: The Child With a Neuroblastoma.* Ongoing support and connection to resources to assist in management of the child's treatment at home will be needed. When the prognosis is poor, parents may appreciate referrals to hospice, to other parents who have experienced similar child illnesses, and to other community resources. See Chapter 13 for additional nursing care for the end of life.

Evaluation

Expected outcomes of nursing care for the child with neuroblastoma include the following:

- Ventilatory exchange is adequate to support daily activities.
- Physical mobility is maintained to the level possible considering developmental age.
- Sensory/perceptual alterations are managed to provide for safety and sensory input.
- Pain is managed to a level of comfort.
- Family members accept and integrate the diagnosis.

Wilms Tumor (Nephroblastoma)

Nephroblastoma, an intrarenal tumor of which the most common type is Wilms tumor, is a common abdominal tumor of childhood and accounts for 6% of all childhood tumors. The incidence

Families Want to Know

The Child With a Neuroblastoma

Surgery Phase

- Teach the parents to observe for signs of infection at the wound site and to take the child's temperature, if necessary.
- Assist the family in providing pain management, including medication administration and various comfort measures.
- Teach the parents the importance of keeping accurate records of urine output and bowel movements and to notify the healthcare provider if the child does not have a bowel movement at least every 3 days.
- Continue with progression to a regular diet.

Chemotherapy Phase

The child frequently has a central line placed early in the chemotherapy phase. The central line greatly reduces the emotional trauma associated with chemotherapy and blood tests.

- Teach the child how to help the parents with cleaning of the central line.
- Teach the child how to protect the central line.
- Teach the parents how to clean and dress the site of the central line.
- Have the parents practice central line care with a model and then on the child before discharge to increase the parents' confidence.
- Give the parents written and illustrated information about care of a central line.
- Arrange for home care dressing supplies before discharge.
- Give the parents detailed chemotherapy information.
- Teach the administration of any medications that the parent will administer via central line or other routes.
- Refer the family to the American Cancer Society for coloring books for children receiving chemotherapy.

is approximately 7.6 cases per million children annually. Wilms tumor occurs most frequently between 2 and 3 years of age, with young ages being more commonly associated with bilateral disease (Buckley, 2011).

ETIOLOGY AND PATHOPHYSIOLOGY

Wilms tumor is associated with several congenital anomalies: aniridia (absence of the iris), hemihypertrophy (abnormal growth of one half of the body or a body structure), genitourinary anomalies, nevi, and hamartomas (benign, nodule-like growths). These connections suggest a genetic link; chromosomal deletions at 11p13 and 11p15 (locations for *WT1* and *WT2* genes) have been associated with Wilms tumor. It has a high incidence in Beckwith-Wiedemann syndrome, which is characterized by macroglossia and hypoglycemia. However, most children with Wilms tumor have no other abnormalities. Wilms tumor grows very quickly, doubling its size in 11 to 13 days. Such fast growth generally contributes to a large tumor by the time of diagnosis. However, chemotherapeutic drugs have significantly increased survival rates for children with Wilms tumor, with 90% survival rates (Anderson, Dhamne, & Huff, 2011; Buckley, 2011; Huff, 2011).

CLINICAL MANIFESTATIONS

Wilms tumor is usually an asymptomatic, firm, lobulated mass located to one side of the midline in the abdomen. Often a parent discovers the mass during the child's bath. Hypertension caused by increased renin activity related to renal damage is reported in 25% of cases. Hematuria or abdominal pain is sometimes present.

CLINICAL THERAPY

The diagnosis of Wilms tumor is based on an ultrasound study of the abdomen and an intravenous pyelogram. CT scanning or MRI of the lungs, liver, spleen, and brain may be performed to identify any metastasis. This information is used in staging the tumor (Table 24–8). A complete blood count is obtained, as well as BUN and creatinine levels. Liver function tests are performed.

Treatment is multifaceted and increasingly successful; about 90% of early stages and 70% of metastatic cases have long-term survival (Anderson et al., 2011). Surgery is performed to remove the affected kidney, to examine the opposite kidney, and to look for other sites of metastasis. Chemotherapy or radiation therapy, alone or in combination, is sometimes used before surgery to reduce the size of the tumor. Radiation, chemotherapy, or both may also follow surgery. Children whose tumors are almost completely excised and who have a favorable prognosis do not require irradiation of the tumor bed and may receive limited chemotherapy.

Long-term complications of treatment include liver damage, portal hypertension, and mild cirrhosis, which may occur in children treated for right-sided Wilms tumor. Radiation damage (such as thinning or weakening) of the skeleton, pelvis, and thorax has been reported. Kyphosis and scoliosis may occur from irradiation of vertebral bodies and the pelvis. Glomerular damage to the remaining kidney may also occur. Second malignancies in the original radiation field have occurred with orthovoltage radiation, but recent changes in radiation therapy have reduced this risk.

Clinical Tip

The following are examples of drugs that may be used to treat Wilms tumor:

- Vincristine
- Actinomycin D
- Doxorubicin
- Cyclophosphamide

TABLE 24–8 National Wilms Tumor Study Staging System

STAGE	DESCRIPTION
I	The tumor is limited to the kidney and completely excised. The surface of the renal capsule is intact. The tumor is not ruptured before or during removal. No residual tumor is apparent beyond the margins of the excision.
II	The tumor extends beyond the kidney but is completely excised. Regional extension of the tumor is present (i.e., penetration through the outer surface of the renal capsule into the perirenal soft tissues). Vessels outside the kidney substance are infiltrated or contain tumor thrombus. Biopsy may have been performed on the tumor, or local spillage of tumor confined to the flank has occurred. No residual tumor is apparent at or beyond the margin of excision.
III	Residual nonhematogenous tumor is confined to the abdomen. Any of the following may occur: • Lymph nodes on biopsy are found to be involved in the hilus, the periaortic chains, or beyond. • Diffuse peritoneal contamination by the tumor has occurred, such as by spillage of tumor beyond the flank before or during surgery, or by tumor growth that has penetrated through the peritoneal surface. • Implants are found on peritoneal surfaces. • The tumor extends beyond the surgical margins either microscopically or grossly. • The tumor is not completely resectable because of local infiltration into vital structures.
IV	Hematogenous metastasis: deposits are present beyond stage III (e.g., lung, liver, bone, and/or brain).
V	Bilateral renal involvement is present at diagnosis. An attempt should be made to stage each side according to the above criteria on the basis of extent of disease before biopsy.

Source: Data from National Cancer Institute. (2011f). *Wilms tumor and other childhood kidney tumors treatment: Stage information.* Retrieved from http://www.cancer.gov/cancertopics/pdq/treatment/wilms/HealthProfessional/page3

Nursing Management

For the Child With Wilms Tumor (Nephroblastoma)

Nursing Assessment and Diagnosis

Perform a thorough baseline assessment of the child. Do not palpate the abdomen because of the potential for spreading the cancerous cells. Monitor the child's blood pressure carefully because hypertension is a common finding that may require treatment.

Nursing diagnoses for a child with Wilms tumor will differ depending on the phase of treatment. Some common nursing diagnoses might include the following (NANDA-I © 2014):

- *Infection, Risk for,* related to inadequate defenses
- *Urinary Elimination, Impaired,* related to anatomic obstruction
- *Tissue Perfusion: Cardiac, Risk for Decreased,* related to hypertension caused by mechanical reduction of blood flow
- *Caregiver Role Strain, Risk for,* related to child's illness severity
- *Home Maintenance, Impaired,* related to child's disease

Planning and Implementation

Nursing management can be divided into two phases: the postrenal surgery phase and the chemotherapy phase. (See Chapter 11 for general care of the child after surgery.) Drawings and special teaching dolls with removable kidneys can be used to teach young children about the surgery. Although chemotherapy may occur at two different times, before and after surgery, nursing management considerations remain the same.

Nursing care during the postrenal surgery phase focuses on pain management and close monitoring of fluid levels. A large incision is necessary to remove the kidney, and the resultant postoperative shift of organs and fluid in the abdominal cavity may create discomfort for the child. Frequently reposition the child and use noninvasive and pharmacologic pain interventions to improve the child's comfort. Gentle handling is important. Monitor fluids closely following surgery to prevent hypovolemia and to assess the shift of fluids out of the third space and out of the body. Assess daily weight, intake and output (I&O), and urine specific gravity. Monitor the function of the remaining kidney. Take blood pressure frequently to watch for signs of shock and to assess the functioning of the remaining kidney.

SAFETY ALERT!

If you feel a mass during palpation of a child's abdomen, stop palpating immediately and report the finding to the child's primary healthcare provider. Never palpate the liver or abdomen of a child with Wilms tumor as this could cause a piece of the tumor to dislodge. Place a sign on the child's bed and in the chart alerting healthcare providers not to palpate the abdomen.

During the chemotherapy phase, monitor the child for side effects of drugs, the potential for infection from the central line site, and the function of the remaining kidney. Advise parents about home care needs, administration of medications, and monitoring for drug side effects and ongoing needs for healthcare monitoring. A long-term complication in children who receive doxorubicin treatment is congestive heart failure, so ongoing periodic healthcare evaluations are needed. Be sure care is well coordinated among all healthcare providers.

Evaluation

Desired outcomes for nursing care of the child with nephroblastoma include balanced intake and output, normal vital signs, recovery from surgery, and successful family management of postsurgical care and ongoing treatments.

Bone Tumors

Osteosarcoma

Osteosarcoma is the most common tumor affecting the skeleton of children, with an incidence of seven cases per million children. Its peak incidence is during the rapid growth years, at age 13 years for girls and age 14 years for boys (Arndt, 2011b). The tumor is usually located at the metaphysis of the distal femur, proximal tibia, or proximal humerus.

ETIOLOGY AND PATHOPHYSIOLOGY

Bone tissue produced by osteosarcoma never matures into compact bone. Although the cause of osteosarcoma is unknown, radiation exposure (either environmental or treatment related) is associated with its development. Survivors of retinoblastoma have a greatly increased incidence of osteosarcoma. An abnormality of gene *p53* has been noted in some cases of this cancer, leading to oncogene malformations and possibly to an absence of tumor suppressor genes (Chen et al., 2014).

CLINICAL MANIFESTATIONS

The common initial symptoms are pain, swelling, and a limp. The pain can be referred to the hip or back, which can delay diagnosis. Deep bone pain causing night awakenings should be investigated (Arndt, 2011b). Pulmonary metastasis occurs in 20% of cases. Other metastatic sites include kidney, adrenals, brain, and pericardium. When lung metastasis is the only site, lung resection may be successful for treatment. Disseminated metastases and bone lesions have poorer prognoses.

CLINICAL THERAPY

Diagnosis is made through radiographic studies of the affected area, bone scan, CT or MRI scans of involved bone, blood test for serum alkaline phosphatase and lactic dehydrogenase (levels may be elevated), and tumor biopsy (to confirm the diagnosis). Arteriography may be performed if limb-sparing surgery is contemplated. Complete blood count, liver studies, and renal studies are performed for information about possible metastases.

Clinical Tip

The following are examples of drugs that may be used to treat osteosarcoma:

- Methotrexate with leucovorin rescue
- Doxorubicin
- Cisplatin
- Ifosfamide with mesna

Treatment involves both surgery and chemotherapy. The surgery is either a limb-salvage procedure or limb amputation. In limb-salvage procedures, the tumor is removed and a bone graft or internal prosthesis is inserted. A limb-salvage procedure is often possible if bone growth has taken place and a neurobundle (area where several nerves converge) is not involved in the tumor (Manfrini, Tiwari, Ham, et al., 2011). Other criteria such as joint involvement and possibility of prosthetic use in the future are weighed in the decision about a salvage procedure or amputation. Physical rehabilitation will be needed after either amputation or limb-salvage procedure. Aggressive chemotherapy following surgery has improved the survival rate. At the time of diagnosis, most children have metastases (even though they may not be identifiable), so chemotherapy is needed. Chemotherapy is started before surgery to shrink the tumor, especially when limb-salvage surgery is planned. It is also given postoperatively to treat and prevent metastasis.

Ewing Sarcoma

Ewing sarcoma is a malignant, small, round cell tumor usually involving the diaphyseal (shaft) portion of the long bones. The most common sites are the femur, pelvis, tibia, fibula, ribs, humerus, scapula, and clavicle, but any bone may be involved. Ewing sarcoma occurs in two children per million, is most common in White and Hispanic children, and is rare in African American and Asian American children. The incidence is highest in children between the ages of 5 and 20 years (HaDuong, Martin, Skapek, et al., 2015; Moore & Haydon, 2014).

Translocations on chromosomes 11 and 22 have been identified in children with Ewing sarcoma; these are t(11;22)(q24;q12). In addition, these tumors express a proto-oncogene, c-*myc*.

The symptoms are similar to those of osteosarcoma and may include pain, swelling, fever, an elevated WBC count, an elevated erythrocyte sedimentation rate, and elevated C-reactive protein. Some children present with a fracture of the affected bone. A tumor biopsy is necessary for diagnosis. Diagnostic tests are the same as those for osteosarcoma.

Initial treatment for Ewing sarcoma is chemotherapy to reduce the tumor, followed by radiation and surgical removal of the tumor and/or bone. Limb-salvage procedures are now commonly performed rather than amputation. Chemotherapy is always used after initial treatment because undetectable metastases are nearly always present.

Clinical Tip

The following are examples of drugs that may be used to treat Ewing sarcoma (Meyer & Grier, 2014):

- Vincristine
- Cyclophosphamide
- Dactinomycin
- Doxorubicin
- Ifosfamide
- Irinotecan
- Etoposide
- Temozolomide
- Topotecan

Nursing Management

For the Child With a Bone Tumor

Nursing Assessment and Diagnosis

Carefully evaluate any child or adolescent who has a limp or complains of pain in an extremity. Confirm the onset and whether the symptoms were associated with injury. Refer for further evaluation if the discomfort persists or is not associated with injury. Physiologic assessment of the child with a bone tumor includes assessment of the site before surgery. Assess the child's pain or discomfort, mobility, and gait. Take careful vital signs, especially noting temperature and respirations. Psychologic assessments of the child and family are needed, especially if amputation is planned. Loss of a limb causes body image disturbances, particularly with school-age children and adolescents. Assess the child's understanding of the treatment and of care after surgery. Find out what support systems are available to the family.

Observe the wound postoperatively for infection and hemorrhage. Assess circulation above and below the operative site. If edema is found, elevate the limb. If a limb-salvage procedure is performed, the child's extremity will remain, but it will not function as before because muscle insertion sites and mass have been removed with the tumor during surgery. Detailed charting of the condition of the surgical site and limb function is important.

If the limb has been amputated, assess the child for the following signs indicating a disturbed body image:

- Refusal to look at or touch the altered or missing body part
- Preoccupation with loss or change
- Feelings of shame or embarrassment, either verbalized or demonstrated
- Distorted perception of normal body (easily seen in the child's drawings of the body)

- Fears of rejection or unwanted attention from others
- Overexposure or hiding of the affected body part
- Actual or perceived change in the structure and function of the body or body parts

Psychosocial assessment of the child and family is discussed in more detail earlier in the general section titled *Childhood Cancer*.

Nursing diagnoses for the child with a bone tumor are based on the treatment and needs of each child. The nursing diagnoses that might be appropriate include the following (NANDA-I © 2014):

- *Infection, Risk for,* related to amputation or limb-salvage procedure
- *Skin Integrity, Impaired,* related to mechanical forces of prosthesis
- *Mobility: Physical, Impaired,* related to musculoskeletal impairment
- *Body Image, Disturbed,* related to treatment and injury
- *Pain, Acute,* related to physical injury of tissues

Planning and Implementation

Care of the child after surgery involves general postoperative care (see Chapter 11). The child who has had an amputation has special needs regarding skin care and rehabilitation. Inspect the tissue at the surgical site, using sterile technique, and turn the child at least every 2 hours. The site needs to heal completely before chemotherapy can begin and a prosthesis can be made. Pain management is a major nursing care need. When amputation has occurred, the adolescent will often experience phantom pain. This is pain that feels as if it were occuring in the amputated extremity and is caused by trauma to the nerves in the area of the amputation. Acknowledge that the pain is real since the nerve endings are intact and the patient is perceiving real discomfort. Medicate adequately and use additional pain control measures such as repositioning the limb using gentle movement, supporting the limb, and using distraction or deep breathing.

Discuss insurance and other financial arrangements with the parents, as prosthetics can be costly. Physical therapy will be needed as well. Referral to a Shriners Hospital is an option for some families.

Implement plans to help the child deal with body image disturbance. Plan for a visit from another child who is well adjusted to a prosthesis. Help the child gradually learn how to care for the stump. Slow progress may be made as the child first looks briefly, then for longer periods, and finally is willing to touch the stump. Show the child how it is possible to continue with sports such as baseball, skiing, or biking with a prosthesis. A discussion group with others can be very useful for adolescents. Plan with the child how to tell friends about the surgery and what issues the child may face upon return to school. Make plans for elevator access if needed and emergency evacuation procedures. Some children or adolescents may need referral for counseling to assist in dealing with body image disturbance.

The child will receive physical rehabilitation while hospitalized and after discharge. When the child is discharged, explain to the family the importance of bringing the child for outpatient chemotherapy and physical rehabilitation visits. Special arrangements may be needed at the child's school to accommodate a wheelchair, crutches, or ambulation with a new prosthesis. Call or visit the school to see whether there are buttons to open doors, wide doorways to facilitate passage, and any limitations of the building. Contact school personnel to plan the child's return.

Follow-up care is needed to monitor for progress and to be alert for signs of metastases. Fracture may be a sign of recurrent tumor. All body systems such as lungs, heart, kidneys, and liver are monitored for signs of recurrence.

Evaluation

Expected outcomes of nursing care for the child with a bone tumor focus on the treatments required and adaptation to changes in lifestyle. Examples include the following:

- The surgical site heals with no signs of infection.
- The child adapts to changes in mobility status.
- The child successfully adjusts to changes required in school settings.
- Skin remains intact.
- Positive body image is achieved.
- Pain is managed to a level of comfort.

Leukemia

Leukemia is the most commonly diagnosed pediatric malignancy in children under 14 years of age. A cancer of the blood-forming organs, leukemia is characterized by a proliferation of abnormal white blood cells in the body. Several types of leukemia are differentiated depending on the blood cells affected. The main types are acute lymphoblastic leukemia (ALL), acute myelogenous leukemia (AML), and the rare chronic leukemias of childhood. Because chronic leukemias such as chronic myelocytic, chronic myelomonocytic, and chronic lymphocytic leukemia are rare in children, the following discussion will focus on ALL and AML.

The most common type of childhood leukemia is acute lymphoblastic leukemia, which accounts for 25% of all childhood cancer and 78% of leukemias in children. The peak age at onset is 2 to 3 years. ALL is more common in White children and in boys (Tubergen, Bleyer, & Ritchey, 2011). Subtypes of ALL are based on the French-American-British (FAB) system of classification. There are three types of ALL in the FAB system: L1, L2, and L3. Rasheed, the 12-year-old boy who is described in the chapter-opening scenario, has ALL.

Acute myelogenous leukemia refers to all leukemias from myeloid cells. About 17% of childhood leukemias are AML. It is most common in children younger than 2 years of age and in adolescents. It is more common in boys than girls and in Asians/Pacific Islanders, Hispanics, and Whites than in African Americans. There are several subtypes of AML in the FAB classification:

M0 = acute nonlymphocytic leukemia without maturation

M1 = acute nonlymphocytic leukemia with poor maturation

M2 = acute nonlymphocytic leukemia with maturation

M3 = acute promyelocytic leukemia

M4 = acute myelomonocytic leukemia

M5 = acute monocytic leukemia

M6 = erythroleukemia

M7 = acute megakaryocytic leukemia

Etiology and Pathophysiology

The causes of leukemia are not well understood. Some investigators theorize that exposure to infectious agents can predispose

Developing Cultural Competence Prevalence of Leukemia

African American, Hispanic, and Native American children have statistically poorer outcomes from leukemia treatment than do White and Asian children. Analysis of 5-year survival rates demonstrated poorer outcomes for African American children than for White children with AML (Bhatia, 2011). It is unclear whether racial and ethnic groups with poorer outcomes have particular genetic characteristics placing them at risk, do not obtain treatment as soon, have more complications from the disease, enroll less often in clinical trials, or have less access to care at oncology centers. Clearly, more research is needed to describe and then eliminate the racial and ethnic disparity in leukemia treatment outcomes.

children to leukemia. Genetic factors are believed to play a role in some types of the disease. For instance, children with chromosomal defects such as Down syndrome, neurofibromatosis type I, Bloom syndrome, and Shwachman syndrome have an increased incidence of ALL (Messinger et al., 2012). Children with immune deficiency states, such as ataxia-telangiectasia, congenital hypogammaglobulinemia, and Wiskott-Aldrich syndrome, have an increased risk of ALL.

Ionizing radiation exposure when in utero and chemical agents such as treatment with chemotherapy for other cancers are thought to play some role in the development of AML. Several chromosomal and genetic abnormalities are associated with AML.

Leukemia occurs when the stem cells in the bone marrow produce immature WBCs that cannot function normally. These cells proliferate rapidly by cloning instead of normal mitosis, causing the bone marrow to fill with abnormal WBCs. The abnormal cells then spill out into the circulatory system where they steadily replace the normally functioning WBCs. As this occurs, the protective lymphocytic functions such as cellular and humoral immunity are reduced, leaving the body vulnerable to infections.

The malignant WBCs rapidly fill the bone marrow, replacing stem cells that produce erythrocytes (red blood cells) and other blood products such as platelets, thereby decreasing the amount of these products in circulation. The stem cells are replaced by leukemic clones, eventually resulting in anemia. Children with leukemia commonly experience abnormal bleeding, ecchymosis, or petechiae because of the reduced amounts of platelets.

Clinical Manifestations

Children with ALL and AML usually have fever, pallor, overt signs of bleeding, lethargy, malaise, anorexia, and large joint or bone pain. Petechiae, frank bleeding, and joint pain are cardinal signs of bone marrow failure. Enlargement of the liver and spleen (hepatosplenomegaly) and changes in the lymph nodes (lymphadenopathy) are common. If the leukemia has infiltrated the central nervous system (entered it by means of the circulatory or lymphoid system), the child may have signs such as headache, vomiting, papilledema, and sixth cranial nerve palsy (inability to move the eye laterally). These findings are caused by the leukemic cells massing and putting pressure on nerves. The testicles, spinal cord, and bone marrow are common sites for infiltration. The leukemic cells in the testicle become a mass that causes the testicle to enlarge, often painlessly.

Clinical Therapy

Diagnosis is based initially on blood counts and bone marrow aspiration. Blood counts commonly reveal a combination of abnormalities such as anemia, thrombocytopenia, and/or neutropenia. Bone marrow aspiration reveals immature and abnormal lymphoblasts and hypercellular marrow and is the differential test. The percentage of blast cells in marrow is measured. Other abnormal laboratory findings include elevated serum uric acid and hypocalcemia, as well as elevated potassium and phosphorus levels. Laboratory studies such as rapid flow cytometric assay are making the measurement of even very small numbers of leukemic cells possible, so that treatment can improve prognosis in children with minimal residual disease. Leukemic cells are examined and classified by FAB type, and DNA analysis may provide clues about genetic changes; all of these considerations are used to establish the protocol for treatment. Blood cells of children with ALL are B cell or T cell; these classifications are also used to establish treatment protocols.

Both ALL and AML are now approached by analysis of molecular targeting for the origin and type of disease identified (Masetti, Kleinschmidt, Biagi, et al., 2011; Pui, Carroll, Meshinchi, et al., 2011). Treatment of ALL involves radiation and chemotherapy (Rabin & Poplack, 2011). Radiation is used for central nervous system (CNS) disease, in T-cell leukemia, and for testicular involvement. Chemotherapy is commonly organized into four phases: (1) induction, (2) consolidation, (3) delayed intensification, and (4) maintenance of remission. Additional drugs may be used for treatment of CNS involvement. Maintenance therapy may continue for 2 to 3 years, causing decreased resistance to infection for this prolonged period. Treatment of AML involves use of a wide variety of drugs during the induction and consolidation phases.

Maximum cell death occurs during the *induction phase*. The cells that remain after this period are more resistant to treatment. After 3 to 4 weeks, bone marrow aspiration is reevaluated. Drugs are used in combination with CNS prophylaxis; cranial irradiation is used in some cases. During the *consolidation phase*, chemotherapy with L-asparaginase is administered. *Delayed intensification* uses additional drugs to target the leukemic cells that have survived. Treatment during the *maintenance phase* is aimed at destroying the remaining leukemic cells. Combinations of active drugs are used to prevent resistance. Occasionally, other drugs are added to the regimen, such as vincristine, prednisone, cyclophosphamide, intravenous methotrexate, cytosine arabinoside, doxorubicin, or anthracyclines.

The prognosis for children with leukemia is much improved with current therapy. An important factor is the initial leukocyte count; the higher the leukocyte count (over 50,000/mm^3) at diagnosis, the worse the prognosis. For children in the low-risk group, the probability of prolonged survival is as high as 90%; even higher risk ALL has a 75% to 80% cure rate with current treatments (Tubergen et al., 2011). Treatment methods and duration are adjusted for each child depending on that child's metabolic analysis and other risk factors (Rabin & Poplack, 2011).

Approximately 15% to 20% of children have a relapse within a year after completing treatment (Tubergen et al., 2011). Treatment for relapse consists of additional chemotherapeutic drugs. The prognosis is best if the relapse occurs late after the initial diagnosis and after the initial treatment is completed. Hematopoietic stem cell transplant (HSCT) is a treatment option for the child who has a relapse with ALL and who then achieves a second remission; the transplant is given when the child is in remission. Transplant is also used for children with AML; they do not need to be in remission for the transplant to be performed.

Clinical Tip

Following are the laboratory values in leukemia:

	Normal	Common Values in Leukemia
Leukocytes	Less than 10,000/mcL	Greater than 10,000/mcL
Platelets	150,000–400,000/mcL	20,000–100,000/mcL
Hemoglobin	12–16 g/dL	7–11 g/dL

Clinical Tip

The following are examples of drugs that may be used to treat acute lymphoblastic leukemia:

Induction Phase
- Prednisone
- Vincristine
- Intrathecal methotrexate (central nervous system prophylaxis)
- L-asparaginase
- Daunorubicin

Consolidation Phase
- L-asparaginase
- Doxorubicin

Delayed Intensification Phase
- Vincristine
- Ara-C
- Cyclophosphamide
- L-asparaginase

Maintenance Phase
- 6-Mercaptopurine or 6-thioguanine
- Methotrexate

Overall, 80% of children with leukemia are cured. Chemotherapy itself can create numerous complications, affecting all body organs. Secondary malignancies sometimes occur later in life. See the section on cancer survival earlier in this chapter.

Clinical Tip

The following are examples of drugs that may be used to treat AML:

Induction Phase
- Daunorubicin
- Doxorubicin
- Mitoxantrone
- Cytarabine

Consolidation Phase
- Etoposide
- Teniposide

Nursing Management
For the Child With Leukemia

Nursing Assessment and Diagnosis

Thorough physical assessment is important to ensure prompt identification of problems without injuring the child who has deficient coagulation and immune function. Perform assessments every 8 hours or more often depending on the chemotherapeutic regimen. Observe carefully for bruising, petechiae, and other signs of bleeding; assess for fever or other signs of infection. Once chemotherapy has begun, closely monitor renal functioning through specific gravity, intake and output, and daily weight measurements. Monitor dietary intake, nausea, vomiting, and constipation. Observe for mucosal ulcers in the mouth. A central line is usually in place for intravenous infusion of medications, so carefully assess the line for proper functioning and for signs of infection. Ask the parents about any behavioral changes. CNS infiltration can affect the child's level of consciousness, causing irritability, vomiting, and lethargy. However, chemotherapeutic drugs and antiemetics can also induce these nonspecific signs. Frequent venipunctures, bone marrow aspirations, and lumbar punctures require pain assessment and an evaluation of the level of knowledge and coping skills of child and family.

Leukemia causes many changes in the body, and confirmation of the disease is difficult for families to face. Among the many nursing diagnoses that might be appropriate for the child with leukemia are the following (NANDA-I © 2014):

- *Nutrition, Imbalanced: Less than Body Requirements,* related to inability to ingest food
- *Infection, Risk for,* related to altered immune system functioning
- *Injury, Risk for,* related to bleeding
- *Activity Intolerance* related to generalized weakness
- *Pain, Acute or Chronic,* related to chemotherapy and disease process
- *Sleep Pattern, Disturbed,* related to chemotherapeutic drugs and disease process
- *Anxiety (Child and Parent)* related to change in health status

Planning and Implementation

Bone marrow suppression may necessitate transmission-based precautions. Instruct parents in the prevention of infection and use nursing care measures to prevent infection also. Perform careful hand hygiene; take temperature frequently; give mouth care with antibacterial mouthwashes; and inspect skin, mouth, rectal area, and central line site for any signs of infection. Care of mouth sores and other side effects of chemotherapy is presented in *Nursing Care Plan: Hospital Care of the Child With Cancer* earlier in this chapter.

Special attention to renal function is needed when the child receives cyclophosphamide. Gross hematuria is a side effect of this drug. Hydration with intravenous fluids to attain a specific gravity of less than 1.010 prevents or reduces the severity of hematuria. It also prepares the kidneys to manage products of tumor cell breakdown. To achieve the desired specific gravity, the child receives intravenous fluids at 1.5 times maintenance volume for at least 6 to 8 hours before and at least 1.5 hours after administration of the drug. Other chemotherapy drugs have different infusion times, and some do not require hydration prior to infusion. Check drug references carefully for recommendations with each drug. Evaluate the infusion site before and frequently during infusion. Although extravasation is not as common with central lines used in cancer treatment as in peripheral lines, it still can occur. Many chemotherapeutic agents are extremely toxic to tissues. In addition, lysis of the cancer cells can produce toxic side effects (see the *Oncologic Emergencies* section earlier in the chapter). Careful monitoring of intake and output is required to record the intravenous fluids, assess kidney functioning, and monitor excretion of by-products from destroyed tumor cells. Monitor specific gravity every 8 hours, as well as before and during administration of the drug, and when the intravenous fluids are reduced to maintenance volume levels. Daily weight measurements are important to assist in planning adequate hydration during chemotherapy, as well as to measure nutritional status.

Drug side effects may necessitate infusion of platelets or packed red blood cells. See the *Clinical Skills Manual* SKILLS for techniques to be used in these situations.

Many children are treated in an oncology clinic, staying in the hospital only on the day of intravenous drug administration and receiving oral medications at home. The time at the hospital is used to assess how the family is managing issues such as nutrition, sleep, medication administration, and obtaining psychosocial support. Careful teaching for the family is needed to ensure safe drug administration and identification of issues requiring further care.

Nurses play a key role in the long-term multidisciplinary treatment of children with leukemia. The impact of a diagnosis of leukemia and the long-term nature of treatment can severely stress the coping abilities of both the child and the family. Ongoing psychosocial assessment and emotional support are essential (see the general discussion of psychosocial assessment in the *Childhood*

Families Want to Know

Chemotherapy for Childhood Leukemia

Physical Care

- Have rest periods each day.
- Avoid exposure to people with illnesses.
- Drink generous amounts of water.
- Eat a healthy diet, using frequent, small, and nutritious meals to obtain enough nutrients.
- Take medicines prescribed to decrease nausea.
- Maintain good oral hygiene with a soft toothbrush and water irrigation device.
- Avoid sun exposure and check skin each day for any signs of bruises, pressure areas, cuts, or scratches.
- Allow time for and eat foods to promote bowel elimination.
- Promote bowel elimination through regular dietary and toileting practices.
- Report any signs of infection, changes in condition, or other concerns.

Emotional Care

- Be prepared for loss of hair with plans for hats, wigs, or other alternatives.
- Continue contact with friends via phone, Internet, and in person when possible.
- Try relaxation techniques to aid in sleep and management of treatments.
- Talk with clergy, teachers, parents, counselors, friends, or other supportive people about the experience of having leukemia.
- Keep a journal to record feelings and experiences.

Sam is a 4-year-old boy recently diagnosed with acute lymphoblastic leukemia. He has been hospitalized for initial diagnostic work and the beginning of chemotherapy. Sam lives about 70 miles from the hospital and his parents have been taking turns staying with him. He has two older siblings at home who are 6 and 9 years old. What are the most urgent needs for the parents? The siblings? What information should you collect to begin planning for psychosocial support for the family?

Cancer section earlier in this chapter). Referral to support groups and social services may be beneficial. Help the family explore alternative therapies such as relaxation, imagery, and nutritional support that may aid the child. Be alert for any interactions that could occur between complementary therapies and the medical regimen.

Evaluation

Expected outcomes for nursing care of the child with leukemia include the following:

- Infection and other secondary complications of chemotherapy are prevented.
- Adequate hydration is maintained.
- Normal urinary output is maintained.
- Blood values are within normal limits.
- The family adapts successfully to parenting a child with chronic illness.
- Parents demonstrate adequate knowledge related to the disease process.

Soft-Tissue Tumors

Hodgkin Disease

Hodgkin disease, a disorder of the lymphoid system, usually arises in a single lymph node or an anatomic group of lymph nodes (see *Pathophysiology Illustrated: Hodgkin Disease*). Hodgkin disease rarely occurs before 10 years of age. It accounts for just 5% of cancers in children under 14 years, but 15% of cancer in youth from 15 to 19 years. The disease has a bimodal peak with higher incidence in the early 20s and after 50 years (Waxman, Hochberg, & Cairo, 2011). Three forms of the disease exist: young person form in those under 14 years, the young adult form in persons from 15 to 34 years, and the older adult form in those over 50 years. There is a slightly increased incidence in males, which is more pronounced in the disease manifested in younger children (Carbone, Spina, Gloghini, et al., 2011).

ETIOLOGY AND PATHOPHYSIOLOGY

Hodgkin disease occurs in clusters and has been reported in families. This suggests a possible genetic link as well as an infectious agent (such as Epstein-Barr virus) or environmental hazard (Waxman et al., 2011).

CLINICAL MANIFESTATIONS

The main symptom of Hodgkin disease is nontender, firm lymphadenopathy, usually in the supraclavicular and cervical nodes but occasionally in the mediastinal area. A mediastinal growth can cause respiratory difficulty because of pressure on the trachea or bronchi. A distinguishing large cell with multiple nuclei, called the

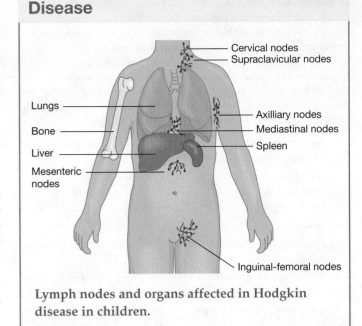

Pathophysiology Illustrated: **Hodgkin Disease**

Cervical nodes
Supraclavicular nodes
Lungs
Bone
Liver
Mesenteric nodes
Axilliary nodes
Mediastinal nodes
Spleen
Inguinal-femoral nodes

Lymph nodes and organs affected in Hodgkin disease in children.

Reed-Sternberg cell, is characteristic of Hodgkin disease, although the cell is found also in infectious mononucleosis and some other lymphomas. Fever, night sweats, and weight loss occur in one third of children with Hodgkin disease and are associated with a more aggressive form of the disease. The leukocyte count and erythrocyte sedimentation rate (ESR) may be elevated.

CLINICAL THERAPY

Diagnosis is based on the presence of Reed-Sternberg cells in a lymph node biopsy. A staging classification is used to determine disease severity (Table 24–9). The basis for staging is data obtained from the history, physical examination, chest x-ray study (for metastasis), chest CT scan, CT or MRI scans of the retroperitoneal nodes, lymphangiogram if there is retroperitoneal involvement, laboratory studies (complete blood count, ESR, serum copper level, C-reactive protein, liver and renal function tests), and a radionuclide scan with gallium. Bone marrow biopsy, bone scan, or a staging laparotomy may be performed if advanced disease is suspected. Minimally invasive surgery can be used to biopsy or remove the spleen for diagnosis, avoiding the potential complications of major surgery (Waxman et al., 2011).

Clinical Tip

The following are examples of drugs that may be used to treat Hodgkin disease:

- Doxorubicin
- Bleomycin
- Vinblastine
- Dacarbazine
- Etoposide
- Prednisone
- Cyclophosphamide
- Procarbazine
- Methotrexate
- Mechlorethamine

TABLE 24–9 Staging System for Hodgkin Disease

STAGE	DESCRIPTION
I	Disease within a single lymph node region
IE	Disease within a single extralymphatic organ or site outside of lymphatic system (extralymphatic organ)
II	Disease within two or more lymph node regions on same side of diaphragm
IIE	Disease within extralymphatic organ, and of one or more lymph node regions on same side of diaphragm
III	Disease of lymph node regions on both sides of diaphragm; stage III(1) indicates involvement of upper abdomen above the renal vein, whereas stage III(2) indicates involvement of pelvic or other lower abdomen nodes
IIIE	Disease of lymph node regions on both sides of the diaphragm with involvement of extralymphatic organ
IIIS	As in III, plus disease within spleen
IIISE	As in III, plus disease in extralymphatic organs and spleen
IV	Disseminated disease within one or more lymphatic organs with or without lymph node involvement

Source: Data from National Cancer Institute. (2011a). *Childhood Hodgkin lymphoma treatment: Staging and diagnostic evaluation.* Retrieved from http://www.cancer.gov/cancertopics/pdq/treatment/childhodgkins/HealthProfessional/page4

Chemotherapy using a four-drug combination has been found to be the most effective drug treatment. Radiation is commonly added, with low doses for children who are still growing, and larger doses for those who are physically mature or those whose disease is more advanced at diagnosis. The 5-year survival rate is approximately 85% to 90%, depending on the stage of the disease at diagnosis.

Autologous stem cell or allogeneic stem cell transplant is a treatment option in children with advanced disease or relapse.

Non-Hodgkin Lymphoma

The four types of pediatric non-Hodgkin lymphoma (NHL) are (1) lymphoblastic lymphoma, (2) small noncleaved cell (Burkitt) lymphoma, (3) diffuse large B-cell lymphoma, and (4) anaplastic large cell lymphoma (Waxman et al., 2011). Lymphomas of all types are the third most common group of malignancies in children, following leukemia and brain tumors. Non-Hodgkin lymphomas are malignant tumors of lymphoreticular (internal framework of the lymph system) origin. The peak incidence for lymphomas occurs between the ages of 7 and 11 years, and they are three times more common in boys than in girls. The cure rate is 85% to 90% (Waxman et al., 2011).

Lymphoblastic non-Hodgkin lymphomas are caused by T-cell abnormalities. These abnormal T cells are diffuse, highly malignant, and very aggressive and do not mature. T-cell lymphomas produced by these cells often occur in children with congenital or acquired immunodeficiency states, chronic immune stimulation, or autoimmune disease. Some lymphomas have B-cell abnormalities, most specifically Burkitt lymphoma; 8q24 chromosomal translocation may be found in these cases (Waxman et al., 2011).

The incidence of lymphomas shows geographic variability. For example, a high incidence of Burkitt lymphoma is found in equatorial Africa, where it causes 50% of childhood cancers. Incidence in Hispanic children is higher than in White children, and African Americans have the lowest incidence. Boys are affected more than girls, sand children with immune system compromise are most commonly affected. Epstein-Barr virus has been associated with Burkitt lymphoma, but in most cases of NHL, there are no known causes (Waxman et al., 2011).

Children with non-Hodgkin lymphoma frequently present with fever and weight loss. The lymph glands are usually enlarged or nodular, with the most frequent sites being the cervical, axillary, inguinal, and femoral nodes. However, the disease may be diffuse, without nodular glands. The anterior mediastinum is the primary site for T-cell lymphomas. Tumors that occur in this area may compress the airway (causing breathing difficulty) or superior vena cava (leading to swelling of the face, neck, or arms), and can cause pain. Jaw involvement is common in Burkitt lymphoma.

A complete blood count is performed; additional blood tests include renal and liver function, electrolytes, uric acid, and LDH. Bone marrow aspiration and lumbar puncture are performed. Chest x-ray, bone scan, gallium scan, CT, and MRI can help to isolate affected body organs. Tissue biopsy confirms the diagnosis.

A staging system is used to describe the tumor mass and extension to other body areas (Table 24–10). Treatment is tailored to the type of cancer and its stage. Stages I and II may be treated with drugs such as vincristine, cyclophosphamide, prednisone, and methotrexate for several months. Intrathecal medication is added if head and neck cancers are present. Stages III and IV are treated with additional drugs (up to nine total) for longer periods (1 to 2 years). Radiation is uncommonly used and may be helpful to treat a tumor that is impinging on a body part. Surgery is used to biopsy the tumor mass and treat any complications caused by the cancer. A hematopoietic stem cell transplant is used for children with recurrent disease.

Rhabdomyosarcoma

Rhabdomyosarcoma is the most common soft-tissue tumor diagnosed in children, and is especially common in children under 5 years of age. The 5-year survival rate is 70% (Egas-Bejar & Huh, 2014). It occurs most often in the muscles around the eyes (extraorbital), in the neck, and less commonly in the abdomen, genitourinary tract, and extremities (Figure 24–10).

The cause of rhabdomyosarcoma is unknown. However, it is more common in children with neurofibromatosis and Li-Fraumeni syndrome. Mutations in tumor suppressor gene *p53* are sometimes seen. The abnormal cells arise from mesenchyme that normally grows into muscle, fat, and bone.

Tumors close to the eye produce swelling, ptosis, visual disturbances, and eye movement abnormalities. When the tumor occurs in the genitourinary tract, the result can be urinary

TABLE 24–10 St. Jude Children's Research Hospital Staging Classification for Non-Hodgkin Lymphoma

STAGE	DESCRIPTION
I	Single tumor or node area involved; no tumor in abdomen or mediastinum
II	Single tumor with lymph node involvement; or two node areas or tumor on same side of diaphragm; or GI tumor in one site
III	Two tumors or node areas on different sides of diaphragm; or a primary mediastinal, intra-abdominal, or epidural tumor
IV	Any involvement with CNS or bone marrow metastases

Source: Adapted from National Cancer Institute. (2011b). *Childhood non-Hodgkin lymphoma treatment: Stage information.* Retrieved from http://www.cancer.gov/cancertopics/pdq/treatment/child-non-hodgkins/HealthProfessional

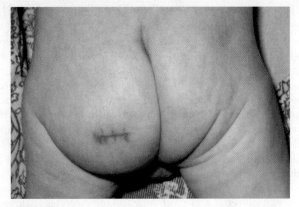

Figure 24–10 Rhabdomyosarcoma can occur in soft tissue throughout the body. Although the areas around eyes and neck are common sites, soft tissue around genitalia, in extremities, and in other sites can also be affected. A biopsy was performed on the buttock of this infant, who will now undergo chemotherapy and surgical removal of the rhabdomyosarcoma tumor, followed by further chemotherapy.

SOURCE: Dr. P. Marazzi/Science Source.

obstruction, hematuria, dysuria, vaginal discharge, and a protruding vaginal mass. Rhabdomyosarcoma occurring in the abdomen may be asymptomatic. There is rapid metastasis to the lungs, bones, bone marrow, and distant lymph nodes.

Diagnosis is confirmed by CT, MRI, PET, bone marrow aspiration, and biopsy. CBC, renal and liver studies, and urinalysis are performed. Lumbar puncture may be used in head and neck tumors. A useful biologic marker, desmin, allows differentiation of rhabdomyosarcoma from other round cell tumors. A significant number of children have metastatic disease at the time of diagnosis, so chest and lung CT scans, as well as regional lymph node biopsies are performed (Arndt, 2011b).

Treatment includes surgical removal of the tumor when possible. However, if the tumor involves other structures, removal may not be possible. Many children have metastasis at the time of diagnosis, so the primary tumor may not be removed. Surgery is followed by wide-field radiation and chemotherapy with a combination of drugs. Some commonly used drugs include the following:

- Vincristine
- Actinomycin
- Cyclophosphamide (VAC therapy)

Prognosis depends on the site, staging (Table 24–11), and histologic findings.

TABLE 24–11 Classification of Rhabdomyosarcoma

STAGE	DESCRIPTION
I	Localized tumor, completely resected disease
II	Total gross resection with regional microscopic spread
III	Locally extensive tumor with residual microscopic spread
IV	Any size primary tumor with distant metastatic disease present

Source: Data from National Cancer Institute. (2011c). *Childhood rhabdomyosarcoma treatment: Stage information.* Retrieved from http://www.cancer.gov/cancertopics/pdq/treatment/childrhabdomyosarcoma/HealthProfessional

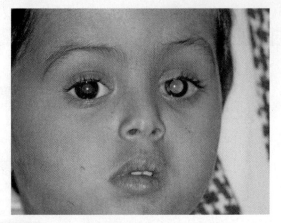

Figure 24–11 Retinoblastoma is characterized by leukokoria, a white reflection in the pupil.

SOURCE: Custom Medical Stock Photo/Newscom.

Retinoblastoma

Retinoblastoma is an intraocular malignancy of the retina. It may be bilateral (20% to 30%) or unilateral. In 40% of children, the disease is inherited by an autosomal dominant gene. Family history is therefore important to collect, although many cases occur with no family history of the cancer (Zage & Herzog, 2011). The tumor arises from embryonic retinal cells. It may be a new mutation or may be passed on to offspring of affected individuals in an autosomal dominant manner. The retinoblastoma gene, *RB1*, is on chromosome 13q14.

The first sign of retinoblastoma is a white pupil, termed *leukokoria* or *cat's-eye reflex* (Figure 24–11). The red reflex is absent, asymmetric, or of a differing color in the affected eye. Other symptoms may include a fixed strabismus (a constant deviation of one eye from the other), orbital inflammation, glaucoma, and heterochromia (irises of different colors).

Retinoblastoma is usually diagnosed when the child is between 1 and 2 years of age. A family history should alert healthcare providers so that regular ophthalmologic examinations can be performed frequently on infants and young children in the family. The appearance of a unilateral tumor demands regular examinations of the healthy eye since bilateral disease can develop. In some children, a pineal gland tumor can also develop, causing CNS symptoms. The overall tumor-free survival rate is 95% (Zage & Herzog, 2011).

Diagnostic tests for the cancer include full ocular examination and CT or MRI scans of the eye orbit. All children with a history of retinoblastoma in the family should be examined by an ophthalmologist after birth, at 6 weeks, every 2 to 3 months until 2 years, every 4 months until 3 years, and then annually to aid in early diagnosis. Tumors are classified according to a staging system, from a very small localized tumor (group I) to tumors involving more than half the retina and with seeding into the vitreous (group V).

Treatment for retinoblastoma may include removal of the eye (enucleation) when there is permanent retinal damage or failure to respond to other treatment. Other surgical treatments involve cryotherapy or photocoagulation (argon laser therapy). Radiation is nearly always used, either as the sole treatment or before surgery to shrink the tumor. Chemotherapy is sometimes used but is frequently ineffective because the drugs often fail to penetrate sufficiently into the eye. Chemotherapeutic drugs include carboplatin, etoposide, vincristine, and cyclosporine. Multiple therapies are more commonly used in children with bilateral retinoblastoma. Children with retinoblastoma are at increased risk of developing a secondary tumor, including another retinoblastoma or a sarcoma, most commonly osteogenic sarcoma. However, most young children who have been treated for the disease have good health and normal mental abilities several years after treatment. The most common sequela of retinoblastoma is decrease in visual acuity.

Nursing Management

For the Child With a Soft-Tissue Tumor

Nursing Assessment and Diagnosis

PHYSIOLOGIC ASSESSMENT

Physiologic assessment of the child with a soft-tissue tumor, such as Hodgkin disease, non-Hodgkin lymphoma, rhabdomyosarcoma, and other lymphomas, focuses on the child's general condition. Accurate height and weight measurements are essential to provide a baseline against which to measure the child's growth during treatment, as well as for calculation of chemotherapeutic drug dosages.

Observe the area of the tumor, such as the face, neck, and abdomen, and describe any changes. Monitor respiratory status if the tumor is in the face or neck. Report any changes in respiratory pattern to the oncology specialist. Avoid palpation of any tumor site or enlarged area; injudicious palpation and manipulation of a tumor site can influence metastasis. Notify the primary healthcare provider of a change in any lymph node or any other area of the body.

Gastrointestinal and genitourinary functions can be altered by the presence of a tumor and by treatment such as chemotherapy and radiation. Careful measurement of the child's intake and output is essential. Abdominal tumors may affect defecation, so charting of all bowel movements is important. Explain to the family and child why keeping accurate records is necessary.

Observe wounds closely for lack of healing as a result of chemotherapy or radiation. Examine the mouth and extremities for wounds or ulcers. Nutritional changes caused by treatment will affect the body's ability to support healthy cells and heal wounds.

A thorough eye examination is warranted for any child who has a family history of retinoblastoma or has undergone treatment for a prior tumor. Assess color and position of the iris and eye movements and perform the cover–uncover test and other eye tests described in Chapter 5. Ask whether the child has been evaluated by an ophthalmologist.

PSYCHOSOCIAL ASSESSMENT

Refer to the general discussion of psychosocial assessment in the *Childhood Cancer* section earlier in this chapter. Assessment of body image is needed when the child has a soft-tissue tumor affecting appearance of the head and neck.

The location and type of a soft-tissue tumor determine the specific nursing diagnoses for a particular child. Common nursing diagnoses might include the following (NANDA-I © 2014):

- *Tissue Perfusion: Peripheral, Risk for Ineffective,* related to interruption of blood flow
- *Breathing Pattern, Ineffective,* related to effect of tumor deformity on neck or chest wall
- *Swallowing, Impaired,* related to tumor or treatment

- *Development: Delayed, Risk for,* related to effects of treatment
- *Body Image, Disturbed,* related to illness and treatment

Planning and Implementation

Nursing management of children with soft-tissue tumors varies depending on the specific tumor. Children with lymphoma affecting the mediastinum may need respiratory support. Position the child so that the head is elevated. Administer chemotherapeutic drugs as ordered, maintaining adequate fluids to facilitate excretion of the resultant breakdown products. Monitor the central line used for chemotherapy administration, and teach parents how to take care of the central line when the child is at home.

For the child with a rhabdomyosarcoma involving the bladder, monitor urinary output carefully. Report hematuria and painful urination. Monitor the changes that occur during therapy. For example, in children with eye tumors, observe for a decrease in ptosis, which may indicate successful treatment. Administer pain medications as needed and use distraction and other techniques to decrease the child's discomfort. Emphasize to parents the need for follow-up CT and MRI scans after completion of treatment.

When the child with retinoblastoma undergoes removal of the eye, the parents and child will need detailed instructions on postsurgical care. Demonstrate to the parents care of the socket and use of a conformer to maintain the eye socket shape. When healing is complete and the child receives a prosthetic eye, instruct parents about its insertion and care. The child can gradually be taught to take over this care when old enough. Encourage periodic healthcare visits to monitor for signs of a tumor in the other eye. Interventions to encourage normal developmental milestones are adapted if sensory alteration has resulted.

Pay attention to the body changes associated with the cancer and its treatment. Children and adolescents may need suggestions to deal with hair loss, disfigurement, and living with serious illness. Referral to other children and teens with similar concerns may be helpful. Parents of all children need help to encourage normal development in the child with cancer.

The child with a soft-tissue tumor often receives chemotherapy or radiation, or sometimes both modalities. Nursing management during chemotherapy and radiation is discussed earlier in this chapter in the general sections on these treatment measures and in *Nursing Care Plan: Hospital Care of the Child With Cancer.* Generally, the family needs help to adjust to the diagnosis of a life-threatening disease and to the care of the ill child. Refer to Chapter 11 for a description of postsurgical care. Consult Chapter 19 for strategies to assist the child and family if the child has a visual impairment resulting from a retinoblastoma. Topics for parent and family teaching and discharge planning are similar to those previously presented.

COMMUNITY-BASED NURSING CARE

Reinforce with families the importance of long-term follow-up after treatment for a soft-tissue tumor. Increased risk for secondary cancers for 2 to 3 decades is possible, and early identification can help with prompt diagnosis. Partner with other healthcare providers to provide instructions to families as the child transitions from oncology treatment back to the pediatrician so they understand the importance of telling all healthcare providers about the cancer and treatment. Establish oncology clinics to track and examine survivors. As children grow into teen and young adult years, help them take over this important task in their care.

Families Want to Know

Care of the Child With a Soft-Tissue Tumor

- Teach the family about the chemotherapeutic drugs and their side effects.
- Teach about the care of surgically placed venous access devices.
- Provide written and illustrated information about the chemotherapy protocol(s).
- Provide the family with radiation and surgery education specific to the tumor treatment.
- Refer the family to nutrition resources such as dietitians for ways to promote the child's adequate intake of food and fluid.

Some recommended annual examinations include the following:

- CBC
- Physical examination with special attention to skin, abdomen, and thyroid
- Monitoring for signs of hypothyroidism and hyperthyroidism
- Neurologic and developmental examinations; monitoring of school performance
- First mammogram at 25 years in those with chest radiation
- Pap and pelvic examinations for teen and young adult women
- Mental status assessment

Evaluation

The following expected outcomes of nursing care for the child with a soft-tissue tumor are examples that illustrate the varied tumor presentations:

- Side effects of treatment are successfully managed.
- The surgical site heals with no signs of infection.
- The child adapts successfully to sensory loss resulting from cancer or treatment.
- The child adapts to an altered self-image.
- The child achieves growth and development to maximum potential.
- In cases of terminal disease, parents receive adequate support for the process of anticipatory grieving.

Chapter Highlights

- Cancer is a leading cause of illness and death among children.
- Cancer may be influenced by chromosomal or genetic messages, environmental carcinogens, or infectious process; often a combination of factors is present.
- Cancer treatments include surgery, chemotherapy, radiation, biotherapy, and alternative therapies. Palliative care is needed when disease has relapsed and cure is no longer possible.
- Oncologic emergencies are life-threatening conditions caused by cancer or its treatment; the main types of emergencies are metabolic, hematologic, or space occupying.
- Key signs of childhood cancer are pain, cachexia, anemia, infection, bruising, petechiae, and neurologic symptoms.
- A protocol is a plan of action for chemotherapy that is based on the type of cancer, its stage, and the particular cell type.
- Nursing assessment for children with cancer involves detailed physical data, as well as psychologic factors, developmental achievements, and family social status.
- Common physical nursing interventions for children with cancer involve nutrition, medication administration, hydration, infection prevention, pain management, and measures to decrease side effects of treatment. Families require ongoing psychosocial support, information, and referral to diverse resources when caring for the child with cancer.
- While the numbers of children who are long-term survivors continue to grow, some of these children experience lasting

effects such as cognitive or behavioral problems, recurrent or secondary cancers, or discrimination.

- Nursing care after cancer treatment is completed includes monitoring for any long-term physiologic or psychosocial sequelae.
- Common brain tumors in children include medulloblastoma, astrocytoma, ependyoma, and glioma; neuroblastoma is a tumor that is located along the sympathetic nervous system chain.
- Headache, vomiting, ataxia, seizures, increased intracranial pressure, hydrocephalus, and sensory disturbances are the major clinical manifestations of brain tumors.
- Nephroblastoma (Wilms tumor) is an intrarenal tumor; when suspected, the abdomen should not be palpated.
- Common bone tumors in childhood are osteosarcoma and Ewing sarcoma; both are most common among adolescents.
- Leukemia is a common childhood malignancy, with the major types being acute lymphoblastic leukemia (ALL) and acute myelogenous leukemia (AML).
- A variety of soft tissue tumors are seen in children and adolescents; they include Hodgkin disease, non-Hodgkin lymphoma, rhabdomyosarcoma, and retinoblastoma.
- Nurses are in a key position to assist families during the cancer diagnosis, treatment during adjustment to school and other life tasks, and in providing palliative care for children who do not survive.

Clinical Reasoning in Action

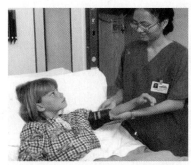

Seven-year-old Christina is brought to the hospital with an unusual rash, lethargy, and fever. Blood work is drawn, and the results are abnormal. The hematologist confirms that Christina has acute lymphoblastic leukemia (ALL), the most common childhood cancer. Her parents are in shock and disbelief about the news; she seems too young. Christina is immediately admitted to the hospital and put on an IV with orders for more blood work.

Christina's blood work demonstrates the following: hemoglobin 9 g/dL, leukocytes 20,000/mm³, and platelets 90,000/mm³.

Chemotherapy was initiated and precautions were taken to avoid infections. Recommendations for Christina include rest times daily, generous amounts of water, intake of healthy foods, and avoidance of sun exposure. The parents are happy when Christina comes home during the chemotherapy. The hematologist advises them it is not uncommon to return to the hospital because of a chemotherapeutic complication. The parents are encouraged to remember to take care of themselves. This will help them deal with Christina's therapy more effectively.

1. What are some of the common side effects of chemotherapy?
2. Why is it important to check Christina's daily weights?
3. What symptoms should Christina's parents report to the doctor while she is on chemotherapy?
4. What are some developmentally appropriate techniques you can encourage that will assist Christina to deal with her illness?

References

American Cancer Society (ACS). (2011). *Cancer in children.* Retrieved from http://www.cancer.org

Anderson, P. M., Dhamne, C. A., & Huff, V. (2011). Wilms tumor. In R. M. Kliegman, B. F. Stanton, J. W. St. Geme, N. F. Schor, & R. E. Behrman (Eds.), *Nelson textbook of pediatrics* (19th ed., pp. 1760–1762). Philadelphia, PA: Elsevier Saunders.

Arndt, C. A. S. (2011a). Neuroblastoma. In R. M. Kliegman, B. F. Stanton, J. W. St. Geme, N. F. Schor, & R. E. Behrman (Eds.), *Nelson textbook of pediatrics* (19th ed., pp. 1763–1768). Philadelphia, PA: Elsevier Saunders.

Arndt, C. A. S. (2011b). Soft tissue sarcomas. In R. M. Kliegman, B. F. Stanton, J. W. St. Geme, N. F. Schor, & R. E. Behrman (Eds.), *Nelson textbook of pediatrics* (19th ed., pp. 1760–1762). Philadelphia, PA: Elsevier Saunders.

Bartel, K. A., Gradisar, M., & Williamson, P. (2014, September). Protective and risk factors for adolescent sleep: A meta-analytic review. *Sleep Medicine Review,* S1087–S0792.

Bhatia, S. (2011). Disparities in cancer outcomes: Lessons learned from children with cancer. *Pediatric Blood & Cancer, 56,* 994–1002.

Bindler, R. M., & Howry, L. B. (2005). *Pediatric drug guide.* Upper Saddle River, NJ: Prentice Hall.

Brain tumor incidence in the U.S. (2011). *Journal of the National Cancer Institute, 103*(9), 707.

Buckley, K. S. (2011). Pediatric genitourinary tumors. *Current Opinion in Oncology, 23,* 297–302.

Burns, R. A., Topoz, I., & Reynolds, S. L. (2014). Tumor lysis syndrome: Risk factors, diagnosis, and management. *Pediatric Emergency Care, 30,* 571–576.

Calzone, K. A., Jenkins, J., Culp, S, Caskey, S., & Badzek, L. (2014). Introducing a new competency into nursing practice. *Journal of Nursing Regulation, 5,* 40–47.

Carbone, A., Spina, M., Gloghini, A., & Tirelli, U. (2011). Classical Hodgkin's lymphoma arising in different host's conditions: Pathobiology parameters, therapeutic options, and outcome. *America Journal of Hematology, 86,* 170–179.

Chen, X., Bahrami, A., Pappo, A., Easton, J., Dalton, J., Hedlund, J., . . . Dyer, M. A. (2014). Recurrent somatic structural variations contribute to tumorigenesis in pediatric osteosarcoma. *Cell Reports, 7,* 104–112.

Clanton, N. R., Klosky, J. L., Jain, N., Srivastava, D. K., Mulrooney, D., Zeltzer, L., . . . Krull, K. R. (2011). Fatigue, vitality, sleep, and neurocognitive functioning in adult survivors of childhood cancer: A report from the childhood cancer survivor study. *Cancer.* doi:10.1002/cncr.25797

Cohen, I. J., & Wolff, J. E. (2013). How long can folinic acid rescue be delayed after high-dose methotrexate without toxicity? *Pediatric Blood & Cancer, 61,* 7–10.

Demirkaya, M., Sevinir, B., Yalcinkaya, U., & Yazici, Z. (2012). Disseminated rhabdomyosarcoma presenting as hypercalcemia. *Indian Pediatrics, 49,* 66–67.

Egas-Bejar, D., & Huh, W. W. (2014). Rhabdomyosarcoma in adolescent and young adult patients: Current perspectives. *Adolescent Health, Medicine and Therapeutics, 5,* 115–125.

Erickson, J. M., Beck, S. L., Christian, B., Dudley, W. N., Hollen, P. J., Albritton, K., . . . Godder, K. (2011). Fatigue, sleep–wake disturbances, and quality of life in adolescents receiving chemotherapy. *Journal of Pediatric Hematology and Oncology, 33,* e17–e25.

Eshelman-Kent, D., Kinahan, K. E., Hobbie, W., Landier, W., Teal, S., Friedman, D., . . . Freyer, D. R. (2011). Cancer survivorship practices, services, and delivery: A report from the Children's Oncology Group (COG) nursing discipline, adolescent/young adult, and late effects committees. *Journal of Cancer Survivorship, 5*(4), 345–357.

Faria, C. M., Rutka, J. T., Smith, C., & Kongkham, P. (2011). Epigenetic mechanisms regulating neural development and pediatric brain tumor formation. *Journal of Neurosurgery: Pediatrics, 8,* 119–132.

Fielding, F., Sanford, T. M., & Davis, M. P. (2013). Achieving effective control in cancer pain: A review of current guidelines. *International Journal of Palliative Nursing, 19,* 584–591.

Greco, K. E., Tinley, S., & Seibert, D. (2011). Development of the essential genetic and genomic competencies for nurses with graduate degrees. *Annual Review of Nursing Research, 29,* 173–190.

Greinert, R., & Boniol, M. (2011). Skin cancer—Primary and secondary prevention (information campaigns and screening)—With a focus on children and sunbeds. *Progress in Biophysics and Molecular Biology, 107*(3), 473–476.

HaDuong, J. H., Martin, A. A., Skapek, S. X., & Mascarenhas, L. (2015). Sarcomas. *Pediatric Clinics of North America, 62,* 179–200.

Henderson, T. O., Bhatia, S., Pinto, N., London, W. B., McGrady, P., Grotty, C., . . . Cohn, S. L. (2011). Racial and ethnic disparities in risk and survival in children with neuroblastoma: A Children's Oncology Group study. *Journal of Clinical Oncology, 29,* 76–82.

Henry, M., & Sung, L. (2015). Supportive care in pediatric oncology: Oncologic emergencies and management of fever and neutropenia. *Pediatric Clinics of North America, 62,* 27–46.

Huff, V. (2011). Wilms tumours: About tumour suppressor genes, an oncogene and a chameleon gene. *Nature Reviews Cancer, 11,* 111–121.

Kirchhoff, A. C., Krull, K. R., Ness, K. K., Armstrong, G. T., Park, E. R., Stovall, M., . . . Leisenring, W. (2011). Physical, mental, and neurocognitive status and employment outcomes in the childhood cancer survivor study cohort. *Cancer Epidemiology and Biomarkers Prevention, 20,* 1838–1849.

Kishimoto, K., Kobayashi, R., Ichikawa, M., Sano, H., Suzuki, D., Yasuda, K., . . . Kobayashi, K. (2014). Risk factors for tumor lysis syndrome in childhood acute myeloid leukemia treated with a uniform protocol without rasburicase prophylaxis. *Leukemia and Lymphoma, 26,* 1–11.

Kolyva, S., Efthymiadou, A., Gkentizi, D., Karana-Ginopoulou, A., & Varvarigou, A. (2014). Hypercalcemia and osteolytic lesions as presenting symptoms of acute lymphoblastic leukemia in childhood. *Journal of Pediatric Endocrinology and Metabolism, 27,* 349–354.

Kuttesch J. F., Rush, S. Z., & Ater, J. L. (2011). Brain tumors in children. In R. M. Kliegman, B. F. Stanton, J. W. St. Geme, N. F. Schor, & R. E. Behrman (Eds.), *Nelson textbook of pediatrics* (19th ed., pp. 1746–1753). Philadelphia, PA: Elsevier Saunders.

Landier, W., Armenian, S., & Bhatia, S. (2015). Late effects of childhood cancer and its treatment. *Pediatric Clinics of North America, 62,* 275–300.

Lewis, M. A., Hendrickson, A. W., & Moynihan, T. J. (2011). Oncologic emergencies: Pathophysiology, presentations, diagnosis, and treatment. *Cancer Journal for Clinicians, 61,* 287–314.

Manfrini, M., Tiwari, A., Ham, J., Colangeli, M., & Mercuri, M. (2011). Evolution of surgical treatment for sarcomas of proximal humerus in children: Retrospective review of a single institute over 30 years. *Journal of Pediatric Orthopedics, 31*, 56–64.

Masetti, R., Kleinschmidt, K., Biagi, C., & Pession, A. (2011). Emerging targeted therapies for pediatric myeloid leukemia. *Recent Patents on Anticancer Drug Discovery, 6*, 354–366.

Matthews, E. E., Neu, M., Cook, P. F., & King, N. (2014). Sleep in mother and child dyads during treatment for pediatric acute lymphoblastic leukemia. *Oncology Nursing Forum, 41*, 599–610.

McLendon, R. E., Adekunle, A., Rajaram, V., Kocak, M., & Blaney, S. M. (2011). Embryonal central nervous system neoplasms arising in infants and young children. *Archives of Pathology and Laboratory Medicine, 135*, 984–993.

Messinger, Y. H., Higgins, R. R., Devidas, M., Hunger, S. P., Carroll, A. J., & Heerema, N. A. (2012). Pediatric acute lymphoblastic leukemia with a t(8;14) (q11.2;q32): B-cell disease with a high proportion of Down syndrome: A Children's Oncology Group study. *Cancer Genetics, 205*, 453–458.

Meyer, W. H., & Grier, H. E. (2014). Comparing oxozophosphorines for treating Ewing sarcoma. *Journal of Clinical Oncology, 32*, 2401–2402.

Moore, D. D., & Haydon, R. C. (2014). Ewing's sarcoma of bone. *Cancer Treatment Research, 162*, 93–115.

National Cancer Institute. (2011a). *Childhood Hodgkin lymphoma treatment: Staging and diagnostic evaluation.* Retrieved from http://www.cancer.gov.cancertopics/pdq/treatment/childhodgkins/HealthProfessional/page4

National Cancer Institute. (2011b). *Childhood non-Hodgkin lymphoma treatment: Stage information.* Retrieved from http://www.cancer.gov.cancertopics/pdq/treatment/child-non-hodgkins/HealthProfessional

National Cancer Institute. (2011c). *Childhood rhabdomyosarcoma treatment: Stage information.* Retrieved from http://www.cancer.gov/cancertopics/pdq/treatment/childrhabdomyosarcoma/HealthProfessional

National Cancer Institute. (2011d). *Pediatric considerations for depression.* Retrieved from http://www.cancer.gov.cancertopics

National Cancer Institute. (2011e). *Stages of neuroblastoma.* Retrieved from http://www.cancer.gov.cancertopics/pdq/treatment/neuroblastoma/HealthProfessional/page2

National Cancer Institute. (2011f). *Wilms tumor and other childhood kidney tumors treatment: Stage information.* Retrieved from http://www.cancer.gov.cancertopics/pdq/treatment/wilms/HealthProfessional/page3

Paisley, M. A., Kang, T. I., Insogna, I. G., & Rheingold, S. R. (2011). Complementary and alternative therapy use in pediatric oncology patients with failure of frontline chemotherapy. *Pediatrics & Blood Cancer, 56*, 1088–1091.

Paldino, M. J., Faerber, E. N., & Poussaint, T. Y. (2011). Imaging tumors of the pediatric central nervous system. *Radiology Clinics of North America, 49*, 589–616.

Pollack, I. F. (2011). Multidisciplinary management of childhood brain tumors: A review of outcomes, recent advances, and challenges. *Journal of Neurosurgery: Pediatrics, 8*, 133–148.

Pollack, I. F., & Jakacki, R. I. (2011). Childhood brain tumors: Epidemiology, current management and future directions. *Nature Reviews Neurology, 7*, 495–506.

Pui, C. H., Carroll, W. L., Meshinchi, S., & Arceci, R. J. (2011). Biology, risk stratification, and therapy of pediatric acute leukemias: An update. *Journal of Clinical Oncology, 29*, 551–565.

Rabin, K. R., & Poplack, D. G. (2011). Management strategies in acute lymphoblastic leukemia. *Oncology, 25*, 328–335.

Reulen, R. C., Frobisher, C., Winter, D. L., Kelly, J., Lancashire, E. R., Stiller, C. A., . . . Hawkins, M. M. (2011). Long-term risks of subsequent primary neoplasms among survivors of childhood cancer. *Journal of the American Medical Association, 305*, 2311–2319.

Roberts, I., & Izraeli, S. (2014). Haemotopoietic development and leukemia in Down syndrome. *British Journal of Haemotology, 167*, 587–599.

Rueegg, C. S., Gianinazzi, M. E., Rischewski, J., Beck Popovic, M., von der Weid, N. X., Michel, G., & Kuehni, C. E. (2013). Health-related quality of life in survivors of childhood cancer: The role of chronic health problems. *Journal of Cancer Survivorship: Research and Practice, 7*, 511–522.

Shuangshoti, S., Shuangshoti, S., Nuchprayoon, I., Kanjanapongkul, S., Marrano, P., Irwin, M. S., & Thorner, P. S. (2011). Natural course of low risk neuroblastoma. *Pediatrics & Blood Cancer.* doi:10.1002/pbc.23325

Sigel, K., Dubrow, R., Silverberg, M., Crothers, K., Braithwaite, S., & Justice, A. (2011). Cancer screening in patients with HIV. *Current HIV/AIDS Report, 8*, 142–152.

Smith, M. A., & Reaman, G. H. (2015). Remaining challenges in childhood cancer and newer targeted therapeutics. *Pediatric Clinics of North America, 62*, 301–312.

Steinberger, J., Sinaiko, A. R., Kelly, A. S., Leisenring, W. M., Steffen, L. M., Goodman, P., . . . Baker, K. S. (2012). Cardiovascular risk and insulin resistance in childhood cancer survivors. *Journal of Pediatrics, 160*(3), 494–499.

Tubergen, D. G., Bleyer, A., & Ritchey, A. K. (2011). The leukemias. In R. M. Kliegman, B. F. Stanton, J. W. St. Geme, N. F. Schor, & R. E. Behrman (Eds.), *Nelson textbook of pediatrics* (19th ed., pp. 1732–1739). Philadelphia, PA: Elsevier Saunders.

Ward, L. D., Haberman, M., & Barbosa-Leiker, C. (2014). Development and psychometric evaluation of the genomic nursing concept inventory. *Journal of Nursing Education, 53*, 511–518.

Waxman, I. M., Hochberg, J., & Cairo, M. S. (2011). Lymphoma. In R. M. Kliegman, B. F. Stanton, J. W. St. Geme, N. F. Schor, & R. E. Behrman (Eds.), *Nelson textbook of pediatrics* (19th ed., pp. 1739–1753). Philadelphia, PA: Elsevier Saunders.

Winick, N. (2011). Neurocognitive outcome in survivors of pediatric cancer. *Current Opinion in Pediatrics, 23*, 27–33.

Zage, P. E., & Ater, J. L. (2011). Neuroblastoma. In R. M. Kliegman, B. F. Stanton, J. W. St. Geme, N. F. Schor, & R. E. Behrman (Eds.), *Nelson textbook of pediatrics* (19th ed., pp. 1753–1757). Philadelphia, PA: Elsevier Saunders.

Zage, P. E., & Herzog, C. E. (2011). Retinoblastoma. In R. M. Kliegman, B. F. Stanton, J. W. St Geme, N. F. Schor, & R. E. Behrman (Eds.), *Nelson textbook of pediatrics* (19th ed., pp. 1768–1769). Philadelphia, PA: Elsevier Saunders.

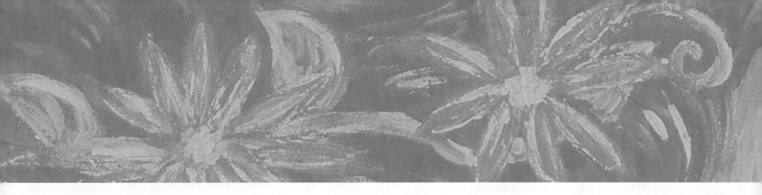

Chapter 25
Alterations in Gastrointestinal Function

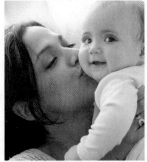

I was so worried when Jerome was born. He had no anal opening and his esophagus did not lead to his stomach. Now that he's had several surgeries, he is growing and doing pretty well, and I'm so happy to see him starting to smile. I can't wait until his final surgery is completed and he no longer has the colostomy.

—Mother of Jerome, 6 months old

Monkey 3000/Fotolia

⌄ Learning Outcomes

25.1 Describe the general function of the gastrointestinal system.

25.2 Discuss the pathophysiologic processes associated with specific gastrointestinal disorders in the pediatric population.

25.3 Identify signs and symptoms that may indicate a disorder of the gastrointestinal system.

25.4 Contrast nursing management and plan care for disorders of the gastrointestinal system

for the child needing abdominal surgery versus the child needing nonoperative management.

25.5 Analyze developmentally appropriate approaches for nursing management of gastrointestinal disorders in the pediatric population.

25.6 Plan nursing care for the child with an injury to the gastrointestinal system.

What causes structural defects of the gastrointestinal tract such as the esophageal atresia and imperforate anus experienced by Jerome? What special care do children with gastrointestinal abnormalities need to promote growth and development during treatment for those anomalies? This chapter discusses the care of infants who have structural defects and those with other common disorders of gastrointestinal functioning.

Structural Defects

Structural defects can involve one or more areas of the gastrointestinal tract. These defects occur when growth and development

of fetal structures are interrupted during the first trimester. This can leave the structure incomplete, resulting in *atresia* (absence or closure of a normal body orifice), malposition, nonclosure, or other abnormalities.

Cleft Lip and Cleft Palate

Cleft lip and cleft palate are two distinct facial defects that can occur singly or in combination (Figure 25–2). Cleft lip with or without cleft palate occurs in 1 out of every 750 to 1000 live births. The incidence is higher in Asian (1 in 500) than in White children (1 in 750). The defect is less common in African Americans, with an incidence of 1 of every 2000 live births. Cleft lip

Text continues on page 658

FOCUS ON:
The Gastrointestinal System

Anatomy and Physiology

The gastrointestinal (GI) tract includes the esophagus, stomach, pancreas, small intestine, and large intestine (Figure 25–1). Through the GI tract, a child ingests and absorbs the foods and fluids necessary to sustain life and promote growth. Elimination of waste products is another role of the GI tract. Other organs located in the abdominal region include the gallbladder, liver, and spleen. The abdomen is generally divided into four quadrants for purposes of assessment. (Refer to Figure 5–25 for the abdominal organs and structures in each quadrant.)

Esophagus and Stomach

The esophagus is a continuous tube that allows food to pass to the stomach. Food enters the esophagus through the mouth, where it is chewed. Initial enzyme secretion then occurs to begin food digestion. (See Chapter 19 for more information related to the mouth and pharynx.) The stomach is located in the left upper quadrant (LUQ) of the abdomen. The role of the stomach is to store food and to secrete enzymes and digestive juices that aid in the digestion of the food. Hydrochloric acid stimulates the stomach's pepsinogens to become pepsins, which break down proteins and are active in acidic levels (pH of 3 or less). The stomach propels food that is partially digested into the duodenum (a part of the small intestine).

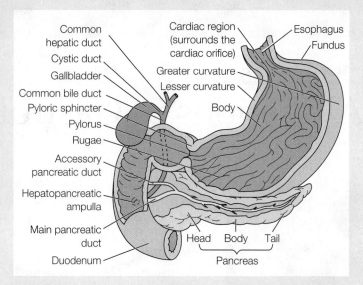

Figure 25–1 The internal anatomic structures of the stomach, including the pancreatic, cystic, and hepatic ducts; the pancreas; and the gallbladder.

As Children Grow: Stomach Capacity

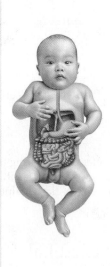

The young infant has a smaller stomach capacity than that of an older child or adolescent. A newborn has a stomach capacity of approximately 20 mL (Bergman, 2013). As infants grow, their stomach capacity increases, decreasing the frequency with which they need to be fed (American Academy of Pediatrics [AAP], 2014). Stomach capacity increases to approximately 90 mL in a 30-day-old term infant and to 360 mL around 1 year of age. An adult stomach holds 2 to 3 L (Collopy & Friese, 2010).

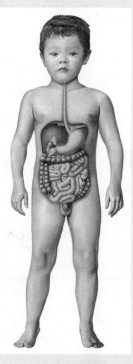

Source: Data from American Academy of Pediatrics. (2014). *Amount and schedule of formula feedings*. Retrieved from healthychildren.org/English/ages-stages/baby/feeding-nutrition/Pages/Amount-and-Schedule-of-Formula-Feedings.aspx; Bergman, N. J. (2013). Neonatal stomach volume and physiology suggest feeding at 1-h intervals. *Acta Paediatrica, 102*, 773–777; Collopy, K., & Friese, G. (2010). Pediatric drug administration. *Emergency Medical Services Magazine, 39*(6), 52–57.

Pancreas

The pancreas is located behind the stomach and has several functions. The pancreas secretes enzymes, electrolytes, and bicarbonate that aid in the digestion and absorption of fats, proteins, and carbohydrates (Werlin & Wilschanski, 2016). Another key function of the pancreas is to regulate blood glucose metabolism through production of insulin, glucagon, and gastrin.

Liver and Gallbladder

The liver, the largest organ in the abdomen, is located in the right upper quadrant (RUQ). Its primary functions include production of blood clotting factors, fibrinogen and prothrombin; secretion of bile and bilirubin (yellow pigment produced from the breakdown of red blood cells); metabolism of fat, protein, and carbohydrates; detoxification of hormones, drugs, and other substances; and storage of vitamins A, D, E, and K and glycogen. The gallbladder is a small organ located behind the liver. The gallbladder stores and concentrates the bile that is produced in the liver. It then releases stored bile as needed into the duodenum. Bile includes a variety of substances such as water, salts, bilirubin, and cholesterol. A major role of bile is to emulsify fats so that fatty acids become soluble and absorbable (Huppert & Balistreri, 2016).

Spleen

The spleen is located in the LUQ of the abdomen and is a highly vascular organ. The spleen contains about 30% of the circulating platelets and is a site for red blood cell production as well. Defense against infection is another key role of the spleen (Brandow & Camitta, 2016).

Small and Large Intestine

The small intestine consists of the duodenum, the jejunum, and the ileum. Each part of the small intestine plays a vital role in the digestion and absorption of carbohydrates, amino acids, and fats. The intestinal wall is covered with small villi, the brush border, through which absorption occurs. Absorption occurs both through diffusion (commonly monosaccharides, amino acids, fatty acids, and glycerol) and active transport (commonly disaccharides, dipeptides, and tripeptides). A complex system of innervation and secretions maintains a basic pH that facilitates metabolism and absorption. The large intestine includes the cecum, the appendix, the colon (consisting of ascending, transverse, descending, and sigmoid portions), and the rectum, which passes to the exterior through the anus. The primary function of the large intestine is reabsorption of fluid and electrolytes from the GI tract and excretion of wastes (Liacouras, 2016). Bacteria in the large intestine synthesize vitamin K and facilitate some vitamin B absorption.

Pediatric Differences

Although the fetus makes sucking and swallowing movements in utero and ingests amniotic fluid, the GI system is immature at birth. The processes of absorption and excretion do not begin until after birth, because the placenta provides nutrients and removes waste. Sucking is a primitive reflex that occurs whenever the lips or cheeks are stroked. The infant does not have voluntary control over swallowing until about 6 weeks of age.

The stomach capacity of the newborn is quite small, and intestinal motility (**peristalsis**) is greater than in older children (see *As Children Grow: Stomach Capacity*). These characteristics explain the newborn's need for small, frequent feedings and the increased frequency and liquid consistency of bowel movements. Because of the relaxed cardiac sphincter, infants frequently regurgitate small amounts of feedings.

Digestion takes place in the duodenum. Infants have a deficiency of several enzymes: amylase (which digests carbohydrates), lipase (which enhances fat absorption), and trypsin (which catabolizes protein into polypeptides and some amino acids). Enzymes are usually not present in sufficient quantities to aid digestion until 4 to 6 months of age. Thus abdominal distention from gas is common.

Liver function is also immature. After the first few weeks of life the liver is able to conjugate bilirubin and excrete bile. The processes of **gluconeogenesis** (formation of glycogen from noncarbohydrates), plasma protein and ketone formation, vitamin storage, and **deamination** (removal of amino group from amino compound) remain immature during the first year of life.

By the second year of life, digestive processes are fairly complete. Stomach capacity increases to accommodate a three-meals-per-day feeding schedule. Around 18 months of age, the child becomes aware of a full rectum and is physically able to have some control over excretory functions (Goldson & Reynolds, 2012).

Use *Assessment Guide: The Child With a Gastrointestinal Condition* to perform a nursing assessment of the gastrointestinal system. A list of diagnostic and laboratory tests used to evaluate gastrointestinal conditions is provided in Table 25–1. See Appendices D and E for further information about lab values and test procedures for the gastrointestinal system.

TABLE 25–1 Diagnostic Tests and Laboratory Procedures for the Gastrointestinal System

DIAGNOSTIC PROCEDURES	LABORATORY TESTS
Abdominal ultrasound	Complete blood count
Barium or contrast enema	Bilirubin
CT of the abdomen	Electrolytes
Endoscopy	Liver enzymes
GI series	Stool for occult blood
Intraesophageal pH probe monitoring	Stool for ova and parasites
Abdominal radiographs	

Note: See Appendices D and E for information about these diagnostic procedures and tests.

(continued)

ASSESSMENT GUIDE | The Child With a Gastrointestinal Condition

Assessment Focus	Assessment Guidelines
Abdomen—inspection	• Observe the shape of the abdomen. • Note any abdominal distention. Measure abdominal girth. • Observe the umbilicus for protrusion. • Observe for peristaltic waves (visible rhythmic contractions of the intestinal wall smooth muscle). • Observe for jaundice, bruising, and increased bleeding.
Abdomen—auscultation	• Auscultate for bowel sounds in all four quadrants prior to palpation.
Abdomen—palpation	• Palpate the abdomen and note if it is soft or firm. • Palpate the size of the umbilical ring. • Does the child complain of pain or tenderness during palpation? Does the infant cry? • Describe any masses palpated by location, shape, size, and consistency. • Palpate the liver for size and tenderness. • Palpate the spleen for size and tenderness.
Mouth and esophagus	• Note the presence of increased oral secretions. • Note the presence of cleft lip or palate.
Nutrition	• Note tolerance of feedings, spitting up, emesis, and recurrent respiratory infections. • Observe amount, color, and frequency of emesis. • Note if emesis is associated with feeding and whether or not it is projectile. • Note amount of intake, frequency of feedings, and growth.
Stool	• Observe color, consistency, and size of stool. Note any changes in stool patterns.
Family history	• Ask about history of gastrointestinal illness with genetic influences such as celiac disease and inflammatory bowel disease.

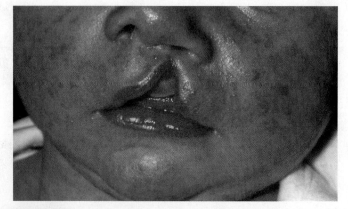

Figure 25–2 Unilateral cleft lip.

SOURCE: Dr. P. Marazzi/Science Source.

and palate occur together in approximately 45% of cases, while cleft palate occurs alone approximately 35% of the time, and cleft lip occurs alone approximately 20% of the time (Patel, Cohen, Ramaswamy, et al., 2014).

ETIOLOGY AND PATHOPHYSIOLOGY

Cleft lip with or without cleft palate results when the maxillary processes fail to fuse with the elevations on the frontal prominence during the sixth week of gestation. Normally, union of the upper lip is complete by the seventh week. Fusion of the secondary palate occurs between 5 and 12 weeks of gestation. Failure of the tongue to move downward at the correct time prevents the palatine processes from fusing.

The intrauterine development of the hard and soft palates is completed in the first trimester. It is during this time that other major organ systems develop. Approximately 30% of children with cleft and/or palate will have another congenital anomaly (Setó-Salvia & Stanier, 2014). There is an increased incidence in families with a prior history of cleft lip or palate. The cause is believed to be multifactorial, involving a combination of environmental and genetic influences. Etiologic factors include smoking during pregnancy, maternal use of alcohol, and use of medications such as anticonvulsants and steroids during pregnancy (Setó-Salvia & Stanier, 2014). Additional studies have suggested that folate intake during pregnancy may reduce the incidence of cleft lip and palate (Blanton et al., 2011; Kelly, O'Dowd, & Reulbach, 2012).

CLINICAL MANIFESTATIONS

A cleft that involves the lip is readily apparent at birth. It may be a simple dimple in the vermilion border of the lip or a complete separation extending to the floor of the nose. The defect may be unilateral or bilateral and may occur alone or in combination with a cleft palate defect. Varying degrees of nasal deformity may also be present.

Cleft palate defects are less obvious when they occur without a cleft lip and may not be detected at birth. Clefts of the hard palate form a continuous opening between the mouth and nasal cavity and may be unilateral or bilateral, involving just the soft palate or both the soft and hard palates.

CLINICAL THERAPY

A multidisciplinary team is involved in cleft lip and palate management since these children have an increased risk for impairment in speech, hearing, and dentition. The team should include the pediatric primary healthcare provider and specialists in plastic and oral surgery, audiology, speech/language pathology, otolaryngology, dentistry, genetics, social work, and psychology (Crockett & Goudy, 2014).

Cleft lip and palate are usually diagnosed at birth or during the newborn assessment, but may be diagnosed in utero. Successful imaging of the face via transabdominal ultrasound can be performed as early as 13 to 14 weeks' gestation. Use of three-dimensional ultrasound or magnetic resonance imaging, if available, allows for a clearer picture of the defect and enhances the ability to detect isolated cleft palate prenatally (Wilkins-Haug, 2014). After the child is born, cleft lip and cleft palate are diagnosed by characteristic physical findings. The upper lip, alveolar arches, nostrils, and primary and secondary palates should be inspected and palpated (Crockett & Goudy, 2014).

The timing of cleft lip repair varies among surgeons. Repair generally occurs between 3 and 5 months of age, but may occur earlier or later depending on surgeon preference (Figure 25–3). If the defect is severe, the child may need more than one operation to achieve total repair. After surgery, soft elbow immobilizers (also known as restraints) are used for 2 weeks to protect the incision. (See the *Clinical Skills Manual* SKILLS .) The child should receive distraction and pain medication as needed because prolonged crying may disrupt the suture line. Antibiotics may also be prescribed (Crockett & Goudy, 2014).

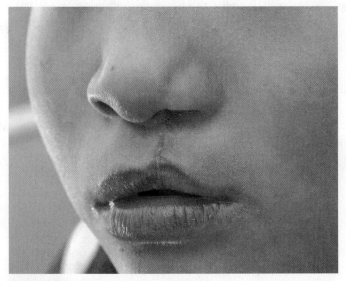

Figure 25–3 **Repaired unilateral cleft lip.**
SOURCE: jorgecachoh/Fotolia.

Early closure of the lip enables the infant to form a better seal around the nipple for feeding. The sucking motion strengthens the muscles necessary for speech. Special feeding devices such as longer nipples with enlarged holes are available to help meet the infant's nutritional needs before surgical correction. A lactation consultant can assist with breastfeeding techniques.

Timing of the cleft palate repair varies among surgeons and depends on the size and severity of the cleft. The palate should be closed by 12 months of age (Wiet, Biavati, & Rocha-Worley, 2013). This protects the formation of tooth buds and allows the infant to develop more normal speech patterns.

Infants with cleft lip and cleft palate are prone to recurrent otitis media, which can lead to hearing problems. (Refer to Chapter 19 for care of the child with chronic otitis media.) The child who has had a cleft palate repair requires orthodontic care. Early visits permit assessment of tooth eruption and the need for future orthodontic work.

Nursing Management

For the Child With Cleft Lip and Cleft Palate

Nursing Assessment and Diagnosis

PHYSIOLOGIC ASSESSMENT

A cleft lip defect is observable at birth. A cleft palate defect is usually noted during the newborn assessment by palpation of the primary and secondary palate (Crockett & Goudy, 2014). A description of the location and extent of the defect helps the nurse determine the correct method of feeding. Thorough and complete physical assessment is required since additional defects are sometimes present.

> ### Developing Cultural Competence Corrective Surgery for Cleft Lip and Palate
> In many developing countries, infants do not have access to surgery for correction of cleft lip and palate. They may grow into childhood and adulthood with these abnormalities. Medical teams from the United States, Canada, and other countries sometimes travel to developing nations for short medical missions, performing surgery on the children and teaching local doctors surgical techniques. Are there medical missions teams from your area that perform these surgeries? What planning is required for such trips to perform surgery safely and care for the children? What is the impact on the communities served?

PSYCHOSOCIAL ASSESSMENT

Assessment of the family's reactions is an integral part of the overall nursing assessment. Physical deformities, especially of the face, can be devastating to parents. A poorly corrected defect can lead to the development of low self-esteem in the older child. Assess the child's developmental level and social interactions with peers.

The accompanying *Nursing Care Plan* lists common nursing diagnoses for the infant with a cleft lip and/or palate. Other diagnoses that might be appropriate include the following (NANDA-I © 2014):

- *Anxiety (Parent)* related to situational crisis and threat to self-concept

- *Attachment, Risk for Impaired (Parent and Infant)*, related to newborn's structural defect
- *Pain, Acute*, related to surgical repair of defect
- *Development: Delayed, Risk for*, related to structural defect and altered nutritional intake

Planning and Implementation

Nursing care involves providing emotional support, performing postsurgical care, educating parents on feeding techniques, helping parents coordinate care and maintain a healthy home environment, and making appropriate referrals. See *Nursing Care Plan: The Infant With a Cleft Lip or Palate* for a summary of nursing care.

Nursing Care Plan: The Infant With a Cleft Lip or Palate

Preoperative Care

1. Nursing Diagnosis: *Aspiration, Risk for,* related to anatomic defect (NANDA-I © 2014)

GOAL: The infant will have no episodes of gagging or aspiration.

INTERVENTION	RATIONALE
• Assess respiratory status and monitor vital signs at least every 2 hr.	• Allows for early identification of problems.
• Keep suction equipment and bulb syringe at bedside.	• Suctioning may be necessary to remove milk or mucus.
• Position upright for feedings.	• Minimizes passage of feedings through cleft.
• Feed slowly and use adaptive equipment as needed.	• Facilitates intake while minimizing risk of aspiration.
• Hold upright for 30 minutes after feeding.	• Prevents aspiration of feedings.
• Burp frequently (after every 15–30 mL of fluid).	• Helps to prevent regurgitation and aspiration.

EXPECTED OUTCOME: Infant will exhibit no signs of respiratory distress.

---

2. Nursing Diagnosis: *Coping: Family, Compromised,* related to birth of a child with a defect (NANDA-I © 2014)

GOAL: Parents will begin bonding process with the infant. The family's coping ability will be maximized. Parents will verbalize the nature and sequelae of the defect.

INTERVENTION	RATIONALE
• Help parents hold the infant and facilitate feeding process.	• Contact is essential for bonding.
• Point out positive attributes of infant (e.g., hair, eyes, alertness.).	• Helps parents see the child as a whole, rather than concentrating on the defect.
• Explain surgical procedure and expected outcome. Show pictures of other children's cleft lip repair.	• Eliminating unknown factors helps to decrease anxiety.
• Assess parents' knowledge of the defect, their degree of anxiety and level of discomfort, and the interpersonal relationships among family members.	• Helps determine the appropriate timing and amount of information to be given regarding the child's defect.
• Provide information about the etiology of cleft lip and palate defects and the special needs of these infants. Encourage questions.	• Concrete information allows parents time to understand the defect and reduces guilt.
• Explore the reactions of extended family members.	• Extended family is an important source of support for most parents of a newborn. Family members can often help promote acceptance and compliance with the treatment plan.
• Support rooming in.	• Rooming in allows parents to continue the bonding process.
• Encourage parents to participate in caretaking activities (holding, diapering, feeding).	• Participation in infant care decreases anxiety and provides parents with a sense of purpose.
• Refer to parent support groups.	• Support groups allow parents to express their feelings and concerns, to find people with concerns similar to their own, and to seek additional information.

EXPECTED OUTCOME: Parents will hold, comfort, and show concern for the infant. Family will demonstrate ability to cope with and manage the infant's care. Parents receive necessary support to care for their infant.

3. Nursing Diagnosis: *Nutrition, Imbalanced: Less than Body Requirements,* **related to the infant's inability to ingest nutrients (NANDA-I © 2014)**

GOAL: The infant will gain weight steadily.

INTERVENTION	RATIONALE
• Assess fluid and calorie intake daily. Assess weight daily (same scale, same time, with infant completely undressed). Teach parents signs of adequate fluid intake such as frequency of wet diapers.	• Provides an objective measurement of whether the infant is receiving sufficient caloric intake to promote growth. Using the same scale and procedure when weighing the infant provides for comparability between daily weights.
• Observe for any respiratory impairment.	• Any symptoms of respiratory compromise will interfere with the infant's ability to suck. Feedings should be initiated only if there are no signs of respiratory distress.
• Provide weight-appropriate calories and fluid amounts. If the infant needs an increased number of calories to grow, referral to a nutritionist should be made. Higher calorie concentration formulas are available.	• Provides optimal calories and fluids for growth and hydration.
• Facilitate breastfeeding.	• Breast milk is recommended as the best food for an infant. The process of breastfeeding helps to promote bonding between mother and infant.
• Hold the infant in an upright position.	• Facilitates swallowing and minimizes the amount of fluid return from the nose.
• Give the mother information on breastfeeding the infant with a cleft lip or palate such as plugging the cleft lip and eliciting a letdown reflex before nursing.	• Information and specific suggestions may encourage the mother to persist with breastfeeding.
• Contact the La Leche League for the name of a support person.	• The La Leche League promotes breastfeeding for all infants. It can provide support people with experience who will aid the mother.
• If the mother is unable to breastfeed (or prefers not to), initiate bottle-feeding:	• Facilitates swallowing and minimizes the amount of fluid return from the nose.
• Place nipple against the inside cheek toward the back of the tongue. If needed, use a premature nipple (slightly longer and softer than regular nipple with a larger opening) or special cleft feeder.	• Use of longer, softer nipples makes it easier for the infant to suck. Special cleft feeders decrease the amount of pressure in the bottle and make the formula flow more easily.
• Initiate nasogastric feedings if the infant is unable to ingest sufficient calories by mouth.	• Adequate nutrition must be maintained. Use of a feeding tube allows the infant who has difficulty with oral feeding to receive adequate nutrition for growth.

EXPECTED OUTCOME: Infant will maintain adequate nutritional intake and gain weight appropriately. Successful breastfeeding will be achieved if desired. Feeding will provide necessary nutrients and will be a positive experience for parents and infant.

Postoperative Care

1. Nursing Diagnosis: *Breathing Pattern, Ineffective,* **related to surgical correction of defect (NANDA-I © 2014)**

GOAL: The infant will maintain an effective breathing pattern.

(continued)

Nursing Care Plan: The Infant With a Cleft Lip or Palate (continued)

INTERVENTION	RATIONALE
• Assess respiratory status and monitor vital signs at least every 2 hr.	• Frequent assessment allows for early identification of problems.
• Apply a cardiorespiratory monitor.	• The monitor enables early detection of abnormal respirations, facilitating prompt intervention.
• Keep suction equipment and bulb syringe at the bedside. Gently suction oropharynx and nasopharynx as needed; avoid suture areas.	• Gentle suctioning will keep the airway clear. Suctioning that is too vigorous can irritate the mucosa.
• Provide cool mist for first 24 hr postoperatively if ordered.	• A mist moisturizes secretions to reduce pooling in the lungs. It also moisturizes the oral cavity.
• Reposition every 2 hr.	• Repositioning ensures expansion of all lung fields.

EXPECTED OUTCOME: Infant will show no signs of respiratory infection or compromise.

---

2. Nursing Diagnosis: *Tissue Integrity, Impaired,* **related to mechanical factors (NANDA-I © 2014)**

GOAL: The infant's lip and/or palate will heal with minimal scarring or disruption.

INTERVENTION	RATIONALE
• Position the infant with cleft lip repair on back.	• Prone positioning would allow the infant to rub the suture line.
• Use soft elbow immobilizers. Remove every 2 hr and replace. Do not leave the infant unattended when immobilizers are removed.	• Immobilizers prevent the infant's hands from rubbing surgical site. Regular removal allows for skin and neurovascular checks.
• Maintain suture line or Steri-Strips placed over cleft lip repair.	• Maintaining suture line will minimize scarring.
• Avoid metal utensils or straws after cleft palate repair.	• These devices may disrupt suture line.
• Do not allow pacifiers.	• Sucking can disrupt suture line.
• Keep the infant well medicated for pain in initial postoperative period. Have parents hold and comfort the infant.	• Good pain management minimizes crying, which can cause stress on the suture line. Increases bonding and soothes the child to decrease crying.
• Provide developmentally appropriate activities (i.e., mobiles, music).	• Appropriate activities soothe and keep the infant calm.

EXPECTED OUTCOME: Lip/palate will heal without complications.

---

3. Nursing Diagnosis: *Nutrition, Imbalanced: Less than Body Requirements,* **related to inability to ingest nutrients (NANDA-I © 2014)**

GOAL: The infant will receive adequate nutritional intake.

INTERVENTION	RATIONALE
• Maintain intravenous infusion as ordered.	• The IV provides fluid when the child is NPO (nothing by mouth).
• Begin with clear liquids, then give half-strength formula or breast milk as ordered.	• Ensures adequate fluids and nutrients.
• Use syringe or dropper inside of mouth.	• Avoids suture line and resultant accumulation of formula in that area.
• Give high-calorie soft foods after cleft palate repair.	• Rough foods, utensils, and straws could disrupt the surgical site.

EXPECTED OUTCOME: Infant will receive adequate nutritional intake. The infant resumes usual feeding patterns and gains weight appropriately.

PROVIDE EMOTIONAL SUPPORT

When a child is born with a cleft lip/cleft palate, parents may grieve the loss of the ideal child that they expected. Parents may need assistance to view their infant as a whole person, rather than focusing solely on the physical defect. Promote parent–infant bonding by explaining the nature of the structural defect and the procedure for correction. Interact and speak to the infant in the parents' presence and point out positive attributes such as alertness, soft skin, or active movements. Self-blame is common among parents. Parents can also be referred to the American Cleft Palate Association for information about the disorder. Pictures of children who have had repair are available at this website. Seeing pictures of children who have had a successful repair offers reassurance to parents.

Parental anxiety is a typical response when children undergo surgery, and it is heightened when the surgery involves an infant. To minimize anxiety, give clear, concise explanations to parents. Allow sufficient time for parents to ask questions. Encourage parents to hold and cuddle the infant before surgery (see Chapter 11).

PROVIDE POSTOPERATIVE CARE

Provide general postoperative care for the infant. (See *Nursing Care Plan: The Infant With a Cleft Lip or Palate* here and *Nursing Care Plan: The Child Undergoing Surgery* in Chapter 11.) Additional postoperative nursing diagnoses may include (NANDA-I © 2014):

- *Infection, Risk for,* related to location of surgical procedure
- *Knowledge, Deficient (Parent),* related to lack of exposure and unfamiliarity with resources

Assess vital signs frequently and maintain the infant's airway. Measure intake and output. When oral fluids with clear liquids are started, they are usually given through a dropper, syringe, or special feeder. Position the infant in a sitting position for the feedings to avoid aspiration. Frequently burp the infant during feedings. The infant then progresses to half-strength formula or breast milk. After each feeding, cleanse the suture line with water or normal saline to avoid accumulation of feedings. In addition, the following specific interventions are necessary to ensure healing of the suture line:

- Prevent the infant from rubbing the suture line on the bedding by positioning the infant in a supine position.
- Maintain soft elbow immobilizers.
- Maintain the suture line or Steri-Strips placed over the incision. Place antibiotic body ointment on the incision site as ordered.
- Medicate the infant as prescribed to control pain and to minimize crying and stress on the suture line.
- After cleft palate surgery, avoid the use of metal utensils or straws, which may disrupt the surgical site.

COMMUNITY-BASED NURSING CARE

Identify and address home care needs well in advance of discharge. Discuss all aspects of the infant's care with the parents throughout hospitalization and after surgery. Involve parents in the infant's care to increase their comfort level before discharge and to promote bonding. Teach feeding techniques, how to recognize signs of infection, how to position the infant, and how to care for the suture line. Breastfeeding is usually possible with some assistance from a lactation specialist, even if the mother pumps her breasts and milk is fed by a special nurser. For infants requiring assistance to feed, several wide-based nipples, squeezable bottles, and other special bottles are available.

Management involves many different healthcare professionals. In addition to hospital, clinic, and home health nurses, members of the healthcare team often include specialists such as a plastic surgeon, orthodontist, dentist, social worker, audiologist, speech pathologist, and pediatrician. The parents are the best coordinators of the child's care. Encourage them to keep a diary listing the professionals with whom they talk and the content of the discussions.

Teach parents how to care for the child after discharge. Teach them how to feed the infant, identify signs of complications (fever, vomiting, respiratory distress), administer any medications as prescribed, and care for the surgical site. Emphasize the importance of soft elbow immobilizers as prescribed.

Discuss with the parents the financial implications of long-term care. Private insurance does not always cover all the costs of care necessary for the child. Refer parents to programs and financial aid for which the parents and child may be eligible. Relief from financial worries enables parents to concentrate on caring for the child. Determine whether additional family supports are necessary.

Growth and Development

An infant who has had a cleft lip repair needs stimulation to provide distraction. This approach will minimize crying, which can damage the suture line. Soft, colorful toys, mobiles, and other visual objects are helpful. Music also can be used to soothe the infant. Parental presence is comforting and reassuring.

Referral to a home healthcare agency for support may be helpful. Encourage follow-up visits with healthcare professionals (see *Health Promotion: The Child With Cleft Lip or Cleft Palate*). The child may need further evaluation of speech development, ear infections, or a recommendation for plastic surgery.

Evaluation

Expected outcomes of nursing care are provided in the accompanying *Nursing Care Plan.*

Esophageal Atresia and Tracheoesophageal Fistula

Esophageal atresia is a malformation that results from failure of the esophagus to develop as a continuous tube during the fourth and fifth weeks of gestation. The defect affects occurs in approximately 1 in 4500 neonates (Liszewski, Bairdain, Buonomo, et al., 2014). At least 90% of those affected also have a tracheoesophageal fistula (Khan & Orenstein, 2016a).

ETIOLOGY AND PATHOPHYSIOLOGY

In esophageal atresia, the foregut fails to lengthen, separate, and fuse into two parallel tubes (the esophagus and trachea) during fetal development. Instead the esophagus may end in a blind pouch or develop as a pouch connected to the trachea by a fistula (tracheoesophageal fistula) (see *Pathophysiology Illustrated: Esophageal Atresia and Tracheoesophageal Fistula*). Esophageal atresia is often associated with a maternal history of polyhydramnios (Khan & Orenstein, 2016a; Saxena, Blair, & Konkin, 2014). Other congenital anomalies occur in greater than 50% of children with esophageal atresia (Barman, Mandal, Shukla, et al., 2014). Jerome, the child described in the quotation at the beginning of the chapter, had esophageal atresia as well as an imperforate anus.

Health Promotion The Child With Cleft Lip or Cleft Palate

The child with cleft lip or cleft palate requires close monitoring and intervention to foster growth and development. The nurse can assist the child and family to achieve healthy outcomes.

Growth and Development Surveillance
- Monitor the child's growth and developmental patterns.
- Monitor for developmental delays.
- Explain to parents that regression following surgery in the toddler or older child is normal.

Nutrition
- Refer the family to sources for nipples, nursers, and other special feeding devices.
- Assist the mother with learning how to express breast milk and facilitate breastfeeding.
- Teach parents to avoid giving foods that can pose a choking hazard to the child.
- Teach parents to feed the infant in an upright position and to burp the child frequently during feedings.

Physical Activity
- Activity for the child having surgical procedures to correct cleft palate is generally restricted for approximately 2 to 3 weeks postsurgery to allow for healing.
- After healing has occurred, encourage the parents to promote the child's activities as they would any child without cleft lip or cleft palate.

Oral Health
- The child should be routinely screened for dental caries. Ask the family about dental visits.
- Teach the parents to provide good dental hygiene to the child.
- Routine dental/orthodontic evaluation is necessary for the child with cleft palate.

Mental and Spiritual Health
- For uncorrected or poorly corrected cleft lip or palate, the child may experience poor self-esteem related to body image.

- Encourage the family to adhere to treatment and surgical correction plan, including staged surgical corrections, dental care, and speech pathology assistance.
- Ask the family about financial ability regarding speech therapy, dental care, and other services that may be required. Financial constraints can impede compliance with recommended therapies.
- Be alert for the child who has had experiences with teasing associated with articulation or physical appearance.
- Refer parents to websites such as Project Smile and other resources.
- Refer the child for counseling if indicated.

Relationships
- Evaluate the parents for parent–infant bonding.
- Promote bonding by encouraging the parents to participate in the infant's care, to hold the infant, and to recognize the infant's positive attributes.

Disease Prevention Strategies
- Teach the family to recognize signs and symptoms of ear or other infections and to seek immediate evaluation. Treatment of acute otitis media is necessary to prevent long-term effects of repeated infections.
- Emphasize to the parents the importance of audiology screening for children with cleft lip and palate to evaluate conductive hearing loss.

Injury Prevention Strategies (Safety)
- Assist parents in properly applying elbow immobilizers to protect the suture line in the postoperative period.
- Ask the parents about eating utensils the child uses.
- Teach parents to avoid straws, metal spoons, and other sharp utensils that may damage the palate.

Pathophysiology Illustrated: **Esophageal Atresia and Tracheoesophageal Fistula**

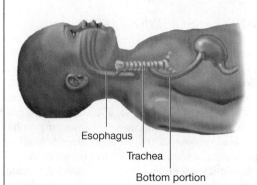

Esophagus

Trachea

Bottom portion
of esophagus

In the most common type of esophageal atresia and tracheoesophageal fistula, the upper segment of the esophagus ends in a blind pouch connected to the trachea; a fistula connects the lower segment to the trachea.

CLINICAL MANIFESTATIONS

Symptoms in the newborn include excessive salivation and drooling, often accompanied by three classic signs for this defect: cyanosis, choking, and coughing. Sneezing may also be noted. During feeding, fluid returns through the infant's nose and mouth. Aspiration places the infant at risk for pneumonia. Depending on the type of defect, the infant's abdomen may be distended because of air trapping.

CLINICAL THERAPY

Esophageal atresia is suspected based on the presence of poly-hydramnios and a small or absent fetal gastric bubble noted on prenatal ultrasound (Garabedian et al., 2014; Nowicki, 2013). After the child is born, passage of a radiopaque tube through the esophagus may be attempted. If the tube meets resistance, a chest and abdominal radiograph can confirm the presence of esophageal atresia. Radiologic examination may also reveal associated anomalies (Nowicki, 2013). Early diagnosis is essential to prevent aspiration of secretions, which can lead to pneumonia (Khan & Orenstein, 2016a).

Primary repair is preferred when possible and involves connecting the two ends of the esophagus and ligating the fistula if present (Nowicki, 2013). If primary repair of the esophageal atresia is not possible in the neonatal period, a gastrostomy tube is placed for feedings and the fistula is ligated (Nowicki, 2013; Saxena et al., 2014). Several procedures have been developed that allow for stretching of the esophagus over a period of time. Once the length of the esophagus is adequate, the two ends are reconnected in a delayed primary repair. The child will generally remain in the hospital setting until the repair. Potential postoperative complications include gastroesophageal reflux, aspiration, stricture formation, leak at the area of anatamosis, and tracheomalacia (Nowicki, 2013).The prognosis is usually good with surgery; however, some conditions are complicated, requiring repeated surgeries and long-term management. In the event that the two ends of the esophagus cannot be reconnected, colonic, jejunal, or gastric segments may be used to lengthen the esophagus (Khan & Orenstein, 2016a).

Nursing Management

The nurse may recognize the signs and symptoms in the immediate newborn period. Assess the infant for difficulty feeding and excessive drooling and the classic signs of choking, coughing, and cyanosis. Assess for respiratory distress and assess the lung sounds carefully.

Esophageal atresia is a surgical emergency. Preoperatively the infant requires close observation and intervention to maintain a patent airway. Specific interventions include:

- Have suction readily available to remove any secretions that accumulate in the nasopharyngeal airway.
- Place the infant with the head of the bed slightly elevated to minimize aspiration of secretions into the trachea.
- Use continuous or low intermittent suction to remove secretions from the blind pouch.
- Withhold oral fluids, and provide maintenance intravenous fluids.
- Constantly monitor the infant's vital signs and overall condition.

After surgery administer intravenous fluids and antibiotics. Monitor strict intake and output. Total parenteral nutrition may be needed until gastrostomy or oral feedings are tolerated.

Monitoring and assessment of feeding tolerance are ongoing. Feedings are introduced slowly and in small amounts. Assess for respiratory difficulty during reintroduction of feedings. Monitor weight, growth, and developmental achievements.

The parents require emotional support throughout the infant's hospitalization. Clearly explain all procedures. Encourage parents to bond with the infant by stroking and talking to the infant. Eliciting questions and allowing parents to participate in the infant's care, especially feeding (when permitted), can facilitate bonding and help to prepare parents for care of the infant after discharge.

The specific details of discharge teaching depend on the types of procedures the child has had. Teach the parents about gastrostomy tube care and feedings if applicable, signs of infection, and how to prevent postoperative complications.

The outcomes of nursing care will depend on the extent of the defect and correction. Examples include the following:

- The child does not experience respiratory distress and maintains normal respirations.
- The child achieves and maintains a normal weight.
- Positive parent–infant bonding is established.
- The parent has knowledge of the defect, its corrections, and the child's needs.

Pyloric Stenosis

Pyloric stenosis is a hypertrophic obstruction of the circular muscle of the pyloric canal. Pyloric stenosis occurs in approximately 2 of every 1000 births (Lin et al., 2014). There is an increased incidence in firstborn males (Hunter & Liacouras, 2016; Taylor, Cass, & Holland, 2013). Pyloric stenosis is more common in the White population (Hunter & Liacouras, 2016; McAteer, Ledbetter, & Goldin, 2013)

ETIOLOGY AND PATHOPHYSIOLOGY

The exact cause of pyloric stenosis is unknown, although frequently there is a family history of the disorder. *Hypergastrinemia* (too much gastrin in the blood) is thought to play a role in the development of pyloric stenosis. Studies have indicated a higher incidence of the disorder in infants who received oral erythromycin before 2 weeks of age (Lozada, Royall, Nylund, et al., 2013).

Hypertrophy of the circular pylorus muscle results in stenosis of the passage between the stomach and the duodenum, partially obstructing the lumen of the stomach (see *Pathophysiology Illustrated: Pyloric Stenosis*). The lumen becomes inflamed and edematous, which narrows the opening until the obstruction becomes complete. At this time, vomiting becomes more forceful. As the obstruction progresses, the infant becomes dehydrated and electrolytes are depleted, resulting in metabolic imbalances.

CLINICAL MANIFESTATIONS

Symptoms usually become evident 2 to 8 weeks after birth, although onset may vary (Taylor et al., 2013). Initially, the infant appears well or regurgitates slightly after feedings. The parents may describe the infant as a "good eater" who vomits occasionally. As the obstruction progresses, the vomiting becomes projectile. In **projectile vomiting**, the contents of the stomach may be ejected up to 3 feet from the infant. The vomitus is non-bilious and may become blood tinged because of repeated irritation to the esophagus. The infant generally appears hungry, especially after emesis; irritable; fails to gain weight; and has

Families Want to Know

Teaching the Family About Gastrostomy Tube Feedings

The infant or child who has difficulty swallowing, consuming oral feedings, or gaining weight may be a candidate for a gastrostomy tube. Indications for a gastrostomy tube placement may include neurologic deficit; avoidant/restrictive food intake disorder (failure to thrive); severe gastroesophageal reflux; feeding aversions; short bowel syndrome; defects of the mouth, esophagus, or stomach; and cerebral palsy (Hannah & John, 2013). Depending on the condition, the child may need the gastrostomy tube for all feedings or supplementary feedings. Research indicates that the use of a standardized education protocol is beneficial. Patient outcomes were improved and caregiver confidence and knowledge increased (Schweitzer et al., 2014). See Chapter 11 for general guidelines related to teaching plans. See also the *Clinical Skills Manual* SKILLS .

General Principles

Preoperatively

- Assess what the family knows about a gastrostomy tube and gastrostomy tube placement.
- Assess what methods will be most effective in teaching care of the gastrostomy tube and enteral feedings.
- Show the family pictures or dolls with gastrostomy tubes and explain what the child's abdomen will look like in the immediate postoperative period.
- Provide the family with a booklet about gastrostomy tubes and enteral feedings.

Postoperatively

- Show the family the child's gastrostomy tube and reassess their understanding of the tube.
- When feedings are ordered, demonstrate the first feeding to the parents while explaining each step.
- Actively involve a family member in the second feeding. With subsequent feedings, have a family member feed the child with the nurse watching.
- Teach the family about:
  - Feeding administration
  - Medication administration
  - Daily care of the tube and the site surrounding the tube
  - How to handle common complications such as blockage, leaking, dislodgement, presence of hypergranulation tissue, and site irritation or infection
  - Phone numbers to call if needed
  - When to seek medical care related to the gastrostomy tube
- All family members who are involved in care of the child should practice feeding the child and administering medications to the child prior to discharge. This allows the nurse to assess for understanding of the procedure and gives the family confidence in their ability to care for the child. Some children will need bolus feedings, others may have continuous feedings via a feeding pump, and yet others may have bolus feedings during the day and continuous feedings at night.

Source: Data from Correa, J. A, Fallon, S. C., Murphy, K. M., Victorian, V. A., Bisset, G. S., Vasudevan, S. A., . . . Lee, T. C. (2014). Resource utilization after gastrostomy tube placement: Defining areas of improvement for future quality improvement projects. *Journal of Pediatric Surgery, 49,* 1598–1601; Hannah, E., & John, R. M. (2013). Everything the nurse practitioner should know about pediatric feeding tubes. *Journal of the American Association of Nurse Practitioners, 25,* 567–577; Schweitzer, M., Aucoin, J., Docherty, S. L., Rice, H. E., Thompson, J., & Sullivan, D. T. (2014). Evaluation of a discharge education protocol for pediatric patients with gastrostomy tubes. *Journal of Pediatric Health Care, 28*(5), 420–428.

fewer and smaller stools. The child may present with dehydration and metabolic alkalosis depending on how long the child has been vomiting (Tigges & Bigham, 2012). On physical examination, peristaltic waves may be observed across the abdomen as the stomach attempts to move contents past the narrowed pyloric canal (Lin et al., 2014). An olive-sized mass in the right upper quadrant may be evident (Lisonkova & Joseph, 2013; Markowitz, 2014).

CLINICAL THERAPY

An abdominal ultrasound to determine the diameter and length of the pyloric muscle is the preferred method performed to confirm the diagnosis (Castellani, Peschaut, Schippinger, et al., 2014; Markowitz, 2014). Blood tests will determine if the child is dehydrated or has an electrolyte or acid–base imbalance (see Chapter 18). Infants with pyloric stenosis are at risk for hypochloremia, hypokalemia, and metabolic alkalosis; however, recent studies show that normal laboratory values are found most often. This could be attributed to earlier diagnosis and the increased use of ultrasound to confirm the diagnosis (Taylor et al., 2013; Tutay, Capraro, Spirko, et al., 2013).

Surgery is performed as soon as possible after the infant's fluid and electrolyte balance is restored. Laparoscopic pyloromyotomy is the preferred surgical method to correct pyloric stenosis (Castellani et al., 2014). In a pyloromyotomy, the pyloric muscle is split to allow the passage of food and fluid. The prognosis is good. The infant is usually taking fluids within a few hours following surgery and discharged on full-strength formula within 24 hours after surgery.

Pathophysiology Illustrated: **Pyloric Stenosis**

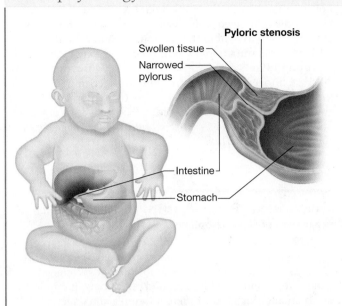

Pyloric stenosis

- Swollen tissue
- Narrowed pylorus
- Intestine
- Stomach

In pyloric stenosis, the hypertrophied pyloric muscle causes symptoms of projectile vomiting and visible peristalsis.

Nursing Management

For the Child With Pyloric Stenosis

Nursing Assessment and Diagnosis

Observe the infant's abdomen for the presence of peristaltic waves. Bowel sounds are hyperactive on auscultation. Auscultate before palpating the abdomen since palpation can cause a change in bowel patterns (see Chapter 5). Palpation reveals an olive-shaped mass in the right upper quadrant of the abdomen.

Assess the infant's history of vomiting, vital signs, weight, and nutritional status. Assess skin turgor, anterior fontanelle, urinary output (weigh diapers), urine specific gravity, and mucous membranes for signs of dehydration. Describe vomiting episodes and estimate emesis amount. Be alert for signs of an electrolyte and/or acid–base imbalance. (See Chapter 18 for a discussion of electrolyte and acid–base imbalances.) Assess parental anxiety related to the child's condition. The child usually appears hungry. Crying and general discomfort are frequently observed.

Nursing diagnoses that might be appropriate for the child with pyloric stenosis include (NANDA-I © 2014):

- *Fluid Volume: Deficient,* related to vomiting
- *Nutrition, Imbalanced: Less than Body Requirements,* related to vomiting and inability to ingest nutrients
- *Sleep Pattern, Disturbed,* related to discomfort and hunger
- *Anxiety (Parents)* related to surgery
- *Pain, Acute,* related to surgical incision

Planning and Implementation

Nursing care focuses on meeting the infant's fluid and electrolyte needs, minimizing weight loss, promoting rest and comfort, preventing infection, and providing supportive care for parents.

MEET FLUID AND ELECTROLYTE NEEDS

Withhold oral feedings preoperatively because projectile vomiting will continue until the obstruction is relieved. Emphasize to the parents the importance of maintaining an NPO status preoperatively. Intravenous therapy is administered to correct fluid and electrolyte imbalances as needed and to maintain adequate hydration. Maintain nasogastric tube to suction if one is present and measure output from the tube. Inform parents that all diapers will be weighed to measure the infant's output of urine and stool.

MINIMIZE WEIGHT LOSS

The infant loses weight because of frequent vomiting. Monitor weight daily both preoperatively and postoperatively. Begin feedings postoperatively according to the healthcare provider's orders. Some surgeons prefer an NPO period following pyloromyotomy, with slow, incremental increases in volume and strength of feedings once feeding has resumed. Others will implement an earlier postoperative feeding approach.

PROMOTE REST AND COMFORT

During the preoperative period, the infant is hungry and cries often. The infant is swaddled to maintain warmth and provide comfort. Encourage the parents to hold and cuddle the infant. Provide a pacifier to meet the infant's need to suck.

Postoperatively, the infant is uncomfortable because of the surgical incision. Analgesics can be administered to relieve discomfort as ordered. (See Chapter 15 for a discussion of pain management.) Instruct parents to avoid pressure on the incision. When diapering the infant, slide the diaper gently under the buttocks rather than lifting the legs. Swaddling, rocking, and use of a pacifier provide comfort to the infant.

PREVENT INFECTION

Postoperatively, the incision is covered with collodion or Steri-Strips and should be kept clean and dry. Inspect the incision site for redness, swelling, or discharge. Monitor the infant's temperature every 4 hours. Auscultate the lungs to assess for any adventitious sounds.

PROVIDE SUPPORTIVE CARE

The need for hospitalization and surgery creates anxiety for parents. Encourage them to participate in the infant's care and to discuss their fears and concerns. Provide simple and clear explanations about the infant's condition and care. Advise parents that occasional vomiting after surgery may occur.

DISCHARGE PLANNING AND HOME CARE TEACHING

Instruct parents to observe the incision for redness, swelling, or discharge and to notify the healthcare provider immediately if these occur or if the infant develops a fever. To reduce the possibility of infection, advise parents to fold the infant's diaper so that it does not touch the incision. Provide instructions about feeding to ensure the infant's intake.

Evaluation

Expected outcomes of care include pain control, intake of recommended fluid and food with absence of vomiting, and manifestation of normal growth patterns.

Gastroesophageal Reflux

Gastroesophageal reflux (GER), the return of gastric contents into the esophagus, is the result of relaxation of the lower esophageal sphincter (Khan & Orenstein, 2016b; Marcdante & Kliegman, 2015). GER is the most common esophageal disorder in children (Khan & Orenstein, 2016b). Approximately 50% of infants have some degree of reflux (Lightdale & Gremse, 2013). Factors that increase the incidence of GER in the pediatric population include a short narrow esophagus, small stomach, large volume feedings, an immature lower esophageal sphincter, a liquid diet, and frequent horizontal position (Marcdante & Kliegman, 2015). Additional factors that increase the incidence of GER include prematurity, neurologic impairment, obesity, chronic respiratory disorders, and a history of repaired esophageal atresia (Lightdale & Gremse, 2013).

The primary symptoms of GER are regurgitation, spitting up, or vomiting (Lightdale & Gremse, 2013). Children with GER are frequently hungry and irritable. They eat often but still lose weight. Infants with reflux are at risk for aspiration and apnea.

Gastroesophageal reflux disease (GERD) is a more serious manifestation of GER. Symptoms of GERD in infants include vomiting or regurgitation associated with irritability, refusal of feedings, poor weight gain, sleep disturbance, respiratory symptoms including coughing, choking and wheezing and arching of the back during feedings (Lightdale & Gremse, 2013; Randel, 2014). Symptoms of GERD in older children include dysphagia, heartburn, and chest pain (Lightdale & Gremse, 2013).

Diagnosis is confirmed by a thorough history of the child's feeding patterns and by diagnostic evaluation. An upper GI series is helpful in assessing anatomy and possibly detecting an alteration in motility. Esophageal pH monitoring and intraluminal esophageal impedance are the preferred diagnostic tools for GER. Upper endoscopy with esophageal biopsy is the method used to determine the amount of damage to the esophagus in the presence of GERD and to rule out other conditions (Lightdale & Gremse, 2013; Randel, 2014).

Treatment depends on the severity of the condition. Generally, feeding modification, thickened feeds, and positioning are effective management for milder cases. A smaller feeding volume and increased frequency of feedings is recommended (Lightdale & Gremse, 2013). The healthcare provider may decide that rice cereal needs to be added to the infant's bottle to thicken feedings (Schwarz & Hebra, 2014). A special nipple may need to be used. Prethickened formulas are commercially available. For example, Enfamil AR contains added rice, is nutritionally balanced, and may be beneficial to young infants who are formula-fed (Schwarz & Hebra, 2014). Children may benefit from smaller, more frequent meals. Greasy and spicy foods, chocolate, peppermint, citrus, and caffeine should be avoided (Schwarz & Hebra, 2014). See *Professionalism in Practice: Guidelines for Management of Gastroesophageal Reflux.*

> **Professionalism in Practice** **Guidelines for Management of Gastroesophageal Reflux**
>
> The American Academy of Pediatrics has established guidelines related to the management of complicated GER and GERD. Included in these guidelines are recommendations related to infant feeding and positioning. Formula-fed infants may need a different formula and maternal diet may need to be modified in breastfed infants. Smaller, more frequent feedings and thickened feedings may decrease symptoms. Upright positioning is recommended. Semisupine positioning in a car seat or infant carrier should be avoided after feedings, as this may exacerbate symptoms (Lightdale & Gremse, 2013). Pediatric nurses care for infants with GER and GERD in both inpatient and outpatient settings. They have the opportunity to help families reduce the symptoms of reflux in the infant by educating parents about strategies related to feeding and positioning.

Use of medications to treat GERD in children varies among healthcare providers. See *Medications Used to Treat: Gastroesophageal Reflux Disease* for examples of medications that may be used.

Treatment for severe cases of GERD may include surgery that involves wrapping the greater curvature of the stomach (fundus) around the distal esophagus (fundoplication) (Khan & Orenstein, 2016b; Lightdale & Gremse, 2013; Randel, 2014). A gastrostomy tube may be inserted during surgery to serve as an access for venting and as a means for feeding if needed (Khan & Orenstein, 2016b).

Nursing Management

Nursing management focuses on supporting the infant's or child's nutritional intake, promoting interventions to reduce associated complications, and supporting the family.

Monitor the infant's weight daily and plot on a growth chart to note progress. Observe for any signs of respiratory distress, and keep the infant's nose and mouth clear of emesis.

Adequate nutrition must be maintained for the child to achieve normal growth and development. Infants receiving oral feedings should be given small, frequent feedings. Elevate the head of the bed to prevent aspiration if vomiting should occur. If the child has a gastrostomy tube, it is important to maintain skin integrity around the stoma site.

Medications Used to Treat: Gastroesophageal Reflux Disease

MEDICATION AND ACTION	NURSING IMPLICATIONS
Histamine H$_2$ Receptor Antagonists Zantac (ranitidine) Pepcid (famotidine) Inhibit the histamine H$_2$ receptor on the gastric parietal cell, thus blocking gastric acid secretion.	May be administered with or without food. Teach parents to avoid OTC medications without checking with healthcare provider. Monitor for side effects: Bradycardia Fatigue Rash Constipation Headache Confusion Nausea Irritability Thrombocytopenia Dizziness Diarrhea
Proton Pump Inhibitors Prevacid (lansoprazole) Prilosec (omeprazole) These powerful inhibitors of gastric acid secretion alleviate symptoms and help to heal esophagitis. Block the final common pathway of acid production by inhibiting activated proton pumps in the gastric parietal cell canaliculus.	Administer in the morning on an empty stomach. Monitor for side effects: Abdominal pain Fatigue Nausea Diarrhea Headache Proteinuria Dizziness Hematuria Rash Constipation Anorexia Teach family to inform primary healthcare provider if severe diarrhea occurs. Teach family to inform primary healthcare provider if changes in urinary elimination, such as pain or discomfort associated with urination, occur.

Source: Data from Blanco, F. C., Davenport, K. P., & Kane, T. D. (2012). Pediatric gastroesophageal disease. *Surgical Clinics of North America, 92*(3), 541–558; Lightdale, J. R., & Gremse, D. A. (2013). Gastroesophageal reflux: Management guidance for the pediatrician. *Pediatrics, 131*(5), e1684–e1695; Wilson, B. A., Shannon, M. T., & Shields, K. M. (2015). *Pearson nurse's drug guide 2015*. Hoboken, NJ: Pearson Education.

Clinical Tip

Parents are encouraged to hold their infant in an upright position for 20 to 30 minutes following feedings. Minimize seated positioning such as in an infant car seat because this increases intra-abdominal pressure and promotes reflux.

Clinical Tip

In older children, a pattern of chronic vomiting (low-grade, nearly daily emesis) or cyclic vomiting (repeated severe vomiting of an episodic nature) can occur. These patterns differ from vomiting seen in colic or gastroesophageal reflux. **Chronic vomiting** is often associated with upper gastrointestinal tract diseases such as gastritis and esophagitis, whereas **cyclic vomiting** (also called *cyclic vomiting syndrome*) is a functional disorder characterized by recurrent episodes of severe nausea and vomiting that last several hours to days. The affected children have symptom-free periods between episodes, in which they are able to participate in normal activities (Tarbell & Li, 2013). Continuous vomiting of any nature should be evaluated.

Discharge planning focuses on instructing parents in how to feed and position the infant, as well as providing comfort and emotional support. Encourage parents to hold and cuddle the infant during all feedings. Providing the infant with a pacifier helps to meet nonnutritive sucking needs. Teach parents how to suction the nose and mouth if vomiting occurs.

Omphalocele and Gastroschisis

Omphaloceles are congenital malformations in which intra-abdominal contents herniate through the umbilical cord (Figure 25–4). An omphalocele results when the intestines fail to return to the abdominal cavity during the 10th to 12th week of gestation (Ledbetter, 2012). The size of the sac varies depending on the extent of the protrusion. Large defects may contain intestines, stomach, liver, and the spleen (Hood & Zimmerman, 2013). The abdominal contents are contained in a sac that is composed of peritoneum, Wharton jelly, and amniotic membrane (Glasser, 2014). Rupture of the sac results in evisceration of the abdominal contents. Omphalocele with herniation of intestines into the umbilical cord occurs in 1 in 5000 births, while omphalocele with herniation of liver and intestines occurs in 1 in 10,000 births (Carlo & Ambalavanan, 2016). Fifty to seventy percent of infants with omphalocele will have an associated anomaly such as bladder exstrophy, cardiac defects, and Meckel diverticulum (Razmus, 2011).

Gastroschisis is a congenital defect of the abdominal wall, characterized by protrusion of bowel through a defect in the abdominal wall to the side (most often to the right) of the umbilicus. Unlike the omphalocele, no membrane covers the organs

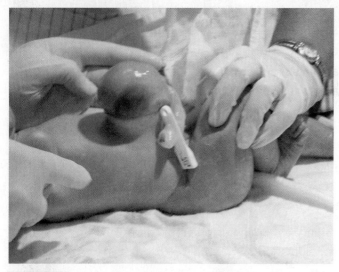

Figure 25-4 In omphalocele, the size of the sack depends on the extent of the protrusion of abdominal contents through the umbilical cord.

SOURCE: Courtesy of Carol Harrigan, RNC, MSN, NNP.

(Corey et al., 2014; Hood & Zimmerman, 2013; Ruano et al., 2011) (Figure 25-5). Gastroschisis occurs in 4 to 5 per 10,000 births (Benjamin & Wilson, 2014). Approximately 20% of infants with gastroschisis have an associated anomaly, most often atresia or intestinal stenosis (Razmus, 2011).

Care of the child with gastroschisis or omphalocele centers on protecting the protruding abdominal organs, correcting the defect, and preventing complications such as hypothermia, infection, and injury to involved organs.

Both gastroschisis and omphalocele are associated with elevation of maternal serum alpha-fetoprotein (MSAFP) (Glasser, 2014). Routine prenatal ultrasonography and determination of MSAFP levels lead to early diagnosis, education of the family, and coordination of the team of specialists needed to manage these congenital anomalies (Razmus, 2011).

The immediate action upon birth is to protect the sac (in omphalocele) or exposed abdominal contents (in gastroschisis) from injury by placing the infant feet first into a bowel bag (large sterile clear bag) that extends to the nipple line and is secured with ties. The bag is filled with warm saline to decrease heat loss, to keep organs moist, and to allow for visualization of the defect (Razmus, 2011). The child will often be transferred to a neonatal intensive care unit (NICU) with surgical capability for this defect.

One surgery may be all that is needed to repair a small defect. For larger defects, the first stage of repair may involve nonoperative placement of the abdominal contents or sac into a Silastic silo. Once the abdominal cavity can accommodate the intestinal contents, the child will have surgery to close the abdominal wall (Razmus, 2011).

Nursing Management

Be alert for signs of associated congenital anomalies. (Refer to the discussion of tracheoesophageal fistula earlier in this chapter, of genitourinary anomalies in Chapter 26, and of congenital heart defects in Chapter 21.)

Immediately after birth, follow healthcare provider protocol for maintaining the omphalocele sac or for the exposed abdominal contents in gastroschisis as discussed previously. Monitor vital signs at least hourly, paying close attention to temperature, as the infant can lose heat through the sac. The child should be in a warmer or isolette for maintenance of temperature control. Inspect the area for signs of infection.

Because the infant is NPO preoperatively, maintain fluid and electrolyte balance with intravenous fluids. Postoperative care includes measures to control pain, prevent infection, maintain fluid and electrolyte balance, and ensure adequate nutritional intake. Attainment of bowel motility and function varies and is often delayed for weeks after surgery. Total parenteral nutrition for the infant is used until full bowel function has returned (Hood & Zimmerman, 2013).

Throughout the infant's hospitalization, parents need clear, accurate explanations about the infant's condition. To help the parents deal with the crisis of an acutely ill newborn, provide emotional support and encourage parents to express their feelings. When the child has multiple anomalies, parents need ongoing support for the lengthy treatment, numerous hospitalizations, and management of nutritional intake.

Expected outcomes of nursing care depend on the severity of the defect and its correction, but may include:

- Fluid volume balance is maintained.
- The incision heals without signs of infection.
- Stable thermoregulatory function is maintained.
- Effective pain management is achieved.
- Parent–infant bonding and attachment are demonstrated.

Intussusception

Intussusception occurs when one portion of the intestine prolapses and then invaginates or telescopes into another. It is one of the most frequent causes of intestinal obstruction during infancy and occurs at a rate of 1 in 2000 infants and children. Intussusception is more common in male babies. An estimated 65% of cases occur in children prior to 1 year of age (Deloach & Farber, 2013).

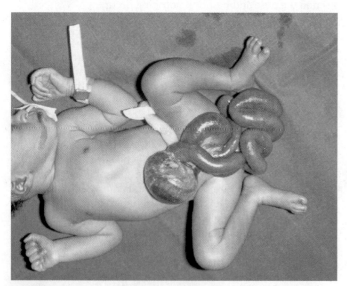

Figure 25-5 The newborn with gastroschisis has abdominal contents located outside the abdominal wall.

SOURCE: Ansary/Custom Medical Stock Photo/Newscom.

ETIOLOGY AND PATHOPHYSIOLOGY

Ninety percent of intussusception cases in children are idiopathic because a direct cause is not generally identified. Although the exact cause is unknown, there is frequently a current or recent enteritis or upper respiratory infection (Pepper, Stanfill, & Pearl, 2012).

The most common site of intussusception is the ileocecal valve (Cochran, Higgins, & Strout, 2011). Telescoping of the intestine obstructs the passage of stool. The walls of the intestine rub together, causing inflammation, edema, and decreased blood flow. This can lead to bowel wall edema, necrosis, and perforation (Territo, Wrotniak, Qiao, et al., 2014) (Figure 25–6).

CLINICAL MANIFESTATIONS

The onset of intussusception is usually abrupt. A previously healthy infant or child suddenly experiences acute abdominal pain with vomiting and passage of brown stool. There may be periods of comfort between acute episodes of pain. As the condition worsens, painful episodes increase. The child may have bilious emesis and a palpable abdominal mass. The stools become red and resemble currant jelly because of the mix of blood and mucus (Cochran et al., 2011; Deloach & Farber, 2013).

CLINICAL THERAPY

Diagnosis is made on the basis of the history and confirmed by radiographs and ultrasound of the abdomen. A contrast enema using air or barium can be both diagnostic and therapeutic. An air (or pneumatic) enema reduces the intussusception in approximately 90% of cases and is considered safer than a barium enema because of the decreased risk of perforation (Pepper et al., 2012).

A nasogastric tube is inserted for gastric decompression. If reduction of the intussusception does not occur during the contrast enema, surgical intervention to reduce the invaginated bowel and remove any necrotic tissue is necessary. Surgery is generally successful in correcting the problem; however, intussusception can recur after hydrostatic reduction or surgical correction.

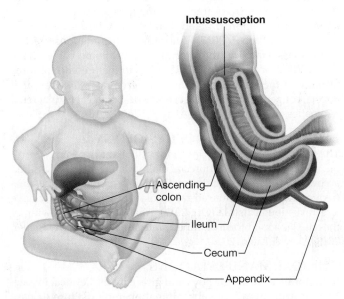

Intussusception

Ascending colon

Ileum

Cecum

Appendix

Figure 25–6 In infants, intussusception is commonly associated with viral illnesses and gastroenteritis.

Nursing Management

Nursing management focuses on maintaining or restoring fluid and electrolyte balance. Intravenous fluids are started immediately. Serum electrolyte monitoring is essential to correct imbalances.

Postoperative care focuses on monitoring for early signs of infection, managing the child's pain, and maintaining nasogastric tube patency. Assess vital signs, check for abdominal distention, and assess for return of bowel function. Feeding protocols vary among practitioners. Generally, after normal bowel function returns, clear liquid feeding or breastfeeding can resume. Feedings are then advanced as the infant or child tolerates them.

Discharge usually occurs shortly after the infant or child begins taking full feedings. Instruct parents to watch for infection and to call the healthcare provider if symptoms recur, a fever develops, or appetite decreases.

Clinical Tip

The passage of a normal brown stool may indicate that an intussusception has been reduced. Report this finding to the primary healthcare provider immediately, as the course of treatment may be altered, especially in the case of a planned surgical reduction.

Volvulus

During the 7th to 12th week of gestation the small intestine undergoes rapid growth. In normal development, the intestine rotates counterclockwise as it settles into its permanent position inside the abdominal cavity. Malrotation of the intestine occurs in approximately 1 of every 500 live births (Shalaby, Kuti, & Walker, 2013). When malrotation of the intestine occurs, the child is at risk for *volvulus*, a twisting of the intestine. Volvulus disrupts blood flow in the intestines and can lead to necrosis of the bowel, short bowel syndrome, and death. Volvulus is considered a surgical emergency. Early diagnosis and treatment is necessary to preserve the bowel and to save the child's life (Hebra & Cuffari, 2012; Shalaby et al., 2013).

Symptoms of volvulus in the infant include bilious vomiting, firm abdomen with distention, irritability secondary to pain, and passage of bloody stools. The diagnosis is confirmed through radiologic studies. Intravenous fluids are given to rehydrate the infant and to correct any electrolyte imbalance. Emergency exploratory surgery to untwist the bowel is essential (Zerpa & Shapiro, 2013). If a portion of the bowel is necrotic, that portion of the bowel is removed. An ostomy may need to be created, depending on the amount of bowel removed. See the section on ostomies later in this chapter. The child is at risk for developing short bowel syndrome if a significant amount of bowel is removed (see discussion later in this chapter).

Nursing Management

The infant or child who presents to the emergency department with bilious vomiting and a firm and distended abdomen should be assessed quickly to determine the cause of the symptoms. Once volvulus has been diagnosed, nursing management focuses on keeping the child NPO, administering intravenous fluids, assessing vital signs, and reporting symptoms of a worsening condition. The child who has had surgery to correct uncomplicated volvulus will need care similar to that described for the child with intussusception. If a necrotic bowel was removed, the child may have an ostomy for a period of time.

Hirschsprung Disease

Hirschsprung disease, also known as *congenital aganglionic megacolon*, is a congenital anomaly in which inadequate motility causes mechanical obstruction of the intestine. The disease occurs in approximately 1 in 5000 live births, and is more common in males than females (Burkhardt, Graham, Short, et al., 2014). Hirschsprung disease can occur as a single anomaly or in combination with other anomalies such as congenital heart defects, Down syndrome, and urinary tract anomalies (Burkhardt et al., 2014; Langer, 2013).

ETIOLOGY AND PATHOPHYSIOLOGY

Hirschsprung disease is the congenital absence of ganglion cells (nerve cells) in the wall of a variable segment of rectum and colon. The absence of autonomic parasympathetic ganglion cells in the colon prevents peristalsis at that portion of the intestine, resulting in the accumulation of intestinal contents and abdominal distention. In most cases, the area lacking ganglion cells is limited to the rectosigmoid region of the colon (Fiorino & Liacouras, 2016).

CLINICAL MANIFESTATIONS

Clinical manifestations of Hirschsprung disease vary depending on the child's age at onset. Symptoms in newborns generally include abdominal distention, feeding intolerance, bilious vomiting, and failure to pass meconium within the first 24 to 48 hours after birth (Holder & Jackson, 2013; Langer, 2013; Nelville, 2014). *Enterocolitis* (inflammation of the intestines) is a complication of Hirschsprung disease that can be fatal if not recognized and treated early. Symptoms of enterocolitis include fever, foul smelling and/or bloody **diarrhea** (frequent, watery stools), abdominal pain, and vomiting (Nelville, 2014).

The older infant or child may have a history of failure to gain weight, malnutrition, and chronic severe **constipation** (difficult and infrequent defecation with passage of hard, dry stool), (Langer, 2013; Nelville, 2014).

CLINICAL THERAPY

Diagnosis is made on the basis of the history, bowel patterns, radiographic contrast studies, and rectal biopsy for presence or absence of ganglion cells. The rectum is small in size on palpation and does not contain stool. Abdominal radiographs generally show a distended bowel with dilated bowel loops throughout the abdomen. Water-soluble contrast studies reveal a transition zone between the normal and aganglionic bowel (Burkhardt et al., 2014; Langer, 2013). Rectal biopsy revealing the absence of ganglionic cells and the presence of hypertrophic nerve bundles has proven to be the most reliable test for confirmation of the diagnosis (Burkhardt et al., 2014; Fiorino & Liacouras, 2016; Langer, 2013).

The primary repair of Hirschsprung disease is to remove the aganglionic portion of the bowel using a pull-through procedure. A primary repair may not be possible in the presence of extensive dilated proximal bowel, enterocolitis, or bowel perforation. In that case, a temporary colostomy is created and is closed when the definitive surgery takes place (Langer, 2013).

The return of normal bowel function depends on the amount of bowel involved. Some fecal incontinence and constipation may persist following surgery. Enterocolitis is a serious complication that can occur before or after surgery, resulting in ischemia and ulceration of the bowel wall. Treatment for enterocolitis associated with Hirschsprung disease includes rectal irrigations and antibiotics (Holder & Jackson, 2013).

Nursing Management

Nursing assessment in the newborn period includes careful observation for the passage of meconium. Because newborns are often discharged within 24 hours of birth, tell parents to notify the healthcare provider if no stool is passed or the abdomen becomes distended. When the disease is diagnosed later in infancy or in childhood, obtain a thorough history of weight gain, nutritional intake, and bowel elimination habits.

When Hirschsprung disease is diagnosed, nursing care includes monitoring for infection, managing pain, maintaining hydration, measuring abdominal circumference to detect any distention, and providing support to the child and family. Preoperative oral intake varies depending on the surgeon; however, intake is generally restricted to clear fluids the day before surgery. Rectal irrigations may be performed to evacuate the bowel prior to surgery.

Initial postoperative nursing care is the same as for any other infant or child having abdominal surgery: Maintain intravenous fluids and nasogastric tube. Monitor intake and output. Administer pain medications as prescribed and assess at least every hour for evidence of pain utilizing a pain scale and documenting assessment. If a colostomy was performed, the stoma should be assessed frequently as well as the return of bowel function. See the section on ostomies later in this chapter.

Children occasionally develop constipation and parents may need guidance to adapt the diet and fluid intake to manage this complication. Because some children develop malabsorption, be alert for signs of poor growth or malnutrition.

Expected outcomes of nursing care include:

- Fluid and electrolyte balance is maintained.
- Adequate nutritional intake to promote growth and development is evident.
- Adequate bowel function is demonstrated.
- The child's pain is managed effectively.
- The parents demonstrate effective coping with stress of the child's condition.

Anorectal Malformations

Anorectal malformations refer to anomalies of the rectum and distal anus, the urinary tract, and the genital tract. They have an incidence of approximately 1 in 5000 live births worldwide (Guardino & Pieper, 2013). Anorectal malformations are frequently associated with other anomalies. Some babies have VACTERL conditions. VACTERL refers to the presence of three or more of the following anomalies: **v**ertebral anomalies, **a**nal atresia, **c**ongenital heart disease, **t**racheo**e**sophageal fistula, **r**enal anomalies, and **l**imb defects (Akay & Klein, 2016).

ETIOLOGY AND PATHOPHYSIOLOGY

The term *imperforate anus* (absence of the anal opening) is frequently used to refer to anorectal malformations and is classified according to the specific defect. Boys with an imperforate anus frequently have a rectourethral fistula and girls generally have a rectovestibular fistula (Orr, 2011). Anal stenosis (narrowing of the anus) is a mild form of imperforate anus (Guardino & Pieper, 2013; Akay & Klein, 2016).

CLINICAL MANIFESTATIONS

Imperforate anus affects boys and girls equally. Perineal inspection at birth reveals the absent anal opening. Failure to pass meconium within the first 24 hours of birth may be indicative of imperforate anus. Stool in the urine usually indicates the presence of a fistula between the colon and urinary tract. Cloacal malformations in girls, in which the urinary tract, vagina, and rectum fuse together, forming a common channel, may occur. The child with a cloacal malformation has one opening in the perineum (Guardino & Pieper, 2013).

Diagnosis of anorectal malformation is usually made at birth or during the newborn assessment of anorectal structures and rectal patency. Ultrasound and lower gastrointestinal radiographic studies are used to confirm the diagnosis and demonstrate the extent of the anomaly.

CLINICAL THERAPY

Management depends on the extent of the malformation and presence of associated conditions. Anal stenosis may be treated with dilation alone. A single operation, anoplasty, may be used to repair rectoperineal defects (previously known as low defects). Higher defects require a three-stage procedure. A temporary colostomy in the newborn period provides for bowel decompression and for protection of the surgical site when the anomaly is repaired. Reconstructive surgery is accomplished via a posterior sagittal anorectoplasty (PSARP). This surgery generally occurs between 3 to 6 months of age, although timing varies among surgeons. When the operative site has healed, approximately 2 weeks after surgery, anal dilations are begun. When the desired size of the anal opening has been achieved, the colostomy is closed (Orr, 2011).

Nursing Management

During the initial newborn assessment, the perineal area is inspected for a poorly developed anal dimple or sacral anomalies. Observe and record passage of meconium.

Once the diagnosis has been made, intravenous fluids are initiated and a nasogastric tube is inserted to decompress the stomach. Monitor the child's intake and output (I&O) and cardiorespiratory functioning. Provide emotional support to the parents and give them information about the upcoming surgery.

Postoperative care specific to the child who has had a PSARP procedure centers on protection of the surgical site. A Foley catheter will be in place for 5 days to protect the new anal opening from urine. The colostomy that is still in place protects the surgical site from stool. The child should have nothing placed in the rectum. Provide adequate pain management for the child. Maintain intravenous fluids until the child is able to take liquids by mouth.

Nursing care for the child who has had colostomy closure is more complex because the bowel has been manipulated during surgery. It is essential to maintain the nasogastric tube to low wall suction until bowel function returns. Provide intravenous fluids or total parenteral nutrition through peripheral or central venous access until the child can tolerate fluids by mouth. Monitor intake and output. The child will frequently have a Foley catheter in place for accurate measurement of urine output.

Care of the operative site may include dressing changes in addition to assessment for signs of infection. As the child begins to pass stool through the anal opening for the first time, skin breakdown is likely. Protect the perineal area with a barrier cream or paste.

Provide intravenous pain medication on a regular basis. The nurse is also responsible for administering prescribed antibiotics that protect the child from infection.

The child with associated abnormalities may need several surgeries and interventions to treat all of the conditions present. Partnering with families and a group of healthcare providers will assist in case management that facilitates the child's health and development. Health promotion and health maintenance that include support of family members, ensuring immunizations, and monitoring developmental status are important.

DISCHARGE PLANNING AND HOME CARE TEACHING

Infants are increasingly discharged shortly after birth, so parents need clear instructions about normal newborn stools and what abnormalities to report. The nurse should:

- Teach parents how to care for the ostomy site if a colostomy is performed in the newborn period (see discussion of ostomies later in this chapter).
- Reassure parents that the colostomy will be closed in the future, and help them plan for that hospitalization.
- Refer parents to ostomy support groups in the community or online.
- Discuss follow-up care and long-term management.
- Arrange follow-up visits and home care visits to evaluate the child's ostomy site and monitor growth.

Clinical Tip

Following colostomy closure in the child who has had a colostomy for several months, the perineal area is not accustomed to contact with stool. Without meticulous skin care, breakdown is very likely. Teach parents to change diapers frequently, clean the perineal area carefully, and apply a protective barrier ointment or cream at each diaper change.

After surgery to create the anal opening, teach parents how to take the infant's temperature using the axillary route (see the *Clinical Skills Manual* SKILLS). Once anal dilations have begun, the family will be taught how to perform them at home. After the final surgical procedure, discuss feeding regimens and bowel habits necessary to maintain adequate nutrition for growth and development. Advise parents that children with anorectal malformations may have difficulty achieving bowel control. Patience in toilet training is important. When the child reaches an age appropriate for toilet training, encourage the family to speak with a healthcare provider to discuss the child's progress.

Clinical Reasoning Imperforate Anus and Esophageal Atresia

Six-month-old Jerome was born with both imperforate anus and esophageal atresia. He had a colostomy created shortly after birth. His esophageal atresia has been repaired. He has just had surgery to create a new anal opening and will have the colostomy closed in approximately 6 weeks. What are the priorities of nursing care after an anorectoplasty? How can the surgical site be protected to ensure healing? What are essential components or preoperative and postoperative teaching related to the colostomy closure? What information related to toilet training should be given to Jerome's parents in the future?

Expected outcomes of nursing care include:

- The child's pain is effectively managed.
- Incisions heal without signs of infection.
- Fluid and electrolyte balance is maintained.
- Adequate bowel function is demonstrated.
- The parents demonstrate an understanding of ostomy care and other treatment protocols.

Hernias

A **hernia** is the protrusion or projection of an organ or a part of an organ through the muscle wall of the cavity that normally contains it. This protrusion may result from the failure of normal openings to close during fetal development or from weakness in the supporting musculature. When intra-abdominal pressure increases (as when the infant cries or strains to pass stool), the weakened area separates, causing a protrusion of underlying organs. Inguinal hernias are the most common type of hernia occurring in children (see Chapter 26). Other hernias that occur frequently in children are diaphragmatic and umbilical.

CONGENITAL DIAPHRAGMATIC HERNIA
In a diaphragmatic hernia, abdominal contents protrude into the thoracic cavity through an opening in the diaphragm. Sites of herniation include the substernal space, the posterolateral region, and the esophageal hiatus. The cause is a delay or failure in closure of the pleuroperitoneal musculature, which forms the diaphragm (Lee, Jun, & Lee, 2014). Intestines and other abdominal structures enter the thoracic cavity through the opening in the diaphragm. The overall incidence of diaphragmatic hernia is 1 in 2200 births (Rollins, 2012). Associated anomalies are present in 40% to 60% of infants born live with diaphragmatic hernia (Sfakianaki, 2012).

A diaphragmatic hernia is a life-threatening condition with an overall mortality rate of 20% to 35% in infants born alive with this condition (Rollins, 2012). Severe respiratory distress secondary to pulmonary hypoplasia occurs shortly after birth. As the infant cries, abdominal organs extend into the thorax, decreasing the size of the thoracic cavity. The infant becomes dyspneic and cyanotic. Characteristic findings include a barrel-shaped chest and sunken abdomen.

Congenital diaphragmatic hernia is diagnosed in utero by ultrasound in approximately two thirds of patients. Prenatal diagnosis improves survival rates, as it allows for early identification of infants who will require complex care after birth (Rollins, 2012).

Immediate respiratory support is essential in a neonatal intensive care unit (NICU). Ventilator support is necessary to manage respiratory compromise. Conventional mechanical ventilation, high-frequency oxygen ventilation, nitric oxide, and extracorporeal membrane oxygenation (ECMO) are the main methods used to treat respiratory failure in these children (Rollins, 2012; Sfakianaki, 2012; Sluiter, van de Ven, Wijnen, et al., 2011).

The infant is positioned with the head and thorax higher than the abdomen to facilitate downward movement of abdominal organs. A nasogastric tube is inserted to decompress the stomach. Intravenous fluids are administered through an umbilical artery catheter.

Once the infant's condition is stabilized, the defect is corrected surgically. The chance for a successful repair and survival is affected by the size of the defect. Children who survive will generally continue to have health concerns and should have continued evaluation of pulmonary, gastrointestinal, nutritional, and neurodevelopmental related problems (Rollins, 2012).

Nursing Management

The infant with a diaphragmatic hernia is admitted to the NICU and requires continuous monitoring. Preoperative management centers on providing supportive care to the infant and parents and includes the following:

- Note the infant's vital signs every 30 minutes on the cardiorespiratory monitor.
- Observe for worsening of respiratory compromise.
- Maintain intravenous fluid administration.
- Promote decreased stimulation to keep the infant calm and thus maintain low abdominal pressure.
- Keep parents informed about the infant's condition, and provide emotional support both before and after surgery.

Postoperative care includes the following:

- Position the infant on the affected side to facilitate expansion of the lung on the unaffected side.
- Observe closely for signs of infection.
- Maintain respiratory support.
- Manage pain.
- Carefully monitor fluid and electrolyte balance.

Before discharge, instruct parents in wound care, prevention of infection, and feeding techniques.

UMBILICAL HERNIA
An umbilical hernia results from a weak or imperfectly closed umbilical ring. Umbilical hernia is a common condition in childhood and occurs more frequently in Black children and low–birth-weight infants (Carlo & Ambalavanan, 2016).

An umbilical hernia appears as a soft swelling covered by skin. Omentum and small intestine herniate or protrude through the opening with coughing, crying, or straining during a bowel movement. It is easily reduced by pushing the bowel back through the fibrous ring. Most defects that appear prior to 6 months of age will resolve spontaneously by 1 year of age. Surgery is indicated in cases of *strangulation* (closure of the muscular ring around a portion of the bowel, preventing it from moving back into the abdomen). Surgery is also recommended if the defect does not resolve by 4 to 5 years of age or if the defect becomes larger after 1 to 2 years of age (Carlo & Ambalavanan, 2016).

Nursing Management

Nursing management is generally supportive. Instruct parents not to apply tape, straps, or coins to reduce the hernia as these methods have not been proven to be effective. If surgery is required, it is usually performed in a short-stay unit. Postoperatively, teach parents how to care for the surgical site, to watch for bleeding, and to recognize signs of infection. Reinforce the importance of returning for follow-up evaluation.

Ostomies

An intestinal **ostomy** is an opening, or **stoma**, into the small or large intestine that diverts fecal matter, providing an outlet when a distal surgical anastomosis, obstruction, or nonfunctioning structure prevents normal elimination (Figure 25–7).

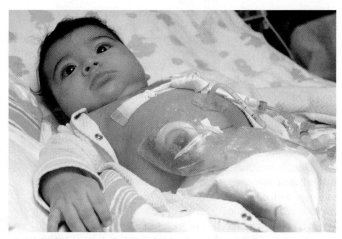

Figure 25–7 This infant has several gastrointestinal problems and requires ostomies for gastric feedings and for drainage of fecal material. Note the appearance of the healthy stoma.

Depending on the integrity and function of anatomic structures, the ostomy may be temporary or permanent. Infants and small children with imperforate anus, necrotizing enterocolitis, Hirschsprung disease, or volvulus may require a temporary or permanent colostomy or ileostomy. Ostomies may also be indicated for children with inflammatory bowel disease, intestinal tumors, or abdominal trauma.

An ostomy may be elective or considered a surgical emergency. In all cases, it affects a child's lifestyle, alters body image, causes anxiety, and increases the risk for alterations in physiologic processes (electrolyte imbalance, increased nutritional requirements). For adolescents, it may also result in dependence at a time when autonomy is a major developmental need.

When assessing the family and child approaching ostomy surgery, it is important to determine their ability to understand and accept the physical changes that will occur. Parents may feel guilt and anger about the need for an ostomy when the child has a genetically transmitted disease, is injured, or has developed an obstruction from necrosis of the bowel. Encourage the parents and child to express their feelings, and correct any misunderstandings. Parents and older children may be referred for counseling and to support groups to help them deal with their feelings. Adolescents often benefit from a visit with an adolescent ostomate (someone who has an ostomy) who can answer questions about living with an ostomy.

PREOPERATIVE CARE

Preoperative education focuses on educating the child and family and preparing them for postoperative management.

Growth and Development

The preschooler has some manual dexterity and can help with some parts of the procedure for changing an ostomy appliance and cleaning the stoma. Teach the child using a doll or stuffed animal. Many school-age children are able to care for their ostomy independently. Teach them how to avoid leakage around the bag, which could be embarrassing. Adolescents are generally totally independent in their self-care of ostomies. However, they may need support to deal with the fact that they are different from their peers.

Discuss how the appliance or ostomy pouch will look, and explain the purpose of the appliance in developmentally appropriate terms. Encourage the parents and child to touch and manipulate all equipment. Show a younger child how to place a pouch on a doll. Older children can practice placing a pouch on their skin. These measures help relieve anxiety by providing information and increasing familiarity with the appliance.

In addition to discussion of the appliance, preoperative education should include discussion of pain control and measures that will be used to prevent postoperative complications (turning, coughing, and breathing deeply). Gear the instructions to the child's developmental level. Encourage parental participation to promote compliance.

POSTOPERATIVE CARE

Postoperative care of a child with an ostomy is similar to that of any child who undergoes abdominal surgery. (See the discussion of nursing management for appendicitis later in this chapter and *Nursing Care Plan: The Child Undergoing Surgery* in Chapter 11.) Management of the stoma may be done by an "ostomy nurse" or other nurses. Major interventions involve ensuring proper function of the stoma, identifying complications, and instituting daily stoma care. Complications include skin breakdown, mucotaneous separation, necrosis, stenosis, prolapse, hernia, retraction, laceration, and leakage (Coha, 2013; Lindholm et al., 2013). Assess the stoma, quality and amount of fecal matter, skin condition, and adherence of the pouch. Evaluate the understanding and ability of the family to care for the ostomy.

Identify and address home care needs well in advance of discharge. Instructions include skin care, care of the stoma, appliance removal and application, and frequency of appliance changes (see the *Clinical Skills Manual* SKILLS). Begin teaching immediately after surgery with responsibility for care transferred gradually to the parents and child as they are ready. Discuss diet, activity level, hygiene, clothing, equipment, and financial considerations. Arrange for home visits to check periodically on the home management program.

Parents and children can be referred to the United Ostomy Association or a local ostomy group for information and support. Make referrals to social service, counseling, and a home health agency, if appropriate.

Expected outcomes of nursing care include successful adjustment to the ostomy, thorough evacuation of the bowel, absence of infection and other complications, intact skin, and formation of a positive self-image in the child.

Clinical Tip

Avoid adhesive enhancers on the skin of newborns and premature infants. Their skin layers are so thin that removal of the appliance can strip off the skin. Remember also that adhesive contains latex and its frequent use is not advised because of the risk of latex allergy development (see Chapter 22).

Inflammatory Disorders

Inflammatory disorders are reactions of specific tissues of the GI tract to trauma caused by injuries, foreign bodies, chemicals, microorganisms, or surgery. These disorders may be acute or chronic and may involve various segments of the GI tract.

Appendicitis

Appendicitis is an inflammation of the vermiform appendix, the small sac near the end of the cecum, and is the most common cause of emergency surgery in children (Hung, Lin, & Chen, 2012; Singh, Kadian, Rattan, et al., 2014). The condition occurs most often in children and adolescents ages 10 to 19 years. While the overall rate of perforated appendix is 20% to 35%, the rate in children less than 3 years of age is 80% to 100% as compared to 10% to 20% in children 10 to 17 years of age (Minkes & Alder, 2014). Other factors may affect the rate of appendiceal perforation. See *Evidence-Based Practice: Perforated Appendix.*

EVIDENCE-BASED PRACTICE | Perforated Appendix

Clinical Question

Early diagnosis and treatment is essential for positive outcomes for the child with appendicitis. Increased morbidity and mortality is associated with a perforated appendix. Young children have a higher rate of perforated appendix than older children. What are other factors that increase the rate of perforated appendix in children?

The Evidence

Ladd et al. (2013) conducted a retrospective study of 667 children who underwent appendectomies to determine if racial and socioeconomic factors were associated with an increased risk of perforated appendix. They also examined whether these factors were associated with symptom duration of greater than 48 hours. Results revealed that symptom duration and age had the strongest effect on the risk of perforated appendix, regardless of the race or ethnicity of the child. Children ages 0 to 4 and those presenting after 2 days of symptoms had significantly higher rates of perforation. Black and Hispanic children had significantly higher rates of perforated appendix than White children. Black children were more likely to have symptom duration of greater than 48 hours, leading the investigators to conclude that the increased incidence of perforated appendix in this population is related to delay in presentation to the hospital for treatment; however, they were not able to conclude that it was related to socioeconomic factors. The investigators found that the incidence of perforated appendix is higher in Hispanics regardless of other factors, leading them to conclude that being of Hispanic origin was a risk factor alone, and that perhaps there might be other cultural or economic factors not examined in this study that might contribute to the higher incidence in this group.

Levas et al. (2014) conducted a multicenter study to determine if there was an association between Hispanic ethnicity and limited English proficiency (LEP) and the rate of perforated appendix and the use of computed tomography (CT) and ultrasound in children presenting with abdominal pain. The sample was comprised of 2590 children ages 3 to 18 presenting with abdominal pain that was concerning for a diagnosis of appendicitis. A diagnosis of appendicitis was made in 1001 of these children. Perforated appendix was diagnosed in 25% of English-speaking non-Hispanics, 31% of English-speaking Hispanics, and 34% of Hispanics with LEP ($p < .01$) English-speaking non-Hispanics had a trend toward a higher incidence of perforated appendix, but it was not statistically significant. Twenty percent of Hispanics with LEP presented with a duration of pain greater than 72 hours, compared with 9.8% of English-speaking non-Hispanics. Hispanics with LEP were less likely to undergo CT or ultrasound. Those with mid-range Pediatric Appendicitis Scores (PAS) were significantly less likely to have these imaging studies, compared with English-speaking non-Hispanics. There was no significant difference in the timing between imaging studies and surgery based on English proficiency or ethnicity.

Lee, Yaghoubian, Stark, et al. (2012) examined whether being treated at a county hospital versus a private hospital affected the rate of perforated appendix, rate of laparoscopic appendectomy, and outcomes in children with appendicitis. For the study, 7902 cases of children treated for appendicitis between 1998 and 2007 were reviewed. Of these, 682 were treated at the county hospital and 7220 were treated at 1 of 11 private medical centers that are part of a larger system. The county hospital in this study was also referred to as a Safety Net hospital, which treats the highest number of uninsured patients and provides care to anyone regardless of financial, immigration, or insurance status. Results of the study showed that patients treated at the county hospital had a lower income, a higher rate of perforated appendix, and longer hospital stays. These patients also had a higher rate of laparoscopic appendectomy and a lower postoperative abscess drainage rate. The study showed that patients treated at the county hospital did not have poorer outcomes than those treated at private hospitals. They did have higher rates of perforated appendix, which the investigators attributed to delayed access to care. These patients had longer hospital stays, even though there was a higher rate of laparoscopic appendectomy, and a lower rate of postoperative abscess drainage. The delay in discharge could be related to fewer resources available, including transportation for discharge or insufficient care available at home for these children because parents are at work. Outcomes within the county hospital were similar regardless of income level or ethnic group. The investigators concluded that the differences in patients at the two hospitals might be related to differences in access to health care and other underlying ethnic and socioeconomic disparities as opposed to hospital type.

Best Practice

Young children have a higher incidence of perforated appendix. This is related to their inability to understand the concept of pain and verbalize this to their parents. Parents must be educated about the importance of recognizing cues in their children that could be indicative of pain. A longer duration of symptoms or delay in seeking health care was also identified as a risk factor for perforated appendix. This could be related to lack of knowledge related to symptoms requiring medical attention or lack of access to health care. Ongoing education for parents related to signs of illness in children is essential. Nurses play a key role in this education, especially in the outpatient clinic setting. Access to health care and resources continues to be a concern and demonstrates the need for improvement in access to all patients regardless of ethnic background, language proficiency, or socioeconomic status. Nurses play an important role in advocating for these patients.

Clinical Reasoning

Give specific examples of how nurses can work with children and families to decrease the incidence of perforated appendix. What are some factors that might attribute to the higher incidence of perforated appendix in Hispanics?

ETIOLOGY AND PATHOPHYSIOLOGY

Appendicitis almost always results from an obstruction in the appendiceal lumen. It can be caused by a fecalith (hard fecal mass), parasitic infestations, stenosis, hyperplasia of lymphoid tissue, or a tumor.

Continued secretion of mucus following acute obstruction of the lumen increases pressure, causing ischemia, cellular death, and ulceration. The appendix may perforate or rupture, resulting in fecal and bacterial contamination of the peritoneum. Peritonitis spreads quickly and if untreated can result in small bowel obstruction, electrolyte imbalances, septicemia, and hypovolemic shock.

CLINICAL MANIFESTATIONS

At onset, symptoms include periumbilical cramps, abdominal tenderness, anorexia, nausea, and fever. In adolescent and young adult females, symptoms must be differentiated from those associated with ruptured ectopic pregnancy, endometriosis, ovarian cysts, and pelvic inflammatory disease (Minkes & Alder, 2014).

As the inflammation progresses, pain in the right lower abdomen becomes constant. Pain is often most intense at the McBurney point, halfway between the anterior superior iliac crest and the umbilicus (see *Pathophysiology Illustrated: Appendicitis*). Symptoms progress to include guarding, rigidity, nausea, vomiting, onset of pain before vomiting, anorexia, and rebound tenderness following palpation over the right lower quadrant (Bishop & Carter, 2013; Minkes & Alder, 2014).

As appendicitis progresses, the child remains motionless, usually in a side-lying position with knees flexed. Sudden relief of pain usually means that the appendix has perforated.

CLINICAL THERAPY

Diagnosis of appendicitis in young children can be difficult because their pain may be less localized and their symptoms more diffuse than in the older child. Continuing evaluations over several hours are often needed to establish the diagnosis. The presence of an elevated white blood cell count (above 10,000/mm^3), increased neutrophil ratio, and an elevated C-reactive protein combined with the symptoms supports a diagnosis of appendicitis (Bishop & Carter, 2013). A white blood cell count greater than 15,000/mm^3 in a patient with appendicitis is a strong indicator that the appendix has perforated (Minkes & Alder, 2014). Abdominal ultrasound is preferred by some healthcare providers as the initial screening tool in the diagnosis of appendicitis; however, CT scans are more sensitive and may be used, especially when the appendix cannot be seen well on ultrasound or the results are inconclusive (Bishop & Carter, 2013; Minkes & Alder, 2014).

Treatment of uncomplicated appendicitis involves immediate surgical removal (appendectomy), generally through a laparoscopic appendectomy (Groves et al., 2013). Preoperatively, the child is kept NPO. Intravenous fluids and electrolytes, and antibiotics are administered (Minkes & Alder, 2014). Postoperatively, the child has an abdominal incision with a dressing covering the incision. Antibiotics may be administered. The child is generally discharged within 24 to 36 hours as long as they have adequate oral intake, are afebrile, and receive effective pain relief with oral pain medication (Bishop & Carter, 2013).

With perforated appendix, laparoscopic appendectomy is generally performed. While open appendectomy has been the treatment of choice in the past, recent studies have indicated that laparoscopic appendectomy is an effective approach for the treatment of perforated appendix as well. With laparascopic appendectomy the abdominal cavity can be explored and lavaged (Groves et al., 2013). Postoperatively, the child with a perforated appendix may have a nasogastric tube to decompress the abdomen and will remain NPO until signs of bowel function return. Bowel function is best indicated by the passage of

Pathophysiology Illustrated: **Appendicitis**

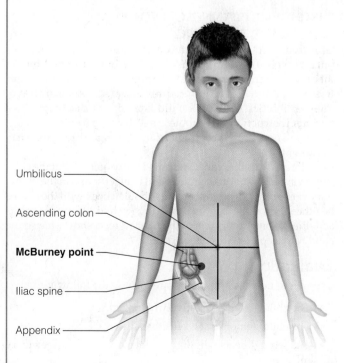

The McBurney point is the common location of pain in children and adolescents with appendicitis.

Umbilicus

Ascending colon

McBurney point

Iliac spine

Appendix

flatus or stool. The child will also have a peripheral or temporary central line for administration of intravenous fluids and medications. After surgery for a perforated appendix, the child will receive antibiotics for several days. Morphine is generally given for pain.

In some cases, where an abscess is formed secondary to rupture of the appendix, the surgeon may choose to place a percutaneous drain, begin broad-spectrum antibiotics, and remove the appendix at a later time. This process is referred to as an interval appendectomy (Santacroce & Ochoa, 2013).

Nursing Management

For the Child With Appendicitis

Nursing Assessment and Diagnosis

PHYSIOLOGIC ASSESSMENT

A detailed assessment of the child's pain is necessary to differentiate appendicitis from other illnesses (see Chapter 15). Ask the child to point to the painful area and describe the pain. Recognize that localizing the pain may be difficult for young children. Note onset, location, and intensity of pain; precipitating factors; and relief measures tried. Remember to inspect, auscultate, and then palpate gently to identify distention and areas of pain. Rebound tenderness can also be assessed. Deep palpation of the left side of the abdomen followed by removing the hand quickly can lead to pain in the area of the appendix (rebound tenderness). However, once appendicitis is suspected or verified, avoid abdominal palpation in order to minimize pain to the child. Assess vital signs to determine baseline values, and monitor every 4 hours thereafter.

PSYCHOSOCIAL ASSESSMENT

Because appendicitis usually occurs in school-age children and adolescents, assessment of the child's coping skills is important. Adolescents, because of their preoccupation with body image, may be concerned about the surgical scar. Assess the parents' and child's anxiety about the sudden hospitalization and need for emergency surgery.

Among the nursing diagnoses that might be appropriate for the child with appendicitis are the following (NANDA-I © 2014):

- *Pain, Acute,* related to inflammation and surgery
- *Fluid Volume: Deficient, Risk for,* related to fluid volume loss and inadequate fluid volume intake
- *Anxiety* related to physical condition
- *Infection, Risk for,* related to bowel trauma
- *Airway Clearance, Ineffective,* related to retained secretions

Planning and Implementation

Nursing management focuses on promoting comfort, maintaining hydration, providing emotional support, supporting respiratory function, providing care of the surgical site, and monitoring for symptoms of infection.

PROMOTE COMFORT

Preoperatively, a right side-lying position with knees bent is usually the most comfortable. If the appendix has perforated, lying on the right side helps the peritoneal cavity drain. Administer analgesics as ordered, and note relief from pain. Postoperatively, the child should be placed in a semi-Fowler or side-lying position on the right side. The child with a perforated appendix will require intravenous pain medication on a regular basis. The child

who has an appendectomy for uncomplicated appendicitis will need oral or intravenous pain management for postoperative pain control.

MAINTAIN HYDRATION

An intravenous infusion is initiated preoperatively and continued until bowel function returns after surgery. Once bowel function returns and after the nasogastric tube has been removed, offer water in small amounts and then other clear fluids. The child should be monitored closely for nausea after beginning to take oral fluids.

PROVIDE EMOTIONAL SUPPORT

For many children, appendicitis may be their first hospitalization and their first experience with healthcare personnel other than their primary healthcare provider. The nurse must elicit a history, perform a physical examination, coordinate diagnostic tests, and prepare the child for surgery in a short period of time. Emotional support is essential for both child and parents. Good preoperative education can reduce anxiety. Answer any questions the child or parents may have.

SUPPORT RESPIRATORY FUNCTION

General anesthesia during surgery compromises respiratory function. It is important for the child to turn, cough, and breathe deeply to prevent atelectasis. Provide adequate analgesia and encourage the child to splint the incision area with a pillow during coughing to decrease pain. Incentive spirometry is frequently ordered for the child. Young children may be resistant to this procedure or may be too young to understand the procedure. An effective alternative approach is to give the child bubbles or a pinwheel to blow.

RECOGNIZE SYMPTOMS OF INFECTION

Assess vital signs and observe the abdominal incision every 4 hours for redness, edema, or drainage. If a drain is present, assess drainage for color, consistency, and amount. The amount of drainage from the wound should decrease gradually as the wound heals. If the appendix perforated, the child is hospitalized for several days of intravenous antibiotics.

DISCHARGE PLANNING AND HOME CARE TEACHING

Children with uncomplicated appendicitis are discharged once bowel function returns and they have a bowel movement. Children with perforated appendix will have a longer hospitalization since they require several days of intravenous antibiotics. When the child is ready for discharge, give parents instructions for home care. Teach parents to recognize the signs and symptoms of infection and to seek early treatment.

Normal activities can be resumed fairly quickly, but the child should avoid strenuous activities and contact sports in the immediate postoperative period. Parents should check with the child's healthcare provider before allowing the child to resume sports activities. Home tutoring may be needed for a short time so the child can keep up with schoolwork.

Evaluation

Expected outcomes of nursing care include the following:

- The child's pain is effectively managed.
- The child demonstrates effective airway clearance.
- The wound heals without the development of a secondary infection.
- Adequate hydration is achieved and maintained.

Necrotizing Enterocolitis

Necrotizing enterocolitis (NEC) is a potentially life-threatening inflammatory disease of the intestinal tract that occurs primarily in premature infants. The overall incidence is 1 in 1000 live births. The disease affects up to 7% of infants of very low–birth-weight infants (weighing less than 1500 g). NEC is associated with a mortality rate of 5% to 24% (Huda, Chaudhery, Ibrahim, et al., 2014). The disease occurs most often in the ileum (Berman & Moss, 2011; Huda et al., 2014).

The etiology of NEC is multifactorial. Intestinal ischemia and inflammation, bacterial or viral infection (a result of the premature infant's decreased immune response and greater risk for infection), enteral feeding, and immaturity of the gastrointestinal mucosa may all be contributing factors (Gregory, DeForge, Natale, et al., 2011; Morgan, Young, & McGuire, 2011).

Manifestations generally occur during the second week of life after enteral feedings are started; however, NEC can develop before feedings are started, after several weeks of life, and long after feedings are started. The infant may initially show signs of feeding intolerance (increased gastric residuals, vomiting, irritability, and abdominal distention). Bloody diarrhea may be present because of the hemorrhagic bowel. The condition progresses to lethargy, periods of apnea and bradycardia, and temperature instability (Berman & Moss, 2011).

Diagnosis is made on the basis of characteristic clinical findings and the presence of free peritoneal gas, dilated bowel loops, bowel distention, and bowel wall thickening on abdominal radiographs. Stools and emesis are monitored for occult blood. Laboratory data reveal anemia, leukopenia, leukocytosis, thrombocytopenia, electrolyte imbalance, and metabolic or respiratory acidosis. Blood cultures are positive for the organism present.

Necrotizing enterocolitis requires prompt intervention to decrease the morbidity and mortality associated with this illness. Treatment includes bowel rest (NPO status), gastric decompression with nasogastric suction, and antibiotic therapy (Gregory et al., 2011; Rapoport & Nishii, 2013; Wright & Miller, 2012). The infant will need central venous access to provide nutrition (Rapoport & Nishii, 2013). Serial radiographs of the abdomen should be performed to detect worsening or resolution of the disease process (Wright & Miller, 2012). Perforation or necrosis of the bowel necessitates surgical resection of the bowel. An ileostomy or colostomy may be performed.

All cases of necrotizing enterocolitis are treated with strict enteric precautions to prevent the spread of infection to other premature infants on the unit.

Long-term complications of necrotizing enterocolitis include short bowel syndrome, strictures, cholestasis, impaired nutrition and growth, and delayed developmental performance.

Nursing Management

Nursing care centers on prevention and early detection of necrotizing enterocolitis to minimize bowel loss, and providing postoperative care. Observe for feeding intolerance by aspirating gastric residual (if the infant is receiving enteral feedings). Measure abdominal circumference and assess bowel sounds in the premature or high-risk infant every 4 to 8 hours. Even minimal changes in circumference can indicate necrotizing enterocolitis and should be reported to the primary care provider.

SAFETY ALERT!
The infant with NEC is at risk to develop sepsis. Signs of sepsis in the newborn or premature infant include:

- Hypothermia or hyperthermia
- Jaundice
- Respiratory distress
- Hepatomegaly
- Abdominal distention
- Poor feeding
- Vomiting
- Lethargy

Report these symptoms to the primary healthcare provider immediately.

Maintaining fluid and electrolyte balance is essential. Provide comfort by holding and cuddling an infant who is NPO, and offer a pacifier to meet nonnutritive sucking needs. Careful assessment for infection and maintenance of skin integrity are essential. Feedings are gradually reestablished once bowel function returns. Because the symptoms of necrotizing enterocolitis may not appear until several days after feedings begin, parents may not be prepared for the infant's decline. Recovery is slow and can be complicated. Give clear explanations and encourage parents to ask questions and express their fears and concerns. If the infant's condition worsens, offer the parents support (see Chapter 13).

After the child is discharged, frequent follow-up is needed. Parents need specific education related to feedings, medications, and any other treatments prescribed. The infant requires regular and thorough physical assessments to check weight gain, assess development, and identify signs of complications. If the child had to have an ostomy created, the family must be taught ostomy care.

The infant requires regular and thorough physical assessments to identify any complications. Growth of the child is monitored and compared with previous findings. Developmental progress is assessed by regular administration of a developmental test such as the Denver II.

Clinical Tip

Cholestasis is a disruption of bile flow and the most common problem in survivors of necrotizing enterocolitis. It is a complication of total parenteral nutrition (TPN) and commonly occurs 2 weeks after TPN therapy has been initiated. It is characterized by hyperbilirubinemia, hepatomegaly, and elevated serum aminotransferase levels (Vitola & Balistreri, 2016).

Expected outcomes of nursing care for the child with necrotizing enterocolitis include:

- The child is free of signs and symptoms of infection.
- Fluid and electrolyte balance is achieved and maintained.
- Tissue perfusion is maintained following surgical removal of necrotic bowel.
- The child consumes adequate nutrition to support growth and development needs.

If surgery is performed, complete healing without infection or other complication is desired. If the infant is not successfully treated, support and comfort for the parents are necessary. When the child survives, desired long-term outcomes include normal developmental progression and nutrition to support growth.

Meckel Diverticulum

Meckel diverticulum results when the omphalomesenteric duct, which connects the midgut to the yolk sac during embryonic development, fails to atrophy. Instead, an outpouching of the ileum remains, usually located near the ileocecal valve. The pouch contains gastric or pancreatic tissue, which secretes acid, causing irritation and ulceration. Meckel diverticulum is the most common GI malformation and occurs in 1% to 4 % of the population (Pepper et al., 2012).

Clinical manifestations usually appear by age 2. Meckel diverticulum most commonly presents as GI bleeding or obstruction. The child generally presents with bloody stool, irritability, fatigue, abdominal pain and distention, nausea, and vomiting (Pepper et al., 2012).

Diagnostic testing for Meckel diverticulum depends on the presentation and includes laboratory analysis to evaluate for the presence of anemia and dehydration (Pepper et al., 2012). Imaging studies are also used to assist in the diagnosis and include radiographs, ultrasound, CT scan, and radionuclide scanning (Kotecha, Bellah, Pena, et al., 2012). Technetium-99*m* pertechnetate nuclear medicine (also called a *Meckel scan*) is the current imaging test of choice for a bleeding diverticulum (Pepper et al., 2012).

Treatment is surgical excision of the diverticulum and removal of any involved bowel. The prognosis is good following surgical excision.

Nursing Management

Preoperatively, an intravenous infusion is initiated to correct fluid and electrolyte imbalances. Monitor intake and output. Observe for rectal bleeding, and test stools for **occult blood** (blood that is present in small quantities and is measurable only by laboratory testing). Keep the child on bed rest. Assess vital signs every 2 hours, and monitor for signs of shock. Postoperative care is similar to that for an infant or child undergoing abdominal surgery. (See the earlier discussion of postsurgical nursing management of appendicitis and *Nursing Care Plan: The Child Undergoing Surgery* in Chapter 11.)

At discharge, parents need instructions on caring for the surgical site, preventing infection, providing an adequate diet, and administering prescribed medications.

Inflammatory Bowel Disease

CROHN DISEASE AND ULCERATIVE COLITIS

Inflammatory bowel disease encompasses two distinct chronic disorders, Crohn disease and ulcerative colitis, that have similar symptoms and treatment. Inflammatory bowel disease differs from irritable bowel syndrome.

Crohn disease is a chronic, inflammatory process. The disorder can occur randomly throughout the GI tract with the ileum, colon, and rectum as the most common sites. A distinct feature of Crohn disease is the development of enteric fistulas between loops of bowel or nearby organs. Mucosal ulcers begin in small locations, and then grow in size and depth into the mucosal wall. Submucosal inflammation can be severe. The etiology is unknown. There is strong evidence to support a genetic association. Crohn disease is more common in Whites than African Americans. It is rare in Asian and Hispanic populations (Grossman & Mamula, 2014). It most often develops in adolescents and young adults. Crohn disease has an incidence of approximately 4.56 per 100,000 (Grossman & Baldassano, 2016). The onset of Crohn disease is subtle. Crampy abdominal pain is usually reported first, followed by diarrhea. Other symptoms include fever, anorexia, growth failure or weight loss, general malaise, and joint pain. Diagnosis is based on laboratory evaluation, diffuse abdominal tenderness, and radiologic and biopsy examinations. Anemia, an elevated erythrocyte sedimentation rate, hypoalbuminemia, and thrombocytosis are other possible findings. Stools are positive for occult blood (Glick & Carvalho, 2011).

Clinical Tip

Irritable bowel syndrome (IBS) refers to a functional disorder of the gastrointestinal tract that is characterized as chronic and episodic. There is no structural cause, but it seems to be triggered by events such as gastroenteritis, major life events or stressors, or dietary intolerance. Other causative factors may include stress, diet, drugs, and alcohol. IBS is characterized by episodes of abdominal cramping and pain, diarrhea or constipation, and bloating (Mason, 2014). Management generally focuses on the symptoms. A change in lifestyle and diet might be effective in decreasing the frequency of symptoms. Medications such as antispasmodics, antimotility agents, and laxatives may also be used (Mason, 2014).

Ulcerative colitis is a chronic recurrent disease of the large intestine and rectal mucosa of unknown etiology. Inflammation is limited to the mucosa, as opposed to Crohn disease, which extends deep into the bowel wall. Ulcerative colitis can involve the entire length of the bowel with varying degrees of inflammation, ulceration, hemorrhage, and edema. Emotional and other psychosocial factors may influence the presentation and course of the disease. It is more prevalent among persons of Jewish heritage. The disease develops before 20 years of age with peak onset at about 12 years. The incidence of pediatric ulcerative colitis in North America is approximately 2 per 100,000 (Grossman & Baldassano, 2016). See Table 25–2 for a comparison of the two diseases.

The first symptom of ulcerative colitis is usually diarrhea. Lower abdominal pain and cramping are present before and during a bowel movement and are relieved by the passage of stool and flatus. The stool is often mixed with blood and mucus. Weight loss or delayed growth, nutritional deficiencies, and arthralgias often occur as effects of the disease.

Diagnosis centers on evaluating the cause and identifying the extent of involved bowel and differentiating an infectious process from ulcerative colitis. Upper endoscopy and colonoscopy are helpful to determine the extent and severity of the inflammatory process. Laboratory studies generally indicate an elevated erythrocyte sedimentation rate, elevated C-reactive protein, hypoalbuminemia, antineutrophil cytoplasmic antibodies (ANCA), and anti–*Saccharomyces cerevisiae* antibodies (ASCA) (Kelsen & Mamula, 2013).

Crohn disease and ulcerative colitis have periods of remission and exacerbation. Treatment for both diseases includes pharmacologic interventions, nutrition therapy, and, in severe cases, surgery. First-line pharmacologic treatment of Crohn disease involves aminosalicylates. Sulfasalazine inhibits prostaglandin synthesis, thereby decreasing inflammation. Corticosteroids and immunosuppressants are used in children with more severe disease. Biologic therapies such as infliximab

TABLE 25–2 Clinical Manifestations of Ulcerative Colitis and Crohn Disease

	ULCERATIVE COLITIS	CROHN DISEASE
Type of lesions	Continuous, superficial involvement	Segmental, transmural (through the wall) involvement
Clinical manifestations		
Anal or perianal lesions	Rare	Common
Anorexia	Mild to moderate	Can be severe
Diarrhea	Often severe	Moderate
Growth retardation	Mild	Significant
Pain	Present	Common
Rectal bleeding	Present	Absent
Weight loss	Moderate	Severe
Risk of cancer	Slightly increased	Greatly increased

(Remicade) have been effective in patients with Crohn disease and ulcerative colitis who fail to respond to other therapies (Glick & Carvalho, 2011).

A nutritionist is part of the team treating the child. The goal of nutrition therapy is to provide adequate caloric intake and nutrients necessary for growth. Vitamin, iron, zinc, and folic acid supplementation is frequently required. Total parenteral nutrition (TPN) is often given to treat nutritional deficiencies and malnutrition, which accompany inflammatory bowel disease (see the *Clinical Skills Manual* SKILLS). A high-protein, high-carbohydrate, low-fiber diet with normal amounts of fat is recommended.

Clinical Tip

The following drugs are used in the treatment of inflammatory bowel disease:

Aminosalicylates

- Sulfasalazine
- Mesalamine

Corticosteroids

- Prednisone
- Prednisolone
- Hydrocortisone
- Budesonide

Biologic Therapies

- Infliximab (Remicade)
- Adalimumab (Humira)
- Certolizumab (Cimzia)

Immunosuppressants

- 6-Mercaptopurine (6-MP)
- Azathioprine
- Cyclosporine
- Methotrexate

Antibiotics

- Metronidazole
- Ciprofloxacin

Source: Data from Glick, S. R., & Carvalho, R. S. (2011). Inflammatory bowel disease. *Pediatrics in Review, 32*(1), 14–25; Peyrin-Biroulet, L. (2011). Why should we define and target early Crohn's disease? *Gastroenterology & Hepatology, 7*(5), 324–326; Triantafillidis, J. K., Merikas, E., & Georgopoulos, F. (2011). Current and emerging drugs for the treatment. *Drug Design, Development and Therapy, 5*, 185–210.

If other treatment measures fail to reduce inflammation, surgery is generally indicated. A temporary colostomy or ileostomy is performed to allow the bowel to rest. However, in Crohn disease, ulcerations tend to recur elsewhere in the GI tract. In ulcerative colitis, removal of the diseased bowel provides a permanent cure.

Nursing Management

Nursing management occurs mainly in the community and home and focuses on helping the child and family adjust to the emotional impact of a chronic disease, administering medications and diet therapy, monitoring nutritional status, and providing appropriate referrals. Provide emotional support and counseling to help the child adjust to feeling "different" from peers. Inability to compete with peers and frequent absences from school can affect the child's self-esteem. Have the parents contact the school district to arrange for tutoring in case extended absences from school become necessary. Encourage the child who is not attending school regularly to maintain contact with friends through telephone calls, cards, and visits.

Body image is a major concern for children and adolescents with inflammatory bowel disease. Corticosteroid therapy causes growth retardation and delayed sexual maturation. Encourage the child to discuss feelings about these side effects. If a permanent colostomy or ileostomy is required, help the child and family understand the need for surgical treatment. (See the discussion of ostomies earlier in this chapter.) Introduce the child and family to other children who have stomas.

If the child is unable to eat or the intake of calories is insufficient to meet basic nutritional and metabolic needs, total parenteral nutrition is ordered (see the *Clinical Skills Manual* SKILLS). If the child is able to eat, parents need instructions about dietary needs. Frequently measure growth and assess nutrition.

Teach parents about medication administration and diet therapy. Reinforce to both the parents and child the importance of adhering to a strict medication regimen. Emphasize that medications should be continued even when the child is asymptomatic. Discuss side effects of the drugs and what to do if any of these symptoms occur. Since immune status may be altered by steroid use, have families avoid contact with infectious diseases when the child is taking steroids. Immunization schedules may need to be altered.

Growth and Development

Providing adequate stress reduction may be helpful in control of inflammatory bowel disease. Teach young children relaxation techniques, such as deep breathing, progressive tensing and relaxing of muscles, and visualization of favorite places. Encourage busy school-age children and teens to have quiet and restful times each day in addition to physical activity periods. Meditation might be effective in older children and teens.

Families Want to Know
Diet Instructions for Inflammatory Bowel Disease

- Several small feedings are usually better tolerated than three meals daily.
- Limiting fiber intake can help decrease intestine motility and inflammation. Peel fruits and avoid large quantities of whole grains and nuts.
- If the child is not eating well, offer high-calorie meals. If lactose intolerance is not a problem for the particular child, cream soups, milkshakes, puddings, and custards can be offered.
- Liquid dietary supplements may be helpful to ensure protein and caloric requirements are met.
- Watch for foods that cause intestinal problems for the individual child, and avoid them in the future.
- Avoid having mealtime become a reason for family strife. Seek help of nurses and dietitians if needed.

Parents need instructions for TPN if this therapy is used, as well as information about care of a central venous catheter, including dressing changes, sterile and nonsterile techniques, signs of infection, how to handle infusion pumps and tubing, and how to measure the child's intake and output. Assist parents in obtaining equipment and supplies necessary for the child's care. Have parents demonstrate their mastery of care for the central venous catheter and their understanding of TPN techniques during home visits and appointments for health care.

Refer parents to social services, the visiting nurse association, and home healthcare agencies, if they are not receiving any of these services. For information about inflammatory bowel disease, refer families to the Crohn's and Colitis Foundation.

Expected outcomes of nursing care for the child with inflammatory bowel disease include the following:

- Normal growth and development are achieved.
- The child demonstrates the ability to cope with episodes of GI distress.
- The child adheres to the medication regimen.
- There is no evidence of central line infection.
- The child has a positive body image.
- The child is able to integrate stress-lowering practices into daily life.

Peptic Ulcer

A peptic ulcer is an erosion of the mucosal tissue in the lower end of the esophagus, in the stomach (usually along the lesser curvature), or in the duodenum. Peptic ulcers occur primarily in individuals receiving nonsteroidal anti-inflammatory drugs and those with *Helicobacter pylori* infection (Chason, Reisch, & Rockey, 2013).

Clinical manifestations vary according to the age of the child and location of the ulcer. The most common symptom is abdominal pain (burning) associated with an empty stomach, which may awaken the child at night. Vomiting and pain after meals, anemia, occult blood in stools, and abdominal distention may also be present.

Diagnosis is based on the history and radiologic studies. Bleeding from peptic ulcer disease is treated with acid-suppressant medications. These medications include histamine-2 receptor antagonists (H2RAs) such as rantidine and famotidine and proton pump inhibitors such as omeprazole, pantoprazole, and lansoprazole. *H. pylori* infection is generally treated with a proton pump inhibitor, amoxicillin, and clarithromycin for 7 to 14 days (Anand, 2015). Follow-up is important to ensure that the organism has been eradicated. The prognosis is usually good with early intervention.

Nursing Management

Assess the child for abdominal pain, vomiting, and abdominal distention. Assess for family history of *H. pylori* infection. Nursing care focuses on interventions to promote adequate nutritional intake, promote healing, and prevent recurrences. Provide a nutritionally sound, age-appropriate diet. Omit foods only if they exacerbate the disorder.

Medications must be given as scheduled. Emphasize the importance of continuing medication therapy as prescribed. The family needs encouragement to continue the medications as ordered and to return for follow-up visits. Children who attend school may prefer to take medications in the form of tablets, which are easier to carry than liquid preparations. The appropriate form must be completed in order for the child to receive medication at school.

Parents should discuss any additional medications with the primary healthcare provider before administering to the child. Caution parents to avoid ibuprofen, which irritates the gastric mucosa. If an antipyretic or pain medication is needed, acetaminophen should be given. Advise parents to read medication labels if they are unsure of product contents.

Because psychologic stress can contribute to peptic ulcer disease, the parents and child should be assisted in identifying sources of stress in the child's life. Assess coping mechanisms and provide referral for psychologic counseling, if appropriate. Teach relaxation techniques and recommend community classes on yoga or other stress reduction.

Disorders of Motility

Fluids are an important part of normal GI functioning. As food passes through the intestines, fluids are reabsorbed and moderately soft stool is formed and evacuated. In disorders such as diarrhea and constipation, fluid balance is altered, causing either more or less fluid to be reabsorbed. This can severely alter the characteristics of the stool. Reabsorption of too little water produces diarrhea and can lead to fluid and electrolyte alterations. Reabsorption of too much fluid can cause constipation, which if untreated can lead to bowel obstruction.

Gastroenteritis (Acute Diarrhea)

Gastroenteritis is an inflammation of the stomach and intestines that may be accompanied by vomiting and diarrhea.

Gastroenteritis can affect any part of the GI tract. It may be an acute problem, caused by viral, bacterial, or parasitic infections, or a chronic problem. Rotavirus is a leading cause of severe gastroenteritis in children less than 5 years of age worldwide. The rotavirus vaccine is recommended for infants in order to decrease the morbidity and mortality related to this organism (Agócs et al., 2014). Infants and small children with gastroenteritis or diarrhea can quickly become dehydrated and are at risk for hypovolemic shock if fluid and electrolyte losses are not replaced (see Chapter 18). A significant number of infants and young children are hospitalized each year for dehydration secondary to gastroenteritis.

ETIOLOGY AND PATHOPHYSIOLOGY

Diarrhea in children is related to many different causes (Table 25–3). The specific etiology is not always identified. The common mechanism is a decrease in the absorptive capacity of the bowel through inflammation, decrease in surface area for absorption, or alteration of parasympathetic innervation. Children in childcare centers and those living in substandard housing with improper sanitation are at increased risk.

Clinical Tip

Carbonated beverages and those containing high amounts of sugar should not be given when a child has diarrhea. Fermentation of sugar in the gastrointestinal tract causes increased gas, abdominal distention, and an increased frequency of diarrhea.

CLINICAL MANIFESTATIONS

Diarrhea may be mild, moderate, or severe. In mild diarrhea, stools are slightly increased in number and have a more liquid consistency. In moderate diarrhea, the child has several loose or watery stools. Other symptoms include irritability, anorexia, nausea, and vomiting. Moderate diarrhea is usually self-limiting, resolving without treatment within 1 or 2 days.

TABLE 25–3 Causes of Diarrhea in Children

ETIOLOGY	BOWEL MANIFESTATIONS
Emotional stress (anxiety, fatigue)	Increased motility
Intestinal infection (bacteria [*Escherichia coli, Salmonella, Shigella*], viral [human rotavirus, enteric adenovirus], fungal overgrowth)	Inflammation of mucosa; increased mucus secretion in colon
Food sensitivity (gluten, cow's milk)	Decreased digestion of food
Food intolerance (lactose, introduction of new foods, overfeeding)	Increased motility; increased mucus secretion in colon
Medications (iron, antibiotics)	Irritation and suprainfection
Colon disease (colitis, necrotizing enterocolitis, enterocolitis)	Inflammation and ulceration of intestinal walls; reduced absorption of fluid; increased intestinal motility
Surgical alterations (short bowel syndrome)	Reduced size of colon; decreased absorption surface

In severe diarrhea, watery stools are continuous. The child exhibits symptoms of fluid and electrolyte imbalance (see Chapter 18), has cramping, and is extremely irritable and difficult to console.

CLINICAL THERAPY

Diagnosis is based on the history, physical examination, and laboratory findings. Physical examination provides a guide to the severity of dehydration (see Chapter 18). The stool can be examined for the presence of ova, parasites, infectious organisms, viruses, fat, and undigested sugars. Laboratory evaluation of serum and urine helps identify electrolyte imbalances and other deficiencies.

Medical management depends on the severity of the diarrhea and fluid and electrolyte imbalances. The goal of treatment is to correct the fluid and electrolyte imbalances. For mild and moderate dehydration, oral rehydration therapy is the first intervention (see Chapter 18). This may be accomplished at home or in the short-stay observation unit in a hospital.

For severe dehydration, rehydration is accomplished by intravenous infusion with a solution chosen to correct the specific electrolyte imbalances. (See Chapter 18 for further information about solutions to correct dehydration.) As soon as possible, introduce clear liquids or breast milk and then encourage the child to progress to a regular diet. Foods generally are not withheld for more than 1 to 2 days.

If the diarrhea is caused by bacteria or parasites, antimicrobial therapy may be prescribed. Antiemetics and antidiarrheals are generally not used in young children since they can mask the signs and symptoms of more serious illness.

Nursing Management

For the Child With Gastroenteritis

Nursing Assessment and Diagnosis

The nurse may encounter the child and family in the emergency department, urgent care center, clinic, or office. The child may be cared for over several hours at a clinic or urgent care center so that dehydration is treated with intravenous infusion and/or oral rehydration, and then sent home with instructions for parents to care for the child. A thorough history may help in identifying the cause.

If the child is hospitalized, it is important to assess onset, frequency, color, amount, and consistency of stools. If the child is also vomiting, monitor the amount and type of vomitus. Initial and ongoing physical assessment of the child focuses on observing for signs and symptoms of dehydration, which reflect underlying fluid and electrolyte status. Evaluate urinary output and specific gravity. An accurate weight must be obtained on admission and daily thereafter. Monitor vital signs every 2 to 4 hours. A febrile child has increased water loss, contributing to the dehydration. Assess skin integrity, especially in the perineal and rectal areas, and note any breakdown or rashes.

The accompanying *Nursing Care Plan* lists common nursing diagnoses for a child with gastroenteritis. The following diagnoses may also be appropriate (NANDA-I © 2014):

- *Anxiety (Child and Parent)* related to change in health status
- *Sleep Pattern, Disturbed,* related to pain
- *Nutrition, Imbalanced: Less than Body Requirements,* related to inability to ingest sufficient nutrients

Nursing Care Plan: The Child Hospitalized With Gastroenteritis

1. Nursing Diagnosis: *Diarrhea* related to infectious process (NANDA-I © 2014)

GOAL: The child's bowel function will be restored to normal.

INTERVENTION	RATIONALE
• Obtain baseline vital signs and monitor every 2–4 hr.	• Fluid and electrolyte imbalances can alter vital body functions.
• Observe stools for amount, color, consistency, odor, and frequency.	• Aids in the diagnosis and in monitoring the child's status.
• Test stools for occult blood.	• Frequent defecation and some infectious organisms can cause bleeding.
• Monitor results of stool culture and sample for ova and parasites.	• Rapid notification of the healthcare provider will facilitate treatment.
• Wash hands well before and after contact with the child.	• Helps prevent transmission of microorganisms.
• Isolate the child until the cause of the diarrhea is determined.	• Prevents exposure of other patients and staff.
• Assist the child with toileting and hygiene.	• The child may be weak, incontinent, physically impaired, or anxious and require assistance to use the bathroom.
• Administer prescribed oral rehydration and intravenous solutions.	• Provides necessary fluids and nutrients.
• Notify the healthcare provider if diarrhea persists, stool characteristics change, or other symptoms of dehydration electrolyte imbalance occur.	• Ensures early intervention.

EXPECTED OUTCOME: Child's bowel function will return to normal.

2. Nursing Diagnosis: *Fluid Volume: Deficient* related to active fluid volume loss (NANDA-I © 2014)

GOAL: The child will remain hydrated and will begin to drink fluids within 24 hours of admission.

INTERVENTION	RATIONALE
• Monitor intake and output. Document time of each voiding. Weigh all diapers.	• Will determine if output exceeds input. Long periods of time without urine output can be an early indicator of poor renal function. A child should produce 1–2 mL of urine/kg/hr.
• Compare admission weight to preadmission weight. Assess weight daily.	• The degree of dehydration can be determined by the percentage of weight loss. Daily weights aid in determining progress toward rehydration.
• Assess level of consciousness, skin turgor, mucous membranes, skin color and temperature, capillary refill, eyes, and fontanelles every 4 hours.	• Will determine degree of hydration and adequacy of interventions.
• Assess for vomiting.	• Vomiting frequently accompanies diarrhea and contributes to the child's fluid loss.
• Provide oral fluid and electrolyte replacement solution if able to tolerate.	• Less invasive than IV fluids. Provides for replacement of essential fluids and electrolytes.
• Provide and maintain IV replacement therapy, as ordered.	• Use of IV replacement is based on the degree of dehydration, ongoing losses, insensible water losses, and electrolyte results.

EXPECTED OUTCOME: Child will have normal fluid and electrolyte balance as indicated by laboratory evaluation and physical examination.

3. Nursing Diagnosis: *Skin Integrity, Risk for Impaired,* **related to altered fluid status (NANDA-I © 2014)**

GOAL: The child will remain free of skin breakdown and rashes.

INTERVENTION	RATIONALE
• Assess skin of perineum and rectum for signs of skin breakdown or irritation.	• Early assessment and intervention can prevent worsening of the condition.
• Provide prevention or restorative care for infants as follows:	
Preventive Care:	
• Change diapers every 2 hr or as needed.	• Minimizes skin contact with chemical irritants from stool and urine.
• Wash diaper area after each soiling.	• Removes traces of stool if present.
• Apply A&D ointment, Aquaphor, or another barrier ointment with each diaper change.	• Provides a barrier and protects intact or reddened skin from becoming excoriated.
Restorative Care:	
• Leave the buttocks open to air for a few minutes several times daily, placing absorbent pads under the infant.	• Promotes air circulation to the area.
• Notify the healthcare provider if the skin is severely broken or peeling or if a rash is present.	• Additional measures such as the use of a barrier cream or paste may be needed to ensure skin healing.
• *For toddlers and older children:* Tub bathe at least daily (if condition allows) in tepid water. Pat the area dry.	• Helps loosen any fecal matter without scrubbing, which can cause additional irritation to the skin.
• Discourage the wearing of underwear if possible.	• Allows air to circulate and prevents accumulation of moisture.
• Apply barrier ointment with each diaper change or as instructed.	• Provides a barrier and protects intact or reddened skin from becoming excoriated.

EXPECTED OUTCOME: Child's perianal and rectal tissue will remain pink and intact.

Planning and Implementation

Nursing care focuses on providing emotional support, promoting rest and comfort, and ensuring adequate nutrition.

PROVIDE EMOTIONAL SUPPORT

The child may have been ill for several days or become suddenly ill a short time before seeking health care. The child and parents are usually anxious, so it is important to allow them to talk and ask questions. The child may require blood tests to help direct rehydration therapy. Most children are cared for at home, although care in a 24-hour monitoring unit may occur. Using therapeutic play techniques, such as allowing the child to manipulate equipment, can reduce anxiety (see Chapter 11).

PROMOTE REST AND COMFORT

Children with gastroenteritis may awaken frequently with periods of vomiting and diarrhea. Provide a quiet, restful environment and cluster nursing care to allow for periods of uninterrupted rest. To reduce the child's anxiety, encourage parents to room-in. Place the child's favorite toys and comfort objects within reach. Keep the child's mouth moistened with a wet washcloth, or an occasional ice chip. Provide skin care after each diarrheal episode to maintain skin integrity. Avoid using commercial baby wipes that contain alcohol as these irritate the skin and cause discomfort for the child.

ENSURE ADEQUATE NUTRITION

Liquids are offered throughout the illness, even if an intravenous infusion is in place. Follow guidelines for oral rehydration therapy in Chapter 18. Small amounts of normal diet for age are provided. Infants are breastfed or given formula. The child's diet progresses according to protocol or the child's tolerance for feedings.

Clinical Tip

Instruct parents in the importance of and techniques for hand hygiene, especially when caring for the child with gastroenteritis. Teach children in childcare centers and school how to wash their hands effectively to prevent spread of infectious diseases.

DISCHARGE PLANNING AND HOME CARE TEACHING

Discharge teaching begins on arrival at the healthcare facility. Teach the parents about the symptoms of dehydration and what actions to take if diarrhea recurs. Be sure that parents understand the recommended diet progression. Emphasize the necessity of good hygiene practices to prevent the spread of microorganisms that can cause gastroenteritis. If the child attends child care, have the parent inform the care center about the infection so the staff can be alerted to watch for other cases and can take steps to prevent the spread of infection.

Evaluation

Expected outcomes of nursing care are provided on the accompanying *Nursing Care Plan*.

Constipation

Constipation is a common complaint in the pediatric population and accounts for 3% of all visits to the pediatric primary care provider (Nurko & Zimmerman, 2014). Up to 30% of the pediatric population experience constipation (Watson, 2014). Most children experience functional constipation. This refers to constipation that cannot be attributed to an underlying physiological or anatomic abnormality (Rogers, 2012).

Because stool patterns vary among children, identification of an abnormal pattern is sometimes difficult. Infants usually have several bowel movements a day. For a young child, one bowel movement a day may be normal. As the child grows, however, three to four bowel movements in a week may be a normal pattern. The diagnosis of constipation must take into account the child's normal stool patterns.

Constipation may be caused by an underlying disease, diet, or psychologic factor. It may result from defects in filling, or more commonly emptying, of the rectum. Pathologic causes of defective filling include ineffective colonic propulsive activity, caused by hypothyroidism or use of medication, and obstruction, caused by a structural anomaly (stricture or stenosis) or by an aganglionic segment (Hirschsprung disease). If the rectum fails to fill, stasis leads to increased water reabsorption and hard, dry stools. Emptying of the rectum depends on the defecation reflex. Lesions of the spinal cord, weakness of the abdominal muscles, and local lesions blocking sphincter relaxation all may impede attempts to defecate.

Constipation during infancy is rare and is most often caused by mismanagement of diet. The transition from formula to cow's milk may cause a transient constipation since the bowel must adjust to the increased protein content of cow's milk.

Constipation occurs most frequently in the toddler and preschool age groups. This increased incidence is often associated with learning to control body functions. Many children do not like the sensations of a bowel movement and may begin withholding stool, which accumulates in and dilates the rectum until the next urge to defecate. The increasingly hard and painful bowel movement reinforces the child's behavior, and a cycle begins (Rogers, 2012).

Constipation in the school-age child, older child, and adolescent is generally related to activity, diet, and toileting habits. The child may not be eating enough fiber and could be eating starchy foods that contribute to constipation. Constipation may occur because of limited time for toileting. The child may not take time during the day to have a bowel movement or may be hesitant to use an unfamiliar bathroom.

Diagnosis is based on a thorough history and physical examination. When constipation occurs along with growth failure, vomiting, or abdominal pain, further investigation is necessary to rule out other disorders. Tests may include thyroid function tests; measurements of calcium, glucose, and electrolytes; a complete blood count; and urinalysis.

CLINICAL THERAPY

Dietary management is the treatment of choice for constipation that has no underlying pathologic cause. Constipation in young infants can usually be corrected by increasing the amount of fluids or adding 2 oz of pear or apple juice to daily intake. Increasing physical activity and fluid intake may be effective for some children.

Removing constipating foods (e.g., bananas, rice, and cheese) from the child's diet often decreases constipation. Increasing the child's intake of high-fiber foods (e.g., whole-grain breads, raw fruits, and vegetables) and fluids also promotes bowel elimination. In older infants, increasing the intake of fluids, cereals, fruits, and vegetables in the diet should correct the problem. A single glycerin suppository or enema may be required to remove hard stool.

Encouragement from parents and relaxation of bathroom privileges at school promote regularity and return of usual bowel patterns within a short time for school-age children. Children may need to get up earlier to have breakfast to allow time for toileting before going to school.

Constipation may follow surgery, especially in children who are immobilized. Stool softeners and a diet high in fiber and fluids prevent and treat constipation. Pharmacologic management of severe constipation usually occurs in two stages. The first stage involves disimpaction, followed by maintenance therapy (Rogers, 2011).

Disimpaction is difficult for the child and those who are managing the child's constipation. Consider the most effective means to evacuate the stool while causing the least amount of stress and anxiety to the child. The oral route is less invasive, but if the child experiences nausea and vomiting, the rectal route might be used. Polyethylene glycol solution with electrolyte solution is recommended for disimpaction (Paul, Dewdney, & Lamb, 2012; Rogers, 2011, 2012). Once the stool has been evacuated, maintenance therapy that may include polyethylene glycol powder, docusate, lactulose, or other products is continued for several weeks after a regular bowel patterns are established (Rogers, 2012).

Behavior modification may prove beneficial to managing constipation and may include having the child sit on the toilet after meals. Providing rewards for toileting at routinely scheduled times is effective (Rogers, 2012).

Nursing Management

Nursing care focuses on teaching parents what constitutes normal bowel patterns in children and the importance of diet in maintaining normal bowel patterns. Assess the child's diet history and obtain a description of bowel patterns from parents. Ask what the family does to treat constipation. Assessment of the child's food likes and dislikes may provide a clue as to the cause of constipation. Regular bowel habits are encouraged by placing the child on the toilet 30 minutes after a meal or around the time defecation usually occurs. Providing positive reinforcement during toilet training helps prevent a withholding pattern.

Teach parents dietary measures to promote regularity of bowel movements. Children can be given a high-fiber diet that includes fruits and vegetables. Cut-up fresh fruits, dried fruits, and fruit juice can be offered as snacks. A glycerin suppository can be used periodically. This is a natural stimulant and lubricant of the bowel. Caution parents to avoid frequent use of laxatives, stool softeners, and enemas since overuse can cause bowel dependency. Herbal stimulant laxatives are discouraged for children younger than 12 years, whereas other intestinal motility aids are not generally harmful. Find out more about any herbs the family commonly uses.

Encopresis

Encopresis is an abnormal elimination pattern characterized by the recurrent soiling or passage of stool at inappropriate times by a child who should have achieved bowel continence. Encopresis is reported to occur in approximately 3% of children ages 3 to 12. Children with primary encopresis have never achieved bowel control. Children with secondary encopresis have been continent of stool for more than 6 months before developing encopresis (Coehlo, 2011).

Encopresis is usually associated with voluntary or involuntary retention of stool in the lower bowel and rectum, leading to constipation, dilation of the lower bowel, and incompetence of the inner sphincter. The retention of stool is usually a result of being "too busy"; the child puts off going to the bathroom because of the inconvenience of leaving an activity. The retention of stool leads to constipation that is untreated and chronic. Loose stool leaks around the hard feces, and the child becomes unaware of a need to eliminate. Soiling may occur during the day or night. Bowel movements are irregular, painful, small, and hard. The child may be ridiculed by peers because of offensive body odor. This rejection leads to withdrawal and behavioral problems, often resulting in altered school performance and attendance. The child continues to hold stool because the passage has become painful. Parents commonly seek health care, believing that the child has diarrhea or constipation.

The underlying constipation that leads to encopresis may be caused by the stress of environmental changes (e.g., birth of a sibling, moving to a new house, attending a new school), issues of anger and control related to bowel training, diet, a full schedule of activities, or a genetic predisposition.

A thorough history, physical examination, and diagnostic studies (possibly including barium or contrast enema) are necessary to rule out organic causes and anatomic abnormalities. Information about the child's toilet training habits and parents' attitudes concerning those habits is obtained. A dietary history, including eating habits and types of foods eaten, is often helpful. Physical examination sometimes reveals a nontender mass in the lower abdomen.

In addition to dietary management and treatment to evacuate the bowel if needed as discussed in the preceding section, bowel training, behavior management, and family support are important components in the management of encopresis. Bowel training involves having the child sit on the toilet for a specific amount of time after breakfast and after dinner. This allows the child to gain or regain control of their bowel and an awareness of a full rectum. Behavior management includes involving the child in their care and provides reward and positive reinforcement for successes. Treatment for encopresis may take 6 to 12 months. The family needs education and support during this process. Long-term management may include oral stool softeners (Coehlo, 2011).

Nursing Management

Prevention of encopresis is the nursing goal. Partner with parents to teach toilet training techniques, emphasizing the child's developmental readiness. Parents are encouraged to praise the child for successes and to avoid punishment and power struggles. Encourage high-fiber diets and regular times for elimination.

Nursing care centers on educating the child and parents about the disorder and its treatment and on providing emotional support. Explain the treatment plan, including dietary changes and use of laxatives or stool softeners. Reassure the child that he or she has a healthy body and, with treatment, will achieve normal functioning. The child is monitored during clinic visits for at least 6 months to be certain new patterns have been established.

Intestinal Parasitic Disorders

Intestinal parasitic disorders occur most frequently in tropical regions. Outbreaks take place where water is not treated, food is incorrectly prepared, or people live in crowded conditions with poor sanitation. In the United States, outbreaks of diseases caused by protozoa or helminths (worms) are increasing. Young children, especially those in day care, are most at risk of infection. Young children often lack good hygiene practices and are likely to put objects and their hands into their mouths. See Table 25–4 for common intestinal parasitic disorders.

Another common cause of young child infection is exposure to pets and wildlife. Pets should be checked regularly for parasites and treated for worms as needed. Sandboxes should be kept covered when not in use, and children should be taught good handwashing techniques after exposure to their pets (CDC, 2014b). Laboratory examination of stool specimens identifies the causative organism (protozoa, worms, larvae, or ova). Treatment usually involves an anthelmintic.

Nursing care centers on preventive teaching. Emphasize the importance of good hygiene practices, especially careful handwashing, after toileting and when handling food. Ensure the family understands proper medication administration. Instruct parents to administer prescribed medications as directed even if the child's condition seems to be improved.

Disorders of Malabsorption

Malabsorption occurs when a child cannot digest or absorb nutrients in the diet. Disorders of malabsorption include celiac disease, lactose intolerance, and short bowel syndrome. Celiac disease and lactose intolerance are discussed in Chapter 14. Cystic fibrosis, a common cause of malabsorption, is discussed in Chapter 20.

Short Bowel Syndrome

Short bowel syndrome is a decreased ability to absorb and digest a regular diet due to a shortened intestine. Loss of intestine may result from extensive bowel resection for treatment of necrotizing enterocolitis or inflammatory disorders or from a congenital bowel anomaly such as intestinal malrotation, gastroschisis, or atresia.

The extent and location of the involved bowel determine the severity of the disorder. Because specific types of absorption occur primarily in certain parts of the bowel, the section lost determines the particular vitamins and other nutrients that are inadequate.

During the first 3 months after bowel resection, watery diarrhea is common. In the transition period, the remaining bowel usually increases its absorptive surface area and partially compensates for the absent intestine. At first, the infant or young child requires nutritional support to provide sufficient nutrients for adequate growth and development. In the initial period, the child only receives total parenteral nutrition (TPN). Once the bowel begins to recover, in addition to TPN, start continuous enteral feedings. Continuous exposure to nutrients allows

TABLE 25–4 Common Intestinal Parasitic Disorders

PARASITIC INFECTION	TRANSMISSION, LIFE CYCLE, PATHOGENESIS	CLINICAL MANIFESTATIONS	CLINICAL THERAPY	COMMENTS
GIARDIASIS Organism: protozoan *Giardia lamblia* 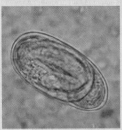 Centers for Disease Control (CDC)	Transmission is through person-to-person contact, unfiltered water, improperly prepared infected food, and contact with animals. Cysts are ingested and passed into the duodenum and proximal jejunum, where they begin actively feeding. They are excreted in the stool.	May be asymptomatic. *Infants:* diarrhea, vomiting, anorexia, avoidant/restrictive food intake disorder (failure to thrive) *Older children:* abdominal cramps; intermittent loose, foul-smelling, watery, pale, and greasy stools	Medications used to treat giardiasis include metronidazole, tinidazole, and nitazoxanide (drugs of choice). Quinacrine, furazolidone, and paromomycin may be used.	Most common intestinal parasitic organism in the United States. Symptoms last 2–6 weeks. Medication may decrease this time frame. Parents or caregivers should wear gloves when handling diapers or stool of an infant or child infected with parasites.
ENTEROBIASIS (PINWORM) Organism: nematode *Enterobius vermicularis* B. G. Partin; Dr. Moore/CDC	Transmission is from discharged eggs inhaled or carried from hand to mouth. Eggs hatch in the upper intestine and mature in 1–2 months. Larvae then migrate to the colon and lay eggs. Movement of worms causes intense itching. Scratching deposits eggs on the hands and under the nails.	Intense perianal itching, irritability, restlessness, and short attention span; in females, can migrate to the vagina and urethra to cause infection. Itching intensifies at night when the female comes to the anal opening to lay eggs.	Medications used to treat enterobiasis include mebendazole, pyrantel pamoate, and albendazole. The child and all household members should be treated at the same time. Treatment may be repeated in 2 weeks.	Most common worm infection in the United States. Transmission is increased in crowded conditions such as housing developments, schools, and childcare centers.
ASCARIASIS (TYPE OF ROUNDWORM) Organism: nematode *Ascaris lumbricoides* James Cavallini/BSIPSA/Alamy	Transmission is from discharged eggs carried from hand to mouth. The adult lays eggs in the small intestine. Eggs are excreted in stool. Swallowed eggs hatch in the small intestine. Larvae may penetrate intestinal villi, entering the portal vein and liver, then moving to the lung. Larvae that ascend to the upper respiratory tract are swallowed and proceed to the small intestine, where they repeat the cycle.	Mild infection may be asymptomatic. Severe infection may result in intestinal obstruction and impaired growth.	Medications used to treat ascariasis include ivermectin, mebendazole, and albendazole.	Most common in warm, moist climates. Associated with poor personal hygiene and poor sanitation.
HOOKWORM DISEASE Organism: nematode *Necator americanus* Centers for Disease Control (CDC)	Transmission is through direct contact with infected soil containing larvae. Worms live in the small intestine and feed on villi, causing bleeding. Eggs are deposited in the bowel and excreted in feces. Eggs hatch in damp, shaded soil. Larvae attach to and penetrate the skin, then enter the bloodstream, migrating to the lungs. Larvae then migrate to the upper respiratory passages and are swallowed.	In healthy individuals, mild infection seldom causes problems. Presence of larvae on the skin may cause itching and a rash. More severe infection may result in diarrhea, abdominal pain, anemia, weight loss, and fatigue.	Medications used to treat hookworm disease include mebendazole, albendazole, and pyrantel pamoate. Iron supplements may also be given.	Children should wear shoes when outdoors. Note, however, that other unprotected areas of the skin may still come in contact with larvae.

PARASITIC INFECTION	TRANSMISSION, LIFE CYCLE, PATHOGENESIS	CLINICAL MANIFESTATIONS	CLINICAL THERAPY	COMMENTS
STRONGYLOIDIASIS (TYPE OF ROUNDWORM)				
Organism: nematode *Strongyloides stercoralis* 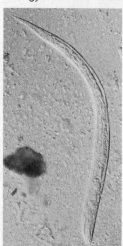 Centers for Disease Control (CDC)	Transmission is from the ingestion of discharged larvae in the soil. Life cycle is similar to that of the hookworm, except this roundworm does not attach to the intestinal mucosa, and feeding larvae (rather than eggs) may be deposited in the soil.	Mild infection may be asymptomatic. Severe infection may result in abdominal pain and distention, nausea, vomiting, diarrhea, dry cough, throat irritation, and itchy rash.	Medications used to treat strongyloidiasis include ivermectin and albendazole. Treatment may need to be repeated if symptoms recur after treatment.	Most common in older children and adolescents.
TOXOCARIASIS (TYPE OF ROUNDWORM)				
Organism: nematode *Toxocara canis* or *T. cati*, commonly found in dogs and cats 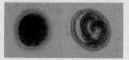 Centers for Disease Control (CDC)	Transmission is through the ingestion of eggs in the soil. Ingested eggs hatch in the intestine. Mobile larvae then migrate to the liver and eventually to all major organs (including the brain). Once migration is complete, they encapsulate in dense fibrous tissue.	Most cases are asymptomatic. Severe symptoms include fever, coughing, pneumonia, and enlarged liver.	Medications used to treat toxocariasis include albendazole and mebendazole. Steroids may also be used.	Deworm household pets on a regular basis. Keep children away from areas contaminated with animal droppings.

Note: Some of the medications listed may not be available in the United States, and some of them may not be approved for use in all age groups.

Source: Data from American Academy of Pediatrics (AAP). (2015). Parasitic diseases. *Red book: 2015 report of the Committee on Infectious Diseases* (30th ed. pp 588–591). Elk Grove Village, IL: Author; Centers for Disease Control and Prevention (CDC). (2014a). *Parasites.* Retrieved from http://www.cdc.gov/parasites; Gershon, A. A., & Hotez, P. J. (2011). Infectious diseases. In C. D. Rudolph, A. M. Rudolph, G. E. Lister, L. R. First, & A. A. Gershon (Eds.), *Rudolph's pediatrics* (22nd ed., pp. 878–1247). New York, NY: McGraw-Hill. Photos of *Giardia lamblia,* strongyloidiasis, hookworm, and toxocariasis are courtesy of the Centers for Disease Control and Prevention, Atlanta, GA.

the bowel to adapt (Cuffari, 2014). It is essential that the child receive the appropriate nutritional components regardless of the method in which nutrition is delivered.

SAFETY ALERT!

The child with short bowel syndrome will receive TPN via a central line. Aseptic technique in the care of the central line is essential to prevent a catheter-associated bloodstream infection and potential sepsis (Gutierrez, Kang, & Jaksic, 2011). Maintaining patency of the central line is also essential because this may be the child's only route for receiving nutrition. It is not uncommon for children with short bowel syndrome to require insertion of multiple central lines over time because of either infection or occlusion of the line, especially if they require long-term TPN. This not only places a stress on the child who must undergo yet another surgical procedure, but it is a stressor for the family as well.

Nursing Management

Nursing care focuses on meeting the child's nutritional and fluid needs and teaching parents how to care for the child at home. Establishing an adequate nutritional intake and bowel pattern is a lengthy process. TPN is provided initially until a feeding regimen can be established. Oral and enteral feedings are instituted gradually to allow the bowel time to compensate. Provide support to the family and child throughout this period. Teach parents how to prepare and administer total parenteral feedings and care for the central line (see the *Clinical Skills Manual* SKILLS). Once enteral or tube feedings have started, teach management of the feeding pump and care of the feeding tube. Ensure regular bowel function and maintain skin integrity. Arrange home visits to monitor the child's growth and development, care of the central line and tube-feeding site, and any side effects such as fluid and electrolyte imbalance and diarrhea.

Hepatic Disorders

The liver is one of the most vital organs in the body. Its primary functions include production of blood clotting factors, fibrinogen, and prothrombin; secretion of bile and *bilirubin* (yellow pigment produced from the breakdown of red blood cells); metabolism of fat, protein, and carbohydrates; detoxification of hormones, drugs, and other substances; and storage of vitamins A, D, E, and K and glycogen. Thus any inflammatory, obstructive, or degenerative disorder that affects liver function can be life threatening. The following discussion focuses on four liver disorders in children: hyperbilirubinemia, biliary atresia, viral hepatitis, and cirrhosis.

Hyperbilirubinemia of the Newborn

Hyperbilirubinemia refers to an elevated serum bilirubin level and occurs in approximately 84% of term newborns (Muchowski, 2014). Jaundice manifests in newborns with total serum bilirubin (TSB) levels greater than 5 mg/dL (Schwartz, Haberman, & Ruddy, 2011).

ETIOLOGY AND PATHOPHYSIOLOGY
Physiologic or *neonatal jaundice* is a normal process that occurs during transition from intrauterine to extrauterine life and is caused by the newborn's shortened red blood cell life span (90 days compared with 120 days in the adult), slower uptake by the liver, lack of intestinal bacteria, and/or established hydration from initial breastfeeding.

CLINICAL MANIFESTATIONS
Jaundice in the newborn is first evident on the face and then progresses to the trunk and finally to the extremities. Jaundice may be difficult to see in babies with dark skin color (Lauer & Spector, 2011). In addition to jaundice, symptoms include lethargy, irritability, and poor feeding (Seagraves, Brulte, McNeely, et al., 2013).

DIAGNOSTIC TESTS
A blood test, performed by heelstick or venipuncture, measures total serum bilirubin (TSB) in the newborn. A transcutaneous bilirubin (TcB) measurement device is a noninvasive method for estimating serum bilirubin in newborns. This method for measuring bilirubin is a screening tool for use in determining if the TSB should be evaluated and is a good estimate of the TSB. A TSB should be obtained when treatment is being considered.

CLINICAL THERAPY
Phototherapy most effectively reduces serum bilirubin in newborns with physiologic jaundice (Wells, Ahmed, & Musser, 2013) Phototherapy is thought to reduce the amount of indirect, or unconjugated, bilirubin in the baby's bloodstream by promoting excretion via the intestines and kidneys. Phototherapy exposes the newborn's skin to blue light, which changes bilirubin into water-soluble forms that can be excreted (Lauer & Spector, 2011). Phototherapy can be provided by conventional banks of fluorescent tube phototherapy lights, by a fiber-optic blanket attached to a halogen light source around the trunk of the newborn, by a fiber-optic mattress placed under the baby, or by a combination of these delivery methods (Bhutani & Committee on Fetus and Newborn, 2011).

Clinical Tip

The newborn's eyes are covered during overhead phototherapy to prevent retinal damage (Hansen, 2014). The eye shields can be removed when the lights are off for feeding (Figure 25–8).

Many newborns with hyperbilirubinemia are also mildly dehydrated. When the newborn is breastfed, supplemental breast milk or formula may be given to improve hydration (Muchowski, 2014). If the newborn is unable to take adequate fluids and is dehydrated, intravenous fluid should be administered.

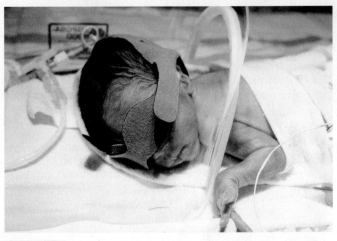

Figure 25–8 Infant receiving phototherapy. The phototherapy light is positioned over the incubator. Bilateral eye patches are always used during photo light therapy to protect the baby's eyes.

SOURCE: Courtesy of Lisa Smith-Pedersen, RNC, MSN, NNP-BC.

Nursing Management
For the Child With Hyperbilirubinemia

The nurse in the newborn nursery and in the outpatient setting plays a critical role in identifying the newborn at risk and providing parent education related to hyperbilirubinemia. Although the nurse in the newborn nursery may be providing care to a baby for a few days after birth, many newborns are discharged home within 24 hours. The newborn may be evaluated for jaundice in the outpatient setting and then admitted to the pediatric unit for treatment. Nurses working in acute care settings must familiarize themselves with the care of very young babies who require treatment for hyperbilirubinemia.

Nursing Assessment and Diagnosis
The newborn should be assessed for jaundice. If the nurse suspects the presence of jaundice, the newborn's primary care provider should be notified so that bilirubin levels can be measured.

FEEDING ASSESSMENT
The mother who is breastfeeding should nurse her newborn at least 8 to 12 times per day for the first several days (Muchowski, 2014; Seagraves et al., 2013). The nurse should be alert to mothers and newborns who are having difficulty and require lactation support during the hospital stay and following discharge. Adequate hydration is essential for adequate elimination of bilirubin from the body. Newborns who are not well hydrated are at increased risk for hyperbilirubinemia (Seagraves et al., 2013). Parents should be educated regarding the number of wet diapers and stools their newborn should have each day. Because many mothers and term newborns are discharged within 24 hours after birth, this is important information to teach parents prior to discharge.

NURSING ASSESSMENT
Nursing diagnoses that may apply to the newborn with hyperbilirubinemia may include the following (NANDA-I © 2014):

- *Fluid Volume: Deficient* related to decreased oral intake and ineffective breastfeeding
- *Attachment, Risk for Impaired,* related to disruption of parental/newborn interaction due to hospitalization and treatment

- *Body Temperature: Imbalanced, Risk for,* related to phototherapy
- *Injury, Risk for,* related to phototherapy

Planning and Implementation

The role of the nurse is to identify the newborn at risk for hyperbilirubinemia, educate parents about newborn jaundice, and care for the newborn and family undergoing treatment for this condition. For the baby undergoing phototherapy, the nurse should monitor the newborn frequently, ensuring that the newborn is receiving the phototherapy properly. Vital signs should be assessed every 4 to 8 hours, especially the newborn's temperature, which might indicate signs of infection or signs of hypothermia in a newborn whose clothing is removed for phototherapy. An accurate measurement of intake and output is essential to make sure the newborn is not dehydrated. Assist the family in breastfeeding or bottle-feeding as appropriate.

SAFETY ALERT!

In cases of severe and untreated hyperbilirubinemia, bilirubin encephalopathy can cause serious neurologic sequelae. The term *acute bilirubin encephalopathy* is used to describe the acute effects of bilirubin toxicity in the first few days to weeks of life. The term *kernicterus* is used when referring to chronic and irreversible effects of bilirubin toxicity (Schwartz, Haberman, & Ruddy, 2011).

DISCHARGE PLANNING AND HOME CARE TEACHING

Problems with breastfeeding in the first week of life can contribute to low caloric intake, dehydration, and subsequent risk of neonatal hyperbilirubinemia (Schwartz, Haberman, & Ruddy, 2011). The nurse assesses adequacy of breastfeeding prior to hospital discharge and coordinates with the newborn's healthcare provider in making appropriate referrals to lactation specialists and support groups in the community when necessary.

For term infants who develop uncomplicated hyperbilirubinemia, home phototherapy may be provided with the use of the fiber-optic pad, also known as a biliblanket. Serum bilirubin levels must be monitored regularly at the physician's office or neighborhood laboratory, or by the home healthcare worker. A visiting or home healthcare nurse often visits the family to establish the phototherapy and inform parents about the care needed. The nurse partners with other professionals such as staff from a medical supply company (to service equipment), a lactation specialist, and a pediatrician (to coordinate services).

Evaluation

Expected outcomes of nursing interventions include:

- The term or near-term newborn at risk for hyperbilirubinemia is identified prior to discharge and receives appropriate follow-up.
- The newborn's parents understand who and when to call if they suspect development of hyperbilirubinemia.
- The newborn receives appropriate intervention if hyperbilirubinemia occurs.
- The newborn's nutritional and fluid intakes are adequate to meet growth and development requirements.
- The newborn does not develop neurologic sequelae as a result of hyperbilirubinemia.

Biliary Atresia

Biliary atresia results when the extrahepatic bile ducts fail to develop or are closed. The disorder leads to cholestasis, cirrhosis, portal hypertension, end-stage liver disease, and death by 2 years of age if left untreated (Flanigan, 2013; Moreira, Cabral, Cowles, et al., 2012; Sira, Taha, & Sira, 2014). Biliary atresia is the leading indication for pediatric liver transplantation (Moreira et al., 2012).

CLINICAL MANIFESTATIONS

Initially, the newborn is asymptomatic. Jaundice may not be detected until 2 to 3 weeks after birth. At that point, bilirubin levels increase, accompanied by abdominal distention and hepatomegaly (see Appendix B for bilirubin levels and other liver function tests). As the disease progresses, splenomegaly occurs. The infant experiences easy bruising, prolonged bleeding time, and intense itching. Stools have putty-like consistency and are white or clay colored because of the absence of bile pigments. Excretion of bilirubin and bile salts results in tea-colored urine. Avoidant/restrictive food intake disorder (failure to thrive) and malnutrition occur as the destructive changes of the disease progress.

The cause of biliary atresia is unknown. Absence or blockage of the extrahepatic bile ducts results in blocked bile flow from the liver to the duodenum. This altered bile flow soon causes inflammation and fibrotic changes in the liver. In addition to blockage, the disease can also be caused by hepatocellular dysfunction. Lack of bile acids also interferes with digestion of fat and absorption of fat-soluble vitamins A, D, E, and K, resulting in steatorrhea and nutritional deficiencies. Without treatment the disease is fatal.

CLINICAL THERAPY

Diagnosis is based on the history, physical examination, and laboratory evaluation. Laboratory findings reveal elevated bilirubin and serum aminotransferase and alkaline phosphatase levels, prolonged prothrombin time, and increased ammonia levels (Schwarz, 2014). Percutaneous liver biopsy suggests biliary atresia, and an exploratory laparotomy and intraoperative cholangiography confirms the diagnosis (Robie, Overfelt, & Xie, 2014).

Treatment involves surgery to attempt correction of the obstruction (hepatoportoenterostomy) and supportive care. In a hepatoportoenterostomy (Kasai procedure), a segment of the intestine is anastomosed to the porta hepatis. The primary purpose of this procedure is to promote bile flow from the liver. Intravenous antibiotics are administered in the postoperative period to prevent cholangitis. Prophylaxis with oral antibiotics is continued for 1 to 2 years after surgery (Flanigan, 2013).

Additional treatment includes administration of intramuscular vitamin K prior to invasive procedures and surgery to decrease the risk of bleeding afterwards and vitamins A, D, E, and K to provide supplementation since absorption of these vitamins is impaired. The infant is breastfed or is given Pregestimil or Nutramigen, formulas that contain medium-chain triglycerides. As the liver disease worsens, the child may need cholestyramine and antihistamines to help decrease itching. Enteral feedings may be needed as well (Flanigan, 2013). Ursodeoxycholic acid (Actigall) may be given to the child to promote bile flow (Schwarz, 2014).

While bile flow is achieved with the Kasai procedure in many children with biliary atresia, approximately 70% to 80% of children having this surgery will eventually need a liver transplant (Mieli-Vergani & Tizzard, 2012). Advances in transplantation surgery now make it possible to perform partial liver transplants from living donor resections. This enables transplantation to be performed before the child develops end-stage liver disease (Flanigan, 2013).

Nursing Management

Nursing care in the initial stages of biliary atresia is the same as that for any healthy newborn. As symptoms develop, the focus of nursing care becomes long-term management and support.

Diagnosis of this potentially fatal disorder can be devastating to parents. Provide emotional support and offer frequent explanations of tests during the initial diagnostic evaluation. As the disease progresses, the infant becomes irritable because of intense itching and the accumulation of toxins. Tepid baths may help to relieve itching and provide comfort. Dry skin by patting rather than rubbing to avoid further skin irritation. Promote rest by grouping nursing activities while the infant is awake. Weigh the infant daily. Administer TPN, lipids, and fat-soluble vitamins A, D, E, and K as prescribed.

Care following a hepatoportoenterostomy is similar to that for a child undergoing abdominal surgery. (See the earlier discussion of postsurgical nursing management for appendicitis and *Nursing Care Plan: The Child Undergoing Surgery* in Chapter 11.) Posttransplant care includes immunosuppressant drugs and close monitoring for vascular complications. Discharge planning focuses on teaching parents how to care for the child's skin, provide for nutritional needs, administer medications, and monitor for increasing symptoms of liver disease. When the child has received a transplant, teach parents how to identify signs of rejection (nausea, vomiting, fever, and jaundice), as well as the administration and side effects of immunosuppressant medications. Refer parents to support groups, clergy, or social services if indicated. They will need ongoing visits from a home healthcare nurse to help them manage the child's complex care. Palliative care may need to be discussed with the family if it becomes evident the child will not survive (see Chapter 13). Expected outcomes for nursing care of the child with biliary atresia are as follows:

- The child consumes adequate nutrition in order to support growth and development.
- Parents cope effectively with stress of the child's condition.
- The child achieves growth and developmental milestones expected for age.

Viral Hepatitis

Hepatitis is an inflammation of the liver caused by a viral infection. Hepatitis may be an acute or chronic disease. Acute hepatitis is rapid in onset and, if untreated, may develop into chronic hepatitis. The most frequently diagnosed causative organisms are hepatitis A virus (HAV), hepatitis B virus (HBV), and hepatitis C virus (HCV). A lesser known type is hepatitis D virus (HDV). Hepatitis E (HEV) occurs primarily in developing countries and is rarely seen in the United States (CDC, 2012a). In 2012, the incidence of hepatitis A declined to 0.5 cases per 100,000 in the United States. The incidence of hepatitis B has also decreased remarkably during the past several years with an incidence of 0.9 cases per 100,000 in 2012 (CDC, 2014c). The decline in both of these illnesses is related to routine vaccine administration, especially in children.

ETIOLOGY AND PATHOPHYSIOLOGY

Hepatitis A is highly contagious and traditionally has been called *infectious hepatitis*. Infection occurs primarily through the fecal–oral route. Transmission is by direct person-to-person spread or through ingestion of contaminated water or food. Hepatitis A frequently occurs in children in childcare settings where hygiene practices are poor. Food handlers can spread hepatitis A if not aware of their infection; it is a common cause of foodborne illness. Because the virus is transmitted in the early stages of the disease when individuals are often asymptomatic or only mildly ill, large numbers of people may be exposed before the diagnosis is confirmed (Table 25–5). Most children recover from hepatitis A; however, in rare instances, acute liver failure may occur (Jensen & Balistreri, 2016).

Hepatitis B can result in acute or chronic infection and is transmitted by the parenteral route through the exchange of blood or any body secretion or fluids, sexual activity, and transmission from mother to fetus in utero (Peate & Jones, 2014). Adolescents who use intravenous drugs and have unprotected sexual intercourse are at risk for contracting hepatitis B. Major sources for the spread of HBV are healthy chronic carriers.

Hepatitis C is the most common chronic bloodborne infection in the United States. The hepatitis C virus is transmitted primarily through intravenous drug use, needlestick injury, and birth to a mother infected with hepatitis C. The virus can also be spread through blood transfusions, but the incidence of this route of transmission in the United States is rare because blood

TABLE 25–5 Comparison of Hepatitis Types

TYPE	IMMUNIZATION AVAILABLE	PROPHYLAXIS	PRIMARY TRANSMISSION	INCUBATION PERIOD
Hepatitis A	Yes	Immune globulin Hepatitis A vaccine	Fecal–oral	15–19 days
Hepatitis B	Yes	Hepatitis B immune globulin Hepatitis B vaccine	Needlesticks or sharps exposure Intravenous drug use During birth Sexual activity	60–180 days
Hepatitis C	No	None	Needlesticks or sharps exposure Intravenous drug use During birth	14–160 days
Hepatitis D	No	Hepatitis B vaccine	Needlesticks or sharps exposure Intravenous drug use During birth Sexual activity	21–42 days
Hepatitis E	No	None	Fecal–oral	21–63 days

Source: Data from Centers for Disease Control and Prevention (CDC). (2012a). *Hepatitis E information for health professionals.* Retrieved from http://www.cdc.gov/hepatitis/HEV/index.htm; CDC. (2012b). *Hepatitis B information for health professionals.* Retrieved from http://www.cdc.gov/hepatitis/HBV/index.htm; CDC. (2014d). *Hepatitis A information for health professionals.* Retrieved from http://www.cdc.gov/hepatitis/HAV/index.htm; CDC. (2014e). *Hepatitis C information for health professionals.* Retrieved from http://www.cdc.gov/hepatitis/HCV/index.htm; CDC. (2014f). *Hepatitis D information for health professionals.* Retrieved from http://www.cdc.gov/hepatitis/HDV/index.htm; Jensen, M. K., & Balistreri, W. F. (2016). Viral hepatitis. In R. M. Kliegman, B. F. Stanton, J. W. St. Geme III, & N. F. Schor (Eds.), *Nelson textbook of pediatrics* (20th ed., pp. 1942–1953). Philadelphia, PA: Elsevier Saunders.

is screened for this infection. Chronic infection occurs in 75% to 85% of those individuals infected with hepatitis C (CDC, 2014e).

Hepatitis D (delta virus) is a defective virus that can gain entry to a human only in connection with hepatitis B (CDC, 2014f). It can occur as a coinfection along with hepatitis B or as a superinfection in someone already infected with hepatitis B.

Hepatitis E infection is primarily transmitted through contaminated water and is most common in developing countries (Jensen & Balistreri, 2016).

The liver's response to injury by the viruses that cause hepatitis is similar (see *Pathophysiology Illustrated: Viral Hepatitis*). Initially, invasion of the parenchymal cells by the virus results in local degeneration and necrosis. Subsequent infiltration of the parenchyma by lymphocytes, macrophages, plasma cells, eosinophils, and neutrophils causes inflammation that heblocks biliary drainage into the intestine. Impaired bile excretion causes a buildup of bile in the blood, urine, and skin (jaundice). Structural changes in the parenchymal cells account for other altered liver functions.

CLINICAL MANIFESTATIONS

Symptoms of acute viral hepatitis infection include nausea, vomiting, fatigue, abdominal pain, joint pain, pruritus, and urticaria in the prodromal phase. In the icteric phase, the child develops jaundice, gray- or pale-colored bowel movements, gastrointestinal symptoms, right upper quadrant pain, and malaise. In the convalescent phase the jaundice resolves and laboratory values return to normal (Buggs, 2014; CDC, 2012c).

CLINICAL THERAPY

Diagnosis is often made on the basis of a thorough history and physical examination. A history of exposure to persons with the disease is significant. Physical examination reveals a tender, enlarged liver. Laboratory evaluation includes serologic testing (to detect the presence of antigens and antibodies to HAV, HBV, HCV, or HDV) liver function studies, serum bilirubin, and prothrombin time (Harris & Crawford, 2013; Jensen & Balistreri, 2016).

Early diagnosis is essential to follow the course of the illness and identify potential complications. Management includes bed rest, hydration, and adequate nutrition.

The spread of viral infections can be interrupted by elimination of the virus from the infected population, institution of proper hygiene, and passive or active immunization. To date, no antiviral agent has been developed to combat the hepatitis viruses. Prevention depends on breaking the cycle of infection.

Active immunization for hepatitis A, a two-dose series, is recommended for all people at increased risk of acquiring infection, for children, and for those who wish to acquire immunity to the illness. The CDC (2012c) recommends that all children receive the first hepatitis A vaccine at 1 year of age.

Hepatitis B immune globulin (HBIG) and the hepatitis B vaccine must be given to infants born to infected mothers within 12 hours of birth to provide protection against the virus. Administration of the first dose of the three-dose series of the hepatitis B vaccine shortly after birth to all infants further reduces the risk of perinatal infection in cases where the mother's status may be unknown or incorrectly documented (CDC, 2012b). (Chapter 16 provides specific information on immunization schedules.)

Individuals who have been exposed to hepatitis A and have not been previously immunized should receive immune globulin or the hepatitis A vaccine within 2 weeks of exposure. Healthy individuals, ages 12 months to 40 years of age, not previously immunized may receive the hepatitis A vaccine instead of immune globulin within 2 weeks of exposure (CDC, 2014d). Passive immunity to HBV can be achieved with hepatitis B immune globulin (HBIG). Used for one-time exposure and for infants of infected mothers, it is given within 12 hours after birth (CDC, 2012b).

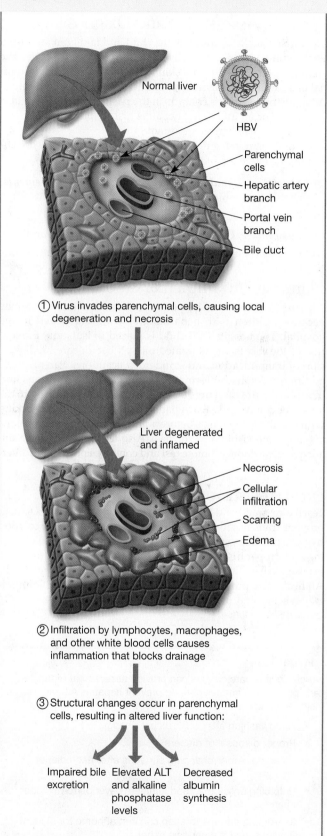

Pathophysiology Illustrated: **Viral Hepatitis**

Normal liver

HBV

Parenchymal cells

Hepatic artery branch

Portal vein branch

Bile duct

① Virus invades parenchymal cells, causing local degeneration and necrosis

Liver degenerated and inflamed

Necrosis

Cellular infiltration

Scarring

Edema

② Infiltration by lymphocytes, macrophages, and other white blood cells causes inflammation that blocks drainage

③ Structural changes occur in parenchymal cells, resulting in altered liver function:

Impaired bile excretion

Elevated ALT and alkaline phosphatase levels

Decreased albumin synthesis

The hepatitis virus causes degeneration and necrosis of the liver, which results in abnormal liver function and illness.

Nursing Management

For the Child With Viral Hepatitis

Nursing Assessment and Diagnosis

The nurse usually encounters the child and family in an outpatient setting. In addition to observing the child for characteristic signs of hepatitis (jaundiced skin and sclera), assess for abdominal pain, anorexia, nausea and vomiting, malaise, and arthralgia. A history of the child's contacts in the past several weeks is also obtained. For an infant, the hepatitis history of the mother and other family members is important.

Common nursing diagnoses for the child with acute hepatitis might include the following (NANDA-I © 2014):

- *Nutrition, Imbalanced: Less than Body Requirements*, related to chronic illness
- *Fatigue* related to disease state
- *Body Image, Disturbed (Older Child)*, related to jaundice
- *Anxiety (Parent and Child)* related to threat to health status

Planning and Implementation

Nursing care involves home and community considerations because children with hepatitis are seldom admitted to the hospital. The hospitalized child is placed in isolation. Prevention of the disease is integrated into all health care by discussion of immunization and standard precautions. Parents need additional detailed information about health precautions and infection control measures if hepatitis cases have occurred in the family or community. Teach parents the importance of checking with health professionals before administering any medications (even nonprescription medicines). Also teach them to maintain adequate nutrition, promote rest and comfort, and provide diversional activities.

PREVENT SPREAD OF INFECTION

Teach the parents and the child infection control measures to help prevent transmission of the virus. For parents, reinforce good hygiene practices, such as washing hands before and after toileting and proper disposal of soiled diapers. Vaccination for those exposed to hepatitis A or B should occur as discussed previously. All healthcare providers should receive the hepatitis B immunization series and use standard precautions at all times (see the *Clinical Skills Manual* SKILLS).

Clinical Tip

Nurses in childcare centers can provide assessment of the center's procedures and teaching to prevent hepatitis A transmission. Help the center to set standards about:

- Handwashing after each diaper change
- Proper disposal of diapers
- Cleaning diaper-changing surfaces after each diaper change
- Enforcing policy that food handlers never perform diaper changes
- Instructing parents to keep children at home for at least 2 weeks after a diagnosis of hepatitis A
- Informing parents of other children attending the childcare center when there is a case of hepatitis A and teaching them the symptoms of the condition

---

MAINTAIN ADEQUATE NUTRITION

Initially, the child is encouraged to eat favorite foods. Once the anorexia and nausea have resolved, a high-protein, high-carbohydrate, low-fat diet is recommended. Increased protein helps maintain protein stores and prevent muscle wasting. Increased carbohydrates ensure adequate caloric intake and prevent protein depletion. The use of low-fat foods lessens stomach distention. Offer the child small, frequent feedings.

PROMOTE REST AND COMFORT

Bed rest is necessary only if the child has severe fatigue and malaise. However, most children voluntarily limit their activities during the initial phase of the disease. Keep the child quiet and comfortable. Offer comfort items such as favorite toys, blankets, and pillows.

ADMINISTER MEDICATIONS

Drug metabolism is altered during hepatitis since the liver cannot detoxify medications readily. As with all liver disorders, medications need to be administered carefully, and the child's condition must be monitored for possible drug side effects, especially since so many drugs are metabolized by the liver. Caution parents to check with healthcare providers before giving any nonprescription medication. For example, acetaminophen is metabolized in the liver, and liver disease can interfere with its breakdown.

PROVIDE DIVERSIONAL ACTIVITIES

Hospitalized children with hepatitis are kept in isolation. Non-hospitalized children with hepatitis do not need to be isolated, but they should be kept at home for 2 weeks following the onset of symptoms. Parents who cannot take time off from work may need to arrange home sitters to stay with the child. Offer suggestions for diversional activities during this period. Young children can be given a new toy or favorite activities. Older children and adolescents can be given board games, puzzles, books or magazines, movies, or video games. Phone calls and short visits from friends help school-age children and adolescents maintain contact with peers.

Evaluation

Expected outcomes of nursing care for hepatitis include the following:

- The child demonstrates adequate nutritional intake to meet growth and development needs.
- The child participates in quiet, nonfatiguing activities and self-care.
- Positive body image is achieved.
- Parents demonstrate effective coping with the stress of the child's condition.
- Hepatitis is not spread to the child's contacts.

Cirrhosis

Cirrhosis is a degenerative disease process that results in fibrotic changes and fatty infiltration in the liver. It can occur in children of any age as the end stage of several disorders such as hepatitis and biliary atresia (Hassan & Balistreri, 2016; Squires & Balistreri, 2016). The diffuse destruction and regeneration of the hepatic parenchymal cells result in an increase in fibrous connective tissue and disorganization of the liver structure. Progressive scarring that occurs in cirrhosis leads to altered blood flow to the liver, which causes further deterioration of liver function (Squires & Balistreri, 2016).

Clinical manifestations of cirrhosis vary. Hepatomegaly may be evident on examination. Jaundice occurs as the disease progresses and is an indication of hyperbilirubinemia. Jaundice is sometimes the only sign of hepatic dysfunction, so its appearance must be investigated. Pruritus is common in children with cirrhosis, although it is not related to the degree of hyperbilirubinemia. Other clinical manifestations of cirrhosis in children include ascites, portal hypertension, encephalopathy, and variceal hemorrhage (Squires & Balistreri, 2016). Severe end-stage complications signaling hepatic failure can occur at any time and with little warning.

Diagnostic evaluation is based on the child's history of infection or disease with liver involvement. Physical examination may reveal jaundice, skin changes, ascites, and hemodynamic changes. Laboratory evaluation reveals abnormal liver function tests. A liver biopsy may help determine the extent of the parenchymal damage.

Medical management focuses on treating the child's symptoms and achieving optimal nutritional status and growth. Liver transplantation is the most common treatment for biliary atresia and metabolic disorders and is the only treatment for end-stage liver disease.

Nursing Management

Nursing care focuses on monitoring physiologic and psychosocial changes to identify early signs of end-stage hepatic failure. Monitor vital signs every 2 to 4 hours. Measure weight daily to assess for fluid retention. Close monitoring of electrolytes and liver function test results helps determine the need for fluid replacement therapy.

Careful administration of medications and monitoring for side effects are necessary because drug metabolism is altered in liver disorders. If ascites is present, provide a low-sodium, low-protein diet and restrict fluids. Remove all water pitchers, glasses, and straws to minimize the child's desire to drink.

Parents of a child with cirrhosis are coping with a life-threatening disorder, and their anxiety and stress are high. The child may be awaiting a liver transplantation that represents the only hope for recovery. Support parents and encourage them to talk about their fears and concerns (see Chapter 13). Encourage parents to participate in the child's care. Referral to a support group or counseling may be beneficial.

Injuries to the Gastrointestinal System

Refer to Chapter 17 for information related to injury to the GI system due to poisoning and ingestion of foreign objects.

Abdominal Trauma

Motor vehicle crashes, falls, and auto–pedestrian injury are the leading causes of blunt abdominal injury in children. Other causes include child abuse, all-terrain vehicle accidents, and bicycle accidents (Mendez, 2014). Although blunt trauma is most common, penetrating injury accounts for 10% to 20% of pediatric trauma admissions. Gunshot wounds are the most common cause of penetrating injury. Other causes include stabbing or impalement on an object (Daley, Raju, & Lee, 2013). Children are more likely than adults to sustain abdominal injuries because of their small pliable rib cage and less developed abdominal muscles, which provide little protection for major solid organs such as the spleen, liver, and kidneys. In addition, the solid organs in children are larger in proportion to their body size compared to adults, so less surface area of the organs is protected by the ribs, making them more exposed and vulnerable to injury (Daley et al., 2013; Mendez, 2014; Saxena, 2013).

The kind of injury determines the extent of organ damage. High-velocity blunt trauma, which may occur in motor vehicle crashes, usually involves multiple organs. Solid organs such as the liver and spleen can be bruised or lacerated. The sudden increase in abdominal pressure that occurs with a lap belt injury causes hollow organs such as the stomach, intestines, and bladder to burst. Sports-related abdominal trauma is often associated with a direct blow to the abdomen, and a single organ is usually injured. Bicycle accidents account for 5% to 14% of blunt abdominal trauma in children. Serious abdominal injury can result if the handlebars hit the child in the abdomen (Alkan et al., 2012; aCevek, Boleken, Sogut, et al., 2013).

Penetrating trauma is generally apparent upon inspection. Blunt trauma may not be as obvious. The abdomen should be inspected for abrasions, bruising, or markings (e.g., tire tracks or lap belt marks) that provide a clue to injury beneath the skin surface (Mendez, 2014). Abrasions, erythema, and ecchymosis in the lower abdominal area are classic visible signs of seat belt trauma (Borgialli et al., 2014). See Chapter 5 for abdominal assessment techniques. Additional clinical manifestations of abdominal injury include pain and tenderness, abdominal distention, and signs of hypovolemic shock such as pallor, altered mental status, hypotension, and tachycardia (Wesson, 2013).

Suspected abdominal trauma in a child necessitates a thorough history and physical examination. The description of the event should be compared with the child's signs and symptoms. Plain abdominal radiographs may reveal air in the abdomen. A focused abdominal ultrasound can reveal free fluid in the abdomen. An abdominal CT scan identifies a solid organ injury. Urinalysis that shows blood in the urine may be indicative of damage to the urinary tract or kidneys (McKenna & Pieper, 2013). Serial hemoglobin and hematocrit evaluation is essential to determine hemodynamic stability. Type and cross-match of blood is also necessary in case the child needs a blood transfusion. In addition, liver function tests and pancreatic enzymes are monitored in the case of injury to the liver and pancreas (Saxena, 2013).

SAFETY ALERT!

The child who is restrained in a motor vehicle with only a lap belt is at high risk for abdominal injury in a crash. As the car stops rapidly, the child's body is restrained and flexes around the lap belt. The sudden increase in abdominal pressure causes injury to hollow organs, and sometimes solid organs. Children no longer using car safety seats should sit in a booster seat so that a shoulder restraint is used in addition to the lap belt. A booster seat should be used until the child is 8 years of age or weighs at least 80 lb.

The spleen and the liver are the organs most commonly injured in blunt abdominal trauma. Nonsurgical management is preferred. The spleen plays a major role in immune function; therefore, the organ is salvaged whenever possible to decrease the risk of infection (Saxena, 2013). Liver lacerations are treated much like spleen lacerations as long as major vessels have not been injured. Exploratory laparotomy is performed to resect hollow organ injuries or to repair liver or spleen lacerations when bleeding is not controlled.

Treatment of an abdominal, liver, or spleen injury takes place in the pediatric intensive care unit (PICU) and focuses on preventing or managing hemorrhage and monitoring for signs of shock. An intravenous infusion is initiated for fluid maintenance and to provide access for blood products. The child is kept NPO. A nasogastric tube is inserted. Blood transfusions and pharmacologic management are used to treat blood loss.

The child is maintained on strict bed rest until bleeding is controlled and the hemoglobin and hematocrit are stable. The length of time the child is hospitalized ranges from 2 to 5 days depending on the severity of the injury. The length of time for activity restrictions after discharge ranges from 3 to 6 weeks and also depends on the severity of the injury (McKenna & Pieper, 2013).

Nursing Management

Nursing care includes initial and ongoing assessments of the child's condition. Assess the abdomen for bruising, pain, guarding, rebound tenderness, distention, and obvious signs of injury such as bruising. Monitor hematocrit and vital signs every hour as warranted to detect hypovolemia (see Chapter 21). Tachycardia and hypotension may indicate hypovolemia or internal bleeding. Strict monitoring of intake and output will provide information about the child's fluid status. Monitor the respiratory status because abdominal injuries may also have thoracic involvement. The child with associated thoracic injuries may not take deep breaths if it is painful.

The child and parents are usually fearful and anxious when the child is admitted to the hospital. If the injury was preventable, parents may have feelings of guilt or anger. Provide emotional support and avoid judgmental comments or statements that assign blame. Additional nursing care includes maintenance of the nasogastric tube, intravenous fluids, and blood, and monitoring of lab studies as appropriate. Any concerns should be reported to the healthcare provider immediately.

Once the child's condition is stabilized, the focus of nursing care shifts to preventive teaching. Parents should be taught safety measures to prevent future injuries. Discuss the use of car safety restraint devices for riding in an automobile (see Chapters 7, 8, and 9). If the child's injury was the result of a bicycle fall or crash, discuss the importance of the proper bicycle size and safety measures such as use of a helmet and proper use of hand signals.

Chapter Highlights

- A variety of structural defects caused by fetal development alterations can affect the gastrointestinal system of infants.

- Cleft lip and palate are structural defects that often involve care by a team of healthcare providers such as a plastic surgeon, pediatrician, nurse, audiologist, speech therapist, and orthodontist.

- A variety of defects of the esophagus and trachea can manifest as mild to life-threatening problems in the newborn period.

- Pyloric stenosis is a common cause of projectile vomiting in the newborn period.

- Gastroesophageal reflux is one of the most common gastrointestinal problems in infants and children.

- Abdominal wall defects and anorectal malformations are serious structural defects of infancy.

- Intussusception is one of the most common causes of intestinal obstruction in the pediatric population and primarily occurs in children less than 1 year of age.

- Hirschsprung disease, or aganglionic megacolon, leads to failure to pass normal stools and distention of the abdomen.

- Several of the intestinal problems of childhood necessitate temporary or permanent ostomy placement.

- Hernias can be present in the diaphragmatic area, umbilicus, or inguinal canal.

- The most common inflammatory disorder of the gastrointestinal tract is appendicitis.

- Necrotizing enterocolitis is a potentially life-threatening inflammatory disease of the intestines seen primarily in premature infants after enteral feedings are begun.

- Common inflammatory bowel diseases affecting primarily adolescent and young adult age groups are Crohn disease and ulcerative colitis.

- Peptic ulcers occur primarily in individuals receiving nonsteroidal anti-inflammatory drugs and those with *Helicobacter pylori* infection.

- Common disorders of motility include diarrhea, constipation, and encopresis.

- Gastroenteritis and parasitic disorders are common causes of gastrointestinal disturbance and distress in children, and may lead to fluid and electrolyte imbalance.

- Short bowel syndrome occurs when surgery is used to treat an intestinal disease and significant sections of the bowel are removed.

- Biliary atresia and hepatitis are the most common liver diseases in young children.

- Abdominal trauma most often occurs to children involved in motor vehicle crashes.

Clinical Reasoning in Action

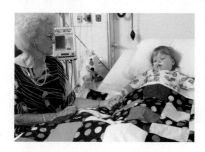

Four-year-old Jenna has just been admitted to the pediatric unit following surgery for a perforated appendix. She complained of her stomach hurting last night, but this morning her condition was worse and she had a temperature of 102°F. Worried that this was not just a virus, Jenna's mother took her to the pediatrician. On the way to the doctor's office Jenna told her mother that her pain "just went away." While at the pediatrician's office she complained of feeling bad all over. On examination, her abdomen was rigid and no bowel sounds were heard. A complete blood count revealed a white blood count (WBC) of 22,000/mm³. The pediatrician diagnosed that Jenna had appendicitis and most likely had a perforated appendix. He referred Jenna to the emergency department for assessment and surgical consultation. A CT scan confirmed a diagnosis of appendicitis. During surgery the appendix was found to have perforated.

Jenna had a laproscopic appendectomy. A dry dressing is in place. She has a peripherally inserted central catheter (PICC) line for fluids, pain medication, and intravenous antibiotics. She also has a nasogastric tube to suction and a Foley catheter.

Jenna's parents are anxious about the surgery. They feel guilty that Jenna became ill so quickly and wonder if they could have done something to prevent it. This is Jenna's first hospitalization. They are worried that she will have a lot of pain and wonder how she will cope with the hospitalization.

1. What is the priority of nursing care for Jenna in the immediate postoperative period?
2. What should the nurse include when teaching Jenna's parents about the postoperative course?
3. Jenna's parents ask why she needs all of the tubes. What information should the nurse include related to the purpose of the nasogastric tube, the Foley catheter, and the central line?
4. Create a concept map for Jenna based on postoperative management of a 4-year-old with a perforated appendix. Include nursing interventions related to fluid and electrolyte balance, pain management, prevention of pulmonary complications, treatment of infection, and developmental and psychosocial care.

References

Agócs, M. M., Serhan, F., Yen, C., Mwenda, J. M., de Oliveira, L. H., Teleb, N., . . . Kang, G. (2014). WHO Global Rotavirus Surveillance Network: A strategic review of the first 5 years, 2008–2012. *Morbidity and Mortality Weekly Report, 63*(29), 634–637.

Akay, B., & Klein, M. D. (2016). Anorectal malformations. In R. M. Kliegman, B. F. Stanton, J. W. St. Geme III, & N. F. Schor (Eds.), *Nelson textbook of pediatrics* (20th ed., pp. 1894–1897). Philadelphia, PA: Elsevier Saunders.

Alkan, M., Iskitt, S. H., Soyupak, S., Tuncer, R., Okur, H., Keskin, E., & Zorludemir, U. (2012). Severe abdominal trauma involving bicycle handlebars in children. *Pediatric Emergency Care, 28*(4), 357–360.

American Academy of Pediatrics (AAP). (2014). *Amount and schedule of formula feedings.* Retrieved from healthychildren.org/English/ages-stages/baby/feeding-nutrition/Pages/Amount-and-Schedule-of-Formula-Feedings.aspx

American Academy of Pediatrics (AAP). (2015). Parasitic diseases. *Red book: 2015 report of the Committee on Infectious Diseases* (30th ed. pp 588–591). Elk Grove Village, IL: Author.

Anand, B. S. (2015). *Peptic ulcer disease treatment & management.* Retrieved from http://emedicine.medscape.com/article/181753-overview

Barman, S., Mandal, K. C., Shukla, R. M., & Mukhopadhyay, B. (2014). Esophageal atresia with tracheoesophageal fistula associated with situs inversus totalis. *Indian Journal of Surgery, 76*(3), 239–240.

Benjamin, B., & Wilson, G. N. (2014). Anomalies associated with gastroschisis and omphalocele: Analysis of 2825 cases from the Texas Birth Defects Registry. *Journal of Pediatric Surgery, 49*, 514–519.

Bergman, N. J. (2013). Neonatal stomach volume and physiology suggest feeding at 1-h intervals. *Acta Paediatrica, 102*, 773–777.

Berman, L., & Moss, R. L. (2011). Necrotizing enterocolitis: An update. *Seminars in Fetal and Neonatal Medicine, 16*, 145–150.

Bhutani, V. K., & Committee on Fetus and Newborn. (2011). Phototherapy to prevent severe neonatal hyperbilirubinemia in the newborn infant 35 or more weeks of gestation. *Pediatrics, 128*(4), e1046–e1052.

Bishop, C. A., & Carter, M. E. (2013). Appendicitis. In N. T. Browne, L. M. Flanigan, C. A. McComiskey, & P. Pieper (Eds.), *Nursing care of the pediatric surgical patient* (3rd ed., pp. 407–416). Burlington, MA: Jones & Bartlett.

Blanco, F. C., Davenport, K. P., & Kane, T. D. (2012). Pediatric gastroesophageal disease. *Surgical Clinics of North America, 92*(3), 541–558.

Blanton, S. H., Henry, R. R., Yuan, Q., Mulliken, J. B., Stal, S., Finnell, R. H., & Hecht, J. T. (2011). Folate pathway and nonsyndromic cleft lip and palate. *Birth Defects Research (Part A): Clinical and Molecular Teratology, 91*, 50–60.

Borgialli, D. A., Ellison, A. M., Ehrlich, P., Bonsu, B., Menaker, J., Wisner, D. H., . . . Holmes, J. F. (2014). Association between the seat belt sign and intra-abdominal injuries in children with blunt torso trauma in motor vehicle collisions. *Academic Emergency Medicine, 21*(11), 1240–1248.

Brandow, A. M., & Camitta, B. M. (2016). Anatomy and function of the spleen. In R. M. Kliegman, B. F. Stanton, J. W. St. Geme III, & N. F. Schor (Eds.), *Nelson textbook of pediatrics* (20th ed., p. 2408). Philadelphia, PA: Elsevier Saunders.

Buggs, A. M. (2014). *Viral hepatitis.* Retrieved from http://emedicine.medscape.com/article/775507-overview

Burkhardt, D. D., Graham, J. M., Short, S. S., & Frykman, P. K. (2014). Advances in Hirschsprung disease genetics and treatment strategies: An update for the primary care pediatrician. *Clinical Pediatrics, 53*(1), 71–81.

Carlo, W. A., & Ambalavanan, N. (2016). The umbilicus. In R. M. Kliegman, B. F. Stanton, J. W. St. Geme III, & N. F. Schor (Eds.), *Nelson textbook of pediatrics* (20th ed., pp. 890–891). Philadelphia, PA: Elsevier Saunders.

Castellani, C., Peschaut, T., Schippinger, M., & Saxena, A. K. (2014). Postoperative emesis after laparoscopic pyloromyotomy in infantile hypertrophic pyloric stenosis. *Acta Paediatrica, 103*(2), e84–87.

Centers for Disease Control and Prevention (CDC). (2012a). *Hepatitis E information for health professionals.* Retrieved from http://www.cdc.gov/hepatitis/HEV/index.htm

Centers for Disease Control and Prevention (CDC). (2012b). *Hepatitis B information for health professionals.* Retrieved from http://www.cdc.gov/hepatitis/HBV/index.htm

Centers for Disease Control and Prevention (CDC). (2012c). *The ABCs of hepatitis.* Retrieved from http://www.cdc.gov/hepatitis/Resources/Professionals/PDFs/ABCTable.pdf

Centers for Disease Control and Prevention (CDC). (2014a). *Parasites.* Retrieved from http://www.cdc.gov/parasites

Centers for Disease Control and Prevention (CDC). (2014b). *Healthy pets, healthy people.* Retrieved from http://www.cdc.gov/Features/HealthyPets

Centers for Disease Control and Prevention (CDC). (2014c). *Viral hepatitis surveillance—United States, 2012.* Retrieved from http://www.cdc.gov/hepatitis/Statistics/2012Surveillance/PDFs/2012HepSurveillanceRpt.pdf

Centers for Disease Control and Prevention (CDC). (2014d). *Hepatitis A information for health professionals*. Retrieved from http://www.cdc.gov/hepatitis/HAV/index.htm

Centers for Disease Control and Prevention (CDC). (2014e). *Hepatitis C information for health professionals*. Retrieved from http://www.cdc.gov/hepatitis/HCV

Centers for Disease Control and Prevention (CDC). (2014f). *Hepatitis D information for health professionals*. Retrieved from http://www.cdc.gov/hepatitis/HDV/index.htm

Cevek, M., Boleken, M. E., Sogut, O., Gokdemir, M. T., & Karakas, E. (2013). Abdominal injuries related to bicycle accidents in children. *Pediatric Surgery International, 29*(5), 459–463.

Chason, R. D., Reisch, J. S., & Rockey, D. C. (2013). More favorable outcomes with peptic ulcer bleeding due to Helicobacter pylori. *The American Journal of Medicine, 126*(9), 811–818.

Cochran, A. A., Higgins, G. L., & Strout, T. D. (2011). Intussusception in traditional pediatric, nontraditional pediatric, and adult patients. *American Journal of Emergency Medicine, 29*, 523–527.

Coehlo, D. P. (2011). Encopresis: A medical and family approach. *Pediatric Nursing, 37*(3), 107–112.

Coha, T. (2013). Care of the child with an ostomy. In N. T. Browne, L. M. Flanigan, C. A. McComiskey, & P. Pieper (Eds.), *Nursing care of the pediatric surgical patient* (3rd ed., pp. 121–148). Burlington, MA: Jones & Bartlett.

Collopy, K., & Friese, G. (2010). Pediatric drug administration. *Emergency Medical Services Magazine, 39*(6), 52–57.

Corey, K. M., Hornik, C. P., Laughon, M. M., McHutchison, K., Clark, R. H., & Smith, P. B. (2014). Frequency of anomalies and hospital outcomes in infants with gastroschisis and omphalocele. *Early Human Development, 90*, 421–424.

Correa, J. A, Fallon, S. C., Murphy, K. M., Victorian, V. A., Bisset, G. S., Vasudevan, S. A., . . . Lee, T. C. (2014). Resource utilization after gastrostomy tube placement: Defining areas of improvement for future quality improvement projects. *Journal of Pediatric Surgery, 49*, 1598–1601.

Crockett, D. J., & Goudy, S. L. (2014). Cleft lip and palate. *Facial Plastic Surgery Clinics of North America, 22*(4), 573–586.

Cuffari, C. (2014). *Pediatric short bowel syndrome*. Retrieved from http://emedicine.medscape.com/article/931855-overview

Daley, B. J., Raju, R., & Lee. S. (2013). *Considerations in pediatric trauma*. Retrieved from http://emedicine.medscape.com/article/435031-overview

Deloach, R., & Farber, L. D. (2013). Intussusception. In N. T. Browne, L. M. Flanigan, C. A. McComiskey, & P. Pieper (Eds.), *Nursing care of the pediatric surgical patient* (3rd ed., pp. 399–406). Burlington, MA: Jones & Bartlett.

Fiorino, K., & Liacouras, C. A. (2016). Congenital aganglionic megacolon (Hirschsprung disease). In R. M. Kliegman, B. F. Stanton, J. W. St. Geme III, & N. F. Schor (Eds.), *Nelson textbook of pediatrics* (20th ed., pp. 1809–1811). Philadelphia, PA: Elsevier Saunders.

Flanigan, L. M. (2013). Biliary atresia and choledochal cyst. In N. T. Browne, L. M. Flanigan, C. A. McComiskey, & P. Pieper (Eds.), *Nursing care of the pediatric surgical patient* (3rd ed., pp. 435–446). Burlington, MA: Jones & Bartlett.

Garabedian, C., Verpillat, P. Czerkiewicz, I., Langlois, C., Muller, F., Avni, F., . . . Houfflin-Debarge, V. (2014). Does a combination of ultrasound, MRI, and biochemical amniotic fluid analysis improve prenatal diagnosis of esophageal atresia? *Prenatal Diagnosis, 34*, 839–842.

Gershon, A. A., & Hotez, P. J. (2011). Infectious diseases. In C. D. Rudolph, A. M. Rudolph, G. E. Lister, L. R. First, & A. A. Gershon (Eds.), *Rudolph's pediatrics* (22nd ed., pp. 878–1247). New York, NY: McGraw-Hill.

Glasser, J. G. (2014). *Pediatric omphalocele and gastroschisis*. Retrieved from http://emedicine.medscape.com/article/975583-overview

Glick, S. R., & Carvalho, R. S. (2011). Inflammatory bowel disease. *Pediatrics in Review, 32*(1), 14–25.

Goldson E., & Reynolds, A. (2012). Child development & behavior. In W. W. Hay, Jr., M. J. Levin, R. R. Deterding, M. J. Abzug, & J. M. Sondheimer (Eds.), *CURRENT diagnosis & treatment: Pediatrics* (21st ed.). New York, NY: McGraw-Hill. Retrieved from http://www.accessmedicine.com

Gregory, K. E., DeForge, C. E., Natale, K. M., Phillips, M., & VanMarter, L. J. (2011). Necrotizing enterocolitis in the premature infant: Neonatal nursing assessment, disease pathogenesis, and clinical presentation. *Advances in Neonatal Care, 11*(3), 155–164.

Grossman, A. B., & Baldassano, R. N. (2016). Inflammatory bowel disease. In R. M. Kliegman, B. F. Stanton, J. W. St. Geme III, & N. F. Schor (Eds.), *Nelson textbook of pediatrics* (20th ed., p. 1819–1831). Philadelphia, PA: Elsevier Saunders.

Grossman, A. B., & Mamula, P. (2014). *Pediatric Crohn disease*. Retrieved from http://emedicine.medscape.com/article/928288-overview

Groves, L. B., Ladd, M. R., Gallaher, J. R., Swanson, J., Becher, R. D., Pranikoff, T., & Neff, L. P. (2013). Comparing the cost and outcomes of laparoscopic versus open appendectomy for perforated appendicitis in children. *The American Surgeon, 79*(9), 861–864.

Guardino, K. O., & Pieper, P. (2013). Anorectal malformations in children. In N. T. Browne, L. M. Flanigan, C. A. McComiskey, & P. Pieper (Eds.), *Nursing care of the pediatric surgical patient* (3rd ed., pp. 359–372). Burlington, MA: Jones & Bartlett.

Gutierrez, I. M., Kang, K. H., & Jaksic, T. (2011). Neonatal short bowel syndrome. *Seminars in Fetal & Neonatal Medicine, 16*, 157–163.

Hannah, E., & John, R. M. (2013). Everything the nurse practitioner should know about pediatric feeding tubes. *Journal of the American Association of Nurse Practitioners, 25*, 567–577.

Hansen, T. W. R. (2014). *Neonatal jaundice*. Retrieved from http://emedicine.medscape.com/article/974786-overview

Harris, H., & Crawford, A. (2013). Hepatitis goes viral. *Nursing 2013, 43*(11), 38–43.

Hassan, H. H. A-K., & Balistreri, W. F. (2016). Neonatal cholestasis. In R. M. Kliegman, B. F. Stanton, J. W. St. Geme III, & N. F. Schor (Eds.), *Nelson textbook of pediatrics* (20th ed., pp. 1928–1932). Philadelphia, PA: Elsevier Saunders.

Hebra, A., & Cuffari, C. (2012). *Intestinal volvulus*. Retrieved from http://emedicine.medscape.com/article/930576-overview

Holder, M., & Jackson, L. (2013). Hirschsprung's disease. In N. T. Browne, L. M. Flanigan, C. A. McComiskey, & P. Pieper (Eds.), *Nursing care of the pediatric surgical patient* (3rd ed., pp. 347–358). Burlington, MA: Jones & Bartlett.

Hood, E., & Zimmerman, B. T. (2013). Abdominal wall defects. In N. T. Browne, L. M. Flanigan, C. A. McComiskey, & P. Pieper (Eds.), *Nursing care of the pediatric surgical patient* (3rd ed., pp. 277–294). Burlington, MA: Jones & Bartlett.

Huda, S., Chaudhery, S., Ibrahim, H., & Pramanik, A. (2014). Neonatal necrotizing enterocolitis: Clinical challenges, pathophysiology and management. *Pathophysiology, 21*, 3–12.

Hung, M.-H., Lin, L.-H., & Chen, D. F. (2012). Clinical manifestations in children with ruptured appendicitis. *Pediatric Emergency Care, 28*(5), 433–435.

Hunter, A. K., & Liacouras, C. A. (2016). Hypertrophic pyloric stenosis. In R. M. Kliegman, B. F. Stanton, J. W. St. Geme III, & N. F. Schor (Eds.), *Nelson textbook of pediatrics* (20th ed., pp. 1797–1799). Philadelphia, PA: Elsevier Saunders.

Huppert, S. S., & Balistreri, W. F. (2016). Morphogenesis of the liver and biliary system. In R. M. Kliegman, B. F. Stanton, J. W. St. Geme III, & N. F. Schor (Eds.), *Nelson textbook of pediatrics* (19th ed., p. 1918–1921). Philadelphia, PA: Elsevier Saunders.

Jensen, M. K., & Balistreri, W. F. (2016). Viral hepatitis. In R. M. Kliegman, B. F. Stanton, J. W. St. Geme III, & N. F. Schor (Eds.), *Nelson textbook of pediatrics* (20th ed., pp. 1942–1953). Philadelphia, PA: Elsevier Saunders.

Kelly, D., O'Dowd, T., & Reulbach, U. (2012). Use of folic acid supplements and risk of cleft lip and palate in infants: A population-based cohort study. *British Journal of General Practice, 62*(600), e466–e472.

Kelsen, J. R., & Mamula, P. (2013). *Ulcerative colitis in children*. Retrieved from http://emedicine.medscape.com/article/930146-overview

Khan, S., & Orenstein, S. R. (2016a). Esophageal atresia and tracheoesophageal fistula. In R. M. Kliegman, B. F. Stanton, J. W. St. Geme III, & N. F. Schor (Eds.), *Nelson textbook of pediatrics* (20th ed., pp. 1783–1784). Philadelphia, PA: Elsevier Saunders.

Khan, S., & Orenstein, S. R. (2016b). Gastroesophageal reflux disease. In R. M. Kliegman, B. F. Stanton, J. W. St. Geme III, & N. F. Schor (Eds.), *Nelson textbook of pediatrics* (20th ed., pp. 1787–1791). Philadelphia, PA: Elsevier Saunders.

Kotecha, M., Bellah, R., Pena, A. H., Jaimes, C., & Mattei, P. (2012). Multimodality imaging manifestations of the Meckel diverticulum in children. *Pediatric Radiology, 42*, 95–103.

Ladd, M. R., Pajewski, N. M., Becher, R. D., Swanson, J. M., Gallaher, J. R., Pranikoff, T., & Neff, L. P. (2013). Delays in treatment of pediatric appendicitis: a more accurate variable for measuring pediatric healthcare inequalities? *The American Surgeon, 79*(9), 875–881.

Langer, J. C. (2013). Hirschsprung disease. *Current Opinion in Pediatrics, 25*(3), 368–374.

Lauer, B. J., & Spector, N. D. (2011). Hyperbilirubinemia in the newborn. *Pediatrics in Review, 32*(8), 341–349.

Ledbetter, D. J. (2012). Congenital abdominal wall defects and reconstruction in pediatric surgery: Gastroschisis and omphalocele. *Surgical Clinics of North America, 92*, 713–727.

Lee, J. Y., Jun, J. K., & Lee, J. (2014). Prenatal prediction of neonatal survival in cases diagnosed with congenital diaphragmatic hernia using abdomen-to-thorax ratio determined by ultrasonography. *Journal of Obstetrics and Gynaecology Research, 40*(9), 2037–2043.

Lee, S. L., Yaghoubian, A., Stark, R., Sydorak, R. M., & Kaji, A. (2012). Are there differences in access to care, treatment, and outcomes for children with appendicitis treated at county versus private hospitals? *The Permanente Journal, 16*(1), 4–6.

Levas, M. N., Dayan, P. S., Mittal, M. K., Stevenson, M. D., Bachur, R. G., Dudley, N. C., . . . Kharbanda, A. B. (2014). Effect of Hispanic ethnicity and language barriers on appendiceal perforation rates and imaging in children. *The Journal of Pediatrics, 164*(6), 1286–1291.

Liacouras, C.A. (2016). Normal development, structure, and function. In R. M. Kliegman, B. F. Stanton, J. W. St. Geme III, & N. F. Schor (Eds.), *Nelson textbook of pediatrics* (20th ed., pp. 1796–1797). Philadelphia, PA: Elsevier Saunders.

Lightdale, J. R., & Gremse, D. A. (2013). Gastroesophageal reflux: Management guidance for the pediatrician. *Pediatrics, 131*(5), e1684–e1695.

Lin, C-Y, Chi, H., Hsu, C-H, Huang, F-Y, Lee, H-C, & Chiu, N-C. (2014). Peristaltic waves in infantile hypertrophic pyloric stenosis. *The Journal of Pediatrics, 164*(2), 423.

Lindholm, E., Persson, E., Carlsson, E., Hallén, A-M., Fingren, J., & Berndtsson, I. (2013). Ostomy-related complications after emergent abdominal surgery: A 2-year follow-up study. *Journal of Wound Ostomy & Continence Nursing, 40*(6), 603–610.

Lisonkova, S., & Joseph, K. S. (2013). Similarities and differences in the epidemiology of pyloric stenosis and SIDS. *Maternal Child Health Journal, 18*(7), 1721–1727.

Liszewski, M. C., Bairdain, S., Buonomo, C., Jennings, R. W. & Taylor, G. A. (2014). Imaging of long gap esophageal atresia and the Foker process: Expected findings and complications. *Pediatric Radiology, 44*(4), 467–475.

Lozada, L. E., Royall, M. J., Nylund, C. M., & Eberly, M. D. (2013). Development of pyloric stenosis after a 4-day course of oral Erythromycin. *Pediatric Emergency Care, 29*(4), 498–499.

Marcdante, K. J., & Kliegman, R. M. (2015). Esophagus and stomach. In K. J. Marcdante & R. M. Kliegman (Eds.), *Nelson essentials of pediatrics* (7th ed., pp. 430–437). Philadelphia, PA: Elsevier Saunders.

Markowitz, R. I. (2014). Olive without a cause: the story of infantile hypertrophic pyloric stenosis. *Pediatric Radiology, 44*(2), 202–211.

Mason, I. (2014). Supporting community patients with irritable bowel syndrome (IBS). *Journal of Community Nursing, 28*(1), 28–33.

McAteer, J. P., Ledbetter, D. J., & Goldin, A. B. (2013). Role of bottle feeding in the etiology of hypertrophic pyloric stenosis. *JAMA Pediatrics, 167*(12), 1143–1149.

McKenna, C., & Pieper, P. (2013). Pediatric trauma. In N. T. Browne, L. M. Flanigan, C. A. McComiskey, & P. Pieper (Eds.), *Nursing care of the pediatric surgical patient* (3rd ed., pp. 513–535). Burlington, MA: Jones & Bartlett.

Mendez, D. R. (2014). *Overview of blunt abdominal trauma in children.* Retrieved from http://www.uptodate.com/contents/overview-of-blunt-abdominal-trauma-in-children

Mieli-Vergani, G., & Tizzard, S. A. (2012). Biliary atresia and Kasai's surgery—When is it too late? *Pediatric OnCall Journal, 9*(9). Retrieved from http://www.pediatriconcall.com/Journal/Article/FullText.aspx?artid=511&type=J&tid=&imgid=&reportid=358&tbltype

Minkes, R. K., & Alder, A. C. (2014). *Pediatric appendicitis.* Retrieved from http://emedicine.medscape.com/article/926795-overview

Moreira, R. K., Cabral, R., Cowles, R. A., & Lobritto, S. J. (2012). Biliary atresia: A multidisciplinary approach to diagnosis and management. *Archives of Pathology and Laboratory Medicine, 136*(7), 746–760.

Morgan, J. A., Young, L., & McGuire, W. (2011). Pathogenesis and prevention of necrotizing enterocolitis. *Current Opinion in Infectious Disease, 24,* 183–189.

Muchowski, K. (2014). Evaluation and treatment of neonatal hyperbilirubinemia. *American Family Physician, 89*(11), 873–878.

Nelville, H. L. (2014). *Pediatric Hirschsprung disease.* Retrieved from http://emedicine.medscape.com/article/929733-overview

Nowicki, D. E. (2013). Esophageal defects. In N. T. Browne, L. M. Flanigan, C. A. McComiskey, & P. Pieper (Eds.), *Nursing care of the pediatric surgical patient* (3rd ed., pp. 219–245). Burlington, MA: Jones & Bartlett.

Nurko, S., & Zimmerman, L. A. (2014). Evaluation and treatment of constipation in children and adolescents. *American Family Physician, 90*(2), 82–90.

Orr, S. (2011). Anal dilatation in children with anorectal malformations. *Gastrointestinal Nursing, 9*(8), 37–40.

Patel, P. K., Cohen, S., Ramaswamy, R., Grasseschi, M. F., & Morris, D. E. (2014). *Unilateral cleft lip repair.* Retrieved from http://emedicine.medscape.com/article/1279641-overview

Paul, S. P., Dewdney, C., & Lam, C. (2012). Managing children with constipation in the community. *Nurse Prescribing, 10*(6), 274–284.

Peate, I., & Jones, N. (2014). Caring for hepatitis B. *British Journal of Healthcare Assistants, 8*(8), 384–389.

Pepper, V. K., Stanfill, A. B., & Pearl, R. H. (2012). Diagnosis and management of pediatric appendicitis, intussusception, and Meckel diverticulum. *Surgical Clinics of North America, 92,* 505–526.

Peyrin-Biroulet, L. (2011). Why should we define and target early Crohn's disease? *Gastroenterology & Hepatology, 7*(5), 324–326.

Randel, A. (2014). AAP releases guideline for the management of gastroesophageal reflux in children. *American Family Physician, 89*(5), 395–397.

Rapoport, K., & Nishii, E. K. (2013). Necrotizing enterocolitis. In N. T. Browne, L. M. Flanigan, C. A. McComiskey, & P. Pieper (Eds.), *Nursing care of the pediatric surgical patient* (3rd ed., pp. 295–311). Burlington, MA: Jones & Bartlett.

Razmus, I. S. (2011). Assessment and management of children with abdominal wall defects. *Journal of Wound, Ostomy, Continence Nursing, 38*(1), 22–26.

Robie, D. K., Overfelt, S. R., & Xie, L. (2014). Differentiating biliary atresia from other causes of cholestatic jaundice. *American Surgeon, 80*(9), 827–831.

Rogers, J. (2011). Functional constipation in childhood. *Nurse Prescribing, 9*(7), 326–331.

Rogers, J. (2012). Assessment, prevention and treatment of constipation in children. *Nursing Standard, 26*(29), 46–52.

Rollins, M. D. (2012). Recent advances in the management of congenital diaphragmatic hernia. *Current Opinion in Pediatrics, 24*(3), 379–385.

Ruano, R., Picone, O., Bernardes, L., Martinovic, J., Dumez, Y., & Benachi, A. (2011). The association of gastroschisis with other congenital anomalies: How important is it? *Prenatal Diagnosis, 31,* 347–350.

Santacroce, L., & Ochoa, J. B. (2013). *Appendectomy.* Retrieved from http://emedicine.medscape.com/article/195778-overview

Saxena, A. K. (2013). *Pediatric abdominal trauma.* Retrieved from http://emedicine.medscape.com/article/1984811-overview

Saxena, A. K., Blair, G., & Konkin, D. E. (2014). *Esophageal atresia with or without tracheoesophageal fistula.* Retrieved from http://emedicine.medscape.com/article/935858-overview

Schwartz, H. P., Haberman, B. E., & Ruddy, R. M. (2011). Hyperbilirubinemia: Current guidelines and emerging therapies. *Pediatric Emergency Care, 27*(9), 884–889.

Schwarz, S. M. (2014). *Pediatric biliary atresia.* Retrieved from http://emedicine.medscape.com/article/927029-overview

Schwarz, S. M., & Hebra, A. (2014). *Pediatric gastroesophageal reflux.* Retrieved from http://emedicine.medscape.com/article/930029-overview

Schweitzer, M., Aucoin, J., Docherty, S. L., Rice, H. E., Thompson, J., & Sullivan, D. T. (2014). Evaluation of a discharge education protocol for pediatric patients with gastrostomy tubes. *Journal of Pediatric Health Care, 28*(5), 420–428.

Seagraves, K., Brulte, A., McNeely, K., & Pritham, U. (2013). Supporting breastfeeding to reduce newborn readmissions for hyperbilirubinemia. *Nursing for Women's Health, 17*(6), 498–507.

Setó-Salvia, N., & Stanier, P. (2014). Genetics of cleft lip and/or cleft palate: Association with other common anomalies. *European Journal of Medical Genetics, 57*(8), 381–393.

Sfakianaki. A. K. (2012). Congenital diaphragmatic hernia. *Contemporary OB/GYN, 57*(9), 26–36.

Shalaby, M. S., Kuti, K., & Walker, G. (2013). Intestinal malrotation and volvulus in infants and children. *British Medical Journal, 347*(7936), 33–35.

Singh, M., Kadian, Y. S., Rattan, K. N., & Jangra, B. (2014). Complicated appendicitis: Analysis of risk factors in children. *African Journal of Paediatric Surgery, 11*(2), 109–113.

Sira, M. M., Taha, M., & Sira, A. M. (2014). Common misdiagnoses of biliary atresia. *European Journal of Gastroenterology & Hepatology, 26*(11), 1300–1305.

Sluiter, I., van de Ven, C. P., Wijnen, R. M. H., & Tibboel, D. (2011). Congenital diaphragmatic hernia: Still a moving target. *Seminars in Fetal & Neonatal Medicine, 16,* 139–144.

Squires, J. E., & Balistreri, W. F. (2016). Manifestations of liver disease. In R. M. Kliegman, B. F. Stanton, J. W. St. Geme III, & N. F. Schor (Eds.), *Nelson textbook of pediatrics* (20th ed., pp. 1922–1928). Philadelphia, PA: Elsevier Saunders.

Tarbell, S. E., & Li, B. U. K. (2013). Health-related quality of life in children and adolescents with cyclic vomiting syndrome: A comparison with published data on youth with irritable bowel syndrome and organic gastrointestinal disorders. *Journal of Pediatrics, 163*(2), 493–497.

Taylor, N. D., Cass, D. T., & Holland, A. J. A. (2013). Infantile hypertrophic pyloric stenosis: Has anything changed? *Journal of Paediatrics and Child Health, 49*(1), 33–37.

Territo, H. M., Wrotniak, B. H., Qiao, H., & Lillis, K. (2014). Clinical signs and symptoms associated with intussusception in young children undergoing ultrasound in the emergency room. *Pediatric Emergency Care, 30*(10), 718–722.

Tigges, C. R., & Bigham, M. T. (2012). Hypertrophic pyloric stenosis: It can take your breath away. *Air Medical Journal, 31*(1), 45–48.

Triantafillidis, J. K., Merikas, E., & Georgopoulos, F. (2011). Current and emerging drugs for the treatment. *Drug Design, Development and Therapy, 5,* 185–210.

Tutay, G. J., Capraro, G., Spirko, B., Garb, J., & Smithline, H. (2013). Electrolyte profile of pediatric patients with hypertrophic pyloric stenosis. *Pediatric Emergency Care, 29*(4), 465–468.

Vitola, B. E., & Balistreri, W. F. (2016). Liver disease associated with systemic disorders. In

R. M. Kliegman, B. F. Stanton, J. W. St. Geme III, & N. F. Schor (Eds.), *Nelson textbook of pediatrics* (20th ed., pp. 1954–1957). Philadelphia, PA: Elsevier Saunders.

Watson, L. (2014). Constipation in children. *Nursing Standard, 28*(41), 18.

Wells, C., Ahmed, A., & Musser, A. (2013). Strategies for neonatal hyperbilirubinemia: A literature review. *MCN: American Journal of Maternal Child Nursing, 38*(6), 377–382.

Werlin, S. L., & Wilschanski, M. (2016). Exocrine pancreas. In R. M. Kliegman, B. F. Stanton, J. W. St. Geme III, & N. F. Schor (Eds.), *Nelson textbook of*

pediatrics (20th ed., pp.1909–1911). Philadelphia, PA: Elsevier Saunders.

Wesson, D. E. (2013). *Liver, spleen, and pancreas injury in children with blunt abdominal trauma.* Retrieved from uptodate.com

Wiet, G. J., Biavati, M. J., & Rocha-Worley, G. (2013). *Reconstructive surgery for cleft palate.* Retrieved from http://emedicine.medscape.com/ article/878062-overview

Wilkins-Haug, L. (2014). *Etiology, prenatal diagnosis, obstetrical management, and recurrence of orofacial clefts.* Retrieved from http://emedicine.medscape. com/article/ 878062-overview

Wilson, B. A., Shannon, M. T., & Shields, K. M. (2015). *Pearson nurse's drug guide 2015.* Hoboken, NJ: Pearson Education.

Wright, K., & Miller, H. D. (2012). Evidence-based findings of necrotizing enterocolitis. *Newborn and Infant Nursing Reviews, 12*(1), 17–20.

Zerpa, J. A., & Shapiro, T. J. (2013). Malrotation and volvulus. In N. T. Browne, L. M. Flanigan, C. A. McComiskey, & P. Pieper (Eds.), *Nursing care of the pediatric surgical patient* (3rd ed., pp. 333–346). Burlington, MA: Jones & Bartlett.

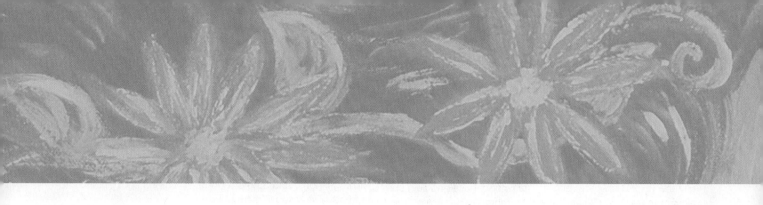

Chapter 26
Alterations in Genitourinary Function

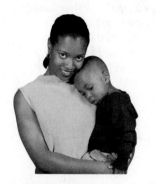

Planning Terrell's day can be a challenge, because his treatment often interferes with his activities. We all hope that Terrell receives a kidney transplant soon so his growth will improve and he will not have to miss school during treatment.
—Aunt of Terrell, 5 years old

Amos Morgan/Getty Images

Learning Outcomes

26.1 Describe the pathophysiologic processes associated with genitourinary disorders in the pediatric population.

26.2 Develop a nursing care plan for the child with a urinary tract infection.

26.3 Discuss the nursing management of a child with a structural defect of the genitourinary system.

26.4 Outline a plan to meet the fluid and dietary restrictions for the child with a renal disorder.

26.5 Identify growth and developmental issues for the child with chronic renal failure.

26.6 Plan nursing care for the child with acute and chronic renal failure.

26.7 Summarize psychosocial issues for the child requiring surgery on the genitourinary system.

Many infections, structural disorders, and disease processes alter genitourinary function. Because the kidneys and other urinary system organs perform several essential body functions, including removal of waste products and maintenance of fluid and electrolyte balance, disorders that affect these organs pose a significant threat to the health of children.

Although the reproductive system is functionally immature until puberty, uncorrected structural defects can have both psychologic and physiologic implications for the developing child.

Urinary Tract Infection

An infection of the urinary tract may be of bacterial, viral, or fungal origin, and can occur in the lower or upper urinary tract. Cystitis is a lower urinary tract infection (UTI) that involves the urethra or bladder. Pyelonephritis is an upper UTI that involves

the ureters, pelvis, and renal parenchyma. UTIs can be acute or chronic (the latter being either recurrent or persistent).

Urinary tract infections are very common in children, with 8% of girls and 2% of boys having at least one UTI by 7 years of age (White, 2011). It is further estimated that 1% of boys and 3% to 5% of girls will have a UTI during childhood and 30% to 50% of them will have at least more than one UTI (Paintsil, 2013).

Etiology and Pathophysiology

Most UTIs in children are caused by *Escherichia coli*, a common gram-negative enteric bacterium (White, 2011). Urinary stasis enhances the risk of UTI. Stasis may be caused by abnormal anatomic structures or abnormal function (e.g., **neurogenic bladder** in which an interrupted nerve supply from myelomeningocele or spinal cord trauma impairs the bladder's voiding function and leads to incomplete bladder emptying). Children normally void 5 to 6 times

Text continues on page 704

FOCUS ON:
The Genitourinary System

Anatomy and Physiology

The genitourinary system is made up of the urinary and reproductive organs. The urinary system—kidneys, ureters, bladder, and urethra—excretes wastes and maintains acid–base and fluid and electrolyte balance (Figure 26–1). The reproductive system consists of internal and external organs that at maturity promote the conception and healthy development of a fetus. Normal renal function requires the following: unimpaired renal blood flow, adequate glomerular ultrafiltration, normal tubular function, and unobstructed urine flow.

The functional unit of the kidney, the nephron, contributes to the formation of urine. The nephron is a tubular structure containing the renal corpuscle, proximal convoluted tubule, loop of Henle, distal convoluted tubule, and collecting duct. The renal corpuscle is composed of the glomerulus (a small group of capillaries) that loops into the Bowman capsule (Figure 26–2). The glomerular capillaries serve as the filtration membrane where metabolic wastes and fluids are separated from the blood cells and plasma proteins to form the urine. The kidney maintains the rate of blood flow to keep the glomerular filtration rate fairly constant. The urine

flows through the proximal convoluted tubule, the loop of Henle, and into the distal convoluted tubule and collecting duct. Water, sodium, potassium, glucose, amino acids, bicarbonate, urea, hydrogen ions, and ammonia ions are among substances reabsorbed or secreted in the tubules.

The presence of antidiuretic hormone (ADH) secreted by the posterior pituitary gland causes more water reabsorption, leading to urine concentration. Absence of ADH leads to dilute urine. See Chapter 18 for more information about fluid and electrolyte physiology.

Urine from the nephron flows into the calyces in the renal pelvis and is funneled into the ureters. The lower end of the ureters connects into the posterior aspect of the bladder. The muscle cells of the ureters move urine to the bladder by peristalsis. Urine collects in the bladder until the internal urethral sphincter relaxes and allows urine to pass into the urethra. Voluntary control of the external urethral sphincter is gained as the child's nervous system matures. Contraction of the bladder during urination compresses the lower end of the ureter and prevents the reflux of urine back into the ureter.

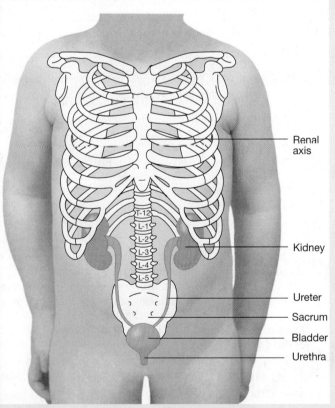

Figure 26–1 **The urinary system is composed of the kidneys, ureters, bladder, and urethra. The kidneys are located between the twelfth thoracic (T12) and third lumbar (L3) vertebrae.**

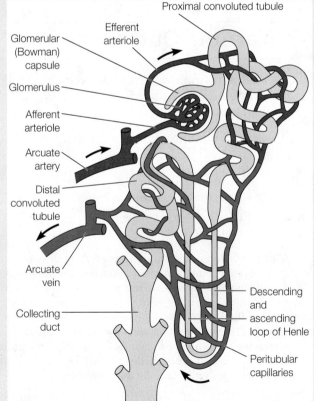

Figure 26–2 **The nephron is the structural and functional unit of the kidneys. A nephron holds six glomeruli, Bowman capsule, proximal tubule, loop of Henle, distal tubule, and the collecting duct.**

The kidney is essential in activating vitamin D, which is needed for the absorption of calcium and phosphorus from the small intestine. The kidney secretes erythropoietin to stimulate the bone marrow to produce red blood cells. The renin-angiotensin system of the kidney is a hormonal regulator that can increase the systemic blood pressure.

The male reproductive system is composed of the testes and scrotum, penis, prostate, and vas deferens, which drains into the urethra. The testes produce the primary male sex hormone, testosterone. The testes produce sperm after puberty.

The female reproductive system is composed of the ovaries, fallopian tubes, uterus, and vagina. The ovaries produce the primary female sex hormone, estrogen. Beginning between 8 and 12 years of age, the ovaries produce increasing amounts of sex hormones to initiate puberty and sexual maturation. After puberty, the ovaries produce the ovum that may be fertilized by the sperm during its passage through the fallopian tube into the uterus. Complex hormonal factors are involved in puberty, the menstrual cycle, and pregnancy.

Pediatric Differences

Urinary System

All the nephrons that will make up the mature kidney are present at birth. The kidneys grow and the tubular system matures gradually during childhood, reaching full size by adolescence.

Most renal growth occurs during the first 5 years of life. This increase in size is due primarily to enlargement of the nephrons. The kidney's efficiency also increases with age. During the first 2 years of life, the kidneys are less efficient at regulating electrolyte and acid–base balance (see Chapter 18) and eliminating some drugs from the body. After the age of 2 years, the kidneys' efficiency markedly increases. Urinary output per kilogram of body weight decreases as the child ages, because the kidney becomes more efficient at concentrating urine. The expected output is as follows:

- Infants—2 mL/kg/hr
- Children—0.5 to 1 mL/kg/hr
- Adolescents—40 to 80 mL per hour

Bladder capacity increases with age from 20 to 50 mL at birth to 700 mL in adulthood. A child's bladder capacity (in ounces) can be estimated by adding 2 to the child's age (e.g., a 4-year-old has a bladder capacity of 6 ounces). Stimulation of "stretch receptors" within the bladder wall initiates urination. Simultaneous contraction of the detrusor muscle of the bladder and relaxation of the internal and external sphincters result in emptying of the bladder. Children less than 2 years of age cannot maintain bladder control because of insufficient nerve development (see *As Children Grow: Development of the Genitourinary System*).

As Children Grow: **Development of the Genitourinary System**

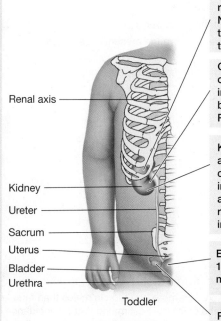

Renal axis

Kidney
Ureter
Sacrum
Uterus
Bladder
Urethra

Toddler

All nephrons are present at birth, the ureters are short, and tubules have a smaller surface area, resulting in diminished water reabsorption. Nephrons grow in size, and the kidneys and the tubule system gradually develop during childhood to reach adult size during adolescence.

Glomerular filtration rate (GFR) in a neonate is one third to one fourth of adult levels. GFR increases progressively and reaches adult levels between 1 and 2 years of age (Otukesh, Hoseini, Rahimzadeh, et al., 2012).

Kidneys are less efficient at regulating electrolyte and acid–base balance, and less able to concentrate urine. Diarrhea, infection, and improper feeding may lead to severe acidosis and fluid imbalance. Efficiency of the kidneys in regulating electrolytes and acid–base balance increases after 2 years of age.

Expected urine output for a neonate and infant is 1–2 mL/kg/hr, while an adult should have 0.5 mL/kg/hr (Alarcon & Fink, 2015).

Reproductive system is immature.

Reproductive system matures after puberty.

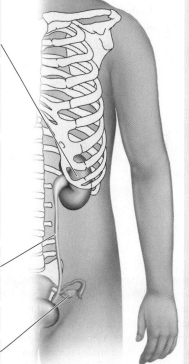

Adolescent

Source: Data from Otukesh, H., Hoseini, R., Rahimzadeh, N., & Hosseini, S. (2012). Glomerular function in neonates. *Iranian Journal of Kidney Diseases, 6*(3), 166–172; Alarcon, L. H., & Fink, M. P. (2015). Physiologic monitoring of the surgical patient. In F. C. Brunicardi, D. K. Andersen, T. R. Billiar, D. L. Dunn, J. G. Hunter, J. B. Matthews, & R. E. Pollock (Eds.), *Schwartz's principles of surgery* (10th ed.). Retrieved from http://www.accessmedicine.com

(continued)

Reproductive System

Throughout childhood the genitalia (with the exception of the clitoris in girls) enlarge gradually. The hormonal changes of puberty accelerate anatomic and functional development (see Chapter 5 for figures illustrating pubertal development). In girls, the mons pubis becomes more prominent, and hair begins to grow. The vagina lengthens, and the epithelial layers thicken. The uterus and ovaries enlarge, and the musculature and vascularization of the uterus also increase. In boys, downy hair begins to appear at the base of the penis, and the scrotum becomes increasingly pendulous as the testes enlarge. The penis increases in length and width.

Use *Assessment Guide: The Child With a Genitourinary Condition* to perform a nursing assessment of the genitourinary system. A list of diagnostic and laboratory tests commonly used to evaluate genitourinary conditions is provided in Table 26–1. See Appendices D and E for expected laboratory values and further information about specific diagnostic procedures.

TABLE 26–1 Diagnostic Tests and Laboratory Procedures for the Genitourinary System

DIAGNOSTIC PROCEDURES	LABORATORY TESTS
Computed tomography (CT)	Blood urea nitrogen (BUN)
Cystoscopy	Creatinine
Diuretic renogram (a type of nuclear scan)	Creatinine clearance
Intravenous pyelogram	Basic metabolic panel (electrolytes)
Magnetic resonance imaging (MRI)	Urinalysis
Radionucleotide renal scan with dimercaptosuccinic acid (DMSA)	Urine culture
Renal biopsy	Urine protein-to-creatinine ratio
Renal or bladder ultrasound	
Voiding cystourethrogram (VCUG) or radionuclide cystography	

Note: See Appendices D and E for information about these diagnostic procedures and tests.

ASSESSMENT GUIDE | The Child With a Genitourinary Condition

Assessment Focus	Assessment Guidelines
Urine characteristics	• Does the urine have a strong odor, a dark or unusual color, or appear cloudy?
Pain or discomfort	• Is there pain or burning with urination? • Is there flank or abdominal pain? • Is there scrotal or testicular pain?
Edema	• Is there generalized edema?
Appearance of genitalia	• What is the location of the urethra on the glans penis? • Is the scrotum large or underdeveloped? Are rugae present? Are testes palpable in the scrotum? • Do the genitalia have characteristic male or female appearance, or are the genitalia ambiguous? • Is there vaginal or urethral discharge? • Are there lesions on the genitalia?
Sexual development	• What is the stage of pubertal development? (See Figures 5–28, 5–29, and 5–30.)

a day. Infrequent voiding, common in school-age children, results in incomplete emptying of the bladder and urinary stasis. Other factors associated with increased risk of UTI include poor hygiene, inadequate cleansing after bowel movements, and an irritated perineum. Uncircumcised males have a higher incidence of UTIs than circumcised males (Dubrovsky, Foster, Jednak, et al., 2012). This increased incidence is highest in the first year of life (Morris & Wiswell, 2013). Constipation in children and sexual activity in adolescent females also contribute to the incidence of UTI in the pediatric population (Fisher et al., 2014). **Vesicoureteral reflux**, the backflow of urine from the bladder into the ureters during voiding, is another cause of UTI and is discussed later in this chapter.

Growth and Development

Urinary tract infections are more common in males than females in the first few months of life. It is estimated that the incidence of UTI in uncircumcised males during the first year of life is 7 to 14 of 1000 as compared to 1 to 2 of 1000 circumcised infants (American Academy of Pediatrics Task Force on Circumcision, 2012). By 1 year of age, the incidence of UTI is much higher in females than males (Fisher et al., 2014). This is related to the shorter female urethra (2 cm [1 in.] in young girls) being closer to the anus and vagina, which increases the risk of contamination by fecal bacteria.

Renal scarring can result from pyelonephritis because of the ischemic effects of infection. It has been associated with hypertension and chronic renal failure (White, 2011). The risk of renal damage increases in the following instances:

- UTI in infant less than 1 year of age
- Delay in diagnosis and effective antibacterial treatment for an upper UTI
- Anatomic obstruction or nerve supply interruption
- Recurrent episodes of upper UTIs

Clinical Manifestations

Symptoms depend on the location of the infection and the age of the child. Symptoms in the newborn period tend to be nonspecific (e.g., unexplained fever, hypothermia, failure to thrive, poor feeding, vomiting and diarrhea, strong-smelling urine, and irritability). Any child under 2 years of age with a fever of unknown origin should be tested for a UTI. The more "classic" symptoms of lower UTI are not seen until the preschool years, as listed in Table 26–2. Many UTIs are asymptomatic and are discovered incidentally on routine examination.

Clinical Therapy

A urine specimen is examined for the presence of bacteria. Dipsticks can be used to screen for urinary tract infection. A dipstick-positive leukocyte esterase test identifies white blood cells and pyuria, and a positive nitrite dipstick detects gram-negative bacteria. The UTI is diagnosed when a midstream clean-catch urine culture yields greater than 100,000 colony-forming units (cfu) of a single bacterium, or when greater than 10,000 cfu of a single bacterium are cultured from a sterile catheterized specimen (Ammenti et al., 2012). See the *Clinical Skills Manual* SKILLS for urine collection methods. Once the presence of bacteria is confirmed, antibiotic sensitivity for the specific organisms cultured is then determined. Urinalysis reveals white blood cells (WBCs) in the urine. A complete blood count reveals an elevated WBC count. A renal ultrasound is recommended after the first urinary tract infection with fever to rule out structural abnormalities (Newman, 2011). A voiding cystourethrogram (VCUG) may be obtained to test for vesicoureteral reflux if the ultrasound results are abnormal or the child has recurrence of a urinary tract infection with fever (Fisher et al., 2014).

Antibiotic therapy is begun as soon as urine samples have been collected. Antibiotics are selected based on the age of the child, sensitivity of the cultured organism, and the child's signs and symptoms. The antibiotic is changed, if necessary, after culture sensitivity is determined. Routine antibiotic prophylaxis is no longer recommended after the first urinary tract infection in infants and children (Paintsil, 2013).

Table 26–1 lists diagnostic tests commonly used to identify urinary tract conditions.

Clinical Tip

Several procedures are available for evaluation of kidney and bladder function. It is important for the patient and family to understand the procedure. Examples of these procedures and their purpose include:

- *Renal ultrasound*—Noninvasive procedure that uses sound waves to visualize the kidneys, ureters, and bladder. Renal ultrasound is useful in determining the size and shape of the kidneys, blood flow to the kidneys, signs of injury or damage, blockage, tumors, or kidney stones.
- *Voiding cystourethrogram*—Determines if there is reflux of urine into the ureters (see the discussion of vesicoureteral reflux later in this chapter). A catheter is placed prior to the procedure so that the bladder may be filled with dye. Radiographs are used to visualize the bladder during the procedure and see if dye moves into the ureters.

Children who appear ill and cannot tolerate oral antibiotics are often hospitalized because they need rehydration and initiation of parenteral antibiotic treatment until afebrile for 24 hours. Infants may develop permanent kidney damage or generalized sepsis if a UTI is not treated aggressively. If a structural defect is identified, surgical correction may be necessary to prevent recurrent infections that could lead to renal damage.

Children treated on an outpatient basis should receive follow-up by phone (or in person if needed) within 24 to 48 hours to validate the child's response to treatment and to make changes to the treatment plan, if needed, based on urine culture sensitivities. A follow-up visit 7 to 10 days after the initiation of treatment is important to see how the patient responded to treatment (Fisher et al., 2014).

Nursing Management

For the Child With Urinary Tract Infection

Nursing Assessment and Diagnosis

PHYSIOLOGIC ASSESSMENT

Obtain a history of urinary symptoms. Assess the infant for toxic (very ill) appearance, fever, and poor feeding. Evaluate the child's oral fluid intake. Assess for quality, quantity, and frequency of voiding. Assess the infant's or child's vital signs, including blood pressure. Palpate the abdomen and suprapubic and costovertebral areas for masses, tenderness, and distention. Assess for abdominal or flank pain, frequency, urgency, and dysuria. Observe the urinary stream, if possible, and perform a urinalysis,

TABLE 26–2 Clinical Manifestations of Urinary Tract Infection

TYPE OF UTI	CLINICAL MANIFESTATIONS
Lower UTI—cystitis	
Infants	Fever, diarrhea, vomiting, irritability, lethargy, foul-smelling diapers, poor feeding, failure to gain weight
Preschooler	Fever, hematuria, urgency, dysuria, frequency, cloudy urine, foul-smelling urine, dehydration, abdominal pain, enuresis
School-age	Fever, hematuria, urgency, dysuria, frequency, cloudy urine, foul-smelling urine, dehydration, abdominal pain, suprapubic or flank pain, enuresis
Upper UTI—pyelonephritis	High fever, chills, abdominal pain, nausea, vomiting, flank pain, costovertebral angle tenderness, moderate to severe dehydration

including specific gravity. Proper collection of the urine specimen is essential. Obtain a clean-catch urine specimen if the child is old enough to do this. If not, get a catheterized sample (see the *Clinical Skills Manual* SKILLS). An early morning urine specimen is preferred because the urine is more concentrated.

PSYCHOSOCIAL ASSESSMENT

Sexually active adolescents may deny having symptoms of a UTI because they fear disclosing their sexual activity to their parents. Careful questioning and a visit alone with the adolescent may be necessary to elicit these concerns. Be open and approachable and give the patient and family the chance to address their concerns.

Common nursing diagnoses for the child with a UTI include the following (NANDA-I © 2014):

- *Urinary Elimination, Impaired,* related to recurrent urinary tract infections
- *Urinary Retention* related to infrequent voiding habits or vesicoureteral reflux
- *Health Management, Family, Ineffective,* related to lack of knowledge of preventive UTI measures
- *Fluid Volume: Deficient, Risk for,* related to fever and inadequate intake

Planning and Implementation

Nursing care for the hospitalized child with a complicated UTI centers on administering prescribed medications, promoting rehydration, assessing renal function, and teaching parents and older children how to minimize the risk of future infection.

Administer antibiotics and antipyretics as prescribed to maintain therapeutic drug levels and reduce fever. Encourage fluid intake to dilute the urine and flush the bladder. Frequent voiding minimizes urinary stasis. Document intake and output. Assess renal function by comparing the child's output to the expected urine output and weigh the child daily.

Because bladder training is such an important milestone for young children, any disorder that affects voiding may have developmental implications. A toddler who has been toilet trained may regress and require diapers temporarily as a result of UTI-related incontinence. An older child may develop enuresis after a prolonged period of being dry at night. Reassure parents that this is normal and emphasize that the child needs support. A preschooler may perceive the infection and any parental disapproval as punishment for an imagined wrong.

DISCHARGE PLANNING AND HOME CARE TEACHING

Children with UTIs are usually cared for at home. Teach parents that all doses of the antibiotic must be taken as prescribed and that they may be continued even after the infection has cleared to prevent a recurrence. Teach prevention through proper hygiene and avoidance of risk behaviors.

Give parents specific guidelines for oral fluid intake. Make sure the amount of fluids recommended for a 24-hour period equals the maintenance fluids needed plus additional fluids required because of fever and diuresis to flush out pathogens (see Chapter 18). Suggest that the parents avoid giving the child caffeinated and carbonated beverages because these have the potential to irritate the bladder mucosa. Teach parents the signs and symptoms of recurrent infection and to seek care promptly.

The child with a neurogenic bladder requires a clean intermittent catheterization to be performed several times a day to reduce urinary stasis and the potential for UTI. Although the procedure for inserting the catheter is the same as that for catheterization using sterile technique, children and families are generally taught to use clean technique. See *Families Want to Know: Prevention of Urinary Tract Infections.*

Evaluation

Expected outcomes of nursing care include:

- The child increases fluid intake and number of times voiding each day.
- Future UTIs are prevented.

Structural Defects of the Urinary System

Bladder Exstrophy

Bladder exstrophy is a rare congenital defect in which the posterior bladder wall extrudes through the lower abdominal wall (Figure 26–3). Failure of the abdominal wall to close during fetal development results in eversion and protuberance of the bladder wall along with a wide separation of the rectus muscles and the symphysis pubis. The upper urinary tract is usually normal. The bladder mucosa appears as a mass of bright-red tissue, and urine continually leaks from the ureters onto the skin (Ring & Huether, 2014). Females have a bifid (split) clitoris. Males have a short, stubby penis, and the glans is flattened with dorsal chordee and a ventral prepuce. Undescended testicles and inguinal hernias are common in children with bladder exstrophy (Elder, 2016a).

The exposed bladder tissue is covered with plastic wrap to keep the bladder mucosa moist until surgery is performed (Elder, 2016a). The goal of primary closure of the bladder and anterior abdominal wall is an acceptable urinary reservoir (Bhatnagar, 2011). Primary closure is generally performed soon after birth but may be delayed if the bladder template is too small or other contraindications are identified (Inouye, Tourchi, DiCarlo, et al., 2014).

Families Want to Know

Prevention of Urinary Tract Infections

- Teach proper perineal hygiene. Girls should always wipe the perineum from front to back after voiding.
- Encourage the child to drink plenty of fluids and avoid long periods of "holding urine."
- Caution against tight underwear; children should wear cotton rather than nylon underwear.
- Encourage the child to void frequently and to fully empty the bladder.
- Discourage bubble baths, bath oils, and hot tubs, which can irritate the urethra.
- Encourage abstinence of sexual activity. However, if girls are sexually active, instruct them to void before and after sexual intercourse to prevent urinary stasis and flush out bacteria introduced during intercourse.

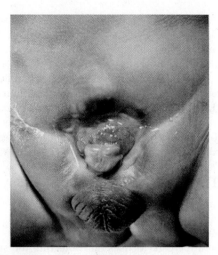

Figure 26–3 This child has bladder exstrophy, noted by extrusion of the posterior bladder wall through the lower abdominal wall.

The wound and pelvis are immobilized to promote healing. An osteotomy (see Chapter 29) to rotate the innominate bones of the pelvis to approximate the symphysis pubis reduces tension on the closed bladder and abdominal wall to promote healing. Epispadias repair is often performed between 1 and 2 years of age or at the same times as a surgical procedure to improve continence. Surgery to reconstruct the bladder neck and reimplant the ureters is performed when the bladder has achieved capacity of 80 to 90 mL (Elder, 2016a). The goals of surgical reconstruction include:

- Closure of the bladder and abdominal wall
- Urinary continence, with preservation of renal function
- Creation of functional and normal-appearing genitalia
- Correction to promote later sexual functioning

Some children require permanent urinary diversion because a functional bladder cannot be reconstructed.

Nursing Management

Preoperative nursing care centers on preventing infection and trauma to the exposed bladder. The bladder mucosa is protected with plastic wrap to keep the bladder mucosa moist (Elder, 2016a). The surrounding area is cleaned daily and protected from leaking urine with a skin sealant.

Postoperatively, the wound and pelvis are immobilized to facilitate healing. Internal and external immobilization techniques are used for pelvic closure (see Chapter 29). In addition to pain assessment and management, nursing care includes maintaining proper alignment, avoiding abduction of the infant's legs, monitoring peripheral circulation, and providing meticulous wound and skin care. Maintain aseptic technique for wound care and monitor for signs of infection including redness, drainage, and edema.

Monitor renal function by assessing the adequacy of urine output and blood and urine chemistries to detect signs of renal damage. Observe for any signs of obstruction in the drainage tubes such as increased intensity of bladder spasms, decreased urine output, or urine or blood draining from the urethral meatus. Promote comfort and give antibiotics as ordered.

Parents need emotional support to help them cope with the disfiguring nature of the infant's defect and the uncertainty of complete repair. To promote parent–infant bonding, encourage parents to participate in all aspects of the infant's care, including bathing, feeding, and wound care. Discharge teaching should include instructions about dressing changes and diapering and the need to immediately report any signs of infection or change in renal function. Emphasize the need for routine follow-up visits after surgery to assess urinary function and to ensure that the next stages of surgery for continence control are performed at the appropriate time in the child's development. The family should be aware that achievement of continence is more difficult in children with bladder exstrophy, and urinary diversion to achieve continence may be necessary if surgical procedures are not successful. Parents may require guidance to promote the child's self-esteem and self-confidence with sexual identity and function. Psychologic counseling may be beneficial to the child during adolescence.

Hypospadias and Epispadias

Hypospadias and epispadias are congenital anomalies involving the abnormal location of the urethral meatus (Figure 26–4). The reported incidence of hypospadias is 1 in 300 male births (Snodgrass & Bush, 2014). The incidence of epispadias is 1 in 40,000 to 118,000 births. Epispadias occurs twice as often in males as females (Ring & Huether, 2014). See the section on bladder exstrophy earlier in this chapter.

In hypospadias, the urethral meatus can be located anywhere along the course of the urethra on the ventral surface of the penile shaft, from the perineum to the tip of the glans. Most cases are mild, with the meatus slightly off center from the tip of the penis; in severe cases, the meatus is located on the scrotum.

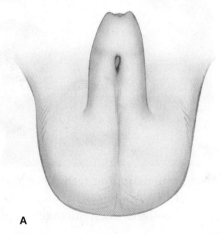

A

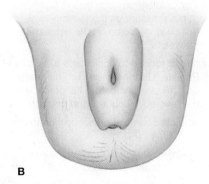

B

Figure 26–4 *A*, In hypospadias, the urethral canal is open on the ventral surface of the penis. *B*, In epispadias, the canal is open on the dorsal surface.

Hypospadias often occurs in conjunction with congenital *chordee*, a fibrous line of tissue that results in ventral curvature of the penile shaft. Associated defects may include inguinal hernia, cryptorchidism (undescended testes), and partial absence of the foreskin (Ring & Huether, 2014).

Clinical Tip

When children are not able to achieve continence, some type of urinary diversion may be created. A *vesicostomy* is a procedure in which an opening is created from the bladder to the skin. The urine drains from the opening (stoma) to the child's diaper or a drainage bag. In the *Mitrofanoff procedure,* a reservoir for urine and a stoma are created so that children can catheterize themselves through the umbilicus (see Chapter 27).

Epispadias and bladder exstrophy are the same condition, but epispadias is the milder expression of the condition. The opening may be small or a fissure may extend the entire length of the penis. Females with epispadias have a cleft of the ventral urethra that generally extends to the bladder neck (Ring & Huether, 2014). The remainder of this discussion will focus on hypospadias and males with distal epispadias because the treatment for severe epispadias in males and epispadias in females is similar to the final stage of repair of bladder exstrophy (Elder, 2016a).

The diagnosis of hypospadias is generally made at birth. If the parents would like to have their son to be circumcised, the procedure should be delayed until surgery to repair the hypospadias is performed (Chalmers, Wiedel, Siparsky, et al., 2014). Hypospadias is corrected surgically, usually during the first year of life, to minimize psychologic effects when the child is older. Surgery is usually performed in a single operation, often as an outpatient procedure. Surgery is recommended between 6 and 12 months of age (Kocherov et al, 2012). The goals of surgical repair are (1) placement of the urethral meatus at the end of the glans penis with satisfactory caliber and configuration for a urinary stream (enabling the child to void in a standing position), (2) release

of chordee to straighten the penis (enabling future sexual function), and (3) satisfactory cosmetic appearance of the penis.

A caudal or penile nerve block is used for intraoperative and postoperative analgesia (Kundra, Yuvaraj, Agrawal, et al., 2011). Anticholinergic medications may be prescribed to relieve bladder spasms. A urethral **stent** (a device used to maintain patency of the urethral canal) or catheter is placed to maintain patency of the new urethral canal opening. The stent or catheter may drain directly into the diaper, using a double-diapering technique, or into a closed drainage collection bag.

Nursing Management

It is important to address parents' concerns at the time of birth. Preoperative teaching can relieve some of their anxiety about the future appearance and functioning of the penis.

Postoperative care focuses on protecting the surgical site from injury. The infant or child returns from surgery with the penis wrapped in a simple dressing, and a urethral stent or catheter for urinary drainage. Plan care to ensure that the stent does not get removed. Refer to the hospital's policy for the appropriate use of immobilizers in this situation.

Encourage fluid intake to maintain adequate urinary output and patency of the stent. Strict documentation of intake and output is essential to detect postoperative complications. Notify the healthcare provider if there is no urine drainage for 1 hour because this may indicate kinks in the system or obstruction. Pain may be associated with bladder spasms. Anticholinergic medications such as oxybutynin may be prescribed. Acetaminophen or other medications may also be given for pain. Antibiotics are often prescribed until the stent is out.

The child is often discharged the day of surgery. Discharge teaching should include instructions for parents about care of the reconstructed area, double-diapering to protect the operative site, fluid intake, medication administration, and signs and symptoms of infection (see *Families Want to Know: Caring for the Child After Hypospadias and Epispadias Repair* and the *Clinical Skills Manual* SKILLS). Tell parents when the child needs to see the healthcare provider for dressing removal.

Families Want to Know

Caring for the Child After Hypospadias and Epispadias Repair

- Use double-diapering to protect the operative site. See the *Clinical Skills Manual* SKILLS .

- Do not bathe the child in a tub until the stent (the small tube that drains the urine) or catheter is removed.

- Restrict the infant or toddler from activities (e.g., playing on riding toys) that put pressure on the surgical site. Avoid holding the infant or child straddled on the hip. Limit the child's activity for 2 weeks.

- Encourage the infant or toddler to drink fluids to ensure adequate hydration. Provide fluids in a pleasant environment or using a special cup. Offer fruit juice, fruit-flavored ice pops, fruit-flavored juices, flavored ice cubes, and gelatin.

- Administer the complete course of prescribed antibiotics to avoid infection.

- Observe for signs of infection: fever, swelling, redness, pain, strong-smelling urine, or change in flow of the urinary stream.

- The urine will be blood tinged for several days. Call the healthcare provider if urine is seen leaking from any area other than the penis.

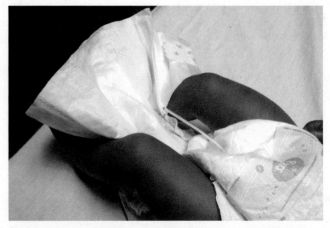

A double-diapering technique protects the operative site after surgery for hypospadias repair. The inner diaper collects stool; the outer diaper, urine.

Obstructive Uropathy

Obstructive uropathy refers to structural or functional abnormalities of the urinary system that interfere with urine flow and result in urine backflow into the kidneys. The pressure caused by urine backup compromises kidney function and often causes **hydronephrosis** (accumulation of urine in the renal pelvis as a result of obstructed outflow). Physiologic changes that may occur as a result of hydronephrosis include the following:

- Cessation of glomerular filtration occurs when the pressure in the kidney pelvis equals the filtration pressure in the glomerular capillaries. To compensate, the blood pressure increases to increase the glomerular filtration pressure; however, increasing pressure on the glomeruli leads to cell death.

- Metabolic acidosis results when the distal nephrons' ability to secrete hydrogen ions is impaired.

- Impairment of the kidney's ability to concentrate urine results in polydipsia and polyuria.

- Obstruction results in urinary stasis, promoting bacterial growth.

- Restriction of urinary outflow causes progressive renal damage and chronic renal failure if untreated.

Obstructive uropathy may be caused by several congenital lesions such as ureteropelvic junction (UPJ) obstruction, posterior urethral valves (PUVs), and stenosis or hypoplasia of the ureterovesicular junction (see *Pathophysiology Illustrated: Obstruction Sites in the Urinary System*). The UPJ is the most common site of obstruction of the upper urinary tract in infants and children. UPJ obstruction occurs in 1 of every 1000 to 2000 newborns, making it the most common cause of hydronephrosis in newborns (Lee, Han, & Rah, 2014). PUVs (abnormal folds of mucosa in the male urethra) occur in 1 of every 5000 children and are a significant cause of end-stage renal disease in children (Kari et al., 2013). Stenosis of the distal ureter at the ureterovesicular junction leads to dilation of the entire ureter, renal pelvis, and kidney (Ring & Huether, 2014).

Clinical manifestations vary depending on the cause and location of the obstruction (Table 26–3). Early diagnosis and treatment prevents kidney damage and deterioration of renal function. Prenatal ultrasound may detect hydronephrosis and PUV. A diuretic-enhanced radionuclide scan and voiding cystourethrogram are performed when UPJ or ureterovesicular obstruction is suspected.

The goals of surgical correction or diversion are to lower the pressure within the collecting system, which reduces renal damage, and to prevent stasis, which decreases the risk of infection. Surgical correction may necessitate **pyeloplasty** (removal of an obstructed segment of the ureter and reimplantation into the renal pelvis) or valve repair or reconstruction depending on the cause of the obstruction. Urinary incontinence resulting from sphincter weakness is a common problem after surgery.

Pathophysiology Illustrated: **Obstruction Sites in the Urinary System**

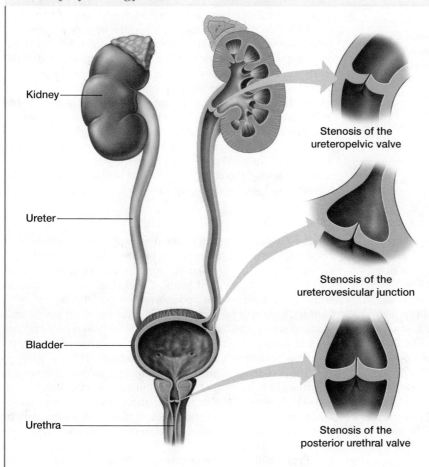

Obstruction may occur in either the upper or lower urinary tract. Common sites of obstruction occur at the ureteropelvic valve, the ureterovesicular junction, or the posterior urethral valve. Renal failure is most likely to occur when both kidneys are affected by hydronephrosis.

Kidney

Ureter

Bladder

Urethra

Stenosis of the ureteropelvic valve

Stenosis of the ureterovesicular junction

Stenosis of the posterior urethral valve

TABLE 26–3 Clinical Manifestations of Obstructive Lesions of the Urinary System

OBSTRUCTIVE LESION	CLINICAL MANIFESTATIONS
Ureteropelvic junction obstruction	*In infants:* Abdominal mass (enlarged kidney), hypertension, urinary tract infection
	In children: Hematuria, pain, intermittent nausea and vomiting
Posterior urethral valves	*In infants:* Abdominal mass (enlarged kidney), distended bladder, poor urinary stream, urinary tract infection, sepsis, low specific gravity, polyuria, increased creatinine level, failure to thrive
	In children: Urinary frequency and incontinence
Ureterovesicular junction obstruction	Urinary tract infection (recurrent or chronic), hematuria, pain, abdominal mass (enlarged kidney), enuresis

Nursing Management

Preoperative nursing care focuses on preparing the parents and child for the procedure and addressing parents' concerns about the postsurgical outcome. Provide parents with an opportunity to discuss concerns about how the disorder will affect the child's long-term renal functioning.

Postoperative care involves monitoring vital signs and intake and output and observing for signs of urine retention, such as decreased output and bladder distention. Many children are discharged with stents or catheters. Teach parents how to change dressings, double-diaper, care for catheters, assess pain and give analgesics, and recognize signs of possible obstruction or infection. Parents should encourage the child to participate in age-appropriate activities. However, children should avoid contact sports because of their potential to injure the bladder.

Vesicoureteral Reflux

In vesicoureteral reflux (VUR), there is a retrograde flow of urine from the bladder into the ureters. Severity ranges from reflux of urine into the ureter only (grade 1) to severe dilation of the ureter and renal pelvis with severely blunted calyces (grade 5) (Estrada & Cendron, 2013). The reflux prevents complete emptying of the bladder, and because urine returns to the bladder, it creates a reservoir for bacterial growth (Ring & Huether, 2014). Bacteria in the urine may be swept up to the kidneys, leading to pyelonephritis, which is the most common cause of kidney damage in children (Wadie & Moriarty, 2012).

Professionalism in Practice Screening Siblings for Vesicoureteral Reflux

Vesicoureteral reflux (VUR) occurs in 1% to 2% of the pediatric population and is present in 30% to 40% of children with a urinary tract infection (UTI). Research has shown that siblings of children with VUR have a much higher risk of having VUR than children without a family history, with a reported incidence of 26% to 50%. The American Urological Association Pediatric Vesicoureteral Reflux Guidelines have been revised to include recommendations related to screening siblings of children with VUR. It is especially important that siblings who present with a UTI be evaluated for VUR with a voiding cystourethrogram (Hunziker, Colhoun, & Puri, 2014). Nurses have opportunities to work with families of children being treated for urinary tract infections and/or VUR. Parents should be made aware of the increased incidence of VUR in siblings and the need for prompt attention to any signs of UTI. It is important that they include in the education of these families the relationship of recurrent UTI and subsequent kidney damage in children.

A renal ultrasound, voiding cystourethrogram (VCUG), and/or dimercaptosuccinic acid (DMSA) scan is used to diagnose, grade, and follow the progression of VUR. Note, however, that VCUG is the only test that provides a definitive diagnosis. The use of prophylactic antibiotics is controversial but may be prescribed to prevent UTIs. Surgical management with ureteral reimplantation may be needed depending on the grade of reflux (Passamaneck, 2011). Endoscopic management with the submucosal injection of Deflux has proven to be a successful alternative for some patients and may be considered as an alternative to surgery (Wadie & Moriarty, 2012).

Nursing Management

Following surgery to reimplant the ureters, a urinary catheter will be in place. The urine will be bloody initially and clear within 2 to 3 days. Intravenous fluids will be administered at a rate sufficient to maintain adequate urine output. Monitor the catheter for patency. Administer medications as prescribed, including antibiotics and antispasmodics such as oxybutynin.

The child can be discharged when the urinary catheter has been removed and the child can void spontaneously. An ultrasound or cystogram may be performed prior to discharge to evaluate the effectiveness of the surgery. Educate the family about the administration of medications including prophylactic antibiotics and antispasmodics if needed. Inform parents of the need for increased fiber in the diet to address the constipating effects of the antispasmodic medication. Guidelines for calling the physician include fever over 38.5°C (101.5°F), abdominal or back pain, or swelling and redness of the incision. The child may take a short shower or tub bath when returning home. The child should avoid active play for 3 weeks following surgery. Provide guidelines for follow-up.

Prune Belly Syndrome

Prune belly syndrome, also known as *Eagle-Barrett syndrome*, is a congenital defect characterized by failure of the abdominal musculature to develop. The skin covering the abdominal wall is thin and resembles a wrinkled prune. Other characteristics include urinary tract anomalies, poor ureteral peristalsis, enlarged bladder, high risk for recurrent UTI, vesicoureteral reflux, and bilateral cryptorchidism in males. Prune belly syndrome occurs predominantly in males (95%), with an incidence of 1 in 29,000 to 40,000 live births (Caldamone & Woodard, 2012).

The etiology of prune belly syndrome is unknown; however, it is thought to be related to a fetal urinary tract obstruction or a specific injury to the mesoderm during the first trimester. In addition to urinary tract anomalies, cardiac, pulmonary, gastrointestinal, and musculoskeletal anomalies also occur (Hassett, Smith, & Holland, 2012).

Prune belly syndrome is frequently diagnosed prenatally by ultrasound. Mortality in the neonatal period is related to pulmonary hypoplasia and severe renal dysfunction (Hassett et al., 2012). Abdominal wall reconstruction and correction of genitourinary defects, including orchiopexy (or orchidopexy), are performed to repair defects. The mortality rate in infants has improved significantly in the past 3 decades with advances in surgical techniques. Approximately 30% of children with prune belly syndrome will develop end-stage renal disease in childhood or adolescence because of inadequate renal function (Elder, 2016b).

Nursing Management

Nursing management for the infant with prune belly syndrome is the same as for other defects of the genitourinary system, including preoperative and postoperative management. Additional management includes psychosocial support for the child and family related to the numerous congenital anomalies, body image concerns, and long-term consequences of the defect.

A discussion of Wilms tumor can be found in Chapter 24.

Enuresis

Enuresis is repeated involuntary voiding by a child old enough that bladder control is expected, usually about 5 to 6 years of age. (See Table 26–4 for bladder control milestones.) Enuresis can occur either at night (nocturnal), during the day (diurnal), or both night and day.

Enuresis is further categorized as primary or secondary:

- *Primary enuresis*—Child has never had a dry night; attributed to maturational delay and small functional bladder; not associated with stress or psychiatric cause.

- *Secondary enuresis*—Child who has been reliably dry for at least 6 months begins bed-wetting; associated with stress, infections, and sleep disorders.

Growth and Development

Nighttime wetting episodes usually decrease as the child ages. An estimated 21% of children ages 4.5 years and 8% of children 9.5 years of age average less than two episodes of nighttime wetting per week. Wetting episodes occur more than 2 times per week in 8% of children ages 4.5 years and 1.5% of children 9.5 years of age (Jacques, 2013).

TABLE 26–4 Milestones in the Development of Bladder Control

AGE	DEVELOPMENTAL MILESTONE
1.5 years	Child passes urine at regular intervals.
2 years	Child announces when voiding is taking place.
2.5 years	Child makes known the need to void; can hold urine.
3 years	Child goes to the bathroom alone; holds urge if preoccupied with play.
2.5–3.5 years	Child achieves nighttime control.
4 years	Child shows great interest in going to bathrooms when away from home (shopping centers, movies).
5 years	Child voids approximately 5 to 6 times a day; prefers privacy; is able to initiate emptying of bladder at any degree of fullness.

Primary nocturnal enuresis is the most common type of enuresis and occurs more frequently in males than females (Elder, 2016c). It occurs more often in children who have a positive family history and generally involves more than one causative factor. Factors may include maturational delay, sleep disorders, and reduced or small functional bladder capacity (Ray, 2011). Nocturnal enuresis is also more prevalent in children with obstructive sleep apnea syndrome (Bascom et al., 2011). Additionally, enuresis frequently occurs in children with constipation. The constipation should be treated prior to the implementation of any treatment for enuresis (Walle et al., 2012).

A thorough history can help identify potential causes of secondary enuresis. The child's lower spine is examined for fistulas, sacral dimples, or tufts of hair that could be signs of spina bifida occulta (see Chapter 27). Diabetes, urinary tract infection, and other conditions should also be ruled out. Prolonged hospitalization, family stressors, and preoccupation with school concerns also have been associated with secondary enuresis.

Clinical Tip

Questions to ask when taking an enuresis history include the following:

Family History

Is there a family history of renal or urinary structural abnormalities?

Is there a family history of bed-wetting? At what age did bed-wetting stop?

Family Management of Enuresis

How serious is the problem for the family?

What happens when the child wets? (Who gets up and changes sheets?)

How is the child treated? Is the child punished or blamed for wetting?

What remedies have been tried?

Toilet Training

When was it initiated and what method was used?

Has the child ever been dry during the day or night for an extended period?

How long was the child's longest dry period?

How often does the child void? Have a bowel movement?

Does the child have a history of constipation or encopresis?

Stressors

How is the child doing in school?

Are any new or chronic stressors present in the child's life?

How does the problem interfere with play and other activities?

Risk Factors

Diabetes—Are there any signs of polyuria or polydipsia?

Urinary tract infection—Does the child have frequency, urgency, burning on urination?

A multitreatment approach is usually most effective. Limiting excessive fluids at night, bladder training, enuresis alarms, and positive reinforcement are common approaches (Table 26–5). Alarms have about a 70% success rate but take 3 to 5 months to be effective (Ray, 2011).

TABLE 26–5 Treatment Approaches for Enuresis

APPROACH	DESCRIPTION
Limiting fluids	Fluid intake is limited in the evening and before the child goes to bed. Fluids with caffeine should be avoided.
Bladder exercises	The child drinks a large amount and then holds urine as long as possible. The child practices stopping voiding midstream. Exercises should continue for at least 6 months.
Timed voiding	The child with diurnal enuresis is instructed to void every 2 hr and to use a double voiding pattern; this trains the bladder to empty completely and avoid overdistention.
Enuresis alarms	A detector strip is attached to the child's pants. The alarm sounds a buzzer that alerts the child when wetting occurs, so the child can get up and finish voiding in the bathroom. This works best for children over 7 years old, and takes 3 to 5 months for success.
Reward system	Set realistic goals for the child and reinforce dry days or nights with stars and stickers on a chart.
Medications	Desmopressin, oxybutynin, and imipramine are used as discussed in the text.

Medications used in the treatment of primary nocturnal enuresis include desmopressin, imipramine, and oxybutynin:

- Desmopressin is the most common medication used for nocturnal enuresis and has an antidiuretic effect. Desmopressin is given at nighttime at the beginning of treatment. Once its effectiveness has been established, it may be used every night or as needed for times when the child is away from home for a short period (e.g., sleepovers or camp) (Nevéus, 2011).

- Oxybutynin, an anticholinergic medication, has an antispasmodic effect, improves storage function of the bladder, and decreases the overactivity of the detrusor muscle. Oxybutynin may also be used in combination with desmopressin in children who have not responded to desmopressin alone or in combination with an alarm (Norfolk & Wootton, 2012).

- Imipramine, a tricyclic antidepressant, has anticholinergic and antispasmodic effects and may be used in children who do not respond to other methods. This medication requires close monitoring because of its effects on mood and the associated danger of overdoses (Nevéus, 2011).

Nursing Management

Teach the child and parents about the physiologic development of bladder control and causes and treatment of enuresis. Explore feelings of guilt or blame. Make sure the parents are aware that the child cannot control the wetting. Psychosocial support is an essential part of care since stress is an important cause of secondary enuresis. Provide emotional support to the parents and child, and encourage the child's participation in the treatment plan. Refer the child for counseling or therapy if appropriate.

Assess the parents' and child's motivation and readiness for interventions. The child needs to be an active participant in the treatment plan for daytime and nighttime wetting. Before parents

buy an enuresis alarm, suggest they use an alarm clock in the child's room for several nights to see if the child will arouse. Find out whether the child shares a room with others who will be disturbed by the alarm. Ask if the child and parents are willing to persist with an enuresis alarm because it may take months to work. Discuss potential strategies with the family to reduce stressors on the child or to help the child cope with the stressors. Expected outcomes of nursing care include:

- The child has an increased number of dry nights.

- The child and family choose one or more interventions that they prefer and persist in using them.

Renal Disorders

Nephrotic Syndrome

Nephrotic syndrome is an alteration in kidney function secondary to increased glomerular basement membrane permeability to plasma protein (see *Pathophysiology Illustrated: Nephrotic Syndrome*). Nephrotic syndrome does not refer to a specific disease, but rather to a clinical state characterized by edema, massive proteinuria, hypoalbuminemia, hypoproteinemia, hyperlipidemia, and altered immunity. Congenital nephrotic syndrome is generally related to a genetic defect (Holmberg & Jalanko, 2014). The term *primary nephrotic syndrome* is used when there is no identifiable cause. *Secondary nephrotic syndrome* results from a systemic disease, drugs, or toxins (Ring & Huether, 2014).

Approximately 85% of children with nephrotic syndrome have a type of primary disease called *minimal change nephrotic syndrome* (MCNS). It is estimated that more than 95% of these children respond to steroid therapy (Pais & Avner, 2016). MCNS derives its name from the normal or only minimally changed appearance of the glomeruli on light microscopic evaluation. MCNS is the focus of the following discussion.

ETIOLOGY AND PATHOPHYSIOLOGY

The cause of primary MCNS is not clearly understood but an immune system role is suspected (Pais & Avner, 2016). The mechanism of increased glomerular permeability is unknown because the glomeruli appear normal (Ring & Huether, 2014). In MCNS, increased permeability of the glomerular membrane permits large, negatively charged molecules such as albumin to pass through the membrane and be excreted in the urine. Proteinuria results in decreased oncotic pressure and edema because fluid remains in the interstitial spaces instead of being pulled back into the vascular compartment (Pais & Avner, 2016). Immunoglobulins are lost, resulting in altered immunity. Loss of protein in the urine, insufficient albumin production by the liver, and a decreased albumin concentration as a result of salt and water retention by the kidney contribute to hypoalbuminemia. Hypercoagulability occurs because of alterations in coagulation factors. The liver responds by increasing synthesis of lipoprotein, resulting in hyperlipidemia (Ring & Huether, 2014). Children who develop steroid-resistant nephrotic syndrome are at risk for end-stage renal disease (Lombel, Hodson, & Gipson, 2013).

CLINICAL MANIFESTATIONS

In most children, edema develops gradually over several weeks. Children may have a history of periorbital edema on waking that resolves during the day as fluid shifts to the abdomen and lower extremities. Other signs include snug fit of clothing and shoes, pallor, hypertension, irritability, anorexia, hematuria, decreased urine output, and nonspecific malaise. The child's urine may be

Pathophysiology Illustrated: **Nephrotic Syndrome**

Note the contrast between the normal glomerular anatomy and the changes that exist in nephrotic syndrome, which permit protein to be excreted in the urine. The lower albumin blood level stimulates the liver to generate lipids and excessive clotting factors. Edema results from decreased oncotic plasma pressure, renin-angiotensin-aldosterone activation, and antidiuretic hormone secretion.

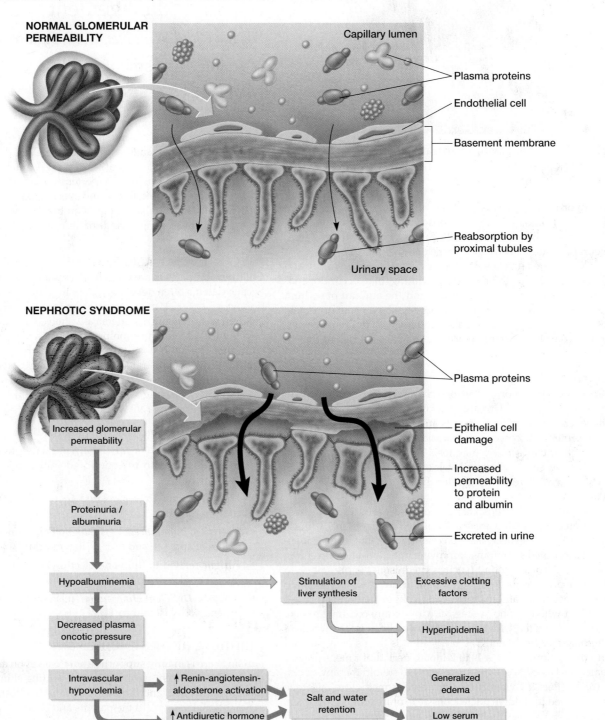

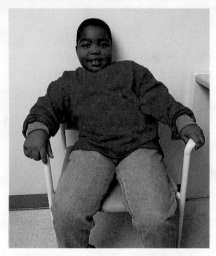

Figure 26–5 This boy has generalized edema, a characteristic finding in nephrotic syndrome.

frothy or foamy. Parents often do not seek medical treatment until generalized edema develops on the child's extremities, abdomen, or genitals (Figure 26–5). Respiratory distress from pleural effusion may occur in some cases.

Massive edema resulting in a dramatic weight gain and abdominal pain, with or without vomiting, may occur depending on the amount of albumin lost and the amount of sodium ingested. The child becomes malnourished as a result of protein loss in the urine. The skin is pale and shiny with prominent veins, and the hair becomes more brittle. An increased risk of thrombosis is present.

CLINICAL THERAPY

Diagnosis is based on the history, characteristic symptoms, and laboratory findings. Urinalysis, serum albumin, sodium, BUN, cholesterol, and electrolytes tests are ordered. Urinalysis shows large protein. Microscopic hematuria may also be present. Other values that confirm the diagnosis include hypoalbuminemia indicated by serum albumin levels of less than 2.5 g/dL and urinary protein excretion of greater than 3.5 grams per 24 hours (Pais & Avner, 2016).

Children may be hospitalized when severe edema or a major infection is present, but are usually treated as outpatients. Clinical therapy focuses on decreasing proteinuria, relieving edema, managing associated symptoms, improving nutrition, and preventing infection. A corticosteroid (such as prednisone) is prescribed to decrease proteinuria. In most children, urine protein levels fall to trace or negative values within 2 to 3 weeks of the start of therapy. Children who respond successfully to therapy continue to take corticosteroids daily for 6 weeks, followed by at least 4 weeks of alternate-day treatment. The medication is then slowly tapered and discontinued over a 1- to 2-month period of time. Approximately 80% to 90% of children respond to steroid therapy within 4 weeks (Pais & Avner, 2016). Intravenous methylprednisolone may be used in children not responsive to oral steroids (Nachman, Jennette, & Falk, 2012). Intravenous administration of albumin followed by furosemide may be ordered in the child with massive edema who is unresponsive to fluid restriction and parenteral diuretics (Pais & Avner, 2016). Analgesics may be ordered for pain related to edema or flank pain from a urinary tract infection.

Relapses occur in many children with nephrotic syndrome (Pais & Avner, 2016). Children who have a relapse after drug therapy is discontinued receive repeat therapy. Other medications used include diuretics, antihypertensive agents, and antibiotics.

Immunosuppressive or immunomodulator medications, including cyclophosphamide, cyclosporine, tacrolimus, and mycophenolate, may be used to prolong remissions in children with nephrotic syndrome who have frequent relapses (Pais & Avner, 2016). Since diuretics can precipitate hypovolemia, hyponatremia, and hypokalemia, electrolyte levels should be carefully monitored.

Nursing Management

For the Child With Nephrotic Syndrome

Nursing Assessment and Diagnosis

PHYSIOLOGIC ASSESSMENT

Careful assessment of the child's hydration status and edema is essential. Carefully monitor intake and output. Weigh the child daily using the same scale, and measure abdominal girth to monitor changes in edema and ascites (see the *Clinical Skills Manual* SKILLS). Monitor vital signs at least every 4 hours to watch for signs of respiratory distress, hypertension, or circulatory overload. Test urine for proteinuria and specific gravity at least once each shift. In addition, assess for skin breakdown from edema, for hypovolemia during periods of diuresis as well as for indications of infection.

PSYCHOSOCIAL ASSESSMENT

Children and parents are often fearful or anxious on admission. Because edema often develops gradually, parents may feel guilty if they did not seek medical attention immediately. School-age children with generalized edema are often concerned about their appearance. Careful questioning may be necessary to elicit these concerns. The child hospitalized for a recurrence of nephrotic syndrome may be frustrated or depressed. Assess individual and family coping mechanisms, support systems, and level of stress.

Common nursing diagnoses for the child with MCNS include the following (NANDA-I © 2014):

- *Infection, Risk for,* related to immunosuppressive therapy
- *Skin Integrity, Risk for Impaired,* related to edema, lowered resistance to infection and injury, immobility, and malnutrition
- *Fluid Volume: Excess* related to renal dysfunction and sodium retention
- *Nutrition, Imbalanced: Less than Body Requirements,* related to loss of appetite and protein loss in urine
- *Fatigue* related to fluid and electrolyte imbalance, albumin loss, altered nutrition, and renal failure
- *Activity, Deficient Diversional,* related to fatigue, immobility, and social isolation

Planning and Implementation

Nursing care is mainly supportive and focuses on administering medications, preventing infection, preventing skin breakdown, meeting nutritional and fluid needs, promoting rest, and providing emotional support to the parents and child.

ADMINISTER MEDICATIONS

It is important to give prescribed medications at the scheduled times. Monitor closely for side effects of corticosteroids such as moon face, increased appetite, increased hair growth, abdominal distention, and mood swings, as well as adverse effects of corticosteroids such as hypertension, nausea, and hyperglycemia. Corticosteroids should be tapered rather than abruptly discontinued. If the child is receiving albumin intravenously, monitor closely for hypertension or signs of volume overload caused by fluid shifts. If diuretics are used, observe for shock. The child may need to have albumin infused simultaneously with diuretics.

PREVENT INFECTION

Children with MCNS are at risk for infection because of the loss of immunoglobulins in the urine and corticosteroid therapy. Implement careful hand hygiene and standard precautions. Strict aseptic technique is essential during invasive procedures. Monitor the child's white blood cell count when cytotoxic drugs are given because bone marrow suppression is a side effect. Monitor vital signs carefully to detect early signs of infection that may be masked by corticosteroid therapy. Decrease the child's social contacts during immunosuppressive treatment, and caution parents and children to avoid exposure to people with respiratory infections and communicable diseases. Emphasize the importance of avoiding shopping malls, sporting arenas, grocery stores, game stores, and other public areas where the risk of exposure to such infections is increased. Provide instructions to the parents on signs of infection, including fever and changes in behavior. Discuss with parents the need for maintenance of annual recommended influenza immunizations and avoiding those who have recently been vaccinated with live viruses.

PREVENT SKIN BREAKDOWN

Meticulous skin care is essential to prevent skin breakdown and potential infection. Assess the skin repeatedly, turn the child frequently, and use therapeutic mattresses (e.g., egg crate, airflow) to help prevent skin breakdown. Keep the skin clean and dry.

MEET NUTRITIONAL AND FLUID NEEDS

Keep the child's food preferences in mind when planning menus. Encourage the child to eat by presenting attractive meals in small portions. Socialization during meals may improve the child's appetite. Fluids are not usually restricted except during severe edema.

PROMOTE REST

Provide opportunities for quiet play as tolerated, such as drawing, playing board games, listening to CDs, and watching movies. Adjust the child's daily schedule to allow rest periods after activities. Signs of fatigue may include irritability, mood swings, or withdrawal. Tell the parents and child about the importance of rest. Limiting visitors during the acute phase of the illness may be necessary. Telephone and computer contacts may be encouraged as an alternative to visitors. To provide a sense of control, encourage these children to set their own limits on activity.

PROVIDE EMOTIONAL SUPPORT

Parents and children often need support to cope with this chronic disease. Thoroughly explain the child's disease and treatment regimen to parents. Parental anxiety in combination with the hospitalization may interfere with the child's independence. Help parents promote the child's independence by allowing the child to choose from the menu or to select the daily activity schedule. This gives the child some sense of control.

Children with MCNS may have a distorted body image because of sudden weight gain and edema. They may refuse to look in the mirror, refuse to participate in care, and take less interest in their appearance. Encourage children to express their feelings. Help them maintain a normal appearance by promoting normal grooming routines. Encourage children to wear their own pajamas rather than hospital gowns. Scarves or hats may be used to lessen the child's edematous appearance. Adolescents can be encouraged to write their feelings in a journal as a coping mechanism. These children may have a long-term psychosocial adjustment because of having a chronic condition with concerns about potential relapse.

DISCHARGE PLANNING AND HOME CARE TEACHING

Explain the disease process, prognosis, and treatment plan to parents and school-age children. Make sure parents know how to administer medications and can identify potential side effects. Inform parents about restricting fluid intake until the edema resolves. Instruct parents about the need to monitor urine daily for protein, and have them keep a diary to record results. Monitoring the child's weight each week may help parents identify early stages of fluid retention and signs of relapse before edema occurs.

Tutoring may be required for a short period after discharge. Encourage parents to allow the child to return to normal activities once the acute episode has resolved. Emphasize the importance of avoiding contact with people with infectious diseases because of the child's reduced immunity. Reinforce to parents that as long as the child is receiving corticosteroid therapy or shows signs of MCNS, a no-added-salt diet should be followed.

Most children do well with corticosteroid therapy; however, relapses are common. These relapses decrease as the child gets older. Children should have periodic bone density evaluations because of the repeated steroid therapy, which can weaken bones and lead to osteoporosis.

Evaluation

Expected outcomes of nursing care may include:

- The child responds to corticosteroid therapy.
- The child does not acquire an infection.
- Fluid, electrolyte, and acid–base balance is restored and maintained.
- Skin integrity is maintained.
- The child meets nutritional requirements and follows dietary guidelines.

Acute Postinfectious Glomerulonephritis

Glomerulonephritis is the most common inflammation of the glomeruli of the kidneys. In children, it is most often a response to a group A beta-hemolytic streptococcal infection of the skin or pharynx. It is also caused by other organisms, including *Staphylococcus* and *Pneumococcus* bacteria and coxsackieviruses. The incidence of acute postinfectious glomerulonephritis (APIGN) is highest in children between 2 and 6 years of age, and the disorder is more common in boys than in girls (Nachman et al., 2012).

ETIOLOGY AND PATHOPHYSIOLOGY

The child with APIGN usually becomes ill after contracting a nephrogenetic strain of group A beta-hemolytic streptococcal infection of the upper respiratory tract or the skin. Often the child contracts a streptococcal infection (e.g., strep throat), recovers, and then develops signs of APIGN after an interval of 10 to 21 days.

Glomerular damage occurs as a result of an immune complex reaction that localizes on the glomerular capillary wall. See *Pathophysiology Illustrated: Acute Postinfectious Glomerulonephritis.* Antibody–antigen complexes become lodged in the glomeruli, leading to inflammation and obstruction. The glomerular membranes thicken, and capillaries in the glomeruli become obstructed by damaged tissue cells, leading to a decreased glomerular filtration rate. Vascular permeability increases, allowing red blood cells and red cell casts to be excreted. Sodium and water are retained, expanding the intravascular and interstitial compartments and resulting in the characteristic finding of edema.

Pathophysiology Illustrated: Acute Postinfectious Glomerulonephritis

Infection from group A beta-hemolytic streptococci causes an immune response that leads to inflammation and damage to the glomeruli. Protein and red blood cells are allowed to pass through the glomeruli. Blood flow to the glomeruli is reduced because of obstruction with damaged cells. Renal insufficiency results, leading to the retention of sodium, water, and waste.

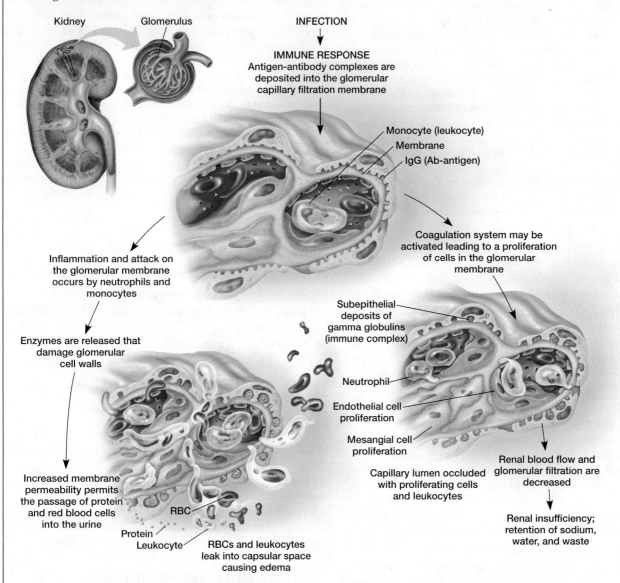

CLINICAL MANIFESTATIONS

Many children are asymptomatic. In other children, the onset is usually abrupt with flank or midabdominal pain, irritability, malaise, and fever. Microscopic hematuria is present in nearly all cases, and gross hematuria, resulting in tea-colored urine, is found in up to 50% of cases. Mild periorbital edema occurs early, along with dependent edema of the feet and ankles. Edema may progress in severity to cause pulmonary congestion or ascites (Nachman et al., 2012). Acute hypertension may lead to headache, nausea, vomiting, lethargy, seizures, and other CNS symptoms. Oliguria may or may not be present (Ring & Huether, 2014).

CLINICAL THERAPY

The serum BUN and creatinine concentrations are elevated. Serum protein is decreased as a result of mild or moderate proteinuria.

The white blood cell count and erythrocyte sedimentation rate may be elevated. An elevated antistreptolysin O (ASO) titer reflects the presence of antibodies from a recent streptococcal respiratory infection, but the ASO level associated with a recent skin infection is low. The anti-DNAse B titer is helpful for detecting antibodies associated with recent skin infections. Most children have a reduced serum complement (C3) level due to the initial infection (Nachman et al., 2012). Urinalysis reveals hematuria, proteinuria, and red blood cell casts. Anemia is common in the acute phase, usually because extracellular fluid dilutes the serum. Hemoglobin and hematocrit levels reveal anemia, which is common in the acute phase and is generally caused by dilution of the serum by the extracellular fluid (Bhimma, 2014).

Treatment focuses on relief of symptoms and supportive therapy. Bed rest is a key component of the treatment plan during the acute phase. Edema and mild to moderate hypertension should be treated with sodium restriction and a diuretic such as furosemide (Nachman et al., 2012; Ring & Huether, 2014). A course of antibiotics may be given to ensure eradication of the original infectious agent. Immediate emergency care is needed for severe hypertension with cerebral dysfunction.

The prognosis for most children with APIGN is good. Clinical signs, proteinuria, and hematuria resolve within several weeks. Over 95% of children recover completely (Ring & Huether, 2014).

Nursing Management

For the Child With Acute Postinfectious Glomerulonephritis

Nursing Assessment and Diagnosis

As with other renal disorders, care of the child with APIGN requires careful monitoring of vital signs and fluid–electrolyte balance to evaluate renal functioning and identify complications. Frequent blood pressure monitoring is required since it can rise as high as 200/120 mmHg. With severe hypertension, assess for signs of central nervous system problems (headache, blurred vision, vomiting, decreased level of consciousness, confusion, and convulsions). Monitor urine for proteinuria and hematuria. Record output. Assess edema, which may be periorbital or dependent and may shift as the child's position is changed. Assess for a pulmonary effusion (crackles, dyspnea, and cough).

Nursing diagnoses may include the following (NANDA-I © 2014):

- *Fluid Volume: Excess* related to decreased glomerular filtration and increased sodium
- *Infection, Risk for,* related to renal impairment and corticosteroid therapy
- *Skin Integrity, Risk for Impaired,* related to tissue edema
- *Nutrition, Imbalanced: Less than Body Requirements,* related to loss of appetite and proteinuria
- *Activity Intolerance* related to fluid and electrolyte imbalance, infectious process, and altered nutrition
- *Health Management, Family, Ineffective,* related to child's medication schedule and treatment regimen after discharge

---

Clinical Tip

Antibiotics are *not* a treatment for APIGN. Instead, antibiotics are prescribed to treat the original infection (such as strep throat) if the infection is still present.

Planning and Implementation

MONITOR FLUID STATUS

Monitor vital signs, fluid and electrolyte status, and intake and output. Hypovolemia can occur as a result of fluid shifting from vascular to interstitial spaces despite the outward clinical signs of excess fluid retention. Monitor the degree of ascites by measuring abdominal girth. Document urine specific gravity. Make sure parents and visitors understand the need to limit fluids to prevent excessive intake.

PREVENT INFECTION

Impaired renal function puts the child at risk for infection. Monitor for signs of infection, including fever, increased malaise, and an elevated white blood cell count. Screen family members for the presence of streptococcal infection and refer for treatment if necessary. Instruct the family in good hand hygiene technique. Limit visitors, and screen for upper respiratory infections.

PREVENT SKIN BREAKDOWN

Bed rest is required during the acute phase. Dependent areas and other pressure areas are vulnerable to skin breakdown. Turn the child frequently. Pad bony prominences or susceptible areas with sheepskin, or protect skin with a transparent dressing. Elevate lower extremities on pillows when in the dependent position or when the child is lying in bed. Make sure the child's bed is free of crumbs or sharp toys. Keep sheets tight and free of wrinkles. Maintain proper hygiene and dry skin.

MEET NUTRITIONAL NEEDS

A team approach (including the nurse, renal dietitian, parents, and child) is often needed to meet the child's nutritional needs. In most cases, the child follows a no-added-salt and low-protein diet. This diet may be challenging since the child may refuse to eat foods that taste different. Anorexia presents the greatest challenge to meeting daily nutritional requirements during the acute phase of the disease. To increase the child's appetite, encourage parents to bring the child's favorite foods from home, serve foods in age-appropriate quantities, and allow the child to eat with other children or with family members.

PROVIDE EMOTIONAL SUPPORT

Parents of a child with APIGN commonly feel guilty. Parents may blame themselves for not responding more quickly to the child's initial symptoms or may believe they could have prevented the development of glomerular damage. Discuss the etiology of the disease and the child's treatment, and correct any misconceptions. Emphasize that it is not possible to predict which of the few children with streptococcal infections will develop APIGN.

DISCHARGE PLANNING AND HOME CARE TEACHING

Children are hospitalized for a few days, although it may require 3 weeks for hypertension and gross hematuria to resolve and longer for the disorder to resolve completely. Discharge planning focuses on teaching parents about the child's medication regimen, potential side effects of medications, dietary restrictions, and signs and symptoms of complications. Teach parents how to take the child's blood pressure and how to test urine for blood or protein. Emphasize that it is important to avoid exposing the child to people with upper respiratory tract infections. Children should be allowed to return to their normal routines and activities after discharge, with periods being allowed for rest.

Evaluation

Expected outcomes of nursing care are the following:

- The child receives appropriate fluid volume each day and maintains normal urine output.
- The child develops no areas of redness, abrasions, or skin breakdown over pressure points.
- The child's temperature remains within normal limits and the child is free of secondary infection.

- The child maintains pre-illness weight and tolerates daily intake that meets nutritional requirements.
- The parents administer medications as prescribed. The child's sodium and potassium levels reflect adherence to dietary restrictions.

Renal Failure

Renal failure, which may be acute or chronic, occurs when the kidney is unable to excrete wastes and concentrate urine. Acute renal failure occurs suddenly (over days or weeks) and may be reversible, whereas in chronic renal failure, kidney function diminishes gradually and permanently over months or years.

Both types of renal failure are characterized by **azotemia** (accumulation of nitrogenous wastes in the blood) and sometimes **oliguria** (reduced urine volume for age), indicating the kidney's inability to excrete metabolic waste products. Chronic renal failure eventually results in **anuria** (absence of urine output).

Acute Renal Failure

Acute renal failure (ARF), also called *acute kidney injury*, is a sudden loss of adequate renal function in which the kidneys are unable to clear metabolic wastes and to regulate extracellular fluid volume, sodium balance, and acid–base homeostasis. Potential causes include hemolytic-uremic syndrome, acute glomerulonephritis, sepsis, poisoning, nephrotoxic medications, hypovolemia, obstructive uropathy, and complication of cardiac surgery.

ETIOLOGY AND PATHOPHYSIOLOGY

Acute renal failure may be caused by prerenal or postrenal factors as well as actual kidney damage. Prerenal ARF is a result of decreased perfusion to an otherwise normal kidney in association with a systemic condition. Hypovolemia secondary to dehydration is generally the cause; however, alterations in renal vasculature or cardiac function may also precipitate prerenal ARF. This is the most common type of ARF in infants and young children (Lum, 2014).

TABLE 26–6 Clinical Manifestations of Acute Versus Chronic Renal Failure

TYPE OF RENAL FAILURE	CLINICAL MANIFESTATIONS
Acute renal failure	Dark urine or gross hematuria, headache, edema, fatigue, crackles, gallop heart rhythm, hypertension, hematuria, lethargy, nausea and vomiting, oliguria
	Mass in flank area if a cyst, tumor, or obstructive lesion is present
Chronic renal failure	Fatigue, malaise, poor appetite, nausea and vomiting, failure to thrive or short stature
	May have oliguria or polyuria
	Headache, decreased mental alertness or ability to concentrate
	Chronic anemia, hypertension, edema
	Fractures with minimal trauma, rickets, valgus deformity

Primary kidney damage (intrinsic factors) may result from infection, diseases such as hemolytic-uremic syndrome, acute glomerulonephritis, and acute tubular necrosis, and nephrotoxic injury (Lum, 2014).

Postrenal ARF is generally found in newborns with urologic anatomic anomalies (Lum, 2014). Children may have oliguria or normal or increased urine output. Renal failure without oliguria usually indicates a less severe renal injury. Children who recover from ARF may have residual kidney damage and compromised renal function.

CLINICAL MANIFESTATIONS

Characteristically, a healthy child suddenly becomes ill with nonspecific symptoms that indicate a significant illness or injury (e.g., nausea, vomiting, lethargy, edema, gross hematuria, oliguria, and hypertension). These symptoms are a result of electrolyte imbalances, uremia, and fluid overload. The child appears pale and lethargic. See Tables 26–6 and 26–7 for more information.

Hyperkalemia is the most life-threatening electrolyte disorder associated with ARF. Hyponatremia affects central nervous system function, resulting in symptoms that range from fatigue to seizures. Edema occurs as a result of sodium and water retention. (Refer to Chapter 18 for a discussion of these fluid and electrolyte alterations.) Children with ARF are also more susceptible to infection because of depressed immune functioning. **Uremia** occurs when there is an excess of urea and other nitrogenous waste products in the blood. Neurologic symptoms from accumulating wastes may include headache, seizures, lethargy, and confusion.

CLINICAL THERAPY

Diagnosis of renal failure is based primarily on urinalysis and blood chemistry results, including BUN, serum creatinine, sodium, potassium, and calcium levels (Table 26–8). The kidneys are normal in size, and no signs of renal **osteodystrophy** (a complex bone disease process of chronic kidney disease in which there is increased resorption of bone caused by chronic hyperparathyroidism) are found on radiography. Various imaging studies to assess kidney structures, renal blood flow, and renal perfusion and function may be performed to determine whether the child has ARF or chronic renal failure. A renal biopsy may be required.

Treatment depends on the underlying cause of the renal failure. The goal is to minimize or prevent permanent renal damage while maintaining fluid and electrolyte balance and managing complications. Initial emergency treatment of children with fluid depletion focuses on rapid fluid replacement of saline or lactated Ringer solution at 20 mL/kg given rapidly over 5 to 10 minutes and repeated as needed to ensure renal perfusion and stabilize blood pressure. Albumin may also be administered when blood loss is the cause of circulatory depletion. If oliguria persists after restoration of adequate fluid volume, intrinsic renal damage is suspected.

Children with fluid overload, such as those with pulmonary edema, require diuretic therapy, and dialysis if they respond poorly to diuretics. Once the child is stabilized, fluid requirements are calculated to maintain zero water balance (intake should equal urine output and insensible fluid loss). All potential sources of potassium should be eliminated until hyperkalemia is controlled. Other electrolyte imbalances are treated. Nutrition must be maintained with extra carbohydrate intake during the catabolic state. Antibiotics are prescribed for infection if applicable. Nephrotoxic antibiotics such as aminoglycosides (e.g., gentamicin, vancomycin) should be avoided.

TABLE 26–7 Clinical Manifestations of Electrolyte Imbalances in Acute and Chronic Renal Failure

ELECTROLYTE IMBALANCE AND CAUSE	CLINICAL MANIFESTATIONS
HYPERKALEMIA Results from inability to adequately excrete potassium derived from diet and catabolized cells. In metabolic acidosis, there is also movement of potassium from intracellular fluid to extracellular fluid.	• Peaked T waves, widening of QRS waves on ECG • Dysrhythmias • Muscle weakness
HYPONATREMIA In the acute oliguric phase, hyponatremia is related to the accumulation of fluid in excess of solute.	• Change in level of consciousness • Muscle cramps • Anorexia • Abdominal reflexes, depressed deep tendon reflexes • Cheyne-Stokes respirations • Seizures
HYPOCALCEMIA Phosphate retention (hyperphosphatemia) depresses the serum calcium ion concentration. Calcium is deposited in injured cells. Hyperkalemia and metabolic acidosis may mask the common clinical manifestations of severe hypocalcemia.	• Muscle tingling • Changes in muscle tone • Seizures • Muscle cramps and twitching • Positive **Chvostek sign** (contraction of facial muscles after tapping facial nerve just anterior to parotid gland)

Note: See Chapter 18 for more information related to these alterations in electrolytes.

Source: Data from Hines, E. Q. (2012). Fluid and electrolytes. In *The Harriet Lane handbook* (19th ed., pp. 271–292). Philadelphia, PA: Elsevier Saunders; Sreedharan, R., & Avner, E. D. (2016). Renal failure. In R. M. Kliegman, B. F. Stanton, J. W. St. Geme, & N. F. Schor (Eds.), *Nelson textbook of pediatrics* (20th ed., pp. 2539–2547). Philadelphia, PA: Elsevier; Verive, M. J. (2013). *Pediatric hyperkalemia*. Retrieved from http://emedicine.medscape.com/article/907543-overview

Some children whose ARF is unresponsive to management require dialysis to correct severe electrolyte imbalances, manage fluid overload, and cleanse the blood of waste products. The clinical situation and age of the child determine whether hemodialysis or peritoneal dialysis is used. Refer to the *Renal Replacement Therapy* section later in this chapter.

Prognosis depends on the cause of ARF. When renal failure results from drug toxicity or dehydration, the prognosis is generally good. However, ARF that results from diseases such as hemolytic-uremic syndrome or acute glomerulonephritis may be associated with residual kidney damage.

TABLE 26–8 Diagnostic Tests for Renal Failure

DIAGNOSTIC TESTS	FINDINGS IN RENAL FAILURE
URINALYSIS	
pH	Acidic urine
Osmolarity	Greater than 500: prerenal ARF Less than 350: intrinsic ARF
Specific gravity	Greater than 1.020: prerenal ARF Less than 1.010: intrinsic ARF
Protein	Positive
Blood	Positive
SERUM CHEMISTRY*	
Potassium	Elevated
Sodium	Normal, low, or high; depends solely on the amount of water in the body
Calcium	Low
Phosphorus	High
Urea nitrogen	Increased
Creatinine	Increased
pH	Low acidic

Note: *Please refer to Appendix D for normal values for various ages.
ARF = acute renal failure.

Source: Data from Sreedharan, R., & Avner, E. D. (2016). Renal failure. In R. M. Kliegman, B. F. Stanton, J. W. St. Geme, N. F. Schor, & R. E. Behrman (Eds.), *Nelson textbook of pediatrics* (20th ed., pp. 2539–2547). Philadelphia, PA: Elsevier; Workeneh, B. T., Agraharkar, M., & Gupta, R. (2014). *Acute kidney injury*. Retrieved from http://emedicine.medscape.com/article/243492-overview

---

SAFETY ALERT!
Nephrotoxic drugs include the following:

• Antimicrobials: aminoglycosides, cephalosporins, tetracycline, sulfonamides
• Radiographic contrast media with iodine (typically used for CT scans)
• Heavy metals: lead, barium, iron
• Nonsteroidal anti-inflammatory drugs: indomethacin, aspirin, ibuprofen

---

Nursing Management

For the Child With Acute Renal Failure

Nursing Assessment and Diagnosis

A complete history and physical examination are necessary to identify progression of symptoms and possible causes of renal failure.

PHYSIOLOGIC ASSESSMENT

Assess vital signs, level of consciousness, and other neurologic indicators to help identify clinical signs of electrolyte imbalance (see Table 26–7). Measure the child's weight on admission to

Pathophysiology Illustrated: **Acute Renal Failure**

The initial kidney injury is usually associated with an acute condition such as sepsis, trauma, or hypotension or is the result of treatment for an acute condition with a nephrotoxic medication. Injury to the kidney can occur because of glomerular injury, vasoconstriction of capillaries, or tubular injury. All consequences of injury lead to decreased glomerular filtration and oliguria.

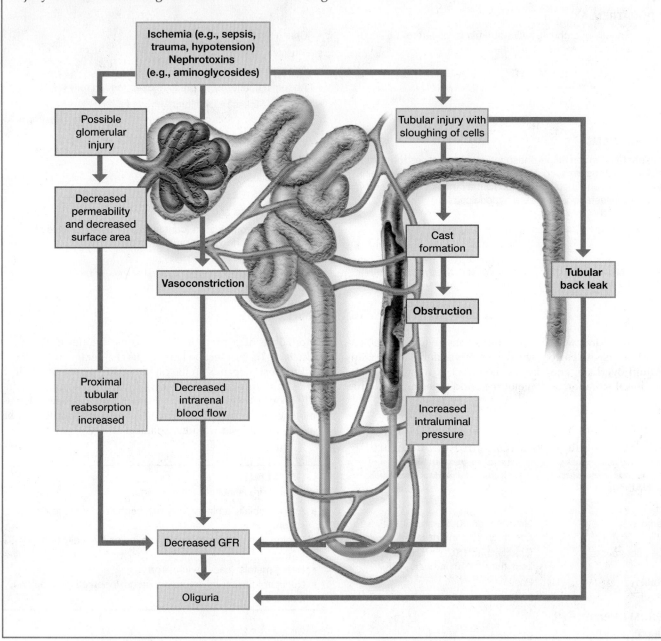

provide a baseline for evaluating changes in fluid status. Monitor urinalysis, urine culture, and blood chemistry studies. Inspect urine for color, specific gravity, amount, and odor. Cloudy urine may indicate infection; tea-colored urine suggests hematuria. Assess urine specific gravity and intake and output.

PSYCHOSOCIAL ASSESSMENT

The unexpected and acute nature of the child's hospitalization creates anxiety for both parents and child. Assess for feelings of anger, guilt, or fear associated with the hospitalization. Such feelings are likely if ARF developed as a result of dehydration,

a preventable injury, or poisoning. Assess coping mechanisms, family support systems, and level of stress.

Several nursing diagnoses may apply to the child with ARF, including the following (NANDA-I © 2014):

- *Perfusion: Renal, Risk for Ineffective,* related to hypovolemia, sepsis, or drug
- *Fluid Volume: Excess* related to renal dysfunction and sodium retention
- *Nutrition, Imbalanced: Less than Body Requirements,* related to anorexia, nausea, vomiting, and catabolic state

- *Infection, Risk for,* related to invasive procedures and monitoring equipment, and diminished immune functioning
- *Coping: Family, Compromised,* related to sudden hospitalization and uncertain prognosis of child

Planning and Implementation

Nursing care focuses on preventing complications, maintaining fluid balance, administering medications, meeting nutritional needs, preventing infection, and providing emotional support to the child and parents.

PREVENT COMPLICATIONS

Complications are best prevented by ensuring compliance with the treatment plan. Careful monitoring of vital signs, intake and output, serum electrolytes, and level of consciousness can alert the nurse to changes that indicate potential complications.

MAINTAIN FLUID BALANCE

Estimate the child's fluid status by monitoring of intake and output and blood pressure 2 or 3 times daily. Also obtain a weight at least daily on the same scale at the same time of day. Monitor serum chemistry values, especially for sodium and potassium.

If the child has oliguria, limit fluid intake (including parenteral nutrition) to replacement of insensible fluid loss (what is excreted by the lungs, skin, and gastrointestinal tract), which is about one third the daily maintenance requirements in afebrile children. If the child is febrile, fluid requirements are increased. See Chapter 18.

Clinical Tip

The child with **renal insufficiency** is at greater risk for fluid loss with illness. In cases of acute gastrointestinal illness, children are at greater risk for dehydration.

ADMINISTER MEDICATIONS

Because the kidney's ability to excrete drugs is impaired in ARF, dosages of all medications should be adjusted. The actual dosage of the drug can be reduced or the time interval between doses may be increased. Check drug levels to monitor for drug toxicity and know the signs of drug toxicity for each medication the child is receiving.

MEET NUTRITIONAL NEEDS

Children are at risk for malnutrition because of their high metabolic rate during ARF. Parenteral or enteral feeding may be used initially to minimize protein catabolism. The diet is tailored to the individual child's need for calories, carbohydrates, fats, and amino acids or protein hydrolysates. Depending on the degree of renal failure, sodium, potassium, and phosphorus may be restricted. Initiate oral feeding as soon as tolerated.

PREVENT INFECTION

The child with ARF is extremely susceptible to hospital-acquired infections because of altered nutritional status, compromised immunity, and numerous invasive procedures. Thorough hand hygiene and standard precautions are imperative to decrease the risk of infection. Use sterile technique for all invasive procedures and when caring for lines. Drainage from catheter sites should be cultured to check for the presence of infectious organisms. Assess vital signs and lung sounds frequently.

PROVIDE EMOTIONAL SUPPORT

The sudden onset of ARF presents parents with an unexpected threat to their child's life. Both the child and the parents experience anxiety because of the unexpected hospitalization and the uncertainty of the prognosis. Parents often feel guilty, regardless of the cause of renal failure. Guilt is intensified if the parents feel there is something they could have done to prevent the condition. Encourage parents to verbalize their fears and help them work through feelings of guilt. Explain procedures and treatment measures to decrease anxiety. Encouraging parents and older siblings to participate in the child's care can increase their sense of control.

Developing Cultural Competence Reducing Sodium in the Child's Diet

Special effort is often needed to reduce the sodium in the diet of an Asian child. Sauces and seasonings for foods (soy sauce, mustards, monosodium glutamate, and garlic salt) are sodium rich even though the foods seasoned (rice, vegetables, shrimp, and chicken) are low in sodium. A child eating a diet of predominantly Mexican cuisine may also require significant modification because many of the foods are high in sodium and potassium. Individualized counseling and motivation are needed to encourage families to reduce the child's sodium intake and to use spices low in sodium when preparing meals.

DISCHARGE PLANNING AND HOME CARE TEACHING

Encourage parental involvement early in the child's hospitalization. Be sure parents understand the importance of administering medications correctly. Teach family members proper technique for measuring blood pressure so they can monitor the child's hypertension, if ordered. Make sure the parents can identify signs of progressive renal failure (see the following chronic renal failure discussion).

Diet counseling is a key component of discharge planning and is usually performed by a renal nutritionist. Depending on the degree of renal failure, the child's diet may include restrictions on protein, water, sodium, potassium, and phosphorus.

The parents should be given written guidelines listing appropriate food choices to assist in menu planning. Ethnic and cultural preferences should be considered when listing menu options.

Continued monitoring of renal function during follow-up examinations is critical as deterioration may occur over time. Referral to support groups can be helpful for both parents and children. The National Kidney Foundation is a source of numerous publications that are helpful to the child and family.

Evaluation

Expected outcomes of nursing care include:

- Kidney function is restored.
- Fluid, electrolyte, and acid–base balance is restored and maintained.
- Nutritional needs are met.
- The child does not acquire a secondary infection.

Chronic Renal Failure

Chronic renal failure (CRF) (also called chronic kidney disease) is a progressive, irreversible reduction in kidney function. The prevalence of CRF in children is approximately 18 per 1 million (Sreedharan & Avner, 2016).

ETIOLOGY AND PATHOPHYSIOLOGY

In children, CRF usually results from developmental abnormalities of the kidney or urinary tract, obstructed urine flow and reflux, hereditary diseases such as polycystic kidney disease, infections such as hemolytic-uremic syndrome, and glomerulonephritis (Lum, 2014).

The gradual, progressive loss of functioning nephrons ultimately results in **end-stage renal disease (ESRD)**. In ESRD, the kidneys can no longer maintain homeostasis and the child requires dialysis (Sreedharan & Avner, 2016).

The kidneys excrete excess acid in the body and regulate the body's fluid and electrolyte balance. Renal failure disrupts this fluid and electrolyte balance. As renal failure progresses, metabolic acidosis occurs because the kidneys cannot excrete the acids that build up in the body. Renal osteodystrophy occurs because the kidneys are unable to produce activated vitamin D or to excrete phosphorus, causing phosphorus levels to rise and serum calcium levels to fall. The parathyroid gland responds by drawing calcium and phosphorus from the bones to maintain the adequate serum calcium and phosphorus levels. Hypocalcemia may occur as the parathyroid glands become less responsive to vitamin D and lower serum calcium levels. Osteodystrophy increases the child's risk for spontaneous fractures (Sreedharan & Avner, 2016).

Growth retardation is caused by disturbances in the metabolism of calcium, phosphorus, and vitamin D; decreased caloric intake; and metabolic acidosis. Healthy kidneys also produce erythropoietin (the growth factor responsible for the production and maturation of red cells); lack of erythropoietin and progressive renal disease are the underlying causes of the anemia of CRF.

CLINICAL MANIFESTATIONS

Children with CRF frequently have no symptoms initially. As progression continues, renal insufficiency occurs with polyuria as the kidneys become unable to concentrate the urine. Symptoms such as pallor, headache, nausea, and fatigue become more common. Decreased mental alertness and ability to concentrate may be seen. The child may have anemia leading to tachycardia, tachypnea, and dyspnea on exertion. As the disease progresses, the child experiences a loss of appetite and has complications of renal impairment, including hypertension, pulmonary edema, growth retardation, osteodystrophy, delayed fine and gross motor development, and delayed sexual maturation. Refer to Table 26–6 to see how these signs contrast with signs of acute renal failure.

In ESRD, renal failure adversely affects all body systems. As the severity of the clinical and biochemical disturbances resulting from progressive renal deterioration increases, uremic symptoms develop. Signs and symptoms of uremic syndrome include nausea and vomiting, progressive anemia, anorexia, dyspnea, malaise, *uremic frost* (urea crystals deposited on the skin), unpleasant (uremic) breath odor, headache, progressive confusion, tremors, pulmonary edema, and congestive heart failure.

CLINICAL THERAPY

Laboratory evaluation, including serum electrolytes, phosphate, BUN, creatinine levels, and pH, is used to confirm the diagnosis of CRF. An early morning urine sample is collected for culture and to calculate the protein-to-creatinine ratio. The child's glomerular filtration rate is calculated from prediction equations using the serum creatinine level and the patient's height and gender. Imaging studies are performed to identify renal diseases that could be causing the renal failure. A renal biopsy may sometimes be performed.

Chronic renal failure is irreversible; however, the course of the disease is variable. Some children progress quickly to renal failure, necessitating dialysis. Other children are managed with a combination of medication and diet therapy for some time before significant renal impairment occurs. Frequent modifications in the treatment plan are often necessary to address the child's changing status.

Dietary management focuses on maximizing caloric intake for growth while limiting phosphorus, potassium, and sodium intake as needed to maintain electrolytes in balance (Sreedharan & Avner, 2016). Adequate calcium needs to be part of the meal plan. Enteral or parenteral feedings may be required to achieve optimal protein intake, especially in children under 1 year of age. Complex carbohydrates should be chosen along with vegetables and fruits that are lower in potassium. Vegetable oils, hard candy, sugar, honey, and jelly may be recommended to add calories to the child's diet. Medications used to treat children with CRF are discussed in the next table.

Children who progress to ESRD require renal replacement therapy. The timetable for dialysis or renal transplantation is different from that of adults; transplantation is the goal so the child has an optimal chance for a more normal childhood. Earlier initiation can prevent some complications of ESRD. In addition to the GFR, nonspecific signs such as uremic syndrome, poorly controlled hypertension, renal osteodystrophy, failure of head circumference measurement to increase normally, developmental delay, and poor growth are used in determining when to initiate renal replacement therapy. (Refer to the *Renal Replacement Therapy* section later in this chapter.)

Nursing Management

For the Child With Chronic Renal Failure

Nursing Assessment and Diagnosis

Nursing assessment focuses on identifying signs and symptoms of renal failure and associated complications as well as assessing the psychosocial effects of renal failure on the child and family.

PHYSIOLOGIC ASSESSMENT

The initial and ongoing assessment of the child focuses on identifying complications of renal failure. Observe for signs of hypertension, edema, poor growth and development, osteodystrophy, and anemia. Assess vital signs, particularly the blood pressure. Observe for signs of alterations in electrolyte balance.

PSYCHOSOCIAL ASSESSMENT

As renal disease progresses, the number of stressors on the child and family increases. Denial and disbelief are commonly the first reactions. A thorough family assessment can help to identify particular needs of the child and family. The development of ESRD is particularly challenging during childhood and adolescence because of differences in appearance and social, psychologic, and physical issues. Nonadherence to treatments can endanger the adolescent's life.

Nursing diagnoses for the child with CRF are similar to those previously listed for ARF. Additional diagnoses might include the following (NANDA-I © 2014):

- *Social Interaction, Impaired,* related to impaired immunity and hemodialysis schedule during school hours
- *Activity Intolerance* related to anemia and fatigue
- *Health Management, Family, Ineffective,* related to complexity of care plan and economic difficulties
- *Body Image, Disturbed,* related to short stature and visible external catheter for dialysis

Medications Used to Treat: Chronic Renal Failure

MEDICATION AND ACTION/INDICATION	NURSING IMPLICATIONS
Vitamin and mineral supplement (Nephrocaps) Adds vitamins and minerals missing from heavily restricted diet.	Only prescribed vitamins should be used; over-the-counter brands may contain elements that are harmful.
Phosphate binding agents: calcium carbonate (Tums), calcium acetate (PhosLo), or sevelamer hydrochloride (Renagel) Reduces absorption of phosphorus from the intestines.	Ensure that phosphate binding agent is aluminum-free.
Calcitriol (Rocaltrol) Replaces the calcitriol that kidneys are no longer producing to keep calcium balance normal.	Monitor serum calcium level. Ensure that calcium supplement is provided.
Epoetin alfa (Epogen, Procrit) Stimulates bone marrow to produce red blood cells, treats anemia due to CRF.	Given by IV or subcutaneous injection. Monitor blood pressure because hypertension is an adverse effect. Monitor hematocrit and serum ferritin levels according to facility guidelines.
Iron supplementation Treats iron deficiency when epoetin alfa is prescribed.	Give without food or other medications to maximize absorption.
Growth hormone (rhGH) Used to stimulate growth in children with CRF.	Record accurate height measurements at regular intervals.
Antihypertensive agents: angiotensin-converting enzyme (ACE) inhibitor (Enalapril, Lisinopril) Used with proteinuric kidney disease because it slows the progression to ESRD.	Monitor blood pressure.
Loop diuretics (Furosemide) Used when volume overload is present.	Monitor urine output and electrolyte balance.

Source: Data from Gulati, S. (2012). *Chronic kidney disease in children*. Retrieved from http://emedicine.medscape.com/article/984358-overview; Lum, G. M. (2014). Kidney & urinary tract. In W. W. Hay, M. J. Levin, R. R. Deterding, & M. J. Abzug, *CURRENT diagnosis and treatment: Pediatrics* (22nd ed.). New York, NY: McGraw-Hill. Retrieved from http://accessmedicine.com; Sreedharan, R., & Avner, E. D. (2016). Renal failure. In R. M. Kliegman, B. F. Stanton, J. W. St. Geme, N. F. Schor, & R. E. Behrman (Eds.), *Nelson textbook of pediatrics* (20th ed., pp. 2539–2547). Philadelphia, PA: Elsevier; Wilson, B. A., Shannon, M. T., & Shields, K. M. (2015). *Pearson nurse's drug guide 2015*. Hoboken, NJ: Pearson Education.

Planning and Implementation

Children with CRF are usually hospitalized for one or more of the following reasons: initial diagnostic evaluation, dialysis treatment initiation, or problems with the treatment plan or infection. Nursing care for the hospitalized child with CRF focuses on monitoring for side effects of medications, preventing infection, meeting nutritional needs, and providing emotional support and anticipatory teaching.

MONITOR FOR SIDE EFFECTS OF MEDICATIONS

Assess for signs of electrolyte imbalance such as weakness, muscle cramps, dizziness, headache, and nausea and vomiting in children who are taking diuretics. Supervise the child's activities closely to prevent falls resulting from dizziness, especially at the beginning of diuretic therapy. If antihypertensive medications such as hydralazine are being administered, monitor the child's weight to detect excessive gain resulting from water and sodium retention.

PREVENT INFECTION

The child with CRF is susceptible to infections. Be alert for signs of infection, such as elevated temperature; cloudy, strong-smelling urine; dysuria; changes in respiratory pattern; or productive cough. Emphasize to the child and family the importance of good hand hygiene practices. Make sure the child receives the 23-valent pneumococcal vaccine and meningococcal vaccines in addition to usual childhood immunizations.

TABLE 26–9 Nutritional Information for the Child With Kidney Disease

Children with kidney disease have restricted diets, generally low in sodium, potassium, and phosphorus. A renal dietitian works with families of children with chronic renal failure to develop meal plans that fit a restricted diet. The nurse can help families remember that certain foods must be avoided or eaten in very small quantities by reviewing this table.

HIGH-SODIUM CONTENT FOODS	HIGH-POTASSIUM CONTENT FOODS	HIGH-PHOSPHORUS CONTENT FOODS
Soups and sauces: e.g., gravy, spaghetti and tomato sauce, barbeque sauce, steak sauce	*Fruit:* apricots, avocados, bananas, citrus fruits, fresh pears, nectarines, dates, figs, cantaloupe and other melons, prunes, and raisins	*Dairy products:* milk, cheese, yogurt, custard, pudding, ice cream
Processed lunch meats: e.g., bologna, ham, salami, hot dogs	*Vegetables:* celery, dried beans, lima beans, potatoes, leafy greens, spinach, tomatoes, winter squash	Dried beans, peas
Smoked meat and fish: bacon, chipped beef, corned beef, ham, lox	*Whole grains:* especially those containing bran	Nuts, peanut butter
Sauerkraut, pickles, and other pickled foods	Sardines, clams	Chocolate
Seasonings: horseradish, soy sauce, Worcestershire sauce, meat tenderizer, and monosodium glutamate (MSG)	Peanuts	Dark cola
	Dairy products: milk, ice cream, pudding, yogurt	Sausage, hot dogs
	Potassium-containing salt substitutes	

MEET NUTRITIONAL NEEDS

Maintaining adequate nutritional intake in a child with CRF who has dietary restrictions is challenging. Provide small, frequent feedings and present meals attractively to encourage the child to eat. A nutritionist works with the child and family to develop meal plans that meet the nutritional requirements and acknowledge the child's preferences. See Table 26–9 for foods that children with CRF should avoid.

MAINTAIN FLUID RESTRICTIONS

Plan the child's oral intake through the entire 24 hours to ensure that the child has some fluids with meals, when taking medications, and when thirsty. Keep in mind that many foods have a high fluid content (gelatin, fruit-flavored ice pops) and must be counted toward the daily fluid allowance. Use medicine cups or small cups for fluids given. Encourage parents and visitors to avoid drinking in the child's presence. Ensure that all visitors know and understand the importance of maintaining the child's fluid restriction.

PROVIDE EMOTIONAL SUPPORT

Progressive CRF requires a total lifestyle change for the child and family. The parents and child need opportunities to express and work through their feelings related to the disease, prognosis, and treatment restrictions. Help children express their feelings through drawings or therapeutic play.

The need for ongoing dialysis treatments and the wait for a suitable donor kidney are stressful for both parents and children. Identify effective coping methods and family support systems to promote treatment compliance. The National Kidney Foundation and local support groups for kidney disease can give the family information or additional support.

DISCHARGE PLANNING AND HOME CARE TEACHING

Parents need to understand the necessity of long-term treatments and follow-up care. Help the family develop a schedule for medication administration that fits with their routine. Emphasize the importance of consistency in administration times. Teach parents how to recognize medication side effects and complications.

Appropriate referrals are made to home care nursing agencies as indicated. Parents of children receiving peritoneal dialysis at home are taught how to perform the treatment and how to identify complications. Strict aseptic technique is necessary to prevent infection at the catheter site and peritonitis.

COMMUNITY-BASED NURSING CARE

Children with CRF require frequent outpatient visits to monitor the progression of signs and symptoms, and to evaluate the effectiveness of current treatments. The blood pressure is monitored. Blood and urine tests are performed to monitor renal function. Radiographs of the bones are often taken at 6-month intervals to assess changes caused by osteodystrophy. See *Health Promotion: The Child With Chronic Renal Failure*.

Encourage parents to register the young child for an early intervention program to promote development and interaction with other children. The dialysis schedule for school-age children should enable the child to participate in school, or home tutoring should be provided.

School-age children and adolescents are often embarrassed about being seen as different from peers. Ask them how they feel about the need to follow a special diet, take medications, and undergo dialysis treatments. To minimize the psychologic consequences of coping with a chronic disease, encourage parents to promote the child's participation in age-appropriate activities. Attendance at school and contact with peers promote normal growth and development. Work to promote the child's self-worth and a healthy self-esteem. Encourage adolescents to participate in a program that helps them transition to adult health services and job skill training. Begin teaching the child during early adolescence about the health condition, about medications taken and their actions, how to access emergency help, and about problems caused by not adhering to treatment. As the adolescent ages, have the family begin giving more responsibility for self-care, such as making appointments for health care, obtaining prescription refills, and seeking out healthcare providers for adult patients and a dialysis program. (See *Evidence-Based Practice: Living With Chronic Kidney Disease*.) As the child's renal impairment progresses, give the parents timely information about the disease process, dialysis treatments, and issues related to renal transplantation.

Health Promotion   The Child With Chronic Renal Failure

Growth and Development Surveillance

- Compare the child's height, weight, and head circumference to age-specific norms to identify growth retardation and to plot progress.
- Assess developmental progress using the Denver II or another screening tool (refer to Chapter 6).
- Educate the parents on normal developmental milestones and measures to promote achieving those milestones.
- Assess the adolescent for signs of delayed sexual maturation and, in girls, amenorrhea.

Nutrition

- Review the dietary restrictions with the child and parents.
- Partner with the family to assist the child to make good food selections and to restrict fluids and sodium as necessary, taking into account the child's likes and dislikes and cultural background. Encourage the child and family to take a list of a few favorite foods to the dietitian to see if they can be integrated into the child's meal plan.
- Make mealtime pleasant and make foods taste more appealing with permitted spices.
- Discuss possible behavioral responses by older children and adolescents to dietary restrictions and limitations imposed by the treatment plan. Involve the child and adolescent in discussions about dietary restrictions, and when possible integrate their recommendations for dietary restrictions and fluid management throughout the day.
- Emphasize to the school-age child that dietary and other restrictions are not punishment.
- Use enteral feeding at night to provide the needed calories for growth.

Physical Activity

- Encourage the child to participate in developmentally appropriate activities as tolerated.
- Partner with the child to establish a routine plan for physical activity as tolerated that will help promote strong bones.

Oral Health

- Promote good dentition and oral hygiene.
- Schedule regular dental visits for examinations and cleaning to reduce infections.
- Partner with the family to ensure they understand the need for antibiotic prophylaxis before certain invasive procedures, including dental care.

Mental and Spiritual Health

- Ask children how they feel about the need to follow a special diet, take medications, and undergo dialysis treatments. Ask what might make it easier for them to cope with the treatments, and integrate at least one idea into the care plan.

- Encourage parents to promote their child's participation in age-appropriate activities to minimize the psychologic consequences of coping with a chronic disease.
- Adolescents often resent the dietary restrictions and ongoing dialysis treatments, which pose a threat to their independence, evolving sense of self, and their need for independence. Noncooperation, depression, and hostility are common responses.
- Assist adolescents to begin the transition to adult health services.

Relationships

- Attendance at school and contacts with peers promote normal growth and development.
- Work to promote the child's self-worth and a healthy self-esteem.
- Prepare the child for peer conflict.
- Ensure that parents understand the importance of encouraging normal socialization of their child.

Disease Prevention Strategies

- Partner with the child and family to establish plans to avoid large crowds, people with infections, or other risks that expose the child to infection.
- If possible, all immunizations should be provided before renal transplantation, as long-term immunosuppressive therapy will then be prescribed.
- Live vaccines should not be given to the child taking immunosuppressive agents.
- Encourage the family to maintain scheduled appointments for routine serum and urine diagnostic tests performed to monitor renal function.

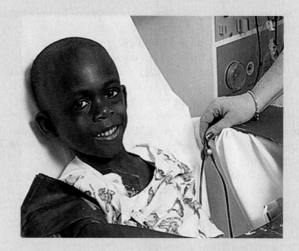

Evaluation

Expected outcomes of nursing care include:

- The child's fluid status is maintained.
- The child eats foods that meet nutritional needs while adhering to dietary restrictions.
- Growth and developmental milestones are achieved.

Renal Replacement Therapy

Renal replacement therapy is the treatment for renal failure and includes both dialysis and renal transplantation. The preferred method of dialysis is generally dependent on the age of the child. Currently, 88% of children 5 years of age and younger are treated with peritoneal dialysis, while 54% of children older than 12 years of age are treated with hemodialysis (Sreedharan & Avner, 2016).

EVIDENCE-BASED PRACTICE | Living With Chronic Kidney Disease

Clinical Question
Chronic kidney disease is a serious chronic condition that requires significant adaptations in lifestyle and complex medical treatments that take a toll on the child and family. What is the impact of this condition on children?

The Evidence
Heath et al. (2011) used the Generic Children's Quality of Life Measure to explore the impact of chronic kidney disease (CKD) on 225 pediatric patients ranging in age from 6 to 18 years. Of these patients, 49 had advanced CKD, 128 were posttransplant, and 47 were on dialysis. Results of the study showed that there was no difference between the mean quality-of-life scores in children who were in different treatment modalities. Age and gender did not affect the mean score. The study also showed that children ages 6 to 14 with CKD had significantly higher quality-of-life scores than children of the same age in the general population. While this was a surprising finding, it emphasized the fact that children with chronic conditions can perceive their quality of life as good despite having challenges with their health. These results could also be related to the psychosocial care provided by the renal team.

Al-Uzri et al. (2013) evaluated the effect of short stature on the health-related quality of life (HRQoL) in children with CKD. Short stature is common in children with CKD. Data collected as part of a larger multicenter Chronic Kidney Disease in Children study was used for the focus of this study. The participants were 483 children and/or parents who were enrolled in the larger study and had completed at least 2 evaluations of their HRQoL. The Pediatric Qualilty of Life Inventory (pedsQL) was used to assess physical, emotional, social, and school functioning. Parents completed the parent proxy version of the form. Results of the study demonstrated that parent-reported physical HRQoL was lower in the short stature group than the normal height group, although this was not statistically significant. Assessment of catch-up growth and its impact on HRQoL revealed that an increase in the height z-score was related to a 7-point increase in the parents' perception of the child's physical and social functioning; however, there was no association between catch-up growth and the child's pedsQL score. Analysis of pedsQL scores in the 58 children who were taking growth hormone versus those who were not did not reveal a relationship; however, there was a significant impact of improved height z-scores with growth hormone use on parents' perceptions of physical and social functioning. Additionally, children ages 15 to 17 with CKD had significantly higher rates on the pedsQL inventory than their parents in all areas except for school functioning. There was a high level of agreement between children ages 8 to 14 and their parents on all aspects of the inventory except emotional functioning, with the child having lower scores than their parents' perception. The results of this study support the need for interventions that improve height in children with CKD. It also demonstrates the importance of evaluating both the perception of the child and the parents.

Research by Kilis-Pstrunsinska et al. (2013) evaluated the HRQoL in Polish children with CKD using the Pediatric Quality of Life Inventory. Participants in the study were 203 children with CKD and 388 parent/proxies. This study found that children with CKD had significantly lower HRQoL scores compared to international population norms for healthy children. Results also showed that children on dialysis had lower scores in physical and social functioning than those treated conservatively. Additionally, patients on hemodialysis had significantly lower overall scores than children treated conservatively or with peritoneal dialysis. In children who were treated conservatively, stage of disease did not affect scores. Differences were also noted between parent/proxy scores and the child. The differences varied depending on the severity of the disease and the intensity of the treatment plan.

Best Practice
Effects of chronic illness in children and adolescents can be both physically and psychosocially overwhelming. It is important to evaluate quality of life in children with chronic illness in order to better understand their responses to the illness and treatment (Heath et al., 2011). Children of different ages may view their quality of life differently. Their view may also be different depending on the severity of their disease, their current treatment plan, and the amount of support they have received. Parents' views of their child's quality of life may vary from that of the child. It is essential that nurses assess each child and family member individually to determine their view of the illness and its impact on their life. This will assist the nurse to develop an effective care plan for the child and family and coordinate additional support for them as needed.

Clinical Reasoning
Initiate a discussion with an older school-age child or adolescent with CKD. Listen to their description of living with the condition. Develop a nursing care plan to help the child take the next steps in self-management.

PERITONEAL DIALYSIS
In peritoneal dialysis, the peritoneum of the abdomen is the membrane through which the body's waste products pass from the blood to the abdominal cavity. A catheter is inserted through the abdominal wall into the peritoneal cavity. In children receiving peritoneal dialysis for ARF, a percutaneously placed catheter can be used for a few weeks. In children with CRF, a catheter is placed surgically for long-term use. The dialysis solution (**dialysate**) that enters the abdomen typically contains dextrose that pulls body wastes and extra fluid into the abdominal cavity. These wastes and extra fluid leave the body with the drained dialysate. This method of dialysis is beneficial to small children since it allows continuous removal of fluids and waste products, decreasing the toxic effects of waste products on the child's developing body. The child can ambulate and interact with the environment. The timing of the treatment can be set to minimize the interruption of school, play, or other social events.

Two types of peritoneal dialysis are commonly used: continuous ambulatory peritoneal dialysis (CAPD) and automated

TABLE 26–10 Complications of Peritoneal Dialysis

COMPLICATIONS AND MANIFESTATIONS	CAUSE
PERITONITIS	
Cloudy dialysate, abdominal pain, tenderness, leukocytosis, fever (neonatal hypothermia), constipation	*Staphylococcus aureus, S. epidermidis,* fungal infections, gram-negative rods (risk is proportional to duration of dialysis and inversely proportional to age)
PAIN	
During inflow	Too rapid a rate of infusion, too large a volume of dialysate, encasement of catheter in a false passage, extremes in temperature of dialysate
During outflow at end of emptying	Omentum entering catheter at end of outflow
LEAKAGE	
Fluid around catheter, edema of penis or scrotum secondary to leakage into abdominal subcutaneous tissue, fluid leakage to pleural spaces through diaphragm	Overfilling of abdomen, catheter that has migrated from peritoneal cavity
RESPIRATORY SYMPTOMS	
Shortness of breath, decreased breath sounds in lower lobes, inadequate chest expansion	Abdominal fullness that compromises diaphragm movement, hole in diaphragm allowing dialysate into chest cavity

peritoneal dialysis (APD). Graduated cylinders are used to monitor the volume of fluid exchanged.

- CAPD uses gravity to instill prefilled bags of dialysate into the peritoneal cavity 4 or 5 times a day. The fluid remains in the cavity for 4 to 8 hours. The attached bag is folded under the child's clothes, permitting normal activity. After the allotted time, the dialysate is drained by hanging the bag lower than the pelvis. The repeated connections and disconnections with this method are time consuming for the child and family and increase the risk of infection.

- APD uses an automatic cycler to instill and drain the dialysate about 5 times over a 10-hour period, usually overnight. One additional exchange may be needed during the day. With this method, the number of connections and disconnections is minimized, which reduces demands on the family as well as the risk of infection. Infants and young children on peritoneal dialysis generally receive APD while they sleep (Zaritsky & Warady, 2011).

Peritonitis is a common complication of peritoneal dialysis. See Table 26–10. Peritonitis is treated with antibiotics infused in the dialysate (Mehrazma, Amini-Alavijeh, & Hooman, 2012).

Teach the family to perform peritoneal dialysis and to use sterile technique when performing dialysis and when doing catheter care. Peritoneal dialysis is time consuming, and family members must be committed to managing this procedure daily. Help the family develop home routines that minimize disruptions to daily family life. For additional information, refer to *Nursing Care Plan: The Child Receiving Home Peritoneal Dialysis*.

HEMODIALYSIS

Hemodialysis is a process in which the blood flows from the patient through a machine with a special filter that removes body wastes and extra fluids. Blood is pumped out of the body and through a dialyzer, where waste products and extra fluids diffuse out across a semipermeable membrane, before the blood is returned to the body. Dialysate is pumped in the direction opposite blood flow to promote waste extraction. Differences in osmolarity and concentration between the child's blood and the dialysate alter the intravascular electrolyte concentration and reduce the intravascular volume.

Clinical Tip
The dominant sign of peritonitis associated with peritoneal dialysis is cloudy dialysate. Other signs and symptoms may include fever, vomiting, diarrhea, abdominal pain, and tenderness. The nurse monitors for these symptoms and ensures that the child and family can recognize the symptoms and report them immediately.

Hemodialysis is used in the critical care setting and for those children with CRF when peritoneal dialysis is not possible for technical reasons, after repeated peritonitis, or when the family is unable to provide peritoneal dialysis safely. Hemodialysis for children is offered in a special dialysis center on an outpatient basis, or it can be performed at bedside during hospitalization. Treatment is usually performed 3 times a week, with each session lasting approximately 3 to 4 hours.

Children over 20 kg (44 lb) often have an arteriovenous (AV) fistula (connection between an artery and a vein) created for long-term vascular access. Alternatively, a synthetic tube can be implanted under the skin, creating a graft between the arterial and venous circulation to provide vascular access. Two needles are inserted into the arteriovenous fistula or the graft: one to carry blood to the dialyzer and one to return cleaned blood to the body. In emergencies and for infants, a double-lumen cannula is inserted into a large vein (e.g., the femoral, jugular, or subclavian vein) for hemodialysis.

Hemodialysis is more efficient than peritoneal dialysis but requires close monitoring for symptoms related to hypotension or rapid changes in fluid and electrolyte balance. Uncommonly, a **disequilibrium syndrome** (rapid changes in the body's water and electrolyte balance during treatment) may occur during or soon after the dialysis procedure is first initiated. Other complications include access thrombosis and infection. Heparin is used to reduce the risk of thrombosis.

Nursing management focuses on care of the child during dialysis and teaching the child and family about the administration of heparin and the control of bleeding from minor trauma. Carefully monitor fluid balance in the child undergoing hemodialysis. Check vital signs and blood pressure every half hour. Monitor oral intake and urinary output every half hour when the child is on the dialysis equipment. Weigh the child before and

Nursing Care Plan: The Child Receiving Home Peritoneal Dialysis

1. Nursing Diagnosis: *Nutrition, Imbalanced: Less than Body Requirements,* related to poor appetite, feeling of fullness after a small amount, and loss of protein in dialysate (NANDA-I © 2014)

GOAL: The child will obtain adequate nutrients each day.

INTERVENTION	RATIONALE
• Develop a meal plan in collaboration with a nutritionist to identify the amounts of essential nutrients needed.	• Parents need concrete guidelines for food preparation.
• Provide small, frequent meals of needed nutrients.	• The child will feel full with smaller amounts of food because of the dialysate.
• Make mealtimes pleasant and avoid battles over the child's intake.	• The child will be more inclined to eat if there is less stress.
• Provide supplements by tube feeding if adequate oral intake is not possible.	• Adequate nutrition is important for growth and development, and must be supported if oral intake is inadequate.

EXPECTED OUTCOME: Child's intake will be adequate to maintain an expected growth pattern.

2. Nursing Diagnosis: *Infection, Risk for,* related to daily invasive procedure (NANDA-I © 2014)

GOAL: The child will not develop peritonitis.

INTERVENTION	RATIONALE
• Wash hands, use sterile gloves and aseptic technique for connection and disconnection of catheters.	• Aseptic technique reduces chance of introducing bacteria into the abdomen.
• Perform daily catheter site care.	• Skin around the catheter site will have fewer organisms that could potentially cause infection.

EXPECTED OUTCOME: Child will not develop peritonitis.

GOAL: If peritonitis occurs, it will be treated appropriately.

INTERVENTION	RATIONALE
• Observe for signs of infection (fever, abdominal pain, cloudy dialysate).	• Early identification of infection will reduce complications.
• Report signs of infection to healthcare provider immediately.	• Rapid intervention may reduce need for hospitalization.

EXPECTED OUTCOME: Hospitalization will not be needed for peritonitis because of early identification and prompt treatment.

3. Nursing Diagnosis: *Caregiver Role Strain* related to daily dialysis treatments (NANDA-I © 2014)

GOAL: The family will cope with daily demands for the child's dialysis treatments.

• Discuss the importance of daily, consistent dialysis treatments for the child's overall health status.	• If parents understand the need for consistent dialysis treatments, they are more likely to adhere to guidelines.
• Collaborate with the family to identify strategies that could reduce the impact of dialysis on the family's life.	• When the family participates in planning care, adherence is more likely.
• Refer the family to local support groups for emotional support, treatment strategies, and respite care.	• Support groups may help the family develop effective coping strategies.

EXPECTED OUTCOME: Family will adhere to daily dialysis treatment guidelines.

after the dialysis to determine any fluid imbalances that require adjustment during the next hemodialysis session.

SAFETY ALERT!

Monitor the child receiving hemodialysis for complications such as these that can occur suddenly:

- Hypotension—sudden nausea and vomiting, abdominal cramping, tachycardia, and dizziness
- Rapid fluid and electrolyte exchange—muscle cramping, nausea and vomiting, and dizziness
- Disequilibrium syndrome—restlessness, headache, nausea and vomiting, blurred vision, muscle twitching, and altered level of consciousness

---

Because fluid and dietary limitations (reduced intake of foods containing potassium, sodium, and phosphorus) are needed more often with hemodialysis than with peritoneal dialysis, make sure the family knows how to plan and provide for the child's daily nutritional needs. Review ways to reduce the risk of infection, including the daily care of the catheter site. Encourage showering rather than tub baths. Activities such as swimming may be discouraged.

KIDNEY TRANSPLANTATION

Kidney transplantation provides the only alternative to long-term dialysis for children with ESRD and generally yields good outcomes. The transplanted kidney can normalize physiology and provide a potential for normal growth. Because of the adverse effects on growth and development resulting from the delay of transplantation, children are given some priority over adults awaiting transplantation. Blood type compatibility between the donor and recipient is essential for a transplant to be successful. A human leukocyte antigen (HLA) system match also improves survival of the graft. A living relative donor kidney has a higher survival rate than a cadaver kidney (Scheinman, 2012). Children and their families are carefully screened prior to transplantation in an effort to identify problems that could lead to rejection of the kidney or infection that could be life threatening if the immune system is suppressed (Figure 26–6).

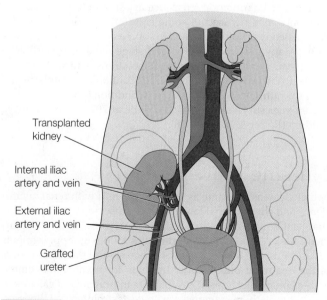

Transplanted kidney

Internal iliac artery and vein

External iliac artery and vein

Grafted ureter

Figure 26–6 **The transplanted kidney is placed in the iliac fossa with anastomosis to the hypogastric artery, iliac vein, and bladder.**

Clinical Reasoning The Child on Hemodialysis

Terrell, who is now 5 years old, was born with posterior urethral valves, which caused damage to his kidneys. Despite undergoing surgery to correct the defect during infancy, his kidney function continued to deteriorate. End-stage renal disease was diagnosed 2 years ago, and dialysis treatment was initiated. Terrell requires a kidney transplant, but in the meantime he is being treated with hemodialysis. He visits the dialysis center 3 afternoons a week for treatments lasting approximately 3 to 4 hours. This schedule permits him to attend kindergarten classes in the morning.

At his scheduled visit to the nephrologist, Terrell has gained weight and is edematous. In talking with him, the nurse discovers that Terrell has been drinking sodas and eating "junk food" at school. Terrell asks the nurse not to tell his mother because she will be mad, but that he just can't help eating and drinking what he isn't supposed to.

How does Terrell's growth and development level affect his adherence to the treatment regimen? What immediate intervention should the nurse take with Terrell? What approach should the nurse take when discussing this nutritional issue with the family?

After transplantation, the child must take immunosuppressive medications such as corticosteroids, azathioprine, cyclosporine, tacrolimus, and monoclonal antibodies to suppress rejection. Immunosuppression regimens use various combinations and sequences of these drugs to reduce the incidence of acute and chronic rejection.

Complications of immunosuppressive therapy include opportunistic infection, lymphomas and skin cancer, and hypertension. Adherence with therapy is essential for survival of the graft and for optimal medical outcomes after transplant. Nonadherence to the medication regimen in pediatric transplant patients ranges; it may be as high as 70% (Guilfoyle, Goebel, & Pai, 2011; Ingerski, Perrazo, Goebel, et al., 2011). Nonadherence is related to several factors, including forgetting to take medication and refusal to take medication because of expected side effects. Family dynamics, functioning, and flexibility also affect adherence (Guilfoyle et al., 2011). Adherence is higher in adolescents when their parents are knowledgeable and supportive, and when they promote the adolescent to become competent in self-care. Some primary kidney diseases, such as glomerulonephritis and hemolytic-uremic syndrome, can also recur in the transplanted kidney.

Nursing management includes teaching parents about the transplantation process before it occurs to help prepare them for the experience. Discuss all aspects of the child's care that will have an impact on the family's life, including follow-up appointments, medications, and general health promotion. Monitor adherence to immunosuppression treatment at each visit in an effort to identify issues early. Teach parents about the signs of acute rejection and infection, including when and how to notify the child's healthcare provider if immediate care is required.

Hemolytic-Uremic Syndrome

Hemolytic-uremic syndrome (HUS) is the most common cause of acute renal failure in young children, occurring primarily in those under 4 years of age (Ring & Huether, 2014). HUS has a classic triad of signs: (1) hemolytic anemia, (2) thrombocytopenia, and (3) acute renal failure (Tan & Silverberg, 2014).

Hemolytic-uremic syndrome is most often caused by *Escherichia coli* strain O157:H7, which is found in undercooked meat and unpasteurized milk and juices (Tan & Silverberg, 2014). The bacteria has also been linked to petting zoos and other animal exhibits (Anderson & Weese, 2012).

E. coli strain O157:H7 produces a toxin that attaches to the glomeruli, collecting ducts, and distal tubules. The toxin damages the lining of the glomerular arterioles, causing the endothelial cells to swell and become occluded with platelets and fibrin clots. This partial occlusion damages the red blood cells, resulting in hemolytic anemia. Platelets cluster in areas of vascular endothelial damage, causing thrombocytopenia. Glomerular filtration is decreased, resulting in hematuria and proteinuria. Oliguria and ARF develop in nearly 50% of children with HUS (Ring & Huether, 2014).

An episode of severe gastroenteritis with diarrhea precedes the development of typical HUS by 1 to 2 weeks followed by 1 to 5 days without symptoms. Signs and symptoms of the onset of HUS include purpura, pallor, bruising, oliguria, and irritability. The child may have a fever, anorexia, abdominal pain, vomiting, watery blood-stained diarrhea, mild jaundice, and circulatory overload. Signs of central nervous involvement include seizures and lethargy (Ring & Huether, 2014).

Treatment focuses on the complications of ARF and includes fluid restrictions and a high-calorie, high-carbohydrate diet that is low in protein, sodium, potassium, and phosphorus. Enteral nutrition is sometimes needed. Medications may include calcium gluconate or calcium chloride, aluminum hydroxide gel to bind to phosphorus, Kayexalate (sodium polystyrene) to remove excess potassium, and antihypertensive agents. Transfusions of fresh-packed red blood cells may be ordered to treat severe anemia. Platelets are given if the child is bleeding or if surgery is needed.

Transfusions are carefully administered to prevent hypertension caused by hypervolemia. Approximately 50% of children with typical HUS will need dialysis in the acute phase (Balestracci, Martin, Toledo, et al., 2012). Peritoneal dialysis is preferred unless the child has severe colitis and abdominal tenderness. Some children may develop chronic renal failure; however, most regain normal renal function (Ring & Huether, 2014).

Nursing Management

Monitor vital signs, neurologic signs, and laboratory values including electrolytes and blood counts. Monitor daily weights and assess intake and output. Observe the child carefully for signs of progressive renal impairment such as oliguria, elevated serum potassium, and elevated creatinine. Monitor for signs of bleeding related to thrombocytopenia, including petechiae and ecchymosis. Monitor the child for abdominal discomfort from diarrhea or other gastrointestinal disturbances.

Discharge planning focuses on teaching parents about medications and dietary and fluid restrictions. Follow-up visits are necessary to evaluate the effectiveness of the treatment plan. Make sure that parents understand that ground beef should be cooked to an internal temperature of 160°F (71°C) (U.S. Department of Agriculture, 2013). Teach the family to wash hands carefully when handling raw ground meats, and to make sure utensils touching raw meat do not come into contact with cooked meats. Encourage the use of a meat thermometer since the absence of pink in the center of the meat does not ensure that the appropriate temperature has been achieved.

Polycystic Kidney Disease

Polycystic kidney disease (PKD) is a genetic disorder that has autosomal recessive and dominant forms. Liver abnormalities are associated with both forms of the disease. The incidence of the autosomal recessive form is 1 per 20,000 live births (Zhou & Pollak, 2015). The autosomal dominant form is one of the most frequently inherited diseases with a prevalence of 1 in 800 live births in the United States (Watnick & Dirkx, 2015).

In PKD, cellular hyperplasia of the collecting ducts causes dilation of the ducts. Fluid secreted into these ducts enables cyst sacs to form. Initially, cysts are usually less than 2 mm in size and do not obstruct urinary flow. As the child grows, however, the cysts become larger and fibrosis occurs. The cysts slowly replace much of the kidney's mass and reduce kidney function. Tubular atrophy may occur in some children, whereas others have minimal changes in renal function. PKD is associated with liver abnormalities that progress in severity with age to fibrosis, portal hypertension, and biliary infection.

Newborns with autosomal recessive PKD may have enlarged kidneys, which are detected at birth. Approximately 60% of neonates with this disorder die within the first month from pulmonary hypoplasia. This complication is a result of deficient amniotic fluid (*oligohydramnios*) in utero secondary to severe intrauterine kidney disease (Zhou & Pollak, 2015).

Clinical manifestations in infants with autosomal recessive PKD include low-set ears, small jaw, and a flattened nose. Hypertension develops in early infancy and is often severe. Infants may have expected urine output or oliguria. Respiratory distress and feeding intolerance may develop from the enlarged kidneys (Porter & Avner, 2016). As uremia develops, infants and children develop renal osteodystrophy and progressive developmental delay and growth failure.

Sonography or renal biopsy confirms the diagnosis. The disease is often diagnosed on prenatal ultrasound. Liver function tests are usually normal initially. A liver biopsy may also be performed. Other family members should be screened for subclinical cases of PKD.

Treatment is supportive. Medications such as diuretics are prescribed for hypertension. Fluid and electrolyte abnormalities are managed. Antibiotics treat urinary tract infection. Growth hormones may be used in some children to promote growth. Renal osteodystrophy is treated to suppress the parathyroid hormone. Many children develop end-stage renal disease (ESRD) by 10 years of age. Dialysis or a kidney transplant will prolong survival; however, liver problems may continue to complicate the child's health, even when the kidney condition is well controlled. Fifteen-year survival is estimated to be at 70% to 80% of these children (Porter & Avner, 2016).

Nursing Management

Nursing care is the same as that for the child with renal insufficiency and chronic renal failure. See the discussion earlier in this chapter. Observe the child for signs of progressive renal impairment. Make sure the family schedules follow-up appointments to assess growth, developmental progress, and the effectiveness of the treatment plan. Family teaching for home management focuses on medications, diet adequate in protein and calories to support growth, management of acute gastrointestinal illnesses, and care for the child with progressive renal insufficiency and a liver disorder. Since the disease is inherited, the family should be referred for genetic counseling.

Structural Defects of the Reproductive System

Phimosis

In **phimosis**, the foreskin over the glans penis cannot be retracted. As a result of natural adhesion, phimosis is a normal finding in uncircumcised infants and young males. Circumcision, surgical removal of the foreskin, has long been a common practice performed in some countries and cultures during the newborn period. It is performed to prevent phimosis, for ease of proper male hygiene, and to prevent urinary tract infections and penile cancer. The procedure removes the skin covering the end of the penis. Circumcision is considered comparatively safe; however, complications such as damage to the urethra and disfigurement to the penis may occur. Nonsurgical treatment of phimosis involves the topical application of steroid cream and is an effective alternative to surgery (Shahid, 2012).

Cryptorchidism

Cryptorchidism (undescended testes) occurs when one or both testes fail to descend through the inguinal canal into the scrotum. Normally, the testes descend during the seventh to ninth month of gestation.

Cryptorchidism may be the result of a congenital defect of the gonads, a narrow inguinal canal, short spermatic cord, adhesions, insensitivity to gonadotropins, or lack of maternal gonadotropins. This disorder occurs in approximately 3% of term male infants and has a higher incidence in premature males (Rodway & McCance, 2014).

The higher temperature in the abdomen than in the scrotum results in morphologic changes to the testis. Complications of cryptorchidism include infertility and malignancy (Connolly & McComiskey, 2013; Lee & Houk, 2013).

Cryptorchidism is usually detected during the newborn examination when palpation of the scrotum fails to reveal one or both testes. It is not unusual for boys with cryptorchidism to have an inguinal hernia as well. In a majority of cases, the testes descend spontaneously by 3 months of age.

Although diagnosis is made on physical examination, diagnostic studies, including ultrasound, CT scan, and MRI, are utilized to determine the location of the testes. A diagnostic laparoscope may also be needed to locate the testis. When neither testis can be palpated, hormonal and chromosomal evaluation may be performed to detect an intersex disorder.

If the testes do not descend spontaneously, an orchiopexy should be performed. Timing of surgery may vary among healthcare providers. The current recommendation is that this procedure be performed at 6 months of age in full-term infants. Surgery may be delayed until 12 months of age in premature infants (Barthoid, 2012).

With an orchiopexy, an incision is made at the location of the testis, either in the abdomen or in the inguinal area. Blood vessels are disentangled to allow the testis to reach into the lower scrotum. A second incision is made in the scrotum at the point where the testis is stitched to the inside wall to keep it in place. A protective sealant is often put over the incision that peels off in 3 to 5 days. If the testis is defective or undeveloped, it may be removed surgically to decrease the risk of later malignancies and a prosthesis may be placed in the scrotum.

The goals of surgery are to repair any existing hernia, improve fertility, decrease the risk of malignancy, prevent testicular torsion, and provide the psychologic benefit of a normal appearing scrotum (Connolly & McComiskey, 2013). The risk of testicular cancer is 35 to 50 times greater in men with a history of cryptorchidism (Rodway & McCance, 2014).

Nursing Management

Preoperative nursing care includes preparing the parents and child for the procedure and addressing parents' concerns about the post-surgical outcome. Orchiopexy is often performed as an outpatient procedure. If the child is hospitalized, postoperative nursing care focuses on maintaining comfort and preventing infection. Encourage bed rest, and monitor voiding. Apply ice to the surgical area, and administer prescribed analgesics to relieve pain.

Discharge instructions should include demonstration of proper incision care. The diaper area should be cleaned well with each diaper change to decrease chances of infection. Sponge bathe the child for 2 days after surgery, and then a tub bath may be given. No medicine or ointment should be placed over the incision. Teach parents to identify signs of infection such as redness, warmth, swelling, and discharge and to notify the healthcare provider if present. Ibuprofen or acetaminophen may be given for pain. Inform parents to avoid straddling the infant across the hip and to permit no strenuous activity or straddle toy riding for 2 weeks after surgery to promote healing and to prevent injury.

Inguinal Hernia and Hydrocele

An **inguinal hernia** is a painless inguinal or scrotal swelling of variable size that occurs when abdominal tissue, such as bowel, extends into the inguinal canal. An inguinal hernia is found in 3.5% to 5.0% of full-term infants and 9% to 11% of preterm infants and occurs more often in boys than girls by an 8:1 ratio (Aiken & Oldham, 2016).

A hydrocele is a fluid-filled mass in the scrotum. The condition is found in 1% to 2% of male neonates. Most hydroceles resolve spontaneously by reabsorption by 1 year of age (Elder, 2016d).

During fetal development a peritoneal sac precedes the testicle's descent to the scrotum. The lower sac enfolds the testis to become the tunica vaginalis, and the upper sac atrophies before birth. Fluid may become trapped in the tunica vaginalis and cause the hydrocele. When the tunica vaginalis does not atrophy, an abdominal structure may move into it. Inguinal hernias are often associated with abdominal wall defects such as bladder exstrophy and prune belly syndrome, and are a common occurrence with undescended testes.

Diagnosis is made by physical examination at birth or in early infancy. Palpation of the scrotum reveals a round, smooth, nontender mass, which is noted with either a hernia or hydrocele. Parents may report an intermittent bulge in the groin or swelling in the scrotum. Swelling associated with a hernia may become more apparent with straining and reduced in size when quiet or asleep.

Outpatient surgery is performed as an elective procedure at an early age (usually after 3 months of age to reduce anesthesia risks) to avoid **incarceration** (hernia cannot be reduced and circulation is impaired), which is a medical emergency. A nerve block may be given in the operating room to reduce postoperative pain. The prognosis is generally excellent.

Nursing care for hydroceles and inguinal hernias includes assessment, explaining the disorder and its treatment, and providing preoperative and postoperative teaching, care, and support.

The incision is covered with a protective sealant rather than a dressing. Provide pain medication as ordered. Inform parents that the scrotum may be edematous and may appear bruised after surgery. Incision care involves careful cleaning of the diaper area.

Inguinal hernias can become incarcerated when a bit of bowel becomes trapped in the inguinal opening and the blood supply is constricted. Symptoms in the infant include irritability, poor feeding, and abdominal distention. An older child may complain of pain. Additional symptoms in infants and children may include an edematous, erythematous scrotum accompanied by fever, vomiting, and bloody stools (Aiken & Oldham, 2016). Efforts are made to reduce the hernia before surgery by applying pressure on the affected side, followed by semiurgent surgery. If the hernia cannot be reduced, emergency surgery is performed (Mishra et al., 2014).

Testicular Torsion

Testicular torsion is an emergency condition in which the testis suddenly rotates on its spermatic cord, cutting off its blood supply. The arteries and veins in the spermatic cord become twisted and interrupt the blood supply, leading to vascular engorgement and ischemia. Testicular torsion occurs in 3.8 per 100,000 males under 18 years of age each year (Sharp, Kieran, & Arlen, 2013). Often the testicles are positioned transversely in the scrotum, secondary to a congenital anomaly known as a *bell clapper deformity*. In this deformity, the tunica vaginalis has an inappropriately high attachment to the testes, allowing them to rotate freely and twist spontaneously on the spermatic cord. Approximately 12% of males have this deformity (Datta, Dhillon, & Voci, 2011; Govindarajan & Nelson, 2013).

Manifestations include severe pain and erythema in the scrotum, nausea and vomiting, abdominal pain, and scrotal swelling that is not relieved by rest or scrotal support. The testes are tender on palpation and become edematous. The cremasteric reflex is absent. Symptoms generally start when the child is sleeping or inactive, but they can occur after trauma, sexual activity, or exercise. Color Doppler ultrasonography is frequently used to confirm the diagnosis (Sharp et al., 2013).

Testicular torsion is a surgical emergency. When surgical treatment is implemented within 6 hours of the onset of symptoms, there is a 90% to 100% chance that the testicle can be saved. During surgery (orchiopexy), the testis is untwisted and stitched to the side of the scrotum in the correct position. The procedure is usually performed bilaterally to prevent future torsion in the other testis. If the testicle does not regain blood flow or is already necrotic, it is removed via orchiectomy (Sharp et al., 2013).

Nursing management involves psychologic support for the child and family related to the need for emergency surgery and concern about the child's future fertility. Reassure parents that because only one testis is usually involved, fertility should not be affected. The child often goes home within a few hours of surgery; thus the child and family need to be taught about proper care of the incision and pain management. Explain to parents that the child should not lift heavy objects for 4 weeks or participate in strenuous activity for 2 weeks after surgery to promote healing. Teach the adolescent testicular self-examination.

Sexually Transmitted Infections

Sexually transmitted infections (STIs) are a major national public health concern, and they pose a significant health risk to children and adolescents. The Centers for Disease Control and Prevention (CDC) reports that approximately 20 million new cases of STIs occur each year, with young people ages 15 to 24 years accounting for almost half the infections (CDC, 2013). Children and adolescents can become infected with sexually transmitted organisms through sexual experimentation, sexual play, molestation, and sexual abuse.

SAFETY ALERT!

When a child younger than 10 years is found to have gonorrhea or another sexually transmitted infection, consider the possibility of sexual abuse. When anorectal symptoms are found, suspect molestation (see Chapter 17).

Results from the CDC National 2011 Youth Risk Behavior Survey revealed that 47.4% of high school students had engaged in sexual intercourse and 60.2% of sexually active adolescents had used a condom at last sexual intercourse (CDC, 2012a). Adolescents are considered an at-risk population because of their inexperience and lack of knowledge about STIs. They may disregard the importance of using barrier protection, may have multiple sexual partners, may have sex frequently, and often do not seek medical treatment until symptoms are well advanced.

Frequently diagnosed STIs include chlamydia, genital herpes (herpes simplex type 2), gonorrhea, genital warts (human papillomavirus), trichomoniasis, and syphilis. Refer to Table 26–11 for more information.

State and local health departments are responsible for controlling the spread of STIs through health promotion programs, staff training, reporting systems, diagnosis, treatment, patient counseling, and the notification of sex partners. To reduce all sexually transmitted infections, the CDC recommends abstinence from sexual contact or a long-term mutually monogamous relationship with a partner who has been tested for STIs and is known to be uninfected (Workowski & Bolan, 2015).

Nursing Management
For the Child With an STI

Nursing Assessment and Diagnosis

Nursing assessment focuses on identifying signs and symptoms indicative of sexually transmitted infections, assessing for the potential for asymptomatic sexually transmitted infections, and assessing the psychosocial impact on the child or adolescent with a sexually transmitted infection.

The nurse usually encounters the child or adolescent and family in the emergency department, outpatient clinic, or nursing unit. Because adolescents are often afraid of the consequences of reporting symptoms, good assessment and communication skills are important considerations for the nurse, particularly when asking questions about sexual activity, partners, and the possibility of abuse. Essential to communication is maintaining a warm, encouraging, nonjudgmental approach and conveying acceptance when discussing sexual health issues with the child or adolescent. In order to achieve the adolescent's cooperation, confidentiality must be ensured. Offer support to the adolescent and encourage the seeking of parental guidance and involvement.

Key areas to discuss when obtaining a sexual history include information related to partners, pregnancy prevention, protection from sexually transmitted infections, sexual practices, and past history of STIs (Workowski & Bolan, 2015).

TABLE 26–11 Clinical Manifestations of Common Sexually Transmitted Infections

SEXUALLY TRANSMITTED INFECTION	CLINICAL MANIFESTATIONS AND COMPLICATIONS	CLINICAL THERAPY AND PATIENT EDUCATION
Chlamydia *Chlamydia trachomatis*	Asymptomatic infection is common in males and females. *Females:* vaginal discharge, dysuria, pelvic pain, mild abdominal pain, vaginal spotting, cervicitis, salpingitis, pelvic inflammatory disease (PID). *Males:* **urethritis** (an infection of the urethra), discharge from the penis, dysuria, proctitis, epididymitis. Complications associated with chlamydia in females include PID, ectopic pregnancy, and infertility. Chlamydia is a leading cause of early pneumonia and conjunctivitis in newborns.	Diagnosis is by culture or a nucleic acid-amplified test on the urine. Recommended medication therapy includes doxycycline twice a day for 7 days or single-dose azithromycin. All sexual partners should be evaluated, tested, and treated. Infected persons should abstain from sexual intercourse until they and their sex partners have completed treatment to prevent reinfection. Encourage use of condoms. All sexually active female adolescents should be screened at least annually for chlamydia.
Genital herpes *Herpes simplex virus 1* (HSV-1) or *2* (HSV-2)	Most infected with HSV-2 are not aware of their infection. Presentation can be variable and ranges from no symptoms to systemic involvement. Common symptoms include dull pain, itching, and small lesions or pimples on genitalia, buttocks, or thighs. Two types of lesions develop, either fluid-filled blisters on an erythematous base or more commonly, painful papules and ulcers. Ulcers can appear between vaginal folds, in posterior cervix, on glans penis, on shaft of penis, in rectum, or in anus. Ulcers heal within 2–4 weeks. Repeat outbreaks are common. Triggers include stress, menses, or trauma.	Diagnosis is confirmed by virology and type-specific serologic tests. There is no permanent cure. Recommended drug therapy includes acyclovir, famciclovir, or valacyclovir for 7–10 days. Antiviral medications can shorten and prevent outbreaks during the period of time the person takes the medication. Daily suppressive therapy for herpes can reduce transmission to partners. A cesarean delivery is usually performed for pregnant women who are infected. Discourage oral sex if ulcers are present in mouth, on lips, in vagina, or on penis. Discourage anal sex when lesions are active. Encourage use of condoms, although they may not prevent transmission. Emphasize that the patient remains contagious, even after lesions are healed.
Gonorrhea *Neisseria gonorrhoeae*	May be asymptomatic. *Females:* symptoms include dysuria, vaginal discharge, vaginal bleeding between periods. *Males:* dysuria, white, yellow, or green discharge from the penis, may have painful or swollen testicles. Complications associated with gonorrhea in females include PID, ectopic pregnancy, and infertility. Gonorrhea can be spread to the infant during childbirth and can result in serious health problems for the infant.	Diagnosed by culture of vaginal or urethral discharge or nucleic acid-amplified test on the urine. Recommended drug therapy includes a single dose of ceftriaxone IM and a single dose of oral azithromycin. Sexual partners should be treated if the adolescent has had sexual contact within 60 days of onset of symptoms. Encourage use of condoms or abstinence. Emphasize the importance of taking all the medication prescribed to cure gonorrhea. The individual and all sex partners must avoid sex until they have completed their treatment for gonorrhea.
Human papillomavirus (HPV)	May be asymptomatic. Males and females may have genital warts. HPV can lead to cervical cancer.	Diagnosis is based on physical findings or biopsy. The Pap smear may be abnormal. No cure exists. Treatment for external genital warts may include patient-applied imiquimod 3.75% or 5% cream, podofilox 0.5% solution or gel, or sinecatechins 15% ointment. Healthcare provider–administered treatments include cryotherapy, surgical removal of anogenital warts, or trichloroacetic acid (TCA) or bichloroacetic acid. Encourage abstinence or condom use, but condoms are not sufficient to prevent contact transmission. The disorder is transmissible even after treatment. HPV vaccine (see Chapter 16).

(continued)

TABLE 26–11 Clinical Manifestations of Common Sexually Transmitted Infections (*continued*)

SEXUALLY TRANSMITTED INFECTION	CLINICAL MANIFESTATIONS AND COMPLICATIONS	CLINICAL THERAPY AND PATIENT EDUCATION
Trichomoniasis *Trichomonas vaginalis*	May be asymptomatic. *Females:* thin discharge that has an unusual odor and is clear, white, yellow or green, dysuria, vulvar pruritus. *Males:* most common site is the urethra; urethral discharge, pruritus, dysuria.	Diagnosis is by culture. Treatment includes metronidazole or tinidazole orally as a single dose or metronidazole orally twice a day for 7 days. Both partners should be treated at the same time to eliminate the parasite. Avoid drinking alcohol during and for several days after treatment if a single dose is used. Sexual contact should be avoided until both partners are cured. No follow-up test is needed if symptoms resolve after treatment.
Syphilis *Treponema pallidum*	Appearance of classic signs and symptoms of syphilis depends on stage of disease. *Primary stage:* Firm, round, painless sore that appears at the location where the infection entered the body. Ulcer spontaneously heals within 3–6 weeks; however, if infection not treated, progresses to secondary stage. *Secondary stage:* Skin rash or sores in mouth, vagina, or anus. Other symptoms include fever, lymphadenopathy, weight loss, headache, muscle aches, fatigue. *Latent stage:* asymptomatic, can last for several years. *Late stage:* Can appear 10–30 years after initial infection. Damage of the internal organs occurs and can lead to death.	Diagnosis is by serologic tests or direct fluorescent antibody tests of lesion exudates. Due to the risk of fetal death, every pregnant woman should have a blood test for syphilis. Syphilis is easy to cure in its early stages. Recommended drug therapy includes single IM injection of penicillin G. Treat all sexual contacts within the past 90 days of diagnosis, depending on stage when diagnosed. During syphilis treatment, abstain from sexual contact with new partners until the syphilis sores are completely healed. Encourage abstinence or the use of condoms plus spermicidal foams, cream, or jelly to prevent infection.

Source: Data from Centers for Disease Control and Prevention (CDC). (2012b). *Trichomoniasis—CDC fact sheet.* Retrieved from http://www.cdc.gov/std/trichomonas/trich-fact-sheet-aug-2012.pdf; Centers for Disease Control and Prevention (CDC). (2014a). *Chlamydia—CDC fact sheet.* Retrieved from http://www.cdc.gov/std/Chlamydia/STDFact-Chlamydia.htm; Centers for Disease Control and Prevention (CDC). (2014b). *Genital herpes—CDC fact sheet.* Retrieved from http://www.cdc.gov/std/herpes/herpes-factsheet-july-2014.pdf; Centers for Disease Control and Prevention (CDC). (2014c). *Gonorrhea—CDC fact sheet.* Retrieved from http://www.cdc.gov/std/gonorrhea/gon-factsheet-july-2014.pdf; Centers for Disease Control and Prevention (CDC). (2014d). *Genital HPV infection—CDC fact sheet.* Retrieved from http://www.cdc.gov/std/hpv/hpv-factsheet-march-2014.pdf; Centers for Disease Control and Prevention (CDC). (2014e). *Syphilis—CDC fact sheet.* Retrieved from http://www.cdc.gov/std/syphilis/STDFact-Syphilis.htm; Workowski, K. A., & Bolan, G. A. (2015). Sexually transmitted diseases treatment guidelines, 2015. *Morbidity and Mortality Weekly Report, 64*(3), 1–134.

Assess the child or adolescent for manifestations as described in Table 26–11. When a child or adolescent is diagnosed with one STI, it is essential to screen for the presence of other STIs, because these diseases may coexist. Adolescents who are symptomatic may postpone care due to feeling uncomfortable about genital examinations. Given that many adolescents have subclinical cases or are asymptomatic, routine screening of sexually active adolescents is recommended.

Nursing diagnoses that may apply to the child or adolescent with a sexually transmitted infection include the following (NANDA-I © 2014):

- *Anxiety* related to presence of sexually transmitted infection
- *Pain, Acute,* related to genital irritation
- *Knowledge, Deficient (Sexually Transmitted Infections),* related to cause, transmission, treatments, and prevention
- *Body Image, Disturbed,* related to genital lesions or presence of genital infection

Planning and Implementation

The nurse focuses on identifying adolescents at risk for STIs, providing appropriate education, and preventing transmission and complications.

When counseling the adolescent, reinforce the importance of treating all sexual partners and modifying high-risk sexual behaviors. Partner notification is essential in order to provide treatment if the partner is infected and to reduce the risk of reinfection. Encourage sexually active adolescents to receive hepatitis B immunization if not already obtained.

CARE IN THE COMMUNITY

Education includes promoting abstinence, which means avoiding *any* type of sexual contact with a partner. (See *Families Want to Know: Preventing STIs and Their Consequences.*) The nurse, in partnership with schools and community organizations, is active in sexual health promotion.

Work with sexually active adolescents to identify methods of reducing the risk of contracting STIs. Suggestions include the use of latex condoms (though the possibility of STI transmission still exists even with the use of latex condoms), voiding immediately after sexual intercourse, and appropriate genital hygiene with soap and water. Assist adolescents to avoid sexual partners who are at higher risk for STIs, such as intravenous drug users and those who have multiple sexual partners. Emphasize to the adolescent that even with applying these measures, there is no guaranteed protection against STIs

Families Want to Know

Preventing STIs and Their Consequences

Collaborate with the child and family to promote the following recommendations in preventing STIs and their consequences:

- Abstinence is the best method to prevent STIs.
- Limit the number of sexual contacts; practice mutual monogamy.
- Always use condoms and spermicidal gels or foams for vaginal and anal intercourse.
- Refrain from oral sex if the partner has active sores in the mouth, vagina, anus, or penis.
- Reduce high-risk sexual behaviors. Use of recreational drugs and alcohol can increase sexual risk taking.
- Seek care as soon as symptoms are noticed and make sure your partner gets treatment.
- Seek annual screening for STIs.

except when using abstinence. Explain to the adolescent that some STIs, such as chlamydia, are asymptomatic.

Additional teaching includes dispelling myths of how STIs are spread. Instruct the child or adolescent that STIs are not contracted from sharing bath towels, clothing, and drinking glasses or from sitting on toilet seats. Inform the female taking contraceptives that birth control offers no protection against STIs.

Evaluation

Expected outcomes for the child or adolescent with a sexually transmitted infection are:

- The child or adolescent remains free from pain.
- An understanding of the transmission, prevention, and treatment of sexually transmitted infections is demonstrated by the adolescent.
- The adolescent has a positive body image.
- Reduced anxiety is displayed by the child or adolescent.

Pelvic Inflammatory Disease (PID)

Pelvic inflammatory disease (PID) is a serious infection of the upper genital tract caused by the ascending spread of organisms in the cervix and vagina. Many cases of PID are caused by complications of sexually transmitted infections, primarily gonorrhea and chlamydia (Workowski & Bolan, 2015).

The infection ascends into the uterus and fallopian tubes during the menses when the cervix mucosal plug is open and retrograde menstrual blood can flow into the fallopian tubes. Signs and symptoms of PID may include fever, mild or dull bilateral lower abdominal pain, dysmenorrhea that is worse or longer lasting than usual, dysuria, vaginal discharge, pain with sexual activity, and prolonged or increased menstrual bleeding. Most cases are mild.

No specific laboratory test exists for PID. During a pelvic examination, uterine or adnexal tenderness or tenderness with cervical motion is present. Other criteria that help support the diagnosis of PID include an elevated erythrocyte sedimentation rate, elevated C-reactive protein level, white blood cells seen on microscopic examination of vaginal secretions, and documented cervical infection with gonorrhea or chlamydia.

A transvaginal sonogram may reveal thickened and fluid-filled fallopian tubes with or without free pelvic fluid (Workowski & Bolan, 2015).

Intravenous cefotetan or cefoxitin plus oral or intravenous doxycycline is recommended as initial treatment for 24–48 hours. With clinical improvement, the patient can be transitioned to oral doxycycline to complete a 14-day course. Another option for treatment is intravenous clindamycin and intravenous or intramuscular gentamicin as initial treatment, followed by oral doxycycline or oral clindamycin to complete a 14-day course. Follow-up physical examination is performed in 72 hours to ensure treatment adherence and to detect improvement in symptoms. Rehospitalization and adjustment of the antibiotic regimen is initiated if no improvement is noted (Workowski & Bolan, 2015).

Nursing Management

A sexual history should be obtained from all adolescent females to identify the risk for sexually transmitted infection and PID. Risk factors for adolescents include those who have a history of an STI, multiple sexual partners, and lack of consistent use of barrier protection (Shepherd, 2013).

Administer medications intravenously for the first 24 hours. Provide education for the ongoing treatment with oral antibiotics, ensuring that the adolescent understands the importance of taking all medications on schedule for the full 14 days. Provide signs of adverse effects and actions to take if they occur.

Determine if the adolescent's parents have been informed about the illness and assist the adolescent in discussing the health problem with the parents. If parents are unaware of the health problem, discuss the importance of telling the parents so that they can help identify any problems that develop during treatment.

Provide counseling about methods to reduce the risk for reinfection with a sexually transmitted infection. Provide information about the potential consequences of infertility, ectopic pregnancy, and chronic abdominal pain for this infection and the increased risk for these consequences with subsequent infections. Encourage regular health visits with screening for sexually transmitted infections, because future chlamydia and gonorrhea infections may be asymptomatic.

Chapter Highlights

- Functions of the urinary system include excretion of wastes, maintenance of acid–base and fluid and electrolyte balance, regulation of blood pressure, production of erythropoietin, and regulation of calcium metabolism.

- Expected urine output for a neonate and infant is 1 to 2 mL/kg per hour while an adult should have 0.5 mL/kg per hour.

- Urinary tract infections are common infections in children. Factors placing the child at risk for a UTI include urinary stasis, infrequent voiding, irritated perineum, constipation, sexual abuse, and sexual activity in adolescent females.

- Structural defects of the urinary system—including bladder exstrophy, hypospadias and epispadias, obstructive uropathy, vesicoureteral reflux, and posterior ureteral valves—generally require surgical treatment.

- Bladder exstrophy is a congenital defect in which the abdominal wall does not fuse during fetal development, leading to exposure of the bladder wall, a separation of the rectus muscles, and widening of the symphysis pubis.

- Surgical correction of hypospadias and epispadias generally occurs during the first year of life to minimize psychologic effects on the child.

- Obstruction of the urinary tract interferes with urine flow and results in hydronephrosis or urine backflow into the kidneys. This results in significant damage to the kidney and is a common cause of renal failure in children.

- Vesicoureteral reflux may result from a structural anomaly in which the ureters insert in an abnormal position into the bladder. Urinary tract infections are often a complication of this disorder.

- Prune belly (Eagle-Barrett) syndrome is a rare congenital disorder in which the skin covering the abdominal wall is thin and resembles a wrinkled prune. Anomalies associated with this syndrome include urinary tract anomalies, poor ureteral peristalsis, enlarged bladder, high risk for recurrent UTI, vesicoureteral reflux, and bilateral cryptorchidism in males.

- Nocturnal enuresis often occurs in children whose parents have a history of enuresis. Very few children have a structural or neurologic cause. Higher rates of enuresis have been noted in children with obstructive sleep apnea and constipation.

- Minimal change nephrotic syndrome is characterized by edema that develops over several weeks, weight gain, hypertension, irritability, hematuria, malaise, anorexia, and foamy or frothy urine.

- Acute postinfectious glomerulonephritis results most often from a beta-hemolytic group A streptococcal infection of the skin or pharynx. It is also caused by other organisms, including *Staphylococcus* and *Pneumococcus* bacteria and coxsackieviruses. Most children have a complete recovery of kidney function.

- Hemolytic-uremic syndrome is often associated with ingestion of *E. coli* strain O157:H7, which produces a toxin that attacks the kidneys. The child develops hemolytic anemia, thrombocytopenia, and acute renal failure that can progress to chronic renal failure.

- Polycystic kidney disease is a genetic disorder with both autosomal recessive and autosomal dominant forms that lead to chronic renal failure. It may be detected prenatally or in young children by ultrasound.

- Acute renal failure occurs when kidney function diminishes abruptly and is often reversible. It may occur as a complication of trauma, sepsis, cardiac surgery, or drug toxicity. It is also seen in critically ill neonates with asphyxia, sepsis, or shock.

- Chronic renal failure is progressive and irreversible reduced function of the kidneys, eventually resulting in end-stage renal disease. It often results from developmental abnormalities of the kidneys or urinary tract.

- Children with end-stage renal disease are treated with renal replacement therapy, including hemodialysis, peritoneal dialysis, or kidney transplant.

- Structural defects of the male reproductive system include phimosis, cryptorchidism, inguinal hernia, hydrocele, and testicular torsion.

- Nursing care of sexually transmitted infections includes identifying the cause and organism, providing appropriate treatment, preventing transmission and complications, and educating the child, adolescent, and family.

- Pelvic inflammatory disease (PID) is an infection of the upper genital tract (uterus and fallopian tubes) caused by the ascending spread of organisms (usually chlamydia or gonorrhea) in the cervix and vagina.

Clinical Reasoning in Action

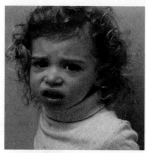

Kendra, a 2-year-old who appears ill, is brought into the urgent care center for a skin rash, fever, irritability, and edema. Her father is concerned she might also be dehydrated because her urine output is decreased. The healthcare provider determines her skin rash does not blanch when pressure is applied and notes a purplish color. Last week, Kendra was treated for an episode of abdominal pain, diarrhea, and vomiting. The healthcare provider immediately admits her to the hospital and orders a urine culture, blood work, and stool tests. The stool comes back positive for the strain of *E. coli* usually found in contaminated hamburger meat. Kendra has hemolytic-uremic syndrome (HUS) and is in acute renal failure (ARF). She also has low hemoglobin, elevated BUN and creatinine, hematuria, and electrolyte imbalances.

Kendra is given medication for her electrolyte imbalances, antihypertensive medications, and is placed on a high-calorie, high-carbohydrate diet with restrictions on protein, sodium, potassium, and phosphorus. You explain to her parents the extreme importance of adhering to her dietary and fluid restrictions to help keep her electrolytes and fluid level balanced. You educate them that in some cases children with HUS need dialysis and some children have long-term kidney damage. You teach them how to take her blood pressure, and how to observe for edema so that Kendra can be monitored after she goes home.

1. How is drug administration adjusted for Kendra since she has ARF? What is an important nursing role when administering various medications to her?
2. What is the reason ARF develops in HUS?
3. What is one way Kendra's condition could have been prevented?
4. Renal failure is characterized by azotemia and oliguria. Describe what these are.

References

Aiken, J. J., & Oldham, K. T. (2016). Inguinal hernias. In R. M. Kliegman, B. F. Stanton, J. W. St. Geme, & N. F. Schor, (Eds.), *Nelson textbook of pediatrics* (20th ed., pp. 1903–1909). Philadelphia, PA: Elsevier.

Alarcon, L. H., & Fink, M. P. (2015). Physiologic monitoring of the surgical patient. In F. C. Brunicardi, D. K. Andersen, T. R. Billiar, D. L. Dunn, J. G. Hunter, J. B. Matthews, & R. E. Pollock (Eds.), *Schwartz's principles of surgery* (10th ed.). Retrieved from http://www.accessmedicine.com

Al-Uzri, A., Matheson, M., Gipson, D. S., Mendley, S. R., Hooper, S. R., Yadin,O., . . . Gerson, R. C. (2013). The impact of short stature on health-related quality of life in children with chronic kidney disease. *The Journal of Pediatrics, 163,* 736–741.

American Academy of Pediatrics Task Force on Circumcision. (2012). Male circumcision. *Pediatrics, 130*(3), e756–e785.

Ammenti, A., Cataldi, L., Chimenz, R., Fanos, V., LaManna, A., Marra, G., . . . Montini, G. (2012). Febrile urinary tract infections in young children: Recommendations for the diagnosis, treatment and follow-up. *Acta Pædiatrica, 101,* 451–457.

Anderson, M. E., & Weese, J. S. (2012). Video observation of hand hygiene practices at a petting zoo and the impact of hand hygiene interventions. *Epidemiology & Infection, 140,* 182–190.

Balestracci, A., Martin., S. M., Toledo, I., Alvarado, C., & Wainsztein, R. E. (2012). Dehydration at admission increased the need for dialysis in hemolytic uremic syndrome children. *Pediatric Nephrology, 27,* 1407–1410.

Barthold, J. S. (2012). Abnormalities of the testis and scrotum and their surgical management. In A. J. Wein, L. R. Kavoussi, A. C. Novick, A. W. Partin, & C. A. Peters (Eds.), *Campbell-Walsh urology* (10th ed., pp. 3557–3596). Philadelphia, PA: Elsevier Saunders.

Bascom, A., Penney, T., Metcalfe, M., Knox, A., Witmans, M., Uweira, T., & Metcalfe, P. D. (2011). High risk of sleep disordered breathing in the enuresis population. *Journal of Urology, 184*(4), 1710–1714.

Bhatnagar, V. (2011). Bladder exstrophy: An overview of the surgical management. *Journal of Indian Association of Pediatric Surgeons, 16*(3), 81–87.

Bhimma, R. (2014). *Acute poststreptococcal glomerulonephritis.* Retrieved from http://emedicine.medscape.com/article/980685-overview

Caldamone, A. A., & Woodard, J. R. (2012). Prune-belly syndrome. In A. J. Wein, L. R. Kavoussi, A. C. Novick, A. W. Partin, & C. A. Peters (Eds.), *Campbell-Walsh urology* (10th ed., pp. 3310–3324). Philadelphia, PA: Elsevier Saunders.

Centers for Disease Control and Prevention (CDC). (2012a). Youth Risk Behavior Surveillance—United States, 2011. *Mortality and Morbidity Weekly Report, 61*(4), 1–162.

Centers for Disease Control and Prevention (CDC). (2012b). *Trichomoniasis—CDC fact sheet.* Retrieved from http://www.cdc.gov/std/trichomonas/trich-fact-sheet-aug-2012.pdf

Centers for Disease Control and Prevention (CDC). (2013). *STD trends in the United States—2011 national data for chlamydia, gonorrhea, and syphilis.* Retrieved from http://www.cdc.gov/std/stats11/trends-2011.pdf

Centers for Disease Control and Prevention (CDC). (2014a). *Chlamydia—CDC fact sheet.* Retrieved from http://www.cdc.gov/std/Chlamydia/STDFact-Chlamydia.htm

Centers for Disease Control and Prevention (CDC). (2014b). *Genital herpes—CDC fact sheet.* Retrieved from http://www.cdc.gov/std/herpes/herpes-factsheet-july-2014.pdf

Centers for Disease Control and Prevention (CDC). (2014c). *Gonorrhea—CDC fact sheet.* Retrieved from http://www.cdc.gov/std/gonorrhea/gon-factsheet-july-2014.pdf

Centers for Disease Control and Prevention (CDC). (2014d). *Genital HPV infection—CDC fact sheet.* Retrieved from http://www.cdc.gov/std/hpv/hpv-factsheet-march-2014.pdf

Centers for Disease Control and Prevention (CDC). (2014e). *Syphilis—CDC fact sheet.* Retrieved from http://www.cdc.gov/std/syphilis/STDFact-Syphilis.htm

Chalmers, D., Wiedel, C.A., Siparsky, G.L. Campbell, J.B., & Wilcox, D.T. (2014). Discovery of hypospadias during newborn circumcision should not preclude completion of the procedure. *Journal of Pediatrics, 164,* 1171–1174.

Connolly, M. E., & McComiskey, C. A. (2013). Common outpatient pediatric surgical procedures: Inguinal and umbilical hernias, hydroceles, undescended testes, and circumcision. In N. T. Browne, L. M. Flanigan, C. A. McComiskey, & P. Pieper (Eds.), *Nursing care of the pediatric surgical patient* (3rd ed., pp. 383–390). Burlington, MA: Jones & Bartlett.

Datta, V., Dhillon, G., & Voci, S. (2011). Testicular torsion/detorsion. *Ultrasound Quarterly, 27*(2), 127–128.

Dubrovsky, A. S., Foster, B. J., Jednak, R., Mok, E., & McGillivray, D. (2012). Visibility of the urethral meatus and risk of urinary tract infections in uncircumcised boys. *Canadian Medical Association Journal, 184*(15), E796–E803.

Elder, J. S. (2016a). Anomalies of the bladder. In R. M. Kliegman, B. F. Stanton, J. W. St. Geme, & N. F. Schor (Eds.), *Nelson textbook of pediatrics* (20th ed., pp. 2575–2578). Philadelphia, PA: Elsevier.

Elder, J. S. (2016b). Obstruction of the urinary tract. In R. M. Kliegman, B. F. Stanton, J. W. St. Geme, & N. F. Schor (Eds.), *Nelson textbook of pediatrics* (20th ed., pp. 2567–2575). Philadelphia, PA: Elsevier.

Elder, J. S. (2016c). Enuresis and voiding dysfunction. In R. M. Kliegman, B. F. Stanton, J. W. St. Geme, & N. F. Schor (Eds.), *Nelson textbook of pediatrics* (20th ed., pp. 2581–2586). Philadelphia, PA: Elsevier.

Elder, J. S. (2016d). Disorders and anomalies of the scrotal contents. In R. M. Kliegman, B. F. Stanton, J. W. St. Geme, & N. F. Schor (Eds.), *Nelson textbook of pediatrics* (20th ed., pp. 2592–2598). Philadelphia, PA: Elsevier.

Estrada, C. R., & Cendron, M. (2013). *Vesicoureteral reflux.* Retrieved from http://emedicine.medscape.com/article/439403-overview

Fisher, D. J., Barton, L. L., Egland, A. G., Egland, T. K., Hellerstein, S., Howes, D. S., . . . Young, G. M. (2014). *Pediatric urinary tract infection.* Retrieved from http://emedicine.medscape.com/article/969643-overview

Govindarajan, K. K., & Nelson C. P. (2013). *Pediatric testicular torsion.* Retrieved from http://emedicine.medscape.com/article/2035074-overview

Guilfoyle, S. M., Goebel, J. W., & Pai, A. L. (2011). Efficacy and flexibility impact perceived adherence barriers in pediatric kidney post-transplantation. *Families, Systems, & Health, 29*(1), 44–54.

Gulati, S. (2012). *Chronic kidney disease in children.* Retrieved from http://emedicine.medscape.com/article/984358-overview

Hassett, S., Smith, G. H. H., & Holland, A. J. A. (2012). Prune belly syndrome. *Pediatric Surgery International, 28,* 219–228.

Heath, J., MacKinlay, D., Watson, A. R., Hames, A., Wirz, L., Scott, S., . . . McHugh, K. (2011). Self-reported quality of life in children and young people with chronic kidney disease. *Pediatric Nephrology, 26,* 767–773.

Hines, E. Q. (2012). Fluid and electrolytes. In *The Harriet Lane handbook* (19th ed., pp. 271–292). Philadelphia, PA: Elsevier.

Holmberg, C., & Jalanko, H. (2014). Congenital nephrotic syndrome and recurrence of proteinuria after renal transplantation. *Pediatric Nephrology, 29,* 2309–2317.

Hunziker, M., Colhoun, E., & Puri, P. (2014). Renal cortical abnormalities in siblings of index patients with vesicoureteral reflux. *Pediatrics, 133*(4), e933–e937.

Ingerski, L., Perrazo, L., Goebel, J., & Pai, A. L. H. (2011). Family strategies for achieving medication adherence in pediatric kidney transplantation. *Nursing Research, 60*(3), 190–196.

Inouye, B. M., Tourchi, A., DiCarlo, H. M., Young, E. E., & Gearhart, J. P. (2014). Modern management of the exstrophy-epispadias complex. *Surgery Research and Practice, 2014.* Retrieved from http://dx.doi.org/10.1155/2014/587064

Jacques, E. (2013). Treating nocturnal enuresis in children and young people. *British Journal of School Nursing, 8*(6), 275–278.

Kari, J. A., El-Desoky, S., Farag, Y., Mosli, H., Altyieb, A. M., Al-Sayad, H., . . . Farsi, H. (2013). Renal impairment in children with posterior urethral valves. *Pediatric Nephrology, 28,* 927–931.

Kilis-Pstrusinska, K., Medynska, A., Chmielewska, I. B., Grenda , R., Kluska-Jozwiak, A., Leszczynska, B., . . . Zwolinska, D. (2013). Perception of health-related quality of life in children with chronic kidney disease by the patients and their caregivers: Multicentre national study results. *Quality of Life Research, 22,* 2889–2897.

Kocherov, S., Prat, D., Koulikov, D., Ioscovich, A., Shenfeld, O. Z., Farkas, A., & Chertin, B. (2012). Outcome of hypospadias repair in toilet-trained children and adolescents. *Pediatric Surgery International, 28,* 429–433.

Kundra, P., Yuvaraj, K., Agrawal, K., Krishnappa, C., & Kumar, L. T. (2011). Surgical outcome in children undergoing hypospadias repair under caudal epidural vs. penile block. *Pediatric Anesthesia, 22,* 707–712.

Lee, H., Han, S. W., & Rah, K. H. (2014). *Pediatric ureteropelvic junction obstruction.* Retrieved from http://emedicine.medscape.com/article/1016988-overview

Lee, P. A., & Houk, C. P. (2013). Cryptorchidism. *Current Opinion in Endocrinology, Diabetes & Obesity, 20*(3), 210–216.

Lombel, R. M., Hodson, E. M., & Gipson, D. S. (2013). Treatment of steroid-resistant nephrotic syndrome

in children: New guidelines from KDIGO. *Pediataric Nephrology, 28,* 409-414.

Lum, G. M. (2014). Kidney & urinary tract. In W. W. Hay, M. J. Levin, R. R. Deterding, & M. J. Abzug (Eds.), *CURRENT diagnosis and treatment: Pediatrics* (22nd ed.). New York, NY: McGraw-Hill. Retrieved from http://accessmedicine.com

Mehrazma, M., Amini-Alavijeh, Z., & Hooman, N. (2012). Prognostic value of dialysis effluent leukocyte count in children on peritoneal dialysis with peritonitis. Iranian Journal of Kidney Diseases, 6(2), 114–118.

Mishra, P. K., Burnand, K., Minocha, A., Mathur, A. B., Kulkarni, M. S., & Tsang, T. (2014). Incarcerated inguinal hernia management in children: A comparison of the open and laparoscopic approach. *Pediatric Surgery International, 30,* 621–624.

Morris, B. J., & Wiswell, T. E. (2013). Circumcision and lifetime risk of urinary tract infection: A systematic review and meta-analysis. *The Journal of Urology, 189*(6), 2118–2124.

Nachman, P. H., Jennette, J. C., & Falk, R. J. (2012). Primary glomerular disease. In M. W. Taal, G. M. Chertow, P. A. Marsden, K. Skorecki, A. S. L. Yu, & B. M. Brenner (Eds.), *Brenner and Rector's the kidney* (9th ed., pp. 1100–1191). Philadelphia, PA: Elsevier Saunders.

Nevéus, T. (2011). Nocturnal enuresis-theoretic background and practical guidelines. *Pediatric Nephrology, 26,* 1207–1214.

Newman, T. B. (2011). The new American Academy of Pediatrics urinary tract infection guidelines. *Pediatrics, 128*(3), 572–575.

Norfolk, S., & Wootton, J. (2012). Nocturnal enuresis in children. *Nursing Standard, 27*(10), 49–56.

Otukesh, H., Hoseini, R., Rahimzadeh, N., & Hosseini, S. (2012). Glomerular function in neonates. *Iranian Journal of Kidney Diseases, 6*(3), 166–172.

Paintsil, E. (2013). Update on recent guidelines for the management of urinary tract infections in children: The shifting paradigm. *Current Opinion in Pediatrics, 25*(1), 88–94.

Pais, P., & Avner, E. D. (2016). Nephrotic syndrome. In R. M. Kliegman, B. F. Stanton, J. W. St. Geme, & N. F. Schor (Eds.), *Nelson textbook of pediatrics* (20th ed., pp. 2521–2528). Philadelphia, PA: Elsevier.

Passamaneck, M. (2011). The changing paradigm for the management of pediatric vesicoureteral reflux. *Urologic Nursing, 31*(6), 363–366.

Porter, C. C., & Avner, E. D. (2016). Autosomal recessive polycystic kidney disease. In R. M. Kliegman, B. F. Stanton, J. W. St. Geme, & N. F. Schor (Eds.), *Nelson textbook of pediatrics* (20th ed., p. 2513). Philadelphia, PA: Elsevier.

Ray, J. (2011). Enuresis. *Al Ameen Journal of Medical Sciences, 4*(2), 104–112.

Ring, R., & Huether, S. E. (2014). Alterations of renal and urinary tract function in children. In K. L. McCance & S. E. Huether (Eds.), *Pathophysiology: The biologic basis for disease in children and adults* (7th ed., pp. 1376–1392). St. Louis, MO: Elsevier Mosby.

Rodway, G., & McCance, K. L. (2014). Alterations of the male reproductive systems. In K. L. McCance & S. E. Huether (Eds.), *Pathophysiology: The biologic basis for disease in children and adults* (7th ed., pp. 885–917). St. Louis, MO: Elsevier Mosby.

Scheinman, J.I. (2012). Pediatric transplantation. In M. W. Taal, G. M. Chertow, P. A. Marsden, K. Skorecki, A. S.

L. Yu, & B. M. Brenner (Eds.), *Brenner and Rector's the kidney* (9th ed., pp. 2694–2718). Philadelphia, PA: Elsevier Saunders.

Shahid, S. K. (2012). Phimosis in children. *ISRN Urology, 2012,* 1–6.

Sharp, V. J., Kieran, K., & Arlen, A. M. (2013). Testicular torsion: Diagnosis, evaluation, and management. *American Family Physician, 88*(12), 835–840.

Shepherd, S. M. (2013). *Pelvic inflammatory disease.* Retrieved from http://emedicine.medscape.com/article/256448-overview

Snodgrass, W., & Bush, N. (2014). Recent advances in understanding/management of hypospadias. *F1000PrimeReports.* Retrieved from http://f1000.com/prime/reports/m/6/101

Sreedharan, R., & Avner, E. D. (2016). Renal failure. In R. M. Kliegman, B. F. Stanton, J. W. St. Geme, & N. F. Schor (Eds.), *Nelson textbook of pediatrics* (20th ed., pp. 2539–2547). Philadelphia, PA: Elsevier.

Tan, A. J., & Silverberg, M. A. (2014). *Hemolytic uremic syndrome in emergency medicine.* Retrieved from http://emedicine.medscape.com/article/779218-overview

U.S. Department of Agriculture. (2013). *Color of cooked ground beef as it relates to doneness.* Retrieved from http://www.fsis.usda.gov/wps/portal/fsis/topics/food-safety-education/get-answers/food-safety-fact-sheets/meat-preparation/color-of-cooked-ground-beef-as-it-relates-to-doneness/ct_index

Verive, M. J. (2013). *Pediatric hyperkalemia.* Retrieved from http://emedicine.medscape.com/article/907543-overview

Wadie, G. M., & Moriarty, K. P. (2012). The impact of vesicoureteral reflux treatment on the incidence of urinary tract infection. *Pediatric Nephrology, 27,* 529–538.

Walle, J., Rittig, S., Bauer, S., Eggert, P., Marschall-Kehrel, D., & Tekgul, S. (2012). Practical consensus guidelines for the management of enuresis. *European Journal of Pediatrics, 171,* 971–983.

Watnick, S., & Dirkx, T. (2015). Kidney disease. In S. J. McPhee, M. A. Papadakis, & M. W. Rabow (Eds.), *Current medical diagnosis and treatment 2015.* New York, NY: McGraw-Hill.

White, B. (2011). Diagnosis and treatment of urinary tract infections in children. *American Family Physician, 83*(4), 409–415.

Wilson, B. A., Shannon, M. T., & Shields, K. M. (2015). *Pearson nurse's drug guide 2015.* Hoboken, NJ: Pearson Education.

Workeneh, B. T., Agraharkar, M., & Gupta, R. (2014). *Acute kidney injury.* Retrieved from http://emedicine.medscape.com/article/243492-overview

Workowski, K. A., & Bolan, G.A. (2015). Sexually transmitted diseases treatment guidelines, 2015. *Morbidity and Mortality Weekly Report, 64*(RR3), 1–137.

Zaritsky, J., & Warady, B. A. (2011). Peritoneal dialysis in infants and young children. *Seminars in Nephrology, 31*(2), 213–224.

Zhou, J., & Pollak, M. R. (2015). Polycystic kidney disease and other inherited tubular disorders. In D. Kasper, A. Fauci, S. Hauser, D. Longo, J. L. Jameson, & J. Loscalzo (Eds.), *Harrison's principles of internal medicine* (19th ed.). New York, NY: McGraw-Hill. Retrieved from http://www.accessmedicine.com

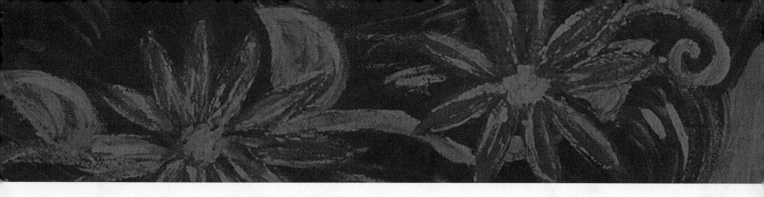

Chapter 27
Alterations in Neurologic Function

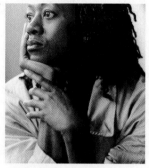

It's so hard to watch your child experience a brain injury and lie in a coma. All we can do is be here every day for Kirani. We keep talking to him and trying to get him to respond to us. We hope he will wake up soon.

—Mother of Kirani, 7 years old

Mel Curtis/Getty Images

Learning Outcomes

27.1 Describe the pediatric differences associated with the anatomy and physiology of the neurologic system.

27.2 Choose the appropriate assessment guidelines and tools to examine infants and children with altered levels of consciousness and other neurologic conditions.

27.3 Differentiate between the signs of a seizure and status epilepticus in infants and children, and describe appropriate nursing management for each condition.

27.4 Differentiate between signs of bacterial meningitis, viral meningitis, encephalitis, and Guillain-Barré syndrome in infants and children.

27.5 Develop a plan of nursing care for the child hospitalized with an acute neurologic condition.

27.6 Develop a nursing care plan for the infant with hydrocephalus and spina bifida.

27.7 Plan family-centered nursing care for the child with cerebral palsy in a community setting.

27.8 Contrast the appropriate initial nursing management for mild versus severe traumatic brain injury.

27.9 Discuss initiatives to prevent drowning in children.

Altered States of Consciousness

Level of consciousness (LOC) is the most important indicator of neurologic dysfunction. *Consciousness* the responsiveness to or awareness of sensory stimuli, has two components: *alertness* or the ability to react to stimuli, and *cognitive power*, or the ability to process the data and respond either verbally or physically. *Unconsciousness* is depressed cerebral function, or the inability of

the brain to respond to stimuli. Altered levels of consciousness can be further categorized as:

- *Confusion:* disorientation to time, place, or person; loss of clear thinking. Answers to simple questions may be correct, but responses to complex ones may be inaccurate.

- *Delirium:* state characterized by disorientation, fear, irritability or agitation, and mental or motor excitement.

Text continues on page 743

FOCUS ON:
The Neurologic System

Anatomy and Physiology

The brain, spinal cord, and nerves are the major structures of the nervous system (Figure 27–1). The brain is protected by the skull and covered by three layers of tissue called the meninges—the dura mater, arachnoid, and pia mater. Cerebrospinal fluid circulates within the ventricles of the brain and around the brain and spinal cord.

The brain is a complex organ that controls, regulates, or coordinates many body functions, including cognition, behaviors, the senses, and motor skills. See Table 27–1 for the primary functions of the brain's structures. Stimuli are received from the environment, and the brain enables response for adaptation, survival, and maintenance of body functions. The 12 cranial nerves arise from the brainstem and have many important sensory and motor functions (Table 27–2).

The spinal cord, covered by the vertebrae, transmits impulses to and from the brain, conveying sensory information and relaying impulses that stimulate motor responses. Spinal nerves send and receive information to specific body locations. Nerve impulses are transmitted by chemical substances (e.g., norepinephrine, acetylcholine, dopamine, histamine, and serotonin) and electrical conduction, enabling the impulse to travel through the synapses from neuron to neuron.

The peripheral nerves transmit impulses from the nerve pathways to the cerebral cortex through simple spinal reflex arcs. The upper motor neurons consist of the fibers originating in the anterior horn of the spinal cord that travel to the brainstem and the nerve cells in the cerebral cortex. The lower motor neurons consist of the peripheral nerves and branches that transmit impulses to the anterior horn of the spinal cord.

The autonomic nervous system maintains a steady state of the internal body organs' and glands' involuntary functions. It is divided into the sympathetic nervous system, which mobilizes the body to respond in times of need or stress, and into the parasympathetic nervous system, which works to conserve and restore energy.

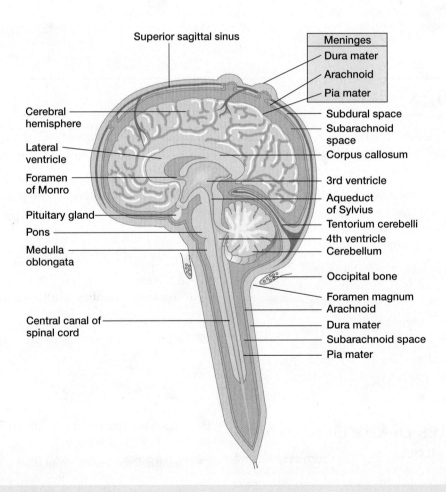

Figure 27–1 Transverse section of the brain and spinal cord. The brain is protected by the skull and covered by three layers of tissue called the *meninges*. Cerebral spinal fluid circulates within the ventricles of the brain and around the brain and spinal cord.

TABLE 27–1 The Primary Functions of Brain Structures

BRAIN STRUCTURE	FUNCTIONS AND CONTROL
Cerebrum	Higher mental functions, general movement, perception, and integration of all functions in lobes below
Frontal lobe	Voluntary skeletal muscle movement, fine repetitive motion, eye movements, motor aspects of speech
Parietal lobe	Interpretation of sensations (taste, visual, smell, hearing, temperature, pressure, pain, texture, and two-point discrimination); recognition of body parts, proprioception
Occipital lobe	Vision center and interpretation of vision
Temporal lobe	Hearing or the perception, reception, and interpretation of sounds, long-term memory
Insula (corpus callosum)	Coordination of activities between the two hemispheres of the cerebrum
Limbic system	Mediation of certain primitive behavior responses, visceral emotional responses, feeding behaviors, biologic rhythms, and sense of smell
Thalamus	Interpretation of most sensations except smell; relay center for sensory motor information
Hypothalamus	Maintenance of temperature, autonomic nervous system function, endocrine function, wakefulness; regulation of emotional expression
Cerebellum	Conscious and reflexive control of muscle tone, maintenance of balance and posture
Brainstem	Location of the descending and ascending motor and sensory pathways; connects the cerebrum, cerebellum, and spinal cord; origin of the 12 cranial nerves

TABLE 27–2 The Cranial Nerves and Their Functions

CRANIAL NERVES	FUNCTION
Olfactory (I)	Reception and interpretation of smell
Optic (II)	Visual acuity, visual fields
Oculomotor (III)	Many eye movements, raise the eyelids, pupil constriction
Trochlear (IV)	Inward and downward eye movement
Trigeminal (V)	Opening and closing the jaw, chewing; eyelid and corneal sensation; sensation of the face, mouth and nose mucosa, tongue, and ear
Abducens (VI)	Lateral eye movement
Facial (VII)	Facial expression, eye closure, and lip speech sounds; taste sensation on anterior two thirds of tongue; pharyngeal sensation
Acoustic (VIII)	Sense of hearing and equilibrium
Glossopharyngeal (IX)	Muscles for swallowing and guttural speech; gag reflex; taste sensation of posterior one third of tongue, nasopharyngeal sensation
Vagus (X)	Sensation behind ear and in a portion of the external ear canal; involuntary control of the heart and lungs
Spinal accessory (XI)	Shrug the shoulders and turn the head
Hypoglossal (XII)	Tongue movement; swallowing, tongue speech sounds

Pediatric Differences

The **neural tube**, the embryonic origin of the central nervous system (CNS), develops by the fourth week of gestation as the neural folds close. The brain forms in the cranial end, and the spinal cord forms in the remainder of the neural tube (Kerr & Huether, 2014). Any insult (such as inadequate folic acid) or critical event (teratogen, infection, substance abuse, or trauma) during this early gestational period can result in a neural tube defect such as spina bifida.

The anatomic and physiologic differences between the nervous systems of children and adults help explain why children and adults have different neurologic problems (see *As Children Grow: Anatomic Differences Between Children's and Adults' Nervous System Structures*). For example, the brain and spinal cord are protected by the skeletal structures of the skull and vertebrae. In infants, however, the cranial bones and vertebrae are not completely ossified. The infant's brain and spinal cord are thus at greater risk for injury. The bones of the skull are separated but held together with bands of connective tissue to allow for normal brain growth. Fontanels are spaces of connective tissue covering the brain at the junction of skull bones that gradually close and ossify. The posterior fontanel closes at 3 months of age, and the anterior fontanel closes by 18 to 24 months of age. (See *As Children Grow: Sutures* in Chapter 5.) The suture lines between the skull bones interlock as early as 6 months of age; by 12 years of age the sutures are completely ossified and cannot be separated (Kerr & Huether, 2014).

A full-term newborn has a complete but immature nervous system. The infant is born with all the nerve cells that will exist

(continued)

As Children Grow: Anatomic Differences Between Children's and Adults' Nervous System Structures

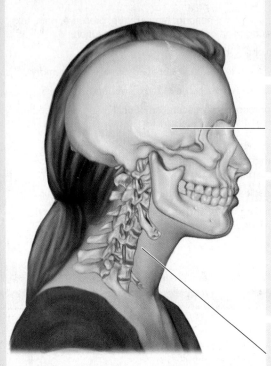

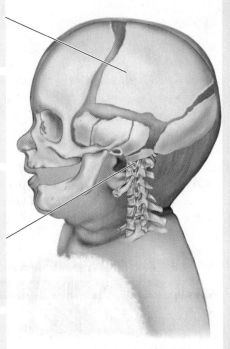

Top heavy, head is large in proportion to body; neck muscles poorly developed; thin cranial bones not well developed; unfused sutures; skull expands until age 2 years. *Prone to brain injury and skull fracture with falls.*

Head size proportional to body; neck muscles well developed, can reduce risk for brain injuries; sutures are ossified by age 12 years; no expansion of skull after 5 years.

Excessive spinal mobility; immature muscles, joint capsule, and ligaments of cervical spine; wedge-shaped, cartilaginous vertebral bodies; incomplete ossification of vertebral bodies. *Greater risk for high cervical spine injury at C1-C2 level or vertebral compression fractures with falls.*

Well-developed muscles and ligaments reduce spinal mobility; vertebral bodies completely formed and ossified.

The skull and brain grow and develop rapidly during early childhood. Infants and young children are at higher risk for injury to the brain and spinal cord because of developing anatomic structures.

throughout life, but maturation of these nerve cells continues after birth. The number of glial cells and dendrites, which enable receipt of nerve impulses, continues to increase until approximately 4 years of age. Brain growth results in increasing head circumference in infants and toddlers and continues until the child is 5 to 8 years of age.

Myelination, the progressive covering of axons with layers of myelin (a lipid protein sheath), is also incomplete at birth. Lack of myelination is associated with the presence of common newborn reflexes (see Table 5–20). As the myelination progresses, the newborn reflexes disappear. The myelination process proceeds in a cephalocaudal direction, and it accounts for the progressive acquisition of fine and gross motor skills and coordination during early childhood; it is ultimately responsible for the speed and accuracy of nerve impulses.

The brain depends on a continuous blood flow to meet its high demands for oxygen. Through an autoregulatory process, the cerebral blood vessels dilate to maintain the cerebral blood flow in response to physiologic changes such as decreased cardiac output, increased intracranial pressure, or constriction of the neck's blood vessels due to positioning. Brain cells become damaged very quickly when blood flow and oxygenation are not maintained. Because the nervous system helps to control and coordinate many body functions, alterations in neurologic function can have widespread effects on the body's metabolism.

Use *Assessment Guide: The Child With a Neurologic Condition* to perform a nursing assessment of the neurologic system. A list of diagnostic and laboratory tests used to evaluate neurologic system function is provided in Table 27–3. See Appendix D for laboratory values and Appendix E for nursing management associated with diagnostic procedures.

TABLE 27–3 Diagnostic Procedures/Laboratory Tests Used to Evaluate Neurologic Conditions*

DIAGNOSTIC PROCEDURES	LABORATORY TESTS
Computed tomography (CT)	Arterial blood gases
Electroencephalogram (EEG)	Complete blood count
Intracranial pressure (ICP) monitoring	Cultures
Lumbar puncture	Toxicology screening
Magnetic resonance imaging (MRI)	
Positron emission tomography (PET) scan	
Radiograph (x-ray)	
Ultrasonography	

*See Appendices D and E for information about these diagnostic procedures and expected laboratory values.

ASSESSMENT GUIDE | The Child With a Neurologic Condition

Assessment Focus	Assessment Guidelines
Level of consciousness	• Is the infant or child lethargic or hard to arouse? • Is the infant or child irritable or difficult to console? • Use the Glasgow Coma Scale when a numeric score is important for future comparison. See Table 27–5.
Cognitive function	• Are the child's verbal skills appropriate for age? Can the child tell you his or her name and age? • Does the child follow directions appropriately?
Cranial nerves	• Assess the cranial nerves. See Table 5–19. See also Table 27–6 for methods to assess cranial nerves in the unconscious child.
Skull	• Palpate the fontanelles for bulging and suture lines for separation.
Pupils	• Check the pupils for size, reaction to light, and accommodation.
Vital signs	• Assess the heart rate, respiratory rate, and blood pressure. • Monitor for late signs of increased ICP (increased systolic blood pressure, a widened pulse pressure, bradycardia, and irregular respirations).
Posture and movement	• Assess the common newborn reflexes in the infant less than 4 months of age to evaluate posture and movement. See Table 5–20. • Observe the child's play or other spontaneous activity to assess strength, coordination, symmetry, and smoothness of movements. Are muscle tone and strength equal bilaterally? Is any weakness present? • Are the child's motor skills developmentally appropriate and acquired at the appropriate age? Has the child lost a previously acquired skill? • Assess the plantar reflex and deep tendon reflexes. See Table 5–21.
Neck stiffness	• Assess for neck stiffness (nuchal rigidity). See Figure 27–6.
Pain	• Assess level of pain when present.
Family history	• Is there a family history of headaches, seizures, neurofibromatosis, or other neurologic conditions?

- *Lethargy:* profound slumber in which speech and movement are limited. The child is aroused with moderate stimulation, but falls asleep easily once stimulation is removed.
- *Stupor:* deep sleep or unresponsiveness; the child is aroused only with repeated vigorous stimulation, but returns to the unresponsive state when the stimulus is removed.
- *Coma:* unconsciousness; cannot be aroused even by painful stimuli.

Etiology and Pathophysiology

Infection of the brain and meninges is a common cause of altered level of consciousness in children. Other causes include trauma, hypoxia, poisoning, seizures, alcohol or substance abuse, endocrine or metabolic disturbances (e.g., diabetic ketoacidosis), electrolyte or acid–base imbalance, brain tumor, stroke, or a congenital structural defect. Any of these pathologic processes can cause increased **intracranial pressure (ICP)** (force exerted by brain tissue, cerebrospinal fluid, and blood within the cranium). The **cerebral perfusion pressure**, the amount of pressure needed to ensure that adequate oxygen and nutrients are delivered by the blood to the brain, can be affected when increased ICP reduces brain arterial blood flow. Rapid diagnosis of the cause of altered consciousness and immediate treatment are essential to prevent poor outcomes.

Clinical Manifestations

Decline in a child's level of consciousness often follows a sequential pattern of deterioration. Initial changes may be subtle: a slight disorientation to time, place, and person. The child may become restless or fussy, and actions that normally calm or soothe only increase irritability. As responsiveness decreases, the child may become drowsy but still respond to loud verbal commands and withdraw from painful stimuli. Keeping the child awake is sometimes difficult. Then response to pain progresses from purposeful to nonpurposeful. The child may exhibit flexor or extensor **posturing**, the abnormal positions sometimes seen after serious injury to the brain (Figure 27–2). Clinical manifestations of increased ICP are provided in Table 27–4.

Clinical Therapy

Clinical therapy focuses on early diagnosis of the cause of altered consciousness and intervention to prevent further insult to the central nervous system (CNS). The Glasgow Coma Scale (GCS) is used to quantify the level of consciousness, most often for acute injury, and pediatric criteria for preverbal children are also available. See Table 27–5.

Laboratory tests may include a complete blood cell count, blood chemistry, clotting factors, and blood culture; toxicology assessments of blood and urine; and urinalysis with culture.

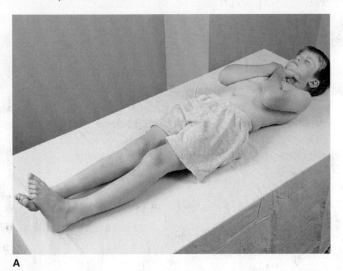
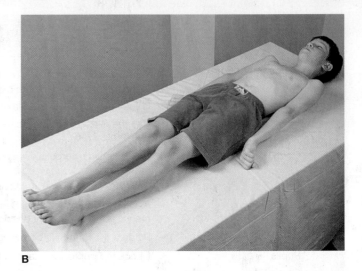

A

B

Figure 27–2 Posturing associated with severe brain injury. *A*, Flexor posturing (decorticate), characterized by rigid flexion, is associated with lesions above the brainstem in the corticospinal tracts. *B*, Extensor posturing (decerebrate), distinguished by rigid extension, is associated with lesions of the brainstem.

A lumbar puncture may be performed if infection is suspected. An electroencephalogram (EEG) identifies damaged or nonfunctioning areas of the brain. Computed tomography (CT) or magnetic resonance imaging (MRI) is used to detect any lesions, structural abnormalities, vascular malformations, or edema. Skull radiographic studies may detect fractures or bony malformations.

SAFETY ALERT!
The lumbar puncture should be postponed if any signs of increased ICP (e.g., papilledema) are present, which could place the child at risk for brain **herniation** (protrusion of brain contents into the brainstem area).

The child is treated with oxygen, and assisted ventilation is provided when gas exchange is inadequate. Any metabolic, acid–base, or electrolyte imbalances are corrected. Antibiotics are initiated for suspected infection.

Maintenance of the cerebral perfusion pressure is important so that adequate oxygen and nutrients are supplied to the brain. Intravenous (IV) fluids or blood products are given if the child is hypovolemic. When poor perfusion and fluid overload exist, a vasopressor medication such as dopamine is administered to increase cardiac output and perfusion of the brain. If the ICP is markedly increased and is a result of obstruction of cerebrospinal fluid (CSF), a ventricular catheter may be inserted to drain CSF to decrease the ICP, temporarily relieving a life-threatening condition. See the *Clinical Skills Manual* SKILLS. See care specific to increased ICP and traumatic brain injury later in this chapter.

Nursing Management
For the Child With Altered Consciousness
Nursing Assessment and Diagnosis

General guidelines for assessing the child with a neurologic condition are provided in the accompanying *Assessment Guide: The Child With a Neurologic Condition*.

When consciousness is altered, initially assess the child's physiologic status, focusing on the child's responsiveness to the environment or stimuli, ability to maintain the airway, vital signs, and breathing patterns. When a cough or gag reflex is present, the child can protect the airway from aspiration. Assess the vital signs, respiratory effort, and color. Monitor pulse oximetry

TABLE 27–4 Signs of Increased Intracranial Pressure

TIMING OF SIGNS	SIGNS
Early signs	Headache
	Visual disturbances, diplopia
	Nausea and vomiting
	Dizziness or vertigo
	Slight change in vital signs
	Pupils not as reactive or equal
	Sunsetting eyes (cranial nerve IV palsy; the iris of eye appears to be setting into the lower eyelid leaving sclera visible above the iris)
	Slight change in level of consciousness, restlessness
Infant has above signs plus:	Irritability
	Bulging fontanelle
	Wide sutures, increased head circumference
	Dilated scalp veins
	High-pitched, catlike cry
Late signs	Significant decrease in level of consciousness
	Seizures
	Cushing triad • Increased systolic blood pressure and widened pulse pressure (systolic pressure increases as the diastolic pressure stays the same or decreases) • Bradycardia • Irregular respirations
	Fixed and dilated pupils, papilledema

TABLE 27–5 Glasgow Coma Scale for Assessment of Coma in Infants and Children

CATEGORY	SCORE*	PREVERBAL CHILD CRITERIA	OLDER CHILD AND ADULT CRITERIA
Eye opening	4	Spontaneous opening	Spontaneous
	3	To voice or sound	To verbal stimuli
	2	To pain	To pressure
	1	No response to painful stimuli	No response
Verbal response	5	Smiles, coos, cries to appropriate stimuli	Oriented; uses appropriate words and phrases
	4	Irritable; spontaneous crying	Confused
	3	Cries to pain	Words
	2	Moans to pain	Sounds
	1	No response	No response
Motor response	6	Spontaneous movement	Obeys commands
	5	Purposeful, localizes pain	Localizes pain
	4	Withdraws to pain	Normal flexion
	3	Flexion to pain	Abnormal flexion; flexor posturing
	2	Extension to pain	Extension; extensor posturing
	1	No response; flaccid	No response; flaccid

*Add the score from each category to get the total. The maximum score is 15, indicating the best level of neurologic functioning. The minimum is 3, indicating total neurologic unresponsiveness.

Source: From Bethel, J. (2012). Emergency care of children and adults with head injury. *Nursing Standard, 26*(43), 49–56; James, H. E. (1986). Neurologic evaluation and support in the child with acute brain insult. *Pediatric Annals, 15*(1), 16–22; Teasdale, G., & Jennett, B. (1974). Assessment of coma and impaired consciousness. *Lancet, 2*, 81–84; Teasdale, G., Allan, D., Brennan, P., McElhinney, E., & Mackinnon, L. (2014). Forty years on: Updating the Glasgow Coma Scale. *Nursing Times, 110*(42), 12–16; Teasdale, G., Maas, A., Lecky, F., Manley, G., Stocchetti, N., & Murray, G. (2014). The Glasgow Coma Scale at 40 years: Standing the test of time. *Lancet Neurology, 13*(8), 844–854; Worrall, K. (2004). Use of the Glasgow Coma Scale in infants. *Paediatric Nursing, 16*(4), 45–47.

and arterial blood gas measurements. Adequate air exchange to keep oxygen and carbon dioxide levels within normal ranges and maintenance of acid–base balance are critical to reduce the risk of hypoxemia and increased ICP.

A baseline neurologic assessment should be performed, including pupils, eye movements, and motor function (Figure 27–3). Assess the cranial nerves; however, be aware that assessment and interpretation may be more challenging in the unconscious child (Table 27–6). Observe for other physiologic signs of increased ICP (Table 27–4). See Table 27–7 for a method to rapidly assess an infant's responsiveness, referred to by the acronym AVPU (alert, verbal, pain response, unresponsive).

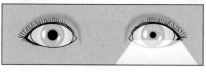

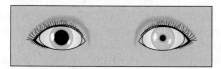

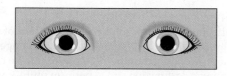

Figure 27–3 **Pupil findings in various neurologic conditions with altered consciousness.** *A,* A unilateral dilated and reactive pupil is associated with an intracranial mass. *B,* A fixed and dilated pupil may be a sign of impending brainstem herniation. *C,* Bilateral fixed and dilated pupils are associated with brainstem herniation from increased intracranial pressure.

TABLE 27–6 Assessment of Cranial Nerves in the Unconscious Child

CRANIAL NERVES	REFLEX	ASSESSMENT PROCEDURE AND NORMAL FINDINGS*
II, III	Pupillary	Shine a light source in eye. *Rapid, concentrically constricting pupils indicate intact cranial nerves II, III.*
II, IV, VI	Oculocephalic	Perform with eyes held open (doll's eyes) and head turned from side to side. *Eyes gazing straight up or lagging slightly behind head motion indicate intact cranial nerves II, IV, VI.* Precaution: Cervical spine injury must be ruled out before this assessment is performed.
III, VIII	Oculovestibular	Place the head in a midline and slightly elevated position. A physician injects ice water into ear canal. *Eyes deviating toward the irrigated ear indicate intact cranial nerves III, VIII.* Precaution: Ensure that the cervical spine is not injured and that the tympanic membranes are intact before this assessment.
V, VII	Corneal	Cornea is gently swabbed with sterile cotton swab. *A blink indicates intact cranial nerves V, VII.*
IX, X	Gag	Pharynx is irritated with tongue depressor or cotton swab. *Gagging response indicates intact cranial nerves IX, X.*

*Italics indicate normal findings.

TABLE 27–7 AVPU—Infant Responsiveness Assessment*

CRITERION	DESCRIPTION
Alert	Responsive to parents; cuddles, coos, or babbles; smiles
Verbal	Responsive to verbal stimulation
Pain response	Responsive to painful stimulation only
Unresponsive	No response to painful stimulation

*AVPU is the acronym formed from the first letter of each criterion.

A cry with a loud, energetic quality, a strong suck and suck–swallowing coordination, and appropriate common newborn reflex responses for age are other signs of an infant's intact mental status.

Among the nursing diagnoses that might be appropriate for the child with an altered level of consciousness are the following (NANDA-I © 2014):

- *Breathing Pattern, Ineffective*, related to neuromuscular dysfunction associated with increased intracranial pressure
- *Aspiration, Risk for*, related to poor control of secretions with decreased level of consciousness
- *Skin Integrity, Risk for Impaired*, related to agitation and skin rubbing against bedding
- *Family Processes, Interrupted*, related to care of a child with an acquired disability

Planning and Implementation

HOSPITAL-BASED NURSING CARE

Nursing care of the child with altered consciousness or increased ICP focuses on maintaining airway patency, monitoring neurologic status, performing routine care, providing adequate nutrition, providing sensory stimulation, and providing emotional support to parents. Nursing care for the child with increased ICP is described later in this chapter.

Make sure the child's airway is patent at all times. If the child has difficulty managing secretions or has no gag reflex, endotracheal intubation or a tracheostomy is performed. Frequent suctioning may be required (see the *Clinical Skills Manual* SKILLS). Keep suction apparatus with catheters, oxygen, resuscitation bag and mask, and extra endotracheal or tracheostomy tubes at the bedside. Pulse oximetry or arterial blood gas measurement is performed at regular intervals to ensure that gas exchange is adequate. Assisted ventilation may be required (see the *Clinical Skills Manual* SKILLS).

Anticipate that seizures may occur. Raise and pad the side rails to protect the child from injury.

Perform routine nursing care. If the corneal reflex is absent, place artificial tears in the eyes and keep them closed with gauze and tape. Perform routine mouth care by brushing the teeth and using swabs with water. Prevent complications associated with immobility (muscle atrophy, contractures, and skin breakdown). See Box 27–1.

Provide adequate nutrition. A nasogastric or transpyloric tube may be inserted if the child remains unconscious or is not alert enough to take food by mouth (see the *Clinical Skills Manual* SKILLS). A gastrostomy tube may be inserted for long-term enteral feeding.

Box 27–1 Care for the Child Who Is Immobile

- Massage child's skin gently using lotion.
- Change the child's position every 2 hours. Use splints or rolls made of towels or blankets to keep the body in proper alignment.
- Place child on a special mattress designed to relieve pressure points (airflow or foam), or use a sheepskin covering when a special mattress is not available.
- Place transparent dressing over skin surfaces exposed to rubbing or friction.
- Support physical therapy efforts with extra passive or gentle range-of-motion (ROM) exercises.
- Use sequential compression devices to prevent deep vein thrombosis.

Provide sensory stimulation. Because children with a severely altered level of consciousness may still be able to hear, talk to them. Listening to music or tapes of family members talking or reading can soothe the child when family members cannot be present. Encourage parents to stroke and touch the child in a soothing manner.

As the child becomes more alert, repeatedly orient the child to time, place, and person, depending on the child's age and level of understanding. Encourage parents to bring objects or toys from home to make the environment more familiar and promote a feeling of security.

Provide emotional support to the child and family. Explain the child's condition in simple terms. Encourage parents to take part in the child's care and therapy as much as possible. Give family members the opportunity to express their feelings. If the child's functioning has been permanently impaired, refer the family to the appropriate psychologic and social services. (See Chapter 13 for information about supporting families during a child's life-threatening illness.)

DISCHARGE PLANNING AND HOME CARE TEACHING

The child's transition from the hospital to home, a long-term care facility, or inpatient rehabilitation center must be planned well in advance of discharge. Identify a case manager or social worker to help plan the child's long-term care needs, including home health nursing and rehabilitation services, modifying the home, and purchasing special equipment.

COMMUNITY-BASED NURSING CARE

Home health nurses play a vital role in the care of the child with acquired neurologic dysfunction and prolonged altered consciousness. Teach the family how to care for the child with severe neurologic dysfunction and to perform routine procedures such as suctioning, maintaining the airway, skin care, feeding, positioning, ROM exercises, and stimulation. Regular follow-up visits are needed to assess the child's progress and to modify the treatment plan.

Link the child and family with community rehabilitation services through an early intervention program or school-based program. The home health nurse or case manager should help the family have an individual education plan (IEP) developed for the child (see Chapter 12).

Evaluation

Expected outcomes of nursing care include the following:

- The child's airway is maintained and the brain is adequately oxygenated.
- Complications of immobility are prevented.
- The family provides appropriate care to the child with prolonged altered consciousness to promote minimal long-term disabilities.

Seizure Disorders

Seizures are periods of abnormal electrical discharges in the brain that cause involuntary movement and behavior and sensory alterations. Epilepsy is a chronic disorder characterized by recurrent, unprovoked seizures, secondary to an underlying brain abnormality. Approximately 326,000 children under the age of 15 years live with epilepsy (Epilepsy Foundation, 2014a). The highest rate of onset occurs during the first 12 months of life (Kerr & Huether, 2014). See *Developing Cultural Competence: Seizures.*

Developing Cultural Competence Seizures

Some cultural groups have misperceptions of the cause of seizures, such as punishment for sins, a lack of spiritual faith, or possession by spirits (Institute of Medicine, 2012, p. 32). For example, the Hmong people of Asia believe the child is experiencing *quag dab peg*, or "the spirit catches you and you fall down." Traditional Hmong view the condition as serious but take pride in the child who has the condition, as they have a link to the spirit world. In 1997, Anne Fadiman wrote a compelling story about the cultural conflict between a Hmong family and healthcare providers over the treatment of their daughter's seizures: *The Spirit Catches You and You Fall Down.*

Etiology and Pathophysiology

When an excessive number of neurons in the brain become overexcited, they discharge abnormally, leading to seizures. An imbalance of exciting and inhibiting mechanisms caused by poor regulation of the gamma-aminobutyric acid ionotropic receptor family A ($GABA_A$) neurotransmitters may be a cause of early childhood seizures (Kerr & Huether, 2014). Rather than being one distinct disorder, epilepsy and seizures are associated with CNS structural defects, or from disorders that affect CNS functioning, such as brain injury, infection, electrolyte disturbance, toxins, and brain tumor. Genetic factors or familial predisposition may lead to seizures. Some seizures have no known cause.

Partial, or **focal**, seizures are caused by abnormal electrical activity in one brain hemisphere or a specific area of the cerebral cortex, most often the temporal, frontal, or parietal lobes. The symptoms depend on the region of the cortex affected.

Generalized seizures are the result of diffuse electrical activity that begins in both brain hemispheres simultaneously, spreading throughout the cortex into the brainstem. The child's movements and spasms are bilateral and symmetric, and consciousness is impaired.

Febrile seizures occur in susceptible infants and children in connection with a rise in temperature to 39.0°C (102.2°F) or higher during the first 24 hours of an associated acute illness.

They occur in 3% to 5% of children (Ismail et al., 2012). No evidence of intracranial infection or systemic metabolic disorder is present. A genetic predisposition may be present. These seizures are usually seen in children between 9 months and 5 years of age (Kerr & Huether, 2014). Simple febrile seizures last less than 15 minutes and do not recur during the same illness. Some children have complex febrile seizures that last 15 minutes or longer and recur within 24 hours, and they may be at greater risk for developing epilepsy.

Status epilepticus is a prolonged continuous seizure of 15 minutes or evidence of intermittent seizures noted from clinical signs or EEG tracings lasting more than 15 minutes without full recovery of consciousness between seizures (Wilkes & Tasker, 2013). Low levels of antiepileptic medications, fever, infection, and a recent medical condition change are risk factors in children. Among children, the highest incidence is in the first 12 months of life (Varelas, Spanaki, & Mirski, 2013). The basal metabolic rate rises during peak seizure activity and increases the demand for oxygen and glucose.

Clinical Manifestations

The symptoms of a seizure depend on the type and duration of the seizure. The characteristics of the various partial and generalized seizures are presented in Table 27–8.

Partial seizures often start with an aura or an abrupt, unprovoked alteration in behavior. The child may have time to get to the floor and avoid injury once the aura pattern is recognized.

Generalized seizures often begin with the **tonic** phase, characterized by unconsciousness, continuous muscular contraction, and sustained stiffness. The **clonic** phase that follows is characterized by alternating muscular contraction and relaxation or repeated rhythmic jerking. During the **postictal period** following seizure activity, the level of consciousness is decreased. The length of the postictal period varies. Children may have a partial seizure that progresses to a generalized seizure.

Growth and Development

Neonatal seizures may be subtle with roving eye movements, repetitive blinking, sucking, lip smacking, tongue thrusting, swimming movements of the arms, leg pedaling movements, and apnea or tachycardia (Beaulieu, 2013).

Simple febrile seizures are generalized seizures with tonic-clonic movements and eye rolling, followed by a brief postictal period. Complex febrile seizures have additional focal signs.

Clinical Therapy

After the child's first seizure, a thorough history is taken from the parent, primary caretaker, or witnesses to the event. The description and length of the seizure, presence or absence of an aura, and whether the child lost consciousness are noted. This information helps to identify the type of seizure according to the International Classification of Epileptic Seizures in Table 27–8.

Based on the physical findings and history, diagnostic tests ordered may include a complete blood cell count, blood chemistry, and urine toxicology. A urine culture, blood culture, and lumbar puncture are performed if meningitis is suspected. A lead level and tests for inborn errors of metabolism may be considered. Radiologic tests such as CT scanning or MRI and angiography may be performed to identify a cerebral lesion or metabolic

TABLE 27–8 Clinical Manifestations of Seizures

TYPE OF SEIZURE AND CAUSE	CLINICAL MANIFESTATIONS
PARTIAL SEIZURES	
***Simple Partial Seizures* (focal seizures)**	
Focal damage (e.g., with cerebral palsy)	Onset: any age
Tumors or lesions	No loss of consciousness; lasts less than 30 sec; no postseizure confusion
Arteriovenous malformation	No **aura** (a visual, auditory, taste, or motor sensation preceding a seizure or migraine headache)
Brain abscesses	Signs depend on section of brain affected: motor activities such as twitching or lost muscle tone (may involve one extremity, part of an extremity, or ipsilateral extremities) or sensory sensations such as tingling, numbness, or a sensation involving sound, smell, or sight
	May progress to a generalized seizure
***Complex Partial Seizures* (psychomotor seizures)**	
Lesions, cysts, or tumors	Onset: 3 years of age to adolescence
Perinatal trauma	Consciousness is impaired immediately; lasts 30 sec to 5 min; postseizure amnesia or confusion
Focal sclerosis (e.g., scarring of the medio-temporal lobe from prolonged febrile seizures)	Aura frequently present
	May have abnormal motor activity, twitching, loss of tone, or posturing; **automatisms** (unusual body movements without purpose, e.g., lip smacking, lip chewing, sucking)
Vascular anomalies (e.g., arteriovenous malformations)	May have sensory changes such as tingling or numbness, feeling of anxiety, fear, or déjà vu (sensation that event occurred before)
Brain trauma	May progress to a generalized seizure
	Abdominal pain
GENERALIZED SEIZURES	
***Tonic-Clonic Seizures* (grand mal seizures)**	
Cerebral damage from perinatal trauma, brain trauma, tumors, structural lesions, metabolic and neuromuscular degenerative disorders	Onset: any age, rare before 6 months of age
	Abrupt onset seizure, 1- to 2-min loss of consciousness, postseizure confusion (few minutes to hours)
Genetic, strong familial incidence	May or may not have aura
Many are idiopathic	Body becomes stiff and rigid when all muscles contract (tonic phase), followed by rhythmic jerking motions (clonic phase)
	Drooling as secretions are not swallowed
	Pupils dilated; eyes roll upward or deviate to one side
	Abdominal or chest wall rigidity with leg, head, and neck extended, and arms flexed or contracted
	Cry or grunt as air is forced out when diaphragm and chest muscles contract
	Urinary or bowel incontinence as muscles become flaccid during clonic phase
	Sleepiness, difficulty in arousal; hypertension; diaphoresis; headache, nausea, vomiting; poor coordination, decreased muscle tone; confusion, amnesia; slurred speech; visual disturbances; combativeness
***Childhood Absence Epilepsy* (petit mal seizures)**	
Hyperventilation for 3 minutes	Onset: ages 4–10 years with remission in adolescence
Genetic (multifactorial) predisposition or mutations	More prevalent in females
	May develop other generalized seizures
	No aura; brief loss of consciousness, usually lasts 5–10 sec, rarely exceeds 30 sec, no postseizure confusion, lethargy, or sleepiness; amnesia regarding the seizure
	Frequent attacks (50–100 or more per day), may cluster, interfere with learning
	Eye blinking, eyelid fluttering, staring, glazed eye appearance, myoclonic jerks; interrupts voluntary activity, slight decrease or loss of muscle tone (head may droop, may drop objects)
	Verbal or touch stimulation does not interrupt seizure
Juvenile Myoclonic Epilepsy	
Genetic disorder	Onset often during puberty
	No loss of consciousness, child recovers in seconds, no postictal period
	Most often occur upon falling asleep or awakening
	Quick involuntary muscle jerks of the neck, shoulders, and arms
	Child usually has normal intelligence

TYPE OF SEIZURE AND CAUSE	CLINICAL MANIFESTATIONS
Infantile Spasms (West syndrome, salaam seizures)	
Tuberous sclerosis (genetic syndrome)	Onset: age 4 and 18 months with peak onset at 3–7 months; more common in males
Mutation of several genes	Severe form of epilepsy; may occur with altered consciousness as part of a complex partial seizure; seizures occur in clusters, 5–150 per day
Intrauterine stroke	
Inborn errors of metabolism	Spasms with abrupt flexion and extension of muscle groups in the neck, trunk, and extremities, involving head nods or jackknife body contractions; occur as infant awakens or falls asleep. Spasms stop by 5 years of age when other seizure types occur.
CNS malformations	
	Developmental delays occur
Lennox-Gastaut Syndrome (akinetic or atonic seizure)	
Gray matter degenerative diseases and subacute seizures	Onset: first seen between 1 and 8 years, predominantly in boys
Sclerosing panencephalitis	Combination of generalized seizures including tonic-clonic, absence, and myoclonic activity; drop attack (falls to ground with sudden loss of postural tone, inability to break fall, is limp for period of time)
Many are idiopathic	
	Associated intellectual disability, delayed psychomotor development, and severe behavior problems

disorder in the brain. An EEG is often performed at a follow-up visit between seizures. If the child is taking any anticonvulsants, a serum drug level is obtained.

Many seizures are self-limiting and require no emergency intervention. When the seizure is prolonged, emergency therapy includes airway management, supplemental oxygen, intravenous benzodiazepines, and careful monitoring of vital signs. Serum electrolytes, glucose, and blood gases may be monitored. The postictal period ranges from 30 minutes to 2 hours. When the child's seizure does not stop as expected with emergency intervention, treatment for status epilepticus is initiated (Table 27–9).

Children with simple febrile seizures are often not treated with an anticonvulsant at the time of the seizure because the seizure has stopped before arrival at the emergency department. Acetaminophen is given to lower the temperature. Long-term antiepileptic medications are not recommended for simple febrile seizures because of their adverse effects.

Most seizure disorders are treated with antiepileptic drugs (AEDs). A single (monotherapy) AED is preferred for seizure control to minimize the side effects such as sleepiness, decreased attention and memory, difficulty with speech, ataxia, and diplopia. A low dose is used initially and gradually increased until seizures are controlled. An alternate AED may be tried if seizure control is not achieved with a high therapeutic dose of the first medication or when unacceptable side effects occur. Some children have refractory or **intractable seizures**, requiring two or more AEDs. See _Medications Used to Treat: Seizures._ Medication dosage adjustments are often needed as the child grows. Blood tests to monitor for liver and hematologic problems and therapeutic drug levels are often performed.

SAFETY ALERT!

Because of the potential adverse effects of medications used to treat seizures, children are monitored for depression, suicidal thinking, and effects on learning. Medications should not be stopped abruptly, and dose is tapered when discontinuation is planned. When starting a new medication, adolescents should not engage in hazardous activities or drive a motorized vehicle until effects of the medication are known. Alcohol intake is contraindicated.

TABLE 27–9 Status Epilepticus Clinical Therapy and Nursing Management

TYPE OF CARE	CLINICAL THERAPY AND NURSING MANAGEMENT
Emergency assessment and management	• Maintain a patent airway. Muscle rigidity may compromise the airway. Keep suction equipment at the bedside in case secretions are excessive. • Give supplemental oxygen because increased metabolic demands deplete oxygen stores. • Monitor vital signs and circulation with pulse oximeter and cardiorespiratory monitor. • Perform neurologic assessments every 5–10 min.
Ongoing urgent management	• Establish an IV line for fluid or medication administration. • Assess blood glucose level; administer glucose if the child is hypoglycemic; the physical stress of the seizure may result in declining glucose levels. • Insert a nasogastric tube to reduce the risk for aspiration due to vomiting. • Protect the child from injury. • Manage thermoregulation.
Medications	• Administer benzodiazepines such as diazepam, lorazepam, or midazolam. If there is no response, the dose may be repeated. Fosphenytoin or phenobarbital may be necessary if seizure activity continues. Cumulative doses of drugs may produce apnea, so be prepared to assist with endotracheal intubation and ventilations.

Source: Data from Shearer, P., & Riviello, J. (2011). Generalized convulsive status epilepticus in adults and children: Treatment guidelines and protocols. _Emergency Care Clinics of North America, 29,_ 51–64; Varelas, P. N., Spanaki M. V., & Mirski, M. A. (2013). Status epilepticus: An update. _Current Neurology and Neuroscience Reports, 13_(7), 357–365; McLauchlan, D. J., & Robertson, N. P. (2012). Management of status epilepticus. _Journal of Neurology, 259,_ 2261–2263.

Medications Used to Treat: Seizures

MEDICATION AND ACTION	NURSING MANAGEMENT
Benzodiazepines (diazepam, lorazepam) CNS depressant, anticonvulsant properties, used for status epilepticus.	• Administer IV push medication very slowly into the IV entry site closest to the child's body. • Monitor for hypotension, tachycardia, and respiratory depression. • The rectal or nasal preparation may be prescribed for home administration to treat prolonged seizures.
Phenobarbital Enhances gamma-aminobutyric acid (GABA) neurotransmitter inhibition by prolonging the time that chloride channels are open in response to GABA.	• Administer IV push medication very slowly into the IV entry site closest to the child's body. • Monitor child's vital signs frequently when given IV. Monitor for excess sedation. • May crush tablets and mix with food or fluid. • Provide vitamin D and folic acid supplements when drug is used long term.
Phenytoin (Dilantin) **Fosphenytoin (Cerebyx)** Reduces voltage, frequency, and spread of electrical discharges within motor cortex to inhibit seizure activity.	• Monitor the child's vital signs frequently after IV dosage for respiratory depression. • Educate family to provide an adequate intake of vitamin D, folic acid, and calcium. • Promote frequent dental care for gingival hyperplasia. • Educate parents that urine may be pink, red, or brown color.
Carbamazepine (Tegretol) Inhibits sustained repetitive impulses and reduces synaptic transmission to the spinal cord, limiting the spread of seizure activity.	• Give with food to enhance absorption. Be aware that grapefruit may increase drug levels. • Educate parents about which tablets can be chewed and not chewed (sustained release). • Do not combine suspension with another liquid medication to prevent precipitation. • Causes photosensitivity reactions when skin is exposed to sunlight.
Valproic acid (Depacon, Depakote) Anticonvulsant; inhibits abnormal neuron discharges in the brain and decreases seizure activity.	• Do not use carbonated beverage to dilute syrup. Educate the child and parents that all tablets and capsules should be swallowed whole, not chewed. • Give with food to decrease gastrointestinal irritation. • Monitor platelet count and bleeding times. • Educate female adolescents about teratogenic effects of the medication, and the importance of contraception and planning pregnancy.
Ethosuximide (Zarontin) Suppresses spike and wave pattern in absence seizures; raises brain's seizure threshold.	• Monitor for weight loss or anorexia. • Give with food if gastrointestinal upset occurs. • Do not expose medication to light. Do not freeze.
Primidone (Mysoline) Raises the seizure threshold and changes seizure patterns.	• Give with food if gastrointestinal upset occurs. • Store medication away from light and moisture.
Felbamate (Felbatol) Blocks repetitive firing of neurons and increases seizure threshold.	• Monitor for weight gain or loss. • Monitor regularly for hematologic and liver problems as well as bruising or bleeding.
Gabapentin (Neurontin) Gamma-aminobutyric acid (GABA) neurotransmitter analog	• Monitor vision, concentration, and coordination as medication may cause impairments. • Do not take medication within 2 hr of an antacid.
Lamotrigine (Lamictal) Inhibits release of glutamate and aspartate in sodium channels to decrease seizure activity.	• Educate family about photosensitivity side effect. • Monitor for dizziness, lack of coordination, drowsiness, or depression if used with valproic acid. • Educate parents to notify the healthcare provider if a skin rash develops because of risk for Stevens–Johnson syndrome.

MEDICATION AND ACTION	NURSING MANAGEMENT
Tiagabine (Gabitril filmtabs) Enhances activity of GABA, making it more available for postsynaptic neurons.	• Give with food. Avoid using with over-the-counter medications that cause drowsiness. • Monitor for signs of dizziness, tremor, and sleepiness.
Topiramate (Topamax) Sodium channel blocker and enhances ability of GABA to move chloride ions into the neurons.	• Monitor for weight loss. • Increase fluid intake to reduce risk of kidney stones. • Monitor mental status and for impaired cognitive function. • Inform parents to report speech and language problems.
Levetiracetam (Keppra) Unknown mechanism of action; inhibits seizure activity.	• Ensure that parents know whether tablet must be swallowed whole or can be chewed or crushed. • Monitor for gait and coordination problems.
Oxcarbazepine (Trileptal) Similar mechanism of action to carbamazepine.	• Monitor for hyponatremia and CNS impairment. • Educate female adolescents that oral contraceptives may be ineffective.
Zonisamide Facilitates dopaminergic and serotonergic transmission between neurons.	• Increase fluid intake to reduce risk of kidney stones. • Capsules should not be broken or crushed.
Rufinamide (Banzel) Modulation of sodium channels inhibits firing of sodium-dependent neuron transmission.	• Tablet may be crushed or swallowed whole. • Give medication with a meal because food increases drug absorption.
Clobazam (Onfi) Binds at GABA$_A$ receptor site to inhibit seizures; used for Lennox-Gastaut syndrome.	• Tablet may be crushed or swallowed whole. • Inform female adolescents that oral contraceptives may be ineffective.

Source: Data from Wilson, B. A., Shannon, M. T., & Shield, K. M. (2015). *Nurse's drug guide 2015*. Hoboken, NJ: Pearson; Taketomo, C. K., Hodding, J. H., & Crause, D. M. (2014). *Pediatric and neonatal dosage handbook* (21st ed.). Hudson, OH: Lexicomp; Zelleke, T. G., Depositario-Cabacar, D. F. T., & Gaillard, W. D. (2013). Epilepsy. In M. L. Batshaw, N. J. Roizen, & G. R. Lotrecchiano (Eds.), *Children with disabilities* (7th ed., pp. 487–506). Baltimore, MD: Paul H. Brookes Publishing Co.

Surgery may be performed to remove a tumor, lesion, or portion of the brain that has been identified as causing the seizures, particularly when seizures do not respond to multiple AEDs. A vagal nerve stimulator with leads wrapped around the left vagus nerve may be implanted in children who are not candidates for surgery and are unable to tolerate multiple medications. The child activates the vagal nerve stimulator after experiencing an aura to reduce the spread of the seizure.

A ketogenic diet may be used for children with seizures that do not respond to AEDs. The diet is customized for the child to have high fat (80% of calories), adequate protein for growth, and very low carbohydrates that will maintain an ideal body weight, maximize ketosis, and achieve optimal seizure control. Each meal typically has about 3 to 4 g of fat for every 1 g of protein and carbohydrate (Epilepsy Foundation, 2014b). Ketosis is believed to produce anticonvulsant effects. Family motivation must be high to maintain the rigid diet for 1 or more years because improved seizure control is directly related to diet compliance. Diet side effects include constipation, kidney stones, and slowed growth. Constipation is treated with medium-chain triglyceride (MCT) oil and increased fluids. Kidney stones are treated by increasing fluids and alkalinizing the urine. Approximately 10% to 15% of children become seizure-free, and nearly half of children have a 50% reduction in number of seizures (Epilepsy Foundation, 2014b).

A trial of medication withdrawal (slowly tapered over a few months) is often attempted for children who have been seizure-free for 2 years or longer. Approximately 25% to 36% of children have seizures recur after discontinuing medications (Zelleke, Depositario-Cabacar, & Gaillard, 2013). Children with epilepsy are more likely to have anxiety, depression, behavior problems, and disabilities (e.g., attention deficit hyperactivity disorder, developmental delay, or autism) than children who do not have epilepsy (Russ, Larson, & Halfon, 2012).

Nursing Management

For the Child With a Seizure Disorder

Nursing Assessment and Diagnosis

Assess and monitor the child's physiologic status. Observe the specific seizure activity, level of consciousness, vital signs, and signs of hypoxia. During the postictal period, monitor the child's vital signs, perform neurologic checks, and keep the environment safe. Once the child is stable, a more definitive assessment can be made. Level of consciousness is one of the most important indicators of neurologic function. Remember that the child's lack of response may be the result of the postictal state. Continuing

TABLE 27–10 Questions to Ask About Seizures

TIME PERIOD	QUESTIONS TO ASK
Just before the seizure	• What was the child doing? • Did the child complain of feeling unwell (headache, nausea, vomiting, muscle pain, fever) or feeling "funny"? • Did the child suffer any trauma? Did the child get into any medications or poisons?
During the seizure	• What movements of the arms and legs were seen? On one or both sides of the body or in one extremity only? • Did the child exhibit any chewing or other automatism? • Were the pupils dilated or the eyes deviated to one side? • Did the child's color change (pale, red, blue)? • Was the child incontinent of urine or stool? • Was the child aware of surroundings or able to respond to questions?
After the seizure	• How long did the episode last? • Was the child lethargic, weak, or uncoordinated when waking up? • Did the child have memory loss or confusion?

motor activity, which may be less intense after benzodiazepines are given, is a potential sign of status epilepticus.

Collect and analyze historical information about the seizure activity. See Table 27–10.

Assess the family's adaptation to the seizure disorder, including how well the family is coping with the uncertainty of when the next seizure will occur.

Common nursing diagnoses for the child with a seizure disorder include the following (NANDA-I © 2014):

- *Breathing Pattern, Ineffective,* related to neuromuscular dysfunction during the tonic phase of a seizure
- *Airway Clearance, Ineffective,* related to inability to control secretions during seizure
- *Trauma, Risk for,* related to falls with seizures
- *Self-Esteem, Chronic Low,* related to refractory seizures and loss of bowel and bladder control during seizure activity
- *Anxiety* related to unpredictable nature of seizure disorder
- *Health Management, Family, Ineffective,* related to poor adherence with medications

Planning and Implementation

Children with a seizure disorder may be hospitalized for another condition. Nursing care focuses on preventing and managing a potential seizure by maintaining airway patency, ensuring safety, administering medications, and providing emotional support. Both acute care and long-term management are involved.

MAINTAIN AIRWAY PATENCY

Place nothing in the child's mouth during a seizure; loose teeth may be knocked out and aspirated. The child is put in side-lying position for secretions to drain. Monitor the child to ensure adequate oxygenation: The child's color should be pink, the heart rate at a normal or slightly above normal rate for age, and the SpO_2 greater than 95%. Oxygen is usually given at SpO_2 levels below 95% (see the *Clinical Skills Manual* SKILLS).

ENSURE SAFETY

Protect the child from self-harm during seizures (Figure 27–4). If the child is in bed, pad the side rails to prevent injury. Children who have frequent, recurrent seizures should wear helmets to protect their heads in case they fall. All children with seizure disorders should wear some form of medical alert identification.

ADMINISTER MEDICATIONS

Take special precautions when administering IV medications (benzodiazepines) for urgent seizure management. Give these medications very slowly over several minutes to minimize the risk of respiratory or circulatory collapse, and carefully monitor the child's vital signs.

Medications for the daily management of seizures are given orally. Ensure that extended-release medications are not crushed or chewed. When a child is NPO because of illness or on the day of surgery, seizure medications are usually given with a swallow of water. Obtain medication orders in these cases.

PROVIDE EMOTIONAL SUPPORT

Seizures are frightening to the child and family because control of body movements and consciousness are often lost. Parents often feel guilty about the child's seizure disorder and need guidance to treat the child as normally as possible. They may perceive that the child is treated differently by family, friends, and peers because of lack of understanding about seizures. Parents need additional support when seizures do not respond to one or more antiepileptic drugs (AEDs) and alternative therapies must be considered. Refer the child and family to support groups and counseling services if indicated. See *Evidence-Based Practice: Supporting Children With Epilepsy and Their Parents.*

Clinical Tip

When the child on a ketogenic diet is hospitalized, limit glucose and dextrose from all sources including IV fluids, elixirs, suspensions, and syrups. Use normal saline IV fluid. Obtain medications in pill form, crush them, and mix with an allowable food approved by the pharmacy.

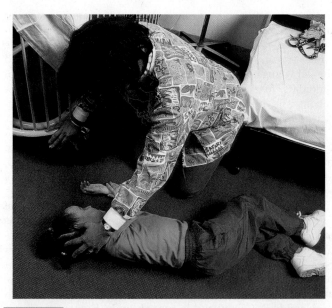

Figure 27–4 **Protect the child from injury during a seizure. The child who is standing should be gently assisted to the floor and placed in a side-lying position. Clear the area of any objects that might cause harm to the child.**

EVIDENCE-BASED PRACTICE | Supporting Children With Epilepsy and Their Parents

Clinical Question

What factors are related to stress and health quality of life for children with epilepsy and their families?

The Evidence

Twenty children, aged 9 to 15 years, and their parents completed a voluntary survey while attending a summer camp for children with epilepsy. The survey asked about seizure control and management, age at diagnosis, the worst thing about having epilepsy, and one thing they could change about having epilepsy. Feeling different or being teased was the most frequent response campers (50%) and parents (27%) gave to the worst thing about epilepsy, followed by the physical act of the seizure (campers, 38%; parents, 40%). Reducing the number or having no seizures was desired by 63% of campers and parents as the one change about having epilepsy. An additional 13% of campers wanted no seizures in public (VanStraten & Ng, 2012). While responses were not statistically significant, they do reveal important information about the impact of the condition on quality of life.

The risk for development of clinical depression among mothers of children with epilepsy participating in a multisite Health-related Quality of Life in Children with Epilepsy Study was identified at time of diagnosis and every 6 months for 24 months. Data were collected using the 20-item Center for Epidemiologic Depression Scale to assess mood, somatic complaints, interactions with others, and motor functioning. Data from several other research instruments helped identify factors such as family functioning, family resources, and epilepsy severity. Of the 338 mothers who agreed to participate in the project, 128 (38%) had a risk for clinical depression at the time of the child's diagnosis and were excluded from further evaluation. Of the remaining 210 mothers, a total of 58 (28%) mothers developed depressive symptoms at some point during the subsequent 24 months. Statistically significant factors associated with risk for clinical depression included a younger mother, the child's prescribed number of antiepileptic drugs,

worse family functioning, fewer family resources, and more family demands (Ferro & Speechley, 2011).

The same multisite Health-related Quality of Life in Children with Epilepsy Study also reported information on child health, well-being, and the impact of illness on life functions during the past 4 weeks for 374 children with a mean age of 7.4 years. The parent form of the Child Health Questionnaire was used at diagnosis and 24 months later for the study. Data from other research instruments helped identify factors such as parent depression, family functioning, family resources, and epilepsy severity. After controlling for physical and psychologic health at diagnosis, multiple regression analysis identified predictors at 24 months of better physical health (less severe cognitive problems and less parental depression) and better psychosocial health (less severe behavior problems, an older parent, better family functioning, and fewer demands) in participating children (Ferro, Landgraf, & Speechley, 2013). These studies further support the important role of the family environment on child health-related quality of life.

Best Practice

Epilepsy is a common neurologic condition that causes families and affected children to have social, psychologic, and physical challenges. Stressors can be related to the stigma associated with epilepsy, the unpredictable nature of when and where seizures may occur, loss of control, and even some of the disabilities associated with epilepsy. Research suggests that intervention programs to improve the family environment and to offer treatment for depression and anxiety may improve the family's healthy adaptation to epilepsy.

Clinical Reasoning

When caring for a child with epilepsy, what questions may help reveal the stressors that the parents and child are experiencing? Once stressors are identified, investigate resources with regard to parent mental health, improved epilepsy management, and support groups for children and their parents.

DISCHARGE PLANNING AND HOME CARE TEACHING

Encourage parents to express their fears and anxieties. Answer their questions honestly, and refer them to organizations such as the Epilepsy Foundation, where they can get more information about the child's disorder. Be sure parents know how to administer medications and keep the child safe. Provide information about whom to call with questions and when to return for follow-up.

COMMUNITY-BASED NURSING CARE

Educate the child and parents about medication regimens. Explain the purpose of each antiepileptic drug (AED), its administration schedule, and the importance of giving all doses. Provide information about the medication side effects, and alert parents to the signs of toxic reactions. Ensure that information is shared directly with older children so that they can begin taking more responsibility for self-care and gain a sense of self-control. A study explored nonadherence to AEDs in 124 newly diagnosed children ages 2 to 12 years. Researchers

discovered that 58% of children had persistent nonadherence and 42% had near perfect adherence during the first 6 months of therapy. The pattern of adherence was established within the first month of therapy. Socioeconomic status was the only factor associated with adherence, and lower socioeconomic status was associated with higher nonadherence (Modi, Rausch, & Glauser, 2011).

Ensure that adolescents understand that alcohol intake is contraindicated and may result in medication toxicity. Ask questions at each visit that may reveal actual medication adherence, such as inquiring about the number of pills remaining or difficulties paying for medications. Monitor the child's growth because a weight change may require dosage adjustment to maintain seizure control. Encourage the family to obtain regular dental care for the child treated with phenytoin and similar AEDs because of their effects on the gingivae.

The parents of children with recurrent febrile seizures should be taught to give the proper dose of acetaminophen or ibuprofen with fever onset. Parents need to know that fever management may not prevent a febrile seizure. Reassure parents that complications from febrile seizures are rare.

Families Want to Know

Safety for the Child With a Seizure Disorder

Children with epilepsy have more injuries of all sorts, including burns and falls. Children are at increased risk for death due to drowning. Planning for safety includes the following:

- Do not leave the child alone in the bathtub.
- Children who bathe alone should use the shower.
- A buddy and lifeguard should always be present when the child swims.
- A life vest should always be worn when boating.
- A child with frequent seizures should wear a helmet to protect the head in case of a fall.
- The child should not play or stand around open flames or outdoor grills.
- The child should avoid areas where fall risks are increased.
- A form of medical identification should be worn, such as a medical alert bracelet.

Educate female adolescents about the potential teratogenicity of some antiepileptic drugs (AEDs). Valproic acid and carbamazepine are associated with neural tube defects. Contraception should be used when the adolescent is sexually active, but ensure that barrier methods are used correctly when AEDs interact with oral contraceptives. When pregnancy is desired, an alternate AED may be prescribed with a lower risk for birth defects.

Teach families about safety guidelines for the child. See *Families Want to Know: Safety for the Child With a Seizure Disorder*. Physical activity and exercise are important for all children. Encourage participation in sports when adequate supervision is provided. Children with well-controlled seizures may participate in most team sports, and activities such as bicycle riding. Activities such as rope climbing, rock or mountain climbing, tree climbing, snow skiing, scuba diving, and skydiving are more dangerous if seizures are not well controlled. Swimming and water sports require one-to-one supervision.

Assist the family to develop an individual health plan so the child can receive medications during school hours, if necessary. Provide information to teachers and school administrators about care of the child during a seizure and what information to report to the parents. Parents may want to provide a towel and clothing change for the child who has incontinence with a seizure.

The child may be afraid of having a seizure in front of friends. Reassure the child and family that taking medications regularly often controls seizures. Children need to be able to explain to peers what a seizure is and what to do if they are present when one occurs . Summer camps for children with seizures can be a safe and comfortable place for the child to enjoy outdoor activities. Teach parents to boost the child's self-image by emphasizing what the child can do, rather than focusing on contraindicated activities. Depending on state laws, most adolescents can drive after they have been seizure-free for at least 2 years.

Evaluation

Expected outcomes of nursing management include the following:

- The child achieves good seizure control with medication, ketogenic diet, or surgical intervention.
- The use of effective safety measures prevents injuries during seizures.

- The child gains enhanced self-esteem through participation in well-supervised sports and activities.

Infectious Diseases

Infections of the central nervous system need to be identified and treated rapidly because they can cause significant consequences in the developing child.

Bacterial Meningitis

Meningitis, an inflammation of the meninges, can be caused by either bacterial or viral agents. Bacterial meningitis is more serious than viral meningitis and is sometimes fatal. Newborns and infants are at greatest risk for bacterial meningitis. Infants and children who develop meningitis may have acute complications and long-term morbidity.

ETIOLOGY AND PATHOPHYSIOLOGY

Meningitis may occur secondary to other infections such as otitis media, sinusitis, pharyngitis, cellulitis, pneumonia, or septic arthritis; brain trauma; or a neurosurgical procedure. *Streptococcus pneumonia*, *Neisseria meningitides*, and staphylococcal and gram-negative microorganisms cause most cases of meningitis in children in the United States. Group B streptococcus causes some cases of meningitis in newborns. Meningitis may also be caused by tuberculosis. Rates of meningitis have fallen for children because of increased protection from several vaccines (Castelblanco, Lee, & Hasbun, 2014). Risk factors for meningitis include immunosuppression, a ventriculoperitoneal shunt, cochlear implant, skull fracture, neurosurgery, or a recent sinus or ear infection (Kerr & Huether, 2014).

In many cases, the infectious organism spreads to the CNS from the bloodstream (see *Pathophysiology Illustrated: Central Nervous System Infection*), triggering an inflammatory response. The brain becomes inflamed and edematous, leading to **cerebral edema** (an increase in intracellular and extracellular fluid in the brain that results from anoxia, vasodilation, or vascular stasis) and increased ICP. If the infection spreads to the ventricles, they can become obstructed and impede the flow of cerebrospinal fluid (CSF), causing cerebral edema and hydrocephalus as acute complications. The infection may trigger the syndrome of inappropriate antidiuretic hormone (SIADH).

Pathophysiology Illustrated: **Central Nervous System Infection**

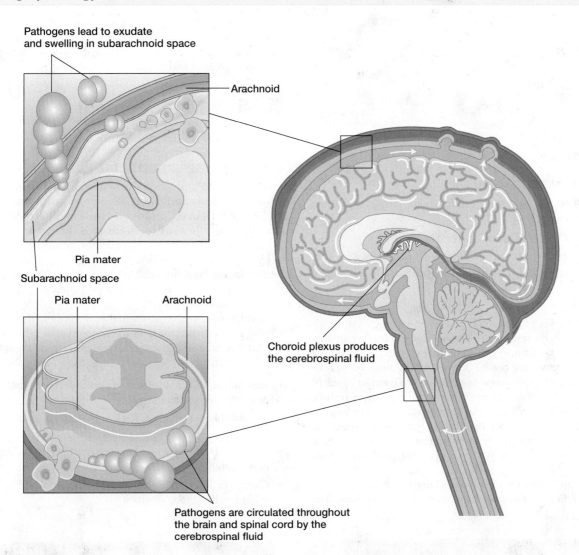

Pathogens lead to exudate and swelling in subarachnoid space

Arachnoid

Pia mater

Subarachnoid space

Pia mater

Arachnoid

Choroid plexus produces the cerebrospinal fluid

Pathogens are circulated throughout the brain and spinal cord by the cerebrospinal fluid

After bacteria reach the central nervous system, the pia mater, the arachnoid, and the cerebrospinal fluid-filled subarachnoid space become infected. The cerebrospinal fluid then circulates the pathogens throughout the brain and spinal cord.

CLINICAL MANIFESTATIONS

Symptoms vary by the child's age, the pathogen, and the length of the illness before diagnosis. Onset may be sudden or develop over 1 to 2 days. Symptoms in the young infant may include fever or hypothermia, change in feeding pattern, vomiting, or diarrhea. The anterior fontanelle may be bulging or flat. The infant may be alert, restless, lethargic, or irritable. Rocking or cuddling, which normally calms a fussy infant, irritates the infant with meningitis.

Older children are usually febrile, have altered consciousness (e.g., confusion, delirium, lethargy, irritability), and may have vomiting and complaints of muscle or joint pain. A hemorrhagic rash of petechiae that changes to purpura or large necrotic patches may be seen in meningococcal meningitis (see Chapter 16). Other symptoms consistent with meningeal irritation may include headache (most often frontal), photophobia, esotropia (inward eye deviation), and **nuchal rigidity** (resistance to neck flexion). The child is often comfortable only in an **opisthotonic position** (hyperextension of the head and neck) (Figure 27–5). The child may have a positive Kernig or Brudzinski sign, or both, on examination (Figure 27–6).

CLINICAL THERAPY

Diagnosis is based on the history, clinical presentation, and laboratory findings. Laboratory tests include a complete blood count, blood cultures, serum electrolytes, blood urea nitrogen, osmolality, and clotting factors. A lumbar puncture is performed to culture the CSF and evaluate it for white blood cells, protein, and glucose levels and also to determine CSF pressure. Real time polymerase chain reaction (PCR) assays of the CSF are also used for diagnosis. CT scanning may be performed when increased ICP or a brain abscess is suspected.

Antibiotics commonly used to treat bacterial meningitis include ampicillin, aminoglycosides, cefotaxime, ceftriaxone, penicillin G, and vancomycin. They are administered as soon

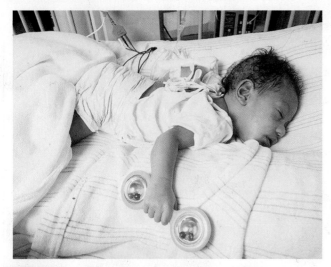

Figure 27-5 The child with bacterial meningitis may assume an opisthotonic position, with the neck and the head hyperextended, to relieve discomfort.

as diagnostic tests are obtained and often changed once culture and sensitivity results are known since many organisms have antibiotic resistance. IV antibiotics are administered for 7 to 21 days, depending on the organism and the child's clinical response. Dexamethasone is given to children in cases of suspected *Haemophilus influenzae* type b infection to reduce the severity of potential sensorineural hearing loss (Le Saux & Canadian Paediatric Society Infectious Diseases and Immunization Committee, 2014). Other treatments include fever and seizure control, increased ICP management, and fluids and electrolytes.

Infants and children receive nothing by mouth and are started on IV fluids to manage cerebral perfusion pressure. The child is carefully monitored for increased ICP and SIADH (see Chapter 30). IV fluid volume is carefully managed to treat cerebral edema.

Approximately 20% of child survivors have significant disabilities (Martin, Sadarangani, Pollard, et al., 2014). Examples of disabilities include hearing impairment, gross neurologic deficits, and behavioral and intellectual disorders.

Nursing Management

For the Child With Bacterial Meningitis

Nursing Assessment and Diagnosis

Assess the child's physiologic status, including vital signs and level of consciousness. Measure head circumference often in hospitalized infants because of the potential for hydrocephalus. Be alert for signs of a change in the child's condition and response to treatment. Monitor the child's ability to control secretions and to drink sufficient fluids. Monitor intake and output. Assess for any sensory deficits. Identify parents' concerns about this potentially life-threatening condition.

Several nursing diagnoses that may apply to the child with bacterial meningitis appear in the accompanying *Nursing Care Plan*. Additional nursing diagnoses might include the following (NANDA-I © 2014):

- *Aspiration, Risk for,* related to altered level of consciousness and poor secretion control
- *Fluid Volume: Deficient, Risk for,* related to poor oral fluid intake
- *Spiritual Distress (Parent)* related to the child's life-threatening condition
- *Caregiver Role Strain* related to a hospitalized child and other family responsibilities

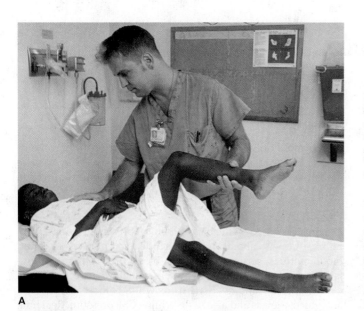

A

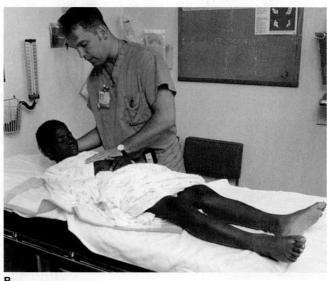

B

Figure 27-6 Testing for Kernig and Brudzinski signs, both common findings with meningitis. *A,* To test for Kernig sign, raise the child's leg with the knee flexed. Then extend the child's leg at the knee. If any resistance is noted or pain is felt, the result is a positive Kernig sign. *B,* To test for Brudzinski sign, flex the child's head while in a supine position. If this action makes the knees or hips flex involuntarily, a positive Brudzinski sign is present.

Nursing Care Plan: The Child With Bacterial Meningitis

1. Nursing Diagnosis: *Injury, Risk for,* related to infection of cerebrospinal fluid and potential sequelae (NANDA-I © 2014)

GOAL: The child will suffer minimal CNS injury secondary to infection.

INTERVENTION	RATIONALE
• Administer antibiotics and corticosteroids as prescribed.	• Antibiotics help eradicate the pathogen and prevent cerebral edema. Corticosteroids reduce inflammation and the chance of neurologic sequelae.
• Note return of fever, nuchal rigidity, or irritability. Monitor vital signs, assess for signs of increased ICP. Measure head circumference once or twice daily. Note changes in responsiveness. Notify the health-care provider immediately if any signs are detected.	• Watching for common sequelae such as subdural effusions, hydrocephalus, or septic arthritis ensures prompt treatment.

EXPECTED OUTCOME: Child's condition will improve significantly within 48–72 hr (fever will decrease and no signs of neurologic sequelae will be detected).

GOAL: The child will not develop cerebral edema as a result of water retention.

INTERVENTION	RATIONALE
• Monitor for signs of increased ICP and SIADH.	• Early recognition is essential for management to be initiated quickly.
• Perform strict intake and output measurements. Determine urine specific gravity. Check electrolytes and osmolality of both serum and urine. Weigh the child daily. Restrict fluids and give sodium chloride as prescribed.	• Low urine output with a high specific gravity is a sign of fluid retention and SIADH. The child is maintained with lower fluids and is provided sodium supplements to reduce the possibility for cerebral edema.

EXPECTED OUTCOME: Cerebral edema will not develop. If SIADH or increased ICP occurs, the condition will be treated promptly so effects are minimized.

GOAL: The child will be free of injury resulting from disseminated intravascular coagulation (DIC).

INTERVENTION	RATIONALE
• Be aware of needlesticks and lesions that continue to bleed. Monitor clotting times.	• Prompt recognition leads to management of the coagulopathy.
• Administer blood products, vitamin K, or heparin as ordered.	• Prompt recognition allows for early initial treatment of DIC. The child may bleed to death if treatment is delayed.

EXPECTED OUTCOME: Child will not sustain injury from DIC.

GOAL: The child with any degree of hearing loss will be identified.

INTERVENTION	RATIONALE
• Arrange for hearing assessment prior to discharge.	• Hearing loss is a common complication. Early intervention is needed to promote growth and development.

EXPECTED OUTCOME: Child with identified hearing loss will be referred to an appropriate specialist or program for intervention.

2. Nursing Diagnosis: *Pain, Acute,* related to meningeal irritation (NANDA-I © 2014)

GOAL: The child will be as comfortable as possible.

INTERVENTION	RATIONALE
• Assess pain with age-appropriate pain scale.	• Pain scales provide ability to quantify pain for future comparison.
• Minimize tactile stimulation.	• Sensory stimulation increases discomfort.

(continued)

Nursing Care Plan: The Child With Bacterial Meningitis (*continued*)

GOAL: The child will be as comfortable as possible. (*continued*)

INTERVENTION	RATIONALE
• Allow the child to assume a comfortable position.	• The child determines the most comfortable position. The opisthotonic position may be the most comfortable.
• Keep the lights dim and maintain a quiet environment.	• Dim lights reduce the discomfort from photophobia. Noise can disturb the child.
• Provide pain medication as prescribed.	• Pain medication is appropriate for acute discomfort associated with illness.

EXPECTED OUTCOME: Child will be calm, and behaviors will indicate increased comfort.

3. Nursing Diagnosis: *Infection, Risk for (Family and Close Contacts)*, related to exposure to child with meningitis (NANDA-I © 2014)

GOAL: Caretakers or family members will have no apparent evidence of infection.

INTERVENTION	RATIONALE
• Explain rationale and dose schedule for taking rifampin or ciprofloxacin.	• Rifampin and ciprofloxacin provide prophylaxis for many bacterial pathogens responsible for meningitis.

EXPECTED OUTCOME: Family members and other close contacts will verbalize the schedule for rifampin or ciprofloxacin therapy.

Planning and Implementation

The accompanying *Nursing Care Plan* summarizes care for the child with bacterial meningitis. Nursing care begins with emergency treatment and continues as the child's condition stabilizes. Monitor respiratory and neurologic status, maintain hydration, administer medications, and prevent complications. Promote the child's comfort with reduced stimulation (dim lights, quiet room) and by placing in a side-lying position. Isolate the child according to hospital protocol until the causative organism is identified and effective treatment has been administered for 24 hours.

SAFETY ALERT!
Monitor the serum sodium concentration and urine specific gravity since the child is at risk for SIADH (see Chapter 30). Maintenance and replacement fluids are usually given to children with bacterial meningitis. If SIADH occurs, moderate fluid restriction with an isotonic solution is ordered until serum sodium levels return to normal.

Monitor the child's response to antibiotic therapy. Observe for signs of gastrointestinal bleeding, which is a potential complication of corticosteroid use.

Respond to parents' concerns about their child's condition, explaining all measures to reduce the child's discomfort and treat the illness. Identify ways parents can help meet the child's comfort needs.

Prevention is a major role for nurses. Encourage parents to get their infants and children fully immunized with the *Haemophilus influenzae*, pneumococcal, and meningococcal vaccines (see Chapter 16).

DISCHARGE PLANNING AND HOME CARE TEACHING

Identify and address home care needs well in advance of discharge. Follow-up visits are important to monitor for complications and sequelae. Help parents deal with any physical requirements resulting from the child's illness and any emotional, social, and financial repercussions of the child's condition. Teach parents what to do if the child has a seizure.

Infants and toddlers with neurologic sequelae should be referred to an early intervention program. Refer the child with a hearing loss to an otolaryngologist and speech and language specialist. Encourage early identification of other neurologic sequelae, such as learning problems. Children with neurologic sequelae need to have an individual education plan (IEP) developed (see Chapter 12), and parents may need help planning for the child's special educational needs. Refer parents to the appropriate social service agencies for support and assistance.

Evaluation

Expected outcomes of nursing care are provided in the accompanying *Nursing Care Plan*.

Viral (Aseptic) Meningitis

Viral meningitis is an inflammatory response of the meninges characterized by an increased number of blood cells and protein in the CSF. In the United States, an enterovirus is the most common cause of viral meningitis in children (Kelesidis, Mastoris, Metsini, et al., 2014).

Generally, the child with aseptic meningitis does not appear as ill as the child with bacterial meningitis. The child may have an abrupt onset of fever of 38.0°C to 40.0°C (100.4°F to 104°F) and have meningeal signs (headache, photophobia, stiff neck, and back pain), myalgia, irritability, and lethargy. Other symptoms include malaise, vomiting and diarrhea, upper respiratory symptoms, and a maculopapular rash. The infant may have a tense anterior fontanelle. Seizures are rare. Symptoms usually resolve spontaneously within 3 to 10 days.

The child with fever and meningeal signs is hospitalized. Blood, urine, and CSF analyses are performed. PCR and DNA testing of the CSF help detect viral meningitis, often within 24 hours. Until the diagnosis of aseptic meningitis is confirmed, the child is treated aggressively for bacterial meningitis. Other treatment is supportive of symptoms. Children usually make a full recovery.

Nursing Management

Initial nursing care focuses on providing supportive care as described for the child with bacterial meningitis. Give acetaminophen or ibuprofen as ordered to reduce fever, headache, and muscle or joint pain. Keep the room dark and quiet (to decrease stimuli and meningeal irritation), give IV or oral fluids, and promote comfort with proper positioning.

The child and family need information about the disease. Explain medical and nursing procedures in terms that the child and family can understand. Keep parents informed about the child's progress. Once the diagnosis of viral meningitis is made, immediately begin discharge planning and teaching for home care. Explain that recovery may take several weeks but that complete recovery is expected.

Encephalitis

Encephalitis is an acute inflammation of the brain often caused by an arbovirus that is transmitted by a mosquito, such as the West Nile, Eastern equine, Western equine, St. Louis, and La Crosse viruses. Other causes of encephalitis include Colorado tick fever, enteroviruses, and Epstein-Barr virus. Inflammation of the meninges is also common. Epidemics occur most often in warm weather seasons.

Encephalitis may occur as a direct or primary infection by an organism (virus, bacteria, fungi, or parasite) that successfully passes through the blood–brain barrier. Some children only have symptoms of a flulike illness after being infected and never develop encephalitis. Signs and symptoms include fever, irritability, severe headache, and bulging fontanelle, followed by altered mental status. The child may have flaccid or spastic paralysis. Meningeal irritation signs such as nuchal rigidity, photophobia, and positive Kernig or Brudzinski signs are common. Focal or generalized seizures may occur. Altered mental status may progress to coma over hours or days.

Diagnosis is based on history and laboratory findings. Information about recent immunizations, insect bites, or residence in or travel to areas where cases of encephalitis are present should be obtained (e.g., West Nile virus or Eastern equine encephalitis). CSF culture and analysis, blood serologic tests, and nasopharyngeal and stool specimens are evaluated to identify viral pathogens. Testing for virus-specific immunoglobulin M antibodies using the enzyme-linked immunosorbent assay (ELISA) test is performed after 5 days of acute illness. The PCR test is used to assay for herpes DNA in the CSF. A CT scan, MRI, and EEG may also be performed. An EEG may help assess seizure activity and help localize the area of the brain affected.

The child with encephalitis is at risk for seizures, respiratory failure, and increased ICP and receives supportive treatment in the intensive care unit (ICU). Physical therapy, occupational therapy, and speech therapy may be prescribed for these children. Children admitted to the ICU with serious symptoms are more likely to have persistent symptoms that last up to 6 months. Some fatalities occur, and significant neurologic sequelae may result.

Nursing Management

Nursing care focuses on monitoring cardiorespiratory function, preventing complications resulting from immobility, reorienting the child, and teaching the parents about the child's condition.

Monitor the child's cardiorespiratory function. Check the child's airway and ability to handle secretions. Assess the child's color, respiratory rate and effort, SpO$_2$, and arterial blood gases. Monitor the heart rate, blood pressure, capillary refill time, and urine output.

Provide seizure precautions. Prevent complications resulting from immobility (see Box 27–1). Maintain skin integrity. Proper positioning with frequent turning is important. When prescribed by the healthcare provider, perform chest physiotherapy to prevent pneumonia.

Give the parents information about their child's condition and prognosis. Provide support to parents as they cope with the serious nature of this condition.

As the level of consciousness begins to improve, the child may at first be confused and disoriented and may have residual effects of the disease. Orient the child to the hospital environment. Have the family take an active role in the child's physical and emotional recovery, such as by bringing favorite stuffed animals or music from home. Engage in therapeutic play (refer to Chapter 11 for techniques). Give the child age-appropriate toys to encourage a return to normal behavior.

Provide parents with instructions for home care. Plan follow-up visits so the child can be evaluated for neurologic sequelae. Ensure that children are referred for physical or speech therapy as needed. Refer parents to home care, social services, family counseling, and support groups as needed.

Reye Syndrome

Reye syndrome is an acute **encephalopathy**, which is a cerebral dysfunction caused by a toxic, inflammatory, or anoxic insult or injury that may result in permanent tissue damage, although the dysfunction may improve over time. In 1980, an association was identified between the use of aspirin for influenza or varicella and Reye syndrome. The condition is now rare in the United States (approximately 35 cases a year) since most parents give children acetaminophen or ibuprofen rather than aspirin for flulike symptoms and varicella (Ibrahim & Balistreri, 2016). The mortality rate associated with Reye syndrome is high.

Reye syndrome is classified as a secondary mitochondrial hepatopathy. It is caused by a drug toxic to the liver or other toxin, metal, or metabolite and results in a poorly functioning organ. In the case of Reye syndrome, an interaction between a viral illness and aspirin occurs in a susceptible individual (Ibrahim & Balistreri, 2016). The disorder is characterized by cerebral edema, hypoglycemia, and an enlarged, fatty, poorly functioning liver (due to an elevation of short-chain fatty acid levels and hyperammonemia).

Reye syndrome begins with a preceding viral illness that seems to be resolving, followed by an acute onset of vomiting, mental status changes, seizures, and progressive unresponsiveness. The condition progresses to cerebral edema and neurologic dysfunction, leading to a final stage with coma, seizures, flaccidity, loss of deep tendon reflexes, and respiratory arrest.

The diagnosis of Reye syndrome is based on an abrupt change in the child's level of consciousness and diagnostic laboratory tests that reveal liver dysfunction and no other identifiable cause. CSF analysis usually reveals white blood cells. Radiographic imaging reveals cerebral edema. Liver enzyme and ammonia levels are elevated, blood glucose levels are below normal, and prothrombin time is prolonged. Serum bilirubin levels are normal. A liver biopsy is sometimes performed to confirm the diagnosis.

The child with Reye syndrome receives supportive care in a pediatric ICU. Efforts are made to prevent the secondary effects of cerebral edema and metabolic injury associated with the elevated short-chain fatty acid and ammonia levels. Mechanical ventilation is often needed once the child is comatose. Arterial and venous blood pressure monitoring is performed. The child is monitored for signs of increased ICP secondary to cerebral edema (see the *Clinical Skills Manual* SKILLS). Hypoglycemia is treated with IV glucose. Electrolytes, blood chemistry, and blood pH are monitored.

Clinical Tip

Make sure all parents know that they should use acetaminophen or ibuprofen rather than aspirin when the child has a viral illness such as influenza to prevent the development of Reye syndrome. Most over-the-counter medications for children are now made with acetaminophen or ibuprofen, but parents should be encouraged to verify this.

Nursing Management

Nursing care focuses on monitoring the child's physical status, providing emotional support, and teaching parents about disease prevention.

Check the child's respiratory and neurologic status frequently, and note any signs of improvement or deterioration. Refer to the discussion of nursing management of altered states of consciousness earlier in this chapter for specific nursing interventions.

Monitor laboratory tests for acidosis, elevation of ammonia levels, or hypoglycemia. Monitor the child's intake and output. Correct imbalances by administering fluids, electrolytes, or medications as ordered. Prevent complications associated with immobility. Support the family faced with the child's life-threatening illness (see Chapter 13).

The child who survives and is discharged is monitored for sequelae. Developmental and neurologic deficits may occur and are more severe in children under 2 years of age. Arrange for home nursing or frequent clinic visits during the recovery period for monitoring. Inform the parents about community resources that can assist them in promoting the child's recovery.

Guillain-Barré Syndrome (Postinfectious Polyneuritis)

Guillain-Barré syndrome is an acute inflammatory peripheral neuropathy with an acute onset of rapidly developing symmetric motor weakness that progresses in an ascending pattern. It is rare in children compared to adults.

Guillain-Barré syndrome is thought to be a postinfectious disorder that affects motor neurons, but may also affect sensory and autonomic neurons. The damaged neurons experience demyelinization. Onset occurs within 6 weeks after an influenza-like or gastrointestinal illness (*Campylobacter jejuni* was the most common organism) in 60% of cases (Shui et al., 2012). An association between immunizations such as for influenza and the disorder has not been confirmed.

Infants have an onset of rapidly progressive severe hypotonia, possible respiratory distress, irritability, and feeding difficulties. Older children initially have pain, numbness, paresthesia, or weakness in all limbs. Weakness progresses bilaterally over days for up to 4 weeks. Maximum weakness is often reached in 2 to 4 weeks. Deep tendon reflexes may be diminished or absent. The child may develop acute ataxia or an inability to walk. Respiratory muscles and cranial nerves may not be affected, but difficulty swallowing and bilateral facial nerve weakness are signs of impending respiratory failure. If the autonomic nervous system is affected, blood pressure fluctuations and episodes of bradycardia and asystole may occur.

Diagnostic criteria of Guillain-Barré syndrome include varying degrees of progressive motor weakness (up to total paralysis of all extremities) and **areflexia** (no reflex response to stimulation). CSF protein levels rise to twice the upper limit of normal, and a few white blood cells are seen in the CSF. Bacterial and viral cultures are usually negative. Electroconduction tests such as electromyography show acute muscle denervation. An MRI of the spinal cord may be requested.

Clinical therapy for Guillain-Barré syndrome is intravenous immune globulin (IVIG) at a dose of 0.4 g/kg/day for 2 to 5 days when ascending paralysis is progressing rapidly. Guidelines for administration of IVIG can be found in Chapter 22. Responses to IVIG are dramatic, often within days. Plasma exchange to remove autoantibodies or immunosuppressive medications are alternate therapies. Corticosteroids are not effective. Pain management is important. Physical therapy and supportive care are initiated early to promote ambulation. The condition is rarely fatal; however, some disability may result.

Nursing Management

Nursing care focuses on monitoring respiratory status, meeting nutritional needs, managing autonomic nervous system dysfunction, preventing complications associated with weakness and immobility, providing emotional support, and teaching the parents how to care for the child after discharge.

Place the child on a cardiorespiratory monitor for continuous assessment in the early phase of the illness. Monitor the child for dyspnea, inability to handle secretions, inadequate respiratory effort, and mucous membrane color changes that may indicate the need for endotracheal intubation and mechanical ventilation.

Monitor the child's vital signs closely for episodes of tachycardia, bradycardia, blood pressure fluctuations, sweating, and bowel and bladder dysfunction. Observe frequently for decreased responsiveness. Promptly report the occurrence of these signs to the child's healthcare provider.

Assess the child's ability to swallow. If the child has no gag reflex, nutrition is provided with IV supplements or nasogastric tube feedings.

Prevent complications associated with immobility (see Box 27–1). Ensure good postural alignment, and turn the child every 2 hours. Maintaining skin integrity is also important.

Evaluate the child's muscle tone, strength, and symmetry. When the child's condition begins to improve, recovery of lost strength is the priority. Active exercise is emphasized in physical therapy. Encourage family members to participate in the child's care, especially during the recovery phase. They can help with the activities of daily living and reinforce what the child has learned in physical therapy.

Explain the progression of Guillain-Barré syndrome to the parents during the initial stages. Witnessing a rapid deterioration in their child's physical status can be frightening; therefore, inform parents that deterioration may continue until the treatment becomes effective. Be honest when discussing recovery and prognosis for the child. Have parents bring in favorite toys, dolls, or books to make the child feel more secure. Playing with or reading to the child can be comforting.

DISCHARGE PLANNING AND HOME CARE TEACHING

Identify and address home care needs well in advance of discharge. Support the parents as they prepare for the child's return home, especially when return to full strength is expected to be slow. Outpatient physical therapy sessions may be needed several times a week in the early recovery stages. Frequent follow-up visits to the health center are essential to monitor the child's recovery. Refer the parents to home health services that can provide guidance for financial assistance.

COMMUNITY-BASED NURSING CARE

Help the child to adjust to any residual effects of Guillain-Barré syndrome. Help the child practice exercises learned in physical therapy sessions, and encourage the child to perform activities of daily living, such as brushing the teeth or combing the hair.

To promote a positive self-image, praise any effort the child makes to be self-sufficient. The child may be frustrated and angry. Allow the child to express these feelings in an appropriate way, either during play or in conversation. Home schooling may be needed until the child has strength to walk and participate in a full school day.

Headaches

An estimated 75% of children experience a headache by age 15 years, and headaches are a major reason for school absence (Antonaci et al., 2014). Up to 20% of children and adolescents experience migraine headaches (Sun et al., 2013). The incidence of headaches increases as children age. Headaches interfere with physical, social, and mental health aspects of daily life.

Etiology and Pathophysiology

Headaches have both benign (migraine, inflammatory, and tension) and structural causes, such as a tumor. See Table 27–11 for headache classifications and clinical manifestations.

- Migraine headaches may be triggered by stress; foods containing nitrates, glutamate, caffeine, tyramine, and salt; menses; fatigue; and hunger. Genetic predisposition may be a factor. Some children may also have abdominal migraine episodes (Catala-Beauchamp & Gleason, 2012).

- Tension headaches may be associated with stress related to school, anxiety, demanding schedules, fasting, and inadequate sleep.

- Medication overuse (rebound) headaches are associated with the frequent use (2 to 3 times a week) of medications for headaches (e.g., acetaminophen, nonsteroidal anti-inflammatory drugs [NSAIDs], decongestants, triptans, opioids, benzodiazepines, and ergotamines).

Clinical Manifestations

Table 27–11 shows the signs and symptoms associated with specific types of headaches.

Clinical Therapy

Diagnosis involves a detailed history of the headache characteristics (onset, duration, pain severity, quality, and location; aura; treatment or medications used) and associated symptoms (abdominal pain, nausea, vomiting). Assessment for neurologic signs such as altered consciousness, abnormal cranial nerves, papilledema, and motor or sensory deficits is performed. Radiologic studies (CT scan or MRI) are used only in cases of abnormal neurologic signs or a suspected structural problem. A lumbar puncture is performed if an infection or inflammatory process is suspected.

Treatment includes relaxation techniques, analgesics, and anti-inflammatory medications. A behavior management program may help reduce common headache triggers (inadequate sleep, stress, missed meals, caffeine, chocolate, or excessive extracurricular activities). Medications to abort migraines (e.g., almotriptan malate and rizatriptan benzoate by mouth) are approved by the U.S. Food and Drug Administration (FDA) for adolescents who can identify an aura or signs of an impending headache. Topiramate was recently approved by the FDA as a prophylactic medication for migraine headaches in adolescents. Medication overuse headaches are treated by withdrawal of all medications used for headaches for a 2- to 4-week period. Limited use of medications may be permitted after that period.

Nursing Management

Assess the child for potential neurologic signs associated with headaches. Encourage the child to keep a headache diary, either written or electronic, that tracks the events and stresses at the time of a headache to help identify patterns and potential triggers. Assist the child and family to see patterns in the headache diary and discuss potential strategies for relieving the headaches. Behavior changes that may reduce headaches include a consistent bedtime and wake-up time 7 days a week, a regular eating schedule, regular physical activity for 30 to 45 minutes at least 5 days a week, and avoidance of hunger, identified food triggers, and smoke and other strong odors.

Teach the child to take the prescribed medications at the first sign of a headache, but no more often than 2 to 3 days a week. See Chapter 24 for care of the child with a brain tumor.

Structural Defects

Common structural defects include microcephaly, hydrocephalus, neural tube defects, craniosynostosis, positional plagiocephaly, and neurofibromatosis.

Microcephaly

Microcephaly is a small brain with a head circumference below the third percentile on growth curves. Causes may include a genetic disorder or destructive insult during infancy, such as an infection, metabolic disorder, or hypoxia-ischemia. Intellectual disability is common (see Chapter 28 for more information).

Hydrocephalus

Hydrocephalus is the body's response to an imbalance between the volume of cerebrospinal fluid (CSF) produced and absorbed. The condition may be congenital or acquired as a result of intraventricular hemorrhage, meningitis, traumatic brain injury, or brain tumor. An estimated 1 to 2 infants per 1000 are born with hydrocephalus (National Institute of Neurological Disorders and Stroke [NINDS], 2014). It is commonly associated with myelomeningocele (described later in this chapter).

TABLE 27–11 Clinical Manifestations of Headaches by Classification

CLASSIFICATION OF HEADACHES	CLINICAL MANIFESTATIONS
MIGRAINE Vascular, acute recurrent	• Unilateral or bilateral pulsatile throbbing pain lasting for hours or days, moderate to severe pain intensity, aggravated by routine activity • Lasts 2–3 hr; may be relieved by sleep, but may last 48–72 hr if untreated • Nausea and vomiting • Photophobia and phonophobia • Visual or motor aura several minutes before headache starts; if no aura may have mood changes, food cravings, or anorexia hours before the attack • Preschool-age children may have irritability, restlessness, malaise, head banging, head holding, and sensitivity to light and sound • Recurrent abdominal pain
TENSION Muscular contraction Acute recurrent (less than 15 days a month)	• Intermittent or constant pain of mild to moderate intensity (may fluctuate), pressure or tightening (nonpulsatile) sensation • May last 30 min to 7 days • Unlikely to have nausea, vomiting, abdominal pain, or visual disturbances • Sensitive to light or sound
REBOUND OR MEDICATION OVERUSE Chronic nonprogressive (more than 15 days a month)	• Pain many be bandlike, over entire head, or crushing; may be bad enough to interfere with academic performance • Occurs at least 2–4 times a week or daily • Usually increases in frequency and severity over time, paralleling the increase in medication use • Recurs when medication wears off
INFLAMMATORY Sinusitis or dental abscess Acute localized	• Facial pain or tenderness over affected sinus, gum, or periorbital area; may be associated with nasal congestion • Dull, constant pressure; severity varies with head position • Fever may be present • No nausea, visual changes, light or sound sensitivity
STRUCTURAL Space-occupying lesion, hemorrhage, increased ICP Chronic progressive	• Severe pain, increases in frequency and severity, often in occipital or frontal location • Pain awakens child or is present in the morning; increases with coughing, sneezing, or straining • Vomiting that is persistent or preceded by recurrent headache • Abnormal neurologic signs (e.g., double vision, papilledema, strabismus, weakness, ataxia)

Source: Data from Blosser, C. G., Albers, A. C., & Reider-Demer, M. (2012). Headache. In C. Burns, A. M. Dunn, M. A. Brady, N. B. Starr, & C. G. Blosser (Eds.), *Pediatric primary care* (5th ed., pp. 606–614). Philadelphia, PA: Elsevier Saunders; Hershey, A. D., Kabbouche, M. A., & O'Brien H. L. (2016). Headaches. In R. M. Kliegman, B. F. Stanton, J. W. St. Geme, & N. F. Schor (Eds.), *Nelson textbook of pediatrics* (20th ed., pp. 2863–2874). Philadelphia: Elsevier; Paul, S. P., Debono, R., & Walker, D. (2013). Clinical update: Recognising brain tumours early in children. *Community Practitioner*, 86(4), 42–45.

ETIOLOGY AND PATHOPHYSIOLOGY

Hydrocephalus may be either communicating or noncommunicating. In communicating hydrocephalus, the CSF flows freely among normal channels and pathways, but CSF absorption in the subarachnoid space and the arachnoid villi is impaired. It may be acquired or caused by a congenital malformation in the subarachnoid spaces.

Noncommunicating hydrocephalus accounts for most cases in children. It results from a blockage in the ventricular system that prevents CSF from entering the subarachnoid space, resulting in enlargement of one or more ventricles (see *Pathophysiology Illustrated: Hydrocephalus*). This obstruction can be caused by infection, hemorrhage, tumor, surgery, or structural deformity. Congenital structural defects include the Chiari type II malformation (found in children with myelomeningocele), aqueduct of Sylvius stenosis, and the Dandy-Walker syndrome (includes hydrocephalus, a posterior fossa cyst, and hypoplasia of the cerebellum).

Pathophysiology Illustrated: **Hydrocephalus**

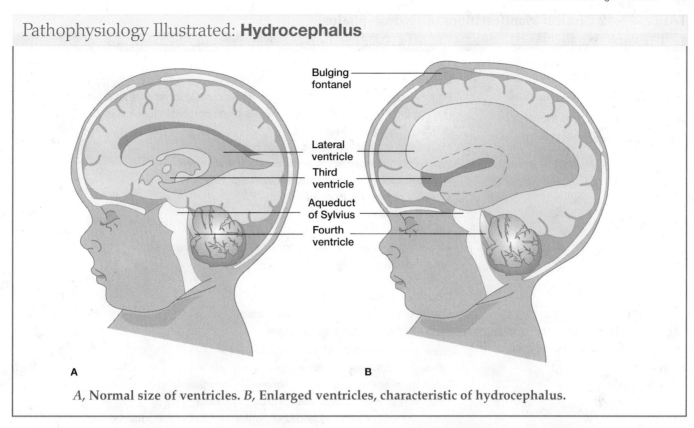

A, Normal size of ventricles. *B*, Enlarged ventricles, characteristic of hydrocephalus.

The Arnold-Chiari malformation (Chiari type II) involves a downward placement of the medulla and lower cerebellum through the foramen magnum of the skull into the cervical vertebrae. This displacement can cause sudden death, respiratory difficulty, swallowing difficulties, and the need for assisted ventilation. Symptoms during infancy may include stridor, a weak cry, and apnea. An older child may have an extremity weakness, difficulty swallowing, choking, hoarseness, vocal cord paralysis, and breath-holding episodes. This defect is also associated with intellectual disability and epilepsy.

CLINICAL MANIFESTATIONS

The signs and symptoms of hydrocephalus vary with the age of the child (Table 27–12). Infants have a rapidly increasing head circumference (Figure 27–7). Older children show signs of increased ICP. Signs of shunt malfunction in infants are nonspecific and include irritability, vomiting, poor appetite, disordered sleep, and fever. Older children with shunt malformation may have a headache, nausea, vomiting, and decreased level of consciousness.

CLINICAL THERAPY

The diagnosis of hydrocephalus may be made prenatally by ultrasound or based on physical findings and neuroimaging studies after birth. Daily head circumference measurements are essential for any infant at risk of developing hydrocephalus. CT and MRI imaging diagnose hydrocephalus, and in some cases reveal the anatomic cause. When the infant's fontanelle is still open, ultrasonography or echoencephalography may be used to confirm the diagnosis. CT and MRI imaging are also used to evaluate shunt failure.

Clinical therapy for hydrocephalus involves surgery to remove the obstruction (e.g., surgical removal of a tumor or endoscopic third ventriculostomy) or to create a pathway to divert excess CSF. A catheter or shunt is placed in the ventricle and passes the CSF to the peritoneal cavity, right atrium of the

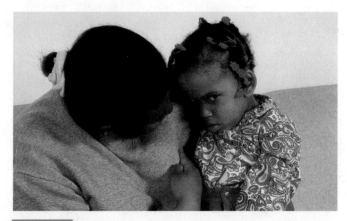

Figure 27–7 In communicating hydrocephalus, an excessive amount of cerebrospinal fluid accumulates in the subarachnoid space, producing the characteristic head enlargement seen here. Note the large forehead and facial features that seem small for the size of the head. When observing the child with hydrocephalus, look for a downward deviation of the eyes in which the lower half of the iris is hidden by the lower eyelid (sunsetting eyes). This finding occurs in severe hydrocephalus, but is not present in this child.

heart, the pleural spaces of the lungs, or the subgaleal space (space between the skull and scalp used for preterm infants with intraventricular hemorrhage) (Figure 27–8). Initial shunt placement is usually performed early in infancy with adequate tubing length for the child's future growth. Shunt revisions are often needed during childhood. Children with ventriculoatrial shunts receive perioperative IV antibiotics to reduce the risk for reinfection.

TABLE 27–12 Clinical Manifestations of Hydrocephalus

CAUSE	CLINICAL MANIFESTATIONS
CONGENITAL STRUCTURAL DEFECT Dandy-Walker syndrome Arnold-Chiari type II malformation **ACQUIRED DEFECT IN INFANCY** Intraventricular hemorrhage	***Early signs*** Rapidly increasing head circumference; tense, bulging fontanelle, split sutures *Bossing* (protrusion) of frontal area, face is disproportionate for skull size Difficulty holding head up Macewen's or "cracked-pot" sign with percussion Prominent, distended scalp veins, translucent scalp skin Increased tone or hyperreflexia, Babinski sign Irritability or lethargy, poor feeding Decline in level of consciousness ***Late signs*** Sunsetting eyes (sclera visible above iris), sixth cranial nerve palsy Apnea spells Shrill, high-pitched cry Difficulty swallowing or feeding; vomiting Cardiopulmonary depression (severe cases)
ACQUIRED HYDROCEPHALUS IN OLDER CHILD AFTER CLOSURE OF SUTURES	
Postinfectious Tumor Hemorrhage	Signs of increased ICP, no head enlargement Headache upon arising with vomiting Irritability, sleepiness, confusion, lethargy, apathy, altered consciousness Personality change, loss of interest in daily activities Poor judgment or verbal incoherence, worsening school performance, memory loss Ataxia, spasticity, or other motor problems Visual defects secondary to pressure on second, third, and sixth cranial nerves

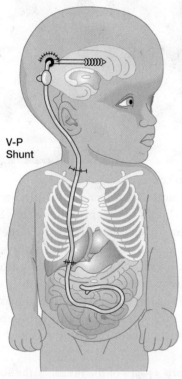

V-P Shunt

Figure 27–8 A ventriculoperitoneal shunt system consists of four parts: a ventricular catheter, a pumping chamber or reservoir, a one-way pressure valve, and a distal catheter. A shunt, commonly used to treat children with hydrocephalus, is often placed at 3 to 4 months of age.

SAFETY ALERT!
Technologic advances have led to the development of shunts with adjustable pressure valves that can be programmed with magnets. If the child receives an MRI, schedule time for the child to have the shunt pressure checked and adjusted as needed because the magnet from the MRI could affect the pressure setting.

Shunt mechanical complications may include a blocked catheter, kinked tube, or valve breakdown. Shunt materials and systems continue to be refined in an attempt to reduce mechanical problems.

Shunt infection is the most serious complication. To confirm the infection, a CSF culture is obtained from the shunt reservoir located in a burr hole placed in the skull. The shunt is surgically removed, and an external drainage device is placed. IV antibiotics are usually prescribed. A new shunt is inserted when the CSF cultures are sterile.

An upper cervical laminectomy may be performed in infants and children with the Arnold-Chiari malformation to prevent an emergency. Alternative treatment includes symptomatic care while maintaining the airway and preventing aspiration. Rapid surgical decompression may be needed to reduce brainstem compression and to prevent death.

Nursing Management

For the Child With Hydrocephalus

Nursing Assessment and Diagnosis

Nurses should assess all infants to promptly identify children with hydrocephalus. Measure the head circumference of all infants at each well-child visit and compare to prior measurements plotted on the growth curve (see the *Clinical Skills Manual* SKILLS). Note any signs of increased ICP, such as irritability, poor appetite, sunsetting eyes, or a shrill cry.

Monitor the child following placement of a ventriculoperitoneal shunt for signs of shunt failure and infection. Signs of infection in infants may include changes in responsiveness, unusual irritability, low-grade fever, diminished appetite, and sleep pattern disturbance. Measure the infant's head circumference daily and compare to prior measurements when shunt failure is suspected. Report any abnormalities to the healthcare provider immediately. Older children will have signs of increased ICP (Table 27–4).

Nursing diagnoses that might be appropriate for the child with hydrocephalus include the following (NANDA-I © 2014):

- *Infection, Risk for,* related to surgical procedure
- *Mobility: Physical, Impaired,* related to insufficient muscle strength to lift the increased weight of head
- *Caregiver Role Strain, Risk for,* related to care of a child with a chronic condition or life-threatening illness
- *Development: Delayed, Risk for,* related to repeated shunt infections and hospitalizations
- *Injury, Risk for,* related to potential shunt failure

Planning and Implementation

HOSPITAL-BASED NURSING CARE

Nursing care focuses on providing preoperative and postoperative care and providing emotional support.

Before surgery, position the infant carefully; do not stretch or strain the neck muscles since they must support the large head. Holding the infant may be difficult because of the additional weight of the head. Reduce the risk for skin breakdown with an airflow mattress or by placing sheepskin under the head. Prevent any other complications associated with immobility (see Box 27–1). Attend to the child's special nutritional needs. Because the infant is prone to vomiting, frequent small feedings and frequent burping are beneficial.

After surgery, the child is usually placed in a flat position to prevent rapid CSF drainage as the shunt begins working. The head of the bed is elevated gradually over a day or 2. Take vital signs, including the assessment of neurologic signs (such as pupil size and response to light, extraocular movements, and change in muscle tone) every 2 to 4 hours. Care for the child's surgical site as directed by healthcare provider order or agency guidelines. Monitor the child carefully for any signs of shunt malfunction, increased ICP, or infection. See Chapter 11 for other postoperative nursing care.

Support the parents and explain the child's condition and all procedures to be performed. Encourage parents and family to help with the child's care in the hospital when appropriate. Be sympathetic and understanding, and allow parents to express their concerns. If hydrocephalus occurs during early infancy, the parents will be anxious about the impact of the chronic condition and subsequent surgical procedures. If hydrocephalus is secondary to neoplasm or other acquired condition, however, the parents' anxieties are compounded by their child's life-threatening illness. Assure parents that most children with shunts lead normal lives, attending school and interacting with others no differently from their peers.

DISCHARGE PLANNING AND HOME CARE TEACHING

Identify and address home care needs well in advance of discharge. Parents must learn how to care for the surgical site until healed. Educate parents and other family members about important signs and symptoms of shunt failure (signs of increased ICP) and infection (changes in responsiveness, irritability, malaise, headache, nausea, and low-grade fever). Provide the telephone numbers of healthcare providers, and reinforce the need to contact a healthcare provider immediately if a problem with the shunt is suspected. Some children experience a seizure after shunt placement. Teach parents how to care for the child if a seizure occurs. Refer families to the appropriate home care, social services, and support groups such as the Hydrocephalus Association.

COMMUNITY-BASED NURSING CARE

Infants and children need frequent monitoring to ensure proper shunt functioning. Head circumference is measured at each visit to monitor growth. After shunt placement in an infant, head circumference may decrease 1 to 2 cm (0.39 to 0.79 in.) as the pressure is relieved. Head growth as a result of brain development may then be noted in 2 to 4 months. Alert the healthcare provider if head growth resumes sooner than 2 to 4 months, as the shunt may have malfunctioned or need a pressure setting change. Assess the child for visual problems and cognitive, speech, and motor developmental delays. Refer the child and family to an early intervention program to promote developmental progress. School-age children may need an IEP (see Chapter 12).

Encourage parents to provide good nutrition and reduce exposure to infections. Teach parents alternate positions for burping infants with an enlarged head and to use an infant seat after feeding to reduce regurgitation. Provide foods with fiber to promote regular bowel movements. Constipation increases abdominal pressure that may interfere with CSF drainage through the ventriculoperitoneal shunt.

Using a childcare setting with a small number of children, such as family or home-based child care, helps decrease exposure to infection. Encourage good hand hygiene by all caregivers.

Teach parents to protect the infant with an enlarged head from injury by using a rear-facing car safety seat regardless of age. This position decreases their risk of cervical spine injury and death in a car crash. Discourage participation in sports with a high potential for head and abdominal impact, but encourage other sports.

Evaluation

Expected outcomes of nursing care include the following:

- The infant develops adequate neck muscle control to interact with the environment.
- Shunt infections and malfunctions are rapidly identified by the parents, and medical attention is sought quickly.
- The child's potential for growth and development is maximized by care and a stimulating environment.

Neural Tube Defects

The neural tube is the tissue that ultimately develops into the CNS, including the brain and spinal cord. **Neural tube defects** occur in about 3000 pregnancies each year in the United States (Kerr & Huether, 2014). Neural tube defects include the following:

- *Anencephaly*—no development of the brain above the brainstem, which is ultimately fatal
- *Encephalocele*—protrusion of meningeal tissue or meninges-covered brain through a defect in the skull

- *Spina bifida occulta*—a vertebral defect in which the posterior vertebral arches fail to fuse (usually the fifth lumbar or first sacral vertebrae), but the spinal cord and meninges are contained in the vertebral canal
- *Spina bifida cystica*—a posterior vertebral arch defect with protrusion of meninges through the bony spine
- *Meningocele*—protrusion of a meningeal sac filled with CSF through a vertebral defect, associated with no abnormalities of the spinal cord
- *Myelodysplasia (spina bifida or meningomyelocele)*—protrusion of a meningeal sac that contains CSF, a portion of the spinal cord, and nerves through a vertebral defect

MYELODYSPLASIA OR SPINA BIFIDA

Myelodysplasia (sometimes called *meningomyelocele*) refers to a malformation of the spinal cord and spinal canal. *Spina bifida* refers to a defect in one or more vertebrae that allows spinal cord contents to protrude. The malformation can occur anywhere along the vertebral column, but is most common at the lumbar or sacral portion of the spine. Each year in the United States, approximately 1500 infants are born with spina bifida (Centers for Disease Control and Prevention [CDC], 2014b). The incidence is higher among newborns of Hispanic women and lowest among non-Hispanic Black women (CDC, 2015).

> ### Developing Cultural Competence Folate Deficiency
>
> Mandatory fortification of all enriched grain products with folate was initiated in 1998. This public health initiative has prevented an estimated 1326 cases of spina bifida and anencephaly annually, a 28% reduction. Hispanic women have a lower intake of folic acid and a higher rate of folate deficiency, potentially because of a genetic susceptibility to folate deficiency or to the greater use of corn masa flour, which is not fortified like other cereal grains (CDC, 2015).

Etiology and Pathophysiology.   The cause of spina bifida is unknown, although environmental factors have been implicated, such as chemicals (excessive use of alcohol), medications (e.g., valproic acid and carbamazepine used for seizures, isotretinoin for acne), genetic factors, and maternal health conditions (diabetes mellitus, gestational diabetes, folic acid deficiency, and maternal obesity). The increased incidence of the condition in families points to a possible genetic influence.

Healthy People 2020

(MICH-28) Reduce occurrence of neural tube defects

Clinical Manifestations.   A saclike protrusion on the infant's back indicates meningocele or myelodysplasia (Figure 27–9). The clinical manifestations (paralysis, weakness, and sensory loss) depend on the location of the defect. The higher the defect on the spinal cord, the greater the neurologic dysfunction:

- *Thoracic level*—paralysis of the legs, weakness and sensory loss in the trunk and lower body region

- *Lumbar 1–2 level*—some hip flexion and adduction, cannot extend knees
- *Lumbar 3 level*—can flex hips and extend the knees; paralyzed ankles and toes
- *Lumbar 4–5 level*—can flex hips and extend the knees; weak or absent ankle extension, toe flexion, and hip extension
- *Sacral level*—mild weakness in ankles and toes

Sensory loss is more pronounced on the back of the legs, and the loss of lower extremity motor and sensory functioning may not be symmetric.

Bowel and bladder incontinence occurs with all but the sacral level lesions, but bowel and bladder function may still be affected at the sacral level. Renal damage may result from neurologic impairment and urinary retention (neurogenic bladder). Hydrocephalus is usually present in children with a myelomeningocele defect above the sacral level, along with the Arnold-Chiari type II malformation (see hydrocephalus earlier in this chapter). The range of problems associated with spina bifida is listed in Table 27–13.

Children with myelodysplasia have mobility problems, intellectual disability, and visual impairment. Additional complications include spinal curvatures, musculoskeletal and joint abnormalities, skin sores, precocious puberty, and sexual dysfunction.

Clinical Therapy.   A high-resolution fetal ultrasound leads to the diagnosis, and an elevated maternal serum alpha-fetoprotein level is present. Fetal surgery prior to 26 weeks' gestation improved cognitive and motor function of infants at 30 months of age. It also reduces the need for a shunt for hydrocephalus; however, the surgery increases the risk for preterm birth (Scully, Mallon, Kerr, et al., 2012). Fetal surgery is becoming more common as maternal-fetal surgery centers are developed.

If fetal surgery is not performed, the lesion is examined after birth and the neurologic status is evaluated. Radiologic imaging by ultrasonography, CT scan, MRI, and flat films of the spinal column can pinpoint the bony defect and nerve

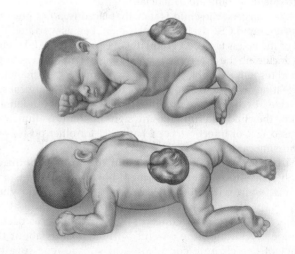

Figure 27–9 **Lumbosacral myelomeningocele is caused by a neural tube defect in which the vertebral column is incompletely closed. The meninges (and sometimes the spinal cord) protrude as a saclike structure. Observe for leakage of cerebrospinal fluid.**

TABLE 27–13 Clinical Manifestations of Myelodysplasia

CAUSE	CLINICAL MANIFESTATIONS
Interruption of the spinal cord at site of the spinal defect	Loss of motor and sensory function of the abdomen and lower extremities, dependent on defect level
	Scoliosis or kyphosis
	Incontinence of urine or urinary retention
	Incontinence of feces or constipation
	Sensory loss around genitalia
Muscle imbalance	Hip abnormalities, hip dysplasia
	Foot deformities (e.g., clubfoot)
Tethered spinal cord (the cord is abnormally attached to tissues around the spine that keeps it from moving freely within the spinal column)	Walking ability deteriorates
	Back pain, increasing scoliosis
	Leg pain, spasticity, progressive foot deformity
	Bladder and bowel function deteriorates
Brain abnormalities	Hydrocephalus, generalized seizures
	Learning problems, attention deficit disorder
	Problems with perceptual motor skills
	Memory and organization problems
	Problems with numeric reasoning

involvement. Subsequent testing is performed to evaluate bowel and bladder function, neurologic and motor function, and cognitive function.

Surgery to close and repair the lesion usually occurs within 24 to 48 hours of the infant's birth to reduce infection risk. As the child grows, braces are used to support joint position and mobility. Assistive devices such as walkers, crutches, and wheelchairs are used to enhance mobility. To minimize the risk for osteoporosis, the diet should ensure adequate calcium and vitamin D, and weight-bearing activities should be encouraged. Surgery to release a tethered spinal cord may be needed. An orthotic jacket may be prescribed to correct spinal deformities that affect lung capacity and interfere with mobility and sitting.

Interventions for a neurogenic bladder are initiated early to prevent kidney damage, to maintain bladder function, and to promote urinary continence. Clean intermittent catheterization is performed on a regular schedule (every 3 to 4 hours) (see Chapter 26). A Mitrofanoff procedure that creates a reservoir for urine and a stoma for catheterization in the umbilicus may be performed.

Dietary fiber, stool softeners, and glycerin or bisacodyl suppositories are prescribed for bowel evacuation and to promote bowel continence. Surgery to create a channel between the skin and bowel using the appendix (Malone antegrade continence enema) is often performed in children with fecal incontinence or severe constipation at the same time as the Mitranoff procedure. This procedure enables a child or adolescent to infuse an enema into the ascending and transverse colon to promote bowel evacuation to eliminate fecal soiling and incontinence.

Prognosis depends on the type of defect, the level of the lesion, and other complicating factors, such as renal dysfunction. In the United States, 90% survive to adulthood, and about 80% have normal intelligence (Spina Bifida Association, 2014).

Children need multiple surgeries and invasive procedures. A team of healthcare providers, nurses, and therapists from the neurosurgery, orthopedic, urology, and physical medicine departments works with the child and family to form a comprehensive care plan.

Nursing Management

For the Child With Myelodysplasia or Spina Bifida

Hospital-Based Nursing Care

The newborn is often transferred to a specialty center or neonatal intensive care unit until surgery is performed. Place the newborn in a prone position with hips slightly flexed and legs abducted to minimize tension on the sac. Monitor the sac for leakage of cerebrospinal fluid (CSF). Assess the extremities for deformities. Frequently assess the vital signs and stay alert for signs of infection, especially meningitis. Encourage the parents to interact with and soothe the newborn while waiting for surgery. Depending on when surgery will be performed, the newborn may be given small frequent feedings in the prone position.

Following surgery, inspect the surgical site for signs of infection and CSF leakage. Manage the infant's postoperative pain. Assess intake and output. Measure the head circumference daily to detect hydrocephalus. If a shunt was placed, provide care as described in the section on hydrocephalus.

Place the infant in a prone or side-lying position for sleep until healing has occurred, after which the supine sleep position may be used. Keep the diaper away from the incision site. Provide incision care according to agency guidelines. Assess the neonate regularly for signs of infection, motor deficits, and bladder and bowel involvement. Perform urinary catheterization on a regular schedule if needed.

Begin gentle range-of-motion (ROM) exercises as soon as possible to prevent muscle contractures and atrophy. Use caution because these children have brittle bones that fracture easily. Splints may be used to maintain extremity alignment.

Support the parents by keeping them informed about their child's status. Allow them to express their frustrations and anger. As soon as parents are able to cope with the child's condition, encourage them to become involved in the infant's care in the hospital.

The child with myelodysplasia may be hospitalized for surgery numerous times to correct deformities. Assess the child's vital signs, responsiveness, and level of pain. Because the child may have decreased pain sensation in the lower extremities, careful assessment is needed. Assess dressing sites for bleeding and drainage. Monitor the distal extremities for swelling and circulation.

SAFETY ALERT!

Children and adolescents with spina bifida are at high risk for latex allergy, thought to be related to frequent and cumulative numbers of exposure over time. See Table 22–10 for a list of products containing latex commonly found in the home.

DISCHARGE PLANNING AND HOME CARE TEACHING

Address home care needs well in advance of discharge. Help parents obtain special devices such as splints, wedges, and rolls, if needed, to prevent complications. Instruct parents how to position, handle, and feed the infant, and to perform ROM exercises. Teach parents to perform intermittent clean catheterization and establish a schedule for catheterization every 3 to 4 hours. See the *Clinical Skills Manual* SKILLS.

Teach parents the symptoms of increased ICP, hydrocephalus, shunt infection or malfunction, and urinary tract infection. Arrange for home care nursing to reinforce skills learned in the hospital as needed. Refer parents to resource groups such as the Spina Bifida Association.

COMMUNITY-BASED NURSING CARE

Because of multiple system involvement and to promote optimal development, children with myelodysplasia need comprehensive care planned and coordinated by a knowledgeable team of healthcare providers (e.g., orthopedics, neurosurgery, urology, developmental pediatrics, rehabilitation medicine, nursing, physical therapy, nutrition, and family support services). This care may be provided in partnership with the primary healthcare provider. A case manager may be helpful to coordinate the health plan coverage and the child's care with numerous healthcare providers. Parents have many financial issues related to the child's need for medical supplies and new adaptive equipment to match growth.

At an appropriate age, teach the child to perform intermittent self-catheterization. When the child begins school, an individualized health plan should be developed so the child has access to the restroom, assistance as needed for toileting, and accommodations for mobility challenges.

Clinical Tip

The child who has clean intermittent catheterization performed usually has some bacteria in the urine. Symptoms indicating a urinary tract infection that should be treated include fever, dysuria, or new-onset incontinence.

Good nutrition planning is important to prevent obesity and to reduce constipation and fecal impaction. Bowel training is initiated to control bowel evacuation. A diet high in fiber helps ensure adequate stool. The child should have a bowel movement at least every 1 to 2 days to avoid impaction. Consistency in time of day for bowel evacuation is important to promote continence. A glycerin or bisacodyl suppository can be given to promote bowel evacuation at the appropriate time.

Promote safety and independent mobility with proper use of braces, walkers, crutches, canes, and in some cases custom-designed wheelchairs and car safety seats (Figure 27–10). For other safety guidelines, see *Families Want to Know: Safety for the Child With Spina Bifida*.

Treat older children according to their intellectual level, not their motor development. Encourage them to take responsibility for self-care, and recognize their need to control their body functions. Monitor adolescents for mental health problems, especially as differences from peers and challenges in lifestyle become of greater concern. Refer for counseling as needed. See *Health Promotion: The Child With Myelodysplasia*.

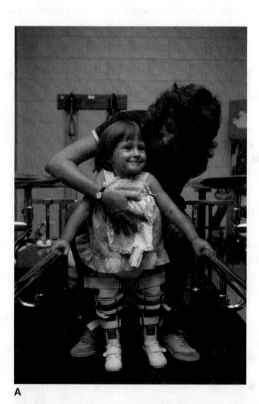
A

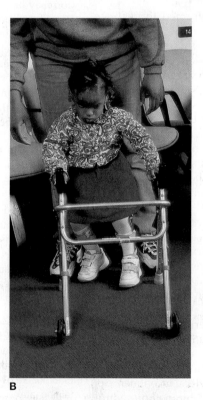
B

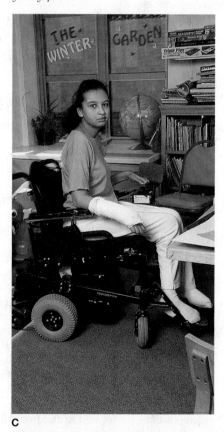
C

Figure 27–10 Help determine the best assistive device for the child to gain the most mobility independence and to promote development. The child may vary the devices used in different settings to promote optimal independence. *A* and *B*, Braces and walkers may be best for young children to promote an upright posture that encourages a normal interaction with the environment. *C*, A motorized wheelchair can assist the child with a significant neurologic impairment to achieve independence and mobility.

SOURCE: *A*, Jaren Wicklund/Fotolia.

Families Want to Know

Safety for the Child With Spina Bifida

Because of the loss of sensation in the lower extremities, injuries to the skin may not be immediately noticed by the child. Several routine actions will help reduce the risk for injury:

- Perform a daily check of all skin surfaces and pressure points associated with sitting, braces, and shoes to identify abrasions, scrapes, reddened areas, and other lesions. Stop using the braces or shoes until the skin heals or redness disappears.
- Keep all skin surfaces clean and dry. Wear socks under braces.
- Use a gel-filled cushion in the wheelchair, and teach the child to shift positions hourly to prevent pressure sores.
- Avoid burns to the lower extremities by checking the temperature of bath water and car safety seats in a hot car.
- Teach parents how to avoid the use of latex products and to inform all healthcare providers about the child's latex allergy or risk.
- Use safe ambulation techniques with walkers, canes, and crutches.

Health Promotion   **The Child With Myelodysplasia**

Preventive Health Care

- Provide all recommended immunizations. If the child has a seizure disorder, alert parents that seizures may occur following immunizations.
- Perform all recommended routine screening procedures (vision, hearing, hematocrit, blood pressure).
- Obtain a urinalysis with culture in the newborn period and when signs of infection are noted.
- Screen for scoliosis annually beginning at birth.

Growth and Development Surveillance

- Monitor the growth of the child (length or height, weight, head circumference) and plot on growth curves. Monitor head circumference growth carefully because of hydrocephalus risk.
- Assess developmental status regularly. Motor skills are often delayed.
- Enroll the infant in an early intervention program to assist the parents to promote the child's development.
- Promote gradual independence in mobility and self-care.

Nutrition

- Teach families appropriate caloric intake and portion control for the child at each age to reduce the risk for obesity.

- Provide guidance about increased fluids and fiber in the diet to reduce the risk for constipation and urinary tract infections.
- Alert parents that allergies to foods such as bananas, avocados, papaya, kiwi, and other foods may occur because of the risk of latex allergy.

Elimination

- Teach families the importance of performing intermittent catheterization on a regular schedule. Teach the child to perform self-catheterization and care for the catheter in preparation for school entry.
- Teach families to initiate bowel training so that a bowel regimen is established.

Sleep and Rest

- Position the child to prevent contractures. Change the child's position during the night to reduce pressure over skin surfaces.
- Teach parents to be alert for apnea spells or snoring that could be related to a Chiari type II malformation.

Relationships

- Encourage interaction with peers.
- Be alert for psychosocial adjustment problems, especially during the adolescent years.

Craniosynostosis

Craniosynostosis is the premature closure of cranial sutures in utero or during the first 18 months of life. This condition occurs in 1 per 1800 to 2200 live births, and boys are affected twice as often as girls (Kerr & Huether, 2014). Craniosynostosis may occur in association with chromosomal abnormality syndromes such as Apert and Crouzon syndromes, but most cases are not related to a syndrome (McCarthy et al., 2012).

When one or more sutures closes too early, bone growth continues in a direction parallel to the suture line. This leads to overgrowth at normal suture lines and classic skull deformities (Figure 27–11). Sagittal synostosis (scaphocephaly) occurs more commonly in males and is the most common form of craniosynostosis (Brown & Proctor, 2011). Bicoronal synostosis is associated with Alpert or Crouzon syndromes.

Diagnosis of craniosynostosis is made by clinical appearance and palpation of a bony ridge along a skull suture line. Detection may occur during fetal ultrasound. Skull measurements, radiographs, and CT imaging confirm the diagnosis. Surgery is performed for cosmetic reasons and when increased ICP occurs. A custom orthotic helmet may be used for several months to promote optimal skull reshaping. Follow-up care is coordinated to manage potential associated problems, such as hypoplasia of the midface, orthodontic or ophthalmologic issues, and obstructive sleep apnea.

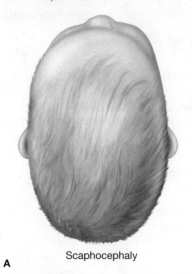

A   Scaphocephaly

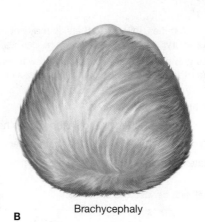

B   Brachycephaly

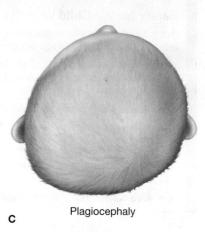

C   Plagiocephaly

Figure 27–11 In craniosynostosis, the head shape is dependent on which sutures are involved. *A,* Scaphocephaly, premature closure of the sagittal suture causes a long, narrow skull, flattened parietal bones with a prominent occiput, a broad forehead, and a small or absent anterior fontanelle. *B,* Brachycephaly, premature closure of the bicoronal suture causes a head shape shortened anterior to posterior, and the occiput is flattened. *C,* Positional plagiocephaly is often asymmetric flattening of the occiput due to preferred sleep position when supine or due to torticollis.

After surgery, nursing care involves keeping the incision dry and intact. Observe the child for symptoms of increased ICP (see Table 27–4). The nurse should monitor intake and output, manage patient positioning, protect skin integrity, and monitor for infection. Explain to parents that surgery will improve the child's appearance. Assure them that most children with craniosynostosis are healthy, and that their brains develop normally.

Positional Plagiocephaly

Positional plagiocephaly (an asymmetric flattening of the skull) is associated with sleep position to prevent sudden infant death syndrome or in infants with neck problems such as congenital torticollis. Some infants have variable tone and developmental delay that reduces development of neck muscles strength (Looman & Flannery, 2012). The sutures do not close prematurely. If the infant's sleep position does not change, the weight of the head flattens the skull (see Figure 27–11C).

If torticollis is a factor in plagiocephaly, a physical therapy referral is important. In cases of severe positional plagiocephaly, a helmet device is used to correct the condition, especially when facial asymmetry is present. The helmet is most effective when treatment is initiated at 6 months of age when the skull bones are most malleable. The helmet is worn for 23 hours a day for 2 to 4 months. Remolding of the head shape continues naturally after that treatment period because the infant spends more time awake and upright.

Clinical Tip

To help prevent positional plagiocephaly, encourage parents to try to reduce the infant's preference for lying supine in one position. Rotate the side of the crib where an interesting toy is placed each day. Alternate the infant between the top and bottom of the crib each day, so the infant must turn the head in a different direction to look at who comes into the room. Put the infant in a bouncy seat while awake. Rotate the arm used for formula feeding the infant. When the child is alert and continuously supervised, place the infant in the prone position on the floor for short periods (tummy time) to promote neck muscle strength and interaction with nearby objects.

Neonatal Abstinence Syndrome

Illicit substances that may cause neonatal abstinence syndrome (NAS) when used by the mother during pregnancy include opioids (heroin, meperidine, methadone), CNS stimulants (cocaine, propoxyphene, amphetamines), CNS depressants (barbiturates, alcohol, and marijuana), as well as antidepressants and benzodiazepines. The overuse of prescription opioids is contributing to an increase in incidence of NAS. It is estimated that 5.4% of women 15 to 44 years of age use illicit drugs during pregnancy, but the rates vary by age: women 15 to 17 years (14.6%), women 18 to 25 years (8.6%), and women 26 to 44 years (3.2%) (Substance Abuse and Mental Health Services Administration, 2014). Among pregnant women 15 to 44 years of age, 8.5% report current alcohol use, and 2.7% report binge drinking (Substance Abuse and Mental Health Services Administration, 2013). See Chapter 28 for information about fetal alcohol syndrome.

Illicit substances readily cross the placenta, enter the fetal circulation, and have the same effects on the fetus that they do on the mother. For example, cocaine decreases placental blood flow, depriving the fetus of essential oxygen and nutrients while elevating the fetal blood pressure and heart rate. The mother's repeated use of opioids and other illicit substances leads to fetal tolerance and physical dependence. Abrupt withdrawal of the illicit substance after birth leads to signs of NAS. See Chapter 15 for information about opioid withdrawal. Withdrawal symptoms for illicit substances usually appear 24 to 72 hours after birth, depending on timing of last exposure prior to birth.

Initial signs of NAS often include irritability, jitteriness, tremors, and excessive crying. Other signs include yawning, diarrhea, vomiting, seizures, inconsolable high-pitched crying, difficulty sleeping, hypertonia, and autonomic nervous system signs (e.g., temperature instability, tachycardia, hypertension, sweating, and sneezing). The skin may become excoriated from continuous movement against bed linens. Severity of signs is associated with number of substances, duration, and total accumulation of exposure. Depending on substances to which the fetus was exposed, signs of NAS may persist for 10 to 30 days after birth (Kocherlakota, 2014).

Diagnosis is based on the history of maternal substance abuse and physical signs in the newborn. Maternal and neonatal urine drug screening identifies substances to which the fetus was exposed a few days before birth. Meconium screening provides information of drug use by the mother for the last half of the pregnancy. Hair and umbilical cord testing may be performed. Neonatal EEG abnormalities may be noted.

Treatment is often supportive when signs and symptoms are mild, minimizing stimulation, swaddling, and gentle handling. Medications are used when supportive treatments do not control signs and symptoms. Medications commonly used include morphine, methadone, phenobarbital, and clonidine to alleviate symptoms of drug withdrawal. The newborn often needs an extended hospital stay. Breastfeeding is encouraged as minimal amounts of most drugs used by the mother cross over into milk. Mothers who breastfeed and misuse prescription opioids should be informed about the sedative effect of these medications. The long-term effects of this condition on cognitive function continue to be studied.

Nursing Management

Prevention and early identification of the newborn with NAS is an important nursing role. Providing information for all parents about the risks and effects of various illicit substances increases the chance that they will avoid these substances in future pregnancies.

High-pitched crying, irritability, tremors, and poor feeding should increase the nurse's suspicion of NAS. Observe the newborn carefully for increased muscle tone, sweating, seizures, vomiting, diarrhea, and tachycardia. Observe the neonate carefully for signs of severe NAS in which diarrhea and vomiting may lead to dehydration and electrolyte disturbances. Monitor the condition of the skin to identify abrasions associated with rubbing against sheets.

Provide frequent, small, high-calorie feedings on demand, which are more readily tolerated by these newborns. Monitor the neonate's weight gain or loss to determine if a change in nutritional approach is needed, such as a formula with 24 calories per ounce or nasogastric feeding (MacMullen, Dulski, & Blobaum, 2014). Support breastfeeding if this is the mother's preference. Patience is needed when feeding these newborns because their sucking and swallowing may be poorly coordinated, and regurgitation is common. Teach parents to use a calm approach and soothing voice when feeding. Newborns may initially feed better in a side-lying position while swaddled. Hold the baby with the spine flexed to decrease extensor tone.

Administer medications, if prescribed, for drug withdrawal and monitor the newborn's response. Keep in mind that many babies are managed without medications, using supportive care. Several techniques are used to calm and soothe the newborn with neonatal abstinence syndrome:

- Keep the newborn in a quiet environment, away from monitors that beep and paging speakers.
- Keep the lighting subdued and minimize stimulation to promote rest and sleep. Cluster nursing care interventions to reduce sleep disruptions.
- Comfort and pacify the newborn with swaddling and a pacifier for sucking needs. Rocking and soothing music may also be calming. Infant massage may be beneficial for some neonates.

Protect the newborn's skin with barrier shields as jitteriness may lead to greater skin surface rubbing against sheets, and apply topical ointments to scratches and abrasions. When diarrhea is present, use a barrier ointment to prevent skin breakdown. Support neonatal rooming-in practices to promote mother–newborn bonding.

Assess the strengths, safety, and competence of the mother and other potential caregivers in preparation for discharge. Determine if the mother is still using illicit drugs and identify other family supports that may help provide the care and safety needed by the newborn. Begin working with the mother and other family members to demonstrate strategies to promote parent–newborn interaction, minimize stimulation, and promote feeding until neonatal withdrawal is completed. Make plans for careful follow-up by healthcare professionals (social services, physicians, and nurses) so that the baby's safety is ensured and growth and development are monitored and promoted.

Long-term follow-up care of the child should be planned to ensure regular developmental testing and assessment for neurobehavioral problems.

Neurofibromatosis

Neurofibromatosis 1 (NF1), or von Recklinghausen disease, is an autosomal dominant genetic disorder in which tumors grow along nerves. One in 3500 individuals develops the disorder, and 50% of new cases result from a mutation (Julian, Edwards, DeCrane, et al., 2014).

The *NF1* gene is located on chromosome 17. Individuals with NF1 do not have adequate neurofibromin to control cell growth, and neurofibromas form from nerve sheath cells along peripheral nerves or at nerve endings. The neurofibroma may be an isolated growth, or extend along the length of a nerve and include nerve branches (plexiform neurofibroma). Dermal neurofibromas, which usually begin to appear around the time of puberty, may reside in the skin or project above the skin surface. Up to 5% of tumors become malignant in the brain or along nerves, and children may be at risk for leukemia, rhabdomyosarcoma, and pheochromocytoma (Julian et al., 2014). A higher prevalence of autism spectrum disorder may also occur in children with NF1 (Garg et al., 2013).

The disorder is characterized by six or more café au lait spots (darker than surrounding skin) 5 mm (0.20 in.) in diameter or larger seen at birth or by 2 years of age. The spots grow to 15 mm (0.6 in.) or larger by adulthood. Freckling in the axillary and inguinal areas is common. Multiple neurofibromas or benign tumors grow on or under the skin beginning during puberty. Pain may occur when a tumor compresses a nerve or grows in the spinal cord. Lisch nodules, tan or brown benign tumors on the iris of the eye, are characteristic. Vision deficits or blindness is found in some children because of a tumor along the optic pathway. Precocious puberty or delayed puberty and menarche may occur when the optic tumor invades the hypothalamus. The child often has a larger than expected head circumference. Other manifestations include thinning or bowing of the tibia, fractures that do not heal properly, and scoliosis. See Figure 27–12.

Diagnosis is made in early childhood by the presence of two or more characteristic physical findings listed in the previous paragraph and a positive family history. Radiologic imaging (MRI of brain and radiographs of the spine and other bones) is performed when problems are detected. Ophthalmologic examinations are performed at least annually. Clinical therapy focuses on monitoring the child for signs of problems associated with the condition. The severity of the condition ranges from mild to severe with disabilities. Surgery may be performed to remove the tumor when neurofibromas become malignant, are painful or disfiguring, cause paralysis, or when life-threatening problems develop.

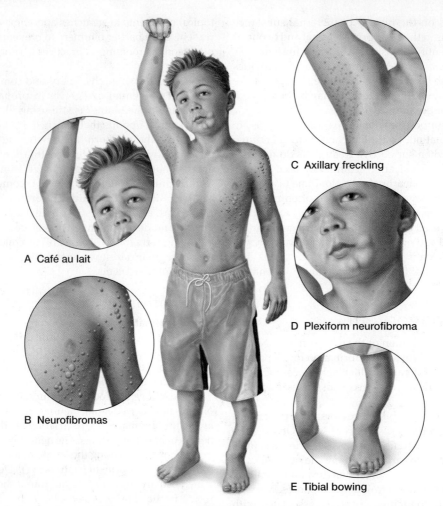

A Café au lait

B Neurofibromas

C Axillary freckling

D Plexiform neurofibroma

E Tibial bowing

Figure 27–12 **Physical signs of neurofibromatosis become more apparent during adolescence. Café au lait spots enlarge, axillary freckling appears, and multiple neurofibromas develop. Some children develop plexiform neurofibromas.**

Nursing Management

Nurses assess the child for signs of neurofibromatosis. Assess the child's growth, pubertal development, vital signs, and vision on a regular basis to detect any problems associated with the disorder. School performance should be monitored as learning disabilities and hyperactivity may occur. Pay attention to any mass that is rapidly enlarging or causing new pain.

Provide psychologic support to the child and family. As tumor development increases during adolescence, problems with self-image and self-esteem are common. Adolescents may fear the response of peers to the tumors and isolate themselves. Identify potential peers or refer the adolescent to a support group.

Cerebral Palsy

Cerebral palsy (CP), a common syndrome of movement and posture development disorders, is caused by a nonprogressive lesion abnormality in the fetal or infant brain that results in activity limitations. The condition may also have associated hearing, vision, communication, perceptual, cognitive, and behavioral problems. An estimated prevalence of CP is 3.9 children per 1000 (Burkhard, 2013). Four types of motor dysfunction seen—spastic, dyskinetic, ataxic, and mixed—are related to the location

of brain insult. Dystonia and athetosis are sometimes categorized together as dyskinesia.

Etiology and Pathophysiology

The majority of cases occur during the prenatal and perinatal periods. Risk factors include low birth weight, placental abnormalities, birth defects, meconium aspiration, birth asphyxia, neonatal seizures, respiratory distress syndrome, hypoglycaemia, and neonatal infections. Postnatal cases are related to meningitis, encephalitis, and traumatic brain injury (Colver, Fairhurst, & Pharoah, 2014).

Healthy People 2020

(MICH-27) Reduce the proportion of children with cerebral palsy born as low-birth-weight infants (less than 2500 grams)

Muscle growth is usually coordinated with bone growth, but muscle spasticity interferes. Contractures can develop that limit joint movement or cause deformities such as scoliosis. Because of more limited weight-bearing activity and potential nutritional problems with swallowing and independent feeding, children with CP are at greater risk for osteoporosis and fractures (Aronson & Stevenson, 2012).

Clinical Manifestations

Cerebral palsy is characterized by abnormal muscle tone and lack of coordination. Children have a variety of symptoms depending on their ages, and the pattern or extremities involved may vary:

- *Diplegia*—both legs are affected
- *Hemiplegia*—one side of the body is involved, the arm is usually more severely affected than the leg
- *Quadriplegia*—all four extremities are affected

All children with CP have motor impairment, with spasticity present more commonly than ataxia or athetosis and dystonia. Even if both sides of the body are affected, the impairment is usually more severe on one side. Spasticity is also associated with muscle weakness that interferes with gross motor activities.

See Table 27–14 for clinical manifestations of CP by type of brain injury. Symptoms are variable for this lifelong disability and depend on the area of the brain involved and the extent of brain injury. Behavioral and emotional problems may result from disruption of nerve pathways that reduce the adaptation of the brain.

Children with CP usually have delayed developmental milestones. The functional consequences of motor deficits become more obvious as the child grows even though the brain injury is nonprogressive. Other complications include intellectual disabilities, vision impairments, hearing loss, speech and language impairments, and seizures. Feeding may be difficult because of oral motor involvement, including hypotonia, with poor sucking and swallowing coordination that may result in aspiration or poor nutrition.

Clinical Therapy

Diagnosis is usually based on clinical findings of delayed development and increased or decreased muscle tone. CP is difficult to diagnose in the early months of life because it must be distinguished from other neurologic conditions and signs may be subtle. Suspicious historical findings include risk factors described in the *Etiology and Pathophysiology* section.

Ultrasonography can be used to detect fetal and neonatal abnormalities of the brain, such as intraventricular hemorrhage. Neuromotor tests are used to evaluate the presence of normal movement patterns, absence of common newborn reflexes, and abnormal tone. Once CP is suspected, CT and MRI imaging provide information about anatomic structures and help identify the cause of CP. Genetic and metabolic tests are performed if congenital anomalies are present. Hearing and vision should be evaluated. Standardized tools, such as the Functional Mobility Scale and Manual Ability Classification System, are used to describe the child's capabilities.

Clinical therapy focuses on helping the child develop to a maximum level of independence and to perform activities of daily living. This involves promoting mobility, an optimal range of motion, muscle control, balance, and communication with braces and splints, serial casting, and positioning devices (prone wedges, standers, and side-lyers). Referrals are made for physical, occupational, and speech therapy, as well as special education to improve motor function and ability.

Orthopedic surgery may be required to improve function by balancing muscle power and stabilizing uncontrollable joints. Surgical interventions may include Achilles tendon lengthening to increase the ankle range of motion, hamstring release to correct knee flexion contractures, procedures to improve hip adduction

TABLE 27–14 Clinical Manifestations of Cerebral Palsy by Type of Insult

CLASSIFICATION AND TYPE OF INSULT	CLINICAL MANIFESTATIONS
SPASTIC	
Cerebral cortex or pyramidal tract injury 75% of cases	Increased muscle tone through a joint's range of motion
	Leads to contractures and abnormal curvature of the spine
	Exaggerated deep tendon reflexes, clonus
	Persistent common newborn reflexes, positive Babinski sign
DYSKINETIC—ATHETOSIS	
Extrapyramidal, basal ganglia injury 10%–15% of cases	Muscle tone abnormalities affecting the entire body
	Difficulty with fine and purposeful movements or coordinating the timing of movement; tremors
	Slow involuntary writhing motions that interfere with ability to maintain a stable posture
DYSKINETIC—DYSTONIA	
Basal ganglia, extrapyramidal injury	Involuntary sustained muscle contractions that lead to sustained or intermittent exaggerated and distorted posturing, twisting, or repetitive movements
	Rigid muscles when awake; normal or decreased muscle tone when asleep
ATAXIC	
Cerebellar (extrapyramidal) injury 5%–10% of cases	Abnormalities of voluntary movement (muscle instability) involving balance and position of the trunk and limbs, difficulty maintaining posture, wide-based unsteady gait
	Difficulty controlling hand and arm movements during reaching
	Increased or decreased muscle tone, hypotonia in first couple of years
MIXED	
Multiple areas of brain are injured	No dominant motor pattern; may have mild spasticity, dystonia, and/or athetoid movement

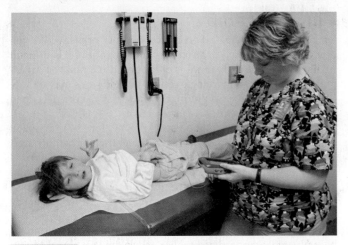

Figure 27–13 **Baclofen may be administered by an intrathecal pump. This child is having the reservoir of the baclofen pump filled.**

or correct spinal deformities, or dorsal rhizotomy (cutting the afferent fibers that contribute to spasticity).

Medications are given to control seizures, to control spasms (skeletal muscle relaxants, baclofen, and benzodiazepines), and to minimize gastrointestinal side effects (cimetidine or ranitidine). Benzodiazepines affect brain control of muscle tone to help control spasticity. Dantrolene is a calcium channel blocker that is a muscle relaxant. Baclofen is administered orally or by intrathecal pump to decrease spasticity. See Figure 27–13. Botulinum toxin injection into specific muscles is a therapy that helps to temporarily control spasticity.

The prognosis for infants and children with CP depends on the level of motor disability and on the presence of intellectual, visual, or hearing deficits. Early intervention programs can help improve performance. Many children with hemiplegia or ataxia show some improvement with maturation and are able to ambulate. Others need assistance with mobility and activities of daily living. Many of these children have difficulty with swallowing and aspiration, making feeding a challenge for families. A gastrostomy tube may ultimately be needed to ensure that the child has adequate nutrition and to prevent aspiration.

Nursing Management

For the Child With Cerebral Palsy

Nursing Assessment and Diagnosis

Be alert for children whose histories indicate an increased risk for CP. Assess all children at each healthcare visit for developmental delays. Note any orthopedic, visual, auditory, or intellectual deficits. When the common newborn reflexes persist beyond the normal age, refer for further evaluation (see Chapter 5). Identify infants who appear to have an abnormal muscle tone or abnormal posture (head lag beyond 6 months of age, arched back, poor trunk control and balance, toe walking or scissoring). Asymmetric or abnormal crawling by using two or three extremities and hand dominance prior to 18 months of age indicates a motor problem. Perform a simple screening test by placing a clean cloth on the infant's face. Infants normally use two hands to remove it. Be concerned if the infant over 6 months of age uses one hand or does not remove the cloth at all. Record dietary intake as well as height and weight percentiles for children suspected to have or diagnosed with the condition.

The child has many potential sources of pain. Pain could be associated with constipation, muscle spasms, physical therapy, bladder spasms, decubitus ulcers, headaches, and dental caries. Anticipate and take a careful history to identify potential causes of pain and pain patterns.

Nursing diagnoses for the child with CP often vary by the type of CP, the child's symptoms and age, and the family situation. *Nursing Care Plan: The Child With Cerebral Palsy* includes several nursing diagnoses. Additional nursing diagnoses might include the following (NANDA-I © 2014):

- *Constipation, Risk for,* related to low intake of fiber and fluids and insufficient physical activity
- *Tissue Integrity, Impaired,* related to decreased physical mobility and limited self-care ability
- *Communication: Verbal, Impaired,* related to hearing and/or motor speech impairment
- *Pain, Chronic,* related to spasticity and stretching exercises to prevent contractures
- *Development: Delayed, Risk for,* related to lack of muscle strength or limited social interaction

Planning and Implementation

The accompanying *Nursing Care Plan* summarizes care for the child with CP. Since the condition varies in severity and manifestations, interventions need to be customized to the child and family. Nursing care focuses on providing adequate nutrition, maintaining skin integrity, promoting physical mobility, promoting safety, promoting growth and development, teaching parents how to care for the child, and providing emotional support.

PROVIDE ADEQUATE NUTRITION

Children with CP require high-calorie diets because of feeding difficulties associated with spasticity or hypotonia. Many children have difficulty chewing and swallowing, and therefore are at risk for aspiration. Give the child small amounts of soft foods at a time. Utensils with large, padded handles may be easier for the child to hold. Make sure the child gets adequate fluids as the child may not be able to communicate thirst. Children with severe CP may need a gastrostomy tube to obtain adequate nutrition and fluids. Adequate fiber is needed to prevent constipation, and some children need a bowel management program to treat chronic constipation.

MAINTAIN SKIN INTEGRITY

Protect bony prominences from skin breakdown. Monitor splints and braces for proper fit and the skin under them for redness. If the skin is red or broken, the braces or splints should be removed and not worn until the skin is healed.

PROMOTE PHYSICAL MOBILITY

Proper body alignment should be maintained at all times. Support the child with pillows, towels, and bolsters whether the child is in bed or in a chair. Use splints and braces to help support joints in extension or a functional position and to reduce the risk for contractures. Support the head and body of a floppy infant. A spastic child with scissored, extended legs or a child with athetosis who writhes constantly is difficult to carry and transport.

Range-of-motion exercises are essential to maintain joint flexibility and to prevent contractures. Consult with the physical therapists who work with the child and assist with recommended exercises. Massage may be helpful when performing stretching exercises. Horseback riding is a therapeutic activity as adjustment to the horse's gait helps improve balance and posture control.

Nursing Care Plan: The Child With Cerebral Palsy

1. Nursing Diagnosis: *Mobility: Physical, Impaired,* related to decreased muscle strength and control (NANDA-I © 2014)

GOAL: The child will attain the maximum physical abilities possible.

INTERVENTION	RATIONALE
• Perform development assessment and record age at which milestones are achieved (e.g., reaching for objects, sitting).	• Delayed development milestones are common with CP. As one milestone is achieved, interventions are revised to focus on the next skill.
• Plan activities to use gross and fine motor skills (e.g., holding eating utensils, toys positioned to encourage reaching). Allow time for the child to complete activities.	• Many activities of daily living and play activities promote physical development. The child may perform tasks more slowly than most children.
• Perform range-of-motion exercises every 4 hours for the child unable to move body parts. Position the child to promote tendon stretching (e.g., foot plantar flexion, legs extended at the knees and hips).	• Exercises and positioning promote mobility and increased circulation, and decrease the risk of contractures.
• Arrange for and encourage parents to keep appointments with a rehabilitation therapist.	• A regular and frequently reevaluated rehabilitation program assists in promoting development.
• Teach the family to use braces and other positioning devices.	• Adaptive devices are often necessary to maximize physical mobility.

EXPECTED OUTCOME: Child will reach maximum physical mobility and achieve developmental milestones.

2. Nursing Diagnosis: *Nutrition, Imbalanced: Less than Body Requirements,* related to difficulty chewing and swallowing and high metabolic needs (NANDA-I © 2014)

GOAL: The child will receive nutrients needed for normal growth.

INTERVENTION	RATIONALE
• Monitor height and weight and plot on a growth grid. Perform hydration status assessment.	• Insufficient intake can lead to impaired growth and dehydration.
• Teach the family techniques to promote caloric and nutrient intake:	• Special techniques can facilitate food intake. Adaptive handles may help the child better manage feeding self.
• Position the child upright for feedings.	
• Place foods far back in the mouth to overcome tongue thrust.	
• Use soft and blended foods. Allow extra time for chewing and swallowing.	
• Obtain adaptive handles for utensils and encourage self-feeding skills.	
• Perform frequent respiratory assessment. Teach the family the preceding techniques to prevent aspiration. Teach care of the gastrostomy and tube-feeding technique as appropriate.	• Aspiration pneumonia is a risk for the child with poor swallowing coordination. Special feeding techniques or tube feeding may be needed.

EXPECTED OUTCOME: Child will show normal growth patterns for height, weight, and other physical parameters.

3. Nursing Diagnosis: *Health Management, Family, Ineffective,* related to excessive demands made on the family for the child's complex care needs (NANDA-I © 2014)

GOAL: The family will adapt to the growth and development needs of the child with CP.

INTERVENTION	RATIONALE
• Allow chances for parents to verbalize the impact of CP on the family. Provide referral to other parents and support groups.	• The family needs to explore the emotional and social impact of the child's care so they can integrate and grow from the experience.

(continued)

Nursing Care Plan: The Child With Cerebral Palsy (*continued*)

GOAL: The family will adapt to the growth and development needs of the child with CP. (*continued*)

INTERVENTION	RATIONALE
• Explore community services for rehabilitation, respite care, child care, early intervention program, and refer family as appropriate.	• Diverse services are available and will be needed because of the multiple impacts of CP on the child.
• During home and office visits, review the child's achievements and praise the family for care provided.	• The child's achievements are positive reinforcement of the family's efforts.
• Teach the family skills needed to manage the child's care (e.g., medication administration, muscle stretching, seizure management).	• Complex skills must be learned before they can be performed efficiently.
• Teach case management techniques.	• The child requires care by many specialists, and many parents become case managers to coordinate care.
• Involve siblings in the care of the child with CP. Review with parents the needs of all children in the family.	• Siblings of the child with CP may feel left out because of the care provided. Special efforts help to meet the developmental needs of all family members.

EXPECTED OUTCOME: Child will demonstrate appropriate growth and developmental progress. Family will successfully support all of its members.

4. Nursing Diagnosis: *Activity, Deficient Diversional (Child)*, related to poor social skills (NANDA-I © 2014)

GOAL: The child will engage in activities that maximize growth and development.

INTERVENTION	RATIONALE
• Refer the family to an early intervention program. Encourage contact with other children.	• The child needs a variety of activities and contact with other children and adults to maximize development.
• Work with the school to develop an individualized education plan that encourages interaction with peers and a variety of activities that support development.	• The education system is obligated to work with families to provide methods to enhance learning, including social interactions.
• Investigate recreational programs for children with disabilities and share information with the parents.	• Recreational programs for children with disabilities may promote social experiences and physical activity.

EXPECTED OUTCOME: Child will engage in activities to maximize development.

Refer parents to the appropriate resources for help getting adaptive devices (Figure 27–14). To enhance interaction with the environment, teach the parents to position the child to foster flexion rather than extension (e.g., the child can bring objects closer to the face). Encourage parents to bring in the child's *adaptive appliances* (braces, positioning devices) for use during a hospitalization; however, secure them as the family may have difficulty replacing them if lost.

PROMOTE SAFETY

Safety belts should be used for children in strollers and wheelchairs (see the *Clinical Skills Manual* SKILLS). Determine if an adaptive car safety seat is needed so the child can be safely transported. A child with chronic seizures should wear a helmet to protect against further injury.

PROMOTE GROWTH AND DEVELOPMENT

Remember that many children with CP are physically but not intellectually disabled. Use terminology appropriate for the child's developmental level. Help the child develop a positive self-image to ensure emotional health and social growth. Children with a hearing impairment may need referral to learn American Sign Language or other communication methods. Provide audio and visual activities for the child who is quadriplegic.

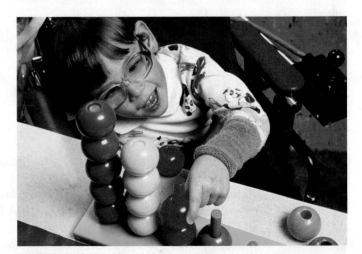

Figure 27–14 This child has cerebral palsy and wears glasses because of vision impairment. She uses a wheelchair for transport to the health center. Notice the planned placement and level of toys to promote her interaction.

SOURCE: Will & Deni McIntyre/Science Source.

Adaptive and assistive technology may be needed to promote mobility and communication. **Assistive technology** is any item, equipment, or product customized for use to promote the functional capabilities and independence of an individual with disabilities. Examples include computers, communication devices, adaptive utensils, and customized wheelchairs.

FOSTER PARENTAL KNOWLEDGE

Teach parents about the disorder and arrange sessions to teach them about all of the child's special needs. Teach administration, desired effects, and side effects of medications prescribed for seizures. Make sure parents are aware of the need for dental care for children because of the enamel defects and malocclusion that commonly occur in children with CP, and the gingival hyperplasia that occurs when taking some antiepileptic medications.

PROVIDE EMOTIONAL SUPPORT

Listen to the parents' concerns and encourage them to express their feelings and ask questions. Explain what they can expect from future treatment. Work with other healthcare providers to help families adjust to this chronic disease. Refer parents to individual and family counseling if appropriate.

COMMUNITY-BASED NURSING CARE

Children with CP need continuous support in the community. A case manager such as the parent or nurse is often needed to coordinate care. Parents may need financial assistance to provide the care that the child needs and to obtain appliances such as braces, wheelchairs, or adaptive utensils. Children need new adaptive devices, ongoing developmental assessment and care planning, and possibly surgery as they grow. Although the brain lesion does not change, it manifests differently as the child grows. For example, once the child begins to walk, the extensor tone may cause Achilles cord tightening. Braces may decrease deformities, but surgery may eventually be needed. Technology offers many new strategies to promote communication and self-care by these children.

Monitor the child's growth. If the child is unable to ambulate, use a scale that accommodates a wheelchair when weighing. Standing height measurements may be inaccurate. Other possible measures for stature include recumbent length, arm span, tibia length, and knee height. Schedule regular vision and hearing screening during health promotion visits. Give immunizations according to the recommended schedule, even though the pertussis, measles, mumps, and rubella vaccines may increase the risk of seizures in children with a seizure disorder. Educate parents about the possible risk for a seizure associated with the vaccines.

Early intervention programs can help parents learn to meet their child's special needs and obtain physical, occupational, and speech therapy. The child often needs an IEP to maximize learning potential (see Chapter 12). The nurse can help parents meet the needs of the child with CP in preschool, school, and healthcare settings. The nurse also makes referrals as appropriate to support groups and organizations such as the United Cerebral Palsy Association and Shriners Hospitals. Recreational activities may be identified through the National Association of Sports for Cerebral Palsy.

An individualized transition plan should be developed during adolescence to assist the family and adolescent with CP with plans for adult living. Vocational training options can be explored. Both the special mobility needs and educational support needed by the child must be addressed. See Chapter 12.

Evaluation

Expected outcomes of nursing care for the child with CP are provided in the *Nursing Care Plan*.

Injuries of the Neurologic System

Injuries to the brain and spinal cord are major causes of disability in previously healthy children. Drowning is another cause of brain injury in children.

Traumatic Brain Injury

A traumatic brain injury (TBI) is a blunt force or penetrating injury to the head that disrupts normal brain functioning, such as a loss of consciousness. More than 2600 children, ages 0 to 14 years, are estimated to die each year as a result of TBI (Brain Injury Association of America, 2014). Adolescents, 15 to 19 years, have the highest rate of death, followed by children less than age 5 years. The highest rate of hospitalization occurs in adolescents 15 to 19 years old, followed by children less than 5 years old (CDC, 2014a). TBI is a leading cause of death and disability in children and adolescents (Geyer, Meller, Kulpan, et al., 2013).

Growth and Development

Leading TBI mechanisms of injury resulting in emergency department visits or hospitalization vary by age (Quayle, Holmes, & Kuppermann, 2014):

- *Children 0 to 2 years old*—falls, usually from elevation or down stairs
- *Children 2 to 12 years old*—falls from elevation or associated with standing, running, or walking at ground level, or struck by or against an object
- *Adolescents 13 to 17 years old*—assault, sports, and motor vehicle related

---

ETIOLOGY AND PATHOPHYSIOLOGY

With a blunt injury the impact transfers energy through the skull and meninges to the brain. Primary injury occurs at the time of the impact when the initial cellular damage takes place, such as skull fracture, bruising, or hemorrhage. See *Pathophysiology Illustrated: Brain Injury* for an explanation of the primary injury. With a penetrating injury, additional brain damage occurs along the track of penetration. The secondary injury for both blunt and penetrating TBI is a biochemical and cellular response to the primary injury. Brain swelling begins immediately, leading to cerebral edema, inflammation, ischemia, and increased ICP. Decreased cerebral perfusion pressure limits the circulation, oxygen and nutrient delivery, and removal of toxins resulting from cell death. Brain cells are further damaged by the release of amino acids and an inflammatory response that increase the permeability of the blood–brain barrier.

CLINICAL MANIFESTATIONS

Traumatic brain injury signs and symptoms in children depend on the pathologic features and severity of the injury. The child with a mild TBI (concussion) may remain conscious or have brief loss of consciousness (seconds to a few minutes). The child with a moderate TBI loses consciousness for 5 to 10 minutes. Following mild or moderate TBI, children may have amnesia about the event, headache, nausea, and vomiting. See Table 27–15 for clinical manifestations of TBI by severity.

Unconsciousness may result from increased ICP, cerebral edema, intracranial hemorrhage, or extensive damage to the cerebral cortex or brainstem. Posttraumatic seizures are common. The presence of retinal hemorrhages, frenulum injuries,

Pathophysiology Illustrated: **Brain Injury**

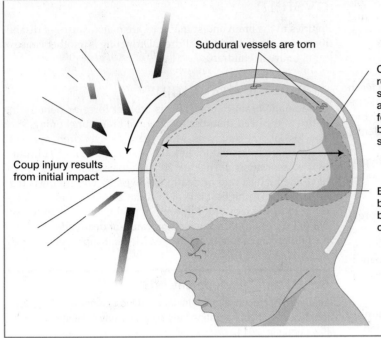

Subdural vessels are torn

Contrecoup injury results from secondary impact as brain moves forward and then backward within skull

Coup injury results from initial impact

Bruising occurs as brain moves over bony prominences on the skull floor

Brain injury can result from a direct blow to the head (coup injury) or the acceleration–deceleration movement of the brain (contrecoup injury) such as occurs from a motor vehicle crash. Movement of the brain in the skull tears nerves, fibers, and blood vessels, causing altered level of consciousness (LOC). Scalp injuries, skull fractures, contusions, and hematomas of brain tissue may also occur if the head experiences a direct blow.

and fractures in an infant should raise the suspicion of child abuse (Fingarson & Pierce, 2012).

SAFETY ALERT!

Any infant who arrives in the emergency department with seizures, failure to thrive, respiratory irregularities, or coma should be evaluated for child abuse (shaken child syndrome). An infant has a large head and relatively weak neck muscles. Shaking an infant causes inertial injuries (acceleration and deceleration) that tear nerve fibers as the brain moves back and forth in the skull. Throwing the infant down onto a mattress further increases the forces with which the brain hits the back of the skull (Dubowitz & Lane, 2016).

Changes in respiratory effort or periods of apnea can occur secondary to shock, injury to the spinal cord above C4, or damage to or pressure on the medulla. Heart rate and blood pressure provide information about brainstem function. Tachycardia can be a sign of blood loss, shock, hypoxia, anxiety, or pain. The Cushing triad (increased systolic blood pressure with a wide pulse pressure, bradycardia, and irregular respirations) is associated with significantly increased ICP, impending herniation, or compromised blood flow to the brainstem. Reflexes may be hyporesponsive, hyperresponsive, or nonexistent. The child may assume a flexor, extensor, areflexic, or flaccid posture (see Figure 27–2). Refer to Table 27–4 for signs of increased ICP. See Table 27–16 for clinical manifestations of specific brain injuries.

TABLE 27–15 Clinical Manifestations of Traumatic Brain Injury by Severity

TYPE OF BRAIN INJURY	CLINICAL MANIFESTATIONS
Concussion or mild brain injury	Low-grade headache that will not go away
	Slowness in thinking, acting, speaking, reading
	Memory problems
	Loss of balance, unsteady walking
	Poor concentration, change in performance at school, lack of motivation or interest in favorite toys
	Feeling tired all the time, change in sleeping pattern
	Change in eating patterns
	Increased sensitivity to lights, sounds, distractions; easily irritated
Moderate brain injury	Glasgow Coma Scale score of 9–12
	Posttraumatic amnesia for 1–24 hr
	Loss of consciousness
Severe brain injury	Glasgow Coma Scale score of 8 or less
	Posttraumatic amnesia lasting longer than 24 hr
	Coma or unconsciousness
	Increased intracranial pressure
	Posttraumatic seizures

TABLE 27–16 Clinical Manifestations of Intracranial Hematomas

TYPE OF HEMATOMA	CLINICAL MANIFESTATIONS
SUBDURAL HEMATOMA Results from severe brain trauma, including shaken child syndrome. Is more common in infants less than age 1 year. Inertial forces tear veins bridging the subdural space; a venous hematoma forms beneath the dura and presses directly on the brain.	Symptoms that may occur 48–72 hr after the injury: • Gradual change in LOC (confusion, agitation, or lethargy) • Hemiparesis or eye deviation • Nausea or vomiting • Headache • Retinal hemorrhages in both eyes • Pupil on side of injury may be fixed and dilated • Seizures
EPIDURAL HEMATOMA Is rare in children, especially those less than 4 years of age. Results from blunt trauma such as falls, assaults, or baseball to temporal area. Arterial or venous bleeding occurs between the skull and the dura; associated with skull fracture.	• Minimal or absent symptoms at time of injury, followed by rapid deterioration in mental status and signs of increased ICP • Headache or full fontanelle • Paresis of cranial nerves III and VI • Papilledema • Fixed and dilated pupil
CEREBRAL CONTUSION Bruising on surface of brain is associated with coup and contre-coup injuries, including the base of the brain as it moves across the bony prominences in the base of the skull. Commonly occurs on frontal and temporal lobes. Is the most common TBI.	• Altered levels of consciousness ranging from confusion and disorientation to being obtunded • Focal symptoms depending on the area of injury
DIFFUSE AXONAL INJURY Results from rapid acceleration-deceleration injuries, such as with motor vehicle crash or shaken child syndrome. Nerve fibers are torn in both cerebral hemispheres and other brain areas. Other organ systems may also be injured.	• Immediate loss of consciousness • Unconsciousness lasting longer than 6 hr • Abnormal movements or posturing • Seizures • Increased ICP • Difficulty regulating blood pressure and breathing
SUBARACHNOID HEMORRHAGE Associated with severe head injuries such as intracranial hematomas or contusions; results from tearing of arteries or veins in the subarachnoid space.	• Progressive decrease in LOC • Severe headache, nausea, and vomiting • Ipsilateral pupil dilation • Diplopia • Hemiparesis • Nuchal rigidity
INTRACEREBRAL HEMATOMA Often results from acceleration-deceleration injury or penetrating injury; hemorrhage to frontal or temporal lobe.	• Focal symptoms depend on size and location of hematoma, such as epilepsy

CLINICAL THERAPY

The severity of a brain injury is diagnosed from the history, physical examination, Glasgow Coma Scale (see Table 27–5), and diagnostic tests. Information about the events associated with and mechanism of injury, the child's initial and current responses, any loss of consciousness, and the child's memory of the event are obtained. The cranial nerves, pupillary response, palpation of the skull for depressions, deep tendon reflexes, and muscle strength are all evaluated.

Laboratory tests include a complete blood cell count, blood chemistry, coagulation tests, toxicology screening, and urinalysis. Radiographs detect fractures of the skull and cervical vertebrae. A CT scan detects fractures, intracranial bleeding, swelling, and diffuse axonal injury. An MRI scan is used during recovery to determine the extent of brain damage. PET scans measure the blood flow in the brain. A fracture indicates a more serious injury. Many children with brain injuries have multiple other injuries. Children with a moderate to severe TBI should be evaluated for a potential cervical spine injury.

The initial management of a child with a severe brain injury is based on the child's physiologic status (see *Concussion* section later in this chapter for management of a mild TBI). The airway must be clear and stable, and hypoxia must be prevented. The child is continuously monitored for hypercapnia, which causes vasodilation and increased ICP. The child may be intubated and mechanically ventilated with 100% oxygen at a slightly increased respiratory rate in the first 24 hours after injury to maintain oxygenation levels and reduce ischemia (see the *Clinical Skills Manual* SKILLS).

Clinical Tip

In the child with moderate head injury, the oxygen saturation should remain over 95%. For the severely injured child who is intubated, monitor arterial blood gas results. A PaO_2 greater than 60 mmHg and a $PaCO_2$ between 35 to 38 mmHg are recommended (Geyer et al., 2013).

An intraventricular catheter (ventriculostomy) may be inserted and attached to a monitor to measure intracranial pressure. Efforts are made to maintain the cerebral perfusion pressure (difference between the mean arterial pressure minus the ICP or central venous pressure) so that the brain circulation is adequate to deliver oxygen and nutrients and to remove neurotoxins. Hypotension is avoided. Hypovolemic shock is treated if present and inotropic medications may be used to maintain the blood pressure. Keep the head of the bed flat until adequate cerebral perfusion pressure is ensured and maintained.

Increased Intracranial Pressure.   Treatment is required when the ICP value is greater than 20 mmHg; it becomes life threatening at 40 mmHg (Geyer et al., 2013). If increased ICP is not relieved, brain shifting begins in the cranium, a precursor of herniation. Invasive procedures may be used to reduce ICP. Burr holes or more extensive surgery may be performed to evacuate a lesion or hematoma. An external ventricular drainage system may be placed to monitor ICP, to drain CSF when brain swelling reaches dangerous heights, and to help maintain CPP (see the *Clinical Skills Manual* SKILLS). Decompressive craniectomy may be considered as a last resort when ICP cannot be otherwise controlled.

Mannitol or IV hypertonic saline (3%) may be administered to decrease the ICP by shifting water out of the brain tissues. When prescribed, serum osmolality and electrolytes should be monitored. Sedation, analgesia, and paralytic agents may be administered to eliminate the child's resistance to mechanical ventilation, relieve pain, and lower the ICP. Medications to prevent seizures may be prescribed. Therapeutic hypothermia may be used. Sometimes despite all efforts, the child dies as a result of the consequences of the TBI.

If there is no cervical spine injury, the head of the bed is elevated up to 30 degrees. The child's head is kept in the midline to promote venous (jugular) drainage. Hip flexion is avoided. Normothermia is maintained. The environment is kept as quiet as possible. A urinary catheter is inserted to monitor output. Enteral nutrition support is started, using a postpyloric feeding tube to reduce the risk for aspiration.

Rehabilitation.   Initial stages of rehabilitation are made during the acute phase of management to prevent complications from immobilization, disuse, and neurologic dysfunction. Physical therapists, occupational therapists, speech-language specialists, and social workers all play vital roles. Moderate and severe TBI may result in a permanent disability, such as epilepsy, motor and cognitive impairments, learning problems, hearing and vision impairment, communication problems, and behavioral or emotional problems. Difficulties with learning skills are common. Reliable predictions of outcome in the child who has experienced a severe brain injury cannot be made until 6 to 12 months postinjury. One study reported that 61.6% of children

with moderate and severe injuries were reported to receive services such as special education, 504 accommodations (see Chapter 12), tutoring, and occupational, physical, and speech therapy for disabilities 12 months after injury (Rivara et al., 2012).

Nursing Management

For the Child With Traumatic Brain Injury

Nursing Assessment and Diagnosis

Frequently assess the child's neurologic status using guidelines in *Assessment Guide: The Child With a Neurologic Condition* at the beginning of this chapter and the Glasgow Coma Scale (see Table 27–5). Compare findings to prior evaluations, and note improvement, stability, or deterioration. Assess the cranial nerves and pupils for size and reactivity. Monitor vital signs, responsiveness, and behavior carefully. Note any irritability or signs that might indicate increased ICP (see Table 27–4). Changes in these signs may indicate hypoxia, decreased perfusion, shock, or increased ICP. When the child has a decreased level of consciousness shortly after a brain injury, consider if a posttraumatic seizure occurred and if the child could still be in the postictal state. The cause of any deterioration must be quickly determined and appropriate interventions taken.

Observe for physiologic and behavioral signs of pain. Assume that the child with increased ICP is in pain, even when unresponsive. Assess the family's coping with the child's life-threatening injury and any support systems available to them (see Chapter 13).

Examples of nursing diagnoses appropriate for the child with TBI include the following (NANDA-I © 2014):

- ***Tissue Perfusion: Cerebral, Risk for Ineffective,*** related to hypoventilation, hypovolemia, and/or reduction of arterial blood flow to the brain due to increased ICP
- ***Aspiration, Risk for,*** related to decreased LOC and loss of protective reflexes
- ***Fluid Volume: Imbalanced, Risk for,*** related to therapies for reducing ICP
- ***Coping: Family, Compromised,*** related to life-threatening injury to child

Planning and Implementation

HOSPITAL-BASED NURSING CARE

The child with a severe TBI is initially cared for in the pediatric ICU. Nursing care focuses on maintaining cerebral perfusion pressure, minimizing increased ICP, reducing stimulation, preventing complications, and providing emotional support.

Once the child is on the general pediatric unit, maintain cardiopulmonary function. In the moderately injured child, observe breathing patterns and check color, neurologic signs, and LOC. The oxygen saturation should remain over 95%. Report any sign of decreased oxygenation or signs and symptoms of increased ICP to the healthcare provider immediately (see Table 27–4). Keep suction equipment at the bedside in case aspiration occurs.

Reduce physiologic stresses on the body that could increase ICP. Minimize unpleasant stimuli when possible, keep the environment quiet, and avoid jarring the bed. Pain management and temperature control are important. Position the child with the bed flat or elevated 15 to 30 degrees to avoid excessive flexion of the hips, and maintain the head and neck in neutral alignment to encourage venous return to the heart. The child may also be placed in a side-lying position with the head neither flexed nor extended. Monitor the effect of nursing procedures on ICP. Determine if clustering procedures is better than spreading procedures over time. Encourage parents to talk to the child and provide comforting touch.

Administer medications as prescribed. When the child is unresponsive, provide oral care to keep mucous membranes moist and intact and to reduce the risk for infection, especially if the child is being ventilated (see the *Clinical Skills Manual* SKILLS). Pad and cushion bony prominences, provide skin care, and change the child's position frequently. Protect the eyes from corneal irritation with ophthalmic ointment and patching.

Enteral feeding may be used initially, slowly progressing to oral foods as tolerated. Fluids are given to meet daily fluid requirements, or to maintain the child's blood pressure within normal ranges for age. Stool softeners and suppositories should be used as needed to prevent constipation. The side rails of the bed should be padded to protect the child if a seizure occurs.

Promote recovery and prevent physical deformities. Perform passive range-of-motion (ROM) exercises to prevent contractures. Splints may be used to position extremities in functional positions. Work with physical, occupational, and speech therapists to reinforce exercises and help teach parents the techniques so they can work with the child in the hospital and at home.

Provide stimulation and promote general awareness when the child is ready, based on the child's age and ability, by using toys, books, music, or games. Assist the family to provide stimulation but also to provide quiet time when the child displays agitation.

Provide emotional support to the family in collaboration with the social workers, healthcare providers, psychologists, rehabilitation therapists, and members of the clergy caring for the child and family. All can help the family adjust to having a child with a new disability.

Sometimes despite all efforts, the child dies as a result of the consequences of the brain injury. Provide support for the family while brain death testing is performed. See Chapter 13 for brain death criteria and methods for supporting the family when termination of life support and organ donation are discussed.

DISCHARGE PLANNING AND HOME CARE TEACHING

Children with serious traumatic brain injuries may be transferred to an inpatient rehabilitation center to promote optimal achievement of function. Other children may have outpatient rehabilitation prescribed, and thus home care needs should be identified and addressed well in advance of discharge. A case manager is often needed to coordinate services and resources during rehabilitation. Social services intervention may be needed when brain injury results from child abuse.

Give parents information about caring for children with mild or moderate TBIs at home and possible behaviors to expect from the child. For children with disabilities, determine what adaptations and assistive technology are needed in the home to care for the child, such as a wheelchair, a walker, braces, or a special bed.

COMMUNITY-BASED NURSING CARE

Home care nursing may be important for the child with an acquired neurologic dysfunction and prolonged altered consciousness. The nurse can teach the family to meet the child's needs, monitor the intake of fluids and foods, position the child, and provide skin care. In-home physical therapists may teach parents to perform ROM exercises and other strategies to prevent contractures. Regular follow-up visits are needed to assess the child's recovery and to modify the treatment plan.

Clinical Reasoning   The Child With Severe Brain Injury

Marcus, 7 years old, was struck by a car and thrown several feet. He was unconscious on admission to the emergency department and showed some signs of increased ICP (dilated and fixed pupils). He was treated for shock, and his neurologic status and vital signs were frequently assessed. Marcus was found to have sustained several contusions of the brain, but no skull fracture. He was intubated and medicated to manage the increased ICP.

Marcus's ICP has now stabilized, but he has not totally regained consciousness. He is restless and agitated, and unable to follow directions. His parents stay at his bedside and provide auditory and tactile stimulation, hoping he will eventually respond. He receives physical therapy to prevent contractures and to maintain function. Marcus will need long-term rehabilitation to achieve the best outcome possible after this injury.

What is the role of the nurse in acute care of the child with a severe brain injury? What support does the family need to contribute to the child's care? How would you work with other healthcare providers to coordinate care during the acute care phase? How would you help plan the long-term care for a child such as Marcus?

Children with moderate brain injuries often have long-term problems with attention, problem solving, speed of information processing, and behavior problems (e.g., impulsivity, irritability, apathy, aggression, and social withdrawal). Neuropsychologic testing is needed to identify subtle learning disabilities that are not usually revealed on standardized school achievement tests. Educational accommodations needed are usually different from those made for children with other learning disabilities.

The child or adolescent facing long-term rehabilitation needs support to adjust to the disability and to find the strength to maximize his or her abilities. Identify recreational opportunities for the child with disabilities to promote exercise and self-esteem. The adolescent may need to gain vocational skills and learn to live independently. Refer parents to the Brain Injury Association for further information.

Prevention of brain injury is another important role of the nurse. Encourage parents to obtain protective helmets and require children to use them for bicycling and skateboarding. Parents should be encouraged to wear a helmet themselves as role models. Encourage parents to monitor playgrounds for appropriate use of wood chips or cushioning tiles to reduce the severity of injuries associated with falls.

Evaluation

Examples of expected outcomes of nursing care for the family and child with TBI include the following:

- Cerebral perfusion pressure is maintained at an adequate rate to sustain oxygenation of the brain.

- Muscle function is maintained and physical deformities are prevented with ROM exercises and splinting during the recovery stages of the brain injury.

- Parents are supported through the child's acute recovery phase and learn to provide care the child will need at home.

- The child's school performance is monitored and appropriate educational resources are provided to support the child's learning.

Concussion

A concussion is a mild TBI that usually results from a direct blow to the head, face, neck, or other part of the body. Nearly a half million emergency department visits per year are associated with a concussion in children under age 15 years (Mason, 2013). Organized sports (football, hockey, rugby, soccer, and basketball) and other activities (snow skiing, skateboarding, falls from bicycles, and horseback riding) are associated with concussion.

The blow causes stretching and bruising of brain tissue that disrupts nerve transmission and metabolic function, but no structural abnormality is seen with radiographic imaging. Most children have concussion symptoms for up to 7 to 10 days, but their cognitive recovery often takes longer.

The child with a concussion has a rapid onset of short-term functional impairment that may or may not involve loss of consciousness and cognitive, physical, emotional, and sleep symptoms that may persist for minutes to months (Meckler, 2014). Signs and symptoms may include the following:

- *Physical*—headache, sensitivity to light or noise, dazed, visual problems, balance problems, fatigue, and nausea and vomiting

- *Cognitive*—feeling foggy or sluggish, difficulty concentrating and remembering, confused about recent events, answers slowly

- *Emotional*—irritable, sad, nervous, more emotional than usual

- *Sleep*—drowsy, sleeps more or less than normal, difficulty falling asleep

Pediatric concussive syndrome is thought to be caused by an injury to the brainstem and occurs in children younger than age 3 years. Toddlers seem stunned at the time of injury, but have no loss of consciousness. Later, these children become pale, clammy, and lethargic, and they may vomit.

Initial sideline evaluation of the child injured in an organized sport involves removing the child from play, and using a checklist to assess orientation, recent and remote memory, new learning, concentration, and balance (Harmon et al., 2013). Questions are asked about events before and after the injury to help identify amnesia, an important sign of a more serious injury. A history is taken and physical examination performed in the health center or emergency department. Because no findings are typically found on CT and MRI, radiologic imaging is not performed unless an intracranial structural injury is suspected. Computerized neuropsychologic tests are available to test a high school athlete's baseline performance for comparison after concussion to monitor recovery.

Treatment is supportive. Children are observed in the emergency department for several hours before being sent home with instructions to the parents to watch them closely for decreased responsiveness. The child who is unconscious for more than 5 minutes or has amnesia of the event may be admitted to the hospital or be observed in a short-stay unit to rule out other injury. All cognitive activities are limited in the first few days after injury, including time out of school, video games, watching television, and using a computer (Meckler, 2014). Before returning to organized sports, the child should be symptom-free and using no analgesia for headache. Symptoms usually disappear within several weeks but may last up to 6 months. Physical activities are gradually increased, and if symptoms recur, return to play is further delayed.

Even though the child looks normal following a brain injury, ensure that parents and teachers know that brain healing takes up to 6 weeks. Typical behaviors during this healing period may include tiring easily, memory loss or forgetfulness, easy distractibility, difficulty concentrating, difficulty following directions, irritability or short temper, and needing help starting and finishing tasks. Return the child to a full school schedule gradually to prevent fatigue and frustration. Educational assessment should be initiated if recovery takes longer than 6 weeks.

Young athletes who return to play too soon may have a delayed reaction time and be at greater risk for a second concussion. Long-term neurologic problems may result from recurrent concussions.

Professionalism in Practice Concussion Management in the School Setting

The American Academy of Neurology recently updated guidelines for evaluation and management of concussions (Giza et al., 2013). Many activities in the school setting (e.g., sports, physical education, and playtime) can place the child at risk for a concussion. School nurses collaborate with school staff members, athletic trainers, and parents to prevent concussions and to assess the child with a potential concussion. Nurses may also coordinate the development of an individualized health plan to accommodate the child's graduated return to school and sports. They also help the teachers understand the emotional and behavioral responses of the child returning to the classroom (National Association of School Nurses [NASN], 2012).

Scalp Injuries

Injuries to the scalp, which can be caused by falls, blunt trauma, or penetration of a foreign body, are usually benign. Bleeding may be extensive, but hypovolemia or shock is uncommon unless the patient is an infant.

Lacerations should be irrigated with copious amounts of sterile normal saline solution and inspected for bony fragments or depressions, CSF leakage with a dural tear, or debris. If the injury is simple, the laceration can be sutured and the child discharged from the emergency department. If more severe, a neurosurgeon should be consulted.

Skull Fractures

A fracture to any of the eight cranial bones requires considerable force:

- *Linear fracture*—most common type of fracture, can potentially be caused by child abuse. May have overlying hematoma or soft tissue swelling; usually no symptoms.

- *Depressed skull fracture*—break in skull itself or an area shattered into many fragments. Pieces of bone may be depressed into brain tissue with hematoma forming on top.

- *Basilar fracture*—fracture at the base of the skull; may involve the frontal, ethmoid, sphenoid, temporal, or occipital bones; a dural tear may be present; increases risk for meningitis. The child may have blood behind the tympanic membranes, CSF leakage (yellow to amber fluid) from the nose or ears, periorbital ecchymosis (raccoon eyes), or bruising of the mastoid (Battle sign).

Any area of the skull with swelling or a hematoma should be evaluated for possible fracture. Diagnosis is made by visual inspection, palpation, skull radiograph, or CT scan.

Treatment includes neurosurgical consultation. Surgery may be required for debridement or to elevate bone fragments of a depressed skull fracture. Tetanus prophylaxis and antibiotic therapy may be prescribed in some cases. Some skull fractures may be associated with intracranial bleeding, cranial nerve injuries, and posttraumatic epilepsy.

Penetrating Injuries

Gunshot wounds to the head can damage brain tissue, bone, and blood vessels. The child's level of consciousness quickly deteriorates because of the edema surrounding the penetration tract.

CT scans evaluate gunshot trauma and pinpoint the location of bullet and bone fragments as well as damaged brain tissue. Surgery is performed to debride the tract, evacuate any hematomas, and remove accessible bone or bullet particles. A high percentage of these children die. Those who survive may suffer multiple focal deficits and seizures.

Impalement injuries may occur in children in association with projectiles, dog bites, or other sharp objects. All objects must be left in place and removed in the operating room by a neurosurgeon. The child is at high risk for focal injury and infection. After surgery, children are managed in the same manner as other postoperative brain injuries, with attention focused on level of consciousness, management of increased ICP, and infection control.

Spinal Cord Injury

Injury to the spinal cord is a rare condition that causes major lifelong disabilities and a shortened life. Only 2% to 5% of spinal cord injuries occur in the pediatric population, and more commonly involve cervical spine injury (Pettiford et al., 2012). Mechanisms of injury in children and adolescents include motor vehicle crashes (passenger and pedestrian), recreational activities, and violence (child abuse, stabbing, and gunshot wounds).

The mechanism of injury and direction of forces determine the type of lesion that occurs (Figure 27–15). Hyperflexion

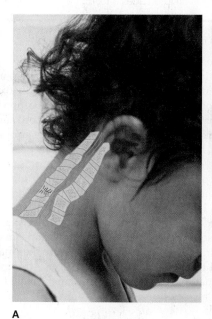
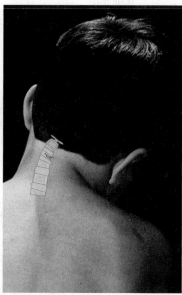
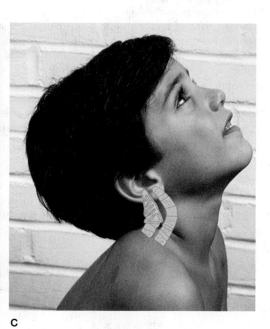

A   B   C

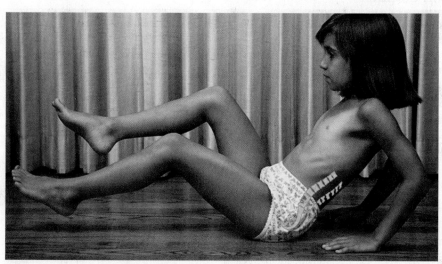
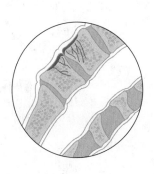

D

Figure 27–15 **Mechanics of injury to the spinal cord.** *A,* **Hyperflexion.** *B,* **Lateral flexion.** *C,* **Hyperextension.** *D,* **Compression.**

injuries (e.g., bending around a car safety seat belt) produce tears or avulsions and fractures of vertebral bodies, as well as subluxation and dislocation. Rotation may cause joint dislocations or unstable spinal fractures. Hyperextension may result in the so-called hangman's fracture, ligament tears, avulsion fractures of vertebral bodies, and central or posterior spinal cord syndrome. Compression injuries may occur when a child falls from a height. Young children are prone to specific kinds of spinal cord injuries because of the mobility and flexibility of their spinal column.

Spinal cord injuries are classified as complete or incomplete. Complete lesions are irreversible and involve a loss of sensory, motor, and autonomic function below the level of the injury. Incomplete lesions involve varying degrees of sensory, motor, and autonomic function below the level of injury. Autonomic dysfunction is associated with hypotension, loss of bladder and bowel control, and loss of environmental thermoregulatory function. The higher the level of spinal cord injury, the more severe the neurologic damage. Table 27–17 describes the spinal cord injuries that occur in children.

At the time of injury due to compression, shear injuries, or other injury, the child is flaccid and loses reflexes below the level of the lesion. Inflammation causes a secondary injury, resulting in ischemia and necrosis. **Spinal shock**, spinal cord concussion resulting in a transient suppression of nerve function below the level of the acute injury, occurs. Some return of function may occur within the first 72 hours of injury in an incomplete lesion. As neurologic recovery begins, spinal reflex activity returns and increasing spasticity is seen below the level of the injury.

The child can experience neurogenic shock in which there is loss of vasomotor tone and sympathetic innervations of the heart, resulting in hypotension, bradycardia, and peripheral vasodilation (a form of distributive shock). See Chapter 21. Priapism may be seen. Respiratory compromise may be present because of paralysis of the diaphragm.

Diagnosis is made by observation, neurologic examination, and radiologic studies of the cervical, thoracic, and lumbosacral spine to determine if a vertebral fracture or compression on the spinal cord is present. When a child with a suspected spinal cord injury was immobilized by prehospital providers, cautious physical and radiologic evaluations are needed before the child is unrestrained. In addition, CT scanning, MRI, fluoroscopy, or myelography may be performed. Some young children have spinal cord injury without radiographic abnormality (SCIWORA) on a plain radiograph, but an MRI can detect the injury to ligaments and soft tissues.

Growth and Development

The vertebrae are not fully ossified in children younger than 9 years. The facet joints are more shallow and horizontal, allowing them to slide over each other more easily as the ligaments stretch. The young child's head is relatively large compared to the strength of the neck muscles. When the neck muscle strength is exceeded, the ligaments supporting the vertebrae can stretch much more than the spinal cord, leading to spinal cord tearing. Injuries to children under age 9 are more likely to occur at the C1 to C3 level, and at the C4 to C6 level in children ages 9 to 15.

Spinal injuries are managed aggressively. The child with a confirmed spinal cord injury may be placed in external immobilization with a halo device. Surgery to reduce and internally fixate the fracture is performed for unstable fractures, dislocations, and progressive deformity. Decompression of the spinal cord and nerve roots may be performed if transection is not complete or if compression by a clot, herniated disk, or other lesion is present and can be relieved.

To decrease neurologic sequelae in children with motor deficits, a high-dose methylprednisolone is often administered intravenously if started within 8 hours of injury. Evidence does not clearly indicate a benefit to this treatment, and adverse effects include increased risk of infection, hyperglycemia, and gastrointestinal bleeding (Pettiford et al., 2012). Gastrointestinal prophylaxis is started to reduce the risk for an ulcer. Atropine and norepinephrine may be given to manage spinal shock. IV fluid resuscitation is also performed if the child could have

TABLE 27–17 Spinal Cord Injuries in Children

SPINE REGION	INJURY CHARACTERISTICS
Cervical	• Site of the majority of spinal injuries in children under 10 years • Injury above C3 segment causes respiratory arrest and death without ventilatory support; many of these injuries are fatal • Diaphragm function is present when injury is at C5 level • **Tetraplegia**, can have loss of sensation and function of the head and neck and upper and lower extremities • Loss of sphincter function • Sensory level lost below the sternum
Thoracic	• More commonly, the site of spinal injuries in children between 8 and 14 years • Full control of upper extremities including hands • Poor trunk balance
Thoracolumbar	• Full control of muscles in abdomen and upper back • Good trunk balance
Lumbar	• Injuries at the L1–L3 level may occur in children 4–8 years using a car lap belt rather than a car safety seat • Below L3 may have functioning of muscles in upper leg • Loss of ankle and foot control

hypovolemic shock from other injuries. Complications of spinal cord injury include:

- Impaired respiratory function due to a paralyzed diaphragm or diminished vital capacity
- Scoliosis if injury occurs before the skeleton is mature
- Hip instability due to poor acetabular development
- Pathologic fractures of the long bones due to immobilization hypercalcemia
- Pressure sores
- Deep vein thrombosis
- Autonomic dysreflexia

Spasticity, muscle atrophy, increased risk of respiratory problems, weight gain, osteoporosis, and other skeletal problems are long-term issues for many children. The goal of rehabilitation is to promote independence in daily activities, as well as mobility, strength, power, and endurance.

SAFETY ALERT!

Autonomic dysreflexia is a condition associated with injuries above the T6 level. It becomes a medical emergency when over-activity of the autonomic nervous system causes an abrupt onset of hypertension, cardiac arrhythmia, pupillary constriction, severe headaches, flushing above the level of the spinal cord lesion, and sweating. Below the level of the lesion, the skin is pale and cool with piloerection. Common triggers are constipation, a full bladder, or a pressure ulcer. Treatment involves positioning the patient upright, loosening tight clothing, emptying the bladder, eliminating any precipitating stimulus, and administering antihypertensive medication. Prevention of autonomic dysreflexia involves an effective bowel and bladder program and prevention of pressure ulcers (Stephenson & Berliner, 2014).

Nursing Management

For the Child With Spinal Cord Injury

HOSPITAL-BASED NURSING CARE

Nursing care focuses on monitoring vital signs, meeting nutritional needs, maintaining skin integrity, promoting independent functioning, providing emotional support, and promoting rehabilitation.

Be alert for any changes in vital signs, especially those that may signify increased respiratory difficulty, neurogenic shock (hypotension, bradycardia, and peripheral vasodilation), increased ICP (see Table 27–4), or autonomic dysreflexia. Monitor intake and output. Monitor bladder and bowel function. Assess the skin for integrity.

With higher cervical injuries, assess the cranial nerves as they may be affected by swelling around the spinal cord. Note the return of reflexes and change from flaccid tone to spasticity. Identify any changes in level of sensation or motor function. Carefully check the immobilizing device to ensure that the spine stays stable.

Some children with cervical lesions have tracheostomies performed to help maintain airway patency; others with high cervical lesions are dependent on ventilators. Keep suctioning equipment and other emergency equipment at the bedside at all times.

Ensure adequate nutrition. A child with complete paralysis may require a gastrostomy tube. When the child begins to eat, feed soft foods slowly as the child may have some swallowing difficulties.

Prevent skin breakdown (see Chapter 31). Observe surgical sites for signs of infection or inflammation. Provide regular traction pin site care according to hospital guidelines. Establish a schedule for patient repositioning.

Promote independent functioning by reinforcing the exercises and skills learned in physical and occupational therapy. Use supports, boots, footboards, splints, and braces as recommended by the therapists to prevent contractures. If hand mobility is limited, explore options for independence. Encourage the child to be as independent as possible in a wheelchair. An important mobility goal is to achieve wheelchair transfer and to perform self-care. Identify adaptive equipment that makes these goals possible.

Achieving bowel and bladder control may be difficult. Regular intermittent catheterizations may be necessary if urinary retention occurs (see the *Clinical Skills Manual* SKILLS). Anticipate that constipation will occur and initiate bowel training with a diet high in fiber and the use of stool softeners.

Therapeutic play appropriate for the child's developmental level is an important part of the healing process. Provide as many normal activities for the child as possible, but do not give the child tasks that will be difficult to complete. Child-life teachers or tutors can help the child keep up with schoolwork.

Television, DVDs, computer games, Internet connections, and music can offer diversion for prolonged hospitalization. Children with paraplegia can learn to use their arms and hands to play interactive games. Devices can also be adapted so that the child can play computer games or manipulate the television or radio. Identify assistive technology that may help the child with tetraplegia gain some level of independence.

Support the child emotionally. Encourage the child to meet small, short-term goals, including those that involve self-care. Encourage the child to express fears and frustrations.

Be compassionate and understanding. Encourage siblings to visit, answer their questions honestly, and help them to discuss their feelings. Involve the parents and siblings in the child's care as much as possible. When appropriate, encourage them to help with activities of daily living.

DISCHARGE PLANNING AND HOME CARE TEACHING

Many children are discharged to inpatient rehabilitation facilities. Assist with arrangements for the transfer. Work closely with the child, parents, and other members of the healthcare team concerning placement. Home care needs, reintegration into educational programs, and safety issues should be identified and addressed well in advance of discharge from the rehabilitation facility. Refer families to social services, family counseling, and support groups if indicated.

Hypoxic-Ischemic Brain Injury (Drowning)

Drowning is defined as the process resulting in primary respiratory impairment from submersion/immersion in a liquid medium. *Submersion injury* is the term used when the child survives. Drowning, a leading cause of unintentional injury death for children of all ages between birth and 19 years, caused 866 deaths in the United States in 2013. Children 1 to 4 years and 15 to 19 years old had the highest rate of drowning deaths in 2013 (National Center for Injury Prevention and Control, 2015). Boys are affected more frequently than girls. For every death, an additional two children are hospitalized for nonfatal drowning events (Bowman, Aiken, Robbins, et al., 2012).

In young children, drowning is associated with bathing and falling in water (e.g., pools or large buckets). Older children are more likely to drown in open water, potentially associated with risk-taking behaviors, seizures, or alcohol use (Bowman et al., 2012).

It takes only enough water to cover the nose and mouth for a child to drown. The child trapped in water panics, struggles, tries to move using swimming motions, and holds the breath. The child aspirates a small amount of water from the oropharynx, causing a laryngospasm that lasts no more than 2 minutes and hypoxia. Because of increasing panic and hypoxia, the child swallows more liquid. As the laryngospasm passes, the child breathes water into the lungs. The child may also vomit and aspirate stomach contents. Aspirated water damages the lung surfactant and impairs alveolar gas exchange. Hypothermia may result because the child's body cools faster in water than in air, and systemic perfusion decreases as a result (see Chapter 31). With increasing hypoxia, the cardiac muscle becomes impaired and ultimately the heart stops.

Anoxia associated with drowning leads to cerebral edema and increased ICP and secondary cerebral injuries. With aggressive cardiopulmonary resuscitation the child may survive, but usually with neurologic impairment.

The signs and symptoms of submersion vary by the length of time underwater, temperature of the water, response to the episode, and the initial scene treatment. The child who has been submerged may be apneic and pulseless. When submerged for short periods (less than 5 to 10 minutes and resuscitated at the scene), children may have few symptoms and fully recover without neurologic impairment. Signs and symptoms in the rescued child may be decreased level of consciousness ranging from stupor to total unresponsiveness, apnea or irregular respirations, gastric distention, and seizures. The child submerged for longer than 10 minutes or who has delayed cardiopulmonary resuscitation is more likely to have neurologic impairment or to die.

Immediate cardiopulmonary resuscitation (CPR) performed at the scene is associated with the best outcomes. Emergency personnel with a defibrillator should assess the heart rhythm and defibrillate if ventricular fibrillation is present. The child should be transported to the hospital even if the child begins breathing spontaneously. Initial emergency treatment is 100% oxygen and rewarming. The airway may be secured with an endotracheal tube.

SAFETY ALERT!

All submersion victims should be observed in the hospital for 6 to 8 hours, even when initially asymptomatic. Signs of respiratory distress and cerebral edema develop within this timeline, and immediate care can be provided as needed.

The child who has a serious anoxic injury is cared for in the ICU. Mechanical ventilation may be used to keep the alveoli open, to promote adequate oxygenation, and to prevent respiratory acidosis. Treatment for cerebral edema is initiated (see the earlier section on care of the child with a traumatic brain injury).

Nursing Management

Nursing care of the child who survives a submersion incident focuses on monitoring the child's neurologic and cardiopulmonary status and providing emotional support to the family.

Assess the child's responsiveness, spontaneous respiratory efforts, oxygenation, and vital signs. Perform frequent neurologic status assessments. Attach a cardiorespiratory monitor and pulse oximeter for continuous patient assessment information.

Implement the nursing interventions for a child with altered states of consciousness as described earlier in this chapter. If cerebral edema develops, implement nursing interventions as described in the earlier section on care of the child with a traumatic brain injury.

Provide emotional support to the family. Be nonjudgmental and provide a forum for parents to express their feelings. Reassure parents who exhibit guilt reactions that their child is receiving all possible medical treatment. Parents may be faced with an unknown prognosis. Encourage them to seek assistance from social workers, members of the clergy, close friends, and relatives. Arrange for appropriate referrals. If the child's prognosis is poor, an ethics consultation may be offered to educate the family about options for decision making regarding sustaining or terminating life support (see Chapter 13).

Identify and address rehabilitation or home care needs well in advance of discharge. Assist with arrangements for the child with minor deficits. Assign a case manager to the child with significant neurologic impairments so that long-term care options can be explored. Inpatient or outpatient rehabilitation options should be matched to the child's needs and family resources.

Drowning can be prevented by education, legislation, and changes in the environment. Pool owners should erect climb-proof 5-foot fences around all four sides of the pool. If fencing is on three sides, with the house serving as the fourth side, the house door to the pool area should be kept locked and have an alarm. Local ordinances may require such fences. Ensure that hot tubs and pools have drain covers or other safety devices that prevent a child from getting a limb or hair entrapped in a drain. Adolescents should learn the dangers of mixing alcohol or drugs and swimming. Keep 5- and 10-gallon buckets empty when not in use. Emphasize the importance of closely supervising children when near or in the water, whether at pools, at the beach, or in the bathtub. Children with seizure disorders should always have a buddy when swimming.

Chapter Highlights

- The nervous system is complete with all nerve cells at birth. Myelination continues throughout childhood.

- Altered level of consciousness is caused by infection, trauma, hypoxia, poisoning, seizures, alcohol or substance abuse, endocrine or metabolic disturbances (e.g. diabetic ketoacidosis), electrolyte or acid–base imbalance, intracranial space-occupying lesion, stroke, and a congenital structural defect.

- Emergency care for the child or adolescent with a prolonged generalized seizure includes airway management, supplemental oxygen, intravenous benzodiazepines, and careful monitoring of vital signs and motor activity. Carefully document the duration of the seizure or series of seizures to detect status epilepticus.

- Neurologic damage from bacterial meningitis often occurs in infants and young children despite early, aggressive management. Complications may include hearing impairment, gross neurologic deficits, and behavioral and intellectual disorders.

- Encephalitis is an acute inflammation of the brain often caused by a virus that is transmitted by a mosquito, such as West Nile virus and Western Equine virus. Presenting signs include a severe headache, fever, irritability, and altered mental status.

- Reye syndrome is an encephalopathy with a high mortality rate that is associated with aspirin use for a mild viral illness. Because most parents give children acetaminophen or ibuprofen rather than aspirin for flulike symptoms and varicella, Reye syndrome has become rare.

- Guillain-Barré syndrome is a disorder of deteriorating motor function and paralysis that progress in an ascending pattern, paresthesia, and areflexia. It may be caused by an autoimmune response to an infectious organism, usually within 1 to 3 weeks of a gastrointestinal or respiratory illness.

- More than 75% of children experience a headache by age 15 years. Types of benign headaches include migraines, inflammatory (sinusitis), and tension.

- Microcephaly is a small brain that may be caused by genetic transmission, fetal or postnatal insult, or intrauterine infection.

- Hydrocephalus is caused by the blockage of cerebrospinal fluid flow through normal channels and pathways or the impaired absorption of cerebrospinal fluid in the subarachnoid space and the arachnoid villi. It can be associated with a congenital condition or acquired from meningitis or intraventricular hemorrhage, tumor, or structural deformity.

- The more common types of neural tube defects include anencephaly (no development of the brain above the brainstem), encephalocele (protrusion of meningeal or skin-covered brain through the skull), and myelomeningocele or spina bifida.

- Myelomeningocele or spina bifida is a malformation of the vertebrae and spinal canal with a protrusion of a meningeal sac filled with a portion of the spinal cord. It is the most common developmental disorder of the CNS.

- Positional plagiocephaly, an asymmetric flattening of the occiput, is associated with sleep position to prevent sudden infant death syndrome or with neck problems such as congenital torticollis. The weight of the infant head sometimes flattens the skull. Strategies to encourage the child to change the position of the head may help reduce its occurrence.

- Neurofibromatosis 1 is characterized by multiple café au lait spots, darker than the surrounding skin, that are 5 mm (0.2 in.) or larger in infants but grow to 15 mm (0.6 in.) in diameter during adolescence. Multiple benign tumors grow on or under the skin beginning during puberty.

- Most cases of cerebral palsy are characterized by spasticity and a lack of coordination. The risk for cerebral palsy is increased with prematurity, intraventricular hemorrhage, intrauterine infection, neonatal sepsis, and hyperbilirubinemia.

- Traumatic brain injury is a leading cause of death and disability during childhood. It results from falls, motor vehicle crashes, sports injuries, and child abuse.

- Concussions result from the stretching, compression, and shearing of nerve fibers after an impact injury to the head that causes signs such as transient altered mental status, amnesia, dizziness, and impairment of memory, orientation, and balance.

- Spinal cord injuries, although relatively rare in children, often result from significant forces such as from motor vehicle crashes. Because of the child's larger and heavier head and weaker neck muscles, cervical spine injuries are more common.

- Children who have the best outcomes following drowning include those submerged less than 5 minutes who receive immediate cardiopulmonary resuscitation.

Clinical Reasoning in Action

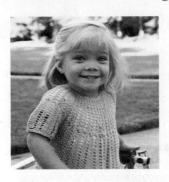

Abigail, a 3-year-old with myelodysplasia, is seen every few months with her parents in the multidisciplinary spina bifida clinic where you work. Her lesion is at the L3 level, so she can flex her hips and extend her knees, but her ankles and toes are paralyzed. She also has a ventriculoperitoneal shunt for hydrocephalus. She uses lower leg braces and a walker to mobilize and has minimal sensation in her lower legs and feet. Her bladder and bowel sphincters are also affected, so Abigail and her parents have worked hard to establish bowel control with a high-fiber diet and by establishing specific times for bowel evacuation. Abigail's parents learned to perform intermittent catheterization for bladder control to reduce the risk for kidney damage.

Her health history reveals she has experienced a case of otitis media since her last visit and responded well to antibiotics. Her legs are well protected by stockings to reduce rubbing by her braces. Her gait is becoming steadier with the walker, and her parents are encouraging exercise of her arms and upper trunk with swimming. You encourage Abigail's parents to promote her cognitive development with age-appropriate games and interaction with siblings. Her parents plan to enroll her in preschool in the fall.

1. What are the safety issues to discuss with Abigail's parents about spina bifida?
2. Describe spina bifida and its relationship with hydrocephalus.
3. Identify important health promotion issues to discuss with Abigail's parents.
4. Describe the issues that need to be addressed in planning for an IEP and individual health plan when Abigail enters preschool.

References

Antonaci, F., Voiticovschi-Iosob, C., Di Stefano, A. L., Galli, F., Ozge, A., & Balottin, U. (2014). The evolution of headache from childhood to adulthood: A review of the literature. *Journal of Headache and Pain, 15*, 15. Retrieved from http://www.thejournalofheadacheandpain.com/content/15/1/15

Aronson, E., & Stevenson, S. B. (2012). Bone health in children with cerebral palsy. *Journal of Pediatric Health Care, 26*(3), 193–199.

Beaulieu, M. J. (2013). Leviteracetam. *Neonatal Network, 32*(4), 285–288.

Bethel, J. (2012). Emergency care of children and adults with head injury. *Nursing Standard, 26*(43), 49–56.

Blosser, C. G., Albers, A. C., & Reider-Demer, M. (2012). Headache. In C. Burns, A. M. Dunn, M. A. Brady, N. B. Starr, & C. G. Blosser (Eds.), *Pediatric primary care* (5th ed., pp. 606–614). Philadelphia, PA: Elsevier Saunders.

Bowman, S. M., Aitken, M. E., Robbins, J. M., & Baker, S. P. (2012). Trends in US pediatric drowning hospitalizations, 1993–2008. *Pediatrics, 129*(2), 275–281.

Brain Injury Association of America. (2014). *Brain injury in children*. Retrieved from http://www.biausa.org/brain-injury-children.htm

Brown, L., & Proctor, M. R. (2011). Endoscopically assisted correction of sagittal craniosynostosis. *AORN Journal, 93*(5), 566–579.

Burkhard, A. (2013). A different life: Caring for an adolescent or young adult with severe cerebral palsy. *Journal of Pediatric Nursing, 28*, 357–363.

Castelblanco, R. L., Lee, M., & Hasbun, R. (2014). Epidemiology of bacterial meningitis in the USA from 1997 to 2010: A population-based observational study. *The Lancet Infectious Diseases, 14*(9), 813–819.

Catala-Beauchamp, A., & Gleason, R. P. (2012). Abdominal migraine in children: Is it all in their heads? *Journal of Nurse Practitioners, 8*(1), 19–26.

Centers for Disease Control and Prevention (CDC). (2014a). *TBI data and statistics*. Retrieved from http://www.cdc.gov/traumaticbraininjury/data/index.html

Centers for Disease Control and Prevention (CDC). (2014b). *Spina bifida*. Retrieved from http://www.cdc.gov/ncbddd/spinabifida/facts.html

Centers for Disease Control and Prevention (CDC). (2015). Updated estimates of neural tube defects prevented by mandatory folic acid fortification—United States, 1995–2011. *Morbidity and Mortality Weekly Report, 64*(1), 1–5.

Colver, A., Fairhurst, C., & Pharoah, P. O. D. (2014). Cerebral palsy. *Lancet, 383*, 1240–1249.

Dubowitz, H., & Lane, W. G. (2016). Abused and neglected children. In R. M. Kliegman, B. F. Stanton, J. W. St. Geme, & N. F. Schor (Eds.) *Nelson textbook of pediatrics* (20th ed., pp. 236–248). Philadelphia: Elsevier Saunders.

Epilepsy Foundation. (2014a). *Seizures in youth*. Retrieved from http://www.epilepsy.com/learn/seizures-youth

Epilepsy Foundation. (2014b). *Ketogenic diet*. Retrieved from http://www.epilepsy.com/learn/seizures-youth/about-kids/dietary-therapy

Fadiman, A. (1997). *The spirit catches you and you fall down*. New York, NY: Farrar, Strauss, Giroux.

Ferro, M. A., Landgraf, J. M., & Speechley, K. N. (2013). Factor structure of the Child Health Questionnaire Parent Form-50 and predictors of health-related quality of life in children with epilepsy. *Quality of Life Research, 22*, 2201–2211.

Ferro, M. A., & Speechley, K. N. (2011). Examining clinically relevant levels of depressive symptoms in mothers following a diagnosis of epilepsy in their children: A prospective analysis. *Social Psychiatry and Psychiatric Epidemiology, 47*, 1419–1428.

Fingarson, A. K., & Pierce, M. C. (2012). Identifying abusive head trauma. *Contemporary Pediatrics, 29*(2), 16–24.

Garg, S., Green, J., Leadbitter, K., Emsley, R., Lehtonen, A., Evans, G., & Huson, S. M. (2013). Neurofibromatosis type 1 and autism spectrum disorder. *Pediatrics, 132*(6), e1642–e1648.

Geyer, K., Meller, K., Kulpan, C., & Mowery, B. D. (2013). Traumatic brain injury in children: Acute care management. *Pediatric Nursing, 39*(6), 283–289.

Giza, C. C., Kutcher, J. S., Ashwall, S., Barth, J., Thomas, S. D., Getchius, T. S. D., Gioia, G. A., . . . Ross Zafonte, R. (2013). Summary of evidence-based guideline update: Evaluation and management of concussion in sports: Report of the Guideline Development Subcommittee of the American Academy of Neurology. *Neurology, 80*(24), 2250–2257.

Harmon, K. G., Drezner, J., Gammons, M., Guskiewicz, K., Halstead, M. Herring, S., . . . Roberts, W. (2013). American Medical Society for Sports Medicine position statement: Concussion in sport. *Clinical Journal of Sport Medicine, 23*(1), 1–18.

Hershey, A. D., Kabbouche, M. A., & O'Brien, H. L. (2016). Headaches. In R. M. Kliegman, B. F. Stanton, J. W. St. Geme, & N. F. Schor (Eds.), *Nelson textbook of pediatrics* (20th ed., pp. 2863–2874). Philadelphia: Elsevier.

Ibrahim, S. H., & Balistreri, W. F. (2016). Mitochondrial hepatopathies. In R. M. Kliegman, B. F. Stanton, J. W. St. Geme, & N. F. Schor (Eds.), *Nelson textbook of pediatrics* (20th ed., pp. 1958–1961). Philadelphia: Elsevier Saunders.

Institute of Medicine. (2012). *Epilepsy across the spectrum: Promoting health and understanding*. Washington, DC: The National Academies Press.

Ismail, S., Lévy, A., Tikkanen, H., Sévère, M., Wolters, F. J., & Carmant, L. (2012). Lack of efficacy of phenytoin in children presenting with febrile status epilepticus. *American Journal of Emergency Medicine, 30*, 2000–2004.

James, H. E. (1986). Neurologic evaluation and support in the child with acute brain insult. *Pediatric Annals, 15*(1), 16–22.

Julian, N., Edwards, N. E., DeCrane, S., & Hingtgen, C. M. (2014). Neurofibromatosis 1: Diagnosis and management. *Journal for Nurse Practitioners, 10*(1), 30–35.

Kelesidis, T., Mastoris, I., Metsini, A., & Tsiodras, S. (2014). How to approach and treat viral infections in ICU patients. *BMC Infectious Diseases, 14*, 32.

Kerr, L. M., & Huether, S. M. (2014). Alterations in neurologic function in children. In K. L. McCance,

S. E. Huether, V. L. Brashers, & N. S. Rote (Eds.), *Pathophysiology: The biologic basis for disease in adults and children* (7th ed., pp. 660–688). St. Louis, MO: Elsevier.

Kocherlakota, P. (2014). Neonatal abstinence syndrome. *Pediatrics, 134*(2), e457–e561.

Le Saux, N., & Canadian Paediatric Society Infectious Diseases and Immunization Committee. (2014). Guidelines for the management of suspected and confirmed bacterial meningitis in Canadian children older than one month of age. *Paediatric Child Health, 19*(3), 141–146.

Looman, W. S., & Flannery, A. B. K. (2012). Evidence-based care of the child with deformational plagiocephaly: Part 1: Assessment and diagnosis. *Journal of Pediatric Health Care, 26*(4), 242–250.

Martin, N. G., Sadarangani, M., Pollard, A. J., & Goldacre, M. J. (2014). Hospital admission rates for meningitis and septicaemia caused by *Haemophilus influenzae, Neisseria meningitidis*, and *Streptococcus pneumoniae* in children in England over five decades: A population-based observational study. *The Lancet Infectious Diseases, 14*(5), 397–405.

MacMullen, N. J., Dulski, L. A., & Blobaum, P. (2014). Evidence-based interventions for neonatal abstinence syndrome, *Pediatric Nursing, 40*(4), 165–172, 203.

Mason, C. N. (2013). Mild traumatic brain injury in children. *Pediatric Nursing, 39*(6), 267–272.

McCarthy, J. G., Warren, S. M., Bernstein, J., Burnett, W., Cunningham, M. L., Edmond, J. C., . . . Yemen, T. A. (2012). Parameters of care for craniosynostosis. *Cleft Palate–Craniofacial Journal, 49*(1), 1S–24S.

Meckler, S. E. (2014). Clinical management of sports-related pediatric concussions. *Clinician Reviews, 24*(9), 24–32.

Modi, A. C., Rausch, J. R., & Glauser, T. A. (2011). Patterns of nonadherence to antiepileptic drug therapy in children with newly diagnosed epilepsy. *Journal of the American Medical Association, 305*(16), 1669–1679.

National Association of School Nurses (NASN). (2012). *Concussions—The role of the school nurse: Position statement.* Retrieved from http://www.nasn.org/portals/0/binder_papers_reports.pdf

National Center for Injury Prevention and Control. (2015). *10 leading causes of unintentional injury deaths, United States 2013, all races, both sexes.* Retrieved from http://webappa.cdc.gov/sasweb/ncipc/leadcaus10_us.html

National Institute of Neurological Disorders and Stroke (NINDS). (2014). *Hydrocephalus fact sheet.* Retrieved from http://www.ninds.nih.gov/disorders/hydrocephalus/detail_hydrocephalus.htm

Paul, S. P., Debono, R., & Walker, D. (2013). Clinical update: Recognising brain tumours early in children. *Community Practitioner, 86*(4), 42–45.

Pettiford, J. N., Bikhchandani, J., Ostlie, D. J., St. Peter, S. D., Sharp, R. J., & Juang, D. (2012). A review: The role of high dose methylprednisolone in spinal cord trauma in children. *Pediatric Surgery International, 28*, 287–294.

Quayle, K. S., Holmes, J. F., & Kuppermann, N. (2014). Epidemiology of blunt head trauma in children in U.S. emergency departments. *New England Journal of Medicine, 371*, 1945–1947.

Rivara, F. P., Koepsell, T. D., Wang, J., Temkin, N., Dorsch, A., Vavilala, M.S., . . . Jaffe, K. M. (2012). Incidence of disability among children 12 months after traumatic brain injury. *American Journal of Public Health, 102*(11), 2074–2079.

Russ, S. A., Larson, K., & Halfon, N. (2012). A national profile of childhood epilepsy and seizure disorder. *Pediatrics, 129*(2), 256–264.

Scully, S. M., Mallon, M., Kerr, J. C., & Ludzia-DeAngelis, A. (2012). Fetal myelomeningocele repair: A new standard of care. *AORN Journal, 96*(2), 176–192.

Shearer, P., & Riviello, J. (2011). Generalized convulsive status epilepticus in adults and children: Treatment guidelines and protocols. *Emergency Medical Clinics of North America, 29*, 51–64.

Shui, I. M., Rett, M. D., Weintraub, E., Marcy, M., Amato, A. A., Sheikh, S. I., . . . Yih, W. K. (2012). Guillain-Barré syndrome incidence in a large United States cohort (2000–2009). *Neuroepidemiology, 39*, 109–115.

Spina Bifida Association. (2014). *What is spina bifida?* Retrieved from http://www.spinabifidaassociation.org/site/c.evKRI7OXIoJ8H/b.8277225/k.5A79/What_is_Spina_Bifida.htm

Stephenson, R. O., & Berliner, J. (2014). *Autonomic dysreflexia in spinal cord injury.* Retrieved from http://emedicine.medscape.com/article/322809-overview\#a30

Substance Abuse and Mental Health Services Administration. (2013). *The NSDUH Report.* Retrieved from http://www.samhsa.gov/data/sites/default/files/spot123-pregnancy-alcohol-2013/spot123-pregnancy-alcohol-2013.pdf

Substance Abuse and Mental Health Services Administration. (2014). *Results from the 2013 National Survey on Drug Use and Health: Summary of national findings.* Retrieved from http://www.samhsa.gov/data/sites/default/files/NSDUHresultsPDFWHTML2013/Web/NSDUHresults2013.pdf

Sun, H., Bastings, E., Temeck, J., Smith, P. B., Men, A., Tandon, V., . . . Rodriguez, W. (2013). Migraine therapeutics in adolescents: A systematic analysis and historic perspectives of triptan trials in adolescents. *JAMA Pediatrics, 167*(3), 243–249.

Taketomo, C. K., Hodding, J. H., & Crause, D. M. (2014). *Pediatric and neonatal dosage handbook* (21st ed.). Hudson, OH: Lexicomp.

Teasdale, G., & Jennett, B. (1974). Assessment of coma and impaired consciousness. *Lancet, 2*, 81–84.

Teasdale, G., Allan, D., Brennan, P., McElhinney, E., & Mackinnon, L. (2014). Forty years on: Updating the Glasgow Coma Scale. *Nursing Times, 110*(42), 12–16.

Teasdale, G., Maas, A., Lecky, F., Manley, G., Stocchetti, N., & Murray, G. (2014). The Glasgow Coma Scale at 40 years: Standing the test of time. *Lancet Neurology, 13*(8), 844–854.

VanStraten, A. F., & Ng, Y. (2012). What is the worst part about having epilepsy? A children's and parents' perspective. *Pediatric Neurology, 47*, 431–435.

Varelas, P. N., Spanaki, M. V., & Mirski, M. A. (2013). Status epilepticus: An update. *Current Neurology and Neuroscience Reports, 13*(7), 357–365.

Wilkes, R., & Tasker, R. C. (2013). Pediatric intensive care treatment of uncontrolled status epilepticus. *Critical Care Clinics, 29*, 239–257

Wilson, B. A., Shannon, M. T., & Shield, K. M. (2015). *Nurse's drug guide 2015.* Hoboken, NJ: Pearson.

Worrall, K. (2004). Use of the Glasgow Coma Scale in infants. *Paediatric Nursing, 16*(4), 45–47.

Zelleke, T. G., Depositario-Cabacar, D. F. T., & Gaillard, W. D. (2013). Epilepsy. In M. L. Batshaw, N. J. Roizen, & G. R. Lotrecchiano (Eds.), *Children with disabilities* (7th ed., pp. 487–506). Baltimore, MD: Paul H. Brookes.

Chapter 28
Alterations in Mental Health and Cognitive Function

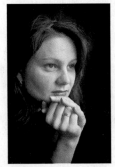

We've been so worried about Cassandra. After being in the car crash, she has become so frightened of everything. She wakes up at night screaming and has lost interest in school and friends. We hope that her work with the therapist will help decrease her fears and get her involved in all of her activities again.

—Mother of Cassandra, 9 years old

Oleg Golovnev/Shutterstock

⌄ Learning Outcomes

28.1 Define mental health and describe major mental health alterations in childhood.

28.2 Discuss the clinical manifestations of the major mental health alterations of childhood and adolescence.

28.3 Plan for the nursing management of children and adolescents with mental health alterations in the hospital and community settings.

28.4 Describe characteristics of common cognitive alterations of childhood.

28.5 Use evidence-based practice to plan nursing management for children with cognitive alterations.

28.6 Establish and evaluate expected outcomes of care for the child with a cognitive alteration.

This chapter will provide the knowledge and tools needed to provide appropriate care for children with alterations in mental health and cognition. Mental health care is provided by psychiatric–mental health specialists, so the nurse's role often centers on identification, support of the therapy, teaching, and referral. Cognitive conditions are commonly managed by the family and the school personnel. The nurse also forms partnerships with families and school personnel to plan and evaluate care for the child with cognitive conditions such as intellectual disability (formerly called *mental retardation*). A thorough knowledge of development is a prerequisite to understanding both mental health alterations and cognitive conditions since developmental status is often altered in both mental health and cognitive conditions. Review Chapter 4 as needed to understand the relationships of development to the conditions described in this chapter.

Mental Health Alterations of Children and Adolescents

Mental health is foundational to a sense of personal well-being, physical health, and psychologic stability. It involves successful engagement in activities and relationships and the ability to

Text continues on page 792

FOCUS ON:
Mental Health and Cognition

Pediatric Differences

Some mental health and cognitive conditions in children originate from a genetic or physiologic cause—for example, intellectual disability (previously called *mental retardation*) and childhood schizophrenia. Often the family and surrounding environments in which children live influence their characteristics and contribute to dysfunctions such as anxiety, depression, and posttraumatic stress disorder. A unique and challenging interplay of genetics and environment influence mental health and cognitive conditions, thus making diagnosis and treatment challenging.

Children differ from adults both in mental health care needs and in the types and progression of mental health disruptions. During childhood, the necessity for bonding and attachment to significant adults forms the foundation of the child's healthy mental development. Therefore, young children rely on adults for establishment of mental health. The child's unique genetic makeup couples with these environmental factors, thereby contributing to a state of mental health. Cognitive disorders are also a result of a unique interplay of genetic and environmental causes. The brain develops from the fetal neural tube early in development, with much critical embryology occurring in the fourth to sixth week of gestation, at which point many women are unaware that they are pregnant. During this time, the brain is not protected by the blood–brain barrier and is at risk for injury from the fetal environment. Environmental conditions such as maternal alcohol ingestion or intake of certain medications can influence the developing fetus's brain.

In addition, children with mental health alterations sometimes display different clinical manifestations for mental illness than adults; therefore, diagnosis is difficult and challenging. For example, a child with a tic syndrome may be mistakenly diagnosed as hyperactive, and the treatment therefore would not be appropriate to the underlying condition.

At birth the brain makes up about 25% of body weight; this percentage decreases to about 2% of weight by adulthood. Most of the brain structure is present at birth, but during the first 5 years of life the brain continues to develop and mature as the young child gains fine and gross motor, social, and language skills. Development and differentiation occur during childhood spurts with fine motor skills improvement and during adolescent years when perception, motor function, and advanced thinking processes further develop. The child remains vulnerable to external forces during periods of brain growth and development. The influence of drugs, poor nutrition, traumatic brain injury, and absence of emotional nurturance are all examples of factors that can interfere with healthy brain and cognitive development.

Examples of diagnostic and laboratory tests used for mental health and cognition include magnetic resonance imaging (MRI), radiograph (x-ray), electroencephalogram, positron emission tomography (PET) scan, neuropsychologic testing, and toxicology screening (see Appendix E). Use *Assessment Guide: The Child With an Alteration in Mental Health or Cognition* to perform a nursing assessment.

The purpose of this chapter is to provide the knowledge and tools that can help you provide appropriate care for children with alterations in mental health or cognition. Much of the care for mental health alterations is provided by psychiatric–mental health specialists, so the nurse collaborates with these specialists to identify problems, support and carry out therapy, provide education for the family, and refer the family to appropriate resources. Children with mental health or cognitive disorders are sometimes hospitalized, visit well-child clinics, and attend schools. Nurses in all settings must gain the skills to provide care for these children. See Chapter 14 for a description of eating disorders.

The nurse collaborates with families and school personnel to plan and evaluate care for the child with cognitive conditions such as intellectual disability. A thorough knowledge of development is a prerequisite to understanding both mental health disruptions and cognitive conditions, because developmental status is often altered in both mental health and cognitive conditions.

Most mental health conditions are treated in community settings, and nurses in these settings play an active role in the treatment and support of the child and family. Nurses may function as case managers, assisting a family to deal with all areas of the child's care. Occasionally a child is hospitalized for treatment of a significant mental health disruption or is hospitalized for treatment of another health problem and requires continued mental health services.

ASSESSMENT GUIDE	The Child With an Alteration in Mental Health or Cognition

Assessment Focus	Assessment Guidelines
History	• Describe prenatal care and problems. Was there any trauma at birth?
	• Is there a diagnosed mental health disorder in the child or other family members?
	• Is there a history of any neurologic injuries or diseases such as cancer?
	• What medications is the child taking? What medications have been taken in the past?
	• Has there been exposure to environmental pesticides or other chemicals?
Growth	• Is growth progressing at a uniform rate so that the child maintains a similar growth percentile?
	• Is head circumference within normal limits?

(continued)

Assessment Focus	Assessment Guidelines
Development	• Perform regular developmental screening to identify any variations from expected developmental milestones. Further testing is required if screening suggests any abnormalities. • What is the progression of skills reported by the family? • Are there any unusual capabilities or deficits? • Inquire about progression in school and extracurricular activities.
Social skills	• Describe the relationship between the child and significant adults. Is close attachment evident? Are there signs of attachment disorders such as lack of eye contact, smiles, or response to others in the environment? • Describe the school-age child's daily schedule, including family and peer activities. Does the child have friends and engage in several activities with them on a regular basis? Does the child generally interact well with others? Has the child recently had a change in school performance? • Ask the teen to describe daily activities and friends. Is there a combination of peer and family influence on personal decision making?
Affect	• Describe facial expression and response to nurse. • Observe body size, position, and posture. • Are interaction behaviors typical for the setting and age of the child? • Does the child display interest in surroundings? • Is the child dressed in an appropriate manner? Does the child establish eye contact?
Appearance	• Is the child's clothing appropriate for age, setting, and developmental level?
Behaviors	• Describe level of consciousness and interaction with surroundings. • Inquire about recent reported changes in behavior (e.g., sleep, eating patterns, communication with others, school performance, friendships, risky activities). • Has the child or parent identified any problem behaviors? • Are any particular events associated with the problem behaviors?
Life events	• Has the child or family experienced recent stress or trauma? • Have there been any changes in family structure? • Evaluate chronic health conditions in family members.

adapt and cope with change. **Cognition** refers to the change in thought, intelligence, and language that occurs over time as brain maturation and life experiences interact to mutually influence child performance (Santrock, 2011).

Approximately 15 million children in the United States suffer from mental illness that is severe enough to impair functioning at home or school. Overall, about 1 in 5 children and adolescents has a mental health disorder, and 1 in 10 has a disorder that profoundly interferes with daily functioning. Up to 75% to 80% of children with mental health disorders do not receive adequate comprehensive or multidisciplinary treatment, leading to unmet mental health needs. (National Center for Children in Poverty, 2014).

Etiology and Pathophysiology

From the ages of 10 to 21 years, mental health issues are among the top two leading causes of hospitalization (see Chapter 1). This high rate of hospitalization suggests that children are not receiving clinical therapy early, when outpatient care is appropriate and prognosis is best.

Certain population groups are at increased risk for mental disorders. Children from homes with low income are twice as likely to have mental health disruptions. Approximately 50% of children in the child welfare system and 70% of youth in the

juvenile justice system have mental disorders (National Center for Children in Poverty, 2014). Children with special healthcare needs and those living in military families have particular barriers to accessing mental health services. More information about military family stress is found in Chapter 17.

There is a wide array of cognitive challenges for children, from conditions that have a genetic basis to those that are caused by prenatal or postnatal trauma or infections. Developmental surveillance often reveals cognitive disorders so that early intervention can be planned in order to maximize potential.

During all healthcare visits, mental health screening should be integrated into care so that alterations can be identified. See Chapters 7, 8, and 9 for specific questions to ask during health promotion and health maintenance visits.

Clinical Manifestations

The manifestations of mental health alterations in children are varied, but most can be identified through careful developmental and behavioral screening. Children with mental health conditions often do not display the usual developmental milestones at the times predicted. They may have social interaction problems with family members or other people, or they may have demonstrated a change in performance from former developmental achievement. Functional patterns of living such as the ability to feed and care for self, regulation of sleep and nutritional intake, and the ability to self-regulate during activities may be lacking. Repetitive actions, behavioral instability and outbursts, and withdrawal are other important signs of mental health disruption.

Clinical Therapy

Diagnosis of mental health conditions involves careful physical and psychologic assessment. Studies such as magnetic resonance imaging (MRI), radiographs, electroencephalograms, and toxicology screening may be useful. Mental health is linked to development so developmental screening tests are administered (see Chapter 6). Mental health status can influence activity level, physiologic parameters, and risk for certain conditions. Therefore, nurses should gather height and weight, review of systems, vital signs, and medication/substance use information. Family interactions, stressors, and methods of coping are assessed. When a potential mental health condition exists, the child receives further assessment from a mental health specialist. A resource commonly used is the *Diagnostic and Statistical Manual of Mental Disorders*, which lists diagnostic criteria for known mental health conditions. The current edition is the *DSM-5* (American Psychiatric Association, 2013).

> **Professionalism in Practice** *Diagnostic and Statistical Manual of Mental Disorders* **(DSM)**
>
> The *DSM-5* is the current compendium of psychiatric conditions, symptoms, and treatment. It includes screening tools and detailed information about pediatric mental health conditions such as attention deficit disorder, intellectual disability, and autism spectrum disorder. The pediatric nurse should access this information for screening tools and current evidence-based practice symptoms, and recognize the importance of acting as a person who identifies mental health disorders and refers children for appropriate care (American Psychiatric Association, 2013; Selekman & Diefenbeck, 2014).

The primary treatment goal for children and adolescents with psychosocial disorders is to assist the child and family to achieve and maintain an optimal level of functioning through interventions designed to reduce the impact of stressors. Therapeutic interventions and communication are based on the principle that feelings motivate behaviors. Parents and others close to the child often fall into the habit of reacting to the child's behaviors rather than trying to find out what feelings may be precipitating the undesirable actions. While behaviors may be considered in treatment, feelings and life experiences are often explored to provide insight and lead to behavior change. Medication may be used to enhance and support other therapy, or it may be the major therapeutic measure.

TREATMENT MODES

Three basic treatment modes are used: individual, family, and group therapy. The choice of treatment mode must take into account the child's age and developmental stage. Most therapists use several intervention strategies simultaneously. Different strategies are more or less effective and appropriate for children and adolescents in various stages of development. A thorough understanding of developmental needs, expectations, and abilities is therefore essential for mental healthcare providers.

Individual Therapy. Individual therapy involves only the child and the therapist. Treatment of specific emotional problems or disorders may involve various techniques such as play therapy, **psychodrama** (being assigned and playing out roles spontaneously in a therapeutic setting to assist in better understanding of the dynamics of a situation), art therapy, and **cognitive therapy** (a technique used to help a person recognize automatic negative thinking). Individual therapy may be short term (four to six sessions) or long term (lasting for several years).

Family Therapy. Family therapy involves the exploration of a particular emotional problem and its manifestations among the family members. Family therapy is based on the idea that the emotional symptoms or problems of an individual are an expression of emotional symptoms or problems in the family. The focus is on the relationships among the family members, not the psychologic conflict within each individual member.

Group Therapy. Group therapy involves an ongoing or limited number of sessions in which several individuals participate. The emphasis is on the interpersonal styles of relating to one another in the group. Group therapy is particularly effective with adolescents because of the importance of the peer group at this age. An advantage of group therapy is that stimuli and feedback come from multiple sources (the group members) instead of just one person (the therapist).

THERAPEUTIC STRATEGIES

Play Therapy. Play is often called the language or work of the child. From a developmental perspective, children progressively learn to express feelings and needs through action, fantasy, and finally language. The special quality of play buffers children against the pressures and demands of daily life. Play helps children master developmental stages by strengthening physical and neurologic processes. Play also assists in cognitive learning, setting the stage for problem solving and creativity.

Play therapy is a technique that reveals problems on a fantasy level through the use of toys, dolls, clay, art, and other creative objects. It is often used with preschool and school-age children who are experiencing anxiety, stress, and other specific nonpsychotic mental disorders. Play therapy encourages children to act out feelings such as anger, hostility, sadness, and fear. It also gives the therapist a chance to help children understand, on a conscious or unconscious level, their own responses and behavior in a safe, supportive environment. This type of therapy was used for Cassandra, described in the chapter-opening quotation, who needed to gain some control over a frightening environment by acting out fears and trying solutions during play with a therapist. Play therapy is different from therapeutic play, which may be used with hospitalized children (see Chapter 11). Only a specialist is qualified to provide play therapy for mental health disorders.

Art Therapy. Children who may be apprehensive about playing can sometimes be encouraged to participate in art therapy, using brief drawing exercises. This technique is appropriate for children of all ages, including adolescents. The drawings can help the therapist gain information about the child, the family, and the interactions between the child and family. However, children's drawings should never be the only basis for a definitive diagnosis.

When used in conjunction with a thorough history and appropriate psychologic testing information, art therapy can guide the child's treatment. These drawing exercises provide an opportunity to help in the healing process. The therapist can assist the child to release feelings of anger, pain, or fear onto paper, where they can be examined objectively. (Figures 28–1 to 28–4 present several examples of this technique.)

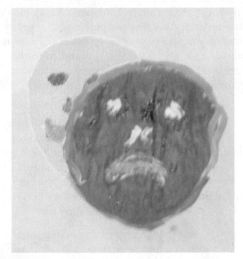

Figure 28–1 "Me." Drawn by a 14-year-old girl with major depression, anxiety, and school phobia who had experienced multiple losses over several years. Her mother had severe chronic lung problems and diabetes, and the girl had stopped attending school for fear that something would happen to her mother. This drawing represents the girl's obvious feelings of sadness and depression but also indicates a glimmer of hope (represented by the yellow mask coming from behind the dark mask of depression).

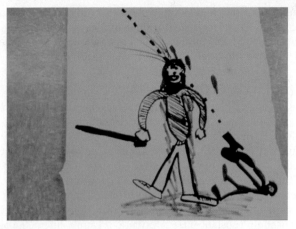

Figure 28–2 "Self-Portrait." Drawn by a 15-year-old boy who was admitted through the emergency department after a failed suicide attempt by hanging. He had a psychiatric diagnosis of depression and polysubstance abuse (including inhalants and alcohol), and he insisted that he was a member of a satanic cult in his hometown. Most of his drawings depicted a preoccupation with violence and suicide. The boy said that he always felt a "darkness" like a shadow that followed him around and wanted him dead. His family history was significant for depression and suicide on both his mother's and his father's side. His father also had a lengthy history of polysubstance abuse and alcoholism. The boy was discharged to a long-term residential treatment facility for adolescents.

Figure 28–3 "An Activity." Drawn by an 8-year-old boy who was initially admitted to the medical–surgical floor of a pediatric hospital for dehydration resulting from vomiting and diarrhea. Psychiatric evaluation was ordered for extreme anxiety. These drawings, completed during the initial interview, led to further investigation, which revealed that the child had started a house fire in which his grandmother (his primary caretaker at the time) was killed. The family's home and all their belongings were lost. No one had known that the child had set the fire. Further sessions indicated that he had been setting neighborhood garage fires and watching them burn from a distance.

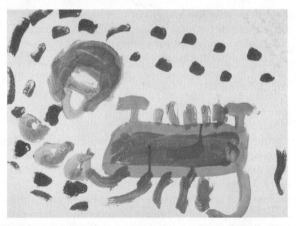

Figure 28–4 "A Family Activity." By the same boy who drew Figure 28–3. This drawing depicts a recurring incident of physical and emotional abuse by his mother's live-in boyfriend. It shows the family bathtub with feces and blood smeared on the floors and walls. The boy reported that when either he or his 3-year-old brother had a toileting accident the boyfriend would make them go into the bathroom and stand in the bathtub while he smeared the feces on the walls. He would then hit the children and make them clean up the mess. The boy had previously been removed from the mother's custody for neglect. He was transferred from the medical–surgical area to the inpatient children's psychiatric unit, where he received a diagnosis of depression, overanxious disorder, and child abuse (physical and emotional). Charges were filed against the mother's boyfriend and custody of both children was temporarily revoked.

Cognitive and Behavioral Therapy (CBT).

A combination of cognitive and behavioral therapy is useful in treating many mental health conditions in children. Cognitive therapy teaches thinking patterns to change reactions to situations that cause anxiety or other undesirable conditions. Children are taught how their brain and body are working; this understanding assists them in having control over the experience and responding with appropriate behaviors (Mayo Clinic, 2013a).

Behavior modification is a therapeutic technique that uses stimulus and response conditioning to alter inappropriate behaviors. It reinforces desirable behaviors, helping the child to replace maladaptive behaviors with more appropriate ones. This technique is based on the assumption that any learned behavior can be unlearned. Thus, if parents, nurses, teachers, and other adults consistently reinforce desirable behaviors, the child will eventually alter or discontinue undesirable behaviors.

Behavior modification may include (1) removing the child from the home to a more structured environment, such as a hospital, for a brief time, and (2) teaching the parents, teachers, and other appropriate adults to be agents of behavioral change. Several ongoing sessions may be required with the adults involved, using role playing and other techniques. Consistency is the most important principle in the success of behavior modification.

Visualization and Guided Imagery.

The techniques of visualization and guided imagery begin with specific directions for progressive relaxation according to the child's ability. This form of therapy uses the child's own imagination and positive thinking to reduce stress and anxiety, decrease the experience of pain or discomfort, and promote healing. The techniques are especially useful for managing anxiety disorders and chronic pain. It is not easy for all children to use their imagination in this way, so the technique may not work or be appropriate for everyone.

Hypnosis.

Hypnosis involves varying degrees of suggestibility and deep relaxation effects. This technique is useful for children and adolescents because they can usually be hypnotized more easily than adults. Hypnosis is especially helpful in treating physical symptoms with a psychologic component, anxiety, and phobias. It is also useful in managing severe physical symptoms or discomfort (pain or nausea) associated with a physiologic disorder or its treatment (e.g., cancer or juvenile rheumatoid arthritis).

Nursing Management

Ongoing assessment of all children and their families for mental health risk should be performed from the beginning of life and throughout childhood and adolescence. When a potential mental health condition exists, the child should receive further assessment from a mental health specialist. Nursing assessment focuses on child behaviors, family interactions, lifestyle routines, developmental progression, and treatment for mental health or cognitive conditions (see *Assessment Guide: The Child With an Alteration in Mental Health or Cognition* earlier in this chapter).

Many mental health disorders are managed effectively with therapy, medication, or both on an outpatient basis, whereas some necessitate admission to an inpatient psychiatric setting. Therefore, the nurse may encounter the child with a mental health disorder in a variety of community settings or during hospitalization for a concurrent psychiatric or physiologic problem.

EVIDENCE-BASED PRACTICE | Pharmacogenetics and the Nursing Role

Clinical Question
Great variability is seen in the response to psychotropic medicines used to treat mental health disorders such as depression. Children and adolescents show even more variability than adults, related to developmental variation in absorption, distribution, metabolism, and elimination; therefore, close monitoring is essential (Madadi, 2015). How can the nurse apply new technologies about individualized treatments to medications when providing mental health care for youth?

The Evidence
The fields of genetics and genomics are growing rapidly (see Chapter 3). Currently, pharmacogenetic testing is being used so that clinicians can select the best psychotropic medications for particular clients. For example, a genetic test for a gene that codes for high manufacture of a body enzyme that metabolizes a particular medication predicts that the client will not respond well to that medication. Another psychotropic can be chosen to enhance response. On the other hand, if the client is a slow metabolizer of the medication, an increased risk of toxicity results. A tailored approach to treatment of attention deficit hyperactivity disorder (ADHD) has the potential to target specific gene patterns rather than using a trial-and-error approach to types of medications tried (Bruxel et al., 2014). Community treatment of mental health disorders has the potential to be enhanced by identification of the best drug to treat a given person. Nurses are called on to collect genetic samples (often from inside the mouth) and explain the procedure and results to families (Bartlett, 2011; Haga, O'Daniel, Tindall, et al., 2012). These roles demand that nurses understand genomics and pharmacogenetics in order to translate concepts to families (Knisely, Carpenter, & Von Ah, 2014).

Best Practice
The nurse in a setting where children and adolescents are treated for psychiatric disorders has an important role in applying new knowledge related to pharmacogenetics. First, the nurse needs to take a careful history of medications, over-the-counter products, and herbal remedies because many of these substances compete with psychotropic medications for metabolism in the body. When a DNA test is recommended prior to beginning medication, families need to understand the reason for the test. They will also need explanations about the test results and how they relate to the specific medication that has been prescribed. It is important that all children and adolescents receiving psychotropic medications be closely monitored for responses and side effects. The nurse is integral to the ongoing evaluation of the prescribed therapy (Kniseley et al., 2014).

Clinical Reasoning
What is the nursing role in history taking and in monitoring for the child or adolescent on psychotropic medication? What questions do you think a family is likely to ask when they learn that a genetic test is recommended before prescribing medication to an adolescent experiencing a mental health disruption such as severe depression? Where will you find the information about pharmacogenetics and pharmacogenomics that will provide necessary background for you and the family? How can pharmacogenetic testing enhance the treatment of individuals by both leading to a therapeutic response in a short time and avoiding serious side effects?

In the hospital, nursing care includes carrying out the prescribed treatment plan and administering psychotropic medications. Evaluate the child's medication regimen for administration schedule, dosage, side effects, and effectiveness. See accompanying *Evidence-Based Practice: Pharmacogenetics and the Nursing Role*.

An important nursing intervention is to ensure safety of the child. Actions begin in the emergency department if a child is admitted for a mental health crisis. Remove or lock up potentially dangerous material such as medications, tubing, and sharps containers that may be in the child's room. A parent, guardian, or healthcare provider should remain with the child at all times. Inform the family member of the need to stay with the child and how to immediately notify the nurse if the adult needs to leave or if the child's condition changes. Part of the initial care is to evaluate risk by asking if the child has tried to hurt himself/herself or has been thinking about it. Ask about recent stresses, thoughts of hurting someone else, and why the child thinks she/he has been brought to the emergency department. If the child is admitted to the psychiatric unit, follow unit policies for ensuring safety for children who are at risk of hurting themselves or others.

Developing Cultural Competence Spiritual Beliefs and Mental Health

In many cultures, care of the "spirit" is believed necessary to promote mental health. An identity with one's community and spiritual wholeness is promoted by storytelling, singing, rites of passage, and use of certain objects such as bags of herbs. Use of healers, family and community support, relaxation or meditation, exorcism, or other procedures may be used by families. Ask what the family believes about mental health, and integrate safe and culturally acceptable practices into the plan of care to enhance the child's mental health.

Psychiatric hospitalization is a stressful event for all families, and both the family and child need supportive care. Continuation of family involvement is critical. The nurse frequently is the liaison between the family and the therapist in making follow-up arrangements at the time of discharge. Be aware of the meaning of mental illness in various cultural groups and the treatments that may be commonly used. Integrate these complementary therapies into the care plan whenever safe. Families must feel that their responses and approaches to the child with a mental disorder are not judged by healthcare providers.

The nurse in the community assesses how a child with a mental health disorder is functioning in each microsystem, such as home, day care, school, and with friends. Assess risk and protective factors of the child and family (see Chapter 4). Evaluate involvement in therapy sessions and ability to manage prescribed pharmacologic interventions.

Developmental and Behavioral Disorders

Autism Spectrum Disorder (Neurodevelopmental Disorder)

An estimated 12% to 16% of children have a developmental or behavioral disorder. The most common group of disorders is called *autism spectrum disorder (ASD)*, which affects about 14.7/1000 children (Centers for Disease Control and Prevention [CDC], 2012a, 2014a). This neurodevelopmental disorder begins in early childhood and is characterized by impaired social interactions and communication, with restricted interests, activities, and behaviors, and repetitive patterns of behavior (American Psychiatric Association, 2013). ASD may be accompanied by other neurodevelopmental, mental, or behavioral conditions, so the manifestations can differ significantly among individuals. ASD is comprised of autism, Asperger syndrome, pervasive developmental disorder not otherwise specified, Rett syndrome, and childhood disintegrative disorder. The present incidence of ASD represents an increase from formerly described levels; before 1985, less than 1 child in 1000 was diagnosed with an autistic disorder. It is unclear whether there is a true increase in cases or simply improved techniques in making the diagnosis, as well as an enlarged diagnostic category that includes more children. The disorder is more common in males than females; peak age at diagnosis is 8 years, but symptoms often begin by 12 to 24 months of age (CDC, 2012a, 2014a).

ETIOLOGY AND PATHOPHYSIOLOGY

The etiology of autism spectrum disorder is unknown. Genes are clearly involved, although a complex array of genes appears to be responsible (Frye, 2014). Immune responses, environmental exposures, certain drugs during pregnancy, and neuroanatomy are being investigated as influences that interact with genetics to cause ASDs (CDC, 2014a; Won, Mah, & Kim, 2013). Neurotransmitters such as dopamine, serotonin, and opioids are abnormal in some children and are a focus of research. Fetal alcohol syndrome, fragile X syndrome, phenylketonuria, Down syndrome, and tuberous sclerosis are all associated with a higher than normal incidence of autism (Won et al., 2013). Despite concern expressed in earlier medical and lay press, no demonstrated relationship has been demonstrated between the measles-mumps-rubella vaccine or thimerosal (mercury-based preservative in some vaccines) and the incidence of ASDs (see Chapter 16 for further information on immunizations) (Maglione et al., 2014).

CLINICAL MANIFESTATIONS

The essential features of autism spectrum disorder typically become apparent by the time a child is 3 years of age. They involve impairments in socialization, communication, and behavior (Harrington, 2013; Webb, 2011). Children with ASD are unable to relate to people in a manner that is common for young children, or to respond to social and emotional cues. In addition, they may engage in **stereotypy**, or rigid, repetitive, and machine-like movement with obsessive behavior (Figure 28–5). Characteristically, these repetitive behaviors in affected children include head banging, twirling in circles, biting themselves, and flapping their hands or arms. Frequently, a child's behavior is self-stimulating or self-destructive. Responses to sensory stimuli are frequently abnormal and include an extreme aversion to touch, loud noises, and bright lights. Emotional lability is common.

Communication difficulties or delays in speech and language are common, and are often the first symptoms that lead to diagnosis. Abnormal communication patterns include both verbal and nonverbal communication. Absence of babbling and other communication by age 1 year, absence of two-word phrases by age 2 years, and deterioration of previous language skills are characteristic. Children with ASD may eventually learn to talk, in some cases well, but their speech is likely to show certain abnormalities: use of *you* in place of *I*; **echolalia** (a compulsive parroting of what is heard); repeating questions rather than answering them; and fascination with rhythmic, repetitive songs and verses.

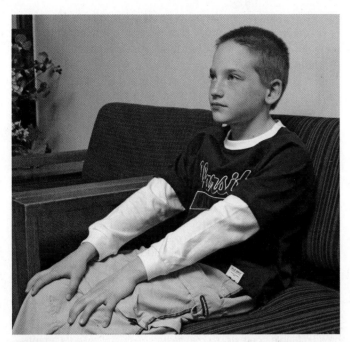

Figure 28–5 **Stereotypy. This child with ASD sits stiffly in the chair and engages in rhythmic rocking behavior. He has a disengaged look and does not readily interact with other children or adults who are in his environment.**

Behaviors of children with ASD show several differences from other children. They do not commonly explore objects but display stereotypy. They may line up objects, play with the same objects over and over, and have certain rituals that must be performed. They often become upset if these normal routines are disrupted. Rituals may involve eating only certain types or colors of foods or eating in specific patterns. Children may manifest disturbances in the rate or sequence of development. They frequently have cognitive impairment but can demonstrate a wide range of intellectual ability and functioning. Cognitive impairment may manifest early in life as slow developmental progression, particularly in social skills. Some children are impaired in particular areas of development, whereas others are above normal.

The clinical manifestations common in autistic spectrum disorder are listed in Table 28–1.

CLINICAL THERAPY

The first step in identifying children at risk of ASD is surveillance at each healthcare visit. Since diagnosis and treatment have often been delayed, the American Academy of Pediatrics has now identified a multistage process for surveillance and screening:

1. Perform surveillance at early healthcare visits to identify if a sibling has ASD, parents or other caregivers are concerned about the developmental progression of the child, or the healthcare provider notes abnormalities in child behavior.

2. The healthcare provider determines if the child appears to be at risk for ASD.

3. The healthcare provider evaluates the risks. If risk exists, the provider administers an age-appropriate and ASD-specific screening tool (e.g., Ages and Stages Questionnaire and Modified Checklist for Autism in Toddlers [M-CHAT]).

4. If no risk exists, an ASD-specific tool is administered at the 18- and 24-month visits.

5. Select appropriate screening tool for age and risk profile of the child.

6. If screening is negative for a child with some risk, provide information to parents and evaluate again in 1 month. If screening is positive, refer for comprehensive ASD evaluation, including audiology, and begin early intervention programs (Harrington, 2013; Johnson et al., 2007, reaffirmed, 2010; Webb, 2011).

Several screening tests are available for use in health maintenance visits if autistic disorder is suspected. Additional testing is performed to rule out other causes of the child's behavior. Tests may include neuroimaging (CT scan or MRI), lead screening,

TABLE 28–1 Clinical Manifestations of Autism Spectrum Disorder

CLINICAL MANIFESTATIONS	CLINICAL THERAPY
Impaired social, communicative, and behavioral development, usually noted in first year of life.	Early intervention is key to maximal performance. Interventions focus on improving behaviors and communication skills, providing physical and occupational therapy, structuring play interactions with other children, and educating parents about the child's needs.
Impaired social interactions with normal language development for age; pitch, tone, and other speech characteristics may be abnormal. Verbal skills involving spelling and vocabulary are high but concept formation, language flexibility, and comprehension are low. Intellectual functioning may be at a high level, particularly in certain areas, whereas social skills are limited.	Social interactions are focus of therapy.
Early development often appears normal, but symptoms emerge at 6–18 months. Ataxia, handwringing, intermittent hyperventilation, dementia, and growth retardation show progressive increase. Appears only in females as an X-linked dominant disorder; mutations occur in the *MeCP2* gene, affecting methyl-CpG–binding protein 2, which is important in brain development.	Early intervention in areas of abnormal behaviors.
First 2–5 years of development appear normal followed by deterioration in many areas of functioning. Behaviors finally stabilize at some point without further deterioration.	Focus on areas of developmental function that show abnormality. Individualized education plans are needed in school to deal with communication, play, physical therapy, and teaching management skills to parents. Regression in toileting and other skills may occur.
Severe social impairment without meeting *DSM* criteria for other types of autistic spectrum disorder.	Behavioral therapy focuses on building social skills.

metabolic studies, DNA analysis, and electroencephalogram. See Chapters 5 and 27 for further descriptions related to neurologic system assessment. Diagnosis is based on the presence of specific criteria, as described in the American Psychiatric Association's *DSM-5* (see Table 28–2).

Early intervention helps maximize the child's potential by improving developmental skills and behaviors, as well as establishing helpful support for parents. Treatment focuses on behavior management to reward appropriate behaviors (called *applied behavior analysis [ABA]*), foster positive or adaptive coping skills, and facilitate effective communication. The goals of treatment are to reduce rigidity or stereotypy and other maladaptive behaviors. Some children must be physically restrained from aggressive or self-destructive behaviors. Speech therapy is an essential part of treatment. Instruction in social skills and occupational therapy to improve fine motor dexterity and sensory integration are provided. Some parents choose to use complementary therapies.

The overall prognosis for children with ASD to become functioning members of society varies. Successful adjustment is more likely for children with higher IQs, adequate speech, and access to specialized programs.

Nursing Management

For the Child With ASD or Neurodevelopmental Disorder

Nursing Assessment and Diagnosis

The nurse may encounter the child with ASD during routine well-child visits, or when parents seek care for a suspected hearing impairment, speech difficulty, or developmental delay. Early and frequent developmental screening of all children can help in referral for thorough assessment and identification of cases. Be alert to parental observations that the baby or young child does

---

TABLE 28–2 *DSM-5* **Diagnostic Criteria for Autistic Spectrum Disorder**

1. Persistent deficits in social communication and social interaction across multiple contexts, as manifested by the following, currently or by history (examples are illustrative, not exhaustive):
   - Deficits in social-emotional reciprocity, ranging, for example, from abnormal social approach and failure of normal back-and-forth conversation; to reduced sharing of interests, emotions, or affect; to failure to initiate or respond to social interactions.
   - Deficits in nonverbal communicative behaviors used for social interaction, ranging, for example, from poorly integrated verbal and nonverbal communication; to abnormalities in eye contact and body language or deficits in understanding and use of gestures; to a total lack of facial expressions and nonverbal communication.
   - Deficits in developing, maintaining, and understanding relationships, ranging, for example, from difficulties adjusting behavior to suit various social contexts; to difficulties in sharing imaginative play or in making friends; to absence of interest in peers.

   Specify current severity:
   - Severity is based on social communication impairments and restricted, repetitive patterns of behavior.

2. Restricted, repetitive patterns of behavior, interests, or activities, as manifested by at least two of the following, currently or by history (examples are illustrative, not exhaustive; see text):
   - Stereotyped or repetitive motor movements, use of objects, or speech (e.g., simple motor stereotypies, lining up toys or flipping objects, echolalia, idiosyncratic phrases).
   - Insistence on sameness, inflexible adherence to routines, or ritualized patterns of verbal or nonverbal behavior (e.g., extreme distress at small changes, difficulties with transitions, rigid thinking patterns, greeting rituals, need to take same route or eat same food every day).
   - Highly restricted, fixated interests that are abnormal in intensity or focus (e.g., strong attachment to or preoccupation with unusual objects, excessively circumscribed or perseverative interests).
   - Hyper- or hyporeactivity to sensory input or unusual interest in sensory aspects of the environment (e.g., apparent indifference to pain/temperature, adverse response to specific sounds or textures, excessive smelling or touching of objects, visual fascination with lights or movement).

   Specify current severity:
   - Severity is based on social communication impairments and restricted, repetitive patterns of behavior.

3. Symptoms must be present in the early developmental period (but may not become fully manifest until social demands exceed limited capacities, or may be masked by learned strategies in later life).
4. Symptoms cause clinically significant impairment in social, occupational, or other important areas of current functioning.
5. These disturbances are not better explained by intellectual disability (intellectual developmental disorder) or global developmental delay. Intellectual disability and autism spectrum disorder frequently co-occur; to make comorbid diagnoses of autism spectrum disorder and intellectual disability, social communication should be below that expected for general developmental level.

Note: Individuals with a well-established *DSM-IV* diagnosis of autistic disorder, Asperger's disorder, or pervasive developmental disorder not otherwise specified should be given the diagnosis of autism spectrum disorder. Individuals who have marked deficits in social communication, but whose symptoms do not otherwise meet criteria for autism spectrum disorder, should be evaluated for social (pragmatic) communication disorder.

Specify if:
- With or without accompanying intellectual impairment
- With or without accompanying language impairment
- Associated with a known medical or genetic condition or environmental factor
- Associated with another neurodevelopmental, mental, or behavioral disorder

Source: Used with permission from American Psychiatric Association. (2013). *Diagnostic and statistical manual of mental disorders* (5th ed.). Washington, DC: Author. Copyright © 2013 American Psychiatric Association.

not look at them or provides other developmental or behavioral cues. Parents may report abnormal interaction such as lack of eye contact, disinterest in cuddling, minimal facial responsiveness, and failure to talk. Be alert for the "red flags": no babbling or communication gestures by 12 months, no single word by 16 months, no spontaneous two-word phrases by 24 months, or loss of language or social skills previously achieved (Johnson et al., 2007, reaffirmed 2010).

Assessment at every healthcare visit focuses on language development, response to others, and hearing acuity (see Chapters 4 and 5). Specialized screening tests for ASD may be administered. Pediatric nurses in outpatient settings should ensure that a variety of autism screening tools for different ages of children are available and used in healthcare settings (Webb, 2011).

When a child with a diagnosis of autistic disorder is hospitalized for a concurrent problem, obtain a history from the parents about the child's routines, rituals, and likes and dislikes, as well as ways to promote interaction and cooperation. Children with ASD may carry a special toy or object that they play with during times of stress. Ask parents about these objects and their use. Document this information in the clinical record.

Ask about the child's behaviors and observe them on admission. Obtain a history of acute and chronic illnesses and injuries. Ask about eating patterns and food restrictions. Inquire about complementary and alternative medicine treatments in a non-judgmental and supportive manner.

Nursing diagnoses must be tailored to fit the individual needs of the child. Examples of nursing diagnoses that might be appropriate for children with ASD include the following (NANDA-I © 2014):

- *Communication: Verbal, Impaired,* related to psychologic condition
- *Social Interaction, Impaired,* related to developmental disability
- *Injury, Risk for,* related to cognitive impairment
- *Caregiver Role Strain, Risk for,* related to chronicity and demands of child's condition
- *Coping: Family, Compromised,* related to having a child with prolonged disability

Planning and Implementation

Nursing care focuses on stabilizing environmental stimuli, providing supportive care, enhancing communication, maintaining a safe environment, giving the parents anticipatory guidance, and providing community-based care.

STABILIZE ENVIRONMENTAL STIMULI

Children with ASD interpret and respond to the environment differently from other individuals. Sounds that are not distressing to the average person may be interpreted by children with ASD as louder, more frightening, and overwhelming. The child needs to be oriented to new settings such as a classroom or the hospital room, and may adjust best to a small classroom or to a hospital room with only one other child. Encourage parents to bring the child's favorite objects from home, and try to keep these objects in the same places because the child does not cope well with changes in the environment.

PROVIDE SUPPORTIVE CARE

Developing a trusting relationship with the child with ASD is often difficult. Adjust communication techniques and teaching to the child's developmental level. Ask parents about the child's usual home routines, and maintain these routines as much as possible when the child is out of the home. Because self-care abilities are often limited, the child may need help meeting basic needs. School programs and individualized education plans (IEPs) (see Chapter 12) can help the child learn self-care skills. When possible, schedule daily care and routine procedures at consistent times to maintain predictability. Encourage parents to remain with the hospitalized child and to participate in daily care planning. Parents are integral parts of the treatment team when the child's learning goals are established in early intervention or school programs. Identify rituals for naptime and bedtime, and maintain them to promote rest and sleep. Establish patterns that help the child eat nutritious foods at mealtimes.

Use of complementary medicine for children with autistic spectrum disorder is common. Parents choose modalities such as special diets, use of supplements and vitamins, herbs, auditory training, hyperbaric treatment, chiropractic manipulation, and nonprescription medications such as melatonin (Valicenti-McDermott et al., 2014). Nurses should inquire about use of complementary therapies and provide information for the family to ensure safe practices.

ENHANCE COMMUNICATION

Since children with ASD have impaired communication, nursing care focuses on using and improving communication with the child. Speech is used when possible; short, direct sentences are usually most effective. When the child responds well to visual cues, pictures, computers, and other visual aids may form an important part of interactions. Some children use sign language.

MAINTAIN A SAFE ENVIRONMENT

Monitor children with ASD at all times, including bath time and bedtime. Close supervision is needed to ensure that the child does not obtain any harmful objects or engage in dangerous behaviors. Bicycle helmets and mittens are sometimes used to protect children with ASD so that they can safely participate in activities.

PROVIDE ANTICIPATORY GUIDANCE

Approximately half of all children with autistic disorder require lifelong supervision and support. This is especially true if the disorder is accompanied by intellectual disability (mental retardation). Some children may grow up to lead independent lives, although they will have social limitations with impaired interpersonal relationships. Encourage parents to promote the child's development through behavior modification and specialized educational programs. The overall goal is to provide the child with the guidance, education, and support necessary for optimal functioning.

COMMUNITY-BASED NURSING CARE

Families need a great deal of support to cope with the challenges of caring for the child with ASD. The diagnosis may trigger feelings of grief and shock. Help the family identify resources for child care, such as special toddler programs, preschools, and parent support groups. The child will need an individualized education and health plan; the school nurse is instrumental in establishing these plans. The parent or primary caretaker often has a hard time getting respite care and may need assistance to find suitable resources. Siblings of the child with ASD may need help explaining the disorder to their friends or teachers. Family support programs are available in some states to provide assistance to parents.

Offer the family resources for genetic counseling. Parents need information about the need for immunizations since they may have heard erroneous information about a connection between immunization and the disorder. Encourage parents to have the child immunized on the recommended schedule. Parents may have questions about where to find information on complementary and alternative therapies.

Local support groups for parents of children with ASD exist in most areas. Parents can also be referred to the Autism Society of America, the American Academy of Pediatrics, and the Centers for Disease Control and Prevention for information.

Evaluation

Expected outcomes of nursing care for the child with ASD include the following:

- Behavioral symptoms are effectively managed.
- The child performs elements of self-care.
- The child remains free from injury.
- Consistent developmental progression is observed.
- The child develops successful communication strategies.

Attention Deficit Disorder and Attention Deficit Hyperactivity Disorder

Attention deficit disorder (ADD) is a variation in central nervous system processing characterized by developmentally inappropriate behaviors involving inattention. When hyperactivity and impulsivity accompany inattention, the disorder is called *attention deficit hyperactivity disorder (ADHD)*. The latter is the more common condition and affects about 11% of school-age children; boys (13.2%) are affected more often than girls (5.6%) (CDC, 2014b). It is also known to affect adolescents and adults, and those with the disorder often continue to manifest at least some of the symptoms as they grow into adulthood. Hyperactivity and impulsivity may improve as the child nears adulthood, with inattentiveness being the most persistent characteristic.

ETIOLOGY AND PATHOPHYSIOLOGY

Although a variety of physical and neurologic disorders are associated with ADHD, children with identifiable causes represent a small proportion of this population. Examples of known associations include exposure to high levels of lead or mercury in childhood and prenatal exposure to alcohol or tobacco smoke. Other prenatal factors associated with a higher incidence of ADHD include preterm labor, impaired placenta functioning, and impaired oxygenation. Seizures and serious head injury are other potential associations. Genetic factors may be important, as well as family dynamics and environmental characteristics. Although ADHD occurs more commonly within families (25% have a first-degree relative with the disorder), a single gene has not been located and a specific mechanism of genetic transmission is not known. It is believed that a genetic predisposition interacts with the child's environment, so that both factors contribute to the appearance of the condition. Family stress, poverty, and poor nutrition may also be contributing factors. Although daily television exposure at ages 1 to 3 years has been associated with attention symptoms of the condition later in childhood, not all studies verify this finding (Ferguson, 2011; van Egmond-Frohlich, Weghuber, & de Zwaan, 2012). It is likely that there are many types of attention deficit, resulting from several different mechanisms that involve interaction of genetic, biologic, and environmental risk factors.

The pathophysiology of ADD/ADHD is not totally known. However, some children exhibit a deficit in the catecholamines dopamine and norepinephrine, lowering the threshold for stimuli input. The disorder is marked by brain maturation delay in the area of self-regulation. Increased input from stimuli and decreased self-regulation cause the hallmark inability to inhibit stimuli and motor activity. Slow brain maturity, in the first 3 years of life, has now been demonstrated on imaging studies. The cortex is particularly affected and may explain the school and concentration difficulty associated with the disorder (National Institutes of Health [NIH], 2012).

CLINICAL MANIFESTATIONS

Children with ADD and ADHD have problems related to decreased attention span, impulsiveness, or increased motor activity. Symptoms can range from mild to severe. The disorders often coexist with various developmental learning disabilities. The child has difficulty completing tasks, fidgets constantly, is frequently loud, and interrupts others. Sleep disturbances are common. Because of these behaviors, the child often has difficulty developing and maintaining social relationships and may be shunned or teased by other children. This only increases the anxiety of the already compromised child, whose behavior is set on a downward-spiraling course.

Typically, girls with ADHD show less aggression and impulsiveness than boys, but far more anxiety, mood swings, social withdrawal, rejection, and cognitive and language problems. Girls tend to be older at the time of diagnosis. Children are frequently diagnosed with the disorder soon after beginning school, with its demands for attentive behavior.

CLINICAL THERAPY

Children are usually brought for evaluation when behaviors escalate to the point of interfering with the daily functioning of teachers or parents. Any child from ages 4 through 18 years who has academic problems, behavior difficulties, inattention, hyperactivity, or impulsivity should be evaluated for ADHD (Subcommittee on Attention-Deficit/Hyperactivity Disorder [Subcommittee on ADHD], 2011). When children have learning disabilities or anxiety disorders, the problem is commonly misdiagnosed as ADHD if full and accurate evaluation of the child's symptoms is not performed. Obtaining an accurate diagnosis after comprehensive testing by a pediatric mental health specialist is vital (NIH, 2012). Specific diagnostic criteria must be applied to all children with the potential diagnosis (see *DSM-5* criteria in Table 28–3). The diagnosis of ADD is often difficult because of the absence of hyperactivity behaviors. Behaviors at home, school, or childcare centers must be evaluated because abnormal patterns in two settings are needed for diagnosis. A variety of tests are available for use by the trained professional in establishing the diagnosis.

Diagnosis begins with a careful history of the child, including family history, birth history, growth and developmental milestones, behaviors such as sleeping and eating patterns, progression and patterns in school, social and environmental conditions, reports from parents and teachers, and any other emotional or behavioral condition (Subcommittee on ADHD, 2011). A physical examination should be performed to rule out neurologic diseases and other health problems. The mental health specialist then performs testing of the child and administers questionnaires to the parent and teacher. It is important to identify other conditions that may either mimic ADD/ADHD or exist in conjunction with the disorders. These might include depression, anxiety, learning disorder, conduct disorder, or oppositional defiant disorder.

Treatment is established to meet the desired behavioral outcomes, and includes a combination of approaches, such as environmental changes, behavior therapy, and pharmacotherapy. The condition is chronic, so assessment should be ongoing for follow-up and evaluation of other mental health conditions (Brown, 2012).

TABLE 28–3 *DSM-5* Diagnostic Criteria for Attention Deficit Hyperactivity Disorder

A. A persistent pattern of inattention and/or hyperactivity-impulsivity that interferes with functioning or development, as characterized by 1 and/or 2:

  1. *Inattention:* Six (or more) of the following symptoms have persisted for at least 6 months to a degree that is inconsistent with developmental level and that negatively impacts directly on social and academic/occupational activities:

    a. **Note:** The symptoms are not solely a manifestation of oppositional behavior, defiance, hostility, or failure to understand tasks or instructions. For older adolescents and adults (age 17 and older), at least five symptoms are required.

    b. Often fails to give close attention to details or makes careless mistakes in schoolwork, at work, or during other activities (e.g., overlooks or misses details, work is inaccurate).

    c. Often has difficulty sustaining attention in tasks or play activities (e.g., has difficulty remaining focused during lectures, conversations, or lengthy reading).

    d. Often does not seem to listen when spoken to directly (e.g., mind seems elsewhere, even in the absence of any obvious distraction).

    e. Often does not follow through on instructions and fails to finish schoolwork, chores, or duties in the workplace (e.g., starts tasks but quickly loses focus and is easily sidetracked).

    f. Often has difficulty organizing tasks and activities (e.g., difficulty managing sequential tasks; difficulty keeping materials and belongings in order; messy, disorganized work; has poor time management; fails to meet deadlines).

    g. Often avoids, dislikes, or is reluctant to engage in tasks that require sustained mental effort (e.g., schoolwork or homework; for older adolescents and adults, preparing reports, completing forms, reviewing lengthy papers).

    h. Often loses things necessary for tasks or activities (e.g., school materials, pencils, books, tools, wallets, keys, paperwork, eyeglasses, mobile telephones).

    i. Is often easily distracted by extraneous stimuli (for older adolescents and adults, may include unrelated thoughts).

    j. Is often forgetful in daily activities (e.g., doing chores, running errands; for older adolescents and adults, returning calls, paying bills, keeping appointments).

  2. *Hyperactivity and impulsivity:* Six (or more) of the following symptoms have persisted for at least 6 months to a degree that is inconsistent with developmental level and that negatively impacts directly on social and academic/occupational activities:

    a. **Note:** The symptoms are not solely a manifestation of oppositional behavior, defiance, hostility, or a failure to understand tasks or instructions. For older adolescents and adults (age 17 and older), at least five symptoms are required.

    b. Often fidgets with or taps hands or feet or squirms in seat.

    c. Often leaves seat in situations when remaining seated is expected (e.g., leaves his or her place in the classroom, in the office or other workplace, or in other situations that require remaining in place).

    d. Often runs about or climbs in situations where it is inappropriate. **(Note:** In adolescents or adults, may be limited to feeling restless.)

    e. Often unable to play or engage in leisure activities quietly.

    f. Is often "on the go," acting as if "driven by a motor" (e.g., is unable to be or uncomfortable being still for extended time, as in restaurants, meetings; may be experienced by others as being restless or difficult to keep up with).

    g. Often talks excessively.

    h. Often blurts out an answer before a question has been completed (e.g., completes people's sentences; cannot wait for turn in conversation).

    i. Often has difficulty waiting his or her turn (e.g., while waiting in line).

    j. Often interrupts or intrudes on others (e.g., butts into conversations, games, or activities; may start using other people's things without asking or receiving permission; for adolescents and adults, may intrude into or take over what others are doing).

B. Several inattentive or hyperactive-impulsive symptoms were present prior to age 12 years.

C. Several inattentive or hyperactive-impulsive symptoms are present in two or more settings (e.g., at home, school, or work; with friends or relatives; in other activities).

D. There is clear evidence that the symptoms interfere with, or reduce the quality of, social, academic, or occupational functioning.

E. The symptoms do not occur exclusively during the course of schizophrenia or another psychotic disorder and are not better explained by another mental disorder (e.g., mood disorder, anxiety disorder, dissociative disorder, personality disorder, substance intoxication or withdrawal).

Specify whether:

- **Combined presentation:** If both Criterion A1 (inattention) and Criterion A2 (hyperactivity-impulsivity) are met for the past 6 months.

- **Predominantly inattentive presentation:** If Criterion A1 (inattention) is met but Criterion A2 (hyperactivity-impulsivity) is not met for the past 6 months.

- **Predominantly hyperactive/impulsive presentation:** If Criterion A2 (hyperactivity-impulsivity) is met and Criterion A1 (inattention) is not met for the past 6 months.

Specify if:

- **In partial remission:** When full criteria were previously met, fewer than the full criteria have been met for the past 6 months, and the symptoms still result in impairment in social, academic, or occupational functioning.

Specify current severity:

- **Mild:** Few, if any, symptoms in excess of those required to make the diagnosis are present, and symptoms result in no more than minor impairments in social or occupational functioning.

- **Moderate:** Symptoms or functional impairment between "mild" and "severe" are present.

- **Severe:** Many symptoms in excess of those required to make the diagnosis, or several symptoms that are particularly severe, are present, or the symptoms result in marked impairment in social or occupational functioning.

Children often benefit from environmental changes. Decreasing stimulation—for example, by turning off television, keeping the environment quiet, and maintaining an orderly and clutter-free desk or study area without distraction—may help the child to stay focused on the task at hand. Another relatively simple change is appropriate classroom placement, preferably in a small class with a teacher who can provide close supervision and a structured daily routine. Consistent limits and expectations should be set for the child. Children living in chaotic homes and communities may function better if the environment can be simplified. When aggressive behaviors occur, therapeutic approaches such as play and group therapy may be useful.

Behavior therapy involves rewarding the child for desired behaviors and applying consequences for undesirable behaviors. Children may be rewarded by praise or earn points toward a movie or other desired outing for staying seated during meals or quietly listening in a classroom. All adults who are in close contact with the child, such as parents and teachers, must be educated to carry out the behavioral program (Subcommittee on ADHD, 2011).

Children with moderate to severe ADHD are treated with pharmacotherapy. Methylphenidate (Ritalin, Concerta) is most often prescribed, with alternatives of dextroamphetamine (Dexedrine or Adderall) and the nonstimulant medication atomoxetine. A skin patch that releases medication transdermally over a 9-hour period is available, facilitating ease of administration; a long-acting liquid medication formulation is also available (Findling & Dinh, 2014). Usually, a favorable response (a decrease in impulsive behaviors and an increase in the ability to sit still and attend to an activity for at least 15 minutes) is seen in the first 10 days of treatment and frequently with the first few doses. Guidelines recommend thorough evaluation of children before stimulant or other medication is prescribed in order to rule out any cardiac condition that could be affected by medication use.

A variety of complementary approaches, in addition to or instead of traditional behavioral therapy and medication, have been tried in children with ADD or ADHD. Chiropractic manipulation, biofeedback, yoga, massage, visual or auditory therapy, and dietary interventions have been used. Dietary therapies include elimination of dietary components such as highly processed foods, sugar, aspartame, or yeast and use of supplements such as omega-3 fatty acids, iron, magnesium, zinc, vitamin B_6, and herbs such as Pycnogenol (pine bark extract), melatonin, *Echinacea*, St. John's wort, and ginkgo biloba. Ask parents about alternative therapies used and investigate what is known about them in order to share this information with parents (Arnold, Hurt, & Lofthouse, 2013; Faraone & Antshel, 2014; Kemper, Gardiner, & Birdee, 2013).

Although ADHD was once thought to be a disorder of childhood that gradually improved with age, it is now known that ADHD is a chronic condition requiring ongoing management; for many individuals, symptoms continue into adulthood (American Psychiatric Association, 2013).

Nursing Management

For the Child With ADD or ADHD

Nursing Assessment and Diagnosis

The nurse often encounters the family who is concerned about the child's behavior before a diagnosis has been made. Ask about family and birth history and have the parents describe the child's behaviors. Perform developmental testing and look specifically for attention span and physical activity. Refer the family to their pediatric healthcare home for further assessment, and then to a mental healthcare specialist who is experienced in diagnosing ADHD. Schedule a visit for complete client and family history, physical examination, and electrocardiogram before medication is begun.

Nurses may encounter the child with ADHD in the hospital when parents bring the child for treatment of an injury (e.g., fracture) or other problem. Explore the parents' report of the child's attention span in detail. Usually within a few minutes in an unstructured setting or waiting area, the child with ADHD becomes restless and searches for distraction. Gather information about the child's activity level and impulsiveness. Be alert for information that reveals a serious problem, such as hurting animals or other children. Find out about distractibility, attention deficit in activities of daily living, characteristic ways of reacting, and the extent of impulsiveness when the child is receiving medication. Find out how the family manages at home. Ask about a family history of the disorder, because that is a common finding among children with ADHD.

Examples of nursing diagnoses that might be appropriate for a child with ADHD include the following (NANDA-I © 2014):

- *Communication: Verbal, Impaired,* related to altered perceptions
- *Social Interaction, Impaired,* related to chronic episodes of impulsive behavior
- *Self-Esteem, Chronic Low,* related to behaviors associated with ADD/ADHD
- *Injury, Risk for,* related to high level of impulsiveness and excitability
- *Caregiver Role Strain, Risk for,* related to management of child with unpredictable moods and high energy

Planning and Implementation

Prevention can focus on discouraging regular television exposure for young children from 1 to 3 years and encouraging daily vigorous physical activity for all children. Nursing care of the hospitalized child with ADD/ADHD focuses on administering medications, minimizing environmental distractions, implementing behavioral management plans, providing emotional support to the child and family, promoting self-esteem, and ensuring ongoing care.

ADMINISTER MEDICATIONS

Stimulant and nonstimulant medications increase the child's attention span and decrease distractibility. Be alert for the common side effects of these medications, including anorexia, insomnia, and tachycardia. Administering medication early in the day helps to alleviate insomnia. Anorexia can be managed by giving medication at mealtimes. Baseline cardiac examinations are needed, as well as periodic reevaluation. Careful monitoring of weight, height, and blood pressure is necessary. Instruct families about the abuse potential of stimulant drugs and teach them to keep the medications locked and to administer them only as directed.

MINIMIZE ENVIRONMENTAL DISTRACTIONS

The child may need an environment with minimal distractions. When hospitalized, this may mean a room with only one other child. Keep potentially harmful equipment out of reach. Monitor and limit television and video game time. Use shades to darken the room at nap- or bedtime, and minimize noise. Teach parents to minimize distractions at home during periods when the child needs to concentrate, for example, when doing schoolwork. Visits to areas such as shopping malls and playgrounds may need to be limited. Plenty of daily exercise and minimal use of television and video games may help the child concentrate when needed for school and other tasks.

IMPLEMENT BEHAVIORAL MANAGEMENT PLANS
Behavioral modification programs can help reduce specific impulsive behaviors. An example is setting up a reward program for the child who has taken medication as ordered or completed a homework assignment. The rewards may be daily as well as weekly or monthly, depending on the child's age. For example, one completed homework assignment might be rewarded with 30 minutes of basketball or a bike ride; assignments completed for a week might be rewarded with an activity of the child's choice on the weekend.

If punishment is necessary, the behavior should be corrected while simultaneously supporting the child as a person. Punishment is generally withdrawal of a privilege, and should follow the offense quickly, as the child may not otherwise connect the punishment with the behavior.

PROVIDE EMOTIONAL SUPPORT
Children with ADD or ADHD offer a special challenge to parents, teachers, and healthcare providers. Parents must cope simultaneously with managing the difficult needs and demands of a hard-to-handle child, obtaining appropriate evaluation and treatment, and understanding and accepting the diagnosis, even when the child exhibits different behaviors with different people. Family support is essential. Educate both the parents and the child about the importance of appropriate expectations and consequences of behaviors. Teach skills that will help as the child grows older: making lists of tasks to accomplish; having routines for eating, sleeping, recreation, and schoolwork; minimizing stimuli in the environment when completing work; and asking teachers and friends to identify when behavior is inappropriate.

PROMOTE SELF-ESTEEM
As the child grows, ask about school and friends in order to assess self-concept and self-esteem. Help the child understand the disorder at an appropriate developmental level, and facilitate a trusting relationship with healthcare providers. Assist the child with social skills through role-play, playing in small groups, and modeling. Promote the child's self-esteem by pointing out the positive aspects of behavior and treating instances of negative behavior as learning opportunities. Help the child to develop ego strengths (the consciousness to be able to screen outside stimuli and control internal demands), which will result in better impulse control and thus increase self-esteem over time (Houck, Kendall, Miller, et al., 2011).

COMMUNITY-BASED NURSING CARE
Most children with ADD or ADHD are hospitalized only when needing care for another condition. Parents need support to understand the diagnosis and to learn how to manage the child. Emphasize the importance of a stable environment, at home as well as at school. At home the child may have difficulty staying on task. Parents need to consider age and developmental appropriateness of tasks, give clear and simple instructions, and provide frequent reminders to ensure completion. Routines in the evening can promote good sleep patterns.

The nurse can serve as a liaison to teachers and school personnel, or as the case manager for the child. An individualized education plan may be needed (see Chapter 12), with clear expected outcomes stated for the child's behaviors. Special classrooms or periods of instruction free from the distractions of the entire class may enable the child to improve school performance. Parents may have difficulty understanding the need for these approaches because the child often tests with above-average intelligence. Reinforce the importance of providing a structured environment free from unnecessary external stimuli. Be sure that parents understand behavioral approaches that will help the child, how to administer prescribed medications, and the importance of returning for healthcare visits to monitor for side effects. Medication should be locked safely away at home to keep it away from other children and prevent illegal use of this controlled substance. An individual school health plan may be needed for medication management.

Parents may have heard about ADHD in the media and often have many questions about its cause and management. Providing information about complementary and alternative treatments is a nursing role.

As the child grows older, explain the disorder and teach about techniques that will assist in dealing with problems. Assist in planning for a quiet environment during work. Encourage children with attention deficits to write down instructions from teachers and to use checklists to help them accomplish specific tasks.

Evaluation
Expected outcomes of nursing care for the child with ADD or ADHD include the following:

- Parents and child demonstrate understanding of the condition.
- Medications are administered and managed safely and as prescribed.
- The child demonstrates increased attentiveness and decreased hyperactivity, impulsivity, and sleep disturbance.
- The child demonstrates formation of a positive self-image.
- Educational performance is achieved to maximum potential.

Mood Disorders
Depression
Depression is psychologic distress that can range from mild to severe. Only in recent years has depression in children been recognized as a clinical condition. Many children referred to child guidance centers and mental healthcare providers because of behavioral difficulties or poor achievement actually suffer from depression. The incidence of major depression is estimated to be about 2% in childhood and up to 8% in adolescence; by age 18 years approximately 11% have had a depressive episode (Chung & Soares, 2012; National Institute of Mental Health [NIMH], n.d.a). A history of substance abuse and anxiety disorder increases risk, and cultural variations in rates exist.

ETIOLOGY AND PATHOPHYSIOLOGY
Theories have been proposed to explain the cause of depression in children and adolescents. Depression may be biologic in origin or a result of learned helplessness, cognitive distortion, social skills deficit, or family dysfunction. The physiologic theory focuses on monoamine neurotransmission. These amines include indolamine, serotonin, norepinephrine, and dopamine, and decreases are sometimes found in depression. Magnetic resonance imaging has identified brain changes in individuals who are depressed, suggesting a biologic basis (NIMH, n.d.a).

Developing Cultural Competence Depression Rates

Ethnic/racial differences in depression rates exist. The highest rates of depression are observed with Hispanic and Native American youth. Although there are scant data with Asian American youth, their rates of depression appear to be low. Data do not provide a clear picture of depression in African American youth as compared to White youth; in some studies, rates are higher and in others they are lower. In general, more female youth than male youth report depression (Lee & Liechty, 2014). It is probable that genetics, environment, and culture interact to influence the differences in prevalence of depression.

Parental depression and stress are predictive of childhood depression. Abuse and neglect, family conflict, parental death, and low socioeconomic status predispose children to depression. Other psychiatric diagnoses are common in children with depression; these include conditions such as ADHD, anxiety disorder, bipolar disease, or substance abuse (Emslie, Kennard, & Mayes, 2011).

CLINICAL MANIFESTATIONS

Characteristic findings of major depression in children and adolescents include declining school performance; withdrawal from social activities; sleep disturbance (either too much or too little); appetite disturbance (too much or too little); multiple somatic complaints, especially headaches and stomachaches; decreased energy; difficulty concentrating and making decisions; low self-esteem; and feelings of hopelessness. There is much variation among children in the symptoms displayed, and they often have some, but not all, of the major criteria. Symptoms vary according to children's developmental levels.

CLINICAL THERAPY

Youth should be screened for depression during well-child examinations or when indicated at other healthcare encounters (Agency for Healthcare Research and Quality [AHRQ], 2014). When depression or major depressive disorder is diagnosed, comprehensive assessment of the child should occur in order to rule out physical illness that can be linked to depressive symptoms, such as diabetes, cancer, and obesity. The child is tested for various mental health problems since comorbidities (combination with other disorders) are common. A history of bullying and substance abuse are examples of these comorbidities.

Initial assessment is performed by a child psychologist or child psychiatrist. A variety of scales and techniques are used; examples of useful tools are the Children's Depression Inventory (CDI), the Revised Children's Manifest Anxiety Scale, the Beck Depression Inventory (BDI-PC), the Guideline for Adolescent Preventive Services Questionnaire, the Patient Health Questionnaire for Adolescents (PHQ-A), the Reynolds Adolescent Depression Scale (RADS), and the Center for Epidemiological Studies Depression Scale for Children (CES-DC) (Stockings et al., 2014).

Treatment may include psychotherapy in combination with psychotropic medication. Often a combination of individual, family, and group therapy provides the greatest benefits for young children and adolescents. Involving parents, other family members, school personnel, and friends in the treatment plan is essential (Hughes & Asarnow, 2011). Group therapy is often effective for adolescents. Cognitive behavioral therapy (CBT) may be used with adolescents, and play therapy with younger children (see discussion of play therapy earlier in this chapter). CBT focuses on identification and restructuring of thoughts, feelings, and behaviors, leading to understanding of negative thoughts and increasing activities that provide pleasure (Mahoney, Kennard, & Mayes, 2011). Supportive interactions with healthcare providers and active problem solving are approaches that improve outcomes in adolescents. Healthcare providers should educate families about depression and counsel as needed. Confidentiality should be ensured. Refer to community resources as needed. Ensure a plan for safety of the adolescent.

Growth and Development

Symptoms of depression in children vary according to their developmental levels. Infants may fail to eat and grow. Toddlers can show regressive behaviors in toileting and other activities. Preschoolers have less symbolic and other play activities, may be irritable, and lack confidence. School-age children may show a decrease in academic performance, increased or decreased activity, somatic complaints, and loss of friends. Adolescents can have a wide array of symptoms such as anxiety, decreased social contact, poor school performance, lack of prior involvement in activities, poor self-care, difficulty with parents and teachers, or focus on violence (NIMH, n.d.a).

Antidepressant medications, most commonly the selective serotonin reuptake inhibitors (SSRIs), imipramine (Tofranil), desipramine (Norpramin), and amitriptyline (Elavil), may be prescribed. The only antidepressant approved to treat major depressive disorders in children and adolescents is fluoxetine HCl (Prozac), but clinicians sometimes use others when the youth does not respond to Prozac.

SAFETY ALERT!

The SSRIs act to block reuptake of serotonin in the synapse, so that serotonin levels (which influence mood) increase. Although the SSRIs are generally considered safer than some other types of antidepressants, their use in children has been limited, so side effects must be monitored. Generally, the child is started with a low dose, which is increased slowly to minimize the chance of side effects. Because of some reports of increased suicidal ideation and the lack of efficacy evidence, a psychiatric-mental health specialist must closely monitor children and adolescents taking SSRIs (AHRQ, 2014; NIMH, 2012a). A patient medication guide with the risks and precautions, as well as drug label information, must be provided for every client and family.

The major serious and life-threatening side effect of SSRIs is serotonin syndrome, a condition characterized by agitation, muscle twitching, gastric upset, chills, fever, confusion, and dizziness. It is more likely to develop when the child or adolescent is also taking St. John's wort, other antidepressants, alcohol, diet pills, or drugs such as ecstasy and LSD (Mayo Clinic, 2013b; Morrison & Schwartz, 2014). Be certain to ask questions in a nonjudgmental way about intake of any alternative therapies, other medications, or substance use to identify those most at risk.

Sudden cardiac death has occurred in several children on tricyclic antidepressants (TCAs). Because of this risk, serum levels should be monitored and electrocardiograms (ECGs) performed. Specific ECG changes along with a resting heart rate above 100, systolic blood pressure above 130 mmHg, and diastolic blood pressure above 85 mmHg necessitate immediate reporting to the prescriber. A narrow margin exists between the therapeutic and lethal doses in children (Weeke et al., 2012).

TABLE 28–4 Risk Factors for Child and Adolescent Depression

CHILD	FAMILY	SCHOOL AND SOCIAL SITUATIONS
• Frequent feelings of sadness, sleep problems, loss of interest in activities • Increase in risk taking and impulsivity • Previous suicide attempt • Alcohol or substance abuse • Diagnosed psychotic disorder • Chronic illness and frequent hospitalization	• Parental neglect, abuse, or loss • Dysfunctional family relationships • Family history of depression, suicide, substance abuse, alcoholism, other psychopathology	• Academic pressures and underachievement • Stressful social relationships • Declining participation in social events

Nursing Management

For the Child With Depression

Nursing Assessment and Diagnosis

Take a thorough history and physical examination, including observation of behavior, at the time of admission. Assess the child for common risk factors for depression (Table 28–4).

Several nursing diagnoses that might be appropriate for the child or adolescent hospitalized with depression are included in the accompanying *Nursing Care Plan*. Other diagnoses might include the following (NANDA-I © 2014):

- *Self Neglect* related to lack of energy and inability to perform daily hygiene
- *Powerlessness* related to sense of helplessness
- *Self-Esteem, Chronic Low,* related to negative self-evaluation

Planning and Implementation

Nursing care of the child or adolescent hospitalized for depression includes administering medications and other therapy and providing supportive care. Monitor vital signs of youth receiving antidepressant medications. Watch for common side effects of the agent(s) used. Carefully monitor for serious side effects of TCAs or SSRIs and be aware that lower doses are used at initiation, with doses increasing slowly to the desired level.

Frequent face-to-face follow-up visits are needed. When dosages are altered, behavior and ideation changes must be closely monitored. Monitor cardiovascular status, including hypertension and tachycardia, observe motor movement, and record dietary intake. Help parents evaluate inpatient settings to be certain the care provided will best meet the needs of the child or adolescent. Refer to accompanying *Nursing Care Plan: The Child or Adolescent Hospitalized With Depression* for specific nursing interventions.

DISCHARGE PLANNING AND HOME CARE TEACHING

When the child has been hospitalized and is returning home, teach parents to recognize signs and symptoms of worsening depression. Also teach them dosages and side effects of any prescribed medications. Refer the family to appropriate healthcare providers and to support groups for family members dealing with depression.

COMMUNITY-BASED NURSING CARE

Most children with depression are cared for in the community. Maintain regular contact with the family through their healthcare visits to outpatient agencies and by making home visits. Monitor the child's affect, activity, and food intake. School teachers and counselors often are aware of the child's ability to perform in the school setting. Have the family schedule after-school care so young children are not left at home alone for extended periods.

Nursing Care Plan: The Child or Adolescent Hospitalized With Depression

1. Nursing Diagnosis: *Hopelessness* related to long-term stress (NANDA-I © 2014)

GOAL: The child or adolescent will discuss feelings of hopelessness.

INTERVENTION	RATIONALE
• Encourage open expression of feelings. Explore hopeless, sad, or lonely feelings. Point out the connection between feelings and behavior. Assess the child or adolescent to identify the precipitating event when feelings of sadness arose. Maintain an accepting and nonjudgmental attitude regarding any feelings expressed by the child.	• Expressing feelings may help relieve sadness, loneliness, despair, and hopelessness.
• Encourage the child or adolescent to take part in self-care and unit activities. Use routines to establish feelings of control.	• An active role in self-care and treatment helps the child or adolescent to feel more in control.
• Medicate as ordered and document results.	• Antidepressants modify mood to a more hopeful outlook.

EXPECTED OUTCOME: By discharge, child or adolescent will express an interest in the future.

(continued)

Nursing Care Plan: The Child or Adolescent Hospitalized With Depression (*continued*)

2. Nursing Diagnosis: *Coping, Ineffective,* related to inadequate social support or disturbance in pattern of appraisal of threat (NANDA-I © 2014)

GOAL: The child or adolescent will use effective coping skills.

INTERVENTION	RATIONALE
• Teach positive, effective coping strategies such as guided imagery and relaxation. Assist the child or adolescent to focus on strengths rather than weaknesses.	• Therapeutic techniques can help the child or adolescent to replace negative thoughts and images with more positive and effective beliefs and images. These interventions foster resilience.
• Assist the child or adolescent to identify friends, family members, and others who are positive and supportive.	• Helps the child or adolescent to become aware that people can be caring and supportive (thus validating self-esteem).

EXPECTED OUTCOME: Child or adolescent will verbalize and demonstrate ability to cope appropriately for his or her age.

3. Nursing Diagnosis: *Social Interaction, Impaired,* related to self-concept disturbance (NANDA-I © 2014)

GOAL: The child or adolescent will participate in and initiate activities and conversation.

INTERVENTION	RATIONALE
• Assist the child or adolescent to identify topics and activities of interest.	• The more the child or adolescent focuses on areas of interest, the less he or she will focus on internal anxiety and depression.
• Encourage interaction with peers and staff.	• Each positive interaction reinforces feelings of success. Each success reinforces the desire for future social interaction.
• Facilitate visits from family and friends.	• Reinforces positive and rewarding relationships.
• Provide guidance to family regarding interaction that promotes self-esteem.	• The family's existing interaction style is often negative.

EXPECTED OUTCOME: By discharge, child or adolescent will initiate conversation and activities with staff and peers.

4. Nursing Diagnosis: *Nutrition, Imbalanced: Less than Body Requirements,* related to loss of appetite secondary to depression (NANDA-I © 2014)

GOAL: The child's or adolescent's daily intake will be adequate to maintain optimal nutritional status.

INTERVENTION	RATIONALE
• Offer nutritious finger foods, sandwiches, and high-calorie liquid supplements frequently throughout the day.	• Convenient easy-to-eat foods encourage the child or adolescent to eat and maintain nutritional status.
• Offer easy-to-carry drinks that are high in vitamins, minerals, and calories.	• These are a convenient method for meeting hydration and electrolyte needs.
• Encourage daily vigorous physical activity of at least 30 min.	• Physical activity stimulates appetite.

EXPECTED OUTCOME: Child or adolescent's daily intake will be adequate to maintain optimal nutritional status by discharge.

Assist the family in finding support for financial and emotional needs related to managing the child's depression. Major expected outcomes for nursing care of the child with depression are found in the accompanying *Nursing Care Plan*.

Bipolar Disorder (Manic Depression)

Bipolar disorder is a mental illness in which extreme changes in affect and energy are manifested. Moods most often alter between mania (high energy and euphoria) and depression. Children often present with irritability or hyperactivity. About 1% of children and adults have bipolar illness, with a high rate of onset from 15 to 19 years, although onset as young as preschool age can occur. There is a high rate of attempted suicide in those with bipolar disease, as well as co-occurrence with other disorders such as ADHD, anxiety, and substance abuse, all of which complicate diagnosis (NIMH, n.d.b).

Families Want to Know

Selecting Residential and Inpatient Care for the Child With Mental Illness

Families need guidelines to help them evaluate inpatient facilities when a child with a mental disorder must be placed in an institution. You can refer them to the National Alliance for the Mentally Ill website. Provide questions for the families to ask:

- What is the staff-to-youth ratio?
- What are the guidelines for chemical and physical restraint?
- Are children isolated when behaviors are inappropriate?
- Are children constantly monitored visually when in restraint or when potentially dangerous to self or others?
- Does the child have a full physical and psychologic evaluation by a specialist within 24 hours of entry to the facility?
- What professionals review the plan of care and how often?
- Who can the family speak to for regular updates on the child?
- How often can the family visit?
- What services will be covered by insurance?
- What subjective feelings do the family members have as they visit the unit and facility?
- What services will be offered on an ongoing basis on discharge?

Bipolar disorder is classified into four types:

- *Bipolar I*—includes a severe manic episode that requires hospitalization or causes functional impairment in life
- *Bipolar II*—at least one episode of mild to moderate mania (hypomania) and one of depression
- *Cyclothymic disorder*—manifests as multiple mild manic and depressive episodes
- *Bipolar not otherwise specified*—rapid mood fluctuations, mania without depressive episodes, or chronic depression with hypomania episodes (NIMH, n.d.b).

When parents or close relatives are affected, the child is more likely to have the disorder. Thus, a genetic etiology is probable. It is believed that genetics and environment interact to create the condition in youth. Brain imaging shows abnormalities of the frontal and prefrontal cortex, the hippocampus, the basal ganglia, and the left amygdala, which is the center for experiencing fear (NIMH, n.d.b).

The manic phase of bipolar illness is characterized by hyperactivity and high energy, irritability, aggression, and sometimes hallucinations. In the depressive phase, the child is sad, has alterations in sleep and eating patterns, and is socially withdrawn, similar to any depressive illness. Mania may be the persistent symptom in children, or rapid cycles of mania and depression can occur throughout the day (Dineen, 2014; Kloos & Robb, 2011; Scrandis, 2014).

Diagnosis and treatment of bipolar disorder should be performed by mental health specialists. Use of alcohol or illegal drugs should be ruled out as a cause of symptoms, even in children. Since the manic phase is often manifested by hyperactivity, the child may incorrectly be treated with stimulants (see treatment of ADHD earlier in this chapter), and the disease can be worsened. Irritability, elation, labile moods, and sleep disturbance are commonly seen in children (Dineen, 2014; Kloos & Robb, 2011; Scrandis, 2014).

The treatment of bipolar disease involves a variety of drugs used to stabilize mood. Lithium, valproate, divalproex, carbamazepine, olanzapine, oxcarbazepine, lamotrigine, quetiapine, and risperidone are examples of drugs used; antidepressants may be prescribed (Blake, 2012; NIMH, 2012a). Only lithium has been approved by the FDA for use in those ages 12 to 18 years. However, clinicians prescribe other drugs with careful monitoring being performed. Early treatment is key to preventing chronic, serious mental illness. Individual and family education and therapy can be helpful.

Nurses are instrumental in identifying children with bipolar disorder, providing information to families, and monitoring the drugs and psychotherapy for the child. Nurses should observe for side effects to the specific drug regimen used and assist parents to find resources for health care since medications and other treatments may be costly. Parents and children need information about the disorder because it may recur several times during the child's life. Nurses can assist the child to find social events and groups that build a sense of self-esteem.

Anxiety and Related Disorders

A large group of anxiety disorders can affect youth as well as adults. Some of the more common types seen in children and adolescents are described in the following sections, with detailed nursing management described for posttraumatic stress disorder.

Generalized Anxiety Disorder

Anxiety is a subjective feeling of uncertainty and helplessness, usually accompanied by central nervous system (CNS) signs, including restlessness, trembling, perspiration, and rapid pulse. Anxiety is second only to substance abuse (see Chapter 17) in incidence for mental disorders and is a common mental disorder among children. From 4% to 20% of youth experience some type of anxiety disorder (Boydston, Hsiao, & Varley, 2012a; Sarvet & Brewer, 2011).

Anxiety disorders are strongly linked to familial and genetic factors. Diagnosis is performed by a mental health specialist, and treatment is usually cognitive behavioral therapy (CBT) and may involve medication. CBT can include child or family interventions that focus on relaxation, recognition of feelings, and self-talking (learned words or phrases said to oneself to aid in management of distress). Medications that have been reported to be successful in children include SSRIs and benzodiazepines (Boydston et al., 2012b).

Separation Anxiety Disorder

Separation anxiety disorder is characterized by an extreme state of uneasiness when in unfamiliar surroundings and often by refusal to visit friends' homes or attend school for at least 2 weeks. It is a common type of anxiety disorder manifested by children (Boydston et al., 2012a). Many children with separation anxiety disorder refuse to attend school at some point (see *School Phobia [Social Phobia]* section later in this chapter). This phobia may be recurrent and become worse at certain times. The condition may be acute in onset (preceded by a traumatic event) or slow in developing over time.

Children with separation anxiety disorder tend to be perfectionistic, overly compliant, and eager to please. They appear to cling to the parent or caretaker. They may use physical complaints such as headaches, abdominal pain, nausea, and vomiting in an attempt to avoid being away from the parent. Depression frequently accompanies separation anxiety disorder. The resulting avoidant behaviors can interfere with personal growth and development, academic achievement, and social functioning.

Diagnosis is made by a mental health specialist. Treatment includes CBT with both child and parents. Parents learn about the disorder and how to structure the setting so that the child is expected to attend school. Consistency in expectations is needed since if the child is permitted to stay home some days or has missed school and other activities for longer periods, treatment is more difficult. The child learns what situations cause anxiety and how to manage the situations and feelings elicited. Both parents and child work out the expectations for behavior for the child with the mental health therapist; school personnel are included in the treatment plan. Medication can be used if CBT is not helpful.

Growth and Development

The separation anxiety commonly experienced by a 2-year-old differs from the psychiatric disorder in age appropriateness, duration, and severity. Separation anxiety disorder affects children of preschool age or older, lasts for at least 2 weeks, and is characterized by excessive anxiety. In contrast, the separation anxiety experienced by the 2-year-old involves a single episode of separation from a familiar caretaker and is a characteristic response in toddlers.

Panic Disorder

Panic disorder is the presence of recurrent, unexpected panic attacks. Panic attacks are periods of intense fear and discomfort in the absence of real danger. The lifetime risk of panic disorder is 2% (Boydston et al., 2012a). Predictive factors for panic attacks in adolescence include a history of separation anxiety or other anxiety disorder in life and a history of parental panic attacks.

Examples of the physical symptoms experienced are palpitations, sweating, chills, hot flashes, shaking, shortness of breath, choking, chest pain, nausea, and dizziness. The person describes feelings of danger or doom. Some people may have accompanying agoraphobia. **Agoraphobia** is anxiety about being in places or situations from which escape may be difficult or embarrassing, or in which help may not be available. The attacks may be continuous or episodic, but generally are chronic.

Diagnosis is made by a mental health specialist. Similar to anxiety, treatment may involve individual and family therapy, with use of medication in some cases. Nurses can help identify the disorder, refer for evaluation, and provide care in the community so that the child attends therapy sessions and takes medication as ordered.

Obsessive-Compulsive Disorder

People with obsessive-compulsive disorder (OCD) may be mildly or severely affected. Up to 2% of children are affected, and about 80% of adults with OCD had the condition in childhood (Boydston et al., 2012a). Affected children have recurrent obsessive thoughts, commonly about contamination, harm, sex, or moral concerns. These obsessions are handled through a series of compulsive behaviors that interfere with daily life. Examples of behaviors are excessive handwashing, counting objects, and

hoarding substances. These practices may take 1 hour or more of time each day. Children with OCD differ from adults in several ways. They have more aggressive obsessions, such as fears of catastrophe, more commonly hoard objects, and are more likely to have religious obsessions. The presence of comorbidity with other mental health disorders is common.

The basal ganglia of the brain are affected and a genetic link is observed. A neurochemical cause may be related to abnormal serotonin metabolism. MRI changes in the globus pallidus and anterior cingulated gyrus of the brain have been noted. Post-streptococcal autoimmune disorder may be a cause in some cases (NIMH, 2012b).

Clinical Tip

Pediatric autoimmune neuropsychiatric disorders (PANDAS) are characterized by obsessive-compulsive and/or tic disorder, childhood onset, association with group A beta-hemolytic streptococcal infection, and neurologic abnormalities. It is believed that in certain children, the strep infection leads to a neural autoimmune response, resulting in the psychiatric disorder. Research continues to identify possible mechanisms, results, and treatments for this cause of OCD (NIMH, 2012b). *Pediatric acute-onset neuropsychiatric syndrome (PANS)* is the term used to refer to all cases of abrupt-onset OCD, not only those following streptococcal infection.

Diagnosis is made by a mental health specialist. Treatment may involve CBT, where the feared occurrence is presented and the person learns that no harm will occur. Involvement of the family in treatment is important so that members learn how to handle the child's ritualistic behaviors. Medications, such as clomipramine and the SSRIs, are effective in most children and adolescents. Nurses can identify cases and refer for mental health evaluation and provide teaching and support for families.

School Phobia (Social Phobia)

School phobia (also called *social phobia, school avoidance,* or *school refusal*) is a persistent, irrational, or excessive fear of negative evaluation or embarrassment in social situations and therefore of attending school. The child may fear being harmed or losing control. Social and school phobias occur in children as young as 5 years of age, often being present at 11 or 12 years, but can occur in children up to 16 years (Boydston et al., 2012a).

Children with social phobia may fear asking for directions, ordering food at a restaurant, and speaking in the classroom. They commonly report that teachers and peers "pick on" them. Somatic complaints are similar to those in children with separation anxiety disorder. Characteristically, symptoms are present only on school days and not on weekends or holidays. The social withdrawal that occurs in this disorder further impairs the child since social interactions are needed for normal developmental progression.

Diagnosis is made by a mental health specialist. Treatment includes the family and child, and establishes firm limits for behavioral expectations and consequences. CBT is used, including education of the youth about the condition, body awareness of symptoms, and methods of changing feelings. SSRI medications may sometimes be needed to lessen anxiety in social situations.

Conversion Reaction

Conversion reaction is a disorder in which a disturbance or loss of sensory, motor, or other physical functions suggests neurologic or other somatic disease. The disturbance or loss cannot be explained by any known pathophysiologic mechanism. Instead, psychologic factors are involved. About 3% of the population experiences conversion reactions at some time. Adolescence and early adulthood are common times for the onset to occur, with onset being rare before 10 years or after 35 years of age (Kozlowska, Scher, & Williams, 2011).

Conversion reactions develop in response to a catastrophic event such as threat, loss, or harm. Clinical manifestations include altered sensations such as blindness or deafness; paralysis or ataxia, including inability to stand or walk and loss of ability to speak (aphonia); involuntary movements, such as pseudo-epileptic convulsions; and constant complaints of pain with no physical basis (psychogenic pain). Children under 10 years old usually present with gait abnormalities or seizures. The onset of conversion symptoms is usually dramatic and sudden. Symptoms often appear to be neurologic, but on careful examination, obvious discrepancies are found. The person is usually calm about the symptoms even though they are serious. Often the child or family members appear indifferent or unconcerned over what healthcare providers consider an overwhelming physical disability.

Children suspected of having a conversion reaction require a complete physical and neurologic evaluation to rule out any possible physiologic basis for the symptoms. Individual and family therapy is usually necessary to identify the source of the psychologic conflict, pain, or need resulting in the conversion symptoms. Pharmacologic approaches may also be used.

Posttraumatic Stress Disorder

Acute stress disorder can occur after any life-threatening event and is manifested in the first month after exposure to the event. Symptoms include repeatedly reliving the traumatic experience, anxiety, and increased arousal. Similarly, people with *posttraumatic stress disorder (PTSD)* have experienced or witnessed a life-threatening event; however, the symptoms of distress continue for more than 1 month and cause impairment in functioning. Estimates of the incidence of PTSD are hard to obtain. It is assumed that about 40% of youth have an episode of trauma that could lead to PTSD, and there is a lifetime risk of 8.7% for the disorder. While 20% of children may experience PTSD after traumatic events, the prevalence rises to 90% when the trauma is severe (Boydston et al., 2012a).

Examples of events associated with posttraumatic stress include sexual or other child abuse, rape, car crash, fire, witnessing violence, and war experiences. Cassandra, described in the chapter-opening quote, was experiencing PTSD resulting from a frightening car crash as she was driven to school. She was too young to describe her feelings verbally to her mother or school personnel; however, she manifested the sleep abnormalities and other complaints common in the disorder.

The disorder involves both a traumatic event and the child's reaction to this event. It is believed that brain changes occur in trauma, leading to neurobiologic alterations that cause dysfunction of memory. Overreactivity of the amygdala, underreactivity of the prefrontal cortex, and increased dopamine in the medial prefrontal cortex are observed. Female gender, having other psychiatric disorders, a family history of psychiatric illness, and severe or lengthy trauma are all risk factors.

Common reactions in persons with PTSD are intrusive symptoms such as negative thoughts and feelings, avoidance of reminders of the event, and arousal or hyperreactivity to events (American Psychiatric Association, 2013). The child with PTSD has feelings of fear, terror, and helplessness, and may relive the event frequently in thought and nightmares. The child may become emotionally numb in a subconscious attempt to protect the self, but may have a persistently increased state of arousal. The child exhibits a state of hypervigilance and an exaggerated startle response, such as to touch or loud noises. The child with PTSD is often irritable, and has sleep problems

Clinical Reasoning Posttraumatic Stress Disorder

Cassandra is a 9-year-old girl who has recently become fearful about attending school and has awakened crying at night. She is in the third grade at a school she has attended for 2 years. A few weeks ago, she was in a car crash as her mother drove her to school. She received only minor injuries and returned to school the next day. However, her mother believes that Cassandra's behavior has been worsening since the car crash. She spoke with the school nurse, who is aware of no trauma at school, but did learn from the teacher that Cassandra has not been paying attention in class recently. Cassandra cannot explain why she does not want to go to school, only that her stomach aches or some other part of her body hurts.

Cassandra visited her pediatrician, who ruled out any physical cause for her complaints, and referred her to a child psychologist. The psychologist has scheduled several sessions with Cassandra to help her learn to verbalize her fears and learn strategies to deal with them. She uses dolls in an attempt to help Cassandra act out her fears and gain some understanding. The psychologist communicates Cassandra's progress to you, the school nurse.

- How can you ensure Cassandra's attendance at school?
- What does the teacher need to know to support Cassandra in the classroom?
- What is your role as liaison between the psychologist, family, and school personnel?
- Parents often feel guilty when a child experiences a mental health disorder. What type of information and support do Cassandra's parents need?

and inattentiveness. The child feels detached from others and alone. Immediately after the event, the child may appear to have adapted and functions normally. However, after several weeks or even months, the symptoms of the disorder begin to appear.

The diagnosis is made by a mental health specialist; a variety of instruments assist in screening for the disorder. Counseling by a mental health specialist is the main therapy for PTSD. Cassandra saw a clinical psychologist who used play therapy to help her communicate her fears related to a car crash (Figure 28–6). CBT is the treatment of choice, with both the child and family members

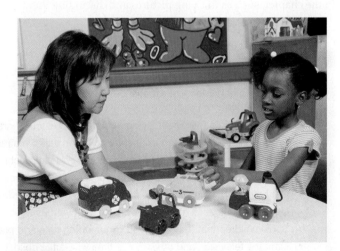

Figure 28–6 The psychologist uses play therapy to help Cassandra reenact her car crash. This helps her gain some control over the event so that it is not so frightening.

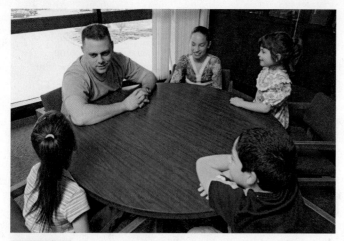 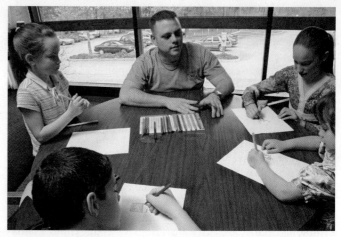

Figure 28–7 This nurse conducts a group therapy session for children who have experienced traumatic events and have resulting anxiety disorders. He is clearly engaged, has a positive rapport, and fosters exchanges among the children. Playing games and drawing are frequent techniques used in the group.

included. Young children show significant improvement in symptoms after a course of CBT (Center for Injury Research and Prevention, 2011). A variety of antidepressants and SSRIs are used for pharmacologic treatment.

Nursing Management

Nurses often help identify PTSD victims so that care can be obtained. Ask about traumatic events in the past and how the child reacted. Inquire about recent changes in the child's behavior. Include school attendance, complaints of physical illness, sleep patterns, and rituals in behavior. A family history of mental disorders may be useful. Youth who run away from home and present at homeless shelters are often suffering from PTSD. Assessment for the condition should be part of the initial history.

Nursing care for anxiety disorders focuses on behavioral and cognitive therapies to enhance coping skills. Mental health nurses may conduct group therapy sessions (Figure 28–7). Group sessions for children often provide a forum for discussion of fears, an opportunity to enhance skills of working together, and an opportunity to learn coping skills. Being a member of a group with other children experiencing anxiety or trauma can remove the stigma and allow the child the freedom to explore the behavior and its causes. Several of the techniques described in the chapter, such as drawing pictures and discussing them or

telling stories, are used by mental health nurses in child therapy groups (Boydston et al., 2012b).

Children need to learn relaxation techniques and nurses may teach such techniques or recommend that the child consider participation in yoga or guided imagery classes. Inquire about alternative therapies that the child and family are using or have an interest in beginning, and refer as needed. Parents or other significant people should be included in the treatment program. Nurses often teach them basic information about the child's diagnosis and therapy. They should be in at least some therapy sessions with the child. Provide the family with resources that will assist with relief from worry about the child, guilt about causing an accident that triggered the child's symptoms, or other feelings related to the diagnosis.

Insurance companies may provide limited payment for mental health services. Help the family to see the importance of recommended therapy and assist them to find resources for care if needed. School personnel may need to know about the child's treatment. Partner with the families to provide needed information. Some schools have counselors that can be instrumental in carrying out treatment plans at school and acting as a resource in that setting. School personnel may be asked to provide feedback about the child's attendance, performance, and social skills as a measure of the success of therapy, and the community or school nurse can relay this information.

Families Want to Know

Talking With Children About Traumatic Events

Whether a child or adolescent experiences trauma from a car crash, abuse, or environmental event, parents can help to decrease the effects of the stress and prevent the appearance of PTSD. Some suggestions for parents include:

- Be sure children feel free to ask parents, teachers, or others about the events and their feelings.
- Assure children that their feelings are common and the stress may return now and then over time.
- Be honest and open in responses, without overloading children with more details than they need.
- Be prepared to repeat answers and discuss the same topics many times.
- Get help from counselors who can suggest how to talk with the child.
- Use communication methods appropriate at various ages, such as reading books, doing art projects, or drawing.
- Show children that they are loved by spending time and planning activities with them.
- Limit the television and other media time where the child is exposed to violence and traumatic events.
- Restore a sense of normal routines into the child's life.
- Be alert for increasing signs of distress and seek care from a professional if they occur.

Nurses often administer medications to children being treated for PTSD and other mental health concerns. Be alert for side effects and ensure the family knows how to safely administer the drugs. These drugs should be kept locked securely. Have the child return for follow-up as needed since some medications may take several weeks to achieve effects, and close monitoring is essential. The child should wear a medication alert identification for drugs being taken.

Other Disorders

Suicide

Suicide is the third leading cause of death in adolescents between 15 and 19 years of age. About 4400 youth commit suicide annually, and an additional 149,000 receive care after attempted suicide. In any 1 year, over 15% of youth admit to contemplating suicide (CDC, 2012b). The prevalence of suicide is about 7.32 per 100,000, with 86% of the deaths among male adolescents. Firearms, suffocation, and poisoning are the most common means of suicide (CDC, 2012b).

Developing Cultural Competence Suicide, **Gender, and Ethnicity**

Some ethnic groups have a high rate of suicide. For example, Native Americans and Alaskan Natives have a rate of suicide of 31/100,000, while for all other youth the rate is 12.2/100,000. The historic pain experienced by this ethnic group and lack of opportunities for many youth may be some of the reasons for a high suicide rate. Hispanic female adolescents have a high rate of suicide attempts. Males have a high rate of suicide at 4 times that of females; males more often use firearms, while females more commonly use poisoning (CDC, 2012b).

Healthy People 2020 goals focus on eliminating such health disparities by finding the causes, decreasing rates of suicide, educating about risk factors, and establishing prevention programs (U.S. Department of Health and Human Services [USDHHS], 2015).

Healthy People 2020

(MHMD-2) Reduce suicide attempts by adolescents from the present 1.9/100 to 1.7/100 (a 10% improvement)

It is not unusual for healthcare providers and parents to label suicide attempts by children and adolescents "accidents." Up to one half of childhood suicides may be recorded as accidents; suicide data for children under age 10 years are not maintained. Adults may have difficulty believing that young children, in particular, would have any reason to want to end their lives. Because of this, many children brought to the emergency department with indications of a suicide attempt are often classified as unintentional injury victims and released without arrangements for appropriate follow-up care. Accurate identification and treatment are needed for youth at risk of suicide.

Many risk factors for suicide exist in children and adolescents, while some protective factors are influential as well (Table 28–5). The most common precursor to adolescent suicide is depression (see earlier discussion in this chapter). Common signs or symptoms of an underlying depression that could

TABLE 28–5 Risk and Protective Factors for Suicide in Children and Adolescents

RISK FACTORS	PROTECTIVE FACTORS
History of previous attempted suicide	Emotional well-being
Friend committed or attempted suicide	Satisfactory school performance
School problems or changes in grades	Participation in sports or other group events
Pregnancy	Weight satisfaction
Drug use or abuse	Parent/family connectedness
Problems with a romantic relationship	Frequent discussions of important issues with family
Minority sexual practice	School connectedness
Loneliness, withdrawal	Safe school
Feelings of anxiety	Safe neighborhood
History of chronic family problems	Caring adult presence at school or elsewhere
Chronic illness	Availability of school counseling
Physical, emotional, or sexual abuse	School policies to limit and cope with fighting, bullying
History of suicide in a family member	
History of depression	
Chronic low self-esteem	
Change in behavior	
Change in weight	
Giving away special possessions	
Access to firearms and ammunition	

lead to suicide include boredom, restlessness, problems with concentration, irritability, lethargy, intentional misbehavior, preoccupation with one's own body or health, and excessive dependence on or isolation from others (especially adults or caregivers).

The child or adolescent at high risk for suicide may be admitted to a mental health unit for care or cared for in a community mental health facility. Treatment may include individual, group, or family therapy. Negotiating a "no suicide" contract is one method that may be used with a suicidal youth. In the contract, the child agrees not to attempt suicide during a specified time period. When a suicide attempt is made, the child or adolescent may be hospitalized for 24 hours, kept in a short-term monitoring unit, or sent home under close observation to ensure adequate assessment and monitoring. It is important to provide crisis intervention at the time of the suicide attempt to minimize the opportunity for repeat attempts and to begin a therapeutic treatment plan.

Nursing Management

The major nursing role is in prevention of suicide. All children and adolescents in health promotion visits and emergency departments should be evaluated for risk. Health promotion visits are an opportunity to be alert for children with depression (see previous discussion in this chapter), substance abuse, recent stresses, and changes in behavior. Inquire about sleep patterns, feelings of sadness, and use of alcohol and other substances. Gather a family history of mental health disorders, suicide attempts, and stresses.

Ask about how often the youth talks with or has meals with the family. Be aware of the risk of self-inflicted strangulation.

SAFETY ALERT!
A tragic cause of unintentional suicide in children is the choking "game." About 25 children with a mean age of 13 years die each year in the United States from this practice. When the blood supply to the brain is interrupted and then rushes back, some people report a feeling of euphoria or a "high." Children and adolescents may seek the experience for the feelings it creates and may even become addicted to it. Unfortunately, some children become unintentionally strangled and die from the experience. Methods that children use to cut off oxygen include using their hands to apply pressure to the carotids in the neck, or tying belts, cords, towels, and other items to the neck and then around doorknobs or other solid objects. Some children perform these rituals with others who then rescue them so that they begin breathing; many of the injuries occur when children are alone and there is no one to perform a rescue. Teachers, parents, and other adults typically have not heard of or are unaware that children are performing these rituals. Adults can watch for signs such as conjunctival hemorrhage, headaches, bruising in the neck area, periods of disorientation, hoarseness, and finding items tied to doors and other solid objects. Parents can also be alert if the history of a family computer has shown the child's entry to a website that describes the practice. Nurses in schools and other settings should educate children about the dangers of strangulation and should provide materials for parents to inform them of the risk (CDC, 2008, 2010; Mechling, Ahern, & McGuinness, 2013).

Recall that all youth who receive medications for treatment of depression should be carefully monitored, especially in the first several weeks in order to identify those who may develop suicide ideation and risk. Although antidepressants have demonstrated efficacy for treating depression in youth, there is an increased risk of suicidal ideation or behaviors in children and adolescents treated with these drugs.

Most suicides are committed with firearms that are usually obtained from the home. Determine at each healthcare visit if the family has firearms. Teach adults to keep the guns unloaded, with ammunition and firearms locked in separate locations. Be sure that children and adolescents do not have access to the keys for the locked firearms. Never underestimate the resourcefulness or abilities of a suicidal child or adolescent, regardless of age, IQ, or physical abilities.

Education in all school settings is appropriate to teach children about resources that can help them if they need it and to identify peers at risk. Mental health services of all types should be available and embedded in schools since that is the setting where youth spend much of their time (USDHHS, 2015). Be alert for children and adolescents at risk for suicide in any setting. Assess children and adolescents in schools, outpatient settings, and emergency departments for the possibility of suicidal behavior. Report threats of suicide and depressive behavior. When a child or adolescent persists in threatening suicide after establishment of a "no suicide" contract, hospitalization is necessary to ensure safety. Recognize that when a child or adolescent has committed suicide, friends of the victim may be at increased risk. Teach students to report to teachers, nurses, or counselors about friends who have threatened suicide or seem depressed or display behaviors different from usual. Nurses often plan with mental health specialists to implement suicide prevention programs in schools and communities. Provide supportive

services to family and friends whenever suicide occurs. Consult websites and refer parents as appropriate. The Suicide Prevention Resource Center has helpful regional offices to facilitate networks at national, state, territorial, community, and tribal levels (Maheshwari & Joshi, 2012).

Professionalism in Practice Suicide Prevention

The U.S. Surgeon General and the National Action Alliance for Suicide Prevention presented the 2012 National Strategy for Suicide Preventions: Goals and Objectives for Action. Major strategies were focused around empowering individuals, families, and communities by increased knowledge; providing comprehensive clinical and community preventive services; providing treatment and support for individuals and families when needed; and conducting surveillance, research, and evaluation (USDHHS, 2012). Nurses have a role in each of these strategies by identifying risk and providing connections to services, integrating suicide prevention in all healthcare settings, and collecting evaluative data from their communities.

Nursing care during hospitalization for suicide centers on taking appropriate precautions to ensure the child's safety. Be alert for children and adolescents in the emergency department who may have attempted suicide (Schmid, Truong, & Damian, 2011). Monitor both the child and the hospital environment for any object that could be used for self-harm. Remove all potentially harmful objects, such as shoestrings, belts, pantyhose, and hair ribbons. Keep all personal care items (including toothbrush and shampoo) locked at the nursing station and monitor them constantly when used by the child.

Children or adolescents considered at high risk for suicidal behaviors are attended to by a nursing staff member at all times, including while using the bathroom and sleeping. It may be necessary for the child to dress in a plain hospital gown, be kept in a visually monitored seclusion room, or (if seriously impaired and self-abusive) be medicated for restraint for a period of time. Restraints are used only when ordered by the youth's physician and collaborative care team. Physical restraint is only a short-term approach to provide immediate safety if necessary. Chemical (medication) restraint may be needed to prevent self-injury by the suicidal person. See *Families Want to Know: Selecting Residential and Inpatient Care for the Child With Mental Illness* earlier in this chapter for information to help families consider when choosing care for their suicidal child.

Hospitalization continues as long as the child's behavior is self-destructive. Children are referred for intensive individual and family therapy. Encourage parents to keep follow-up clinic appointments, to watch for self-destructive behaviors, and to administer any prescribed medications according to the treatment schedule. Arrange home visits and other community resources for families. Desired outcomes include an increase in coping skills for the child, no further suicide attempts, and an improved sense of well-being.

Tic Disorders and Tourette Syndrome

Tics are sudden, rapid, recurrent, nonrhythmic, and brief motor movements or vocalizations. They may involve movement of the head or upper body, blinking of eyes, or a variety of verbal noises. They may be worse during periods of stress or tiredness. Many children have mild motor tics at some time that gradually disappear with no intervention. When the tics are severe or last more than 1 year, they are considered chronic and may require attention from a mental healthcare provider.

Severe motor tics accompanied by verbal utterances are known as *Tourette syndrome*. The syndrome is often accompanied by other diagnoses such as attention deficit and learning disabilities. Children with Tourette syndrome may exhibit coprolalia, the involuntary utterance of obscenities, profanities, and racial slurs, or copropraxia, the involuntary use of obscene gestures. Tic disorders are characterized by disruptions in the levels of dopamine, serotonin, and other neurotransmitter and neuropeptide levels (National Institute of Neurological Disorders and Stroke, 2014).

Nursing care involves supporting parents and encouraging normal developmental progression for the child. Nurses should carefully monitor symptoms after medication is begun, minimize stress, and teach relaxation techniques.

Schizophrenia

Schizophrenia is a psychotic disorder that is relatively rare in young children and adolescents, occurring in 1 in 10,000 children. The condition can manifest in childhood but is more common in adolescence (Lachman, 2014; Mayo Clinic, 2014).

The cause of schizophrenia is unknown, but genetic predisposition or neurointegration deficits are suspected causes (Mayo Clinic, 2014). The brain is altered in the disease, with progressively enlarged ventricles and nervous system arousal. Impaired glucose metabolism is often present. Onset is usually slow with increasing intensity. Most often the child demonstrates restlessness, poor appetite, and social withdrawal over several weeks to months. Behavioral problems, slowed development, and minor neurologic symptoms may occur.

The clinical manifestations of schizophrenia are the same in children as in adults. Characteristic behaviors include social withdrawal, impaired social relationships, flat **affect** (outward appearance of feeling or emotion), regression, loose associations (thought characterized by speech in which ideas shift from one subject to another that is unrelated), poor judgment and problem solving, anxiety, delusions, and hallucinations. Motor abnormalities may include rocking and arm flapping.

During adolescence, acute schizophrenia can occur suddenly while the teenager is making plans to leave home and family to attend college, marry, or work in another area. Onset of symptoms may be triggered by an important loss (death of a significant other, parent, child, or friend).

Prompt diagnosis can lead to early treatment and more positive outcomes. Clinical therapy for childhood schizophrenia is multifaceted, including individual psychotherapy, family therapy, and various psychotropic medications (antipsychotics such as haloperidol [Haldol], clozapine, olanzapine, risperidone, antianxiety agents such as lorazepam [Ativan], and antidepressants such as imipramine [Tofranil]) (Lachman, 2014; Mayo Clinic, 2014). Drugs are only moderately effective at controlling hallucinations and delusions. Responses vary considerably, and children may have different responses than adults. Side effects determine what drugs are used and for how long. Antipsychotic medication is continued for at least 4 to 6 weeks before effectiveness can be determined. Medications often must be continued for several months or years after recovery from an acute schizophrenic episode, although medication-free trials may be tried in children who have not shown symptoms for 6 to 12 months.

Episodes of acute schizophrenia may require inpatient hospitalization on a psychiatric unit for thorough diagnosis and beginning management. Treatment may include an intensive school-based program in a structured, supervised setting with specially trained professionals. The goal of initial treatment is to reduce or control schizophrenic episodes and provide a safe, structured environment for the child or adolescent, enabling the child to live each day at an optimal level of functioning. Outpatient care is provided in the community following initial diagnosis and establishment of a treatment regimen.

Most children with acute schizophrenia require long-term treatment, including intermittent periods of hospitalization. Children or adolescents whose symptoms are difficult to control and who present a safety risk to themselves or others may require long-term residential treatment. Earlier age at diagnosis and delay in treatment lead to poorer prognosis.

Nursing Management

The nurse may encounter the child or adolescent with schizophrenia during hospitalization for an acute episode, for treatment of another problem, or while working with the individual in the community. Nursing care centers on providing for physical safety and psychologic care, and normal growth and development for the child.

Family education and involvement in the treatment plan are essential. Teach the family to monitor the child's symptoms and progression. Educating the child and parents about the risk of recurrence and methods to alleviate side effects of prescribed medications may increase compliance with the treatment plan. Assess the child for common medication side effects. For example, when excess weight is a potential side effect, frequent growth measurements are made. Neurologic assessment and laboratory studies may be needed with some medications. Help the family establish educational plans and integration within the school system. Communicate with school personnel to ensure understanding of the child's condition and ongoing management of the individualized education plan.

Cognitive Alterations

A wide array of cognitive conditions occur in childhood. Some are mild and not diagnosed until a child has difficulty in school, whereas others may be associated with physical signs that are visible at birth. Two common conditions, learning disabilities and intellectual disabilities (mental retardation), are discussed in this section.

Learning Disabilities

Learning disabilities are a common problem of young children, affecting about 5% to 10% of school children (Boyle et al., 2011; CDC, 2013). They involve neurologic conditions in which the brain cannot receive or process information in the normal manner. Often the impairment is only in one or two types of learning, making diagnosis difficult. Common types of learning disorders are listed in Table 28–6.

Children may have difficulty processing visual information, which may be manifested in reading, writing, and mathematics performance. Others may have difficulty with oral information, leading to problems in language development and reading.

TABLE 28–6 Examples of Learning Disabilities

DISORDER	CLINICAL MANIFESTATIONS
Dyslexia	Difficulty with writing, reading, spelling
Dyscalculia	Mathematics and computation problems
Dysgraphia	Difficulty with writing, spelling, and composition
Dyspraxia	Problems with manual dexterity and coordination

The causes of learning disorders are complex. Sometimes they are related to low birth weight or problems during the perinatal period. There may be a genetic component since their occurrence is more common when other family members are affected.

Learning disabilities should be diagnosed by a learning specialist such as a psychologist with special training. A series of cognitive and developmental tests are commonly used; magnetic resonance imaging (MRI) is sometimes used. Treatments involve learning how to compensate for the difficulties by using capabilities that are intact. Some children need to have all material written for them, and others need to have verbal presentations. Specific learning goals are established with the assistance of learning specialists. Children with learning disabilities should have individualized education plans (IEPs) established with realistic goals for school performance. (See Chapter 12 for further information about IEPs.)

Nurses play a major role in identifying children with learning disabilities. The nurse may be in contact with families during health promotion visits or in other settings when parents relay concern about the child's performance or difficulty in some aspect of school. Nurses should assess the child for the following developmental milestones, which can indicate learning disability (National Joint Committee on Learning Disabilities, 2015):

- Tasks such as tying shoes, buttoning, or hopping
- Expressive and receptive speech
- Naming objects or reading
- Fine and gross motor milestones
- Following simple instructions

When a child may have a learning disability, the nurse should refer the family to the school or other testing resource. The nurse should partner with the family to plan for the child's learning needs, help the family work closely with the child, suggest providing a setting at home to maximize potential for learning, and offer suggestions for building healthy self-esteem in the child. The nurse should assist the family to work with the school to establish annual goals for the child. Most children with learning disabilities can learn to perform well in their areas of strength and compensate for areas of difficulty. Early intervention is key to success and building a positive self-image regarding abilities.

Intellectual Disability (Formerly Called Mental Retardation)

Intellectual disability is now the preferred term for what was previously called *mental retardation*. **Intellectual disability** is defined as significant limitation in intellectual functioning and adaptive behavior. It is manifested as differences in conceptual, social, and practical adaptive skills, beginning before the age of 18 years (American Association on Intellectual and Developmental Disabilities, 2013). Later events that lead to limitations in function are commonly referred to as *brain injury*. Intellectual functioning is generally characterized by an intelligence quotient (IQ) below 70 to 75, accompanied by significant impairments in **adaptive functioning** (the ability to meet the standards expected for a cultural group). The child with intellectual disability has adaptive deficits in at least two areas such as communication, self-care, home living, social/interpersonal skills, use of community resources, self-direction, functional academic skills, work, leisure, health, or safety. A low IQ score by itself does not necessarily correlate with an impaired ability to carry out adaptive skills. The child should be evaluated within the contexts of the individual cultural and community environment. The IQ score and the level of adaptive skills together determine the degree of severity of intellectual disability.

Intellectual disability is one type of **developmental disability**, any of a variety of chronic conditions that are characterized by mental or physical impairments. Other examples include pervasive developmental disorder, cerebral palsy, and sensory loss. A developmental disability begins by age 21 years and lasts throughout life.

ETIOLOGY AND PATHOPHYSIOLOGY

Intellectual disability occurs in 12 per 1000 children, a decrease from 15.5 per 1000 a decade ago (CDC, n.d.). Its causes can be grouped into three general categories: prenatal errors in the development of the central nervous system, prenatal or postnatal changes in the person's biologic environment, and external forces leading to central nervous system damage. In each instance, the precipitating factor changes the form, function, and adaptation of the central nervous system. Table 28–7 provides examples of common conditions associated with intellectual disability.

SAFETY ALERT!

Zika virus is transferred to humans by the bite of the *Aedes* mosquito, which is most common in tropical, moist climates. An infected sexual partner can also transfer the virus. The symptoms found in most people with Zika virus disease are common to many viral illnesses: fever, rash, fatigue, conjunctivitis, and muscle aches. Since 2015, an increase in disabilities to women who contracted Zika virus in pregnancy was noted in Brazil. Further studies indicate that fetuses exposed to Zika virus have a higher risk than normal of being born with microcephaly (small head and brain), hearing problems, vision disabilities, and growth dysplasia. Much research is being carried out to learn about the disease, its transmission, and its effects on the fetus. No immunization is available against the virus, so protection from mosquito bites, ensuring protected sex with partners who have been exposed or infected, or delaying pregnancy if exposed to geographic areas where the virus is common are the only methods of known prevention (CDC, 2015).

Three conditions from prenatal life that are associated with intellectual disability are Down syndrome, fragile X syndrome, and fetal alcohol syndrome. In the United States, about 1 in 700 infants, or 5500 infants each year, are born with Down syndrome (CDC, 2014c). The syndrome is caused by an extra chromosome; the child has 47 rather than 46 chromosomes. (See discussion of genetic transmission in Chapter 3.) The most common chromosome affected is 21 so that the child often has "trisomy 21," or three instead of two copies of number 21 chromosome. In addition to intellectual disability and physical signs, the child with Down syndrome is at higher risk of developing other conditions such as cardiac defects, hearing loss, gastrointestinal problems, orthodontic conditions, thyroid disease, dermatologic conditions, and leukemia (CDC, 2014c).

TABLE 28–7 Common Conditions Associated With Intellectual Disability

PRENATAL CONDITIONS	BIOLOGIC ENVIRONMENT	EXTERNAL FORCES
Down syndrome	Inborn errors of metabolism (e.g., phenylketonuria, hypothyroidism)	Traumatic brain injury (e.g., accident)
Fragile X syndrome		Poison ingestion (acute or chronic)
Fetal alcohol syndrome		Hypoxia/anoxic insult
Maternal infection (e.g., rubella, cytomegalovirus)		Infection (e.g., meningitis)
		Environmental deprivation

Fragile X syndrome is caused by a single recessive gene abnormality on the X chromosome. A permutation to the X chromosome may occur in males or females. When a father or mother passes the faulty X chromosome to a daughter, it may remain as a permutation or may change into a true mutation. The daughter has two X chromosomes and therefore does not manifest this recessive disorder. However, she can pass the mutated X chromosome to her son who becomes affected with fragile X. The mutation of fragile X is on gene *FMRP-1*, which instructs cells to make a protein necessary for normal brain development. The faulty gene creates a deficiency in the FMRI protein that leads to brain changes. The condition is often associated with other conditions such as sudden death heart disease (SDHD), anxiety, and autism (CDC, 2014d).

Fetal alcohol spectrum disorder (FASD) describes the wide range of effects of ethyl alcohol on the developing fetus. The condition ranges from alcohol-related birth defects (ARBDs), such as disorders of the heart, kidneys, bones, or hearing; to alcohol-related neurodevelopment disorder (ARND), such as intellectual disability; to fetal alcohol syndrome, which is the most severe end of the spectrum, leading to a combination of mental health and intellectual and physical problems (CDC, 2014e). Alcohol ingestion by the pregnant woman can influence development of many body organs, and effects can range from mild to severe. Despite many years of public health education, alcohol use remains a leading cause of intellectual disability. From 0.3 to 1.5 per 1000 births are affected by fetal alcohol syndrome (CDC, 2014e).

For a discussion of phenylketonuria and hypothyroidism, two common biochemical causes of intellectual disability, see Chapter 30. Other causes involve traumatic brain injury and infections of the central nervous system (see Chapter 27). Intellectual disability is more common in children born prematurely.

CLINICAL MANIFESTATIONS

Mild intellectual disability was originally described as an IQ between 50 and 70, moderate disability with IQ of 35 to 50, severe disability with IQ 20 to 35, and profound disability below 20. Although an IQ below 70 is generally considered indicative of intellectual disability, the functional assessment of the child is now considered a more accurate identification of children's performance and needs. Children who have intellectual disabilities manifest delays in all areas of development, including motor movement, language, and adaptive behavior. They usually achieve developmental milestones more slowly than the average child. These developmental delays may be the first indication to parents, teachers, and healthcare providers of the child's condition.

Intellectual disability is sometimes accompanied by sensory impairment, speech problems, motor and orthopedic disabilities, and seizure disorders. Of children with the disability, 10% to 30% manifest one of these other disorders. Table 28–8 lists several physical characteristics associated with Down syndrome, fragile X syndrome, and fetal alcohol syndrome.

Developing Cultural Competence Fetal Alcohol Syndrome

Fetal alcohol syndrome is more common in groups with higher intake of alcohol. Because some Native American tribes have a high rate of alcoholism, the federal government and some tribes have joined together to lower that risk among this ethnic group. Some reservations, such as the Yakama Nation in Washington State, do not sell alcoholic beverages and have put educational programs in place.

TABLE 28–8 Characteristics Associated With Three Common Types of Intellectual Disability

SYNDROME	CHARACTERISTICS
Down syndrome (see Figures 5–8 and 5–33)	Small head (microcephaly)
	Flattened forehead
	Wide, short neck
	Epicanthal eye folds
	White spots on eye iris (Brushfield spots)
	Congenital cataracts
	Flat nose
	Small, low-set ears
	Protruding tongue
	Short broad hands
	Simian line on palm
	Wide space between first and second toes
	Hearing loss
	Increased incidence of diabetes, congenital heart defect, and leukemia
	Hypotonia
Fragile X syndrome	Long face
	Prominent jaw
	Large ears
	Frequent otitis media
	Large testicles
	Epicanthal eye folds
	Strabismus
	High arched palate
	Scoliosis
Fetal alcohol syndrome (see Figure 4–4)	Flat midface
	Low nasal bridge
	Long philtrum with narrow upper lip
	Short upturned nose
	Poor coordination
	Failure to thrive
	Skeletal and joint abnormalities
	Hearing loss

CLINICAL THERAPY

Intellectual disability is diagnosed and initial treatment is planned in a multistep process, and by involving a collaborative care team. Team members may include a developmental specialist, physician, geneticist, nurse, teacher, language therapist, occupational therapist, and physical rehabilitation specialist. See Table 28–9 for a description of the *DSM-5* diagnostic criteria for intellectual disability. Diagnosis begins with a comprehensive history and evaluation of the child's physical characteristics, developmental level, and intellectual and adaptive functioning. Laboratory tests such as chromosome analysis, blood enzyme levels, lead levels, or cranial imaging provide valuable information in some circumstances. A three-generation family history is performed.

Developmental screening (see Chapter 6) can help identify children at risk. Tests of intellectual and adaptive functioning are performed when disability is suspected. A neurologic examination may indicate asymmetry of movement or strength, irritability or lethargy, or abnormal pitch to an infant's cry. Because intellectual disability may be accompanied by physical abnormalities, it is important to observe the child for facial symmetry, distance between the eyes, level of the ears, hair growth, and palmar creases. These abnormalities may be clues to other health problems.

TABLE 28–9 *DSM-5* Diagnostic Criteria for Intellectual Disability

Intellectual disability (intellectual developmental disorder) is a disorder with onset during the developmental period that includes both intellectual and adaptive functioning deficits in conceptual, social, and practical domains. The following three criteria must be met:

1. Deficits in intellectual functions, such as reasoning, problem solving, planning, abstract thinking, judgment, academic learning, and learning from experience, confirmed by both clinical assessment and individualized, standardized intelligence testing.

2. Deficits in adaptive functioning that result in failure to meet developmental and sociocultural standards for personal independence and social responsibility. Without ongoing support, the adaptive deficits limit functioning in one or more activities of daily life, such as communication, social participation, and independent living, across multiple environments, such as home, school, work, and community.

3. Onset of intellectual and adaptive deficits during the developmental period.

Note: The diagnostic term *intellectual disability* is the equivalent term for the diagnosis of *intellectual developmental disorders*. Moreover, a federal statute in the United States (Public Law 111-256, Rosa's Law) replaces the term *mental retardation* with *intellectual disability*, and research journals use the term *intellectual disability*. Thus, *intellectual disability* is the term in common use by medical, educational, and other professions and by the lay public and advocacy groups.

Specify current severity as:

- Mild
- Moderate
- Severe
- Profound

Source: Used with permission from American Psychiatric Association. (2013). *Diagnostic and statistical manual of mental disorders* (5th ed.). Washington, DC: Author. Copyright © 2013 American Psychiatric Association.

Based on the results of the evaluation, a multidisciplinary team plans the support needed to maximize the child's potential for development. Management focuses on early intervention to improve the degree of adaptive functioning. Associated physical, emotional, and behavioral problems are treated simultaneously. Depending on the child's condition, special education programs and physical or occupational therapy may be necessary (Figure 28–8). The Education for All Handicapped Children Act (PL 94-142) provides free appropriate education to all handicapped children between 2 and 21 years of age. Amendments to this act in 1986 (PL 99-457) encouraged states to provide early intervention services for infants and toddlers with developmental delay conditions through federal funding.

The child may require supportive care and assistance with activities of daily living. The plans for intervention need to change as the child grows and the family situation alters. Classes and special services are needed for youth and families when the adolescent with intellectual disability transitions into young adulthood.

Nursing Management

For the Child With Intellectual Disability

Nursing Assessment and Diagnosis

Nurses can help identify children with intellectual disability through history taking, observation, and developmental screening during early childhood. The history should provide information about the mental and adaptive functioning of birth parents and other family members, as intellectual disability may cluster in some families, and conditions such as fragile X syndrome are genetic in origin. The pregnancy and birth history can provide important information about the mother's alcohol and drug use during pregnancy. Be alert for a history of difficult pregnancy

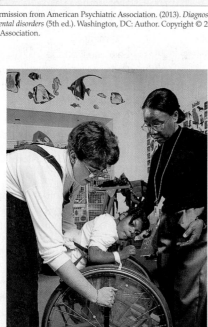

A

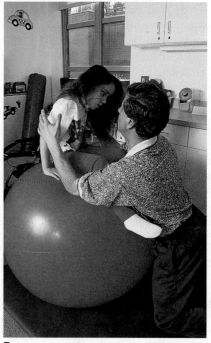

B

Figure 28–8 **Physical therapy is an important component of medical management for many children who have intellectual disabilities.** *A,* **This girl, who is severely intellectually disabled and uses a wheelchair, is being positioned in a mobile prone stander, which enables her to interact in a different manner with her therapists and the environment.** *B,* **Physical therapists also provide outpatient care in the community to children with varying degrees of disability.**

and problems during birth. Prematurity places the child at risk of below-normal cognitive development. Frequent developmental testing during early childhood is needed for infants born prematurely. When genetic conditions in the family predispose family members to intellectual disability, assess the child carefully. Children from deprived environments or those at risk because of environmental factors such as lead poisoning (see Chapter 17) are more likely to manifest intellectual disability.

Many children with intellectual disability are not diagnosed until they reach school age, particularly if the condition is mild. Early intervention, however, can help enhance the child's functioning later. During home visits, during clinic appointments, in childcare centers, and during hospitalization, be alert for signs such as developmental delays, multiple (more than three) physical anomalies associated with a specific condition (see Table 28–8), or neurologic alterations. Developmental assessment should be part of each healthcare visit; see Chapters 7, 8, and 9 for developmental surveillance recommended at each age.

When the diagnosis of intellectual disability has been made, assess the adaptive functioning of the child and family. Perform a functional assessment of the child, including toileting, dressing, and feeding skills. Assess the child's language, sensory, and psychomotor functioning. Assess the home and community for safety hazards. Observe how the family is managing with the child. Ask about family activities that include the child, community and school attitudes and support, and care management as well as planning for the future. Assess the availability of services such as groups for parents and special education opportunities for children. Evaluate the coping skills of family members.

Several nursing diagnoses may be appropriate for the child with intellectual disability, depending on the degree, cause, and outcome of the child's condition. Some of these diagnoses relate to impairments in adaptive functioning; others relate to the impact on the family. Examples include the following (NANDA-I © 2014):

- *Development: Delayed, Risk for,* related to neonatal disease or condition
- *Nutrition, Imbalanced: Less than Body Requirements,* related to inability to ingest sufficient food
- *Self-care Deficit: Dressing, Toileting, Bathing,* related to developmental disability
- *Communication: Verbal, Impaired,* related to developmental disability
- *Injury, Risk for,* related to lack of understanding of environmental hazards
- *Coping: Family, Compromised,* related to the child's developmental variations

Planning and Implementation

Nearly all children with intellectual disability are cared for in the community. However, they may have conditions that require periodic hospitalization or frequent healthcare visits. Nursing care focuses on providing emotional support and information to family members, maintaining a safe environment, assisting the child with adaptive functioning, and fostering parental management of the child's activities. Whenever possible, the nurse uses preventive teaching to lower the risk of disability. For example, nurses can integrate teaching into care for all women about the importance of avoiding all alcohol during any times when they might become pregnant. This helps prevent fetal alcohol syndrome, especially in early pregnancy when women may not know they are pregnant.

PROVIDE EMOTIONAL SUPPORT AND INFORMATION

Family members need empathy and support both at the time of diagnosis and in the ensuing years. Parents may be in an acute or chronic state of grief over the loss of the healthy child. Encourage them to verbalize their feelings. Introducing them to parents of other children who have intellectual disabilities may help and support them as they learn how to manage the child's needs. Discuss the availability of respite care to provide parents with a break from caretaking. Other family members such as grandparents and siblings may also feel grief or guilt and should be given an opportunity to talk about their feelings.

Parents need honest information and answers to their questions about the child's condition. Reinforce information provided by genetic counselors and other healthcare professionals. Parents need to know about community resources designed to assist children with intellectual disability. As mentioned earlier, the Education for All Handicapped Children Act (PL 94-142) provides free appropriate education to all handicapped children between 2 and 21 years of age. States and local communities may provide early intervention services for infants and toddlers with disabilities. Examples of programs include the Zero to Three early intervention programs, special education preschools and schools, county health services, and respite care. Ask parents if they have questions about IEPs and refer them to Internet sources if that is helpful. Review federal and state laws and services that might be helpful to the family, and help them interpret information they find to analyze its strengths and limitations.

MAINTAIN A SAFE ENVIRONMENT

Children with intellectual disabilities require close supervision because they may not understand common hazards. Ensure safety in the hospital. Assist parents in providing safety at home and school, and teaching the child necessary skills such as pedestrian safety. Consider both physical and emotional safety. The child may be indiscriminately trusting and sometimes is at risk for physical or sexual abuse.

PROVIDE ASSISTANCE WITH ADAPTIVE FUNCTIONING

Encourage parents' efforts to maximize the child's areas of strength and identify needs related to adaptive behaviors. Refer them to resources to help with the child's impaired areas of adaptive functioning, such as communication, self-care, or social skills. During hospitalization, support parents' efforts to maintain the child's skills in toileting, dressing, and self-care by planning interventions to use the skills being taught at home.

COMMUNITY-BASED NURSING CARE

The child with intellectual disability needs ongoing care throughout childhood; interventions must be adapted as the child develops and the family's needs evolve. Parents often act as case managers for the child's care. Assist parents as necessary to acquire the skills required to coordinate the child's plan of care. Evaluate the child's needs regularly and help parents with the treatment plan as necessary. Provision of education including services such as physical or speech therapy is a primary goal. Most children with intellectual disability have an IEP designed to meet their specific learning needs. Parents, nurses, and others such as teachers and language therapists are part of the team that establishes the child's IEP. Promote optimal development and socialization. As the child reaches adolescence, education is directed toward a vocation, issues of sexuality, and the goal of independent living, when appropriate. Transition classes for adolescents with intellectual disability can teach self-care skills that may enable some to live in group homes or other community settings. Parents need help planning for the child's future and their own retirement.

Specific guidelines for care are available for the child with Down syndrome (Bull & Committee on Genetics, 2011). These guidelines suggest times for evaluation of hearing, growth, cardiac function, and other areas designed for early identification and treatment of associated disorders. There are growth grids for children with Down syndrome, and specific topics to suggest for anticipatory guidance during healthcare visits.

Evaluation

The expected outcomes of nursing care depend on the child's needs and developmental level. Early in the diagnostic phase, desired outcomes may involve the family's understanding of the diagnosis and the child's special needs. Later outcomes may focus on the child's communication of self-help skills. Outcomes related to cognitive performance and adaptive skills may be developed during childhood. Successful transition into adulthood at the maximal level of function is the ultimate desired outcome.

Chapter Highlights

- Major treatment modes for children with mental health disorders include individual therapy, family therapy, and group therapy.

- Therapeutic strategies for treatment of children and adolescents with mental health disorders include play therapy, art therapy, cognitive behavioral therapy (CBT), visualization, and hypnosis.

- Nurses conduct mental health assessments, prevent disorders when possible, participate in intervention to treat disorders, and evaluate outcomes of treatment.

- Autism spectrum disorder is the major type of pervasive developmental disorder and is manifested by abnormal behavior, social interaction, and communication.

- Attention deficit hyperactivity disorder is characterized by developmentally altered behaviors involving inattention and hyperactivity.

- Mood disorders in childhood and adolescence are commonly manifested as depression or bipolar disorder.

- Several anxiety disorders occur in children and adolescents, most notably generalized anxiety, separation anxiety, panic,

obsessive-compulsive disorder, social phobia, conversion reaction, and posttraumatic stress disorder (PTSD).

- Behavioral therapy and selective serotonin reuptake inhibitors (SSRIs) are used in treatment of anxiety; prescription drug use in children must be closely monitored.

- Suicide is a significant cause of death among youth; nurses play a key role in identifying youth at risk, instituting prevention programs, and counseling families and friends of suicide victims.

- Nurses play a role in identifying children with potential learning disabilities, referring for diagnosis, and partnering with the family to provide a positive learning experience for the child.

- Intellectual disability is subaverage intellectual and adaptive functioning, and may be caused by chromosomal, genetic, or environmental factors.

- A multidisciplinary team plans the care for children with intellectual disability and periodically evaluates the child's progress and the family's needs.

Clinical Reasoning in Action

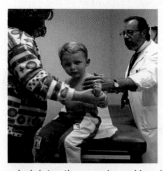

Cooper, a 5-year-old child with autism spectrum disorder, comes into the office for his annual checkup and school immunizations of diphtheria, tetanus, and acellular pertussis (DTaP); inactivated polio vaccine (IPV); and measles-mumps-rubella (MMR). He is very combative and it takes four people to help hold him and administer the vaccines. He will be attending a special school for children with autism spectrum and related disorders. Diagnosed at 3 years old, he has never been in the hospital or had surgery. It is extremely difficult to examine him as he does not like to be touched. During prior visits in the office, Cooper has stood facing the wall and twisting his hands. He continues to be combative for most of the examination, even with the use of

decreased stimuli, communication, and slow movements, but you are able to assess that his blood pressure is 95/53 mmHg. He is in the 50th percentile for both height and weight and his temperature is 99°F.

You give Cooper's mother information about local support groups for children with autism spectrum disorder and about local psychiatrists who can treat the condition with medication that helps control aggressive behavior. You also supply her with contact information for counselors in the area to help her deal with her own stress. She is appreciative of your help and support and looks forward to being able to send Cooper to school.

1. The mother has questions about the MMR vaccine and whether it causes autism. What can you tell her about that? Would you administer the vaccine today?

2. What can you tell the mother about safety issues with Cooper?

3. How can you enhance communication with Cooper when he comes into the office?

References

Agency for Healthcare Research and Quality (AHRQ). (2014). *Recommendations for children and adolescents: Guide to clinical preventive services.* Retrieved from http://www.ahrq.gov/professionals/clinicians-providers/guidelines-recommendations/guide/section3.html

American Association on Intellectual and Developmental Disabilities. (2013). *Definition of intellectual disability.* Retrieved from http://www.aaidd.org/content_100.cfm

American Psychiatric Association. (2013). *Diagnostic and statistical manual of mental disorders (DSM-5)* (5th ed.). Washington, DC: Author.

Arnold, L. E., Hurt, E., & Lofthouse, N. (2013). Attention-deficit/hyperactivity disorder: Dietary and nutritional treatments. *Child and Adolescent Psychiatric Clinics of North America, 22,* 381–402.

Bartlett, D. (2011). Drug therapy gets personal with genetic profiling. *American Nurse Today, 6*(5). Retrieved from http://www.americannursetoday.com/article.aspx?id=7814&fid=7770

Blake, T. (2012). Three medication pathways for bipolar disorder. *Nursing 2012, 42*(5), 28–35.

Boydston, L, Hsiao, R. C., & Varley, C. K. (2012a). Identifying anxiety disorders in the primary care setting. *Contemporary Pediatrics, 29*(6), 28–34.

Boydston, L, Hsiao, R. C., & Varley, C. K. (2012b). Anxiety disorders in adolescents: Assessment and treatment. *Contemporary Pediatrics, 29*(7), 36–42.

Boyle, C. A., Boulet, S., Schieve, L. A., Cohen, R. A., Blumberg, S. J., Yeargin-Allsop, M., . . . Kogan, M. D. (2011), Trends in the prevalence of developmental disabilities in U.S. children, 1997–2008. *Pediatrics.* doi:10.1542/peds.2010-2989

Brown, P. (2012). ADHD guidelines: An update for your practice. *Consultant for Pediatricians, October Supplement,* S3–S7.

Bruxel, E. M., Akutagava-Martins, G. C., Salatno-Oliveira, A., Contini, V., Kieling, C., Hutz, M. H., & Rohde, L. A. (2014). ADHD pharmacogenetics across the life cycle: New findings and perspectives. *American Journal of Medical Genetics, 165B,* 263–282.

Bull, M. J., & Committee on Genetics. (2011). Clinical report—Health supervision for children with Down syndrome. *Pediatrics, 128,* 393–406.

Center for Injury Research and Prevention. (2011). *PTSD in children and parents.* Retrieved from http://injury.research.chop.edu/our_research/carit_research.php

Centers for Disease Control and Prevention (CDC). (n.d.). *Intellectual disabilities among children.* Retrieved from http://www.cdc.gov

Centers for Disease Control and Prevention. (CDC). (2008). Unintentional strangulation deaths from the "choking game" among youths ages 6–19 years—United States 1995–2007. *Morbidity and Mortality Weekly Report, 57,* 141–146.

Centers for Disease Control and Prevention (CDC). (2010). *The choking game: Risky youth behavior.* Retrieved from http://www.cdc.gov

Centers for Disease Control and Prevention (CDC). (2012a). Prevalence of autism spectrum disorder among children aged 8 years—Autism and developmental disabilities monitoring network, 14 sites, United States, 2008. *Morbidity and Mortality Weekly Report (MMWR) Surveillance Summary, 61*(SS03), 1–19.

Centers for Disease Control and Prevention (CDC). (2012b). *Suicide.* Retrieved from http://www.cdc.gov/violenceprevention/pdf/Suicide-DataSheet-a.pdf

Centers for Disease Control and Prevention (CDC). (2013). *Developmental disabilities.* Retrieved from http://www.cdc.gov/ncbddd/developmentaldisabilities/index.html

Centers for Disease Control and Prevention (CDC). (2014a). Prevalence of autism spectrum disorder among children aged 8 years—Autism and developmental disabilities monitoring network, 11 sites, United States, 2010. *Morbidity and Mortality Weekly Report (MMWR) Surveillance Summary, 63*(2), 1–21.

Centers for Disease Control and Prevention (CDC). (2014b). *Attention-deficit/hyperactivity disorder.* Retrieved from http://www.cdc.gov/ncbddd/adhd/data.html

Centers for Disease Control and Prevention (CDC). (2014c). *Occurrence of Down syndrome.* Retrieved from http://www.cdc.gov/ncbddd/birthdefects/downsyndrome/data.html

Centers for Disease Control and Prevention (CDC). (2014d). *Facts about fragile X syndrome.* Retrieved from http://www.cdc.gov/ncbddd/fxs/facts.html

Centers for Disease Control and Prevention (CDC). (2014e). *Facts about FASDs.* Retrieved from http://www.cdc.gov/ncbddd/fasd/facts.html

Centers for Disease Control and Prevention (CDC). (2015). *About Zika virus disease.* Retrieved from http://www.cdc.gov/zika/about/

Chung, P. J., & Soares, N. S. (2012). Childhood depression: Recognition and management. *Consultant for Pediatricians, September,* 259–267.

Dineen, W. K. (2014). Timely topics in pediatric psychiatry. *Journal of Clinical Psychiatry, 75,* 1224–1225.

Emslie, G. J., Kennard, B. D., & Mayes, T. L. (2011). Predictors of treatment response in adolescent depression. *Pediatric Annals, 40,* 300–306.

Faraone, S. V., & Antshel, K. M. (2014). Towards an evidence-based taxonomy of nonpharmacologic treatments for ADHD. *Child and Adolescent Psychiatric Clinics of North America, 23,* 965–972.

Ferguson, C. J. (2011). The influence of television and video game use on attention and school problems: A multivariate analysis with other risk factors controlled. *Journal of Psychiatric Research, 45,* 808–813.

Findling, R. L., & Dinh, S. (2014). Transdermal therapy for attention-deficit hyperactivity disorder with the methylphenidate patch (MTS). *CNS Drugs, 28,* 217–228.

Frye, R. E. (2014). Metabolic and mitochondrial disorders associated with epilepsy in children with autism spectrum disorder. *Epilepsy Behavior.* doi:10.1016/j.yebeh.2014.08.134

Haga, S. B., O'Daniel, J. M., Tindall, G. M., Lipkus, I. R., & Agans, R. (2012). Survey of US public attitudes toward pharmacogenetic testing. *Pharmacogenomics Journal, 12,* 197–204.

Harrington, J. W. (2013, January). Autism in the school-aged child: Diagnostic dilemma, comorbid condition—or both? *Consultant for Pediatricians,* 13–17.

Houck, G., Kendall, J., Miller, A., Mirrell, P., & Wiebe, G. (2011). Self-concept in children and adolescents with attention deficit hyperactivity disorder. *Journal of Pediatric Nursing, 26,* 239–247.

Hughes, J. L., & Asarnow, J. R. (2011). Family intervention strategies for adolescent depression. *Pediatric Annals, 40,* 314–318.

Johnson, C. P., Myers, S. M., & Council on Children with Disabilities. (2007, reaffirmed 2010). Identification and evaluation of children with autism spectrum disorders. *Pediatrics, 120,* 1183–1215.

Kemper, K. J., Gardiner, P., & Birdee, G. S. (2013). Use of complementary and alternative medical therapies among youth with mental health concerns. *Academic Pediatrics, 13,* 540–545.

Kloos, A. L., & Robb, A. S. (2011). Bipolar disorder in children and adolescents. *Pediatric Annals, 40,* 481–487.

Knisely, M. R., Carpenter, J. S., & Von Ah, D. (2014). Pharmacogenomics in the nursing literature: An integrative review. *Nursing Outlook, 62,* 285–296.

Kozlowska, K., Scher, S., & Williams, L. M. (2011). Patterns of emotional-cognitive functioning in pediatric conversion patients: Implications for the conceptualization of conversion disorders. *Psychosomatic Medicine, 73*(9), 775–788.

Lachman, A. (2014). New developments in diagnosis and treatment update: Schizophrenia/first episode psychosis in children and adolescents. *Journal of Child and Adolescent Mental Health, 26,* 109–124.

Lee, M. J., & Liechty, J. M. (2014, May 7). Longitudinal associations between immigrant ethnic density, neighborhood processes, and Latino immigrant youth depression. *Journal of Immigrant and Minority Health.* doi:10.1007/s10903-014-0029-4

Madadi, P. (2015). Ethical perspectives on translational pharmacogenetic research involving children. *Paediatric Drugs, 17*(1), 91–95. doi:10.1007/s40272-014-0111-3

Maglione, M. S., Das, Raaen, L., Smith, A., Chari, R., Newberry, S., . . . Gidengil, C. (2014). Safety of vaccines used for routine immunization of U.S. children: A systematic review. *Pediatrics, 134,* 325–337.

Maheshwari, R., & Joshi, P. (2012). Assessment, referral, and treatment of suicidal adolescents. *Pediatric Annals, 41,* 516–521.

Mahoney, J. R., Kennard, B. D., & Mayes, T. L. (2011). Cognitive behavioral treatment of depression in youth. *Pediatric Annals, 40,* 307–313.

Mayo Clinic. (2013a). *Cognitive behavioral therapy.* Retrieved from http://www.mayoclinic.org/tests-procedures/cognitive-behavioral-therapy/basics/definition/prc-20013594

Mayo Clinic. (2013b). *Depression (major depressive disorder).* Retrieved from http://www.mayoclinic.org/diseases-conditions/depression/in-depth/ssris/ART-20044825?pg=2

Mayo Clinic. (2014). *Childhood schizophrenia.* Retrieved from http://www.mayoclinic.org/diseases-conditions/childhood-schizophrenia/basics/causes/con-20029260

Mechling, G., Ahern, N. R., & McGuinness, T. M. (2013). The choking game: A risky behavior for youth. *Journal of Psychosocial Nursing and Mental Health Services, 51*(12), 15–20.

Morrison, J., & Schwartz, T. L. (2014). Adolescent angst or true intent: Suicidal behavior, risk and neurological mechanisms in depressed children and teenagers taking antidepressants. *International Journal of Emergency Mental Health, 16,* 247–250.

National Center for Children in Poverty. (2014). *Children's mental health.* Retrieved from http://www.nccp.org/topics/mentalhealth.html

National Institute of Mental Health (NIMH). (n.d.a). *Depression in children and adolescents.* Retrieved from http://www.nimh.nih.gov/health/publications/depression-in-children-and-adolescents/index.shtml

National Institute of Mental Health (NIMH). (n.d.b). *Bipolar disorder.* Retrieved from http://www.nimh.nih.gov/health/topics/bipolar-disorder/index.shtml

National Institute of Mental Health (NIMH). (2012a). *Mental health medications.* Retrieved from http://www.nimh.nih.gov/health/publications/mental-health-medications/what-medications-are-used-to-treat-bipolar-disorder.shtml

National Institute of Mental Health (NIMH). (2012b). *Information about PANDAS.* Retrieved from http://www.nimh.nih.gov/labs-at-nimh/research-areas/clinics-and-labs/pdnb/web.shtml

National Institute of Neurological Disorders and Stroke. (2014). *Tourette syndrome fact sheet.* Retrieved from http://www.ninds.nih.gov/disorders/tourette/detail_tourette.htm

National Institutes of Health (NIH). (2012). *Attention deficit hyperactivity disorder (ADHD).* Retrieved from http://www.nimh.nih.gov/health/publications/attention-deficit-hyperactivity-disorder/index.shtml

National Joint Committee on Learning Disabilities. (2015). *What is a learning disability?* Retrieved from http://www.ldonline.org/ldbasics/whatisld

Santrock, J. W. (2011). *Child development* (13th ed.). Boston, MA: McGraw-Hill.

Sarvet, B., & Brewer, S. (2011). Anxiety disorders in pediatric primary care. *Pediatric Annals, 40,* 499–505.

Schmid, A. M., Truong, A. W., & Damian, F. J. (2011). Care of the suicidal pediatric patient in the ED: A case study. *American Journal of Nursing, 111*(9), 34–43.

Scrandis, D. A. (2014). Identification and management of bipolar disorder. *Nurse Practitioner, 39*(10). 30–37.

Selekman, J., & Diefenbeck, C. (2014). The new DSM-5 and its impact on the mental health care of children. *Journal of Pediatric Nursing, 29,* 442–450.

Stockings, E., Degenhardt, L., Lee, Y. Y., Mihalopoulos, C., Liu, A., Hobbs, M., & Patton, G. (2014). Symptom screening scales for detecting major depressive disorder in children and adolescents: A systematic review and meta-analysis of reliability, validity and diagnostic utility. *Journal of Affective Disorders, 174C,* 447–463.

Subcommittee on Attention-Deficit/Hyperactivity Disorder, Steering Committee on Quality Improvement and Management. (2011). ADHD: Clinical practice guideline for the diagnosis, evaluation, and treatment of attention-deficit/hyperactivity disorder in children and adolescents. *Pediatrics.* doi:10.1542/peds.2011-2654

U.S. Department of Health and Human Services (USDHHS). (2012). *2012 national strategy for suicide prevention: Goals and objectives for action.* Washington, DC: Author

U.S. Department of Health and Human Services (USDHHS). (2015). *Healthy People 2020.* Retrieved from http://www.healthypeople.gov

Valicenti-McDermott, M., Burrows, B., Bernstein, L., Hottinger, K., Lawson, K., Seijo, R., . . . Shinnar, S. (2014). Use of complementary and alternative medicine in children with autism and other developmental disabilities: Associations with ethnicity, child comorbid symptoms, and parental stress. *Journal of Child Neurology, 29,* 360–367.

Van Egmond-Frohlich, A. W., Weghuber, D., & de Zwaan, M. (2012). Association of symptoms of attention-deficit/hyperactivity disorder and childhood overweight adjusted for confounding parental variables. *International Journal of Obesity, 36,* 963–968.

Webb, P. L. (2011). Screening for autism spectrum disorders during well-child visits in a primary care setting. *Journal for Nurse Practitioners, 7,* 229–237.

Weeke, P., Jensen, A., Folke, F., Gislason, G. H., Olesen, J. B., Andersson, C., . . . Torp-Pedersen, C. (2012). Antidepressant use and risk of out-of-hospital cardiac arrest: A nationwide case-time-control study. *Clinical Pharmacology and Therapeutics, 92,* 72–79.

Won, H., Mah, W., & Kim, E. (2013). Autism spectrum disorder causes, mechanisms and treatments: Focus on neuronal synapses. *Frontiers in Molecular Neuroscience.* doi:10.3389/fnmol.2013.00019

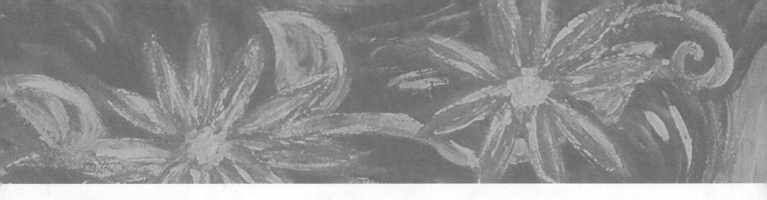

Chapter 29
Alterations in Musculoskeletal Function

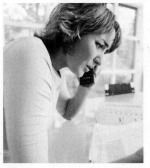

When I got the call that Douglass was in the emergency room I was so scared. I guess we're lucky it was just a broken leg. I've never had a cast. What do you need to do with it? I also wonder if it's safe for him go back to his friend's house where he broke his leg on a trampoline. Should I tell him not to use the trampoline when he heals? It's hard to decide.

—Mother of Douglass, 12 years old

OMG/The Image Bank/Getty Images

∨ Learning Outcomes

29.1 Describe pediatric variations in the musculoskeletal system.

29.2 Plan nursing care for children with structural deformities of the foot, leg, hip, and spine.

29.3 Recognize signs and symptoms of infectious musculoskeletal disorders and refer for appropriate care.

29.4 Partner with families to plan care for children with musculoskeletal conditions that are chronic or require long-term care.

29.5 Prioritize nursing interventions to promote safety and developmental progression in children who require braces, casts, traction, and surgery.

29.6 Develop a nursing care plan for fractures, including teaching for injury prevention and nursing implementations for the child who has sustained a fracture.

The musculoskeletal system helps the body protect its vital organs, support weight, control motion, store minerals, and supply red blood cells. Bones provide a rigid framework for the body, muscles provide for active movement, and tendons and ligaments hold the bones and muscles together. Therefore, alterations in musculoskeletal functioning can have a significant impact on a child's growth and development.

What concerns do parents and children have when a child has musculoskeletal conditions? Will the child need any special adaptations in the home and school? Can musculoskeletal injuries be prevented? The information in this chapter will answer these questions and enable nurses to provide effective care for children who have musculoskeletal disorders.

Musculoskeletal disorders may be congenital, such as clubfoot, or acquired, such as osteomyelitis. They may require short- or long-term management, and may be treated on an outpatient basis or require hospitalization.

Text continues on page 826

FOCUS ON:
The Musculoskeletal System

Anatomy and Physiology

The musculoskeletal system is composed of the bones and muscles; joints, the supporting structures that facilitate movement; and tendons and ligaments that connect parts of the system. Cartilage is the connective tissue precursor to bone and remains in some structures such as ears and ribs throughout life. Bone formation is a dynamic system at any age, but particularly so in children and adolescents. Children depend on a functioning musculoskeletal system to enable support and movement, which in turn ensures that exposure to various stimuli and normal development can occur.

Bones are composed of osseous or dense connective tissue; they contain an exterior shell or cortex and an inner, primarily protein, matrix (Figure 29–1). The cells covering the cortex are called lining cells or compact bone, and they protect the bone from penetration by circulating blood cells and other components of circulation; this covering is called the periosteum. The inner matrix is composed of a series of interconnected plates called cancellous, trabecular, or spongy bone. Spaces between these plates are called bone marrow, and this is the area where hematopoiesis (production and development of blood cells) occurs. In addition to the lining cells found on the bone exterior, other types of cells include osteoblasts, which synthesize and lay down bone and then attract calcium and phosphates to strengthen the bone; osteoclasts, which resorb bone in the constant process of bone formation and breakdown; and osteocytes, which are special osteoblasts that sense and respond to bone pressure and bending to direct the process of bone remodeling. The process of bone growth and remodeling is influenced by factors such as pressure (via physical activity), hormones (parathyroid hormone, glucocorticoids, insulin-like growth factor, and calcitonin), and external factors (dietary intake of calcium and phosphorus, bisphosphonate drugs, gallium, and so on).

The 206 bones of the human body include several types:

- *Long bones* such as the fibula, tibia, femur, humerus, and ulna; most childhood growth occurs in these bones
- *Short bones* such as those in the wrist and ankle
- *Flat bones* such as the skull, sternum, and ribs; the ribs retain large components of cartilage even when mature
- *Irregular bones* that have a variety of shapes and sizes, such as vertebrae, pelvic bones, and scapula

Muscles are collections of cells that can contract, causing the accompanying skeleton to move. Muscle fibers require a supply of blood and nerves and vary from small to quite large in size. Muscle cells develop in response to the stimulation of activity. Types of muscle cells include:

- *Skeletal* (striated) or *voluntary* muscles that involve the biceps, triceps, deltoid, gluteus maximus, and others
- *Smooth* (short-fibered) or *involuntary* muscles such as those in the gastrointestinal tract, lungs, and pupils of the eye
- *Cardiac* (striated, special-function) muscles that ensure the heart's constant contraction and relaxation

Muscles enable parts of the body to flex and extend, abduct and adduct, and carry out other motions (Figure 29–2). As one muscle flexes, the opposing muscle must extend to allow the movement.

Several other structures enable the musculoskeletal system to function. The joints are articulations or connections between bones. Fibrous joints provide for little movement (e.g., those in the skull), cartilaginous joints allow for slight movement (e.g., vertebral joints), and synovial joints are movable within certain limits (e.g., knee, hip, elbow, and shoulder). Joints are complex in structure and function, containing the fibrous end of the bone, synovial membrane and fluid, other sacs called bursae, and ligaments. Ligaments are tough fibers that bind the ends of bones together. Tendons are fibrous bands that connect bone to its accompanying muscles, allowing the bone to move when a muscle contracts or relaxes.

Pediatric Differences

Bones

Several differences exist between the bones of children and those of adults. Although primary centers of **ossification** (bone formation) are nearly complete at birth, a fibrous membrane still exists between the cranial bones (fontanelles). (See *As Children Grow: Sutures* in Chapter 5.) The posterior fontanelle closes

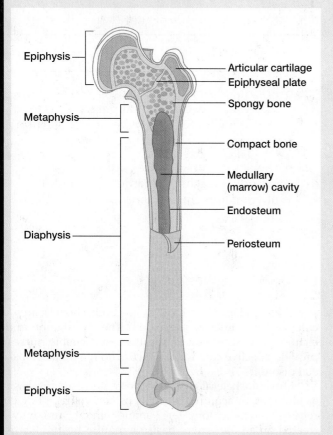

Epiphysis
Metaphysis
Diaphysis
Metaphysis
Epiphysis

Articular cartilage
Epiphyseal plate
Spongy bone
Compact bone
Medullary (marrow) cavity
Endosteum
Periosteum

Figure 29–1 **The parts of long bones.**

Varus
An abnormal position of a limb that involves bending inward toward the midline of the body

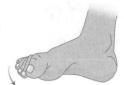

Valgus
An abnormal position of a limb that involves bending outward away from the midline of the body

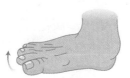

Supination
Lying on the back or placing the hand so that palm faces upward

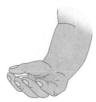

Pronation
Lying on the stomach or placing the hand so the palm faces downward

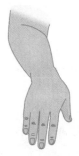

Adduction
Lateral movement of limbs toward the midline of the body

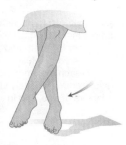

Abduction
Lateral movement of limbs away from the midline of the body

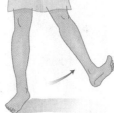

Flexion
A decrease in angle between bones forming a joint

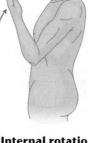

Extension
A movement that brings a limb into a straight position

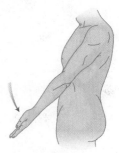

Inversion
Turning inward, usually more than normal

Eversion
Turning outward

Internal rotation
Rotation of a body part toward the midline of the body

External rotation
Rotation of a body segment away from the midline of the body

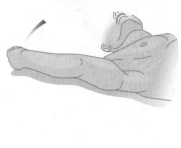

Figure 29–2 Musculoskeletal positions and joint motions.

TABLE 29–1 Diagnostic and Laboratory Procedures/Tests for the Musculoskeletal System

DIAGNOSTIC PROCEDURES	LABORATORY TESTS
Arthrogram	Alkaline phosphatase (ALP)
Bone scan	C-reactive protein (CRP)
Computed tomography (CT)	Erythrocyte sedimentation rate (ESR or sed rate)
Dual energy x-ray absorptiometry (DEXA)	Rheumatoid factor (RF)
Electromyelogram	
Evoked potential	
Magnetic resonance imaging (MRI)	
Radiograph (x-ray)	
Ultrasound	

(continued)

As Children Grow: **Musculoskeletal System**

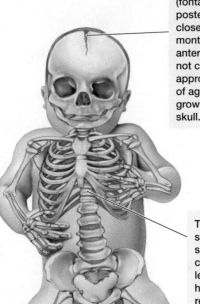

A fibrous membrane still exists between the cranial bones (fontanelles). The posterior fontanelle closes between 2 and 3 months of age. The anterior fontanelle does not close until approximately 18 months of age, allowing for growth of the brain and skull.

The thoracic and sacral regions of the spine are convex curves. As the infant learns to hold up the head, the cervical region becomes concave.

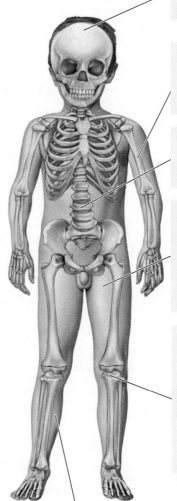

Most growth of the skull occurs by 2 years of age, with the skull reaching full size by 16 years.

The long bones of children are porous and less dense than those of adults, leading to higher rates of fracture.

When the child learns to stand, the lumbar region becomes concave in shape.

As a child grows, muscles do not increase in number, but rather in length and circumference. Muscle fibers reach maximum diameter in girls at about 10 years of age, and in boys at 14 years.

During childhood, cartilage cells at the epiphyses (an area enriched with blood cells) are replaced by osteoblasts (immature bone cells), which push the end of the bone away from the shaft and engineer the deposition of calcium within the newly formed bone.

The rapid bone growth of childhood facilitates healing after fractures, but may also lead to "growing pains" as muscles are pulled when bones grow quickly.

between 2 and 3 months of age. The anterior fontanelle does not close until approximately 7 to 19 months of age, allowing for growth of the brain and skull (National Institutes of Health, 2012a). Most growth of the skull occurs by 2 years of age, with the skull reaching full size by 16 years.

Secondary ossification occurs as the long bones grow. Cartilage cells at the epiphyses (an area enriched with blood cells) are replaced by osteoblasts (immature bone cells), which push the end of the bone away from the shaft and engineer the deposition of calcium within the newly formed bone. Calcium intake during childhood and adolescence is essential to

provide adequate bone density that will prevent osteoporosis and fractures in adulthood. See Chapter 14 for a discussion of inadequate calcium intake during school age and adolescence. Because growth takes place at the epiphyseal plates, injuries to this portion of a long bone are of particular concern in young children. The rapid bone growth of childhood facilitates healing after fractures but may also lead to "growing pains," as muscles are pulled when bones grow quickly. The ends of the long bones (epiphyses) remain cartilaginous, allowing growth, until approximately age 20 years, when skeletal maturation is complete. At this time, the epiphyseal plate

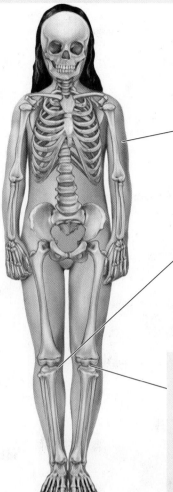

Muscle strength continues to increase until about 25–30 years of age.

The ends of long bones (epiphyses) remain cartilaginous, allowing growth, until approximately age 20 years, when skeletal maturation is complete. At this time the epiphyseal plate closes, cartilage at the site is replaced by bone, and only an epiphyseal line remains.

Until puberty, both ligaments and tendons are stronger than bone. As the child ages and cartilage is replaced by bone, the resulting bone is stronger than ligaments or tendons. Rates of fractures decrease while injuries to ligaments and tendons increase.

closes, cartilage at the site is replaced by bone, and only an epiphyseal line remains.

Children and adolescents may sustain injury to the musculoskeletal system from falls, car crashes, and sports. Fractures are one type of common injury. The long bones of children are porous and less dense than those of adults. For this reason, children's bones can bend, buckle, or break as a result of a simple fall. In addition to the structural differences between the bones of children and adults, there are functional differences in the skeletal system of children. Before birth, the thoracic and sacral regions of the spine are convex curves. As the infant learns to hold up the head, the cervical region becomes concave. When the child learns to stand, the lumbar region also becomes concave. Failure of the spine to assume these final curves results in an abnormal curvature of the spine (kyphosis or lordosis).

Muscles, Tendons, and Ligaments

The muscular system, unlike the skeletal system, is almost completely formed at birth, with any remaining increase achieved in the first year of life. As a child grows, muscles do not increase in number, but rather in length and circumference. Muscle fibers reach maximum diameter in girls at about 10 years of age, and in boys at 14 years. Muscle strength continues to increase until about 25–30 years of age.

Until puberty, both ligaments and tendons are stronger than bone. When these structural differences are not recognized, a childhood fracture is sometimes mistaken for a sprain. A **sprain** is a tearing of ligaments, the structural support connecting bones, usually caused when a joint is twisted or otherwise traumatized. Tendons, which connect bones to muscles, grow in length and fibrous tissue as mechanical pressure is placed on them.

Use the *Assessment Guide* to perform a nursing assessment of the musculoskeletal system. Many diagnostic and laboratory tests are used for the musculoskeletal system. Examples can be found in Table 29–1; see Appendices D and E for more information about these tests and procedures.

Figure 29–2 reviews several terms that will be used throughout this chapter in describing the positioning of a child's limbs. See *Assessment Guide: The Child With a Musculoskeletal System Alteration*.

ASSESSMENT GUIDE	The Child With a Musculoskeletal System Alteration

Assessment Focus	Assessment Guidelines
Muscles	• Is muscle mass symmetric?
	• Do fine and gross motor movements correspond to developmental expectations?
	• Can you identify any abnormal signs such as asymmetry of movement, tenderness, masses, weakness, hypotonia, hypertonia?
	• Can the school-age child get up from a lying or sitting position in the usual manner?
	• Can you describe the child's usual daily physical activity?
	• Has there been a loss of ability to perform developmental milestones?

(continued)

Assessment Focus	Assessment Guidelines
Joints	• Are movements smooth and symmetric?
	• Are there any signs of tenderness, decreased range of motion, inflammation, crepitus/grinding, or masses?
	• Do the hips of newborns and infants manifest symmetric full range of motion?
	• Were there recent events of trauma such as in sports or a fall?
Bones	• Are any masses noted?
	• Are arms and legs the same length?
	• Is there a recent decrease or change in mobility, such as limping?
	• Are bones in alignment, or are abnormalities noted such as bowlegs or knock-knees?
	• Upon spinal screening, is the spine properly aligned (see screening procedure within this chapter)?
	• In what sports does the child participate? Is recommended protective gear worn?
Tendons and ligaments	• Do all joints move through full range of motion?
	• Is there any pain upon joint motion or palpation?
	• Are there feelings of grinding or crepitus as the joint moves?
	• Has there been a recent sports or other injury?
	• In what sports does the child participate?
Family history	• Is there a family history of disorders of the muscular or skeletal systems?

Some disorders affect other body systems as well; for example, see cerebral palsy in Chapter 27. Many musculoskeletal disorders require surgical correction, casting, or braces.

Disorders of the Feet and Legs

Metatarsus Adductus

Metatarsus adductus, the most common congenital foot deformity, is characterized by an inward turning of the forefoot at the tarsometatarsal joints (Figure 29–3). Often referred to as "intoeing," metatarsus adductus affects male and female infants equally and occurs in approximately 1 in 1000 births, with more common incidence being in first births and in families with prior cases of the disorder. It is sometimes accompanied by other problems such as developmental dysplasia of the hip (described later in this chapter) (Gilmore & Thompson, 2013; National Institutes of Health, 2012b). This condition is most likely caused by both intrauterine positioning and genetic factors. Metatarsus adductus is differentiated from other causes of intoeing, such as internal tibial torsion (more common in children ages 12 to 18 months who are learning to walk) and femoral anteversion (seen more often in preschool-age children).

Treatment depends on the degree of foot flexibility. If the foot can be readily maneuvered past the neutral position, simple exercises may correct the problem. Most cases resolve spontaneously by the time the infant is about 3 months of age. Serial casting is the treatment of choice for curvature angles greater than 15 degrees, or in cases that do not improve. The infant's feet are placed in a position as close to neutral as possible and are held secure with casts. Casts are changed weekly until the desired correction is achieved. Braces and orthopedic shoes may also be used to maintain correction after casting.

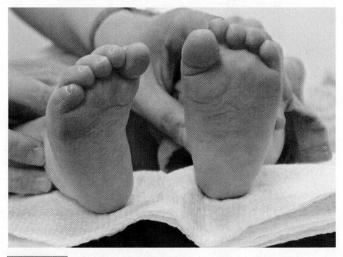

Figure 29–3 **Metatarsus adductus. This disorder is characterized by convexity (curvature) of the lateral border of the foot. The child's right foot demonstrates the disorder. Note that the forefoot turns inward and appears out of alignment with the remainder of the foot.**

Nursing Management

Reassure parents that the child's condition can be corrected. If the child's deformity is mild, teach parents simple stretching exercises to perform at each diaper change. The foot is held securely by the heel, and the forefoot is moved outward from the body with the other hand. The position is maintained for 5 seconds, and repeated 5 times at each diaper change. If casting is necessary, provide cast care as outlined in Table 29–2 and teach parents how to care for the child in a cast at home. If metatarsus adductus persists into childhood without correction, the challenge is to find shoes that accommodate the unusual shape of the foot.

Clinical Tip

Casts are made out of plaster or fiberglass material. The former is durable and may be chosen for applications that will last for a long time. Plaster casts must be kept dry or they will deteriorate. Fiberglass casts are lighter and available in various colors and are therefore popular with children. While the outside of the cast can become moist without breakdown, the lining underside is not waterproof, so caution is still followed to preserve the cast integrity.

Clubfoot

Clubfoot is a congenital abnormality in which the foot is twisted out of its normal position. It occurs in approximately 1 to 2 in 1000 births, affects boys nearly twice as often as girls, and is bilateral in about half of affected infants (Gilmore & Thompson, 2013).

ETIOLOGY AND PATHOPHYSIOLOGY

The exact cause of clubfoot is unknown; however, several possible etiologies have been proposed. Some authorities believe abnormal intrauterine positioning causes the deformity. Others suspect neuromuscular or vascular problems as causes. There is a genetic component in some cases because the risk of having a second child with clubfoot when an earlier child is affected is 25% (Gilmore & Thompson, 2013).

CLINICAL MANIFESTATIONS

A clubfoot (talipes equinovarus) involves three areas of deformity: The midfoot is directed downward (**equinus**), the hindfoot turns inward (**varus**), and the forefoot curls toward the heel (adduction) and turns upward in partial supination. Muscles, tendons, and bones are all involved in the abnormality, and it cannot be corrected by exercise. Most children have this combination of findings. The foot is small with a shortened Achilles tendon. Muscles in the lower leg are atrophied, but leg lengths are generally normal (see *Pathophysiology Illustrated: Clubfoot*).

TABLE 29–2 Nursing Care of the Child in a Cast

- A plaster cast takes anywhere from 24–48 hr to dry. When handling the wet cast, be gentle and use the palms of your hands, as fingertips can indent plaster and create pressure areas.

- After the cast is applied, elevate the extremity on a pillow above the level of the heart. Elevation helps reduce swelling and increases venous return.

- If the cast is applied after surgery, there may be drainage or bleeding through the cast material. Circle the stain and note the date and time on the cast to provide a way to assess the amount of fluid lost.

- Assess the distal pulses, and check the fingers and toes for color, warmth, capillary refill, and edema. Assess sensation as well as movement. Any deviation from normal may indicate nerve damage or decreased blood supply.

- During the first 24 hr, check the casted extremity every 15–30 min for 2 hr, then every 1–2 hr thereafter. The skin should be warm. It should blanch when slight pressure is applied and then return to its normal color within 3 sec (**A**). For the next 2 days, assess the casted extremity at least every 4 hr.

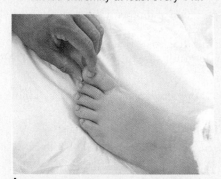

- Check the edges of the cast for roughness or crumbling. If necessary, pull the inner stockinette over the edge of the cast and tape in place.

- The rough edges of the cast may also be alleviated by "petaling." This is done by securing tape or padding to the inside of the cast and pulling it over the edge, covering the jagged or broken pieces of plaster, and securing it to the outer surface of the cast (**B, C, D**). Moleskin may be used on the cast as well.

- Keep the cast as clean and dry as possible. Cover the cast with plastic when the child bathes. Never leave the child alone to bathe, and discard the plastic safely so that the child cannot reach it because of suffocation hazard.

- The skin under the cast may itch; however, do not use powders or lotions near the edges or under the cast as they can cause skin irritation.

- Be sure that children do not put small objects between the casts and their extremities; that can cause skin irritation as well as neurovascular compromise.

A

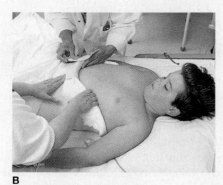

B

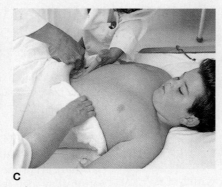

C

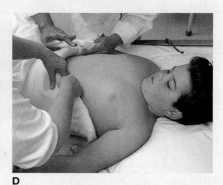

D

Pathophysiology Illustrated: **Clubfoot**

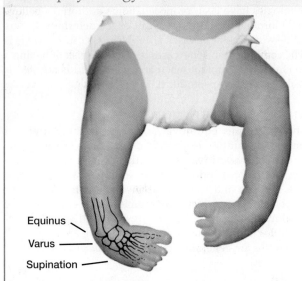

Equinus
Varus
Supination

Bilateral clubfoot deformity. Parents of a child with clubfoot will have many questions. Can the condition be treated? Will the child be able to walk normally after surgery? Will they need help caring for the infant? How much will surgery and other care cost? Will any subsequent children have a clubfoot?

CLINICAL THERAPY

Diagnosis is made at birth on the basis of visual inspection. Radiographs are used to confirm the severity of the condition.

Early treatment is essential to achieve successful correction and reduce the chance of complications. Serial casting is the treatment of choice. Casting should begin as soon as possible after birth. Timing is critical because the short bones of the foot, which are primarily cartilaginous at birth, begin to ossify shortly thereafter. The foot is manipulated to achieve maximum correction first of the varus deformity and then of the equinus deformity. A long leg cast holds the foot in the desired position (Figure 29–4). The cast is changed every 1 to 2 weeks. This regimen of

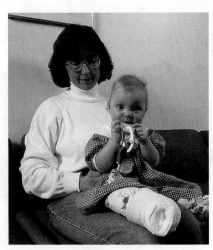

Figure 29–4   **This girl has a long leg cast, which was applied after surgery to correct her clubfoot deformity.**

manipulation and casting continues for approximately 8 to 12 weeks until maximum correction is achieved. If the deformity has been corrected, the child may begin wearing a splint or reverse cast (shaped so that the foot turns outward away from the body instead of the normal inward turn) or corrective shoes to maintain the correction. If the deformity has not been corrected, surgery is required. Casting holds the foot in position until surgery is performed.

The age at which a child undergoes clubfoot surgery varies among surgeons. However, most children have surgery between 3 and 12 months of age. The one-stage posteromedial release procedure, which involves realignment of the bones of the foot and release of the constricting soft tissue, is most common. The foot is held in the proper position by one or more stainless steel pins. A cast is then applied with the knee flexed to prevent damage to the pin and to discourage weight bearing. Casting continues for 6 to 12 weeks. The child may then need to wear a brace or corrective shoes, depending on the severity of the deformity and the surgeon's preference (Gilmore & Thompson, 2013).

More severe cases or those not corrected in infancy may require more than one surgery to correct the foot.

Nursing Management
For the Child With Clubfoot

Nursing Assessment and Diagnosis

Nursing assessment, which begins at birth and continues throughout the child's subsequent outpatient casting visits and hospitalization for surgery, includes taking a genetic and birth history, performing a physical examination (including position and appearance of the foot), and assessing the child's motor development and family's coping mechanisms. Because parents will need to bring the child for frequent cast changes, assess access to transportation and other arrangements needed for these visits.

Among the nursing diagnoses that might apply to the child with a clubfoot deformity are the following (NANDA-I © 2014):

- *Mobility: Physical, Impaired,* related to prescribed movement restriction of cast
- *Skin Integrity, Risk for Impaired,* related to cast
- *Parenting, Impaired,* related to birth of a child with a physical defect
- *Health Maintenance, Ineffective,* related to lack of information about deformity, treatment, and home care

Planning and Implementation

Nursing management involves providing emotional support, educating the family about home care of the child in a cast and the importance of keeping appointments at the outpatient facility for cast changes, preparing the family for the child's hospitalization if surgery is to occur, and providing postsurgical care.

PROVIDE EMOTIONAL SUPPORT

Clubfoot affects both the child and the family. The child's foot deformity is upsetting to parents, and they need emotional support to allay their fears. Helping parents understand the condition and its treatment is essential.

Families Want to Know

Care of the Child With a Cast

Skin Care

- Check the skin around the cast edges for irritation, rubbing, or blistering. The skin should be clean and dry.
- Cleanse the skin just under the cast edges and between the toes or fingers with a cotton-tipped applicator and rubbing alcohol. Avoid using lotions, oils, and powders near the cast as they may cause caking.
- Avoid poking sharp objects down inside the cast as this may result in sores.

Cast Care

- Keep the cast dry. Protect plaster with a cast shoe, thick sock, or sling.
- Allow a new, wet cast to air-dry for 24 hours. Raise it on pillows just above heart level to prevent swelling.
- Begin walking on a leg cast only when the physician gives permission.

Be Alert for Possible Complications

- Toes or fingers should be pink, not blue or white.
- Skin should be warm and the tips of the toes should blanch when pinched.

Notify Your Healthcare Provider if Any of the Following Occurs

- Unusual odor beneath the cast
- Burning, tingling, or numbness in the casted arm or leg
- Drainage through the cast
- Swelling or inability to move the fingers or toes
- Slippage of the cast
- Cast cracked, soft, or loose
- Sudden unexplained fever
- Unusual fussiness or irritability in an infant or child
- Fingers or toes that are blue or white
- Pain that is not relieved by any comfort measures (e.g., repositioning or pain medication)

Source: Courtesy of Shriners Hospital for Children, Spokane, WA.

Promote bonding by encouraging parents to hold and cuddle the child and to take an active role in the child's care. Explain that, with treatment, the child is expected to grow and develop normally.

PROVIDE CAST AND BRACE CARE

Routine cast care, earlier outlined in Table 29–2, is important to ensure skin and neurovascular integrity. After serial casting is complete, or after surgery, the child may progress to wearing a brace or special shoe for 6 to 12 months. Braces should fit snugly but should not interfere with neurovascular function. Before the child begins to wear a brace, check the skin for any areas of redness or breakdown. Give parents guidelines for brace wear. Emphasize that proper skin care is essential. If skin redness develops, arrange to have the fit of the brace evaluated and modified if necessary.

PROVIDE POSTSURGICAL CARE

Routine postoperative care after surgical correction includes neurovascular status checks every 2 hours for the first 24 hours and observing for any swelling around the cast edges (see Table 29–2). Apply ice bags to the foot, and keep the ankle and foot elevated on a pillow for 24 hours. This promotes healing and helps with venous return. Check for drainage or bleeding. Administer pain medication routinely for 24 to 48 hours. Popliteal or epidural blocks may be placed during surgery and used in the immediate postsurgical period for

pain control. Monitor these blocks for effectiveness and any undesired effects. (See Chapter 15 for detailed instructions on pain management.)

SAFETY ALERT!

The most serious complication of a cast is the obstruction to normal blood flow and nerve innervation. Monitoring of the child's distal extremity is important to identify this complication. If color, temperature, or other abnormalities are present, inform the nursing supervisor or physician immediately. Have a cast cutter readily available on the unit in case the cast needs to be removed. See the section on compartment syndrome later in this chapter.

DISCHARGE PLANNING AND HOME CARE TEACHING

Give parents written instructions for care of the child with a cast (see *Families Want to Know: Care of the Child With a Cast*). In addition, assist them in the following ways:

- Demonstrate the use of a sponge bath to protect the cast from water breakdown. Have parents contact the healthcare provider if the cast gets wet with water or urine.
- Discuss options for clothing that accommodate a cast, for example, one-piece snap suits or sweatpants.

Families Want to Know

Guidelines for Brace Wear

- Braces should be as comfortable as possible and the child should have adequate mobility while wearing the brace.
- Begin wearing the brace for periods of 1 to 2 hours and then progress to 2 to 4 hours.
- Check the skin at 1- to 2-hour intervals initially, then every 4 hours once skin has been clear for several days. If redness is apparent, leave the brace off and allow the skin to clear. If breakdown has occurred, the brace cannot be replaced until healing is complete. (See Chapter 31 for a discussion of pressure ulcers.)
- Always have the child wear a clean white sock, T-shirt, or other thin white liner beneath the brace. Be sure the liner is wrinkle-free under the brace. Avoid using powders or lotions that can cause skin to break down. Toughen any sensitive areas using alcohol wipes 3 to 4 times daily.
- Reapply the brace when the skin returns to its normal color.
- Return to the orthotic specialist or other specified healthcare provider if discomfort or red areas persist or if the brace needs adjustment or repair or is outgrown.
- Check the brace daily for rough edges.

- Discuss potential safety hazards that may result from awkward positioning. Be sure the child is properly situated in a car safety seat for the trip home.
- Provide resources for strollers and other equipment that will support the cast so it does not hang down during the baby's activities.
- Suggest that parents try to place toys within the child's reach, since the movements of a child in a cast may be slowed.

Evaluation

Expected outcomes of nursing care include maintenance of skin integrity, recovery without complications after surgery, normal developmental progression of the child, and demonstrated parental knowledge of care of braces or casts, as needed.

Genu Varum and Genu Valgum

Genu varum (bowlegs) is a deformity in which the knees are widely separated while the ankles are close together and the lower legs are turned inward (varus). In genu valgum (knock-knees), the knees are close together and the lower legs are directed outward (valgus) (Figure 29–5). Chapter 5 discusses the assessment of bowlegs and knock-knees in children.

At certain stages of a child's development, the appearance of bowlegs or knock-knees is normal. Until 2 to 3 years of age, the knees are normally bowed, showing varus alignment, and by 4 to 5 years, some knock-knee or valgus alignment is common. However, the persistence of knock-knees beyond the age of 4 to 5 years necessitates further evaluation. The most common pathologic causes of bowed legs are Blount disease and rickets (see Chapter 14). Blount disease is characterized by abnormal growth on the medial side of the proximal tibia, which causes an increasing varus deformity. It is believed to be caused by increasing compression forces across the medial knee; is more common in overweight, Black, and female children; and has been associated with low serum vitamin D levels (Sabharwal, 2015). Rickets is a result of inadequate bone mineralization, usually caused by a deficiency of calcium, vitamin D, or both. Because the bones are decalcified or softened, long bones such as those in the legs may bend into a bowed position. Occasionally, rickets is congenital and is caused by an X-linked autosomal dominant or recessive gene with the chromosomal location Xp22.31-p21.3. It results in an enzyme deficiency of alkaline phosphatase, which in turn leads to excessive inhibitors of bone

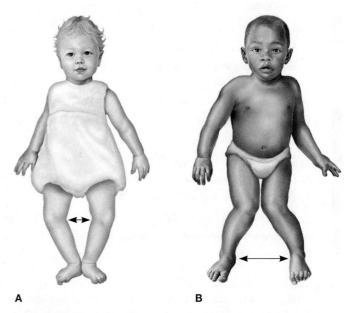

A   **B**

Figure 29–5 Genu varum and genu valgum. *A*, Genu varum, or bowlegs. The legs are bowed so that the knees are far apart as the child stands. *B*, Genu valgum, or knock-knees. Note that the ankles are far apart when the knees are together.

mineralization. This type of rickets is rare and is called *familial hypophosphatemic rickets (FHR)*.

Measurements, radiographs, arthrography (joint radiograph), magnetic resonance imaging (MRI), and computed tomography (CT) imaging may be used for accurate diagnosis. Braces are often used to correct mild deformities that could worsen as the child grows. Braces for bowlegs are worn at night; those for knock-knees both day and night. Duration of brace wear is determined by the severity of the deformity, which is usually evaluated by radiographs. If the deformity continues to worsen, surgery is necessary. Surgery is common in treatment of Blount disease. An **osteotomy** (cutting of the bone) is performed and the tibiofemoral angle surgically corrected. The child is then placed in a cast for approximately 6 to 10 weeks, or until completely healed (Birch, 2013). When dietary rickets is the cause of varus deformity, supplementation with calcium and vitamin D is needed. FHR is treated with calcium and phosphorus in 5 to 6 daily doses.

Nursing Management

Reassure parents that bowlegs and knock-knees are usually a normal part of a child's growth and development. These conditions often resolve spontaneously and need no treatment other than continued observation.

Nursing care focuses on educating the parents and child about the condition and its treatment. Give the child and family guidelines for brace wear and maintenance (see *Families Want to Know: Guidelines for Brace Wear*).

Disorders of the Hip

Developmental Dysplasia of the Hip

Developmental dysplasia of the hip (DDH) refers to a variety of conditions in which the femoral head and the acetabulum are improperly aligned. These conditions include hip instability, **dislocation** (displacement of the bone from its normal articulation with the joint), **subluxation** (in this instance, a partial dislocation), and acetabular **dysplasia** (abnormal cellular or structural development leading to instability) (Schwend, Shaw, & Segal, 2014). In the past, DDH was referred to as *congenital dislocated hip (CDH)*. The revised name of the disorder emphasizes that many cases of dislocation, subluxation, and dysplasia occur well after the neonatal period and involve more than a simple dislocation.

One in 100 newborns has hip instability, while dislocation occurs in 1.5 to 20 in 1000 births, depending on the studies examined. The condition affects girls four times as often as boys. It is unilateral in 80% of affected children, and the left hip is affected three times as often as the right (Roof, Jinguji, & White, 2013).

ETIOLOGY AND PATHOPHYSIOLOGY

Although the exact cause of DDH is unknown, genetic factors appear to play a role. The condition is 20 to 50 times more common in first-degree relatives of an infant with the condition than in the general population. If one child of a set of identical twins has DDH, the other twin is affected 30% to 40% of the time. Some types of DDH are linked to early gestational events at 12 and 18 weeks' gestation, as the lower limbs rotate and surrounding muscles develop. On the other hand, milder cases may be influenced by mechanical forces in the last month of pregnancy such as breech position, oligohydramnios, or fetal size, and can occur after birth as the hip assumes an extended rather than flexed posture (National Institutes of Health, 2013). The left hip is involved more often than the right hip as a result of intrauterine

positioning of the left side of the fetus against the mother's sacrum. Maternal estrogen may cause laxity of the hip joint and capsule, leading to joint instability, especially in female infants who respond to these estrogen levels. Carrying infants with legs predominantly in extended position rather than with hips flexed may also be associated with DDH.

CLINICAL MANIFESTATIONS

Common signs and symptoms of DDH include limited abduction of the affected hip, asymmetry of the gluteal and thigh skinfolds, and telescoping or pistoning of the thigh (Figure 29–6). The older child with untreated DDH walks with a significant limp, which results from telescoping of the femoral head into the pelvis. The longer the disorder goes untreated and the more pronounced the clinical manifestations become, the more difficult the treatment.

CLINICAL THERAPY

From 60% to 80% of hip abnormalities noted in infants resolve by 2 months of age, so practitioners use care and caution in diagnosing DDH. However, only 15% to 25% of infants have known risk factors for the disorder. Therefore, the Pediatric Orthopaedic Society of North America recommends that all infants and young children should be screened for DDH until walking is well established at about 1 to 2 years of age (American Academy of Orthopaedic Surgeons [AAOS], 2014a; Roof et al., 2013). Physical examination reveals an Allis sign (one knee lower than the other when the knees are flexed) and positive Ortolani and Barlow maneuvers in babies under 8 to 12 weeks of age. Refer to Chapter 5 for a discussion of the assessment of hip dysplasia in newborns and infants. Radiographs are generally not reliable until approximately 4 months of age because the pelvis in a newborn is still primarily cartilaginous. Before 4 months of age, ultrasonography may be useful for diagnosis. Family history of DDH and a female baby in the breech position necessitate careful evaluation (AAOS, 2014a).

Treatment plans vary according to the child's age. For infants younger than 3 months, the Pavlik harness is the most commonly used method for hip reduction (Figure 29–7). The Pavlik harness is a dynamic splint—a splint that allows movement. It ensures hip flexion and abduction and does not allow hip extension or adduction. For infants older than 6 months of

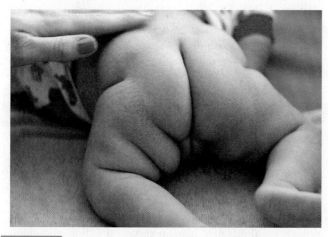

Figure 29–6 Common signs of developmental dysplasia of the hip (DDH). The asymmetry of the gluteal and thigh skinfolds is easy to see in this child with DDH.

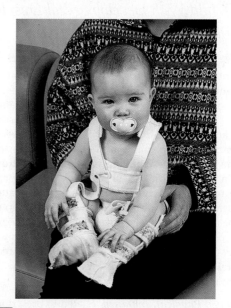

Figure 29–7 The most common treatment for DDH in a child under 3 months is a Pavlik harness. A shirt should be worn under the harness to prevent skin irritation. (It was omitted for clarity in this photograph.)

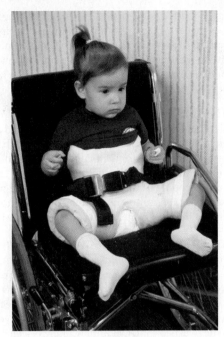

Figure 29–8 Surgery followed by spica cast application is commonly used in treatment of DDH.

age, surgery with closed reduction is generally performed (positioning of the head of the femur into the acetabulum without an incision of the skin) followed by the application of a spica cast (Figure 29–8). Surgery may be preceded by a course of Bryant traction to facilitate stretching of the tissues that will promote positive surgical outcomes. In children over 18 months of age, open or closed reduction surgery and casting are usually necessary and bracing may also be required.

Early screening, detection, and treatment enable most affected children to attain normal hip function. A late diagnosis results in a lowered prognosis for full function.

Nursing Management

For the Child With Developmental Dysplasia of the Hip

Nursing Assessment and Diagnosis

Assessment for DDH begins at birth and continues through all health promotion visits during the first 2 years of life. The family history or birth data may indicate a high-risk infant. Instructions for performing the physical examination to assess the infant for DDH are provided in Chapter 5. Once treatment begins, assessments are performed based on risks of the treatment. Assess the skin of the child in traction or a cast every few minutes in the immediate postoperative period, progressing to once or twice daily at home. Include respiratory and circulatory assessments when the child is immobilized. Ongoing assessment of the child's growth and development is needed. Weigh the child in a cast once the cast is dry so a baseline casted weight can be used for comparison while the cast remains in place.

Several nursing diagnoses that may apply to the child with DDH include the following (NANDA-I © 2014):

- *Mobility: Physical, Impaired,* related to prescribed movement restriction (Pavlik harness, traction, spica cast, brace)
- *Skin Integrity, Risk for Impaired,* related to irritation from harness straps or skin traction

- *Urinary Elimination, Impaired or Constipation,* related to immobility caused by treatment
- *Nutrition, Imbalanced: Less than Body Requirements,* related to decreased appetite
- *Development: Delayed, Risk for,* related to limited mobility and potential decreased exposure to stimulation
- *Knowledge, Readiness for Enhanced (Parental),* related to lack of information about disease process and treatment

Planning and Implementation

The infant with DDH is often cared for at home and in outpatient facilities. If surgery is performed, the child is hospitalized for surgery and the immediate postoperative period. Nursing care varies according to the medical treatment and the child's age. Management includes maintaining traction, if ordered; providing cast care; preventing complications resulting from immobility; promoting normal growth and development; and teaching parents about the condition and care (e.g., management of a cast or a Pavlik harness). Because treatment may interfere with the child's normal movement, the treatment plan should take into consideration the age and developmental stage of the child in order to substitute activities to stimulate development.

PROVIDE CAST CARE AND CORRECT HARNESS ALIGNMENT

The principles of routine cast care presented in Table 29–2 apply to the care of spica casts. Special techniques should be used to help keep the cast clean and dry in children who are not toilet trained. Female and male urinals can be used for older children. Use a plastic lining to protect the cast edges during elimination for older children and use a small disposable diaper to cover the perineum in babies, tucking edges beneath the cast. Be sure to change the diaper frequently to prevent soiling of the cast.

The child in a Pavlik harness will have the harness applied in the healthcare facility. Parents need instructions on maintaining the child in the harness at all times. Return visits will be scheduled to ensure proper fit, maintenance of hip position, and skin condition.

PREVENT COMPLICATIONS RESULTING FROM IMMOBILITY

Immobilization from traction or a cast can cause alterations in physiologic functioning. To prevent complications:

- Assess breathing patterns and lung sounds frequently for congestion or respiratory compromise.
- Perform skin and neurovascular assessments approximately every 2 hours.
- Use adequate padding and skin wrapping to avoid placing pressure on the popliteal space. Such pressure could lead to nerve damage.
- For the child in a cast, change the child's position every 2 to 3 hours while awake to help avoid areas of pressure and promote increased circulation. The child can be placed either prone or supine or positioned on the floor and supported with pillows.
- Help prevent skin irritation and breakdown in the child with a cast. Use moleskin to protect from rough edges. Place tape around the perineal opening of the cast to prevent soiling.
- Increase fluids and fiber in the child's diet, as a change in bowel or bladder status is commonly associated with immobility.

Families Want to Know

Transporting the Child With Orthopedic Devices

The American Academy of Pediatrics and the National Center for the Safe Transportation of Children with Special Health Care Needs have established guidelines for transporting children with special healthcare needs:

- Riding in the rear seat is preferable.
- If the front seat must be used, the front passenger airbag should be disconnected. The National Highway and Traffic Safety Administration provides information and assistance (1-888-327-4236 or www.nhtsa.dot.gov) on how to make the disconnection.
- Use only car seat transport systems approved for use with children who have special needs.
- Install and use seats as instructed. Never alter a car safety seat to transport a child.
- Move a child from a wheelchair or other special device to the vehicle safety seat whenever this is reasonable.
- Pieces of medical equipment required during transportation (such as monitors or oxygen) or that are being transported with the child (such as wheelchair or walker) should be secured to the floor of the vehicle.
- If the child is transported by school bus, follow state and federal recommendations for school bus transportation of children with special needs.
- Keep a cellular phone and emergency equipment in the vehicle.

Source: Data from American Academy of Pediatrics, Committee on Injury and Poison Prevention. (1999, reaffirmed 2013). Transporting children with special health care needs. *Pediatrics, 104*, 988–992 (original policy); *Pediatrics, 132*, e281–e282 (reaffirmation).

- If permitted by physician orders, release the child from traction for meals and daily care. The time out of traction should not exceed 1 hour per day. Encourage parents to hold and cuddle the child at this time to promote comfort and bonding.

PROMOTE NORMAL GROWTH AND DEVELOPMENT

Engage the child in activities that stimulate the upper extremities and all five senses. Provide stimulating toys such as stacking blocks, brightly colored mobiles, soft balls, or musical toys. Position toys within the child's reach and interact with the child as much as possible. See Chapter 11 for specific recommendations for stimulating activities.

DISCHARGE PLANNING AND HOME CARE TEACHING

Teach parents how to care for a child in traction or a spica cast at home. Family members' active participation in the child's daily care during hospitalization gradually increases their confidence in their ability to provide care once home. Identify and address home care needs well in advance of discharge. Before discharge, be sure the parents have:

- Information about general cast care (see Table 29–2), positioning, bathing, toileting, and age-appropriate diversional activities. Include body mechanics for the adults moving the child.
- Knowledge of the importance of performing neurovascular checks and reporting any abnormalities immediately. Teach them circulation, motion, and sensitivity checks.
- An understanding that the bar between the legs on the cast is not to be used for holding or turning the child. The bar is used to position the legs at the proper distance; using it to lift can cause the cast to fracture, weaken, or disintegrate.
- Information on feeding the child.
- Safety teaching to minimize chance of injury to a casted child.

- Instruction about types of toys that are age appropriate and measures to prevent them from being placed into the cast (a T-shirt should be placed over the cast, covering its edges).
- Appropriate referrals for periodic assessment by a visiting nurse or home health nurse.
- Family resources to care for the child.

Before discharge, have parents demonstrate how to dress and feed a child in a spica cast. Ensure that safe travel arrangements have been made for the day of discharge. Help parents get an appropriate car safety seat in advance of discharge. Encourage parents to let the child interact with other children at home, and to provide the child in a cast with similar opportunities for play and social activities.

COMMUNITY-BASED NURSING CARE

Have parents of an infant in a Pavlik harness demonstrate care of the infant while in the harness. Teach family members about daily care (bathing, dressing, and feeding) of the infant. The harness is worn full time; instructions generally include sponge bathing while it is in place, although some physicians may allow it to be removed briefly each day for bathing. One shoulder strap is removed at a time to change a T-shirt while the legs are held in proper position. The hips and buttocks should be supported carefully in the abducted position at all times. Demonstrate how to feed the infant in an upright position to maintain abduction and how to change a diaper without removing the harness.

Instruct the parents of an infant with a harness or a child in a cast to look for any reddened or irritated areas near the harness or cast edges and to check toes frequently for proper circulation. Frequent repositioning reduces the risk of pressure sores or circulatory compromise. The infant should wear an undershirt and socks under the harness to prevent rubbing of the skin.

Safety precautions are important as the child will not have normal mobility. Parents will need to use a specially designed car seat that accommodates the child with abducted hips. Strollers and cribs should provide sufficient room to protect the legs from injury and to prevent hip adduction.

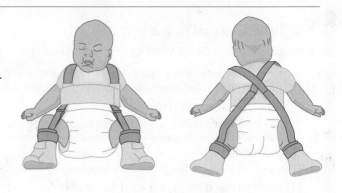
Evaluation

Expected outcomes for nursing care of the child with developmental dysplasia of the hip include the following:

- The skin remains intact.
- The child has no complications due to immobility.
- Parents demonstrate adequate knowledge regarding the condition, treatment, and necessary home care.
- A safe environment is maintained for the child.
- The child regains normal mobility.

Legg-Calvé-Perthes Disease

Legg-Calvé-Perthes disease (or simply Perthes disease) is a self-limiting condition in which there is avascular necrosis of the femoral head. The disease occurs in approximately 1 in 12,000 children and affects boys 4 times more often than girls. It usually occurs between the ages of 2 and 12 years, with an average age of 7 years at onset. The disease can be unilateral or bilateral (Kannu & Howard, 2014; Perry & Hall, 2011).

ETIOLOGY AND PATHOPHYSIOLOGY

The necrosis associated with Legg-Calvé-Perthes disease results from an interruption of the blood supply to the femoral epiphysis. How and why this occurs is not completely understood, but several predisposing factors have been identified. A coagulation system disorder causes repeated vascular interruptions to the proximal femur. Disturbed blood supply to the epiphyseal plate of the femoral bone is noted, leading to necrosis of the femoral head. The incidence of the condition is increased in families with a history of the disease, which suggests that genetic factors may play a role. In 17% of cases, onset of the disease is preceded by a mild traumatic injury, and 10% of children affected have a history of breech birth (Mazloumi, Ebrahimzadeh, & Kachooei, 2014). Trauma may cause a subchondral fracture and resultant synovitis, which in turn causes pressure that occludes the blood supply. Children with Legg-Calvé-Perthes disease often have delayed skeletal maturation, increased thyroid levels, and low somatomedin C (insulin-like growth factor). It is more common in those with low birth weight, increased parental age, and exposure to environmental tobacco smoke (Mazloumi et al., 2014).

CLINICAL MANIFESTATIONS

Legg-Calvé-Perthes disease progresses through four distinct stages, over a period of 1 to 4 years, after the original insult (usually unidentified) occurs (Table 29–3). Early symptoms of Perthes disease include a mild pain in the hip or anterior thigh and a limp, which are aggravated by increased activity and relieved by rest. The child favors the affected hip and limits hip movement to avoid discomfort.

As the disease progresses, range of motion becomes limited and weakness and muscle wasting develop. The affected thigh is 2 to 3 cm (0.8 to 1.2 in.) smaller than the unaffected thigh. Prolonged hip irritability may produce muscle spasms and increased pain. This period of the disease varies from 1 to 4 years. Gradually, revascularization begins and pain decreases.

CLINICAL THERAPY

Because the child's initial symptoms are mild, parents often do not seek medical attention until symptoms have been present for several months. Diagnosis is made using standard anteroposterior and frog-leg radiographs. However, radiographs taken

TABLE 29–3 Clinical Manifestations of Legg-Calvé-Perthes Disease

STAGE	CLINICAL MANIFESTATIONS
Prenecrosis	An insult causes loss of blood supply to the femoral head.
I—Necrosis	Avascular stage (3–6 months); the child is asymptomatic, bone radiographs are normal, and the head of the femur is structurally intact but avascular.
II—Revascularization	Period of 1–4 years characterized by pain and limitation of movement. Bone radiographs show new bone deposition and dead bone resorption. Fracture and deformity of the head of the femur can occur.
III—Bone healing	Reossification takes place; pain decreases.
IV—Remodeling	The disease process is over, pain is absent, and improvement in joint function occurs.

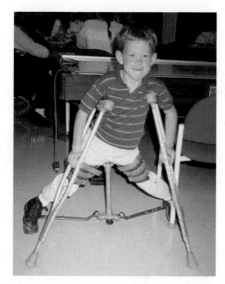

Figure 29–9 Although the Toronto brace may seem formidable for a child to wear, you can see by this photograph that, as usual, children adapt quite well to it.

early in the course of the disease may be normal or show vague widening of the cartilage space. Bone scans, MRI, and arthrography may be used in diagnosis. Laboratory studies of the blood, such as white blood cell count, help to rule out inflammatory synovitis of the hip. Protein C, protein S, and APC-R (resistance to activated protein C) may sometimes be performed to evaluate if a coagulation abnormality is present (de Sanctis, 2011; Milani & Dobashi, 2011).

Medical management and prognosis depend on the degree of femoral involvement. Early detection is important. The desired outcome is a pain-free hip that functions properly. To promote healing and prevent deformity, the femoral head must be contained within the hip socket until ossification is complete. This can happen only if the hips remain in an abducted position. At the beginning of treatment, traction can be used to maintain the hips in an abducted and internally rotated position. Once abduction is accomplished, treatment consists of Petrie (leg abduction) casting, or surgical soft-tissue releases such as adductor tenotomy, followed by bracing. Toronto (Figure 29–9) and Scottish Rite braces are most commonly used. Prognosis is good if the femoral head can be contained long enough for proper healing to occur. Severe disease may be treated by surgery to release adductor muscles, treat the acetabulum or femur, and restore range of motion. Children with untreated disease or those diagnosed late in the disease process occasionally develop osteoarthritis, leg length discrepancy, or hip dysfunction later in life (Nakamura et al., 2015).

Nursing Management

For the Child With Legg-Calvé-Perthes Disease

Nursing Assessment and Diagnosis

Suspect Legg-Calvé-Perthes disease in any child, especially a boy 2 to 12 years of age, who complains of hip discomfort accompanied by a limp. The school nurse may be the first person to observe the child with symptoms of Legg-Calvé-Perthes disease. The child may complain of pain and have to rest during physical education classes. Refer the child to the healthcare provider immediately. Question the child who has an apparent limp about pain, and assess the child's range of motion. Ask if the child injured the hip at some time in the past.

Nursing diagnoses, which center on altered activities and compliance, might include the following (NANDA-I © 2014):

- *Mobility: Physical, Impaired,* related to restriction of brace or cast
- *Injury, Risk for,* related to potential complications resulting from noncompliance with the treatment regimen
- *Activity, Deficient Diversional,* related to forced inactivity
- *Body Image, Disturbed,* related to brace

Planning and Implementation

Children with Legg-Calvé-Perthes disease often receive all of their treatment at home. Helping the child and family comply with the prescribed treatment plan may be challenging because children develop the disease at an age when they are usually very active. The child, who may have little pain, often finds immobilization difficult.

PROMOTE NORMAL GROWTH AND DEVELOPMENT

Give parents suggestions to help redirect the child's energy within the limitations in mobility imposed by treatment. A return to school promotes a feeling of normality. Coordinate the return to school by facilitating the child's use of an elevator or ramp as needed in that setting. Partner with the family to provide instruction for school personnel and other children to foster understanding of the child's condition and treatment. Activities that involve peers also help the child achieve developmental milestones. Help the child adjust to wearing a brace.

Growth and Development

Legg-Calvé-Perthes disease primarily affects boys with an average age of 7 years. These school-age children are industrious and independent. Suggest activities that redirect energy and promote normal development. These may include horseback riding, which promotes hip abduction; swimming to increase mobility; handcrafts to promote fine motor skills; and computer activities to stimulate cognitive development.

COMMUNITY-BASED NURSING CARE

Both the child and the family should be aware that treatment generally takes more than 2 years. Emphasize the importance of following the treatment plan to ensure adequate hip containment and proper healing. Teach the family how to care for a child in traction and how to check the child's skin for breakdown (see Table 29–11 later in this chapter). Follow-up visits should be arranged at regular intervals in addition to home care visits during the period of traction.

Evaluation

Expected outcomes of nursing care are elimination of hip pain and discomfort, normal development during the period of immobilization, absence of complications, and parent and child knowledge of the treatment regimen.

Slipped Capital Femoral Epiphysis

Slipped capital femoral epiphysis (SCFE) occurs when the femoral head is displaced from the femoral neck. This condition is seen in 10 of 100,000 adolescents, commonly in the prepubertal growth spurt, between the ages of 12 to 15 years in boys and 10 to 13 years in girls. Boys are more often affected than girls. Black children and those with predisposing factors are affected more often than other children (Georgiadis & Zaltz, 2014).

ETIOLOGY AND PATHOPHYSIOLOGY

The cause of SCFE is unknown. Predisposing factors include obesity, a recent growth spurt, and endocrine disorders such as hypothyroidism and hypogonadism.

Slippage of the femoral head occurs at the proximal epiphyseal plate, and the femur displaces from the epiphysis (see *Pathophysiology Illustrated: Slipped Epiphysis*). Slippage is usually gradual (chronic), but may also result from acute trauma. The synovial membrane becomes inflamed, edematous, and painful. If untreated, callous formation occurs, resulting in a deformed hip with limited range of motion.

Growth and Development

Obesity is a known risk factor for SCFE. Increasing rates of obesity among children contribute to an increasing risk for the disorder. Research continues to demonstrate a relationship between body mass index (BMI) and SCFE. High rates of elevated BMI likely play a role in both bilateral SCFE occurrences and increasing incidence of the condition (Compton, 2014; Witbreuk et al., 2013). Nurses are well positioned to work with children and families to teach weight reduction strategies and to share information about the numerous health risks associated with elevated BMI.

CLINICAL MANIFESTATIONS

Symptoms include a limp knee; thigh, groin, or hip pain; and loss of hip motion. Out-toeing, decreased internal rotation, and external rotation with flexion of the leg are symptomatic (Georgiadis & Zaltz, 2014). The condition is categorized as *acute* (sudden onset with less than 3 weeks' duration), *chronic* (longer than 3 weeks' duration), or *acute-on-chronic* (an additional slippage in a child with a chronic condition), depending on the onset and severity of symptoms. The child with an acute slip has sudden, severe pain and cannot bear weight. An acute slip may be associated with traumatic injury. The youth may be able to walk (stable) or unable to bear weight (unstable).

CLINICAL THERAPY

A complete history provides information about risk factors and the development of the condition. Radiographs confirm the diagnosis. A bone scan, ultrasound, CT, and MRI may also be performed.

The goal of medical management is to stabilize the femoral head while keeping displacement to a minimum and retaining as much hip function as possible. Surgical treatment is usually necessary; this involves fixation of the epiphysis with screws or pins. If the condition is stable, a single screw into the hip in an outpatient procedure is sufficient for stabilization; if unstable, surgical treatment may include traction and surgery.

Prognosis is related to the severity of the deformity and the occurrence of complications, such as avascular necrosis of the femoral head or **chondrolysis** (the breaking down and absorption of cartilage).

Nursing Management

For the Child With Slipped Capital Femoral Epiphysis

Nursing Assessment and Diagnosis

The child usually presents with hip pain or referred pain to the groin, thigh, or knee and limited mobility. A thorough history is needed to assess for injury as a cause. Assess the child's range of motion, pain, and limp, if apparent. Refer the child for treatment immediately if SCFE is suspected. This condition is considered to be an emergency, and it is essential that the child be treated immediately to keep weight off the affected joint (Georgiadis & Zaltz, 2014).

Among the nursing diagnoses that may apply to the child with SCFE are the following (NANDA-I © 2014):

- *Mobility: Physical, Impaired,* related to treatment
- *Pain, Acute,* related to hip injury
- *Body Image, Disturbed,* related to treatment
- *Development: Delayed, Risk for,* related to mobility restrictions
- *Obesity* related to immobility

Pathophysiology Illustrated: **Slipped Epiphysis**

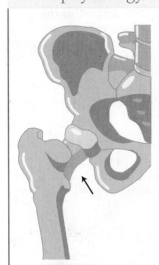 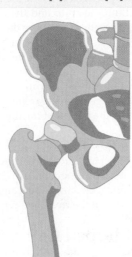

In slipped capital femoral epiphysis, the femoral head is displaced from the femoral neck at the proximal epiphyseal plate.

Slipped epiphysis   Normal hip

- *Tissue Perfusion: Peripheral, Ineffective,* related to traction, casting, and other treatments
- *Knowledge, Readiness for Enhanced (Child and Parent),* related to disease process and treatment

Planning and Implementation

Nursing management involves caring for the child in traction or after surgery, administering medications and other pain-control interventions, maintaining mobility within the limits imposed by treatment, providing adequate nutrition, educating the child and family about the disorder, providing emotional support, and promoting compliance with the treatment plan.

ENCOURAGE APPROPRIATE NUTRITIONAL INTAKE AND PHYSICAL ACTIVITY

A growing adolescent needs increased amounts of proteins, carbohydrates, and calcium to promote skeletal healing. Provide written instructions about nutritional requirements to promote bone healing and maintain an ideal body weight. If a child is overweight, encourage weight loss by decreasing the percentage of fat and sugar in the diet and by increasing physical activity that is safe to do. Weight loss decreases pressure on the femoral epiphysis and can also lead to a more positive self-image. Incorporate upper body exercises into treatment, both to assist in weight control and to build muscle. A few visits to physical therapy may facilitate a program of upper body exercise and teach safe ways of increasing the total amount of physical activity.

PROVIDE EMOTIONAL SUPPORT

Because the onset of SCFE is usually unexpected, the child and family may find themselves facing surgery with little warning. Explain the treatment plan simply and thoroughly. Reassure the child and family that with proper compliance, treatment should be successful.

DISCHARGE PLANNING AND HOME CARE TEACHING

Help the family plan for the child's return to school. If attendance is not possible for a time because of traction or surgery, arrange for tutors and computer communication with school as needed. Follow-up visits are necessary until the child's epiphyseal plates close. It is not uncommon for SCFE to occur in the other hip. Make sure the child and family are aware of symptoms such as decreased range of motion or pain that could indicate onset of the disorder in the other hip. Tell parents to contact their healthcare provider immediately if these symptoms occur.

Evaluation

Expected outcomes of nursing care for the child with slipped capital femoral epiphysis include maintenance of normal weight and recommended nutritional intake, absence of complications of immobility, successful adaptation to school following treatment, and family recognition of the need for ongoing monitoring for complications.

Disorders of the Spine

Scoliosis

Scoliosis is a lateral S- or C-shaped curvature of the spine that is often associated with a rotational deformity of the spine and ribs. Many people exhibit some degree of spinal curvature; curvatures of more than 10 degrees are considered abnormal. Curves are either idiopathic or compensatory, the latter occurring as the spine curves to compensate for a structural deformity such as leg length discrepancy. Idiopathic scoliosis occurs most often in girls, especially during the growth spurt between the ages of 10 and 13 years. From 1% to 3% of adolescents manifest with idiopathic scoliosis of greater than 10 degrees. A smaller number of children manifest infantile scoliosis before 3 years of age or juvenile scoliosis from 3 to 10 years (Lombardi, Akoume, Colombini, et al., 2011).

ETIOLOGY AND PATHOPHYSIOLOGY

The cause of scoliosis is complex. Structural scoliosis may be congenital, idiopathic, or acquired (associated with neuromuscular disorders such as muscular dystrophy or myelodysplasia, or secondary to spinal cord injuries).

In idiopathic structural scoliosis (the most common type), the spine for unknown reasons begins to curve laterally, with vertebral rotation. The most common curve is a right thoracic and left lumbar deformity. As the curve progresses, structural changes occur. The ribs on the concave side (inside of the curve) are forced closer together, while the ribs on the convex side separate widely, causing narrowing of the thoracic cage and formation of the rib hump. The lateral curvature affects the vertebral structure. Disc spaces are narrowed on the concave side and spread wider on the convex side, resulting in an asymmetric vertebral canal (Figure 29–10).

Scoliosis can also occur in congenital diseases involving the spinal structure and in the musculoskeletal changes seen in conditions such as myelomeningocele, cerebral palsy (see Chapter 27), or muscular dystrophy. Disturbances in platelet function, melatonin levels, and bone-related trace substances are sometimes evident (Lombardi et al., 2011). Scoliosis can also be acquired after injury to the spinal cord.

CLINICAL MANIFESTATIONS

The classic signs of scoliosis include truncal asymmetry, uneven shoulder and hip height, a one-sided rib hump, and a prominent scapula. The child does not usually complain of pain or discomfort.

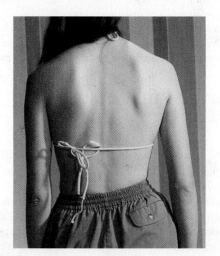

Figure 29–10 Clues for early detection of scoliosis. A child may have varying degrees of scoliosis. For mild forms, treatment will focus on strengthening and stretching. Moderate forms will require bracing. Severe forms may necessitate surgery and fusion. Clothes that fit at an angle, such as this teenage girl's shorts, and anatomic asymmetry of the back provide clues for early detection.

CLINICAL THERAPY

Generally, observation and radiographic examination are used to diagnose scoliosis. Additional diagnostic studies include MRI, CT, and bone scanning, which are used occasionally to assess the degree of curvature. The goal of medical management is to limit or stop progression of the curvature.

Early detection is essential to successful treatment. Adequate treatment and follow-up maximize the child's chances for proper spinal alignment. The treatment regimen chosen depends on the degree and progression of the curvature and the reaction of the child and family to medical management.

Treatment of children with mild scoliosis (curvatures of 10 to 20 degrees) consists of exercises to improve posture and muscle tone and to maintain, or possibly increase, flexibility of the spine. Emphasis is placed on building strength toward the outside of the curve while stretching the inside of the curve. However, these exercises are not a cure, and the child should be evaluated by a physician at 3-month intervals, with radiographic evaluation every 6 months.

Medical management of moderate scoliosis (curvatures of 20 to 40 degrees) includes bracing with a Boston brace. The goal of wearing a brace is to maintain the existing spinal curvature with no increase. Brace wear begins immediately after diagnosis. To achieve maximum effectiveness, the brace should be worn 23 hours per day. Brace treatment is lengthy, favorite sports may not be allowed, it can affect body image, and it requires a high degree of compliance, all of which can be difficult for adolescents.

Children with severe scoliosis (curvatures of 40 to 50 degrees or more) generally require surgery, which involves spinal fusion. The majority of spinal fusions are performed using segmental instrumentation of the spinal cord with hooks, wires, rods, and screws (Lubicky, Hanson, Riley, et al., 2011; Scottish Rite Hospital, 2011). Examples of surgical approaches include Luque wires, Cotrel-Dubousset (CD) instrumentation, Texas Scottish Rite Hospital system, and Moss-Miami system. These treatments stabilize the spine well during surgery, may be accompanied by bone grafting to the spine, and require no long-term therapy or postoperative casting; instrumentation remains permanently in the back. Following surgery with wires or instrumentation, the child is on bed rest during a recovery period and then is generally fitted with anteroposterior plastic shells (also called thoracolumbar sacral orthotics) that are worn for several months to provide stability for the spine.

Nursing Management

For the Child With Scoliosis

Nursing Assessment and Diagnosis

School nurses often screen children for scoliosis, generally in the fifth and seventh grades. Several states mandate this screening, but it is not universal in all states, nor is it now recommended for all children (U.S. Preventive Services Task Force, 2014). When abnormalities are noted, refer the child to an orthopedic center for further evaluation. Children should be examined every 6 to 9 months thereafter. If scoliosis is detected, the child's brothers and sisters should be examined and observed closely. Scoliosis screening involves visual observations of the following:

From the front:

- Is the head midline?
- Are the shoulders at the same height?
- Is there the same amount of space between the arms and body on each side?

From the back:

- Is the head midline?
- Are the shoulders at the same height?
- Are the scapulae equally prominent and at the same height?
- Is the spine straight?
- Is there the same amount of space between the arms and body on each side?
- Are the hips at the same height?

With the adolescent holding hands together and bent over slightly:

- Are the scapula humps even?

With the adolescent holding hands together and bent over toward the floor:

- Are the flank humps even?
- Is the spine straight?
- Is there a marked roundness when viewed from the side? (evidence of kyphosis)

Once scoliosis has been identified, the focus becomes education and follow-up. Any child with scoliosis should have a comprehensive neurologic, cardiac, and respiratory examination, since the rib cage deformity can influence the functioning of these systems.

Professionalism in Practice Scoliosis Screening of Adolescents

The U.S. Preventive Services Task Force previously recommended screening of all young adolescents for scoliosis, generally in the school and/or office setting. However, analysis of research studies has not shown that screening of all adolescents aids in the identification or treatment of this condition, and it may be costly and difficult in the school setting and lead to unnecessary health referrals. Therefore, the 2014 guidelines did not recommend screening of all adolescents for scoliosis (U.S. Preventive Services Task Force, 2014). School nurses can work with administration in their districts to make decisions about whether or not scoliosis screening should be done on children in the school setting. The decision and information about scoliosis should be communicated with families.

The following nursing diagnoses may apply to the child with scoliosis (NANDA-I © 2014):

- *Health Behavior, Risk-Prone,* related to duration and intensity of exercise prescription
- *Mobility: Physical, Impaired,* related to brace or movement restrictions and pain following surgery
- *Skin Integrity, Risk for Impaired,* related to brace
- *Knowledge, Deficient,* related to unfamiliarity with disease process and home care
- *Body Image, Disturbed,* related to deformity and brace wear

Common nursing diagnoses for the child having surgery can be found in the accompanying *Nursing Care Plan.*

Nursing Care Plan: The Child Undergoing Surgery for Scoliosis

1. Nursing Diagnosis: *Knowledge, Deficient (Child and Parents),* related to lack of information about surgery (NANDA-I © 2014)

GOAL: The child and parents will verbalize understanding of the disease, its treatment, and the surgical procedure.

INTERVENTION	RATIONALE
• Teach the child and family about the course of the disease, its signs and symptoms, and treatment. Provide appropriate handouts. Encourage the child and parents to ask questions.	• Understanding and involvement increase motivation and compliance while reducing fear.
• Begin preoperative teaching at the time of admission. Orient the child to hospital and postoperative procedures. Before surgery, have the child demonstrate log-rolling, range-of-motion (ROM) exercises, and the use of an incentive spirometer. Discuss pain management.	• Preoperative teaching and familiarity with hospital procedures reduce the stress related to surgery and postoperative complications.

EXPECTED OUTCOME: Child and family will accurately verbalize knowledge about the disease and its treatment. Child and family will ask appropriate questions about postoperative care.

2. Nursing Diagnosis: *Breathing Pattern, Ineffective,* related to hypoventilation syndrome (NANDA-I © 2014)

GOAL: The child will show no signs of respiratory compromise.

INTERVENTION	RATIONALE
• Monitor respiratory status, especially after the administration of analgesics. Apply pulse oximeter.	• Evaluation of the child's respiratory condition anticipates and avoids complications. Analgesics such as morphine may increase or potentiate respiratory compromise.
• Administer oxygen if ordered.	• Oxygen increases peripheral oxygen saturation to 95%–100%.
• Have the child use an incentive spirometer.	• Spirometry increases lung expansion and aeration of the alveoli.
• Monitor intake and output.	• Adequate hydration promotes loose secretions and helps prevent infection.
• Reposition the child at least every 2 hr.	• Repositioning ensures inflation of the lung fields.

EXPECTED OUTCOME: Child will have normal respiratory patterns.

3. Nursing Diagnosis: *Injury, Risk for,* related to neurovascular deficit secondary to instrumentation (NANDA-I © 2014)

GOAL: The child's neurovascular system will remain intact as evidenced by circulation, sensation, and motor assessments. The child will feel no numbness or tingling.

INTERVENTION	RATIONALE
• Monitor the child's color, circulation, capillary refill, warmth, sensation, and motion in all extremities. Perform neurovascular assessments every 2 hr for the first 24 hr and then every 4 hr for the next 48 hr. Record presence of pedal and distal tibial pulses every hour for 48 hr. Report changes and abnormal findings immediately.	• When the spinal column is manipulated during surgery, altered neurovascular status, thrombosis formation, and paralysis are possible complications. Postoperative risks include loss of bowel or bladder control, weakness or paralysis, and impaired vision or sensation.
• Have the child wear antiembolism stockings until ambulatory. The stockings may be removed for 1 hr 2–3 times daily.	• Antiembolism stockings prevent blood clots and promote venous return. Thrombus formation is a postoperative risk.
• Check for any pain, swelling, or a positive Homans sign (pain in the calf of the leg when the toes are dorsiflexed). Record any evidence of edema.	• Swelling may indicate a tight dressing and tissue damage. A positive Homans sign and pain may indicate thrombus formation.
• Monitor input and output.	• Abnormalities may indicate a fluid shift problem.
• Log roll while on bed rest. Encourage and assist the child with ROM exercises, both passive and active as prescribed.	• Log rolling maintains a straight spine. Exercises promote mobility and reduce risk of thrombus formation.

(continued)

Nursing Care Plan: The Child Undergoing Surgery for Scoliosis (*continued*)

EXPECTED OUTCOME: Child will exhibit only temporary alteration (pale skin, faint pulse, and edema occur but they resolve within the initial postoperative phase). Child will return to the preoperative baseline state by discharge.

4. Nursing Diagnosis: *Pain, Acute*, related to spinal fusion with instrumentation (NANDA-I © 2014)

GOAL: The child will verbalize an adequate level of comfort or show absence of pain behavior within 1 hour of a specific nursing intervention.

INTERVENTION	RATIONALE
• Assess the level of pain and initiate pain management strategies as soon as possible. Use patient-controlled analgesia if ordered.	• Adequate pain management allows for faster healing and a more cooperative patient. Patient-controlled analgesics may be effective.
• Administer pain medication around-the-clock to help ensure pain relief, especially during the first 48 hours. Monitor epidural blocks and patient-controlled analgesia or other methods used for pain control.	• Medicating around-the-clock helps to maintain comfort. Monitoring ensures patient safety.
• Use nonpharmacologic pain management techniques, such as imagery, relaxation, touch, music, application of heat and cold, and reduced environmental stimulation to supplement medications (see Chapter 15).	• Alternative treatments also interrupt the pain stimulus and provide relief. Nonpharmacologic methods can be an effective adjunct to pain management.
• Document pain assessment interventions and the child's response.	• Proper documentation guides the selection of the most effective means of pain control.
• Reassure the child that some discomfort is expected and that a variety of measures can be tried to reduce discomfort.	• Realistic expectations decrease anxiety and give the child a sense of control.

EXPECTED OUTCOME: Child will experience pain relief early in the postoperative period.

Planning and Implementation

An important aspect of nursing care is client education. Client adherence to prescribed measures is critical to the success of treatment. Children and their families need to understand the condition and the stages of treatment; this is particularly true for adolescents undergoing treatment for scoliosis.

Children or adolescents facing surgery require education, reassurance, and support. Teach about pain control and the patient-controlled analgesia (PCA) pump. Often children donate some of their own blood prior to surgery, and the family may also donate so blood transfused in surgery is the children's or a family member's. Teach the child the safety that this ensures. The adolescent will benefit from learning about deep breathing, positioning, surgical incision, and all other aspects of postoperative care. The *Nursing Care Plan* summarizes nursing care for the child undergoing surgery for scoliosis.

PROMOTE ACCEPTANCE OF THE TREATMENT PLAN

Provide instructions about exercises that will help decrease the severity of the spinal curvature, and obtain baseline exercise levels. Demonstrate the exercises, and explain their purpose (i.e., to strengthen back muscles). Help the child adjust to wearing a brace. Adolescents, in particular, may be reluctant to wear an external device such as a brace. To promote a sense of control, allow the adolescent to choose when to exercise and when to be out of the brace, within the treatment guidelines. Provide reassurance and encouragement and promote interaction with peers. Suggest that the adolescent work with a peer support person who is being treated for scoliosis or has had the condition in the past. Provide information about fashionable clothing that can be worn with the brace and facilitate visits to department stores that will help the teen shop for clothing.

DISCHARGE PLANNING AND HOME CARE TEACHING

Identify and address home care needs well in advance of discharge after spinal surgery. The child will need to adapt to a new set of body mechanics. Show the child how to do simple tasks without bending or twisting the torso. Have the child demonstrate the ability to perform activities of daily living before discharge from the hospital. Partner with physical therapy/rehabilitation personnel to plan for the youth's needs related to safe and effective movement with the brace.

Activities for the child who has had spinal surgery are commonly limited for a period of time. The child can usually walk and perform physical activity such as gentle swimming, but lifting heavy loads, bending or twisting at the waist, or engaging in activities such as skiing, rollerblading, bicycle riding, and many other sports may not be allowed. Restrictions usually should be followed for 6 to 8 months, depending on the type of surgery and the surgeon. Emphasize to both the child and the family the importance of compliance. Give written discharge instructions to the child and family. Follow-up visits are important. The child should be examined 4 to 6 weeks after discharge, then every 3 to 4 months for 1 year, and every 1 to 2 years thereafter. The metal hardware in the back will set off metal detectors at airports. The teen should be prepared to tell screeners about the implants so that alternative screening methods can be used.

Several organizations provide information and assistance to families of children with scoliosis. Make referrals as appropriate.

Evaluation

Expected outcomes of nursing care for the child with scoliosis treated by brace are maintenance of intact skin and compliance with prescribed therapy. Expected outcomes after surgical correction are given in the accompanying *Nursing Care Plan*.

Clinical Reasoning Adolescent Braces for Scoliosis

It is common knowledge that adolescents are concerned about body image and that wearing a brace can be challenging. Although there has been controversy about the efficacy of braces for scoliosis treatment, studies have found that bracing significantly decreases the progression of high-risk curves to the need for surgery (Brox, Lange, Gunderson, et al., 2012; Weinstein, Dolan, Wright, et al., 2013). Healthcare providers may need to address psychosocial coping issues in order to ensure compliance with brace therapy for scoliosis. What assessments can assist you in learning about the activity level, social interactions, and well-being of adolescents beginning scoliosis treatment?

Torticollis, Kyphosis, and Lordosis

Torticollis is tilt of the head caused by rotation of the cervical spine. The cause is generally an injury sustained to the sternocleidomastoid muscle at the time of birth or to a cervical spine abnormality. Stretching exercises or surgical lengthening of the sternocleidomastoid muscle are usual treatments. Occasionally, the cause of torticollis is visual impairment, leading to constant turning in one direction to see with the better eye.

Kyphosis (hunchback) and lordosis (swayback) are two other types of spinal curvature that may occur in children. Clinical therapy depends on the cause and degree of the curvature, and the age of the child at onset. Nurses can perform thorough musculoskeletal assessments of children (see Chapter 5) and refer any children with abnormalities for further evaluation. (See Table 29–4.)

Growth and Development

Postural lordosis is a characteristic finding in toddlers but should disappear by the school-age years.

Additional Disorders of the Bones and Joints

Osteoporosis and Osteopenia

Osteoporosis, a condition in which there is decreased density and mass of bone, promotes the risk of fractures and is commonly associated with aging. However, children can have osteoporosis (also known as *metabolic bone disease* or a bone mineral density more than 2.5 standard deviations below the norm) related to imbalanced nutrition or other pathologic conditions. Osteoporosis is preceded by osteopenia or low bone mass, which is between 1.0 and 2.5 standard deviations below the norm (Szadek & Scharer, 2014).

ETIOLOGY AND PATHOPHYSIOLOGY

Very-low–birth-weight infants who are premature often have osteopenia of prematurity because much of the bone mass is usually acquired in the latter weeks of pregnancy. In addition, they may have other health problems after birth and be unable to ingest enough nutrients to meet metabolic needs for bone growth. Premature infants are often less active than others, which decreases the amount of mechanical loading on their bones, a factor known to increase bone resorption and decrease bone mass (Rack et al., 2011).

A group of children who may show signs of osteoporosis are those who have decreased mechanical loading. Children with spina bifida or cerebral palsy, conditions that interfere with ambulation, have limited pressure on bones and resultant lowered bone mass in affected extremities and spine. Some

---

TABLE 29–4 Clinical Manifestations of Kyphosis and Lordosis

CONDITION	CLINICAL MANIFESTATIONS	DIAGNOSTIC TESTS AND CLINICAL THERAPY	NURSING MANAGEMENT
KYPHOSIS			
Excessive convex curvature of the cervical thoracic spine	Visible hunchback or rounded shoulders; shortness of breath or fatigue; abdominal creases and tight hamstrings in severe cases	*Diagnostic tests:* Spinal curvature is assessed by having the child bend 90 degrees at the waist and looking at the scapular area from the side. Diagnosis is confirmed by radiograph. *Clinical therapy:* Exercises are prescribed for mild condition; bracing is commonly used; surgery is performed in severe cases.	Provide support. Encourage exercises and diligent brace wear. Help the child to deal with the psychologic stress of altered body image.
LORDOSIS			
Excessive concave curvature of the lumbar spine with an angle of more than 60 degrees; most common in prepubescent girls and African Americans	Presence of swayback; prominent buttocks; hip flexion contractures; tight hamstrings	*Diagnostic tests:* Spinal curvature is assessed by looking at the standing child from the side. Lumbar lordosis is confirmed by visualizing the spine on standing, lateral radiograph. *Clinical therapy:* Treatment focuses on exercises and postural awareness. Bracing and surgery are rarely prescribed.	Provide support. Reassure the child and family that the condition is often outgrown as the child matures. Encourage physical conditioning exercises and follow-up examinations on a yearly basis.

Pathophysiology Illustrated: **Effects of Immobility**

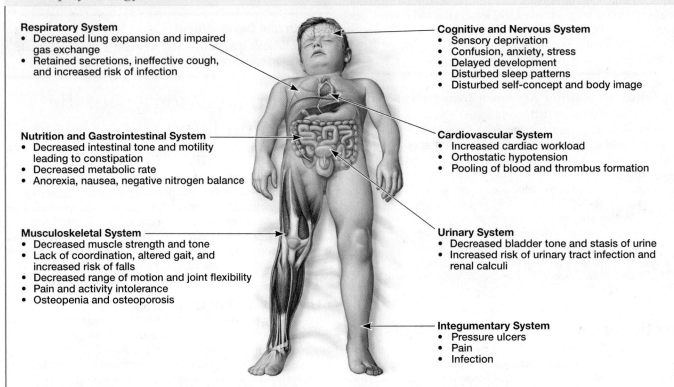

Respiratory System
- Decreased lung expansion and impaired gas exchange
- Retained secretions, ineffective cough, and increased risk of infection

Nutrition and Gastrointestinal System
- Decreased intestinal tone and motility leading to constipation
- Decreased metabolic rate
- Anorexia, nausea, negative nitrogen balance

Musculoskeletal System
- Decreased muscle strength and tone
- Lack of coordination, altered gait, and increased risk of falls
- Decreased range of motion and joint flexibility
- Pain and activity intolerance
- Osteopenia and osteoporosis

Cognitive and Nervous System
- Sensory deprivation
- Confusion, anxiety, stress
- Delayed development
- Disturbed sleep patterns
- Disturbed self-concept and body image

Cardiovascular System
- Increased cardiac workload
- Orthostatic hypotension
- Pooling of blood and thrombus formation

Urinary System
- Decreased bladder tone and stasis of urine
- Increased risk of urinary tract infection and renal calculi

Integumentary System
- Pressure ulcers
- Pain
- Infection

For older children at risk of developing osteoporosis, calcium and vitamin D intake is encouraged and oral supplements may be given. Standing therapy for those who are nonambulatory can provide mechanical weight and enhance bone density. Bisphosphonates, calcitonin, fluoride, and parathyroid hormone may be used to treat children and adolescents with osteoporosis (Szadek & Scharer, 2014). When a cast or other immobilizing device is removed from a child, a program of gradually increasing exercise in collaboration with physical rehabilitation professionals promotes bone strengthening and lowered risk for fractures or related sequelae.

other conditions are associated with lower bone mass, including Turner syndrome, growth hormone deficiency, osteogenesis imperfecta, juvenile rheumatoid arthritis, and diabetes. Children who are treated for disorders or injuries with casting and bracing are also at high risk of osteoporosis due to immobilization.

Finally, adolescence is a period when adequate intakes of calcium and vitamin D are needed to maximize bone formation and prevent osteoporosis later in life. Adolescents, particularly females, often do not meet the recommended daily allowance (RDA) for these nutrients and are at risk for osteoporosis even though it may not be manifested for years. Other lifestyle patterns of youth that decrease bone formation are smoking, alcohol use, excessive soda intake, and keeping weight at a very low level. Those with anorexia nervosa are at risk for osteoporosis and increased risk of fractures (Mehler, Cleary, & Guadiani, 2011).

CLINICAL MANIFESTATIONS
Osteoporosis is a silent disease, as is its precursor osteopenia; those who have the disorders are often without signs or symptoms for years. It may become apparent when a baby or child has a fracture and radiologic studies make the problem evident.

CLINICAL THERAPY
Bone mineral content and density are measured by single-photon absorptiometry (SPA), dual-photon absorptiometry (DPA), and dual-energy x-ray absorptiometry (DEXA); ultrasound may be used to assess preterm infants (Rack et al., 2011). Serum studies

such as thyroid, bone-specific alkaline phosphatase, phosphorus, and type I collagen studies can be used to measure osteoblastic and osteoclastic activity. Vitamin D and calcium are measured, but since over 90% of the body's calcium is stored in bone, serum calcium is not accurately reflective of bone density.

Premature newborns at risk of osteopenia of prematurity need collaborative management by neonatologists, neonatal nutritionists, and neonatal nurses. Breast milk is enhanced by adding special fortifiers; premature formula should be used rather than regular baby formula. When infants need enteral or parenteral feedings, calcium-to-phosphorus ratios are carefully balanced to enhance osteoblastic activity. There is evidence to suggest that assisted range-of-motion exercise can promote weight gain and bone mineralization in premature infants (Schulzke, Kaempfen, Trachsel, et al., 2014).

Nursing Management

For the Child With Osteoporosis or Osteopenia

Nursing Assessment and Diagnosis

Nurses identify newborns, children, and adolescents at risk of developing low bone mass and density. This is accomplished by identifying diseases and medications putting the child at risk, as well as history of fractures or malabsorption disorder. Ask about exercise and activity patterns, and physical therapy for children who are nonambulatory. Dietary intake is measured periodically for all youth at health promotion visits, and RDAs for calcium, phosphorus, and vitamin D are compared to intake.

Nursing diagnoses that may apply to the child with osteoporosis include the following (NANDA-I © 2014):

- *Nutrition, Imbalanced: Less than Body Requirements,* related to inability to consume essential nutrients
- *Injury, Risk for,* to bones related to decreased bone mass and density
- *Health Maintenance, Ineffective,* related to inadequate dietary intake

Planning and Implementation

Perform a dietary analysis of children at risk. (See Chapter 14 for detailed methods for diet assessment.) Refer children at risk to nutritionists and a physician for further education and diagnosis. Suggest referrals to physical rehabilitation to recommend weight-bearing exercise. Administer nutritional supplements when prescribed, and teach families how to give these medications. Partner with families to provide therapy that stimulates weight bearing for nonambulatory children. Teach parents how to recognize fractures in children who may not have normal sensation and are unable to report them. Edema, unusual shape of a limb, fussiness of the child, and falls should be reported promptly.

When osteoporosis is caused by immobility, many other symptoms occur as well. Be alert for these problems and integrate physical activity into care as much as possible to minimize their effects.

Evaluation

Expected outcomes of nursing care for the child with a potential for osteoporosis include adequate intake of recommended amounts of nutrients, absence of fractures, and normal findings on studies of bone mineral content and density.

Osteomyelitis

Osteomyelitis is an infection of the bone, most often one of the long bones of the lower extremity. It may be acute or chronic and may spread into surrounding tissues. Although osteomyelitis may occur at any age, it is most common in children between the ages of 1 and 12 years. Boys are affected 2 to 3 times as often as girls, primarily because they have a greater incidence of trauma. Overall incidence is 5 in 10,000 youth (Thomsen & Creech, 2011).

ETIOLOGY AND PATHOPHYSIOLOGY

Osteomyelitis is caused by a microorganism, usually bacterial but possibly viral or fungal. *Staphylococcus aureus* is the most common causative pathogen; others include *Escherichia coli, Neisseria meningitidis, Streptococcus pneumoniae, Mycobacterium tuberculosis, Borrelia burgdorferi,* and *Kingella kingae* (Bautista, Gholve, & Dormans, 2011; Thomsen & Creech, 2011). Common sources of infection are upper respiratory infection, trauma to the bone, and surgery.

The infecting organism spreads through the bloodstream or through a penetrating injury to the bone, where it becomes established. Infections in children often begin in the metaphysis (see Figure 29–1), which has a sluggish blood supply (Bautista et al., 2011). Eventually the infection may penetrate the bone cortex and periosteum. Inflammation and abscess formation can interrupt the blood supply to the underlying bone, affect the surrounding soft tissue, and, if the infection is left untreated, lead to necrosis.

CLINICAL MANIFESTATIONS

Symptoms include pain and tenderness with swelling, decreased mobility of the infected joint, and fever. Redness over the area may occur. The child may refuse to walk or may limp. The onset of acute osteomyelitis is generally rapid and is therefore sometimes misdiagnosed as a sports injury.

CLINICAL THERAPY

A history suggestive of osteomyelitis includes an upper respiratory infection or blunt trauma followed by pain at the area of a growth plate. Laboratory evaluation shows leukocytosis and an elevated erythrocyte sedimentation rate (ESR) and C-reactive protein. Radiographs and bone scans may identify the area of involvement. A needle aspiration of the site or a blood culture can confirm the diagnosis and provide a culture of the causative organism. Other studies may include enzyme-linked immunosorbent assay (ELISA) for Lyme antibody titer, antistreptolysin-O for recent streptococcal infections, or purified protein derivative (PPD) for exposure to tuberculosis (Thomsen & Creech, 2011).

Medical management begins with the intravenous administration of a broad-spectrum antibiotic, even before culture results are available. Since *S. aureus* is a common cause of infection, the antibiotic should be effective against this organism. Treatment is influenced by the possibility of methicillin-resistant *S. aureus* (MRSA), so intravenous antibiotics are usually vancomycin or clindamycin, drugs effective against MRSA (see Chapter 16). After the culture results are obtained, the antibiotic may be altered. Oral antibiotics are given once an adequate response has occurred. However, extended intravenous home therapy may be used. Antibiotic therapy continues for about 3 to 6 weeks. The cause of infection is not always identified from culture, so ESR and C-protein levels are followed carefully in these cases to identify if treatment is successful. When an adequate response is not obtained within 2 to 3 days, the area may be aspirated again or surgically drained. Intravenous fluids may be administered to ensure adequate hydration. In children with extensive orthopedic surgery or in those with immunosuppression, a short course of prophylactic antibiotic may be administered after surgery.

Growth and Development

Osteomyelitis in a newborn is of great concern because before 18 months of age the blood vessels cross the growth plates. This creates a higher risk of epiphyseal involvement with resultant limb length discrepancy. Poor feeding, crying when moved, and refusal to move a limb may indicate osteomyelitis.

Prompt diagnosis and treatment usually completely resolve the infection. The prognosis is related to the initiation of therapy—the earlier treatment begins, the better the outcome. Long-term unfavorable outcomes include disruption of the growth plate, which can interrupt growth, and damage to the joints from septic arthritis.

Nursing Management

For the Child With Osteomyelitis

Nursing Assessment and Diagnosis

A thorough history, including information about the onset of symptoms and a history of recent infections or puncture wounds, is essential. Ask about immunization status, especially tetanus vaccine. Assess the affected area for signs of redness, swelling, pain, and decreased range of motion. Measure vital signs; increased temperature and pulse in particular may provide clues about worsening infection. When osteomyelitis is possible, all cultures of blood or wound must be taken before antibiotic therapy is started.

Among the nursing diagnoses that may apply to the child with osteomyelitis are the following (NANDA-I © 2014):

- *Pain, Acute,* related to biologic injury
- *Mobility: Physical, Impaired,* related to discomfort
- *Infection, Risk for (Sepsis),* related to spread of infection
- *Imbalanced Nutrition: Less than Body Requirements,* related to loss of appetite
- *Knowledge, Readiness for Enhanced (Child and Parent),* related to lack of information about disease process

Planning and Implementation

Nursing management focuses on administering antibiotics, protecting the child from spread of the infection, and encouraging a well-balanced diet. Use standard precautions, with transmission-based precautions for any drainage from the site of infection.

OBTAIN CULTURES AND BLOOD WORK

Blood cultures and cultures of any open wound must be performed before the first dose of antibiotic when osteomyelitis is suspected. Obtain continuing blood samples as needed to monitor ESR and C-reactive protein levels. See the *Clinical Skills Manual* SKILLS.

ADMINISTER FLUIDS AND MEDICATIONS

Administer intravenous fluids as ordered to maintain the child's hydration status. Antibiotics are administered intravenously, at first, then orally. Monitor the intravenous site and provide care for the central line, if one is used. See the *Clinical Skills Manual* SKILLS.

In the early stages of the infection, analgesics are prescribed to relieve the associated pain and joint tenderness.

PROTECT FROM THE SPREAD OF INFECTION

Strict aseptic technique and transmission-based precautions should be used during all dressing changes. Children and family members should avoid direct contact with any dressings or drainage. Teach good hygiene practices, including hand hygiene, to maintain infection control. Take vital signs and evaluate the child frequently for symptoms indicating the spread of infection (e.g., increasing pain, difficulty breathing, increased pulse rate, fever).

ENCOURAGE A WELL-BALANCED DIET

Educate both the child and the parents about healthy dietary choices that promote healing. A high-protein diet and extra vitamin C will contribute to this process. Encourage increased fluid intake to provide adequate hydration and circulation.

DISCHARGE PLANNING AND HOME CARE TEACHING

Emphasize the importance of completing the full course of antibiotic therapy, especially for children who have had an abscess or lesion surgically drained. Some children may be discharged on intravenous antibiotics if the family is willing to learn the procedure for medication administration and care of the central line. Several sessions of demonstration and return demonstration are needed to ensure safe administration. If the family is unable to perform antibiotic therapy, a home infusion company may be available to come to the home and administer the medication. Explain that failure to follow the prescribed antibiotic therapy may result in chronic infection. Emphasize the importance of returning for blood analysis to monitor progression of healing.

Consider the child's age and developmental level and partner with the family to plan quiet activities and access to schoolwork. Provide suggestions for the family if the child will be immobilized at home.

Clinical Tip

If the child needs to remain home for a period of time during treatment for osteomyelitis, help the family plan for completion of school tasks. The nurse can partner with other health disciplines that are available to plan for the following:

- Contact the school and ask that work be sent home.
- Arrange for a tutor if needed.
- Facilitate computer communication between child, teacher, and other students.
- Help the family plan for help at home to monitor the child when the family needs to be at work or performing other tasks.
- Refer families to financial resources as appropriate for the services the child needs.
- Suggest activities that the child can do at home that foster developmental progress.

Evaluation

Expected outcomes of nursing care for the child with osteomyelitis include the following:

- The child has no signs of infection or sepsis.
- The child completes the prescribed course of antibiotics.
- Intake of fluids and nutrients is adequate for good health.
- The child's pain is effectively managed.
- The child is able to return to normal activities of daily living.

Skeletal Tuberculosis and Septic Arthritis

Skeletal tuberculosis (Figure 29–11) and septic arthritis are two infections that, although infrequent, may affect children and adolescents. See Table 29–5 for diagnostic tests and medical and nursing management for these infections.

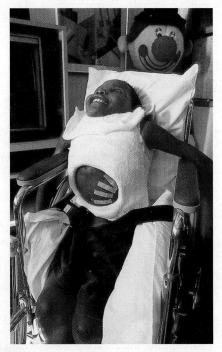

Figure 29–11 This boy from Kenya had surgery to correct severe kyphosis and scoliosis caused by tuberculosis of the spine. A Risser cast has been applied to maintain stability of the spine and thoracic cage during healing. Notice the area cut out of the cast to allow for auscultation of the abdomen, as well as to facilitate the child's comfort and adequate intake of food.

TABLE 29–5 Clinical Manifestations of Skeletal Tuberculosis and Septic Arthritis

CONDITION	CLINICAL MANIFESTATIONS	DIAGNOSTIC TESTS AND CLINICAL THERAPY	NURSING MANAGEMENT
SKELETAL TUBERCULOSIS			
Rare microbacterial infection that can be very destructive. The spine is the most frequent site of infection (Pott disease), with joints and other sites sometimes affected.	Depending on the site, pain, limp, severe muscle spasms, kyphosis, muscle atrophy, "doughy" swelling of joints, decreased joint motion, changes in reflexes, low-grade fever	*Diagnostic tests:* Diagnostic studies include tuberculosis skin test, complete blood count, synovial fluid analysis, and radiographs of affected limb or joint. *Clinical therapy:* Antibiotic therapy (using a combination of drugs) for 6–9 months is the treatment of choice. The affected site is immobilized. Disease may become resistant to these drugs, and additional drug therapy may be necessary.	Educate the child and family about the disorder and stress the importance of complying with long-term antibiotic therapy. Test all members of the family for tuberculosis. Report the disease to the local health department. Facilitate the immobilization and physical therapy of the child at home.
SEPTIC ARTHRITIS			
Joint infection of the synovial space most often caused by *Haemophilus influenzae, Staphylococcus,* and *Streptococcus.* The most common site of infection is the knee, followed by the hip, ankle, and elbow.	Fever, pain and local inflammation, joint tenderness, swelling, loss of spontaneous movement	*Diagnostic tests:* CBC with differential, ESR, blood cultures. Diagnosis is made based on joint aspiration findings. Results are commonly 100,000 WBCs and 75% neutrophils, ESR greater than 44 mm/hr. Radiographic changes may not be evident until later in the disease process. *Clinical therapy:* This is a medical emergency requiring prompt treatment to avoid permanent disability. Treatment involves joint aspiration, open drainage, and irrigation, followed by intravenous antibiotic therapy for 3–4 weeks and then oral antibiotics. If the full course of antibiotic treatment is not completed, the child risks recurrent infection and further degeneration of the infected joint.	Educate the child and family about the disorder and emphasize the importance of proper antibiotic therapy. Carefully position the painful joint. Administer antibiotics as prescribed. Use transmission-based precautions. Encourage fluids to ensure adequate hydration. Support and rest the joint; provide activities that do not require joint movement.

Achondroplasia

Dwarfism is a genetic condition usually resulting in an adult height of 58 inches or less. The most common cause of dwarfism is achondroplasia, which causes short arms and legs. The torso and head are approximately normal size, but decreased growth of long bones causes short stature. This is known as *disproportionate short stature*. Achondroplasia is caused by an abnormal gene of chromosome 4 and occurs in 1 in 15,000 to 40,000 births (March of Dimes, 2012). The gene is coded to produce proteins called *fibroblast growth factor receptors*. When fewer receptors are produced, the cells cannot respond normally to signals from growth factors. Achondroplasia may occur as a new genetic mutation with no previous family history or can occur when one or both parents are also dwarfs. There are other less common forms of dwarfism with about 200 identified types. (Refer to Chapter 3 for further information about genetic disease transmission.)

Children with achondroplasia have short legs and arms, short fingers with a separation between middle and ring fingers, and a large, prominent forehead. Hydrocephalus sometimes occurs in children with achondroplasia. (See Chapter 27 for a description of hydrocephalus.) Most children with the disorder inherit the gene from one parent. Since only one faulty gene must be present for manifestation of the disorder, it is a dominant characteristic. When a child inherits two copies of the gene from two affected parents, a fatal form of achondroplasia occurs, which is characterized by a small thorax, respiratory failure, and death in infancy.

Children with the disorder are diagnosed prenatally, at birth, or shortly after. When there is a family history, genetic testing before or after birth identifies the presence of the fibroplast growth factor receptor 3 (*FGFR3*) gene on chromosome 4. Characteristics common in the growth disorder include frequent otitis media, dental malocclusion, short fingers, bowing of legs, marked lordosis, and sleep apnea. The child may be slow at meeting gross motor developmental milestones (Ireland et al., 2012).

There is no treatment for the disorder at this time. Gene therapy and growth plate targeting are being explored as possible future treatments (Laederich & Horton, 2012). Some children and adults with dwarfism have undergone limb-lengthening procedures such as that described later in this chapter. Other orthopedic intervention may be needed to treat back pain or bone problems. For those children who develop hydrocephalus, insertion of a shunt to divert excess fluid may be needed. Treatment of conditions such as otitis media and malocclusion of teeth is provided.

Nursing Management

Nurses play an important role in helping families when a child is diagnosed with achondroplasia. If a parent is a dwarf or there is a positive family history of dwarfism, genetic counseling should be offered prenatally. Explain findings of testing and provide assistance with decision making about pregnancy if needed. Nurses assist parents who have a child with achondroplasia to adjust to the diagnosis, particularly if the parents have had no previous experience with the condition. They may feel guilt and anxiety; contact with other families who have children with achondroplasia can be a supportive intervention.

Nurses help the child with achondroplasia to develop a positive self-concept during childhood. Many resources, such as the organizations listed in the next paragraph, provide suggestions about how to foster a positive self-concept, adjust the home to facilitate the dwarf, and assist the child with adjustments in school settings. Partner with school nurses or counselors to ensure the child's successful inclusion in all school facilities and an individualized education plan. While some families decide to explore limb-lengthening procedures, most organizations state that focus should be placed on development of a healthy self-image rather than encouraging limb lengthening.

Nurses provide careful assessments of children throughout childhood. Head circumference is especially important in early childhood to identify hydrocephalus if it should occur. Carefully evaluate growth with specialized growth grids for achondroplasia, evaluate dental health at each visit, and perform developmental assessment with special emphasis on gross motor skills. Suggest activities such as swimming and biking that provide activity with little stress on bones. Assist the family by providing resources that assist with planning for car safety seats, methods of adjusting the home, and partnering with the school to provide a supportive atmosphere for the child. Some helpful organizations include Little People of America, Dwarf Athletic Association of America, Human Growth Foundation, Magic Foundation for Children's Growth and Related Adult Disorders, and March of Dimes. Refer for care for otitis media and provide postoperative care if tympanostomy tubes are inserted (see Chapter 19). Refer to dentists and orthodontists and encourage regular dental care.

Marfan Syndrome

Marfan syndrome is another example of a condition inherited in an autosomal dominant manner. About 1 in 5000 to 10,000 children are affected with the syndrome, which manifests with several conditions of connective tissue (Kumar & Agarwal, 2014; Rosenbush & Parker, 2014). The most common problems are cardiac (mitral valve prolapse, aortic regurgitation, abnormal aortic root dimensions), skeletal (pectus excavatum, long arms and digits, scoliosis, elongated head, high arched palate), ocular (lens subluxation), and respiratory (pneumothorax). The woman with Marfan syndrome has an increased risk of complications during pregnancy, primarily related to the extra requirements placed on the heart. The average age for diagnosis is 3 years, with a heart murmur as the usual finding. Careful assessment identifies additional characteristics of the condition along with a positive family history.

Diagnosis is made after a complete family history, a detailed physical examination, an eye examination, a thorough heart examination, radiographs of the chest, and MRI or CT.

There is no treatment for the syndrome, which causes abnormal formation of fibrillin matrix in connective tissue. However, early diagnosis can be successful in treating the cardiac abnormalities with medication or surgery to prevent dissection of the aorta, the major cause of death. Diagnosis in children is often difficult because many features of Marfan syndrome are not apparent until adolescence. Surgery may be needed to correct scoliosis, pectus excavatum, or pneumothorax. Careful monitoring throughout life is needed to prevent and treat abnormalities associated with the disorder.

Nursing Management

Nursing management of Marfan syndrome begins with identification of infants and children with symptoms of the disorder. Once diagnosed, collaboration with a cardiologist, ophthalmologist, and orthopedist is needed throughout the child's life. The child may require surgery for one or more conditions, can require antibiotics during elective procedures or dental care if the mitral valve is affected, and needs echocardiogram and other cardiac studies regularly. The nurse may need to explain the disorder to the family and provide referrals for genetic counseling. Case management for the numerous medical specialists will be advantageous. The child needs support during childhood to learn about the disorder and to manage the medication and monitoring required.

> **Clinical Reasoning** Autosomal Dominant Disorders
>
> Both achondroplasia and Marfan syndrome are autosomal dominant disorders. Does this mean that the child needs one or two genes to manifest the disorders? If one parent has the disorder, what is the chance that a pregnancy will result in an affected child? Will there ever be a carrier who does not manifest the disease? See Chapter 3 for further information about autosomal dominant inheritance.

Osteogenesis Imperfecta

Osteogenesis imperfecta (OI), also known as *brittle bone disease*, is a connective tissue disorder that primarily affects the bones. Children with this condition have fragile bones that are more likely to fracture. Osteogenesis imperfecta occurs in 1 in 10,000 to 15,000 live births and affects boys and girls equally (van Dijk et al., 2011).

The underlying disorder is a biochemical defect in the production of collagen. The disease is genetically transmitted, generally in an autosomal dominant inheritance pattern, although some types are transmitted in a recessive pattern. The most common types are caused by mutations on the *COL1A 1* or *COL1A 2* genes on chromosomes 17 and 7, respectively (van Dijk et al., 2011).

Clinical manifestations include multiple and frequent fractures; blue sclerae; thin, soft skin; altered joint flexibility; short stature; enlargement of the anterior fontanelle; weak muscles; soft, pliable, brittle bones; and short stature. Conductive hearing loss can occur by adolescence or young adulthood.

Osteogenesis imperfecta is classified into four main types. In type I disease, the most common form, children have fragile bones, blue sclerae, weakened tooth dentin, and possible hearing loss that manifests in adolescence. In type II disease, the ribs and skeleton are extensively involved; most children with this form of the disease die in utero or shortly after birth. Type III disease is identified in the newborn period or in infancy when the child sustains numerous fractures and manifests blue sclerae.

Severe bone fragility and kyphoscoliosis are observed. Type IV disease is characterized by fractures without other symptoms of the disease. Bowing of the legs and other structural deformities can occur; however, the incidence of fractures decreases beginning in puberty. Recent genetic research has identified up to 11 different genetic mutations leading to various types of OI (Ben Amor, Rauch, Monti, et al., 2013; Womack, 2014).

Improved knowledge about the genetic transmission of this disease means that some cases of OI can be identified before birth using ultrasound or collagen analysis of chorionic villus cells or genetic testing. In many cases, however, diagnosis of OI is made only when the child has a delay in walking or sustains a fracture. Radiographic evaluation may detect old as well as new fractures. This may lead to an erroneous diagnosis of child abuse. Tests such as DEXA can be used to measure bone density. Serum alkaline phosphatase may be elevated; other measures of bone metabolism such as serum osteocalcin, procollagen 1 C-terminal peptide, collagen 1 teleopeptide, and urine deoxypyridinoline studies may be performed occasionally to measure effects of medication.

There is no cure for OI. Medical management consists primarily of fracture care and prevention of deformities. The goal is to maximize the child's independence and mobility while minimizing the risk of fractures. Treatment includes physical therapy; casting, bracing, or splinting; surgical stabilization; nutritional management with high vitamin D and calcium; and bisphosphonate medication such as pamidronate. Health supervision that includes dental examinations and hearing screening is important. Hematologic stem cell transplant has been used successfully in some children with severe OI and is under further research.

Nursing Management

Nursing care is primarily supportive and focuses on educating the parents and child about the disease and its treatment. The family may have been suspected of child abuse before the disease was diagnosed; explain the similar presenting symptoms of these cases. Ask about favorite activities of the child since these will need to be integrated into plans for physical activity and developmental progression. Perform careful growth measurements and developmental screening; ensure health promotion visits include dental and hearing screening.

To prevent fractures, children with osteogenesis imperfecta must be handled gently. Support the trunk and extremities using a blanket whenever moving the child. Tasks such as bathing and diapering may cause fractures and should be performed carefully. Never pull the legs upward during diaper changes, but slip a hand gently under the hips to raise them.

Children commonly have several fractures during childhood. The period of immobility and casting causes further bone breakdown due to decreased weight bearing, further increasing the chance of fracture. Children should have a well-balanced diet with additional vitamin C, vitamin D, and calcium to encourage healing and bone growth. Calories should be limited to maintain weight at recommended levels since immobility can lead to overweight and these children are generally short for their age. Partner with parents if the child is receiving experimental bisphosphonate medication so that doses are properly administered and serum/urine samples are obtained for monitoring.

When the child needs a fracture stabilized in surgery, or is having rods inserted to strengthen bones, surgical care management is important. Assess the child's vital signs and growth measurements. Obtain accurate weight before surgery and again after with the cast in place. Administer fluids and use pain-control techniques such as medication and other comfort measures. Be alert for signs of infection such as osteomyelitis, or respiratory or urinary tract infection. Begin fluids and perform dietary teaching before discharge to promote intake that fosters healing. Follow activity orders precisely to minimize safety hazards for the child. Partner with physical and occupational therapists to plan for the child's return to home and school, and to ensure the family can perform ROM exercises and other therapies. Ensure that the family has an approved car safety seat to transport the child.

Emphasize the importance of maintaining normal patterns of growth and development. Help toddlers explore and interact safely in their environment. Socialization is essential during the school-age and adolescent years. Encourage exercise, such as swimming, to improve muscle tone and prevent obesity. Adaptive equipment and motorized wheelchairs promote independent functioning. Maintenance of function can depend on proper rehabilitation services. Arrange and manage such services for the family.

The Osteogenesis Imperfecta Foundation provides information about the disease and can put families in touch with others who have the disease. Parents should receive genetic counseling. For parents who have a child with type II or III osteogenesis imperfecta, the terminal nature of the condition necessitates psychologic support, links to potential resources, and assistance with managing other tasks of family life. (See Chapter 13 for management of end-of-life care.) The siblings and extended family will need support to understand the disease and deal with their feelings and the affected child.

Expected outcomes include minimal fractures with optimal healing, normal range of motion, maintenance of a healthy diet and recommended weight, achievement of developmental milestones, family support, and adequate resources to provide necessary treatments for the child.

Muscular Dystrophies

The muscular dystrophies are a group of inherited diseases characterized by muscle fiber degeneration and muscle wasting. These disorders can begin early or late in life, and onset can be at birth or gradual. They are all terminal disorders, but the progression can vary from a few to many years.

Many types of muscular dystrophies affect children and adults. The most common form of childhood muscular dystrophy is Duchenne muscular dystrophy (pseudohypertrophic), which occurs in 1 per 3500 live male births (Theadom et al., 2014). **Pseudohypertrophy** refers to enlargement of the muscles as a result of their infiltration with fatty tissue. The gene for Duchenne muscular dystrophy was identified in 1987; it is carried in the Xp21.2 region of the chromosome and is either absent or deleted in affected children. This area codes for a protein called *dystrophin*, which is needed as a muscle membrane stabilizer. In the absence of dystrophin, a cascade of cellular events occurs, leading to necrosis in the fibers and their replacement by connective tissue. Since this is an X-linked disorder, it is seen only in males. There is similar incidence in various ethnic groups.

Becker muscular dystrophy is also X-linked and affects 1 in 30,000 boys (Becker Muscular Dystrophy, n.d.). Although the gene mutation is similar to Duchenne, it is milder in form. Other rare muscular dystrophies manifest in infancy, later childhood, or adolescence. There are a variety of genetic mutations ranging from X linked to autosomal.

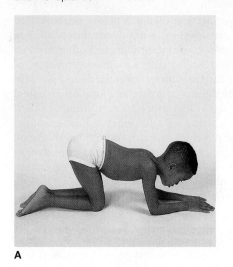

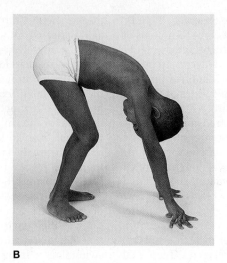

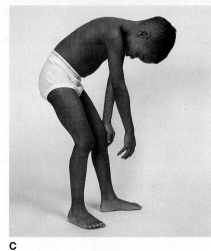

A

B

C

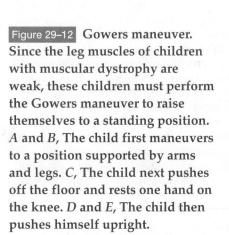

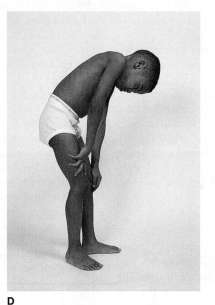

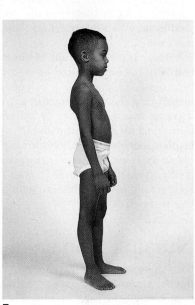

Figure 29–12 Gowers maneuver. Since the leg muscles of children with muscular dystrophy are weak, these children must perform the Gowers maneuver to raise themselves to a standing position. *A* and *B*, The child first maneuvers to a position supported by arms and legs. *C*, The child next pushes off the floor and rests one hand on the knee. *D* and *E*, The child then pushes himself upright.

D

E

Children with muscular dystrophy have generalized muscle weakness. They compensate for weak lower extremities by using the upper extremity muscles to raise themselves to a standing position (Gowers maneuver) (Figure 29–12). (See Table 29–6.)

Diagnosis and classification are most often based on clinical signs and the pattern of muscle involvement. Biochemical examinations such as serum enzyme assay, muscle biopsy, and electromyography confirm the diagnosis. Serum creatine kinase (CK) is elevated early in the disease. Muscle biopsy can measure dystrophin, the muscle protein that is deficient in muscular dystrophy. Genetic testing establishes the specific abnormality and type of disease present. Testing of newborns may be offered to families who have one child with the disease since this helps some families to adapt and prepare for the care the child will need. Respiratory function is measured periodically with pulmonary function tests and overnight pulse oximetry.

There is no effective treatment for childhood muscular dystrophy. Research is being directed at several techniques to repair mutations by gene therapy, override the genetic error in order to produce dystrophin, and apply stem cell therapy (Goyenvaile, Seto, Davies, et al., 2011). The steroids prednisone and deflazacort may preserve muscle function, preserving walking for a longer period. Rehabilitative therapy is needed to maximize independence and physical activity and to decrease hazards of immobility. Children and families can benefit from mental health support to help them in adapting to the progressive and terminal nature of the disease. A common complementary care used for muscular dystrophy is dietary enhancement. This enhancement includes giving vitamins A, C, E, D, and B-complex; minerals such as calcium, magnesium, zinc, and selenium; probiotic supplement; omega-3 fatty acids; herbal remedies such as green and rhodiola rosea teas; muscular and immunologic enzymes such as coenzyme Q10, N-acetyl cysteine, acetyl-L-carnitine, creatine, L-theanine; and melatonin to promote sleep. Massage is often used to assist with reduction of muscle spasms (University of Maryland Medical Center, 2011).

Progressive weakness and muscle deformity result in chronic disability (Figure 29–13). Respiratory infections are vigorously treated with deep breathing, coughing, nebulizer treatments, and antibiotics. Comprehensive and regular cardiac evaluations are recommended. The team approach to managing the child with muscular dystrophy ensures a comprehensive management plan. Team members should include physicians (pediatrician, orthopedic surgeon, neurologist), nurses, physical and occupational therapists, a nutritionist, psychologist or mental health therapist, and a social worker.

TABLE 29–6 Clinical Manifestations of Muscular Dystrophies of Childhood

TYPE OF DYSTROPHY	CLINICAL MANIFESTATIONS	CLINICAL THERAPY
DUCHENNE MUSCULAR DYSTROPHY		
X-linked recessive disorder seen in boys (on *Xp21* gene); however, 30%–50% of affected children have no family history *Onset:* within the first 3–4 years of life	Delayed walking; frequent falls; easily tired when walking, running, or climbing stairs; toe walking, hypertrophied calves; waddling gait; lordosis; positive Gowers maneuver; intellectual disability frequently seen	Supportive care; physical therapy and braces to help maintain mobility and prevent contractures Most children are wheelchair bound by 12 years of age; death usually occurs during adolescence from respiratory or cardiac failure
BECKER MUSCULAR DYSTROPHY		
X-linked recessive disorder *Onset:* usually after 5 years	Symptoms are similar to those of Duchenne muscular dystrophy, but milder and delayed; child is mobile until late teens; normal intelligence; congestive heart failure; contractures	Supportive care, same as for Duchenne muscular dystrophy Slow progression; death usually occurs from the third to the fifth decade of life
FACIOSCAPULOHUMERAL MUSCULAR DYSTROPHY		
Autosomal dominant disorder (on 4q35 chromosome) *Onset:* later childhood and adolescence	Face, shoulder girdle, lower limbs affected; unable to raise arms over head; lordosis; cannot close eyes, whistle, smile, or drink from a straw because of inability to move face; characteristic appearance includes facial weakness, winging of the scapula, thin arms, well-developed forearms	Physical therapy Slow progression; confined to wheelchair as older adult, but usually attains normal life span
EMERY-DREIFUSS MUSCULAR DYSTROPHY		
X-linked recessive disorder (on *Xq28* gene) *Onset:* childhood	Early onset of contractures followed by weakness; Achilles tendon, elbow, and spine affected; muscle weakness in upper body follows, with lower body weakness occurring later; cardiac conduction defect may occur	Physical therapy Surgery Pacemaker insertion
CONGENITAL MUSCULAR DYSTROPHIES		
Autosomal recessive group of disorders *Onset:* present at birth	Muscle weaknesses present at birth; motor development delay; contractures and joint deformities; hypotonia	Correction of skeletal deformity (orthosis or surgery) Usually nonprogressive

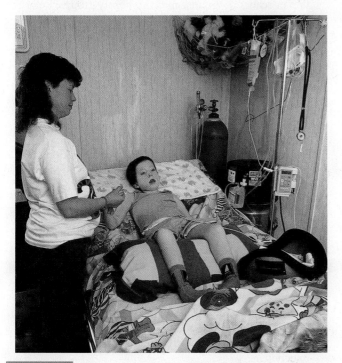

Figure 29–13 This young boy with muscular dystrophy needs to receive tube feedings and home nursing care. He attends school when possible and is able to use an adapted computer.

Nursing Management

Nursing care focuses on promoting independence and mobility and providing psychosocial support that helps the child and family deal with this progressive, incapacitating disease. Nearly all body systems become involved in the disease, and emotional care is important as well for child and family.

Monitor cardiac and respiratory functioning frequently. Assess urinary function and frequency of bowel movements. Periodically measure strength and range of motion. Assess mobility via ambulation or assisted device. Perform periodic developmental and nutritional assessments. Meet with teachers to evaluate the child's learning needs and functional level in the classroom. Evaluate the family's risk and protective factors for managing this chronic and fatal disorder.

Administer oxygen or respiratory therapy as ordered. Encourage the child to be independent for as long as possible. Concentrate on what the child can accomplish, and do not ask the child to complete tasks that may prove frustrating. Encourage parents to establish an individualized education plan with the school system. Reading books to the child, listening to tapes, and watching television offer the child stimulation during hospitalization. Exercise as tolerated contributes to muscle strength. Physical therapy helps the child ambulate and prevents joint contractures. It is important to provide back support and recommended posture by keeping the child's body in alignment when confined to a wheelchair. Provide information about complementary care that the family chooses to use.

Health Promotion The Child With Muscular Dystrophy

The child with muscular dystrophy needs close monitoring and intervention to foster growth and development in spite of a chronic and terminal disease. The nurse in health promotion can assist the child and family in many ways.

Growth and Development Surveillance

- Perform developmental screening of the young child.
- Refer to early intervention programs that establish educational plans to foster development.
- Provide resources and ideas for the parents based on the child's status rather than expected age norms. Plan interventions to maximize the highest level of function possible.
- Measure growth at each healthcare visit and plot on growth grids. Be alert for the child who is gaining weight related to decreased activity.
- Ensure visits with specialists in respiratory medicine and cardiology as recommended.

Nutrition

- Perform 24-hour analysis and evaluate for all essential nutrients. Base the analysis on the child's height and weight rather than chronologic age.
- Ask about appetite and food likes and dislikes.
- Encourage adequate fluid, whole grains, fruits, and vegetables to maintain bowel function.
- For the infant with muscular dystrophy, evaluate intake carefully; gavage feeding or nutritional supplementation such as with high-calorie formula may be needed.

Physical Activity

- Carefully monitor physical ability at each visit. Observe for decreases in movement, difficulty ambulating, or a history of falls.
- Partner with physical therapists to ensure range of motion and proper positioning of extremities.
- Explore activities that the child can do as mobility decreases. Swimming and upper body exercise may be good options.
- If the child is using a wheelchair, evaluate fit, safety, and ability to move the chair by arm controls.
- Physical activity should be regular and daily. Ensure that the family has resources to accomplish this need.

Activities of Daily Living

- Partner with occupational therapy to evaluate the child's ability to feed, bathe, dress, and provide own oral care. Provide adaptive devices as needed.
- Encourage the family to provide time for the child to perform own self-care as much as possible.
- Make a home visit or discuss with the family adaptations that could make it easier for the child to be independent in activities of daily living. Low drawers for clothing or open shelves that do not require pulling out to get items are examples of important adaptations.

Mental and Spiritual Health

- Inquire about the child's general mood.

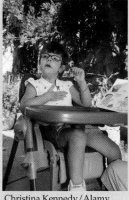
Christina Kennedy/Alamy

- Ask the parents what is best and worst about their lives at this time. Use the information to establish a list of their meaningful activities and to identify the areas most in need of support.
- Ask about sources of support such as a group for parents of a child with muscular dystrophy, family participation in faith-based activity, and extended family or neighbors.
- Be alert for signs of depression in child or family (see Chapter 28).
- Assist the family to establish activities to increase self-esteem in the youth. The youth should be able to make choices appropriate for developmental age.
- If the child was diagnosed at a younger age, ask what the parents have now told the child about the disease. Provide support and role-playing opportunities for parents who wish to tell the child about the terminal nature of the disorder.
- Refer for services such as genetic counseling, grief counseling, or other supportive interventions.

Relationships

- Ask about siblings and their relationship with the child with muscular dystrophy.
- Inquire about the child's participation in early intervention or school programs, and community groups. Refer the family to resources that encourage the child's interactions with peers. This is particularly important for teens.
- Ask the parents if and how often they are able to spend time with other adults.

Disease Prevention Strategies

- Immunize the child at recommended times. If the child is ill and immunization is delayed, be sure to call the family back promptly to reschedule administration of vaccines so that infectious diseases can be avoided. Annual influenza vaccine is needed. If the child is treated with steroids for the disease, follow recommendations for immunization of children on steroids.
- Teach the family to avoid crowds and known infectious persons. The child may need to be out of school for a few days or weeks if there is an influenza or other disease outbreak in the school population.
- Teach the family signs of infection, especially of the respiratory tract. Have them report these symptoms promptly.
- Monitor effects of antibiotics when administered for infection.
- Encourage daily activities that encourage deep breathing. Swimming, blowing into an incentive spirometer, or playing with a pinwheel are examples.

Parents may feel guilty and hopeless; encourage them to express their feelings. Genetic counseling is recommended for the entire family, and it is especially important to identify female relatives who are carriers of one of the X-linked disorders. Siblings may feel neglected because their brother or sister is receiving so much attention. They may be concerned that they will develop the disease, and in some families, this indeed occurs. Encourage the parents to spend individual time with each child and to involve siblings in the child's care.

Refer family members to resource and support groups such as the Muscular Dystrophy Association. Provide ongoing support during hospitalizations, management of home care, and the child's changes in condition.

Injuries to the Musculoskeletal System

Musculoskeletal injuries are classified according to the mechanism, the location, and the force of the injury. Strains, sprains, dislocations, and fractures are the most common musculoskeletal injuries in children; athletic participation and injuries from car crashes are frequent causes. Distinguishing among these injuries is often difficult. See Table 29–7. See accompanying *Evidence-Based Practice* for a discussion of backpack use by children. A detailed discussion of fractures follows.

Fractures

A fracture is a break in a bone that occurs when more stress is placed on the bone than the bone can withstand. Fractures may occur at any age; they are frequent in children because their bones are less dense and more porous than those of adults (see *Pathophysiology Illustrated: Classification and Types of Fractures*).

ETIOLOGY AND PATHOPHYSIOLOGY

Fractures in children may result from direct trauma to a bone (falls, sports injuries, abuse, motor vehicle crashes) or bone diseases that result in weakening of the bone (osteogenesis imperfecta). Children with osteoporosis or osteopenia are more prone to fractures (see description of these conditions earlier in the chapter). Trauma may be caused by an acute injury, by direct and forceful impact, or by overuse such as in chronic and repetitive

TABLE 29–7 Clinical Manifestations of Strains, Sprains, and Dislocations

CONDITION	CLINICAL MANIFESTATIONS	CLINICAL THERAPY
STRAIN • Stretching or tearing of either a muscle or a tendon, usually from overuse (example: back strain resulting from improper or overly heavy lifting).	• Vary according to the type and severity of the strain. Pain can be acute or chronic.	• Rest and support of the injured part until the muscle or tendon heals and normal activity can occur.
SPRAIN • Stretching or tearing of a ligament, usually caused by falls, sports injuries, or motor vehicle crashes. For example, an anterior cruciate ligament (ACL) tear is a severe sprain requiring reconstruction.	• Edema, joint immobility, and pain.	• For the first 24–36 hr: **R**est **I**ce **C**ompression **E**levation • After the first 24–36 hr, mobility is gradually increased.
DISLOCATION • Complete displacement of an articular joint surface, usually associated with falls, sports injuries, or motor vehicle crashes. Although almost any joint may be dislocated, most dislocations occur in the shoulder, knee, and hip.	• Pain and tenderness, swelling and obvious deformity, and instability of the joint.	• Varies according to the site and severity of the injury, and consists of: Shoulder: open or closed reduction followed by the application of a sling Knee: closed reduction with gentle traction, then immobilization with a splint Hip (posterior): immediate closed reduction or possibly open reduction, traction, or hip spica cast Hip (anterior): immediate closed reduction, extension traction, and hip spica cast

EVIDENCE-BASED PRACTICE | Do Heavy Backpacks Cause Back Pain?

Clinical Question

Many children wear backpacks that are heavy and are carried for large parts of the day. Low back, neck, and shoulder pain are prevalent in children, and a possible connection with backpacks has been suggested (Dockrell, Simms, & Blake, 2013). What can nurses do to reduce risk of back pain related to backpacks in children?

The Evidence

Several studies have investigated the relationships between backpack use and complaints of pain. Carrying a backpack over one shoulder, having heavier backpacks, and carrying the pack lower rather than higher were associated with greater back and shoulder pressure. Postural angle and lumbar curvature are altered by heavy backpacks. Children carrying backpacks that exceeded 10% of their body weight had a 50% increased chance of back pain, and girls more commonly experienced back pain (Rodriguez-Oviedo et al., 2012). Design, fit, and weight all may play a part in discomfort related to backpacks (Amiri, Dezfooli, & Mortezaei, 2012).

Best Practice

An association between backpack use and weight and complaints of pain appears to be evident, especially among girls.

Therefore, nurses should ask about backpack use at health promotion visits and advise on how to wear them. Encourage children to store backpacks in lockers when available throughout the day in order to decrease wearing time. The American Academy of Pediatrics and North American Spine Society list recommendations for backpack use:

- Have wide, padded shoulder straps and wear the pack on both shoulders, close to the body.
- Use a padded back and waist strap.
- Be sure the backpack is lightweight (no more than 10% to 15% of the youth's weight) or consider a rolling pack if it is heavy.
- Practice back strengthening exercises and learn to bend at the knees when lifting objects.

Clinical Reasoning

How will you partner with youth who are in sports after school to plan how to carry school items and sports gear safely? What exercises can you plan to help strengthen the back and thighs for carrying a pack? Which children are most at risk for back pain from heavy backpacks (consider gender and weight)?

Pathophysiology Illustrated: **Classification and Types of Fractures**

Complete (transverse) fracture

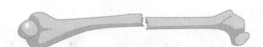

Break across entire section of a bone at a right angle to the bone shaft resulting in two or more fragments

Spiral fracture

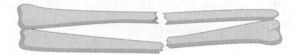

Associated with twisting force; fracture coils around the bone

Open fracture

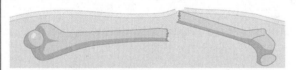

Broken bone protrudes through the skin leaving a path to the fracture site; high risk of infection exists

Closed fracture

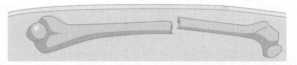

Broken bone does not protrude through the skin

Greenstick fracture

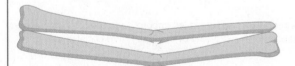

Caused by compression force; often seen in young children

Comminuted fracture

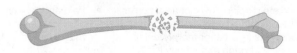

Associated with high-impact forces; bone breaks into three or more segments

Additional types of fractures include incomplete, in which the break occurs in only one side of the cortex; oblique, in which the fracture slants across the long axis of the bone; compression, in which two bones are jammed together (usually occurs in spinal area); and compacted, in which one bone fragment is wedged into another.

activities. Child abuse is a cause of fracture and should be suspected when the type of fracture is uncommon for a given age (see Chapter 17).

CLINICAL MANIFESTATIONS

Signs and symptoms of fractures vary depending on the location, type, and nature of the causative injury. Fractures are generally characterized by pain, abnormal positioning, edema, immobility or decreased range of motion, ecchymosis, guarding, and crepitus. Childhood fractures most often involve the clavicle, tibia, ulna, and femur, with distal forearm fractures the most common type. Stress fractures are most common in the tibia, fibula, metatarsals, and calcaneus, while regular exercise can encourage bone development and be protective against fractures (Farr, Laddu, & Going, 2014; Harrington, Sochett, & Howard, 2014). Douglass, described in the chapter-opening vignette, had a fracture of his tibia. Fractures to the pelvis are often associated with motor vehicle crashes. Epiphyseal injuries are dangerous in children as they can interfere with bone growth at the site. These injuries are described using the Salter-Harris classification system (Figure 29–14).

CLINICAL THERAPY

Emergency care focuses on accurate diagnosis, pain management, and establishment of a treatment plan. Radiographs are useful for determining the exact location and type of the fracture. Medical management consists of two basic steps: (1) reduction to realign displaced or fragmented bones and (2) immobilization so that healing can take place.

A closed reduction aligns the bone by manual manipulation or traction. Sedation and additional pain management techniques will be used during closed reduction. An open reduction requires surgical alignment of the bone, often using pins, plates, wires, or screws. For open fractures, surgery must also be performed for debridement, to remove dead tissue and clean the wound. Casting is the most common external method of immobilization. Casts may be placed on extremities (short or long leg or arm cast), the upper body to immobilize the spine, or from chest to legs to stabilize pelvis or hips (spica cast). Leg casts may be walking or nonwalking casts. Cast material is either plaster or a synthetic fabric. Other external methods of stabilization include traction and splinting (later in the chapter, see Table 29–10 for types of traction). Pins may be inserted to stabilize the fracture, and can be used with or without casts or traction. A child with multiple fractures following a car crash or other trauma may need a combination of treatments.

Growth and Development

Stress fractures are becoming more common in adolescents and are most common in those who limit their intake of calories and calcium in an attempt to remain lean for sports such as distance running, cheerleading, or gymnastics (Field, Gordon, Pierce, et al., 2011). These fractures may present with chronic pain that changes in intensity. Be alert to this possibility when teenagers' diets and athletic activities place them at risk. The risk of bone fractures is increased with high cola consumption and television viewing time and with lower levels of physical activity and lower milk intake. Teach healthy diet and activity patterns to youth and their families to decrease these health risks.

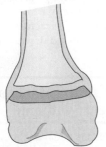

Type I
Common
Growth plate undisturbed
Growth disturbances rare

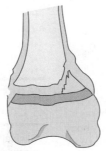

Type II
Most common
Growth disturbances rare

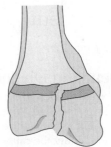

Type III
Less common
Serious threat to growth
  and joint

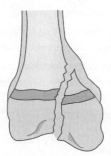

Type IV
Serious threat to growth

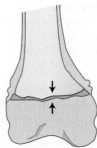

Type V
Rare
Crush injury causes cell death in growth plate,
  resulting in arrested growth and limited
  bone length
If growth plate is partially destroyed, angular
  deformities may result

Figure 29–14 The Salter-Harris classification system is based on the angle of the fracture in relation to the epiphysis.

TABLE 29–8 Complications of Fracture Reduction

COMPLICATION	CLINICAL THERAPY
Infection Acute (may occur with open fractures) Chronic (osteomyelitis)	Debridement, drainage, culture, and treatment with antibiotics
Neurovascular injury resulting from physical nerve damage	Nerve repair
Vascular injury	Vascular repair, amputation, tendon lengthening
Malunion (undesired healed alignment of bone) or delayed union	Corrective osteotomy; prolonged immobilization
Nonunion	Surgical intervention; internal fixation
Leg length discrepancy	Shoe lift

Immobilization is essential for the bone-healing process. Healing of fractures is influenced by factors including age, size of the involved bone, and fracture site. Fractures heal more quickly in children than in adults because the periosteum or vascular outer layer of bone is thicker and remains intact even during a fracture (AAOS, 2014b). If a fracture is properly reduced, complications should be minimal (Table 29–8). Fractures involving the epiphyseal growth plate must be treated properly to minimize the chance for limb length discrepancy, joint incongruity, and angular deformities.

Nursing Management

For the Child With a Fracture

Nursing Assessment and Diagnosis

When assessing an injured child, be alert to the signs and symptoms of fractures before moving the child. When in doubt about the type of injury, apply a splint to immobilize the joints above and below the injury. Try to identify the cause of the injury by asking the child, parents, or other family members what happened. Evaluate pain, edema, and any abnormal positioning of the injured area. When a child is admitted to the emergency department or hospital, nursing assessment includes the extent of the injury, the degree of pain, and the child's vital signs (respiratory status, pulse, and blood pressure). Monitor all systems since infection, fat emboli, and other problems can emerge during the treatment period.

Several nursing diagnoses may apply to the child with a fracture. They include the following (NANDA-I © 2014):

- *Pain, Acute*, related to injury
- *Skin Integrity, Risk for Impaired*, related to treatment
- *Infection, Risk for*, related to open fracture or trauma
- *Mobility: Physical, Impaired*, related to treatment
- *Health Behavior, Risk-Prone*, related to peer group influence and chosen activities

Planning and Implementation

Nurses may be in community settings when children experience a fracture and may need to provide emergency care and arrange for transport. Inform emergency personnel of the assessment data to provide for safe care. In addition, be aware that repeated fractures in the same child can be a sign of other healthcare conditions. Young children may have osteogenesis imperfecta, an older child may be experimenting with risky behavior, and child abuse may have occurred if there are several fractures in various states of healing or if the parental explanation does not match the clinical presentation. Nursing care focuses on care of the child before and after fracture reduction, encouraging mobility as ordered, maintaining skin integrity, preventing infection, and teaching the parents and child how to care for the fracture. If sedation or pain blocks are used, nursing care for these procedures is needed. See the *Clinical Skills Manual* SKILLS .

When caring for a child who has undergone fracture reduction, it is important to know the signs of complications and follow protocols for assessment. Notify the physician immediately if these signs occur. The major serious complication is **compartment syndrome**, or a condition of increased pressure in a limited space such as the soft tissue of an extremity, which compromises circulation and nervous innervation (Schaffzin et al., 2013). (See Table 29–9.)

MAINTAIN PROPER ALIGNMENT

Immobilization maintains proper alignment of the fracture. Casts and traction are methods used for immobilizing an injured child. Cast care guidelines are included in Table 29–2, earlier in this chapter.

Different types of traction are used, depending on the location and type of fracture (Table 29–10). Nursing care for the child in traction is described in Table 29–11.

MONITOR NEUROVASCULAR STATUS

Neurovascular assessment is used for early detection of compartment syndrome. Compartment syndrome may occur with a crush injury or when a fracture is reduced. The swelling of inflammation reduces blood flow to the affected area, and casting

TABLE 29–9 Clinical Manifestations of Compartment Syndrome

Clinical manifestations begin about 30 min after tissue ischemia starts. Major manifestations include the following:

- Paresthesia (tingling, burning, loss of 2-point discrimination)
- Pain (unrelieved by medication, characterized by crying in the young child)
- Pressure (skin is tense, cast appears tight)
- Pallor (pale, gray or white skin tone)
- Paralysis (weakness or inability to move extremity)
- Pulselessness (weak or absent pulse)
- Poikilothermia (skin temperature assumes that of the environment)

Check extremities for:

• Color	• Edema
• Temperature	• Sensation
• Capillary refill	• Motor ability
• Peripheral pulses	• Pain

Document results and report changes or abnormal results immediately. Changes are a medical emergency.

Source: Data from Tschudy, M. M., & Arcara, K. M. (Eds.). (2012). *The Harriet Lane handbook.* Philadelphia: Mosby Elsevier; Schaffzin, J. K., Prichard, H., Bisig, J., Gainor, P., Wolfe, K., Solan, L. G., . . . McCarthy, J. J. (2013). A collaborative system to improve compartment syndrome recognition. *Pediatrics, 132*, e1672–e1679; Wright, E. (2009). Neurovascular impairment and compartment syndrome. *Paediatric Nursing, 21*(3), 26–29.

TABLE 29–10 Types of Traction

SKIN TRACTION

Pull is applied to the skin surface, which puts traction directly on the bones and muscles. Traction is attached to the skin with adhesive materials or straps, or foam boots, belts, or halters.

DUNLOP TRACTION (CAN BE EITHER SKELETAL OR SKIN)

Used for fracture of the humerus. The flexed arm is suspended horizontally with straps placed on both the upper and lower portions for pull from both sides.

SKELETAL TRACTION

Pull is directly applied to the bone by pins, wires, tongs, or other apparatus that have been surgically placed through the distal end of the bone.

SKELETAL CERVICAL TRACTION

Used for cervical spine injuries to reduce fractures and dislocations. Crutchfield, Gardner-Wells, or Vinke tongs are placed in the skull with bur holes. Weights are attached to the apparatus with a rope and pulley system to the hyperextended head.

HALO TRACTION

Used to immobilize the head and neck after cervical injury or dislocation. Also used for positioning and immobilization after cervical injury.

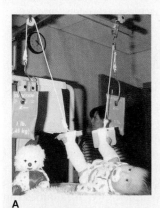

A

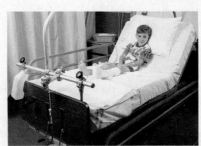

B

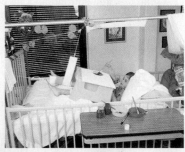

C

BRYANT TRACTION (A)

Used specifically for the child under 3 years of age and weighing less than 35.0 lb (17.5 kg) who has developmental dysplasia of the hip or a fractured femur. This bilateral traction is applied to the child's legs and kept in place by wrapping the legs from foot to thigh with elastic bandages. The hips are flexed at a 90-degree angle, with knees extended. This position is maintained by attaching the traction appliance to weights and pulleys suspended above the crib. The buttocks do not rest on the mattress, but are slightly elevated off the bed.

BUCK TRACTION (B)

Used for knee immobilization; to correct contractures or deformities; or for short-term immobilization of a fracture. It keeps the leg in an extended position, without hip flexion. Traction is applied to the extremity in one direction (straight line) with a single pulley system.

RUSSELL TRACTION (C)

Used for fractures of the femur and lower leg. Traction is placed on the lower leg while the knee is suspended in a padded sling. The slightly flexed hips and knees are immobilized. One force is applied by a double pulley to the foot and another force is applied upward using a sling under the knee and an overhead pulley.

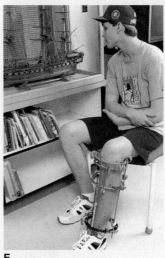

E

EXTERNAL FIXATORS (E)

These devices can be used in the treatment of simple fractures, both open and closed; complex fractures with extensive soft tissue involvement; correction of bony or soft-tissue deformities; pseudoarthroses; and limb length discrepancies. They are attached to the extremity by percutaneous transfixing of pins or wires to the bone. When used to lengthen an extremity, the device can be "distracted" or turned as ordered by the surgeon for a very small amount several times daily. This separates the bone and allows new growth, gradually lengthening the extremity.

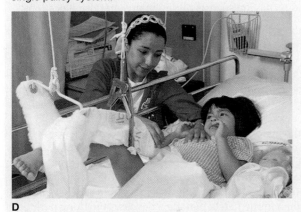

D

90–90 TRACTION (D)

Used for fractures of the femur or tibia. A skeletal pin or wire is surgically placed through the distal part of the femur, while the lower part of the extremity is in a boot cast. Traction ropes and pulleys are applied at the pin site and on the boot cast to maintain the flexion of both the hip and knee at 90 degrees. This traction can also be used for treatment of an upper extremity fracture.

TABLE 29–11 Care of the Child With Traction or External Fixator

1. Assess the child in traction by first checking the equipment. Make sure that the equipment is in the proper position. Observe both the body appliance and the attached weights and pulleys. Make certain that the child's body is in proper alignment.

2. Assess the skin under the straps and pin insertion sites for any signs of redness, edema, or skin breakdown.

3. Assess the extremity by checking neurovascular status frequently (check warmth, color, distal pulses, capillary refill time, movement, sensation).

4. Provide pin care when ordered using sterile technique. Clean the area surrounding the pin with cotton-tipped applicators saturated with normal saline or half-strength hydrogen peroxide. Clean the area again with sterile water or more saline. Apply an antibacterial ointment, if ordered, using another cotton-tipped applicator.

5. When external skin traction is used, perform skin care every 4 hr when the traction device is removed.

6. Place a sheepskin pad under the child's extremity if prescriptions permit.

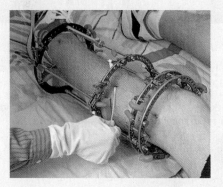

causes further constriction of blood flow. Douglass, who was described in the chapter-opening quotation, had a splint applied for several days, with casting later, to allow swelling to decrease and to minimize risk for compartment syndrome. Monitor the child's sensation to touch, temperature, movement, strength of the pulse, and capillary refill time in the extremity distal to the injury. Monitor every 15 minutes after the cast is applied for at least 2 hours and then every 1 to 2 hours, depending on the facility's policy and the child's condition. Keep the cast elevated above heart level to minimize edema. Report symptoms of compartment syndrome immediately as permanent damage to nerves and circulatory system can occur.

PROMOTE MOBILITY

The amount of mobility the child is allowed is ordered by the physician; restrictions depend on the extent and site of the fracture. Fractures of the hip or pelvis may involve body casts; wheeled carts make mobility possible. Children with leg fractures can sometimes bear weight on the cast, but if they cannot, they move around with crutches, walkers, or wheelchairs. See the *Clinical Skills Manual* SKILLS .

DISCHARGE PLANNING AND HOME CARE TEACHING

Most fractures can be easily managed at home. Activities are generally limited for approximately 8 weeks. Teach the parents and child cast care, activity restrictions, and how to identify problems that should be reported (see Table 29–2). Help parents identify any modifications that may be needed at home and school. The child who has to manage steps at home or school may need special training with crutches or a temporary ramp. Refer parents to home health nurses or home teaching services if indicated. Provide pertinent teaching to prevent future injuries. Reinforce the need for protective gear for many sports (see Chapter 17).

Evaluation

Desired outcomes for treatment of injuries is proper healing of the body parts affected, return to usual strength and range of motion, and no impairment of musculoskeletal development.

Sports Injuries

Sports injuries are the most common type of injury in youth from 13 to 19 years of age. Football, soccer, cycling, and basketball are sports commonly associated with injury, and foot–ankle injuries are most common (Atay, 2014). Fractures, described earlier, are common sports injuries of young athletes, and may be treated on an outpatient basis or may require surgery and hospitalization. Douglass, in the opening scenario, is a good example of a youth with this type of injury. However, a variety of other injuries that affect the musculoskeletal system are common in sports; strains and sprains are examples. Overuse injuries can occur when tendons, muscles, or bones are stressed excessively without adequate rest periods (Luke et al., 2011). Children and adolescents have characteristics that put them at risk for injury. These include:

- Vulnerability of growth plates to injury, especially the distal tibia and fibula

- Increased joint mobility from lax tendons and ligaments, leading to injury of the knee, ankle, and hip

- More porous bones, leading to fractures and to more common injury to underlying organs

- Lack of experience in the sport and inadequate training

- Lack of acceptance of protective gear

- Impatience with taking the time to heal after injury

- Vulnerability to spinal injury related to high-impact sports and recreation such as diving in unsupervised locations

Common sports injuries are listed in Table 29–12. Treatments for sprains, strains, dislocations, and fractures are described in the preceding sections. Head and neck injuries are discussed in Chapter 27 and dental emergencies in Chapter 19. Clear guidelines for concussion injuries have been established (Harmon et al., 2013) and are discussed in Chapter 27. General approaches to minimize and treat injuries for youth athletes follow.

Athletes can benefit from teaching that enhances performance of their sports and also minimizes chance of injury. They should receive instruction in correct techniques from a person qualified to coach and supervise children. Nurses should encourage youths to gradually increase time and intensity at a sport, rather than immediately playing a new sport for long periods of time. Parents should be encouraged to inquire about the coach's experience and also verify that the coaching staff is prepared in emergency care.

The nurse should be alert for sports injuries during contacts with children and adolescents in health promotion visits. The nurse should ask about sports participation for all youths, but especially when there are complaints of sore muscles, edema of body parts, and bruises. Neurovascular assessment of extremities,

TABLE 29–12 Common Sports Injuries

SPORT	TYPE OF INJURIES
Baseball/ basketball	• Hand and finger fractures and sprains • Contusions and sprains of upper or lower extremities; wrists, elbows, knees, and ankles are common sites • Injury to body parts when hit by a ball (e.g., broken teeth, face, head, eye, and chest injuries)
Football	• Head and neck injuries such as skull or cervical vertebrae fracture • Pulled muscles or dislocations in shoulders and legs
Gymnastics	• Wrist and elbow fractures and strains • Tendonitis in elbows and ankles/legs
Hockey (ice and inline)	• Dental injury • Leg fractures • Head and neck injuries
Soccer	• Head and neck injury • Strains and fractures of legs
Wrestling	• Fractures and dislocations of upper and lower extremities

Clinical Reasoning The Child Wearing a Cast

Douglass was admitted to the clinic today for application of a short leg cast. He fractured his tibia nearly a week ago when he was on a trampoline with three friends, trying to see who could jump the highest. Douglass slipped and his leg hit the frame on the side. His friends helped him off the trampoline and found someone to transport Douglass to the emergency department. They then reached his mother by phone, who rushed to the hospital when she heard the news.

His mother states that he is now 12 years old and in middle school. He has been going to a friend's house nearly every day after school and spending time on activities such as the trampoline and rollerblading, as well as watching television and playing video games. She felt this was safer than him being at home alone during her work hours, but is now starting to wonder about whether to allow Douglass to engage in activities with his friend.

A splint has provided support for several days and has allowed the swelling to decrease before today's cast application. Douglass has been non–weight bearing on his leg and has been using crutches. He returned to school yesterday for part of the day and found it was hard to get to all of his classes.

• What teaching should you provide to help him keep the cast intact to ensure his safety and to alert him to signs of compartment syndrome?

including color, temperature, capillary refill time, edema, pulses, sensation, and pain, should be performed. Questions should be phrased so that sports such as skateboarding or snowboarding, which might not be performed under supervision or in organized sports programs, can be identified. Youths might not consider these "sports."

Teach the importance of warming up for 10 to 15 minutes before participation and cooling down for a corresponding period at the end of activity. Encourage wearing recommended safety gear for the sport, including equipment such as a well-fitted protective helmet, face masks, eye protection, mouth guards, elbow and wrist guards, gloves, knee pads, and shin pads. Parents may need assistance to learn about the recommended equipment and resources for purchase. Frequent updates are needed as the child grows. The child should be taught not to ignore pain.

Injuries such as muscle strains should be treated promptly. They involve several steps:

• Resting the injury for 24 to 48 hours, applying ice for 20 minutes 4 times daily, compression with an elastic wrap to provide comfort and decrease edema, and elevating the affected part above heart level

• Gradually increasing motion to the part

• Adding flexibility and resistance or strengthening exercises

• Returning gradually to the sport, usually in 2 to 3 weeks after injury

The nurse should partner with the child, family, and other health professionals to plan for activity whenever an injury has occurred. Praise the family and youth for physical activity, an important part of a healthy lifestyle. Provide community resources to foster sports participation.

Amputations

Amputation—the complete absence of a body extremity—can be either congenital or acquired. Approximately two thirds of amputations in children are congenital and one third are acquired. Congenital amputations can be caused by constrictive amniotic bands, drugs, or irradiation. Acquired amputations are generally associated with trauma or the result of a disease or disorder. Children are prone to such injuries because of their small extremities and limited skeletal mass. Lawn mower injury, exercise equipment, and motor vehicle crashes are common causes. Most common traumatic amputations involve fingers or toes but hands and limbs are also at risk.

The child with an absent limb should be fitted with a prosthesis as soon as feasible and encouraged to use it several hours daily. This fosters a positive body image, independence, and self-confidence, and also ensures that motor skills develop as normally as possible (Ulger & Sener, 2011). The prosthetic device should be reevaluated as the child progresses physically and developmentally. Children with traumatic amputations may need frequent stump reconstructions because as children grow, so do their bones, and the skin tends to adhere to the bone. Bone may need to be cut and soft tissue added to keep the stump rounded. Joint fusions or stump lengthenings may also be needed to allow the effective use of a prosthesis. Several prosthetic revisions will be needed as the child grows and develops.

Nursing Management

Nursing care focuses on providing emotional support regarding altered body image, managing pain, maintaining skin integrity, and encouraging maximal independent functioning.

Recovering from the loss of a limb is one of the most difficult challenges facing children. Emphasize what children can do rather than what they cannot do. Good listening skills are important.

The child who has had surgery or a traumatic injury experiences pain. Many techniques discussed in Chapter 15 are useful interventions. After surgery, an epidural may be the treatment of choice. Oral analgesics are used during the period of adaptation to a prosthesis if the stump is tender. Children may have "phantom" limb pain in the lost extremity, although this phenomenon decreases significantly in the first year after amputation (Burgoyne et al., 2012; Wolff et al., 2011). The child usually begins wearing the prosthetic device for 1- to 2-hour intervals. Check the skin for any redness or breakdown. If redness or breakdown develops, leave the prosthesis off and allow the skin to clear before reapplying. Have the prosthesis adjusted if necessary, and increase wearing time as tolerated by the child.

Children with amputated limbs quickly learn how to accommodate to the prosthetic device. Use physical therapy programs specifically designed to help the child perform activities of daily living.

DISCHARGE PLANNING AND HOME CARE TEACHING

Answer any questions the family has about how to care for the prosthetic device and how to perform skin checks. Encourage parents to allow the child to participate in physically and emotionally challenging peer activities. Sporting activities that enable the child to participate using modified equipment are a good way to build self-confidence and motivation. For example, ski centers may offer programs that teach children with physical disabilities how to ski, or the Paralympics may be motivating for some children. Assess the need for counseling and offer referrals as appropriate.

Chapter Highlights

- Children may develop musculoskeletal conditions as a result of congenital conditions, developmental variations, or trauma.
- Talipes equinovarus (clubfoot) is a common unilateral or bilateral variation in newborns that is treated by casting, traction, and/or surgery.
- Genu varum and genu valgum are normal variations at certain times in development that may need treatment if they persist.
- The nurse may identify developmental dysplasia of the hip (DDH) during newborn assessments and must refer the child for care to a specialist.
- Mild DDH is treated by a harness, but more severe cases may require surgery for the child to walk normally.
- Legg-Calvé-Perthes is a reversible disease most commonly seen in school-age boys, and causes necrosis of the femoral head.
- Slipped capital femoral epiphysis is treated by casting, tractions, or more commonly surgery with pinning, to stabilize the epiphysis.
- Scoliosis is a lateral curvature of the spine, and nurses commonly screen adolescents to identify the disorder.

- Scoliosis may require exercises, bracing, or surgery with instrumentation and spinal fusion.
- Osteoporosis can occur in premature infants, in children with conditions that lead to immobility and decreased weight bearing, and in youth with inadequate calcium or vitamin D intake.
- Osteomyelitis most commonly follows another infection and requires prompt treatment to prevent sepsis and serious injury to the bone.
- The child with osteogenesis imperfecta (brittle bone disease) requires careful handling by the nurse and parents to prevent fractures while fostering developmental progression.
- Muscular dystrophies are inherited diseases characterized by muscle wasting and degeneration.
- Children can experience a variety of fractures due to sports, car crashes, and other injuries.
- Many sports injuries experienced by youth can be avoided with proper equipment.
- Casts, braces, and traction are common interventions for musculoskeletal disorders; nursing interventions minimize development of complications related to these treatments.

Clinical Reasoning in Action

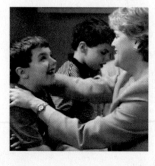

Peter, now 7 years old, was diagnosed at 5 years old with Duchenne muscular dystrophy. His parents are well informed about the disease since they had an older son who died of the disorder at 19 years. At the present time, he walks on his toes but is able to ambulate well with leg braces. Today, Peter is visiting the specialty clinic for children with muscular dystrophies. His braces will be checked for fit and performance, physical therapy will be performed, and he will attend a group session with other school-age children. During these visits, the parents also meet in a support group with other families and receive instruction and resources to help them with Peter's health management. As a nurse in the clinic you perform a physical and mental assessment on Peter. All findings are within normal limits, although he has had some constipation and several upper respiratory infections. You learn that he has an individualized education plan (IEP) in place at school that allows for periods of rest and physical therapy; the parents report that he is at grade level and excels at computer skills.

1. What are the main roles of the nurse working with Peter in the specialty clinic?

2. Children with muscular dystrophy often get to a standing position by mainly using arm muscles. What is the name of the maneuver?

3. What are some of the tests performed to see if a child has muscular dystrophy, and what are the expected results?

4. Who can Peter expect to meet with on the days he goes to the specialty clinic for muscular dystrophy?

5. Construct a concept map for Peter that demonstrates the multisystem involvement of his disease and how his developmental needs can be met in spite of his disability.

References

American Academy of Orthopaedic Surgeons (AAOS). (2014a). *Detection and management of pediatric developmental dysplasia of the hip in infants up to six months of age: Evidence-based clinical practice guideline.* Retrieved from http://www.aaos.org/research/guidelines/DDHGuidelineFINAL.pdf

American Academy of Orthopaedic Surgeons (AAOS). (2014b). *Forearm fractures in children.* Retrieved from http://orthoinfo.aaos.org/topic.cfm?topic=A00039

American Academy of Pediatrics. (1999, reaffirmed 2013). Transporting children with special health care needs. *Pediatrics, 104,* 988–992 (original policy); *Pediatrics, 132,* e281–e282 (reaffirmation).

Amiri, M., Dezfooli, M. S., & Mortezaei, S. R. (2012). Designing and ergonomics backpack for student aged 7–9 with user centred design approach. *Work, 41*(Suppl 1), 1193–1201.

Atay, E. (2014). Prevalence of sport injuries among middle school children and suggestions for their prevention. *Journal of Physical Therapy Science, 26,* 1455–1457.

Bautista, S. R., Gholve, P., & Dormans, J. P. (2011). Pediatric musculoskeletal infections: Managing the significant organisms. *Consultant for Pediatricians, 10*(2), 41–45.

Becker Muscular Dystrophy. (n.d.). *Becker muscular dystrophy.* Retrieved from http//www.beckermusculardystrophy.org

Ben Amor, M., Rauch, F., Monti, E., & Antoniazzi, F. (2013). Osteogenesis imperfecta. *Pediatric Endocrinology Reviews, 10*(Suppl 2), 397–405.

Birch, J. G. (2013). Blount disease. *Journal of American Academy of Orthopaedic Surgery, 21,* 408–418.

Brox, J. I., Lange, J. E., Gunderson, R. B., & Steen, H. (2012). Good brace compliance reduced curve progression and surgical rates in patients with idiopathic scoliosis. *European Spine Journal, 21,* 1957–1963.

Burgoyne, L. L., Billups, C. A., Jiron, J. L., Kaddoum, R. N., Wright, B. B., Bikhazi, G. B., . . . Pereiras, L. A. (2012). Phantom limb pain in young cancer-related amputees: Recent experience at St. Jude Children's Research Hospital. *Clinical Journal of Pain, 28*(3), 222–225.

Compton, S. (2014). Childhood obesity and slipped capital femoral epiphysis. *Radiologic Technology, 85,* 321–324.

de Sanctis, N. (2011). Magnetic resonance imaging in Legg-Calvé-Perthes disease: Review of literature. *Journal of Pediatric Orthopaedics, 31*(2 Suppl.), S163–S167.

Dockrell, S., Simms, C., & Blake, C. (2013). Schoolbag weight limit: Can it be defined? *Journal of School Health, 83,* 368–377.

Farr, J. N., Laddu, D. R., & Going, S. B. (2014). Exercise, hormones and skeletal adaptation during childhood and adolescence. *Pediatric Exercise Science, 26,* 384–391.

Field, A. E., Gordon, C. M., Pierce, L. M., Ramappa, A., & Kocher, M. S. (2011). Prospective study of physical activity and risk of developing a stress fracture among preadolescent and adolescent girls. *Archives of Pediatrics and Adolescent Medicine, 165,* 723–728.

Flaherty, E. G., Perez-Rossello, J. M., Levine, M. A., Hennrikus, W. L., & the American Academy of Pediatrics Committee on Child Abuse and Neglect. (2014). Evaluating children with fractures for child physical abuse. *Pediatrics, 133*(2), e477–e489.

Georgiadis, A. G., & Zaltz, I. (2014). Slipped capital femoral epiphysis: How to evaluate with a review and update of treatment. *Pediatric Clinics of North America, 61,* 1119–1135.

Gilmore, A., & Thompson, G. H. (2013, January). Common childhood foot deformities. *Consultant for Pediatricians, 28–34.*

Goyenvaile, A., Seto, J. T., Davies, K. E., & Chamberlain, J. (2011). Therapeutic approaches to muscular dystrophy. *Human Molecular Genetics, 20*(Review Issue I), R69–R78.

Harmon, K. G., Drezner, J. A., Gammons, M., Guskiewicz, K. M., Halstead, M., Herring, S. A., . . . Roberts, W. O. (2013). American Medical Society for Sports Medicine position statement: Concussion in sport. *British Journal of Sports Medicine, 47,* 15–26.

Harrington, J., Sochett, E., & Howard, A. (2014). Update on the evaluation and treatment of osteogenesis imperfecta. *Pediatric Clinics of North America, 61,* 1243–1247.

Ireland, P. J., Donaghey, S., McGill, J., Zankl, A., Ware, R. S., Pacey, V., . . . Johnston, L. M. (2012). Development in children with achondroplasia: A prospective clinical cohort study. *Developmental Medicine Child Neurology, 54,* 532–537.

Kannu, P., & Howard, P. (2014). Perthes disease. *British Medical Journal.* doi:10.1136/bmj.g5584

Kumar, A., & Agarwal, S. (2014). Marfan syndrome: An eyesight of syndrome. *Meta Gene, 2,* 96–105.

Laederich, M. B., & Horton, W. A. (2012). FGFR3 targeting strategies for achondroplasia. *Expert Reviews in Molecular Science, 19,* e11.

Lombardi, G., Akoume, M. Y., Colombini, A., Moreau, A., & Banfi, G. (2011). Biochemistry of adolescent idiopathic scoliosis. *Advances in Clinical Chemistry, 54,* 165–182.

Lubicky, J. P., Hanson, J. E., Riley, E., & Spinal Deformity Study Group. (2011). Instrumentation constructs in pediatric patients undergoing deformity correction correlated with Scoliosis Research Society scores. *Spine, 36,* 1692–1700.

Luke, A., Lazaro, R. M., Bergeron, M. F., Keyser, L., Benjamin, H., Brenner, J., . . . Smith, A. (2011).

Sports-related injuries in youth athletes: Is over-scheduling a risk factor? *Clinical Journal of Sports Medicine, 21,* 307–314.

March of Dimes. (2012). *Achondroplasia.* Retrieved from http://www.marchofdimes.com/search.html

Mazloumi, S. M., Ebrahimzadeh, M. H., & Kachooei, A. R. (2014). Evolution in diagnosis and treatment of Legg-Calve-Perthes disease. *Archives of Bone and Joint Surgery, 2,* 86–92.

Mehler, P. S., Cleary, B. S., & Guadiani, J. L. (2011). Osteoporosis in anorexia nervosa. *Eating Disorders, 19,* 194–202.

Milani, C., & Dobashi, E. T. (2011). Arthrogram in Legg-Calve-Perthes disease. *Journal of Pediatric Orthopaedics, 31*(2 Suppl.), S156–S162.

Nakamura, J., Kamegaya, M., Saisu, T., Kakizaki, J., Hagiwara, S., Ohtori, S., . . . Takahashik, K. (2015). Outcome of patients with Legg-Calve-Perthes onset before 6 years of age. *Journal of Pediatric Orthopedics, 35,* 144–150. doi:10.1097/BPO.0000000000000246

National Institutes of Health. (2012a). *Fontanelles.* Retrieved from http://www.nlm.nih.gov/medlineplus/ency/article/003310.htm

National Institutes of Health. (2012b). *Metatarsus adductus.* Retrieved from http://www.nlm.nih.gov/medlineplus/ency/article/001601.htm

National Institutes of Health. (2013). *Developmental dysplasia of the hip.* Retrieved from http://www.ncbi.nlm.nih.gov/pubmedhealth/PMH0001966/

Perry, D. C., & Hall, A. J. (2011). The epidemiology and etiology of Perthes disease. *Orthopedic Clinics of North America, 42,* 279–283.

Rack, B., Lochmuller, E. M., Janni, W., Lipowsky, G., Engelsberger, I., Friese, K., & Kuster, H. (2011). Ultrasound for the assessment of bone quality in preterm and term infants. *Journal of Perinatology.* doi:10.1038/jp.2011.82

Rodriguez-Oviedo, P., Ruano-Ravina, A., Perez-Rios, M., Garcia, F. B., Gomez-Fernandez, D., Fernandez-Alonso, A., . . . Turiso, J. (2012). School children's backpacks, back pain and back pathologies. *Archives of Disease in Childhood, 97,* 730–732.

Roof, A. C., Jinguji, T. M., & White, K. K. (2013). Musculoskeletal screening: Developmental dysplasia of the hip. *Pediatric Annals, 42,* 229–235.

Rosenbush, S. W., & Parker, J. M. (2014). Height and heart disease. *Reviews in Cardiovascular Medicine, 15,* 102–108.

Sabharwal, S. (2015). Blount disease: An update. *Orthopedic Clinics of North America, 46,* 37–47.

Schaffzin, J. K., Prichard, H., Bisig, J., Gainor, P., Wolfe, K., Solan, L. G., . . . McCarthy, J. J. (2013). A collaborative system to improve compartment syndrome recognition. *Pediatrics, 132,* e1672–e1679.

Schulzke, S. M., Kaempfen, S., Trachsel, D., & Patole, S. K. (2014). Physical activity programs for promoting bone mineralization and growth in preterm infants. *Cochrane Database Systematic Reviews*, *22*, 4:CD005387.

Schwend, R. M., Shaw, B. A., & Segal, L. S. (2014). Evaluation and treatment of developmental hip dysplasia in the newborn and infant. *Pediatric Clinics of North America*, *61*, 1095–1107.

Scottish Rite Hospital. (2011). *Scoliosis and spine.* Retrieved from http://www.tsrhc.org/scoliosis-scoliometer.htm

Szadek, L. L., & Scharer, K. (2014). Identification, prevention, and treatment of children with decreased bone mineral density. *Journal of Pediatric Nursing*, *29*, e3–e14.

Theadom, A., Rodrigues, M., Roxburgh, R., Balalla, S., Higgins, C., Bhattacharjee, R., . . . Feigin, V. (2014). Prevalence of muscular dystrophies: A systematic literature review. *Neuroepidemiology*, *43*, 259–268.

Thomsen, K., & Creech, C. B. (2011). Advances in the diagnosis and management of pediatric osteomyelitis. *Current Infectious Disease Reports*, *13*, 451–460.

Tschudy, M. M., & Arcara, K. M. (Eds.). (2012). *The Harriet Lane handbook* (19th ed.). St. Louis, MO: Elsevier Mosby.

Ulger, O., & Sener, G. (2011). Functional outcome after prosthetic rehabilitation of children with acquired and congenital lower limb loss. *Journal of Pediatric Orthopaedics*, *20*, 178–183.

University of Maryland Medical Center. (2011). *Muscular dystrophy.* Retrieved from http://www.wmm.edu/altmed/articles/musculardystrophy-000113.htm

U.S. Preventive Services Task Force. (2014). *Idiopathic scoliosis in adolescents: Screening.* Retrieved from http://www.uspreventiveservicestaskforce.org/Page/Document/RecommendationStatementFinal/idiopathic-scoliosis-in-adolescents-screening

van Dijk, F. S., Cobben, J. M., Kariminijad, A., Maugeri, A., Nikkels, P. G., van Rijn, R. R., & Pals, G. (2011). Osteogenesis imperfect: A review with clinical examples. *Molecular Syndromology*, *2*, 1–20.

Weinstein, S. L., Dolan, L. A., Wright, J. G., & Dobbs, M. B. (2013). Effects of bracing in adolescents with idiopathic scoliosis. *New England Journal of Medicine*, *369*, 1512–1521.

Witbreuk, M., van Kemenade, F. J., van der Sluijs, J. A., Jansma, E. P., Rottefeel, J., & van Royen, B. J. (2013). Slipped capital femoral epiphysis and its association with endocrine, metabolic and chronic diseases: A systematic review of the literature. *Journal of Children's Orthopaedics*, *7*, 213–223.

Wolff, A., Vanduynhover, E., van Kleef, M., Huygen, F., Pope, J. E., & Mehhail, N. (2011). Phantom pain. *Pain Practice*, *11*, 403–413.

Womack, J. (2014). Osteogenesis imperfect types I-XI: Implications for the neonatal nurse. *Advances in Neonatal Care*, *14*, 309–315.

Wright, E. (2009). Neurovascular impairment and compartment syndrome. *Paediatric Nursing*, *21*(3), 26–29.

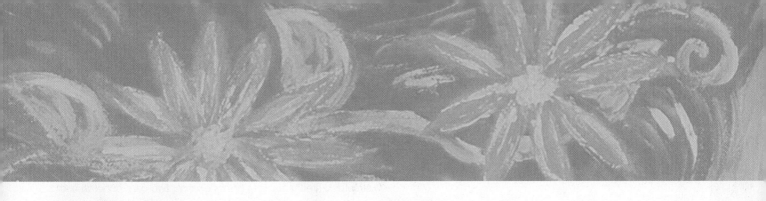

Chapter 30
Alterations in Endocrine Function

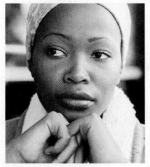

I am really worried about how Anthony is going to learn to manage all these aspects of diabetes care. Learning to check his blood sugar is pretty easy compared to counting calories and figuring out how much insulin to take and when to take it. I hope we have some time to get into a routine with his diabetes management before he gets sick. We have to work hard to keep the diabetes under control.

—Mother of Anthony, 12 years old

Stockbyte/Getty Images

∨ Learning Outcomes

30.1 Identify the function of important hormones of the endocrine system.

30.2 Summarize signs and symptoms that may indicate a disorder of the endocrine system.

30.3 Identify all conditions for which short stature is a sign.

30.4 Prioritize nursing care for each type of acquired metabolic disorder.

30.5 Develop a family education plan for the child who needs lifelong cortisol replacement.

30.6 Distinguish between the nursing care of the child with type 1 and type 2 diabetes.

30.7 Plan care for the child with an inherited metabolic disorder.

Disorders of Pituitary Function

Pituitary disorders such as growth hormone deficiency, hyperpituitarism, and precocious puberty directly affect a child's growth, while diabetes insipidus and the syndrome of inappropriate antidiuretic hormone are disorders affecting fluid balance. These disorders are discussed in the following subsections.

Growth Hormone Deficiency (Hypopituitarism)

Growth hormone deficiency (GHD) is a disorder caused by decreased activity of the pituitary gland. Because most children with this disorder secrete inadequate amounts of growth hormone, the term *growth hormone deficiency* is often preferred to *hypopituitarism.* The disorder is estimated to occur in 1 of 4000 to 1 of 10,000 people (Stanley, 2012).

ETIOLOGY AND PATHOPHYSIOLOGY

The release of growth hormone from the anterior pituitary gland is controlled by the hypothalamus, which secretes releasing and inhibitory factors (somatostatin). Growth hormone (GH) (somatotropin) stimulates linear growth and bone mineral density, as well as the growth of all body tissues. Growth hormone also stimulates the synthesis of proteins in the liver, among them the somatomedins, or insulin-like growth factors (IGFs), which promote glucose utilization by the cells and cell proliferation.

Infarction of the pituitary gland (related to sickle cell disease), central nervous system disease, tumors of the pituitary gland or hypothalamus (primarily craniopharyngiomas and gliomas), other brain tumors, cranial irradiation, brain trauma, chemotherapy, and psychosocial deprivation may cause GHD by interfering with the production or release of growth hormone. Other major causes of short stature include familial short stature, hypothyroidism, Turner

Text continues on page 866

FOCUS ON:
The Endocrine System

The endocrine system controls the cellular activity that regulates growth and body metabolism through the release of hormones. Hormones are chemical messengers secreted by various glands that exert controlling effects on the cells of the body.

- Differentiation of the reproductive and central nervous systems in the fetus
- Regulation of the pace of growth and development in concert with the central nervous system throughout childhood and adolescence
- Coordination of the male and female reproductive systems, enabling sexual reproduction
- Maintenance of an optimal level of hormones for body functioning
- Maintenance of homeostasis, a healthy internal environment, in the presence of a constantly changing external environment

Anatomy and Physiology

The endocrine and nervous systems interact to regulate responses within the body and with the external environment. The hypothalamic-pituitary axis (or system) produces a number of releasing and inhibiting hormones that regulate the function of many endocrine glands, including the thyroid, adrenal, and male and female reproductive glands. The hypothalamus synthesizes many hormones, and the pituitary gland works by stimulating or inhibiting the release of these hormones. The pituitary gland also secretes certain hormones. Hormones originating from this axis regulate growth. Other endocrine glands include the parathyroid glands and the islets of Langerhans in the pancreas (Figure 30–1). All of these glands secrete hormones into the bloodstream, which carries them to target organs or tissues. Most hormones exert their influence through interaction with receptors in the target cells of specific tissues (Table 30–1).

Hormone secretion regulation occurs through a *negative feedback* mechanism that maintains an optimal internal body environment (Figure 30–2). Negative feedback occurs when an endocrine gland or secretory tissue receives a message that the target cells have received an adequate amount of hormone. In response, further secretion is inhibited. Secretion is resumed only when the secretory tissue receives another message indicating that levels of the hormone are low.

Pediatric Differences

The endocrine system is responsible for sexual differentiation during fetal development. As the embryo develops, the initial reproductive structures are the same (a pair of gonads, two pairs of ducts, and the genital tubercle). Beginning at 7 to 8 weeks of gestation, the male embryo begins secreting testosterone, which causes the gonads to differentiate into testes. The pairs of ducts develop into the vas deferens. The female embryo begins secreting estrogen, causing the gonads to differentiate into ovaries, while the ducts develop into the uterus and the fallopian tubes. The genital tubercle also differentiates and develops the male and female external genitalia.

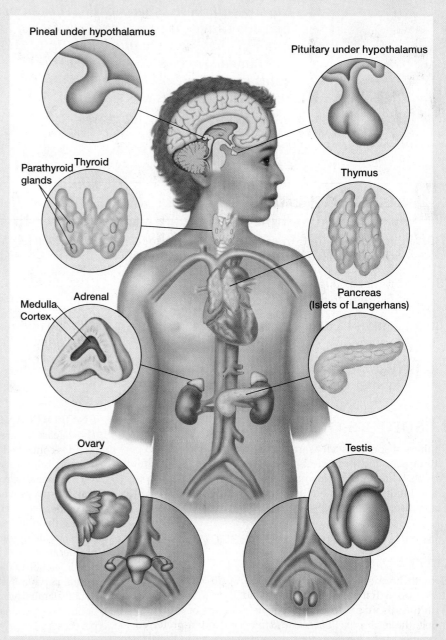

Pineal under hypothalamus

Pituitary under hypothalamus

Parathyroid glands

Thyroid

Thymus

Medulla
Cortex

Adrenal

Pancreas
(Islets of Langerhans)

Ovary

Testis

Figure 30–1 Major organs and glands of the endocrine system.

TABLE 30–1 Endocrine Glands and Their Functions

GLAND/HORMONE	FUNCTION
ANTERIOR PITUITARY	
Growth hormone (somatotropin)	Regulates metabolic process related to growth.
Thyroid-stimulating hormone (TSH)	Stimulates thyroid hormone secretion.
Adrenocorticotropic hormone (ACTH) (corticotropin)	Stimulates secretion of glucocorticoids and androgens.
Follicle-stimulating hormone (FSH) (a gonadotropin)	Stimulates secretion of estrogen; stimulates follicle maturation in ovaries. Also critical for sperm production in males.
Luteinizing hormone (LH) and interstitial cell-stimulating hormone (ICSH) (male analog) (a gonadotropin)	Stimulates secretion of androgens in males and progesterone in females.
Prolactin-releasing hormone (PRH)	Stimulates secretion of prolactin, which stimulates the secretion of milk during lactation.
Melanocyte-stimulating hormone (MSH)	Stimulates skin pigmentation.
Beta endorphins	Involved with pleasure during exercise and the alleviation of pain.
POSTERIOR PITUITARY	
Antidiuretic hormone (ADH)	Promotes water reabsorption back into blood, decreasing urine output.
Oxytocin	Stimulates uterine contractions and breast milk let-down reflex.
HYPOTHALAMUS	
Corticotropin-releasing hormone (CRH)	Regulates the release of ACTH from the pituitary gland.
Gonadotropin-releasing hormone (GnRH)	Stimulates the anterior pituitary gland to secrete luteinizing hormone (LH) and follicle-stimulating hormone (FSH).
Growth hormone-releasing hormone (GHRH)	Stimulates the anterior pituitary gland to secrete growth hormone.
Somatostatin	Inhibits the pituitary gland's secretion of growth hormone and TSH.
Thyrotropin releasing hormone (TRH)	Stimulates release of TSH and prolactin from the anterior pituitary gland.
Prolactin inhibiting hormone (PIH) (dopamine)	Inhibits prolactin, which inhibits milk production.
THYROID	
Thyroxine (T_4) and triiodothyronine (T_3)	Regulates metabolic rate of all cells, body heat production; protein, fat, and carbohydrate catabolism in all cells.
Thyrocalcitonin	Stimulates bone ossification and development.
PARATHYROID	
Parathyroid hormone	Regulates serum calcium levels and excretion of phosphorus.
ADRENAL	
Aldosterone	Increases sodium ion reabsorption, and increases potassium and hydrogen ion excretion in the kidneys.
Androgens	Stimulate bone development and secondary sexual characteristics.
Cortisol	Stimulates anti-inflammatory reactions; protects from harmful stress responses.
Epinephrine	Activates sympathetic nervous system; stimulates increase in heart rate, blood pressure, and blood glucose levels; opens airways and reduces swelling.
PANCREAS (ISLETS OF LANGERHANS)	
Insulin	Facilitates cellular glucose utilization.
Glucagon	Increases blood glucose when low by stimulating glycogenolysis.
Somatostatin	Inhibits insulin and glucagon secretion; may prevent excess insulin secretion.
OVARIES	
Estrogen	Stimulates development of breasts and ova.
Progesterone	Stimulates breast glandular development; acts to maintain pregnancy.
TESTES	
Testosterone	Stimulates production of sperm, development of secondary sexual characteristics, and closure of epiphysis.

(continued)

GHRF = Growth Hormone Releasing Factor

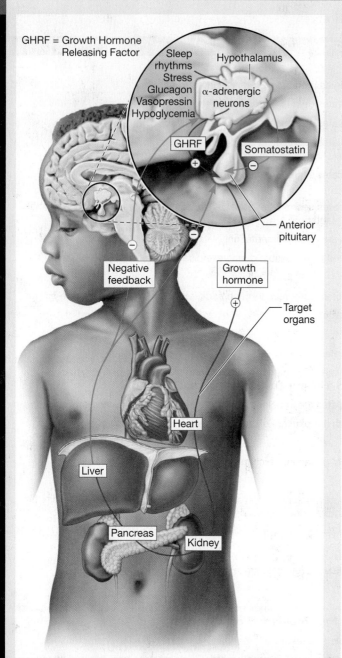

Figure 30–2 **Feedback mechanism in hormonal stimulation of the gonads during puberty.**

The endocrine system is also responsible for stimulating growth and development during childhood and adolescence. Multiple hormones in the endocrine system, including the growth hormone, thyroid hormone, adrenal and gonadal androgens, and estrogen, are responsible for skeletal growth and maturation. (Carroll & Kerr, 2014). Skeletal maturity can be detected by examining the child's **bone age** (stage of bone ossification) (see *As Children Grow: Bone Age*).

During childhood, the production of sex hormones (estrogen, progesterone, and testosterone) is low. **Puberty** (sexual maturation, lasting an average of 4.5 years) occurs when the gonads begin to secrete increased amounts of the sex hormones estrogen and androgens. At the average age of 9 years in girls and 11 years in boys, the hypothalamus produces increased amounts of gonadotropin-releasing hormone (GnRH). This hormone stimulates the anterior

As Children Grow: **Bone Age**

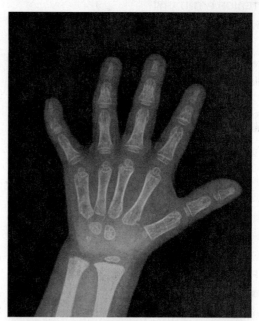

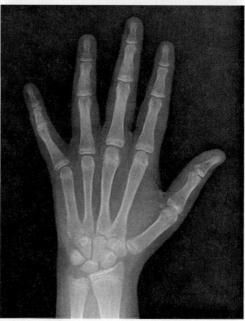

The radiographs of the hand and wrist of a 3-year-old girl and a 14-year-old girl reveal significant differences in skeletal maturation that are closely tied to physiologic maturation. The 3-year-old has many bones in the hand and wrist that have not fully developed. The secretion of estrogen during puberty has resulted in the development and calcification of secondary ossification centers of most of the bones in the hand and wrist of the 14-year old.

Source: Photos courtesy of Dr. Evelyn Anthony, MD, Department of Radiology, Brenner Children's Hospital, Wake Forest University Health System.

pituitary gland to secrete luteinizing hormone (LH) and follicle-stimulating hormone (FSH). In boys, LH stimulates testosterone production and FSH stimulates sperm production. In girls, LH and FSH stimulate development and maturation of the ova and ovulation. These hormones in turn stimulate the gonads to secrete more sex hormones, resulting in the development of primary and secondary sex characteristics. They also stimulate the genitalia to grow to adult proportions. **Adrenarche** refers to the onset of adrenal androgen production. These adrenal hormones lead to the development of acne, pubic hair, and adult body odor (Bordini & Rosenfield, 2011a). Pubertal development usually follows a specific sequence (breast development, pubic hair growth, and menarche in females; testicular enlargement, pubic hair growth, appearance of spermatozoa in seminal fluid, facial hair, and voice change in males) (Bordini & Rosenfield, 2011b). See Figures 5–28, 5–29, and 5–30 for the development of secondary sexual characteristics in males and females.

Menarche, the onset of menstruation, occurs at an average age of 12.1 years in African American girls and 12.6 years in White girls (Bordini & Rosenfield, 2011b). Menstruation is controlled by several hormones (FSH, LH, estrogen, and progesterone). For 1 to 2 years, cycles are anovulatory of variable duration. In contrast, males begin producing sperm once testicular and penile growth has occurred, during genital stages 3 and 4 (Bordini & Rosenfield, 2011b).

Use *Assessment Guide: The Child With an Endocrine Condition* to perform a nursing assessment. Examples of diagnostic and laboratory tests used to evaluate endocrine conditions are provided in Table 30–2.

Endocrine disturbances result in alterations in metabolism, growth and development, and behavior that may have significant implications for children. If not diagnosed and treated early, these conditions can result in delays in growth and development, intellectual disability (previously called mental retardation), and, occasionally, death. However, treatment, which usually consists of supplementation of missing hormones, adjustment of hormone levels, or dietary measures, allows most children to live a normal life.

Inborn errors of metabolism—inherited biochemical abnormalities of the urea cycle and amino acid and organic acid metabolism—often have a significant impact on the endocrine system's ability to support growth and development. Some chromosomal abnormalities also result in disturbances in growth and sexual development.

TABLE 30–2 Diagnostic Tests and Laboratory Procedures for the Endocrine System

DIAGNOSTIC PROCEDURES	LABORATORY TESTS
ACTH stimulation test	Fasting plasma glucose
Adrenal (ACTH) suppression test	Hemoglobin A_{1c}
Bone age	Hormone levels
Computed tomography (CT)	Insulin-like growth factor (IGF-1) and insulin-like growth factor-binding protein 3 (IGFBP-3)
Fluid deprivation test	Newborn metabolic screening
Karyotype	Provocative growth hormone testing
Magnetic resonance imaging (MRI)	Thyroid antibodies
Thyroid radioactive iodine uptake (RAIU) scan	

Note: See Appendices D and E for more information about these tests and procedures.

ASSESSMENT GUIDE | The Child With an Endocrine Condition

Assessment Focus	Assessment Guidelines
Growth	• Carefully measure weight, length, or height and plot on a growth curve.
	• Compare measurements at different ages to assess the growth pattern over time and to assess the growth velocity.
Blood pressure	• Assess blood pressure and compare to expected norms for age. See Appendix B.
Facial characteristics	• Inspect the face for unusual features such as a protuberant tongue, protuberant eyes, or moon face.
Neck	• Palpate the neck for an enlarged thyroid or goiter.
Muscles	• Assess strength and muscle tone.
Genitalia and secondary sexual characteristics	• Assess external genitalia for signs of ambiguous genitalia or inappropriate development for age.
	• Determine the child's stage of development for each characteristic (breast and pubic hair for girls, genital and pubic hair for boys) by comparing to the images in Figures 5–28, 5–29, and 5–30.
	• Assess the sexual maturity rating with information given in Chapter 5 (Table 5–13). Compare the stage of development to the age of the boy or girl to determine early or delayed onset of puberty.
Body odor	• Assess body odor for unusual smell (e.g., sweet, musty, cheesy, sweaty feet).
Skin	• Assess skin color, noting areas of unusual pigmentation.
Family history	• Assess for family history of metabolic or endocrine disorders.

syndrome, *constitutional growth delay* (delayed pubertal hormone secretion causes a late pubertal growth spurt), chronic renal failure, malnutrition, Cushing syndrome, Down syndrome, inborn error of metabolism, and severe cardiac, pulmonary, immunologic, or gastrointestinal disease. Psychosocial dwarfism is a syndrome of emotional deprivation that causes transient growth hormone deficiency; it is reversed by placing the child in a nurturing environment (Sirotnak, 2013). Refer to Chapter 29 for information about achondroplastic dwarfism.

CLINICAL MANIFESTATIONS

Children with GHD have normal birth weights and length. However, by the age of 1 year, they are below the 3rd percentile on the growth chart. The child characteristically grows at a rate of less than 5 cm (2 in.) per year. Other characteristic findings in infants include hypoglycemic seizures, hyponatremia, neonatal jaundice, pale optic discs, micropenis, and undescended testicles. Children with GHD tend to appear "cherubic" and exhibit youthful facial features, higher pitched voices, delayed dentition, "ripply" abdominal fat, decreased muscle mass, delayed skeletal maturation, and delayed sexual maturation. Slipped capital femoral epiphysis (see Chapter 29) has been associated with growth hormone therapy. Any child receiving growth hormone treatment who complains of hip pain or knee pain, or who manifests a limp, must be evaluated for this disorder (Cooke, Divall, & Radovick, 2011).

Any child whose height is 2 to 3 standard deviations below the mean height for age or whose measurement is falling off the normal growth chart should be evaluated for short stature (Table 30–3). A child whose screening tests reveal low levels of insulin-like growth factor (IGF-1) requires further evaluation by a pediatric endocrinologist. A careful history, physical examination, assessment of pubertal development and unusual facies, and radiologic studies are necessary to rule out familial short stature and constitutional growth delay, which are normal variants; skeletal dysplasias; or psychosocial short stature, which requires further evaluation.

CLINICAL THERAPY

Radiographic imaging of the hand or wrist bone is used to evaluate the stage of bone ossification and thus the bone age of the child. Using standardized norms for bone ossification, it can be determined if the child's chronologic and bone ages match. Significantly delayed (less than the child's age) or advanced (greater than the child's age) bone age may be indicative of the possibility of a systemic chronic disease or hormone abnormality requiring investigation (see *As Children Grow: Bone Age* earlier in this chapter).

Provocative growth hormone testing, in which various medications (arginine, clonidine, glucagon, insulin, L-dopa) are administered to stimulate release of growth hormone, is a diagnostic test that may be used to confirm growth hormone deficiency (Guo, 2013).

For growth hormone deficiency, replacement therapy with growth hormone (GH) is administered to promote growth and development. Growth hormone replacement requires subcutaneous injections 6 to 7 times per week and generally continues for several years until growth is complete. The pediatric endocrinologist adjusts the dosage based on response to treatment (Ferguson, 2011).

The child usually experiences increased growth velocity for the first year of treatment, followed by a gradual decrease in growth for subsequent months or years. Growth should progress at least at the normal rate for age while the child continues on growth hormone treatment. If growth is slower than anticipated, compliance with therapy must be considered before the dosage is increased. Replacement therapy is continued until either the child achieves an acceptable height or growth velocity drops to less than 2 cm (1 in.) per year. Additionally, a bone age of greater than 14 years in girls and 16 years in boys is the criterion to stop treatment. In some cases, the onset of puberty is delayed with GnRH analogs to provide more time for growth hormone therapy to stimulate growth (Parks & Felner, 2016).

Nursing Management

Nursing care consists of monitoring growth, teaching the child and family about the disorder and its treatment, and providing emotional support. Collect blood samples in the manner and time ordered. Carefully measure the child's height and weight and plot them on a growth chart (see Appendix A and the *Clinical Skills Manual* SKILLS).

Teach the parents and child about the GH replacement therapy, preparation and administration of subcutaneous injections, rotating injection sites, potential side effects, and actions to take if any side effects are noticed. Provide the parents with ideas about how to minimize the child's stress associated with daily injections. Give parents educational resources, such as information from the Magic Foundation and the Human Growth Foundation. Replacement therapy is expensive and may not be covered by insurance (Ferguson, 2011).

Children with GHD, especially those whose deficiency is caused by tumors and trauma from radiation or surgery, may have academic problems because of acquired learning disabilities. Before the child enters or returns to school, a comprehensive evaluation should be performed to identify potential problems.

TABLE 30–3 Diagnostic Tests for Short Stature

TEST	PURPOSE RELATED TO SHORT STATURE
IGF-1 (insulin-like growth factor) and IGFBP-3 (insulin-like growth factor-binding protein 3)	Screens for growth hormone deficiency
MRI of the pituitary gland	Detects pituitary malformation or tumor
Provocative growth hormone testing	Tests for growth hormone deficiency
Bone age	Identifies skeletal maturation compared to chronological age
Karyotype (girls)	Detects Turner syndrome
Thyroid function studies	Detects hypothyroidism
ACTH and cortisol levels	Detects other pituitary hormonal deficiencies
Urine creatinine, pH, specific gravity, urea nitrogen, electrolytes	Detects chronic renal failure (see Chapter 26)
Complete blood count and erythrocyte sedimentation rate	Screens for inflammatory bowel disease with anemia
Antigliadin antibodies	Screens for celiac disease

Source: Data from Parks, J. S., & Felner, E. I. (2016). Hypopituitarism. In R. M. Kliegman, B. F. Stanton, J. W. St. Geme, & N. F. Schor (Eds.), *Nelson textbook of pediatrics* (20th ed., pp. 2637–2644). Philadelphia, PA: Elsevier; Cooke, D. W., Divall, S. A., & Radovick, S. (2011). Normal and aberrant growth. In S. Melmed, K. S. Polonsky, P. R. Larsen, & H. M. Kronenberg (Eds.), *Williams textbook of endocrinology* (12th ed., pp. 935–1053). Philadelphia, PA: Elsevier Saunders.

Encourage parents and teachers to treat the child in an age-appropriate manner. The child should dress in clothing that reflects chronologic age. Emphasize the child's strengths, support independence, and encourage participation in age-appropriate activities to aid in the development of a positive self-image. Suggest that the child take part in sports in which ability does not depend on size (e.g., swimming, gymnastics, wrestling, ice skating, and martial arts). Identifying positive role models, short people who accomplish their goals, also promotes a positive image. Refer the child for counseling if appropriate.

The best results occur when treatment begins at an early age, before the psychologic effects of short stature become apparent and when attainment of near-normal height is reached. People often treat short children on the basis of their size rather than their age, and such children experience social prejudice about height. Teasing is a common problem. The teenage years may be particularly stressful because of adolescents' characteristic preoccupation with body image.

Growth Hormone Excess (Hyperpituitarism)

Hyperpituitarism, a disorder in which excessive secretion of growth hormone increases the growth rate, is rare in children. If combined with precocious puberty, a tumor of the hypothalamus may be present. Affected children can grow to 7 or 8 feet in height when oversecretion occurs before closure of the epiphyseal plates. If the disorder occurs after closure of the epiphyseal plates, acromegaly occurs.

Because tall stature is valued in our society, assessment of children (particularly males) with accelerated linear growth is often delayed. Any child whose predicted height exceeds that consistent with parental height should be evaluated for possible growth problems and underlying pathologic conditions.

A complete history is obtained, and physical examination and laboratory testing are performed. Increased levels of insulin-like growth factor (IGF-1) establish the diagnosis of hyperpituitarism. Radiologic examination for bone age is obtained to determine if the epiphyseal plates have begun to fuse. Radiologic studies are used to detect a tumor. Thorough evaluation is required to differentiate hyperpituitarism from familial tall stature.

Treatment depends on the cause of the excessive growth and may involve surgical removal of a tumor or pituitary gland (hypophysectomy), radiation therapy, or radioactive implants. High doses of sex steroids are given to close the epiphyseal plates. The child may need lifelong pituitary hormone replacement following surgery.

Nursing Management

Tall stature, like short stature, can be stressful for children. Tall children are often treated as if they are older than their chronologic age. Tall adolescents may have problems with self-image, and girls in particular may worry about their appearance.

Nursing care focuses on teaching the parents and child about the disorder and its treatment, providing emotional support, and, if surgery is required, providing preoperative and postoperative teaching and care (see Chapter 11).

Diabetes Insipidus

Diabetes insipidus is a disorder of the posterior pituitary gland and is defined as an inability of the kidneys to concentrate urine. Two forms of diabetes insipidus occur: central (neurogenic) and nephrogenic diabetes insipidus. Central diabetes insipidus results from inadequate production of vasopressin (antidiuretic hormone), and nephrogenic diabetes insipidus results from ineffective action of vasopressin in the kidneys (Di lorgi et al., 2012; McHugo & Harden, 2011).

Antidiuretic hormone facilitates concentration of the urine by stimulating reabsorption of water from the distal tubule of the kidney. When ADH is inadequate, the tubules do not resorb, leading to **polyuria** (passage of a large volume of urine in a given period). Therefore, the body is unable to conserve water, resulting in severe dehydration.

The cause of 20% to 50% of cases of central diabetes insipidus is unknown and is classified as being idiopathic (Di lorgi et al., 2012). Known causes of central diabetes insipidus include brain tumors, brain trauma, central nervous system infection, and neurosurgery (McHugo & Harden, 2011). Genetic nephrogenic diabetes insipidus is not as common as the acquired type, but its presentation is more severe. Acquired nephrogenic diabetes insipidus may be caused by drug toxicity, an adverse drug reaction, or illnesses that impair the ability of the kidneys to concentrate urine (Breault & Majzoub, 2016).

Polyuria and **polydipsia** (excessive thirst) are the cardinal signs of diabetes insipidus. Enuresis is common in children. Polydipsia is the body's attempt to preserve fluid balance. Additional manifestations observed in children with diabetes insipidus include hypernatremia, dilute urine, and dehydration (Table 30–4).

Clinical Tip

During the fluid deprivation test, advise parents that the child will be frustrated and irritable from thirst. No one should drink in front of the child during the testing period. Monitor the child's vital signs, intake, output, and weight carefully (McHugo & Harden, 2011).

TABLE 30–4 Clinical Manifestations of Diabetes Insipidus

CAUSE	CLINICAL MANIFESTATIONS	CLINICAL THERAPY
CENTRAL DIABETES INSIPIDUS		
ADH (vasopressin) deficiency	Polyuria, polydipsia	Desmopressin acetate
Familial or idiopathic	Nocturia, enuresis	
	Thirsty at night	
	Irritable if fluids withheld	
	Constipation, fever, dehydration	
NEPHROGENIC DIABETES INSIPIDUS		
Inherited or acquired	Polyuria, polydipsia	Diuretics
Decreased responsiveness of kidneys to ADH (vasopressin)	Hypernatremia in neonatal period	High fluid intake
	Dehydration, fever, vomiting	Salt- and protein-restricted diet
	Mental status changes	

Although the onset of symptoms is usually sudden, diagnosis is often delayed. Children who can quench their thirst may not complain to parents about symptoms. In infants, symptoms may include irritability, lethargy, vomiting, poor feeding, failure to thrive, and constipation (McHugo & Harden, 2011; Walsh & March, 2013).

In all forms of diabetes insipidus, the urine cannot be concentrated no matter how dehydrated the child becomes. A dehydration episode usually leads to the diagnosis. Serum sodium concentration and osmolality increase rapidly to pathologic levels. Often an unconscious child is admitted to the emergency department with dehydration and hypernatremia.

Initial testing involves serum electrolyte concentrations and a urinalysis including specific gravity and osmolality. Serum osmolality is increased (greater than 300 mOsm/kg), and urine osmolality is decreased (less than 300 mOsm/kg). Urine specific gravity is decreased (less than 1.005), and serum sodium is elevated (greater than 145 mEq/L). A CT scan or MRI may be ordered to visualize the pituitary gland to detect a tumor. A fluid-deprivation test evaluates the level of ADH and helps to confirm the diagnosis (Walsh & March, 2013).

Central ADH deficiency is treated by intranasal or oral desmopressin acetate (DDAVP). The medication reduces urinary output, enabling the child to live a more normal life with a decrease in thirst, urinary output, and nocturia. The dose of DDAVP is based on route of administration, age, and response to therapy (McHugo & Harden, 2011). Nephrogenic diabetes insipidus is treated with thiazide diuretics, which promote sodium excretion and stimulate the proximal tubule to reabsorb water. Indomethacin and amiloride may also be prescribed to have an additive effect on decreased water excretion (Breault & Majzoub, 2016). The child's sodium and potassium levels must be carefully monitored to prevent hypernatremia and hypokalemia (McHugo & Harden, 2011) (see Chapter 18).

Nursing Management

Educate parents about making fluids available to the child as needed, administering DDAVP, obtaining and recording daily weights, measuring intake and output, and recognizing signs of dehydration. Parents may need to weigh diapers to monitor urine output in infants. Cold fluids are often preferred and help relieve thirst. The child's fluid intake will need to be adjusted to prevent dehydration during an illness. Children often wake to drink fluids at night, but infants will need to have fluids provided. Many infants have coexisting brain damage and need nasogastric or gastrostomy feeding to maintain adequate hydration and nutrition. However, care should be taken to avoid the intake of excessive fluid as the child will not be able to excrete the excess water load with DDAVP treatment.

The child with chronic diabetes insipidus should always wear a medical alert identification (tag, bracelet, or necklace) to indicate the presence of the disorder. Partner with the parents and school officials to make arrangements to provide the child unrestricted access to toilet facilities and water.

Syndrome of Inappropriate Antidiuretic Hormone (SIADH)

Syndrome of inappropriate antidiuretic hormone (SIADH) results from an excessive amount of serum ADH. It is seen in children with central nervous system infections, brain tumors, and brain trauma; in children with pulmonary disorders such as pneumonia, asthma, or cystic fibrosis; and in children

receiving positive-pressure ventilation. Some medications, including diuretics and chemotherapy, have been associated with SIADH.

Failure of normal feedback mechanisms from the hypothalamus, pituitary gland, and kidney results in excessive secretion of ADH, leading to water reabsorption despite the presence of low serum osmolality. ADH secretion causes increased permeability of the distal renal tubules and collecting ducts and resulting in water reabsorption (Thomas & Fraer, 2014). Elevated ADH also causes suppression of the renin-angiotensin mechanism and sodium excretion. The outcome is **water intoxication** (an abnormal proportion of water to sodium in the extracellular fluid) and hyponatremia.

Signs of SIADH are related to water intoxication and hyponatremia, and include elevated blood pressure, distended jugular veins, crackles in lung fields, weight gain without edema, fluid and electrolyte imbalance, and concentrated urine with decreased urine output. As serum sodium levels continue to fall, lethargy, confusion, headache, altered level of consciousness, seizures, and coma occur because of cerebral edema.

Laboratory findings include a high urine osmolality, low serum osmolality, low serum sodium, high urine sodium, and decreased blood urea nitrogen (Pillai, Unnikrishnan, & Pavithran, 2011; Shoback & Funk, 2011).

Fluids are restricted to prevent further dilution of the blood. Medications include diuretics, demeclocycline to block action of ADH at the renal collecting tubules, and hypertonic saline IV fluids (Robinson & Verbalis, 2011; Shoback & Funk, 2011).

Nursing Management

Nursing care focuses on preventing injury, monitoring fluid balance, administering medications, and managing nutritional intake. Monitor intake and output, serum sodium, urine osmolality, and specific gravity. Educate the parents about the child's fluid restrictions and the hidden sources of water and fluids in foods to help avoid excessive fluid intake.

Teach the importance of checking weight daily and reporting weight gain, which may indicate fluid retention. Refer the family to a registered dietician to assist in identifying hidden sources of water and fluids, such as fruit-flavored ice pops, gelatin, watermelon, and citrus fruit, to prevent excessive fluid intake.

Depending on the cause of the disorder, lifelong medication may be required. If the child is prescribed demeclocycline, emphasize to the family the importance of follow-up care since the drug has nephrotoxic side effects. The child should wear a medical identification alert tag, bracelet, or necklace identifying the disorder and treatment.

Precocious Puberty

Precocious puberty is defined as the appearance of any secondary sexual characteristics before 8 years of age in girls (breast development or pubic hair) and 9 years of age in boys (pubic hair or genital development) (Bordini & Rosenfield, 2011b).

Earlier than expected secretion of the normal hormones responsible for pubertal changes is not usually associated with an endocrine system abnormality (an idiopathic problem). External sources of hormones such as anabolic steroids or estrogen may be identified. Central precocious puberty or true precocious puberty occurs when the hypothalamus is activated to secrete gonadotropin-releasing hormone. Other potential causes of precocious puberty include tumors of the ovary or adrenal gland and a rare genetic condition known as McCune-Albright syndrome (Fuqua, 2013).

Isolated signs of premature sexual development such as **thelarche** (breast development), menarche (vaginal bleeding without other signs of sexual development), and adrenarche (leading to development of pubic and axillary hair) before 8 years of age in girls and 9 years in boys often needs no treatment.

Children with precocious puberty have an advanced bone age (premature skeletal maturation) and may appear unusually tall for their age. However, their growth ceases prematurely as the hormones stimulate closure of the epiphyseal plates, resulting in short stature. Behavioral changes may include mood swings and emotional lability. Early menarche also increases the risk for breast cancer because of prolonged exposure to estrogen (Collaborative Group on Hormonal Factors in Breast Cancer, 2012).

Serum diagnostic studies include LH, FSH, testosterone, or estradiol. Provocative testing includes gonadotropin-releasing hormone (GnRH) stimulation to confirm the diagnosis. Radiologic imaging of the brain, as well as bone age tests, may be performed.

Treatment for central precocious puberty includes a GnRH analog to maintain a constant serum level of GnRH (Fuqua, 2013). Treatment often continues until a more normal age for puberty is reached (e.g., 11 years in girls and 12 years in boys). Simple monitoring of growth patterns may be the only intervention for children closer to the lower than expected age for puberty to begin. Tumors require surgery, radiation, and/or chemotherapy.

Nursing Management

Nursing care should focus on teaching the child and parents about the condition and its treatment, promoting growth, and providing emotional support. Inform the child in age-appropriate terms that the physiologic changes are normal but are occurring at an earlier than usual age. Reassure the child that friends will experience the same stages of development eventually. Emphasize to the family that the child's social, cognitive, and emotional development matches the child's age even though physical development is advanced.

> ## Developing Cultural Competence Onset of Puberty
>
> Differences exist by race in the onset of thelarche in girls of normal weight. Non-Hispanic African American girls and Mexican American girls normally undergo breast development during the seventh year, about 1 year earlier than non-Hispanic White girls (Bordini & Rosenfield, 2011b).

Children with precocious puberty become self-conscious as body changes occur. Provide the child opportunities to express concerns and discuss issues related to body changes. The child may need to practice role-playing as a coping mechanism to manage teasing by other children. Partner with the family to encourage dressing the child in a manner appropriate to the child's chronologic age even though the child may look older. Provide privacy during physical examinations. Advise parents that they may need to discuss issues of sexuality with the child at an earlier age than normal. Refer the child and family for counseling if appropriate.

Teach the family proper medication administration and adherence to the treatment regimen. Determine the family's ability to financially manage the cost of treatment. Assistance in covering the cost of therapy may be available through pharmaceutical companies and third-party payers.

Disorders of Thyroid Function
Hypothyroidism

Hypothyroidism is a disorder in which levels of active thyroid hormones are decreased. It may be congenital or acquired. Congenital hypothyroidism occurs in approximately 1 in 3000 to 1 in 4000 live births worldwide (Seth & Maheshwari, 2013). It is twice as common in females as it is in males. In comparison to White infants, congenital hypothyroidism is less prevalent among Black infants but more prevalent in Hispanic, Asian American, Pacific Islander, and Native American infants (LaFranchi & Huang, 2016).

ETIOLOGY AND PATHOPHYSIOLOGY

Thyroid hormones are important for growth and development and for metabolizing nutrients and energy. When these hormones are not available to stimulate other hormones or specific target cells, growth is delayed and intellectual disability develops.

Congenital hypothyroidism is usually caused by a spontaneous gene mutation, an autosomal recessive genetic transmission of an enzyme deficiency, hypoplasia or aplasia of the thyroid gland, failure of the CNS–thyroid feedback mechanism to develop, or iodine deficiency. Intellectual disability is irreversible if the disorder is not treated.

Acquired hypothyroidism can be idiopathic or result from autoimmune thyroiditis (Hashimoto thyroiditis), late-onset thyroid dysfunction, isolated thyroid-stimulating hormone (TSH) deficiency caused by pituitary or hypothalamic dysfunction, or exposure to drugs or substances such as lithium that interfere with thyroid hormone synthesis. In the case of Hashimoto thyroiditis, the thyroid is infiltrated by lymphocytes that cause an autoimmune reaction and an enlarged thyroid. A genetic predisposition to autoimmune thyroiditis and an autosomal dominant inheritance of thyroid antibodies has been identified (LaFranchi & Huang, 2016).

CLINICAL MANIFESTATIONS

Infants with congenital hypothyroidism have few clinical signs of the disorder in the first weeks of life. Symptoms may include jaundice, thick tongue, hypotonia, umbilical hernia, hoarse cry, dry skin, constipation, and large fontanelles (Zeitler et al., 2014) (Figure 30–3).

Children with acquired hypothyroidism have many of the same signs as adults: decreased appetite; dry, cool skin; thinning hair or hair loss; depressed deep tendon reflexes; bradycardia; constipation; sensitivity to cold temperatures; abnormal menses; and a **goiter** (a nontender enlarged thyroid gland).

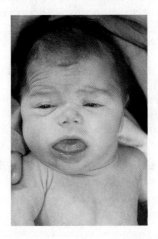

Figure 30–3 **Child with congenital hypothyroidism.**
SOURCE: Mediscan/Alamy.

Manifestations unique to children include change in past normal growth patterns with a weight increase, decreased height velocity, delayed bone and dental age, hypotonia with poor muscle tone, and delayed or precocious puberty.

CLINICAL THERAPY

Congenital hypothyroidism is usually detected during newborn screening, which is mandatory in all 50 states (National Newborn Screening and Genetics Resource Center, 2014). Newborn screening has greatly reduced the incidence of intellectual disability associated with this disorder (Shanholtz, 2013). A decreased T_4, normal T_3, and elevated thyroid-stimulating hormone level indicate hypothyroidism. An elevated TSH level indicates that the disease originated in the thyroid, not the pituitary. The two tests used to identify the disorder should occur: (1) before the newborn leaves the hospital and (2) at the first healthcare visit at 1 to 2 weeks of age. Rapid response from the laboratory testing the samples is important to reduce the time to diagnosis and the effects of hypothyroidism on the infant's development.

Levothyroxine is the drug of choice for newborns with congenital hypothyroidism. The recommended starting dose is 10 to 15 mcg/kg per day (Zeitler et al., 2014). The dose is increased gradually as the child grows to ensure a **euthyroid** (thyroid hormones in appropriate balance) state. A pediatric endocrinologist monitors treatment. To ensure an adequate growth rate and prevent intellectual disability, the hormone must be taken throughout life. Periodic evaluation of T_4 and TSH serum levels, bone age, and growth parameters is necessary to assess for signs of excess or inadequate thyroid hormone.

Antithyroid antibodies are measured in children with a goiter and suspected Hashimoto thyroiditis because increased titers of antithyroglobulin and antimicrosomal antibodies are often found.

Children with congenital hypothyroidism that are diagnosed before 3 months of age have the best prognosis for optimal mental development. Children with acquired hypothyroidism usually have normal growth following a period of catch-up growth. Many adolescents with Hashimoto thyroiditis have a spontaneous remission.

Nursing Management

For the Child With Hypothyroidism

Nursing Assessment and Diagnosis

Routine neonatal screening is performed before discharge from the hospital and is often repeated at the infant's first health visit to evaluate levels of circulating thyroid hormones (see the *Clinical Skills Manual* SKILLS).

Record the length or height and weight at each follow-up visit and plot on a growth curve. The child is assessed for signs of inadequate growth to determine if the dose of thyroid hormone needs to be adjusted and to monitor compliance with medication. Conduct developmental screening to detect delays in developmental milestones.

Among the nursing diagnoses that might be appropriate for the child with hypothyroidism are the following (NANDA-I © 2014):

- *Development: Delayed, Risk for,* related to delayed initiation of thyroid replacement therapy
- *Growth: Disproportionate, Risk for,* related to poor adherence to thyroid hormone therapy
- *Body Image, Disturbed,* related to physical changes associated with condition
- *Fatigue* related to inadequate dose of thyroid medication

Planning and Implementation

Nursing care focuses on teaching the parents and child about the disorder and its treatment and monitoring the child's growth rate. Explain how to administer thyroid hormone (e.g., tablets can be crushed and mixed in a small amount of formula or applesauce as long as the child gets all of the medication). Advise parents that the child may experience temporary sleep disturbances or behavioral changes in response to therapy. Teach the parents how to assess for an increased pulse rate, which could indicate the presence of too much thyroid hormone, and advise them to report problems such as fatigue, which could indicate an improper drug dose that needs to be adjusted.

Caution parents to dress the child appropriately for the season to prevent hypothermia. Modify the child's diet by increasing the amount of fruits and bulk if constipation is a problem.

Reassure the family that the child has the best chance of normal development when the hormone replacement therapy is given as prescribed. Reinforce the importance of follow-up visits to assess growth rate and response to therapy and to regulate drug dosages as the child grows. Periodic assessments of educational achievement are needed. Even with good control, adolescents have persistent visual-spatial deficits and memory and attention problems. Parents should be informed that therapy will be lifelong and is needed to promote the child's mental development. When the cause is genetic, make a referral for genetic counseling.

Evaluation

Expected outcomes of nursing care of the child with hypothyroidism include the following:

- The child maintains adequate growth of height and weight, following a percentile curve throughout childhood.
- The child's diet contains adequate fruits and bulk to prevent constipation.
- The child's cognitive development is appropriate for age.

Hyperthyroidism

Hyperthyroidism occurs when thyroid hormone levels are increased, resulting in excessive levels of circulating thyroid hormones. Graves disease is the most common cause of hyperthyroidism in children, occurring more often in females and in children ages 11 to 15 years (Gastaldi et al., 2014).

ETIOLOGY AND PATHOPHYSIOLOGY

Graves disease is an autoimmune disorder. Immunoglobulins produced by the B lymphocytes stimulate oversecretion of thyroid hormones, resulting in the clinical symptoms. It has a high familial incidence.

Other less common causes of hyperthyroidism result from thyroiditis and thyroid hormone–producing tumors, including thyroid adenomas and carcinomas, and pituitary adenomas. Congenital hyperthyroidism can occur in infants of mothers with Graves disease as a result of transplacental transfer of immunoglobulins. This condition generally resolves by 6 to 12 weeks of age but can last longer (Huang & LaFranchi, 2016).

CLINICAL MANIFESTATIONS

Signs and symptoms are caused by hyperactivity of the sympathetic nervous system and may include an enlarged, nontender thyroid gland (goiter), prominent or bulging eyes (**exophthalmos**) (Figure 30–4), eyelid lag, tachycardia, nervousness, increased appetite with weight loss, emotional lability, moodiness, heat

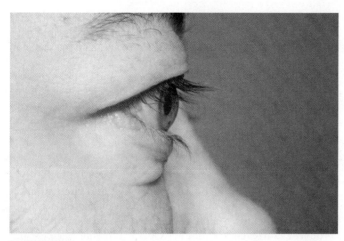

Figure 30–4 **Exophthalmos in an adolescent with Graves disease.**

SOURCE: Biophoto Associates/Science Source.

intolerance, hypertension, hyperactivity, irregular menses, insomnia, tremor, and muscle weakness (Bauer, 2011; Gastaldi et al., 2014). The thyroid gland may be slightly enlarged or grow to 3 to 4 times its normal size; feel warm, soft, and fleshy; and have an auditory bruit on auscultation. Onset is subtle, and the condition often goes unrecognized for 1 to 2 years.

Children with Graves disease usually have difficulty concentrating, behavioral problems, and declining performance in school. They become easily frustrated in the classroom and overheated and fatigued during physical education class. Children with this disorder find it difficult to relax or sleep. These symptoms usually prompt parents to seek medical treatment for the child.

The most serious complication of hyperthyroidism is severe **thyrotoxicosis**, also called *thyroid crisis* or *thyroid storm*. It is a life-threatening emergency resulting from extreme hyperthyroidism, in which elevated circulating levels of TH result in a hypermetabolic state. Symptoms include muscle weakness, diaphoresis, tachycardia, tremor, palpitations, diarrhea, irritability, nervousness, and anxiety (Bahn et al., 2011; Bauer, 2011; Fitzgerald, 2015).

CLINICAL THERAPY

Diagnostic studies include laboratory evaluation of serum TSH, T_3, and T_4 levels and a thyroid scan. T_3 and T_4 levels are markedly elevated, whereas the TSH level is decreased. Serum studies are also performed to detect thyroid autoantibodies anti-TG (antithyroglobulin) and anti-TPO (antiperoxidase), usually present in Graves disease and Hashimoto thyroiditis. A thyroid scan is performed to identify nodules or to confirm the high uptake of radioactive iodine associated with Graves disease.

The goal of clinical therapy is to inhibit excessive secretion of thyroid hormones. Treatment may include medication therapy, radiation therapy, or surgery. Medication therapy is most often the initial treatment, but compliance is often a problem because of side effects. Methimazole (Tapazole) and propylthiouracil (PTU) are antithyroid drugs that are used in children with hyperthyroidism. Because of the concern for severe liver disease with the administration of PTU, current recommendations are that children with hyperthyroidism receive methimazole instead (Bauer, 2011; Huang & LaFranchi, 2016; Rivkees, 2014).

Symptoms usually improve within weeks of starting treatment. Adjunct therapy with beta-adrenergic blocking agents such as propranolol or atenolol may be administered to relieve symptoms of tremors, tachycardia, lid lag, and excessive sweating (Bahn et al., 2011; Huang & LaFranchi, 2016).

Less than 30% of children achieve remission after a 2-year course of treatment with medication. Radiation therapy or thyroidectomy are other options if medication therapy is not effective (Leger et al., 2012). Thyroidectomy (removal of most of the thyroid) provides an immediate cure and avoids radiation and possible long-term complications of radioactive iodine. Removal of the thyroid gland results in hypothyroidism. Complications of thyroidectomy include hemorrhage, hypocalcemia, and damage to the laryngeal nerve paresis (Rivkees, 2014).

Nursing Management

For the Child With Hyperthyroidism

Nursing Assessment and Diagnosis

Assess the child's vital signs, as blood pressure and pulse may be elevated. Keep a record of food intake. Accurate measurement and recording of height and weight are important to establish baselines and identify patterns of growth. Observe the child's behavior, activity, and level of fatigue.

Common nursing diagnoses for the child with hyperthyroidism include the following (NANDA-I © 2014):

- *Thermoregulation, Ineffective,* related to illness and excessive activity of the sympathetic nervous system
- *Nutrition, Imbalanced: Less than Body Requirements,* related to high metabolic needs
- *Body Image, Disturbed,* related to physical changes caused by illness (prominent eyes, excessive perspiration, and tremors)
- *Fatigue* related to hypermetabolic state and sleep deprivation

Planning and Implementation

Nursing care focuses on teaching the child and parents about the disorder and its treatment, promoting rest, providing emotional support, and, if the child needs surgery, providing preoperative and postoperative teaching and care. Promote increased caloric intake by providing five or six moderate meals per day. Encourage the child and family to express their feelings and concerns about the disorder. Pointing out even slight improvements in the child's condition increases adherence with therapy.

Children with hyperthyroidism are easily fatigued. Rest periods should be scheduled at school and home and physical activities kept to a minimum until symptoms resolve. Encourage parents to provide a cool environment and allow the child to wear fewer clothes until symptoms subside.

Children who have partial or total removal of the thyroid gland receive antithyroid drugs, such as iodine, for approximately 2 weeks before surgery to reduce the vascularity and size of the thyroid gland and to decrease the risk of thyroid storm.

Teach the child and parents about drug therapy and instruct parents to watch for side effects of antithyroid drugs, including fever, urticaria, and lymphadenopathy. Provide preoperative teaching (see Chapter 11). Young children in particular may be fearful about having their throat "cut."

Postoperatively, elevate the head of bed to 30 degrees to promote patent airway. A tracheostomy kit, suction supplies, and IV calcium gluconate should be immediately available for emergency treatment of hypocalcemia and respiratory distress. If thyroidectomy is performed, thyrotoxicosis develops, and it does not immediately resolve because the half-life of T_4 is 7 to 8 days. Antithyroid medications should be slowly tapered (Sharma, 2014).

Teach the family about the need for lifelong thyroid hormone replacement if radiation or surgery is performed. The child should wear a medical alert identification bracelet, tag, or necklace. Make sure the child is monitored regularly to ensure that the T_4 level is adequate to sustain growth.

Evaluation

Expected outcomes of nursing care for the child with hyperthyroidism include the following:

- The child achieves balanced thermoregulation.
- The child participates in daily activities without experiencing fatigue.
- The child demonstrates a positive body image.

Disorders of the Parathyroid

Children usually have four parathyroid glands located posterior to the thyroid gland. Their primary function is to work in conjunction with vitamin D to regulate total body calcium.

Hyperparathyroidism

Primary hyperparathyroidism, rare during childhood, may result from a tumor (adenoma) or hyperplasia (Doyle, 2016a). Secondary hyperparathyroidism is due to disease outside of the parathyroid gland, leading to excessive secretion of parathyroid hormone. This is commonly seen in chronic renal failure when the kidneys are unable to reabsorb calcium, causing low serum calcium levels and stimulating continual secretion of parathyroid hormone (Kemper & van Husen, 2014). See Chapter 26.

At any age, symptoms of primary hyperparathyroidism may include bone pain, nephrolithiasis (kidney stones), and pathologic bone fractures. For primary hyperparathyroidism, unilateral surgical parathyroid exploration is recommended to remove the affected gland and biopsy the other gland on the same side. If bilateral disease is suspected, both sides are explored surgically (Belcher, Metrailer, Bodenner, et al., 2013). Treatment of secondary hyperparathyroidism focuses on prevention of hypercalcemia using vitamin D replacement and phosphorus binders (Kemper & van Husen, 2014).

Nursing Management

Nursing care centers on fluid management and electrolyte monitoring. In children who require surgery, assess for respiratory distress and a potential airway obstruction due to edema and a potential hematoma around the tracheal space. Monitor for signs of infection.

Following surgery, educate the child and parents to recognize signs of hypocalcemia and to provide appropriate amounts of calcium supplementation. After diagnosis or after surgical intervention, follow-up is important to monitor serum calcium and phosphorus levels to detect persistence of hyperparathyroidism.

Hypoparathyroidism

Primary hypoparathyroidism is rare, but it may result from congenital disorders (parathyroid aplasia, DiGeorge syndrome), surgical removal of the parathyroid glands (e.g., parathyroid adenoma, thyroidectomy), disease processes that destroy the parathyroid glands (Wilson disease, hemochromatosis), or medications (e.g., aluminum, asparagine, doxorubicin, cytosine, and arabinoside). Hypoparathyroidism can also be idiopathic. The primary result is hypocalcemia and hyperphosphatemia.

Infants may display hyperirritability, muscle rigidity, seizures, vomiting, abdominal distention, apneic episodes, intermittent cyanosis, or twitching. Muscle pain and cramps may progress to numbness, stiffness, and tingling of the hands and feet. A positive **Chvostek sign** (spasm of facial muscles after tapping facial nerve) may be present. Tetany and convulsions may occur with hypocalcemia (Doyle, 2016b).

Serum calcium and PTH levels are low and serum phosphorus is elevated. Radiographs often demonstrate increased bone density. Oral calcitriol and calcium are prescribed. Foods with high phosphorus content (dairy products and eggs) are limited (Doyle, 2016b).

Nursing Management

Assess and stabilize the airway, breathing, and circulation. In the acute care setting, children should be placed on a cardiorespiratory monitor. Maintain seizure precautions until normal serum calcium levels are attained. Obtain intravenous access and administer calcium supplementation as ordered.

SAFETY ALERT!

Dilute intravenous calcium per hospital protocol. Infiltration of IV calcium can cause extravasation and tissue sloughing. Always check the patency of the IV prior to administration. Monitor ECG during administration. Evaluate for hypocalcemia and hypercalcemia after administration.

Partner with the family to ensure their understanding of the need for calcium supplementation and reduced intake of phosphorus. Teach the family that periodic monitoring of calcium levels is important. Inform the family that hypoparathyroidism may require lifelong therapy.

Disorders of Adrenal Function

Cushing Syndrome and Cushing Disease

Cushing syndrome, also called *adrenocortical hyperfunction*, is characterized by a group of symptoms resulting from excess blood levels of glucocorticoids (especially cortisol). The most common cause of Cushing syndrome is the prolonged administration of glucocorticoid hormones (White, 2016a). Cushing disease is a type of Cushing syndrome and is caused by a pituitary tumor (Shah & Lila, 2011). During infancy most cases of endogenous Cushing disease are caused by a functioning adrenocortical tumor. The most common cause of endogenous Cushing syndrome in children older than 7 years of age is Cushing disease in which a pituitary tumor (adenoma) secretes excessive ACTH. This leads to bilateral adrenal hyperplasia (White, 2016a). The remainder of this discussion will focus on the child with Cushing syndrome caused by a pituitary tumor (Cushing disease). See *Clinical Tip* and *Safety Alert!* for discussions of Cushing syndrome caused by corticosteroid administration.

Clinical Tip

Cushingoid features occur most often in children receiving high doses of corticosteroids or corticosteroids over a prolonged period of time. Cushingoid features may develop in a shorter time than occurs with Cushing disease. Corticosteroids suppress adrenal function when administered long term. These children have exogenous Cushing syndrome and are at increased risk of hypertension, hyperglycemia, weight gain, linear growth retardation, and fractures (White, 2016a). These children may also exhibit mood swings and are at increased risk for infection (Wilson, Shannon, & Shields, 2016).

Obesity is common in children with Cushing syndrome. Excessive weight gain is followed by slowed linear growth. The child develops the characteristic cushingoid features, which include a rounded (moon) face with prominent cheeks. Additional manifestations include hirsutism, acne, deepening of the voice, and hypertension (White, 2016a). Older children may also experience delayed puberty, irregular menstrual periods, headaches, weakness, pathologic fractures, emotional problems, and hyperglycemia (Pluta, Burke, & Golub, 2011; White, 2016a).

Diagnosis is based on characteristic physical findings and laboratory values, including increased 24-hour urinary levels of free cortisol and elevated nighttime salivary cortisol level. The child will also have an abnormal glucose tolerance test (White, 2016a). See Appendix D for laboratory values.

The adrenal-suppression test using an 11 p.m. dose of dexamethasone reveals that adrenal cortisol output is not suppressed overnight as would occur normally in children. Computed tomography (CT) and magnetic resonance imaging (MRI) are used to detect the specific location of tumors in the adrenal and pituitary glands.

Surgical removal of the pituitary adenoma is the current treatment of choice when this is the cause of Cushing syndrome. Irradiation of the pituitary is performed when surgical removal of the adenoma does not substantially reduce cortisol levels. Bilateral removal of the adrenal glands may be necessary in some cases to stop the excessive secretion of cortisol. Lifelong hormone replacement is required when both adrenal glands are removed (Pluta et al., 2011; White, 2016a).

Nursing Management

Nursing assessment includes monitoring the child's vital signs, fluid status, nutritional status, and weight. Additional assessment includes monitoring muscle strength and endurance during hospital play activities.

Teach the child and family about the disorder and its treatment. For children undergoing surgery, provide preoperative and postoperative teaching and care. Answer any questions the child and family may have and explain all laboratory and diagnostic tests. Explain to parents that the child's cushingoid appearance is reversible with treatment. Refer to Chapter 24 for general nursing care of the child with cancer. Provide nutritional guidance or refer the child and parents to a registered dietician to promote maintenance of an appropriate weight. Encourage the child to discuss feelings regarding changes in physical appearance. Assist the child and family to identify effective coping strategies.

For children who need cortisol replacement therapy following the surgical removal of both adrenal glands, administering the medication early in the morning or every other day causes fewer symptoms and mimics the normal diurnal pattern of cortisol secretion. Cortisol replacement in the postoperative period must be explained carefully to the parents. Hydrocortisone (Cortef, Solu-Cortef, cortisone acetate) is available in liquid, tablet, or injectable form. Parents may need to crush the tablet and mix with a small amount of applesauce, but the entire dose of medication must be taken. The oral preparations of cortisone have a bitter taste and can cause gastric irritation. Giving the dose at mealtimes and using antacids between meals help reduce these side effects. Teach parents how and when to administer the injectable form—usually when the child is vomiting, has diarrhea, or cannot take the oral medication. Failure to give medication when the child is ill may lead to severe illness and cardiovascular collapse.

Congenital Adrenal Hyperplasia

Congenital adrenal hyperplasia (CAH) is an autosomal recessive disorder occurring in 1 in 10,000 to 1 in 20,000 births (Boyse, Gardner, Marvicsin, et al., 2014). CAH is considered to be an inborn error of metabolism.

ETIOLOGY AND PATHOPHYSIOLOGY

Approximately 90% to 95% of children with congenital adrenal hyperplasia have a deficiency in 21-hydroxylase (Hird, Tetlow, Tobi, et al., 2015). Children with CAH have insufficient production of aldosterone and cortisol and an overproduction of androgen (Boyse et al., 2014; Hird et al., 2015).

Of the two classic forms of the disorder, 75% are salt-losing, caused by aldosterone deficiency and overproduction of androgen, and 25% are non–salt-losing with **virilization** (the production of masculine secondary sexual characteristics in females). In all forms, increased secretion of ACTH occurs in response to diminished cortisol levels (Nimkarn, Lin-Su, & New, 2011).

Families Want to Know

Hydrocortisone Administration

Teach the family the following tips regarding hydrocortisone administration:

- Always give the medication at the times prescribed since the schedule follows the body's normal cortisol release pattern.

- Never abruptly discontinue the medication.

- Have the child wear a medical alert ID.

- If the child has vomiting or diarrhea and is unable to take the medication by mouth, administer the injections to replace oral doses as instructed and notify the healthcare provider immediately. Higher doses of hydrocortisone are needed when the child is ill.

- Always have injectable hydrocortisone available at home, at school, and everywhere the child travels. An emergency kit should be available at all times to supply cortisol to the child during acute illnesses and stressful situations. Check expiration dates frequently and maintain current medications in the emergency kit.

During fetal development the lack of cortisol triggers the pituitary to continue secretion of ACTH. This in turn stimulates overproduction of the adrenal androgens. Virilization of the female external genitalia begins in week 10 of gestation. If untreated, the overproduction of androgens results in accelerated height, early closure of the epiphyseal plates, and premature sexual development with both pubic and axillary hair.

CLINICAL MANIFESTATIONS

Congenital adrenal hyperplasia is the most common cause of **pseudohermaphroditism** (ambiguous genitalia) in newborn girls (see Figure 30–5). The female baby is born with an enlarged clitoris and partial or complete labial fusion. Females who are severely virilized may be mistaken for males with cryptorchidism, hypospadias, or micropenis (see Chapter 26). The uterus, ovaries, and fallopian tubes are normal. The male newborn may look normal at birth or may have a slightly enlarged penis and hyperpigmented scrotum. The boy may have tall stature and an adult-sized penis by school age, but the testes are appropriately sized for age. Partial enzyme deficiency produces less obvious symptoms. Precocious puberty, tall stature for age, acne, and excessive muscle development may be noted in both males and females as the child grows. As a result of early epiphyseal fusion, adult stature is shorter.

Signs of adrenal insufficiency may be the first indication of the disorder. Recurrent vomiting, dehydration, weakness, metabolic acidosis, hypotension, hypoglycemia, hyponatremia, and hyperkalemia are characteristic signs of the salt-wasting form of the disorder (White, 2016b).

CLINICAL THERAPY

Diagnosis in infants and children is usually confirmed by laboratory evaluation of the serum 17-hydroxyprogesterone (17-OHP) level (Hird et al., 2015). Routine newborn screening for congenital adrenal hyperplasia is performed in all 50 states (National Newborn Screening and Genetics Resource Center, 2014). Prenatal diagnosis is available. In instances of ambiguous genitalia, a karyotype determines the infant's gender (see Chapter 3). Ultrasonography may be used to visualize pelvic structures.

In the salt-wasting form of the disorder, the child may have hyponatremia, hyperkalemia, acidosis, hypoglycemia, a high urine sodium level, and low serum and urinary aldosterone levels. Serum concentrations of testosterone in girls and

androstenedione in boys and girls are elevated in affected infants. Measurement of ACTH and 17-hydroxyprogesterone levels reveals high readings, while the serum cortisol level is inappropriately low in comparison to ACTH (White, 2016b).

The goal of treatment is to suppress adrenal secretion of androgens by replacing deficient hormones. This is accomplished by the lifelong use of oral glucocorticoids (dexamethasone, prednisone, or hydrocortisone). The glucocorticoid replacement reduces secretion of ACTH, which had overstimulated the adrenal cortex. As a result, excessive adrenal androgen production is suppressed. The dose is individualized by monitoring growth parameters, bone age, and hormone levels. If the infant has the salt-wasting form of the disorder, salt is added to the infant's formula, and a mineralocorticoid is given to replace the missing hormone. Hormone dosage must be doubled or tripled during acute illnesses or injury and for surgery. Injectable hydrocortisone is used for severe stress. Generally, there are no side effects to the hormone; however, elevated doses can result in hypertension and growth impairment. Adrenalectomy is recommended only in cases when medical therapy is ineffective (Sharma & Seth, 2014; White, 2016b).

Reconstructive surgery of the enlarged clitoris is often performed on girls during the first year of life; however, some centers support waiting until adolescence, allowing the girl to participate in the decision for surgery.

Nursing Management

For the Child With Congenital Adrenal Hyperplasia

Nursing Assessment and Diagnosis

Assess the infant and child for signs of dehydration, electrolyte imbalance, and hypovolemic shock in the salt-wasting form of the disease (see the *Clinical Skills Manual* SKILLS). Monitor the airway, breathing, circulation, and responsiveness. Assess vital signs and peripheral perfusion (capillary refill, distal pulses, color and temperature of the extremities) frequently to detect early changes in condition such as hypovolemia.

Assess the parents' emotional response to a child with ambiguous genitalia and a chronic condition. Explore their values and beliefs regarding gender roles and sexuality while awaiting results of the karyotype.

Nursing diagnoses for the child with congenital adrenal hyperplasia might include the following (NANDA-I © 2014):

- *Parenting, Impaired,* related to a child with undetermined gender identity
- *Caregiver Role Strain* related to care of a child with a chronic, potentially life-threatening condition
- *Fluid Volume: Deficient, Risk for,* related to failure of regulatory mechanisms and excess excretion of salt by the kidneys
- *Growth: Disproportionate, Risk for,* related to accelerated growth and premature closure of epiphyseal plates

Planning and Implementation

Nursing care of the newborn with CAH focuses on teaching parents about the disorder and its treatment, offering emotional support, and providing preoperative and postoperative teaching for parents of infants undergoing reconstructive surgery. The administration of glucocorticoids and mineralocorticoids must be carefully controlled.

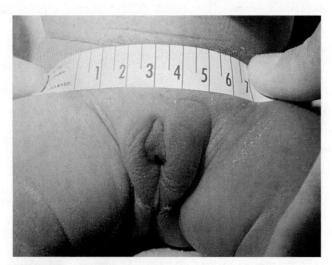

Figure 30–5 **Newborn girl with ambiguous genitalia.**

SOURCE: Courtesy of Patrick C. Walsh, MD.

It is often difficult for parents to accept that their infant, whose genitalia look male, is really female. Reassure parents that with medication and surgery, the genitalia assume a female appearance and all organs necessary for future childbearing are usually functional. Several surgeries may be performed before 2 years of age and then during adolescence to dilate the vagina. Because of the risk for adrenal insufficiency, the child will most likely be hospitalized for surgery rather than having outpatient surgery.

Nurses can assist parents in educating the child's siblings, grandparents, other family members, and childcare workers about the condition. In the newborn nursery, the infant should be referred to as "your beautiful infant," not "your son" or "your daughter," until gender identity is confirmed.

Inform parents that genetic counseling should be provided for the child during adolescence. Inform parents considering a future pregnancy that prenatal testing may detect congenital adrenal hyperplasia in the fetus. Refer the family for counseling if indicated.

COMMUNITY-BASED NURSING CARE

Teach parents about the special problems that develop in the salt-wasting form of the disease during acute illness. Explain the medication regimen and help the family develop an emergency care plan. The child should wear a medical alert identification. Teach parents how to administer intramuscular injections of hydrocortisone. If injectable hydrocortisone is not available, the child needs urgent treatment in an emergency department. The child may become dehydrated quickly and need intravenous fluid and electrolyte replacement in addition to higher doses of hydrocortisone.

Evaluation

Expected outcomes of nursing care for congenital adrenal hyperplasia include the following:

- Parent–newborn attachment is achieved.
- The child maintains fluid volume balance.
- The child achieves age-appropriate growth and developmental milestones.
- The parents demonstrate understanding of treatment and respond appropriately when injectable medication is needed.

Adrenal Insufficiency (Addison Disease)

Adrenal insufficiency, also known as *Addison disease*, is a rare disorder in childhood characterized by a deficiency of glucocorticoids (cortisone) and mineralocorticoids (aldosterone). The lack of glucocorticoids affects the body's ability to handle stress. The majority of cases of Addison disease are caused by an autoimmune process. Other causes include infection, hemorrhage, medication use, and metastatic cancer (Michels & Michels, 2014).

Adrenal insufficiency usually develops slowly as the adrenal glands deteriorate. Symptoms generally worsen over a period of years. The early signs may not be noticed initially but include weakness, fatigue, weight loss, and gastrointestinal symptoms such as nausea, vomiting, diarrhea, constipation, and abdominal pain. Other symptoms include hyperpigmentation, hypotension, dizziness, joint pain, salt cravings, and hypoglycemia (Michels & Michels, 2014; National Endocrine and Metabolic Diseases Information Service, 2014).

CLINICAL THERAPY

The ACTH stimulation test is used to determine if the levels of cortisol are adequate. Serum cortisol is measured in the early morning. Low levels of serum cortisol are associated with adrenal insufficiency. The diagnostic workup also includes a complete blood count, serum electrolytes, and thyroid function tests. Hyponatremia and hyperkalemia are common in Addison disease. A CT scan may be used to visualize the adrenal glands (Ficorelli, 2013).

Treatment involves replacement of the deficient hormones with an oral glucocorticoid such as hydrocortisone, prednisone, or dexamethasone. Fludrocortisone acetate (Florinef), a mineralocorticoid, is given for aldosterone deficiency (Ficorelli, 2013).

Adrenal crisis (also called *Addisonian crisis* and *acute adrenal insufficiciency*) may be caused by stressors such as infection, surgery, trauma, vomiting, and diarrhea. Noncompliance with the treatment plan may also be a precipitating factor (Ficorelli, 2013). The crisis is treated with aggressive fluid resuscitation, intravenous glucose, and intravenous glucocorticoids such as hydrocortisone. Children will also need increased doses of steroids during periods of increased physiologic stress, such as surgery, stressful procedures, and febrile illnesses. In these cases, the dose of hydrocortisone should be tripled and given every 6 to 8 hours while the stressor is present. Injectable hydrocortisone should always be available in case the child is vomiting or unable to take oral fluids (Speiser & Wilson, 2014).

Nursing Management

Nursing management focuses on restoring hemodynamic homeostasis in the child with Addison disease who is acutely ill. Educating the child and parents about the disorder, providing emotional support, and caring for the child during acute episodes are other aspects of nursing management. See the earlier discussion of congenital adrenal hyperplasia for further detail.

Pheochromocytoma

Pheochromocytoma is a tumor that arises from the adrenal gland. Tumors that are extra-adrenal with no anatomic connection are called *paragangliomas* (Mishra, Mehrotra, Agarwal, et al., 2014). In most cases, these tumors are benign and curable. They can occur in a familial pattern (autosomal dominant trait) with a male-to-female ratio of 3:2. Most tumors diagnosed in children are identified between the ages of 6 and 14 years; however, this accounts for only 10% of these tumors as most are identified during adult years (White, 2016c). Pheochromocytomas may also be associated with neurofibromatosis (see Chapter 27).

The tumor causes an excessive release of catecholamines. Clinical manifestations include hypertension, palpitations, sweating, anxiety, tremors, and headache for those with symptomatic pheochromocytoma. Twenty to 30% of these tumors are detected incidentally without a history of symptoms (Shuch, Ricketts, Metwalli, et al., 2014)

CLINICAL THERAPY

Diagnosis is based on biochemical studies measuring catecholamines in the blood and urine. Radiologic imaging with CT or MRI is used to provide the location of the tumor.

The treatment of choice is curative surgical removal of all identified tumors; however, the procedure is dangerous and may result in pheochromocytoma crisis. Removal of the tumor during surgery may cause a release of stored epinephrine and norepinephrine, leading to elevated blood pressure and changes in heart rate (pheochromocytoma crisis). If this occurs, alpha-adrenergic blocking agents are administered.

Medications to control hypertension, tachycardia, and catecholamine release are given for 7 to 21 days before surgery (Tsirlin, Oo, Sharma, et al., 2014). Plasma catecholamines are used to measure the effectiveness of the preoperative adrenergic blockade. Postoperatively, for several days, a 24-hour urine collection is measured for catecholamines to determine if all tumor sites were removed. With successful removal of all tumor sites, the prognosis is generally good. Follow-up is important to assess for recurrence.

Nursing Management

Nursing care is mainly supportive. Provide preoperative and postoperative teaching and care (see Chapter 11). Preoperatively, monitor vital signs and observe for signs of complications associated with pheochromocytoma crisis. Administer antihypertensives and watch for any signs of hyperglycemia, as discussed later in this chapter. Postoperatively, the child may be managed initially in an intensive care unit. Monitor blood pressure and glucose levels. Hypoglycemia and hypotension may occur following the withdrawal of excessive amounts of catecholamines. Observe for changes in neurologic status, respiratory distress, and signs of shock. Lifelong follow-up care with screening for hypertension and increased urinary catecholamine levels is required as symptoms recur if the child has other tumors not yet detected that activate at a later age (Tsirlin et al., 2014; White, 2016c).

Disorders of Pancreatic Function

Diabetes Mellitus

Diabetes mellitus, the most common metabolic disease in children, is a disorder of hyperglycemia resulting from defects in insulin secretion, insulin action, or both, leading to abnormalities in carbohydrate, protein, and fat metabolism (American Diabetes Association [ADA], 2014a). There are two main types of diabetes. Most children have immune-mediated type 1 diabetes, formerly called *insulin-dependent diabetes mellitus* or *juvenile diabetes*.

Type 1 Diabetes

In the United States, approximately 1 in every 400 to 600 children and adolescents have type 1 diabetes (Monaghan, Hoffman, & Cogen, 2013). According to the SEARCH for Diabetes in Youth Study, an estimated 18,436 people less than 20 years of age were diagnosed during 2008 to 2009. Non-Hispanic White children and adolescents had a higher incidence of new-onset type 1 diabetes than other groups (Centers for Disease Control and Prevention [CDC], 2014).

ETIOLOGY AND PATHOPHYSIOLOGY

Type 1 diabetes results from destruction of pancreatic islet beta cells, which fail to secrete insulin. The body becomes dependent on exogenous sources of insulin. Type 1 diabetes is a multifactorial disease caused by autoimmune destruction of insulin-producing pancreatic beta cells in individuals who are genetically predisposed (ADA, 2014a).

Type 1 diabetes has familial tendencies but does not show any specific pattern of inheritance. The number of autoantibodies helps predict the risk of developing type 1 diabetes. For children with one antibody, the risk is only 10% to 15%, while those with three or more antibodies have a risk of 55% to 90% (Marcdante & Kliegman, 2015). The child inherits a susceptibility to the disease rather than the disease itself. It is believed that an event such as a virus or other environmental factors trigger the inflammatory process, resulting in development of islet cell serum antibodies. These antibodies can be detected in the blood months to years before the onset of beta cell destruction (Marcdante & Kliegman, 2015).

Insulin helps transport glucose into the cells so that the body can use it as an energy source. It also prevents the outflow of glucose from the liver to the general circulation. Environmental factors such as enteroviruses or toxins are believed to lead to an autoimmune destruction of the beta cells in the islets of Langerhans (see *Pathophysiology Illustrated: Mechanism of Diabetes Mellitus*). Antigens are generated, leading to production of antibodies that indicate ongoing destruction of the islet cells. Chronic immune-mediated destruction of the beta cells continues over a period of time. Symptoms of type 1 diabetes are evident when approximately 90% of the beta cells have been destroyed (Craig et al., 2014)

As the secretion of insulin decreases, the blood glucose level rises and the glucose level inside the cells decreases. When the renal threshold for glucose (180 mg/dL) is exceeded, **glycosuria** (abnormal amount of glucose in the urine) occurs as a result of osmotic diuresis (Svoren & Jospe, 2016). Fluids follow the highly osmotic glucose and water is excreted in large volumes of urine (polyuria).

When glucose is unavailable to the cells for metabolism, free fatty acids provide an alternate source of energy. The liver metabolizes fatty acids at an increased rate, producing acetyl coenzyme A (CoA). The by-products of acetyl CoA metabolism (ketone bodies) accumulate in the body, resulting in a state of metabolic acidosis, or ketoacidosis. (Refer to Chapter 18 for a discussion of metabolic acidosis.)

CLINICAL MANIFESTATIONS

Children with type 1 diabetes generally present with polyuria, polydipsia, and weight loss. **Polyphagia** (excessive appetite) may be present. Enuresis may also occur in a previously toilet-trained child (Craig et al., 2014). The child may also present with a history of fatigue (Table 30–5). Children with new-onset diabetes may present with diabetic ketoacidosis (DKA). The prevalence varies but is higher in children less than 5 years of age with a reported incidence of 17.3% to 54.5% in that age group (Larsson et al., 2011). Other investigators report an overall incidence of DKA in youth at the time of diagnosis as being 15% to 67% (Szypowska & Skora, 2011). See the following *Clinical Tip* for information about cystic fibrosis–related diabetes.

Clinical Tip

Cystic fibrosis–related diabetes (CFRD) has similar features of types 1 and 2 diabetes; however, it is considered to be a separate condition. In cystic fibrosis, the pancreas is scarred and does not produce sufficient insulin (as in type 1 diabetes), which is referred to as **insulin deficiency**. Another mechanism of CFRD is **insulin resistance**, an impairment in insulin receptors on cell membranes, leading to inability to transfer sufficient amounts of glucose into cells, requiring higher levels of insulin for metabolism. Insulin deficiency and insulin resistance combined can lead to the development of diabetes more frequently in these patients than in the general population (Cystic Fibrosis Foundation, 2012).

Pathophysiology Illustrated: **Mechanism of Diabetes Mellitus**

Destruction of the alpha and beta cells in the islets of Langerhans produces multiple metabolic changes. Acute signs and symptoms are followed by short-term and long-term complications if the disease is not well managed.

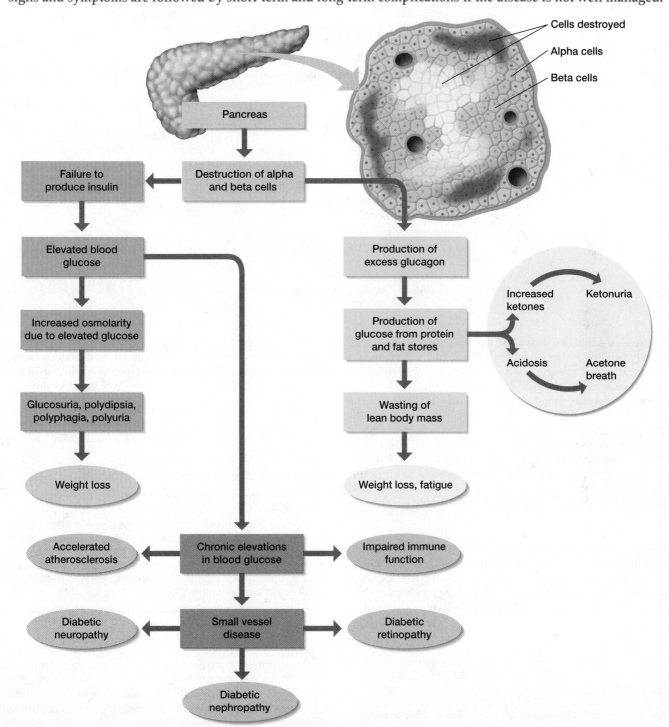

CLINICAL THERAPY

Diagnosis is based on the presence of classic symptoms and one of the following plasma glucose levels (ADA, 2014a, p. S88; 2014b, p. S15):

- A_{1c} greater than or equal to 6.5%
- Fasting plasma glucose greater than or equal to 126 mg/dL (7 mmol/L), no caloric intake for at least 8 hours

- Two-hour plasma glucose greater than or equal to 200 mg/dL (11.1 mmol/L) during an oral glucose tolerance test
- Random plasma glucose concentration greater than or equal to 200 mg/dL (11.1 mmol/L) in a patient with classic symptoms of hyperglycemia

When an asymptomatic child's screening test reveals an elevated glucose level, confirmation of a second fasting plasma

TABLE 30–5 Clinical Manifestations of Diabetes by Type

CAUSE	CLINICAL MANIFESTATIONS	CLINICAL THERAPY
Type 1—immune mediated, insulin deficiency due to pancreatic beta-cell destruction	Polyuria, polydipsia May have polyphagia Weight loss Ketoacidosis may be present at diagnosis, at continued risk for ketoacidosis Short duration of symptoms Initial period of decreased insulin requirement, then need insulin for survival	Blood glucose monitoring Insulin Dietary management, balancing carbohydrate intake to insulin Exercise
Type 2—insulin resistance with relative insulin secretory defect	Obese, little or no weight loss, or may have significant weight loss Acanthosis nigricans Long duration of symptoms Polyuria, polydipsia, may be mild or absent Glycosuria with or without ketonuria Ketoacidosis may be present Lipid disorders Hypertension Androgen-mediated problems such as acne, hirsutism, menstrual disturbances, polycystic ovary disease Excessive weight gain and fatigue due to insulin resistance	Diet with decreased calories and low-fat foods Decrease sedentary activity time or increase routine physical activity Blood glucose monitoring Oral medication (metformin) to improve insulin sensitivity May need insulin

glucose level should be performed. An oral glucose tolerance test is rarely required. Other laboratory tests for known autoantibodies can indicate an autoimmune attack against the insulin-producing beta cells of the pancreas, and may be helpful in some cases to distinguish between types 1 and 2 diabetes. Plasma C-peptide levels are low or undetectable in type 1 diabetes, indicating little or no insulin secretion (ADA, 2014a). A careful history is necessary to rule out a stress-related illness, corticosteroid use, fracture, acute infection, cystic fibrosis, pancreatitis, or liver disease.

Clinical therapy for type 1 diabetes combines insulin, nutrition management to support growth and maintain blood glucose at near-normal levels, an exercise regimen, and psychosocial support.

Insulin Therapy. Multiple approaches to insulin therapy for children and adolescents are available, and an approach that works for the child and family should be selected. Children often need several daily injections of insulin before meals and at bedtime to maintain an optimal blood glucose level.

Clinical Tip

The American Diabetes Association (2014b) considers a fasting glucose level of 100 to 125 mg/dL (5.6 to 6.9 mmol/L) to be an *impaired fasting glucose (IFG)*, and a 2-hour postload glucose level of 140 to 199 mg/dL (7.8 to 11.0 mmol/L) to be an *impaired glucose tolerance (IGT)*. Individuals with IFG or IGT are considered at increased risk for developing diabetes. A hemoglobin A_{1c} value of 5.7% to 6.4% is an additional risk factor for the development of diabetes.

A basal-bolus insulin regimen has resulted in improved glycemic control in the pediatric population (ADA, 2014b). When multiple injections are used, basal insulin is administered once a day using a very long-acting insulin (Glargine or Detemir). A bolus of rapid-acting insulin (insulin lispro, insulin glulisine, or insulin aspart) is administered with each meal and snack based on the carbohydrate grams consumed and the blood glucose level.

This means that a child may get six to seven injections a day. Stress, infection, and illness may either increase or decrease insulin needs. If basal-bolus therapy for type 1 diabetes is to be effective, the child and family need to do each of the following:

- Monitor the blood glucose appropriately to establish insulin requirements. For example, test glucose before and 2 hours after meals, as well as once a week at midnight and 3 a.m.
- Count carbohydrates consumed.
- Incorporate exercise into the daily routine.

Clinical Tip

Insulin is usually provided in prepackaged doses of 100 units/mL. Diluted insulin prepared by a pharmacist may be used for infants and toddlers who require a small insulin dosage. Insulin cartridges, disposable pens, and other devices are available, making insulin easy to carry by older children and adolescents who need frequent insulin injections during the day.

Continuous subcutaneous insulin infusion (CSII) pump therapy is being increasingly used by children and adolescents as the technology makes it possible to more closely match the plasma insulin levels found in children who do not have diabetes. CSII pump therapy has been used successfully in children of all ages and has been found to improve glycemic control with less hypoglycemia. Pump therapy requires the willingness of the patient or parent (with young children) to monitor blood glucose frequently, practice advanced insulin management skills, learn how to troubleshoot the pump, and be technology capable (Carchidi, Holland, Minnock, et al., 2011). Advantages and disadvantages of an insulin pump are outlined in Table 30–6.

Clinical Tip

Very long-acting insulins (Glargine and Detemir) cannot be mixed with other insulins.

TABLE 30–6 Advantages and Disadvantages of an External Insulin Infusion Pump

ADVANTAGES	DISADVANTAGES
• Delivers a continuous infusion of insulin to match the basal rate needed plus an insulin bolus at mealtime to more closely simulate normal pancreatic function. • Helps maintain blood glucose control between meals. • Decreases HbA$_{1c}$ level. • Improves glycemic control. • Improves growth in children. • Reduces number of injections. • New pumps calculate bolus insulin dose to number of carbohydrates consumed. • Allows child to eat with less adherence to a schedule and have a more flexible lifestyle. • Reduces number of injection sites, so variation in absorption decreases. • Results in fewer incidences of diabetic ketoacidosis. • Improves quality of life and psychosocial functioning.	• Requires constant vigilance and adherence, including frequent blood sugar testing, carbohydrate counting, and dose calculations. • Requires willingness to live connected to a device (can be disconnected for short periods by removing or clamping the catheter; however, DKA can occur within hours of interruption of insulin flow). • Pump visibility and size. • Requires site to be changed every 2 to 3 days. • Can increase risk of infection at the injection site. • Overuse of catheter-site locations may occur. • Possible weight gain can occur when blood glucose control improves. • Costs more than other insulin therapies. • Can increase risk of DKA and ketonuria secondary to pump failure.

Source: Data from Alsaleh, F. M., Smith, F. J., & Taylor, K. M. (2012). Experiences of children/young people and their parents, using insulin pump therapy for the management of type 1 diabetes: Qualitative review. *Journal of Clinical Pharmacy and Therapeutics, 37*, 140–147; Blackman, S. M., Raghinaru, D., Adi, S., Simmons, J. H., Ebner-Lyon, L., Chase, H.P., . . . DiMeglio, L. A. (2014). Insulin pump use in young children in the T1D Exchange clinic registry is associated with lower hemoglobin A1c levels than injection therapy. *Pediatric Diabetes, 15*, 564–572; Carchidi, C., Holland, C., Minnock, P., & Boyle, D. (2011). New technologies in pediatric diabetes care. *MCN, 36*(1), 32–39; Woerner, S. (2014). The benefits of insulin pump therapy in children and adolescents with type 1 diabetes. *Journal of Pediatric Nursing, 29*(6), 712–713.

Tight blood glucose control has long-term benefits and is becoming a standard of care for children of all ages. Maintaining tight control for young children is challenging because of the erratic eating patterns and difficulty in recognizing symptoms of hypoglycemia (Blackman et al., 2014). In the past, target blood glucose levels were higher in younger children because of these challenges and concerns over complications of hypoglycemia. While there are still concerns, better tools are available now to detect hypoglycemia. Additionally, there is now evidence that prolonged hyperglycemia in children can lead to early development of complications such as cardiovascular and renal disease. Based on this evidence, the American Diabetes Association (2014c) now recommends a target HbA$_{1c}$] goal of 7.5% across all pediatric age groups. It is important however that targets for blood glucose and HbA$_{1c}$] be individualized to achieve the best control and minimize the risk of both hypoglycemia and hyperglycemia (Chiang, Kirkman, Laffel, et al., 2014). The HbA$_{1c}$] is a predictor of the average blood glucose over the past 3 months (National Diabetes Information Clearinghouse, 2014).

Complications of type 1 diabetes (retinopathy, heart disease, renal failure, and peripheral vascular disease) result from long-term hyperglycemic effects on the blood vessels. Without careful management, children with diabetes may develop renal failure and loss of vision in adulthood. Intensive therapy is expected to reduce the risk for or delay the development of these complications. Risk may be further reduced if the adolescent does not begin smoking and if the blood pressure is controlled.

Nutrition Therapy. The goal of nutrition therapy is to provide adequate calories for the child's normal growth and development. An evaluation of the child's food intake, metabolic status, and lifestyle is necessary before establishing a nutrition plan. Daily caloric requirements are individualized for each child according to need. To facilitate adherence to the nutritional plan, an individualized approach with consideration of the child's and family's culture, lifestyle, and financial means should be incorporated. Careful instruction by a registered dietician or certified nurse educator is essential in the management of diabetes.

Carbohydrate counting provides flexibility in meal planning and is simple for children and adolescents to use. One carbohydrate choice equals 15 g of carbohydrates. The number of carbohydrate choices needed at meals and snacks varies depending on the child's individualized nutrition plan. Generally, 1 unit of insulin covers 15 g of carbohydrates, making insulin dosage calculation for meal coverage relatively easy; however, a different ratio of insulin to carbohydrates may be calculated for individual children. If additional carbohydrates are eaten at a meal or snack, the number of insulin units can also be adjusted, providing further flexibility. A high-fiber diet is also recommended for improved control of blood glucose.

Exercise Program. Physical activity is associated with increased insulin sensitivity. Regular exercise and fitness improve glucose control, reduce cardiovascular risk factors, contribute to weight loss, and improve overall well-being. Blood lipid levels are also positively affected. However, the child must have an adequate caloric intake to prevent hypoglycemia. Excessive exercise associated with sports requires careful planning and management.

Nursing Management

For the Child With Type 1 Diabetes

Nursing Assessment and Diagnosis

PHYSIOLOGIC ASSESSMENT

Children with type 1 diabetes are frequently admitted to the hospital at the time of diagnosis. Assess the child's physiologic status, focusing on vital signs and level of consciousness. Assess hydration by checking mucous membranes, skin turgor, and urine output. Blood initially is collected to monitor blood gases, glucose, and electrolytes. The frequency of blood collection will depend on whether the child is in diabetic ketoacidosis. When the child is stable, assess dietary and caloric intake and the ability of the child or family to manage care.

PSYCHOSOCIAL ASSESSMENT

Parents may feel guilty at the time of diagnosis if they waited to seek care until the child began to experience symptoms of diabetic ketoacidosis. Assess coping mechanisms, family strengths and resources, ability to manage the disease, and educational needs of both the child and parents. Examples of questions to ask in assessing the family's strengths and limitations in the child's disease management include:

- Do both parents or the single parent work? What hours?
- Who else is involved in the child's care?
- What is the child's usual daily schedule? Does the schedule vary on the weekend or any other days of the week?
- Does the child have health insurance? What coverage exists for diabetes education, treatment, and home management?
- Does the child have any cognitive, behavioral, motor, or visual problems coexisting with this condition?
- What other family stressors coexist with the diagnosis?

Clinical Reasoning Managing Adolescent Diabetes

Anthony, 12 years old, has just been diagnosed with diabetes mellitus. His parents took him to their family healthcare provider after Anthony complained of being constantly thirsty and hungry for over a week. Despite this, he has lost 5 lb. They note that he had a viral illness about 1 month ago but seemed to recover from it. His mother says that Anthony seemed lethargic for several days.

Anthony and his family must now learn to manage his diabetes using the combination of diet, exercise, and insulin therapy. Monitoring his blood glucose level is important in determining how much insulin he will need every day. Anthony's meals and activity will need to be coordinated with the insulin doses. Anthony and his parents will need to watch closely for signs of hypoglycemia. Develop a teaching plan that includes the following information:

- What causes diabetes?
- What potential problems need prompt treatment?
- What does Anthony need to monitor for when he gets sick?
- Intensive therapy will be a goal of Anthony's treatment. How can you help Anthony and his family decide if this should be accomplished with insulin injections or an insulin pump?
- What are some strategies to help an adolescent actively participate in his disease management and maintain optimal diabetic control?

DEVELOPMENTAL ASSESSMENT

Assess the child's developmental level, particularly fine motor skills and cognitive level. The child will need to learn how to obtain and read a blood glucose sample and how to inject insulin (see the *Clinical Skills Manual* SKILLS). Children can usually perform some of these tasks with supervision by 6 to 8 years of age.

Adolescents often perceive type 1 diabetes as a disability and may deny having the disease so they can be like their peers when eating and exercising. Talk with the adolescent and assess problem-solving skills associated with daily condition management, and the ability to manage special circumstances such as illness or changes in exercise. Self-management is the eventual goal, and the child's responsibilities are gradually increased.

Several diagnoses that may apply to the child newly diagnosed with type 1 diabetes are provided in the accompanying *Nursing Care Plans.* Additional diagnoses that may be appropriate include the following (NANDA-I © 2014):

- *Fluid Volume: Deficient, Risk for,* related to active fluid loss associated with hyperglycemia
- *Breathing Pattern, Ineffective,* related to metabolic acidosis
- *Coping, Ineffective,* related to inability to admit impact of disease on lifestyle

Planning and Implementation

Nursing care focuses on teaching the child and parents about the disease and its management, planning dietary intake, providing emotional support, and planning strategies for daily management in the community. Refer to the accompanying *Nursing Care Plans,* which summarize nursing care for the child who is hospitalized with newly diagnosed type 1 diabetes and the child who is receiving care in the community.

PROVIDE EDUCATION

The nurse is an important member of the management team (physician, nurse, registered dietician, certified nurse educator, and social worker) and is usually responsible for educating the child and family. The majority of teaching may be performed by an advanced practice nurse or a certified diabetes nurse educator in the clinic setting, since children may be hospitalized only briefly following diagnosis.

The timing and amount of information provided are especially important in the first days following diagnosis. Both the child and parents are very tired, and they are often in a state of shock and disbelief. Information presented during this period needs to be repeated. This time should be used to assess learning needs and to answer the family's questions. Initial teaching focuses on the survival skills necessary for home management, including insulin administration, blood glucose testing, meal planning, and the recognition and treatment of both hypoglycemia and hyperglycemia (Figure 30–6). Partner with the child and family to identify barriers to management.

Explain the goals of insulin therapy. Teach the parents and child (if appropriate) how to draw up and administer insulin or how to use an insulin pen. Insulin pens might be accepted more readily than the traditional syringe and vial method; they are

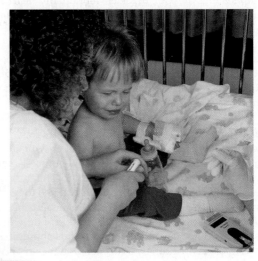

Figure 30–6 **This mother is learning how to test her child's blood glucose level.**

Nursing Care Plan: The Child Hospitalized With Newly Diagnosed Type 1 Diabetes Mellitus

1. Nursing Diagnosis: *Knowledge, Deficient (Survival Skills),* **related to lack of exposure to diabetic management in the newly diagnosed child (NANDA-I © 2014)**

GOAL: The child and parents will acquire survival skills for home management.

INTERVENTION	RATIONALE
• Assess the child's developmental level and select an educational approach and self-care activities to match.	• Learning goals for the child must match knowledge and skill expectations appropriate for developmental stage.
• Teach blood glucose monitoring, drawing up and injecting insulin, urine testing for ketones, record keeping, survival food guidelines, and when to call the healthcare provider.	• Diabetic management survival skills are needed for initial home management until more extensive education can be completed that permits more independent management.
• Use demonstration/return demonstration until the child and family are comfortable with procedures.	• Return demonstration permits evaluation, positive reinforcement and guidance for modification of techniques.

EXPECTED OUTCOME: Child and parents will demonstrate proper technique for blood glucose monitoring, urine testing for ketones, drawing up and injecting insulin doses, survival food guidelines, and record keeping.

GOAL: The child and parents will recognize signs and symptoms of hypoglycemia and hyperglycemia.

INTERVENTION	RATIONALE
• Teach signs and symptoms of hypoglycemic and hyperglycemic reactions.	• Recognition of and treatment of poor glucose control will prevent progression of symptoms.
• Teach the child to test blood glucose when feeling different than usual, and record the reading and symptoms felt.	• Permits child to learn his/her specific symptoms of hyperglycemia and hypoglycemia.

EXPECTED OUTCOME: Child and family will be able to describe symptoms of hypoglycemia and hyperglycemia.

2. Nursing Diagnosis: *Injury, Risk for (Complication),* **related to potential episodes of hypoglycemia and diabetic ketoacidosis (NANDA-I © 2014)**

GOAL: The child will experience few episodes of hypoglycemia during hospitalization.

INTERVENTION	RATIONALE
• Assess the child at least every 2 hr for signs of hypoglycemia. If signs are present, check blood glucose to verify and administer source of quick sugar.	• Hypoglycemia commonly occurs during hospitalization because of change in diet, lack of food intake, or illness.
• When the child is NPO for a special procedure, verify with healthcare provider when food, fluids, and insulin are to be given, or if an intravenous infusion with dextrose is to be given.	• Giving insulin without food intake can lead to hypoglycemia. Intravenous dextrose and insulin can be used when the child must be NPO.
• Have glucose paste or 50% dextrose solution readily available.	• Glucose paste is used for oral treatment. Dextrose is used for emergency intravenous treatment of severe hypoglycemia.

EXPECTED OUTCOME: Child and staff will manage episodes of hypoglycemia without a crisis developing.

GOAL: The child's condition will be treated slowly to gradually reverse hyperglycemia and ketoacidosis and to prevent cerebral edema.

INTERVENTION	RATIONALE
• Assess the child's mental status for improvement or deterioration.	• Improvement in mental status may indicate successful treatment. Deterioration may indicate onset of cerebral edema.

(continued)

Nursing Care Plan: The Child Hospitalized With Newly Diagnosed Type 1 Diabetes Mellitus (continued)

GOAL: The child's condition will be treated slowly to gradually reverse hyperglycemia and ketoacidosis and to prevent cerebral edema. (continued)

INTERVENTION	RATIONALE
• Check blood glucose and urine ketones frequently to confirm reduction in blood glucose level and ketosis, and to identify the insulin dose for administration.	• Frequent blood glucose and ketone level determination helps assess progress in treating ketoacidosis.
• Monitor and control IV fluid intake. Measure output.	• The child with ketoacidosis will be dehydrated. IV fluid intake needs to be carefully controlled to prevent cerebral edema.
• Have insulin doses checked by a second nurse.	• Doses are frequently small, and the possibility of error is great.

EXPECTED OUTCOME: Child's hyperglycemia and ketoacidosis will resolve without additional complications.

GOAL: The child and parents will demonstrate emergency management of hypoglycemia.

INTERVENTION	RATIONALE
• Identify sources of glucose to give in case of hypoglycemic reaction. Tell the child and parent to carry glucose tablets or paste with them at all times.	• Access to sources of glucose and its rapid administration are important for emergency care.

EXPECTED OUTCOME: Child and family will be able to identify several glucose sources for emergencies. The child and family have a source of glucose with them at each visit.

GOAL: The child and parents will demonstrate management of sick days.

INTERVENTION	RATIONALE
• Teach the child and family to test blood glucose and urine for ketones with acute symptoms and notify the healthcare provider.	• When the child is ill, hyperglycemia needs special management to prevent progression to ketoacidosis.

EXPECTED OUTCOME: Child's hyperglycemic episodes will not progress to ketoacidosis.

3. Nursing Diagnosis: _Nutrition, Imbalanced: Less than Body Requirements,_ related to disorder of glucose and insulin (NANDA-I © 2014)

GOAL: The child will eat a well-balanced diet and maintain normal height and weight proportions.

INTERVENTION	RATIONALE
• Encourage and serve meals and snacks with consistent carbohydrates at the same time each day.	• Keeps blood glucose levels stable during initial disease management stages.
• Provide a calorie nonrestricted diet.	• Enables weight lost during onset of diabetes to be regained.

EXPECTED OUTCOME: Child will regain weight lost and demonstrate normal growth and stable blood glucose levels.

GOAL: The child and parents will state understanding of dietary management of diabetes mellitus.

INTERVENTION	RATIONALE
• Make an appointment with a registered dietician or certified nurse educator who can assess the child's favorite foods and promote their integration into the child's diet. Reinforce the dietary information taught.	• The registered dietician or certified nurse educator can develop dietary recommendations that fit the specific needs of the child and include favorite foods, thereby increasing compliance with the diet.
• Provide sample menus and teach the use of carbohydrate counting.	• Assists the family and adolescent with diet planning.

EXPECTED OUTCOME: Child and parents will describe nutritional needs of the child and select the dietary management best suited to the family's and child's eating habits.

Nursing Care Plan: The Child With Previously Diagnosed Type 1 Diabetes Being Cared for at Home

1. Nursing Diagnosis: *Nutrition, Imbalanced: Less than Body Requirements,* **related to chronic illness (type 1 diabetes) (NANDA-I © 2014)**

GOAL: The child will eat a well-balanced diet that maintains weight proportional to height.

INTERVENTION	RATIONALE
• Assess height and weight regularly and plot on growth chart.	• Assesses change in body mass index to identify potential weight problem early.
• Make an appointment with a registered dietician or certified nurse educator who can assess the child's favorite foods and integrate them into a food plan that controls caloric intake. Encourage the child to keep a food diary.	• Inclusion of child's favorite foods helps child adapt to changes in the food plan.

EXPECTED OUTCOME: Diet records will indicate meals and snacks have the appropriate distribution of carbohydrates, protein, and fats, and daily caloric intake goals will be met.

2. Nursing Diagnosis: *Family Processes, Readiness for Enhanced,* **related to management of a chronic disease (NANDA-I © 2014)**

GOAL: The child and family will manage the food plan, exercise, blood glucose monitoring, and medication regimen.

INTERVENTION	RATIONALE
• Assess the family's lifestyle and attempt to fit the child's care needs into the family's schedule.	• Fitting the care to the family's lifestyle promotes adherence with the regimen.
• Discuss the family's routines for special occasions and vacations. Identify ways to modify the child's management for these occasions.	• It is important for the child to participate in special events with the family and peers as a normal child to promote psychologic development.

EXPECTED OUTCOME: Child and family will make minimal changes in usual lifestyle while managing the type 1 diabetes.

3. Nursing Diagnosis: *Coping, Ineffective (Individual),* **related to inadequate level of confidence in ability to cope (NANDA-I © 2014)**

GOAL: The child will demonstrate enhanced coping skills.

INTERVENTION	RATIONALE
• Ask how the child has solved problems in the past. Review possible problems the child may encounter. Together evaluate the effectiveness of solutions. Suggest other solutions to consider.	• Children's success in mastering maturational conflicts and daily psychosocial problems will influence their pattern of coping.

EXPECTED OUTCOME: Child will demonstrate enhanced coping skills and express positive attitude toward self. Child will display warmth and affection toward family.

GOAL: The child will develop positive self-esteem.

INTERVENTION	RATIONALE
• Role-play ways to talk about diabetes with friends and teachers. Encourage the child to express feelings about diabetes to those who the child trusts.	• Sharing information about the condition helps others understand changes in lifestyle needed by the child. Expressing feelings decreases anxiety.
• Encourage the child to attend diabetes camp.	• Learning and support networks developed at camp can promote self-esteem.
• Encourage the child to continue previous social activities and hobbies.	• Increased social interaction, especially in group sessions, improves self-esteem.

EXPECTED OUTCOME: Child will demonstrate confidence in interactions with peers and maintain social network.

easier to transport, they provide more accurate dosing, and they decrease anxiety associated with needles and insulin administration in public (Hanas, de Beaufort, Hoey, et al., 2011). Rotating the injection sites is important to decrease the chances of *lipoatrophy,* loss of subcutaneous tissue, or hypertrophy in which collagen is replaced by fat cells (Figure 30–7). The absorption rate of insulin varies by the site used. Insulin is usually absorbed most rapidly from the abdomen; however, insulin absorption is increased in the extremities with exercise. An understanding of the different types of insulin and their actions is essential.

Once the child and parents demonstrate understanding of this information, teach guidelines for managing episodes of hyperglycemia during acute illness and using an insulin correction scale. A correction scale indicates specific insulin dosages appropriate for a particular blood glucose level. The family also needs to learn "sick day" care guidelines to prevent diabetic ketoacidosis.

Initial teaching related to dietary management may be taught by the registered dietician. The nurse needs to assess understanding and reinforce principles taught. Assist the parent and child (if appropriate) to learn carbohydrate counting and how to plan nutritious meals for the child. See the accompanying *Nursing Care Plans* for additional guidelines.

Eating at consistent intervals is important for glycemic control, whether counting carbohydrates or following a conventional meal plan (three meals a day and three snacks a day). Although the child with diabetes is not restricted from eating any food, the child and parents need to learn about the relationship between foods eaten and insulin needed. Meal plans also need to be adjusted for exercise. Nonnutritive sweeteners such as aspartame and saccharin may be used in moderation. The child and family should learn how to read food labels. The meal plan should be customized, with the assistance of a registered dietician to the child's age, cultural and family food preferences, and activity level.

PROVIDE EMOTIONAL SUPPORT
The diagnosis of type 1 diabetes often comes as a shock to the family. If there is a familial history, parents may feel guilty about having caused the disease. The diagnosis of a chronic disease that requires daily management can be difficult to accept. Provide the family with information about diabetes education programs, refer them to support groups with other parents of children with diabetes, and assist them in learning the role of disease management. Support for the child depends on age and developmental stage. Encourage the child to express feelings about the disease and its management. The adolescent may benefit from contact with other adolescents who have diabetes.

DISCHARGE PLANNING AND HOME CARE TEACHING
Home care needs should be identified and addressed before discharge. Initial survival skills described earlier are taught with the plans for ongoing outpatient education.

Make every effort to incorporate the diabetic regimen (insulin administration, food plan, blood glucose monitoring, and exercise) into the family's present lifestyle. The fewer changes the family has to make, the greater the chance of adherence.

The family and child newly diagnosed with diabetes should be made aware of the "honeymoon phase." This is a period during new-onset diabetes when the child has some residual beta-cell function, which reduces exogenous insulin requirements. The child and family may assume this is an indication that the diabetes "is better." However, the insulin requirement does eventually return. The duration of this phase varies among individuals.

Provide written materials and refer parents to books and other materials they can use in teaching the child about diabetes. The Juvenile Diabetes Research Foundation and the American Diabetes Association are excellent sources of information.

COMMUNITY-BASED NURSING CARE
During follow-up visits, ask the child or parents about signs indicating problems with diabetic control. Questions to ask that could help identify such problems include:

- Is the child hungry at meals? Between meals?
- How much fluid is the child drinking?
- Has the child been going to the bathroom frequently or had episodes of bed-wetting?
- Does the child have dry skin?
- Are there sores on the feet? Do scratches or scrapes take a long time to heal?
- Has the child had any skin infections?

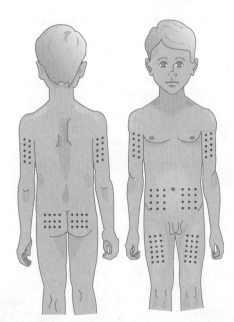

Figure 30–7 **Insulin injection sites. Give all morning insulin in one site (e.g., arms) and all evening insulin in another (e.g., legs) because of different rates of absorption from these sites. Space injections about 1.25 cm (0.5 in.) apart.**

Families Want to Know

Sick Day Guidelines

Parents should receive written guidelines specific to their child related to sick-day management. Some general guidelines include the following (American Diabetes Association, 2013; Brink et al., 2014):

- Monitor the blood glucose levels every 2 to 3 hours or as instructed.
- Test urine ketones every 4 hours or as instructed by the healthcare provider.
- The usual dose of insulin may be increased for high blood glucose levels.
- Notify the healthcare provider if the child has fever or other signs of infection, is unable to tolerate fluids, has ketones in the urine, has blood glucose levels that are out of target range, or has signs of dehydration.

- Does the child have changes in mood (depression, unexplained sadness, irritability) or energy level from day to day or throughout the day?
- Have there been any changes in vision?

Maintain a record of the child's growth measurements and vital signs. Review the child's typical dietary intake and exercise regimens. Assess the child's sexual development using Tanner staging guidelines (see Chapter 5). Puberty may be delayed if diabetic control is inadequate. Evaluation for the potential complications of diabetes should be performed annually, including blood for lipid levels, blood pressure, liver and renal function, urine for albumin, an ophthalmologic examination for retinopathy, and a neurologic examination of the extremities for neuropathies.

Education is ongoing, especially for children who develop diabetes at a young age. As they grow and assume more responsibility for their care, they need to learn more about the pathophysiology of the disease and the rationale for its management.

The child with diabetes should be treated as any other child without a chronic condition, including limit setting and consistent discipline for unacceptable behavior. Children with type 1 diabetes may learn maladaptive behaviors, using their disease to obtain something they want. Teach parents to be alert to signs of maladaption, such as helpless, demanding, or whining behaviors, and any evidence of poor coping. Additional behaviors may include skipping blood glucose testing and losing or damaging equipment. Food may become a battleground for toddlers who are picky eaters, but must eat enough for the insulin dose. Referral for counseling may be appropriate for some families.

Continually work with the child to encourage responsibility for self-care and with parents to promote the child's self-care (Figure 30–8). The child's developmental stage and cognitive level influence readiness to take on responsibility for self-care. Summer camps and other programs for children with diabetes are often helpful in providing education and support.

The preschool child's need for autonomy and control can be met by allowing the child to choose snacks or to pick which finger to stick for glucose testing and by helping parents to gather necessary supplies. School-age children can learn to test blood glucose, administer insulin, and keep records. They should be taught how to select foods and portion sizes appropriate for dietary management and how to plan food intake for an exercise program. School-age children need to learn to recognize the signs of hypoglycemia and hyperglycemia, and understand the importance of carrying a rapidly absorbed sugar product.

Although adolescents understand explanations about the potential complications of diabetes, they are present-time oriented and may rebel against the daily regimen of insulin injections, the food plan, and the exercise plan. Successful self-care depends in part on the adolescent's adjustment to the chronic nature of the

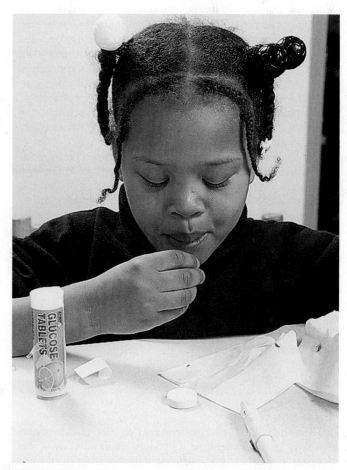

Figure 30–8 This girl is old enough to understand the need to take glucose tablets or another form of a rapidly absorbed sugar when her blood glucose level is low.

disease and feelings of being different from peers. Although adolescents are able to manage self-care, the desire to be like peers may interfere with treatment adherence. Talk with adolescents to assess their mood and to evaluate their motivation to manage the meal plan, exercise regimen, blood glucose monitoring, and insulin therapy. Discuss how carbohydrate counting and insulin dose adjustment may provide the flexibility to participate in activities with peers. Collaborate with the adolescent in preparation to assume care, and assist parents in accepting the growing independence from adult supervision. A discussion of the hazards associated with having diabetes and the use of alcohol, drugs, and tobacco should occur. At every subsequent healthcare visit, the adolescent should be asked about alcohol intake. See *Evidence-Based Practice: Coping With Type 1 Diabetes in Adolescents.*

Clinical Question

What factors are associated with how adolescents cope with type 1 diabetes?

The Evidence

Jaser and White (2011) explored how coping strategies affect resilience in adolescents with type 1 diabetes. Thirty participants ages 10 to 16 years with type 1 diabetes and their mothers completed questionnaires that focused on the teens' use of coping strategies, competence, and quality of life. Hemoglobin A_{1c} measurements were obtained from each teen's medical record. The study examined how adolescents use primary control and secondary control engagement strategies and/or disengagement strategies to cope with stress related to diabetes. Primary control coping strategies such as problem solving and emotional expression and secondary control coping strategies such as acceptance and distraction were associated with better metabolic control, better quality of life, and higher social competence. Use of disengagement strategies such as withdrawal or denial were associated with poorer metabolic control and lower social competence.

Jaser et al. (2012) studied the relationship of coping and stress reactivity with metabolic control, quality of life, and self-management in adolescents with type 1 diabetes. An ethnically diverse sample of 327 adolescents ages 11 to 14 with type 1 diabetes completed questionnaires about coping and stress reactivity, self-management, and quality of life. Hemoglobin A_{1c} measurements were obtained from medical records. Participants from low-income families and minority status had lower levels of primary control coping such as problem solving and secondary control coping such as acceptance. This group also had higher levels of disengagement coping such as avoidance. Results of the study also revealed that the use of primary and secondary control strategies to cope with stress related to diabetes was correlated with better self-management and better adaptation. The investigators concluded that there are differences in coping related to income and ethnicity and that coping strategies impact self-management and metabolic control in adolescents with diabetes.

Iafusco et al. (2011) evaluated the effectiveness of a chat line for adolescents with type 1 diabetes on quality of life and metabolic control. The participants were 193 children and adolescents 10 to 18 years of age. Computer-based chats, moderated by a physician, took place once a week and covered topics such as diabetes management, fears related to hypoglycemia, anxiety related to the future, and relationships. At routine office visits, a research assistant gathered demographic data and assessed management of diabetes. Questionnaires, including the Diabetes Quality of Life for Youth Inventory (DQOLY), were completed at baseline, 1, and 2 years. A control group consisted of 203 adolescents who did not participate in the chat line. Results of the study found that participation at least once a month in the chat group improved well-being and metabolic control.

Best Practice

Adolescents with type 1 diabetes must cope with the increasing responsibility for complex self-management, including insulin administration, blood glucose testing, exercise, and nutrition. The types of coping strategies that are used affect the adolescent's quality of life and metabolic control. It is important that these adolescents learn effective coping strategies such as problem solving and distraction. Interventions that involve group discussions about concerns related to diabetes and routine follow-up to assess coping strategies, quality of life, and metabolic control are essential in maximizing outcomes for these adolescents with diabetes.

Clinical Reasoning

How can you address coping strategies and quality of life issues in adolescents with diabetes? What interventions can you think of that may improve quality of life and metabolic control in these adolescents?

The child with type 1 diabetes may develop circulatory and neurologic changes over time. Emphasize the importance of good foot care from an early age—for example, wearing clean cotton socks, changing socks and shoes when they are damp, washing and drying feet, and keeping toenails short. Adolescents getting pedicures should inform the person performing them that they have diabetes.

Explain to parents that the child should wear some type of medical alert identification. Help them have an individualized school health plan developed (see Chapter 12) to ensure that school administrators and teachers can identify the signs of hypoglycemia or hyperglycemia and provide emergency management.

Evaluation

Expected outcomes of nursing care for children with type 1 diabetes can be found in the *Nursing Care Plans* in this chapter.

Diabetic Ketoacidosis

Diabetic ketoacidosis (DKA) is a common and potentially life-threatening condition that occurs primarily in children with type 1 diabetes. Potential causes of DKA include incorrect or missed insulin doses, incorrect administration of insulin, or an illness, trauma, or surgery. DKA may be present in children with new-onset diabetes.

Professionalism in Practice **Management of Diabetes in the School Setting**

Section 504 of the Rehabilitation Act of 1973 and the Americans with Disabilities Act of 1990 are federal laws that require that students with disabilities, including those with diabetes, be given an equal opportunity to participate in school activities. The position statement of the National Association of School Nurses states that a school nurse is required to develop an individualized health plan from the child's diabetes medical management plan. The school nurse oversees the implementation and evaluation of the plan (Butler, Fekaris, Pontius, et al., 2012). It is essential for the school nurse to work with parents to ensure that equipment and medications needed at school are provided so that children with disabilities are able to receive the care they need.

Health Promotion The Child With Diabetes Mellitus

Growth and Development Surveillance

- Compare the child's height, weight, and head circumference to age-specific norms to determine if growth is meeting expectations for age. Monitor body mass index (BMI) percentile at each healthcare visit.
- Assess developmental progress using the Denver II or another screening tool (refer to Chapter 6). Assess school performance.
- Assess for delays in development of secondary sexual characteristics and pubertal changes.

Nutrition

- Promote adherence to nutrition guidelines by including the child's personal preferences in the food plan.

Physical Activity

- Encourage regular physical activity and educate the child to modify insulin dosage or food intake for extra physical activity periods.
- Encourage the child to participate in sports when interested and work to balance exercise, food intake, and insulin dosage.

Oral Health

- Promote good dentition and oral hygiene.
- Regular dental visits are important to reduce risk of infections.
- The child with poorly controlled diabetes is at risk of gingivitis and cavities.

Mental and Spiritual Health

- Provide the child and adolescent an opportunity to discuss feelings regarding diabetes.

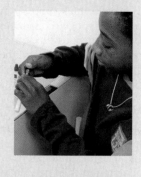

- Assess the adolescent for evidence of depression.

Relationships

- The child should attend school or child care as any other child. Parents may need support to find facilities able to monitor the child as needed and to provide the teaching required for facility employees.
- Encourage the development of special friends who can be informed about the child's disorder and seek help when the child has signs of hypoglycemia or hyperglycemia.

Disease Prevention Strategies

- Encourage the family to ensure that the child receives all recommended immunizations, including an annual influenza vaccine.
- Refer the child for an annual ophthalmologic examination.
- Maintain appointments for regular evaluation of HbA_{1c} to monitor glycemic control.

Injury Prevention Strategies

- Encourage the child to wear a medical alert identification.
- Encourage daily inspection of feet and foot care.
- Provide the family with strategies for safe disposal of needles and syringes.

Insulin deficiency is accompanied by a compensatory increase in hormones (epinephrine, norepinephrine, cortisol, growth hormone, and glucagon) that are released when inadequate glucose is delivered to the cells. The muscle cells break down protein into amino acids that are then converted to glucose by the liver, leading to hyperglycemia. The adipose tissue releases fatty acids that are transformed by the liver into ketone bodies. Their accumulation leads to ketoacidosis. The hyperglycemia causes an osmotic diuresis resulting in dehydration, acidosis, and hyperosmolality. The rising ketones lead to metabolic acidosis. DKA is associated with severe metabolic, electrolyte, and fluid imbalances.

Characteristic signs of DKA include polyuria, polydipsia, weight loss, abdominal pain, nausea and vomiting, tachycardia, signs of dehydration, flushed ears and cheeks, Kussmaul respirations, acetone breath (fruity smell), altered level of consciousness, and hypotension. Hyperglycemia, glycosuria, and ketonuria are also present. In response to metabolic acidosis, children complain of abdominal or chest pain, nausea, and vomiting. The disorder may progress to electrolyte disturbances, arrhythmias, altered consciousness, pupillary changes, irregular respirations, inappropriate slowing of the heart rate, and widening pulse pressure. See Table 30–7 for clinical manifestations of hypoglycemia and hyperglycemia.

Diabetic ketoacidosis is present with the following findings: blood glucose level greater than 250 mg/dL, serum ketones, acidosis (pH less than 7.3 and bicarbonate less than 15 mEq/L),

and ketonuria. Alteration in electrolytes occur. The blood urea nitrogen (BUN) and creatinine are elevated (Masharani, 2015).

The child with ketoacidosis is hospitalized. Medical management includes isotonic intravenous fluids and electrolytes for dehydration and acidosis. Intravenous insulin (0.1 unit/kg per hour) is administered by continuous infusion pump to decrease the serum glucose level at a rate not to exceed 100 mg/dL/hr. Faster reduction of hyperglycemia and serum osmolality increases the risk for cerebral edema. When glucose is lowered too rapidly, water is freed and attracted to the glucose, which has accumulated in large quantities in the brain. Cerebral edema is the most common complication of DKA and the most common cause of death in children with diabetes (Bialo, Agrawal, Boney, et al., 2015). As insulin and fluids are administered, potassium shifts to the cells, resulting in hypokalemia. Potassium replacement is needed as hypokalemia can lead to cardiac arrhythmia (McFarlane, 2011). See Chapter 27 for information about cerebral edema.

Nursing Management

Continuously monitor the child's vital signs, respiratory status, perfusion, and mental status. Assess for changes in neurologic status, respiratory pattern, blood pressure, and heart rate. Monitor for cardiac arrhythmias associated with hypokalemia. Assess for signs of dehydration, including dry skin and mucous membranes and depressed fontanelles in infants. Monitor blood glucose levels hourly or as indicated. Frequently monitor the electrolytes and acid–base status, as well as urine glucose and ketone levels as indicated. Intake and output are monitored hourly. Assess for signs of hypoglycemia that may occur during insulin infusion.

Intravenous fluids are given in boluses of 10 to 20 mL/kg rapidly over 5 minutes if the child is in hypovolemic shock. Adequate fluids are given to reverse the fluid deficit. The insulin infusion must be carefully titrated to control the gradual reduction in hyperglycemia. The child is tapered off intravenous insulin and transitioned to subcutaneous insulin when clinically stable. Oral feedings are reintroduced when the child is alert and the glucose level is stabilized.

The prevention of future episodes of DKA is important. The parents and child need to learn strategies to keep hyperglycemic episodes from progressing to DKA. Parents should have specific instructions on how often to check the blood glucose and when to check the urine for ketones when the child is sick. If the child has an elevated blood glucose and moderate or large amounts of ketones, treatment with extra insulin and fluids can be initiated. Increased attention to blood glucose and urine ketone monitoring

is especially important when the child has significant stressors such as an illness. It is important for the child and family to understand that insulin is required even when the child is not eating to counter the hormones secreted in response to the stressor.

SAFETY ALERT!
Only regular insulin is administered intravenously for treatment of hyperglycemia or diabetic ketoacidosis. Do not use other insulin types as they may lower the blood glucose too rapidly or too slowly.

Hypoglycemia in the Child With Diabetes

Hypoglycemia can develop within minutes in children with type 1 diabetes mellitus. The symptoms outlined in Table 30–7 may occur when blood glucose levels suddenly drop or fall below 70 mg/dL. Children are at risk of hypoglycemia because of their rapid growth rates and unpredictable eating habits and physical activity.

Families Want to Know

Preventing DKA

When to Monitor for DKA

- Abdominal pain
- Nausea, vomiting, and anorexia
- 1- or 2-day history of polyuria and polydipsia
- Has illness (e.g., viral or other) and is unable to eat

Recognizing Signs of DKA

- Change in mental status
- Blood glucose greater than 250 mg/dL
- Moderate to large ketones present in urine
- Fruity breath odor
- Rapid, deep respirations
- Decreased urine output

Source: Data from Masharani, U. (2015). Diabetes mellitus & hypoglycemia. In M. A. Papadakis, S. J. McPhee, & M. W. Rabow (Eds.), *CURRENT medical diagnosis & treatment 2015*. New York, NY: McGraw-Hill; McFarlane, K. (2011). An overview of diabetic ketoacidosis in children. *Paediatric Nursing, 23*(1), 14–19.

Families Want to Know

Treating Hypoglycemic Episodes

- If the child shows signs of hypoglycemia (pallor, sweating, tremors, dizziness, numb lips or mouth, confusion, irritability, altered mental status), test the blood glucose level.
- Assist the child to perform the test. Skills needed to get an accurate reading deteriorate with altered mental status.
- If the blood glucose reading is less than or equal to 70 mg/dL, give glucose rapidly. Use one of the following to give 15 g of rapid-acting glucose to raise the blood sugar level:
  - $\frac{1}{2}$ cup fruit juice
  - $\frac{1}{2}$ cup of regular cola or soda
  - 1 small box raisins
  - 3 to 4 glucose tablets
- Wait 15 minutes and recheck the blood glucose level. Repeat the 15 g of rapid-acting glucose if it is still less than or equal to 70 mg/dL. Recheck the blood glucose level in another 15 minutes.
- When blood sugar has returned to at least 80 mg/dL, give a more substantial snack such as cheese and crackers if the next meal will be more than 30 minutes later or an activity or exercise is planned.
- If the child is unconscious, administer glucagon by injection or spread glucose paste on the gums.

TABLE 30–7 Clinical Manifestations of Hypoglycemia and Hyperglycemia

CAUSE	CLINICAL MANIFESTATIONS	CLINICAL THERAPY
HYPOGLYCEMIA		
• Insulin dose too high for food eaten • Insulin injection into muscle • Too much exercise for insulin dose • Too long between meals/snacks • Too few carbohydrates eaten • Illness, stress	Rapid onset Irritability, nervousness, tremors, shaky feeling, difficulty concentrating or speaking, behavior change, confusion, repeating something over and over Unconsciousness, seizure, shallow breathing, tachycardia Pallor, sweating Moist mucous membranes, hunger Headache, dizziness, blurred vision, double vision, photophobia Numb lips or mouth	If conscious, give 15 g of carbohydrate. Wait 15 minutes and recheck blood glucose level. Give another 15 g of carbohydrate if 70 mg/dL or below. Recheck the blood glucose level in 15 minutes. If unconscious, give glucagon by injection.
HYPERGLYCEMIA		
• Insulin dose too low for food eaten • Illness or injury, stress • Too many carbohydrates eaten • Meals/snacks too close together • Insulin injected just under skin or injected into hypertrophied areas • Decreased activity	Gradual onset Lethargy, sleepiness, slowed responses, or confusion Deep, rapid breathing Flushed skin, dry skin Dry mucous membranes, thirst, hunger, dehydration Weakness, fatigue Headache, abdominal pain, nausea, vomiting Blurred vision Shock	Give additional insulin at usual injection time. Give correction scale insulin doses for specific blood glucose levels when ill or injured. Give extra injections if hyperglycemia and moderate to large ketones. Increase fluids.

Severe hypoglycemic episodes may occur at night in children who are treated with two to three injections per day. Other common causes include an error in insulin dosage, errors in injection technique, inadequate calories because of missed meals, or exercise without a corresponding increase in caloric intake. Severe hypoglycemia can cause seizures.

Hypoglycemia can be diagnosed on the basis of the sudden onset of signs and symptoms. A blood glucose reading should be taken to confirm a low blood sugar is possible if equipment is readily available. Give a glucose source immediately by mouth. If the child becomes unconscious, administer an injection of glucagon, or, if unavailable, administer sugar gel or glucose paste squeezed onto the gums. In the hospital setting, administer an intravenous infusion of dextrose to prevent progression of symptoms. Since the effects of dextrose and glucagon are temporary, additional snacks or a meal is provided. The child should be continually observed for several hours after treatment.

Nursing Management

Teach parents and children to recognize the signs of hypoglycemia and take appropriate action. Parents are taught to give **glucagon** (a hormone produced by the pancreas that helps release stored glucose from the liver) by injection for cases of severe hypoglycemia and to activate the emergency medical system (9-1-1). Reinforce the importance of balancing dietary intake, insulin, and exercise every day.

Type 2 Diabetes

Type 2 diabetes is a disease associated with insulin resistance (an alteration of the insulin receptor that signals the presence of insulin in the interior of cells). Significant risk factors for type 2 diabetes includes obesity, low levels of physical activity, intake of high-energy foods, low socioeconomic status, ethnicity, and family history of diabetes (Bacon, 2013; Dea, 2011; Svoren & Jospe, 2016). Over 75% of children with type 2 diabetes have a first- or second-degree relative with diabetes (Dea, 2011).

The increasing number of children being diagnosed with type 2 diabetes has caused significant concern in the healthcare community. According to the SEARCH for Diabetes in Youth Study, an estimated 5089 people younger than 20 years were newly diagnosed with type 2 diabetes annually during 2008 to 2009. The incidence was highest in children ages 10 to 19 and in U.S. minority populations (CDC, 2014). The true incidence is unknown because many children are undiagnosed.

Developing Cultural Competence Type 2 Diabetes Risk

Children of African American, Native American, Hispanic/Latino, and Asian/Pacific Islander origins are at greater risk for developing type 2 diabetes (American Diabetes Association, 2015).

ETIOLOGY AND PATHOPHYSIOLOGY

Children who are obese are at risk to develop type 2 diabetes because the excess body fat decreases the body's ability to use insulin (Bacon, 2013). The onset of puberty and increased secretion of growth hormone are believed to be contributing factors in the development of insulin resistance (Dea, 2011). The pancreatic cells produce more insulin in an attempt to overcome the insulin resistance and maintain a normal glucose tolerance. When the beta cells are not able to produce enough insulin, blood glucose levels increase (Khan, Cooper, & Del Prato, 2014).

CLINICAL MANIFESTATIONS

Signs and symptoms of type 2 diabetes vary. The child may not have any symptoms or may present with polydipsia, polyuria, blurred vision, and fatigue (American Diabetes Association, 2015). **Acanthosis nigricans** is described as a hyperpigmentation and thickening of the skin with velvety irregularities in the skin folds of the back of the neck, axillae, and flexor skin surfaces. It has been established as a risk factor for the development of type 2 diabetes and is associated with insulin resistance (Abraham & Rozmus, 2012) (see Figure 30–9). The child with type 2 diabetes is usually obese with a high waist circumference. Approximately 5% to 25% of children with type 2 diabetes present with ketoacidosis at the time of diagnosis (Dea, 2011).

CLINICAL THERAPY

Blood glucose levels of 200 mg/dL or greater without fasting or a fasting glucose of 126 mg/dL or greater, are diagnostic of diabetes (ADA, 2014b). HbA$_{1c}$] predicts the average blood glucose over the past 3 months (National Diabetes Information Clearinghouse, 2014). Islet cell autoantibodies, fasting insulin levels, and C-peptide levels are used to help differentiate between type 1 and type 2 diabetes but are not definitive. Islet cell autoantibodies (GAD-65, islet cell antibodies, insulin) are suggestive for type 1 diabetes; however, autoantibodies specific to a certain antigen are not present in approximately 15% of children with type 1 diabetes. Additionally, some children with type 2 diabetes will have detectable autoantibodies. While insulin and C-peptide levels are usually low in children with type 1 diabetes, there is some overlap with type 2, so these values are not helpful with the initial classification (Cohee, 2012). A fasting lipid profile is obtained since dyslipidemia (primarily elevated triglycerides and LDL cholesterol) is usually present (Svoren & Jospe, 2016). High blood pressure for age, gender, and height percentile is also seen (see Appendix B).

The multiple goals for managing the child with type 2 diabetes include the following: normalizing the blood glucose and HbA$_{1c}$ levels, decreasing weight, increasing exercise, normalizing lipid profile and blood pressure, and preventing complications. Nutrition education and weight loss make up the major therapy.

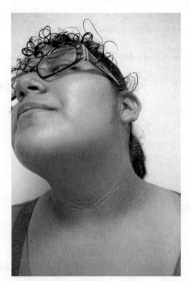

Figure 30–9 **Acanthosis nigricans.**

SOURCE: Benedicte Desrus/Alamy.

The child needs to have gradual, sustained weight loss, metabolic control of blood glucose levels, exercise, and emotional support.

If the child or adolescent presents with severe hyperglycemia or diabetic ketoacidosis, insulin will be required to gain initial glycemic control. When metabolic control is achieved, oral medication (metformin) is initiated as the child is weaned off of insulin. Metformin is used when diet and exercise efforts are inadequate to control hyperglycemia. Metformin improves the sensitivity of target cells to insulin, slows the gastrointestinal absorption of glucose, and reduces hepatic and renal glucose production. It can be used when there is normal liver and kidney function and no ketosis. The dosage may be gradually increased to improve metabolic control. If additional medication is needed, sulfonylureas may be used if metformin alone is not adequate or is contraindicated, but their use in pediatrics is limited. Thiazolidinediones are not approved for use in children but may be used if metformin is contraindicated. Some children ultimately require insulin for glycemic control (Svoren & Jospe, 2016).

Nursing Management

For the Child With Type 2 Diabetes

Nursing Assessment and Diagnosis

Because the child with type 2 diabetes does not often have an acute onset, assess any child with a body mass index (BMI) greater than 85th percentile for age and gender for signs of insulin resistance (acanthosis nigricans, hypertension, and dyslipidemia). Family history of diabetes in an overweight child is a reason to begin screening for the condition. Once the child has been diagnosed, monitor the child's blood glucose levels and blood pressure. Assess the child's diet and activity patterns to determine appropriate changes for disease management. Consider evaluating the siblings for diabetes.

Nursing diagnoses that may apply to the child with type 2 diabetes include the following (NANDA-I © 2014):

- *Activity Intolerance* related to sedentary lifestyle and disease state (insulin resistance)
- *Health Management, Family, Ineffective,* related to family conflict over changing eating patterns
- *Self-Esteem, Situational Low,* related to situational crisis associated with diagnosis of new-onset chronic illness

Planning and Implementation

The child with type 2 diabetes may be hospitalized at the time of diagnosis because of ketoacidosis. However, the nurse in an inpatient setting is more likely to encounter this child when hospitalized for another condition or during visits for health care in clinics or schools. Nursing care focuses on managing the child's blood glucose levels and hypertension during the hospitalization, assessing growth and dietary intake, evaluating goals for weight loss and exercise programs, and reviewing the child's knowledge about diabetes and strategies for management at home.

COMMUNITY-BASED NURSING CARE

Since the child is initially diagnosed with type 2 diabetes and managed on an outpatient basis, nursing care focuses on teaching the child and parents about the disease and its management, managing dietary intake, providing emotional support, and planning strategies for daily management in the community.

Educate the child and family about the disease and lifestyle changes required for effective management of the condition. Focus on the need to increase activity with routine exercise of at least 30 to 60 minutes daily and to decrease sedentary activity time, such as computer and television viewing time to no more than 2 hours daily. Customize the activity strategy for each child with motivation to develop a regular routine.

Work with the family to substitute high-calorie and high-fat foods with a meal plan sensitive to the family's resources and ethnic preferences. Suggestions include limiting fast food and snacking on fruits and vegetables rather than foods high in fat and sugar. Assess the child's height, weight, and BMI on each visit, and plot on the appropriate growth curve for age and gender. A gradual sustained weight loss or decrease in BMI is the goal. If the child is experiencing a height growth spurt, maintenance of weight rather than weight loss is the goal. Encourage the entire family to make dietary changes, especially since other family members are also at risk for the condition.

Teach the child and family to perform home blood glucose testing to monitor glycemic control. This will let the child and family know that efforts to manage the disease are successful. Take HbA$_{1c}$ levels at each visit to determine the average blood glucose level for the past 3 months. When dietary control and exercise are not successful in reducing blood glucose levels, teach the child and family about the prescribed oral medication.

Give the child and family opportunities to talk about the impact of the disease on their lives. Identify resources for information about strategies that have worked for other families. Identify local support groups and peer groups for the family and child. Suggest weekly activities, summer camps, and other ongoing programs to provide necessary support and motivation.

Make sure the child gets annual evaluations for potential complications of diabetes. The tests to be performed include blood for lipid levels, blood pressure, liver and renal function, urine for albumin, an eye examination for retinopathy, and a neurologic examination of the extremities for neuropathies. The child with type 2 diabetes has the same risk for developing long-term vascular complications as the child with type 1 diabetes when hyperglycemia is poorly controlled.

Evaluation

Examples of expected outcomes of nursing care include the following:

- The child decreases sedentary activity time to less than 2 hours a day.
- The child's daily intake of fruits and vegetables increases to five to eight servings daily, and total fat intake decreases to less than 30% of total calories.
- The child's BMI slowly and consistently decreases.

Disorders of Gonadal Function

Gynecomastia

Gynecomastia is a proliferation of glandular breast tissue in males that occurs in approximately 40% to 65% of adolescent boys. Gynecomastia results from an imbalance in estrogens and androgens in the breast tissue. Gynecomastia is generally idiopathic, although it can be associated with a chronic disorders, tumors, or drug use (Saito et al., 2014). The condition disappears in 75% of cases. If gynecomastia is causing pain or psychologic distress to the adolescent, treatment with a medication such as tamoxifen or surgical intervention with a minimally invasive approach may be indicated (Fischer et al., 2014).

Nursing care focuses on reassuring the child and his parents that gynecomastia is common and transient. Because of the body image concerns common during adolescence, embarrassment is a frequent problem. Recommend clothing styles and other methods to camouflage the enlarged breasts. If treatment is indicated, education regarding medication use or surgery is needed.

Amenorrhea

Amenorrhea, or lack of menstruation, may be primary or secondary. Criteria for primary amenorrhea include absence of menarche by age 14.5 years in association with no growth or development of secondary sexual characteristics, or absence of menses by age 16 when secondary sexual characteristics and growth are present.

Secondary amenorrhea is the cessation of menstrual periods 6 months or 3 cycles after menstruation has begun; it is characterized by an absence of spontaneous bleeding for at least 120 days. Pregnancy is the most common cause of secondary amenorrhea in adolescents. It is common for adolescents to have irregular menstrual cycles and duration of the menstrual period for 1 to 2 years after menarche. A large number of cycles are anovulatory for the first 2 years after menarche.

Primary amenorrhea is most often caused by structural defects of the reproductive system; chromosomal abnormalities (such as Turner syndrome); hypothalamic or pituitary tumors; thyroid dysfunction; or polycystic ovary syndrome. No underlying pathologic condition is found in some adolescents. Primary or secondary amenorrhea may be found in competitive athletes and in youth with anorexia nervosa (see Chapter 14).

A thorough history (including sexual activity), physical examination, and laboratory evaluation are required to determine the cause of amenorrhea. The history focuses on asking questions about recent excessive weight loss or gain; excessive physical activity or sports training; chronic illness; use of illegal drugs, birth control pills, or phenothiazines; emotional problems; and age of the mother at menarche. A family history helps to identify other female family members with similar issues. The physical examination focuses on evaluating the adolescent's stage of sexual development and assessing for hirsutism (see Chapter 5). A vaginal exam is performed to determine vaginal patency and if the vaginal mucosa is estrogenized. A pregnancy test is performed. Bone age and hormone levels are evaluated (estrogen, LH, FSH, and prolactin).

Growth and Development

Girls competing in sports such as long-distance running and track and field may be at increased risk for musculoskeletal injury. The female athlete triad places the runner at increased risk for injury such as stress fractures and comprises these three components: low energy availability (with or without disordered eating), low bone mineral density, and menstrual dysfunction. Research indicates that oligomenorrhea (infrequent menstruation) or amenorrhea (lack of menstruation) and low bone mineral density are associated with injury in the lower extremities (Rauh, Barrack, & Nichols, 2014) (see Chapter 29).

Treatment of amenorrhea depends on the specific cause. The most common approach is to prescribe birth control pills containing both estrogen and progesterone. Athletic teenagers are encouraged to eat a well-balanced, high-calorie diet. Calcium supplements may be ordered. Estrogen with progesterone in low doses may be prescribed for athletes to reduce the risk for osteoporosis. Nursing management centers on patient education and emotional support. The goal is to maintain normal growth and development.

Dysmenorrhea

Dysmenorrhea (menstrual pain or cramping) is a common problem in adolescent females. Primary dysmenorrhea refers to painful menstrual cramps that occur without any underlying disease process and affects 80% to 90% of female adolescents and women who are menstruating (Maruf, Ezenwafor, Moroof, et al., 2013). Primary dysmenorrhea is usually caused by an increased secretion of prostaglandins that are produced during the ovulatory cycle. Prostaglandin causes smooth muscle contraction in the uterus, leading to pain (Calis, Erogul, Popat, et al., 2015). Dysmenorrhea is the leading cause of school absence in the female adolescent population (Maruf et al., 2013; Wong, Ip, Choi, et al., 2015).

Dysmenorrhea usually occurs just prior to or at the beginning of the menstrual period and decreases over 1 to 3 days. The cramping pain ranges from mild to severe and varies with the individual. Other symptoms may include dizziness, syncope, nausea, vomiting, diarrhea, headache, lightheadedness, and fatigue (Maruf et al., 2013).

The treatment of choice for primary dysmenorrhea is non-steroidal anti-inflammatory drugs (NSAIDs), such as ibuprofen and naproxen sodium. These drugs inhibit prostaglandin synthesis, which leads to a reduction in uterine activity and pain. Oral contraceptives may be prescribed to prevent ovulation and to decrease prostaglandin production. A gynecologic examination may be conducted to rule out any structural abnormalities.

Secondary dysmenorrhea is defined as painful menstruation associated with pelvic abnormalities. Common causes of secondary dysmenorrhea include endometriosis, uterine fibroids, pelvic inflammatory disease, tubo-ovarian abscess, ovarian torsion, ovarian cyst, and presence of an intrauterine device (Calis et al., 2015). Vaginal and cervical cultures are taken when a sexually transmitted infection is possible. See Chapter 26.

Nursing Management

Nursing care centers on providing patient education and emotional support. Instruct the adolescent with chronic dysmenorrhea to keep a calendar and begin taking NSAIDs 1 day before the onset of the menstrual period. The medications should be taken with food to minimize side effects.

Disorders Related to Sex Chromosome Abnormalities

Turner Syndrome

In Turner syndrome, girls have a missing or partial absence of one X chromosome. This condition occurs in approximately 1 in 2000 to 1 in 5000 live female births (Oliveira, Ribeiro, Lago, et al., 2013). An estimated 90% of fetuses with Turner syndrome are spontaneously aborted during the first trimester. Turner syndrome is primarily associated with short stature and infertility (Martin & Smyth, 2012).

Characteristic clinical findings in the newborn include edema of the hands and feet, a webbed neck, a low hairline, a high-arched palate, a small jaw, low-set ears, droopy eyelids, a short fourth toe, short fingers, a broad chest, and widely separated nipples (Figure 30–10). Some children may have only one or two mild symptoms, and the diagnosis may not be made until adolescence when pubertal delay and lack of the onset of menstruation are apparent (Martin & Smyth, 2012).

Growth usually proceeds at a normal rate until around years of life and then slows, ceasing after puberty (Walker, 2014).

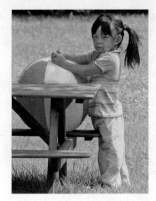

Figure 30–10 What characteristic physical manifestations of Turner syndrome can you identify in this girl?

SOURCE: Ed Suba Jr./Akron Beacon Journal/AP Photo.

Congenital heart defects frequently associated with Turner syndrome include coarctation of the aorta and bicuspid aortic valve (Levitsky, Luria, Hayes, et al., 2015). Other associated conditions include hearing loss, structural abnormalities of the kidney, and ophthalmic abnormalities (Martin & Smyth, 2012). Musculoskeletal disorders may include scoliosis and osteoporosis (Walker, 2014).

Diagnosis of Turner syndrome may be determined prenatally by amniocentesis or chorionic villi sampling (Martin & Smyth, 2012). The condition is diagnosed definitively by a karyotype. The most common phenotype is 45,X, indicating an absent X chromosome, which occurs in 40% to 60% of girls with Turner syndrome (Oliveira et al., 2013). Other types of Turner syndrome occur when the X chromosome is partially missing or rearranged, or when there are chromosomal changes in some of the cells (mosaicism) (Genetics Home Reference, 2012).

Treatment involves careful monitoring of the child's growth. A growth chart made especially for girls with Turner syndrome is available from the Turner Syndrome Society. Growth hormone therapy may be prescribed to promote growth during childhood. With treatment, final height generally reaches approximately 5 feet 2 inches; without treatment, the final height is approximately 4 feet 8 inches (Martin & Smyth, 2012). Estrogen and progesterone therapy are generally prescribed to promote breast development and decrease the risk of osteoporosis (Walker, 2014).

Nursing Management

Nursing assessment is focused on monitoring growth rates and observing for signs of cardiac, renal, gastrointestinal, vision, hearing, musculoskeletal, or thyroid dysfunction. Carefully measure the child's height and plot on the growth curve. Teach the family the correct administration of growth hormone and potential side effects.

The lack of growth and sexual development associated with Turner syndrome presents problems not only for physical growth but also for psychosocial development. The girl's perception of her body and how she differs from peers affects self-image, self-consciousness, and self-esteem. In the United States, cultural values place importance on attaining normal to tall stature. Short children tend to be treated according to their size rather than their age. Emphasis is also placed on sexual maturity. Encourage parents to treat the child by her chronologic age rather than size. Even though the child's intelligence is generally normal, learning disabilities are common (Saenz, Tsai, Manchester, et. al., 2014).

Klinefelter Syndrome

Klinefelter syndrome is a genetic condition that occurs in boys who have an extra X chromosome (usually 47,XXY). It occurs in approximately 1 in 450 males. Klinefelter syndrome is associated with androgen deficiency, infertility in males, and tall stature (Bourke, Herlihy, Snow, et al., 2014).

Klinefelter syndrome may be diagnosed when the onset of puberty is delayed or an abnormal progression is evident. Testes are small and firm. Less facial and body hair may develop. Gynecomastia is a characteristic finding (Bourke et al., 2014).

Klinefelter syndrome may also be diagnosed during the school-age years when the child is having difficulty at school. The child may have delayed developmental milestones and a low verbal IQ. Language and learning problems including difficulty reading may be present. The child may have difficulty socializing with others and body image issues (Bourke et al., 2014).

Chromosomal analysis revealing one or more extra X chromosomes confirms the diagnosis. The goal of treatment is to stimulate masculinization and the development of secondary sex characteristics when adolescence is delayed. Testosterone replacement is begun at puberty when the male is 11 or 12 years of age. A testosterone preparation is given by intramuscular injection every 3 to 4 weeks to maintain serum testosterone levels within the normal range. The dose is increased gradually every 6 to 9 months until a maintenance dose is achieved in adults (Ali & Donohoue, 2016).

Nursing Management

Nursing care consists of educating the parents and child about the syndrome, evaluating the child's and family's coping mechanisms, assisting with school problems, and reinforcing the child's strengths. Encourage parents to channel their son's energy into areas that will provide opportunities for success and productive experiences. Emphasize the importance of rewarding the boy's successes in school, sports, or hobbies. Make genetic counseling available to adolescents, if indicated, because sexual functioning and fertility may be impaired.

Inborn Errors of Metabolism

Inborn errors of metabolism are inherited biochemical abnormalities of the urea cycle, amino acid, or organic acid metabolism. Therefore, protein, carbohydrate, fat, electrolyte, blood, and respiratory metabolism can be affected. Individually they are rare disorders; however, as a group they are a significant health problem in infancy.

The biochemical defect usually causes an abnormal chemical by-product to accumulate in the blood, urine, or tissues or results in a decreased amount of normal enzymes. Most disorders are associated with protein intolerance with symptoms developing shortly after formula or breast milk feedings begin.

Clinical manifestations usually occur within days or weeks of birth. Signs and symptoms may include lethargy and poor feeding, persistent vomiting, abnormal muscle tone and seizures, apnea and tachycardia, and an unusual urine or body odor (musty, sweet odor of maple syrup or burnt sugar, or cheesy or sweaty feet).

Newborn screening has been demonstrated to save lives and to prevent serious disability. The March of Dimes (2012) recommends newborn screening tests for 31 health conditions. In most states, newborn screening programs lead to the detection of several conditions before symptoms develop.

In some cases, disorders associated with inborn errors of metabolism are not detected until signs and symptoms are present. Initial laboratory tests include measurement of serum glucose, electrolytes, blood gases, and serum ammonia. Tests results make it possible to classify the disorder by the presence of hypoglycemia, metabolic acidosis, hyperammonemia, or liver dysfunction. Further diagnostic laboratory tests are then performed on newborns with positive results.

Treatment, when available, focuses on replacing or reducing the amount of the substance causing the biochemical abnormality.

Four of the more common inborn errors of metabolism—phenylketonuria, galactosemia, mitochondrial diseases, and maple syrup urine disease—are presented in this section. Congenital hypothyroidism and congenital adrenal hyperplasia, which are also considered inborn errors of metabolism, were discussed earlier in this chapter.

Phenylketonuria

Phenylketonuria (PKU) is an autosomal recessive inherited disorder of amino acid metabolism that affects the body's use of protein. It is caused by a mutation of the phenylalanine hydroxylase gene. The incidence is approximately 1 in 15,000 newborns in the United States (Araujo et al., 2013; Brosco & Paul, 2013). Approximately 275 children are born with PKU each year in the United States (Brosco & Paul, 2013). The defect results in an accumulation of phenylalanine in the blood or phenylalanine metabolites in the urine. If untreated, this disease leads to irreversible brain damage and severe intellectual disability. Phenylalanine levels above 20 mg/dL are indicative of classic PKU (Rezvani & Ficicioglu, 2016).

Children with PKU have a deficiency of the liver enzyme phenylalanine hydroxylase that normally breaks down the essential amino acid phenylalanine into tyrosine. As a result, phenylalanine accumulates in the blood, causing a musty or mousey body and urine odor, irritability, vomiting, hyperactivity, hypertonia, hyperreflexive deep tendon reflexes, seizures, and an eczema-like rash (Rezvani & Ficicioglu, 2016). Persistence of elevated phenylalanine leads to disruption of cellular processes of myelination and protein synthesis, and results in a seizure disorder and untreatable intellectual disability.

Babies appear normal at birth except for lighter skin complexion than their nonaffected siblings. If diagnosis is delayed, a mousy or musty body odor is noticed and intellectual disability may be severe. Other common findings in untreated children include microcephaly, growth retardation, enamel hypoplasia, prominent maxilla, and widely spaced teeth (Rezvani & Ficicioglu, 2016).

Screening for PKU is required by state law in all 50 states. For best results, the newborn should have begun formula or breast milk feeding before specimen collection. Early hospital discharge places newborns at risk for false-negative screening tests if screened within 24 hours of birth. Screening needs to occur no sooner than 48 hours after birth, or the test should be repeated at 1 to 2 weeks of age. If the test shows elevated levels of plasma phenylalanine, a repeat quantitative test is performed. If the second test is positive, the family is referred to an outpatient treatment center. Serum levels of phenylalanine should be measured periodically throughout life.

Phenylketonuria is treated using special formulas and a diet low in phenylalanine to keep plasma phenylalanine levels between 2 and 6 mg/dL. The diet must also meet the child's needs for optimal growth. High-protein foods (meats and dairy products) are avoided because they contain large amounts of phenylalanine. Elemental medical foods (modified protein hydrolysates in which the phenylalanine has been removed) are used instead. The low-phenylalanine diet should be maintained throughout life for the best outcomes (Marcason, 2013).

Nursing Management

Nursing care is mainly supportive and focuses on teaching parents about the disorder and its management. The low-phenylalanine diet is a rigid, strict diet that excludes many foods. Educate the family about sources of phenylalanine, and refer the family to a registered dietician to establish an appropriate meal plan. Parents and children need a great deal of support to promote compliance. The formula and elemental medical food costs are relatively expensive. The formula is usually reimbursed by insurance, but negotiations with health plans may help parents obtain some support for medical foods. Parents of an affected child who are considering a future pregnancy and adolescents with the disorder should be referred for genetic counseling.

Galactosemia

Galactosemia, a disorder of carbohydrate metabolism, has an autosomal recessive inheritance pattern. It occurs in approximately 1 in 30,000 to 60,000 births in the United States (Screening, Technology, and Research in Genetics [STRG], 2012).

Galactosemia results from a deficiency of the liver enzyme galactose 1-phosphate uridyltransferase (GALT), one of three enzymes needed to convert galactose to glucose. The lack of enzyme leads to an accumulation of galactose metabolites in the eyes, liver, kidney, and brain, rapidly damaging the organs and causing life-threatening problems. Affected children become susceptible to gram-negative sepsis.

Early signs include poor sucking, failure to gain weight due to vomiting followed by diarrhea, hypoglycemia, and an enlarged liver. Later signs include intellectual disability, jaundice, ascites, sepsis, lethargy, seizures, hypotonia, cataracts, and coma. Babies may die within 1 month of birth without treatment, usually because of sepsis. When diagnosis is not made at birth, cirrhosis of the liver and intellectual disability progresses and becomes irreversible (Kishnani & Chen, 2016).

Routine newborn screening for galactosemia is performed in all 50 states (National Newborn Screening and Genetics Resource Center, 2014). (See the *Clinical Skills Manual* SKILLS .) Infants who are not screened at birth are identified once they become symptomatic. The diagnosis is based on history, physical examination, and laboratory tests (galactose, aspartate aminotransferase [AST], and alanine aminotransferase [ALT] levels are abnormally high). Urine specimens are checked for reducing substances (the Clinitest is positive and the Clinistix is negative) in several specimens while the infant is receiving human milk or formula with lactose.

Treatment involves placing infants on a lactose- or galactose-free formula. A lactose- and galactose-free diet must be followed for life. Calcium, vitamin D, and vitamin K supplements may be prescribed as well (STRG, 2012).

Despite compliance with the diet, complications (learning disabilities, speech defects, ovarian failure, and neurologic syndromes) develop in many children (Kishnani & Chen, 2016).

Nursing Management

Nursing management focuses on educating the parents and child about the disorder and required diet, assessing coping abilities, and providing emotional support. Refer the family to a registered dietician for diet counseling. Families must learn to screen foods for added milk solids and to avoid medications, such as antibiotics, that have lactose fillers. Calcium supplementation may be needed. Advise parents that several galactose-free cheeses are sold commercially. Because the disorder is inherited, refer the family for genetic counseling.

Mitochondrial Diseases

Mitochondrial diseases are a heterogeneous group of genetic disorders that result from a mutation in the nuclear or mitochondrial genes (Codier & Codier, 2014). It is estimated that 1 in 300 people have a genetic mutation that could affect mitochondrial function, but only a small fraction (1:5000) will develop mitochondrial disease (Codier & Codier, 2014).

Mitochondria are the cell's energy "powerhouses," producing energy through a process called *oxidative phosphorylation*, which uses glucose and oxygen to produce adenosine triphosphate (ATP) through the respiratory electron transport chain complexes I to V of the Krebs cycle (Codier & Codier, 2014). Point mutations, deletions, or duplications in mitochondrial DNA (mtDNA) can cause mitochondrial disorders that are transmitted from mothers to their children. Mitochondrial disorders can also result from mutations in the nuclear DNA (nDNA) of either parent and follow an autosomal recessive Mendelian pattern of inheritance (United Mitochondrial Disease Foundation [UMDF], 2011) (see Chapter 3 for further information about inheritance). Malfunction of the mitochondria results in the inability of the cell to produce sufficient energy and maintain metabolic regulation. Numerous mutations are known to cause mitochondrial disease. Some of the more common disorders are Leigh syndrome, Barth syndrome, Kearns-Sayers syndrome, fatty acid oxidation disease, mitochondrial encephalopathy with lactic acidosis and stroke-like episodes (MELAS), neurogenic weakness with ataxia and retinitis pigmentosa (NAEP), and Pearson syndrome (Dassler & Allen, 2014).

Mitochondrial disease may present at any age, ranging from the newborn period into childhood and adulthood, with a spectrum of possible signs and symptoms (see Table 30–8). Clinical presentation is very diverse but affects "high energy demand" organs (Codier & Codier, 2014). Hallmarks of mitochondrial disease include (1) more than one organ system involved, (2) atypical features of another type of known disease, and (3) recurrent setbacks or flare-ups during an infection or stress. Mitochondrial disease should be considered in any patient with unexplained multisystem involvement and progressive deterioration (UMDF, 2011). A single organ may be predominately affected, but a combination of dysfunction in unrelated organs, unexplained multisystem symptoms, or involvement of three or more organ systems without a unifying diagnosis should raise concern for mitochondrial disease (Codier & Codier, 2014).

Diagnosis is elusive, time consuming, laborious, and expensive, with limited evidence-based guidelines or biomarkers (Dassler & Allen, 2014). Clinical symptoms, family history, age of symptom onset, muscle biopsy, imaging, and genetic testing are considered in making a diagnosis (Dassler & Allen, 2014). Genetic testing is still in its infancy, remains expensive, and may not be covered by insurance. Many patients have delayed diagnoses or diagnoses of probable or possible mitochondrial disease.

There is no cure or well-studied pharmacologic treatment for mitochondrial disease. Treatment focuses on conserving energy; frequent intake of nutrients; regular sleep; maintaining health; maximizing mitochondrial function; symptom management; nutrition therapy; physical therapy; reducing physiologic stressors such as extremes in cold or heat; avoiding known mitochondrial toxins such as alcohol, cigarette smoke, and

TABLE 30–8 Affected Systems and Associated Symptoms of Mitochondrial Disease

SYSTEM	SYMPTOMS
Cardiovascular	Cardiomyopathy, heart block, arrhythmias, tachycardia, bradycardia
Endocrine	Short stature, diabetes mellitus, exocrine pancreatic failure, thyroid dysfunction, hypoglycemia
Eyes and ears	Vision loss and blindness, droopy eyelids, paralysis or weakness of the eye muscles, optic atrophy, degenerative eye disease, acquired strabismus, hearing loss, deafness
Gastrointestinal	Anorexia, vomiting, diarrhea, constipation, pseudo-obstruction, irritable bowel syndrome, dysphagia, dysmotility, gastroesophageal reflux, delayed gastric emptying
Genitourinary/renal	Glomerular disease, renal tubular acidosis, frequency, urgency, urinary retention
Hematologic	Bruising, bleeding, anemia, pancytopenia
Musculoskeletal	Exercise intolerance, low muscle tone, weakness, muscle pain
Neurologic	Developmental delay, cognitive disabilities, seizures, migraines, strokes, ataxia, spasticity, temperature instability, fainting, absent reflexes
Respiratory	Obstructive sleep apnea, tachypnea, dyspnea
Systemic	Fatigue, failure to gain weight

Source: Data from Dassler A., & Allen, P. (2014). Mitochondrial disease in children and adolescents. *Pediatric Nursing, 40*(3), 150–154; Klehm, M., & Korson, M. (2014). *A clinician's guide to the management of mitochondrial disease.* Retrieved from http://www.mitoaction.org/guide/table-contents; United Mitochondrial Disease Foundation (UMDF). (2011). *MitoFIRST handbook: An introductory guide.* Retrieved from http://www.kintera.org/atf/cf/%7B858ACD34-ECC3-472A-8794-39B92E103561%7D/mito_first.pdf

monosodium glutamate (MSG); and providing emotional care and family support (Codier & Codier, 2014; Dassler & Allen, 2014; UMDF, 2011). Nutritious foods and frequent hydration provide cells with nutrients to support mitochondrial function, while prolonged periods of fasting produce mitochondrial stress and should be avoided (Dassler & Allen, 2014). The only current pharmacologic treatments available consist of vitamin and dietary supplementation, known as a "mitochondrial cocktail" (Dassler & Allen, 2014). This cocktail often contains antioxidants such as thiamine, vitamin C, vitamin E, and alphalipoic acid, along with coenzyme Q10 (CoQ10) and levo-carnitine (Carnitor) as essential components of mitochondrial electron transport (UMDF, 2011).

Nursing Management

Nursing management for mitochondrial disease is multifaceted and includes physiologic, emotional, and spiritual care while educating parents about energy and fatigue management, nutritional support, physical therapy, acute and long-term symptom management, physiologic stress reduction, and immunizations (Codier & Codier, 2014). Multisystem care must be individualized to meet the needs of the patient. During an acute phase, nursing care involves extensive neurologic support, seizure management, cardiac respiratory support, tube feedings, nutritional supplementation, and frequent hydration. Children with the disease should usually go no longer than 8 to 12 hours without food. Infants should be fed around the clock every 2 to 4 hours. Small frequent meals are a better choice than three full meals a day. Consumption of a complex carbohydrate or protein before bed will help prevent overnight hypoglycemia. Children who are unable to sustain oral intake during an acute illness must be referred to the hospital for intravenous dextrose supplementation. Specialists should manage care during hospitalizations or surgery, especially the administration of anesthesia. Even simple infections such as otitis media or influenza can become life threatening. Long-term management includes assessment for mobility aids, home environment adaptations, educational care plans, vision and hearing aids, assessment of family functioning, stress and coping, genetic

counseling, and end-of-life care. Nursing care also involves assisting parents to navigate the complex healthcare system and coordinate visits involving multiple specialists. Nurses should inquire about specific stressors related to travel, frequent hospitalizations, medical visits, school accommodations, care for siblings, and parental guilt, and suggest effective coping strategies to manage the many aspects of mitochondrial disease (Senger, 2013). If one child in the family is diagnosed with the disorder, the siblings should also be monitored or tested even if they are asymptomatic.

Maple Syrup Urine Disease

Maple syrup urine disease (MSUD) is a disorder of amino acid metabolism that has an autosomal recessive inheritance pattern (Cole, 2014). It is rare, occurring in approximately 1 in 150,000 to 1 in 185,000 of the general population, but it occurs as often as 1 in 760 in Mennonites (Burfield, Hussa, & Randall, 2012).

In MSUD leucine, isoleucine, and valine cannot be metabolized because of an enzyme defect in the branched chain of these three essential amino acids. All three amino acids are essential to form normal structures such as the hair, skin, and muscle. Accumulation of these three amino acids leads to encephalopathy and progressive neurologic impairment if left untreated (Bodamer & Lee, 2014).

Within 5 to 7 days of life, the newborn develops symptoms of poor sucking, irregular respirations, and rigidity with alternating flaccidity (Burfield et al, 2012). Ketosis and a sweet odor of maple syrup in urine are generally present when symptoms develop (Bodamer & Lee, 2014). If the child is not treated, symptoms progress to seizures, apnea, and death (Burfield et al., 2012).

All states require newborn screening for this condition (National Newborn Screening and Genetics Resource Center, 2014). Diagnosis is made with laboratory tests of the urine for positive ketones and blood tests for elevated levels of leucine, isoleucine, alloisoleucine, and valine.

Treatment during the acute stage involves removal of the branched-chain amino acids and their metabolites from the tissues and body fluids. Some critically ill infants may require dialysis to remove these compounds because their renal clearance is poor.

Lifelong treatment includes specially designed medical formulas and foods rich in amino acids, calories, vitamins, minerals, and other nutrients as prescribed. These special medical foods have the three amino acids removed. The child needs special low-protein foods that are adequate for growth with enough calories to support twice the child's basal metabolic rate. Daily urine testing is required to determine if ketones are being excreted, an indication that the body is in a catabolic state. Liver transplants have been performed in a few affected children who were subsequently able to tolerate a normal diet. The long-term prognosis of children with MSUD is guarded (Rezvani & Rosenblatt, 2016).

Nursing Management

Nursing care includes educating the family about the disorder and special dietary requirements. The parents need to learn how to mix the child's special formula with a natural protein source, amino acid supplements, and water. The child needs formula even when ill. Parents should have a sick-day plan to prevent ketoacidosis. The child should be permitted moderate exercise only to prevent increases in leucine levels. Help families identify sources of information or support groups who can share recipes and tips for managing the child's condition.

Chapter Highlights

- The hypothalamic-pituitary axis produces several releasing and inhibiting hormones that regulate the function of many endocrine glands.

- Puberty is the process of sexual maturation that occurs when the gonads secrete increased amounts of the sex hormones estrogen and testosterone, resulting in the development of primary and secondary sexual characteristics.

- Children with hypopituitarism have short stature as a result of growth hormone deficiency. Treatment with growth hormone early in life enables these children to potentially attain genetically appropriate heights.

- An excessive secretion of growth hormone or hyperpituitarism may cause children to have tall stature, growing up to 7 or 8 feet in height if no intervention is provided before the epiphyseal plates close.

- Diabetes insipidus is a disorder of the posterior pituitary gland and is defined as an inability of the kidneys to concentrate urine.

- Syndrome of inappropriate antidiuretic hormone (SIADH) results from an excessive amount of serum antidiuretic hormone (ADH), leading to water intoxication and hyponatremia.

- Precocious puberty is defined as the appearance of any secondary sexual characteristics before 8 years in girls and 9 years in boys. If no treatment is provided, the hormones will stimulate closure of the epiphyseal plates and the child will have short stature as an adult.

- Untreated or ineffectively treated congenital hypothyroidism results in impaired growth and intellectual disability.

- Signs of hyperthyroidism include an enlarged, nontender thyroid gland (goiter), prominent or bulging eyes , eyelid lag, tachycardia, nervousness, increased appetite with weight loss, emotional lability, moodiness, heat intolerance, hypertension, hyperactivity, irregular menses, insomnia, tremor, and muscle weakness.

- During infancy, most cases of endogenous Cushing disease are due to a functioning adrenocortical tumor. The most common cause of endogenous Cushing syndrome in children older than 7 years of age is Cushing disease, in which a pituitary tumor (adenoma) secretes excess ACTH.

- Congenital adrenal hyperplasia has two forms, salt-losing or non–salt-losing with virilization. The salt-losing form accounts for 75% of cases and is caused by aldosterone deficiency and overproduction of androgen. The non–salt-losing form accounts for the other 25% of cases.

- Congenital adrenal hyperplasia is the most common cause of pseudohermaphroditism (ambiguous genitalia) in newborn girls.

- Adrenal insufficiency, also known as *Addison disease*, is a rare disorder in childhood characterized by a deficiency of glucocorticoids (cortisone) and mineralocorticoids (aldosterone). Symptoms include weakness, fatigue, weight loss, and gastrointestinal symptoms such as nausea, vomiting, diarrhea, constipation, and abdominal pain. Other symptoms include hyperpigmentation, hypotension, dizziness, joint pain, salt cravings, and hypoglycemia.

- Pheochromocytoma is a tumor that arises from the adrenal gland and causes an excessive release of catecholamines. Clinical manifestations include hypertension, palpitations sweating, anxiety, tremors, and headache.

- Diabetes mellitus type 1 is the most common metabolic disease in children and one of the most common chronic diseases in school-age children. It is a disorder of carbohydrate, protein, and fat metabolism.

- Treatment of the child with diabetic ketoacidosis includes intravenous fluids and electrolytes for dehydration and acidosis. Insulin is given by continuous infusion pump to decrease the serum glucose level at a slow but steady rate to prevent the development of cerebral edema.

- Common causes of hypoglycemia in children with type 1 diabetes include an error in insulin dosage, inadequate calories because of missed meals, or exercise without a corresponding increase in caloric intake.

- Type 2 diabetes mellitus is a condition that results from insulin resistance. Children most commonly affected are obese, and many have family members with the same type of diabetes.

- Secondary amenorrhea is the cessation of spontaneous menstrual periods for at least 120 days and occurs 6 months or 3 cycles after menarche.

- Turner syndrome is diagnosed definitively by a karyotype. The most common and most severe phenotype is 45,X indicating an absent X chromosome.

- Signs of Klinefelter syndrome include gynecomastia, delayed onset of puberty with an abnormal progression, decreased testicular size, and less facial and body hair than normal.

- Inborn errors of metabolism—inherited biochemical abnormalities of the urea cycle and amino acid and organic acid metabolism—often have a significant impact on the endocrine system's ability to support growth and development. These disorders include phenylketonuria, galactosemia, defects in mitochondrial diseases, and maple syrup urine disease.

- Children with phenylketonuria (PKU) have a deficiency of the liver enzyme phenylalanine hydroxylase that normally breaks down the essential amino acid phenylalanine into tyrosine.

- Galactosemia results from a deficiency of a liver enzyme needed to convert galactose to glucose. This leads to an accumulation of galactose metabolites in the eyes, liver, kidney, and brain, rapidly damaging the organs and causing life-threatening problems.

- Mitochondrial diseases are a group of genetic disorders resulting from a mutation in the nuclear or mitochondrial genes.

- Maple syrup urine disease is a rare disorder in which leucine, isoleucine, and valine cannot be metabolized because of an enzyme defect in the branched chain of these three essential amino acids.

Clinical Reasoning in Action

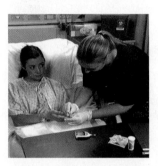

Fourteen-year-old Amanda is admitted to the hospital with newly diagnosed type 1 diabetes mellitus. She had initially been taken to her healthcare providers's office for enuresis, polyphagia, polydipsia, and lethargy, but when assessed, her urinalysis had glucose and ketones, and she had a weight loss of 15 lb.

Upon admission to the hospital, a full assessment is performed and the following vital signs are documented: weight 115 lb, temperature 98.8°F, respiratory rate 40 breaths per minute, heart rate 90 beats per minute, and blood pressure 106/63 mmHg. She has dry mucous membranes, but skin turgor is brisk. Blood is drawn immediately and will continue to be drawn every hour until she is stable.

After Amanda's condition stabilizes, education related to management of type 1 diabetes is initiated for Amanda and her parents. Amanda understands the nutritional guidelines associated with type 1 diabetes and how, under adult supervision, to perform blood glucose monitoring as well as how to draw up and administer insulin. Amanda and her parents spend most of the time in the hospital learning survival skills for managing her diabetes. Daily education and monitoring will occur in the diabetes clinic until the family is confident about taking care of Amanda. Regular follow-up visits will be scheduled with the diabetes nurse educator and endocrinologist.

1. What is the blood work most likely to be done on Amanda when admitted to the hospital for type 1 diabetes?

2. How should the family be told to manage hypoglycemic episodes?

3. What should the parents be told about preventing diabetic ketoacidosis in Amanda?

4. How often should blood glucose monitoring be performed once the condition is stabilized?

References

Abraham, C., & Rozmus, C. L. (2012). Is acanthosis nigricans a reliable indicator for risk of type 2 diabetes in obese children and adolescents? A systematic review. *The Journal of School Nursing, 28*(3), 195–205.

Ali, O., & Donohoue, P. A. (2016). Hypofunction of the testes. In R. M. Kliegman, B. F. Stanton, J. W. St. Geme, & N. F. Schor (Eds.), *Nelson textbook of pediatrics* (20th ed., pp. 2735–2741). Philadelphia, PA: Elsevier.

Alsaleh, F. M., Smith, F. J., & Taylor, K. M. (2012). Experiences of children/young people and their parents, using insulin pump therapy for the management of type 1 diabetes: Qualitative review. *Journal of Clinical Pharmacy and Therapeutics, 37*, 140–147.

American Diabetes Association (ADA). (2013). *Sick days*. Retrieved from http://www.diabetes.org/living-with-diabetes/parents-and-kids/everyday-life/sick-days.html

American Diabetes Association (ADA). (2014a). Diagnosis and classification of diabetes mellitus. *Diabetes Care, 37*(Suppl. 1), S81–S90.

American Diabetes Association (ADA). (2014b). Standards of medical care in diabetes—2014. *Diabetes Care, 37*(Suppl. 1), S14–S80.

American Diabetes Association (ADA). (2014c). *Diabetes association sets new A1C target for children with type 1 diabetes*. Retrieved from http://www.diabetes.org/newsroom/press-releases/2014/diabetes-association-sets-new-a1c-target-for-children-with-type-1-diabetes.html

American Diabetes Association (ADA). (2015). *Preventing type 2 in children*. Retrieved from http://www.diabetes.org/living-with-diabetes/parents-and-kids/children-and-type-2/preventing-type-2-in-children.html

Araujo, G. C., Christ, S. E., Grange, D. K., Steiner, R. D., Coleman, C., Timmerman, E., & White, D. A. (2013). Executive response monitoring and inhibitory control in children with phenylketonuria: Effects of expectancy. *Developmental Neuropsychology, 38*(3), 139–152.

Bacon, C. (2013). Supporting children and young people diagnosed with type 2 diabetes in school. *British Journal of School Nursing, 8*(5), 222–226.

Bahn, R. S., Burch, H. B., Cooper, D. S., Garber, J. R., Greenlee, C., Klein, I., . . . Stan, M. N. (2011). Hyperthyroidism and other causes of thyrotoxicosis: Management guidelines of the American Thyroid Association and American Association of Clinical Endocrinologists. *Thyroid, 21*(6), 593–646.

Bauer, A. J. (2011). Approach to the pediatric patient with Graves' disease: When is definitive therapy warranted? *Journal of Clinical Endocrinology and Metabolism, 96*(3), 580–588.

Belcher, R., Metrailer, A. M., Bodenner, D. L., & Stack, B. C. (2013). Characterization of hyperparathyroidism in youth and adolescents: A literature review. *International Journal of Pediatric Otorhinolaryngology, 77*, 318–322.

Bialo, S. R., Agrawal, S., Boney, C. M., & Qunitos, J. B. (2015). Rare complications of pediatric diabetic ketoacidosis. *World Journal of Diabetes, 6*(1), 167–174.

Blackman, S. M., Raghinaru, D., Adi, S., Simmons, J. H., Ebner-Lyon, L., Chase, H. P., . . . DiMeglio, L. A. (2014). Insulin pump use in young children in the T1D Exchange clinic registry is associated with lower hemoglobin A1c levels than injection therapy. *Pediatric Diabetes, 15*, 564–572.

Bodamer, O. A., & Lee, B. (2014). *Maple syrup urine disease*. Retrieved from http://emedicine.medscape.com/article/946234-overview

Bordini, B., & Rosenfield, R. L. (2011a). Normal pubertal development: Part I: The endocrine basis of puberty. *Pediatrics in Review, 32*(6), 223–229.

Bordini, B., & Rosenfield, R. L. (2011b). Normal pubertal development: Part II: Clinical aspects of puberty. *Pediatrics in Review, 32*(7), 281–292.

Bourke, E., Herlihy, A., Snow, P., Metcalfe, S., & Amor, D. (2014). Klinefelter syndrome: A general practice perspective. *Australian Family Physician, 43*(1), 38–41.

Boyse, K. L., Garnder, M., Marvicsin, D. J., & Sandberg, D. E. (2014). "It was an overwhelming thing": Parents' needs after infant diagnosis with congenital adrenal hyperplasia. *Journal of Pediatric Nursing, 29,* 436–441.

Breault, D. T., & Majzoub, J. A. (2016). Diabetes insipidus. In R. M. Kliegman, B. F. Stanton, J. W. St. Geme, & N. F. Schor (Eds.), *Nelson textbook of pediatrics* (20th ed., pp. 2644–2646). Philadelphia, PA: Elsevier.

Brink, S., Joel, D., Laffel, L., Lee, W. W. R., Olsen, B., Phelan, H., & Hanas, R. (2014). Sick day management in children and adolescents with diabetes. *Pediatric Diabetes, 15*(Suppl. 20), 193–202.

Brosco, J. P., & Paul, D. B. (2013). The political history of PKU: Reflections on 50 years of newborn screening. *Pediatrics, 132*(6), 987–989.

Burfield, J., Hussa, C., & Randall, R. (2012). Hot topics in metabolism: A focus on phenylketonuria, liver transplantation, and galactosemia. *Topics in Clinical Nutrition, 27*(3), 181–195.

Butler, S., Fekaris, N., Pontius, D., & Zacharski, S. (2012). *Diabetes management in the school setting.* Retrieved from http://www.nasn.org/PolicyAdvocacy/PositionPapersandReports/NASN-PositionStatementsArticleView/tabid/462/ArticleId/22/Diabetes-in-the-School-Setting-School-Nurse-Role-in-Care-and-Management-of-the-Child-with-Revised-20

Calis, K. A., Erogul, M., Popat, V., Kalantaridou, S. N., & Dang, D. K. (2015). *Dysmenorrhea.* Retrieved from http://emedicine.medscape.com/article/253812-overview

Carchidi, C., Holland, C., Minnock, P., & Boyle, D. (2011). New technologies in pediatric diabetes care. *MCN, 36*(1), 32–39.

Carroll, K. L., & Kerr, L. M. (2014). Alterations of musculoskeletal function in children. In K. L. McCance & S. E. Huether (Eds.), *Pathophysiology: The biologic basis for disease in adults and children* (7th ed., pp. 1591–1615). St. Louis, MO: Elsevier Mosby.

Centers for Disease Control and Prevention (CDC). (2014). *National diabetes statistics report, 2014.* Retrieved from http://www.cdc.gov/diabetes/pubs/statsreport14/national-diabetes-report-web.pdf

Chiang, J. L., Kirkman, M. S., Laffel, L. M. B., & Peters, A. L. (2014). Type 1 diabetes through the life span: A position statement of the American Diabetes Association. *Diabetes Care, 37,* 2034–2054.

Codier, E., & Codier, D. (2014). Understanding mitochondrial disease and goals for its treatment. *British Journal of Nursing, 23*(5), 254–258.

Cohee, L. (2012). Endocrinology. In *The Harriet Lane handbook* (19th ed., pp. 243–270). Philadelphia, PA: Elsevier.

Cole, C. (2014). Successful pregnancy and delivery with maple syrup urine disease. *Journal of Obstetric, Gynecologic & Neonatal Nursing, 43*(Suppl. 1), S95–S96.

Collaborative Group on Hormonal Factors in Breast Cancer. (2012). Menarche, menopause, and breast cancer risk: Individual participant meta-analysis, including 118,964 women with breast cancer from 117 epidemiological studies. *The Lancet Oncology, 13*(11), 1141–1151.

Cooke, D. W., Divall, S. A., & Radovick, S. (2011). Normal and aberrant growth. In S. Melmed, K. S. Polonsky, P. R. Larsen, & H. M. Kronenberg (Eds.), *Williams textbook of endocrinology* (12th ed., pp. 935–1053). Philadelphia, PA: Elsevier Saunders.

Craig, M. E., Jefferies, C., Dabelea, D., Balde, N., Seth, A., & Donaghue, K. C. (2014). Definition, epidemiology, and classification of diabetes in children and adolescents. *Pediatric Diabetes, 15*(Suppl. 20), 4–17.

Cystic Fibrosis Foundation. (2012). *Cystic fibrosis-related diabetes.* Retrieved from http://www.cff.org/LivingWithCF/StayingHealthy/Diet/Diabetes/

Dassler A., & Allen, P. (2014). Mitochondrial disease in children and adolescents. *Pediatric Nursing, 40*(3), 150–154.

Dea, T. L. (2011). Pediatric obesity & type 2 diabetes. *MCN, 36*(1), 42–48.

Di Iorgi, N., Napoli, F., Allegri, A. E. M., Olivieri, I., Bertelli, E., Gallazia, A., . . . Maghnie, M. (2012). Diabetes insipidus—Diagnosis and management. *Hormone Research in Paediatrics, 77,* 69–84.

Doyle, D. A. (2016a). Hyperparathyroidism. In R. M. Kliegman, B. F. Stanton, J. W. St. Geme, & N. F. Schor (Eds.), *Nelson textbook of pediatrics* (20th ed., pp. 2694–2697). Philadelphia, PA: Elsevier.

Doyle, D. A. (2016b). Hypoparathyroidism. In R. M. Kliegman, B. F. Stanton, J. W. St. Geme, & N. F. Schor (Eds.), *Nelson textbook of pediatrics* (20th ed., pp. 2690–2693). Philadelphia, PA: Elsevier.

Ferguson, L. A. (2011). Growth hormone use in children: Necessary or designer therapy? *Journal of Pediatric Health Care, 25*(1), 24–30.

Ficorelli, C. T. (2013). Addison disease: The importance of early diagnosis. *Nursing Made Incredibly Easy!, 11*(2), 11–15.

Fischer, S., Hirsch, T., Hirche, C., Kiefer, J., Kueckelhaus, M., Germann, G., & Reichenberger, M. A. (2014). Surgical treatment of primary gynecomastia in children and adolescents. *Pediatric Surgery International, 20,* 641–647.

Fitzgerald, P. A. (2015). Endocrine disorders. In M. A. Papadakis, S. J. McPhee, & M. W. Rabow (Eds.), *CURRENT Medical Diagnosis & Treatment 2015.* New York, NY: McGraw-Hill.

Fuqua, J. S. (2013). Treatment and outcomes of precocious puberty: An update. *Journal of Clinical Endocrinology & Metabolism, 98*(6), 2198–2207.

Gastaldi, R., Poggi, E., Mussa, A., Webber, G., Vigone, M. C., Salerno, M., . . . Corrias, A. (2014). Graves disease in children: Thyroid-stimulating hormone receptor antibodies as remission markers. *The Journal of Pediatrics, 164*(5) 1189–1194.

Genetics Home Reference. (2012). *Turner syndrome.* Retrieved from http://ghr.nlm.nih.gov/condition/turner-syndrome

Guo, C. (2013). Diagnostic value of provocative test by insulin combined with clonidine for growth hormone deficiency in children. *Iranian Journal of Pediatrics, 23*(3), 315–320.

Hanas, R., de Beaufort, C., Hoey, H., & Anderson, B. (2011). Insulin delivery by injection in children and adolescents. *Pediatric Diabetes, 12,* 518–526.

Hird, B. E., Tetlow, L., Tobi, S., Patel, L., & Clayton, P. E. (2015). No evidence of an increase in early infant mortality from congenital adrenal hyperplasia in the absence of screening. *Archives of Disease in Childhood, 99,* 158–164.

Ho, C. W., Loke, K. Y., Lim, Y. L., & Lee, Y. S. (2014). Exogenous Cushing syndrome: A lesson of diaper rash cream. *Hormone Research in Paediatrics, 82,* 415–418.

Huang, S. A., & LaFranchi, S. (2016). Hyperthyroidism. In R. M. Kliegman, B. F. Stanton, J. W. St. Geme, & N. F. Schor (Eds.), *Nelson textbook of pediatrics* (20th ed., pp. 2680–2685). Philadelphia, PA: Elsevier.

Iafusco, D., Galderisi, A., Nocerino, I., Cocca, A., Zuccotti, G., Prisco, F., & Scaramuzza, A. (2011). Chat line for adolescents with type 1 diabetes: A useful tool to improve coping with diabetes: A 2-year follow-up study. *Diabetes Technology & Therapeutics, 13*(5), 551–555.

Jaser, S. S., Faulkner, M. S., Whittemore, R., Jeon, S., Delamater, A., & Grey, M. (2012). Coping, self-management, and adaptation in adolescents with type 1 diabetes. *Annals of Behavioral Medicine, 43,* 311–319.

Jaser, S. S., & White, L. E. (2011). Coping and resilience in adolescents with type 1 diabetes. *Child: Care Health and Development, 37*(3), 335–342.

Kemper, M. J., & van Husen, M. (2014). Renal osteodystrophy in children: Pathogenesis, diagnosis and treatment. *Current Opinion in Pediatrics, 26*(2), 180–186.

Khan, S. E., Cooper, M. E., & Del Prato, S. (2014). Pathophysiology and treatment of type 2 diabetes: Perspectives on the past, present, and future. *Lancet, 383,* 1068–1083.

Kishnani, P. S., & Chen, Y. (2016). Defects in metabolism of carbohydrates. In R. M. Kliegman, B. F. Stanton, J. W. St. Geme, & N. F. Schor (Eds.), *Nelson textbook of pediatrics* (20th ed., pp. 715–737). Philadelphia, PA: Elsevier.

Klehm, M., & Korson, M. (2014). *A clinician's guide to the management of mitochondrial disease.* Retrieved from http://www.mitoaction.org/guide/table-contents

LaFranchi, S., & Huang, S. A. (2016). Hypothyroidism. In R. M. Kliegman, B. F. Stanton, J. W. St. Geme, & N. F. Schor (Eds.), *Nelson textbook of pediatrics* (20th ed., pp. 2665–2675). Philadelphia, PA: Elsevier.

Larsson, H. E., Vehik, K., Bell, R., Dabelea, D., Dolan, L., Pihoker, C., . . . Haller, M. J. (2011). Reduced prevalence of diabetic ketoacidosis at diagnosis of type 1 diabetes in young children participating in longitudinal follow-up. *Diabetes Care, 34,* 2347–2352.

Leger, J., Gelwane, G., Kaguelidou, F., Benmerad, M., Alberti, C., & French Childhood Graves' Disease Study Group. (2012). Positive impact of long-term antithyroid drug treatment on the outcome of children with Graves' disease: National long-term cohort study. *Journal of Clinical Endocrinology and Metabolism, 97*(1), 1–10.

Levitsky, L. L., Luria, A. H. O., Hayes, F. J., & Lin, A. E. (2015). Turner syndrome: Update on biology and management across the life span. *Current Opinion in Endocrinology, Diabetes, & Obesity, 22*(1), 65–72.

Marcason, W. (2013). Is there a standard meal plan for phenylketonuria (PKU)? *Journal of the Academy Of Nutrition And Dietetics, 113*(8), 1124.

Marcdante, K. J., & Kliegman, R. M (2015). Diabetes mellitus. In K. J. Marcdante & R. M. Kliegman (Eds.), *Nelson essentials of pediatrics* (7th ed., pp. 572–579). Philadelphia, PA: Elsevier Saunders.

March of Dimes. (2012). *Newborn screening.* Retrieved from http://www.marchofdimes.org/baby/newborn-screening-tests-for-your-baby.aspx

Martin, C. J. H., & Smyth, A. (2012). A midwives' guide to Turner syndrome. *British Journal of Midwifery, 20*(9), 628–631.

Maruf, F. A., Ezenwafor, N. V., Moroof, S. O., Adeniyi, A. F., & Okoye, E. C. (2013). Physical activity level and adiposity: Are they associated with primary dysmenorrhea in school adolescents? *African Journal of Reproductive Health, 17*(4), 167–174.

Masharani, U. (2015). Diabetes mellitus & hypoglycemia. In M. A. Papadakis, S. J. McPhee, & M. W. Rabow (Eds.), *CURRENT medical diagnosis & treatment 2015*. New York, NY: McGraw-Hill.

McFarlane, K. (2011). An overview of diabetic ketoacidosis in children. *Paediatric Nursing, 23*(1), 14–19.

McHugo, J., & Harden, A. (2011). Diabetes insipidus: Navigating troubled waters. *Advance for NPs and PAs, 2*(4), 20–24.

Michels, A., & Michels, N. (2014). Addison disease: Early detection and treatment principles. *American Family Physician, 89*(7), 563–568.

Mishra, A., Mehrotra, P. K., Agarwal, G., Agarwal, A., & Mishra, S. K. (2014). Pediatric and adolescent pheochromocytoma: Clinical presentation and outcome of surgery. *Indian Pediatrics, 51,* 299–302.

Monaghan, M., Hoffman, K. M., & Cogen, F. R. (2013). License to drive: Type 1 diabetes management and obtaining a learner's permit in Maryland and Virginia. *Diabetes Spectrum, 26*(3), 194–199.

National Diabetes Information Clearinghouse. (2014). *The A1C test and diabetes.* Retrieved from http://diabetes.niddk.nih.gov/dm/pubs/A1CTest/#1

National Endocrine and Metabolic Diseases Information Service (NEMDIS). (2014). *Adrenal insufficiency and Addison's disease.* Retrieved from http://endocrine.niddk.nih.gov/pubs/addison/addison.aspx

National Newborn Screening and Genetics Resource Center. (2014). *National newborn screening status report.* Retrieved from https://genes-r-us.uthscsa.edu/sites/genes-r-us/files/nbsdisorders.pdf

Nimkarn, S., Lin-Su, K., & New, M. I. (2011). Steroid 21 hydroxylase deficiency congenital adrenal hyperplasia. *Pediatric Clinics of North America, 58,* 1281–1300.

Oliveira, C. S., Ribeiro, F. M., Lago, R., & Alves, C. (2013). Audiological abnormalities in patients with Turner syndrome. *American Journal of Audiology, 22,* 226–232.

Parks, J. S., & Felner, E. I. (2016). Hypopituitarism. In R. M. Kliegman, B. F. Stanton, J. W. St. Geme, & N. F. Schor (Eds.), *Nelson textbook of pediatrics* (20th ed., pp. 2637–2644). Philadelphia, PA: Elsevier.

Pillai, B. P., Unnikrishnan, A. G., & Pavithran, P. V. (2011). Syndrome of inappropriate antidiuretic hormone secretion: Revisiting a classical endocrine disorder. *Indian Journal of Endocrinology and Metabolism, 15* (Suppl. 3), S208–S215.

Pluta, R. M., Burke, A. E., & Golub, R. M. (2011). Cushing syndrome and Cushing disease. *Journal of the American Medical Association, 306*(24), 2742.

Rauh, M. J., Barrack, M., & Nichols, J. F. (2014). Associations between the female athlete triad and injury among high school runners. *The International Journal of Sports Physical Therapy, 9*(7), 948–958.

Rezvani, I., & Ficicioglu, C. (2016). Phenylalanine. In R. M. Kliegman, B. F. Stanton, J. W. St. Geme, & N. F. Schor (Eds.), *Nelson textbook of pediatrics* (20th ed., pp. 636–640). Philadelphia, PA: Elsevier.

Rezvani, I., & Rosenblatt, D. S. (2016). Valine, leucine, isoleucine and related organic acidemias. In R. M. Kliegman, B. F. Stanton, J. W. St. Geme, & N. F. Schor (Eds.), *Nelson textbook of pediatrics* (20th ed., p. 649). Philadelphia, PA: Elsevier.

Rivkees, S. A. (2014). Pediatric Graves' disease: Management in the post–propylthiouracil era. *International Journal of Pediatric Endocrinology. 2014*(1), 1–23.

Robinson, A. G., & Verbalis, J. G. (2011). Posterior pituitary. In S. Melmed, K. S. Polonsky, P. R. Larsen, & H. M. Kronenberg (Eds.), *Williams textbook of endocrinology* (12th ed., pp. 292–323). Philadelphia, PA: Elsevier Saunders.

Saenz, M., Tsai, A. C., Manchester, D. K., & Elias, E. R. (2014). Genetics & dysmorphology. In W. W. Hay, M. J. Levin, R. R. Deterding, & M. J. Abzug (Eds.), *CURRENT diagnosis and treatment: Pediatrics* (22th ed.). New York, NY: McGraw-Hill. Retrieved from http://accessmedicine.com

Saito, R., Yamamoto, Y., Goto, M., Araki, S., Kubo, K., Kawagoe, R., . . . Fukami, M. (2014). Tamoxifen treatment for pubertal gynecomastia in two siblings with partial androgen insensitivity syndrome. *Hormone Research in Paediatrics, 81,* 211–216.

Screening, Technology, and Research in Genetics (STRG). (2012). *Galactosemia.* Retrieved from http://www.newbornscreening.info/Parents/otherdisorders/Galactosemia.html

Senger, B. (2013). *Identifying disease characteristics, parent experience, and coping strategies when predicting pediatric illness-related stress in parents of children with mitochondrial disease* (doctoral dissertation). Retrieved from Washington State University Research Exchange, http://hdl.handle.net/2376/5035

Seth, A., & Maheshwari, A. (2013). Common endocrine problems in children (hypothyroidism and type 1 diabetes mellitus). *Indian Journal of Pediatrics, 80*(8), 681–687.

Shah, N. S., & Lila, A. (2011). Childhood Cushing disease: A challenge in diagnosis and management. *Hormone Research in Paediatrics, 76*(Suppl 1), 65–70.

Shanholtz, H. J. (2013). Congenital hypothyroidism. *Journal of Pediatric Nursing, 28*(2), 200–202.

Sharma, P. K. (2014). *Complications of thyroid surgery.* Retrieved from http://emedicine.medscape.com/article/852184-overview

Sharma, R., & Seth. A. (2014). Congenital adrenal hyperplasia: issues in diagnosis and treatment in children. *Indian Journal of Pediatrics, 81*(2), 178–185.

Shoback, D., & Funk J. L., (2011). Humoral manifestations of malignancy. In D. G. Gardner & D. Shoback (Eds.), *Greenspan's basic & clinical endocrinology* (9th ed.). Retrieved from http://www.accessmedicine.com

Shuch, B., Ricketts, C. J., Metwalli, A. R., Pacak, K., & Linehan, W. M. (2014). The genetic basis of pheochromocytoma and paraganglioma: Implications for management. *Urology, 83,* 1225–1232.

Sirotnak, A. P. (2013). *Psychosocial dwarfism.* Retrieved from http://emedicine.medscape.com/article/913843-overview

Speiser, P. W., & Wilson, T. A. (2014). *Pediatric adrenal insufficiency (Addison disease).* Retrieved from http://emedicine.medscape.com/article/919077-overview

Stanley, T. (2012). Diagnosis of growth hormone deficiency in childhood. *Current Opinion in Endocrinology, Diabetes and Obesity, 19*(1), 47–52.

Svoren, B. M., & Jospe, N. (2016). Diabetes mellitus. In R. M. Kliegman, B. F. Stanton, J. W. St. Geme, & N. F. Schor (Eds.), *Nelson textbook of pediatrics* (20th ed., pp. 2760–2790). Philadelphia, PA: Elsevier.

Szypowska, A., & Skora, A. (2011). The risk factors of ketoacidosis in children with newly diagnosed type 1 diabetes mellitus. *Pediatric Diabetes, 12,* 302–306.

Thomas, C. P., & Fraer, M. (2014). *Syndrome of inappropriate antidiuretic hormone secretion.* Retrieved from http://emedicine.medscape.com/article/246650-overview

Tsirlin, A., Oo, Y., Sharma, R., Kansara, A., Gliwa, A., & Banerji, M. A. (2014). Pheochromocytoma: A review. *Maturitas, 77,* 229–238.

United Mitochondrial Disease Foundation (UMDF). (2011). *MitoFIRST handbook: An introductory guide* (web pamphlet). Retrieved from http://www.kintera.org/atf/cf/%7B858ACD34-ECC3-472A-8794-39B92E103561%7D/mito_first.pdf

Walker, K. A. B. (2014). Oral manifestations of Turner syndrome. *Access, 28*(5), 32–34.

Walsh, K., & March, P. (2013, August). Diabetes insipidus. *CINAHL Information Systems.*

White, P. C. (2016a). Cushing syndrome. In R. M. Kliegman, B. F. Stanton, J. W. St. Geme, & N. F. Schor (Eds.), *Nelson textbook of pediatrics* (20th ed., pp. 2723–2725). Philadelphia, PA: Elsevier.

White, P. C. (2016b). Congenital adrenal hyperplasia and related disorders. In R. M. Kliegman, B. F. Stanton, J. W. St. Geme, & N. F. Schor (Eds.), *Nelson textbook of pediatrics* (20th ed., pp. 2714–2723). Philadelphia, PA: Elsevier.

White, P. C. (2016c). Pheochromocytoma. In R. M. Kliegman, B. F. Stanton, J. W. St. Geme, & N. F. Schor (Eds.), *Nelson textbook of pediatrics* (20th ed., pp. 2727–2729). Philadelphia, PA: Elsevier.

Wilson, B. A., Shannon, M. T., & Shields, K. M. (2016). *Pearson nurse's drug guide 2016.* Hoboken, NJ: Pearson Education.

Wong, C. L., Ip, W. Y., Choi, K. C., & Lam, L. W. (2015). Examining self-care behaviors and their associated factors among adolescent girls with dysmenorrhea: An application of Orem's self-care deficit nursing theory. *Journal of Nursing Scholarship, 47*(3), 219–227.

Woerner, S. (2014). The benefits of insulin pump therapy in children and adolescents with type 1 diabetes. *Journal of Pediatric Nursing, 29*(6), 712–713.

Zeitler, P. S., Travers, S. H., Nadeau, K., Barker, J. M., Kelsey, M. M., & Kappy, M. S. (2014). Endocrine disorders. In W. W. Hay, M. J. Levin, R. R. Deterding, & M.J. Abzug (Eds.), *CURRENT diagnosis and treatment: Pediatrics* (22th ed.). New York, NY: McGraw-Hill. Retrieved from http://accessmedicine.com

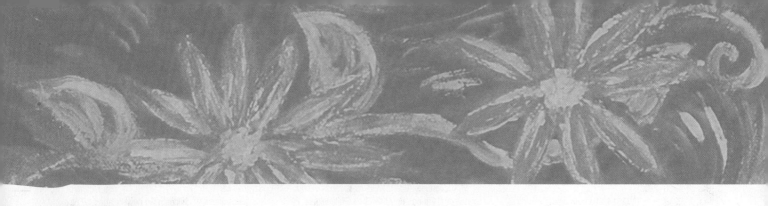

Chapter 31
Alterations in Skin Integrity

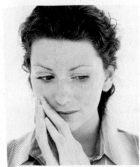

I didn't know that hot soup could cause such a bad injury. I am worried about the scars Shanelle might have over her chest from this scald burn.

—Mother of Shanelle, 1 year old

George Doyle/Getty Images

✓ Learning Outcomes

31.1 Classify the characteristics of skin lesions caused by irritants, drug reactions, mites, infection, and injury.

31.2 Differentiate among the stages of wound healing.

31.3 Compare skin conditions that have a hereditary cause or predisposition.

31.4 Plan the nursing care for the child with alterations in skin integrity, including dermatitis, infectious disorders, and infestations.

31.5 Prepare an education plan for adolescents with acne to promote self-care.

31.6 Summarize the process to measure the extent of burns and burn severity in children.

31.7 Develop a nursing care plan for the child with a full-thickness burn injury.

31.8 Contrast preventive strategies to reduce the risk of injury from burns, hypothermia, bites, and stings.

Skin Lesions

Skin lesions vary in size, shape, color, and texture. The two major types of skin lesions are primary lesions and secondary lesions. Primary lesions arise from previously healthy skin and include macules, patches, papules, nodules, tumors, vesicles, pustules, bullae, and wheals. (See *Pathophysiology Illustrated: Common Primary Skin Lesions and Associated Conditions* in Chapter 5.) Secondary lesions result from changes in primary lesions. They include crusts, scales, **lichenification** (thickening of the skin with more visible skin furrows), scars, keloids, excoriation, fissures, erosion, and ulcers. It is important for the nurse to be able to identify and describe the primary and secondary skin lesions and understand their underlying cause and treatment.

Text continues on page 903

FOCUS ON:
The Integumentary System

Anatomy and Physiology

The skin is the largest organ in the body and performs several essential functions. The skin protects underlying tissues from invasion by microorganisms and from trauma. The nerves in the skin enable the perception of touch, pain, pressure, heat, and cold. The skin also assists the body to conserve heat by constricting blood vessels. Dilation of blood vessels and the secretion of sweat by the eccrine sweat glands enable the body to release excess heat. The sweat glands, secreting a solution of water, electrolytes, and urea, also help rid the body of toxins. The skin supplements the body's intake of vitamin D by synthesizing this vitamin from ultraviolet light.

The skin has three distinct layers: the epidermis, the dermis, and the subcutaneous fatty layer that separates the skin from the underlying tissue (Figure 31–1). The epidermis is the thin, rapidly growing, outermost layer of skin. Skin is continually shed by the stratum corneum, the superficial layer of the epidermis. The thickness of the epidermis varies by location on the body (e.g., 0.3 mm on the eyelids and 1.5 mm on the soles of the feet) (Rote, Huether, & McCance, 2014). The epidermis contains the melanocytes that synthesize and secrete melanin when the skin is exposed to ultraviolet light. The Langerhans cells within the epidermis initiate the skin's immune response when exposed to environmental antigens.

The dermis, the middle layer of the skin, is mostly composed of connective tissue, which allows the skin to stretch and contract with movement. Nerves, muscles, hair follicles, sebaceous and sweat glands, lymph channels, and blood vessels are all contained within the dermis. Mast cells located within the dermis play a role in the skin's hypersensitivity reactions.

The third skin layer, the subcutaneous layer, connects the dermis to the muscle below. This layer of fat cells helps insulate the body from cold temperatures. The sebaceous glands appear all over the body except on the palms of the hands and the soles of the feet and are connected with hair follicles in most cases. Sebum, a lipid substance produced and secreted into the hair follicle or directly onto the skin, lubricates the skin and hair.

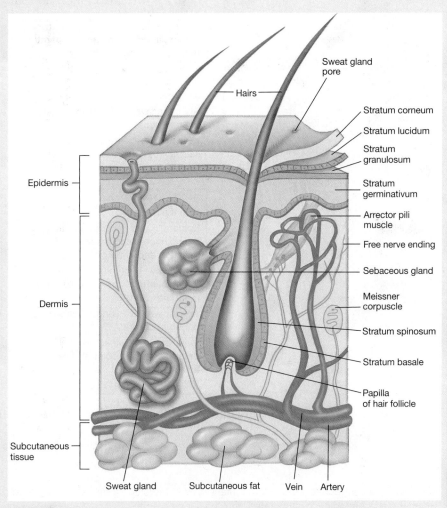

Figure 31–1 **Layers of the skin with accessory structures.**

Eccrine sweat glands, located in the dermis, open onto the skin's surface. They secrete sweat, an odorless, watery fluid containing sodium, chloride, urea, and other body wastes. As the body temperature elevates, an increased production of sweat evaporates and cools the body.

Apocrine sweat glands are primarily located in the axillary and genital areas, and their secretions contain more lipids and proteins. Decomposition of the fluid secreted by these glands leads to body odor.

Pediatric Differences

The newborn's skin is the largest organ of the body, but it is thinner and more fragile than adult skin. With thinner skin and less subcutaneous fat, the infant loses heat more rapidly, has greater difficulty regulating body temperature, and becomes more easily chilled than an older child or an adult. The thinner skin also increases the potential absorption of topical medications. The infant's skin contains more water than an adult's

As Children Grow: Integumentary System Changes

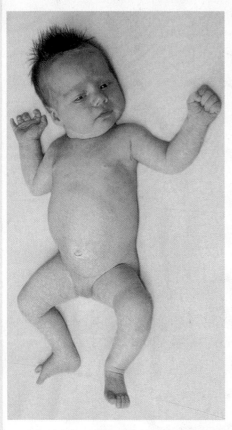

Newborns
Skin is very thin
Epidermis is loosely bound to the dermis, friction can cause separation of the layers with blistering
Eccrine sweat glands function, produce sweat in response to heat and emotional stimuli
Apocrine sweat glands are small and nonfunctional
Less melanin is present at birth so skin is lighter colored

Adolescents
Skin thickens
Epidermis and dermis are tightly bound, increasing resistance to infection and irritation
Eccrine sweat glands achieve full function, after puberty males sweat more than females
Apocrine sweat glands mature during puberty
Melanin is at adult levels, determining skin color and serving as a shield against ultraviolet radiation

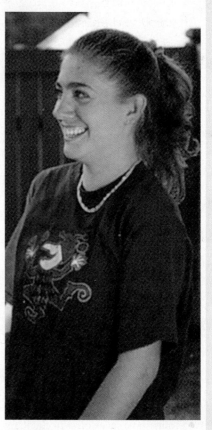

The structures of the skin mature during childhood, reaching adult function at puberty.

and has loosely attached cells. As the infant grows, the skin toughens and becomes less hydrated, making it less susceptible to bacteria (see *As Children Grow: Integumentary System Changes*).

Melanin, a peptide synthesized by an enzyme in melanocytes, influences skin color. Melanin production is low at birth and during the newborn period, accounting for the lighter skin in newborns of all races. Newborns and young infants are therefore more susceptible to damage from the sun and ultraviolet light.

Sebaceous glands and eccrine sweat glands are functional at birth in a term infant, although somewhat immaturely. The apocrine glands do not function until puberty.

Use *Assessment Guide: The Child With a Skin Condition* to perform a nursing assessment of the integumentary system. A list of diagnostic and laboratory tests used to evaluate skin conditions is provided in Table 31–1.

TABLE 31–1 Diagnostic Tests and Procedures for Integument Evaluation

DIAGNOSTIC PROCEDURES	LABORATORY TESTS
Culture of wound or skin drainage	Complete blood count
Tissue biopsy	Immunoglobulin E
Computed tomography (CT)	Potassium hydroxide on skin scrapings
Radiograph	
Ultrasound	

Note: See Appendices D and E for more information about these tests and procedures.

ASSESSMENT GUIDE | The Child With a Skin Condition

Assessment Focus	Assessment Guidelines*
Skin characteristics	• Inspect the skin for color, elevations, and imperfections. • Palpate the skin for texture, moisture, temperature, turgor, and edema.
Hair	• Inspect the scalp hair for color, distribution, and cleanliness. Inspect for nits (lice eggs) that adhere to the hair. • Inspect for areas of hair loss, bald spots, or broken hairs.
Lesions	• Describe skin lesions according to the characteristics listed in *Pathophysiology Illustrated: Common Primary Skin Lesions and Associated Conditions* in Chapter 5 and Table 31–2. Note erythema, signs of scratching (excoriation), or secondary infection. • Identify the location and distribution of lesions on the body (e.g., generalized, diaper area, flexor surfaces). • Palpate lesions for induration and temperature. • Measure the size of lesions (length, width, and height when appropriate).
Pain	• Assess level of pain when present.
Temperature	• Assess the body temperature.
Family history	• Identify family members with allergies or chronic skin conditions.

*See Chapter 5 for examination techniques.

TABLE 31–2 Common Secondary Skin Lesions and Associated Conditions

LESION NAME	DESCRIPTION	EXAMPLE
Burrow	A narrow, raised irregular channel caused by a parasite	Scabies
Comedone	A plug of sebaceous and keratin material in a hair follicle	Acne
Crust	Dried residue of serum, pus, or blood	Impetigo
Erosion	Loss of superficial epidermis; moist but does not bleed	Ruptured chickenpox vesicle
Excoriation	Abrasion or scratch mark	Scratched insect bite
Fissure	Linear crack in skin	Tinea pedis (athlete's foot)
Keloid	Overdevelopment or hypertrophy of scar that extends beyond wound edges and above skin line because of excess collagen	Healed skin area following traumatic injury
Lichenification	Thickening of skin with increased visibility of normal skin furrows	Atopic dermatitis (eczema)
Scale	Thin flake of exfoliated epidermis	Dandruff, psoriasis
Scar	Replacement of destroyed tissue with fibrous tissue	Healed surgical incision
Telangiectasia	Dilated, superficial blood vessels	Birthmark
Ulcer	Deeper loss of skin surface; bleeding or scarring may ensue	Pressure ulcer

Wound Healing

Wound healing occurs in three overlapping phases: hemostasis and inflammation, tissue formation, and maturation (see *Pathophysiology Illustrated: Phases of Wound Healing*).

Nursing responsibilities include wound cleansing and dressing changes. Wound cleansing is important because it removes loose material and bacteria from the site. Common cleansers are sterile water, normal saline, and commercial products that help loosen and suspend contaminants in water. Wound dressings have various properties that promote wound healing. See Table 31–3 for examples of primary dressings. Most primary dressings need a cover or secondary dressing. As the wound heals, the scar eventually achieves about 80% of the tissue's preinjury strength (Rote et al., 2014). A keloid results from an imbalance between collagen synthesis and collagen breakdown. The cause is unknown, but there is a familial tendency. A hypertrophic scar is raised but stays within the original wound boundaries.

Dermatitis

Many skin inflammations occur in early childhood. Most are easily treated and have no long-term consequences. Dermatitis is a condition in which skin changes occur in response to external stimuli. The three most common types of acute

Pathophysiology Illustrated: **Phases of Wound Healing**

Wound healing occurs in three overlapping phases:

Hemostasis and Inflammation (3–5 days)

Platelets flow to site and form a clot to stop bleeding, sealing the wound with fibrin, trapped cells, and platelets.

Platelets release inflammatory mediators (cytokines, chemokines, and growth factors).

Increased blood flow to area delivers leukocytes, phagocytes, and lymphocytes.

Increased capillary permeability causes swelling and erythema.

Bacteria are destroyed and cellular debris and foreign particles are removed.

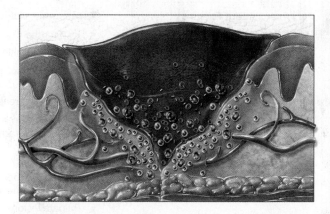

Tissue Formation (4 days to 2 weeks)

Natural debridement with fibrinolytic enzymes dissolves the fibrin clots.

Fibroblasts and endothelial cells in surrounding tissue direct the migration of cells to the newly developed fibrin matrix (replacing the clot), so remodeling can begin.

Granulation tissue forms and the wound is closed.

Capillary budding occurs for development of new blood vessels.

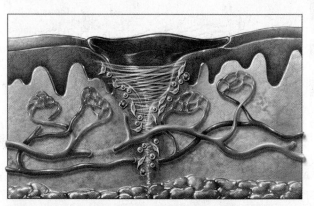

Maturation (months to 2 years)

Wound contraction occurs.

Epithelial cells migrate from the peripheral areas.

Collagen development leads to scar formation and strengthening.

Capillaries disappear from the scar tissue, returning the tissue to its original blood supply.

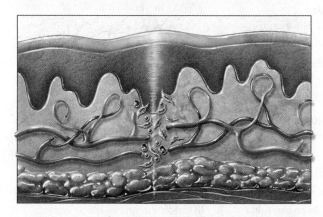

Source: Data from Reinke, J. M., & Sorg, H. (2012). Wound repair and regeneration. *European Surgical Research, 49,* 35–43; Yao, K., Bae, L., & Yew, W. P. (2013). Postoperative wound management. *Australian Family Physician, 42*(12), 867–870; Rote, N. S., Huether, S. E., & McCance, K. L. (2014). Innate immunity: Inflammation. In K. L. McCance, S. E. Huether, V. L. Brashers, & N. S. Rote (Eds.), *Pathophysiology: The biologic basis for disease in adults and children* (7th ed., pp. 191–223). St. Louis, MO: Elsevier.

dermatitis in infants, children, and adolescents are contact dermatitis, diaper dermatitis, and seborrheic dermatitis. See information on atopic dermatitis later in this chapter. These skin disorders may cause an emotional response in the child and family. Be supportive and reassure the family that the child is not infectious.

Contact Dermatitis

Contact dermatitis is an inflammation of the skin that occurs in response to direct contact with an allergen or irritant.

When an external irritant causes contact dermatitis, an inflammatory response occurs without an immune response. Common irritants include soaps, detergents, fabric softeners, bleaches, lotions, urine, and stool. An irritant can affect the skin any time there is adequate concentration and contact duration. Sweating and friction enhance the exposure to an irritant. Children with atopic dermatitis may be at risk for irritant contact dermatitis because of decreased skin barrier function.

Phytophotodermatitis can result when the child has skin contact with certain citrus fruits, celery, parsley, fennel, fig leaves, or ragweed. These plants have a chemical (furocoumarin) that

TABLE 31–3 Primary Wound Dressings

DRESSING TYPE	PROPERTIES	NURSING MANAGEMENT
Hydrocolloid—semiocclusive	Uses wound exudates to form a gel-like cover that adheres and protects wound bed from contaminants Maintains moist environment Promotes autolytic debridement	Use for granulating and epithelializing wounds with low or moderate amount of exudates. Use with caution in infected wounds. Cover at least 1 in. of intact skin around the wound.
Hydrogel—semiocclusive	Increases and maintains moisture content Promotes autolytic debridement Does not adhere, reducing pain with removal	Use with minimal or moderate exudate as limited exudates absorption. Cover at least 1 in. of intact skin around the wound.
Foam—semiocclusive	Absorbent—used for moderate to heavy exudate Nonadherent	Use for packing deep wounds. Use for heavy exudate when drainage is at peak.
Alginates—semiocclusive	Absorbs exudate and converts it to a gel Provides a moist environment	Use for moderate to heavy exudate. Use to pack wounds.
Transparent film—occlusive	Permeable to oxygen and water vapor Maintains moist environment Nonabsorbent Protects wound from contamination	Its use provides visible wound evaluation. Use on superficial wounds with little or no drainage or on areas of friction. Use care when removing film to prevent skin tearing.

Source: Data from Rolstad, B. S., Bryant, R. A., & Nix, D. P. (2012). Topical management. In R. A. Bryant & D. P. Nix (Eds.), *Acute & chronic wounds: Current management concepts* (4th ed., pp. 289–295). St. Louis, MO: Elsevier Mosby; Wound Care Information Network. (2013). *Wound care product and category index*. Retrieved from http://www.medicaledu.com/prodindx.htm; Wound Educators. (2015). *Wound dressings*. Retrieved from http://woundeducators.com/resources/wound-dressings/

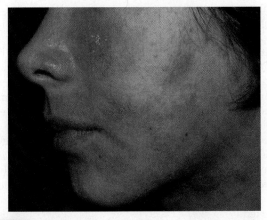

Figure 31–2 **Contact dermatitis caused by poison ivy. Note the clustered tiny erythematous papules involving the face and neck. In some areas (particularly the neck), lesions are distributed in a linear fashion.**

SOURCE: Courtesy of Daniel P. Krowchuk, MD, Professor of Pediatrics and Dermatology, Wake Forest School of Medicine, Winston-Salem, NC.

sensitizes the skin to sunlight. Following sun exposure the child develops erythema and blistering at the site of the contact, and the skin then becomes hyperpigmented 1 to 2 weeks later. The hyperpigmentation fades over several months (Shulstad, 2012).

Allergic contact dermatitis is a delayed T-cell–mediated hypersensitivity reaction. An antigen is absorbed from the skin surface during the initial sensitization phase, and an immune memory is created. A repeated exposure or a long-term exposure is required to cause the immune response and the dermatitis. See Chapter 22 to review the immune response to allergens. Common allergens include poison ivy, poison oak, lanolin, neomycin, rubber, chemicals in shoe leather, nickel, fragrances, and latex (Figure 31–2). Children may have both irritant and allergic

reactions to latex, which is found in many types of hospital equipment and supplies and products in the home.

With irritant contact dermatitis, a discrete area of redness is seen that corresponds to the exposure location, and severity is related to duration of exposure. The rash usually develops within a few hours of contact, peaks within 24 hours, and quickly resolves with removal of the irritant. With longer exposure, reactions may include painful erythema, edema, vesicles, and exudate.

Allergic contact dermatitis is characterized by erythema, edema, pruritus, vesicles, or bullae that rupture, ooze, and crust. The rash is usually limited to the area of contact (Table 31–4). Symptoms of allergic contact dermatitis can develop several hours following exposure, after the immune response has been activated. Symptoms can last 3 to 4 weeks without treatment.

The history of potential exposures and distribution of lesions provide clues about the source and identity of the allergen or irritant. Secondary infection may occur. For irritant contact dermatitis, treatment involves removing the offending agent (e.g., clothes, plant, soap). Use emollients to restore the skin barrier. Decrease inflammation with hydrocortisone cream or ointment. Antihistamines may help relieve itching or be given for their sedative effect.

SAFETY ALERT!

Some children have allergic contact dermatitis associated with spices such as vanilla, clove, and cinnamon, as well as citrus peels. These children may develop systemic contact dermatitis through oral ingestion of these products that are in the Balsam of Peru family of flavorings in chewing gum, toothpaste, baked goods, and food condiments. These children may need special dietary guidelines to reduce exposure to Balsam of Peru products (Fonacier et al., 2012).

TABLE 31–4 Distribution of Lesions by Type of Allergen

DISTRIBUTION OF LESION	ALLERGEN
Face, eyelids, neck	Cosmetics, hair and skin care products, nail polish and cosmetics, fragrances, eyeglasses with nickel
Earlobes, area with body piercing	Jewelry with nickel, cell phone
Lips, mouth	Oral hygiene products, bubblegum, lipstick
Hands	Rubber or neoprene gloves, mouse pad
Dorsal aspects of toes and feet	Rubber or leather chemical in shoes, metal buckles on sandals
Trunk	Snaps or other metal fasteners on clothing, belt buckles, moisturizers, cleansers, sunscreen products

Source: Data from Kwan, J. M., & Jacob, S. E. (2012). Contact dermatitis in the atopic child. *Pediatric Annals, 41*(10), 422–428; Fonacier, L. S., Aquino, M. R., & Mucci, T. (2012). Current strategies in treating severe contact dermatitis in pediatric patients. *Current Allergy and Asthma Reports, 12*, 599–606; Krowchuk, D. P., & Mancini, A. J. (2012). *Pediatric dermatology: A quick reference guide* (2nd ed., pp. 43–53). Elk Grove, IL: American Academy of Pediatrics; Halloran, L. (2014). Developing dermatology detective powers: Allergic contact dermatitis. *Journal for Nurse Practitioners, 10*(4), 284–285.

Acute allergic contact dermatitis is managed with medium-potency topical corticosteroids when less than 10% of the body surface area is affected. The topical corticosteroids are applied to the affected area twice a day for 2 to 3 weeks. Do not apply the medication to open lesions. Rebound dermatitis may occur if treatment is stopped early. Reactions to poison ivy or other allergens covering more than 10% of the body surface area require oral corticosteroid treatment for 7 to 14 days and a tapered dose for 7 to 10 additional days.

Nursing Management

Assess the child's skin using guidelines found earlier in the chapter in *Assessment Guide: The Child With a Skin Condition*. Family education for home care management focuses on care of the skin and prevention of future exposures. Teach parents how to apply topical corticosteroids and to keep using the medication for 2 to 3 weeks even when the skin shows signs of healing. Wet dressings may be soothing and help loosen crusts. Burow solution used as a soak helps dry lesions. Familiarize parents with the symptoms of infection in the affected area (i.e., increased redness, oozing, fever) and tell them when to return for follow-up care.

Teach parents to avoid exposure to allergens or irritants. Advise parents to wash all clothes before the first wearing and to rinse clothes an extra time to remove all the soap. Mild soap should be used to clean the skin. An emollient may be used for dry skin. Place a barrier between the irritant (e.g., metal, shoe leather) and the skin. If a nickel allergy exists, avoid use of nickel jewelry and belt buckles.

Diaper Dermatitis

Diaper dermatitis, a common cause of irritant contact dermatitis, occurs in approximately one third of young children, usually in a mild form. It is more common in infants from 9 to 12 months and toddlers.

Diaper dermatitis is a primary reaction to urine, feces, moisture, or friction. Urine and feces interact with the skin to cause dermatitis. The urine increases the wetness and pH of the skin, increasing abrasion and its permeability to irritants and microbes. Urine also metabolizes to ammonia, producing another irritant. Fecal organisms provide more irritants.

Infection with *Candida albicans* is a common complication of diaper dermatitis or antibiotic therapy for another condition. It is frequently the underlying cause of severe diaper rash. Diaper candidiasis often occurs simultaneously with oral candidiasis.

The rash is characterized by raw, moist, or weeping macules and papules of the skin in direct contact with the diaper. The skinfolds are usually spared. In severe cases, the infant develops a rash that is fiery red, raised, and confluent (Figure 31–3). Pustules with tenderness can also be present. When a *C. albicans* infection occurs, the rash has bright-red beefy plaques with sharp margins that may rupture and leave scales. Small papules and pustules may be seen, along with satellite lesions. Skinfolds may be affected.

Families Want to Know

Exposure to Poison Ivy or Poison Oak

- The rash is caused by contact with urushiol, a resin of the plants, either directly or indirectly, such as transfer from an animal or clothing. Avoid hugging a pet exposed to poison ivy until after the pet has been bathed. Once the rash develops, it is not contagious.

- Wash exposed skin with soap and water, and scrub under the nails as soon as possible after contact. Zanfel and Ivy X are over-the-counter products that remove urushiol after poison ivy exposure to reduce itching and severity of rash if used promptly.

- Do not rub fingers exposed to poison ivy against broken skin or the eyes.

- Launder clothing worn during exposure, and wash hands after handling exposed clothing.

- Wear vinyl gloves to handle plants (cloth and rubber gloves allow sap to penetrate).

- Search the yard and remove all plants. Do not burn plants removed. A person with a sensitivity may inhale the smoke and develop severe airway inflammation.

- For children with sensitivity to poison ivy, an over-the-counter barrier cream such as Ivy X preexposure solution can be applied to help prevent skin penetration of plant oil.

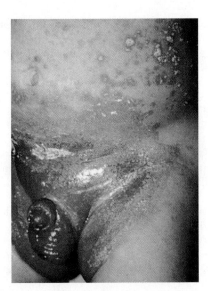

Figure 31–3 **Diaper dermatitis. Note the skinfold that is free of inflammation.**

SOURCE: Courtesy of the Centers for Disease Control and Prevention, Atlanta, GA.

Mild diaper dermatitis is treated with a water-impermeable barrier or protective sealant such as zinc oxide, Aquaphor, Desitin, or Balmex after every diaper change. In some cases, a diaper ointment combined with a protective powder (e.g., karaya powder) may be effective. An antifungal topical medication (e.g., nystatin) is applied to the skin before the barrier product when *C. albicans* is present, and is continued for 3 days after the rash clears. Topical corticosteroids are often avoided for diaper dermatitis because occlusion in the diaper area increases corticosteroid systemic absorption. If topical corticosteroids are necessary, a low- potency product is used.

Nursing Management

Diaper dermatitis can be a major source of stress for parents when the child is in constant discomfort. Instruct parents to change the diaper as soon as the infant is wet, or at least every 2 hours during the day and once during the night to minimize contact with urine and fecal irritants. Teach parents to apply barrier products and to remove them once or twice a day so fresh medication can be applied. Mineral oil and a soft cloth are effective for removing pastes. Encourage the parents to return for further care if the infant's skin is not greatly improved within a week.

Encourage parents to use superabsorbent disposable diapers, which tend to reduce the frequency and severity of diaper dermatitis. When wet, these diapers form a gel that keeps the skin drier than cloth diapers; however, diapers should still be changed every 2 to 3 hours. Exposing the diaper area to air aids healing. For example, allow the infant to go without a diaper while lying on an absorbent pad or cloth.

Advise parents to wash the perianal area with warm water or a waterless cleanser (Aquanil HC lotion or Cetaphil) after a bowel movement. Advise parents to use soft cloths or paper towels with warm tap water or to use baby wipes without alcohol if baby wipes are preferred. Pat the skin dry to reduce friction and skin injury. Avoid using powder or cornstarch because they may increase friction.

Seborrheic Dermatitis

Seborrheic dermatitis is a recurrent inflammatory skin condition thought to be caused by an overgrowth of a yeast, *Malassezia furfur* (formerly *Pityrosporum ovale*). The condition is thought to be influenced by hormones. The rash is found over the areas of the body where the sebaceous glands are most plentiful: scalp (cradle cap), face, and postauricular and periorbital areas. The condition is frequently seen in infants up to 3 months of age and in adolescents.

Common symptoms are pruritus and a mildly erythematous, adherent, waxy scaling of the scalp (or "dandruff"). Yellow-red patches with greasy scaling may be present, typically on the scalp and nasolabial folds on the face, behind the ears, on the upper chest, and sometimes on the **intertriginous** (skinfolds of the neck, axillae, antecubital fossa) areas (Figure 31–4). Itching is less intense than with atopic eczema.

Treatment for young infants consists of daily shampooing with baby shampoo. An **emollient**, a topical product that soothes and softens the skin, such as warm mineral or olive oil, is left on the scalp for about 20 minutes to soften the crusts after shampooing. The scales are removed by brushing with the fingertips or a soft toothbrush. The hair is then shampooed again and rinsed thoroughly. A shampoo with 2% ketoconazole may be used in infants if baby shampoo is not effective (Ooi & Tidman, 2014).

Lesions on the body of adolescents can be treated with shampoos containing selenium sulfide or salicylic acid. Use baby shampoo to wash lesions on the eyelids and eyelashes. Treatments are continued for several days after the lesions disappear and may be repeated weekly to prevent recurrence. Topical corticosteroids are used to treat seborrhea that is not on the scalp, but avoid its use around the eyes.

Nursing Management

Teach new parents to wash the infant's hair daily with each bath. Reassure parents that gentle cleansing will not harm the infant's "soft spot." Demonstrate bathing to show them the proper technique, if necessary. Follow-up is seldom necessary, as the condition resolves with treatment. Advise

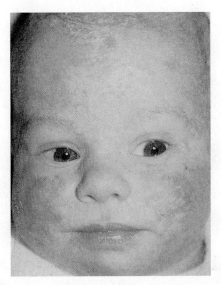

Figure 31–4 Seborrheic dermatitis. Note the extensive red patches with scales over the forehead and face.

adolescents that emotional distress may trigger future flare-ups and to initiate treatment promptly when symptoms begin.

Bacterial Infections

Impetigo

Impetigo, the most common bacterial skin condition, is a highly contagious, superficial (epidermal) infection. The most common sites are the face, around the mouth, the hands, the neck, and the extremities. Minor skin injuries, insect bites, and dermatitis provide the portal for the infectious agent. Impetigo occurs more commonly in children who are in close physical contact with others, such as in childcare settings, or in those who have poor hygiene.

Either group A beta-hemolytic streptococcus, *Staphylococcus aureus*, or both together are usually responsible. *S. aureus*, the more common organism, colonizes on the skin and in the nose and throat. Some children will pick their nose and infect themselves. Bullous impetigo results from a strain of *S. aureus* that produces an exfoliative toxin that blisters the epidermis.

The impetigo lesion begins as a papule that turns into a vesicle at the injury site. The vesicle ruptures and forms an erosion, and serous fluid forms the characteristic honey-colored crusts. Pruritus and regional lymphadenopathy may be present. The rash may spread to the face and extremities by self-inoculation (Figure 31–5). In bullous impetigo, vesicles stimulated by a toxin enlarge and coalesce to form bullae with sharp margins and no surrounding erythema. A thin honey-colored crust forms when the bullae rupture. When the crust is removed, a moist, erythematous lesion with a collar of skin around the erosion is seen. These lesions occur more commonly in moist skinfold areas. Impetigo is diagnosed by appearance or lesions or by bacterial culture.

Local treatment of nonbullous impetigo involves removal of the crusts and application of a topical antibiotic. A topical bactericidal ointment such as mupirocin or retapamulin is applied 3 times a day for 5 days (Stevens et al., 2014). Oral antibiotics are prescribed for bullous impetigo. Skin generally heals without scars. The infection is communicable for 24 hours after antibiotic ointment treatment is begun.

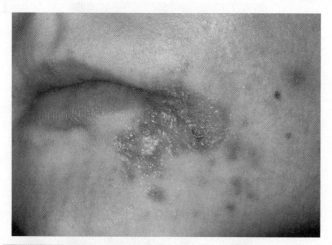

Figure 31–5 Impetigo. Note the honey-colored crusts over the lesion.

SOURCE: Dr. P. Marazzi/Science Source.

Potential complications are postinfectious streptococcal glomerulonephritis (see Chapter 26) and cellulitis.

Nursing Management

Teach parents to soak crusts in warm water and gently scrub them off with a gauze pad and antiseptic soap prior to using topical ointment. Teach parents to dispose of the gauze pad in a plastic bag to avoid spreading the infection to other family members. Advise parents to continue using the topical or oral medication for the full number of days prescribed. Inform the parents to observe all close contacts and family members for lesions. The infected child should not share towels or toiletries with others, and all linens and clothing used by the child should be washed separately with detergent and hot water. Keep fingernails short and clean to prevent spreading infection by scratching. Inform the childcare center about the infection, so staff can sanitize toys and surfaces.

Community-Acquired Methicillin-Resistant *Staphylococcus aureus*

Community-acquired, methicillin-resistant *Staphylococcus aureus* (CA-MRSA) may cause a severe and aggressive skin and soft-tissue infection in healthy children. CA-MRSA is colonized on the skin, the mucous membranes, and nares of healthy individual carriers. Direct contact transmission and respiratory droplet transmission occur. Athletes are at high risk because of their potential for frequent skin-to-skin contact, cuts or abrasions, wound contact, and shared items.

Clinical manifestations include furuncles or abscesses that may invade deeper tissues. Localized swelling, redness, warmth, purulent drainage, fever, and pain may be present.

Incised abscesses are cultured to diagnose CA-MRSA. Simple abscesses are treated with incision, drainage, wound care, and systemic antibiotics. Children with repeated CA-MRSA infections may be encouraged to decolonize the skin to reduce the number of infections.

Clinical Tip

When the child has recurrent CA-MRSA infections, the child or family member may be a nasal carrier of *S. aureus*. All household members may be treated with nasal application of mupiricin 2 times a day for 5 days and bathe with diluted bleach solution (one half cup to a tub one quarter full) or chlorhexidine scrub for 5 days. Surfaces frequently touched and bed linens must be decontaminated. A second round of household treatment may be needed (Fritz et al., 2012).

Nursing Management

Ensure that parents and adolescents understand the importance of taking the full course of the prescribed antibiotic. Educate parents about meticulous wound care to prevent the spread of CA-MRSA:

- Keep the wound and drainage completely covered at all times.
- Change the dressing twice a day using vinyl gloves. Use good hand hygiene before and after dressing changes.

- Dispose of used dressings in a tightly closed plastic bag.
- Disinfect surfaces that come into contact with the wound or wound drainage using a bleach solution.
- Use hot water to wash linens and clothing used by the child, and dry clothes in a hot dryer.

Nurses have a major role in prevention of CA-MRSA infections. Nurses in contact with the wound should remove gloves before touching and contaminating surfaces in the examining room. Ensure that any equipment and linen used by the child are appropriately managed and the examining room is cleaned with an effective agent.

Educate parents, adolescents, coaches, and teachers about the importance of a regular schedule for cleaning equipment and having athletes take showers with soap and water after all practice sessions. Discourage athletes from sharing towels and clothing. Cover minor wounds to reduce exposure to other athletes. Skin infections that worsen rather than heal with regular topical antibiotics should be seen by a healthcare provider.

Folliculitis

Folliculitis is a superficial inflammation of the pilosebaceous follicle caused by infection, trauma, or irritation. The causative organism is usually *Staphylococcus aureus*. The condition is common in children and teenagers because of increased sweat production. Folliculitis may be associated with *Pseudomonas aeruginosa* exposure in a poorly chlorinated pool or hot tub.

Symptoms include pain or pruritus, localized swelling, and the formation of tiny dome-shaped, yellowish pustules and red papules at follicular openings with surrounding erythema. Individual lesions may become deeper and form an abscess (furuncle). Lesions are usually seen in clusters on the face, scalp, trunk, and extremities. Some children have fever, aching, and flulike symptoms. If associated with *Pseudomonas* exposure in a pool or hot tub, lesions may develop on areas covered by bathing suits.

Folliculitis is treated by washing the affected area with a topical antibacterial cleanser (e.g., chlorhexidine) and water. A benzoyl peroxide gel or wash or another drying agent will also help clear the infection. Ruptured lesions heal with hyperpigmentation and no scarring. Complications are rare. If the child or adolescent has systemic symptoms, oral antibiotics (e.g., clindamycin or doxycycline) may be prescribed. If a furuncle develops, incision and drainage may be needed. Children who are immunocompromised should not use hot tubs because of the potential for complications from *Pseudomonas*.

Nursing Management

Nursing management focuses on educating the parents and child about prevention. Advise children to shower daily and shortly after exercise, to cleanse with an antibacterial soap, and to wear loose cotton clothing. Talk with parents about the importance of maintaining the correct pH level and chlorine concentration in swimming pools and hot tubs. Bathing suits of affected children should be laundered and dried well before the next use.

Cellulitis

Cellulitis is an acute inflammation of the loose connective and subcutaneous tissues and the dermis. The condition usually occurs on the face and extremities as a result of trauma or a compromised skin barrier.

ETIOLOGY AND PATHOPHYSIOLOGY

The child may have a history of trauma, surgery, or skin lesions. Common causative organisms are *Staphylococcus aureus* and *Streptococcus pyogenes*. The condition may also result from a nearby abscess or sinusitis. Onset is usually rapid.

CLINICAL MANIFESTATIONS

Children with cellulitis have a rapid onset and they appear ill. Classic signs and symptoms include red or lilac, tender, warm, edematous skin around the infected site (Figure 31–6). The border is often indistinct because the infection is deep in the tissue. Other symptoms include fever, chills, malaise, and enlargement and tenderness of regional lymph nodes. **Lymphangitis**, inflammation of the lymphatic system draining the site of infection (seen as tender, erythematous streaks extending in a proximal direction), may be present.

CLINICAL THERAPY

Blood studies may show an increase in white blood cells. Cultures are taken by needle aspiration to identify the causative organisms. Blood cultures and a lumbar puncture are performed if the child has a toxic (very ill) appearance (see the *Clinical Skills Manual* SKILLS).

Children with severe cases or involvement of the face or a large affected surface area are hospitalized and treated aggressively with IV antibiotics and analgesics to avoid serious complications, such as sepsis, necrotizing fasciitis, or osteomyelitis. Children with less severe cellulitis on the trunk, limbs, or perianal area may be treated on an outpatient basis with oral antibiotics. Recovery begins within 48 hours, but therapy should continue for at least 10 days (Juern & Drolet, 2016). See Chapter 19 for treatment of periorbital cellulitis.

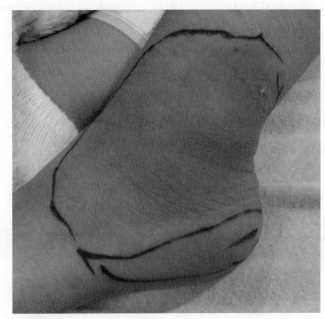

Figure 31–6 Characteristic appearance of cellulitis with borders of extensive inflammation outlined.

SOURCE: Courtesy of Daniel P. Krowchuk, MD, Professor of Pediatrics and Dermatology, Wake Forest School of Medicine, Winston-Salem, NC.

Nursing Management

Assessment centers on recognition of the severity of infection, documentation of location and related symptoms, and monitoring of vital signs. Administer prescribed oral or IV antibiotics as scheduled. Supportive care includes warm compresses to the affected area 4 times daily, elevation of the affected limb, and bed rest. Outpatient follow-up is crucial to ensure response to therapy.

Advise parents about possible complications, such as abscess formation. Instruct parents of children treated at home to contact their healthcare provider if the child has any of the following signs:

- Spread of the infected area in the 24- to 48-hour period after the start of treatment
- Temperature over 38.3°C (101.0°F)
- Increased lethargy

Reinforce to parents the importance of compliance with the treatment regimen and the seriousness of the possible complications.

Viral Infections

Molluscum Contagiosum

Molluscum contagiosum is a skin infection caused by a poxvirus. It is transmitted by direct contact, contact with contaminated objects, or sexual contact. Spread occurs by autoinoculation. The incubation period is 2 to 7 weeks (American Academy of Pediatrics [AAP], 2015, p. 561. Children 2 to 11 years of age are most commonly affected, but increased risk is believed to be associated with atopic eczema and immunodeficiency.

Multiple pearl-like flesh-colored smooth papules (usually less than 30) are about 2 to 5 mm (0.08 to 0.2 in.) in size. The lesion has a central depression, and a plug of cheesy material can be expressed when punctured. Lesions may appear anywhere on the body, but are more often found on the face, trunk, and extremities. Adolescents may have lesions on the genital mucous membranes. If children have genital lesions, consider sexual abuse as a possible source of infection.

Supportive care is often preferred because aggressive treatments frequently cause scars or hyperpigmentation in children with darker skin. A single lesion may be present for 2 months, but the usual duration of the condition is 8 to 12 months, resolving spontaneously. Emollients, topical corticosteroids, or oral antihistamines are used for pruritus. When treatment is provided, options to destroy lesions include curettage, **cryotherapy** (freezing each lesion with liquid nitrogen), or pulsed-dye laser. Topical anesthesia is needed for curettage. Other treatment options include chemical treatment (e.g., salicylic acid or cantharidin), an immune modulator (e.g., imiquimod), or antiviral medication. No one treatment has demonstrated better effectiveness (Chen, Anstey, & Bugert, 2013). Secondary infections are a potential complication.

Nursing Management

Nursing education focuses on reducing disease transmission. Infected children should not use public swimming pools, hot tubs, or bathe with other children because the virus is more easily transmitted when the skin is wet. Transmission of the virus among household members is high. Towels, sponges, and clothing should not be shared. Wash the skin daily with gentle fragrance-free cleansers. Apply a hypoallergenic moisturizer or emollient to the entire skin surface. Teach parents to recognize potential secondary infections.

When intervention such as curettage or cryotherapy is performed, ensure that adequate topical anesthetic is used to minimize pain. Inform the child about what will happen, and provide distraction during the procedure to reduce anxiety.

Warts (Papillomavirus)

Warts commonly are found in children between 1 and 17 years, with a prevalence of 3.3% in the United States. The peak age is 9 to 10 years when 8.6% of children are affected (Silverberg & Silverberg, 2013). Several types of human papillomavirus infect epithelial cells and cause warts. Common warts appear on any skin surface, and plantar warts are found on the feet. The virus is commonly transmitted by direct skin-to-skin contact or mucous membrane contact. It also survives on various surfaces, and transmission can occur with contact, such as plantar warts from locker room floors. The incubation period may be 2 to 6 months; however, a latency period may exist in some cases. Children with immune compromise are more susceptible and often have numerous warts.

Common warts appear as skin-colored, rough, scaly papules and nodules on exposed skin surfaces. Individual and multiple warts may be seen, or large plaques may form if autoinoculation occurs. Warts usually cause no pain or itching unless on skin surface areas that becomes irritated. Plantar warts appear as papules and plaques on the bottom of feet that grow inward and cause pain. Small black dots result from thrombosed vessels on the surface of the warts caused by weight bearing.

No intervention may be recommended as warts often resolve spontaneously over a couple of years. Warts do not produce scarring unless treated surgically or in an aggressive manner. If warts cause pain or a social stigma, clinical therapy may be initiated. Treatment usually involves destruction by daily home application of salicylic acid plasters, and occlusion with tape is sometimes recommended. Other treatments include liquid nitrogen or pulsed-dye laser. No one treatment is fully effective. A keratolytic agent (imiquimod) may be used to treat external anogenital warts. Immunotherapy may also be used.

Nursing Management

Educate the parents and child about how warts are spread by picking at it or chewing on it. If the child will not stop sucking or chewing on the wart, bitter apple or a pepper solution may discourage the child. Teach parents about the application of peeling agents when prescribed for home use. If the reaction to the treatment is painful, encourage the parents to reduce the frequency of the treatment until the pain subsides and then to resume the original treatment schedule. Successful treatment may take several months, and parents may need encouragement to continue the therapy and remain optimistic.

Other viral skin conditions are described in Chapter 16.

Fungal Infections

Oral Candidal Infection (Thrush)

Thrush is a fungal infection, usually caused by *Candida albicans*. An acute infection may occur in newborns or in children who regularly use a corticosteroid inhaler or have received

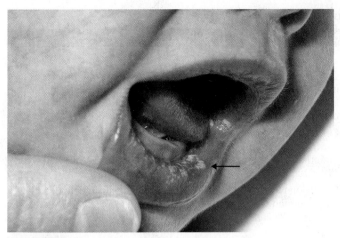

Figure 31–7 Oral thrush is an acute pseudomembranous form of candidiasis. It is a common fungal infection in infants and children.

SOURCE: Alamy.

antibiotics that disturb normal flora. An invasive *C. albicans* infection may occur in children with either an impaired immune status (immunodeficiency) or a central venous catheter receiving long-term parenteral alimentation therapy (AAP, 2015, p. 275).

Oral thrush is characterized by white patches that look like coagulated milk on the oral mucosa and may bleed when removed (Figure 31–7). Gentle attempts to remove patches are unsuccessful, while actual milk residue can be removed with gentle swabbing. The infant may refuse to nurse or feed because of discomfort and pain. The infant may also have diaper dermatitis. Fever is usually not present.

Diagnosis is made by clinical appearance, microscopic examination of a skin scraping suspended in potassium hydroxide, or fungal culture. Treatment involves oral nystatin suspension or clotrimazole applied to the mouth and tongue after feedings. Fluconazole or itraconazole may be used for immunocompromised patients with oropharyngeal candidiasis. Intravenous amphotericin B may be used for invasive and systemic *Candida* infections.

Nursing Management

Teach parents to give the medication by swabbing the suspension on the buccal mucosa and tongue surfaces, allowing the infant to swallow the remaining suspension. Teach older children to swish the solution around in the mouth before swallowing it.

To help prevent a reinfection, educate parents to use good hand hygiene and to sterilize bottle nipples and pacifiers. Teach parents and older children with asthma to rinse the mouth well with water after using a corticosteroid inhaler. If a spacer is used, it should also be rinsed with water after use. A commercial antiseptic spray may be used on toys put in the mouth that cannot be autoclaved, but follow directions carefully so the child does not ingest any harmful residue.

Dermatophytoses (Ringworm)

Dermatophytoses are fungal infections that commonly affect the skin, hair, or nails. Children of all ages may be affected. Dermatophytoses may be spread from another person or animal or by

contact with a contaminated object. See Table 31–5 for the clinical manifestations of tinea infections.

Diagnosis is confirmed through microscopic examination of the hair and scalp scrapings using a potassium hydroxide (KOH) wet mount to reveal rows and chains of spores within the hair shaft. A fungal culture can also be taken from a scalp lesion by rubbing a cotton-tipped applicator across the scalp or body lesion. Shining a Wood lamp on the lesion helps identify some forms of tinea (e.g., microsporum fluoresces a brilliant green). The most common cause of tinea, *Trichophyton tonsurans*, does not fluoresce (AAP, 2015, p. 780). See Table 31–5 for clinical therapy.

Clinical Tip

Some children treated for tinea capitis develop an "id" reaction, an extensive, itchy papulovesicular rash on the trunk, extremities, and face similar to atopic dermatitis. This is a hypersensitivity reaction to the fungal antigen, not an allergic reaction to the oral medication (AAP, 2015, p. 779). Antifungal therapy must be continued to resolve the infection.

Nursing Management

Assess all members of the family and household pets for fungal lesions. Since person-to-person transmission is common, family members should not share hair accessories, brushes, and hats. Because a family member may be an asymptomatic carrier, all family members should be treated with selenium shampoo. Teach parents and older children or teenagers that fungi are found in soil and animals and are transmitted through direct contact.

Advise parents to give oral griseofulvin with fatty foods such as whole milk or peanut butter to enhance absorption. To prevent recurrence of the infection, the medications must be used for the entire prescribed period, even if the lesions are gone. Advise parents about the possibility of the "id" reaction so they will continue to give the medication.

Parents of children with tinea capitis should be told that hair regrowth is slow and may take 6 to 12 months. In rare cases, hair loss is permanent, which can be particularly stressful for older children or adolescents. Provide emotional support. Encourage children to wear shower shoes in public showers and locker rooms to prevent tinea pedis.

Drug Reactions

Adverse reactions to over-the-counter or prescription medications are relatively common. Children with drug allergies usually have reactions after ingestion (e.g., aspirin, antibiotics, sedatives), injection (e.g., penicillin), or direct skin contact with medications. Drug sensitivities may result from variations in an individual's ability to tolerate a particular drug or concentration of a drug or from allergic responses. (See Chapter 22 for a description of allergic reactions.)

Sensitivity reactions may occur after 1 or 2 doses when the child has previously taken the drug, but it may take up to 7 days for sensitivity to occur to a drug not previously administered. The most common reactions in children are erythematous macules and papules or urticaria, which may be pruritic. Drugs that may cause a sensitivity reaction include the following: sulfonamides, anticonvulsants, antibiotics, and nonsteroidal anti-inflammatory drugs (NSAIDs). Be alert to the possibility of serious drug reactions that may become a medical emergency. See Table 31–6 for clinical manifestations of drug reactions.

TABLE 31–5 Clinical Manifestations of Tinea Infections

INFECTION SITE AND CLINICAL MANIFESTATIONS	CLINICAL THERAPY

TINEA CAPITIS (SCALP)

Scaly pustular bald areas with indistinct margins; may appear as seborrhea, with yellow, greasy scales; erythema or lesion lighter than skin color

Broken hairs; black dotted stubbed appearance where weakened hair has broken off

Mild itching

Kerion—large purulent tender boggy mass on scalp with drainage

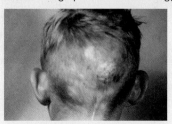

Tinea capitis.
Source: Centers for Disease Control and Prevention.

Oral griseofulvin for 8–12 weeks, OR oral terbinafine for 6 weeks in children over age 4 years. Fluconazole and itraconazole are not U.S. Food and Drug Administration (FDA) approved in children under 12 years of age.

Selenium sulfide or ketoconazole shampoo 2–3 times weekly, leaving the shampoo on the scalp for 10 min before rinsing. Encourage family members to use the shampoo 2–3 times a week to reduce the number of fungal spores in the household.

For kerions with evidence of secondary bacterial infection, antibiotics are added to oral antifungal agents (AAP, Committee on Infectious Disease, 2015, p. 781).

TINEA CORPORIS (TRUNK)

Pink, scaly circular patch with an expanding border, may be scaly or erythematous throughout; slightly raised borders with a clearing center

Usually acquired from contact with infected human, animal, or contaminated object (e.g., hat)

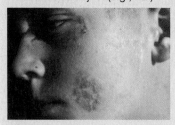

Tinea corporis.
Source: Centers for Disease Control and Prevention.

Topical cream (e.g., clotrimazole, miconazole, ketoconazole, terbinafine if 12 years and older or tolnaftate, naftifine, or ciclopirox if 10 years and older) twice a day for 4–6 weeks. Do not use a topical corticosteroid to prevent a persistent or recurrent infection.

Selenium sulfide shampoo 2 times a week on the child's body to help reduce the number of spores. Family members may also use the shampoo.

An oral antifungal agent when no response to topical therapy.

TINEA CRURIS ("JOCK ITCH")

Scaly, erythematous annular lesions on groin and upper thighs, may spread to the abdomen and buttocks; usually spares the penis and scrotum

May have elevated lesions, papules, or vesicles

Topical antifungal agent (e.g., clotrimazole, miconazole, and terbinafine for ages 12 years and older, tolnaftate or ciclopirox for 10 years and older) for 4–6 weeks.

Topical corticosteroids are not used.

Wash body area with selenium sulfide shampoo.

Wear loose clothing to promote dryness in the groin area.

TINEA PEDIS ("ATHLETE'S FOOT")

Vesicles or erosions on instep or between toes (fissures, red scaly); dry scaly patches or plaques with erythema on plantar and lateral surfaces of foot

Peeling maceration and fissures in lateral toe web spaces indicate secondary bacterial involvement

Pruritus

Broad-spectrum topical antifungal agent with antibacterial properties (e.g., econazole or ciclopirox)

Allow feet to air dry.

Use 100% cotton socks, change twice daily; put socks on before other clothing to reduce transmission of fungus to groin.

Source: Data from American Academy of Pediatrics, Committee on Infectious Disease. (2015). *Red book: Report of the Committee on Infectious Diseases* (30th ed., pp. 778–786). Elk Grove Village, IL: Author; Krowchuk, D. P., & Mancini, A. J. (2012). *Pediatric dermatology: A quick reference guide* (2nd ed., pp. 233–245). Elk Grove Village, IL: American Academy of Pediatrics; Wyatt, H. (2013). Common skin infections in children. *Nursing Standard, 27*(46), 43–48.

The treatment of choice for most drug sensitivity reactions is discontinuation of the causative drug. In rare cases, a drug may be continued with careful monitoring when the child has a less severe sensitivity reaction because it is the best treatment choice. Supportive measures should be taken to decrease the intensity of the reaction. An antihistamine may be used to block the release of histamine, which causes the rash. Topical corticosteroids, cool compresses, and baths may also be prescribed for pruritus. For some severe drug reactions, the child must be hospitalized and treated on a burn unit.

TABLE 31–6 Clinical Manifestations of Drug Reactions

TYPE OF REACTION	CLINICAL MANIFESTATIONS
ALLERGIC DRUG REACTION	
Most commonly caused by sulfonamides, tetracyclines, NSAIDs, oral contraceptives, barbiturates, phenytoin, carbamazepine, benzodiazepines, and morphine	Erythematous, pruritic macules and papules; urticaria (hives) begins on the trunk and extends in a symmetric fashion, often sparing mucous membranes. Affected area darkens over 1–2 weeks, and skin peeling may occur. May heal with pigment changes.
ERYTHEMA MULTIFORME MINOR	
Hypersensitivity reaction to anticonvulsants, penicillins, salicylates, sulfa antibiotics, barbiturates, and phenytoin; infectious agents (e.g., herpes simplex virus)	Skin lesions may be preceded by fever, malaise, and upper respiratory symptoms. Widespread erythematous macules progress to target lesions (papules, vesicles, or bullae in a pale ring with an erythematous border). May progress to blisters and bullous lesions. Lesions may itch or burn. Lesions common on palms and soles, elbows, extensor surface of forearms and legs.
STEVENS–JOHNSON SYNDROME (SJS) AND TOXIC EPIDERMAL NECROLYSIS (TEN)	
Potentially life-threatening hypersensitivity reaction to penicillins, sulfonamides, cephalosporins, fluoroquinolones, antiepileptic medications, NSAIDs, acetaminophen, or reaction to infectious disease such as *Mycoplasma pneumoniae* Believed to be forms of the same disease and the most severe form of erythema multiforme.	Prodromal infection for 1–7 days with low-grade fever, sore throat, or malaise. Headache, muscle aches, joint pain, and vomiting and diarrhea may be seen. Erythematous skin is tender, progressing to blisters and bullae, and then to necrotic epidermis that sheds and weeps. Mucous membranes have blisters, erosions, ulcerations, and hemorrhagic crusting. Painful crusting and sloughing of the lips and oral membranes occur. Respiratory and gastrointestinal mucosa may also be affected. Erosions (similar to partial-thickness burns) may spread to cover up to 10% of the skin surface in SJS, 10%–30% in overlapping SJS and TEN, and more than 30% in TEN. Corneal blistering can lead to scarring and blindness.

Source: Data from Nicol, N. H., & Huether, S. E. (2014). Alterations in the integument in children. In K. L. McCance, S. E. Huether, V. L. Brashers, & N. S. Rote (Eds.), *Pathophysiology: The biologic basis for disease in adults and children* (7th ed., pp. 1653–1667), St. Louis, MO: Elsevier; Joyce, J. C. (2016). Vesiculobullous disorders. In R. M. Kliegman, B. F. Stanton, J. W. St. Geme, & N. F. Schor (Eds.), *Nelson textbook of pediatrics* (20th ed., pp. 3140–3150). St. Louis, MO: Elsevier; Feinberg, A. N., Shwayder, T. A., Ruqiya, T., & Therdpong, T. (2014). Pediatric dermatologic disorders. *Journal of Alternative Medicine Research, 6*(2), 95–137; Yang, M., Kang, M., Jung, J., Song, W., Kang, H., Cho, S., & Min, K. (2013). Clinical features and prognostic factors in severe cutaneous drug reactions. *International Archives of Allergy and Immunology, 162*(4) 346–354.

Nursing Management

Teach parents to be alert for the signs of drug sensitivity reactions. Obtain a careful history of the child's past reactions to medications before starting new therapies. If a reaction occurs, discontinue the medication until the healthcare provider is notified. See the section on burns later in this chapter for nursing care for the child with a severe drug reaction.

SAFETY ALERT!

Children with a true drug allergy (having a past serious systemic reaction) should never be treated with that drug again. Prominently mark the child's records so that all allergies are easily identified. The child should wear some type of medical alert identification.

Chronic Skin Conditions

Atopic Dermatitis

Atopic dermatitis (eczema) is a chronic, relapsing, superficial inflammatory skin disorder characterized by intense pruritus (Figure 31–8). The condition affects approximately 20% of infants, children, and adolescents (Nicol & Huether, 2014). Up to 60% of children who develop the condition do so during the first year of life (Roduit et al., 2012). Most children have or develop allergic conditions such as asthma or food allergy.

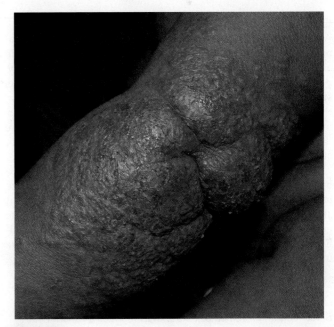

Figure 31–8   **Severe atopic dermatitis in an infant. Note the thick (i.e., lichenified), hyperpigmented plaque on the extensor surface of the elbow.**

SOURCE: Courtesy of Daniel P. Krowchuk, MD, Professor of Pediatrics and Dermatology, Wake Forest School of Medicine, Winston-Salem, NC.

ETIOLOGY AND PATHOPHYSIOLOGY

It is believed that mutations in the *filaggrin* gene are associated with a defective skin barrier that allows epidermal water loss that leads to **xerosis**, generally dry skin that is likely to crack and fissure. This also permits the penetration of allergens, irritants, and organisms. Both an IgE-mediated immediate immune response and T-cell–mediated delayed immune response are involved. The inflammatory response with cytokines, T-lymphocytes, and other cells plus scratching further damages the skin barrier (Tom, 2012). Although food allergies often occur in children with atopic dermatitis, food allergies do not cause the condition (Tollefson, Bruckner, & Section on Dermatology, 2014).

Decreased recognition of pathogens by immune receptors and decreased response by neutrophils and natural killer cells after an infectious agent enters the skin leads to more skin infections, such as *Staphylococcus aureus*, which is colonized on the skin of 90% of affected children (Tollefson et al., 2014; Tom, 2012).

CLINICAL MANIFESTATIONS

Acute atopic dermatitis is characterized by patches with papules, vesicles, exudate, crusts, and excoriation. Some patches may weep. Chronic atopic dermatitis characteristics include darkened, thickened skin with prominent skin lines (lichenification), excoriation, dryness, and scaling. Inflammation usually occurs on the face, neck, and extensor surfaces in infants. The diaper area is usually spared in infants because the skin is damp and protected from scratching. The antecubital and popliteal skinfolds are often affected after age 2 years. Adolescents may additionally have these areas affected: the eyelids, where the earlobe touches the face, fingertips, toes, nipples, and the vulva.

The itching interferes with sleep and causes irritability. The child moves so much because of the itching discomfort that a perception of hyperactivity may occur. Erythema and warmth may indicate a secondary bacterial infection. Some children have repeated flares or chronic atopic dermatitis that persists into adulthood. Other children may have skin resolution when respiratory symptoms such as asthma develop.

CLINICAL THERAPY

Atopic dermatitis is distinguished by its history and clinical manifestations. Diagnostic features of atopic dermatitis include an early age of onset, parent or sibling with history of atopy, pruritus, dry skin, and the typical distribution of lesions for age, such as the cheeks, scalp, trunk, and extremities during infancy, the flexural areas during childhood, and the hands and feet during adolescence (Tollefson et al., 2014). No laboratory tests are diagnostic; however, children have an elevated IgE level. A skin culture may be obtained when secondary infection occurs.

Because there is no cure, the goals of treatment are to hydrate and lubricate the skin, reduce pruritus, minimize inflammatory responses, manage infectious triggers, and treat skin infections. The skin is hydrated by bathing, and then the entire body is lubricated by applying occlusive topical emollients within 3 minutes of leaving the water. This traps moisture in the skin and promotes flexibility of the skin without cracking.

Clinical Tip

Select fragrance-free emollients with a cream or ointment base that have the fewest preservatives. Lotions contain alcohol that will further dry the skin. Examples of emollients include Eucerin cream, Aveeno cream, Vanicream, Cetaphil cream, SBR-Lipo-cream, and petroleum jelly. Petroleum jelly (e.g., Vaseline) has the benefit of lower cost, especially since so much of the emollient must be used to cover the entire body each day.

Moisturizing ointments and creams are applied 3 to 4 times a day, or when the skin feels dry.

Topical corticosteroids reduce inflammation and achieve quick control. Ointments are preferred over creams because of their occlusive effect, which ensures a stronger barrier and absorption into the skin. Many different preparations and seven categories of corticosteroid strength exist. Moderate-strength corticosteroids are used twice daily for 2 weeks under the emollient. Low-strength corticosteroids are used for thinner skin areas, such as the face, diaper area, and skinfolds. When the inflammation resolves, topical corticosteroids are tapered in frequency of application and potency and then discontinued. To reduce the risk for steroid side effects, topical steroids are not used on healthy skin. Oral corticosteroids are not commonly used because of a rebound effect may occur in which a more severe rash returns after the medication is discontinued (Tollefson et al., 2014).

SAFETY ALERT!

The potency or strength of a topical corticosteroid is based on whether it is fluorinated and contains other ingredients. Refer to a drug manual to identify the corticosteroid potency, not the percentage listed on the medication label. Avoid the use of higher potency corticosteroids on the face, genitalia, and skinfolds where absorption of the medication is increased because of the thinness of the skin. Intraocular hypertension, cataracts, skin atrophy, and adrenal suppression are potential adverse effects of higher potency topical corticosteroids.

Immunomodulator ointments such as tacrolimus (Protopic) and pimecrolimus (Elidel) are increasingly used as a second-line treatment for some children. Disadvantages include the cost of these medications and burning with application as perceived by some children. The medications are approved by the U.S. Food and Drug Administration (FDA) for children over 2 years of age, for short-term or intermittent treatment, who are not responsive to conventional therapy. The FDA has placed a black box warning on both drugs because of rare cases of malignancy (Tom, 2012).

The *Staphylococcus aureus* colonization on the child's skin may trigger an immune cascade that increases pruritus. Topical, oral, or IV antibiotics may be selected depending on severity of infection. Cephalexin is a common oral antibiotic used to treat *S. aureus* when CA-MRSA is not involved. When the child's skin condition does not respond, a skin culture may be needed to identify the correct antibiotic. Superinfections with herpes simplex may be treated with oral or intravenous acyclovir, depending on the severity of the infection. Children may be encouraged to soak in a tub with dilute chlorine bleach (one half cup to a tub one quarter full) once or twice a week to help reduce the number of *S. aureus* bacteria on the skin (Tollefson et al., 2014).

Pruritus is a significant problem, and treatment of flare-ups is the best way to reduce itching. Oral antihistamines have a limited effect on itching, but the sedative effect may help promote sleep. Tolerance to the sedating effects of these medications occurs, so their use is limited to 2 to 7 nights during a flare-up, when scratching interferes with sleep. Topical antihistamines are not recommended because of the potential for hypersensitivity reactions and contact dermatitis. Environmental control may be helpful. A humidifier in the winter counteracts dryness of the surrounding air, minimizing loss of skin moisture. Air conditioning in the summer limits unnecessary sweating that can exacerbate inflamed areas.

Food allergies causing urticaria and pruritus may aggravate atopic dermatitis. When the child younger than age 5 years has atopic dermatitis that does not respond to optimal management, efforts may be made to identify specific allergies to foods such as

Noah, 15 months of age, has had atopic dermatitis since 6 months of age. Today, he has skin lesions on his face, neck, elbows, and knees. The patches on his elbows and knees are weeping, and he is very uncomfortable because of the itching. His mother has worked hard to treat his skin and is very frustrated at this latest flare-up. She has run out of the corticosteroid ointment.

When talking with Noah's mother, the nurse reviews the daily routine for his care and identifies some changes that may help reduce the number of flare-ups. The nurse recommends the following daily skin care routine: Let Noah soak for 10 to 15 minutes in a warm bath and use mild soap only on skin that is dirty. Pat dry and immediately put the corticosteroid ointment over skin lesions and then petroleum jelly over his entire body. Apply petroleum jelly or other moisturizer every morning to skin that is dry.

- What signs of infection should the nurse and mother be observing for?

- What information can you provide to Noah's mother regarding the role of food allergies in causing atopic dermatitis?

- Contrast the treatment of acute flare-ups with daily maintenance care for atopic dermatitis.

eggs, cow's milk, wheat, soy, and peanuts (Tollefson et al., 2014). See Chapter 14 for more information on food allergies and food elimination trials to identify food allergies.

Nursing Management

For the Child With Atopic Dermatitis

Nursing Assessment and Diagnosis

Take a thorough history, including any family history of allergy, environmental or dietary factors, past exacerbations, and what triggers a flare. For example, common triggers include harsh soaps and detergents, fragrances, rough nonbreathable clothing, sweat, and psychosocial stress. Note distribution and type of lesions, presence of weeping, or signs of infection.

Identify the impact that the skin disorder is having on the child and family. How much is the sleep of the child, siblings, or other family members disturbed? Is the child's self-esteem disturbed? What other stresses has the child's skin disorder placed on the family? Does the family have concerns about topical steroid medication use?

Common nursing diagnoses that may be appropriate for the child with atopic dermatitis include the following (NANDA-I © 2014):

- *Tissue Integrity, Impaired,* related to chemical irritants and mechanical factors (abrasive clothing)

- *Insomnia* related to prolonged physical discomfort (itching)

- *Infection, Risk for,* related to breaks in skin barrier

- *Self-Esteem, Chronic Low,* related to peer reaction to visible skin lesions

- *Health Management, Family, Ineffective,* related to excessive demands made on the family to keep the condition under control

Planning and Implementation

Nursing management focuses on education and emotional support. Atopic dermatitis can be controlled, but there is no cure. Advise parents that the lesions are not contagious and usually do not scar. Daily optimal management often reduces flares, but the time it takes is a family stressor. Emphasize the importance of following the daily treatment plan to promote healing of existing lesions and to reduce the risk of secondary infections. See *Families Want to Know: Atopic Dermatitis Daily Skin Care.* Help parents and adolescents deal with the frustration of the acute flare-ups of the condition by reinforcing that remissions do occur with good home care.

Clinical Tip

Daily application of emollients to the entire body of newborns with a parent or sibling with atopic dermatitis or atopic condition has been suggested as a strategy to postpone the onset of atopic dermatitis. A pilot study involving 124 families demonstrated reduced incidence in newborns with daily emollient treatment compared to babies with routine newborn skin care (Simpson et al., 2014). This may be a potential future strategy for newborns at high risk of atopic dermatitis.

The child, parents, and siblings are often tired because of lost sleep when the child scratches at night during an acute flare-up. School performance may be affected if the child has sleep deprivation or if the child is experiencing physical discomfort that interferes with learning. The itching and scratching may cause constant movement similar to attention-deficit hyperactivity. If an oral antihistamine has been ordered, make sure the parents understand when to give the medication to maximize its effectiveness for better sleep.

Atopic dermatitis produces visible changes that can affect a child's self-confidence and self-esteem. Identify activities that the child can participate in to improve self-esteem. Even though humidity and sweating can make eczema worse, encourage the child to participate in sports. The child should shower as soon as possible after strenuous activity and then apply needed medications and emollients.

Provide encouragement and positive reinforcement for improvements in the child's skin during healthcare visits. Ensure that a focus is on the child's health promotion during visits. See *Health Promotion: The Child With Atopic Dermatitis.* Encourage the parents to support the child's self-esteem. Atopic dermatitis is difficult to manage and may have a more profound effect on the child's and family's quality of life.

When atopic dermatitis is under control, educate parents that increased itching within hours of eating a food may be associated with a food allergy that aggravates atopic dermatitis. If a specific food allergy, such as eggs, has been identified, educate the parents about strategies for avoidance of food products that contain the allergen. Nutritional counseling may be needed to make sure the child has food options that meet daily nutritional requirements.

Evaluation

Expected outcomes of nursing care include the following:

- The child's atopic dermatitis is controlled and no infection occurs.

- Parents identify triggers of the child's atopic dermatitis and avoid or eliminate them.

- The child's sleep is minimally disturbed by itching.

Families Want to Know

Atopic Dermatitis Daily Skin Care

- Have the child soak in the bathtub 10–15 minutes or shower once a day. Use mild, unscented soap only on dirty areas. Salt or baking soda added to the bath water may help if water stings the child's open lesions. Rinse and pat excess water from the skin and apply adequate emollient to the entire body within 3 minutes to trap moisture in the skin.

- Help the parents select an unscented emollient ointment or cream (Eucerin, Aveeno, Vanicream, Cetaphil, SBR Lipocream, or petroleum jelly) that fits into the family's budget. Large quantities are needed to cover the entire body twice a day. Petroleum jelly is inexpensive, safe, and easily applied.

- In regions with low humidity, apply emollients to the skin more frequently.

- Help ensure that parents receive adequate amounts of topical corticosteroids for effective treatment of a flare-up. When the child has a flare-up, bathe the child twice a day and apply the topical medications on inflamed areas, spreading thinly and rubbing in. Emollients are applied on top of medications as well as over the rest of the body.

- If immunomodulators are prescribed rather than topical corticosteroids, spread a pea-size amount to cover a 2-in. (5-cm) circle over the inflamed area. Apply emollients as for topical corticosteroids.

- Encourage the child to wear loose cotton clothing rather than wool or other irritating fabrics.

- Keep the child's fingernails trimmed and use clean cotton gloves or socks over the infant's or child's hands to decrease scratching and reduce the chance of secondary infection.

- Contact the child's healthcare provider if signs of infection are noted so that antibiotic treatment can be started.

Health Promotion The Child With Atopic Dermatitis

Growth and Development Surveillance

- Assess growth measurements and plot on a growth chart. Identify any changes that could be related to an altered meal plan due to food allergies.
- Assess developmental progress for age.

Nutrition

- Postpone adding eggs to the infant's diet if atopic dermatitis develops early in infancy. Provide nutritional counseling to ensure the child gets all essential nutrients when foods must be avoided.

Physical Activity

- Encourage physical activity, but have the child bathe and apply emollients soon afterwards.
- After swimming have the child immediately rinse off chlorine after leaving the pool and apply emollients.

Family Interactions

- Identify how frequently the sleep of the child and other family members is disturbed by scratching. Encourage the use of an antihistamine to promote sleep when a skin flare-up occurs.
- Discuss strategies to effectively use time for daily skin care.

Mental and Spiritual Health

- Assess the child's self-esteem and impact of skin lesions on relationships with peers.
- Identify how disturbed sleep affects behavior and learning.

Disease Prevention Strategies

- Provide all immunizations on schedule.
- Encourage good hand hygiene to reduce the risk of infection.
- Educate the child and parents to provide skin care as described in *Families Want to Know: Atopic Dermatitis Daily Skin Care* to reduce skin inflammation and the risk for secondary infection.

Acne

Acne is a chronic inflammatory disorder of the pilosebaceous hair follicles on the face and trunk. It is the most common skin disorder in the pediatric population, affecting 85% of the population ages 12 to 25 years (Nicol & Huether, 2014). Acne is found in all ethnic groups, and occurs equally in male and female adolescents. Severe acne is more common in male adolescents. Adolescents with severe acne often have a genetic predisposition.

ETIOLOGY AND PATHOPHYSIOLOGY

Keratin and sebum usually flow to the skin surface through the hair follicles. Androgens, released as puberty begins, trigger the sebaceous glands to increase the production of sebum. When the extra sebum mixes with the keratinocytes and causes them to clump together, the hair follicle canal becomes obstructed by **comedones** (whiteheads and blackheads). The sebum behind the comedone is an ideal environment for the anaerobic bacterium *Propionibacterium acnes,* which metabolizes the sebum, leading to an increased response by inflammatory mediators (Kim & Mancini, 2013). When the inflammatory reaction is close to the surface, a papule or pustule develops. If the inflammatory reaction is deeper, a larger papule or nodule develops. When the follicles rupture, bacteria spreads and the resulting inflammation in the deeper tissues leads to nodules and cysts that can result in scars.

Acne may occur in neonates in response to maternal androgen hormones and androgens produced by the fetal adrenal glands. Neonatal acne usually resolves spontaneously in a few months. When acne occurs in children between 1 and 7 years, it may be associated with true precocious puberty or an androgen-secreting tumor (Kim & Mancini, 2013).

CLINICAL MANIFESTATIONS

Lesions occur most often on the face, upper chest, shoulders, and back. Comedones are initial skin lesions. Closed comedones are whiteheads or flesh-colored papules with tiny follicular openings. Open comedones are blackheads in which the follicular plug has enlarged and dilated the follicular opening. As inflammation occurs, papules and pustules develop (Figure 31–9). Nodules are larger areas of inflammation that may involve more than one hair follicle. Cysts are compressible nodules without overlying inflammation. Scars form when the surrounding dermis is damaged and may be pitted, atrophic, or hypertrophic (keloid).

CLINICAL THERAPY

Diagnosis is based on the examination of the skin. Treatment is customized to the predominant type of lesion present and severity of the lesions. The goal of treatment is to suppress lesions until the condition is outgrown, thus preventing infection and scarring, and minimizing psychologic distress. A variety of topical and oral medications are prescribed (see *Medications Used to Treat: Acne*). Acne will recur gradually if the treatment is stopped, so maintenance therapy with topical retinoids is recommended once acne is controlled.

Skin irritation related to topical preparations may occur in adolescents with sensitive skin. Using a lower-concentration product and removing it after a few hours may reduce the initial irritation. With continued use the skin adapts, permitting the product concentration to be changed. Creams are used when skin is more sensitive, and gels are used when skin is oilier. (See *Developing Cultural Competence: Acne Lesions in Individuals With Dark Skin*.)

Isotretinoin (Accutane) is reserved for severe acne that is not responsive to other therapies. The daily 16- to 20-week course of treatment results in a dramatic improvement for up to 90%

of patients (Studor-Heikenfeld & Colella, 2014). An intermittent lower-dose schedule over 6 to 18 months is also effective and has fewer side effects. Because isotretinoin is a teratogen, the FDA established the iPLEDGE program, a mandatory Internet-based registry for prescribers, patients, and pharmacies. See *Medications Used to Treat: Acne* for important guidelines. Inquire about prior episodes of depression and suicide attempts because of isotretinoin's potential association with both problems.

> **Developing Cultural Competence** Acne Lesions in Individuals With Dark Skin
>
> Inflammatory acne in adolescents with darker skin color is associated with a dark discoloration as extra pigment gets deposited in the areas of inflammation. If protected from sun exposure, this darker coloration fades over 3 to 18 months. Encourage adolescents with dark skin to use noncomedonic sunscreen (SPF 30 or higher) whenever sun exposure is likely.

Nursing Management

For the Child With Acne

Nursing Assessment and Diagnosis

Physical assessment should include documentation regarding distribution, type, and severity of acne lesions. Assess the adolescent's and parents' knowledge about the cause and treatment of acne. Also explore the extent of emotional distress and low self-esteem that acne may be causing.

The accompanying *Nursing Care Plan: The Adolescent With Acne* lists common nursing diagnoses and summarizes nursing care.

Planning and Implementation

Nursing management focuses on educating the adolescent and parents about acne and its treatment. Encourage good hand hygiene before touching affected areas. Educate adolescents that picking and squeezing lesions may increase the inflammation when lesions rupture below the skin surface and may cause scarring. Excoriated acne lesions do not respond as well to the treatment used for the primary acne lesions. Inform the adolescent to avoid cleansing products with a greasy base, to shampoo the hair regularly, and to treat seborrheic dermatitis that can accompany acne. Correct misconceptions about dietary causes. Although no food is known to cause acne or increase the severity of lesions, good nutrition is important.

Topical medications should be spread in a thin film over the skin, according to directions. Inform the adolescent that treatment may seem to worsen acne as the comedones are being pushed out, and this is a sign that the medication is working. Emphasize that treatment is often long term. It may take at least 6 to 12 weeks for significant improvement to be seen after beginning treatment. Educate adolescents that healing lesions initially look like fading red areas, and, in some cases, hyperpigmented areas. Flare-ups are expected despite treatment, potentially caused by increased sweating, heat, humidity, and emotional stress.

Tretinoin is **phototoxic** (a rapid nonimmunologic reaction of the skin when exposed to sunlight), causing sunburn with even minimal exposure. Encourage adolescents to limit sun exposure

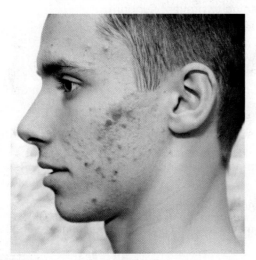

Figure 31–9 Note the comedones, papules, pustules, and healing lesions. Acne can have a significant effect on an adolescent's self-esteem.

SOURCE: bluecinema/Getty Images.

(continued on p. 920)

Medications Used to Treat: Acne

MEDICATION AND ACTION	NURSING MANAGEMENT
Topical retinoids (tretinoin [Retin-A], adapalene, tazarotene) For mild or moderate papulopustular acne Regulates follicular keratinocyte shedding, has anti-inflammatory properties, helps to prevent new lesions, enhances penetration of topical antibiotics	• Use lower concentrations initially as skin irritation is common. • Divide and spread a pea-sized amount over the entire face. Do not use as spot therapy. • Apply at night to reduce photosensitivity effect. • Use long term between flares for maintenance.
Benzoyl peroxide For mild or moderate papulopustular acne Topical antimicrobial with bacteriocidal action	• A lower strength may be used initially if skin irritation occurs. • Apply in the morning. • Inform clients that the product can bleach fabric.
Antibiotics (tetracycline, minocycline, erythromycin, doxycycline) Topical for mild inflammatory acne; oral for moderate to severe inflammatory acne Antimicrobial action reduces resident skin bacterial colonization	• Combined with topical retinoid and benzoyl peroxide to reduce antibiotic resistance. • Takes 6–8 weeks to see improvement; antibiotic is changed if no response. Use is evaluated after 3 months to determine need for longer treatment. Avoid long-term use to reduce risk for antibiotic resistance.
Azelaic acid For mild or moderate papulopustular acne Keratolytic and anti-inflammatory properties	• Used in patients who cannot tolerate topical retinoids. • Apply twice daily.
Isotretinoin (Accutane) For severe nodular acne, especially when resistant to other treatment Causes sebaceous gland atrophy and decreases sebum production; reduces excess desquamation, bacteriocidal action, reduces inflammatory response, reverses effect of androgens on sebaceous glands	• Requires informed consent. • Females need a monthly pregnancy test before each prescription refill as well as monthly tests for blood counts, lipid levels, and liver enzymes. • Females must use 2 forms of contraception, beginning 1 month prior to treatment, during treatment, and for 1 month after completing treatment to prevent pregnancy that would expose the fetus to teratogenic effects of the drug. • Take medication with food to increase oral absorption. • Encourage the use of sunscreen and protective clothing to prevent sunburn.
Oral contraceptives For persistent inflammatory papules and nodules Suppresses gonadotropin secretion and reduces ovarian androgen production	• Use as an adjunct to other acne treatments. • May cause red, dry, and itching skin that can be treated with emollients. • Inform adolescent that acne may worsen during the first 3–6 weeks of treatment.
Spironolactone For severe acne. Blocks the androgen receptor on the sebaceous gland	• Prescribed for 1–3 months along with an antibiotic. • Not FDA approved for acne treatment, but commonly prescribed for that purpose.

Source: Data from Kim, W., & Mancini, A. J. (2013). Acne in childhood: An update. *Pediatric Annals, 42*(10), 418–427; Weinstein, M. (2013). Acne and the adolescent: A practical approach to management. *Contemporary Pediatrics, 30*(5), 30–36; Studor-Heikenfeld, J., & Colella, C. (2014). Isotretinoin: Reconsidering management of acne vulgaris in primary care. *Journal for Nurse Practitioners, 10*(9), 714–720.

Nursing Care Plan: The Adolescent With Acne

1. Nursing Diagnosis: *Health Maintenance, Ineffective,* related to daily hygiene and skin care (NANDA-I © 2014)

GOAL: The adolescent will verbalize proper hygiene, nutrition, and treatment of acne.

INTERVENTION	RATIONALE

• Teach good skin care:
  • Wash skin with mild soap and water twice a day.
  • Do not use astringents or abrasive cleansers.
  • Wash hands frequently, especially after eating greasy foods.
  • Apply topical retinoid 20 min after washing and drying face.
	• Good hygiene and appropriate skin care reduces irritation, surface oils, and bacteria, which intensify inflammatory reactions. Astringents and aftershave may contain alcohol and further dry the skin.

• Praise good habits.	• Positive reinforcement encourages continued effort.
• Advise the adolescent to wash hair with antiseborrheic shampoo and to avoid oil-based cosmetics, pomades, or petroleum-based hair products.	• Seborrhea frequently accompanies acne. Oil-based products can obstruct sebaceous glands, exacerbating acne.
• Encourage the adolescent to keep a diary of skin care, menses, and diet habits.	• A record may help identify associations with flares that can be managed in the future.

EXPECTED OUTCOME: Adolescent will exhibit good hygiene habits and nutrition.

GOAL: The adolescent will verbalize understanding of treatment regimen.

INTERVENTION	RATIONALE
• Educate the adolescent about medications (action, side effects, dosage, method of application).	• Proper application of medication enhances healing of lesions.
• Encourage application of tretinoin at night. Encourage use of noncomedonic sunscreens of at least SPF 30 during the day.	• Nighttime application helps reduce sensitivity to sun and sunscreen helps to avoid sunburn.
• Educate the adolescent about time needed for a therapeutic response and importance of adhering to daily regimen.	• Up to 3 months may be needed for significant improvement. The adolescent needs a reason to continue with the care plan.
• Encourage continuation of daily therapies even when acne has improved significantly.	• Acne will return if treatment stops.

EXPECTED OUTCOME: Adolescent will implement the treatment regimen as outlined, resulting in a noticeable reduction in lesions.

2. Nursing Diagnosis: *Body Image, Disturbed,* related to biophysical factors (visible facial lesions) (NANDA-I © 2014)

GOAL: The adolescent will demonstrate increased self-confidence and self-esteem.

INTERVENTION	RATIONALE
• Establish a rapport with the adolescent.	• A trusting relationship promotes verbalization of concerns and fears.
• Provide education about the condition and therapy modalities.	• Providing information better enables the adolescent to take control of the condition.
• Encourage the adolescent to be responsible for treatment and follow-up, and give positive reinforcement.	• Responsibility reinforces sense of self-esteem.
• Encourage the adolescent to become involved with school activities and peers.	• Involvement in activities helps enhance self-esteem and allows the adolescent to explore new experiences and friendships.

EXPECTED OUTCOME: Adolescent will freely discuss concerns and fears. Adolescent will demonstrate active involvement in own care. Adolescent will show increased confidence, as demonstrated by involvement in extracurricular activities.

and to use noncomedonic sunscreen products. Review instructions for taking other prescribed drugs, such as tetracycline and isotretinoin (Accutane), and discuss possible side effects. Emphasize the importance of return visits to the adolescent's healthcare provider to monitor medication side effects.

Psychologic support is an important aspect of care. Because adolescents are preoccupied with their body image and peer relationships, they often find having acne embarrassing. Monitor for signs of anxiety or depression. Encourage them to express their feelings and refer for counseling, if necessary.

Evaluation

Expected outcomes of nursing care can be found in *Nursing Care Plan: The Adolescent With Acne.*

Psoriasis

Psoriasis is a chronic, relapsing, pruritic, papulosquamous condition that affects the skin, scalp, and nails. It begins during childhood or adolescence in a third of cases (Bhutani, Kamangar, & Cordoro, 2012). A family history of psoriasis is often present, but a multifactorial inheritance is suspected.

Psoriasis is a T-helper cell–mediated autoimmune disease. Inflammatory cytokines from activated T cells cause chronic inflammation and are responsible for the skin changes (McCann & Huether, 2014). Cells proliferate so rapidly they do not mature and fully keratinize, leading to thickened epidermis and plaque formation. The onset of psoriasis may be triggered in children, particularly guttate-type psoriasis, by a streptococcal infection. Other triggers may include trauma, stress, and recent withdrawal from oral corticosteroids (Bhutani et al., 2012).

The typical psoriatic lesion is a thick, silvery, scaly erythematous plaque with an irregular border, surrounded by normal skin. Pruritus is often present. These lesions commonly are found on the scalp, elbows, knees, umbilicus, and genitals, or at the site of trauma. Nails may also be involved. Small points of bleeding may be noted when a scale is removed. Guttate psoriasis is characterized by an eruption of small round or oval papules on the trunk, face, and extremities. Some children also develop psoriatic arthritis.

Diagnosis is based on skin lesion characteristics or microscopic examination. Treatment includes topical steroids twice a day. Care must be taken to use lower-potency steroids in the diaper area and the face, and to switch from higher-potency to lower-potency steroids when lesions thin. Other topical medications include vitamin D, a retinoid, and tacrolimus or pimecrolimus. A tar shampoo may be used to clear scales in the scalp prior to topical steroid application. Salicylic acid may be used to remove some layers of plaques. Ultraviolet B phototherapy is used for children who do not respond to topical therapy. Systemic therapy with drugs such as methotrexate, oral retinoids, and cyclosporine is reserved for children with severe psoriasis. No cure exists, and lifelong relapses and remissions occur.

Nursing Management

Assess the child's skin for extent of the lesions and response to therapy. Spend time talking with the child and family to learn how the condition affects them. Educate them about the condition and reasonable expectations related to treatment. Families need to understand that lesions are not contagious, and periods of remissions and flare-ups are common. Actively involve the family and child in decision making regarding the treatment plan, such as the type of topical products (e.g., lotion, cream,

ointment) they prefer to use. Teach them how to apply topical medications. Encourage the child to avoid situations in which chemical and physical trauma to the skin could occur.

Children and adolescents may have feelings of embarrassment, anger, and frustration related to their visible skin lesions. Psoriasis may impact their daily lives causing problems at school, with personal relationships, and with social acceptance. Children may anticipate rejection and withdraw from physical activities that require them to expose affected skin areas, such as swimming. The mental health of adolescents should be monitored to identify psychologic distress, depression, or substance abuse.

Epidermolysis Bullosa

Epidermolysis bullosa (EB) is a rare and severe chronic blistering skin disorder that occurs with minor trauma. EB is most often inherited in an autosomal dominant pattern (see Chapter 3). The incidence of the most common and least severe form, EB simplex (EBS), is estimated to be 1 per 25,000 live births (Coulombe & Lee, 2012).

Genetic changes in the intracellular proteins compromise their ability to provide structural support in keratinocytes of the epidermis. The basal keratinocytes are fragile and rupture easily with any mechanical injury trauma. One variant of EBS is localized to blistering of the hands, and another variant leads to more generalized blistering. It is often diagnosed when the child begins to walk or during puberty. With severe forms of EB, blistering and skin erosions are seen at birth and occur on all parts of the body, including the respiratory, gastrointestinal, and urologic systems. These children lose protein and have electrolyte and fluid imbalances, malnutrition, and anemia. Severe EB has a high mortality rate due to secondary infection.

Children with EB have extremely fragile skin, and blisters form with minor trauma, friction, or heat applied to the skin. In severe forms, the blistering can be extensive and damage to the skin is apparent. Fingers and toes may fuse with healing, leading to malformations. Children experience pain with blisters and may have difficulty walking when feet are affected. In the more common form of EB, blisters generally heal without scarring.

Diagnosis can be made prenatally by amniocentesis or chorionic villus sampling or by skin biopsy. The condition is managed by prevention of new blisters, wound care, good nutrition, and minimizing the risk for infection. Wound care is important to reduce the risk of infection. Blisters are pricked on two sides with a sterile needle each day and drained so that they do not extend. The blister roof is kept intact to act as a natural biologic dressing. Antibiotic ointments are applied to wounds, and changed monthly to reduce the risk for bacterial resistance. Wounds are covered, and care is taken to avoid placing adhesives directly on the skin. Biologic dressings may be used to cover larger wounds in some cases. Infants and children need additional protein and calories to support chronic wound healing. Pain management is customized to the severity of the child's condition and wound care provided.

Nursing Management

Teach the family to provide daily wound care at home. Wound care can be quite time consuming, so help the parents select the best time to do routine dressing changes. Perform dressing changes in a location without air currents to reduce pain from exposed wounds. Determine if financial support is needed to ensure that parents have the dressing supplies needed to effectively manage the child's wounds. Provide parents with guidance on all aspects of dressing changes.

- Precut dressings to reduce the wound exposure time.
- Gather all supplies and have an assistant present. Ask the assistant to gently hold the child's extremities to prevent movement of the extremity during blister lancing and dressing changes. Holding or grabbing the extremity too tightly can cause friction injury.
- Use soft music and distraction to help calm the infant.
- Soak off dressings that are stuck to the skin. Remove dressings from one area at a time as air exposure may cause pain.
- Inspect the skin each day for signs of infection.
- Use nonadherent dressings that can absorb the blister fluid to help prevent dressings from sticking to the skin. Place a bulky cover over the dressing to protect the skin and promote healing. Wrap fingers and toes separately so they do not fuse together with healing.

Help the parents identify ways to protect the skin but still permit the child to interact with other children and have opportunities for development. Dress the child in soft cotton clothing that covers the skin, placing rough seams that can irritate the skin on the outside. Foam padding can be sewn into clothing over the knees and elbows for the infant who is crawling or walking. Shoes without seams on the inside should be worn with seamless cotton socks. Cotton socks can be used to mitten the infant's hands during sleep. The child should also avoid sun exposure and stay where temperatures are cool.

Because protein is lost with blisters, and chronic wound healing requires extra calories, it is important to promote good nutrition with adequate calories and high protein to meet the child's growth and healing requirements. In infants, blistering in the mouth may interfere with feeding. A soft nipple with a larger hole may be easier for the infant to use. Vaseline on the lips may help reduce trauma to the mouth. Food temperature should be cool or room temperature and nonacidic to prevent injury to the gastrointestinal tract. In some cases, a gastrostomy tube is inserted for nutritional supplementation. Regularly measure height and weight and plot measurements on a growth curve to monitor growth and to identify growth deficiencies early.

Help parents and the child manage the psychologic impact of this disfiguring disorder and the inability to fully participate in all activities. An individualized health plan with educational accommodations will be necessary. Because the hands and feet are often involved, writing and test taking may be challenging. Mobility and walking throughout the school may also be a problem. Information needs to be provided to classroom teachers and classmates to help minimize injury.

Infestations

Pediculosis Capitis (Lice)

Pediculosis capitis is a lice infestation of the hair and scalp. Infestation occurs among children from all socioeconomic levels, and it is most common in children ages 3 to 11 years (Eisenhower & Farrington, 2012). Parents or teachers may be the first to notice lice, or healthcare providers may spot them during routine examination (see Chapter 5). Outbreaks occur periodically among children in child care and elementary school.

Head lice live and reproduce only on humans and are transmitted by direct hair-to-hair contact or indirect contact such as

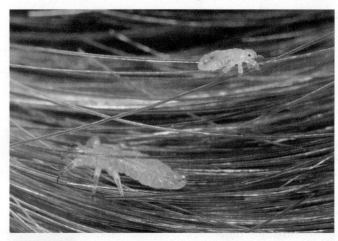

Figure 31–10 Note the presence of lice (highly magnified) crawling through the hair.

SOURCE: Darlyne A. Marawski / National Geographic Image Collection.

sharing of hair accessories, hats, towels, and bedding. Lice do not fly or jump, but they can crawl quickly. The female louse can lay up to 10 eggs (nits) a day on the hair shaft, close to the scalp. The incubation period for eggs to hatch is 7 to 10 days. Lice feed on human blood, sensitizing the child with their saliva to cause pruritus.

The child has intense pruritus and complaints of "dandruff" that sticks to the hair (actually the nits) and "bugs" in the hair. Nits look like silvery white, yellow, or darker 1-mm teardrops adhering to one side of the hair shaft, often near the scalp. Lice are wingless insects (2 to 3 mm long) that move away from light and are not easily seen (Figure 31–10). Scratching may lead to inflammation, pustules, and bacterial infection. Occipital and posterior cervical nodes are frequently palpable.

Treatment involves a pediculicide shampoo, such as pyrethrin within an enzymatic lice egg remover, or an ovicidal rinse, such as permethrin (Nix); however, resistance to these products has increased. Permethrin cream rinse is applied to dry hair and left in place for 10 minutes, before rinsing. The hair is towel-dried, and the nits are removed with a fine-toothed comb. A second treatment is needed in 7 to 10 days because the neurotoxin is not effective on nits. If live lice still persist after two treatments, a prescription ovicide such as malathion may be ordered. Some newer agents are available. See *Medications Used to Treat: Head Lice.*

SAFETY ALERT!

Lindane is no longer recommended for treatment of head lice. However, it is still classified as a second-line treatment for head lice. It must be used with caution in any child weighing less than 50 kg (110 lb) because of neurotoxicity and potential to cause seizures. High levels of resistance by lice have been documented (AAP, 2015, p. 600).

Nursing Management

Carefully assess children exposed to head lice using a bright light and magnifying glass to look for lice and nits along the hair shaft close to the scalp. To avoid potential infestation, change gloves with each child when assessing several children in a classroom setting.

Infestation with lice can be upsetting for both the child and family. Emphasize to the family that anyone can get lice. All

Medications Used to Treat: Head Lice

NAME OF MEDICATION/PREPARATION	NURSING MANAGEMENT
First-line pesticide treatment	
Permethrin 1% Crème Rinse—Nix	• Apply to the hair after shampooing and towel drying the hair. Leave on 10 min and rinse. Repeat in 7–10 days.
Pyrethrin shampoo (0.33%) or piperonyl butoxide (Rid, A-200, Bayer, and generic brands)	• Apply to *dry hair and scalp*. Lather, leave on 10 min, and rinse with cool water. Wet hair dilutes the product and may contribute to treatment failure.
	• Permethrin is approved for children 2 months of age and older.
Benzyl alcohol 5% (Ulesfia)—FDA-approved nonneurotoxic treatment for children ages 6 months and older; lice die by suffocation	• Apply to *dry hair*, saturating the hair and scalp. Rinse after 10 min. Repeat in 7 days. Protect eyes during use. Available by prescription.
Spinosad (Natroba)—FDA-approved for children 4 years and older; lice become paralyzed and die, ovicidal	• Apply topical suspension to *dry hair*, saturating the scalp and all hair. Rinse off after 10 min. May repeat in 7 days. Available by prescription and is expensive.
Sklice—FDA-approved 0.5% ivermectin lotion for children ages 6 months and older	• Apply to *dry hair*, completely covering the scalp and all hair. Leave on 10 min and rinse only with water; *do not* shampoo. No retreatment needed in most cases.
Second-line pesticide treatment	
Malathion 0.5%—Ovide lotion	• Apply to *dry hair*. Leave on 4 minutes and rinse. No retreatment is needed. May cause stinging sensation. Has potential to cause chemical burns.
	• Treatment is flammable; do not expose the child to electric heat sources.

Source: Data from Eisenhower, C., & Farrington, E. A., (2012). Advances in the treatment of head lice in pediatrics. *Journal of Pediatric Health Care, 26*(6), 451–461; Pariser, D. M., Meinking, T. L., Bell, M., & Ryan, W. G. (2012). Topical 0.5% Ivermectin lotion for treatment of head lice. *New England Journal of Medicine, 367*(18), 1687–1693; Bowden, V. R. (2012). Losing the louse: How to manage this common infestation in children. *Pediatric Nursing, 38*(5), 253–254, 277.

family members and contacts of the child should be examined for infestation and treated as necessary. Teach the child not to share clothing, headwear, or combs.

Explain to parents that the shampoo and rinses prescribed are pesticides and must be used for the time specified and as directed. An extra bottle of the product may be needed if the child has extra-long hair. Inform parents that in order to avoid treatment failure no other shampoo or conditioner should be used before the lice shampoo or lotion. Do not wash the hair for 1 to 2 days after the pediculicide treatment. Keep these products out of the eyes and mouth of the child because they will irritate mucous membranes.

To remove nits, use a fine-toothed comb, tweezers, and a basin filled with water or isopropyl alcohol to dip and clean the comb and tweezers. Comb 1-inch sections from the scalp outward and pin these out of the way when done. Nits adhere to the hair shaft and must be manually pulled down the shaft with the comb, tweezers, or fingernails. All nits should be removed. Have blunt-nosed scissors available to cut a hair below the level of the nit when the nit cannot be removed. Put the child under a bright light and use distractions such as a video to keep the child entertained during the procedure. Check the hair every 2 to 3 days and remove any lice or nits seen. Giving boys a buzz haircut is one alternative. A shorter hair cut for girls may help with nit removal. Both the American Academy of Pediatrics and the National Association of School Nurses have policies that allow the child to stay in school even if all nits have not been removed.

Lice survive only about 3 days away from a human host, but nits may hatch after 8 to 10 days. For this reason, the child's bedding, towels, and clothing should be changed daily, laundered in hot water with detergent, and dried in a hot dryer for 20 minutes. Store nonessential bedding and clothing in a tightly sealed bag for 2 to 3 weeks and then wash. Discard hair accessories, brushes, and combs or soak them in hot soapy water (54.4°C [130.0°F]) for 10 minutes. Vacuum furniture and carpets and treat them with a hot iron when possible. Use of an insecticide in the home to kill the lice on carpets, furniture, and other items is not recommended when young children and pets may be exposed. Seal toys and other personal items that cannot be washed or dry-cleaned in a plastic bag for 2 weeks.

Scabies

Scabies is a highly contagious infestation caused by the mite *Sarcoptes scabiei*. It is spread by skin-to-skin and sexual contact. Transmission within a household is common. Children of all ages and both sexes can be affected. Because the mite usually takes at least 45 minutes to burrow into the skin, transient contact is unlikely to cause infestation.

The female mite burrows into the outer layer of the epidermis (stratum corneum) to lay her eggs, leaving a trail of debris and feces under the skin. The larvae hatch in approximately 3 to 4 days and proceed toward the surface of the skin. The cycle is repeated 14 to 17 days later. A delayed type IV hypersensitivity reaction to the mites, debris, and feces occurs within

4 weeks of infestation, causing irritation and intense pruritus (Cohen, 2014). Hypersensitivity response to reinfestation can occur within 24 hours.

Symptoms include a rash with papules and pustules, restlessness, and severe pruritus that worsens at night. Lesions may appear as linear, threadlike, grayish burrows 1 to 10 cm (0.4 to 4.0 in.) in length, which may end in a pinpoint vesicle. Lesions are usually located in the webs of the fingers, in the intergluteal folds, around the axillae, or on the palms, wrists, head, neck, legs, buttocks, chest, abdomen, and waist. In children under age 2 years, the head, neck, face, palms, and feet can be affected. The child's scratching and secondary infection often obliterate the linear burrow lesions. Nodules 2 to 20 mm (0.08 to 0.6 in.) in size occasionally develop as a granulomatous response to the dead mite antigens and feces and can persist for weeks after effective treatment.

Diagnosis is confirmed by microscopic examination of scrapings from a burrow, which reveals actively moving mites, fecal pellets, eggs, or nits. Treatment involves application of a scabicide, such as 5% permethrin lotion, over the entire body except the face, with special attention to the hands, fingers, feet, toes, and skin under the nails. Application of 5% permethrin lotion or malathion is preceded by a warm soap-and-water bath. When the skin is cool and dry, apply the lotion. The lotion is left in place for 8 to 48 hours before washing off. A second treatment is used 1 week later. Treat all members of the household and childcare contacts at the same time, even if they have no symptoms.

An oral antihistamine (e.g., Benadryl, Atarax) may be prescribed to help relieve itching. Antibiotics may be needed when a secondary infection occurs. Oral ivermectin, a new antiparasitic product with FDA approval for children weighing more than 15 kg, may be prescribed when treatment failure occurs.

Nursing Management

Advise parents that scabies is transmitted by close contact and is very contagious. All clothing, bedding, and pillowcases used by the child should be changed daily, washed with hot water, and ironed before reuse. Nonwashable toys and other items should be sealed in plastic bags for 5 to 7 days.

Educate the parents about the proper application of the scabicide. The child should have the scabicide reapplied to the hands if hands are washed or the child sucks the fingers or thumb. Socks over the young child's hands may reduce ingestion of the scabicide.

Treat all household members simultaneously. Uninfested individuals should avoid touching the affected child until after treatment is completed. If contact is made, they should wash their hands well. Inform the parents about signs of secondary infections and that itching and nodules may persist for weeks after effective treatment. Encourage the use of emollients because the treatment dries the skin.

Scabies, like pediculosis, can be embarrassing or upsetting for the child and family. Educate the child and parents about the condition, its spread, and treatment measures to prevent recurrence.

Vascular Tumors (Hemangiomas)

Vascular tumors, or hemangiomas, occur in 4% to 5% of infants (Lauren & Garzon, 2012). An increased incidence has been noted in female infants who are non-Hispanic, White, low birth weight, and of multiple births (Chung & Cohen, 2014). An increased incidence is found in infants with fetal exposure to chorionic villus sampling, placental complications, or preeclampsia (Uihlein, Liang, & Mulliken, 2012).

Hemangiomas are vascular tumors believed to result from the proliferation of endothelium-like cells that could be caused by a mutation and some type of environmental exposure. These tumors undergo rapid growth and attain 80% of full size by age 3 months, and most growth will be completed by age 5 months (Chung & Cohen, 2014). This phase is followed by a slow **involution** (process of decreasing in size) phase that may take years. Hemangiomas may be superficial (in the epidermis), deep (in the dermis or subcutaneous tissue), or mixed superficial and deep. When multiple hemangiomas are found, some may be in major organs, such as the liver. Complications caused by the rapid growth pressure against or obstruction of vital structures (e.g., airway, eye, or ear canal) may occur.

Infantile hemangiomas begin as barely visible **telangiectasias** (dilated superficial blood vessels) or red macules that begin to grow rapidly and become bright red and compressible. Some lesions ulcerate with rapid growth. Superficial hemangiomas are bright-red vascular cutaneous plaques that resemble strawberries. Deep hemangiomas appear as bluish tumors covered with normal-appearing epidermis. Mixed hemangiomas have features of both superficial and deep tumors. The lesions, appearing any place on the body, are minimally compressible and have no bruit or thrill. As the vascular tumor involutes, signs of tissue atrophy, wrinkles, telangiectasias, and hypopigmentation may be noted.

Initial diagnosis is by physical examination and monitoring the growth of the vascular tumor. When a vital organ could become obstructed or a large facial hemangioma is present, ultrasound, computed tomography, or magnetic resonance imaging may be performed.

Simple hemangiomas are monitored and receive no treatment. Hemangiomas in problem areas may be treated with oral propranolol at 1 mg/kg twice daily. Vital signs are checked prior to first dose and at 1 and 2 hours after the first dose. The child is checked again at 1 week and then monthly with vital signs being checked each visit. If the child has cardiovascular, respiratory, or endocrine conditions, or hemangioma in a vital organ, the child may be admitted for initial propranolol dosing because of potential adverse effects. The medication may be stopped temporarily if the infant has wheezing or severe cough because it may worsen wheezing associated with asthma (Block & Blackmon, 2013). Photos are taken of lesions at each visit to document changes in the lesion.

Pulsed-dye laser treatment may be used after involution for residual telangiectasia. Light energy pulses target the lesion's oxyhemoglobin, which is heated after absorbing the wavelength of light. This ruptures the lesion's blood vessels. Provide topical anesthesia and eye protection. The lesion may darken for 1 to 2 weeks, as red blood cells are released from ruptured blood vessels. The treated skin surface eventually lightens. Surgical removal of ulcerated hemangiomatous tissue may be considered if a poor cosmetic outcome is expected.

Nursing Management

Assess the distribution of the hemangioma and consider the potential for complications as it goes through a rapid growth stage, such as potential compression of the airway for a hemangioma in the neck area. Monitor the child for signs of any complications, such as ulceration. Assess the parents' response to the infant's appearance and how they are managing interactions with friends and family about the infant's changing appearance.

Take photos of the infant at each visit so that parents have a record of improvements once therapy is initiated.

Educate the parents about the type of vascular lesion and the time when growth is most rapid. Inform parents about the possible ulceration, if a hemangioma is rapidly growing, and what signs to expect. Parents should return for care when concerned about the lesion, if watchful waiting has been selected.

When propranolol medication is administered in the outpatient setting, monitor the pulse and blood pressure as directed for the first dose to detect adverse effects such as hypotension, bradycardia, or arrhythmia. Vital signs are taken on each subsequent visit. Educate the parents that propranolol should be given with or after meals to prevent hypoglycemia. Inform parents about the need to wake the infant to feed once or twice during the night to prevent hypoglycemia. Educate them about the signs of hypoglycemia to watch for and if seen to feed the infant before the blood sugar drops lower. Other adverse effects include restless sleep, cold extremities, and delayed capillary refill time.

Talk with parents about comments people make about the infant's appearance and provide some possible responses that parents can make. To promote attachment, help the parents see the infant's positive characteristics, such as responsiveness and smiling. Show photos of other children with similar lesions who have completed therapy to show that improvements in appearance are gradual, but possible.

Prepare parents for the changes in the child's appearance with pulsed-dye laser therapy. Some swelling may occur after the treatment, so the application of ice packs for 10 minutes every hour during the first day may help. Teach parents to protect the skin surface from trauma after pulsed-dye laser treatments and to keep the infant's nails short to prevent scratching. Cleanse the area treated with water and pat it dry. Inform parents to avoid sun exposure for several weeks after the treatments, and to use sunscreen in the future.

Injuries to the Skin

Pressure Ulcers

Many children with disabilities are cared for in hospital, community, and home care settings, and they are at risk for skin breakdown and pressure ulcers. Children at greatest risk are those with limited mobility, the inability to change positions, sensory deficits, or incontinence. Infants and children at higher risk in hospital settings are those cared for in neonatal and pediatric intensive care units, sometimes associated with mechanical devices.

Soft tissues and capillary beds can be compressed between a bony prominence and an external surface. Tissue ischemia occurs when compression slows blood flow to the skin and deeper tissues. The cells are deprived of oxygen and nutrients, and metabolic waste products accumulate, resulting in hypoxia and soft-tissue injury. If compression is not relieved, the injury progresses rapidly and a pressure ulcer forms.

Stages 1 and 2 are the most common stages of pressure ulcers in children (Figure 31–11). In stage 3, an ulcer forms as the subcutaneous tissue is exposed, causing a full-thickness injury. In stage 4, the ulcer deepens and extends to muscle, bone, or supporting tissues. See Table 31–7 for common sites and potential causes of pressure ulcers in children.

Clinical Tip

The site of greatest pressure in infants and young children is the occiput. Older children have increased pressure on the sacral and occipital areas.

Initial treatment for early stages of skin damage is removing pressure from the affected site until the skin has healed. Children who use leg braces for alignment and mobility are often put in

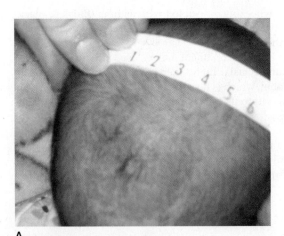

A

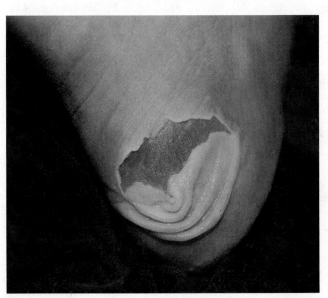

B

Figure 31–11 The initial stages of pressure ulcer formation. *A*, Stage 1, an area of redness does not go away within 30 minutes of removing the pressure or skin irritant. Children with dark skin may have persistent red, blue, or purple discoloration. *B*, Stage 2, the skin looks rubbed or raw like a blister or abrasion, a partial-thickness injury with damage through epidermis, dermis, or both.

SOURCE: Courtesy of Sandra Quigley, Children's Hospital, Boston, MA.

TABLE 31–7 Sites and Potential Causes of Skin Breakdown

SITES	POTENTIAL CAUSES
Occipital region of scalp	Inability to lift head
Sacrum and buttocks	Confinement to bed or wheelchair
Legs and feet	Orthotics, leg braces, casts
Spine and neck	Scoliosis brace
Knees, elbows, heels of feet	Rubbing against bed sheet
Sternum, iliac crest	Prone positioning for mechanical ventilation

wheelchairs. Children who use wheelchairs may be put on bed rest with a pressure-reducing surface. Frequent repositioning is needed. A transparent film may be applied to affected red skin to minimize friction. Pressure ulcers are treated with dressings, such as hydrocolloids, gels or hydrogels, and calcium alginates that do not adhere to the wound.

Nursing Management

The Braden Q Scale (for children under age 5 years) or the Braden Scale are tools to assess the child's risk for pressure ulcers when hospitalized and when the child has a chronic condition with limited mobility. The nurse should assess the child for each of the following risk factors:

- Ability to change and control body position
- Amount of physical activity
- Ability to respond to the discomfort associated with pressure
- Degree to which the skin is exposed to moisture
- Movement of the skin against surfaces
- Food intake pattern
- Tissue perfusion and oxygenation

Carefully inspect the dependent skin surfaces of all infants and children confined to bed at least 3 times in each 24-hour period. Identify the size (length, width, and depth) and character of any skin lesion. Note any signs of infection, the appearance of wound edges, type of tissue at the wound base, and drainage. Describe any drainage amount, color, and type.

Develop protocols for pressure ulcer prevention so that children at high risk are identified and have appropriate interventions initiated (e.g., increased ambulation, frequent position changes, pressure-reducing surfaces, and moisture barriers). If the child is incontinent, change the diaper frequently to keep the skin clean and dry. Ensure an adequate intake of fluids, proteins, and vitamins to keep the skin healthy.

Moist wounds heal more rapidly than dry wounds because cell migration across the moist wound bed more effectively fights infection and removes cellular debris. Provide wound care and dressing changes according to agency guidelines. These guidelines may include saline irrigation, debridement, and a dressing appropriate for the wound condition. See Table 31–3 for types of wound dressings (see the *Clinical Skills Manual* SKILLS). Gauze wraps to hold the dressing in place help prevent skin damage caused by adhesives.

Teach parents of children with braces to inspect the skin under the braces every day for irritation (redness or blisters).

Help the child use a mirror with a long handle to inspect skin on the bottom and sides of the feet, behind the knees, and on the lower legs. Check all edges of the braces for roughness or breakage that can pinch or scrape the skin. If any skin irritation is seen and redness does not go away within 30 minutes, do not put the brace back on until the skin heals. Inform the child's healthcare provider so that treatment can be started immediately. To reduce irritation, have the child wear cotton socks under the braces and make sure the shoes are large enough to accommodate the brace, socks, and the foot. Advise parents to return to a prosthetist regularly for brace refitting as the child grows.

Children who use a wheelchair are at risk for skin breakdown on the buttocks and lower back from the pressure of sitting for hours. A wheelchair cushion can distribute and shift the child's weight when sitting in the chair. Teach the child to change position frequently by doing wheelchair push-ups or by shifting the weight (leaning to the side or forward) for several minutes every 10 to 15 minutes. Make sure the child wears a safety belt when sitting in the wheelchair. Teach school personnel about the child's recommended protocol so they can provide opportunities in school to change positions and reinforce the routine.

Burns

Burns are among the top five leading causes of injury and death in children between 1 and 14 years of age (National Center for Health Statistics, National Vital Statistics System, 2015). In the United States, 128,765 children and adolescents under age 19 years were treated for burns in 2013 (Centers for Disease Control and Prevention [CDC], 2015). Of these children, the majority were less than age 5 years (Vloemans, Hermans, van der Wal, et al., 2014).

The four main types of burns are thermal, chemical, electrical, and radioactive. Thermal burns, the most common in children, result from flames, scalds (such as coffee or grease), or contact with hot objects (such as a wood stove or curling iron). Chemical burns occur when children touch or ingest caustic agents. Electrical burns are caused by direct or alternating current in electrical wires, appliances, or high-voltage wires. Radiation burns result from exposure to radioactive substances or sunlight. Burns are also found in 10% of cases of child abuse (Hazinski, Mondozzi, & Baker, 2014). See Chapter 17 for more information about child abuse.

ETIOLOGY AND PATHOPHYSIOLOGY

Children at different developmental stages are at risk for different types of burns:

- Infants are most often injured by thermal burns (scalding liquids, house fires).
- Toddlers are at risk for thermal burns (pulling hot liquids or grease onto themselves), electrical burns (biting electrical cords), contact burns, and chemical burns (ingesting cleaning agents, button batteries, and other substances) associated with exploring the environment (Figure 31–12).
- Preschool-age children are most often injured by scalding or contact with hot appliances (curling irons, ovens).
- School-age children are at risk for thermal burns (playing with matches, fireworks), electrical burns (climbing high-voltage towers, climbing trees, and contact with electrical wires), and chemical burns (combustion experiments).
- Adolescents also experience thermal, chemical, and electrical burns, as well as radiation burns associated with sunbathing.

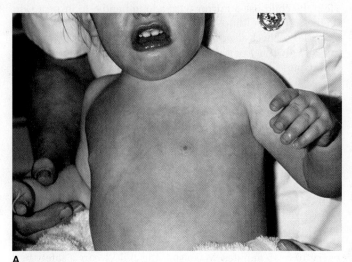

A

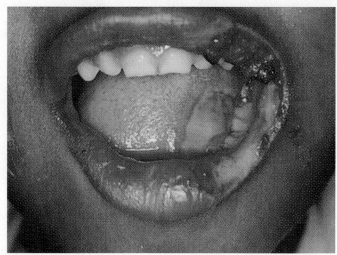

B

Figure 31–12   *A*, Scald injury from hot liquid is a common thermal burn injury in infants and toddlers. Notice the distribution of the burned skin, a wide area on the upper chest where the hottest liquid fell, with a narrower area indicating the liquid cooled as it traveled down the chest. *B*, Electrical burn caused by biting on electrical cord. The burn is caused when the current arcs through the lips, often causing a full-thickness injury through the mucosa, muscle, nerves, and blood vessels. The labial artery may be injured and cause significant bleeding once the eschar falls off after 2 to 3 weeks.

SOURCE: *A*, Dr. P. Marazzi/Science Source. *B*, Courtesy of Dr. Lezley McIveen, Department of Dentistry, Children's National Medical Center, Washington, DC.

The depth of the burn depends on the temperature and duration of the heat application, and on the ability of tissues to dissipate the transferred energy. Immediately after the burn, the cell membranes are altered, leading to increased capillary permeability and extracellular fluid loss. Fluid and plasma shift into the interstitial spaces, causing edema and decreased circulating volume in the blood vessels. Capillary perfusion to most capillaries is decreased because of myocardial depression, leading to tissue ischemia. The child loses increased water, electrolytes, and heat through the injured epidermis. A hypermetabolic state develops from the stress response, and severe alterations in glucose, lipid, and amino-acid metabolism may last for months after the burn injury (Jeschke & Herndon, 2014). A high number of calories are needed in an effort to maintain body temperature and begin healing. Immunosuppression also occurs, which increases the risk for infection.

SAFETY ALERT!
Coffee, tea, soup, and other hot beverages are often served at temperatures high enough to cause a serious scald injury. To prevent scald injuries, adults should not hold infants in their laps while drinking hot beverages.

CLINICAL MANIFESTATIONS

Burns are classified by the depth of penetration into the skin layers. Partial-thickness burns, in which the injured tissue can regenerate and heal, may be either first or second degree. Full-thickness burns, in which the injured tissue cannot regenerate, are also known as third-degree burns. See *Pathophysiology Illustrated: Classification of Burns by Depth* for clinical manifestations by burn depth.

Signs of infection include purulent drainage, swelling, erythema, discoloration of wound margins, and pain in the uninjured skin around the wound.

CLINICAL THERAPY

Assessment of Burn Severity.   Burn severity is determined by the burn depth, percentage of body surface area (BSA) affected, and involvement of specific body parts. A Lund and Browder chart with BSA distributions for various body parts at different ages is used to calculate the total area affected by the burn injury (Figure 31–13). The palm of a child's hand (without fingers and thumb) is 1% of the child's BSA and can be used to make a quick estimate of the burn size. Reassessment of the extent of burn injury is performed 24 to 48 hours after the injury. The true extent of BSA burned and depth of burns may not be apparent for several days.

Criteria for pediatric burns that should be referred to a specialized burn center include (American College of Surgeons, Committee on Trauma, 2014, p. 101):

- Partial-thickness burn greater than 10% BSA and full-thickness burns of any size

- Burns involving the hands, face, eyes, ears, feet, genitalia, perineum, and skin over major joints

- Electrical burns, including lightning injury

- Chemical or inhalation injury

- Burns in a child with another medical condition or additional trauma that increases the risk for death or increased morbidity

- Need for special social and emotional or long-term rehabilitation support, including cases of suspected child maltreatment

Initial Treatment.   The first step is to ensure that the child has an airway, is breathing, and has a pulse. Then stop the burning process by removing jewelry and clothing. Moist soaks or ice (if a small surface area is affected) is used to stop the burning process and to relieve pain. A tetanus vaccine booster is given if

Pathophysiology Illustrated: **Classification of Burns by Depth**

SUPERFICIAL PARTIAL THICKNESS (FIRST DEGREE)	**PARTIAL THICKNESS (SECOND DEGREE)**	**FULL THICKNESS (THIRD DEGREE)**

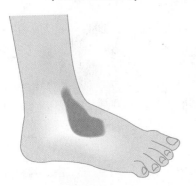
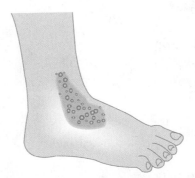
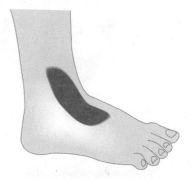

Damages only outer layer of skin; burn is painful and red; heals in a few days (e.g., sunburn)	Involves epidermis and upper layers of dermis; may have sparing of sweat glands and sebaceous glands; heals in 10–14 days	Involves all of epidermis and dermis; may also involve underlying tissue; nerve endings usually destroyed; requires skin grafting
Erythema, blanches on pressure, no bullae, peeling after a few days due to premature cell death	Blisters or bullae, erythema, blanches on pressure, pain and sensitivity to cold air, minimal scar formation	Skin may appear brown, black, deep cherry red, white to gray, waxy or translucent; usually no pain, injured area may appear sunken

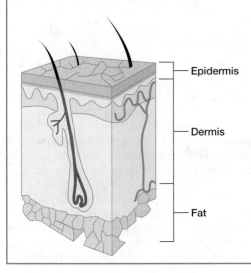
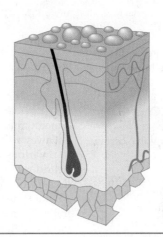
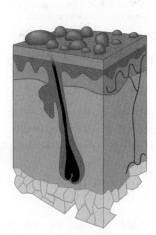

Epidermis

Dermis

Fat

---

more than 5 years have passed since the last vaccine, or when the child has not completed the full vaccine series.

Treatment of Major Burns. The goals of treatment include decreasing burn fluid losses, preventing infection, controlling pain, promoting nutrition, and salvaging all viable tissue. Fluid resuscitation is necessary to maintain the cardiovascular and renal systems. Fluid shifts from the vasculature to the interstitial spaces (third spacing) soon after the burn and can cause hypovolemic shock. Fluid replacement for the first 24 hours after the injury is based on a fluid volume formula calculated from the child's body weight, affected BSA, and normal maintenance needs (e.g., the Parkland and Galveston formulas):

- *Parkland formula:* 4 mL × body weight (kg) × percentage of total BSA burned = total 24-hour fluid requirement in milliliters. Maintenance fluids must be added to the amount of fluid calculated with this formula.

- *Galveston or Shriners Burn Hospital formula:* 5000 mL/m^2 burned area + 2000 mL/m^2 of total BSA = total 24-hour fluid requirement in milliliters.

Lactated Ringer or normal saline solution is the preferred IV fluid. Half of the total volume calculated for the 24-hour period is infused over the first 8 hours, starting at the time of the burn rather than emergency department arrival time. The remainder is distributed evenly over the next 16 hours. Urine output is used to monitor end-organ perfusion. When the urine output reaches 1 mL/kg/hr in children weighing less than 30 kg or 50 mL/kg/hr in heavier children, the fluid rate is reduced (Hazinski et al., 2014). Efforts are also focused on maintaining the child's temperature because heat is lost rapidly through burned skin.

A temperature elevation to 38.0°C (100.4°F) is expected because of the high metabolic rate, not always a sign of infection. A lower temperature is of concern as a possible sign of sepsis or physiologic reserves are exhausted for temperature maintenance (Hazinski et al., 2014). Infection is a frequent complication and wounds are cultured to identify specific organisms and sensitivities before prescribing antibiotic therapy.

Aggressive pain management with intravenous opioids is needed around the clock and for all procedures. The burns cause

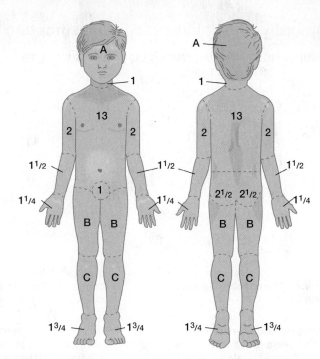

Relative Percentages of Areas Affected by Growth

Area	0	1	5	10	15	Adult
			Age in years			
A = $1/2$ of head	$9^1/2$	$8^1/2$	$6^1/2$	$5^1/2$	$4^1/2$	$3^1/2$
B = $1/2$ of one thigh	$2^3/4$	$3^1/4$	4	$4^1/2$	$4^1/2$	$4^3/4$
C = $1/2$ of one lower leg	$2^1/2$	$2^1/2$	$2^3/4$	3	$3^1/4$	$3^1/2$

Figure 31–13 Body surface area (BSA) percentages for estimating pediatric burn injuries by age group. The extent of burn injury is calculated by adding BSAs affected for each body region.

SOURCE: Data from Artz, C. P., & Moncrief, J. A. (1969). *The treatment of burns* (2nd ed.). Philadelphia: Saunders; Fenlon, S., & Nene, S. (2007). Burns in children. *Continuing Education in Anaesthesia, Critical Care & Pain, 7*(3), 76–80; Tschudy, M. M., & Arcara, K. M. (2012). *The Harriet Lane handbook* (19th ed., p. 99). Philadelphia, PA: Elsevier Saunders.

a significant emotional distress that increases the perception of pain. See Chapter 15 for pain management information. Cimetidine or other H_2 blockers may be ordered to prevent a burn stress ulcer. Medications to help manage the hypermetabolic state may include propranolol, oxandrolone, and insulin (D'Cruz, Martin, & Holland, 2013).

Special consideration is needed when burns involve certain areas of the body:

- Deep partial-thickness and full-thickness burns develop **eschar** (the tough leathery scab that forms over severely burned areas) with no elasticity. When the burn is **circumferential** (surrounds the chest or an extremity), blood flow can become restricted as a result of edema, leading to tissue hypoxia. An **escharotomy** (incision into the constricting tissue) may be necessary to restore peripheral circulation.

- Facial burns usually cause significant edema. Care must be taken to ensure airway patency. An ophthalmologist should assess burns to the eye and prescribe treatment. If the lips are burned, an infant may be unable to suck.

- Burns of the hands require careful management to maintain function. Special splinting and physical therapy are usually necessary.

- Perineal burns are at higher risk for infection because of frequent contamination with urine and stool. Frequent dressing changes are required. A urinary catheter is usually inserted but is removed once hydration status is stable to minimize the risk of urinary tract infection.

Wound Management. Burn wound care has several goals: (1) to remove necrotic tissue and speed wound debridement, (2) to maintain moist wound conditions and adequate circulation, (3) to conserve body heat and fluids, (4) to protect from infection, and (5) to control scarring and prevent scar contracture. Several treatment regimens are used to achieve these goals.

When the burn is extensive, the entire body is bathed to initiate debridement. Sedation, pain management, and anesthesiology support are used during debridement sessions. Intact blisters provide a natural, pain-free, sterile dressing. However, some healthcare providers break blisters open, believing that the fluid provides a medium for bacterial infection. The tissues should be carefully cut away when the wound is being prepared for skin grafting.

Various options are used for wound management after debridement. Traditional burn care for a partial-thickness injury involved the application of antibacterial agents, such as silver sulfadiazine (Silvadene) or mafenide acetate (Sulfamylon) after initial cleansing, followed by a dressing that was changed once or twice daily. However, silver sulfadiazine was found to be cytotoxic (Kim, Martin, & Holland, 2012).

Silver-based antimicrobial dressings (e.g., Aquacel, Acticoat) provide a sustained-release delivery of silver, valued for its antimicrobial property. These dressings also absorb exudate from the wound and can be left in place several days (Figure 31–14). When the dressing is removed, a layer of eschar may also be debrided. These dressing changes are often painful, so pain management is needed (see Chapter 15).

Hydrotherapy (whirlpool bath or shower) may be used to cleanse extensive wounds before debridement, to increase vasodilation and circulation, and to speed healing. The water loosens exudate, topical medications, and dead tissue, and it may help soak off dressings that adhere to the skin. Gentle washing is necessary to protect new epithelial cells. Superficial partial-thickness burns reepithelialize within 3 weeks.

Skin grafting is necessary with any deep partial-thickness or full-thickness burn. Often a biologic dressing (e.g., Integra or Biobrane) or **allograft** (cadaver skin from a skin bank) is used to cover deep burns until an **autograft** (healthy skin taken from a nonburned area of the child's body) can be performed. The biologic dressing or allograft is effective in decreasing infection risk and pain, protecting against fluid loss, and promoting

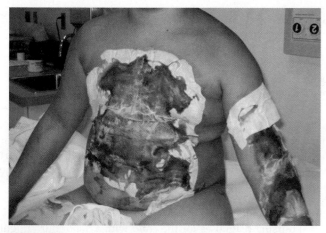

Figure 31–14 This child's scald burn is being treated with an Aquacel AG dressing, a silver-embedded dressing. Note the absorbed exudate that is visible through the burn dressing.

SOURCE: Courtesy of Martin Eichelberger, MD, and Lisa Ring, RN, PNP, Children's National Medical Center, Washington, DC.

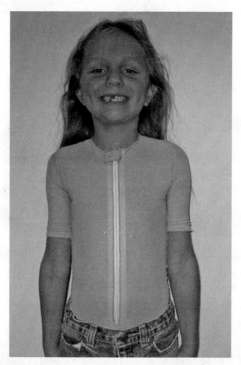

Figure 31–15 Pressure garment used to reduce hypertrophic scarring from a burn to the chest and upper arms.

SOURCE: Courtesy of Martin R. Eichelberger, MD, and Lisa Ring, RN, PNP, Children's National Medical Center, Washington, DC.

revascularization. An autograft is permanent. The autograft is placed after the wound is debrided in the operating room to reveal healthy, bleeding tissue. The donor site (where the autograft was harvested) is a new wound, causing pain and requiring close monitoring for signs of infection.

Vacuum-assisted wound closure (negative pressure wound therapy) is sometimes used for management of partial-thickness burns, graft sites, and other complex wounds. A pump generates a vacuum or suction to remove waste materials from the wound area. Once the burn site is debrided, a foam dressing is applied and sealed with adhesive before the device is attached. The vacuum over the surface of the wound draws out fluids, increases blood perfusion, decreases bacterial colonization, and draws wound edges together to speed healing. These devices are being used more often, but the U.S. Food and Drug Administration has not yet approved them for use in infants and children (U.S. FDA, 2014).

During the rehabilitation stage, pressure garments (e.g., Jobst) are used to reduce development of hypertrophic scarring and contractures. Such garments are worn 23 hours a day for 6 to 8 months to shorten the time of scar maturation and to reduce the thickness of the scars (Figure 31–15).

Severe morbidity is likely to occur with major burns. Significant scarring may occur despite the use of autografting and pressure garments. Contractures and loss of function are also possible. Children with major burns require comprehensive follow-up, sometimes involving repeated hospitalizations for surgery to release burn contractures or perform new grafting, or cosmetic surgery for scar revision.

Nursing Management

For the Child With a Burn Injury

Nursing Assessment and Diagnosis

Emergency assessment first focuses on the potential for life-threatening injuries that need immediate response. Assessment of the airway is necessary, especially when signs of smoke inhalation or burns to the face and neck are noted. Other potential injuries are important to identify when the mechanism of injury also includes a fall or explosion. Identify signs of respiratory distress and any potential bleeding source. A weak, thready pulse, tachycardia, and pallor are important signs of early shock that may provide clues to an internal injury.

Obtain information about the type of burn, when and how it happened, and first aid provided, along with a complete history. If a burn injury was preventable, parents may be emotionally stressed by feelings of guilt. Take care to avoid sounding accusatory when questioning parents about the injury. Be alert to signs of child abuse when the history does not match the injury (e.g., glove and stocking burns, popliteal or antecubital areas spared from burns where the child flexed the knees or elbows, contact burns from cigarettes or irons, and zebra burn lines from contact with a hot grate) (Figure 31–16). Photographs are often taken to document these injuries. Child neglect can be a factor in the burn of an inadequately supervised child.

Assess the extent of burn injury (BSA and depth). Frequently monitor the vital signs and pain control. Monitor the child's circulatory and respiratory status to identify signs of hypovolemia in the first 24 hours or fluid overload as capillary integrity is restored. A head-to-toe assessment is performed at the beginning of every shift, followed by system-specific assessments, depending on clinical findings and changes in the child's status. A urinary catheter may be inserted to enable close monitoring of urine output (see the *Clinical Skills Manual* SKILLS). Weigh the child daily, as the hypermetabolic state may result in weight loss if nutritional intake is inadequate. Be alert to signs of infection such as purulent drainage and edematous, red, or discolored wound margins.

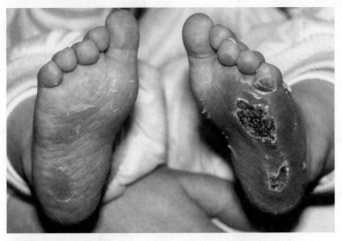

Figure 31–16 **Burns of the hands or feet distributed like gloves or stockings are associated with child abuse. Contact burns on the soles of the feet in a pattern are also suspicious. Note the similar burn pattern on each foot.**

SOURCE: SPL/Science Source.

SAFETY ALERT!
If a burn is circumferential, completely surrounding an extremity, compartment syndrome often occurs. Assess for an increase in cyanosis, deep tissue pain, capillary refill time, and a decreased pulse distal to the burn. If these signs are detected, notify the healthcare provider immediately.

Assess the child's concerns over appearance and the stress of hospitalization. Determine if the child has memories or nightmares about the burn and arrange psychologic support as needed. Identify any family stressors that might need to be addressed during the child's care.

Common nursing diagnoses for the child with a major burn injury are included in the accompanying *Nursing Care Plan*. Additional nursing diagnoses for the child with a major burn might include the following (NANDA-I © 2014):

- *Hyperthermia* related to hypermetabolic state
- *Body Image, Disturbed,* related to burn injury
- *Anxiety* related to situational crisis and threat of death or disfigurement

Nursing Care Plan: The Child With a Major Burn Injury

1. Nursing Diagnosis: *Pain, Acute,* related to physical injury agents (NANDA-I © 2014)

GOAL: The child will verbalize adequate relief from pain and will be able to perform activities of daily living (ADLs).

INTERVENTION	RATIONALE
• Assess the level of pain frequently using pain scales (see Chapter 15).	• Provides objective pain measurement. Changes in pain location and intensity may indicate complications.
• Cover burns as much as possible.	• Temperature change or air movement causes pain.
• Change the child's position frequently. Perform range-of-motion (ROM) exercises.	• Reduces joint stiffness and prevents contractures and increases comfort.
• Provide diversional activities.	• Helps lessen focus on pain.
• Promote uninterrupted sleep with use of medications and comfort measures.	• Sleep deprivation can increase pain perception.
• Use analgesics and sedation (as appropriate) before all dressing changes and burn care. Use sedation when appropriate for major debridement.	• Helps to reduce pain and decreases anxiety for subsequent dressing changes.

EXPECTED OUTCOME: Child will verbalize adequate relief from pain and be able to perform ADLs.

2. Nursing Diagnosis: *Infection, Risk for,* related to trauma and destruction of skin barrier (NANDA-I © 2014)

GOAL: The child will have reduced risk for infection or have secondary infection identified early.

INTERVENTION	RATIONALE
• Take vital signs frequently.	• Increased temperature may be an early sign of infection, but it is also a common with the hypermetabolic state. A normal or decreased temperature may be a sign of sepsis.
• Use standard precautions (gown, gloves, mask) when wounds of a major burn are exposed. Do not allow anyone with an infectious disease to visit.	• Reduces risk of wound contamination.
• Clip hair around burns.	• Hair harbors bacteria and can irritate the wound.
• Keep burn dressing clean and intact.	• Helps reduce the number of bacteria introduced to the burned site.
• Do not place the IV in any burned area.	• Reduces risk of wound contamination.
• Administer oral or IV antibiotics for diagnosed infections as prescribed.	• Antibiotics help to clear the infection quickly.

EXPECTED OUTCOME: Child will have infection risk reduced, and secondary infections are diagnosed and treated promptly.

3. Nursing Diagnosis: *Fluid Volume: Imbalanced, Risk for,* **related to loss of fluids through wounds and to subsequent excess fluid intake (NANDA-I © 2014)**

GOAL: The child will maintain adequate urine output.

INTERVENTION	RATIONALE
• Monitor vital signs, capillary refill time, and pulses.	• The child is initially at risk for hypovolemic shock and needs fluid resuscitation (see Chapter 21).
• Administer IV and oral fluids as ordered.	• Careful calculation of fluid needs and ensuring proper intake helps keep the child properly hydrated.
• Monitor intake and output.	• The child is initially at risk for hypovolemia and then overhydration during fluid resuscitation.
• Weigh child daily using the same scale and amount of clothing.	• Significant weight loss or gain can help determine fluid imbalances.
• Insert urinary catheter if prescribed.	• Helps maintain accurate output measurement during critical care stage.
• Monitor for hyponatremia and hypercalcemia (see Chapter 18).	• Sodium is lost with burn fluid and potassium is lost from damaged cells, causing electrolyte imbalances.

EXPECTED OUTCOME: Child will achieve the expected urine output for age during each stage of acute burn treatment.

4. Nursing Diagnosis: *Mobility: Physical, Impaired,* **related to joint stiffness due to burns (NANDA-I © 2014)**

GOAL: The child will maintain maximum range of motion.

INTERVENTION	RATIONALE
• Arrange physical and occupational therapy twice daily for stretching and ROM exercises. Splint as ordered.	• Positioning in alignment and ROM exercises help to prevent contractures.
• Encourage activities to promote range of motion (toss a bean bag, mimic animal movements).	• Fun activities help the child with diversion and provide movement.

EXPECTED OUTCOME: Child will maintain maximum range of motion without contractures.

5. Nursing Diagnosis: *Nutrition, Imbalanced: Less than Body Requirements,* **related to high metabolic needs (NANDA-I © 2014)**

GOAL: The child will maintain weight and demonstrate adequate serum albumin and hydration.

INTERVENTION	RATIONALE
• Provide an opportunity to choose meals and snacks. Offer a variety of high-protein and high-calorie foods. Provide small frequent feedings.	• Encourages intake. General malaise and anorexia lead to poor healing.
• Encourage the child to have meals with other children.	• Socialization improves intake.
• Provide a multivitamin supplement.	• Vitamin C aids zinc absorption; zinc aids in healing.
• Provide enteral feedings as needed.	• A child with a burn greater than 10% of BSA cannot usually meet nutrition requirements without assistance.
• Weigh the child daily.	• Provides objective evaluation.

EXPECTED OUTCOME: Child will maintain weight, adequate hydration, and normal serum albumin.

Planning and Implementation

Care of the burned child involves various treatments designed to promote healing and prevent complications. These include analgesia and comfort measures, wound management, infection control, fluid and nutrition management, physical therapy, and psychologic support. See the *Nursing Care Plan* for several of these topics.

PROMOTE COMFORT

Assess the child's pain frequently and provide pain management around the clock with intravenous opioids (see Chapter 15). To reduce stress on the child, begin pain and sedation management as soon as possible for the initial debridement. Promote the child's comfort during periods of elevated temperature while keeping burns covered to reduce pain. Fluids should be administered at the rate prescribed for resuscitation for the first 24 hours, and then adjusted as prescribed. Keep the room temperature at a comfortable level. Change bed linens as needed when the child perspires heavily.

PROVIDE WOUND CARE

The burned area is debrided and cleaned, often with a chemical enzyme in a whirlpool bath or shower. An antibacterial/antimicrobial dressing is applied. In some cases, a semipermeable wound membrane is applied to superficial partial-thickness burns. At each dressing change, the wound needs to be assessed for appearance, exudate, odor, appearance of surrounding tissue, and presence of granulation tissue.

Allografts or autografts may be put in place in the operating room after debridement to prepare the burned tissue for the graft. Following the grafting process, vacuum-assisted wound closure may be used over graft sites to maintain a moist environment for healing. Donor sites are treated as separate wounds. Splints may be required to promote healing when the skin over a joint is burned. The child may be kept on bed rest for several days following an autograft to protect the graft until it has a vascular supply.

PREVENT COMPLICATIONS

The healthcare team's goal is to prevent complications. Severe complications of burns include infections, pneumonia, and renal failure, as well as possible irreversible loss of function of the burned area. Significant scarring may occur regardless of autografting. Contractures and loss of function are also possible.

PROVIDE EMOTIONAL SUPPORT

Children with burns have received a profound insult to their body and their self-image. Fear and anxiety about disfigurement and scarring are common, especially among adolescents. The shock and pain of the injury cause increased stress, as do the unfamiliar surroundings and presence of healthcare providers.

Psychologic support is essential to the child's recovery. Continuity of healthcare providers is important in developing a trusting relationship with the child and family. Orient the child to their surroundings and give ample preparation for procedures, when possible. Encourage the child and parents to voice concerns, and show understanding and support for their concerns. Make appropriate referrals to social workers, chaplains, and child-life specialists to ensure that the child and family receive necessary services. See *Evidence-Based Practice: Psychologic Impact of Burn Injury.*

EVIDENCE-BASED PRACTICE | Psychologic Impact of Burn Injury

Clinical Question
How do the intensive treatments and long rehabilitation associated with a severe burn impact the child survivor and the family?

The Evidence
A qualitative review of 75 articles focused on the psychologic consequences of pediatric burns for the child and family. Findings revealed that injured children had anxiety, traumatic stress reactions, and behavior problems in the first months after the burn event, whereas parents had high rates of posttraumatic stress, depressive symptoms, and guilt feelings. After recovery, child survivors as a group had few differences (feelings of self-worth, body image, and social competence) from populations on which assessment tools were normalized. Some children had problems with social functioning and feeling stigmatized. A lower body image was noted more often in girls and those with more severe visible scarring. Family functioning was found to be comparable to norms, but parental stress was apparent. Reviewed studies linked the psychologic responses of parents and family functioning as important factors in the child's psychologic outcome (Bakker, Maertens, Van Son, et al., 2013).

A study was conducted to determine the prevalence of posttraumatic stress disorder (PTSD), depression, anxiety, and stress among parents (n = 120) and the child in the first 6 months after the burn injury. Signs of PTSD in the child were determined from an interview with the parent and the Child Behavior Checklist. Tools administered to parents included the Posttraumatic Diagnostic Scale, Depression Anxiety Stress Scale-21, and a scale to assess coping styles used in stressful situations. During the first month after burn injury, parents scored in the moderate to extremely severe range for depression, anxiety, and stress, but these scores lowered to normal or to mild range 6 months after the injury. During the first month, 25 (22%) parents had a probable PTSD diagnosis, but at 6 months, 28 (24%) parents had moderate to moderately severe posttraumatic stress syndrome (PTSS) or impaired functioning. Presence of PTSS in the child was a factor associated with PTSS in parents at 1 month and 6 months postinjury (De Young, Hendrikz, Kenardy, et al., 2014).

A study of 98 child survivors of a burn injury greater than 30% BSA before age 16 years and treated in a Shriners' burn center investigated the potential for development of personality disorders after the injury (mean = 13.9 years later). A structured clinical interview tool and the 16 Personality Factor Fifth Edition Questionnaire were used to identify personality disorders. Half of the survivors (n = 49, 51%) did not have a personality disorder. The most common personality disorders found were paranoid (19.4%), passive aggressive (18.4% and more common in women [27.5%]), and antisocial personality disorder (17.3% and more common in men [22.4%]). Development of a personality disorder was not associated with age at time of burn, burn severity, or facial or other visible burn scars. However, the overall prevalence of personality disorders was higher in these burn survivors than in the general population (Thomas et al., 2012).

Best Practice
Concern about the parents' psychologic response to the child's acute burn is important because higher levels of distress may impact the parents' ability to be emotionally available to help their child manage distress. Young children may also model their responses to the parents' behavior. All children with severe burns and their families need psychologic support to improve coping during the acute and rehabilitation phases of care and to achieve the best social and psychologic functioning. Such support involves nurses, child-life therapists, and mental health professionals.

Clinical Reasoning
When caring for a child with burns in a clinic setting, investigate the resources available for ongoing mental health support for the child and parents. Is attention being paid to the child's behavioral symptoms? What support is provided to parents? What additional resources could help children with acute burn care in the clinic setting?

Play therapy is encouraged for children, even if they can only observe initially. Play therapy serves several purposes for the child with a major burn:

- It provides an outlet for frustration, independence, and creativity.
- It promotes activities that challenge range of motion.
- It normalizes the child's daily routine.
- It encourages the child, who sees the progress other children make day by day.

Families are at risk for emotional stress. Forewarn them about the expected edema and the changes in the child's body. Parents often feel guilty and responsible for the child's injury. Help parents focus on recovery rather than past actions. Anxiety usually results from lack of knowledge about the severity of the burn and the child's status, especially in the early stages of burn care and admission to the hospital ICU or burn center. Include the family in the child's care whenever possible. Involve parents in their child's care so they learn how to change dressings, assess for infection and dehydration, and perform range-of-motion exercises to aid in the child's recovery.

DISCHARGE PLANNING AND HOME CARE TEACHING

Identify and address home care needs well in advance of discharge. Discharge planning may include instructing parents in nutrition and diet needs, safety in the home, protection of the burned area, wound care, signs of infection and actions to take, use of pressure garments, and range-of-motion exercises to prevent contractures. Provide support and encouragement to parents as they learn how to care for the child with a burn injury.

COMMUNITY-BASED NURSING CARE

Care of the child with a serious burn requires long-term therapy and rehabilitation. Long-term care commonly occurs in the home. Many burn centers use silver-embedded burn dressings to reduce the frequency of dressing changes needed. After discharge, visits to the burn clinic are needed 2 to 3 times a week for dressing changes. Sedation may be necessary, depending on the extent of injury and debridement needed. Parents may be instructed to give pain medication prior to arrival at the clinic to ensure that the child has good pain management.

Children with extensive burns or with burns in locations where scarring may limit function must often wear a pressure garment, and sometimes a face mask if the face was burned. The garment is removed only for bathing and laundering. The pressure garment may present a threat to the child's body image, but it is an important way to decrease scarring. Help families understand the need for the special garments and masks, and how to clean and care for them.

Clinical Tip

Moisturizing creams can be used after burns heal to relieve drying. The healed skin is highly sensitive to sunburn, so cover the area or use a sunscreen. The sunscreen will also help prevent hyperpigmentation after burn healing.

Continued physical therapy and occupational therapy are often needed to regain strength and dexterity for self-care skills and to prevent contractures. Emphasis is placed on returning to normal activities of daily living as soon as possible, such as returning to school. Some children have home tutors or computer connections to school for a time to ensure opportunities for learning while decreasing their risk of exposure to infection.

School reentry is often a traumatic experience, especially for older children and adolescents, because of the fear of rejection, decreased self-esteem, and impaired body image. In some cases, the child's primary nurse may visit the school of a child with a burn injury before the child returns to school—bringing photographs of the child, pressure garments, or other items—to inform classmates and allow them to explore their feelings about the child's burn injury. Some communities may offer support groups for families and children with burn injuries. Referral to these groups may be beneficial.

A major role of nurses in the community is prevention. Provide burn prevention information to parents at each health promotion visit. Become involved with a Safe Kids coalition or with local firefighters to help educate families and caregivers about ways to prevent scald burns and house fires. Examples of prevention messages include the following:

- Appropriate temperature settings for hot water heaters
- Keeping the handles of pots on the stove turned toward the wall and dishes with hot liquids out of the toddler's reach
- Keeping infants and toddlers off the lap when drinking hot beverages or eating soup
- Keeping matches, lighters, and flammable materials away from children
- Installing smoke detectors and replacing the batteries annually

MANAGEMENT OF MINOR BURNS

Many children with minor burns are cared for at home after an initial visit to the emergency department or urgent care clinic. Discuss home remedies for minor burn care. For superficial burns covering a small area, use moist soaks to stop the burning process and to relieve pain. Any open blisters are debrided, and a thin layer of antibiotic medication (e.g., Bacitracin, silver sulfadiazine) is applied over the burn. Do not place this medication close to the eyes or mouth. The burn is then covered with one or two layers of gauze. Acetaminophen with codeine may be prescribed for burn dressing changes at home. Burn dressings should be changed twice daily. The child should be seen within 48 hours of initial treatment to monitor progress. Alternatively, a burn dressing may be applied and changed every few days in the clinical setting so the wound can be monitored. See *Families Want to Know: Caring for Minor Burns*.

Evaluation

Examples of expected outcomes of nursing management are included in the *Nursing Care Plan*. Some additional outcomes include the following:

- The child expresses and shows signs of reduced anxiety.
- Effective pain management is provided for dressing changes.

Sunburn

Sunburn is a burn injury to the outer layer of skin caused by excess ultraviolet light exposure, or sun exposure after taking phototoxic drugs (acne medication, sulfonamides, tetracycline, nonsteroidal anti-inflammatory drugs, and birth control pills). Young children have less melanin to protect their skin against harmful ultraviolet (UV) rays. It is estimated more than 25% of a person's lifetime exposure to sunburns occurs before 18 years

Families Want to Know

Caring for Minor Burns

- Place burn under cool, running water to stop the burning process and to help reduce pain. Do not use ice, as it can cause more damage to the injured skin.

- Remove all clothing and jewelry from the burned area.

- Do not use butter or margarine on the burn as it may introduce bacteria into the wound.

- Topical application of gel from the leaf of an aloe vera plant may help promote healing (National Center for Complementary and Alternative Medicine [NCCAM], 2012).

- Apply a topical antibiotic such as bacitracin to the burned area and cover the area with a couple of layers of gauze. Keep the area clean and dry.

- Clean and change the dressing twice daily. The pain medication may be given about an hour before the dressing change is planned. The dressing may be saturated with sterile normal saline and gently removed if it adheres to the burn area. Reapply the antibiotic cream and cover.

- Monitor for signs of infection, such as odor, increased drainage, and increasing redness of the skin around the burn. Contact the healthcare provider if infection is suspected.

of age (Gupta & Cohen, 2012). A childhood sun exposure history that includes intense repeated sunburns and chronic overexposure to UV radiation for the purpose of tanning is strongly associated with the development of all three types of skin cancer (basal cell, squamous cell, and melanoma) in future years (Gupta & Cohen, 2012). Avoiding sunburn during childhood is believed to be more important than protecting skin during adulthood. Use of indoor tanning beds and facilities increases the risk for developing melanoma by 74% (Gupta & Cohen, 2012).

SAFETY ALERT!
Behaviors and skin characteristics that increase the risk for pediatric melanoma include light skin and eyes, freckling, skin with an inability to tan, family history of melanoma, immunosuppression, and ultraviolet radiation treatment for psoriasis (Gupta & Cohen, 2012). Other factors include intermittent intense sun exposure (e.g., blistering sunburns before 20 years of age) and frequent sun exposure without use of sunscreen.

Erythema, pain, skin tenderness, swelling, blistering, and itching usually develop between 3 and 5 hours after exposure to ultraviolet B (UVB) rays. Solar UVA rays penetrate more deeply into the skin. Increased vasodilation and vascular permeability result in the extravasation of fluid to the tissues (edema, vesicles, and bullae) and white blood cell migration to the damaged skin. The erythema peaks at 12 to 24 hours and subsides after 72 hours. Systemic complaints include malaise, poor sleep due to

Professionalism in Practice Sun Tanning
The American Academy of Pediatrics policy statement on ultraviolet radiation (UVR) states that the deliberate exposure to artificial sources of UVR (e.g., tanning beds and facilities) and overexposure to the sun to increase vitamin D concentrations should be avoided (AAP, 2011). Nurses have an important role in educating adolescents about the risks for skin cancer and damage to the eyes from UVR exposure. Nurses can also work with community leaders to develop local policies that ban adolescents under age 18 years from using tanning facilities or tanning beds.

skin tenderness, fatigue, headaches, and chilling resulting from rapid heat loss.

Treatment is generally supportive. Pain can be relieved by cool compresses, local anesthetic sprays or creams, and an emollient to help keep skin from drying out. Nonsteroidal anti-inflammatory drugs (NSAIDs) may be used for pain relief and to reduce inflammation. See Chapter 15 for information on NSAIDs. Skin exposed by broken blisters is gently washed 2 to 3 times a day and covered with clean clothing or a sterile dressing if the sunburned skin is limited to a small area.

Nursing Management

Educate parents and children about preventing sunburn. Advise parents and children that repeated sunburns may lead to permanent skin damage, skin cancer, cataracts, and premature aging of the skin. See *Families Want to Know: Preventing Sunburn.*

Healthy People 2020

(C-20) Increase the proportion of persons who participate in behaviors that reduce their exposure to harmful ultraviolet (UV) irradiation and avoid sunburn

---

Hypothermia

Hypothermia is a condition in which the core body temperature falls below 35°C (95°F). This occurs when the heat produced by the body is less than the heat lost. Hypothermia is a life-threatening emergency that can occur in any season and any geographic location. Infants and young children are at risk because of immature temperature regulatory mechanisms, thinner skin, limited subcutaneous fat, and a high skin surface area-to-body mass ratio. Adolescents are at risk because of risk-taking behaviors such as drug and alcohol use and engaging in remote outdoor activities without proper equipment.

Primary hypothermia results from environmental exposure. As with newborns, heat is lost through radiation, conduction, convection, and evaporation. As the core body temperature falls, the body tries to conserve body heat and to rewarm the blood by vasoconstriction (to shunt blood to the body core). The body generates heat by increasing muscle tone and shivering. Hypothermia leads to increased blood viscosity, slower blood flow through the capillaries, and the potential for blood coagulation.

Families Want to Know

Preventing Sunburn

- Keep children out of direct sunlight as much as possible, especially between 10 a.m. and 4 p.m. Encourage children to play in the shade.

- Be aware that water, concrete, and sand reflect sunlight and increase exposure by reflecting UV rays up toward the skin.

- Minimize sun exposure by wearing a hat with a 3-inch brim, closely woven cotton long-sleeved clothing and pants, and wraparound UV blocking sunglasses with 99% UV blockage. Wear a T-shirt while swimming.

- Use sunscreen with a sun protection factor (SPF) of 30 or higher. Apply thickly to all exposed areas 30 minutes before sun exposure. Reapply 15 to 20 minutes after first sun exposure, and then again every 2 hours as needed. Reapply sooner if swimming, toweling off, or perspiring heavily.

- Use a waterproof sunscreen when swimming for protection in water that lasts 60 to 80 minutes. Then reapply. Avoid placing it near the eyes as it causes a chemical burn and pain. Call the poison control center immediately if eyes are exposed.

- Use UV blocking agents such as zinc oxide or titanium oxide for infants under 6 months of age because infants may absorb sunscreen chemical through their skin.

- If the child is taking any medications, check with the healthcare provider before exposure (some medications cause hypersensitivity to sunlight).

- Adolescents should avoid indoor tanning facilities and artificial tanning devices because the rays are as damaging to the skin as the sun.

Symptoms of mild hypothermia (32 to 35°C [89.6 to 95.0°F]) include slurred speech, poor coordination, poor judgment and inappropriate behavior, shivering, and muscle stiffness. Symptoms of moderate hypothermia (28 to 32°C [82.4 to 89.6°F]) include depressed respirations, slow pulse, low blood pressure, pale or cyanotic color, shivering, and dilated pupils. Lethargy, mental impairment, irrational thinking, hallucinations, and coma develop as the central nervous system becomes depressed. Profound hypothermia (body temperature below 28°C [82.4°F]) is characterized by apnea, no shivering, low blood pressure, ventricular fibrillation, dilated and unresponsive pupils, and coma.

Clinical therapy focuses on resuscitation, if necessary, and gradual core body rewarming. The child who has profound hypothermia should receive cardiopulmonary resuscitation until the body temperature returns to normal because the hypothermia may have preserved vital organs. Aggressive techniques for rewarming may include humidified, warm oxygen; warmed intravenous fluids; warm packs to the core circulation areas (axillae, groin, and neck); and peritoneal lavage and dialysis. Hypoglycemia is a common complication and is treated with IV glucose.

For mild hypothermia (temperature above 35°C [95°F]), external heat lamps, immersion in warm water, and an electric blanket are used.

Nursing Management

Monitor vital signs and urine output during rewarming. Educate parents to layer children's clothing in cold climates, recognize signs of hypothermia, decrease time of exposure to cold, and know how to treat mild hypothermia. Teach school-age children and adolescents who go on camping and hunting trips how to recognize and manage hypothermia in themselves and others. Teach preventive techniques such as avoiding riding snowmobiles or walking on ice that is not known to be deep enough to support the weight.

First aid for hypothermia includes moving the child to a dry area and removing any wet clothing. Replace with warm, dry clothing, and encourage the child to drink a warm, high-calorie liquid, if possible. If a child becomes hypothermic during a camping trip or other outing, a warm person should get into a sleeping bag (or under the blankets) next to the child after any wet or heavy clothing is removed. This action will trap heat the child's body generates and provide passive rewarming by the other person.

Frostbite

Frostbite is a cold injury in which the skin tissue is exposed to temperatures below freezing for more than an hour when environmental protection is inadequate. Areas of the body at high risk for frostbite include the hands, feet, cheeks, nose, and ears. Ice crystallizes in the tissues, resulting in dehydration of the cells and ischemic damage. Frostbite can also occur if a chemical cold pack used for first aid is left in contact with the skin for an extended period.

Clinical manifestations vary by the severity of injury. In mild or superficial frostbite, the skin appears reddened or mottled, edematous, and stiff, and transient tingling or burning is present. In severe or deeper frostbite, the skin is gray or mottled, edematous, hard with no rebounding, and numb.

With superficial injury, rapid rewarming causes a flush and the sensation of tingling, burning, or prickling in the affected area. With deeper injury, the skin may appear mottled and cyanotic followed by erythema, swelling, and burning pain with rewarming. Vesicles and bullae develop in 24 to 48 hours, which slowly heal. The extent of injury is not initially apparent.

If frostbite is suspected, get the child to a warmer environment and remove any wet clothes. Because the frostbitten area may be numb, protect it from trauma. Slowly rewarm the area to decrease the chance of cellular damage by immersing the affected part in warm water between 40°C and 42°C (104.0°F and 107.6°F) until thawed. Analgesics are given to treat pain caused by thawing. Gently clean the affected skin with saline and cover it with sterile dressings. Wound care may be similar to that provided to a child with burns. Physical therapy may be important to improve circulation and maintain function.

Nursing Management

As with hypothermia, the goal of management is prevention. Teach parents to layer children's clothing for warmth and to pack extra blankets and clothing if cold temperatures are expected during outdoor activities. Teach adolescents how to avoid frostbite during hunting and other cold weather expeditions. Wet clothing and gloves should be changed quickly.

Early care is instrumental in minimizing permanent injury. Severe frostbite requires hospitalization, fluid management, dressing changes, and careful attention to diet. Provide emotional support to the child and family while they wait to learn the full extent of injury and disability.

Bites

ANIMAL BITES

Dog bites accounted for nearly 134,000 emergency department visits in 2013 for children and youth less than age 20 years (National Center for Injury Prevention and Control, 2015). Children, and especially boys, ages 5 to 9 years have the highest rate of dog bites (CDC, 2014). In many cases, the child knows the dog or cat, and most bites occur in the home or a familiar place. Bites are often associated with the child's inappropriate behavior, such as teasing, rough play, or interfering with feeding or care of puppies. Other animals that may bite include cats, birds, turtles, and wild animals such as bats, squirrels, and raccoons.

Assessment includes noting the location and number of puncture wounds, abrasions, lacerations, and crushing injuries; redness or swelling at entry sites; redness extending out from site (possible cellulitis); and any drainage related to the bite. Damage to nerves, muscles, tendons, and vascular structures is identified. Dog bites tend to be crushing rather than clean, sharp lacerations. Cat bites tend to be puncture wounds; 50% become infected (AAP, 2015, p. 205). Head and neck bites require radiographic examination to rule out any associated injury, such as trauma to the airway or a depressed skull fracture.

Initial treatment involves irrigation of the wound, removal of devitalized tissue, and application of a clean dressing. Povidone-iodine solution (a virucidal agent) may be used in some cases to irrigate the wound. Sedation and pain management may be needed for some children. Puncture wounds may be debrided in the operating room. Prophylactic antibiotics may be prescribed to reduce the risk for infections. A delay in seeking care after the bite is associated with a greater risk for infection.

Wounds may be closed with adhesive strips rather than suturing because of the potential for infection. Severe bites sometimes require surgical closure or reconstruction. Wounds over joints should be immobilized and elevated. The major complication of bites is infection (such as cellulitis, septic arthritis, or osteomyelitis), which may require hospitalization.

Dog bites should be reported to animal control, and the dog should be confined and observed for 10 days for signs of rabies. Cat bites are also dangerous because cats are less commonly immunized against rabies. If the animal develops rabies during that interval, human rabies immune globulin (HRIG) and rabies vaccine is administered immediately, followed by a rabies vaccine injection on days 3, 7, and 14 following the first injection. HRIG and rabies vaccine are given immediately to all children bitten by wild animals in which rabies cannot be excluded. See Chapter 16 for a description of rabies treatment.

Nursing Management

If a child is bitten by an animal, obtain information about the extent of the injury, circumstances surrounding the attack, present location of the animal, and attempts to assess the animal's health.

To decrease infection, the wound is gently washed with antibacterial soap and water followed by high-pressure irrigation (unless it is a puncture wound) with large quantities of sterile saline or lactated Ringer solution. An 18-gauge needle on a 60-mL syringe may be used to provide high-pressure irrigation. A clean dressing is applied and the affected body part is elevated to reduce bleeding. Check the child's immunization record to determine whether a tetanus booster is necessary. Teach parents how to care for the wound and signs of infection that indicate a need to return for care.

Prevention of animal bites is another important nursing role (see *Families Want to Know: Preventing Animal Bites*).

HUMAN BITES

Human bites are more common than most people realize. Toddlers, young children, and adolescents often receive human bites during altercations. The skin may be broken, with erythema, abrasion, bruising, or laceration. Because the mouth harbors many bacteria, infection is fairly common. Assess the risk for hepatitis B and HIV infection. Initial treatment includes irrigating with sterile saline and debridement. Antibiotics may be prescribed to prevent systemic complications. Parents should be instructed about how to care for the wound and to observe for infection.

Families Want to Know

Preventing Animal Bites

General Guidelines for Pets in the Home

- Never leave a young child alone with an animal.
- Do not buy or adopt a pet unless you are confident of your child's ability to respect it.
- Spay or neuter the pet to reduce aggression.

Teach Children the Following Rules

- Avoid all unfamiliar animals and report them to a parent.
- Avoid contact with all wild animals. If an animal (wild or unknown) is sick or acting strangely, notify the health department.
- Do not touch an animal when it is eating, sleeping, or nursing.
- Never overexcite an animal, even in play. Do not roughhouse or play games that stimulate aggressive behavior. Do not tease or throw objects at an animal.
- Never put your face close to an animal. Seek permission before hugging or petting an animal.
- If approached by a dog, stay calm, stand still, talk softly, and back away slowly until the dog loses interest; do not run.
- If attacked, pretend to be a tree or a log and protect the face. If knocked down, curl into a ball and protect the face and neck.

INSECT BITES AND STINGS

Insect bites and stings occur frequently in children and usually are not a cause for concern. Exceptions include bites or stings by insects that carry parasites or communicable diseases (ticks, mosquitos), those of a venomous nature (spiders), and those that produce an allergic reaction. A small percentage of the population is sensitized to *Hymenoptera* (bee, wasps, fire ants) stings and has a generalized response. See Table 31–8 for clinical manifestations of insect bites and stings. For a discussion of communicable diseases carried by ticks and mosquitoes (e.g., Lyme disease, Rocky Mountain spotted fever, West Nile virus, malaria), see Chapter 16.

Nursing Management

The goal of nursing care is prevention. Become familiar with the harmful insects in your area, so you can identify them and recognize their effects. Teach children to avoid spiders and other biting or stinging insects. Also, teach children to stay calm when a bee or wasp approaches and to slowly walk away without swatting. Many commercial repellents (OFF, Cutter's, Deep Woods OFF) are available. Most products contain DEET (diethyltoluamide) or oil of lemon eucalyptus. They are effective against many insects, including mosquitoes, fleas, ticks, and chiggers, but do not repel stinging insects.

Warn parents against using heavily perfumed shampoos, powders, soaps, or lotions. Do not dress children in bright-colored or floral print clothing when outdoors, as these may attract insects. Avoid eating sweet foods and beverages outdoors as these will attract bees and wasps. Bees and wasps may crawl into a canned beverage and not be seen. Pour beverages into a cup rather than drinking from a can to prevent stings to the mouth and lips.

Household pets may be a source of fleas or ticks. Encourage frequent inspection of pets and preventive treatments against fleas and ticks before pets are allowed prolonged contact with children.

When a systemic reaction to *Hymenoptera* has occurred, the child should wear a medical alert identification and carry an emergency kit with epinephrine (see Chapter 22). Teach parents and school personnel how to administer epinephrine. Desensitization injections may be given.

SNAKE BITES

Venomous snakes are found in most areas of the country. During warm months, snakes are active and likely to bite if disturbed. Fortunately, many bites are dry, delivering no venom. Fatalities are rare.

Rattlesnake, copperhead, and cottonmouth venom is composed of enzymes and toxins that cause hemolysis and tissue necrosis. Coral snake venom causes neuromuscular paralysis that can affect breathing and lead to respiratory arrest (Wilbeck, & Gresham, 2013). The amount and toxicity of the venom injected has an impact on the consequences of the snakebite. Because children usually receive a higher amount of venom relative to body mass, their response may be greater than that of an adult.

Puncture marks, white wheal, and burning sensation appear at the site of the bite. With envenomation erythema, bruising and edema rapidly develop and extend from the site for up to 24 hours. Systemic signs include dizziness, tachycardia, nausea, vomiting, diarrhea, sweating, chills, and muscle twitching. Signs of a severe response may include hypotension, altered consciousness, bleeding from multiple sites (disseminated intravascular coagulation), pulmonary edema, and renal failure. Coral snake neurologic signs may include diplopia and ptosis, difficulty speaking and swallowing, hypersalivation, and altered mental status (lethargy, drowsiness, or euphoria).

Clinical therapy involves immobilization of the extremity and a cold compress to slow the spread of the venom. Laboratory studies include complete blood count, platelet count, coagulation studies, electrolytes, and renal function. Attempts to identify the snake causing the bite should be made to determine if it is venomous. A cell phone photograph of the snake is useful in identifying whether the snake is venomous. The poison control center is contacted to obtain treatment guidelines. Specific antivenom (often made with horse serum) is usually administered within 4 to 6 hours. CroFab, a newer antivenom used for cottonmouth, copperhead, and rattlesnake bites, has a lower rate of hypersensitivity reactions. Children at risk for severe hypersensitivity reaction are pretreated with antihistamines and corticosteroids. Monitor children treated with CroFab for thrombocytopenia, bleeding, or development of coagulopathy due to hemolytic effect of venom. Acetaminophen and codeine may be prescribed for pain management. A tetanus booster is given if vaccination status is unknown or the tetanus series is incomplete.

Nursing Management

Nursing care involves assessing the child for initial and progressive signs of envenomation. Try to keep the child calm to slow the circulation. First aid involves immobilizing the extremity, keeping it in a dependent position to slow the spread of venom, and cold compresses. Hands with a bite should be elevated after splinting in functional position. Ice should not be used. Rings or constricting items should be quickly removed from the injured extremity. Monitor the distal extremity's color, pulse, and sensation, and measure the circumference of the extremity above and below the affected extremity; reassess every 15 to 30 minutes to track progression of edema and response to treatment. Clean the wound with germicidal soap and water.

The child receiving antivenom may be cared for in the critical care unit. The antivenom is diluted in saline and slowly administered intravenously as ordered. Administer the antihistamines after tests for sensitivity to horse serum are completed. Have resuscitation equipment on hand in preparation for an anaphylactic reaction. Help locate additional antivenom if the hospital does not have an adequate supply. At time of discharge, educate parents of children who receive antivenom to monitor for unusual bleeding and to contact the health professional if noted. NSAIDs should not be used for 2 weeks after discharge because of increased bleeding risk.

Provide emotional support to the child and family. Teach children and their families to avoid future snakebites.

Contusions

Contusions are soft-tissue injuries that have a variety of causes. Often it is difficult to assess whether an injury has caused underlying tissue damage. An injury does not have to break the skin to result in internal damage. Radiographic examination may be necessary to rule out broken bones or further tissue damage. Signs and symptoms that indicate a need for treatment include swelling that does not subside within 72 hours, intense pain, inability to move the injured part, and infection. Elevate the injured extremity and apply ice as soon as possible after injury. This can reduce inflammation and swelling in the area.

Foreign Bodies

Many skin injuries result from penetration of foreign particles. Common substances include gravel from abrasions, bee stingers,

TABLE 31–8 Clinical Manifestations of Insect Bites and Stings

TYPE OF BITE AND CLINICAL MANIFESTATIONS	CLINICAL THERAPY
MOSQUITOES AND FLEAS Local inflammation results from injected foreign protein or chemicals. • Local reaction: discrete, red papules and edema at the bite site with itching, burning, pain, and hives; minimal discomfort; pruritic wheals and bullae tend to develop with repeat exposure. • Systemic reaction: wheezing, urticaria; laryngeal edema; shock.	Local reactions: • Apply cold compresses or ice to the site. • Antihistamine medication. Systemic reactions need emergency medical treatment.
BED BUGS Local inflammation results from injected saliva, an anesthetic and anticoagulant. • Local reaction: numerous pruritic papules, often in pattern of three papules; child often wakes up with numerous lesions on exposed skin areas that were not present the night before. • Systemic reaction: rare severe allergic reaction.	Local reactions: • Keep skin clean. • Topical corticosteroids may be applied. • Antihistamines may be prescribed. • Oral corticosteroids may be prescribed for severe allergic reaction. • Treat infested areas, and discard infested bedding.
BEE OR WASP STING Venoms contain enzymes that affect vascular tone and permeability. • Local reaction: mild, local pain; erythema and edema. • Systemic reaction: generalized urticaria, flushing, angioedema, pruritus; wheezing; dizziness, hypotension; abdominal pain, vomiting, diarrhea; anaphylaxis is rare.	Local reactions: • Remove stinger as soon as possible. • Apply cold compresses and elevate extremity. • A dash of meat tenderizer (papain powder) and a drop of water massaged into the skin for 5 minutes relieve the pain. • Antihistamine medication. Systemic reactions are treated with glucocorticoids and antihistamines or epinephrine. Desensitization for severe reactions.
FIRE ANTS Venom is hemolytic and neurotoxic, causing a histamine-like response. • Local reaction: a black center at the point of the bite, or trail of lesions across skin; initial wheal becomes a vesicle in a few hours; in 24 hr the fluid is cloudy, and the vesicle has a red halo; pruritus, erythema, edema, induration. • Systemic and anaphylactic reactions can occur.	Local reactions: • Ice or cold compresses. • Antihistamine medication. • Elevate extremity. Systemic reactions—same as bees and wasps.
BLACK WIDOW SPIDER Venom is neurotoxic. • Local reaction: stinging sensation at time of bite; localized edema and erythema, two fang marks, petechiae branching from site. • Systemic reaction in 1–3 hr, symptoms peak in 3–12 hr, diminish in 72 hr; muscle rigidity of torso and abdomen, priapism, muscle cramps near the bite; malaise, sweating, nausea, vomiting, dizziness, restlessness, insomnia, and diaphoresis; hypertension and arrhythmias; oliguria.	Ice Diazepam and opioids for pain management. Antihistamine medication. Hydrocortisone may decrease the inflammatory response. Antivenom IV is used in severe reactions after negative skin test for hypersensitivity to horse serum.
BROWN RECLUSE SPIDER Venom contains proteolytic enzymes and sphingomyelinase D, a cytotoxic factor. • Local reaction: within 2 hr, sinking blue macule with a halo of inflammation at the bite site; pain; a hemorrhagic blister forms in 1–2 days with a necrotic ulcer seen when it breaks. Most ulcers are 1–2 cm (0.4 to 0.8 in.) in meter, but some progress to 15 cm (6 in.) in meter with full-thickness injury. • Systemic reaction: fever, chills, nausea and vomiting, and hemolysis.	Ice Cleanse the wound and good wound care. Elevate extremity. Analgesics. Oral anti-inflammatory agent. Antibiotics for secondary infection. Excision and skin grafting in cases of severe necrosis.

Source: Data from Krau, S. D. (2013). Bites and stings: Epidemiology and treatment. *Critical Care Nursing Clinics of North America, 25,* 143–150; Barnes, E. R., & Murray, B. S. (2013). Bedbugs: What nurses need to know. *American Journal of Nursing, 113*(10), 58–62; Camp, N. E. (2014). Black widow spider envenomation. *Journal of Emergency Nursing, 40*(2), 193–194.

and splinters. Treatment of superficial foreign bodies involves irrigating the wound to try to forcibly dislodge the debris. A deeply embedded foreign body is best removed under medical supervision to avoid permanent injury or scarring.

Lacerations

Lacerations are cuts or tears to the skin. In many cases, the cut is minor and can be managed at home with gentle cleansing, antibiotic ointment, and a bandage. More extensive lacerations and those on the face or over joints often need suturing to promote healing and reduce scarring. Laceration repair is performed after wound cleansing and appropriate local analgesia to control pain. Sutures or dermal adhesive may be used. Sutures are usually removed about 7 days later.

Chapter Highlights

- Wound healing has three overlapping phases: hemostasis and inflammation, tissue formation, and maturation.

- Contact dermatitis is a skin inflammation that occurs following direct contact with an allergen that causes an immune response, or with an irritant that causes no immune response.

- Superabsorbent disposable diapers reduce the frequency and severity of diaper dermatitis because, when wet, a gel forms inside the diaper keeping moisture away from the skin.

- Seborrheic dermatitis is an inflammatory skin condition due to an overgrowth of *Malassezia furfur* yeast in areas of sebaceous gland activity. Lesions are commonly found on the scalp, nasolabial folds, behind the ears, and intertriginous areas.

- The classic impetigo lesion begins as a vesicle surrounded by edema and redness. The vesicle fluid turns cloudy and ruptures, leaving a honey-colored crust on an ulcerated base.

- Athletes are at high risk for community-acquired methicillin-resistant *Staphylococcus aureus* because of their potential for frequent skin-to-skin contact, cuts or abrasions, wound contact, and shared items.

- Folliculitis, a superficial inflammation of the pilosebaceous follicle, may be associated with *Pseudomonas* exposure in a poorly chlorinated pool or hot tub.

- Children with cellulitis appear ill with fever, chills, malaise, and enlarged lymph nodes. The infected site is red or lilac in color, warm, edematous, and tender with an indistinct border.

- Viral skin infections include molluscum contagiosum and warts (papillomavirus).

- Oral thrush (candidiasis), a fungal infection, is characterized by white patches that resemble coagulated milk on the oral mucosa and may bleed when removed.

- Children being treated for tinea capitis may develop an "id" hypersensitivity reaction rash to the fungal antigen, and this is not an allergic reaction to the medication.

- Drug reactions vary in severity from a simple allergic reaction and erythema multiforme minor to potential life-threatening conditions, such as Stevens–Johnson syndrome and toxic epidermal necrolysis.

- Treatment of atopic eczema involves hydration and lubrication of the skin by bathing followed by emollients to trap in skin moisture. Topical corticosteroids are used to treat skin flares and then discontinued.

- Acne medications, tretinoin or isotretinoin, are phototoxic, resulting in sunburn with even minimal exposure. Protection with sunscreen or protective clothing is important to prevent significant sunburn.

- Psoriasis is chronic skin condition with pruritic, thick, silvery, scaly erythematous plaques that have irregular borders surrounded by normal skin.

- Epidermolysis bullosa is a rare, autosomal dominant, severe chronic blistering skin disorder that occurs with minor trauma.

- Treatment for lice includes a pediculicide applied to the hair and combing the hair with a fine-toothed comb to remove all the nits. Depending on product used, a second treatment may be needed in 7 days.

- Scabies is a mite infestation in which the female mite burrows under the skin to lay eggs, which causes irritation and intense itching.

- Hemangiomas undergo a period of rapid growth during infancy before involuting. The rapid growth may cause significant complications, such as pressure on the airway, eye, or ear canal.

- Children at greatest risk for pressure ulcers are those with limited mobility, sensory deficits, or the inability to change positions. Tissue ischemia occurs when the soft tissues and capillary beds are compressed between a bony prominence and another surface.

- Of the four main types of burns (thermal, chemical, electrical, and radioactive), thermal burns are most common in children. Infants, toddlers, and preschool-age children most commonly suffer scald burns. Other types of thermal burns include flames and contact with a hot object.

- Initial treatment for a child with a significant burn injury includes emergency assessment of the airway, breathing, and circulation and stopping the burning process by removing jewelry and clothing, and applying moist soaks or ice.

- More than 25% of a person's lifetime exposure to the sun occurs by 18 years of age. Repeated blistering sunburns during childhood increase the risk for development of melanoma.

- Children are at greater risk for hypothermia because of their thinner skin, limited subcutaneous fat, and high surface area to body mass ratio. Body heat is lost more quickly in water or when clothing is wet.

- Frostbite occurs when ice crystallizes in the tissues, causing cellular dehydration and ischemic damage.

- Children at highest risk for dog bites are those 5 to 9 years old. Most children know the dog that bites them.

- Insects and spiders with venomous bites include bees, fire ants, black widow spiders, and brown recluse spiders.

- Venomous snakes living in the wild in the United States include rattlesnakes, copperheads, water moccasins, and coral snakes. Initial treatment includes calming the child, immobilization of the extremity, and applying cold compresses to slow the spreasd of the venom.

Clinical Reasoning in Action

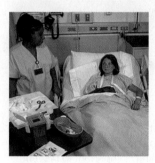

Twelve-year-old Rebecca is admitted to the burn unit with a scald burn from spilling a pot of boiling spaghetti water on her chest, abdomen, and legs. The burn is classified as a partial-thickness burn covering 12% of her body surface area (BSA) and full-thickness burn covering 3% of BSA. IV fluids are started in the emergency department and a continuous infusion of morphine is given for pain. Her temperature is 101.0°F (38.3°C). The initial debridement of the burns is performed in the operating room so that Rebecca is anesthetized and does not feel pain from the procedure. A silver-embedded dressing is applied to her partial-thickness burns, and a biologic dressing is placed over the full-thickness injury. Following debridement, Rebecca is put on a high-calorie, high-protein diet to help meet her increased nutritional requirements. Her parents are encouraged to bring in foods Rebecca enjoys to encourage her to eat. Wound care around the biologic dressing is performed twice a day, and all burn sites are inspected for signs of infection. The dressing over the partial-thickness burns is replaced every 3 days. Pain medication for wound care is provided through the IV. After several days, Rebecca is scheduled for an autograft for the full-thickness injury. Rebecca's nutritional intake and urine output are carefully monitored while she is hospitalized. Physical therapy is initiated to maintain range of motion and to prevent contractures.

The nurse talks with Rebecca and her family about what to expect as the burns heal. Education of the family includes signs and symptoms of infection and the care of the graft donor site and the graft site. After a few days in the hospital, Rebecca is discharged with daily follow-up in the burn clinic for wound care.

1. Which IV fluid is most likely used to treat Rebecca when she is admitted to the emergency department? Why?

2. Why is it important to monitor Rebecca's urine output?

3. What are the advantages of the type of dressing used for Rebecca's partial-thickness burns?

4. What regular assessments of Rebecca's burn sites should be performed?

5. What are some high-protein, high-calorie foods that might appeal to Rebecca?

References

American Academy of Pediatrics (AAP), Committee on Infectious Disease. (2015). *Red book: Report of the Committee on Infectious Disease* (30th ed.). Elk Grove Village, IL: Author.

American Academy of Pediatrics Council on Environmental Health and Section on Dermatology. (2011). Policy statement—Ultraviolet radiation: A hazard to children and adolescents. *Pediatrics, 127*(3), 588–597.

American College of Surgeons, Committee on Trauma. (2014). *Resources for the optimal care of the injured patient, 2014*. Chicago, IL: Author.

Artz, C. P., & Moncrief, J. A. (1969). *The treatment of burns* (2nd ed.). Philadelphia, PA: Elsevier Saunders.

Bakker, A., Maertens, K. J. P., Van Son, M. J. M., & Van Loey, N. E. E. (2013). Psychological consequences of pediatric burns from a child and family perspective: A review of the empirical literature. *Clinical Psychology Review, 33*, 361–371.

Barnes, E. R., & Murray, B. S. (2013). Bedbugs: What nurses need to know. *American Journal of Nursing, 113*(10), 58–62.

Bhutani, T., Kamangar, F., & Cordoro, K. M. (2012). Management of pediatric psoriasis. *Pediatric Annals, 41*(1), e11–e17.

Block, S. L., & Blackmon, L. (2013). Treating infantile hemangiomatosis: A case study. *Pediatric Annals, 42*(6), 230–233.

Bowden, V. R. (2012). Losing the louse: How to manage this common infestation in children. *Pediatric Nursing, 38*(5), 253–254, 277.

Camp, N. E. (2014). Black widow spider envenomation. *Journal of Emergency Nursing, 40*(2), 193–194.

Centers for Disease Control and Prevention (CDC). (2014). *Dog bites*. Retrieved from http://www.cdc.gov/HomeandRecreationalSafety/Dog-Bites/index.html

Centers for Disease Control and Prevention (CDC). (2015). *Overall fire/burn nonfatal injuries and rates per 100,000, 2013, United States*. Retrieved from http://www.cdc.gov/injury/wisqars/nonfatal.html

Chen, X., Anstey, A. V., & Bugert, J. J. (2013). Molluscum contagiosum virus infection. *Lancet Infectious Diseases, 13*, 877–888.

Chung, J., & Cohen, B. A. (2014). Infant's growing birthmark causes blurry vision. *Contemporary Pediatrics, 31*(9), 58–59.

Cohen, B. A. (2014). Infant with a persistent nodular rash. *Contemporary Pediatrics, 31*(1), 32, 35.

Coulombe, P. A., & Lee, C. (2012). Defining keratin protein function in skin epithelia: Epidermolysis bullosa simplex and its aftermath. *Journal of Investigative Dermatology, 132*, 763–775.

D'Cruz, R., Martin, H. C. O., & Holland, A. J. A. (2013). Medical management of paediatric burn injuries: Best practice, Part 2. *Journal of Paediatrics and Child Health, 49*, e397–e404.

De Young, A. C., Hendrikz, J., Kenardy, J. A., Cobham, V. E., & Kimble, R. M. (2014). Prospective evaluation of parent distress following pediatric burns and identification of risk factors for young child and parent posttraumatic stress disorder. *Journal of Child and Adolescent Psychopharmacology, 24*(1), 9–17.

Eisenhower, C., & Farrington, E. A. (2012). Advancements in the treatment of head lice in pediatrics. *Journal of Pediatric Health Care, 26*(6), 451–461.

Feinberg, A. N., Shwayder, T. A., Ruqiya, T., & Therdpong, T. (2014). Pediatric dermatologic disorders. *Journal of Alternative Medicine Research, 6*(2), 95–137.

Fenlon, S., & Nene, S. (2007). Burns in children. *Continuing Education in Anaesthesia, Critical Care & Pain, 7*(3), 76–80.

Fonacier, L. S., Aquino, M. R., & Mucci, T. (2012). Current strategies in treating severe contact dermatitis in pediatric patients. *Current Allergy and Asthma Reports, 12*, 599–606.

Fritz, S. A., Hogan, P. G., Hyack, G., Eisenstein, K. A., Rodriguez, M., Epplin, E. K., . . . Fraser, V. J. (2012). Household versus individual approaches to eradication of community-associated *Staphylococcus aureus* in children: A randomized trial. *Clinical Infectious Diseases, 54*, 743–751.

Gupta, A., & Cohen, B. (2012). Ultraviolet radiation exposure and melanoma. *Contemporary Pediatrics, 29*(5), 10–14.

Halloran, L. (2014). Developing dermatology detective powers: Allergic contact dermatitis. *Journal for Nurse Practitioners, 10*(4), 284–285.

Hazinski, M. F., Mondozzi, M. A., & Baker, R. A. U. (2014). Shock, multiple organ dysfunction syndrome, and burns in children. In K. L. McCance, S. E. Huether, V. L. Brashers, & N. S. Rote (Eds.), *Pathophysiology: The biologic basis for disease in adults and children* (7th ed., pp. 1699–1727). St. Louis, MO: Elsevier.

Jeschke, M. G., & Herndon, D. N. (2014). Burns in children: Standard and new treatments. *Lancet, 383*, 1168–1178.

Joyce, J. C. (2016). Vesiculobullous disorders. In R. M. Kliegman, B. F. Stanton, J. W. St. Geme, & N. F. Schor (Eds.), *Nelson textbook of pediatrics* (20th ed., pp. 3140–3150). St. Louis, MO: Elsevier.

Juern, A. M., & Drolet, B. A. (2016). Cutaneous bacterial infections. In R. M. Kliegman, B. F. Stanton, J. W. St. Geme, & N. F. Schor (Eds.), *Nelson textbook of pediatrics* (20th ed., pp. 3203–3213). Philadelphia, PA: Elsevier.

Kim, L. K. P., Martin, H. C. O., & Holland, A. J. A. (2012). Medical management of paediatric burn injuries: Best practice. *Journal of Paediatrics and Child Health, 48*, 290–295.

Kim, W., & Mancini, A. J. (2013). Acne in childhood: An update. *Pediatric Annals, 42*(10), 418–427.

Krau, S. D. (2013). Bites and stings: Epidemiology and treatment. *Critical Care Nursing Clinics of North America, 25*, 143–150.

Krowchuk, D. P., & Mancini, A. J. (2012). *Pediatric dermatology: A quick reference guide* (2nd ed.). Oak Grove, IL: American Academy of Pediatrics.

Kwan, J. M., & Jacob, S. E. (2012). Contact dermatitis in the atopic child. *Pediatric Annals, 41*(10), 422–428.

Lauren, C., & Garzon, M. C. (2012). Treatment of infantile hemangiomas. *Pediatric Annals, 41*(8), e167–e173.

McCann, S. A., & Huether, S. E. (2014). Structure, function, and disorders of the integument. In K. L. McCance, S. E. Huether, V. L. Brashers, & N. S. Rote (Eds.), *Pathophysiology: The biologic basis for disease in adults and children* (7th ed., pp. 1616–1652). St. Louis, MO: Elsevier.

National Center for Complementary and Alternative Medicine (NCCAM). (2012). *Aloe vera*. Retrieved from http://nccam.nih.gov/health/aloevera

National Center for Health Statistics, National Vital Statistics System. (2015). *Ten leading causes of unintentional injury deaths, United States, 2013, all races, both sexes*. Retrieved from http://www.cdc.gov/injury/wisqars/leading_causes_death.html

National Center for Injury Prevention and Control. (2015). *Overall dog bite nonfatal injuries and rates per 100,000, 2013, United States, all races, both sexes*. Retrieved from http://www.cdc.gov/injury/wisqars/nonfatal.html

Nicol, N. H., & Huether, S. E. (2014). Alterations in the integument in children. In K. L. McCance, S. E. Huether, V. L. Brashers, & N. S. Rote (Eds.), *Pathophysiology: The biologic basis for disease in adults and children* (7th ed., pp. 1653–1667), St. Louis, MO: Elsevier.

Ooi, E. T., & Tidman, M. J. (2014). Improving the management of seborrhoeic dermatitis. *The Practitioner, 258*(1768), 23–26.

Pariser, D. M., Meinking, T. L., Bell, M., & Ryan, W. G. (2012). Topical 0.5% ivermectin lotion for treatment of head lice. *New England Journal of Medicine, 367*(18), 1687–1693.

Reinke, J. M., & Sorg, H. (2012). Wound repair and regeneration. *European Surgical Research, 49*, 35–43.

Roduit, C., Frei, R., Loss, G., Buchele, G., Weber, J., Depner, M., . . . Lauener, R. (2012). Development of atopic dermatitis according to age of onset and association with early-life exposures. *Journal of Allergy and Clinical Immunology, 130*, 130–136.

Rolstad, B. S., Bryant, R. A., & Nix, D. P. (2012). Topical management. In R. A. Bryant & D. P. Nix (Eds.), *Acute & chronic wounds: Current management concepts* (4th ed., pp. 289–295). St. Louis, MO: Elsevier Mosby.

Rote, N. S., Huether, S. E., & McCance, K. L. (2014). Innate immunity: Inflammation. In K. L. McCance, S. E. Huether, V. L Brashers, & N. S. Rote (Eds.), *Pathophysiology: The biologic basis for disease in adults and children* (7th ed., pp. 191–223). St. Louis, MO: Elsevier.

Shulstad, R. M. (2012). Rash causing no fun in the sun. *Journal for Nurse Practitioners, 8*(9), 755–756.

Silverberg, J. I., & Silverberg, N. B. (2013). The US prevalence of common warts in childhood: A population-based study. *Journal of Investigative Dermatology, 133*, 2788–2790.

Simpson, E. L., Chalmers, J. R., Hanifin, J. M., Thomas, K. S., Cork, M. J., McLean, W. H. I., . . . Williams, H. C. (2014). Emollient enhancement of the skin barrier from birth offers effective atopic dermatitis prevention. *Journal of Allergy and Clinical Immunology, 134*, 818–823.

Stevens, D. L., Bisno, A. L., Chambers, H. F., Dellinger, E. P., Goldstein, E. J. C., Gorbach, S. L., . . . Wade, J. C. (2014). *Practice guidelines for the diagnosis and management of skin and soft tissue infections: 2014 update by the Infectious Diseases Society of America.*

Retrieved from http://cid.oxfordjournals.org/content/early/2014/06/14/cid.ciu296.full.pdf+html

Studor-Heikenfeld, J., & Colella, C. (2014). Isotretinoin: Reconsidering management of acne vulgaris in primary care. *Journal for Nurse Practitioners, 10*(9), 714–720.

Thomas, C. R., Russell, W., Robert, R. S., Holzer, C. E., Blakeney, P., & Meyer, W. J. (2012). Personality disorders in young adult survivors of pediatric burn injury. *Journal of Personality Disorders, 26*(2), 255–266.

Tollefson, M. M., Bruckner, A. L., & Section on Dermatology. (2014). Atopic dermatitis: Skin-directed management. *Pediatrics, 134*(6), e1735–e1744.

Tom, W. L. (2012). Atopic dermatitis: Recent findings and insights. *Pediatric Annals, 41*(1), e1–e5.

Tschudy, M. M., & Arcara, K. M. (2012). *The Harriet Lane handbook* (19th ed., p. 99). Philadelphia, PA: Elsevier Saunders.

Uihlein, L. C., Liang, M., G., & Mulliken, J. B. (2012). Pathogenesis of infantile hemangiomas. *Pediatric Annals, 41*(8), e154–e159.

U.S. Food and Drug Administration (FDA). (2014). *FDA safety communication: Update on serious complications associated with negative pressure wound therapy systems*. Retrieved from http://www.fda.gov/MedicalDevices/Safety/AlertsandNotices/ucm244211.htm#pediatric

Vloemans, A. F. P. M, Hermans, M. H. E., van der Wal, M. B. A., Liebregts J., & Middelkoop, E. (2014). Optimal treatment of partial thickness burns in children: A systematic review. *Burns, 40*, 177–190.

Weinstein, M. (2013). Acne and the adolescent: A practical approach to management. *Contemporary Pediatrics, 30*(5), 30–36.

Wilbeck, J., & Gresham, C. (2013). North American snake and scorpion envenomations. *Critical Care Nursing Clinics of North America, 25*, 173–190.

Wound Care Information Network. (2013). *Wound care product and category index*. Retrieved from http://www.medicaledu.com/prodindx.htm

Wound Educators. (2015). *Wound dressings*. Retrieved from http://woundeducators.com/resources/wound-dressings/

Wyatt, H. (2013). Common skin infections in children. *Nursing Standard, 27*(46), 43–48.

Yao, K., Bae, L., & Yew, W. P. (2013). Post-operative wound management. *Australian Family Physician, 42*(12), 867–870.

Yang, M., Kang, M., Jung, J., Song, W., Kang, H., Cho, S., & Min, K. (2013). Clinical features and prognostic factors in severe cutaneous drug reactions. *International Archives of Allergy and Immunology, 162*(4), 346–354.

Appendix A
Physical Growth Charts

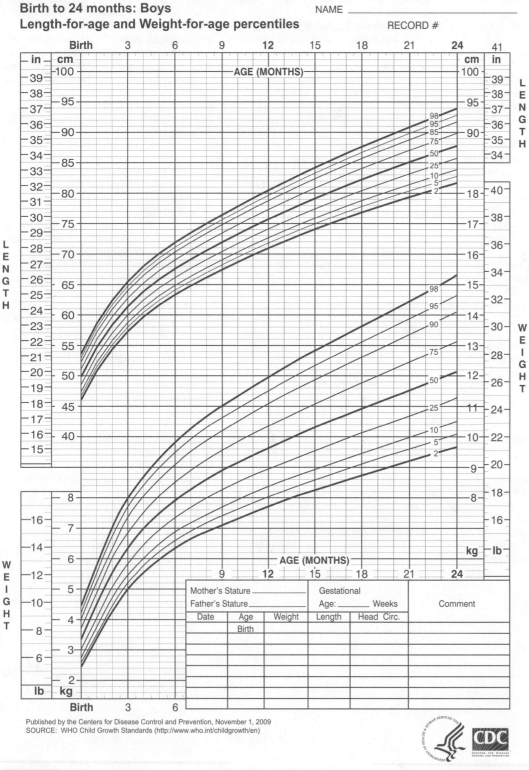

Birth to 24 months: Boys
Length-for-age and Weight-for-age percentiles

NAME _____

RECORD # _____

Published by the Centers for Disease Control and Prevention, November 1, 2009
SOURCE: WHO Child Growth Standards (http://www.who.int/childgrowth/en)

Figure A–1 Physical growth percentiles for length and weight—boys: birth to 24 months.

From WHO Child Growth Standards, http://www.who.int/childgrowth/en

Birth to 24 months: Boys
Head circumference-for-age and
Weight-for-length percentiles

NAME _____

RECORD # _____

Published by the Centers for Disease Control and Prevention, November 1, 2009
SOURCE: WHO Child Growth Standards (http://www.who.int/childgrowth/en)

Figure A–2 Physical growth percentiles for head circumference, weight for length—boys: birth to 24 months.

From WHO Child Growth Standards, http://www.who.int/childgrowth/en

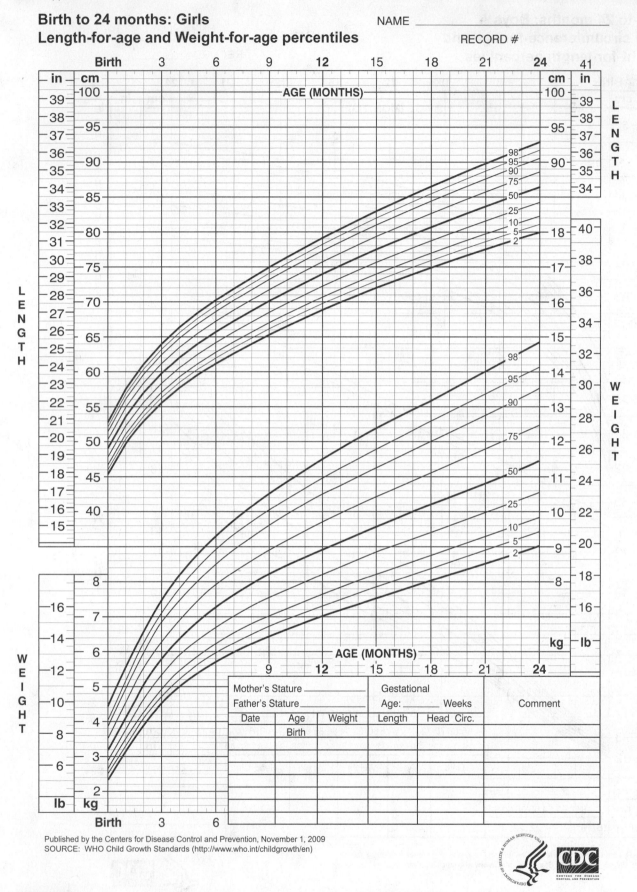

Birth to 24 months: Girls
Length-for-age and Weight-for-age percentiles

NAME _____

RECORD # _____

Published by the Centers for Disease Control and Prevention, November 1, 2009
SOURCE: WHO Child Growth Standards (http://www.who.int/childgrowth/en)

Figure A–3 Physical growth percentiles for length and weight—girls: birth to 24 months.

From WHO Child Growth Standards, http://www.who.int/childgrowth/en

**Birth to 24 months: Girls
Head circumference-for-age and
Weight-for-length percentiles**

NAME _____

RECORD # _____

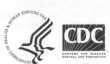

Published by the Centers for Disease Control and Prevention, November 1, 2009
SOURCE: WHO Child Growth Standards (http://www.who.int/childgrowth/en)

Figure A–4 Physical growth percentiles for head circumference, weight for length—girls: birth to 24 months.

From WHO Child Growth Standards, http://www.who.int/childgrowth/en

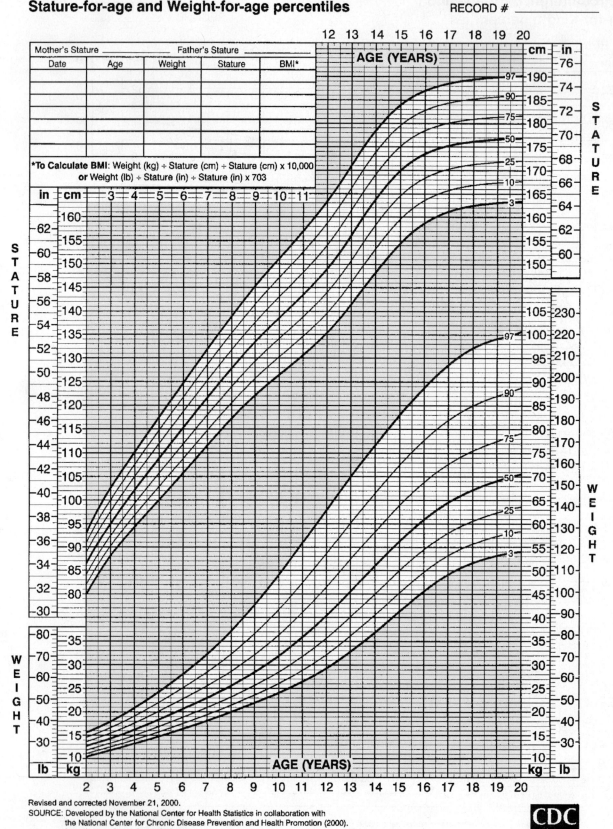

Figure A–5 Physical growth percentiles for stature and weight according to age—boys: 2 to 20 years.

From CDC, 2001, http://www.cdc.gov/growthcharts

2 to 20 years: Boys
Body mass index-for-age percentiles

NAME _____

RECORD # _____

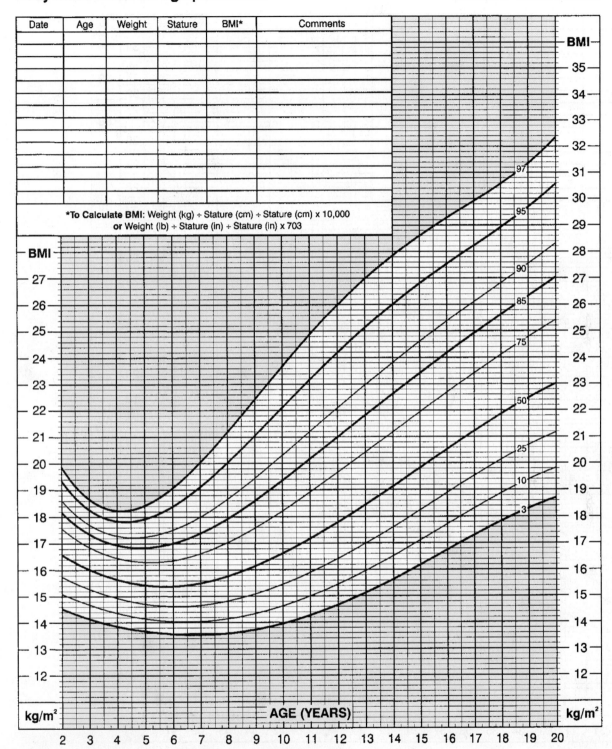

Date	Age	Weight	Stature	BMI*	Comments

*To Calculate BMI: Weight (kg) ÷ Stature (cm) ÷ Stature (cm) x 10,000
or Weight (lb) ÷ Stature (in) ÷ Stature (in) x 703

SOURCE: Developed by the National Center for Health Statistics in collaboration with
the National Center for Chronic Disease Prevention and Health Promotion (2000).
http://www.cdc.gov/growthcharts

Figure A-6   **Physical growth percentiles for body mass index according to age—boys: 2 to 20 years.**

From CDC, 2001, http://www.cdc.gov/growthcharts

Weight-for-stature percentiles: Boys

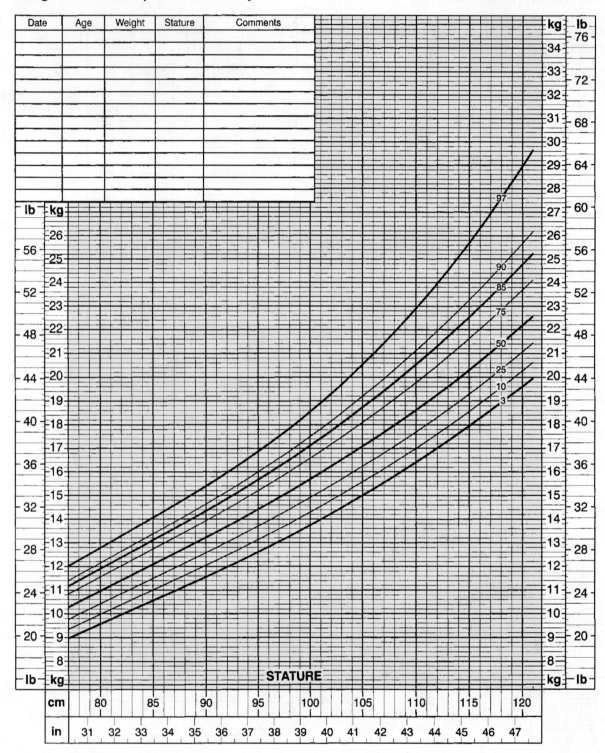

NAME _____

RECORD # _____

SOURCE: Developed by the National Center for Health Statistics in collaboration with
the National Center for Chronic Disease Prevention and Health Promotion (2000).
http://www.cdc.gov/growthcharts

Figure A–7 Physical growth percentiles for weight for stature—boys: 2 to 20 years.

From CDC, 2001, http://www.cdc.gov/growthcharts

2 to 20 years: Girls
Stature-for-age and Weight-for-age percentiles

NAME _____

RECORD # _____

Revised and corrected November 21, 2000.
SOURCE: Developed by the National Center for Health Statistics in collaboration with
the National Center for Chronic Disease Prevention and Health Promotion (2000).
http://www.cdc.gov/growthcharts

CDC

Figure A–8 Physical growth percentiles for stature and weight according to age—girls: 2 to 20 years.

From CDC, 2001, http://www.cdc.gov/growthcharts

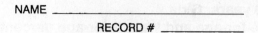

2 to 20 years: Girls
Body mass index-for-age percentiles

NAME _____

RECORD # _____

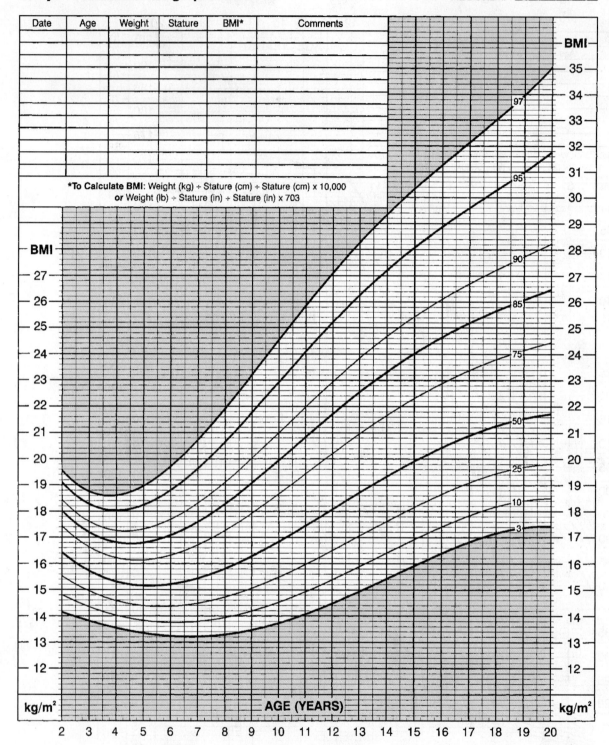

Figure A–9 Physical growth percentiles for body mass index according to age—girls: 2 to 20 years.

From CDC, 2001, http://www.cdc.gov/growthcharts

NAME _____

Weight-for-stature percentiles: Girls

RECORD # _____

Date	Age	Weight	Stature	Comments

STATURE

cm | 80 | 85 | 90 | 95 | 100 | 105 | 110 | 115 | 120

in | 31 32 33 34 35 36 37 38 39 40 41 42 43 44 45 46 47

SOURCE: Developed by the National Center for Health Statistics in collaboration with the National Center for Chronic Disease Prevention and Health Promotion (2000).
http://www.cdc.gov/growthcharts

Figure A–10 Physical growth percentiles for weight for stature—girls: 2 to 20 years.

From CDC, 2001, http://www.cdc.gov/growthcharts

Appendix B
Blood Pressure Tables

TABLE B–1 Blood Pressure Levels for Boys by Age and Height Percentile

Use the child's height percentile for the age and gender from the standard growth charts found in Appendix A. A blood pressure value at the 50th percentile for the child's age, gender, and height percentile is considered the midpoint of the normal range. A reading at or above the 95th percentile indicates hypertension.

Age (Year)	BP Percentile	SYSTOLIC BP (mmHg) PERCENTILE OF HEIGHT							DIASTOLIC BP (mmHg) PERCENTILE OF HEIGHT						
		5th	10th	25th	50th	75th	90th	95th	5th	10th	25th	50th	75th	90th	95th
1	50th	80	81	83	85	87	88	89	34	35	36	37	38	39	39
	95th	98	99	101	103	104	106	106	54	54	55	56	57	58	58
2	50th	84	85	87	88	90	92	92	39	40	41	42	43	44	44
	95th	101	102	104	106	108	109	110	59	59	60	61	62	63	63
3	50th	86	87	89	91	93	94	95	44	44	45	46	47	48	48
	95th	104	105	107	109	110	112	113	63	63	64	65	66	67	67
4	50th	88	89	91	93	95	96	97	47	48	49	50	51	51	52
	95th	106	107	109	111	112	114	115	66	67	68	69	70	71	71
5	50th	90	91	93	95	96	98	98	50	51	52	53	54	55	55
	95th	108	109	110	112	114	115	116	69	70	71	72	73	74	74
6	50th	91	92	94	96	98	99	100	53	53	54	55	56	57	57
	95th	109	110	112	114	115	117	117	72	72	73	74	75	76	76
7	50th	92	94	95	97	99	100	101	55	55	56	57	58	59	59
	95th	110	111	113	115	117	118	119	74	74	75	76	77	78	78
8	50th	94	95	97	99	100	102	102	56	57	58	59	60	60	61
	95th	111	112	114	116	118	119	120	75	76	77	78	79	79	80
9	50th	95	96	98	100	102	103	104	57	58	59	60	61	61	62
	95th	113	114	116	118	119	121	121	76	77	78	79	80	81	81
10	50th	97	98	100	102	103	105	106	58	59	60	61	61	62	63
	95th	115	116	117	119	121	122	123	77	78	79	80	81	81	82
11	50th	99	100	102	104	105	107	107	59	59	60	61	62	63	63
	95th	117	118	119	121	123	124	125	78	78	79	80	81	82	82
12	50th	101	102	104	106	108	109	110	59	60	61	62	63	63	64
	95th	119	120	122	123	125	127	127	78	79	80	81	82	82	83
13	50th	104	105	106	108	110	111	112	60	60	61	62	63	64	64
	95th	121	122	124	126	128	129	130	79	79	80	81	82	83	83
14	50th	106	107	109	111	113	114	115	60	61	62	63	64	65	65
	95th	124	125	127	128	130	132	132	80	80	81	82	83	84	84
15	50th	109	110	112	113	115	117	117	61	62	63	64	65	66	66
	95th	126	127	129	131	133	134	135	81	81	82	83	84	85	85
16	50th	111	112	114	116	118	119	120	63	63	64	65	66	67	67
	95th	129	130	132	134	135	137	137	82	83	83	84	85	86	87
17	50th	114	115	116	118	120	121	122	65	66	66	67	68	69	70
	95th	131	132	134	136	138	139	140	84	85	86	87	87	88	89

Source: National Heart, Lung, and Blood Institute. (2004). *Blood pressure tables for children and adolescents from the fourth report on the diagnosis, evaluation, and treatment of high blood pressure in children and adolescents*. Retrieved from http://www.nhlbi.nih.gov/guidelines/hypertension/child_tbl.htm, accessed 6/11/2016.

Key: BP = blood pressure.

*The 95th percentile is 1.645 SD over the mean.

TABLE B–2 Blood Pressure Levels for Girls by Age and Height Percentile

Use the child's height percentile for the age and gender from the standard growth charts found in Appendix A. A blood pressure value at 50th percentile for the child's age, gender, and height percentile is considered the midpoint of the normal range. A reading at or above the 95th percentile indicates hypertension.

Age (Year)	BP Percentile	SYSTOLIC BP (mmHg) PERCENTILE OF HEIGHT							DIASTOLIC BP (mmHg) PERCENTILE OF HEIGHT						
		5th	10th	25th	50th	75th	90th	95th	5th	10th	25th	50th	75th	90th	95th
1	50th	83	84	85	86	88	89	90	38	39	39	40	41	41	42
	95th	100	101	102	104	105	106	107	56	57	57	58	59	59	60
2	50th	85	85	87	88	89	91	91	43	44	44	45	46	46	47
	95th	102	103	104	105	107	108	109	61	62	62	63	64	65	65
3	50th	86	87	88	89	91	92	93	47	48	48	49	50	50	51
	95th	104	104	105	107	108	109	110	65	66	66	67	68	68	69
4	50th	88	88	90	91	92	94	94	50	50	51	52	52	53	54
	95th	105	106	107	108	110	111	112	68	68	69	70	71	71	72
5	50th	89	90	91	93	94	95	96	52	53	53	54	55	55	56
	95th	107	107	108	110	111	112	113	70	71	71	72	73	73	74
6	50th	91	92	93	94	96	97	98	54	54	55	56	56	57	58
	95th	108	109	110	111	113	114	115	72	72	73	74	74	75	76
7	50th	93	93	95	96	97	99	99	55	56	56	57	58	58	59
	95th	110	111	112	113	115	116	116	73	74	74	75	76	76	77
8	50th	95	95	96	98	99	100	101	57	57	57	58	59	60	60
	95th	112	112	114	115	116	118	118	75	75	75	76	77	78	78
9	50th	96	97	98	100	101	102	103	58	58	58	59	60	61	61
	95th	114	114	115	117	118	119	120	76	76	76	77	78	79	79
10	50th	98	99	100	102	103	104	105	59	59	59	60	61	62	62
	95th	116	116	117	119	120	121	122	77	77	77	78	79	80	80
11	50th	100	101	102	103	105	106	107	60	60	60	61	62	63	63
	95th	118	118	119	121	122	123	124	78	78	78	79	80	81	81
12	50th	102	103	104	105	107	108	109	61	61	61	62	63	64	64
	95th	119	120	121	123	124	125	126	79	79	79	80	81	82	82
13	50th	104	105	106	107	109	110	110	62	62	62	63	64	65	65
	95th	121	122	123	124	126	127	128	80	80	80	81	82	83	83
14	50th	106	106	107	109	110	111	112	63	63	63	64	65	66	66
	95th	123	123	125	126	127	129	129	81	81	81	82	83	84	84
15	50th	107	108	109	110	111	113	113	64	64	64	65	66	67	67
	95th	124	125	126	127	129	130	131	82	82	82	83	84	85	85
16	50th	108	108	110	111	112	114	114	64	64	65	66	66	67	68
	95th	125	126	127	128	130	131	132	82	82	83	84	85	85	86
17	50th	108	109	110	111	113	114	115	64	65	65	66	67	67	68
	95th	125	126	127	129	130	131	132	82	83	83	84	85	85	86

Source: National Heart, Lung, and Blood Institute. (2004). *Blood pressure tables for children and adolescents from the fourth report on the diagnosis, evaluation, and treatment of high blood pressure in children and adolescents*. Retrieved from http://www.nhlbi.nih.gov/guidelines/hypertension/child_tbl.htm, accessed 6/11/2016.

Key: BP = blood pressure.

*The 95th percentile is 1.645 SD over the mean.

Appendix C
Dietary Reference Intakes

TABLE C–1 Dietary Reference Intakes for Infants, Children, and Adolescents

	Age	Vitamin A (mcg/d)	Vitamin D (mcg/d)	Vitamin E (mg/d α-tocopherol)	Vitamin K (mcg/d)	Vitamin C (mg/d)	Thiamin (mg/d)	Riboflavin (mg/d)	Niacin (mg/d)	Vitamin B₆ (mg/d)
Infants	0–6 months	400*	10*	4*	2.0*	40*	0.2*	0.3*	~0.2*	0.1*
	7–12 months	500*	10*	5*	2.5*	50*	0.3*	0.4*	~0.4*	0.3*
Children	1–3 years	300	15	6	30*	15	0.5	0.5	6	0.5
	4–8 years	400	15	7	55*	25	0.6	0.6	8	0.6
Males	9–13 years	600	15	11	60*	45	0.9	0.9	12	1.0
	14–18 years	900	15	15	75*	75	1.2	1.3	16	1.3
Females	9–13 years	600	15	11	60*	45	0.9	0.9	12	1.0
	14–18 years	700	15	15	75*	65	1.0	1.0	14	1.2

Source: Data from Otten, J. J., Hellwig, J. P., & Meyers, L. D. (Eds.). (2006). *Dietary reference intakes: The essential guide to nutrient requirements.* Washington, DC: National Academies Press; Wagner, C. L., Greer, F. R., & Section on Breastfeeding and Committee on Nutrition. (2008). Prevention of rickets and vitamin D deficiency in infants, children, and adolescents. *Pediatrics, 122*(5), 1142–1152; Ross, A. C., Taylor, C. L. O., Yaldine, A. L., & Del Valle, H. B. (Eds.). (2011). *Dietary reference intakes for calcium and vitamin D.* Washington, DC: Institute of Medicine.

*Values are Adequate Intakes (AIs) rather than Recommended Dietary Allowances (RDAs). All other values on chart are RDAs. See Chapter 14 for a discussion of nutrient requirements.

TABLE C–2 Recommended Dietary Allowances

	Age	Protein	Carbohydrate	Polyunsaturated Fatty Acids N-6	Polyunsaturated Fatty Acids N-3	Total Fat	Fiber
Infants	0–6 months	9.1 g/d or 1.52 g/kg/d*	60 g/d*	4.4 g/d	0.5 g/d	31 g/d	NE
	7–12 months	1.5 g/kg/d	95 g/d*	4.6 g/d	0.5 g/d	30 g/d	NE
Children	1–3 years	1.1 g/kg/d or 13 g/d	130 g/d	7 g/d (linoleic)	0.7 g/d (α-linolenic)	NE	19 g/d
	4–8 years	0.95 g/kg/d or 19 g/d	130 g/d	10 g/d (linoleic)	0.9 g/d (α-linolenic)	NE	25 g/d
Males	9–13 years	0.95 g/kg/d or 34 g/d	130 g/d	12 g/d (linoleic)	1.2 g/d (α-linolenic)	NE	31 g/d
	14–18 years	0.85 g/kg/d or 52 g/d	130 g/d	16 g/d (linoleic)	1.6 g/d (α-linolenic)	NE	38 g/d
Females	9–13 years	0.95 g/kg/d or 34 g/d	130 g/d	10 g/d (linoleic)	1.0 g/d (α-linolenic)	NE	26 g/d
	14–18 years	0.85 g/kg/d or 46 g/d	130 g/d	11 g/d (linoleic)	1.1 g/d (α-linolenic)	NE	26 g/d

Source: Data from Institute of Medicine. (2002). *Dietary reference intakes.* Washington, DC: National Academies Press.

*Values are Adequate Intakes (AIs) rather than Recommended Dietary Allowances (RDAs). All other values on charts are RDAs.

Key: NE = not established.

Folate (mcg/d)	Vitamin B$_{12}$ (mcg/d)	Calcium (mg/d)	Phosphorus (mg/d)	Magnesium (mg/d)	Iron (mg/d)	Zinc (mg/d)	Iodine (mcg/d)	Selenium (mcg/d)
65*	0.4*	200*	100*	30*	0.27*	2*	110*	15*
80*	0.5*	260*	275*	75*	11	3	130*	20*
150	0.9	700	460	80	7	3	90	20
200	1.2	1000	500	130	10	5	90	30
300	1.8	1300	1250	240	8	8	120	40
400	2.4	1300	1250	240	11	11	150	55
300	1.8	1300	1250	410	8	8	120	40
400	2.4	1300	1250	360	15	9	150	55

Appendix D
Selected Pediatric Laboratory Values

All laboratory value intervals listed are approximate. Consult your local laboratory for guidelines as to normal values for the specific testing procedures used.

Normal Blood Chemistry and Hematology Value Intervals

Albumin (S)[1]

1 month–1 year:	2.8–4.8 g/dL
1–18 years:	3.2–4.7 g/dL

Alkaline Phosphatase (S)[1]

Age	Male Units/L	Female Units/L
1–30 days	75–316	48–406
1–3 years	104–345	108–317
4–6 years	93–309	96–297
7–9 years	86–315	69–325
10–12 years	42–362	51–332
13–15 years	74–390	50–162
16–18 years	52–171	47–119

α-Fetoprotein (AFP) (S)[1]

Newborn:	50–100,000 ng/mL
1–3 months:	40–1000 ng/mL
4 months–18 years:	0–12 ng/mL

Bilirubin (S)[1]

Conjugated:	Newborn: Less than 0.6 mg/dL
Total:	Birth–5 days: Less than 11.7 mg/dL

Blood Gases

CARBON DIOXIDE, PARTIAL PRESSURE (PCO_2) (B)[1]

Infants:	27–41 mmHg (3.6–5.5 kPa)
Children:	32–48 mmHg (4.3–6.4 kPa)

OXYGEN, PARTIAL PRESSURE (PO_2) (B)[1]

Greater than 1 day:	83–108 mmHg (11–14.4 kPa)

BICARBONATE, ACTUAL (P)[3]

22–29 mmol/L

Key for type of specimen: *S = serum; B = whole blood; P = plasma.*

pH (B)[1]

0–6 months:	7.18–7.50
6–12 months:	7.27–7.49
Children:	7.37–7.43
Adolescents:	7.35–7.41

BASE EXCESS (B)[1]

Infants:	–7 to –1 mmol/L
Children:	–4 to +2 mmol/L
Thereafter:	–3 to +3 mmol/L

OXYGEN SATURATION (B)[1]

Newborns:	85%–90%
Thereafter:	95%–99%

BUN—see Electrolytes, Urea Nitrogen

Coagulation Values[4]

Fibrinogen:	175–400 mg/dL
Partial thromboplastin time, activated (aPTT):	22.1–34.1 seconds
Prothrombin time (PT):	11.2–13.2 seconds
International normalized ratio (INR):	2–3

C-Reactive Protein (CRP) (P, S)[1]

0.08–1.8 mg/L

Creatinine (S, P)[1]

1–7 days:	0.7–1.2 mg/dL
7 days–1 year:	0.2–0.5 mg/dL
1–9 years:	0.2–0.8 mg/dL
10–18 years:	0.5–1.1 mg/dL

Electrolytes[1]

CALCIUM (S, P)

Newborn:	7.9–10.7 mg/dL
Thereafter:	8.7–10.7 mg/dL

CHLORIDE (S, P)

102–112 mmol/L

GLUCOSE, FASTING (S, P)[1]

Newborn:	55–117 mg/dL (3.1–6.4 mmol/L)
After 1 month of age:	70–126 mg/dL (3.9–7 mmol/L)

MAGNESIUM (P, S)

1.6–2.4 mg/dL (0.66–0.99 mmol/L)

OSMOLALITY (S)

280–300 mOsm/kg

PHOSPHORUS, INORGANIC (S, P)

2.8–5.6 mg/dL (0.91–1.8 mmol)

POTASSIUM (S, P)

3.7–5 mmol/L

SODIUM (P, S)

134–143 mmol/L

UREA NITROGEN (S, P)

| 1–13 years: | 5–17 mg/dL (1.8–6 mmol/L) |
| 14–19 years: | 8–21 mg/dL (2.9–7.5 mmol/L) |

Hematology Values (B)

Values are for children 2 to 12 years.

HEMATOCRIT (HCT)[1]

31.7%–39.8%

HEMOGLOBIN (HGB)[1]

10.2–13.4 g/dL

MEAN CORPUSCULAR HEMOGLOBIN (MCH)[1]

23.7–29.5 pg

MEAN CORPUSCULAR HEMOGLOBIN CONCENTRATION (MCHC)[1]

31.8%–34.9%

MEAN CORPUSCULAR VOLUME (MCV)[1]

71.3–87.6 mm^3

RED BLOOD CELL (RBC)[1]

$3.89–5.03 \times 10^{12}$/L

WHITE BLOOD CELL (WBC)[1]

$4.86–11.4 \times 10^9$/L

DIFFERENTIAL[1]

Neutrophils	22.4%–74.7%
Eosinophils	0%–4.7%
Basophils	0.1%–0.6%
Lymphocytes	18.1%–57.8%
Atypical lymphocytes	2%–4%
Monocytes	4.1%–12.3%

Key for type of specimen: *S = serum; B = whole blood; P = plasma.*

PLATELET COUNT[3]

$202–367 \times 10^9$/L

RETICULOCYTE COUNT[1]

0.82%–1.49%

Erythrocyte Sedimentation Rate (Micro)[4]

1–13 mm/hr

Growth Hormone (P, S)[1]

0–6.9 years:	Less than 13.7 mcg/L
7–10.9 years:	Less than 16.5 mcg/L
11–14.9 years:	Less than 14.5 mcg/L
15–18.9 years:	Less than 13.5 mcg/L

Hemoglobin A$_{1c}$ (B)[1]

| Normal: | 4%–6% |

Hemoglobin Fetal (B)[5]

| 1–30 days: | 2.8%–92% |
| Decreases to adult levels by 12 months: | 0%–0.9% |

Iron-Related Values

FERRITIN (P, S)[1]

1–5 years:	6–24 ng/mL
6–9 years:	10–55 ng/mL
10–19 years:	Males: 23–70 ng/mL
	Females: 6–40 ng/mL

IRON (S, P)[1]

| 1–14 years: | 22–136 mcg/dL (4–25 micromol/L) |
| 14–19 years: | 34–162 mcg/dL (6–29 micromol/L) |

IRON-BINDING CAPACITY (S, P)[1]

1–5 years:	268–441 mcg/dL (48–79 micromol/L)
6–9 years:	240–508 mcg/dL (43–91 micromol/L)
10–19 years:	290–570 mcg/dL (52–102 micromol/L)

Lead (B)[3]

Less than 5 mcg/dL

Lipids (S)[2]

TOTAL CHOLESTEROL

| Acceptable: | Less than 170 mg/dL |
| Elevated: | Greater than 200 mg/dL |

HIGH-DENSITY LIPOPROTEIN

| Acceptable: | Greater than 45 mg/dL or higher |
| Low: | Less than 40 mg/dL |

LOW-DENSITY LIPOPROTEIN

Acceptable:	Less than 110 mg/dL
High:	130 mg/dL and higher

TRIGLYCERIDES

Acceptable	0–9 years: Less than 75 mg/dL
	10–19 years: Less than 90 mg/dL
High	0–9 years: Greater than 100 mg/dL
	10–19 years: Greater than 130 mg/dL

Thyroid Hormones

THYROID-STIMULATING HORMONE (TSH) (P, S)[1]
(in milli-International Units/L)

Age	Males	Females
1–30 days	0.7–16.1	1.0–13.7
1 month–5 years	0.8–7.5	0.7–8.6
6–18 years	0.6–6.4	0.6–6.2

THYROXINE (T_4) (S, P)[1]

1–5 years:	5–14.45 mcg/dL
6–20 years:	4.4–12.1 mcg/dL

THYROXINE, "FREE" (Free T_4) (S, P)[1]

Under 1 year:	1.3–2.8 ng/dL (16.8–36.1 pmol/L)
1–18 years:	1.3–2.42 ng/mL (16.8–31 pmol/L)

THYROXINE-BINDING GLOBULIN (TBG) (P)[1]
(in mg/L)

Age	Males	Females
Cord blood	19–39	19–39
1–11 months	16–36	17–37
1–9 years	12–28	15–27
10–19 years	14–26	14–30

TRIIODOTHYRONINE (T_3) (S)[1]

1–5 years:	106–203 ng/dL
6–10 years:	104–183 ng/dL
11–14 years:	68–186 ng/dL
15–20 years:	71–175 ng/dL

Normal Value Ranges: Urine

Albumin[4]

Less than 1 mg/dL

Catecholamines (Norepinephrine, Epinephrine)[1]
(in mmol/mol creatinine)

Age	Norepinephrine	Epinephrine
0–24 months	0–0.28	0–0.46
2–4 years	0–0.8	0–0.035
5–9 years	0–0.059	0–0.022
10–19 years	0–0.055	0–0.021

Creatinine[1]

3–8 years:	0.11–0.68 g/24 hr
9–12 years:	0.17–1.41 g/24 hr
13–17 years:	0.29–1.87 g/24 hr
Adults:	0.63–2.5 g/24 hr

Osmolality[4]

500–800 mOsm/kg water

Should be higher than serum osmolality.

Protein[4]

Less than 150 mg/24 hr

Specific Gravity[4]

Birth–2 years:	1.001–1.018
Over 2 years:	1.001–1.03

Normal Value Ranges: Sweat

Electrolytes[1]

Sodium and chloride: under 40 mmol/L

Normal Value Ranges: Cerebrospinal Fluid

Protein[1]

Under 1 month:	15–153 mg/dL
Over 1 month:	15–48 mg/dL

Glucose[1]

All ages: 41–84 mg/dL (60%–80% of blood glucose)

Key for type of specimen: *S = serum; B = whole blood; P = plasma.*
[1]Adapted from Soldin, S. J., Wong, E. C., Brugnara, C., & Soldin, O. P. (2011). *Pediatric reference intervals* (7th ed.). Washington, DC: American Association for Clinical Chemistry Press.
[2]National Heart Lung and Blood Institute. (2012). *Expert panel on integrated guidelines for cardiovascular health and risk reduction in children and adolescents: Summary report.* Retrieved from http://www.nhlbi.nih.gov/files/docs/peds_guidelines_sum.pdf
[3]Data from Kliegman, R. M., Stanton, B. F., St. Geme, J. W., & Schor, N. F. (2016). *Nelson textbook of pediatrics* (20th ed., Table 727-5). Philadelphia, PA: Elsevier Saunders.
[4]Data from Corbett, J.V. (2013). *Laboratory tests and diagnostic procedures with nursing diagnoses* (8th ed.). Upper Saddle River, NJ: Pearson Education.
[5]Data from Mayo Clinic Mayo Medical Laboratories. (2014). *Test ID: Hemoglobin F.* Retrieved from http://www.mayomedicallaboratories.com/test-catalog/Clinical + and + Interpretive/8269

Appendix E
Diagnostic Tests and Procedures

Consider the growth and developmental level of the child when preparing the child for a procedure, and support the child during and after the procedure. See Chapter 11 for more information about preparing a child for procedures. Parents need to complete a signed consent after making sure they have an understanding of the procedure, results, and risk factors. When possible, allow the parents to remain with the child during the procedure.

PROCEDURE, DESCRIPTION, AND PURPOSE	NURSING MANAGEMENT
ACTH Stimulation Test A drug, metyrapone, is administered to block the production of cortisol. In persons with pituitary insufficiency, the ACTH level does not increase as expected.	• Phenytoin and estrogen compounds interfere with the test results. • Contact the laboratory for timing of the blood specimens to be collected.
ACTH Suppression Test Dexamethosone, a potent corticosteroid, is administered to suppress the pituitary and ACTH production. In cases of Cushing syndrome, high levels of serum cortisol continue to be produced.	• Administer dexamethosone in the dose and at the time prescribed. • Contact the laboratory for timing of the blood specimens to be collected. A plastic tube is used rather than glass. Urine may also be collected to test the level of cortisol.
Arteriography/Angiogram A contrast dye is injected to allow visualization of blood vessels. Useful in evaluating patency of blood vessels and blood flow to parts of the body and in identifying abnormal vasculature.	• Obtain history of hypersensitivity to iodine, seafood, or radiographic contrast dye. Antihistamines and/or steroids may be prescribed if allergy is suspected. • Administer sedation as prescribed, and follow assessment guidelines to monitor the child during and after the procedure; assess for vasovagal and allergic reactions. • Tell the child to expect a warm, flushing feeling that could last a few minutes.
Arthrogram After a local anesthetic, a needle is inserted into a joint (e.g., knee or shoulder). Samples of joint fluid may be aspirated, and then air or contrast medium is injected into the joint cavity. The joint is moved to spread the dye. Radiographs are taken with the joint in various positions to detect injuries to cartilage or ligaments and to visualize the joint capsule.	• Prepare the child and family for the procedure. • Local anesthesia is often used with general anesthesia for very young children. Support the child when the local anesthetic is inserted. • Rest, ice on the joint, elevation, and an analgesic may be needed for discomfort after the procedure.
Barium or Contrast Enema Barium or barium and air are administered via a tube through the rectum to the colon. The large intestine is visualized to detect any abnormalities. Fluoroscopy is used to monitor the process and radiographs are taken.	• Give parents preprocedure instructions regarding diet, laxatives, and/or enemas so that the colon is clear. • Prepare the child and parents for the procedure and to expect the sensation of fluid entering the rectum. Tell the child of the need to not have a bowel movement until told it is okay to do so. • Ensure that the child holds still while the radiographs are taken.
Biopsy Removal and examination of tissue from the body organs or skin to detect malignancies or the presence of disease. Biopsies can be obtained in several ways: • Surgical excision at tissue site • Needle aspiration at tissue site, with or without ultrasound • Needle insertion into skin • Brush method, scraping cells and tissue with stiff bristles as is done with a Pap smear • Punch, using an instrument to excise a small area of tissue	• Prepare necessary instruments and specimen containers. Assist with preparation of biopsy site. • Monitor the child receiving sedation and analgesia according to protocol. • Ensure that the child remains still during the procedure. • Apply dressing, if appropriate, to the site after the procedure. • Label specimens accurately and arrange for specimen transport as recommended. • Teach family to care for wound and to monitor site for infection.
Bone Marrow Aspiration Marrow is removed from pelvic or iliac crest bones through a large gauge needle with a syringe used for aspiration. The test is diagnostic for leukemia, metastatic tumors, and some anemias, and it tests for response to treatment. Marrow may also be harvested for transplant.	• The child is usually given anesthesia, or sedation and analgesia. Follow monitoring guidelines during and after the procedure. • The site is prepped with a cleansing agent according to agency protocol. • Positioning is determined by the site used (e.g., side-lying for the iliac crest). • After the procedure, maintain the child on bed rest for at least 1 hour. • Mild analgesics are provided for pain at the harvest site.

PROCEDURE, DESCRIPTION, AND PURPOSE	NURSING MANAGEMENT
Bronchoscopy A flexible fiber-optic bronchoscope is used to visualize the trachea and bronchi to identify and extract foreign objects in the airway, or for a biopsy.	• Maintain NPO status preprocedure according to agency guidelines. • The child will often be sedated for the procedure; if the child is not sedated, a local anesthetic spray is used prior to passing the bronchoscope. Monitor the child according to agency guidelines. • Monitor vital signs per protocol postprocedure. Resume oral feedings as prescribed.
Cardiac Catheterization A radiopaque catheter is passed through a large vein or artery in an arm or leg to the heart. It is then threaded to the heart chambers or coronary arteries, or both, guided by fluoroscopy. The procedure enables precise measurement of oxygen saturation within the heart's chambers and great arteries and pressure gradients in the pulmonary vessels or heart chambers. This helps assess for: • Congenital heart defects • Cardiac valvular disease • Coronary artery disease • Evaluation of artificial valves Other purposes of cardiac catheterization include heart muscle biopsy, tissue sampling for heart transplant rejection, or radiofrequency ablation for a heart rhythm disturbance.	• Preparation includes discontinuation of anticoagulant therapy a week prior to the test and no food or fluid 6 to 8 hours preprocedure (may be a shorter interval for infants). Have the child void. • Prepare the child about the equipment to be used and sensations that will be felt. • Obtain history of hypersensitivity to iodine, seafood, or radiographic contrast dye. Antihistamines and/or steroids may be ordered if allergy is suspected. Assess for allergic reaction during procedure. • An IV is started for sedation administration, and to provide access for emergency drugs if needed. • ECG leads are applied to the chest to monitor heart activity. Baseline vital signs, extremity circulation, and pulses are assessed and documented. Vital signs, heart rhythm, and the pulse strength and neurovascular assessment of the affected extremity are monitored according to agency protocol. • See Chapter 21 for nursing management after the procedure.
Computed Tomography (CT) The CT scan is a radiographic procedure that examines body sections from 360 degrees, producing cross-section images that build into a two-dimensional image of any body structure. It may be performed with or without contrast dye. Multislice CT is performed with a greater number of images obtained simultaneously for a more rapid procedure so that moving organs are not blurred. CT is used to screen for head, liver, abdominal, and renal lesions; tumors; edema; abscesses; and bone destruction. It is also used to locate foreign objects in soft tissue, such as the eye.	• If contrast dye is required, the infant or child may be NPO. CT must be performed 4 days after any other barium studies of abdomen. • If contrast dye is to be used, obtain a history about any hypersensitivity to iodine, seafood, or radiographic contrast dye. If allergy is suspected, antihistamines and/or steroids may be ordered prior to procedure. Assess for allergic reaction during procedure. • Prepare child for the procedure by describing the equipment, noises, and other expected sensations, and how the child can help during the procedure by not moving. • If sedation is ordered for infants and small children to keep them still, monitor them according to protocol. • If contrast dye is used, encourage fluids after the procedure.
Cultures Cultures are taken to isolate and identify microorganisms causing infection, and often to identify the specific antibiotics to which the organisms are sensitive. Cultures commonly used with children include: blood, throat, sputum, stool, wound, urine, and cerebrospinal fluid.	• Collect culture specimens before administering new antimicrobials to prevent false results. List any antimicrobials given on laboratory slip. • Send all specimens immediately to the laboratory, or refrigerate the specimen. • Use strict aseptic technique to handle the specimen. Keep lids on sterile specimen containers.
Cystoscopy A flexible fiber-optic scope is inserted through the urethra into the bladder to inspect the interior urethra and bladder for inflammation, tumors, stones, or structural abnormalities. The procedure may be done simultaneously with a voiding cystourethrogram (see Voiding cystourethrogram later in this table).	• Keep infants and children NPO prior to the study if sedation will be used. • Administer sedation and/or analgesia as prescribed, and monitor the child according to protocol. • Encourage fluids after the procedure to detect problems with voiding. • Inform the child and parents that dysuria and frequency may occur for a short time following the procedure.
Dual Energy X-ray Absorptiometry (DEXA) DEXA is radiographic procedure emitting two photon energy beams used to measures bone mineral density in children at risk for glucocorticoid-induced osteoporosis.	• Identify factors increasing a child's risk for osteoporosis or skeletal problems. • Explain the procedure and equipment to be used to the child and parents. • Inform the child of the need to not move, and let the child know the test does not cause pain.
Echocardiography An ultrasound study of the heart used to identify the heart size, structure, pattern of movement, hemodynamics, valvular disease, blood flow, and blood flow disturbances. The ultrasound probe (transducer) is held over the chest (transthoracic) or inserted through the esophagus (transesophageal) to send an ultrasound beam to the tissues. The reflected sound waves are then transformed into scans, graphs, or sounds (Doppler).	• Explain the procedure to the parents and child. Inform the child of the need to hold still for the procedure. • Inform the child that patches and a gel will be applied to the skin and a transducer will move over the area with some pressure, but that the test should cause no pain.

PROCEDURE, DESCRIPTION, AND PURPOSE	NURSING MANAGEMENT
Electrocardiography (ECG or EKG) and Ambulatory Electrocardiography An (ECG) records the electrical impulses of the heart via electrodes and a galvanometer (ECG machine). Eight electrodes are placed on the chest and an electrode is placed on each extremity. The lead selector is turned to read the 12 standard leads. A Holter monitor may be attached to capture ambulatory ECG readings over a 24-hour period. An ECG is used to detect cardiac arrhythmias, identify electrolyte imbalances, or to monitor ECG changes during an exercise or stress test.	• Obtain list of current medications and when they were last taken. • Inform the child that patches will be applied to the chest, arms, and legs. Then wires will be attached to the patches. Tell the child that the test causes no pain. • Ask the child to hold still for a brief time. A pacifier or bottle may help the infant be still. • Encourage the child with a Holter to engage in usual activities, but no swimming or bathing in a tub or shower is allowed until electrodes are removed. • Ask the parents of the child wearing a Holter monitor to keep a diary of any events or emotional stress that cause symptoms. A daily schedule of sleep, eating, exercise, and other activities may be requested.
Electroencephalogram (EEG) Approximately 20 electrodes are applied to the scalp to record cerebral cortex electrical activity over 1 to 2 hours. In some cases an EEG is performed when the child is asleep. An EEG is used to identify the potential for seizures, to determine brain death, and to detect other abnormalities such as a tumor, abscess, or intracranial hemorrhage.	• Inform the parents and child about all medications and other substance (e.g., cola, tea, or coffee) to withhold for 24 to 48 hours. • Ensure that the hair is clean, and dry, and no hair products (e.g., oil, gel, spray) have been applied. • Do not permit infants or children to nap before the test. • Explain that the procedure is not painful as electrodes are applied. • Explain that washing the child's hair will remove the electrode gel.
Electromyography (EMG) Needle electrodes are inserted into skeletal muscles, and muscle activity is measured during rest, voluntary activity, and electrical stimulation. The test is useful in assisting with diagnosis of muscular dystrophy and to differentiate muscle diseases and lower motor neuron neuropathies such as those caused by hypothyroidism or diabetes.	• Be alert to medications (muscle relaxants, antiholinergics, and cholinergics) or caffeine use that could affect EMG results, and whether they should be withheld. • Inform the child that there may be slight pain when the needle electrodes are inserted. Support the child with age-appropriate relaxation techniques or distraction techniques. If pain persists, inform technician. Pain may cause false reports. • Administer analgesic as needed for residual pain.
Esophagogastroduodenoscopy/Esophagastroscopy A flexible fiber-optic endoscope is used to visualize the internal structures of the esophagus, stomach, and duodenum. This procedure is also used to collect cytology specimens and to confirm gastrointestinal pathology (e.g., tumors, ulcerations, bleeding).	• Keep the child NPO prior to the procedure. • Administer sedation as prescribed and monitor the child during and postprocedure according to protocol. • Inform children that they may be asked to swallow and may feel some pressure when the endoscope is inserted. • Resume oral feedings as prescribed. Explain that some burping may occur, which helps remove air inserted to visualize the GI tract.
Evoked Potential A child who is awake is monitored by electrodes measuring brain (e.g., electroencephalogram) and related muscle activity. The baseline of electrical activity obtained is then used during later surgery, such as a spinal fusion for scoliosis, in order to monitor innervation to muscle groups and avoid injury to the spinal cord during the surgical procedure.	• Prepare the child for the procedure, including the size of equipment, sounds, and time it will take. • Assist the child to relax with quiet music during the test.
Exercise Testing A test performed with a treadmill or stationary bicycle to evaluate exercise tolerance. ECG leads, a blood pressure cuff, and sometimes an oxygen consumption monitor are attached. Acceleration and pitch of the treadmill or bicycle are increased at intervals until the patient is fatigued, symptomatic, or a predetermined endpoint is reached. An ECG recording with a controlled activity increase helps identify significant cardiac compensation or inadequate cardiac output.	• Prepare the adolescent for the test, what to expect, and that the test can be stopped at any time. • Instruct the adolescent to report vertigo, extreme shortness of breath, chest pain, and excessive fatigue. • Ensure that the adolescent understands that the test is of greater value when the exercise continues until the predetermined stopping level is reached. • Take baseline vital sign measurements prior to the exercise and throughout according to agency guidelines.
GI Series Upper GI and small bowel series are fluoroscopic and radiographic examinations of the esophagus, stomach, and small intestine as ingested oral barium or water-soluble contrast agent passes through the digestive tract. This series identifies ulcers; gastroesophageal reflux; polyps, tumors, or hiatal hernias in the GI tract; pyloric stenosis; and foreign bodies, varices, or strictures.	• Keep child NPO after midnight or for the number of hours according to agency guidelines. A low-residue diet may be ordered for the night before the test. • Withhold medications as ordered. • Record vital signs; note epigastric pain or discomfort. • Inform child that all the liquid must be swallowed, but that the test will not cause pain or discomfort. • Inform the child that the room will be dark and the table on which the child is lying may be tilted. • Inform parents that the stool will be light colored after the test.

PROCEDURE, DESCRIPTION, AND PURPOSE	NURSING MANAGEMENT
Hyperoxitest Arterial blood is collected before and at least 10 minutes after giving the infant 100% oxygen to see how the child's PO_2 level responds to the oxygen. Differences between the arterial blood gas levels when an infant has central cyanosis help distinguish between cardiac disease and pulmonary disease (Park, 2014).	• Follow guidelines for arterial blood collection from the upper right side of the body. • Administer oxygen through a plastic hood for at least 10 minutes to replace all alveolar air with oxygen.
Intraesophageal pH Probe Monitoring A probe is placed in the distal esophagus for 24 hours to detect pH changes below 4. The pH is measured and recorded every 4 to 8 seconds. The test determines how frequently stomach acid enters the esophagus and how long it stays there. It is used to diagnose gastroesophageal reflux disease and to evaluate atypical symptoms such as apnea, stridor, or cough.	• Inform the family of medications that must be withheld before and during the test (e.g., antacids, H2 inhibitors, proton pump inhibitors). • Prevent the infant or child from inadvertent removal of the probe. Use soft mittens on the child's hands if necessary. • Monitor and record pH measurements per protocol. • Instruct parents to keep a diary of the child's activities while probe is in place (e.g., feeding or sleeping).
Intravenous Pyelogram A contrast dye is administered by IV and excreted by the urinary system. A series of radiographs is taken at various intervals over an hour to evaluate the entire urinary system, including the kidney cortex, kidney pelvis, ureters, and bladder. A post-void radiograph is taken to see how well the bladder empties. The test is used to diagnose structural defects and tumors in the urinary system.	• Assess for potential allergy to the contrast dye. An antihistamine or corticosteroid may be given to children with a potential allergy. Monitor the child carefully for an allergic reaction. • Obtain a serum creatinine and BUN prior to the test to assess renal function. • Follow orders for an NPO or clear liquid diet prior to the study, in addition to the cleansing enema the morning of the test. • Encourage fluids after the procedure to flush out the contrast media, and monitor urinary output.
Lumbar Puncture A lumbar puncture is performed at the L3–L4 or L4–L5 level to obtain a specimen of cerebrospinal fluid (CSF) and to measure the CSF pressure. CSF is cultured and analyzed for glucose and protein content, and the number of lymphocytes present.	• Obtain a blood glucose level prior to the test for comparison with the CSF glucose level. • Hold the infant or child in knee-chest position and keep the child still during the procedure. • Label the tubes of CSF obtained by numerical sequence. • Assess breathing and any changes in neurological function during the test. • Administer analgesics as ordered for headache.
Magnetic Resonance Imaging (MRI) A radiographic examination that uses a large magnet to produce a magnetic field and radio waves to produce detailed images without ionizing radiation. The MRI scanner is a large, doughnut-shaped cylinder and the child lies on a table in the cylinder. An intravenous contrast dye often used. An MRI provides detailed images of internal organ structure, blood flow patterns, and abnormalities in soft tissues.	• Prepare the child for loud sounds, the size of the equipment, and the tunnel. Cardiorespiratory leads are often placed on the chest when contrast dye is used. • Assess the child for potential allergy to the contrast dye. An antihistamine or corticosteroid may be ordered if the child is at risk for allergy. Monitor the child for allergy during the procedure. • Carefully check for and remove all metal objects from the body. Only preapproved medical equipment can be in the room. • Sedation may be needed to keep the infant or child still. Headphones with music may help older children to cooperate. Monitor the child according to agency guidelines. Commonly, the examiner can talk with the child via a speaker system to provide information and reassurance.
Nuclear Scan or Radionuclide Imaging A radionuclide (an unstable radioisotope that decays or disintegrates, emitting radiation) is given by mouth or IV, which concentrates in certain parts of the body. Scintillation (gamma) camera detectors are used to create a two-dimensional image of an organ in gray tones or color that is sent to a computer. The scans may be taken in several minutes, hours, or 24 hours later. The test may identify a functional (rather than a structural) problem in the bone, brain, gastrointestinal tract, or kidney, or a thyroid scan may diagnose hyperthyroidism or hypothyroidism.	• Explain the procedure to the parents and child. Inform them that the amount of radiation received from radionuclide imaging is usually less than that received from a radiograph, and that there will be no discomfort. • The child may be NPO for several hours before the initial scan. • The nurse should wear two pairs of disposable gloves when in direct contact with the child's wastes for several hours. Follow agency guidelines for handling waste products. • Inform the child and family that radionuclide is excreted from the body in 6 to 24 hours. Ask the child and family to flush the toilet 3 times after voiding. Ask parents to schedule the test when airline travel is not planned for several days as the radioactive substance may set off security scanners.
Polysomnography (Sleep Study) Electrodes are attached to the head and chest, and a pulse oximeter is used. Recordings of brain activity, eye movement, apnea episodes, oxygen desaturation, and sleep disturbances are taken during sleep over an 8-hour period. The test is used to identify apnea during sleep and to determine the cause of sleep disorders.	• Instruct family to keep sleep log 1 to 2 weeks prior to sleep studies, including notes about snoring and sleepiness during the day. Review the sleep log. • Instruct patient/family to avoid caffeine products, sedatives, and naps for 1 to 2 days prior to testing. • Obtain a history related to medications, head injury, headache, and seizures. Caffeine and sedatives may be withheld. • Explain the procedure to the parents and child. • Monitor vital signs and observe for respiratory distress during the test.

PROCEDURE, DESCRIPTION, AND PURPOSE	NURSING MANAGEMENT
Positron Emission Tomography (PET) Scan and Single Photon Emission Computed Tomography (SPECT)	
PET alone or in combination with CT uses an intravenous radioisotope to measure emission of positive electrons in body organs, such as the brain or heart, or detect tumors and metastases. PET is effective in evaluating cerebral blood flow and myocardial perfusion as well as detecting recurrent cancer. SPECT is used to measure blood perfusion in the brain and evaluate central nervous system disorders.	• Inform the child and family if food and fluids must be withheld. • Prepare the child for the procedure in order to reduce anxiety. • Start two IVs, one for the radioisotope and the other for serial blood gases. • Monitor vital signs. • Assess for potential allergies to the radioisotope medium.
Pulmonary Function Tests (Spirometry)	
The patient breathes into a spirometer connected to a computer, and the results are analyzed. The vital capacity (maximum amount of air that can be expired after a normal inspiration) and forced expiratory volume (FEV), the percentage of air expired at 1, 2, and 3 seconds, can be calculated. Pulmonary function tests are used to assess pulmonary function and to identify the severity of obstructive airway disease.	• Obtain a list of any bronchodilators and steroids the child is taking. • Record child's age, gender, height, weight, and vital signs. • Assess for signs and symptoms of respiratory distress. • Explain the purpose of the tests and procedures. • Help the child practice breathing patterns required for the test. • Take two readings and average the values; compare to expected values for age, gender, and height.
Pulse Oximetry	
Pulse oximetry provides an estimate of the hemoglobin saturated by oxygen, measured percutaneously (SpO_2). It serves as an alternate to the direct measurement of PaO_2 (SaO_2) through arterial blood gas analysis.	• Explain that the sensor needs to be over a finger or nailbed. • Monitor the skin under the sensor regularly if it is kept in place for a constant measurement.
Radiograph (X-ray)	
The most common form of imaging, radiographs use electromagnetic radiation to obtain images of body structures on film for diagnostic purposes. Radiographs are commonly used to detect abnormalities in the size, structure, and shape of bone and body structures, or to detect abnormalities of the chest, such as air trapping in the alveoli (hyperinflation), consolidation of lung tissue (pneumonia), or lung collapse.	• Determine if any other radiographic procedures have been performed recently, as the contrast dye used may distort radiograph images. • Explain the procedure to the parents and child and the need for a lead apron. Explain that one or more films will be taken in about 5 to 10 minutes. Explain that modern equipment decreases radiation exposure. • Prepare the child. Have the child practice holding still and holding a breath in preparation for the test.
Sweat Chloride Test	
Gel pads containing pilocarpine are placed on the child's arms. A small electrode is attached to the pads to stimulate sweating until enough sweat is collected. The arms are covered with plastic. Sweat is collected and analyzed for the concentration of chloride and osmolality. The test is used to diagnose cystic fibrosis.	• Explain the purpose of the test to the parents and child. • Explain the need for the child to keep the plastic covering over the lower arms in place for the duration of test (about 30 minutes).
Tympanogram	
The procedure provides an estimate of middle ear pressure and an indirect measure of tympanic membrane movement. This helps identify the presence of fluid accumulation in the middle ear.	• Explain the procedure to the parents and child. The young child should be held still by a parent. • Insert the earpiece with the probe into the auditory canal until the canal is sealed tightly. • Use the machine according to the manufacturer's instructions. • Repeat the test in the other ear.
Ultrasound	
An ultrasound probe (transducer) is held over the skin or body cavity to transmit ultrasound waves to the tissues and receives deflected sound waves as they bounce off various body structures. The computer transforms the deflected sound waves into two-dimensional electronic scans or audible sounds (Doppler). Ultrasound is usually a noninvasive procedure used to detect tissue abnormalities.	• Explain the procedure to the parents and child. Inform them that the procedure is painless, and there is no exposure to radiation. • Maintain NPO status preprocedure for abdominal studies. • Confirm the child has not received any tests that will interfere with results (e.g., upper GI series). • Instruct the child to remain still during the procedure.
Voiding Cystourethrogram or Radionuclide Cystography	
A cystoscopy procedure is combined with a radionucleotide scan to examine bladder structure and function, urethral anatomy, and bladder masses. The test may detect vesicoureteral reflux.	• Assess for potential allergies to radioisotope medium. • Explain catheterization to the child and that the bladder will be filled. • Provide coaching strategies for parents accompanying the child to help the child cooperate and cope during the test. • Encourage fluids after the procedure to flush out the contrast media.

Source: Data from Corbett, J.V., & Banks, A. D. (2013). *Laboratory tests and diagnostic procedures with nursing diagnosis* (8th ed.). Upper Saddle River, NJ: Pearson; Kee, J. L. (2014). *Laboratory and diagnostic tests with nursing implications* (9th ed.). Upper Saddle River, NJ: Pearson; Park, M. (2014). *Pediatric cardiology for practitioners* (6th ed., pp. 207–208). Philadelphia, PA: Elsevier Saunders; Bindler, R. C., & Ball, J. W. (2012). *Clinical skills manual for principles of pediatric nursing: Caring for children* (5th ed.). Upper Saddle River, NJ: Pearson; U.S. National Library of Medicine. (2012). *Esophageal pH monitoring.* Retrieved from http://www.nlm.nih.gov/medlineplus/ency/article/003401.htm

Appendix F
Body Surface Area Nomogram

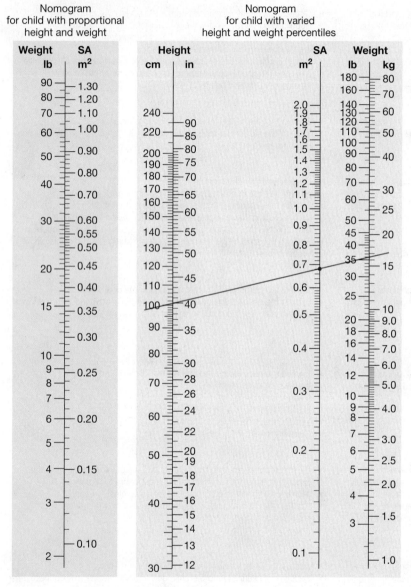

Nomogram for child with proportional height and weight

Nomogram for child with varied height and weight percentiles

Figure F–1 The proportion between height and weight in children is different from the proportion in adults. These differences are most manifest in newborns, infants, and young children. Therefore, dosages of drugs that have been established for adults cannot simply be reduced and, correspondingly, be safe for young children. Weight is used as a better method of calculating drug dosage in children and is used when medications have a dose of drug recommended in mg/kg.

Weight alone, however, is not always accurate as a method of calculating a drug dosage for a child. Another more accurate method is that of body surface area (BSA). BSA is a relationship of height to weight and is measured in square meters. It increases about 7 times from birth to adulthood. It is a good reflection of many physiologic processes significant in metabolizing, transporting, and eliminating drugs, such as metabolic rate, extracellular fluid and total fluid volumes, cardiac output, and glomerular filtration rate. BSA is calculated by the formula:

$$\text{Surface area(m}^2) = \sqrt{\frac{\text{height(cm)} \times \text{weight(kg)}}{3600}}$$

A nomogram or graph has been developed to calculate BSA quickly and accurately. The nomogram on the left in Figure F–1 can be used when a child has height and weight in proportion, or in the same percentile range. (See Chapter 14 for a description of growth measurements and percentiles.) When the percentiles for height and weight differ, the nomogram on the right can be used. To calculate a child's BSA, draw a straight line from the height to the weight. The point at which the line intersects the surface area (SA) column is the BSA (measured in square meters, m²). Medications that are prescribed using the BSA system are dosed in mg/m².

Appendix G
Conversions and Equivalents

Temperature Conversion

(Fahrenheit temperature – 32) × 5/9 = Centigrade temperature
(Centigrade temperature × 9/5) + 32 = Fahrenheit temperature

Selected Conversion to Metric Measures

KNOWN VALUE	MULTIPLY BY	TO FIND
inches	2.54	centimeters
ounces	28	grams
pounds	454	grams
pounds	0.45	kilograms

Selected Conversion From Metric Measures

KNOWN VALUE	MULTIPLY BY	TO FIND
centimeters	0.4	inches
grams	0.035	ounces
grams	0.0022	pounds
kilograms	2.2	pounds

Conversion of Pounds and Ounces to Grams

	OUNCES															
POUNDS	**0**	**1**	**2**	**3**	**4**	**5**	**6**	**7**	**8**	**9**	**10**	**11**	**12**	**13**	**14**	**15**
0	—	28	57	85	113	142	170	198	227	255	283	312	340	369	397	425
1	454	482	510	539	567	595	624	652	680	709	737	765	794	822	850	879
2	907	936	964	992	1021	1049	1077	1106	1134	1162	1191	1219	1247	1276	1304	1332
3	1361	1389	1417	1446	1474	1503	1531	1559	1588	1616	1644	1673	1701	1729	1758	1786
4	1814	1843	1871	1899	1928	1956	1984	2013	2041	2070	2098	2126	2155	2183	2211	2240
5	2268	2296	2325	2353	2381	2410	2438	2466	2495	2523	2551	2580	2608	2637	2665	2693
6	2722	2750	2778	2807	2835	2863	2892	2920	2948	2977	3005	3033	3062	3090	3118	3147
7	3175	3203	3232	3260	3289	3317	3345	3374	3402	3430	3459	3487	3515	3544	3572	3600
8	3629	3657	3685	3714	3742	3770	3799	3827	3856	3884	3912	3941	3969	3997	4026	4054
9	4082	4111	4139	4167	4196	4224	4252	4281	4309	4337	4366	4394	4423	4451	4479	4508
10	4536	4564	4593	4621	4649	4678	4706	4734	4763	4791	4819	4848	4876	4904	4933	4961
11	4990	5018	5046	5075	5103	5131	5160	5188	5216	5245	5273	5301	5330	5358	5386	5415
12	5443	5471	5500	5528	5557	5585	5613	5642	5670	5698	5727	5755	5783	5812	5840	5868
13	5897	5925	5953	5982	6010	6038	6067	6095	6123	6152	6180	6209	6237	6265	6294	6322
14	6350	6379	6407	6435	6464	6492	6520	6549	6577	6605	6634	6662	6690	6719	6747	6776
15	6804	6832	6860	6889	6917	6945	6973	7002	7030	7059	7087	7115	7144	7172	7201	7228
16	7257	7286	7313	7342	7371	7399	7427	7456	7484	7512	7541	7569	7597	7626	7654	7682
17	7711	7739	7768	7796	7824	7853	7881	7909	7938	7966	7994	8023	8051	8079	8108	8136
18	8165	8192	8221	8249	8278	8306	8335	8363	8391	8420	8448	8476	8504	8533	8561	8590
19	8618	8646	8675	8703	8731	8760	8788	8816	8845	8873	8902	8930	8958	8987	9015	9043
20	9072	9100	9128	9157	9185	9213	9242	9270	9298	9327	9355	9383	9412	9440	9469	9497
21	9525	9554	9582	9610	9639	9667	9695	9724	9752	9780	9809	9837	9865	9894	9922	9950
22	9979	10007	10036	10064	10092	10120	10149	10177	10206	10234	10262	10291	10319	10347	10376	10404

Glossary

A

Acanthosis nigricans Hyperpigmentation and thickening of the skin associated with chronic hyperinsulinemia.

Accommodation The process of changing one's cognitive structures to include data from recent experiences.

Accommodations Services or special assistance provided in the school setting to ensure that a student with a physical or mental impairment has access to an appropriate education and is able to participate as fully as possible in school activities.

Acculturation The process of modifying one's culture to fit within the new or dominant culture.

Acellular pertussis vaccine A vaccine that uses pertussis proteins rather than the whole cell to stimulate active immunity.

Acidemia Decreased blood pH.

Acidosis Condition caused by excess acid in the blood.

Acquired immunity Humoral (antibody-mediated) and cell-mediated immunity that is not fully developed until a child is about 6 years of age.

Active immunity Stimulation of antibody production without causing clinical disease; antibody development for specific infections through immunization or exposure to the natural disease.

Acute pain Sudden pain of short duration, associated with a tissue-damaging stimulus.

Adaptation phase Period during a crisis when the child and family meet the challenge and use resources effectively.

Adaptive functioning The ability of an individual to meet the standards expected for his or her age by his or her cultural group.

Adherence The extent to which a client or parent follows recommended care for the health problem.

Adjustment phase Period just after a family is confronted by a crisis; characterized by disorganization and unsuccessful attempts to deal with the problem.

Adoption A legal relationship between the child and parents not related by birth in which the adoptive parents assume all legal and financial responsibility for the child.

Adrenarche The development of pubic and axillary sexual hair.

Advance directives A client's living will or appointed durable power of attorney for healthcare decisions.

Adventitious sounds Breath sounds that are not normally heard, such as wheezes, crackles, and rhonchi.

Advocacy Acting to safeguard and advance the interests of another.

Affect Outward manifestation of feeling or emotion; the tone of a person's reaction or response to people or events.

Agoraphobia Anxiety of being in places or situations from which escape may be difficult or embarrassing, or in which help may not be available.

Air hunger The most severe form of dyspnea, when a person or child looks panicked, gasps for breath, and sits upright.

Airway resistance The effort or force needed to move oxygen through the trachea to the lungs.

Alkalemia Increased blood pH.

Alkalosis Condition caused by too little acid in the blood.

Alleles Different forms of a gene or DNA occupying the same place on a pair of chromosomes; an allele for each gene is inherited from each parent.

Allergen An antigen capable of inducing hypersensitivity.

Allergy An abnormal or altered reaction to an antigen.

Allogeneic transplantation A procedure in which a donor (often a sibling [related] or sometimes someone unrelated) with a compatible human leukocyte antigen (HLA) gives bone marrow to a child with an immune or hematologic disease needing restoration of normal cells.

Allograft Cadaver skin from a skin bank used to temporarily cover a full-thickness burn.

Allow natural death (AND) Continuation of ongoing care, managing pain, and choosing not to initiate cardiopulmonary resuscitation if the child stops breathing or the heart stops beating.

Alternative therapy A substance or procedure that is used in place of conventional medicine.

Amenorrhea Lack of menstruation.

Anemia Reduction in the number of red blood cells, the quantity of hemoglobin, and the volume of packed red cells per 100 mL of blood to below-normal levels.

Aneuploidy An increase or decrease in chromosome number that is the result of an error during cell division, most often when nondisjunction occurs during meiosis.

Animal-assisted therapy A form of therapy used in hospitals and units in which specially trained animals (commonly dogs) provide diversion, distraction, comfort, and relaxation during health care.

Anthropometric measurement The term used to refer to growth assessment of various parts of the body.

Antibodies Proteins capable of responding to specific infectious agents (antigens).

Anticipation The tendency for certain genetic disorders to display earlier onset and increased severity in successive generations of a family.

Anticipatory guidance The process of understanding upcoming developmental needs and then teaching caretakers to meet those needs.

Antigen A foreign substance that triggers an immune system response.

Anuria Absence of urine output.

Apical impulse Also called the point of maximum intensity; is located where the left ventricle taps the chest wall during contraction. The apical impulse is usually seen in thin children.

Apnea Cessation of respiration lasting longer than 20 seconds.

Apoptosis Programmed cell death. When the cell "realizes" something is wrong and destroys itself.

Areflexia A lack of reflex response to verbal, sensory, or pain stimulation.

Arrhythmias Abnormal heart rhythms or dysrhythmias.

Asplenia Loss of the spleen due to surgery or nonfunctioning due to sickle cell disease.

Assent Voluntary agreement to accept treatment or to participate in a research project.

Assimilation   The process of incorporating new experiences into an individual's cognitive awareness; the process of incorporating traits of the new culture within one's practice.

Assistive technology   Any item, equipment, or product customized for use to promote the functional capabilities and independence of an individual with disabilities.

Association   A group of abnormalities of unknown cause that is seen together more often than would be expected by chance.

Associative play   A type of play that emerges in preschool years when children interact with one another, engaging in similar activities and participating in groups.

Atopy   A hereditary allergic tendency.

Audiography   A test used to assess hearing in which sounds of various pitches and intensity are presented to children through earphones.

Aura   A visual, auditory, taste, or motor sensation that gives warning of an impending seizure or migraine headache.

Auscultation   The technique of listening to sounds produced by the airway, lungs, stomach, heart, and blood vessels to identify their characteristics. Auscultation is usually performed with the stethoscope to enhance the sounds heard.

Autograft   Use of healthy skin taken from a nonburned area of the child's body to cover an area with a full-thickness burn.

Autologous transplantation   A procedure in which the child's own marrow is taken, treated, stored, and reinfused after the child has received chemotherapy.

Automatism   Unusual body movement without purpose (e.g., lip smacking, lip chewing, and sucking).

Autonomic dysreflexia   Condition in which hypertension, bradycardia, severe headaches, pallor below and flushing above the level of the spinal cord lesion, and seizures occur due to an impaired autonomic nervous system, triggered by simultaneous sympathetic and parasympathetic activity.

Autosome   Chromosome other than the sex chromosome.

Azotemia   Accumulation of nitrogenous wastes in the blood.

B

Behavior modification   A therapeutic technique used to reinforce desirable behaviors, helping the child replace maladaptive behaviors with more appropriate ones.

Benign   Describing a growth that does not endanger life or health.

Binge eating   A compulsion to consume large quantities of food in a short period of time.

Binocularity   Ability of the eyes to function together.

Biotherapy   A treatment that uses and/or enhances the body's abilities to fight disease, particularly by using biologic agents to promote an immune response.

Bisexual   Sexual attraction to both men and women.

Body fluid   Body water that has substances (solutes) dissolved in it.

Body image   The idea that one forms about one's body.

Body mass index (BMI)   A calculation (kilograms of weight/m2 of height) used to determine the proportion between a child's or adult's height and weight.

Bone age   Stage of bone ossification.

Brain death   The irreversible cessation of all functions of the brain, including the cerebral cortex and brainstem.

Breakthrough pain   Pain that emerges as the pain medication wears off, resulting in the loss of pain control.

Bronchiectasis   A persistent abnormal dilation of the bronchi.

Bronchophony   Change in vocal resonance in the presence of a lung consolidation, in which there is increased intensity and clarity of sounds while the words remain indistinct.

Buffer   Related acid–base pair that gives up or takes up hydrogen ions as needed to prevent large changes in the pH of a solution; a compound that binds hydrogen ions when their concentration rises and releases them when their concentration falls..

Bullying   Repeatedly aggressive behavior intended to cause physical or emotional harm that exists in a relationship with an imbalance of power.

C

Carcinogens   Chemicals or processes that, when combined with genetic traits and in interaction with one another, cause cancer.

Cardiac output   Volume of blood ejected from the left ventricle each minute.

Cardiomegaly   Enlargement (hypertrophy) of the heart muscle.

Care coordination   The process of planning and integrating healthcare services among providers in an effort to achieve and promote good health in the child.

Caregiver burden   The unrelenting pressure and anxiety related to providing daily care to a child with disabilities while meeting other family obligations.

Carrier   Any individual who carries a single copy of an altered gene or mutation for a recessive condition on one chromosome of a chromosome pair and an unaltered form of that gene on the other chromosome; a carrier generally is not affected by the gene alteration; on the average, each person in the general population is a carrier of five or six gene mutations for recessive disorders.

Case management   A process that involves the assessment, planning, facilitation, and delivery of healthcare services, which includes healthcare options by the interprofessional team to promote quality and cost effectiveness of care.

Case manager   Person who coordinates health care to prevent gaps or overlaps.

Cell   The basic unit of life and the working unit of all living systems.

Cephalocaudal development   The process by which development proceeds from the head downward through the body and toward the feet.

Cerebral edema   An increase in intracellular and extracellular fluid in the brain that results from anoxia, vasodilation, or vascular stasis.

Cerebral perfusion pressure   Amount of pressure needed to ensure that adequate oxygen and nutrients are delivered by the blood to the brain.

Chelation   A reaction in which an organic compound, containing carbonyl (CO) and hydroxyl (OH) groups, coordinates with a metal to form a firmly bound ringlike structure.

Chemotherapy   Treatment to combat cancer that involves drugs taken orally, intravenously, intrathecally, or by injection, which kill both normal and cancerous cells.

Child-life specialist   Trained professional who plans age-appropriate therapeutic activities for hospitalized children.

Child sexual abuse   The exploitation of a child for the sexual gratification of an adult or older child.

Children with special healthcare needs (CSHCN)   Children who have or are at increased risk for a chronic physical, developmental, behavioral, or emotional condition and who also require health and related services of a type or amount beyond that required by children generally.

Cholestasis   Disruption of bile flow.

Chondrolysis   The breaking down and absorption of cartilage.

Chronic condition   A health condition that lasts or is expected to last 3 months or more.

Chronic pain   Persistent pain lasting longer than 3 months, generally associated with a prolonged disease process.

Chronic vomiting   Low-grade, nearly daily emesis.

Chvostek sign   Contraction of facial muscles after tapping the facial nerve just anterior to the parotid gland.

Circumferential   Injury completely surrounding the thorax or an extremity.

Clinical practice guideline   A consensus of evidence-based and expert opinion statements about the care for a specific diagnosis used to assist the interprofessional team of healthcare providers to make decisions about the appropriate care of a child with that condition.

Clinical reasoning   The analytical process used when assessing client cues and information, synthesizing that information and applying it to understand a child's or family's problem or concern, and then using the nursing process to plan and evaluate the child's care.

Clonic   Alternating muscular contraction and relaxation; often used to describe seizure activity.

Clubbing   A widening of the nail bed with an increased angle between the proximal nail fold and nail.

Cognition   The change in thought, intelligence, and language that occurs from the mutual interaction of brain maturation with life experiences.

Cognitive therapy   A therapeutic approach that attempts to help the person recognize automatic thought patterns that lead to unpleasant feelings (automatic negative thinking).

Collaborative practice   A comprehensive model of health care that uses an interprofessional team of health professionals to provide high-quality, cost-effective care.

Coloboma   A keyhole-shaped pupil caused by a notch in the iris.

Coma   State of unconsciousness in which the child cannot be aroused, even by powerful stimuli.

Comedone   A plug of sebaceous and keratin material in a hair follicle; commonly known as *whiteheads* and *blackheads*.

Communicable disease   An illness that is transmitted directly or indirectly from one person to another.

Community assessment   A process of compiling data about a community's health status and resources for the purpose of developing a public health plan to address the priority health needs of a target population within that community.

Compartment syndrome   A condition of increased pressure in a limited space that compromises circulation and tissue function.

Complementary therapy   Any procedure or product that is used as an adjunct to conventional medical treatment.

Compliance   Amount of expansion the ventricles can achieve to increase stroke volume.

Conductive hearing loss   Hearing loss caused by inadequate conduction of sound from the outer to the middle ear.

Confidentiality   An agreement between a client and a provider that information discussed during the healthcare encounter will not be shared without the client's permission.

Conjugated forms   An altered organism is joined with another substance in a vaccine to increase the immune response to the vaccine.

Consanguinity   Related by having a common ancestor; close blood relationship.

Consciousness   The responsiveness to or awareness of sensory stimuli, including the ability to process the data and respond either verbally or physically.

Conservation   The knowledge that matter is not changed when its form is altered.

Constipation   Difficult and infrequent defecation with passage of hard, dry stool.

Consultand   A designated "index" patient who seeks genetic counseling without being known to have a given genetic disorder, around which a pedigree is often constructed.

Continuity of care   The process of facilitating a patient's care between and among healthcare providers and settings based on health needs and available resources.

Cooperative play   A type of play that emerges in school years when children join into groups to achieve a goal or play a game.

Coping   The use of learned behavioral and cognitive strategies to manage or relieve perceived stress; the cognitive and behavioral responses that help a person manage specific internal and external demands that exceed personal resources, enabling the person to solve problems and to respond appropriately.

Copy number variation   An additional source of human genetic variation in which stretches of DNA of variable size are replicated one or more times.

Cor pulmonale   Obstruction of pulmonary blood flow that leads to right ventricular hypertrophy and heart failure.

Crepitus   A crinkly sensation palpated on the chest surface caused by air escaping into the subcutaneous tissues.

Critical thinking   An individualized, creative thinking or reasoning process that nurses use to solve problems.

Crossing over   A process that occurs during meiosis in which homologous maternal and paternal chromosomes break and exchange corresponding sections of DNA and then rejoin; this process can cause an exchange of alleles between chromosomes and provides human diversity.

Cryotherapy   The use of cold or cold agents (liquid nitrogen) to treat specific injuries or conditions. Often used for treating warts and other skin conditions.

Cultural competence   The ability to understand and effectively respond to the needs of patients and families from different cultural backgrounds.

Culture   The beliefs, values, attitudes, and practices that are accepted by a population, community, or an individual.

Cushing triad   Reflex response associated with increased intracranial pressure or compromised blood flow to the brainstem; characterized by hypertension, increased systolic pressure with wide pulse pressure, bradycardia, and irregular respirations.

Cyberbullying   A situation in which a child or adolescent is targeted by another via Internet posting or other digital technology and threatened, tormented, harassed, humiliated, or embarrassed.

Cyclic vomiting   Repeated severe vomiting of an episodic nature.

Cytogenetics   The study of chromosomes and alterations to health caused by abnormalities in the number or structure of chromosomes.

D

Deamination   Removal of an amino group from an amino compound.

Death anxiety   A feeling of apprehension or fear of death.

Death imagery   Any reference to death or death-related topics, such as going away, separation, funerals, and dying, given in response to a picture or story that would not usually stimulate other children to discuss death-related topics.

Debridement   Enzyme action to clean a lesion and dissolve fibrin clots or scabs; or removal of dead tissue to speed the healing process.

Decibels   Units used to measure the loudness of sounds.

Deciduous teeth   Primary set of 20 teeth that is complete by about 2 years of age and will be lost during childhood, beginning at about 6 years.

Decontamination   The removal of chemicals and nerve agents from the skin.

Deep sedation   A controlled state of depressed consciousness or unconsciousness in which the child may experience partial or complete loss of protective airway reflexes.

Defense mechanisms   Techniques used by the ego to unconsciously change reality, thereby protecting itself from excessive anxiety.

Dehydration   The state of body water deficit.

Dermatophytoses   Fungal infections that affect primarily the skin, but also may affect the hair and nails.

Desaturated blood   Blood with a lower than normal oxygen level resulting when a heart defect causes oxygenated and unoxygenated blood to mix.

Development   The process of increasing capability or function.

Developmental delay   A delay in mastering functions, such as motor coordination and behavioral skills.

Developmental disability   Any of a variety of chronic conditions that are characterized by mental or physical impairments. Intellectual disability, pervasive developmental disorder, cerebral palsy, and sensory loss are examples of developmental disabilities.

Developmental surveillance   A flexible, continuous process of skilled observations that provides data about the child's capabilities, allows for early identification of any neurologic problems, and helps to verify that the home environment is stimulating.

Dialysate   The solution used in dialysis.

Diarrhea   Frequent passage of abnormally watery stool.

Dietary Reference Intakes (DRIs)   A set of nutrient values established by the Food and Nutrition Board of the Institute of Medicine (IOM) and the National Academy of Science that can be used to assess and plan intake for individuals of different ages.

Diffusion   Movement of molecules across a membrane from an area of higher concentration to lower concentration.

Direct transmission   The passage of an infectious disease through physical contact between the source of the pathogen and a new host.

Disability   A limitation that interferes with a child's ability to fully participate in society, which can be related to medical impairment (chronic health condition), functional limitation (mobility, self-care, communication, or learning behavior impairment), or a mental condition that interferes with social interactions.

Disaster   A serious and massive event that impacts many people and causes extensive damage, hardship, death, injuries, and psychologic trauma.

Disaster preparedness   Community planning for responses to natural and man-made disasters that involve multiple casualties.

Discipline   A method for teaching the rules that govern behavior or conduct.

Disequilibrium syndrome   Rapid changes in the body's water and electrolyte balance during treatment.

Dislocation   Displacement of a bone from its normal articulation with a joint.

Distraction   The ability to focus attention on something other than pain, such as an activity, music, or a story.

Dominant   A characteristic or gene that is apparent even when the relevant gene is present in only one copy; a person with a dominant gene usually expresses that gene trait.

Dramatic play   A type of play in which a child acts out the drama of daily life or in which medical situations encountered are reenacted by the child.

Dwarfism   A genetic condition usually resulting in an adult height of 58 inches or less. The most common cause of dwarfism is achondroplasia, which causes short arms and legs. The torso and head are approximately normal size, but decreased growth of long bones causes short stature.

Dysmenorrhea   Menstrual pain or cramping.

Dysmorphology   The study of human congenital defects or abnormalities of body structure that begin before birth.

Dysphagia   Difficulty in swallowing.

Dysphonia   Muffled, hoarse, or absent voice sounds.

Dysplasia   Abnormal development resulting in altered size, shape, and cell organization.

Dyspnea   Shortness of breath; difficulty breathing.

E

Early childhood caries (ECC)   The presence of one or more decayed, missing, or filled tooth surfaces in primary teeth in a child 71 months of age or younger; frequently caused by drinking from a bottle or nursing for prolonged periods, especially when sleeping; previously referred to as *nursing bottle mouth syndrome* and *baby bottle tooth decay.*

Early intervention   Special services provided by state or local education programs for infants and toddlers up to age 3 years who have a developmental delay or are at risk for developmental delay in the hopes that these children will have a lowered total cost of educational services.

Ecchymosis   Bruising.

Echolalia   A compulsive parroting or repetition of what is heard.

Ecologic theory   A theory of development that emphasizes the importance of interactions between the developing child and the settings in which the child lives.

Ecomap   An illustration of a family's relationships and social networks.

Edema   An accumulation of excess fluid in the interstitial spaces.

Electroanalgesia   A method of delivering electrical stimulation to the skin by electrodes, to compete with pain stimuli for transmission to the spinal cord; also known as *transcutaneous electrical nerve stimulation (TENS).*

Electrolytes   Charged particles (ions) dissolved in body fluid.

Emancipated minors   Economically self-supporting adolescents under 18 years of age not subject to parental control (e.g., married, pregnant, enlisted, or incarcerated).

Emergency preparedness   Readiness to manage a healthcare emergency that involves planning, equipment and supplies for responses, and provider training and guidelines for action when an emergency occurs.

Emollient   A topical product that soothes and softens the skin.

Emotional abuse   Shaming, ridiculing, embarrassing, or insulting a child.

Emotional neglect   A caretaker's inability to meet the psychosocial needs of a child.

Encephalopathy   Cerebral dysfunction resulting from an insult (e.g., toxin, injury, inflammation, or anoxic event) of limited duration; the tissue damage is often permanent, but the dysfunction may improve over time.

Endogenous pyrogens Pyrogens (chemicals, interleukins, interferons, and tumor necrosis factor) released in response to an invasive organism that travel through the circulatory system to the hypothalamus, where they trigger the production and release of prostaglandins, resulting in the fever response.

Endorphins Opioidlike substances produced by the body.

End-stage renal disease (ESRD) Irreversible kidney failure.

Enteral therapy Nutrition introduced through the intestinal tract, including oral or tube feedings.

Enuresis Repeated involuntary voiding by a child who has reached the age at which bladder control is expected.

Epicanthal fold An extra fold of skin covering all or part of the lacrimal caruncle of the medial canthus (nasal side) of the eye.

Epidemiologist A specialist with training in the study of patterns of diseases or health risks in a population.

Epigenetic Describes any factor that can affect gene function (usually by changing gene expression, or translation) without changing the DNA sequence.

Equianalgesic dose The amount of a drug, when administered orally, that produces the same level of analgesia as when it is administered parenterally.

Equinus A condition that limits dorsiflexion to less than normal; usually associated with clubfoot.

Ergogenic aids Products that enhance physical performance.

Erythropoiesis Formation of red blood cells.

Eschar Slough or layer of dead skin or tissue; the tough leathery scab that forms over severely burned areas.

Escharotomy Incision into constricting dead tissue of a burn injury to restore peripheral circulation.

Esotropia Momentary inward deviation of the eyes.

Ethics The philosophic study of morality, and the analysis of moral problems and moral judgments.

Ethnicity A social identity that is associated with shared beliefs, behaviors, patterns, and cultural heritage.

Euthyroid Normal thyroid state; thyroid hormones in appropriate balance.

Evidence-based practice An approach to problem solving and decision making that is based on the consideration of data from research, statistical analysis, quality measures, risk management measurements, and other sources of reliable information.

Exophthalmos Prominent or bulging eyes.

Exotropia Outward deviation of the eyes ("wall-eyes").

Expressive jargon Use of unintelligible words with normal speech intonations as if truly communicating in words; common in toddlerhood.

Extracellular fluid The fluid in the body that is outside the cells.

Extravasation Damage that occurs when a chemotherapeutic drug leaks into the soft tissue surrounding the infusion site.

F

Faith-based belief An organized system of shared beliefs regarding the significance of the nature, cause, and purpose of life and the universe.

Family Refers to two or more persons who are joined together by marriage, birth, or adoption and live together in the same household.

Family-centered care The effort to address and meet the emotional, social, and developmental needs of children and families seeking health care in all settings.

Family crisis An event that causes problems for a family that for a time seem insurmountable and with which the family is unable to cope in its usual ways.

Family strengths Relationships, processes, and resources that families can use during times of adversity and change to manage stressors.

Fever An increased body temperature of 38.0°C (100.4°F) or higher taken by rectal or tympanic route, and 37.8°C (100°F) or higher by the oral or temporal route.

Filtration Movement of fluid into or out of capillaries as the net result of several opposing forces.

Focal Specific area of the brain; often used to describe seizures or neurologic deficits.

Food allergy An IgE-mediated reaction to a given food that is potentially systemic, characteristically rapid in onset, and may be manifested as swelling of the lips, mouth, uvula or glottis, generalized urticaria, and, in severe reactions, anaphylaxis.

Food insecurity An inability or uncertainty that one will be able to acquire or consume adequate quality or quantity of foods in socially acceptable ways.

Food intolerance An abnormal physiologic response (flatulence, sweating, hives, indigestion) to a food that is not immunoglobulin E (IgE)–mediated.

Food jags Eating only a few foods for several days or weeks.

Food security Access at all times to enough nourishment for an active, healthy life.

Foster care The provision of protection and shelter for a child in an approved living situation away from the family of origin.

Futility A situation in which treatments do not provide a clear clinical benefit.

G

Gamete Female or male germ cell; contains a haploid number of chromosomes.

Gay An adjective used to describe or refer to a homosexual male.

Gene A sequence of DNA on a chromosome that represents a fundamental unit of heredity; occupies a specific spot on a chromosome (gene locus).

Gene expression When the protein product of a gene is visible (presence of a body structure or identifiable through biochemical tests such as insulin or phenylalanine levels).

Genetic disease Any disease associated with gene dysfunction. Genetic diseases have traditionally been thought of as relatively rare inherited diseases, but it is now known that nearly all diseases have a genetic component.

Genogram A pedigree that displays information about a family's health history over at least three generations.

Genome The entire DNA sequence that makes up the complete genetic information of a gamete, an individual, a population, or a species.

Genomewide association study A rapid examination of many common genetic variations in DNA or genomes, in different individuals, to identify genetic variations associated with a certain disease.

Genomics The study of all the genes in the human genome together, including their interactions with each other, the environment, and the influence of other psychosocial and cultural factors.

Genotype The genetic composition of an individual.

Glucagon A hormone produced by the pancreas that helps release stored glucose from the liver.

Gluconeogenesis Formation of glycogen from noncarbohydrate sources such as protein or fat.

Glycosuria Abnormal amount of glucose in the urine.

Goiter Enlargement of the thyroid gland.

Graft-versus-host disease A series of immunologic responses mounted by the host of a transplanted organ with the purpose of destroying the transplant cells.

Growth An increase in physical size.

H

Hazing An activity that is forced on an individual that causes humiliation and is required for membership in an organization or group. It can sometimes be harmful.

Health A state of complete physical, mental, and social well-being and not merely the absence of disease and infirmity.

Health maintenance Activities that preserve an individual's present state of health and prevent disease or injury occurrence.

Health promotion Activities that increase well-being, enhance wellness or health, and lead to actualization of positive health potential; strategies that seek to foster conditions to allow populations to be healthy and to make healthy choices.

Health supervision The process of health promotion services, growth and development monitoring, and disease and injury prevention at key intervals throughout the child's life.

Heaving Lifting of the chest wall during contraction.

Hemarthrosis Bleeding into joint spaces.

Hematopoiesis Blood cell production.

Hemodynamics Passage of blood through the heart and pulmonary system and pressures generated by the blood.

Hemoglobinopathy Disease characterized by abnormal hemoglobin.

Hemoptysis Coughing up blood from the respiratory tract.

Hemosiderosis Increased storage of iron in body tissues; associated with diseases involving the destruction of red blood cells.

Herd immunity The protection provided by a large group of persons who have immunity to a disease and indirectly protect others without immunity by reducing the risk for exposure and infection.

Hernia The protrusion or projection of a body part or structure through the muscle wall of the cavity that normally contains it.

Herniation Protrusion of brain contents through the cranial vault at the base of the skull into the brainstem area.

Heterozygous Nonidentical copies of a particular gene (different alleles) on the paired chromosomes.

Homologous chromosomes Chromosomes that are members of the same pair and normally have the same number and arrangement of genes; usually one copy is from the mother and the other copy is from the father.

Homosexuality Sexual attraction to people of the same sex.

Homozygous A genotypic situation in which two similar genes occur at a given locus on homologous chromosomes.

Hospice A philosophy of care that focuses on helping persons with short life expectancies to live their remaining lives to the fullest—without pain and with choices and dignity.

Human genome The entire DNA sequence of an individual.

Hydronephrosis Accumulation of urine in the renal pelvis as a result of obstructed outflow.

Hyperbilirubinemia An abnormally elevated serum bilirubin level.

Hypercapnia Greater than normal amounts of carbon dioxide in the blood.

Hypersensitivity response An overreaction of the immune system, responsible for allergic reactions.

Hypersplenism A syndrome characterized by splenomegaly and blood cell deficiencies.

Hypertelorism Widely spaced eyes.

Hypertonic dehydration (or hypernatremic dehydration) Fluid loss characterized by a proportionately greater loss of water than sodium.

Hypertonic saline Fluid more concentrated with salt than body fluid.

Hypoplastic Small and nonfunctional.

Hypotonic dehydration (or hyponatremic dehydration) Fluid loss characterized by a proportionately greater loss of sodium than water.

Hypotonic fluid Fluid that is more dilute (contains less salt) than normal body fluid.

Hypoxemia Lower than normal amounts of oxygen in the blood.

Hypoxia Lower than normal amounts of oxygen in the tissues.

I

Immunodeficiency A state of the immune system in which it cannot cope effectively with foreign antigens; a state of decreased responsiveness of the immune system.

Immunoglobulin A protein that functions as an antibody. Immunoglobulins are responsible for humoral immunity.

Inborn errors of metabolism Hereditary deficiencies of a specific enzyme needed for normal metabolism of specific chemicals.

Incarceration Occurs when the presence of intestine in the groin causes constriction of the blood supply to the scrotal sac, leading to intestinal strangulation and testicular ischemia.

Incest Sexual activity between family members close enough that marriage between them would be legally or culturally prohibited.

Incidental findings Unanticipated, abnormal results of genetic testing that are not relevant to the diagnostic indication for which the test was ordered.

Incubation period The time interval between exposure to an infectious disease and development of symptoms.

Independent assortment The random distribution of different combinations of parental genes to gametes.

Indirect transmission The passage of an infectious disease (to a person by contact with contaminated objects or by vectors) involving survival of pathogens outside humans before they invade a new host.

Individualized approach An assessment approach that involves measuring individual children seen in a clinic, sharing results with the family, and addressing appropriate teaching about weight control and nutritious intake.

Individualized education plan (IEP) A form of education planning/intervention that is developed for a child with cognitive, motor, social, and communication impairments who needs special education services. The IEP is jointly planned with the school administrator, teacher, parents, and other special support professionals as appropriate for the child's condition.

Individualized family service plan (IFSP) A form of education planning/intervention that is developed for early intervention with infants with special healthcare needs and their families. The IFSP contains information about the services required to support a child's development and enhance the family's capacity to facilitate the child's development. The family and education service providers work as a team to plan, implement, and evaluate services specific to the family's unique concerns, priorities, and resources.

Individualized health plan (IHP)   A formal mechanism to ensure that the child's health needs are managed in the school setting.

Individualized transition plan (ITP)   A plan that focuses on assisting the adolescent with special healthcare needs in moving successfully from school into the community.

Induration   An area of extra firmness on the skin with a distinct border.

Infant mortality   Death in infants less than 12 months of age.

Infectious disease   Any communicable disease caused by microorganisms transmitted from one person to another or from an animal to a person.

Informed consent   A legal concept that protects a person's rights to autonomy and self-determination by specifying that no action may be taken without that person's prior understanding and freely given consent; a formal authorization by the child's parent or guardian allowing an invasive procedure to be performed or for participation in research.

Inguinal hernia   A painless inguinal or scrotal swelling of variable size that occurs when abdominal tissue, such as bowel, extends into the inguinal canal.

Insensible fluid loss   Fluid loss not directly measurable or observable, such as through skin and the respiratory tract.

Inspection   The technique of purposeful observation by carefully looking at the characteristics of the child's physical features and behaviors. Physical feature characteristics include size, shape, color, movement, position, and location.

Insulin deficiency   A condition in which the pancreas does not produce sufficient insulin (as in type 1 diabetes).

Insulin resistance   An alteration of the insulin receptor that signals the presence of insulin in the interior of cells.

Intellectual disability   Significant limitation in intellectual functioning and adaptive behavior, manifested by differences in conceptual, social, and practical adaptive skills, beginning before the age of 18 years.

Interstitial fluid   That portion of the extracellular fluid that is between the cells and outside the blood and lymphatic vessels.

Intertriginous areas   Areas where skin is in contact with other skin, (e.g., between fingers, and within skinfolds of the neck, axillae, or antecubital fossa).

Intracellular fluid   The fluid in the body that is inside the cells.

Intracranial pressure   Force exerted by brain tissue, cerebrospinal fluid, and blood within the cranium.

Intractable seizure   A seizure that continues to occur even with optimal medical management.

Intrathecal   A method of drug or medication delivery in which the drug is introduced into the spinal canal.

Intravascular fluid   The portion of the extracellular fluid that is in the blood vessels.

Inversion   A chromosomal alteration in which a gene or DNA sequence in a segment of a chromosome has been reversed.

Involution   Rolling or turning inward; the process of decreasing in size; the reduction in size of the uterus following childbirth.

Isotonic dehydration (or isonatremic dehydration)   Fluid loss that is not balanced by intake; the loss of water and sodium are in proportion.

Isotonic fluid   Fluid that has the same osmolality as normal body fluid.

J

Joint custody   A legal situation in which both parents have equal responsibility and legal rights for a child, regardless of where the child lives.

K

Karyotype   A picture of an individual's chromosomes arranged in a standard order.

Keloid   Overdevelopment or hypertrophy of a scar that extends beyond the wound edges and above the skin line because of excess collagen.

Kerion   A large tender boggy mass on the scalp with drainage; associated with tinea capitis.

Killed virus vaccine   A vaccine that contains a killed microorganism that is still capable of inducing the human body to produce antibodies to the disease.

Kinesthesia   The sense of one's body position and movement.

Kussmaul respirations   Increased rate and depth of respirations (hyperventilation).

L

Lacto-ovovegetarians   Vegetarians who eat eggs and dairy products.

Lactovegetarians   Vegetarians who eat dairy products but not eggs.

Laryngospasms   Spasmodic vibrations of the larynx, which create sudden, violent, unpredictable, involuntary contraction of airway muscles.

Legal guardianship   A permanent placement option for the child, often with relatives, in which parental rights are not terminated.

Lesbian   An adjective used to describe or refer to a homosexual female.

Leukocytosis   A higher than normal leukocyte count.

Leukopenia   A lower than normal white blood cell (leukocyte) count.

Level of consciousness   The most important indicator of neurologic dysfunction. Consciousness, the responsiveness to or awareness of sensory stimuli, has two components: alertness, or the ability to react to stimuli, and cognitive power, or the ability to process the data and respond either verbally or physically.

Lichenification   Thickening of the skin with more visible skin furrows.

Life-threatening condition   A condition in which there is a likelihood that the child will die prematurely.

Limit setting   Established rules or guidelines for behavior.

Live virus vaccine   A vaccine that contains the microorganism in a live but attenuated, or weakened, form.

Lymphangitis   Inflammation of the lymphoid system draining the site of infection that is seen as tender, erythematous streaks extending in a proximal direction from the site of injury.

M

Macronutrients   The major building blocks of the body: carbohydrates, protein, and fat.

Major anomaly   A serious structural defect present at birth that may have severe medical or cosmetic consequences that interfere with normal functioning of body systems, lead to a lifelong disability, or even cause early death.

Malignant   The progressive growth of a tumor that will, if not checked by treatment, spread to other sites in the body and result in death.

Mature minors   Adolescents between 14 and 18 years of age who are able to understand treatment risks and who in some states can consent to or refuse treatment.

Medically fragile   Having a complex chronic health condition that requires skilled nursing and often technology support for vital functions.

Meiosis The process of cell division that occurs in the maturation of sperm and ova that decreases their number of chromosomes by one half.

Menorrhagia Heavy menstrual bleeding.

Mental health Foundational to a sense of personal well-being, physical health, and psychologic stability; it involves successful engagement in activities and relationships and the ability to adapt and cope with change.

Metastasis The spread of cancer cells to other sites in the body.

Microarray analysis A laboratory method in which labeled RNA from a specimen is added to a glass slide or other platform on which DNA fragments are arranged. Useful for identifying and quantifying mRNA and indicating which genes are actively expressed in a tissue.

Microcephaly A small brain with a head circumference below the third percentile on growth curves.

Micronutrients Substances needed in small quantities for healthy body functioning; vitamins and minerals are micronutrients.

Minor anomaly An unusual morphologic feature that is of no serious medical or cosmetic concern.

Mitosis Process of cell division whereby both daughter cells have the same number and pattern of chromosomes as the original cell.

Mixed hearing loss Hearing loss having a combination of conductive and sensorineural causes.

Modeling Imitating the behavior of someone else.

Moderate sedation A lower dose of a sedative that enables the child to maintain protective reflexes independently, continuously maintain a patent airway, and respond to tactile and verbal stimuli.

Monosomic (monosomy) Genetic condition that occurs when a normal gamete unites with a gamete that is missing a chromosome.

Moral dilemma A conflict involving individual beliefs, social values, and ethical principles.

Morbidity An illness or injury that limits activity, requires medical attention or hospitalization, or results in a chronic condition; incidence and prevalence of certain diseases.

Mosaicism Condition of an individual who has at least two cell lines with differing karyotypes.

Multifactorial Health conditions determined by multiple factors, including genetic and environmental factors, each having an additive effect.

Myelodysplasia Any malformation of the spinal cord and spinal canal.

Myelosuppression A decreased production of blood cells in the bone marrow.

Myringotomy A procedure whereby an incision is made in the tympanic membrane to drain fluid.

N

Nadir The lowest point, such as for a laboratory value or serum blood titer.

Nasal flaring A sign of respiratory distress; an effort the child makes to widen the airway by widening the nares with breathing.

Natural immunity The body's defenses present at birth, such as intact skin, body pH, natural antibodies from the mother, and inflammatory and phagocytic properties.

Nature The genetic or hereditary capability of an individual.

Neoplasms Cancerous growths.

Nephrotic syndrome An alteration in kidney function secondary to increased glomerular basement membrane permeability to plasma protein.

Neural tube Cell tissue that ultimately develops into the central nervous system, including the brain and spinal cord.

Neural tube defect Malformation of embryonic tissue that develops into the central nervous system and includes anencephaly, encephalocele, spina bifida, and myelodysplasia.

Neurogenic bladder The result of urinary tract obstruction related to an interrupted nerve supply to the bladder.

Neuropathic pain A form of chronic pain, initiated or caused by a primary lesion or dysfunction of the nervous system; an abnormal processing of pain stimuli by the peripheral or central nervous system.

Neutropenia A low neutrophil count.

Nightmares Frightening dreams that awaken the child, who is often crying and upset.

Night terrors (or sleep terrors) A situation in which the child cries out, appears frightened, and has tachycardia and tachypnea while sleeping, but in contrast to nightmares, the child having a night terror is not fully awake and may appear disoriented.

Nociceptive pain The perception of pain; the normal processing of pain stimuli caused by tissue injury or damage.

Nociceptors Free nerve endings at the site of tissue damage that are able to detect and respond to chemical, mechanical, and thermal stimuli.

Nondisjunction An error in cell division in which a pair of homologous chromosomes does not separate as expected, resulting in monosomy or trisomy in gametes.

Nonsteroidal anti-inflammatory drugs (NSAIDs) Drugs that are effective for the relief of mild to moderate pain and chronic pain.

Nosocomial infection An infection acquired in a healthcare agency, not present at the time of entrance to the agency.

Nuchal rigidity Resistance to neck flexion.

Nurture The effects of environment on an individual's performance.

Nutrition Taking in of food and assimilating it metabolically for use by the body.

O

Object permanence The knowledge that an object or person continues to exist when not seen, heard, or felt.

Occult blood Blood that is present in small quantities and is measurable only by laboratory testing.

Oliguria Diminished urine output (less than 0.5 to 1 mL/kg/hr).

Oncogene A portion of the DNA that is altered and, when duplicated, causes uncontrolled cellular division.

Oncotic pressure The part of the blood osmotic pressure that results from plasma proteins; also called blood colloid osmotic pressure.

Opioids Analgesics commonly given for severe pain, such as after surgery or a severe injury.

Opisthotonic position Rigid hyperextension of the head and neck.

Opisthotonos Rigid hyperextension of the entire body.

Opportunistic infection An infection that is often caused by normally nonpathogenic organisms in persons who lack normal immunity.

Orchitis Inflammation of the epididymis, pain on testicular palpation, and scrotal swelling, often associated with mumps infection in postpubertal males.

Organelle A small cellular structure such as a ribosome or mitochondria that performs specific cellular functions.

Osmolality The amount of concentration of a fluid; technically, the number of moles of particles per kilogram of water in the solution.

Osmosis Movement of water across a semipermeable membrane into an area of higher particle concentration.

Ossification Formation of bone from fibrous tissue or cartilage.

Osteodystrophy A complex bone disease process of chronic kidney disease in which there is increased resorption of bone caused by chronic hyperparathyroidism.

Osteotomy Surgical cutting of bone.

Ostomy An artificial abdominal opening into the urinary or gastro-intestinal canal that provides an outlet for the diversion of urine or fecal matter.

Outcome expectancy What a person expects to get from performing a certain behavior.

P

Pain An unpleasant sensory and emotional experience associated with actual or potential tissue damage. Pain exists when the patient says it does.

Palliative care A multidisciplinary care approach for children with life-shortening disorders and their families. It is intended to relieve suffering of all types (physical, psychologic, spiritual, and social); to enhance quality of life for patients and their families; to facilitate informed decision making by the patient, family, and healthcare professionals; and to improve care coordination.

Palliative procedure Intervention used to preserve life in children with a potentially fatal or lethal condition; a surgical procedure that does not create normal anatomic or hemodynamic results.

Palpation The technique of touch to identify characteristics of the skin, internal organs, and masses. Characteristics include texture, moistness, tenderness, temperature, position, shape, consistency, and mobility of masses and organs.

Pancytopenia A decreased number of blood cell components.

Pandemic flu A worldwide influenza epidemic.

Paradoxical breathing Severe respiratory distress in which the chest falls and the abdomen rises on inspiration.

Parallel play A type of play that emerges in toddlerhood when children play side by side with similar or different toys, demonstrating little or no social interaction.

Parenting A leadership role in the family in which children are guided to learn acceptable behaviors, beliefs, morals, and rituals of the family and to become socially responsible contributing members of society.

Partnership A relationship in which participants join together to ensure healthcare delivery in a way that recognizes the critical roles and contributions of each partner in promoting health, preventing illness, and managing healthcare conditions.

Passive immunity Immunity produced through introduction of specific antibodies to the disease, which are usually obtained from the blood or serum of immune persons and animals. Does not confer lasting immunity.

Patient-controlled analgesia (PCA) A method of pain control in which anesthesia, usually morphine, is initially administered by the anesthesiologist and subsequent doses are self-administered by pushing a button controlled by a special IV pump system.

Patient safety The freedom from unintentional injury caused by medical care, including such injuries that could be related to adverse drug events, misidentification of the patient, and healthcare-associated infections

Pediatric healthcare home The site of comprehensive, family-centered, continuous, culturally sensitive, coordinated, and compassionate health care by a pediatric healthcare professional focused on the overall well-being of children and families.

Pedigree Graphic representation of a family tree.

Penetrance The percentage or likelihood that an individual who has inherited a gene mutation will actually express the disease signs and symptoms in his or her lifetime.

Percussion The technique of striking the surface of the body, either directly or indirectly, to set up vibrations that reveal the density of underlying tissues and borders of internal organs.

Periodic breathing Sporadic episodes of apnea, not associated with cyanosis, that last for about 10 seconds and commonly occur in preterm infants.

Peristalsis A progressive, wavelike muscular movement that occurs involuntarily throughout the gastrointestinal tract.

Petechiae Small pinpoint red or purple spots on the mucous membranes or skin.

pH Negative logarithm of the hydrogen ion concentration; used to monitor the acidity of body fluid.

Pharmacogenomics The study of how an individual's genotype affects his or her response to medications.

Phenotype The whole physical, biochemical, and physiologic makeup of an individual as determined both genetically and environmentally.

Phimosis A structural defect in which the foreskin over the glans penis cannot be retracted.

Phototoxic A rapid nonimmunologic reaction of the skin when exposed to sunlight.

Physical abuse The deliberate maltreatment of another individual that inflicts pain or injury and may result in permanent or temporary disfigurement or even death.

Physical dependence The physiologic adaptation to an analgesic or sedative drug at the level of the peripheral and central neurons that may lead to withdrawal.

Physical neglect The deliberate withholding of or failure to provide the necessary and available resources to a child.

Physiologic anorexia A decrease in appetite manifested when the extremely high metabolic demands of infancy slow to keep pace with the more moderate growth rate of toddlerhood.

Pica An eating disorder characterized by ingestion of nonfood items or food items consumed in abnormal quantities or forms.

Pitting edema A "pit" or concave indentation that remains after an edematous area is pressed downward by the examiner's fingers.

Play therapy A therapeutic intervention often used with preschool and school-aged children. The child reveals conflicts, wishes, and fears on an unconscious level while playing with dolls, toys, clay, and other objects.

Polycythemia An abnormal increase in the number of total red blood cells in the body's circulation.

Polydipsia Excessive thirst.

Polyphagia Excessive or voracious eating.

Polypharmacy A term used to describe the act of taking multiple drugs at one time to treat multiple health conditions.

Polysomnography A sleep study that simultaneously records the sleep state, gas exchange, breathing efforts, cardiac rhythm, and muscle activity and movement.

Polyuria Passage of a large volume of urine in a given period.

Population-based approach Health assessment and intervention performed with a group of children.

Postictal period Period after seizure activity during which the level of consciousness is decreased.

Postpartum The period after giving birth.

Posturing Abnormal position assumed after injury or damage to the brain that may be seen as extreme flexion or extension of the limbs.

Practice guideline A consensus of evidence-based and expert opinion statements about the appropriate care for a child with a specific diagnosis that is used to assist healthcare providers to make decisions about the care of a child with that condition.

Prebiotic   A nondigestible food ingredient that can stimulate growth or activity of probiotic bacteria.

Preload   Volume of blood in the ventricle at the end of diastole that stretches the heart muscle before contraction.

Primary care   The range of healthcare services that include health promotion, health maintenance, episodic acute care, and health maintenance care for children with chronic conditions.

Primary immune deficiency   Congenital immunodeficiency.

Primary immune response   The process in which B lymphocytes produce antibodies specific to a particular antigen on first exposure.

Proband   The family member around whom a family history is collected.

Probiotic   A food supplement containing a live microorganism that alters the balance of gut microflora, thereby providing a health benefit.

Prodrome   The phase of early manifestations of the infection until the development of the overt clinical syndrome.

Projectile vomiting   Vomiting in which the stomach contents are ejected with great force.

Prostration   Extreme exhaustion.

Protective factors   Characteristics of a child and family that provide strength and assistance when dealing with a crisis.

Protocol   A plan of action for chemotherapy that is based on the type of cancer, its stage, and the particular cell type.

Proto-oncogene   A gene that regulates cellular growth and development but can become an oncogene, capable of causing cancerous growth.

Proximodistal development   The process by which development proceeds from the center of the body outward to the extremities.

Pseudohermaphroditism   Ambiguous development of the external genitalia.

Pseudohypertrophy   Enlargement of the muscles as a result of infiltration by fatty tissue.

Psychodrama   Being assigned and playing out roles spontaneously in a therapeutic setting to assist in understanding of the dynamics of the situation.

Puberty   The developmental period between childhood and attainment of adult sexual characteristics and functioning.

Punishment   The action taken to enforce the rules when the child misbehaves.

Purpura   Bleeding into the tissues, particularly beneath the skin and mucous membranes, causing lesions that vary from red to bluish purple.

Pyeloplasty   Removal of an obstructed segment of the ureter and reimplantation into the renal pelvis.

Q

Quality improvement   The continuous study of systems, services, and processes of care, and using that information to improve healthcare processes, services, and patient outcomes.

R

Race   A group of people who share biologic similarities such as skin color, bone structure, and genetic traits. Examples of races include White (sometimes called Caucasian or European American), Black (sometimes called African American in the United States), Hispanic, Natives (such as Native Americans, Alaskan Native, Hawaiian Native, and First Nation people of Canada), and Asian.

Radiation   A therapy that involves unstable isotopes that release varying levels of energy to cause breaks in the DNA molecule and thereby destroy cells. It is often used for the local and regional control of cancer, and in combination with surgery and chemotherapy; it may be curative or palliative.

Radioallergosorbent test (RAST)   A technique in which radioimmunoassay is used to measure the presence in the blood of IgE antibodies to specific allergens.

Radio-frequency ablation   The use of radio energy (heat) to destroy a very small section of the myocardium through which an accessory conduction pathway passes.

Recessive   A characteristic that is apparent only when two copies of the gene encoding it are present, one from the mother and one from the father.

Recombinant forms   Genetically altered organisms used in a vaccine to produce immunity with a minimum of side effects.

Red reflex   The orange-red glow of the vascular retina seen as a light shines through the cornea, aqueous humor, lens, and vitreous humor to the retina.

Regression   Return to an earlier behavior; a defense mechanism that may be displayed by children during times of stress.

Rehabilitation   Assisting a child with physical or mental challenges to reach full potential through therapy and education that considers the physiologic, psychologic, and environmental strengths and limitations of the child.

Reliability   When consistent results are obtained when measured by the same rater or other raters.

Religion   An organized system of shared beliefs regarding the significance of the nature, cause, and purpose of life and of the universe.

Renal insufficiency   Any degree of renal failure in which the kidneys' ability to conserve sodium and concentrate the urine decreases.

Repression   Involuntary forgetting; a defense mechanism often displayed by children with life-threatening or mortal illness.

Resilience   The family's capacity to develop strengths and abilities to "bounce back" from stress and challenges.

Resiliency theory   An assessment theory that states that all individuals experience crises that lead to adaptation and development of inner strengths and the ability to handle future crises.

Respiratory depression   An unresponsiveness and progressively decreasing respiratory rate that may progress to respiratory arrest.

Respite care   Short-term home care to relieve the primary caregiver and allow time away from home.

Retractions   A visible "drawing in" of the skin of the neck and chest that occurs on inspiration in infants and young children in respiratory distress; visible depression of tissue is seen between the ribs of the chest wall with each inspiration.

Risk factors   Characteristics of a child and family that promote or contribute to their challenges when dealing with a crisis.

Risk management   A process established by a healthcare institution to identify, evaluate, and reduce the risk of injury to patients, staff, and visitors, and thereby reduce the institution's liability.

Rooming in   Practice in which parents stay in the child's hospital room during the course of the child's hospitalization.

S

Saline   A mixture of salt and water; normal saline refers to the mixture of salt and water in equal concentration in body fluids.

Screening   Procedures used to detect the presence of a health condition before symptoms are apparent.

Secondary cancers Cancers (most commonly solid tumors) that appear subsequent to the primary cancer and treatment but are of a different histologic type. Also called *second malignant neoplasms (SMNs)*.

Secondary immune deficiency Acquired immunodeficiency.

Secondary immune response The body's response to an antigen at any time other than the initial exposure.

Sedation A medically controlled state of depressed consciousness used for painful diagnostic and therapeutic procedures.

Self-concept Evaluation of the self in certain specific areas, such as those related to academic achievement, athletic ability, physical appearance, and social interactions.

Self-efficacy A person's belief in the ability to perform a behavior to produce a desired outcome.

Self-esteem Feelings and beliefs of competence and worth as an individual, ability to meet challenges, and ability to learn lessons from success and failure; feelings of self-worth or value.

Self-regulation Infant's ability to maintain state and self-console (e.g., by sucking the fingers to stay calm instead of crying).

Sensible fluid loss Fluid loss that is measurable and observable, such as urine and wound drainage from tubes.

Sensorineural hearing loss Hearing loss caused by damage to the inner ear structures or the auditory nerve.

Separation anxiety Distress behaviors observed in young children separated from familiar caregivers.

Sequelae A chronic condition resulting as a complication of a disorder.

Sequence A cascade of events that are initiated by a single factor and lead to birth defects or congenital abnormalities.

Sex chromosome The X or Y chromosomes, which are responsible for gender determination.

Sexuality A person's view of self as a sexual being.

Shock An acute, complex state of circulatory dysfunction resulting in failure to deliver sufficient oxygen and other nutrients to meet cell and tissue demands.

Shunt An abnormal anatomic or surgically created opening in the septum between the systemic and pulmonary circulation.

Single nucleotide polymorphism (SNP) A variation in DNA sequence in which a single nucleotide base (A, T, C, or G) is substituted for another.

Sleep hygiene Behaviors that foster a regular and sufficient sleep pattern and daytime alertness.

Solitary play When infants play by themselves.

Spinal shock A concussion of the spinal cord resulting in the transient suppression of nerve function below the level of the acute injury.

Spiritual dimension A connection with a greater power than that in the self that guides a person to strive for life purpose, joy, peace, and fulfillment.

Spiritual health The ability to develop a spiritual nature, including awareness of a life purpose or meaning, a sustaining power during times of stress, a feeling of harmony with the universe, and a sense of fulfillment.

Spirituality An individual's experience and own interpretation of a relationship with a Supreme Being.

Sprain A tearing of ligaments usually caused when a joint is twisted or otherwise traumatized.

Stakeholders All community residents, policy makers, health providers, and funders concerned with the outcome of the community assessment.

Status epilepticus A prolonged continuous seizure of 15 minutes or evidence of intermittent seizures noted from clinical signs or EEG

tracings lasting more than 15 minutes without full recovery of consciousness between seizures.

Stenosis Narrowing of a valve or valve area below the valve or in the blood vessel.

Stent A device used to maintain patency of the urethral canal after surgery.

Stereotyping The assumption that all members of a cultural, ethnic, or racial group are alike and share the same characteristics.

Stereotypy Repetitive, obsessive, machine-like movements, commonly seen in autistic or schizophrenic children.

Stoma An opening, commonly in the abdominal wall, to provide for drainage from the intestinal or urinary systems.

Stranger anxiety Wariness of strange people and places, often shown by infants between 6 and 18 months of age.

Stridor An abnormal, high-pitched, crow-like respiratory sound caused when air moves through a narrowed larynx or trachea.

Stroke volume The amount of blood ejected with each ventricular contraction.

Subluxation Partial or complete dislocation of a joint.

Support systems The extended network of family, friends, and religious and community contacts that provide nurturance, emotional support, and direct assistance to parents.

Syncope Transient loss of consciousness and muscle tone.

Syndrome A collection of anomalies that occur in a consistent pattern and have a common cause.

T

Tachypnea An abnormally rapid rate of respiration.

Tactile fremitus Producing vibrations by either crying or talking that can be palpated on the chest.

Technology-assisted State of depending on a medical device that is required to sustain life (mechanical ventilators, intravenous nutrition or drugs, tracheostomy, suctioning, oxygen, or nutritional support with tube feedings).

Telangiectasia Permanent dilation of superficial capillaries and blood vessels.

Tetraplegia A loss of sensation and function of the head and neck and upper and lower extremities.

Thelarche Breast development.

Therapeutic play Planned play techniques that provide an opportunity for children to deal with their fears, concerns, and stressors of health experiences related to illness or hospitalization.

Thrill A vibration that may feel like a cat's purr while palpating the precordium. It is caused by turbulent blood flow from a defective heart valve and a heart murmur.

Thrombocytopenia A low platelet count.

Thyrotoxicosis A condition that can occur when thyroid hormone is suddenly released into the bloodstream during surgery or in cases of extreme hyperthyroidism. The child experiences fever, diaphoresis, and tachycardia, progressing to shock and, if untreated, death.

Tinnitus Ringing in the ears.

Tolerance Adaptation to an opioid dosage that results in a shorter duration of drug effectiveness over time.

Tonic Continuous muscular contraction; often used to describe seizure activity.

Total parenteral nutrition (TPN) A feeding regimen accomplished entirely by intravenous injection or other nongastrointestinal route.

Toxic appearance   Lethargy, poor perfusion, hypoventilation or hyperventilation, and cyanosis.

Toxicants   Harmful natural or synthetic chemicals not metabolically produced by an organism.

Toxins   Harmful or poisonous chemicals produced by metabolism or an organism (e.g., ricin).

Toxoid   A toxin that has been treated (by heat or chemical) to weaken its toxic effects but retain its antigenicity.

Tracheostomy   The creation of a surgical opening into the trachea through the anterior neck at the cricoid cartilage when long-term airway management is needed.

Transgendered   An adjective used to describe or refer to someone who chooses to dress and act like a member of the opposite sex from that assigned at birth; some transgendered persons choose to have surgery and take medications to facilitate their appearance in the chosen gender.

Translocation   The joining of a part of or a whole chromosome to another separate chromosome.

Transplacental immunity   Passive immunity that is transferred from mother to infant.

Treatment room   In a hospital or medical center, a room designated for performing treatments such as intravenous starts, blood drawing, and lumbar punctures to promote children's sense of security that their own room is a "safe" and relatively pain-free site.

Trigger   An inflammatory or noninflammatory stimulus that initiates an asthmatic episode; a substance or condition, including exercise, infectious agents, allergens, fragrances, food additives, pollutants, weather changes, emotions, and stress.

Tripod position   Sitting forward with arms on knees for support and extending the neck.

Trisomic (trisomy)   The presence of three homologous chromosomes rather than the usual two.

Tumor suppressor genes   Genetic material that controls the growth of cells, decreasing the effects of oncogenes.

Tympanogram   A graph showing the ability of the middle ear to transmit sound energy; measured by inserting an airtight probe into the external ear entrance and emitting a tone.

Tympanostomy tubes   Pressure-equalizing tubes inserted to drain fluid from the middle ear.

U

Uremia   Toxicity resulting from the buildup of urea and nitrogenous waste in the blood.

Urethritis   An infection of the urethra.

Uveitis   Inflammation of the middle layer of the eye.

V

Vacuum-assisted wound closure   Negative pressure wound therapy in a pump generates a vacuum or suction to remove waste materials from the wound area.

Validity   When a scale or tool accurately measures the concept it was designed to measure.

Varus   A condition in which the hindfoot turns inward; usually associated with clubfoot.

Vaso-occlusion   Blockage of a blood vessel.

Vegan   Strict vegetarian who eats no animal products.

Vegetarian   One who eats no poultry, meat, or fish.

Vertical transmission   The passage of disease from the mother to the fetus during the period of pregnancy.

Vesicoureteral reflux   The backflow of urine from the bladder into the ureters during voiding.

Violence   Threatened or actual use of physical force or power that leads to potential or actual physical or emotional trauma.

Virilization   The production of masculine secondary sexual characteristics in females.

Vision   A complex process of acquiring meaning from what is seen, involving the eye, brain, and related neurologic and physiologic structures.

Visual acuity   Measurement of the ability to discriminate a letter or other object to test sight.

Vocal resonance   How well voice sounds are transmitted over the chest.

W

Water intoxication   An abnormal proportion of water to sodium in the extracellular fluid.

Wheezing   A noise resulting from the passage of air through mucus or fluids in a narrowed lower airway.

Wild type gene   The most common type of gene; designated as normal.

Windshield survey   A walking or driving tour around a neighborhood or community for the purpose of identifying resources and characteristics of the community.

Withdrawal   The physical signs and symptoms that occur when a sedative or pain drug is suddenly stopped in a patient who is physically dependent.

X

Xerosis   Generally dry skin that is likely to crack and fissure.

X-linked   Any gene found on the X chromosome, or traits determined by such genes; also refers to the specific mode of inheritance of such genes; one altered gene on an X chromosome in a male can produce disease, such as hemophilia.

Z

Zygote   A fertilized egg.

Index

Note: Page numbers with *t* indicate tables, those with *f* indicate figures, and those with *b* indicate boxes.

Special Features